SINGLE PC LICENSE AGREEMENT AND LIMITED WAI

READ THIS LICENSE CAREFULLY BEFORE OPENING TI YOU ARE AGREEING TO THE TERMS AND CONDITION DO NOT OPEN THE PACKAGE. PROMPTLY RETURN COMPANYING ITEMS TO THE PLACE YOU OBTAINI CENSED SOFTWARE ON THE CD EXCEPT THAT THE FREEWARE ON THE CD ARE AS SET FORTH IN THE ELECTRONIC LICENSE LOCATED ON THE CD.

110639325

1. GRANT OF LICENSE and OWNERSHIP: The enclosed computer programs ("Software") are licensed, not sold, to you by Pearson Education, Inc. ("We" or the "Company") and in consideration of your purchase or adoption of the accompanying Company textbooks and/or other materials, and your agreement to these terms. We reserve any rights not granted to you. You own only the disc(s) but we and/or our licensors own the Software itself. This license allows you to use and display your copy of the Software on a single computer (i.e., with a single CPU) at a single location for academic use only, so long as you comply with the terms of this Agreement. You may make one copy for back up, or transfer your copy to another CPU, provided that the Software is usable on only one computer.

2. RESTRICTIONS: You may not transfer or distribute the Software or documentation to anyone else. Except for backup, you may not copy the documentation or the Software. You may not network the Software or otherwise use it on more than one computer or computer terminal at the same time. You may not reverse engineer, disassemble, decompile, modify, adapt, translate, or create derivative works based on the Software or the Documentation. You may be held legally responsible for any copying or copyright infringement which is caused by your failure to abide by the terms of these restrictions.

3. TERMINATION: This license is effective until terminated. This license will terminate automatically without notice from the Company if you fail to comply with any provisions or limitations of this license. Upon termination, you shall destroy the Documentation and all copies of the Software. All provisions of this Agreement as to limitation and disclaimer of warranties, limitation of liability, remedies or damages, and our ownership rights shall survive termination.

4. LIMITED WARRANTY AND DISCLAIMER OF WARRANTY: Company warrants that for a period of 60 days from the date you purchase this SOFTWARE (or purchase or adopt the accompanying textbook), the Software, when properly installed and used in accordance with the Documentation, will operate in substantial conformity with the description of the Software set forth in the Documentation, and that for a period of 30 days the disk(s) on which the Software is delivered shall be free from defects in materials and workmanship under normal use. The Company does not warrant that the Software will meet your requirements or that the operation of the Software will be uninterrupted or error-free. Your only remedy and the Company's only obligation under these limited warranties is, at the Company's option, return of the disk for a refund of any amounts paid for it by you or replacement of the disk. THIS LIMITED WARRANTY IS THE ONLY WARRANTY PROVIDED BY THE COMPANY AND ITS LICENSORS, AND THE COMPANY AND ITS LICENSORS DISCLAIM ALL OTHER WARRANTIES, EXPRESS OR IMPLIED, INCLUDING WITHOUT LIMITATION, THE IMPLIED WARRANTIES OF MERCHANTABILITY AND FITNESS FOR A PARTICULAR PURPOSE. THE COMPANY DOES NOT WARRANT, GUARANTEE OR MAKE ANY REPRESENTATION REGARDING THE ACCURACY, RELIABILITY, CURRENTNESS, USE, OR RESULTS OF USE, OF THE SOFTWARE.

5. LIMITATION OF REMEDIES AND DAMAGES: IN NO EVENT, SHALL THE COMPANY OR ITS EMPLOYEES, AGENTS, LICENSORS, OR CONTRACTORS BE LIABLE FOR ANY INCIDENTAL, INDIRECT, SPECIAL, OR CONSEQUENTIAL DAMAGES ARISING OUT OF OR IN CONNECTION WITH THIS LICENSE OR THE SOFTWARE, INCLUDING FOR LOSS OF USE, LOSS OF DATA, LOSS OF INCOME OR PROFIT, OR OTHER LOSSES, SUSTAINED AS A RESULT OF INJURY TO ANY PERSON, OR LOSS OF OR DAMAGE TO PROPERTY, OR CLAIMS OF THIRD PARTIES, EVEN IF THE COMPANY OR AN AUTHORIZED REPRESENTATIVE OF THE COMPANY HAS BEEN ADVISED OF THE POSSIBILITY OF SUCH DAMAGES. IN NO EVENT SHALL THE LIABILITY OF THE COMPANY FOR DAMAGES WITH RESPECT TO THE SOFTWARE EXCEED THE AMOUNTS ACTUALLY PAID BY YOU, IF ANY, FOR THE SOFTWARE OR THE ACCOMPANYING TEXTBOOK. BECAUSE SOME JURISDICTIONS DO NOT ALLOW THE LIMITATION OF LIABILITY IN CERTAIN CIRCUMSTANCES, THE ABOVE LIMITATIONS MAY NOT ALWAYS APPLY TO YOU.

6. GENERAL: THIS AGREEMENT SHALL BE CONSTRUED IN ACCORDANCE WITH THE LAWS OF THE UNITED STATES OF AMERICA AND THE STATE OF NEW YORK, APPLICABLE TO CONTRACTS MADE IN NEW YORK, AND SHALL BENEFIT THE COMPANY, ITS AFFILIATES AND ASSIGNEES. HIS AGREEMENT IS THE COMPLETE AND EXCLUSIVE STATEMENT OF THE AGREEMENT BETWEEN YOU AND THE COMPANY AND SUPERSEDES ALL PROPOSALS OR PRIOR AGREEMENTS, ORAL, OR WRITTEN, AND ANY OTHER COMMUNICATIONS BETWEEN YOU AND THE COMPANY OR ANY REPRESENTATIVE OF THE COMPANY RELATING TO THE SUBJECT MATTER OF THIS AGREEMENT. If you are a U.S. Government user, this Software is licensed with "restricted rights" as set forth in subparagraphs (a)-(d) of the Commercial Computer-Restricted Rights clause at FAR 52.227-19 or in subparagraphs (c)(1)(ii) of the Rights in Technical Data and Computer Software clause at DFARS 252.227-7013, and similar clauses, as applicable.

Should you have any questions concerning this agreement or if you wish to contact the Company for any reason, please contact in writing: Pearson Education, Inc. 1 Lake Street, Upper Saddle River, NJ 07458.

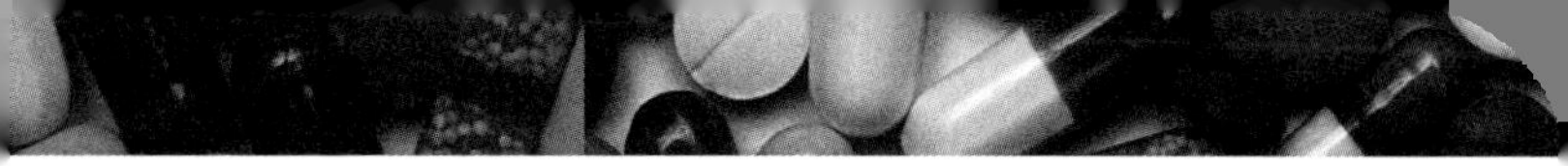

GUIDE TO USING
the Prentice Hall Nurse's Drug Guide 2006

Classifications and Prototype Drugs

> **CIMETIDINE**
> (sye-met'i-deen)
> **Novocimetine ✦, Peptol ✦, Tagamet, Tagamet HB**
> **Classifications:** GASTROINTESTINAL AGENT; ANTISECRETORY (H_2-RECEPTOR ANTAGONIST)
> **Pregnancy Category:** B

The classifications used in this book are based upon the classification scheme used by the American Hospital Formulary Service (AHFS), which classifies drugs by pharmacological and therapeutic categories. This enables the nurse to identify different classes of drugs that have similar therapeutic implications or that primarily affect the same physiologic system. In general, all drugs in a class will have similar actions, uses, side effects, and nursing implications. Therefore, we have selected certain drugs that are representative of a class—**prototype drugs**—and discuss them in more detail than the other drugs in that class. Throughout the book, prototype drug monographs are identified with a small icon, e.g., Acetaminophen. The user can refer to the prototype drug to obtain in-depth information on those drugs in the class that may not be as extensively discussed in their monographs. When a drug belongs to a classification that has a designated prototype drug, that prototype is identified directly below the classification. The table on pages x–xvi outlines the classification scheme and lists the drug prototype considered to be representative of each class. All prototype drugs are highlighted in **bold** type in the index for quick identification. Finally, not every drug has a prototype. Some drugs have a unique therapeutic effect or mechanism of action. In these cases, no prototype drug will be identified.

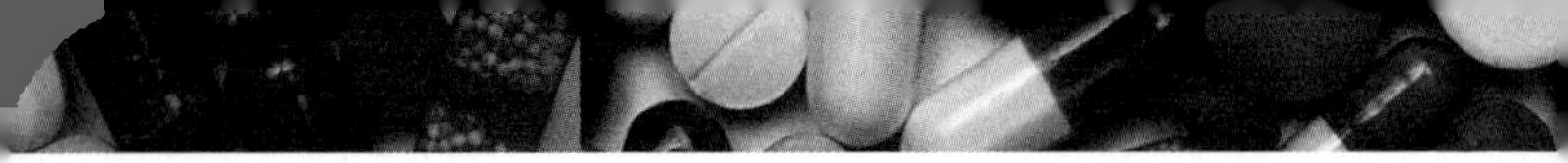

Pregnancy Category

Drugs may be described as category A, B, C, D, or X according to the risk–benefit ratio for the mother and the fetus, with A being the lowest and X the highest risk. If the FDA pregnancy category is known, it will be indicated after the classifications and prototype in each monograph. Refer to Appendix C, FDA Pregnancy Categories, for a more complete description of each category.

Controlled Substances

In the United States, controlled substances, such as narcotics, are classified as belonging to one of five schedules (I to V) according to abuse potential. Schedule I has the highest, and Schedule V has the lowest potential for abuse. Refer to Appendix B, U.S. Schedules of Controlled Substances, for a more complete description of each schedule.

Availability

Since drugs come in a variety of dosages and forms, the authors have added a *new* section to each monograph. This section identifies the available forms, e.g., tablets, capsules, etc., and the available dosage amounts for every drug.

> **AVAILABILITY** 100 mg, 200 mg, 400 mg, 800 mg tablets; 300 mg/5 mL liquid; 150 mg/mL injection

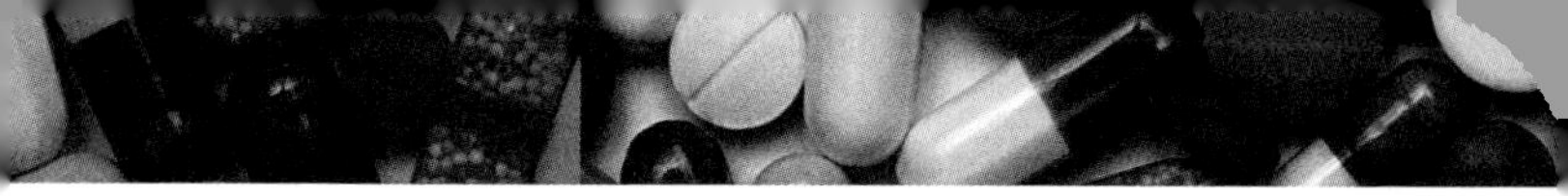

Actions and Therapeutic Effects

This entry in each monograph describes the mechanism by which the specific drug produces physiologic and biochemical changes at the cellular, tissue, and organ levels. This information helps the user understand how the drug works in the body and makes it easier to learn its side effects, adverse reactions, and cautions. The therapeutic effects are the reasons why a drug is prescribed. Therapeutic effectiveness of the drug can be determined by monitoring improvement in the condition for which the drug is prescribed.

ACTIONS Enzyme inhibitor structurally similar to histamine. Belongs to the antihistamine group with high selectivity for histamine H_2-receptors on parietal cells of the stomach (minimal effect on H_1-receptors). By reversible competitive inhibition of histamine at the H_2-receptor sites, it suppresses all phases of daytime and nocturnal basal gastric acid secretion in the stomach. Indirectly reduces pepsin secretion; it is not a cholinergic. Has no effect on lower esophageal sphincter pressure, gastric motility or emptying, biliary or pancreatic secretion.

THERAPEUTIC EFFECTS Cimetidine blocks the H_2-receptor on the parietal cells of the stomach, thus decreasing gastric acid secretion, raises the pH of the stomach and, thereby, reduces pepsin secretion.

Uses and Unlabeled Uses

USES Short-term treatment of active duodenal ulcer and prevention of ulcer recurrence (at reduced dosage) after it is healed. Also used for short-term treatment of active benign gastric ulcer, pathologic hypersecretory conditions such as Zollinger-Ellison syndrome, and heartburn.

UNLABELED USES Prophylaxis of stress-induced ulcers, upper GI bleeding, and aspiration pneumonitis; gastroesophageal reflux; chronic urticaria; acetaminophen toxicity.

The therapeutic applications of each drug are described in terms of approved, or labeled, uses and unlabeled uses. An unlabeled use is literally one that does not appear on the drug label or in the manufacturer's literature on the use of the drug. The unlabeled use is, nevertheless, an accepted use for the drug supported by the medical literature.

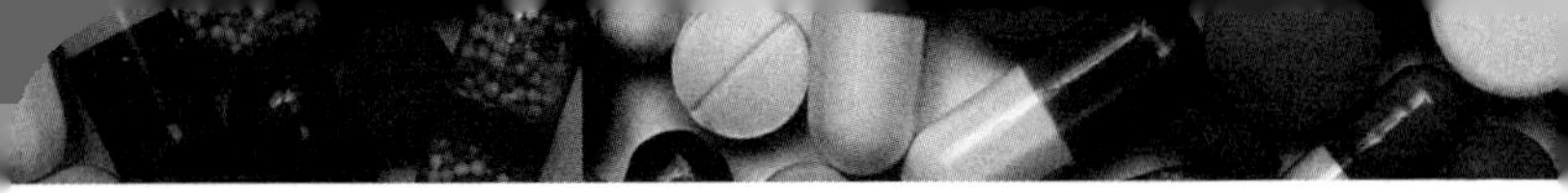

Contraindications and Cautious Use

Many drugs have contraindications and therefore should not be used in specific conditions, such as during pregnancy, or with particular drugs or foods. In other cases, the drug should be used with great caution because of a greater than average risk of untoward effects.

> **CONTRAINDICATIONS** Known hypersensitivity to cimetidine or other H_2 receptor antagonists; lactation, pregnancy (category B). Safe use in children <16 y not established.
> **CAUTIOUS USE** Older adults or critically ill patients; impaired renal or hepatic function; organic brain syndrome; gastric ulcers; immunocompromised patients.

Route and Dosages

> **ROUTE & DOSAGE**
>
> **Duodenal Ulcer**
> *Adult:* **PO** 300 mg q.i.d. *or* 400 mg b.i.d. *or* 800 mg h.s. **IM/IV** 300 mg q6–8h
> *Child:* **PO/IM/IV** 20–40 mg/kg/d in 4 divided doses
> *Neonate:* **PO/IM/IV** 5–10 mg/kg/d divided q8–12h
> *Infant:* **PO/IM/IV** 10–20 mg/kg/d divided q6–12h

Route of administration is specified as SC, IM, IV, PO, PR, nasal, ophthalmic, vaginal, topical, aural, intradermal, or intrathecal. Dosages are listed according to indication, or use. One of the hallmarks of this drug guide is the comprehensive dosage information it provides. The guide includes adult, geriatric, and pediatric dosages, as well as dosages for neonates and infants. This section also indicates dosage adjustments for renal impairment (based on creatinine clearance) and for impaired hepatic function whenever applicable. In all monographs, the routes and dosages are highlighted in a gray box to facilitate quick reference.

Administration

Since drug administration is an important primary role for the nurse, the authors have reorganized this section in every monograph. Organized by different routes, this section lists comprehensive instructions for administering, handling, and storing medications.

> **ADMINISTRATION**
>
> **Oral**
> - Give 1 h before or 2 h after an antacid.

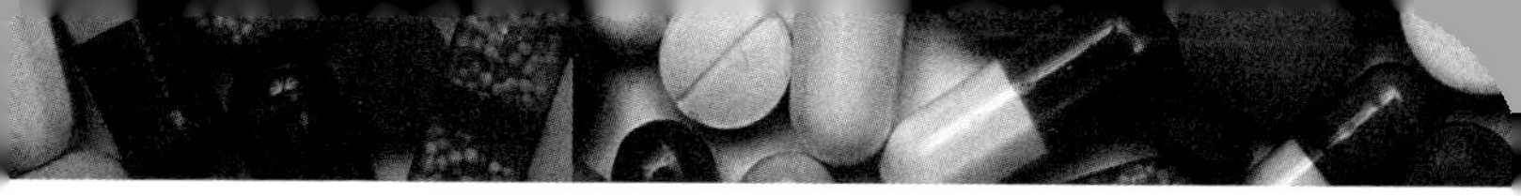

Intravenous Drug Administration

Within the Administration section of each monograph, the authors have added a new section highlighting intravenous drugs. Indicated by a vertical red bar, this section provides users with comprehensive instructions on how to Prepare and Administer direct, intermittent, and continuous intravenous medications. It also includes Solution/Additive and Y-Site incompatibility for every monograph where appropriate to indicate which drugs and solutions should not be mixed with the intravenous drug. This is crucial information for drug administration. Additionally, a chart for Y-Site compatibility for intravenous drugs is located inside the back cover of this drug guide. With these enhancements, this new drug guide eliminates the need for additional resources for intravenous administration.

Intravenous

- IV administration to neonates, infants and children: Verify correct IV concentration and rate of infusion/injection with physician.

PREPARE: **Direct:** Dilute 300 mg in 18 mL D5W or NS to yield 300 mg/20 mL. **Intermittent:** Dilute 300 mg in 50 mL D5W or NS. **Continuous:** Further dilute in up to 1000 mL of selected IV solution.

ADMINISTER: **Direct:** Give 300 mg or fraction thereof over at least 5 min. **Intermittent:** Give over 15–20 min. **Continuous:** Give a loading dose of 150 mg at the intermittent infusion rate; then give continuous infusion equally spaced over 24 h.

INCOMPATIBILITIES **Solution/additive: Amphotericin B, atropine, cefamandole, cefazolin, chlorpromazine, pentobarbital, secobarbital. Y-site: Allopurinol, amphotericin B cholesteryl complex, amsacrine, cefepime, indomethacin, warfarin.**

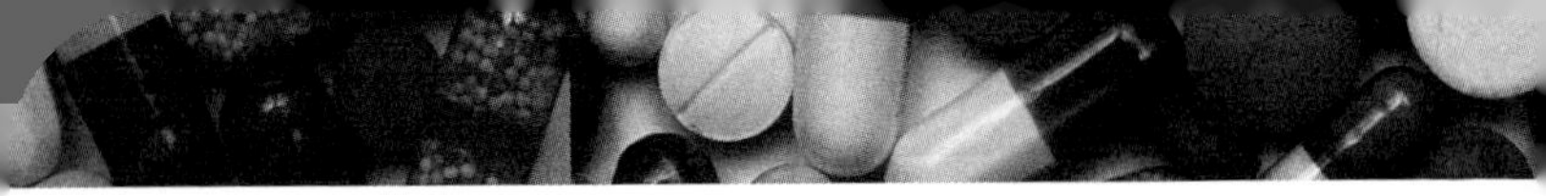

Adverse Effects

Virtually all drugs have adverse side effects that may be bothersome to some individuals but not to others. In each monograph, adverse effects with an incidence of ≥1% are listed by body system or organs. The most common adverse effects appear in *italic* type, while those that are life-threatening are underlined. Users of the drug guide will find a key at the bottom of every page as a quick reminder.

> **ADVERSE EFFECTS** (≥1%) **Body as a Whole:** Fever. **CV (rare):** Cardiac arrhythmias and cardiac arrest after rapid IV bolus dose. **GI:** Mild transient diarrhea; severe diarrhea, constipation, abdominal discomfort. **Hematologic:** Increased prothrombin time; neutropenia (rare), thrombocytopenia (rare), aplastic anemia. **Metabolic:** Slight increase in serum uric acid, BUN, creatinine; transient pain at IM site; hypospermia. **Musculoskeletal:** Exacerbation of joint symptoms in patients with preexisting arthritis. **CNS:** Drowsiness, dizziness, lightheadedness, depression, headache, reversible confusional states, paranoid psychosis. **Skin:** Rash, Stevens-Johnson syndrome, reversible alopecia. **Urogenital:** Gynecomastia and breast soreness, galactorrhea, reversible impotence.

Diagnostic Test Interference

> **DIAGNOSTIC TEST INTERFERENCE** Cimetidine may cause false-positive ***Hemoccult test for gastric bleeding*** if test is performed within 15 min of oral cimetidine administration.

This section describes the effect of the drug on various diagnostic tests and alerts the nurse to possible misinterpretations of test results when applicable. The specific altered element is highlighted in ***bold italic*** type.

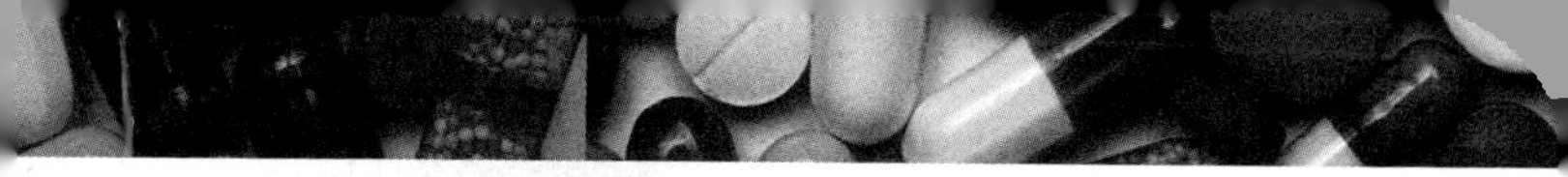

Interactions

The authors have expanded this section to include herbal interactions. Whenever appropriate, this section will list individual drugs, drug classes, foods, and herbs that interact with the drug discussed in the monograph. Drugs may interact to inhibit or enhance one another. Thus, drug interactions may improve the therapeutic response, lead to therapeutic failure, or produce specific adverse reactions. Only drugs that have been shown to cause clinically significant interactions with the drug discussed in the monograph are listed in this section. Note that generic drugs appear in **bold** type, and drug classes appear in small caps.

> **INTERACTIONS Drug:** Cimetidine decreases the hepatic metabolism of **warfarin, phenobarbital, phenytoin, diazepam, propranolol, lidocaine, theophylline,** thus increasing their activity and toxicity; ANTACIDS may decrease absorption of cimetidine.

Pharmacokinetics

This section identifies how the drug moves throughout the body. It lists the mechanisms of absorption, distribution, metabolism, elimination, and half-life when known. It also provides information about onset, peak, and duration of the drug action.

> **PHARMACOKINETICS Absorption:** 70% of oral dose absorbed from GI tract. **Peak:** 1–1.5 h. **Distribution:** Widely distributed; crosses blood-brain barrier and placenta. **Metabolism:** Metabolized in liver. **Elimination:** Most of drug excreted in urine in 24 h; excreted in breast milk. **Half-Life:** 2 h.

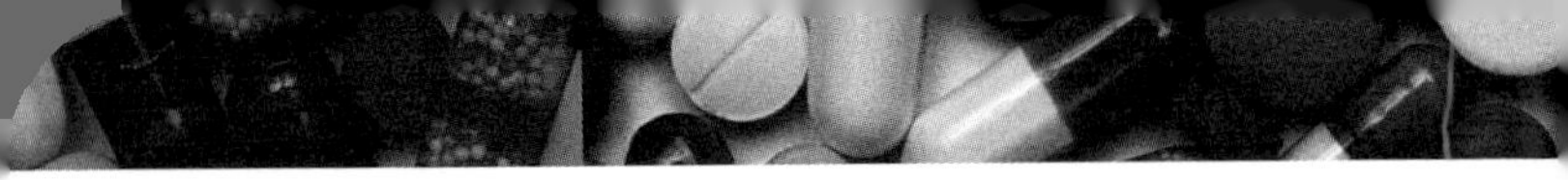

Nursing Implications

The Nursing Implications section of each drug monograph is formatted in an easy-to-use manner so that all the pertinent information that nurses need is listed under two headings: Assessment & Drug Effects and Patient & Family Education. Under these headings, the user can quickly and easily identify needed information and incorporate it into the appropriate steps of the nursing process. Before administering a drug, the nurse should read both sections to determine the assessments that should be made before and after administration of the drug, the indicators of drug effectiveness, laboratory tests recommended for individual drugs, and the essential patient or family education related to the drug.

> **NURSING IMPLICATIONS**
>
> **Assessment & Drug Effects**
>
> - Ulcer healing may occur within the first 2 wk of therapy but generally requires at least 4 wk in most patients. Short-term (i.e., 8 wk) therapy of active duodenal ulcer does not prevent ulcer recurrence when drug is discontinued.
> - Monitor pulse of patient during first few days of drug regimen. Bradycardia after PO as well as IV administration should be reported. Pulse usually returns to normal within 24 h after drug discontinuation.
>
> **Patient & Family Education**
>
> - Cimetidine must be taken exactly as prescribed. Sudden discontinuation of therapy reportedly has caused perforation of chronic peptic ulcer.
> - Seek advice about self-medication with any OTC drug.
> - Report breast tenderness or enlargement. Mild bilateral gynecomastia and breast soreness may occur after ≥1 mo of therapy. It may disappear spontaneously or remain throughout therapy.

Therapeutic Effectiveness

Therapeutic effectiveness of the drug can be determined by monitoring improvement in the condition for which the drug is prescribed, and by using the Assessment & Drug Effects section of the Nursing Implications. Drugs have multiple uses or indications. Therefore, it is important to know why a drug is being prescribed for a specific client. In many monograghs specific indicators of drug effectiveness are provided for reference.

PRENTICE HALL

Nurse's Drug Guide 2006

Billie Ann Wilson, RN, PhD

Professor and Director
Department of Nursing
Loyola University New Orleans
New Orleans, Louisiana

Margaret T. Shannon, RN, PhD

Professor Emeritus of Nursing
Our Lady of Holy Cross College
New Orleans, Louisiana

Carolyn L. Stang, PharmD

Vice President, Clinical Program Development
Caremark Inc.
Northbrook, Illinois

PEARSON
Prentice Hall

Upper Saddle River, New Jersey 07458

Notice: The authors and the publisher of this volume have taken care to make certain that the doses of drugs and schedules of treatment are correct and compatible with the standards generally accepted at the time of publication. Nevertheless, as new information becomes available, changes in treatment and in the use of drugs become necessary. The reader is advised to carefully consult the instruction and information material included in the package insert of each drug or therapeutic agent before administration. This advice is especially important when using, administering, or recommending new and infrequently used drugs. The authors and publisher disclaim all responsibility for any liability, loss, injury, or damage incurred as a consequence, directly or indirectly, of the use and application of any of the contents of this volume.

www.prenhall.com/drugguides

05 06 07 / 10 9 8 7 6 5 4 3 2 1

Pearson Education Ltd.
Pearson Education Australia Pty, Limited
Pearson Education Singapore, Pte. Ltd.
Pearson Education North Asia Ltd.
Pearson Education Canada, Ltd.
Pearson Educación de Mexico, S.A. de C.V.
Pearson Education—Japan
Pearson Education Malaysia, Pte. Ltd.

ISBN 0-13-171358-2
[retail] ISBN 0-13-171361-2

PRINTED IN THE UNITED STATES OF AMERICA

CONTENTS

To

Alvin, Theresa, Ellen, and

Michael, Bob, Mary Elizabeth, and Richard

without whom this work would not have been possible

♦

ABOUT THE AUTHORS

Billie Ann Wilson is currently Professor and Director of the Department of Nursing at Loyola University in New Orleans, Louisiana. Prior to entering nursing, she taught natural and physical sciences at the secondary and collegiate levels. She holds a Bachelor of Science in Biology from Boston College, a Master of Science in Biology from Purdue University, a Bachelor of Science in Nursing from Northwestern State University of Louisiana, a Master of Nursing from Louisiana State University Health Sciences Center, and a PhD in Curriculum and Instruction from the University of New Orleans.

Margaret T. Shannon is currently Professor Emeritus of Nursing at Our Lady of Holy Cross College, New Orleans, Louisiana. Her educational preparation includes a Bachelor of Science in Chemistry and a Master of Science in Chemistry, both from Saint Louis University; a Master of Arts in Teaching Biology from Saint Mary's College, a Bachelor of Science in Nursing from Northwestern State University of Louisiana, a Master of Nursing from Louisiana State University Health Sciences Center, and a PhD in Curriculum and Instruction from the University of New Orleans. Prior to entering nursing, she taught physical science, natural science, and mathematics at the secondary and collegiate levels.

Carolyn L. Stang is currently Vice President for Clinical Program Development at Caremark Inc. She has worked in hospital and community pharmacies, home health care, and the pharmaceutical industry. Dr. Stang has been a freelance medical writer and an assistant professor at Rutgers University College of Pharmacy. She holds a Bachelor of Science in Pharmacy from The Ohio State University and a Doctor of Pharmacy from the University of Tennessee, Memphis, and completed a fellowship in Family Medicine at the Medical University of South Carolina, Charleston.

CONSULTANT REVIEWERS

Marianne Adam, RN, MSN
St. Luke's Hospital School of Nursing
Bethlehem, PA

June Alberto, DNS, RN
School of Nursing
Georgia Southern University
Statesboro, GA

Susan Buchholtz, RN, MSN
School of Nursing
Georgia Perimeter College
Clarkston, GA

Judy Davidson, RN, MSN
Division of Nursing and Health Professions
Columbus State University
Columbus, GA

Heather Davis, PharmD
College of Pharmacy
University of Washington Medical Center
Seattle, WA

Frederica Gould, MS, RPh, BCPS
College of Pharmacy
Idaho State University
Pocatello, ID

Ruth Grendell, DNSc, RN
School of Nursing
Point Loma Nazarene
San Diego, CA

Lemont B. Kier, PhD
School of Pharmacy
Virginia Commonwealth University
Richmond, VA

Patricia Marken, PharmD, BCPP
Division of Pharmacy Practice
University of Missouri
Kansas City, MO

Corinne Wilhoit, RN, MSN
School of Nursing
University of Central Oklahoma
Edmond, OK

STUDENT REVIEWERS

Jolene Agosta
Worcester State College
Worcester, MA

Mikal Black
Boise State University
Boise, ID

Amy Harrison
Washburn University
Topeka, KS

Tina Kunze
University of Maryland
Baltimore, MD

Traci Kauffman
Grand View College
Des Moines, IA

Julia Kimmey Lynch
University of New Hampshire
Durham, NH

Angie Metcalf
Boise State University
Boise, ID

Ann Marie Momenee
Widener University
Chester, PA

John Risner
Wesley College
Dover, DE

Kimberly Romano
Salisbury State University
Salisbury, MD

PREFACE

Prentice Hall Nurse's Drug Guide 2006 is a current and reliable reference designed to provide comprehensive information needed to make appropriate decisions regarding drug administration. This new edition includes 22 monographs for new drugs recently approved by the FDA, and several drugs removed from the market have been eliminated and archived on the Companion Website accompanying this handbook. The new drugs are also included on the CD-ROM packaged in the back of this drug guide. On pages x–xvi, the user will find a current listing of drug classifications and their associated drug prototypes with page references to those drug entries. Prototype drugs are representative of all drugs in a particular classification. The classification list serves as a valuable tool, especially to students learning pharmacology and familiarizing themselves with drug families and prototypes.

Each drug monograph provides the necessary information for safe and effective drug administration. The user should read all the information provided. Occasionally, the user will be referred to Appendix F, Glossary of Key Terms, Clinical Conditions, and Associated Signs and Symptoms. This unique glossary provides valuable information regarding common assessment findings related to therapeutic effectiveness or ineffectiveness of specific drugs.

The authors recognize that the decision-making process related to drug administration is a cyclical one. For example, assessments are made both prior to and after drug administration. Thus, nursing diagnoses and interventions may change as a result of an *achieved therapeutic effect, therapeutic failure, manifestation of an adverse effect,* or *demonstration of a learning need.* The authors believe that the users of this drug reference will find that the clear and logical design of the drug monographs facilitates decision making and supports the nursing process.

While some advanced practice nurses and other health professionals now have prescriptive privileges, the term physician is used throughout this book to designate the prescriber of medications.

ORGANIZATION

The ***Prentice Hall Nurse's Drug Guide 2006*** is user friendly. Nurses in clinical practice, nursing professors, pharmacists, and nursing students from across the country reviewed the content of this handbook and provided helpful suggestions on how it could be made more useful. Based upon these comments, the authors organized monographs and added new elements to every monograph in the book. To help readers better understand how to use the drug guide, the authors illustrate and describe all the components of a drug monograph in the next section.

In this drug guide, all drugs are listed alphabetically according to their generic names. However, each drug is indexed by both its generic and trade names in the back of the guide to make it easier for the user to locate individual drug monographs. Trade names followed by a maple leaf indicate that brand of the drug is available only in Canada. If a drug is not listed in the alphabetical section, it may be a combination drug, which is a drug made up of more than one generic component. These combination drugs are listed under their trade names in the index and in Appendix E, Prescription Combination Drugs. The appendix identifies the generic components and the amount of each generic drug contained in the combination.

Appendixes

This edition of the drug guide includes several helpful tables and charts in the appendixes, including Appendix A, Ocular Medications, Low Molecular Weight Heparins, Inhaled Corticosteroids, and Topical Corticosteroids; Appendix B, U.S. Schedules of Controlled Substances; Appendix C, FDA Pregnancy Categories; Appendix D, Oral Dosage Forms That Should Not Be Crushed; Appendix E, Prescription Combination Drugs; Appendix F, Glossary of Key Terms, Clinical Conditions, and Associated Signs and Symptoms; and Appendix G, Abbreviations.

Index

The index in the ***Prentice Hall Nurse's Drug Guide 2006*** is perhaps the most often-used section in the entire book. All generic, trade, and combination drugs are listed in this index. Whenever a trade name is listed, the generic drug monograph is listed in parentheses. Additionally, classifications are listed and identified in SMALL CAPS, while all prototype drugs are highlighted in **bold** type.

CD-ROM

The CD-ROM inside the ***Prentice Hall Nurse's Drug Guide 2006*** runs on all Windows-based computers. It is designed to assist nurses in providing drug information and nursing implications for patients in hospitals, clinics, and all community settings. The

CD-ROM contains monographs from the book, including prototypes and new drugs approved by the FDA. Students and nurses may print these monographs for use in patient teaching or for quick reference.

Companion Website – www.prenhall.com/drugguides

The Companion Website for the ***Prentice Hall Nurse's Drug Guide 2006*** is a free online resource that offers additional information and is updated periodically. Go to **www.prenhall.com/drugguides** to access drug updates, links to drug-related sites, drug-related tools and updates, medication administration techniques, drug classifications, principles of pharmacology, common herbal remedies, archived drug monographs for rarely used and discontinued drugs, and more. You can also send the authors your feedback about the drug guide through this website.

PDA Version

With the touch of a stylus, you can search for and access drug information quickly and easily, right at the point of care. Like the handbook, you can jump to availability, route & dosages, administration, adverse effects, contraindications, interactions, uses, drug action therapeutic effects, pharmacokinetics, and nursing implications, including assessment & drug effects, monitoring, laboratory tests, and patient & family education. There is even a toolbox with appendixes, glossary of signs & symptoms, abbreviations, list of Do Not Crush drugs, and more. Compatible with Palm® OS 3.1 or higher and PocketPC 2002 or later.

To register your PDA and to receive free update notifications regularly via email, go to **www.prenhall.com/drugguides.** Your own Drug Home Page includes drug information updates, newly approved drugs, links to drug-related websites, illustrated medication administration techniques, common herbal remedies, and much more.

ACKNOWLEDGMENTS

We wish to express our appreciation to our past and present students who have provided the inspiration for this work. It is for these individuals and all who strive for excellence in patient care that this work was undertaken.

Billie Ann Wilson, RN, PhD
Margaret T. Shannon, RN, PhD
Carolyn L. Stang, PharmD

Classifications	Prototype
ANTIGOUT AGENT	Colchicine
ANTIHISTAMINES	
ANTIHISTAMINES (H_1-RECEPTOR ANTAGONIST)	Diphenhydramine HCl
NON-SEDATING	Loratidine
ANTIPRURITIC	Hydroxyzine HCl
ANTIVERTIGO AGENT	Meclizine HCl
ANTI-INFECTIVES	
ANTIBIOTICS	
AMEBICIDE	Paromomycin Sulfate
ANTHELMINTIC	Mebendazole
AMINOGLYCOSIDES	Gentamicin Sulfate
ANTIFUNGALS	Amphotericin B
AZOLE ANTIFUNGAL	Fluconazole
BETA-LACTAM	Imipenem-Cilastatin
CEPHALOSPORIN	
FIRST GENERATION	Cefazolin Sodium
SECOND GENERATION	Cefonicid Sodium
THIRD GENERATION	Cefotaxime Sodium
CLINDAMYCIN	Clindamycin HCl
MACROLIDES	Erythromycin
PENICILLIN	
AMINOPENICILLIN	Ampicillin
ANTIPSEUDOMONAL PENICILLIN	Mezlocillin Sodium
NATURAL PENICILLIN	Penicillin G Potassium
QUINOLONES	Ciprofloxacin HCl
SULFONAMIDES	Sulfisoxazole
TETRACYCLINE	Tetracycline HCl
ANTILEPROSY (SULFONE) AGENT	Dapsone
ANTIMALARIAL	Chloroquine HCl
ANTIPROTOZOAL	Metronidazole
ANTITUBERCULOSIS AGENTS	Isoniazid
ANTIVIRAL AGENTS	
ANTIVIRAL AGENTS	Acyclovir
ANTIRETROVIRAL AGENTS	
NUCLEOSIDE REVERSE TRANSCRIPTASE INHIBITOR	Zidovudine
NONNUCLEOSIDE REVERSE TRANSCRIPTASE INHIBITOR	Nevirapine
PROTEASE INHIBITOR	Saquinavir

*Based on the American Hospital Formulary Service Pharmacologic–Therapeutic Classification
†Prototype drugs are highlighted in tinted boxes in this book.
Complete list of drugs for each classification found in classification index starting on p. 1777.

Classifications	Prototype
URINARY TRACT ANTI-INFECTIVE	Trimethoprim
VACCINE	Hepatitis B
ANTINEOPLASTICS	
ALKYLATING AGENT	Cyclophosphamide
ANTIBIOTIC	Doxorubicin HCl
ANTIMETABOLITE	Fluorouracil
CAMPTOTHECIN	Topotecan HCl
AROMATASE INHIBITOR	Anastrozole
EPIDERMAL GROWTH FACTOR RECEPTOR INHIBITOR	Gefitinib
HORMONE, ANTIESTROGEN	Tamoxifen Citrate
MITOTIC INHIBITOR	Vincristine Sulfate
NITROGEN MUSTARD	Mechlorethamine HCl
TAXANE	Paclitaxel
ANTITUSSIVES, EXPECTORANTS, & MUCOLYTICS	
ANTITUSSIVE	Benzonatate
EXPECTORANT	Guaifenesin
MUCOLYTIC	Acetylcysteine
AUTONOMIC NERVOUS SYSTEM AGENTS	
ADRENERGIC AGONISTS (SYMPATHOMIMETICS)	
ALPHA-ADRENERGIC AGONIST	Methoxamine HCl
ALPHA- & BETA-ADRENERGIC AGONIST	Epinephrine
BETA-ADRENERGIC AGONIST	Albuterol
ADRENERGIC ANTAGONISTS (SYMPATHOLYTICS)	
ALPHA ANTAGONISTS (BLOCKING AGENT)	Prazosin HCl
BETA ANTAGONISTS	Propranolol HCl
ERGOT ALKALOID	Ergotamine Tartrate
5-HT_1 SEROTONIN AGONISTS	Sumatriptan
ANTICHOLINERGICS (PARASYMPATHOLYTICS)	
ANTIPARKINSON AGENTS	Levodopa
CATECHOLAMINE O-METHYL TRANSFERASE (COMT) INHIBITOR	Tolcapone
ANTIMUSCARINIC, ANTISPASMODIC	Atropine Sulfate
CHOLINERGICS (PARASYMPATHOMIMETICS)	
CHOLINESTERASE INHIBITOR	Neostigmine
CENTRAL-ACTING	Donepezil
DIRECT-ACTING CHOLINERGIC	Bethanechol Chloride

Classifications	Prototype
BENZODIAZEPINE ANTAGONIST	Flumazenil
BIOLOGIC RESPONSE MODIFIERS	
MONOCLONAL ANTIBODY	Basiliximab
IMMUNOSUPPRESSANT	Cyclosporine
IMMUNOGLOBULIN	Immune Globulin
TUMOR NECROSIS FACTOR MODIFIER	Etanercept
FUSION PROTEIN	Alefacept
BLOOD DERIVATIVE, PLASMA VOLUME, EXPANDER	Normal Serum Albumin
BLOOD FORMERS, COAGULATORS, & ANTICOAGULANTS	
ANTICOAGULANT	Heparin Sodium
DIRECT THROMBIN INHIBITOR	Lepirudin
LOW MOLECULAR WEIGHT HEPARIN	Enoxaparin
ANTIPLATELET AGENTS	Ticlopidine
GLYCOPROTEIN IIb/IIIa INHIBITOR	Abciximab
HEMATOPOIETIC GROWTH FACTOR	Epoetin Alpha
HEMOSTATIC	Aminocaproic Acid
IRON PREPARATION	Ferrous Sulfate
THROMBOLYTIC ENZYME	Alteplase
BRONCHODILATORS (RESPIRATORY SMOOTH MUSCLE RELAXANT)	
BETA-ADRENERGIC AGONIST	Isoproterenol HCl
XANTHINE	Theophylline
LEUKOTRIENE INHIBITOR	Zafirlukast
CARDIOVASCULAR AGENTS	
ANGIOTENSIN II RECEPTOR ANTAGONISTS	Losartan Potassium
ANGIOTENSIN-CONVERTING ENZYME INHIBITORS	Captopril
ANTIARRHYTHMIC AGENTS	
CLASS IA	Procainamide HCl
CLASS IB	Lidocaine HCl
CLASS IC	Flecainide
CLASS II	Propranolol HCl
CLASS III	Amiodarone HCl
ANTILIPEMICS	
BILE ACID SEQUESTRANT	Cholestyramine
FIBRATES	Clofibrate

Classifications	Prototype
HMG-CoA REDUCTASE INHIBITOR (STATIN)	Lovastatin
CALCIUM CHANNEL BLOCKER	Nifedipine
CARDIAC GLYCOSIDE	Digoxin
CENTRAL-ACTING ANTIHYPERTENSIVE	Methyldopa
INOTROPIC AGENT	Inamrinone
NITRATE VASODILATOR	Nitroglycerin
NONNITRATE VASODILATOR	Hydralazine HCl
RAUWOLFIA ALKALOID	Reserpine
CENTRAL NERVOUS SYSTEM AGENTS	
ANALGESICS, ANTIPYRETICS	
NARCOTIC (OPIATE) AGONISTS	Morphine
NARCOTIC (OPIATE) AGONIST-ANTAGONIST	Pentazocine HCl
NARCOTIC (OPIATE) ANTAGONIST	Naloxone HCl
NONNARCOTIC ANALGESICS	Acetaminophen
NONSTEROIDAL ANTI-INFLAMMATORY DRUGS (NSAID) COX-1	Ibuprofen
COX-2	Celecoxib
SALICYLATE	Aspirin
ANESTHETIC	
GENERAL	Thiopental Sodium
LOCAL (ESTER TYPE)	Procaine HCl
LOCAL (AMIDE TYPE)	Lidocaine HCl
ANTICONVULSANTS	
BARBITURATE	Phenobarbital
BENZODIAZEPINE	Diazepam
GABA INHIBITOR	Valproic Acid Sodium
HYDANTOIN	Phenytoin
SUCCINIMIDE	Ethosuximide
SULFONAMIDE	Zonisamide
TRICYCLIC	Carbamazepine
ANXIOLYTICS, SEDATIVE-HYPNOTICS	
BARBITURATE	Secobarbital
BENZODIAZEPINE	Lorazepam
NONBENZODIAZEPINE	Zolpidem
CARBAMATE	Meprobamate
PSYCHOTHERAPEUTIC	
ANTIDEPRESSANTS	
SELECTIVE SEROTONIN-REUPTAKE INHIBITORS (SSRI)	Fluoxetine HCl
SEROTONIN NOREPINEPHRINE REUPTAKE INHIBITORS	Venlafaxine
MONOAMINE OXIDASE (MAO) INHIBITORS	Phenelzine Sulfate

Classifications	Prototype
TETRACYCLIC ANTIDEPRESSANTS	Mirtazapine
TRICYCLIC ANTIDEPRESSANTS	Imipramine HCl
ANTIPSYCHOTIC AGENT	
BUTYROPHENONE	Haloperidol
PHENOTHIAZINE	Chlorpromazine
ATYPICAL	Clozapine
MOOD STABILIZER	Lithium Carbonate
CEREBRAL STIMULANT	
AMPHETAMINE	Amphetamine Sulfate
XANTHINE	Caffeine
ELECTROLYTIC & WATER BALANCE AGENTS	
DIURETIC	
LOOP	Furosemide
OSMOTIC	Mannitol
POTASSIUM-SPARING	Spironolactone
THIAZIDE	Hydrochlorothiazide
PHOSPHATE BINDER	Sevelamer HCl
REPLACEMENT SOLUTION	Calcium Gluconate
ENZYMES	
ENZYME REPLACEMENT	Pancrelipase
ENZYME INHIBITOR	Alpha$_1$-Proteinase Inhibitor
EYE, EAR, NOSE, & THROAT (EENT) PREPARATIONS	
ANTIHISTAMINE, OCULAR	Levocabastine HCl
CARBONIC ANHYDRASE INHIBITOR	Acetazolamide
CYCLOPLEGIC	Cyclopentolate HCl
MIOTIC (ANTIGLAUCOMA AGENT)	Pilocarpine HCl
MYDRIATIC	Homatropine HBr
PROSTAGLANDIN	Latanoprost
VASOCONSTRICTOR, DECONGESTANT	Naphazoline HCl
GASTROINTESTINAL AGENTS	
ANORECTANT	Diethylpropion HCl
ANTACID, ADSORBENT	Aluminum Hydroxide
ANTIDIARRHEAL	Diphenoxylate HCl with Atropine Sulfate
ANTIEMETIC	Prochlorperazine
ANTIEMETIC (5-HT$_3$ ANTAGONIST)	Ondansetron HCl
ANTISECRETORY (H$_2$-RECEPTOR ANTAGONIST)	Cimetidine
BULK LAXATIVE	Psyllium Hydrophilic Mucilloid
MUCOUS MEMBRANE ANTI-INFLAMMATORY	Mesalamine

Classifications	Prototype
PROKINETIC AGENT (GI STIMULANT)	Metoclopramide HCl
PROTON PUMP INHIBITORS	Omeprazole
SALINE CATHARTIC	Magnesium Hydroxide
STIMULANT LAXATIVE	Bisacodyl
STOOL SOFTENER	Docusate Calcium
GOLD COMPOUND	Aurothioglucose
HORMONES & SYNTHETIC SUBSTITUTES	
ADRENAL CORTICOSTEROID	
GLUCOCORTICOSTEROID	Prednisone
MINERALOCORTICOID	Fludrocortisone Acetate
ANDROGEN/ANABOLIC STEROIDS	Testosterone
ANTIANDROGENS	
5-ALPHA REDUCTASE INHIBITORS	Finasteride
ANTIDIABETIC AGENTS	
ALPHA-GLUCOSIDASE INHIBITOR	Acarbose
BIGUANIDES	Metformin
INSULIN	Insulin injection
MEGLITINIDES	Repaglinide
SULFONYLUREAS	Glyburide
THIAZOLIDINEDIONES	Rosiglitazone
ESTROGENS	Estradiol
GONADOTROPIN-RELEASING HORMONE ANALOGS	Leuprolide Acetate
GROWTH HORMONE	Somatropin
OXYTOCIC	Oxytocin Injection
PITUITARY (ANTIDIURETIC)	Vasopressin Injection
PROGESTINS	Progesterone
THYROID AGENTS	
ANTITHYROID AGENT	Propylthiouracil
THYROID	Levothyroxine Sodium
VITAMIN D ANALOG	Calcitriol
IMMUNOMODULATORS	
INTERFERONS	Interferon Alfa-2a
IMPOTENCE AGENT	
PHOSPHDIESTERASE INHIBITOR	Sildenafil
LUNG SURFACTANT	Beractant
MAST CELL STABILIZER	Cromolyn Sodium
PROSTAGLANDIN	Dinoprostone
BISPHOSPHONATE (REGULATOR, BONE METABOLISM)	Etidronate Disodium

Classifications	Prototype
SKIN & MUCOUS MEMBRANE AGENTS	
ANTIACNE (RETINOID)	Isotretinoin
ANTI-INFLAMMATORY STEROID	Hydrocortisone
PEDICULICIDE	Permethrin
PSORALEN	Methoxsalen
SCABICIDE	Lindane
SOMATIC NERVOUS SYSTEM AGENTS	
SKELETAL MUSCLE RELAXANTS	
CENTRAL-ACTING	Cyclobenzaprine HCl
DEPOLARIZING	Succinylcholine Chloride
NONDEPOLARIZING	Tubocurarine Chloride

ABACAVIR SULFATE

(a-ba'ca-vir)
Ziagen
Classifications: ANTIINFECTIVE; ANTIVIRAL AGENT; ANTIRETROVIRAL AGENT; NUCLEOSIDE REVERSE TRANSCRIPTASE INHIBITOR (NRTI)
Prototype: Zidovudine
Pregnancy Category: C

AVAILABILITY 300 mg tablets; 20 mg/mL oral solution

ACTIONS Abacavir is a synthetic nucleoside analogue with inhibitory activity against HIV. It inhibits the activity of HIV-1 reverse transcriptase (RT) both by competing with the natural DNA nucleoside and by incorporation into viral DNA.
THERAPEUTIC EFFECTS Abacavir prevents the formation of viral DNA replication. Therefore the viral load decreases as measured by an increased CD_4 lymphocyte cell count and suppression of HIV RNA, indicated by decreased HIV RNA copies, in HIV-positive individuals with little or no exposure to zidovudine (AZT).

USES Treatment of HIV infection in combination with other antiretroviral agents.

CONTRAINDICATIONS Hypersensitivity to abacavir (fatal rechallenge reactions reported); lactic acidosis; creatinine clearance of <50 mL/min; severe hepatomegaly, pregnancy (category C); lactation.
CAUTIOUS USE Prior resistance to another nucleoside reverse transcriptase inhibitor (NRTI); hepatic dysfunction; older adults.

ROUTE & DOSAGE

HIV Infection
Adult: **PO** 300 mg b.i.d.
Child: **PO** *3 mo–16 y,* 8 mg/kg b.i.d. (max: 300 mg b.i.d.)

ADMINISTRATION

Oral
- Tablets & oral solution are interchangeable on a mg-for-mg basis.
- Store tablets and liquid at 20°–25° C (68°–77° F). Liquid may be refrigerated.

ADVERSE EFFECTS (≥1%) **Body as a Whole:** Hypersensitivity reactions (including fever, skin rash, fatigue, nausea, vomiting, diarrhea, abdominal pain); malaise; lethargy; myalgia; arthralgia; paresthesia; edema; shortness of breath. **CNS:** Insomnia, *headache, fever.* **CV:** Hypotension (associated with hypersensitivity reaction). **GI:** <u>Hepatomegaly</u> with steatosis, *nausea, vomiting, diarrhea, anorexia,* pancreatitis, increased GGT, increased liver function tests. **Skin:** *Rash.* **Other:** Lactic acidosis, renal insufficiency.

INTERACTIONS Drug: Alcohol may increase abacavir blood levels.

PHARMACOKINETICS Absorption: Rapidly absorbed, 83% bioavailable. **Distribution:** Distributes into extravascular space and erythrocytes; 50% protein bound. **Metabolism:** Metabolized by alcohol dehydrogenase and glucuronyl transferase to inactive metabolites. **Elimination:** 84% excreted in urine, primarily as inactive metabolites; 16% excreted in feces. **Half-Life:** 1.5 h.

NURSING IMPLICATIONS

Assessment & Drug Effects
- Monitor for S&S of hypersensitivity: fever, skin rash, fatigue, GI distress (nausea, vomiting, diarrhea, abdominal pain). Withhold drug immediately & notify physician if hypersensitivity develops.

- Lab tests: Periodically monitor liver function, BUN and creatinine, CBC with differential, triglyceride levels, and blood glucose, especially in diabetics.
- Withhold drug & notify physician for S&S of acidosis, hepatotoxicity, or renal insufficiency.

Patient & Family Education

- Take drug exactly as prescribed at indicated times. Missed dose: Take immediately, then resume dosing schedule. Do not double a dose.
- Withhold drug immediately & notify physician at first sign of hypersensitivity reaction (see Assessment & Drug Effects).
- Carry Warning Card provided with drug at all times.
- Do not breast feed while taking this drug.

ABARELIX

(a-ba-re'lix)

Plenaxis

Classifications: HORMONES AND SYNTHETIC SUBSTITUTES; GONADOTROPIN-RELEASING HORMONE (GNRH) ANALOG

Prototype: Leuprolide acetate

Pregnancy Category: X

AVAILABILITY 50 mg/mL injection

ACTIONS A synthetic antagonist of gonadotropin-releasing hormone (GnRH), also known as luteinizing hormone-releasing hormone (LHRH), that inhibits the hypothalamic-pituitary-gonadal axis and blocks GnRH receptors in the pituitary, thus blocking gonadotropin and related androgen production.

THERAPEUTIC EFFECTS Causes rapid sex hormone suppression without an initial increase in serum testosterone concentration.

USES Palliative treatment of men with advanced symptomatic prostate cancer in whom LHRH agonist therapy is not appropriate and who refuse surgical castration, and have one or more of the following: (1) risk of neurological compromise due to metastases, (2) ureteral or bladder outlet obstruction due to local encroachment or metastatic disease, or (3) severe bone pain from skeletal metastases persisting with narcotic analgesia.

CONTRAINDICATIONS A known hypersensitivity to any of the drug components, women, pregnancy (category X), lactation, and children.

CAUTIOUS USE Patients with baseline QTc values >450 msec (e.g., congenital QT prolongation) and those taking Class IA (e.g., quinidine, procainamide) or Class III (e.g., amiodarone, sotalol) antiarrhythmic medications.

ROUTE & DOSAGE

Prostate Cancer

Adult: **IM** 100 mg to the buttock on day 1, 15, 29 (week 4) and every 4 wk thereafter

ADMINISTRATION

Intramuscular

- Hold vial at 45° angle and tap lightly on table to break up caking. To reconstitute, use diluent and syringes provided with drug. **Step 1:** Inject 2.2 mL diluent (NS injection) and discard remaining diluent; keep vial **upright,** insert needle all the way into vial, then inject diluent **quickly;** before withdrawing needle, remove 2.2 mL of air. **Step 2:** Keeping vial upright, shake immediately for about 15 sec; allow vial to stand for about 2 min, swirl occasionally and tap to reduce foaming. Repeat Step 2. **Step 3:** Locate a second injection spot on vial stopper and insert the 18 G needle. Invert vial and draw up some of the suspension into syringe and, **without removing needle from the vial,** reinject it at any remaining solids in vial. Repeat process until all solids are dispersed. Swirl vial before withdrawal, then withdraw **entire contents** from inverted vial by positioning the needle at a 45° angle. Monitor for anaphylaxis for at least 30 min following injection.

- Exchange the 18 G × 1½" needle with the enclosed 22 G × 1½" Safety Glide™ injection needle. Inject immediately into the ventral or dorsal gluteal muscle in buttock.
- Observe patient for 30 min for any sign of an allergic-type response.
- Store at 25° C (77° F), excursions permitted to 15°–30° C (59°–86° F).

ADVERSE EFFECTS (≥1%) **Body as a Whole:** Immediate-onset systemic allergic reactions, some resulting in hypotension and syncope, can happen after any dose, *hot flushes, pain, back pain, peripheral edema, fatigue.* **CNS:** *Sleep disturbance, dizziness, headache.* **GI:** *Constipation, diarrhea, nausea.* **Endocrine:** *Breast enlargement, breast pain/nipple tenderness.* **Respiratory:** *URI.* **Urogenital:** *Dysuria, frequent micturition, urinary retention, UTI.*

INTERACTIONS Drug: No drug interaction studies have been performed.

PHARMACOKINETICS Absorption: Slowly absorbed from IM site. **Peak:** 3 d. **Metabolism:** Metabolized by hydrolysis of peptide bonds. **Elimination:** Renally eliminated. **Half-Life:** 13 d.

NURSING IMPLICATIONS

Assessment & Drug Effects

- Observe closely for at least 30 min following every injection for a systemic allergic response (e.g., anaphylaxis, hypotension, syncope, urticaria, and pruritis). Note that risk of an allergic reaction increases with each successive injection.
- Monitor ECG and CV status for any patient with prolonged QT syndrome or arrythmia.
- Lab tests: Baseline and periodic LFTs; total testosterone levels just prior to administration on day 29 and q8wk thereafter; more frequent serum testosterone levels in patients weighing >225 lbs; periodic serum PSA; periodic Hgb and triglyceride levels; BMD (Bone Mineral Density) with extended treatment.

Patient & Family Education

- Report immediately itching, rash, difficulty breathing, swelling about the face and neck, faintness or any other unusual feelings or reactions following injection of drug.
- Inform physician of all other medicines you are taking, including nonprescription medicines, nutritional supplements, or herbal products.

ABCIXIMAB (Pr)

(ab-cix′i-mab)

ReoPro

Classifications: BLOOD FORMERS AND COAGULANTS; ANTITHROMBOTIC; ANTIPLATELET; GLYCOPROTEIN IIB/IIIA INHIBITOR

Pregnancy Category: C

AVAILABILITY 2 mg/mL in 5 mL vials

ACTIONS Abciximab is a human–murine monoclonal antibody Fab (fragment antigen binding) fragment that binds to the glycoprotein IIb/IIIa (GPIIb/IIIa) receptor sites of platelets.

THERAPEUTIC EFFECTS Abciximab inhibits platelet aggregation by preventing fibrinogen, von Willebrand's factor, and other molecules from adhering to GPIIb/IIIa receptor sites of the platelets.

USES Adjunct to aspirin and heparin for the prevention of acute cardiac ischemic complications in patients undergoing percutaneous transluminal coronary angioplasty (PTCA).

CONTRAINDICATIONS Hypersensitivity to abciximab or to murine proteins; active internal bleeding; GI or GU bleeding within 6 wk; history of CVA within 2 y or a CVA with severe neurologic deficit; administration of oral anticoagulants unless PT <1.2 times control; thrombocytopenia (<100,000 cells/mL); recent major surgery or trauma; intracranial neoplasm, aneurysm, severe hypertension; history of vasculitis; use of dextran before or during PTCA.

CAUTIOUS USE Pregnancy (category C); lactation; patients weighing <75 kg; older adults; history of previous GI disease; recent thrombolytic therapy; PTCA within 12 h of MI; unsuccessful PTCA; PTCA procedure lasting >70 min.

ROUTE & DOSAGE

PTCA

Adult: **IV** Starting 10–60 min prior to start of angioplasty, 0.25 mg/kg bolus over 5 min followed by continuous infusion of 10 mg/min for next 12 h

ADMINISTRATION

Intravenous

Do not shake vial. Discard if visible opaque particles are noted.

- Use a nonpyrogenic low protein-binding 0.2- or 0.22-µm filter when withdrawing drug into a syringe from the 2 mg/mL vial and when infusing as continuous IV.

PREPARE: **Direct:** No dilution required. **Continuous:** Inject 4.5 mL of drug into 250 mL of NS or D5W.

ADMINISTER: **Direct:** Give undiluted bolus dose over 5 min. **Continuous:** Infuse at 17 mL/h (10 mg/min) via an infusion pump; add no other drugs to the solution or IV line.

INCOMPATIBILITIES **Solution/additive:** Infuse through separate IV line. **Y-site:** Infuse through separate IV line.

- Discard any unused drug at the end of the 12-h infusion as well as any unused portion left in vial.
- Store vials at 2°–8° C (36°–46° F).

ADVERSE EFFECTS (≥1%) **Hematologic:** *Bleeding*, including intracranial, retroperitoneal, and hematemesis; thrombocytopenia.

INTERACTIONS Drug: ORAL ANTICOAGULANTS, NSAIDS, **dipyridamole, ticlopidine, dextran** may increase risk of bleeding.

PHARMACOKINETICS Onset: >90% inhibition of platelet aggregation within 2 h. **Duration:** Approximately 48 h. **Half-Life:** 30 min.

NURSING IMPLICATIONS

Assessment & Drug Effects

- Monitor for S&S of: bleeding at all potential sites (e.g., catheter insertion, needle puncture, or cutdown sites; GI, GU, or retroperitoneal sites); hypersensitivity that may occur any time during administration.
- Lab tests: Monitor Hgb, Hct, platelet count, PT, APTT, INR, and acti-

vated clotting time, every 2–4 h during first 24 h.

- Avoid or minimize unnecessary invasive procedures and devices to reduce risk of bleeding.
- Elevate head of bed ≤30° and keep limb straight when femoral artery access is used; following sheath removal, apply pressure for 30 min.
- Stop infusion immediately & notify physician if bleeding or S&S of hypersensitivity occurs.

Patient & Family Education

- Report any S&S of bleeding immediately.
- Do not breast feed while taking this drug without consulting physician.

ACAMPROSATE CALCIUM

(a-cam-pro′sate)

Classifications: CENTRAL NERVOUS SYSTEM AGENT; SUBSTANCE ABUSE DETERRENT

Pregnancy Category: C

AVAILABILITY 333 mg delayed-release tablets

ACTIONS May interact with CNS glutamate and GABA neurotransmitter systems and help restore normal balance between neuronal excitation and inhibition. Acamprosate is a neurotransmitter analog.

THERAPEUTIC EFFECTS Reduces craving for alcohol intake due to chronic use, but does not cause alcohol aversion or a disulfiram-like reaction as a result of ethanol ingestion.

USES Maintenance of abstinence from alcohol in patients with alcoholism

CONTRAINDICATIONS Hypersensitivity to acamprosate calcium or any of its components; suicidal ideation; pregnancy (category C). Safety and efficacy in patients with severe renal impairment (Cl_{cr} ~30 mL/min) have not been established.

CAUTIOUS USE Moderate renal impairment; depression; lactation. Safety and efficacy of acamprosate have not been established in adolescents or children <18 y.

ROUTE & DOSAGE

Maintenance of Alcohol Abstinence

Adult: **PO** 666 mg t.i.d.

Renal Impairment

Adult: **PO** Cl_{cr} 30–50 mL/min: 333 mg t.i.d.; Cl_{cr} <30 mL/min: do not use

ADMINISTRATION

Oral

- Ensure that the drug is not chewed or crushed. It must be swallowed whole.
- Store at 15°–30° C (59°–86° F).

ADVERSE EFFECTS (≥1%) **Body as a Whole:** Flu syndrome, chills. **CNS:** Depression, anxiety, insomnia, asthenia, dizziness, paresthesia, headache, somnolence, decreased libido, amnesia, abnormal thinking, tremor. **CV:** Palpitation, syncope. **GI:** *Diarrhea,* nausea, vomiting, anorexia, flatulence, dry mouth, abdominal pain, dyspepsia, constipation, increased appetite. **Metabolic:** Peripheral edema, weight gain. **Musculoskeletal:** Musculoskeletal pain. **Respiratory:** Rhinitis, cough, dyspnea, pharyngitis, bronchitis. **Skin:** Pruritus, diaphoresis, rash. **Special Senses:** Abnormal vision, taste perversion. **Urogenital:** Impotence.

INTERACTIONS Drug: None reported.

PHARMACOKINETICS Absorption: 11% bioavailability. **Metabolism:** Not metabolized. **Elimination:** Renal. **Half-Life:** 20–33 h.

NURSING IMPLICATIONS

Assessment & Drug Effects

- Monitor for S&S depression or suicidal thinking.
- Monitor for dizziness or impaired judgment, thinking, and motor skills; take appropriate protective measures.

Patient & Family Education

- Report any alcohol consumption while taking acamprosate.
- Report promptly any of the following: unusual anxiousness or nervousness; depression or suicidal thoughts; burning or tingling sensations in arms, legs, hands, or feet; chest pains or palpitations; difficulty urinating.
- Do not drive or engage in other hazardous activities until reaction to the drug is known.
- Do not breast feed while taking this drug.

ACARBOSE (Pr)

(a-car'bose)

Precose

Classifications: HORMONE AND SYNTHETIC SUBSTITUTES; ANTIDIABETIC AGENT; ALPHA-GLUCOSIDASE INHIBITOR

Pregnancy Category: B

AVAILABILITY 50 mg, 100 mg tablets

ACTIONS Acarbose is an oral alpha-glucosidase inhibitor. It inhibits or delays the absorption of sugars from the intestinal tract. The inhibitory effect of acarbose varies according to which enzymes are involved; from most to least inhibited are glucoamylase, sucrase, maltase, and isomaltase. Lactase is not affected by acarbose.

THERAPEUTIC EFFECTS Acarbose reduces blood sugar by interfering with carbohydrate absorption from the GI tract.

USES As monotherapy or in combination with a sulfonylurea in patients with type 2 diabetes mellitus.

UNLABELED USES In combination with insulin and metformin in patients with type 1 diabetes mellitus.

CONTRAINDICATIONS Inflammatory bowel disease, colon ulcers, partial bowel obstruction, predisposition for obstruction; patients <18 y; lactation.

CAUTIOUS USE GI distress or liver disorders, pregnancy (category B).

ROUTE & DOSAGE

Diabetes Mellitus

Adult: **PO** Initiate with 25 mg q.d. to t.i.d. with meals, may increase q4–8wk up to 50–100 mg t.i.d. with meals (max: 150 mg/d for ≤60 kg, 300 mg/d for >60 kg)

ADMINISTRATION

Oral

- Remove drug from foil wrapper immediately before administration.
- Give drug with first bite at each of the three main meals.
- Do not store above 25° C (77° F). Keep tightly closed and protect from moisture.

ADVERSE EFFECTS (≥1%) **CNS:** Sleepiness, weakness, dizziness, headache, vertigo (may be due to poor diabetic control). **Endocrine:** Hypoglycemia (especially in combination with sulfonylureas and insulin). **GI:** *Diarrhea, flatulence, abdominal distention,* borborygmi, increased liver function tests. **Hematologic:** Anemia (especially iron deficiency). **Skin:** Erythema, exanthema, urticaria.

INTERACTIONS Drug: SULFONYLUREAS may increase hypoglycemic effects. Drugs that induce hyperglycemia (e.g., THIAZIDES, CORTICOSTEROIDS, PHENOTHIAZINES, ESTROGENS, **phenytoin, isoniazid**) may decrease effectiveness of acarbose. **Herbal: Garlic, ginseng** may increase hypoglycemic effects.

PHARMACOKINETICS Absorption: Only 0.5%–2% is absorbed intact from GI tract. After degradation by intestinal bacteria, up to 35% of dose may be absorbed. **Peak:** Peak blood glucose reduction approximately 70 min after dose. **Metabolism:** Metabolized in GI tract by intestinal bacteria and digestive enzymes. **Elimination:** 35% excreted in urine, 51% excreted in feces, and 5% excreted in air as CO_2. **Half-Life:** 2 h.

NURSING IMPLICATIONS

Assessment & Drug Effects

- Lab tests: Periodically monitor blood glucose, HbA_{1C} liver, enzymes, Hct and Hgb.
- Treat hypoglycemia with dextrose; not with sucrose (table sugar).

Patient & Family Education

- Note: Acarbose prevents the breakdown of table sugar. Have a source of dextrose, such as dextrose paste, available to treat low blood sugar.
- Monitor closely blood glucose especially following dosage changes.
- Report abdominal distress; dietary adjustment or dosage reduction may be warranted.
- Monitor weight and report significant changes.
- Do not breast feed while taking this drug.

ACEBUTOLOL HYDROCHLORIDE

(a-se-byoo-toe'lole)

Monitan ✦, Sectral

Classifications: AUTONOMIC NERVOUS SYSTEM AGENT; BETA-ADRENERGIC ANTAGONIST (BLOCKING AGENT, SYMPATHOLYTIC); CARDIOVASCULAR AGENT; ANTIHYPERTENSIVE; ANTIARRHYTHMIC, CLASS II AGENT

Prototype: Propranolol

Pregnancy Category: B

AVAILABILITY 200 mg, 400 mg capsules

ACTIONS $Beta_1$-selective adrenergic blocking agent with mild intrinsic sympathomimetic activity (partial beta-agonist activity). Exhibits antiarrhythmic activity (class II antiarrhythmic agent). Produces negative chronotropic and inotropic activity (i.e., decreases exercise-induced heart rate, inhibits reflex orthostatic tachycardia, and decreases cardiac output at rest and during exercise).

THERAPEUTIC EFFECTS Decreases both systolic and diastolic BP at rest and during exercise.

USES Treatment of mild to moderate hypertension. Management of recurrent stable ventricular arrhythmias.

UNLABELED USES Supraventricular arrhythmias, chronic stable angina pectoris.

CONTRAINDICATIONS Overt CHF, second- or third-degree AV block, severe bradycardia, cardiogenic shock; lactation; children <12 y.

CAUTIOUS USE Impaired cardiac function, well-compensated CHF, mesenteric or peripheral vascular disease; patients undergoing major surgery involving general anesthesia; renal or hepatic impairment; labile diabetes mellitus; hyperthyroidism; bronchospastic disease (asthma, emphysema); avoid abrupt withdrawal; pregnancy (category B).

ROUTE & DOSAGE

Hypertension

Adult: **PO** 400–800 mg/d in 1–2 divided doses (max: 1200 mg/d)
Geriatric: **PO** 200–400 mg/d (max: 800 mg/d)

Ventricular Arrhythmias

Adult: **PO** 200 mg b.i.d. increased to 600–1200 mg/d

Angina Pectoris

Adult: **PO** 300–400 mg t.i.d.

Renal Impairment

Cl_{cr} <50 mL/min: reduce dose by 50%; <25 mL/min: reduce dose by 75%

ADMINISTRATION

Oral

- Check apical pulse before administration. If <60 bpm or other ordered parameter, consult physician.
- Discontinue gradually over a period of 2 wk.
- Store at 15°–30° C (59°–86° F).

ADVERSE EFFECTS (≥1%) **Body as a Whole:** *Fatigue.* **CNS:** Dizziness, insomnia, drowsiness, confusion, fainting. **CV:** *Bradycardia*, hypotension, CHF. **GI:** Nausea, *diarrhea, constipation,* flatulence. **Hematologic:** Agranulocytosis, *antinuclear antibodies (ANA).* **Metabolic:** hypoglycemia (may mask symptoms of a hypoglycemic reaction). **Respiratory:** Bronchospasm, pulmonary edema, dyspnea. **Urogenital:** Decreased libido; impotence.

DIAGNOSTIC TEST INTERFERENCE False-negative test results possible (see **propranolol**).

INTERACTIONS Drug: Other HYPOTENSIVE AGENTS, DIURETICS increase hypotensive effect; with **albuterol, metaproterenol, terbutaline,** or **pirbuterol,** there is mutual antagonism with acebutolol; NSAIDS blunt hypotensive effect; decreases hypoglycemic effect of **glyburide;** increases bradycardia and sinus arrest with **amiodarone.**

PHARMACOKINETICS Absorption: Well absorbed after PO administration; undergoes extensive first-pass metabolism in liver with an average bioavailability of 40%. (In geriatric patients, bioavailability increases twofold). **Peak:** 3 h. **Distribution:** Minimally into CSF; crosses placenta; is excreted in breast milk. **Metabolism:** Metabolized in liver to diacetolol with activity equipotent to parent compound. **Elimination:** Metabolite 8–13 h; 50%–60% excreted via bile into feces, and 30%–40% excreted in urine. **Half-Life:** 3–4 h.

NURSING IMPLICATIONS

Assessment & Drug Effects

- Monitor BP and cardiac status throughout therapy. Observe for and report marked bradycardia or hypotension, especially when patient is also receiving a catecholamine-depleting drug (e.g., reserpine).

- Monitor I&O ratio and pattern and report changes to physician (e.g., dysuria, nocturia, oliguria, weight change).
- Monitor for S&S of CHF, especially peripheral edema, dyspnea, activity intolerance.
- Lab tests: Monitor for drug-induced positive ANA titer during long-term therapy, especially in women and older adults; periodic CBC with long-term therapy.

Patient & Family Education

- Know parameters for withholding drug (e.g., pulse less than 60).
- Note: Common adverse effects include insomnia, drowsiness, and confusion.
- Do not drive or engage in potentially hazardous activities until response to drug is known.
- Do not increase, decrease, omit, or discontinue drug regimen without advice from the physician. Abrupt withdrawal may worsen angina or precipitate MI in patient with heart disease.
- Contact physician promptly at the first signs or symptoms of CHF (see Appendix F).
- Report muscle and joint pain to physician. Discontinuation of drug therapy usually reverses these adverse effects.
- Monitor for loss of glycemic control if diabetic.
- Note: Drug may mask symptoms of hypoglycemia (see Appendix F) and potentiate insulin-induced hypoglycemia in diabetics.
- Avoid use of OTC oral cold preparations and topical nasal decongestants unless approved by the physician.
- Do not breast feed while taking this drug without consulting physician.

ACETAMINOPHEN, PARACETAMOL (Pr)

(a-seat-a-mee′noe-fen)

Abenol ♣, A'Cenol, Acephen, Anacin-3, Anuphen, APAP, Atasol ♣, Campain ♣, Datril Extra Strength, Dolanex, Exdol ♣, Halenol, Liquiprin, Panadol, Pedric, Robigesic ♣, Rounox ♣, Tapar, Tempra, Tylenol, Valadol

Classifications: CENTRAL NERVOUS SYSTEM AGENT; NONNARCOTIC ANALGESIC, ANTIPYRETIC

Pregnancy Category: B

AVAILABILITY 80 mg, 120 mg, 125 mg, 300 mg, 325 mg, 650 mg suppositories; 80 mg, 160 mg, 325 mg, 500 mg tablets; 80 mg/0.8 mL, 80 mg/2.5 mL, 80 mg/5 mL, 120 mg/5 mL, 160 mg/5 mL, 500 mg/5 mL liquid

ACTIONS Produces analgesia by unknown mechanism, perhaps by action on peripheral nervous system. Reduces fever by direct action on hypothalamus heat-regulating center with consequent peripheral vasodilation, sweating, and dissipation of heat. Unlike aspirin, acetaminophen has little effect on platelet aggregation, does not affect bleeding time, and generally produces no gastric bleeding.

THERAPEUTIC EFFECTS It provides temporary analgesia for mild to moderate pain. In addition, acetaminophen lowers body temperature in individuals with a fever.

USES Fever reduction. Temporary relief of mild to moderate pain. Generally as substitute for aspirin when the latter is not tolerated or is contraindicated.

CONTRAINDICATIONS Hypersensitivity to acetaminophen or phenacetin; use with alcohol.

CAUTIOUS USE Children <3 y unless directed by a physician; repeated administration to patients with anemia or hepatic disease; arthritic or rheumatoid conditions affecting children <12 y; alcoholism; malnutrition; thrombocytopenia. Safety during pregnancy (category B) or lactation is not established.

ROUTE & DOSAGE

Mild to Moderate Pain, Fever

Adult: **PO** 325–650 mg q4–6h (max: 4 g/d) **PR** 650 mg q4–6h (max: 4 g/d)
Child: **PO** *0–3 mo,* 40 mg q4–6h; *4–11 mo,* 80 mg q4–6h; *1–2 y,* 120 mg q4–6h; *2–3 y,* 160 mg q4–6h; *4–5 y,* 240 mg q4–6h; *6–8 y,* 320 mg q4–6h; *9–10 y,* 400 mg q4–6h; *11–12 y,* 480 mg q4–6h **PR** *2–5 y,* 120 mg q4–6h (max: 720 mg/d); *6–12 y,* 325 mg q4–6h (max: 2.6 g/d)
Neonate: **PO** 10–15 mg/kg q6–8h

ADMINISTRATION

Oral

- Administer tablets or caplets whole or crushed and give with fluid of patient's choice.
- Chewable tablets should be thoroughly chewed and wetted before they are swallowed.
- Do not coadminister with a high carbohydrate meal; absorption rate may be significantly retarded.
- Store in light-resistant containers at room temperature, preferably between 15°–30° C (59°–86° F).

Rectal

- Insert suppositories beyond the rectal sphincter.

ADVERSE EFFECTS (≥1%) **Body as a Whole:** Negligible with recommended dosage; rash. **Acute poisoning:** Anorexia, nausea, vomiting, dizziness, lethargy, diaphoresis, chills, epigastric or abdominal pain, diarrhea; onset of hepatotoxicity—elevation of serum transaminases (ALT, AST) and bilirubin; hypoglycemia, hepatic coma, acute renal failure (rare). **Chronic ingestion:** Neutropenia, pancytopenia, leukopenia, thrombocytopenic purpura, *hepatotoxicity in alcoholics,* renal damage.

DIAGNOSTIC TEST INTERFERENCE False increases in ***urinary 5-HIAA*** (5-hydroxyindoleacetic acid) by-product of serotonin; false decreases in ***blood glucose*** (by ***glucose oxidase–peroxidase procedure***); false increases in ***urinary glucose*** (with certain instruments in glucose analyses); and false increases in ***serum uric acid*** (with ***phosphotungstate method***). High doses or long-term therapy: hepatic, renal, and hematopoietic function (periodically).

INTERACTIONS Drug: Cholestyramine may decrease acetaminophen absorption. With chronic coadministration, BARBITURATES, **carbamazepine, phenytoin,** and **rifampin** may increase potential for chronic hepatotoxicity. Chronic, excessive ingestion of **alcohol** will increase risk of hepatotoxicity.

PHARMACOKINETICS Absorption: Rapid and almost complete absorption from GI tract; less complete absorption from rectal suppository. **Peak:** 0.5–2 h. **Duration:** 3–4 h. **Distribution:** Well distributed in all body fluids; crosses placenta. **Metabolism:** Extensively metabolized in liver. **Elimination:** 90%–100% of drug excreted as metabolites in urine; excreted in breast milk. **Half-Life:** 1–3 h.

NURSING IMPLICATIONS

Assessment & Drug Effects

- Monitor for S&S of: hepatotoxicity, even with moderate acetaminophen doses, especially in individuals with poor nutrition or who have ingested alcohol over prolonged periods; poisoning, usually from accidental ingestion or suicide attempts; potential abuse from psychological dependence (withdrawal has been associated with restless and excited responses).

Patient & Family Education

- Do not take other medications (e.g., cold preparations) containing acetaminophen without medical advice; overdosing and chronic use can cause liver damage and other toxic effects.
- Do not self-medicate adults for pain more than 10 d (5 d in children) without consulting a physician.
- Do not use this medication without medical direction for: fever persisting longer than 3 d, fever over 39.5° C (103° F), or recurrent fever.
- Do not give children more than 5 doses in 24 h unless prescribed by physician.
- Do not breast feed while taking this drug without consulting physician.

ACETAZOLAMIDE (Pr)

(a-set-a-zole'a-mide)

Acetazolam ♣, AkZol, Apo-Acetazolamide ♣, Dazamide, Diamox, Diamox Sequels

ACETAZOLAMIDE SODIUM

(a-set-a-zole'a-mide)

Diamox Parenteral

Classifications: EYE PREPARATION; CARBONIC ANHYDRASE INHIBITOR; DIURETIC; CENTRAL NERVOUS SYSTEM AGENT; ANTICONVULSANT

Pregnancy Category: C

AVAILABILITY 125 mg, 250 mg tablets; 500 mg sustained-release capsules; 500 mg powder for injection

ACTIONS The mechanism of anticonvulsant action with acetazolamide is unknown but thought to involve inhibition of CNS carbonic anhydrase, which retards abnormal paroxysmal discharge from CNS neurons. Diuretic effect is due to inhibition of carbonic anhydrase activity in proximal renal tubule, preventing formation of carbonic acid. Inhibition of carbonic anhydrase in eye reduces rate of aqueous humor formation with consequent lowering of intraocular pressure.

THERAPEUTIC EFFECTS Reduces seizure activity and intraocular pressure. Additionally, Diamox has a diuretic effect.

USES Treatment of seizures: absence or petit mal, generalized tonic-clonic (grand mal), and focal; reduction of intraocular pressure in open-angle glaucoma and secondary glaucoma; preoperative treatment of acute closed-angle glaucoma; drug-induced edema and as adjunct in treatment of edema due to congestive heart failure; acute high-altitude sickness.

UNLABELED USES Prevent uric acid or cystine renal calculi; to treat acute pancreatitis, premenstrual syndrome (PMS), metabolic alkalosis, and hypokalemic and hyperkalemic forms of familial periodic paralysis; to increase secretion of phenobarbital or lithium; hydrocephalus.

CONTRAINDICATIONS Hypersensitivity to sulfonamides and derivatives (e.g., thiazides), marked renal and hepatic dysfunction; Addison's disease or other types of adrenocortical insufficiency; hyponatremia, hypokalemia, hyperchloremic acidosis; prolonged administration to patients with hyphema or chronic noncongestive angle-closure glaucoma. Safety during pregnancy (category C) or lactation is not established.

CAUTIOUS USE History of hypercalciuria; diabetes mellitus, gout, patients receiving digitalis, obstructive pulmonary disease, respiratory acidosis.

ROUTE & DOSAGE

Glaucoma

Adult: **PO** 250 mg 1–4 times/d, 500 mg sustained release b.i.d. **IM/IV** 500 mg, may repeat in 2–4 h
Child: **PO** 8–30 mg/kg/d in 3 doses **IM/IV** 5–10 mg/kg q6h

Epilepsy

Adult/Child: **PO** 8–30 mg/kg/d in 1–4 doses

Edema

Adult: **PO** 250–375 mg every AM (5 mg/kg)
Child: **PO/IM/IV** 5 mg/kg or 150 mg/m^2/every AM

High Altitude Sickness

Adult: **PO** 250 mg q8–12h or 500 mg sustained release q12–24h, starting 24–48 h before climb and continuing for 48 h at high altitude

Treatment Hydrocephalus

Neonate/Infant: **PO/IV** 5 mg/kg q6h, may increase by 25 mg/kg/d (max: of 100 mg/kg/d)

Renal Impairment

Cl_{cr} 10–50 mL/min: dose q12h; <10 mL/min: use not recommended

ADMINISTRATION

Oral

- Administer diuretic dose in morning to avoid interrupted sleep.
- Give with food or meals to minimize GI upset.
- Note: If tablet(s) cannot be swallowed, soften tablet(s) (not sustained release form) in 2 tsp of hot water and add to 2 tsp of honey/syrup to disguise bitter taste; avoid syrups containing alcohol or glycerin, or crush tablet(s) and suspend in syrup (250–500 mg/5 mL syrup). Prepare just before administration. Drug does not dissolve in fruit juices.
- Store oral preparations at 15°–30° C (59°–86° F) unless otherwise directed.

Intramuscular

- Reconstitute as for IV administration. See PREPARE Direct.
- Give IM for rapid lowering of intraocular pressure or in patients unable to take oral dosage.
- Note: The intramuscular dosage is not the route of choice because the alkalinity of the solution makes the injection painful.

Intravenous

- IV administration to neonates, infants, and children: Verify correct IV concentration and rate of infusion/injection with physician.

PREPARE: **Direct:** Reconstitute each 500 mg vial with at least 5 mL of sterile water for injection. **IV Infusion:** Reconstituted solution may be further diluted with D5W or NS. Use within 24 h of reconstitution.

ADMINISTER: **Direct:** Give at a rate of 500 mg or fraction thereof over 1 min. **IV Infusion:** Give as a continuous infusion over 4–8 h.

ADVERSE EFFECTS (≥1%) **CNS:** Paresthesias, sedation, malaise, disorientation, depression, fatigue, muscle weakness, flaccid paralysis. **GI:** Anorexia, nausea, vomiting, weight loss, dry mouth, thirst, diarrhea. **Hematologic:** Bone marrow depression with agranulocytosis, hemolytic anemia, aplastic anemia, leukopenia, pancytopenia. **Metabolic:** Increased excretion of calcium, potassium, magnesium, and sodium; metabolic acidosis; hyperglycemia; hyperuricemia. **Urogenital:** Glycosuria, urinary frequency, polyuria, dysuria, hematuria, crystalluria. **Other:** Exacerbation of gout, hepatic dysfunction.

DIAGNOSTIC TEST INTERFERENCE Monitor for false-positive ***urinary protein*** determinations; falsely high values for ***urine urobilinogen;*** depressed ***iodine uptake*** values (exception: hypothyroidism).

INTERACTIONS Drug: Renal excretion of AMPHETAMINES, **ephedrine, flecainide, quinidine, procainamide,** TRICYCLIC ANTIDEPRESSANTS may be decreased, thereby enhancing or prolonging their effects. Renal excretion of **lithium** is increased. Excretion of **phenobarbital** may be increased. **Amphotericin B** and CORTICOSTEROIDS may accelerate **potassium** loss. DIGITALIS GLYCOSIDES may predispose persons with hypokalemia to **digitalis** toxicity; puts patients on high doses of SALICYLATES at high risk for SALICYLATE toxicity.

PHARMACOKINETICS Absorption: Well absorbed from GI tract. **Onset:** 1 h regular release; 2 h sustained release; 2 min IV. **Peak:** 2–4 h reg; 8–18 h sustained; 15 min IV. **Duration:** 8–12 h reg; 18–24 h sustained; 4–5 h IV. **Distribution:** Distributed throughout body, concentrating in RBCs, plasma, and kidneys; crosses placenta. **Elimination:** Excreted primarily in urine. **Half-Life:** 2.4–5.8 h.

NURSING IMPLICATIONS

Assessment & Drug Effects

- Establish baseline weight before initial therapy and weigh daily thereafter when used to treat edema.
- Monitor for S&S of: mild to severe metabolic acidosis; potassium loss which is greatest early in therapy (see hypokalemia in Appendix F).
- Monitor I&O especially when used with other diuretics.
- Lab tests: Blood pH, blood gases, urinalysis, CBC, and serum electrolytes (initially and periodically during prolonged therapy or concomitant therapy with other diuretics or digitalis).

Patient & Family Education

- Maintain adequate fluid intake (1.5–2.5 L/24 h; 1 liter is approximately equal to 1 quart) to reduce risk of kidney stones.
- Report any of the following: numbness, tingling, burning, drowsiness, and visual problems, sore throat or mouth, unusual bleeding, fever, skin or renal problems.
- Eat potassium-rich diet and take potassium supplement when taking this drug in high doses or for prolonged periods.
- Do not breast feed while taking this drug without consulting physician.

ACETOHEXAMIDE

(a-seat-oh-hex'a-mide)

Dimelor ✤, Dymelor

Classifications: HORMONE AND SYNTHETIC SUBSTITUTE; SULFONYLUREA ANTIDIABETIC AGENTS
Prototype: Glyburide
Pregnancy Category: C

AVAILABILITY 250 mg, 500 mg tablets

ACTIONS Lowers blood glucose by stimulating pancreatic beta cells to secrete insulin.
THERAPEUTIC EFFECTS More potent and has longer action than tolbutamide. Promotes increased effectiveness of endogenous insulin.

USES Mild to moderately severe stable type 2 diabetes mellitus. Preferred by some clinicians for patients who also have gout.

CONTRAINDICATIONS Hypersensitivity to sulfonylureas; severe impairment of hepatic, renal, thyroid, or other endocrine function; as sole therapy for type 1 diabetes mellitus and in diabetes complicated by ketosis, acidosis, coma, infection, trauma, hyperglycemia, and glycosuria associated with primary renal disease. Safety during pregnancy (category C), lactation, or in children is not established.
CAUTIOUS USE Renal insufficiency, history of hepatic porphyria.

ROUTE & DOSAGE

Diabetes
Adult: **PO** 250 mg/d before breakfast, may be increased by 250–500 mg q5–7d (max: 1.5 g/d)

ADMINISTRATION

Oral
- Administer daily dose before breakfast.
- Divided doses are given before breakfast and dinner.
- Store at 15°–30° C (59°–86° F), unless otherwise directed.

ADVERSE EFFECTS (≥1%) **Body as a Whole:** Generally dose-related. Erythema, urticaria, pruritus, rash, photosensitivity. **GI:** Nausea, vomiting, epigastric fullness, anorexia, stomach pain or discomfort, heartburn, diarrhea. **Hematologic:** <u>Agranulocytosis, aplastic anemia, severe hypoglycemia</u>, thrombocytopenia. **CNS:** Headache, dizziness.

DIAGNOSTIC TEST INTERFERENCE ***Serum uric acid*** levels may be appreciably reduced.

INTERACTIONS Drug: Alcohol may elicit **disulfiram** reaction; **warfarin, aspirin** and other SALICYLATES, **chloramphenicol, clofibrate, fenfluramine, guanethidine,** MAO INHIBITORS, **oxytetracycline, phenylbutazone, probenecid, sulfinpyrazone,** and SULFONAMIDES may enhance hypoglycemic effects; with **diazoxide** there is mutual antagonism and effects of both drugs are reduced; THIAZIDE DIURETICS may exacerbate hyperglycemia, resulting in need for increased acetohexamide doses; **phenytoin** may decrease effects of acetohexamide; BETA-ADRENERGIC BLOCKERS may mask symptoms of hypoglycemia. **Herbal: Garlic, ginseng** may increase hypoglycemic effects.

PHARMACOKINETICS Absorption: Rapidly absorbed from GI tract. **Onset:** 1 h. **Peak:** 2–4 h. **Duration:** 12–24 h. **Distribution:** Breast milk. **Metabolism:** Metabolized in liver to active metabolite. **Elimination:** 80%–95% eliminated in urine; 15% in bile. **Half-Life:** 5–6 h.

NURSING IMPLICATIONS

Assessment & Drug Effects

- Monitor blood glucose levels closely during first 24–48 h after therapy is initiated or the dose is changed.
- Monitor for S&S of hypoglycemia/ exaggerated hypoglycemic response, particularly in older adults, malnourished, and debilitated patients or those with impaired hepatic, renal function, adrenal, or pituitary insufficiency.
- Lab tests: Periodic blood glucose, hemoglobin $A_{1\text{-}C}$, and liver functions.

Patient & Family Education

- Ingest some form of sugar (e.g., orange juice, dissolved table sugar, corn syrup, honey) if symptoms of hypoglycemia develop, and seek medical assistance.
- Check blood glucose as prescribed.
- Do not take any other medication unless approved by physician.
- Alcoholic beverages may produce a disulfiram-type reaction (see Appendix F).
- Avoid prolonged direct exposure to sun to prevent photosensitivity reaction.
- Report dermatologic reactions such as rash or itching.
- Do not breast feed while taking this drug without consulting physician.

ACETYLCYSTEINE Pr

(a-se-til-sis'tay-een)

Airbron ♣, Mucomyst, Mucosol, *N*-Acetylcysteine, Acetadote, Acys-5

Classifications: SKIN AND MUCOUS MEMBRANE AGENT; MUCOLYTIC; ANTIDOTE

Pregnancy Category: B

AVAILABILITY 10%, 20% solution for inhalation; 20% solution for injection; 500 mg tablet

ACTIONS Acetylcysteine probably acts by disrupting disulfide linkages of mucoproteins in purulent and nonpurulent secretions.

THERAPEUTIC EFFECTS Acetylcysteine lowers viscosity and facilitates the removal of secretions.

USES Adjuvant therapy in patients with abnormal, viscid, or inspissated mucous secretions in acute and chronic bronchopulmonary diseases, and in pulmonary complications of cystic fibrosis and surgery, tracheostomy, and atelectasis. Also used in diagnostic bronchial studies and as an antidote for acute acetaminophen poisoning.

UNLABELED USES As an ophthalmic solution for treatment of dry eye (keratoconjunctivitis sicca); as an enema to treat bowel obstruction due to meconium ileus.

CONTRAINDICATIONS Hypersensitivity to acetylcysteine; patients at risk of gastric hemorrhage.

CAUTIOUS USE Patients with asthma, older adults, severe hepatic disease, esophageal varices, peptic ulcer disease; debilitated patients with severe respiratory insufficiency, pregnancy (category B), lactation.

ROUTE & DOSAGE

Mucolytic

Adult: **Inhalation** 1–10 mL of 20% solution q4–6h or 2–20 mL of 10% solution q4–6h **Direct Instillation** 1–2 mL of 10%–20% solution q1–4h **PO** 200 mg 2–3 times/d; 300 mg b.i.d.; or 600 mg once daily, twice daily, or 3 times/wk

Child: **Inhalation** 3–5 mL of 20% solution or 6–10 mL of 10% solution 3–4 times/d
Infant: **Inhalation** 1–2 mL 20% solution or 2–4 mL of 10% solution 3–4 times/d

Acetaminophen Toxicity

Adult/Child: **PO** 140 mg/kg followed by 70 mg/kg q4h for 17 doses (use a 5% solution)
Adult/Adolescent: **IV** 150 mg/kg infused over 15 min, followed by 50 mg/kg over 4 h, then 100 mg/kg over 16 h; OR 140 mg/kg infused over 1 h, then, 4 h after the loading dose, give 70 mg/kg q4h × 12 doses

ADMINISTRATION

Inhalation and Instillation

- Prepare dilution within 1 h of use; drug does not contain an antimicrobial agent. A light purple discoloration does not significantly impair drug's effectiveness.
- Dilute the 20% solution with NS or water for injection. The 10% solution may be used undiluted.
- Give by direct instillation into tracheostomy (1–2 mL of 10%–20% solution).
- Instruct patient to clear airway, if possible, coughing productively prior to aerosol administration to ensure maximum effect.
- Store opened vial in refrigerator to retard oxidation; use within 96 h.
- Store unopened vial at 15°–30° C (59°–86° F), unless otherwise directed.

Oral

- Dilute the 20% solution 1:3 with cola, orange juice, or other soft drink to make a 5% solution. If administered via a gastric tube, water may be used as the diluent.
- Freshly prepare all diluted solutions and use within 1 hour of preparation.

Intravenous

PREPARE: **IV Infusion:** Acetylcysteine reacts with certain metals and rubber; use IV equipment made of plastic or glass. Dilute all required doses in D5W as follows: for loading dose, add a dose equal to 150 mg/kg to 200 mL; for first maintenance dose, add a dose equal to 50 mg/kg to 500 mL; for second maintenance dose, add a dose equal to 100 mg/kg to 1000 mL. Note: The total IV volume should be reduced for patients <40 kg and for those with fluid restriction. In small children, individualize the total IV volume to avoid water intoxication and hyponatremia.

ADMINISTER: **IV Infusion:** Give loading dose over 15 min, maintenance dose 1 over 4 h, maintenance dose 2 over 16 h.

- Store reconstituted solution for up to 24 h at 15°–30° C (59°–86° F).

ADVERSE EFFECTS (≥1%) **CNS:** Dizziness, drowsiness. **GI:** Nausea, *vomiting,* stomatitis, hepatotoxicity (urticaria). **Respiratory:** Bronchospasm, rhinorrhea, burning sensation in upper respiratory passages, epistaxis.

PHARMACOKINETICS Onset: 1 min after inhalation or instillation. **Peak:** 5–10 min. **Metabolism:** Deacetylated in liver to cysteine and subsequently metabolized.

NURSING IMPLICATIONS

Assessment & Drug Effects

- During IV infusion, carefully monitor for fluid overload and signs of hyponatremia (i.e., changes in mental status).

- Monitor for S&S of aspiration of excess secretions, and for bronchospasm (unpredictable); withhold drug and notify physician immediately if either occurs.
- Lab tests: Monitor ABGs, pulmonary functions and pulse oximetry as indicated.
- Have suction apparatus immediately available. Increased volume of respiratory tract fluid may be liberated; suction or endotracheal aspiration may be necessary to establish and maintain an open airway. Older adults and debilitated patients are particularly at risk.
- Nausea and vomiting may occur, particularly when face mask is used, due to unpleasant odor of drug and excess volume of liquefied bronchial secretions.

Patient & Family Education

- Report difficulty with clearing the airway or any other respiratory distress.
- Report nausea, as an antiemetic may be indicated.
- Note: Unpleasant odor of inhaled drug becomes less noticeable with continued use.
- Do not breast feed while taking this drug without consulting physician.

ACITRETIN

(a-ci-tree'tin)

Soriatane

Classifications: SKIN AND MUCOUS MEMBRANE AGENT; ANTIACNE; RETINOID

Prototype: Isotretinoin

Pregnancy Category: X

AVAILABILITY 10 mg, 20 mg capsules

ACTIONS The mechanism of action of acitretin is unknown.

THERAPEUTIC EFFECTS Acitretin is a highly toxic metabolite of retinol (vitamin A).

USES Treatment of severe psoriasis in adults.

CONTRAINDICATIONS Pregnancy (category X), sensitivity to parabens, lactation.

CAUTIOUS USE Patients with impaired hepatic function, hepatitis, diabetes mellitus, obesity, alcoholism, history of pancreatitis, hypertriglyceridemia, hypercholesterolemia, coronary artery disease, retinal disease, degenerative joint disease.

ROUTE & DOSAGE

Psoriasis

Adult: **PO** 10–50 mg q.d. with main meal

ADMINISTRATION

Oral

- Administer as single dose with main meal because food enhances absorption.
- Store at 15°–25° C (59°–77° F) and protect from light. After opening, avoid exposure to high temperatures and humidity.

ADVERSE EFFECTS (≥1%) **Body as a Whole:** *Hyperesthesia, paresthesias, arthralgia, progression of existing spinal hyperostosis, rigors,* back pain, hypertonia, myalgia, fatigue, hot flashes, increased appetite. **CNS:** Headache, depression, aggressive feelings and thoughts of self-harm, insomnia, somnolence. **CV:** Flushing, edema. **GI:** *Dry mouth, increased liver function tests, increased triglycerides and cholesterol,* hepatitis, gingival bleeding, gingivitis, increased saliva, stomatitis, thirst, ulcerative stomatitis, abdominal pain, diarrhea, nausea, tongue disorder. **Special Senses:** Blurred vision, blepharitis, conjunctivitis, decreased night vision/night blindness, eye pain, photophobia; earache, tinnitus; taste perversion. **Respiratory:** Sinusitis. **Skin:** *Alopecia, skin peeling, dry skin, nail disorders, pruritus, rash, cheilitis, skin atrophy, paronychia,* abnormal skin odor and hair texture, cold/clammy skin, increased sweating, purpura, seborrhea, skin ulceration, sunburn. **Other:** *Rhinitis, epistaxis, xerophthalmia.*

INTERACTIONS Drug: Combination with **ethanol** can create **etretinate,** which has a significantly longer half-life than acitretin; interferes with the contraceptive efficacy of **progestin**-only ORAL CONTRACEPTIVES.

PHARMACOKINETICS Absorption: Rapidly absorbed from GI tract, optimal absorption when taken with food. **Peak:** 2–5 h. **Distribution:** Crosses placenta, distributed into breast milk. **Metabolism:** Metabolized active metabolite, *cis*-acitretin. **Elimination:** Excreted in both urine and feces. **Half-Life:** 49 h acitretin, 63 h *cis*-acitretin.

NURSING IMPLICATIONS

Assessment & Drug Effects

- Monitor for S&S of pancreatitis or loss of glycemic control in diabetics. Report either condition immediately to physician.
- Lab tests: Before initiating therapy and at 1- to 2-wk intervals until response to drug is known, do lipid profile and liver function tests. Monitor blood glucose and HbA_{1-C} periodically.

Patient & Family Education

- Note: Transient worsening of psoriasis may occur during early therapy.
- Review common adverse effects of drug; lag time of 2–3 mo may be necessary before drug effect is evident.
- Discontinue drug and report immediately to physician if visual problems develop.
- Note: Dry eyes with decreased tolerance for contact lenses may occur.
- Do not drink alcohol while taking this drug; it increases risk of hepatotoxicity and hypertriglyceridemia; females should avoid alcohol during and for 2 mo following therapy.
- Do not donate blood for 3 y following therapy.
- Avoid excessive exposure to sunlight or UV light.
- Use two forms of effective contraception for 1 mo before and at least 3 y following therapy because of the serious risk of fetal deformities that could result from exposure to this medication.
- Do not breast feed while taking this drug

ACRIVASTINE/ PSEUDOEPHEDRINE

(a-cri-vas′teen)

Semprex-D (combination with pseudoephedrine)

Classifications: ANTIHISTAMINE; H_1-RECEPTOR ANTAGONIST; DECONGESTANT

Prototype: Diphenhydramine

Pregnancy Category: B

AVAILABILITY Acrivastine 8 mg/pseudoephedrine 60 mg capsules

ACTIONS Acrivastine is an H_1-receptor histamine antagonist that controls histamine-mediated symptoms and acts on sympathetic nerve endings. Pseudoephedrine produces

decongestion of the respiratory tract mucosa.
THERAPEUTIC EFFECTS It is effective in allergic rhinitis and dermatologic disorders.

USES Seasonal and perennial allergic rhinitis with nasal congestion.

CONTRAINDICATIONS Hypersensitivity to acrivastine, triprolidine, pseudoephedrine, or ephedrine; severe hypertension or severe coronary artery disease; patients on MAO inhibitor drugs; lactation.
CAUTIOUS USE Renal insufficiency, hypertension, DM, ischemic heart disease, increased intraocular pressure, hyperthyroidism, BPH, GI disorders, older adults, pregnancy (category B). Safety and effectiveness in children <2 y is not established.

ROUTE & DOSAGE

Allergic Rhinitis
Adult: **PO** 1 tab (8 mg acrivastine/60 mg pseudoephedrine) t.i.d.

ADMINISTRATION

Oral
- Do not give to patients with a creatinine clearance of 48 mL/min or less.
- Store at 15°–25° C (59°–77° F); protect from light and moisture.

ADVERSE EFFECTS (≥1%) **CNS:** Headache, vertigo, dizziness, insomnia, jitteriness, *drowsiness*. **GI:** Nausea, diarrhea, dry mouth, dyspepsia.

INTERACTIONS Drug: Alcohol may increase psychomotor impairment.

PHARMACOKINETICS Absorption: Rapidly absorbed from GI tract. **Onset:** 1 h. **Duration:** Approximately 12 h. **Metabolism:** Metabolized in liver. **Elimination:** Approximately 65% excreted unchanged in urine. **Half-Life:** 1.5 h.

NURSING IMPLICATIONS

Assessment & Drug Effects
- Monitor for dizziness, sedation, urinary obstruction, and hypotension, especially in older adults.
- Assess for significant drowsiness, which may necessitate drug discontinuation.

Patient & Family Education
- Do not use this drug in combination with other OTC antihistamines or decongestants.
- Do not drive or engage in potentially hazardous activities until response to drug is known.
- Do not take alcohol or other CNS depressants while taking this drug.
- Do not breast feed infants while taking this drug.

ACYCLOVIR, ACYCLOVIR SODIUM (Pr)

(ay-sye'kloe-ver)
Acycloguanosine, Zovirax
Classifications: ANTIINFECTIVE; ANTIVIRAL
Pregnancy Category: C

AVAILABILITY 200 mg capsules; 400 mg, 800 mg tablets; 200 mg/5 mL suspension; 50 mg/mL injection; 5% ointment, cream

ACTIONS Acyclovir is a synthetic acyclic purine nucleoside analog, derived from guanine. It reduces viral shedding and formation of new lesions and speeds healing time. Acyclovir triphosphate preferentially interferes with DNA synthesis of herpes simplex virus types 1 and 2 (HSV-1 and HSV-2) and varicella-zoster virus, thereby inhibiting viral replication.

THERAPEUTIC EFFECTS Acyclovir demonstrates antiviral activity against herpes virus simiae (B virus), Epstein-Barr (infectious mononucleosis), varicella-zoster and cytomegalovirus, but does not eradicate the latent herpes virus.

USES Parenterally for treatment of initial and recurrent mucosal and cutaneous herpes simplex virus (HSV-1 and HSV-2) infections in immunocompromised adults and children and for severe initial episodes of herpes genitalis in immunocompetent (normal immune system) patients. Used orally for treatment of initial episodes of genital herpes, for management of selected patients with severe recurrent episodes, and for prophylaxis to reduce frequency and severity of recurrent infections. Also used orally in varicella-zoster (chickenpox) in immunocompetent children and adolescents. Used topically for herpes labialis (cold sores), initial episodes of herpes genitalis and in non-life-threatening mucocutaneous herpes simplex virus infections in immunocompromised patients.

UNLABELED USES Treatment of eczema herpeticum caused by HSV localized and disseminated herpes zoster.

CONTRAINDICATIONS Safety during pregnancy (category C) or in children is not established.

CAUTIOUS USE Lactation, renal insufficiency, dehydration.

ROUTE & DOSAGE

Cold Sores

Adult/Adolescents: **Topical** ≥*12 y* Apply 5 times/d for 4 d

Genital Herpes Simplex

Adult: **PO** 200 mg q4h 5 times/d, 400 mg t.i.d. for 7–10 d cycle **IV** 5 mg/kg q8h **Topical** Apply q3h 6 times/d for 7 d

Child: **IV** *<12 y,* 250 mg/m^2 q8h, 80 mg/kg/d in 2–5 doses

Herpes Simplex Immunocompromised Patient

Adult: **IV** 15 mg/kg/d divided q8h for 5–7 d cycle

Child: **IV** *<1 y,* 15–30 mg/kg/d divided q8h for 7–14 d cycle; *≥1 y,* 750–1500 mg/m^2/d, 15–30 mg/kg/d divided q8h for 7–14 d cycle

Prophylaxis for Genital Herpes Simplex

Adult: **PO** 200 mg 2–5 times/d, 400 mg t.i.d., 800 mg b.i.d.

Child: **PO** 80 mg/kg/d in 2–5 divided doses

Herpes Zoster

Adult: **PO** 800 mg q4h 5 times/d

Child: **PO** 80 mg/kg/d in 5 divided doses

Herpes Simplex Encephalitis

Adult/Child: **IV** 15 mg/kg q8h for 14–21 d cycle

Neonate: **IV** 30 mg/kg/d divided q8h for 14–21 d cycle

Premature neonate: **IV** 20 mg/kg/d divided q12h for 14–21 d cycle

Varicella Zoster

Child/Adolescent: **PO** 20 mg/kg (max: 800 mg) q.i.d. for 5 d cycle initiated within 24 h of onset of rash

Renal Impairment

Cl_{cr} 25–50 mL/min: same dose q12h; 10–25 mL/min: same dose q24h

ADMINISTRATION

Oral

- Shake suspension well prior to use.
- Store capsules in tight, light-resistant containers at 15°–30° C (59°–86° F) unless otherwise directed.

Topical

- Wash hands thoroughly before and after treatment of lesions and after handling and disposition of secretions.
- Apply approximately 1/2 inch of cream or ointment ribbon for each 4 square inches of surface area. Use sufficient ointment or cream to completely cover lesions.
- Apply topical preparation with finger cot or surgical glove.
- Store at 15°–25° C (59°–78° F) unless otherwise directed.

Intravenous

Verify correct IV concentration and rate of infusion with physician for neonates, infants, children. ▪ Note: Solutions containing benzyl alcohol are toxic to neonates. ▪ Directions for administration to adults follow.

PREPARE: **Intermittent:** Reconstitute by adding 10 mL sterile water for injection to 500-mg vial to yield 50 mg/mL. Shake well. ▪Use reconstituted solution within 12 h. ▪Dilute to ≤7 mg/mL to reduce risk of renal injury and phlebitis. Example: Add 1 mL of reconstituted solution to 9 mL of diluent to yield 5 mg/mL. ▪Use standard electrolyte and glucose solutions (e.g., NS, RL, D5W) for dilution. Diluted solution should be used within 24 h.

ADMINISTER: **Intermittent:** Administer over at least 1 h to prevent renal tubular damage. Rapid or bolus IV administration must be avoided. ▪ Monitor IV flow rate carefully; infusion pump or microdrip infusion set preferred.

INCOMPATIBILITIES **Solution/additive: Bacteriostatic water for injection, albumin, hetastarch, dopamine, dobutamine**. **Y-site: Foscarnet, TPN.**

- Refrigerated reconstituted solution may precipitate; however, crystals will redissolve at room temperature. ▪Store acyclovir powder and reconstituted solutions at controlled room temperature preferably at 15°–30° C (59°–86° F) unless otherwise directed by manufacturer.

ADVERSE EFFECTS (≥1%) **Body as a Whole:** Generally minimal and infrequent. **CNS:** *Headache,* lightheadedness, lethargy, fatigue, tremors, confusion, seizures, dizziness. **GI:** *Nausea, vomiting, diarrhea.* **Urogenital:** Glomerulonephritis, renal tubular damage, <u>acute renal failure</u>. **Skin:** Rash, urticaria, pruritus, burning, stinging sensation, irritation, sensitization. **Other:** Inflammation or phlebitis at IV injection site, sloughing (with extravasation), <u>thrombocytopenic purpura/hemolytic uremic syndrome</u>.

INTERACTIONS Drug: Probenecid decreases acyclovir elimination; **zidovudine** may cause increased drowsiness and lethargy.

PHARMACOKINETICS Absorption: Oral dose is 15%–30% absorbed. **Peak:** 1.5–2 h after oral dose. **Distribution:** Distributes into most tissues with lower levels in the CNS; crosses placenta. **Metabolism:** Drug is primarily excreted unchanged.

Elimination: Renally eliminated; also excreted in breast milk. **Half-Life:** 2.5–5 h.

NURSING IMPLICATIONS

Assessment & Drug Effects

- Observe infusion site during infusion and for a few days following infusion for signs of tissue damage.
- Monitor I&O and hydration status. Keep patient adequately hydrated during first 2 h after infusion to maintain sufficient urinary flow and thus prevent precipitation of drug in renal tubules. Consult physician about amount and length of time oral fluids need to be pushed after IV drug treatment.
- Monitor for S&S of: reinfection in pregnant patients; acyclovir-induced neurologic symptoms in patients with history of neurologic problems; drug resistance in immunocompromised patients receiving prolonged or repeated therapy; acute renal failure with concomitant use with other nephrotoxic drugs or preexisting renal disease.
- Lab tests: Monitor baseline and periodic renal function studies, particularly with IV administration. Elevations of BUN and serum creatinine and decreases in creatinine clearance indicate need for dosage adjustment, discontinuation of drug, or correction of fluid and electrolyte balance.
- Monitor for adverse effects and viral resistance with long-term prophylactic use of the oral drug.

Patient & Family Education

- Start therapy as soon as possible after onset of S&S for best results.
- Do not exceed recommended dosage, frequency of drug administration, or specified duration of therapy. Contact physician if relief is not obtained or adverse effects appear.
- Cleanse affected areas with soap and water 3–4 times daily prior to topical application; dry well before application. With application to genitals, wear loose-fitting clothes over affected areas.
- Note: Even after HSV infection is controlled, latent virus can be activated by stress, trauma, fever, exposure to sunlight, sexual intercourse, menstruation, treatment with immunosuppressive drugs.
- Refrain from sexual intercourse if either partner has S&S of herpes infection; neither topical nor systemic drug prevents transmission to other individuals.
- Avoid topical drug contact in or around eyes. Report unexplained eye symptoms to physician immediately (e.g., redness, pain); untreated infection can lead to corneal keratitis and blindness.
- Do not breast feed while taking this drug without consulting physician.

ADALIMUMAB (D2E7)

(a-da-lim′u-mab)

Humira

Classifications: BIOLOGIC RESPONSE MODIFIER; TUMOR NECROSIS FACTOR MODIFIER

Prototype: Etanercept

Pregnancy Category: B

AVAILABILITY 40 mg/0.8 mL injection

ACTIONS Adalimumab is a DNA recombinant cytokine that binds to tumor necrosis factor (TNF)-alpha and blocks its interaction with cell surface TNF receptors. Adalimumab also modulates changes in levels of cell adhesion molecules needed for WBC migration out of the circulatory system to sites of inflammation. In the presence of complement, adalimumab may also lyse TNF-expressing cells.

THERAPEUTIC EFFECTS Reduces the levels of acute phase inflammatory reactants (C-reactive protein, ESR, interleukin-6) thus decreasing overall joint inflammation; also reduces levels of enzymes that produce tissue remodeling responsible for cartilage destruction. In RA, adalimumab reduces the numerous inflammatory events of polyarthritis. It reduces the overproduction of TNF-alpha principally by macrophages in rheumatoid joints.

USES Treatment of moderate to severe rheumatoid arthritis and to reduce progression of the disease in patients that have had an inadequate response to at least one disease-modifying antirheumatic drug (DMARD).

UNLABELED USE IV administration.

CONTRAINDICATIONS Hypersensitivity to adalimumab or mannitol; active infection, either chronic or acute; neoplastic disease; sepsis; lactation. Safe use in children has not been established.

CAUTIOUS USE History of recurrent infection or conditions predisposing to infection; recurrent history of sensitivity to monoclonal antibodies; cardiovascular disease; neurological disease; patients residing in areas with endemic TB or histoplasmosis; active or latent TB infection prior to therapy; demyelinating disorders; concurrent administration of immunosuppressants; surgery; pregnancy (category B).

ROUTE & DOSAGE

Rheumatoid Arthritis

Adult: **SC** 40 mg every other wk (may use 40 mg every wk if not on concomitant methotrexate)

ADMINISTRATION

Subcutaneous

- Do not administer to persons with active infections. Evaluate for latent TB with TB skin test prior to initiation of therapy.
- Inspect prefilled syringe for particulate matter and discoloration prior to SC injection.
- Rotate injection sites and do not inject into skin that is red, bruised, tender, or hard. After injecting the drug, do not rub the site.
- Discard any remaining solution in prefilled syringe, as it contains no preservatives.
- Store in original carton at 2°–4° C (38°–48° F). Protect from light. Do not use beyond the expiration date.

ADVERSE EFFECTS (≥1%) **Body as a Whole:** Infections (especially reactivation of latent tuberculosis), sepsis, may see increase in malignancies (lymphoma), back pain, fever, allergic reactions (including anaphylactic shock), *flu-like symptoms, fatigue.* **CNS:** *Headache.* **CV:** Hypertension. **GI:** *Nausea, vomiting,* abdominal pain. **Hematologic:** Development of ANA antibodies. **Respiratory:** *Upper respiratory infection, sinusitis.* **Skin:** *Injection site reactions (erythema, itching, hemorrhage, pain, swelling), rash,* urticaria, fixed drug reaction. **Urogenital:** Urinary tract infection.

INTERACTIONS Drug: Do not give LIVE VIRUS VACCINES to patient on adalimumab; not recommended for use with other TNF BLOCKERS (**etanercept, infliximab, anakinra**).

PHARMACOKINETICS Absorption: 64% absorbed from SC injection site. **Peak:** 131 h. **Distribution:** Minimal distribution beyond vascular/synovial space. **Elimination:** Higher clearance in presence of antiadalimumab antibodies, lower clearance with increasing age. **Half-Life:** 11.8 d (10–20 d).

NURSING IMPLICATIONS

Assessment & Drug Effects

- Monitor for and report lupus-like syndrome (e.g., joint pain, rash on cheeks or arms that is sensitive to sun).
- Monitor for and report promptly S&S of infection.
- Monitor neurological status closely. Report any change in status such as blurred vision or paresthesia.

Patient & Family Education

- Live vaccines should not be accepted by persons taking this drug.
- Report promptly any of the following to the physician: unexplained joint pain, rash on cheeks or arms, fever, sore throat or other signs of infection, changes in vision, numbness or tingling in extremities.
- Do not breast feed without consulting physician.

ADAPALENE

(a-da'pa-leen)
Differin
Classifications: SKIN AND MUCOUS MEMBRANE AGENT; ANTIACNE; RETINOID
Prototype: Isotretinoin
Pregnancy Category: C

AVAILABILITY 0.1% gel

ACTIONS Adapalene is a topical retinoid-like compound that modulates cellular differentiation, keratinization, and inflammatory processes related to the pathology of acne vulgaris. Topical adapalene may normalize the differentiation of epithelial follicular cells.

THERAPEUTIC EFFECTS Adapalene decreases inflammatory process and acne formation.

USES Topical treatment of acne vulgaris.

CONTRAINDICATIONS Hypersensitivity to adapalene or any of the components of the gel, irritating topical products, and sunburn.
CAUTIOUS USE Pregnancy (category C), lactation. Safety and effectiveness in children <12 y is not established.

ROUTE & DOSAGE

Acne
Adult: Apply once daily to affected areas in evening

ADMINISTRATION

Topical

- Apply a thin film to clean skin, avoiding eyes, lips, mucous membranes, cuts, abrasions, eczematous or sunburned skin.
- Do not apply to skin recently treated with preparations containing sulfur, resorcinol, or salicylic acid.
- Store at 20°–25° C (68°–77° F).

ADVERSE EFFECTS (≥1%) **Skin:** *Erythema, scaling, dryness, pruritus, burning*, skin irritation, stinging, sunburn, acne flares.

PHARMACOKINETICS Absorption: Minimal absorption through intact skin. **Elimination:** Excreted primarily in bile.

NURSING IMPLICATIONS

Assessment & Drug Effects

- Monitor therapeutic effectiveness, which is indicated by improvement after 8–12 wk of treatment; early therapy may be marked by apparent worsening of acne.

- Note: Cutaneous reactions (e.g., erythema, scaling, pruritus) are common and normally diminish after first month of therapy.

Patient & Family Education

- Apply only as directed; excessive application will not result in faster healing but will cause marked redness, peeling, and discomfort.
- Minimize exposure to sunlight and sunlamps, and use sunscreen and protective clothing as needed.
- Do not breast feed while using this drug without consulting physician.

ADEFOVIR DIPIVOXIL

(a-de'fo-vir)

Hepsera

Classifications: ANTIVIRAL AGENT; NUCLEOTIDE ANALOG

Pregnancy Category: C

AVAILABILITY 10 mg tablets

ACTIONS Inhibits HBV DNA polymerase (reverse transcriptase) by competing with the natural substrate deoxyadenosine triphosphate and by causing DNA chain termination after its incorporation into viral DNA.

THERAPEUTIC EFFECTS A nucleotide analog with activity against human hepatitis B virus (HBV).

USES Treatment of chronic hepatitis B.

CONTRAINDICATIONS Hypersensitivity to adefovir; untreated or unknown human immunodeficiency virus (HIV); exacerbations of hepatitis B, especially in patients who have discontinued anti-hepatitis B therapy; pregnancy (category C); lactation. Safety and efficacy in children are not established. Appropriate infant immunizations should be used to prevent neonatal acquisition of the hepatitis B virus.

CAUTIOUS USE Decreased cardiac function due to concomitant disease or other drug therapy; elderly; concomitant use of highly nephrotoxic drugs; renal dysfunction; co-administration with drugs that reduce renal function or compete for active tubular secretion.

ROUTE & DOSAGE

Hepatitis B

Adult: **PO** 10 mg q.d.

Renal Insufficiency

Cl_{cr} 20–49 mL/min, 10 mg q48h; 10–19 mL/min, 10 mg q72h; hemodialysis, 10 mg q7d following dialysis

ADMINISTRATION

Oral

- Note that the dosing interval of adefovir should be adjusted in patients with baseline creatinine clearance <50 mL/min.
- Store in original container at 15°–30° C (59°–86° F).

ADVERSE EFFECTS (≥1%) **CNS:** *Asthenia,* headache. **GI:** Abdominal pain, nausea, flatulence, diarrhea, dyspepsia, exacerbation of hepatitis after discontinuation of therapy, hepatomegaly. **Metabolic:** *Increased ALT, AST,* increased creatine kinase, amylase, lactic acidosis. **Urogenital:** *Hematuria,* glycosuria, increased serum creatinine, nephrotoxicity. **Other:** HIV resistance in patient with unrecognized HIV.

INTERACTIONS Drug: No clinically significant interactions established.

ACTIONS Fabry disease is caused by a deficiency of alpha-galactosidase A resulting in an accumulation of glycosphinolipids in body tissues causing cardiomyopathy, renal failure, and CVA. Agalsidase beta provides an exogenous source of K-galactosidase A that catalyzes the breakdown of glycosphingolipids including GL-3.

THERAPEUTIC EFFECTS Reduces globotriaosylceramide (GL-3) deposition in capillary endothelium of the kidney and certain other cell types.

USES Treatment of Fabry disease.

CONTRAINDICATIONS Safety and efficacy in children <16 y have not been established.

CAUTIOUS USE Hypersensitivity reaction to agalsidase beta or mannitol; compromised cardiac function, mild to severe hypertension; renal impairment; pregnancy (category B), lactation.

ROUTE & DOSAGE

Fabry Disease
Adult: **IV** 1 mg/kg q2wk

ADMINISTRATION

Intravenous

- Give antipyretics prior to infusion.

PREPARE: **Infusion:** Bring Fabrazyme vials and supplied sterile water for injection to room temperature prior to reconstitution. Reconstitute each 35 mg vial slowly injecting 7.2 mL of sterile water for injection down inside wall of vial. Roll and tilt vial gently to mix but do not shake. Reconstituted vial contains 5.0 mg/mL of clear, colorless solution. Do not use if there is particulate matter or if discolored. Further dilute in NS to a final total volume of 500 mL; prior to adding the volume of reconstituted Fabrazyme required for the dose, remove an equal volume of NS from the 500 mL infusion bag.

ADMINISTER: **Infusion:** Initial rate should not exceed 0.25 mg/min (15 mg/h; give more slowly if infusion-associated reactions occur). After tolerance to infusion is established, may increase rate in increments of 0.05–0.08 mg/min (increments of 3 to 5 mg/h) for each subsequent infusion.

- Store refrigerated until needed. Vials are for single use. Discard any unused portion. Do NOT use after expiration date.

ADVERSE EFFECTS (≥1%) **Body as a Whole:** *Fever, pain, pallor, rigors, temperature change sensation,* ataxia, stroke. **CNS:** *Dizziness, headache, paresthesia, anxiety, depression,* vertigo. **CV:** *Chest pain, cardiomegaly, hypertension, hypotension, dependent edema,* bradycardia, heart failure, exacerbation of preexisting arrhythmias. **GI:** *Dyspepsia, nausea, abdominal pain.* **Metabolic:** *Antibody development.* **Musculoskeletal:** *Arthrosis, skeletal pain.* **Respiratory:** *Bronchitis,* bronchospasm, laryngitis, *pharyngitis, rhinitis,* sinusitis, dyspnea. **Skin:** Pruritus, urticaria. **Special Senses:** Hearing loss. **Urogenital:** Testicular pain, nephrotic syndrome.

INTERACTIONS Drug: Coadministration with **amiodarone, chloroquine, hydroxychloroquine, gentamicin** is not recommended due to potential of decreased response to agalsidase beta therapy.

PHARMACOKINETICS Metabolism: Degraded through peptide hydrolysis. **Elimination:** Renal elimination expected to be a minor pathway. **Half-Life:** 45–102 min.

NURSING IMPLICATIONS

Assessment & Drug Effects

- During infusion, monitor for infusion-related reactions such as hypertension or hypotension, chest pain or chest tightness, dyspnea, fever and chills, headache, abdominal pain, pruritus and urticaria.
- Slow infusion and notify physician immediately if infusion reaction occurs. Note that additional antipyretic and/or an antihistamine and oral steroid may reduce the symptoms.
- Monitor cardiac status closely, especially with preexisting heart disease.

Patient & Family Education

- Notify physician if you have experienced an unusual reaction to agalsidase beta, agalsidase alfa, mannitol, other drugs, foods, or preservatives.
- Report any of the following to physician immediately: chest pain or chest tightness, rapid heartbeat, shortness of breath or difficulty breathing; depression; dizziness; skin rash, hives or itching; throat tightness; swelling of the face, lips, neck, ears, or extremities.
- Do not drive or engage in other hazardous activities until reaction to drug is known.
- Do not breast feed without consulting physician.

ALBENDAZOLE

(al-ben′da-zole)
Albenza
Classifications: ANTIINFECTIVE; ANTHELMINTIC AGENT
Prototype: Mebendazole
Pregnancy Category: C

AVAILABILITY 200 mg tablets

ACTIONS Albendazole is a broad-spectrum oral anthelmintic agent. It is the only anthelmintic drug active against all stages of the helminth life cycle (ova, larvae, and adult worms). Its mechanism of action is unclear, but it appears to cause selective degeneration of cytoplasmic microtubules in the intestinal cells of the helminths and larvae.
THERAPEUTIC EFFECTS Albendazole ultimately causes decreased ATP production in the helminths, resulting in energy depletion, which kills the worms.

USES Treatment of neurocysticercosis caused by the larval form of pork tapeworm (*Taenia solium*), hydatid disease caused by the larval form of dog tapeworm (*Echinococcus granulosus*).

CONTRAINDICATIONS Hypersensitivity to the benzimidazole class of compounds or any components of albendazole; pregnancy (category C).
CAUTIOUS USE Retinal lesions, lactation.

ROUTE & DOSAGE

Neurocysticercosis
Adult/Child: **PO** >6 y, weight <60 kg, 15 mg/kg/d divided b.i.d. for 8–30 d cycle (max: 800 mg/d); weight ≥60 kg, 400 mg b.i.d. for 8–30 d cycle

Hydatid Disease
Adult/Child: **PO** >6 y, weight <60 kg, 15 mg/kg/d divided b.i.d. (max: 800 mg/d); weight ≥60 kg, 400 mg b.i.d. for 28 d cycle (then 14 d without drug & repeat regimen for 3 cycles)

ADMINISTRATION

Oral

- Give with meals. Absorption is significantly increased with a fatty meal.
- Do not exceed maximum total daily dose of 800 mg.
- Store at 20°–25° C (68°–77° F).

ADVERSE EFFECTS (≥1%) **Body as a Whole:** Hypersensitivity reactions. **CNS:** *Headache,* dizziness, vertigo, increased intracranial pressure, meningeal signs, alopecia (reversible), fever. **GI:** *Abnormal liver function tests,* abdominal pain, nausea, vomiting. **Hematologic:** (Rare) Leukopenia, granulocytopenia, pancytopenia, agranulocytosis. **Skin:** Rash, urticaria.

INTERACTIONS Drug: Cimetidine, dexamethasone, praziquantel increase albendazole levels.

PHARMACOKINETICS Absorption: Poorly absorbed from GI tract, absorption enhanced with a fatty meal. **Peak:** 2–5 h. **Distribution:** 70% bound to plasma proteins; widely distributed throughout body including cyst fluid and CSF; secreted into animal breast milk. **Metabolism:** Metabolized in liver to active metabolite, albendazole sulfoxide. **Elimination:** Excreted in bile. **Half-Life:** 8–12 h.

NURSING IMPLICATIONS

Assessment & Drug Effects

- Lab tests: Monitor WBC count, absolute neutrophil count, and liver function tests at start of each 28-d cycle and q2wk during cycle.
- Withhold drug and notify physician if WBC count falls below normal or liver enzymes are elevated.
- Note: Patients should be concurrently treated with appropriate steroid and anticonvulsant therapy.

Patient & Family Education

- Take with meals (see ADMINISTRATION).
- Do not become pregnant during or for at least 1 mo after therapy.
- Do not breast feed while taking this drug without consulting physician.

ALBUTEROL Pr

(al-byoo'ter-ole)

Accuneb, Novosalmol ✦, Proventil, Proventil HFA, Proventil Repetabs, Salbutamol, Ventolin, Ventolin Rotocaps, Volmax

Classifications: AUTONOMIC NERVOUS SYSTEM AGENT; BETA-ADRENERGIC AGONIST (SYMPATHOMIMETIC); BRONCHODILATOR (RESPIRATORY SMOOTH MUSCLE RELAXANT)

Pregnancy Category: C

AVAILABILITY 2 mg, 4 mg tablets; 4 mg, 8 mg, extended-release tablets; 2 mg/5 mL syrup; 200 mcg capsules for inhalation; 0.083%, 0.5% solution for inhalation

ACTIONS Synthetic sympathomimetic amine and moderately selective $beta_2$-adrenergic agonist with comparatively long action. Acts more prominently on $beta_2$ receptors (particularly smooth muscles of bronchi, uterus, and vascular supply to skeletal muscles) than on $beta_1$ (heart) receptors. Minimal or no effect on alpha-adrenergic receptors. Inhibits histamine release by mast cells.

THERAPEUTIC EFFECTS Produces bronchodilation, regardless of administration route, by relaxing smooth muscles of bronchial tree. This decreases airway resistance, facilitates mucus drainage, and increases vital capacity.

USES To relieve bronchospasm associated with acute or chronic

Common adverse effects in *italic*, life-threatening effects underlined: generic names in **bold**; classifications in SMALL CAPS; ✦ Canadian drug name; Pr Prototype drug

asthma, bronchitis, or other reversible obstructive airway diseases. Also used to prevent exercise-induced bronchospasm.

UNLABELED USES Adjunct in treatment of refractory heart failure and to stimulate intracellular transport of potassium in hyperkalemic familial periodic paralysis.

CONTRAINDICATIONS Pregnancy (category C), lactation. Use of oral syrup in children <2 y.

CAUTIOUS USE Cardiovascular disease, hypertension, hyperthyroidism, diabetes mellitus, hypersensitivity to sympathomimetic amines or to fluorocarbon propellant used in inhalation aerosols.

ROUTE & DOSAGE

Bronchospasm

Adult: **PO** 2–4 mg 3–4 times/d, 4–8 mg sustained release 2 times/d **Inhaled** 1–2 inhalations q4–6h

Child: **PO** *2–6 y,* 0.1–0.2 mg/kg t.i.d. (max: 4 mg/dose); *6–12 y,* 2 mg 3–4 times/d; **Inhaled** *6–12 y,* 1–2 inhalations q4–6h

ADMINISTRATION

Oral

- Do not crush extended release tablets. Scored tablets may be broken in half.
- Note: An initial dose of 2 mg t.i.d. or q.i.d. is recommended for older adult patients.
- Store tablets and syrup between 2°–25° C (36°–77° F) in tight, light-resistant container.

Inhalation

- Administer albuterol 20–30 min before concomitant beclomethasone (Vanceril) inhalation treatments to allow deeper penetration of beclomethasone into lungs, unless otherwise directed by physician.
- Store canisters between 15°–30° C (59°–86° F) away from heat and direct sunlight.

ADVERSE EFFECTS (≥1%) **Body as a Whole:** Hypersensitivity reaction. **CNS:** *Tremor,* anxiety, nervousness, restlessness, convulsions, weakness, headache, hallucinations. **CV:** Palpitation, hypertension, hypotension, bradycardia, reflex tachycardia. **Special Senses:** Blurred vision, dilated pupils. **GI:** Nausea, vomiting. **Other:** Muscle cramps, hoarseness.

DIAGNOSTIC TEST INTERFERENCE Transient small increases in ***plasma glucose*** may occur.

INTERACTIONS Drug: With **epinephrine,** other SYMPATHOMIMETIC BRONCHODILATORS, possible additive effects; MAO INHIBITORS, TRICYCLIC ANTIDEPRESSANTS potentiate action on vascular system; BETA-ADRENERGIC BLOCKERS antagonize the effects of both drugs.

PHARMACOKINETICS Onset: Inhaled: 5–15 min; PO 30 min. **Peak:** Inhaled: 0.5–2 h; PO 2.5 h. **Duration:** Inhaled: 3–6 h; PO 4–6 h (8–12 h with sustained release). **Metabolism:** Metabolized in liver; may cross the placenta. **Elimination:** 76% of dose eliminated in urine in 3 d. **Half-Life:** 2.75 h.

NURSING IMPLICATIONS

Assessment & Drug Effects

- Monitor therapeutic effectiveness which is indicated by significant subjective improvement in pulmonary function within 60–90 min after drug administration.
- Monitor for: S&S of fine tremor in fingers, which may interfere with precision handwork; CNS stimulation, particularly in children 2–6 y,

(hyperactivity, excitement, nervousness, insomnia), tachycardia, GI symptoms. Report promptly to physician.

- Lab tests: Periodic ABGs, pulmonary functions, and pulse oximetry.
- Consult physician about giving last albuterol dose several hours before bedtime, if drug-induced insomnia is a problem.

Patient & Family Education

- Review directions for correct use of medication and inhaler (see ADMINISTRATION).
- Avoid contact of inhalation drug with eyes.
- Do not increase number or frequency of inhalations without advice of physician.
- Notify physician if albuterol fails to provide relief because this can signify worsening of pulmonary function and a reevaluation of condition/therapy may be indicated.
- Note: Albuterol can cause dizziness or vertigo; take necessary precautions.
- Do not use OTC drugs without physician approval. Many medications (e.g., cold remedies) contain drugs that may intensify albuterol action.
- Do not breast feed while taking this drug without consulting physician.

ALCLOMETASONE DIPROPIONATE

(al-clo-met′a-sone)
Alclovate
Classifications: SKIN AND MUCOUS MEMBRANE AGENT; ANTIINFLAMMATORY; STEROID
Prototype: Hydrocortisone
Pregnancy Category: C

AVAILABILITY 0.05% ointment or cream
See Appendix A-4.

ALEFACEPT (Pr)

(a-le′fa-cept)
Amevive
Classifications: BIOLOGIC RESPONSE MODIFIER; FUSION PROTEIN
Pregnancy Category: B

AVAILABILITY 7.5 mg, 15 mg vials

ACTIONS Activation of T cells plays a role in chronic plaque psoriasis. Alefacept is thought to bind to CD2 receptors found on all peripheral T cells and to immunoglobulin receptors on cytotoxic cells, such as natural killer cells. Alefacept blocks further activation of T cells and reduces cellular-mediated apoptosis of T cells.
THERAPEUTIC EFFECTS Alefacept modulates the immune response by decreasing activation of T cells that are believed to be the key mediators of psoriasis.

USES Treatment of moderate to severe chronic plaque psoriasis.
UNLABELED USES Treatment of psoriatic arthritis.

CONTRAINDICATIONS Hypersensitivity to alefacept; CD4+ T lymphocyte count below normal; history of systemic malignancies; patients with a clinically important infection; serious infections; live or attenuated vaccines; lactation.
CAUTIOUS USE Patients at high risk for malignancies; pregnancy (category B); elderly.

ROUTE & DOSAGE

Chronic Plaque Psoriasis

Adult: **IM** 15 mg once/wk × 12 wk, may repeat course after 12 wk off therapy. **IV** 7.5 mg once/wk × 12 wk, may repeat course after 12 wk off therapy

Psoriatic Arthritis

Adult: **IV** 7.5 mg once/wk × 12 wk

ADMINISTRATION

- Administer only if CD4+ T lymphocyte count is ≥250 cells/µL.
- Reconstituted alefacept should be clear and colorless to slightly yellow.

Intramuscular

- Reconstitute the 15 mg vial IM administration with 0.6 mL of the supplied diluent to yield 15 mg/0.5 mL. Gently swirl vial for about 2 min to mix, but do not shake.
- Rotate the injection sites and space at least 1 inch from an old site.
- Never inject into areas where the skin is tender, bruised, red, or hard.

Intravenous

PREPARE: **Direct:** Reconstitute the 7.5 mg vial for IV administration with 0.6 mL of the supplied diluent to yield 7.5 mg/0.5 mL. Gently swirl vial for about 2 min to mix, but do not shake.

ADMINISTER: **Direct:** Prime supplied infusion set with 3.0 mL of supplied diluent and insert into vein. Give reconstituted solution over ≤5 sec and do not use a filter. Follow with flush using 3 mL of supplied diluent.

INCOMPATIBILITIES **Solution/additive:** No data available at this time.

- Store vials of powder away from light at 15°–30° C (59°–86° F).
- Store reconstituted solution for up to 4 h between 2°–8° C (36°–46° F); discard solution not used within 4 h of reconstitution.

ADVERSE EFFECTS (≥1%) **Body as a Whole:** Secondary malignancies, serious infections, chills, *injection site pain,* injection site inflammation. **CNS:** Dizziness, headache. **GI:** Nausea, vomiting. **Hematologic:** *Lymphopenia,* alefacept antibody formation. **Musculoskeletal:** Myalgia. **Respiratory:** Pharyngitis, increased cough. **Skin:** Pruritus.

INTERACTIONS Drug: Additive immunosuppression with other immunosuppressant drugs (e.g., CORTICOSTEROIDS); LIVE VACCINES increase risk of secondary transmission of infection.

PHARMACOKINETICS Absorption: 63% absorbed from IM injection. **Metabolism:** Presumed to be broken down in plasma. **Half-Life:** 270 h.

NURSING IMPLICATIONS

Assessment & Drug Effects

- Discontinue drug immediately and institute supportive measures if a serious hypersensitivity reaction occurs.
- Note: Drug should be discontinued if CD4+ T lymphocyte counts remain below 250 cells/µL for one month.
- Lab tests: Weekly WBC with differential during 12-wk dosing period; periodic liver enzymes.
- Monitor for and promptly report S&S of infection.

Patient & Family Education

- Report any of the following promptly: chest pain or tightness, rapid or irregular heart beat; difficulty breathing or swallowing;

swelling of face, tongue, hands, feet or ankles; rapid weight gain; signs of infection (e.g., fever, chills, cough, sore throat, pain or difficulty passing urine); skin rash or itchy skin; severe stomach pain.
- Do not accept live or live-attenuated vaccines while taking this drug.
- Notify physician if you become pregnant while taking this drug or within 8 wk of discontinuing drug.
- Do not breast feed without consulting physician.

ALEMTUZUMAB
(a-lem′tu-zu-mab)
Campath
Classifications: IMMUNOMODULATOR; MONOCLONAL ANTIBODY
Prototype: Basiliximab
Pregnancy Category: C

AVAILABILITY 30 mg/3 mL injection

ACTIONS Recombinant DNA monoclonal antibody that attaches to CD52 cell surface antigens expressed on a variety of leukocytes, including normal and malignant B and T lymphocytes, monocytes, and some granulocytes. Proposed mechanism of action is antibody-dependent lysis of leukemic cells following cell surface binding.
THERAPEUTIC EFFECTS Initiates antibody dependent cell lysis, thus inhibiting cell proliferation in chronic lymphocytic leukemia.

USES Treatment of B-cell chronic lymphocytic leukemia in patients who have failed fludarabine therapy.
UNLABELED USES Treatment of mycosis fungoides, non-Hodgkin's lymphoma.

CONTRAINDICATIONS Type I hypersensitivity to alemtuzumab or its components, hamster protein hypersensitivity; serious infection or exposure to viral infections (i.e., herpes or chickenpox), HIV infection, dental work; infection; pregnancy (category C), lactation.
CAUTIOUS USE History of hypersensitivity to other monoclonal antibodies; ischemic cardiac disease, angina, coronary artery disease; dental disease; history of varicella disease; females of childbearing age. Safety and efficacy in children are not established.

ROUTE & DOSAGE

B-Cell Chronic Lymphocytic Leukemia
Adult: **IV** Start with 3 mg/d infused over 2 h; when 3 mg/d is tolerated, increase dose over next 3–7 d to 10 mg/d, when 10 mg/d is tolerated, increase to maintenance dose of 30 mg/d (give 30 mg/d 3 times/wk)

ADMINISTRATION

Note: Premedication with antihistamines, acetaminophen, antiemetics, and corticosteroids prior to infusion may reduce the severity of adverse side effects.

Intravenous

PREPARE: **IV Infusion:** Do NOT shake ampule prior to use. Withdraw required dose into a syringe and filter with a sterile, low-protein binding, non-fiber releasing 5 micron filter prior to dilution. Inject into 100 mL NS or D5W. Gently invert bag to mix. Infuse within 8 h of mixing. Protect from light. Discard any unused solution.
ADMINISTER: **IV Infusion:** Infuse each dose over 2 h. Do NOT give single doses >30 mg or cumulative weekly doses >90 mg.

INCOMPATIBILITIES **Solution/additive:** Do not infuse or mix with other drugs.

- Store at 2°–8° C (36°–46° F). Discard if ampule has been frozen. Protect from direct light.

ADVERSE EFFECTS (≥1%) **Body as a Whole:** *Infusion reactions (rigors, fever, nausea, vomiting, hypotension, rash, shortness of breath, bronchospasm, chills), fatigue, pain, sepsis, asthenia, edema, herpes simplex, myalgias,* malaise, moniliasis, temperature change sensation, coma, seizures. **CNS:** *Headache, dysesthesias, dizziness, insomnia,* depression, tremor, somnolence, cerebrovascular accident, subarachnoid hemorrhage. **CV:** *Hypotension, tachycardia, hypertension,* cardiac failure, arrhythmias, MI. **GI:** *Diarrhea, nausea, vomiting, stomatitis, abdominal pain, dyspepsia, anorexia,* constipation. **Hematologic:** *Neutropenia, anemia, thrombocytopenia,* purpura, epistaxis, pancytopenia. **Respiratory:** *Dyspnea, cough, bronchitis, pneumonia, pharyngitis,* bronchospasm, rhinitis. **Skin:** *Rash, urticaria, pruritus, increased sweating.*

INTERACTIONS Drug: Additive risk of bleeding with ANTICOAGULANTS, NSAIDS, PLATELET INHIBITORS, SALICYLATES increased risk of opportunistic infections with **fludarabine. Herbal: Feverfew, garlic, ginger, ginkgo** may increase risk of bleeding.

PHARMACOKINETICS Peak: Steady-state levels in approximately 6 wk. **Half-Life:** 12 d.

NURSING IMPLICATIONS

Assessment & Drug Effects

- Monitor for acute infusion-related events, including hypotension, rigors, fever, shortness of breath, bronchospasm, chills, and/or rash. If such a reaction occurs, the infusion should be discontinued and the physician notified.
- Withhold drug and notify physician if absolute neutrophil count <250/microliter or platelet count ≤25,000/microliter.
- Monitor BP closely during infusion period. Careful monitoring of BP and hypotensive symptoms is especially important in patients with ischemic heart disease and those on antihypertensives.
- Discontinue infusion and notify physician immediately if any of the following occurs: hypotension, fever, chills, shortness of breath, bronchospasm, or rash.
- Withhold drug during any serious infection. Therapy may be reinstituted following resolution of the infection.
- Lab tests: CBS with differential and platelet counts weekly or more frequently in the presence of anemia, thrombocytopenia, or neutropenia; periodic blood glucose, serum electrolytes, and alkaline phosphatase.
- Monitor diabetics closely for loss of glycemic control.
- Monitor for S&S of dehydration especially with severe vomiting.

Patient & Family Education

- Do not accept immunizations with live viral vaccines during therapy or if therapy has been recently terminated.
- Use effective methods of contraception to prevent pregnancy during therapy and for at least 6 mo following therapy.
- Report any of the following to physician immediately: Unexplained bleeding, fever, sore throat, flu-like symptoms, S&S of an infection, difficulty breathing,

significant GI distress, abdominal pain, fluid retention, or changes in mental status.

- Diabetics should monitor blood glucose levels carefully since loss of glycemic control is a possible adverse reaction.
- Do not breast feed while taking this drug.

ALENDRONATE SODIUM

(a-len'dro-nate)

Fosamax

Classifications: BISPHOSPHONATE; REGULATOR, BONE METABOLISM

Prototype: Etidronate

Pregnancy Category: C

AVAILABILITY 5 mg, 10 mg, 35 mg, 40 mg, 70 mg tablets; 70 mg/ 75 mL oral solution

ACTIONS Alendronate is a bisphosphonate that inhibits osteoclast-mediated bone resorption. Antiresorption mechanism is not fully understood. It does, however, localize preferentially to resorption sites of active bone turnover and has minimal to no interference with bone mineralization.

THERAPEUTIC EFFECTS Alendronate decreases bone resorption thus minimizing loss of bone density.

USES Prevention and treatment of osteoporosis in postmenopausal women, Paget's disease. Treatment of glucocorticoid-induced osteoporosis.

CONTRAINDICATIONS Hypersensitivity to alendronate or other bisphosphonates; severe renal impairment (Cl_{cr} 35 mL/min); hypocalcemia; abnormalities; lactation, pregnancy (category C).

CAUTIOUS USE Renal impairment, CHF, hyperphosphatemia, liver disease, fever or infection, active upper GI problems.

ROUTE & DOSAGE

Treatment of Osteoporosis

Adult: **PO** 10 mg once/d (max: 40 mg/d) or 70 mg q wk

Prevention of Osteoporosis, Treatment of Steroid-induced Osteoporosis

Adult: **PO** 5 mg q.d. or 35 mg q wk

Treatment of Paget's Disease

Adult: **PO** 40 mg once/d for 6 mo

Renal Impairment

Cl_{cr} <35 mL/min use not recommended

ADMINISTRATION

Oral

- Correct hypocalcemia before administering alendronate.
- Administer in the morning at least 30 min before the first food, beverage, or medication. Do not administer within 2 h of calcium-containing foods, beverages, or medications. At least 30 min should elapse after alendronate dose before taking any other drugs.
- *Oral Solution:* Use oral syringe for accurate dosage. Give with at least 60 cc (2 oz) of plain water.
- *Tablet:* Give with 8 oz of plain water.
- Keep patient sitting up or ambulating for 30 min after taking drug.
- Store according to manufacturer's directions.

ADVERSE EFFECTS (≥1%) **Endocrine:** Hypocalcemia. **GI:** Esophageal irritation and *ulceration, nausea, vomiting, abdominal pain, dyspepsia,* diarrhea, constipation, flatulence. **Other:** Arthralgias, myalgias, headache, rash.

INTERACTIONS Food: Calcium and food (especially dairy products) reduce alendronate absorption.

PHARMACOKINETICS Absorption: 0.5%–1% absorbed from GI tract (absorption significantly decreased by calcium and food). **Onset:** 3–6 wk. **Duration:** 12 wk after discontinuation. **Distribution:** Rapid skeletal uptake. **Metabolism:** Not metabolized. **Elimination:** Up to 50% excreted unchanged in urine. **Half-Life:** Up to 10 h.

NURSING IMPLICATIONS

Assessment & Drug Effects

- Lab tests: Monitor albumin-adjusted serum calcium, serum phosphate, serum alkaline phosphatase, fasting and 24 h urinary calcium, and serum electrolytes. Periodically monitor renal and liver functions.
- Diagnostic test: Bone density scan every 12–18 mo.
- Discontinue drug if the Cl_{cr} <35 mL/min.

Patient & Family Education

- Review directions for taking drug correctly (see ADMINISTRATION).
- Report fever, especially when accompanied by arthralgia and myalgia.
- Do not breast feed while taking this drug.

ALFENTANIL HYDROCHLORIDE

(al-fen′ta-nill)

Alfenta

Classifications: CENTRAL NERVOUS SYSTEM AGENT; NARCOTIC (OPIATE) AGONIST ANALGESIC; GENERAL ANESTHETIC

Prototype: Morphine

Pregnancy Category: C

Controlled Substance: Schedule II

AVAILABILITY 500 mcg/mL injection

ACTIONS Alfentanil is a narcotic agonist analgesic with rapid onset and short duration of action. CNS effects of alfentanil appear to be related to interaction of drug with opiate receptors.

THERAPEUTIC EFFECTS Brief duration is advantageous for short surgical procedures but necessitates incremental injections or continuous infusion for long operations.

USES Major component of balanced anesthesia; analgesic, analgesic supplement, and primary anesthetic for induction of anesthesia when endotracheal and mechanical ventilation are required.

CONTRAINDICATIONS Safety during pregnancy (category C), lactation, or in children <12 y is not established.

CAUTIOUS USE Older adults, history of pulmonary disease.

ROUTE & DOSAGE

Anesthesia Induction

Adult: **IV** 8–20 mcg/kg for surgery lasting <30 min, maintenance anesthesia can be maintained with incremental doses of 3–5 mcg/kg, continuous infusion of 0.5–1 mcg/kg/min (total dose of 8–40 mcg/kg)

ADMINISTRATION

Intravenous

PREPARE: **Direct or Continuous:** Alfentanil is available in concentrations of 500 mcg/mL.
- Add 20 mL of alfentanil to 230 mL of compatible IV solution to yield 40 mcg/mL. Compatible IV

solutions include NS, D5/NS, D5W, and RL. ▪ Note: Alfentanil may be diluted to concentrations of 25–80 mcg/mL.

ADMINISTER: **Direct:** Administer over at least 3 min. Do not administer more rapidly. **Continuous:** Administer at a rate of 0.5–1 mcg/kg/min. Note: Dose may be individualized.

- Store at 15°–30° C (59°–86° F). Avoid freezing.

ADVERSE EFFECTS (≥1%) **Body as a Whole:** Thoracic muscle rigidity, flushing, diaphoresis; extremities feel heavy and warm. **CNS:** Dizziness, euphoria, drowsiness. **CV:** Hypotension, hypertension, tachycardia, bradycardia. **GI:** *Nausea,* vomiting, anorexia, constipation, cramps. **Respiratory:** Apnea, respiratory depression, dyspnea.

INTERACTIONS Drug: BETA-ADRENERGIC BLOCKERS increase incidence of bradycardia; CNS DEPRESSANTS such as BARBITURATES, TRANQUILIZERS, NEUROMUSCULAR BLOCKING AGENTS, OPIATES, and INHALATION GENERAL ANESTHETICS may enhance the cardiovascular and CNS effects of alfentanil in both magnitude and duration; enhancement or prolongation of postoperative respiratory depression also may result from concomitant administration of any of these agents with alfentanil.

PHARMACOKINETICS Onset: 2 min. **Duration:** Injection 30 min; continuous infusion 45 min. **Distribution:** Crosses placenta. **Metabolism:** Completely metabolized in liver. **Elimination:** Excreted in breast milk. **Half-Life:** 46–213 min.

NURSING IMPLICATIONS

Assessment & Drug Effects

- Monitor for S&S of increased sympathetic stimulation (arrhythmias) and evidence of depressed postoperative analgesia (tachycardia, pain, pupillary dilation, spontaneous muscle movement) if a narcotic antagonist has been administered to overcome residual effects of alfentanil.
- Evaluate adequacy of spontaneous ventilation carefully during postoperative period.
- Monitor vital signs carefully during postoperative period; check for bradycardia, especially if patient is also taking a beta blocker.
- Note: Narcotic effects wear off quickly with negligible residual effects.
- Note: Dizziness, sedation, nausea, and vomiting are common when drug is used as a postoperative analgesic.

Patient & Family Education

- Report unpleasant adverse effects when drug is used for patient-controlled analgesia.
- Do not breast feed infants while taking this drug without consulting physician.

ALFUZOSIN

(al-fuz′o-sin)

UroXatral

Classifications: AUTONOMIC NERVOUS SYSTEM AGENT; ALPHA-ADRENERGIC ANTAGONIST (BLOCKING AGENT, SYMPATHOLYTIC)

Prototype: Prazosin

Pregnancy Category: B

AVAILABILITY 10 mg extended-release tablet

ACTIONS Alfuzosin is a short-acting, selective antagonist at alpha-1 receptors with a low incidence of hypotension and sexual dysfunction at therapeutic doses. Alpha-1 receptors cause contraction of smooth muscle in the prostate, prostatic capsule, prostatic urethra, bladder base, and bladder neck. Both alpha-1a (70%) and alpha-1b receptors exist in the prostate.

THERAPEUTIC EFFECTS Blockade of alpha-1 receptors by alfuzosin causes smooth muscles in the bladder neck and prostate to relax, thereby reducing pressure on the urethra and improving urine flow rate. This results in a reduction in BPH symptoms.

USES Treatment of symptomatic benign prostatic hypertrophy (BPH).

CONTRAINDICATIONS Hypersensitivity to alfuzosin; lactation; moderate or severe hepatic insufficiency; concurrent treatment with potent CYP3A4 inhibitors (e.g., ketoconazole, itraconazole, and ritonavir).

CAUTIOUS USE Pregnancy (category B); coronary artery disease; hepatic disease; dizziness, light-headedness, orthostatic hypotension.

ROUTE & DOSAGE

Benign Prostatic Hypertrophy
Adult: **PO** 10 mg q.d.

ADMINISTRATION

Oral

- Give immediately after same meal each day.
- Ensure that extended-release tablet is not crushed or chewed. It must be swallowed whole.
- Store at 15°–30° C (59°–86° F). Protect from light and moisture.

ADVERSE EFFECTS (≥1%) **Body as a Whole:** Fatigue, pain. **CNS:** Dizziness, headache. **GI:** Abdominal pain, dyspepsia, constipation, nausea. **Respiratory:** Upper respiratory infection, bronchitis, sinusitis, pharyngitis. **Urogenital:** Impotence.

INTERACTIONS Drug: Increased risk of hypotension with other ANTIHYPERTENSIVE AGENTS; **ketoconazole, itraconazole,** PROTEASE INHIBITORS may increase alfuzosin levels and toxicity. **Food: Grapefruit juice** may decrease metabolism of alfuzosin. **Herbal: Hawthorn** may increase risk of hypotension.

PHARMACOKINETICS Absorption: 49% absorbed when taken with food. **Peak:** 8 h. **Metabolism:** Metabolized in liver by CYP3A4. **Elimination:** 69% excreted in feces, 24% excreted in urine. **Half-Life:** 10 h.

NURSING IMPLICATIONS

Assessment & Drug Effects

- Monitor CV status and BP, especially if on concurrent treatment with antihypertensive drugs or inhibitors of CYP3A4. See INTERACTIONS.
- Check postural vital signs to evaluate for orthostatic hypotension within a few hours following administration.
- Withhold drug and report new or worsening angina to physician.
- Lab tests: Baseline and periodic LFTs.

Patient & Family Education

- Inform physician about all other prescription, nonprescription, or herbal drugs being taken.
- Make position changes slowly to minimize dizziness.
- Do not drive or engage in other hazardous activities until reaction to drug is known.
- Moderate or eliminate grapefruit juice consumption while on this drug.

ALITRETINOIN (9-*cis*-RETINOIC ACID)

(a-li-tre′ti-noyne)

Panretin

Classifications: SKIN AND MUCOUS MEMBRANE AGENT; ANTIACNE (RETINOID)

Prototype: Isotretinoin

Pregnancy Category: D

AVAILABILITY 0.1% gel

ACTIONS Naturally occurring retinoid that binds to and activates all known retinoid receptors in cells, which regulate cellular differentiation and proliferation in both healthy and neoplastic cells.

THERAPEUTIC EFFECTS Inhibits the growth of Kaposi's sarcoma (KS) in HIV patients. It does not prevent the development of new KS lesions.

USES Treatment of cutaneous lesions of AIDS-related Kaposi's sarcoma.

CONTRAINDICATIONS Hypersensitivity to alitretinoin or other retinoids including vitamin A; when systemic anti-KS therapy is required; pregnancy (category D), lactation.

CAUTIOUS USE Safety & efficacy in children <18 y, or older adults ≥65 y are unknown; cutaneous T-cell lymphoma.

ROUTE & DOSAGE

Cutaneous Kaposi's Sarcoma

Adult: **Topical** Apply sufficient gel to cover lesions b.i.d., may increase application to 3–4 times daily if tolerated

ADMINISTRATION

Topical

- Apply gel liberally over lesions; avoid unaffected skin and mucus membranes.
- Dry 3–5 min before covering with clothes. Do not cover with occlusive dressing.
- Store at 15°–30° C (59°–86° F).

ADVERSE EFFECTS (≥1%) **Skin:** Erythema, edema, vesiculation, *rash, burning pain,* pruritus, exfoliative dermatitis, excoriation, paresthesia.

INTERACTIONS Drug: Increased toxicity with insect repellents containing DEET.

PHARMACOKINETICS Absorption: Minimal absorption.

NURSING IMPLICATIONS

Assessment & Drug Effects

- Monitor for S&S of dermal toxicity (e.g., erythema, edema, vesiculation).

Patient & Family Education

- Allow up to 14 wk for therapeutic response.
- Avoid exposure of medicated skin to sunlight or sun lamps.
- Contact physician if inflammation, swelling, or blisters appear on medicated areas.
- Do not breast feed while using this drug.

ALLOPURINOL

(al-oh-pure′i-nole)

Alloprin A ♣, Alloprim, Apo-allopurinol-A ♣, Lopurin, Novo-purinol A, Purinol ♣, Zyloprim

Classification: ANTIGOUT AGENT

Prototype: Colchicine

Pregnancy Category: C

AVAILABILITY 100 mg, 300 mg tablets; 500 mg vial

ACTIONS Allopurinol reduces endogenous uric acid by selectively inhibiting action of xanthine oxi-

dase, the enzyme responsible for converting hypoxanthine to xanthine and xanthine to uric acid (end product of purine catabolism). Has no analgesic, antiinflammatory, or uricosuric actions.
THERAPEUTIC EFFECTS Thus, urate pool is decreased by the lowering of both serum and urinary uric acid levels, and hyperuricemia is prevented.

USES To control primary hyperuricemia that accompanies severe gout and to prevent possibility of flare-up of acute gouty attack; to prevent recurrent calcium oxalate stones; prophylactically to reduce severity of hyperuricemia associated with antineoplastic and radiation therapies, both of which greatly increase plasma uric acid levels by promoting nucleic acid degradation.
UNLABELED USES To reduce hyperuricemia secondary to Lesch–Nyhan syndrome, polycythemia vera, G6PD deficiency, sarcoidosis, and therapy with thiazides or ethambutol.

CONTRAINDICATIONS Hypersensitivity to allopurinol; as initial treatment for acute gouty attacks; idiopathic hemochromatosis (or those with family history); children (except those with hyperuricemia secondary to neoplastic disease and chemotherapy). Safety during pregnancy (category C) or lactation is not established.
CAUTIOUS USE Impaired hepatic or renal function, history of peptic ulcer, lower GI tract disease, bone marrow depression.

ROUTE & DOSAGE

Treatment Hyperuricemia
Adult: **PO** 100 mg/d, may increase by 100 mg/wk (max: 800 mg/d), divide doses >300 mg/d **IV** 200–400 mg/m²/d (max: 600 mg/d) in 1–4 divided doses
Child: **PO** *≤10 y,* 10 mg/kg/d in 2–3 divided doses (max: 800 mg/d) **IV** 200 mg/m²/d in 1–4 divided doses

Treatment Secondary Hyperuricemia
Adult: **PO** 200–800 mg/d for 2–3 d or longer, divide doses >300 mg/d
Child: **PO** *6–10 y,* 100 mg t.i.d., *<6 y,* 50 mg t.i.d.

Renal Impairment
Cl_{cr}: 80 mL/min: 250 mg/d; 60 mL/min: 200 mg/d; 40 mL/min: 150 mg/d; 20 mL/min: 100 mg/d; 10 mL/min: 100 mg q2d; 0 mL/min: 100 mg q3d

ADMINISTRATION

Oral
- Give after meals for best toleration; tablet may be crushed and taken with fluid or mixed with food.
- Store at 15°–30° C (59°–86° F) in a tightly closed container.

Intravenous

PREPARE: **Intermittent:** Reconstitute a single dose vial (500 mg) with 25 mL of sterile water for injection to yield 20 mg/mL. ▪ Further dilute with NS or D5W to a concentration of ≤6 mg/mL. ▪ Note: Adding 2.3 mL of diluent yields 6 mg/mL.
ADMINISTER: **Intermittent:** Usually administered over 30–60 min.
INCOMPATIBILITIES **Solution/Additive: Amikacin, amphotericin B, carmustine, cefotaxime, chlorpromazine, cimetidine, clindamycin, cytarabine, da-**

carbazine, daunorubicin, doxycycline, droperidol, floxuridine, gentamicin, haloperidol, hydroxyzine, idarubicin, imipenem-cilastatin, mechlorethamine, meperidine, metoclopramide, methylprednisolone, minocycline, nalbuphine, netilmicin, ondansetron, prochlorperazine, promethazine, sodium bicarbonate, streptozocin, tobramycin, vinorelbine.

ADVERSE EFFECTS (≥1%) **CNS:** Drowsiness, headache, vertigo. **GI:** Nausea, vomiting, diarrhea, abdominal discomfort, indigestion, malaise. **Hematologic:** (Rare) Agranulocytosis, aplastic anemia, bone marrow depression, thrombocytopenia. **Skin:** Urticaria or pruritus, pruritic maculopapular rash, toxic epidermal necrolysis. **Other:** Hepatotoxicity, renal insufficiency.

DIAGNOSTIC TEST INTERFERENCE Possibility of elevated blood levels of ***alkaline phosphatase*** and ***serum transaminases (AST, ALT),*** and decreased blood ***Hct, Hgb, leukocytes.***

INTERACTIONS Drug: Alcohol may inhibit renal excretion of uric acid; **ampicillin, amoxicillin** increase risk of skin rash; enhances anticoagulant effect of **warfarin;** toxicity from **azathioprine, mercaptopurine, cyclophosphamide, cyclosporin** increased; increases hypoglycemic effects of **chlorpropamide**; THIAZIDES increase risk of allopurinol toxicity and hypersensitivity (especially with impaired renal function).

PHARMACOKINETICS Absorption: 80%–90% absorbed from GI tract. **Onset:** 24–48 h. **Peak:** 2–6 h. **Metabolism:** 75%–80% metabolizes to the active metabolite oxypurinol. **Elimination:** Slowly excreted in urine; excreted in breast milk. **Half-Life:** 1–3 h; oxypurinol, 18–30 h.

NURSING IMPLICATIONS

Assessment & Drug Effects

- Monitor for therapeutic effectiveness which is indicated by normal serum and urinary uric acid levels usually by 1–3 wk (aim of therapy is to lower serum uric acid level gradually to about 6 mg/dL), gradual decrease in size of tophi, absence of new tophaceous deposits (after approximately 6 mo), with consequent relief of joint pain and increased joint mobility.
- Monitor for S&S of an acute gouty attack which is most likely to occur during first 6 wk of therapy.
- Lab tests: Monitor serum uric acid levels q1–2wk to check adequacy of dosage. Perform baseline CBC, liver and kidney function tests before therapy is initiated and then monthly, particularly during first few months. Check urinary pH at regular intervals.
- Monitor patients with renal disorders more often; they tend to have a higher incidence of renal stones and drug toxicity problems.
- Report onset of rash or fever immediately to physician; withdraw drug. Life-threatening toxicity syndrome can occur 2–4 wk after initiation of therapy (more common with impaired renal function) and is generally accompanied by malaise, fever, and aching, a diffuse erythematous, desquamating rash, hepatic dysfunction, eosinophilia, and worsening of renal function.

Patient & Family Education

- Drink enough fluid to produce urinary output of at least 2000 mL/d (fluid intake of at least

3000 mL/d). (Note that 1000 mL is approximately equal to 1 quart.) Report diminishing urinary output, cloudy urine, unusual color or odor to urine, pain or discomfort on urination.

- Report promptly the onset of itching or rash. Stop drug if a skin rash appears, even after 5 or more wk (and reportedly as long as 2 y) of therapy.
- Minimize exposure of eyes to ultraviolet or sunlight which may stimulate the development of cataracts.
- Do not drive or engage in potentially hazardous activities until response to drug is known.
- Remain under medical supervision while taking allopurinol (generally continued indefinitely); drug can cause severe adverse reactions.
- Do not breast feed while taking this drug without consulting physician.

ALMOTRIPTAN

(al-mo-trip'tan)

Axert

Classifications: AUTONOMIC NERVOUS SYSTEM AGENT; ADRENERGIC AGONIST (SYMPATHOMIMETIC); SEROTONIN 5-HT_1-RECEPTOR AGONIST

Prototype: Sumatriptan

Pregnancy Category: C

AVAILABILITY 6.25 mg, 12.5 mg tablets

ACTIONS Selective agonist that binds with high affinity to 5-HT_{1D}, 5-HT_{1B}, 5-HT_{1F} serotonin receptors which are found on extracerebral and intracranial blood vessels, and on other structures in the central nervous system.

THERAPEUTIC EFFECTS Due primarily to agonist effects on 5-HT_{1D} and 5-HT_{1B} serotonin receptors on cranial blood vessels resulting in vasoconstriction and agonist effects on nerve terminals in the trigeminal system. Activation of these receptors results in constriction of cranial vessels which become dilated during a migraine attack, inhibition of neuropeptide release, and reduced signal transmission in the pain pathways.

USES Treatment of migraine headache with or without aura.

CONTRAINDICATIONS Hypersensitivity to almotriptan malate. Significant cardiovascular disease such as ischemic heart disease, coronary artery vasospasms, MI, angina, arteriosclerosis, cardiac arrhythmias, diabetes mellitus, colitis, history of cerebrovascular events, or uncontrolled hypertension; stroke, smoking, Wolff-Parkinson-White syndrome, within 24 h of receiving another 5-HT_1 agonist or an ergotamine-containing or ergot-type drug; basilar or hemiplegic migraine, pregnancy (category C).

CAUTIOUS USE Significant risk factors for coronary artery disease unless a cardiac evaluation has been done; hypertension; risk factors for cerebrovascular accident; peripheral vascular disease, impaired liver or kidney function, Raynaud's disease, children, elderly, lactation.

ROUTE & DOSAGE

Migraine Headache

Adult: **PO** 6.25–12.5 mg. If headache returns, may repeat after at least 2 h (max: 2 tabs/24 h)

Renal Impairment

Cl_{cr} <10 mL/min: 6.25 mg (max: 12.5 mg/d)

ADMINISTRATION

Oral

- Do not give within 24 h of an ergot-containing drug.
- Administer any time after symptoms of migraine appear.
- Do not administer a second dose without consulting the physician for any attack during which the FIRST dose did NOT work.
- Give a second dose if headache was relieved by first dose but symptoms return; however, wait at least 2 h after the first dose before giving a second dose.
- Do not give more than two doses in 24 h.
- Store at 15°–30° C (59°–86° F).

ADVERSE EFFECTS (≥1%) **Body as a Whole:** Flushing. **CNS:** Drowsiness, headache, paresthesia. **CV:** Palpitations, tachycardia, serious cardiac events (including MI) have been reported within a few hours after administration. **GI:** Nausea, vomiting, dry mouth.

INTERACTIONS Drug: Dihydroergotamine, methysergide, other 5-HT1 AGONISTS may cause prolonged vasospastic reactions; SSRIS, **sibutramine** have rarely caused weakness, hyperreflexia, and incoordination; MAOIS should not be used with 5-HT1 AGONISTS. **Herbal: Gingko, ginseng, echinacea, St. John's wort** may increase triptan toxicity.

PHARMACOKINETICS Absorption: Well absorbed, 70% reaches systemic circulation. **Peak:** 1–3 h. **Distribution:** 35% protein bound. **Metabolism:** 27% metabolized by monoamine oxidase. **Elimination:** 75% excreted renally, 13% excreted in feces. **Half-Life:** 3–4 h.

NURSING IMPLICATIONS

Assessment & Drug Effects

- Monitor cardiovascular status carefully following first dose in patients at relatively high risk for coronary artery disease (e.g., postmenopausal women, men over 40 years old, persons with known CAD risk factors) or who have coronary artery vasospasms.
- Report to physician immediately chest pain or tightness in chest or throat that is severe or does not quickly resolve following a dose of almotriptan.
- Pain relief usually begins within 10 min of ingestion, with complete relief in approximately 65% of all patients within 2 h.
- Monitor BP, especially in those being treated for hypertension.

Patient & Family Education

- Review patient information leaflet provided by the manufacturer carefully.
- Notify physician immediately if symptoms of severe angina (e.g., severe or persistent pain or tightness in chest, back, neck, or throat) or hypersensitivity (e.g., wheezing, facial swelling, skin rash, or hives) occur.
- Do not take any other serotonin receptor agonist (e.g., Imitrex, Maxalt, Zomig, Amerge) within 24 h of taking almotriptan.
- Advise physician of any drugs taken within 1 wk of beginning almotriptan.
- Check with physician regarding drug interactions before taking any new OTC or prescription drugs.
- Report any other adverse effects (e.g., tingling, flushing, dizziness) at next physician visit.
- Do not breast feed while taking this drug without consulting physician.

ALOSETRON

(a-lo′se-tron)

Lotronex

Classification: SEROTONIN 5-HT_3 RECEPTOR ANTAGONIST

Prototype: Ondansetron

Pregnancy Category: B

AVAILABILITY 1 mg tablets

ACTIONS Potent and selective serotonin (5-HT_3) receptor antagonist. Serotonin 5-HT_3 receptors are extensively located on enteric neurons of the GI tract. Activation of these receptors affects amount of visceral pain experienced, transit time in the colon, and GI secretions.

THERAPEUTIC EFFECTS Blockage of the serotonin 5-HT_3 receptors by alosetron results in significant control of GI pain, and severe diarrhea related to irritable bowel syndrome.

USES Treatment of severe irritable bowel syndrome (IBS) in women whose predominant symptom is diarrhea and whose symptoms have lasted >6 mo and have failed to respond to conventional therapy.

CONTRAINDICATIONS Constipation, ischemic colitis, development of ischemic bowel symptoms such as sudden onset of rectal bleeding, bloody diarrhea, new or sudden worsening of abdominal pain; history of chronic or severe constipation, intestinal obstruction, toxic megacolon, GI adhesions, GI perforation, active diverticulitis, history of, or current Crohn's disease or ulcerative colitis; hypersensitivity to alosetron; thrombophlebitis, hypercoagulable state, inability to comply with Patient–Physician Agreement.

CAUTIOUS USE Hepatic insufficiency; pregnancy (category B), lactation; elderly. Safety and efficacy in children are not established.

ROUTE & DOSAGE

Irritable Bowel Syndrome

Adult: **PO** Start with 1 mg q.d. for 4 wk, may increase to 1 mg b.i.d. if tolerated

ADMINISTRATION

Oral

- Ensure that the patient has signed the Patient–Physician Agreement prior to administering alosetron.
- Do not give this drug if the patient has constipation.
- Review the contraindications for this drug and ensure that the patient has none of the conditions for which the drug is contraindicated.
- Store at 25° C (77° F).

ADVERSE EFFECTS (≥1%) **Body as a Whole:** Malaise, fatigue, cramps, pain. **CNS:** Anxiety. **CV:** Tachyarrhythmias. **GI:** *Constipation*, abdominal pain, nausea, distention, reflux, hemorrhoids, hyposalivation, dyspepsia, ischemic colitis. **Skin:** Sweating, urticaria. **Urogenital:** Urinary frequency.

INTERACTIONS Drug: No clinically significant interactions established.

PHARMACOKINETICS Absorption: Rapidly absorbed, average bioavailability of 50–60%. **Peak:** 1 h. **Distribution:** 82% protein bound. **Metabolism:** Extensively metabolized in liver. **Elimination:** 73% excreted in urine, 24% excreted in feces. **Half-Life:** 1.5 h.

NURSING IMPLICATIONS

Assessment & Drug Effects

- Monitor for and report immediately signs of ischemic colitis such as new or worsening abdominal pain, bloody diarrhea, or blood in the stool.

- Withhold drug and notify physician if patient has not had adequate control of IBS symptoms after 4 weeks of treatment with 1 mg twice a day.
- Monitor carefully patients who have decreased GI motility (e.g., older adults, persons receiving other drugs which may decrease GI motility) as they may be at greater risk of serious complications of constipation.
- Monitor carefully patients with any degree of hepatic insufficiency as they may be more susceptible to adverse drug effects.
- Monitor periodically for cardiac arrythmias, especially with preexisting cardiovascular disease.

Patient & Family Education

- Read the Medication Guide before starting alosetron and each time you refill your prescription.
- Do not start taking alosetron if you are constipated.
- Discontinue alosetron immediately and contact your physician if you experience any of the following: constipation, new or worsening abdominal pain, bloody diarrhea, or blood in the stool.
- Contact your physician immediately if constipation does not resolve after discontinuation of alosetron. Resume alosetron again only if constipation has resolved and your physician directs you to begin taking the medication again.
- Stop taking alosetron and contact your physician if IBS symptoms are not adequately controlled after 4 weeks of taking 1 tablet twice a day.
- Do not breast feed while taking this drug without consulting physician

ALPHA1-PROTEINASE INHIBITOR (HUMAN)

(pro′ten-ase)
Prolastin, Aralast, Zemaira
Classifications: HORMONES AND SYNTHETIC SUBSTITUTES; ENZYME INHIBITOR
Pregnancy Category: C

AVAILABILITY Prolastin: 20 mg/mL; Aralast: 0.5 g/25 mL, 1 g/50 mL vial; Zemaira: 20 mL vial

ACTIONS Alpha$_1$-proteinase inhibitor (alpha$_1$-PI; alpha$_1$-antitrypsin) is extracted from plasma and used in patients with panacinar emphysema who have alpha$_1$-antitrypsin deficiency. Alpha$_1$-antitrypsin deficiency is a chronic, hereditary, and usually fatal autosomal recessive disorder that results in a slowly progressive, panacinar emphysema.
THERAPEUTIC EFFECTS Prevents the progressive breakdown of elastin tissues in the alveoli, thus showing panacinar emphysema progression.

USES Indicated for chronic replacement therapy in patients with alpha$_1$-antitrypsin deficiency and demonstrable panacinar emphysema.

CONTRAINDICATIONS Individuals with selective IgA deficiencies; pregnancy (category C), lactation.
CAUTIOUS USE Patients with significant heart disease or other conditions that may be aggravated with slight increases in plasma volume. Safety and efficacy in children are not established.

ROUTE & DOSAGE

Panacinar Emphysema
Adult: **IV** 60 mg/kg once/wk administered at a rate of ≥0.08 mL/kg/min

ADMINISTRATION

Intravenous

Give hepatitis B vaccine prior to utilizing this drug.

PREPARE: **IV Infusion:** Warm unopened diluent and concentrate to room temperature. ▪ Reconstitute with sterile water for injection supplied by manufacturer to yield a concentration of 20 mg/mL.

ADMINISTER: **IV Infusion:** Give within 3 h after reconstitution. ▪ Give alone, without mixing with other agents. ▪ Administer at rate of at least 0.08 mL/kg/min. ▪ Note: The recommended dosage takes about 30 min to administer to a 70 kg person.

▪ Store unreconstituted drug at 2°–8° C (35°–46° F). Do not refrigerate after reconstitution. Discard unused solution.

ADVERSE EFFECTS (≥1%) **Hematologic:** Leukocytosis. **CNS:** Dizziness, fever (may be delayed). **Other:** Hepatitis B if not immunized.

PHARMACOKINETICS Distribution: Crosses placenta; distributed into breast milk. **Metabolism:** Undergoes catabolism in the intravascular space; approximately 33% is catabolized per day, with estimated production levels of 34 mg/kg/d. **Half-Life:** 4.5–5.2 d.

NURSING IMPLICATIONS

Assessment & Drug Effects

- Administer with caution in patients at risk for circulatory overload. Monitor cardiac status.
- Monitor respiratory status (rate, dyspnea, lung sounds) throughout therapy.
- Lab tests: Monitor serum alpha$_1$-PI level (minimum serum concentration level should be 80 mg/mL); periodic pulmonary functions and ABGs.

Patient & Family Education

- Avoid smoking and notify physician of any changes in respiratory pattern.
- Do not breast feed while taking this drug.

ALPRAZOLAM

(al-pray′zoe-lam)

Xanax, Xanax XR

Classifications: CENTRAL NERVOUS SYSTEM AGENT; ANXIOLYTIC; SEDATIVE-HYPNOTIC; BENZODIAZEPINE

Prototype: Lorazepam

Pregnancy Category: D

Controlled Substance: Schedule IV

AVAILABILITY 0.25 mg, 0.5 mg, 1 mg, 2 mg tablets; 0.5 mg, 1 mg, 2 mg, 3 mg sustained-release tabs; 0.5 mg/5 mL, 1 mg/mL oral solution

ACTIONS CNS depressant. Mode of action not known, but appears to act at the limbic, thalamic, and hypothalamic levels of the CNS. It is associated with significantly less drowsiness.

THERAPEUTIC EFFECTS Drug has antidepressant as well as antianxiety actions.

USES Management of anxiety disorders or for short-term relief of anxiety symptoms. Also used as adjunct in management of anxiety associated with depression and agitation, and for panic disorders, such as agoraphobia.

CONTRAINDICATIONS Sensitivity to benzodiazepines; acute narrow angle glaucoma; pulmonary disease; use alone in primary depression or psychotic disorders; during pregnancy (category D), lactation; children <18 y.

CAUTIOUS USE Impaired renal or hepatic function; history of alcoholism; geriatric and debilitated patients. Effectiveness for long-term treatment (>4 mo) not established.

ROUTE & DOSAGE

Anxiety Disorders

Adult: **PO** 0.25–0.5 mg t.i.d. (max: 4 mg/d)
Geriatric: **PO** 0.125–0.25 mg b.i.d.

Panic Attacks

Adult: **PO** 1–2 mg t.i.d. (max: 8 mg/d); sustained release: initiate with 0.5 mg to 1 mg once/d. Depending on the response, the dose may be increased at intervals of 3 to 4 days in increments of no more than 1 mg/d. Target range 3–6 mg/d (max: 10 mg/d)

ADMINISTRATION

Oral

- Reduce drug gradually when discontinuing drug.
- Store in light-resistant containers at 15°–30° C (59°–86° F), unless otherwise directed.

ADVERSE EFFECTS (≥1%) **CNS:** *Drowsiness, sedation,* light-headedness, dizziness, syncope, depression, headache, confusion, insomnia, nervousness, fatigue, clumsiness, unsteadiness, rigidity, tremor, restlessness, paradoxical excitement, hallucinations. **CV:** Tachycardia, hypotension, ECG changes. **Special Senses:** Blurred vision. **Respiratory:** Dyspnea.

INTERACTIONS Drug: Alcohol and other CNS DEPRESSANTS, ANTICONVULSANTS, ANTIHISTAMINES, BARBITURATES, NARCOTIC ANALGESICS, BENZODIAZEPINES, compound CNS depressant effects; **cimetidine, disulfiram** increase alprazolam effects (decreased metabolism); ORAL CONTRACEPTIVES may increase or decrease alprazolam effects. **Herbal: Kava-kava, valerian** may potentiate sedation.

PHARMACOKINETICS Absorption: Rapidly absorbed. **Peak:** 1–2 h. **Distribution:** Crosses placenta. **Metabolism:** Oxidized in liver to inactive metabolites. **Elimination:** Renal elimination. **Half-Life:** 12–15 h.

NURSING IMPLICATIONS

Assessment & Drug Effects

- Monitor for S&S of drowsiness and sedation, especially in older adults or the debilitated; they may require supervised ambulation and/or side rails.
- Lab tests: Monitor periodic blood counts, urinalyses, and blood chemistry studies, particularly during continuing therapy.

Patient & Family Education

- Note: Adverse reactions that may occur during early high-dose therapy. These usually disappear with continuing therapy, but dosage adjustments may be indicated.
- Make position changes slowly and in stages to prevent dizziness.
- Do not use alcohol, other CNS depressants, or OTC medications containing antihistamines (e.g., sleep aids, cold, hay fever, or allergy remedies) without consulting physician.
- Do not drive or engage in potentially hazardous activities until response to drug is known.

- Taper dosage following continuous use; abrupt discontinuation of drug may cause withdrawal symptoms: nausea, vomiting, abdominal and muscle cramps, sweating, confusion, tremors, convulsions.
- Do not breast feed while taking this drug.

ALPROSTADIL (PGE_1)

(al-pross'ta-dil)

Prostin VR Pediatric, Caverject, Muse, Edex

Classification: PROSTAGLANDIN
Prototype: Dinoprostone
Pregnancy Category: C

AVAILABILITY 500 mcg/mL injection; 5 mcg/mL, 10 mcg/mL, 20 mcg/mL, 40 mcg/mL powder for injection; 125 mcg, 250 mcg, 500 mcg, 1000 mcg pellets

ACTIONS Actions include vasodilation, inhibition of platelet aggregation, and stimulation of intestinal and uterine smooth muscles.

THERAPEUTIC EFFECTS Preserves ductal patency by relaxing smooth muscle of ductus arteriosus. Alprostadil induces penile erection by relaxing the smooth muscles of the corpus cavernosum and dilating the cavernosal arteries and their penile arterioles. Sufficient rigidity of the penis also requires increased venous outflow resistance, thus resulting in penile blood engorgement and erection.

USES Temporary measure to maintain patency of ductus arteriosus in infants with ductal-dependent congenital heart defects until corrective surgery can be performed. Also used in erectile dysfunction.

CONTRAINDICATIONS Ductus arteriosus respiratory distress syndrome (hyaline membrane disease); hypersensitivity to alprostadil; patients with penile implants. *Muse, Edex:* Women, children, and newborns; lactation. *Muse:* Patients with urethral stricture, inflammation/infection of glans of penis, severe hypospadias, acute or chronic urethritis; sickle cell anemia or trait, thrombocytopenia, polycythemia, multiple myeloma.

CAUTIOUS USE Ductus arteriosus; bleeding tendencies; erectile dysfunction; hypersensitivity to alprostadil; sickle cell anemia or trait; multiple myeloma or leukemia; penile anatomic deformations; patients on anticoagulants, vasoactive or antihypertensive drugs.

ROUTE & DOSAGE

To Maintain Patency of Ductus Arteriosus

Neonate: **IV/Intraarterial/Intraaortic** 0.05–0.1 mcg/kg/min, may increase gradually (max: 0.4 mcg/kg/min if necessary)

Erectile Dysfunction of Vasculogenic, Psychogenic, or Mixed Etiology

Adult: **Intracavernosal** initiate with 2.5 mcg; if inadequate response, increase dose by 2.5 mcg. May then increase dose in 5- to 10-mcg increments until a suitable erection occurs, not exceeding 1 h in duration. Doses >60 mcg not recommended

Erectile Dysfunction of Pure Neurogenic Etiology

Adult: **Intracavernosal** initiate with 1.25 mcg; if inadequate response, increase dose by 1.25 mcg, then increase by 2.5 mcg, may then increase dose in 5 mcg increments until a suitable erection occurs, not exceeding 1 h in duration. Doses >60 mcg not recommended

ADMINISTRATION

Intracavernosal Injection

- Administer only after proper training in the penile injection technique. Refer to information on administration provided to the patient by the manufacturer.
- Use reconstituted solutions immediately.
- Store dry powder at or below 25° C (77° F) for up to 3 mo. Do not freeze.

Transurethral Insertion

- Refer to information on insertion into the urethra provided to the patient by the manufacturer.

Intravenous

PREPARE: **Continuous:** Dilute 500 mg alprostadil with NS or D5W to volume appropriate for pump delivery system. ▪ Prepare fresh solution q24h. Discard unused portions. ▪ A 500 mg ampule diluted in 250 mL yields a concentration of 2 mg/mL.

ADMINISTER: **Continuous:** Infuse at rate of 0.05–0.1 mg/kg/min up to a maximum of 0.4 mg/kg/min. ▪ Reduce infusion rate immediately if arterial pressure drops significantly or if fever occurs. ▪ Discontinue promptly, if apnea or bradycardia occurs.

- Store at 2°–8° C (36°–46° F) unless otherwise directed by manufacturer. Protect from freezing.

ADVERSE EFFECTS (≥1%) **CNS:** *Fever,* seizures, lethargy. **CV:** *Flushing,* bradycardia, hypotension, syncope, tachycardia; CHF, ventricular fibrillation, shock. **GI:** Diarrhea, gastric regurgitation. **Hematologic:** Disseminated intravascular coagulation (DIC), thrombocytopenia. **Respiratory:** Apnea. **Urogenital:** Oliguria, anuria. *Penile pain,* prolonged erection, priapism, penile fibrosis, injection site hematoma/ecchymosis, penile rash and edema, prostatitis, perineal pain. **Skin:** Rash on face and arms, alopecia. **Other:** Leg pain.

INTERACTIONS **Drug:** May increase anticoagulant properties of **warfarin;** ANTIHYPERTENSIVE AGENTS increase risk of hypotension.

PHARMACOKINETICS **Onset:** 15 min to 3 h. **Metabolism:** Rapidly metabolized in lungs. **Elimination:** Metabolites excreted through kidneys. **Half-Life:** 5–10 min.

NURSING IMPLICATIONS

Assessment & Drug Effects

Ductus Arteriosus

- Monitor therapeutic effectiveness which is indicated by increase in blood oxygenation (Po_2), usually evident within 30 min, in infants with cyanotic heart disease (restricted pulmonary blood flow). Normal Po_2 for neonates is 60–70 mm Hg. Indicated by increased pH in those with acidosis, increased systemic BP and urinary output, return of palpable pulses, and decreased ratio of pulmonary artery to aortic pressure in infants with restricted systemic blood flow.
- Monitor for arterial pressure, ECG, heart rate, BP, respiratory rate, and rectal temperature, intermittently throughout the infusion.
- Lab tests: Monitor arterial blood gases and arterial blood pH intermittently throughout the infusion.
- Monitor: Systemic BP, pulmonary artery and descending aorta pressures, femoral pulse, and urinary output.

Patient & Family Education

Erectile Dysfunction

- Follow carefully directions for penile injection provided by the manufacturer.
- Do not change dose without consulting the physician.
- Do not use intracavernosal injection more often than 3 times/wk; allow at least 24 h between uses.
- Do not use more than 2 urethral suppository systems in a 24 h period.
- Report nodules or hard tissue in penis; penile pain, redness, swelling, tenderness; or curvature of the erect penis to the physician as soon as possible.
- Seek immediate medical attention if an erection persists longer than 6 h.

ALTEPLASE RECOMBINANT Pr

(al'te-plase)

Actilyse, Activase, Cathflo Activase

Classifications: BLOOD FORMERS, COAGULATORS, AND ANTICOAGULANTS; THROMBOLYTIC ENZYME

Pregnancy Category: C

AVAILABILITY 50 mg, 100 mg vials

ACTIONS This recombinant DNA-derived form of human tissue-type plasminogen activator (t-PA) is a thrombolytic agent.

THERAPEUTIC EFFECTS The agent t-PA promotes thrombolysis by forming the active proteolytic enzyme plasmin. Plasmin is capable of degrading fibrin, fibrinogen, and factors V, VIII, and XII.

USES Indicated in selective cases of acute MI, preferably within 6 h of attack for recanalization of the coronary artery; lysis of acute pulmonary emboli; acute ischemic stroke or thrombotic stroke (within 3 h of onset); treatment of acute coronary artery thrombosis in the setting of percutaneous coronary intervention (PCI); reestablishing patency of occluded IV catheter.

UNLABELED USES Lysis of arterial occlusions in peripheral and bypass vessels; DVT.

CONTRAINDICATIONS Active internal bleeding, history of cerebrovascular accident, recent (within 2 mo) intracranial or interspinal surgery or trauma, intracranial neoplasm, arteriovenous malformation, bleeding disorders, severe uncontrolled hypertension, likelihood of left heart thrombus, acute pericarditis, bacterial endocarditis, severe liver dysfunction, age >75, pregnancy (category C), septic thrombophlebitis, current use of oral anticoagulants.

CAUTIOUS USE Recent major surgery (within 10 d), cerebral vascular disease, recent GI or GU bleeding, recent trauma, hypertension, lactation, hemorrhagic ophthalmic conditions. Safety and effectiveness in children are not established.

ROUTE & DOSAGE

Acute MI

Adult: **IV** ≥65 kg: 60 mg over first hour, with 6–10 mg infused over first 1–2 min; then 20 mg/h over the second hour and 20 mg over the third hour (100 mg over 3 h); <65 kg: Infuse 1.25 mg/kg over 3 h (60%; h1; 20%; h2, 20%; h3) *accelerated schedule,* 15-mg bolus, then 0.75 mg/kg (up to 50 mg) over 30 min, then 0.5 mg/kg (up to 35 mg) over 60 min

Acute Ischemic Stroke/ Thrombotic Stroke

Adult: **IV** 0.9 mg/kg over 60 min with 10% of dose as an initial bolus over 1 min (max: 90 mg)

Pulmonary Embolism

Adult: **IV** 100 mg infused over 2 h
Child: **IV** 0.1–0.6 mg/kg/hr × 6 h

Reopen Occluded IV Catheter

Adult/Child: **IV** *>30 kg:* Instill 2 mg/2 mL into dysfunctional catheter for 2 h. May repeat once if needed.
Child: **IV** *>2 y, 10–29 kg:* Instill 110% of internal lumen volume with 1 mg/mL concentration (max 2 mg). May repeat if function not restored within 2 h. **IV** *< 2 y, <10 kg:* 0.5 mg diluted in a volume to fill the lumen of the catheter.

ADMINISTRATION

Intravenous

PREPARE: **IV Infusion:** Reconstitute the 50-mg vial as follows: Do not use if vacuum in vial has been broken. Use a large-bore needle (e.g., 18 gauge) and do not prime needle with air. ▪ Dilute contents of vial with sterile water for injection supplied by manufacturer. ▪ Direct stream of sterile water into the lyophilized cake. Slight foaming is usual. Allow to stand until bubbles dissipate. Resulting concentration is 1 mg/mL. ▪ Reconstitute the 100-mg vial as follows: The 100-mg vial does not contain a vacuum. Use supplied transfer device for reconstitution and follow manufacturer's directions.

ADMINISTER: **IV Infusion:** Start IV infusion as soon as possible after the thrombolytic event, preferably within 6 h. ▪ Administer drug as reconstituted (1 mg/mL) or further diluted with an equal volume of NS or D5W to yield 0.5 mg/mL. ▪ **Acute MI:** Administer 60% of total dose in the first hour for acute MI, with 6–10% given as a bolus dose over 1–2 min and remainder of first dose infused over hour 1. Follow with second dose (20% of total) over hour 2, and third dose (20% of total) over hour 3. ▪ For patients weighing <65 kg calculate dose using 1.25 mg/kg over 3 h. See accelerated schedule under Route & Dosage. ▪ **Pulmonary embolism:** Administer entire dose over a 2 h period. ▪ **Acute ischemic stroke:** Give 5 mg as an initial bolus over 1 min, then give the remainder of the 0.75 mg/kg dose over 60 min. ▪ Do not exceed a total dose of 100 mg. Higher doses have been associated with intracranial bleeding. ▪ Follow infusion of drug by flushing IV tubing with 30–50 mL of NS or D5W. ▪ Reconstituted drug is stable for 8 h in above solutions at room temperature (2°–30° C; 36°–86° F). Since there are no preservatives, discard any unused solution after that time.

▪ Store above reconstituted solutions at room temperature 2°–30° C (36°–86° F) for no longer than 8 h. Discard any unused solution after that time.

ADVERSE EFFECTS (≥1%) **Hematologic:** Internal and superficial bleeding (cerebral, retroperitoneal, GU, GI).

PHARMACOKINETICS Peak: 5–10 min after infusion completed. **Duration:** Baseline values restored in 3 h. **Metabolism:** Metabolized in liver.

Elimination: Excreted in urine. **Half-Life:** 26.5 min.

NURSING IMPLICATIONS

Assessment & Drug Effects

- Monitor for S&S of excess bleeding q15min for the first hour of therapy, q30min for second to eighth hour, then q8h. Monitor neurological checks throughout drug infusion q30min and qh for the first 8 h after infusion.
- Protect patient from invasive procedures because spontaneous bleeding occurs twice as often with alteplase as with heparin. IM injections are contraindicated. Also prevent physical manipulation of patient during thrombolytic therapy to prevent bruising.
- Lab tests: Coagulation tests including APTT, bleeding time, PT, TT, INR, must be done before administration of drug. Also check *baseline* Hct, Hgb, and platelet counts, in case of bleeding. Draw Hct following drug administration to detect possible blood loss.
- Keep patient in bed while receiving this medication.
- Check vital signs frequently. Be alert to changes in cardiac rhythm.
- Stop therapy immediately if dysrhythmias occur.
- Report signs of bleeding: gum bleeding, epistaxis, hematoma, spontaneous ecchymoses, oozing at catheter site, increased pain from internal bleeding. Stop the infusion, then resume when bleeding stops.
- Use the radial artery to draw ABGs. Pressure to puncture sites, if necessary, should be maintained for up to 30 min.
- Continue monitoring vital signs until laboratory reports confirm anticoagulant control; patient is at risk for postthrombolytic bleeding for 2–4 d after intracoronary alteplase treatment.

Patient & Family Education

- Report immediately a sudden severe headache.
- Report blood in urine and bloody or tarry stools.
- Report any signs of bleeding or oozing from cuts or places of injection.
- Remain quiet and on bedrest while receiving this medicine.

ALTRETAMINE, HEXAMETHYLMELAMINE

(al-tre′ta-meen)

Hexalen

Classifications: ANTINEOPLASTIC; ALKYLATING AGENT

Prototype: Cyclophosphamide

Pregnancy Category: D

AVAILABILITY 50 mg capsules

ACTIONS Altretamine, formally hexamethylmelamine, is a synthetic cytotoxic antineoplastic drug. The mechanism of action is not clearly understood. Altretamine probably requires the liver enzyme system for activation of its cytotoxic properties. **THERAPEUTIC EFFECTS** Altretamine has demonstrated neoplastic activity in patients resistant to alkylating agents.

USES Ovarian cancer.
UNLABELED USES Breast, cervical, colon, endometrial, head, and neck cancer; small-cell lung cancers and lymphomas.

CONTRAINDICATIONS Hypersensitivity to altretamine, severe bone marrow depression, neurologic toxicity, pregnancy (category D), lactation.

CAUTIOUS USE Safety and efficacy in children are not established.

ROUTE & DOSAGE

Ovarian Cancer

Adult: **PO** 260 mg/m²/d for 14 or 21 consecutive d in a 28-d cycle

ADMINISTRATION

Oral

- Give only under supervision of a qualified physician experienced in the use of antineoplastics.
- Give in 4 divided doses after meals and at bedtime.
- Discontinue altretamine for 14 d or longer and restart at 200 mg/m²/d if any of the following occur: severe GI intolerance; WBC count <2000/mm³, granulocyte count <1000/mm³; or progressive neurotoxicity.
- Store at room temperature, 15°–30° C (59°–86° F).

ADVERSE EFFECTS (≥1%) **CNS:** *Paresthesias, hyporeflexia, muscle weakness, peripheral numbness, ataxia, Parkinson-like tremors.* **GI:** *Nausea, vomiting.* **Hematologic:** *Leukopenia, thrombocytopenia.* **Urogenital:** Slight increase in serum creatinine. **Skin:** Alopecia and eczema.

INTERACTIONS Drug: Concomitant administration of altretamine and TRICYCLIC ANTIDEPRESSANTS (**imipramine, amitriptyline**), MONOAMINE OXIDASE INHIBITORS, or **selegiline** have been reported to result in incapacitating dizziness and syncopal episodes during the first week of altretamine treatment. Patients became asymptomatic 24–96 h after discontinuing ANTIDEPRESSANTS.

PHARMACOKINETICS Absorption: Rapidly absorbed from GI tract. Approximately 25% reaches systemic circulation due to extensive hepatic first-pass metabolism. **Metabolism:** Rapidly demethylated in the liver to 5 minor and 4 major metabolites. **Elimination:** 62% of the dose is excreted in the urine in 24 h. A small amount of altretamine is excreted through the lungs. **Half-Life:** 13 h.

NURSING IMPLICATIONS

Assessment & Drug Effects

- Lab tests: Monitor blood counts at least monthly and prior to each course of therapy.
- Perform a neurologic examination regularly; question patient about the presence of: paresthesias, hypoesthesias, muscle weakness, peripheral numbness, ataxia, decreased sensations, and alterations in mood or consciousness.
- Withhold medication if neurologic symptoms fail to resolve with dose reduction. Notify physician. Note: Concurrent administration of vitamin B_6, 100 mg b.i.d., may allow altretamine therapy to continue.
- Monitor for nausea and vomiting, which are related to the cumulative dose of altretamine. After several weeks some patients develop tolerance to the GI effects. Antiemetics may be required to control GI distress.

Patient & Family Education

- Taking altretamine after meals or with food or milk may decrease nausea.
- Report symptoms indicative of neurotoxicity to physician (paresthesias, hypoesthesias, muscle weakness, peripheral numbness, ataxia, decreased sensations, and alterations in mood or consciousness).

- Note: GI, hematologic, and neurologic adverse effects may be severe.
- Do not breast feed while taking this drug.

ALUMINUM HYDROXIDE (Pr)

(a-lu′mi-num)

ALternaGEL, Alu-Cap, Alugel, Alu-Tab, Amphojel, Dialume

ALUMINUM CARBONATE, BASIC

Basaljel

ALUMINUM PHOSPHATE

Phosphaljel

Classifications: GASTROINTESTINAL AGENT; ANTACID; ADSORBENT

Pregnancy Category: C

AVAILABILITY Aluminum Hydroxide 300 mg, 400 mg, 500 mg, 600 mg tablets; 300 mg, 400 mg, 500 mg, 600 mg capsules; 320 mg/5 mL, 450 mg/5 mL, 600 mg/5 mL, 675 mg/5 mL suspension **Aluminum Carbonate, Basic** 608 mg tablets; 608 mg capsules; 400 mg/5 mL suspension **Aluminum Phosphate** 608 mg tablets; 608 mg capsules; 400 mg/5 mL suspension

ACTIONS Nonsystemic antacid with moderate neutralizing action. Decreases rate of gastric emptying and has demulcent, adsorbent, and mild astringent properties. Reduces acid concentration and pepsin activity by raising pH of gastric and intraesophageal secretions.

THERAPEUTIC EFFECTS Reduces gastric acidity by neutralizing the stomach acid content. Aluminum carbonate lowers serum phosphate by binding dietary phosphate to form insoluble aluminum phosphate, which is excreted in feces.

USES Symptomatic relief of gastric hyperacidity associated with gastritis, esophageal reflux, and hiatal hernia; adjunct in treatment of gastric and duodenal ulcer. More commonly used in combination with other antacids. Aluminum carbonate is used primarily in conjunction with a low phosphate diet to reduce hyperphosphatemia in patients with renal insufficiency and for prophylaxis and treatment of phosphatic renal calculi.

CONTRAINDICATIONS Prolonged use of high doses in presence of low serum phosphate; pregnancy (category C).

CAUTIOUS USE Renal impairment; gastric outlet obstruction; older adults; decreased bowel activity (e.g., patients receiving anticholinergic, antidiarrheal, or antispasmodic agents); patients who are dehydrated or on fluid restriction.

ROUTE & DOSAGE

Antacid (hydroxide & phosphate)

Adult: **PO** 600 mg t.i.d. or q.i.d.

Antacid (carbonate)

Adult: **PO** 10–30 mL of regular suspension or 5–15 mL of extra strength suspension or 2 capsules or tablets q2h

Phosphate Lowering (carbonate)

Adult: **PO** 10–30 mL of regular suspension or 5–15 mL of extra strength suspension or 2–6 capsules or tablets 1h p.c. and h.s.

ADMINISTRATION

Oral

- Tablet must be chewed until it is thoroughly wetted before swallowing.
- Note for antacid use: Follow well-chewed tablet with one-half

glass of water or milk; follow liquid preparation (suspension) with water to ensure passage into stomach. For phosphate lowering: follow tablet, capsule, or suspension with full glass of water or fruit juice.

- Store between 15°–30° C (59°–86° F) in tightly closed container.

ADVERSE EFFECTS (≥1%) **GI:** *Constipation*, fecal impaction, intestinal obstruction. **CNS:** Dialysis dementia (thought to be due to aluminum intoxication). **Metabolic:** Hypophosphatemia, hypomagnesemia.

INTERACTIONS Drug: Aluminum will decrease absorption of **chloroquine, cimetidine, ciprofloxacin, digoxin, isoniazid,** IRON SALTS, NSAIDS, **norfloxacin, ofloxacin, phenytoin, phenothiazines, quinidine, tetracycline, thyroxine. Sodium polystyrene sulfonate** may cause systemic alkalosis.

PHARMACOKINETICS Absorption: Minimal absorption. **Peak:** Slow onset. **Duration:** 2 h when taken with food; 3 h when taken 1 h after food. **Elimination:** Excreted in feces as insoluble phosphates.

NURSING IMPLICATIONS

Assessment & Drug Effects

- Note number and consistency of stools. Constipation is common and dose related. Intestinal obstruction from fecal concretions has been reported.
- Lab tests: Monitor periodic serum calcium and phosphorus levels with prolonged high-dose therapy or impaired renal function.

Patient & Family Education

- Increase phosphorus in diet when taking large doses of these antacids for prolonged periods; hypophosphatemia can develop within 2 wk of continuous use of these antacids. The older adult in a poor nutritional state is at high risk.
- Note: Antacid may cause stools to appear speckled or whitish.
- Report epigastric or abdominal pain; it is a clinical guide for adjusting dosage. Keep physician informed. Pain that persists beyond 72 h may signify serious complications.
- Seek medical help if indigestion is accompanied by shortness of breath, sweating, or chest pain, if stools are dark or tarry, or if symptoms are recurrent when taking this medication.
- Seek medical advice and supervision if self-prescribed antacid use exceeds 2 wk.

AMANTADINE HYDROCHLORIDE

(a-man'ta-deen)

Symmetrel

Classifications: ANTIINFECTIVE; ANTIVIRAL; AUTONOMIC NERVOUS SYSTEM AGENT; ANTICHOLINERGIC (PARASYMPATHOLYTIC); ANTIPARKINSONISM AGENT

Prototype: Acyclovir

Pregnancy Category: C

AVAILABILITY 100 mg capsules; 50 mg/5 mL syrup

ACTIONS Because it does not suppress antibody formation, it can be administered for interim protection in combination with influenza A virus vaccine until antibody titer is adequate or to augment prophylaxis in a previously vaccinated individual. Mechanism of action in parkinsonism not understood, but may be related to release of dopamine and other catecholamines from neuronal storage sites.

THERAPEUTIC EFFECTS Active against several strains of influenza A virus; not effective against influenza B infections. Also provides anticholinergic effects.

USES In initial therapy or as adjunct with anticholinergic drugs or levodopa in treatment of all forms of parkinsonism (arteriosclerotic, idiopathic, postencephalitic) and for relief of drug-induced extrapyramidal reactions and symptomatic parkinsonism caused by carbon monoxide poisoning. Also used for prophylaxis and symptomatic treatment of influenza A infections.

UNLABELED USES Primary enuresis, pseudosclerosis, neuroleptic malignant syndrome (NMS), management of cocaine dependency and withdrawal.

CONTRAINDICATIONS Safety during pregnancy (category C), lactation, and in children <1 y is not established.

CAUTIOUS USE History of epilepsy or other types of seizures; CHF, peripheral edema, orthostatic hypotension; recurrent eczematoid dermatitis; psychoses, severe psychoneuroses; hepatic disease; renal impairment; older adults with cerebral arteriosclerosis.

ROUTE & DOSAGE

Influenza A

Adult: **PO** 200 mg once/d or 100 mg q12h
Child: **PO** *1–9 y,* 4.4–8.8 mg/kg in 2–3 equal doses (max: 150 mg/d)

Parkinsonism

Adult: **PO** 100 mg 1–2 times/d, start with 100 mg/d if patient is on other antiparkinsonism medications

Drug-induced Extrapyramidal Symptoms

Adult: **PO** 100 mg b.i.d. (max: 400 mg/d if needed)

Renal Impairment

Cl_{cr} 40–60 mL/min: 100 mg/d; 30–40 mL/min: 200 mg 2 times/wk; 10–20 mL/min: 100 mg 3 times/wk

ADMINISTRATION

Oral

- Give with water, milk, or food.
- Use supplied calibrated device for measuring syrup formulation.
- Influenza prophylaxis: Drug should be initiated when exposure is anticipated and continued for at least 10 d.
- Note: Used in conjunction with influenza A vaccine (generally in high-risk patients who have not been vaccinated previously) until protective antibodies develop (10–21 d) after vaccine administration.
- Schedule medication in the morning or, with q12h dosing, schedule 2nd dose several hours before bedtime. If insomnia is a problem, suggest patient limit number of daytime naps.
- Store in tightly closed container preferably at 15°–30° C (59°–86° F) unless otherwise directed by manufacturer. Avoid freezing.

ADVERSE EFFECTS (≥1%) **CNS:** *Dizziness, light-headedness,* headache, ataxia, irritability, anxiety, *nervousness, difficulty in concentrating,* mood or other mental changes, confusion, visual and auditory hallucinations, *insomnia*, nightmares, convulsions. **CV:** Orthostatic hypotension, peripheral edema, dyspnea. **Special Senses:** Blurring or loss of vision. **GI:** Anorexia, *nausea,* vomiting, dry mouth. **Hematologic:** Leukopenia.

INTERACTIONS Drug: Alcohol enhances CNS effects; may potentiate effects of ANTICHOLINERGICS.

PHARMACOKINETICS Absorption: Readily and almost completely absorbed from GI tract. **Onset:** Within 48 h. **Peak:** 1–4 h. **Distribution:** Distributed to saliva, nasal secretions, breast milk, placenta, CSF. **Metabolism:** Not metabolized. **Elimination:** 90% excreted unchanged in urine. **Half-Life:** 9–37 h (prolonged in renal insufficiency).

NURSING IMPLICATIONS

Assessment & Drug Effects

- Monitor effectiveness. Note that with parkinsonism, maximum response occurs within 2 wk–3 mo. Effectiveness may wane after 6–8 wk of treatment; report change to physician.
- Monitor and report: Mental status changes; nervousness, difficulty concentrating, or insomnia; loss of seizure control; S&S of toxicity, especially with doses above 200 mg/d.
- Establish a baseline profile of the patient's disabilities to accurately differentiate disease symptoms and drug-induced neuropsychiatric adverse reactions.
- Monitor vital signs for at least 3 or 4 d after increases in dosage; also monitor urinary output.
- Lab tests: pH and serum electrolytes.
- Monitor for and report reduced salivation, increased akinesia or rigidity, and psychological disturbances that may develop within 4–48 h after initiation of therapy and after dosage increases with parkinsonism.

Patient & Family Education

- Note: For influenza take within 24 h but no later than 48 h after onset of symptoms for effective response and continue for 24–48 h after symptoms disappear; contact physician if no improvement within this time.
- Make all position changes slowly, particularly from recumbent to upright position, in order to minimize dizziness.
- Report any of the following to physician: Shortness of breath, peripheral edema, significant weight gain, dizziness or lightheadedness, inability to concentrate, and other changes in mental status, difficulty urinating, and visual impairment.
- Do not drive and exercise caution with potentially hazardous activities until response to the drug is known.
- Note: People with Parkinson's disease should not discontinue therapy abruptly; doing so may precipitate a parkinsonian crisis with severe akinesia, rigidity, tremor, and psychic disturbances. Adhere to established dosage regimen.
- Do not breast feed while taking this drug without consulting physician.

AMBENONIUM CHLORIDE

(am-be-noe′nee-um)

Mytelase

Classifications: AUTONOMIC NERVOUS SYSTEM AGENT; CHOLINERGIC (PARASYMPATHOMIMETIC); CHOLINESTERASE INHIBITOR

Prototype: Neostigmine

Pregnancy Category: C

AVAILABILITY 10 mg tablets

ACTIONS Indirect-acting and a slowly reversible cholinesterase inhibitor approximately six times more potent than neostigmine.

THERAPEUTIC EFFECTS Inhibits destruction of acetylcholine (ACh) by cholinesterase, thereby prolonging effects of ACh (neurotransmitter) at postsynaptic receptor sites. Has direct stimulant effect on striated muscles.

USES Symptomatic treatment of myasthenia gravis for patients who cannot tolerate neostigmine bromide or pyridostigmine bromide because of bromide sensitivity. Has been used in conjunction with corticosteroids, ephedrine sulfate, and potassium chloride to increase muscle strength.

CONTRAINDICATIONS Intestinal or urinary tract obstruction; patients receiving mecamylamine. Safety during pregnancy (category C) and lactation is not established.

CAUTIOUS USE Epilepsy, bradycardia, cardiac arrhythmias, recent coronary occlusion; bronchial asthma; hyperthyroidism; vagotonia; peptic ulcer, megacolon.

ROUTE & DOSAGE

Myasthenia Gravis

Adult: **PO** 2.5–5 mg t.i.d. or q.i.d., may increase q1–2d to 50–75 mg t.i.d. or q.i.d. if necessary

Child: **PO** 0.3 mg/kg/d in 3–4 divided doses, may need up to 1.5 mg/kg/d in 3–4 divided doses

ADMINISTRATION

Oral

- Give with food or milk to minimize adverse effects.
- Schedule larger doses when patient experiences the most fatigue or muscle weakness; to improve ability to eat, give drug 30–45 min before meals.
- Store at 15°–30° C (59°–86° F) unless otherwise directed.

ADVERSE EFFECTS (≥1%) **CNS:** Exaggerated cholinergic (muscarinic) effects; muscle cramps, headache, confusion, dizziness, incoordination, fasciculations, agitation, restlessness, muscle weakness, paralysis, slurred speech, convulsions, respiratory depression. **CV:** Bradycardia. **GI:** Nausea, vomiting, diarrhea, abdominal cramps, excessive salivation. **Special Senses:** Blurred vision, lacrimation. **Respiratory:** Bronchospasm, increased bronchial secretions, dyspnea. **Other:** Diaphoresis.

INTERACTIONS Drug: Demecarium and other CHOLINESTERASE INHIBITORS possibly compound toxicity; **mecamylamine, succinylcholine, procainamide, quinidine,** AMINOGLYCOSIDES increase neuromuscular blocking effects with possibility of respiratory depression; atropine antagonizes effects of ambenonium.

PHARMACOKINETICS Absorption: Poorly absorbed from GI tract. **Onset:** 20–30 min. **Duration:** 3–8 h. **Metabolism:** Unknown. **Elimination:** Unknown.

NURSING IMPLICATIONS

Assessment & Drug Effects

- Therapeutic effect may not be apparent for several days after initiation of therapy.
- Keep atropine sulfate immediately available to treat severe cholinergic reactions.

- Monitor for S&S of overdosage (muscle weakness within 1 h; headache, weakness of muscles of neck, chewing, and swallowing, increased salivation) and inadequate ventilation (unusual apprehension, restlessness, rapid pulse and respirations, rising BP).
- Monitor vital signs during dosage adjustment periods.
- Note: Muscle weakness beginning 3 h or more after drug administration is probably due to underdosage or drug resistance.

Patient & Family Education

- Follow directions for taking this drug (see ADMINISTRATION).
- Learn to recognize adverse effects, how to modify the doses accordingly, and when to take atropine.
- Note: During long-term therapy the drug may become ineffective; responsiveness usually returns when dosage is reduced or drug is withdrawn for several days.
- Carry medical identification indicating medical diagnosis and medication(s) being taken.
- Do not breast feed while taking this drug without consulting physician.

AMCINONIDE

(am-sin'oh-nide)

Cyclocort

Classifications: SKIN AND MUCOUS MEMBRANE AGENT; ANTIINFLAMMATORY; STEROID

Prototype: Hydrocortisone

Pregnancy Category: C

AVAILABILITY 0.1% ointment, cream, lotion

See Appendix A-4.

AMIFOSTINE

(am-i-fos'teen)

Ethyol

Classification: CYTOPROTECTIVE AGENT

Pregnancy Category: C

AVAILABILITY 500 mg vial

ACTIONS Amifostine reduces cytotoxic damage induced by radiation or alkylating agents in well-oxygenated cells. Protective effects appear to be mediated by the formation of a thiol metabolite of amifostine (WR-1065), which removes free radicals from normal cells, and by promotion of the repair of macromolecules. The higher concentration of WR-1065, the metabolite, in normal tissues is available to bind to metabolites produced by cisplatin and also to remove free radicals that are generated in tissues exposed to cisplatin.

THERAPEUTIC EFFECTS Amifostine is cytoprotective in the kidney, bone marrow, and GI mucosa, but not in the brain or spinal cord. The cytoprotection results in decreased myelosuppression and peripheral neuropathy.

USE Reduction of the cumulative renal toxicity associated with cisplatin.

CONTRAINDICATIONS Sensitivity to aminothiol compounds or mannitol, patients with potentially curable malignancies, hypotensive patients or those who are dehydrated, pregnancy (category C), lactation.

CAUTIOUS USE Patients at risk for hypocalcemia, cardiovascular disease (i.e., arrhythmias, CHF, TIA, CVA).

ROUTE & DOSAGE

Renal Protection
Adult: **IV** 910 mg/m² once daily

ADMINISTRATION

Intravenous

Give antiemetics, adequately hydrate, and defer antihypertensives for 24 h prior to administration.

PREPARE: **IV Infusion:** Reconstitute IV solution by adding 9.5 mL of NS injection to a single-dose vial.

ADMINISTER: **IV Infusion:** Infuse over no more than 15 min, beginning 30 min before chemotherapy; place patient in supine position prior to and during infusion.

INCOMPATIBILITIES **Solution/Additive:** Do not mix with any solutions other than NS.

- Store reconstituted solution at 15°–30° C (59°–86° F) for 5 h or refrigerate up to 24 h.

ADVERSE EFFECTS (≥1%) **CV:** *Transient reduction in blood pressure.* **GI:** *Nausea, vomiting.* **Other:** Infusion reactions (flushing, feeling of warmth or coldness, chills, dizziness, somnolence, hiccups, sneezing), hypocalcemia, hypersensitivity reactions.

INTERACTIONS Drug: No clinically significant interactions established.

PHARMACOKINETICS Onset: 5–8 min. **Metabolism:** Rapidly metabolized in liver to active free thiol metabolite. **Elimination:** Renally excreted. **Half-Life:** 8 min.

NURSING IMPLICATIONS

Assessment & Drug Effects

- Monitor for S&S of hypocalcemia and fluid balance if vomiting is significant.
- Monitor BP every 5 min during infusion. Stop infusion if systolic BP drops significantly from baseline (e.g., baseline[drop]: <100[20], 100–119[25], 120–139[30], 140–179[40], >80[50]) and place patient flat with legs raised. Restart infusion if BP returns to normal in 5 min.

Patient & Family Education

- Know and understand adverse effects.
- Do not breast feed while taking this drug.

AMIKACIN SULFATE

(am-i-kay′sin)
Amikin
Classifications: ANTIINFECTIVE; AMINOGLYCOSIDE ANTIBIOTIC
Prototype: Gentamicin
Pregnancy Category: C

AVAILABILITY 250 mg/mL, 50 mg/mL injection

ACTIONS Semisynthetic derivative of kanamycin with broad range of antimicrobial activity that includes many strains resistant to other aminoglycosides. Pharmacologic properties are essentially the same as those of gentamicin. Appears to inhibit protein synthesis in bacterial cell and is usually bactericidal.

THERAPEUTIC EFFECTS Effective against a wide variety of gram-negative bacteria including *Escherichia coli, Enterobacter, Klebsiella pneumoniae,* most strains of *Pseudomonas aeruginosa,* and many strains of *Proteus species, Serratia, Providencia stuartii, Citrobacter freundii, Acinetobacter.* Also effective against penicillinase- and non-penicillinase-producing *Staphylococcus* species, and against *Mycobacterium tuberculosis* and atypical mycobacteria.

USES Primarily for short-term treatment of serious infections of respiratory tract, bones, joints, skin, and soft tissue, CNS (including meningitis), peritonitis burns, recurrent urinary tract infections (UTIs).

UNLABELED USES Intrathecal or intraventricular administration, in conjunction with IM or IV dosage.

CONTRAINDICATIONS History of hypersensitivity or toxic reaction with an aminoglycoside antibiotic. Safety during pregnancy (category C), lactation, neonates and infants, or use period exceeding 14 d is not established.

CAUTIOUS USE Impaired renal function; eighth cranial (auditory) nerve impairment; preexisting vertigo or dizziness, tinnitus, or dehydration; fever; older adults, premature infants, neonates and infants; myasthenia gravis; parkinsonism; hypocalcemia.

ROUTE & DOSAGE

Moderate to Severe Infections

Adult: **IV/IM** 5–7.5 mg/kg loading dose, then 7.5 mg/kg q12h
Child: **IV/IM** 5–7.5 mg/kg loading dose, then 5 mg/kg q8h or 7.5 mg/kg q12h
Neonate: **IV/IM** 10 mg/kg loading dose, then 7.5 mg/kg q12–24h

Uncomplicated UTI

Adult: **IV/IM** 250 mg q12h

ADMINISTRATION

Intramuscular

Use the 250 mg/mL vials for IM injection. Calculate the required dose and withdraw the equivalent number of mLs from the vial.
▪ Give deep IM into a large muscle.

Intravenous

Verify correct IV concentration and rate of infusion with physician for neonates, infants, and children.

PREPARE: **Intermittent:** Add contents of 500 mg vial to 100 or 200 mL D5W, NS injection, or other diluent recommended by manufacturer. ▪ For pediatric patients, volume of diluent depends on patient's fluid tolerance. ▪ Note: Color of solution may vary from colorless to light straw color or very pale yellow. Discard solutions that appear discolored or that contain particulate matter.

ADMINISTER: **Intermittent:** Give a single adult dose (including loading dose) over at least 30–60 min by IV infusion. ▪ Increase infusion time to 1–2 h for infants. ▪ Monitor drip rate carefully. A rapid rise in serum amikacin level can cause respiratory depression (neuromuscular blockade) and other signs of toxicity.

INCOMPATIBILITIES **Solution/additive: aminophylline, amphotericin B,** CEPHALOSPORINS, **chlorothiazide, erythromycin, heparin, oxytetracycline,** PENICILLINS, **phenytoin, thiopental, vitamin B complex with C, warfarin. Y-site: amphotericin B, heparin, phenytoin, thiopental.**

▪ Store at 15°–30° C (59°–86° F) unless otherwise directed.

ADVERSE EFFECTS (≥1%) **CNS:** Neurotoxicity: drowsiness, unsteady gait, weakness, clumsiness, paresthesias, tremors, convulsions, peripheral neuritis. **Special Senses:** *Auditory–ototoxicity*, high-frequency hearing loss, complete hearing loss (occasionally permanent); tinnitus; ringing or buzzing in ears; *Vestibular:* dizziness, ataxia. **GI:** Nausea, vomiting, hepatotoxicity. **Metabolic:** Hypokalemia, hypomagnesemia. **Skin:** Skin rash, urticaria, pruritus, redness. **Urogenital:** Oliguria, urinary frequency, hematuria, tubular necrosis, azotemia. **Other:** Superinfections.

INTERACTIONS Drug: ANESTHETICS, SKELETAL MUSCLE RELAXANTS have additive neuromuscular blocking effects; **acyclovir, amphotericin B, bacitracin, capreomycin, cephalosporins, colistin, cisplatin, carboplatin, methoxyflurane, polymyxin B, vancomycin, furosemide, ethacrynic acid** increase risk of ototoxicity and nephrotoxicity.

PHARMACOKINETICS Peak: 30 min IV; 45 min to 2 h IM. **Distribution:** Does not cross blood–brain barrier; crosses placenta; accumulates in renal cortex. **Elimination:** 94%–98% excreted renally in 24 h, remainder in 10–30 d. **Half-Life:** 2–3 h in adults, 4–8 h in neonates.

NURSING IMPLICATIONS

Assessment & Drug Effects

- Baseline tests: Before initial dose, C&S; renal function and vestibulocochlear nerve function (and at regular intervals during therapy; closely monitor in the older adult, patients with documented ear problems, renal impairment, or during high dose or prolonged therapy).
- Monitor peak and trough amikacin blood levels: Draw blood 1 h after IM or immediately after completion of IV infusion; draw trough levels immediately before the next IM or IV dose.
- Lab tests: Periodic serum creatinine and BUN, complete urinalysis. With treatment over 10 d, daily tests of renal function, weekly audiograms, and vestibular tests are strongly advised.
- Monitor serum creatinine or creatinine clearance (generally preferred) more often, in the presence of impaired renal function, in neonates, and in the older adult; note that prolonged high trough (>8 mg/mL) or peak (>30–35 mg/mL) levels are associated with toxicity.
- Monitor S&S of ototoxicity (primarily involves the cochlear (auditory) branch; high-frequency deafness usually appears first and can be detected only by audiometer); indicators of declining renal function; respiratory tract infections and other symptoms indicative of superinfections and notify physician should they occur.
- Monitor for and report auditory symptoms (tinnitus, roaring noises, sensation of fullness in ears, hearing loss) and vestibular disturbances (dizziness or vertigo, nystagmus, ataxia).
- Monitor & report any changes in I&O, oliguria, hematuria, or cloudy urine. Keeping patient well hydrated reduces risk of nephrotoxicity; consult physician regarding optimum fluid intake.

Patient & Family Education

- Report immediately any changes in hearing or unexplained ringing/roaring noises or dizziness, and problems with balance or coordination.
- Do not breast feed while taking this drug without consulting physician.

AMILORIDE HYDROCHLORIDE

(a-mill'oh-ride)
Midamor
Classifications: ELECTROLYTE AND WATER BALANCE AGENTS; DIURETICS, POTASSIUM-SPARING
Prototype: Spironolactone
Pregnancy Category: B

AVAILABILITY 5 mg tablets

ACTIONS Potassium-sparing diuretic with mild diuretic and antihypertensive action. Diuretic action is independent of aldosterone and carbonic anhydrase.
THERAPEUTIC EFFECTS Induces urinary excretion of sodium and reduces excretion of potassium and hydrogen ions by direct action on distal renal tubules.

USES Potassium-sparing effect in prevention or treatment of diuretic-induced hypokalemia in patients with CHF, hepatic cirrhosis, or hypertension. Also used in management of primary hyperaldosteronism. Usually combined with a potassium-wasting (kaliuretic) diuretic such as a thiazide or loop diuretic.
UNLABELED USES With hydrochlorothiazide for recurrent calcium nephrolithiasis, lithium-induced polyuria.

CONTRAINDICATIONS Elevated serum potassium (>5.5 mEq/L), concomitant use of other potassium-sparing diuretics; anuria, acute or chronic renal insufficiency; evidence of diabetic nephropathy; type 1 diabetes mellitus; metabolic or respiratory acidosis; hepatic function impairment. Safety during pregnancy (category B), lactation, or in children is not established.
CAUTIOUS USE Debilitated patients; diet-controlled or uncontrolled diabetes mellitus; cardiopulmonary disease; the older adult.

ROUTE & DOSAGE

Diuretic
Adult: **PO** 5 mg/d, may increase up to 20 mg/d in 1–2 divided doses

ADMINISTRATION

Oral
- Give once/d dose in the morning and schedule the second b.i.d. dose early to avoid interrupting sleep.
- Give with food to reduce possibility of gastric distress.
- Store at 15°–30° C (59°–86° F) in a tightly closed container unless otherwise directed.

ADVERSE EFFECTS (≥1%) **Body as a Whole:** Generally well tolerated. **CNS:** *Headache,* dizziness, nervousness, confusion, paresthesias, drowsiness. **CV:** Cardiac arrhythmias. **Metabolic:** Hyperkalemia, hyponatremia, positive Coombs' test. **Hematologic:** <u>Aplastic anemia</u>. **Special Senses:** Tinnitus; nasal congestion. Visual disturbances, increased intraocular pressure. **GI:** *Diarrhea* or constipation, anorexia, *nausea,* vomiting, abdominal cramps, dry mouth, thirst. **Urogenital:** Polyuria, dysuria, bladder spasms, urinary frequency, impotence, decreased libido. **Respiratory:** Dyspnea, shortness of breath. **Skin:** Rash, pruritus, photosensitivity reactions. **Other:** Weakness, fatigue, muscle cramps.

DIAGNOSTIC TEST INTERFERENCE Manufacturer advises discontinuing amiloride in patients with diabetes mellitus at least 3 d before ***glucose tolerance*** test.

INTERACTIONS Drug: Blood from blood banks, ACE INHIBITORS (e.g., **captopril**), **spironolactone, triamterene,** POTASSIUM SUPPLEMENTS may cause hyperkalemia with cardiac arrhythmias; possibility of increased **lithium** toxicity (decreased renal elimination); possibility of altered **digoxin** response; NSAIDS may attenuate antihypertensive effects. **Food:** POTASSIUM-CONTAINING SALT SUBSTITUTES increase risk of hyperkalemia.

PHARMACOKINETICS Absorption: 50% absorbed from GI tract. **Onset:** 2 h. **Peak:** 6–10 h. **Duration:** 24 h. **Elimination:** 20%–50% excreted unchanged in urine, 40% in feces. **Half-Life:** 6–9 h.

NURSING IMPLICATIONS

Assessment & Drug Effects

- Monitor for S&S of hyperkalemia and hyponatremia (see Appendix F). Hyperkalemia occurs in about 10% of patients receiving amiloride and serum potassium can rise suddenly and without warning. It is more common in older adults and patients with diabetes or renal disease.
- Lab tests: Serum potassium levels, particularly when therapy is initiated, whenever dosage adjustments are made, and during any illness that may affect kidney function. Intermittent evaluations of BUN, creatinine, and ECG for patients with renal or hepatic dysfunction, diabetes mellitus, older adults, or the debilitated.

Patient & Family Education

- Learn S&S of hyperkalemia and hyponatremia (see Appendix F) and report to physician immediately.
- Do not take potassium supplements, salt substitutes, high intake of dietary potassium unless prescribed by physician.
- Do not drive or engage in potentially hazardous activities until response to drug is known.
- Do not breast feed while taking this drug without consulting physician.

AMINOCAPROIC ACID (Pr)

(a-mee-noe-ka-proe'ik)

Amicar, EACA (epsilon-aminocaproic acid)

Classifications: BLOOD FORMERS, COAGULATORS, AND ANTICOAGULANTS; HEMOSTATIC

Pregnancy Category: C

AVAILABILITY 250 mg/mL injection; 500 mg tablets; 250 mg/mL syrup

ACTIONS Synthetic hemostatic with specific antifibrinolysis action. Acts principally by inhibiting plasminogen activator substance; to a lesser degree slightly inhibits activity of plasmin (fibrinolysin), which is concerned with destruction of clots. Does not control bleeding caused by loss of vascular integrity.

THERAPEUTIC EFFECTS Acts as an inhibitor of fibrinolytic bleeding.

USES To control excessive bleeding resulting from systemic hyperfibrinolysis, a pathologic condition that may accompany heart surgery, portocaval shunt, abruptio placentae, aplastic anemia, and carcinoma of lung, prostate, cervix, and stomach. Also used in urinary fibrinolysis associated with severe trauma, anoxia, shock, urologic surgery, and neoplastic diseases of GU tract.

UNLABELED USES To prevent hemorrhage in hemophiliacs undergoing dental extraction; as a specific antidote for streptokinase or urokinase toxicity; to prevent recurrence of subarachnoid hemorrhage, especially when surgery is delayed; for management of amegakaryocytic thrombocytopenia; and to prevent or abort hereditary angioedema episodes.

CONTRAINDICATIONS Severe renal impairment; active disseminated intravascular clotting (DIC); upper urinary tract bleeding (hematuria); hemophilia; benzyl alcohol hypersensitivity, especially in neonates; paraban hypersensitivity; pregnancy (category C), lactation. Safety and efficacy in children have not been established.

CAUTIOUS USE Cardiac, renal, or hepatic disease; renal impairment; history of pulmonary embolus or other thrombotic diseases; hypovolemia.

ROUTE & DOSAGE

Hemostatic

Adult: **PO/IV** 4–5 g during first hour, then 1–1.25 g qh for 8 h or until bleeding is controlled (max: 30 g/24h)
Child: **PO/IV** 100 mg/kg during first hour, then 33.3 mg/kg qh (max: 18 g/m^2/24 h)

ADMINISTRATION

Oral

- Note: May need to give patient as many as 10 tablets or 4 tsp for a 5 g dose during the first hour of treatment (each tablet contains 500 mg, syrup contains 250 mg/mL).

Intravenous

PREPARE: **IV Infusion:** Dilute parenteral aminocaproic acid before use. Each 4 mL (1 g) is diluted with 50 mL of NS, D5W, or RL.

ADMINISTER: **IV Infusion:** Physician orders specific IV flow rate. ▪ Usual rate is 5 g or a fraction thereof over first hour (5 g/250 mL). ▪ Give each additional gram over 1 h. Avoid rapid infusion to prevent hypotension, faintness, and bradycardia or other arrhythmias.

- Store in tightly closed containers at 15°–30° C (59°–86° F) unless otherwise directed. Avoid freezing.

ADVERSE EFFECTS (≥1%) **CNS:** Dizziness, malaise, headache, seizures. **CV:** Faintness, orthostatic hypotension; dysrhythmias; thrombophlebitis, thromboses. **Special Senses:** Tinnitus, nasal congestion. Conjunctival erythema. **GI:** Nausea, vomiting, cramps, diarrhea, anorexia. **Urogenital:** Diuresis, dysuria, urinary frequency, oliguria, reddish-brown urine (myoglobinuria), <u>acute renal failure</u>. Prolonged menstruation with cramping. **Skin:** Rash.

DIAGNOSTIC TEST INTERFERENCE ***Serum potassium*** may be elevated (especially in patients with impaired renal function).

INTERACTIONS Drug: ESTROGENS, ORAL CONTRACEPTIVES may cause hypercoagulation.

PHARMACOKINETICS Absorption: Rapidly absorbed from GI tract. **Peak:** 2 h. **Distribution:** Readily penetrates RBCs and other body cells. **Elimination:** 80% excreted as unmetabolized drug in 12 h.

NURSING IMPLICATIONS

Assessment & Drug Effects

- Check IV site at frequent intervals for extravasation.
- Observe for signs of thrombophlebitis. Change site immediately if

extravasation or thrombophlebitis occurs (see Appendix F).

- Monitor & report S&S of myopathy: muscle weakness, myalgia, diaphoresis, fever, reddish-brown urine (myoglobinuria), oliguria, as well as thrombotic complications: arm or leg pain, tenderness or swelling, Homan's sign, prominence of superficial veins, chest pain, breathlessness, dyspnea. Drug should be discontinued promptly.
- Monitor vital signs and urine output.
- Lab tests: with prolonged therapy, monitor creatine phosphokinase activity and urinalyses for early detection of myopathy.

Patient & Family Education

- Report difficulty urinating or reddish-brown urine.
- Report arm or leg pain, chest pain, or difficulty breathing.

AMINOGLUTETHIMIDE

(a-mee-noe-gloo-teth′i-mide)

Cytadren

Classifications: ANTINEOPLASTIC; HORMONE ANTAGONIST

Pregnancy Category: D

AVAILABILITY 250 mg tablets

ACTIONS Blocks adrenal corticosteroid biosynthesis by inhibiting enzymatic conversion of cholesterol to precursors of cortisol and aldosterone. Also blocks aromatase, thereby preventing conversion of androgens to estrogens in peripheral tissues.

THERAPEUTIC EFFECTS Because estrogens are supplied principally by the adrenals in postmenopausal and oophorectomized women, aminoglutethimide-induced lowering of plasma estrogen levels (by adrenal suppression) is reportedly as effective as that produced by surgical adrenalectomy.

USES Temporary treatment of selected patients with Cushing's syndrome associated with adrenal carcinoma, ectopic ACTH-producing tumors, or adrenal hyperplasia.

UNLABELED USES To produce medical adrenalectomy in postmenopausal women with positive estrogen receptor test, metastatic breast cancer, or who fail or relapse with tamoxifen (Nolvadex), and for patients with prostatic carcinoma.

CONTRAINDICATIONS Hypothyroidism; infection. Safety during pregnancy (category D), lactation, and in children is not established.

CAUTIOUS USE Older adults.

ROUTE & DOSAGE

Cushing's Disease

Adult: **PO** 250 mg q6h, may be increased 250 mg/d q1–2wk if needed (max: 2 g/d)

Breast Cancer

Adult: **PO** 250 mg b.i.d. and hydrocortisone 60 mg h.s., 20 mg in a.m., and 20 mg at 2 p.m. daily for 2 wk, then 250 mg q.i.d. and hydrocortisone 20 mg h.s., 10 mg in a.m., and 10 mg at 2 p.m. thereafter

ADMINISTRATION

Oral

- Note: For breast cancer, 40 mg of hydrocortisone daily, in divided doses is usually ordered to be given concurrently.
- Store at 15°–30° C (59°–86° F) in tightly closed containers unless otherwise directed.

ADVERSE EFFECTS (≥1%) **CNS:** Lethargy, drowsiness, *dizziness,* uncontrolled eye movements (dose related); clumsiness, *headache*. **CV:** *Hypotension, tachycardia*. **Endocrine:** Masculinization. **GI:** Nausea, vomiting, anorexia, hepatotoxicity. **Hematologic:** (Rare) Neutropenia, leukopenia, thrombocytopenia, pancytopenia, agranulocytosis, decreased Hgb and Hct, anemia, Coombs' negative hemolytic anemia. **Skin:** *Measles-like (morbilliform) rash*, pruritus.

INTERACTIONS Drug: Dexamethasone decreases pharmacologic effects of aminoglutethimide; decreases anticoagulant response to **warfarin**.

PHARMACOKINETICS Onset: 3–5 d. **Distribution:** Crosses placenta. **Metabolism:** Hepatic metabolism. **Elimination:** Excreted by kidneys; recovery of adrenal responsiveness to stress occurs 36–72 h after discontinuation. **Half-Life:** 13 h (7 h with long-term use).

NURSING IMPLICATIONS

Assessment & Drug Effects

- Monitor & report S&S of: Adrenal insufficiency or hypothyroidism (see Appendix F); in older adults, CNS effects (e.g., lethargy, ataxia, orthostatic dizziness, lightheadedness).
- Lab tests: Baseline & periodic fasting plasma cortisol levels, periodic CBC with differential, serum electrolytes, serum alkaline phosphate, liver functions, and thyroid function.
- Monitor BP in the recumbent and upright positions to evaluate fluid volume status and presence of orthostatic hypotension.
- Note: Dose reduction or temporary discontinuation may be indicated by: extreme drowsiness, severe skin rash, extremely low cortisol levels.
- Note: Patients with Cushing's syndrome may show reduced effect with continuing therapy and generally are not treated beyond 3 mo with this drug.

Patient & Family Education

- Change positions gradually, pausing between each change. Do not stand still for prolonged periods.
- Note: Lethargy, drowsiness, dizziness, and other adverse effects often disappear during the first few weeks of therapy. Inform physician if adverse effects persist or become bothersome.
- Report skin rash that persists beyond 5–8 d.
- Contact physician immediately in times of physical and emotional distress (e.g., acute illness, dental work). Steroid supplements may be indicated.
- Do not drive or engage in potentially hazardous activities until response to drug is known.
- Carry medical identification indicating medical diagnosis, medication(s), physician's name, address, and telephone number.
- Notify physician immediately if pregnancy is suspected.
- Do not breast feed while taking this drug without consulting physician.

AMINOPHYLLINE (theophylline ethylenediamide)

(am-in-off'i-lin)

Corophyllin ✦, Paladron ✦, Phyllocontin, Somophyllin, Somophyllin-DF, Truphylline

Classifications: BRONCHODILATOR (RESPIRATORY SMOOTH MUSCLE RELAXANT); XANTHINE

Prototype: Theophylline

Pregnancy Category: C

AVAILABILITY 100 mg, 200 mg tablets; 225 mg sustained release tablets; 105 mg/5 mL oral liquid; 250 mg/10 mL injection; 250 mg, 500 mg suppositories

ACTIONS Aminophylline is a salt of theophylline with effects similar to those of other xanthines (e.g., caffeine and theobromine). Action is dependent on theophylline content (approximately 80%) and is measured as theophylline in the serum.
THERAPEUTIC EFFECTS It is a respiratory smooth muscle relaxant that results in bronchodilation.

USES To prevent and relieve symptoms of acute bronchial asthma and treatment of bronchospasm associated with chronic bronchitis and emphysema.
UNLABELED USES As a respiratory stimulant in Cheyne-Stokes respiration; for treatment of apnea and bradycardia in premature infants; as cardiac stimulant and diuretic in treatment of CHF.

CONTRAINDICATIONS Hypersensitivity to xanthine derivatives or to ethylenediamine component; cardiac arrhythmias. Safety during pregnancy (category C) or lactation is not established.
CAUTIOUS USE Severe hypertension, cardiac disease, arrhythmias; impaired hepatic function; diabetes mellitus; hyperthyroidism; glaucoma; prostatic hypertrophy; fibrocystic breast disease; history of peptic ulcer; neonates and young children, patients over 55 y; COPD, acute influenza or patients receiving influenza immunization.

ROUTE & DOSAGE

Bronchospasm
Adult: **IV Loading Dose** 6 mg/kg over 30 min **IV Maintenance Dose** *nonsmoker,* 0.5 mg/kg/h; *smoker,* 0.75 mg/kg/h; *CHF or cirrhosis,* 0.25 mg/kg/h **PO** *nonsmoker,* 0.5 mg/kg/h times 24 h in 4 divided doses; *smoker,* 0.75 mg/kg/h times 24 h in 4 divided doses; *CHF or cirrhosis,* 0.25 mg/kg/h times 24 h in 4 divided doses
Child: **IV Loading Dose** 6 mg/kg IV over 30 min **IV Maintenance Dose** *1–9 y,* 1 mg/kg/h; *>9 y,* 0.75 mg/kg/h **PO** *1–9 y,* 1 mg/kg/h times 24 h in 4 divided doses; *>9 y,* 0.75 mg/kg/h times 24 h in 4 divided doses
Infant: **PO/IV** *6–11 mo,* 0.87 g/kg/h; *2–6 mo,* 0.5 mg/kg/h
Neonate: **PO/IV** 0.16 mg/kg/h

Neonatal Apnea
Neonate: **PO/IV Loading Dose** 5 mg/kg **PO/IV Maintenance Dose** 5 mg/kg/d divided q12h

ADMINISTRATION

Note: All doses based on ideal body weight.

Oral
- Give with a full glass of water on an empty stomach (1/2–1 h before or 2 h after meals) for faster absorption, which is delayed but is not reduced with food.
- Minimize GI symptoms by taking immediately after a meal or with food.
- Do not chew or crush extended (controlled) release preparations before swallowing; however, if tablet is scored, it can be broken in half, then swallowed.
- Do mix contents of extended release capsules with soft, moist food to promote swallowing.

Suppository
- Note: Rectal preparations may be ordered when patient must fast or cannot tolerate the drug orally;

absorption is enhanced if rectum is empty.

Intravenous

Verify correct IV concentration and rate of infusion with physician for neonates, infants, and children.

PREPARE: **IV Infusion:** Dilute loading dose in 100–200 mL NS, D5W, D5/NS, or RL. For continuous or intermittent infusion dilute in 500–1000 mL. ▪ Do not use aminophylline solutions if discolored or if crystals are present.

ADMINISTER: **IV Infusion:** Infuse at a rate not to exceed 25 mg/min.

INCOMPATIBILITIES **Solution/additive:** **amikacin, bleomycin,** CEPHALOSPORINS, **chlorpromazine, ciprofloxacin, clindamycin, codeine phosphate, dimenhydrinate, dobutamine, dopamine, doxapram, doxorubicin, epinephrine, hydralazine, hydroxyzine, insulin, isoproterenol, levor phanol, meperidine, methadone, methylprednisolone, morphine, nafcillin, norepinephrine, oxytetracycline, papaverine, penicillin G, pentazocine, procaine, prochlorperazine, promazine, promethazine, tetracycline, verapamil, vitamin B complex with C.** **Y-site:** **amiodarone, codeine phosphate, ciprofloxacin, clindamycin,** PHENOTHIAZINES (**chlorpromazine, prochlorperazine,** etc.), **epinephrine, dobutamine, dopamine, levorphanol, morphine, meperidine, methadone, norepinephrine, verapamil.**

▪ Store at 15°–30° C (59°–86° F) in tightly closed containers unless otherwise directed. ▪ Follow manufacturer's directions regarding storage of suppositories; some can be stored at room temperature; others must be refrigerated.

ADVERSE EFFECTS (≥1%) **CNS:** *Nervousness*, restlessness, depression, insomnia, irritability, headache, dizziness, muscle hyperactivity, convulsions. **CV:** Cardiac arrhythmias, tachycardia (with rapid IV), hyperventilation, chest pain, <u>severe hypotension, cardiac arrest</u>. **GI:** *Nausea, vomiting, anorexia*, hematemesis, diarrhea, epigastric pain.

INTERACTIONS Drug: Increases **lithium** excretion, lowering **lithium** levels; **cimetidine,** high-dose **allopurinol** (600 mg/d), **ciprofloxacin, erythromycin, troleandomycin** can significantly increase **theophylline** levels.

PHARMACOKINETICS Absorption: Most products are 100% absorbed from GI tract. **Peak:** IV 30 min; uncoated tablet 1 h; sustained release 4–6 h. **Duration:** 4–8 h; varies with age, smoking, and liver function. **Distribution:** Crosses placenta. **Metabolism:** Extensively metabolized in liver. **Elimination:** Parent drug and metabolites excreted by kidneys; excreted in breast milk.

NURSING IMPLICATIONS

Assessment & Drug Effects

- Monitor for S&S of toxicity (generally related to theophylline serum levels over 20 mg/mL). Observe patients receiving parenteral drug closely for signs of hypotension, arrhythmias, and convulsions until serum theophylline stabilizes within the therapeutic range.
- Note: High incidence of toxicity is associated with rectal suppository use due to erratic rate of absorption.

- Monitor & record vital signs and I&O. A sudden, sharp, unexplained rise in heart rate may indicate toxicity.
- Lab tests: Monitor serum theophylline levels.
- Note: Older adults, acutely ill, and patients with severe respiratory problems, liver dysfunction, or pulmonary edema are at greater risk of toxicity due to reduced drug clearance.
- Note: Children appear more susceptible to CNS stimulating effects of xanthines (nervousness, restlessness, insomnia, hyperactive reflexes, twitching, convulsions). Dosage reduction may be indicated.

Patient & Family Education

- Note: Use of tobacco tends to increase elimination of this drug (shortens half-life), necessitating higher dosage or shorter intervals than in nonsmokers.
- Report excessive nervousness or insomnia. Dosage reduction may be indicated.
- Note: Dizziness is a relatively common side effect, particularly in older adults; take necessary safety precautions.
- Do not take OTC remedies for treatment of asthma or cough unless approved by physician.
- Do not breast feed while taking this drug without consulting physician.

AMINOSALICYLIC ACID (*PARA*-AMINOSALICYLIC ACID)

(a-mee-noe-sal-i-sil′ik)

Paser

Classifications: ANTIINFECTIVE; ANTITUBERCULOSIS AGENT

Prototype: Isoniazid

Pregnancy Category: C

AVAILABILITY 4 g packets

ACTIONS Aminosalicylic acid and salts are highly specific bacteriostatic agents that suppress growth and multiplication of *Mycobacterium tuberculosis* by preventing folic acid synthesis. Their mechanism of action resembles that of sulfonamides. Aminosalicylates also reportedly have potent hypolipemic action.

THERAPEUTIC EFFECTS Aminosalicylates are an effective antiinfective alone or in combined therapy and reduce serum cholesterol and triglycerides by lowering LDL and VLDL.

USES In combination with streptomycin or isoniazid or both in treatment of pulmonary and extrapulmonary tuberculosis to delay emergence of strains resistant to these drugs.

UNLABELED USES Documented for lipid-lowering effect.

CONTRAINDICATIONS Hypersensitivity to aminosalicylates, salicylates, or to compounds containing *para*-aminophenyl groups (e.g., sulfonamides, certain hair dyes), G6PD deficiency, use of the sodium salt in patients on sodium restriction or CHF. Safety during pregnancy (category C) or lactation is not established.

CAUTIOUS USE Impaired renal and hepatic function; blood dyscrasias; goiter; gastric ulcer.

ROUTE & DOSAGE

Tuberculosis

Adult: **PO** 10–12 g/d in 2–3 divided doses
Child: **PO** 150–300 mg/kg/d in 3–4 divided doses

ADMINISTRATION

Oral

- Give with or immediately following meals to reduce irritative gastric effects. Physician may order an antacid to be given concomitantly. Generally, GI adverse effects disappear after a few days of therapy.

- Store in tight, light-resistant containers in a cool, dry place, preferably at 15°–30° C (59°–86° F), unless otherwise directed.

ADVERSE EFFECTS (≥1%) **Body as a Whole:** Fever, chills, generalized malaise, joint pain, rash, fixed-drug eruptions, pruritus; vasculitis; Loeffler's syndrome. **CNS:** Psychotic reactions. **GI:** *Anorexia, nausea, vomiting, abdominal distress, diarrhea*, peptic ulceration, acute hepatitis, malabsorption. **Hematologic:** Leukopenia, agranulocytosis, eosinophilia, lymphocytosis, thrombocytopenia, hemolytic anemia; (G6PD deficiency), prothrombinemia. **Urogenital:** Renal (irritation), crystalluria. **Other:** With long-term administration, goiter.

DIAGNOSTIC TEST INTERFERENCE Aminosalicylates may interfere with urine ***urobilinogen*** determinations (using ***Ehrlich's reagent***), and may cause false-positive ***urinary protein*** and ***VMA*** determinations (with ***diazoreagent***); false-positive ***urine glucose*** may result with ***cupric sulfate tests,*** e.g., ***Benedict's solution,*** but reportedly not with ***glucose oxidase reagents,*** e.g., ***TesTape, Clinistix.*** Reduces ***serum cholesterol,*** and possibly ***serum potassium, serum PBI,*** and 24-hour ***I-131 thyroidal uptake*** (effect may last almost 14 days).

INTERACTIONS Drug: Increases hypoprothrombinemic effects of ORAL ANTICOAGULANTS; increased risk of crystalluria with **ammonium chloride, ascorbic acid;** decreased intestinal absorption of **cyanocobalamin, folic acid;** may decrease absorption of **digoxin;** ANTIHISTAMINES may inhibit PAS absorption; may increase or decrease **phenytoin** levels; **probenecid, sulfinpyrazone** decrease PAS elimination.

PHARMACOKINETICS Absorption: Readily and almost completely absorbed from GI tract; aminosalicylate sodium is more rapidly and completely absorbed than the acid. **Peak:** 1.5–2 h. **Duration:** 4 h. **Distribution:** Well distributed to most tissue and body fluids except CSF unless meninges are inflamed. **Metabolism:** Metabolized in liver. **Elimination:** >80% excreted in urine in 7–10 h. **Half-Life:** 1 h.

NURSING IMPLICATIONS

Assessment & Drug Effects

- Monitor for abrupt onset of fever, particularly during the early weeks of therapy, and clinical picture resembling that of infectious mononucleosis (malaise, fatigue, generalized lymphadenopathy, splenomegaly, sore throat), as well as minor complaints of pruritus, joint pains, and headache, which strongly suggest hypersensitivity; report these symptoms promptly.
- Monitor I&O and encourage fluids. High concentrations of drug are excreted in urine, and this can cause crystalluria and hematuria.
- Note: To minimize crystalluria, keep urine neutral or alkaline with adjunctive drugs, such as antacids or with diet.

Patient & Family Education

- Rinse mouth with clear water or chew sugar-free gum or candy to relieve the mildly sour or bitter aftertaste of aminosalicylic acid.
- Note: Hypersensitivity reactions may occur after a few days, but

most commonly in the fourth or fifth week; report promptly.

- Notify physician if sore throat or mouth, malaise, unusual fatigue, bleeding or bruising occurs (symptoms of blood dyscrasia).
- Note: Therapy generally lasts about 2 y. Adhere to the established drug regimen, and remain under close medical supervision to detect possible adverse drug effects during the treatment period. Resistant TB strains develop more rapidly when drug regimen is interrupted or is sporadic.
- Note: Urine may turn red on contact with bleach used in commercial toilet bowl cleaners.
- Do not take aspirin or other OTC drugs without physician's approval.
- Discard drug if it discolors (brownish or purplish); this signifies decomposition.
- Do not breast feed while taking this drug without consulting physician.

AMIODARONE HYDROCHLORIDE (Pr)

(a-mee′oh-da-rone)

Cordarone, Amio-Aqueous, Pacerone

Classifications: CARDIOVASCULAR AGENT; ANTIARRHYTHMIC, CLASS III

Pregnancy Category: D

AVAILABILITY 200 mg tablets; 50 mg/mL injection

ACTIONS Structurally related to thyroxine. Class III antiarrhythmic; also has antianginal and antiadrenergic properties. Totally unrelated to other antiarrhythmics. Acts directly on all cardiac tissues. Prolongs duration of action potential and refractory period without significantly affecting resting membrane potential.

THERAPEUTIC EFFECTS By direct action on smooth muscle, decreases peripheral resistance and increases coronary blood flow. Blocks effects of sympathetic stimulation.

USES Prophylaxis and treatment of life-threatening ventricular arrhythmias and supraventricular arrhythmias, particularly with atrial fibrillation.

UNLABELED USES Treatment of nonexertional angina.

CONTRAINDICATIONS Hypersensitivity to amiodarone, or benzyl alcohol; cardiogenic shock, severe sinus bradycardia, advanced AV block unless a pacemaker is available, severe sinus-node dysfunction or sick sinus syndrome, bradycardia, congenital or acquired QR prolongation syndromes, or history of torsade de pointes; severe liver disease, children. Safety during pregnancy (category D) or lactation is not established.

CAUTIOUS USE Hepatic disease, cirrhosis; Hashimoto's thyroiditis, goiter, thyrotoxicosis, or history of other thyroid dysfunction; CHF, left ventricular dysfunction; hypersensitivity to iodine; older adults; Fabry disease, especially with visual disturbances; electrolyte imbalance, hypokalemia, hypomagnesemia, hypovolemia; preexisting lung disease, COPD; open heart surgery.

ROUTE & DOSAGE

Arrhythmias

Adult: **PO Loading Dose** 800–1600 mg/d in 1–2 doses for 1–3 wk **PO Maintenance Dose** 400–600 mg/d in 1–2 doses **IV Loading Dose** 150 mg over 10 min followed by 360 mg over next 6 h **IV Maintenance Dose** 540 mg over 18 h (0.5 mg/min), may continue at 0.5 mg/min

Convert IV to PO Duration of infusion <1 wk use 800–1600 mg PO, 1–3 wk use 600–800 mg PO, >3 wk use 400 mg PO
Child: **PO Loading Dose** 10–15 mg/kg/d or 600–800 mg/1.73 m^2/d, in 1–2 divided doses for 4–14 d cycle or until adequate control of arrhythmia **PO Maintenance Dose** 5 mg/kg/d or 200–400 mg/1.73 m^2/d once daily, may be able to reduce to 2–5 mg/kg/d 5 d per week

ADMINISTRATION

Note: Correct hypokalemia and hypomagnesemia prior to initiation of therapy.

Oral

- Give consistently with respect to meals.
- Note: Only a physician experienced with the drug and treatment of life-threatening arrhythmias should give loading doses.
- Note: GI symptoms commonly occur during high-dose therapy, especially with loading doses. Symptoms usually respond to dose reduction or divided dose given with food, including milk.

Intravenous

PREPARE: **IV Infusion: First rapid loading dose infusion:** Add 150 mg (3 mL) amiodarone to 100 mL D5W to yield 1.5 mg/mL. **Second infusion during first 24 h (slow loading dose and maintenance infusion):** Add 900 mg (18 mL) amiodarone to 500 mL D5W to yield 1.8 mg/mL. **Maintenance infusions after the first 24 h:** Prepare concentrations of 1–6 mg/mL amiodarone. Note: (Use central line to give concentrations >2 mg/mL).

ADMINISTER: **IV Infusion:** Rapidly infuse initial 150 mg dose over the first 10 min at a rate of 15 mg/min. Over next 6 h, infuse 360 mg at a rate of 1 mg/min. Over the remaining 18 h, infuse 540 mg at a rate of 0.5 mg/min. After the first 24 h, infuse maintenance doses of 720 mg/24 h at a rate of 0.5 mg/min.

INCOMPATIBILITIES **Solution/additive: sodium bicarbonate. Y-site: aminophylline, cefamandole, cefazolin, heparin; mezlocillin, sodium bicarbonate.**

- Store at 15°–30° C (59°–86° F) protected from light, unless otherwise directed.

ADVERSE EFFECTS (≥1%) **CNS:** Peripheral neuropathy (*muscle weakness,* wasting numbness, tingling), *fatigue,* abnormal gait, dyskinesias, *dizziness,* paresthesia, headache. **CV:** Bradycardia, *hypotension* (IV), sinus arrest, cardiogenic shock, CHF, arrhythmias; AV block. **Special Senses:** *Corneal microdeposits,* blurred vision, optic neuritis, optic neuropathy, permanent blindness, corneal degeneration, macular degeneration, photosensitivity. **GI:** *Anorexia, nausea, vomiting, constipation,* hepatotoxicity. **Metabolic:** Hyperthyroidism or hypothyroidism; may cause neonatal hypo- or hyperthyroidism if taken during pregnancy. **Respiratory:** (Pulmonary toxicity) Alveolitis, pneumonitis (fever, dry cough, dyspnea), interstitial pulmonary fibrosis, *fatal gasping syndrome* with IV in children. **Skin:** Slate-blue pigmentation, *photosensitivity,* rash. **Other:** With chronic use, angioedema.

INTERACTIONS Drug: Significantly increases **digoxin** levels; enhances pharmacologic effects and toxicities of **disopyramide,**

procainamide, quinidine, flecainide, lidocaine; anticoagulant effects of ORAL ANTICOAGULANTS enhanced; **verapamil, diltiazem,** BETA-ADRENERGIC BLOCKING AGENTS may potentiate sinus bradycardia, sinus arrest, or AV block; may increase **phenytoin** levels 2- to 3-fold; **cholestyramine** may decrease amiodarone levels; **fentanyl** may cause bradycardia, hypotension, or decreased output; may increase **cyclosporine** levels and toxicity; **cimetidine** may increase amiodarone levels; **ritonavir** may increase risk of amiodarone toxicity, including cardiotoxicity. **Herbal: Echinacea** possible increase in hepatotoxicity.

PHARMACOKINETICS Absorption: Approximately 50% absorbed (22%–86%). **Onset:** 2–3 d to 1–3 wk. **Peak:** 3–7 h. **Distribution:** Concentrates in adipose tissue, lungs, kidneys, spleen; crosses placenta. **Metabolism:** Extensively hepatically metabolized; undergoes some enterohepatic cycling. **Elimination:** Excreted chiefly in bile and feces; also excreted in breast milk. **Half-Life:** Biphasic, initial 2.5–10 d, terminal 40–55 d.

NURSING IMPLICATIONS

Assessment & Drug Effects

- Monitor BP carefully during infusion and slow the infusion if significant hypotension occurs; bradycardia should be treated by slowing the infusion or discontinuing if necessary. Monitor heart rate and rhythm and BP until drug response has stabilized; report promptly symptomatic bradycardia. Sustained monitoring is essential because drug has an unusually long half-life.
- Monitor for S&S of: Adverse effects, particularly conduction disturbances and exacerbation of arrhythmias, in patients receiving concomitant antiarrhythmic therapy (reduce dosage of previous agent by 30%–50% several days after amiodarone therapy is started); drug-induced hypothyroidism or hyperthyroidism (see Appendix F), especially during early treatment period; pulmonary toxicity (progressive dyspnea, fatigue, cough, pleuritic pain, fever) throughout therapy.
- Lab tests: Baseline and periodic assessments should be made of liver, lung, thyroid, neurologic, and GI function. Drug may cause thyroid function test abnormalities in the absence of thyroid function impairment.
- Monitor for elevations of AST and ALT. If elevations persist or if they are 2–3 times above normal baseline readings, reduce dosage or withdraw drug promptly to prevent hepatotoxicity and liver damage.
- Auscultate chest periodically or when patient complains of respiratory symptoms. Check for diminished breath sounds, rales, pleuritic friction rub; observe breathing pattern. Drug-induced pulmonary function problems must be distinguished from CHF or pneumonia. Keep physician informed.
- Anticipate possible CNS symptoms within a week after amiodarone therapy begins. Proximal muscle weakness, a common side effect, intensified by tremors presents a great hazard to the ambulating patient. Assess severity of symptoms. Supervision of ambulation may be indicated.

Patient & Family Education

- Check pulse daily once stabilized, or as prescribed. Report a pulse <60.

- Take oral drug consistently with respect to meals.
- Become familiar with potential adverse reactions and report those that are bothersome to the physician.
- Use dark glasses to ease photophobia; some patients may not be able to go outdoors in the daytime even with such protection.
- Follow recommendation for regular ophthalmic exams, including funduscopy and slit-lamp exam.
- Wear protective clothing and a barrier-type sunscreen that physically blocks penetration of skin by ultraviolet light (e.g., titanium oxide or zinc formulations) to prevent a photosensitivity reaction (erythema, pruritus); avoid exposure to sun and sunlamps.
- Do not breast feed while taking this drug without consulting physician.

AMITRIPTYLINE HYDROCHLORIDE

(a-mee-trip'ti-leen)

Amitril, Apo-Amitriptyline ♣, Elavil, Emitrip, Endep, Enovil, Levate ♣, Meravil, Novotriptyn ♣, SK-Amitriptyline

Classifications: CENTRAL NERVOUS SYSTEM AGENT; PSYCHOTHERAPEUTIC; TRICYCLIC ANTIDEPRESSANT

Prototype: Imipramine

Pregnancy Category: C

AVAILABILITY 10 mg, 25 mg, 50 mg, 75 mg, 100 mg, 150 mg tablets; 10 mg/mL injection

ACTIONS Among the most active of the tricyclic antidepressants (TCAs) in inhibition of serotonin uptake from synaptic gap; also inhibits norepinephrine reuptake to a moderate degree. Restoration of the levels of these neurotransmitters is a proposed mechanism of antidepressant action.

THERAPEUTIC EFFECTS Interference with the reuptake of serotonin and norepinephrine results in the antidepressant activity of amitriptyline.

USE Endogenous depression.

UNLABELED USES Prophylaxis for cluster, migraine, and chronic tension headaches; intractable pain, peptic ulcer disease, to increase muscle strength in myotonic dystrophy, to treat pathologic weeping and laughing secondary to forebrain disease, for eating disorders associated with depression (anorexia or bulimia), and as sedative for nondepressed patients.

CONTRAINDICATIONS Acute recovery period after MI, history of seizure disorders, pregnancy (category C), lactation, children <12 y.

CAUTIOUS USE Prostatic hypertrophy, history of urinary retention or obstruction; angle-closure glaucoma; diabetes mellitus; hyperthyroidism; patient with cardiovascular, hepatic, or renal dysfunction; patient with suicidal tendency, electroshock therapy; elective surgery; schizophrenia; respiratory disorders; older adults, adolescents.

ROUTE & DOSAGE

Antidepressant

Adult: **PO** 75–100 mg/d, may gradually increase to 150–300 mg/d (use lower doses in outpatients) **IM** 20–30 mg q.i.d. until patient can take PO

Adolescent: **PO** 25–50 mg/d in divided doses, may gradually increase to 100 mg/d (max: 200 mg/d)

Geriatric: **PO** 10–25 mg h.s., may gradually increase to 25–150 mg/d

ADMINISTRATION

Oral

- Give with or immediately after food to reduce possibility of GI irritation. Tablet may be crushed if patient is unable to take it whole; administer with food or fluid.
- Give increased doses preferably in late afternoon or at bedtime due to sedative action that precedes antidepressant effect.
- Give as single dose at bedtime to promote sleep or for patients with dizziness or when daytime sedation interferes with work productivity.
- Note that dose is usually tapered over 2 wk at discontinuation to prevent withdrawal symptoms (headache, nausea, malaise, musculoskeletal pain, panic attack, weakness).

Intramuscular

- Reserve IM injections for patients unable or unwilling to take oral drug.
- Inject deep IM into a large muscle.
- Store drug at 15°–30° C (59°–86° F) and protect from light unless otherwise directed by manufacturer.

ADVERSE EFFECTS (≥1%) **CNS:** *Drowsiness, sedation, dizziness,* nervousness, restlessness, fatigue, headache, insomnia, abnormal movements (extrapyramidal symptoms), seizures. **CV:** *Orthostatic hypotension,* tachycardia, palpitation, ECG changes. **Special Senses:** Blurred vision, mydriasis. **GI:** *Dry mouth,* increased appetite especially for sweets, *constipation,* weight gain, sour or metallic taste, nausea, vomiting. **Urogenital:** *Urinary retention.* **Other:** (Rare) <u>Bone marrow depression</u>.

INTERACTIONS Drug: ANTIHYPERTENSIVES may decrease some antihypertensive response; CNS DEPRESSANTS, **alcohol,** HYPNOTICS, BARBITURATES, SEDATIVES potentiate CNS depression; ANTICOAGULANTS, ORAL, may increase hypoprothrombinemic effect; **ethchlorvynol,** transient delirium; **levodopa,** SYMPATHOMIMETICS (e.g., **epinephrine, norepinephrine**), possibility of sympathetic hyperactivity with hypertension and hyperpyrexia; MAO INHIBITORS, possibility of severe reactions, toxic psychosis, cardiovascular instability; **methylphenidate** increases plasma TCA levels; THYROID DRUGS may increase possibility of arrhythmias; **cimetidine** may increase plasma TCA levels. **Herbal: Ginkgo** may decrease seizure threshold, **St. John's wort** may cause serotonin syndrome.

PHARMACOKINETICS Absorption: Rapidly absorbed from GI and injection sites. **Peak:** 2–12 h. **Distribution:** Crosses placenta. **Metabolism:** Metabolized in liver to active metabolite. **Elimination:** Primarily excreted in urine; enters breast milk. **Half-Life:** 10–50 h.

NURSING IMPLICATIONS

Assessment & Drug Effects

- Monitor therapeutic effectiveness. It may take 1–6 wk to reduce attacks when used for migraine prophylaxis.
- Monitor for S&S of drowsiness and dizziness (initial stages of therapy); institute measures to prevent falling. Also monitor for overdose or suicide ideation in patients who use excessive amounts of alcohol.
- Lab tests: Baseline and periodic leukocyte and differential counts; renal and hepatic function tests;

eye examinations (including glaucoma testing); recommended particularly for older adults, adolescents, and patients receiving high doses/prolonged therapy.

- Monitor BP and pulse rate in patients with preexisting cardiovascular disease. Assess for orthostatic hypotension especially in older adults. Withhold drug if there is a rise or fall in systolic BP (by 10–20 mm Hg), or a sudden increase or a significant change in pulse rate or rhythm. Notify physician.
- Monitor I&O, including bowel elimination pattern.

Patient & Family Education

- Monitor weight; drug may increase appetite or a craving for sweets.
- Understand that tolerance/adaptation to anticholinergic actions (see Appendix F) usually develops with maintenance regimen. Keep physician informed.
- Relieve dry mouth by taking frequent sips of water and increasing total fluid intake.
- Make position change slowly and in stages to prevent dizziness.
- Do not drive or engage in potentially hazardous activities until response to drug is known.
- Do not use OTC drugs without consulting physician while on TCA therapy; many preparations contain sympathomimetic amines.
- Note: Amitriptyline may turn urine blue-green.
- Do not breast feed while taking this drug.

AMLEXANOX

(am-lex'a-nox)

Aphthasol, OraDisc A

Classification: SKIN AND MUCOUS MEMBRANE AGENT

Pregnancy Category: B

AVAILABILITY 5% paste; 2 mg mucoadhesive disc

ACTIONS Mechanism of action by which healing of aphthous ulcers occurs is unknown.

THERAPEUTIC EFFECTS Amlexanox reduces healing time and pain related to aphthous ulcers or canker sores.

USES Treatment of aphthous ulcers in patients with normal immune systems.

CONTRAINDICATIONS Sensitivity to amlexanox.

CAUTIOUS USE Pregnancy (category B), lactation. Safety and efficacy in children are not established.

ROUTE & DOSAGE

Aphthous Ulcers

Adult: **Topical** Apply 1/4 in. (0.5 cm) to finger and dab onto each mouth ulcer q.i.d. (after oral hygiene p.c. and h.s.) for 10 d cycle; apply disc to each mouth ulcer and allow to dissolve

ADMINISTRATION

Topical

- Apply after oral hygiene following each meal and before bedtime.
- Avoid prolonged contact with skin and wash off skin if contact occurs.
- Store at 15°–30° C (59°–86° F) away from heat and moisture. Do not freeze.

ADVERSE EFFECTS (≥1%) **Body as a Whole:** Transient pain, stinging, or burning at application site.

PHARMACOKINETICS Absorption: Minimally absorbed through ulcer. **Onset:** Approximately 3 d.

Elimination: 17% of orally absorbed dose excreted in urine. **Half-Life:** 3.5 h.

NURSING IMPLICATIONS

Assessment & Drug Effects

- Discontinue use if rash or inflamed membranes develop.

Patient & Family Education

- Use at first sign of canker sore. Wash hands before and immediately after application.
- Flush eyes immediately with large amount of cold water if paste accidentally comes in contact with eyes or eye area.
- Contact physician if healing does not result after 10 d of therapy.
- Do not breast feed while taking this drug without consulting physician.

AMLODIPINE

(am-lo′di-peen)
Norvasc
Classifications: CARDIOVASCULAR AGENT; CALCIUM CHANNEL BLOCKER; ANTIHYPERTENSIVE AGENT
Prototype: Nifedipine
Pregnancy Category: C

AVAILABILITY 2.5 mg, 5 mg, 10 mg tablets

ACTIONS Amlodipine is a calcium channel blocking agent that selectively blocks calcium ion reflux across cell membranes of cardiac and vascular smooth muscle without changing serum calcium concentrations. It predominantly acts on the peripheral circulation, decreasing peripheral vascular resistance, and increases cardiac output.
THERAPEUTIC EFFECTS Amlodipine reduces systolic, diastolic, and mean arterial blood pressure.

USES Treatment of mild to moderate hypertension and angina.

CONTRAINDICATIONS Hypersensitivity to amlodipine; pregnancy (category C).
CAUTIOUS USE Liver disease; concomitant use with hypotension; CHF; lactation; older adults.

ROUTE & DOSAGE

Hypertension
Adult: **PO** 5–10 mg once daily
Geriatric: Start with 2.5 mg, adjust dose at intervals of not less than 2 wk

Hepatic Impairment
Start with 2.5 mg, adjust dose at intervals of not less than 2 wk

ADMINISTRATION

Oral

- Give drug without regard to meals.
- Prescribed initial dosages of 2.5 mg daily are common if added to a regimen including other antihypertensive drugs.
- Note: Doses are usually titrated over a period of 14 d or more rapidly if warranted.
- Store at 15°–30° C (59°–86° F).

ADVERSE EFFECTS (≥1%) **CV:** Palpitations, flushing tachycardia, *peripheral or facial edema*, bradycardia, chest pain, syncope, postural hypotension. **CNS:** Lightheadedness, fatigue, *headache*. **GI:** Abdominal pain, nausea, anorexia, constipation, dyspepsia, dysphagia, diarrhea, flatulence, vomiting. **Urogenital:** Sexual dysfunction, frequency, nocturia. **Respiratory:** Dyspnea. **Skin:** Flushing, rash. **Other:** Arthralgia, cramps, myalgia.

INTERACTIONS Drug: Adenosine may increase the risk of bradycardia; **bosentan** may decrease efficacy of amlodipine; additive hypotensive effects with other ANTIHYPERTENSIVE AGENTS; AZOLE ANTIFUNGALS (e.g., **fluconazole, itraconazole**) may inhibit metabolism of amlodipine; **itraconazole** may increase edema. **Food: Grapefruit juice** may increase amlodipine levels. **Herbal: Ephedra, Ma Huang, melatonin** may antagonize antihypertensive effects.

PHARMACOKINETICS Absorption: >90% absorbed from GI tract. **Onset:** Gradual. **Peak:** 6–9 h. **Duration:** 24 h. **Distribution:** >95% protein bound. **Metabolism:** Extensively metabolized in the liver to inactive metabolites. **Elimination:** Inactive metabolites primarily excreted in urine (<5%–10% excreted unchanged), 20%–25% excreted in feces. **Half-Life:** <45 y: 28–69 h; >60 y: 40–120 h.

NURSING IMPLICATIONS

Assessment & Drug Effects

- Monitor BP for therapeutic effectiveness. BP reduction is greatest after peak levels of amlodipine are achieved 6–9 h following oral doses.
- Monitor for S&S of dose-related peripheral or facial edema that may not be accompanied by weight gain; rarely, severe edema may cause discontinuation of drug.
- Monitor BP with postural changes. Report postural hypotension. Monitor more frequently when additional antihypertensives or diuretics are added.
- Monitor heart rate; dose-related palpitations (more common in women) may occur.

Patient & Family Education

- Report significant swelling of face or extremities.
- Take care to have support when standing & walking due to possible dose-related light-headedness/ dizziness.
- Report shortness of breath, palpitations, irregular heartbeat, nausea, or constipation to physician.
- Do not breast feed while taking this drug without consulting physician.

AMMONIUM CHLORIDE

(ah-mo'ni-um)

Classification: ELECTROLYTIC BALANCE AND WATER BALANCE AGENTS

Pregnancy Category: B

AVAILABILITY 26.75% or 5 mEq/mL solution; 500 mg tablets; 486 mg enteric-coated tablets

ACTIONS Acidifying property is due to conversion of ammonium ion (NH_4^+) to urea in liver with liberation of H^+ and Cl^-. Potassium excretion also increases acid, but to a lesser extent. Tolerance to diuretic effect occurs within 2–3 d.

THERAPEUTIC EFFECTS Systemic acidifier in metabolic alkalosis by releasing H+ ions which lower pH.

USES Treatment of hypochloremic states and metabolic alkalosis. Diuretic or urinary acidifying agent.

CONTRAINDICATIONS Severe renal or hepatic insufficiency; primary respiratory acidosis. Safety during pregnancy (category B) or lactation is not established.

CAUTIOUS USE Cardiac edema, pulmonary insufficiency.

ROUTE & DOSAGE

Urine Acidifier, Diuretic

Adult: **PO** 4–12 g/d divided q4–6h
Child: **PO** 75 mg/kg/d in 4 divided doses

Metabolic Alkalosis and Hypochloremic States

Adult/Child: **IV** Dose calculated on basis of CO_2 combining power or serum Cl deficit, 50% of calculated deficit is administered slowly

ADMINISTRATION

Oral

- Give after meals for best tolerance or use enteric-coated tablets. Tablets should be swallowed whole.
- Store in airtight container.

Intravenous

Check with physician for slower rate for infants.

PREPARE: **Intermittent:** Dilute each 20 ml vial in 500 mL NS. Do not exceed a concentration of 1%–2%.

ADMINISTER: **Intermittent:** Give slowly to avoid serious adverse effects (ammonia toxicity) and local irritation and pain. Give at a rate not to exceed 5 mL/min.

INCOMPATIBILITIES **Solution/additive: Codeine phosphate, levorphanol, methadone, nitrofurantoin, warfarin**.

- Avoid freezing. ▪ Concentrated solutions crystallize at low temperatures. ▪ Crystals can be dissolved by placing intact container in a warm water bath and warming to room temperature.

ADVERSE EFFECTS (≥1%) **Body as a Whole:** Most secondary to ammonia toxicity. **CNS:** Headache, depression, drowsiness, twitching, excitability; EEG abnormalities. **CV:** Bradycardia and other arrhythmias. **GI:** Gastric irritation, nausea, vomiting, anorexia. **Metabolic:** Metabolic acidosis, hyperammonia. **Skin:** Rash. **Respiratory:** Hyperventilation. **Skin:** Rash. **Urogenital:** Glycosuria **Other:** Pain and irritation at IV site.

DIAGNOSTIC TEST INTERFERENCE Ammonium chloride may increase ***blood ammonia*** and ***AST,*** decrease ***serum magnesium*** (by increasing urinary magnesium excretion), and decrease ***urine urobilinogen.***

INTERACTIONS Drug: Aminosalicylic acid may cause crystalluria; increases urinary excretion of AMPHETAMINES, **flecainide, mexiletine, methadone, ephedrine, pseudoephedrine;** decreased urinary excretion of SULFONYLUREAS, SALICYLATES.

PHARMACOKINETICS Absorption: Completely absorbed in 3–6 h. **Metabolism:** Metabolized in liver to HCl and urea. **Elimination:** Primarily excreted in urine.

NURSING IMPLICATIONS

Assessment & Drug Effects

- Assess IV infusion site frequently for signs of irritation. Change site as warranted.
- Monitor for S&S of: metabolic acidosis (mental status changes including confusion, disorientation, coma, respiratory changes including increased respiratory rate and depth, exertional dyspnea); ammonium toxicity (cardiac arrhythmias including bradycardia, irregular respirations, twitching, seizures).
- Monitor I&O ratio and pattern. The diuretic effect of ammonium chloride is compensatory and lasts only 1–2 d.

- Lab tests: Baseline and periodic determinations of CO_2 combining power, serum electrolytes, and urinary and arterial pH during therapy to avoid serious acidosis.

Patient & Family Education

- Report pain at IV injection site.
- Do not breast feed while taking this drug without consulting physician.

AMOBARBITAL

(am-oh-bar'bi-tal)
Amytal, Isobec, Novamobarb

AMOBARBITAL SODIUM

Amytal Sodium

Classifications: CENTRAL NERVOUS SYSTEM AGENT; ANTICONVULSANT; BARBITURATE; SEDATIVE-HYPNOTIC
Prototype: Phenobarbital
Pregnancy Category: D
Controlled Substance: Schedule II

AVAILABILITY 30 mg, 50 mg, 100 mg capsules; 250 mg, 500 mg vials

ACTIONS Intermediate-acting barbiturate similar to phenobarbital. CNS depressant action appears to be related to ability to interfere with ascending impulse transmission from reticular activating system (concerned with alertness) to cerebral cortex. Does not impair pain perception.

THERAPEUTIC EFFECTS Controls seizure activity by increasing the threshold for motor cortex stimuli.

USES Sedative, to relieve anxiety, and as short-term hypnotic to treat insomnia. Also used parenterally to control status epilepticus or acute convulsive episodes, agitated behavior, and for narcoanalysis and narcotherapy.

CONTRAINDICATIONS Hypersensitivity to barbiturates; history of addiction; family or patient history of porphyria; severe respiratory, hepatic, or renal disease. Safety during pregnancy (category D), lactation, or in children <6 y is not established.

CAUTIOUS USE Hypotension, hypertension, cardiac disease; acute or chronic pain; older adults.

ROUTE & DOSAGE

Sedative

Adult: **PO** 30–50 mg b.i.d. or t.i.d.
Child: **PO** 2 mg/kg or 70 mg/m^2/d in 4 divided doses

Preoperative Sedation

Adult: **PO/IM** 200 mg 1 h before surgery

Labor

Adult: **PO** 200–400 mg repeated at 1–3 h intervals (max: 1 g)

Hypnotic

Adult: **PO/IM** 65–200 mg (max: 500 mg)
Child: **IM** 2–3 mg/kg

Anticonvulsant, Agitated Behavior, Hypnotic

Adult/Child: **IV** 65–500 mg, not to exceed 1 g

ADMINISTRATION

Oral

- Give on an empty stomach to increase rate of absorption.
- Give hypnotic dose 30–60 min before bedtime. Hypnotic use should be limited to 2 wk.

Intramuscular

- Give injection within 30 min after vial is opened.
- Inject deep IM in a large muscle mass (e.g., upper outer quadrant of gluteus maximus). Superficial

injections are painful and can cause sterile abscess or sloughing.
- Do not inject more than 5 mL into any one site.

Intravenous

PREPARE: **Direct:** Dilute each 125 mg with 1.25 mL of sterile water for injection. ▪ Add diluent slowly, rotate vial to dissolve but do not shake. ▪ Do not use if solution does not clear within 5 min or contains a precipitate. ▪ Consult manufacturer's package insert for reconstitution directions to prepare specific concentrations.
ADMINISTER: **Direct:** Give at rate not to exceed 100 mg/min for adults or 60 mg/m^2/min for children. ▪ Do not give >1 mL of a 10% solution/min.
INCOMPATIBILITIES **Solution/additive: Codeine phosphate, dimenhydrinate, phenytoin, hydrocortisone, hydroxyzine, insulin, levophanol, meperidine, methadone, morphine, norepinephrine, pentazocine, procaine, streptomycin, tetracycline, vancomycin, penicillin G,** PHENOTHIAZINES, **cimetidine, pancuronium.**

- Store at 15°–30° C (59°–86° F) unless otherwise directed. Avoid freezing. Discard any vial which has been opened ≥30 min.

ADVERSE EFFECTS (≥1%) **CNS:** Drowsiness, dizziness, hangover, unsteadiness, lethargy, paradoxical excitement. **Hematologic:** Agranulocytosis & thrombocytopenia (rare). **Body as a Whole:** Rash, angioedema. **Other:** Pain at IM injection site, Stevens-Johnson syndrome, hypotension, respiratory depression.

INTERACTIONS Drug: Antagonizes effects of **phenmetrazine;** CNS DEPRESSANTS, **alcohol,** SEDATIVES compound CNS depression; MAO INHIBITORS cause excessive CNS depression; **methoxyflurane** presents risk of nephrotoxicity. **Herbal: Kava-kava, valerian** may potentiate sedation.

PHARMACOKINETICS Onset: 1 h PO; 5 min IV. **Duration:** 6–8 h PO; 3–6 h IV. **Distribution:** Crosses placenta; appears in breast milk. **Metabolism:** Metabolized primarily in liver. **Elimination:** 40%–50% of dose excreted in urine. **Half-Life:** 20–25 h.

NURSING IMPLICATIONS

Assessment & Drug Effects

- Observe IV injection site during and after administration. Extravasation can cause thrombophlebitis and tissue necrosis.
- Monitor vital signs during IV infusion and for several hours after drug administration. Caution patient not to get out of bed without assistance.
- Note: Personnel and equipment for management of respiratory depression and hypotension must be immediately available when IV drug is administered.
- Monitor for S&S of paradoxical restlessness, excitement, confusion, and depression in older adults and children. Dosage adjustments may be required.

Patient & Family Education

- Do not take alcoholic beverages or other CNS depressants while taking this drug.
- Note: Excitement may occur with onset of pain while taking this drug. Report to your physician immediately.
- Do not drive or perform other potentially hazardous tasks until response to drug is known.

- Note: Prolonged use may lead to tolerance and dependence; take only as prescribed.
- Do not breast feed while taking this drug without consulting physician.

AMOXAPINE

(a-mox'a-peen)
Asendin
Classifications: CENTRAL NERVOUS SYSTEM AGENT; PSYCHOTHERAPEUTIC; TRICYCLIC ANTIDEPRESSANT
Prototype: Imipramine
Pregnancy Category: C

AVAILABILITY 25 mg, 50 mg, 100 mg, 150 mg tablets

ACTIONS Tricyclic antidepressant (TCA) and secondary amine with mixed antidepressant and neuroleptic tranquilizing properties. Unlike some TCAs, not associated with severe cardiotoxicity, has mild sedative action, and causes slight orthostatic hypotension.
THERAPEUTIC EFFECTS Antidepressant activity is thought to be due to reduced reuptake of norepinephrine and serotonin. Also blocks response to dopamine by dopaminergic receptors.

USES Neurotic and endogenous depression accompanied by anxiety or agitation.

CONTRAINDICATIONS Hypersensitivity to other tricyclic compounds; acute recovery period after MI. Safety during pregnancy (category C), lactation, or children <16 y of age is not established.
CAUTIOUS USE History of convulsive disorders, schizophrenia, manic depression, electroshock therapy; alcohol abuse; history of urinary retention, benign prostatic hypertrophy; angle-closure glaucoma or increased intraocular pressure; cardiovascular disorders; impaired renal or hepatic function; elective surgery.

ROUTE & DOSAGE

Antidepressant
Adult: **PO** Start at 50 mg b.i.d. or t.i.d., may increase on third day to 100 mg t.i.d. Maintenance doses ≤300 mg/d as single dose at bedtime
Geriatric: **PO** 25 mg h.s., may increase q3–7d to 50–150 mg/d in divided doses (max: 300 mg/d)

ADMINISTRATION

Oral
- Give with or after food to reduce GI irritation; tablet may be crushed and taken with fluid or mixed with food.
- Give maintenance dose as a single dose at bedtime to minimize daytime sedation and other annoying drug adverse effects.
- Do not abruptly discontinue drug. Doses should be tapered over 2 wk.
- Store at 15°–30° C (59°–86° F) in tightly closed container unless otherwise directed.

ADVERSE EFFECTS (≥1%) **CNS:** *Drowsiness,* dizziness, headache, fatigue, *sedation,* lethargy; extrapyramidal effects (acute dystonic reactions, panic attacks, parkinsonism, tardive dyskinesia), seizures (over-dosage). **CV:** Orthostatic hypotension; arrhythmias. **GI:** Constipation, diarrhea, flatulence, *dry mouth,* peculiar taste, nausea, heartburn. **Special Senses:** Blurred vision, dry eyes. Urogenital: nephrotoxicity (overdosage).

INTERACTIONS Drug: May decrease response to ANTIHYPERTENSIVES; CNS DEPRESSANTS, **alcohol,** HYPNOTICS, BARBITURATES, SEDATIVES potentiate CNS depression; may increase hypoprothrombinemic effect of ORAL ANTICOAGULANTS; **ethchlorvynol,** transient delirium; with **levodopa,** SYMPATHOMIMETICS (e.g., **epinephrine, norepinephrine**), possibility of sympathetic hyperactivity with hypertension and hyperpyrexia; with MAO INHIBITORS, possibility of severe reactions: toxic psychosis, cardiovascular instability; **methylphenidate** increases plasma TCA levels; thyroid drugs may increase possibility of arrhythmias; **cimetidine** may increase plasma TCA levels. **Herbal: Ginkgo** may decrease seizure threshold, **St. John's wort** may cause serotonin syndrome.

PHARMACOKINETICS Absorption: Rapidly absorbed. **Peak:** 1–2 h. **Distribution:** Probably crosses placenta; distributed into breast milk. **Metabolism:** Metabolized active metabolite. **Elimination:** 60% excreted in urine in 6 d; 7%–18% excreted in feces. **Half-Life:** 8 h parent drug, 30 h metabolite.

NURSING IMPLICATIONS

Assessment & Drug Effects

- Monitor therapeutic effectiveness. Initial antidepressant effect (mild euphoria, increased energy) may occur within 4–7 d; however, in most patients clinical response does not occur until after 2–3 wk of drug therapy.
- Supervise patient closely during therapy for suicidal ideation and potential serious adverse effects.
- Report immediately signs of neuroleptic malignant syndrome: fever, sweating, rigidity (catatonia), unstable BP, rapid, irregular pulse; changes in level of consciousness, coma. Although rare, it can be life-threatening if drug is not stopped immediately. Death can result from acute respiratory, renal, or cardiovascular failure.
- Report immediately the onset of signs of tardive dyskinesia (see Appendix F); careful observation/reporting may prevent irreversibility.
- Monitor I&O ratio and bowel elimination pattern. Report continuing constipation.

Patient & Family Education

- Follow directions for taking this drug (see ADMINISTRATION).
- Do not abruptly discontinue drug. Dosage should be tapered over 2 wks. Maintain established dosage regimen. Do not skip, reduce, or double doses or change dose intervals.
- Minimize alcohol intake as it may potentiate drug effects, thus increasing the dangers of overdosage or suicidal ideation.
- Drink at least 2000 mL (approximately 2 qts) fluid daily and eat foods with high fiber content (if allowed) to provide needed roughage.
- Monitor weight at least weekly and report significant weight gain.
- Do not drive or engage in potentially hazardous tasks until response to drug is known.
- Rinse mouth frequently with clear water, especially after eating, to relieve mouth dryness.
- Do not take any prescription or OTC drugs without consulting physician.
- Do not breast feed while taking this drug without consulting physician.

AMOXICILLIN

(a-mox-i-sill'in)

Amoxil, Apo-Amoxi ✦, Larotid, Novamoxin, Polymox, Sumox, Trimox, Utimox, Wymox, DisperMox

Classifications: ANTIINFECTIVE; ANTIBIOTIC; AMINOPENICILLIN

Prototype: Ampicillin

Pregnancy Category: B

AVAILABILITY 125 mg, 250 mg, 500 mg tablets; 250 mg, 500 mg capsules; 50 mg/mL, 125 mg/5 mL, 250 mg/5 mL powder for suspension; 200 mg, 400 mg, 600 mg dispersible tablets

ACTIONS Broad-spectrum, acid-stable, semisynthetic aminopenicillin and analogue of ampicillin. Acts by inhibiting mucoprotein synthesis in cell wall of rapidly multiplying bacteria. It is bactericidal and is inactivated by penicillinase.

THERAPEUTIC EFFECTS Active against both aerobic gram positive and aerobic gram negative bacteria including: *Enterococcus faecalis, Streptococcus pneumonia, Escherichia coli, Haemophilus influenzae, Helicobacter pylori*.

USES Infections of ear, nose, throat, GU tract, skin, and soft tissue caused by susceptible bacteria. Also used in uncomplicated gonorrhea. Available in combination with potassium clavulanate, which extends antibacterial spectrum of amoxicillin to include beta-lactamase-producing strains.

CONTRAINDICATIONS Hypersensitivity to penicillins; infectious mononucleosis.

CAUTIOUS USE History of or suspected atopy or allergy (hives, eczema, hay fever, asthma); history of cephalosporin or carbapenem hypersensitivity; colitis, dialysis, diarrhea, GI disease; infants, neonates; viral infection, syphilis, renal impairment or failure, diabetes mellitus, leukemia, pregnancy (category B), or lactation.

ROUTE & DOSAGE

Mild to Moderate Infections

Adult: **PO** 250–500 mg q8h
Child: **PO** 25–50 mg/kg/d (max: 60–80 mg/kg/d) divided q8h or 200–400 mg q12h

Gonorrhea

Adult: **PO** 3 g as single dose with 1 g probenecid
Child: **PO** ≥2 y, 50 mg/kg as single dose with probenecid 25 mg/kg

ADMINISTRATION

Oral

- Ensure that chewable tablets are chewed or crushed before being swallowed with a liquid.
- Place reconstituted pediatric drops directly on child's tongue or add to formula, milk, fruit juice, water, ginger ale, or other soft drink. Have child drink all the prepared dose promptly.
- Store in tightly covered containers at 15°–30° C (59°–86° F) unless otherwise directed. Reconstituted oral suspensions are stable for 7 d at room temperature.

ADVERSE EFFECTS (≥1%) **Body as a Whole:** As with other penicillins. Hypersensitivity (rash, anaphylaxis), superinfections. **GI:** Diarrhea, nausea, vomiting, pseudo-membranous colitis (rare). **Hematologic:** Hemolytic anemia, eosinophilia,

Common adverse effects in *italic*, life-threatening effects underlined: generic names in **bold**; classifications in SMALL CAPS; ✦ Canadian drug name; ● Prototype drug

agranulocytosis (rare). **Skin:** Pruritus, urticaria, or other skin eruptions. **Special Senses:** Conjunctival ecchymosis.

INTERACTIONS TETRACYCLINES may inhibit activity of amoxicillin; **probenecid** prolongs the activity of amoxicillin.

PHARMACOKINETICS Absorption: Rapid and nearly complete absorption. **Peak:** 1–2 h. **Distribution:** Diffuses into most tissues and body fluids, except synovial fluid and CSF (unless meninges are inflamed); crosses placenta; distributed into breast milk in small amounts. **Metabolism:** Metabolized in liver. **Elimination:** 60% of dose excreted in urine in 6–8 h. **Half-Life:** 1–1.3 h.

NURSING IMPLICATIONS

Assessment & Drug Effects

- Determine previous hypersensitivity reactions to penicillins, cephalosporins, and other allergens prior to therapy.
- Lab tests: Baseline C&S tests prior to initiation of therapy, start drug pending results; periodic assessments of renal, hepatic, and hematologic functions should be made during prolonged therapy.
- Monitor for S&S of an urticarial rash (usually occurring within a few days after start of drug) suggestive of a hypersensitivity reaction. If it occurs, look for other signs of hypersensitivity (fever, wheezing, generalized itching, dyspnea), and report to physician immediately.
- Report onset of generalized, erythematous, maculopapular rash (ampicillin rash) to physician. Ampicillin rash is not due to hypersensitivity; however, hypersensitivity should be ruled out.
- Closely monitor diarrhea to rule out pseudomembranous colitis.

Patient & Family Education

- Take drug around the clock, do not miss a dose, and continue therapy until all medication is taken, unless otherwise directed by physician.
- Report onset of diarrhea and other possible symptoms of superinfection to physician (see Appendix F).
- Do not breast feed while taking this drug without consulting physician.

AMOXICILLIN AND CLAVULANATE POTASSIUM

(a-mox-i-sill′in)

Augmentin, Augmentin-ES600, Augmentin XR, Clavulin ♣

Classifications: ANTIINFECTIVE; BETA-LACTAM ANTIBIOTIC; AMINOPENICILLIN

Prototype: Ampicillin

Pregnancy Category: B

AVAILABILITY 250 mg, 500 mg, 875 mg tablets; 125 mg, 200 mg, 400 mg chewable tablets; 125 mg/5 mL, 200 mg/5 mL, 250 mg/5 mL, 400 mg/5 mL, 600 mg/5 mL oral suspension; 1000 mg amoxicillin/62.5 mg clavulanate sustained-release tablets

ACTIONS Used alone, clavulanic acid antibacterial activity is weak. In combination, it inhibits enzyme (beta-lactamase) degradation of amoxicillin and by synergism extends both spectrum of activity and bactericidal effect of amoxicillin against many strains of beta-lactamase-producing bacteria resistant to amoxicillin alone.

THERAPEUTIC EFFECTS Semisynthetic broad-spectrum antibiotic with fixed combination of amoxicillin, an aminopenicillin, and the potassium salt to clavulanic acid, a competitive beta-lactamase inhibitor. Active against gram-positive bacteria including *Staphylococcus aureus, Streptococcus pneumoniae, Clostridium, Peptococcus, Bacteroides fragilis* group, and many gram-negative organisms including *Branhamella catarrhalis* (formerly *Neisseria catarrhalis), Haemophilus influenzae, Proteus mirabilis; Salmonella, Shigella,* and *Klebsiella sp.* Generally inactive against *Pseudomonas.*

USES Infections caused by susceptible beta-lactamase-producing organisms: lower respiratory tract infections, acute bacterial sinusitis, community acquired pneumonia, otitis media, sinusitis, skin and skin structure infections, and UTI.

CONTRAINDICATIONS Combination shares toxic potential of ampicillin. Hypersensitivity to penicillins; infectious mononucleosis.

CAUTIOUS USE Pregnancy (category B), lactation.

ROUTE & DOSAGE

Mild to Moderate Infections

Adult: **PO** 250 or 500 mg tablet (each with 125 mg clavulanic acid) q8–12h; Sustained-release tabs: 2 tablets (2000 mg amoxicillin/125 mg clavulanate) q12h × 7–10 d
Child: **PO** *<40 kg,* 20–40 mg/kg/d (based on amoxicillin component) divided q8–12h; *>3 mo,* 90 mg/kg/d of 600 ES divided q12h × 10 d
Neonate/Infant: **PO** *<3 mo,* 30 mg/kg/d (amoxicillin) divided q12h

ADMINISTRATION

Oral

- Give at the start of a meal to minimize GI upset and enhance absorption.
- Note that both 250- and 500-mg tablets contain the exact amount of clavulanic acid (125 mg and potassium salt); therefore, two 250-mg tablets are not equivalent to one 500-mg tablet.
- Reconstitute oral suspension by adding amount of water specified on container to provide a 5 mL suspension. Tap bottle before adding water to loosen powder, then add water in 2 portions, agitating suspension well before each addition.
- Agitate suspension well just before administration of each dose.
- Give dialysis patient an additional 2 doses on the day of dialysis; one dose before and another dose after dialysis.
- Store tablets in tight containers at <24° C (71° F). Reconstituted oral suspension should be refrigerated at 2°–8° C (36°–46° F), then discarded after 10 d.

ADVERSE EFFECTS (≥1%) **GI:** *Diarrhea,* nausea, vomiting. **Skin:** Rash, urticaria. **Other:** Candidal vaginitis; moderate increases in serum ALT, AST; glomerulonephritis; <u>agranulocytosis</u> (rare).

DIAGNOSTIC TEST INTERFERENCE May interfere with ***urinary glucose*** determinations using ***cupric sulfate, Benedict's solution, Clinitest;*** does not affect ***glucose oxidase methods*** (e.g., Clinistix, TesTape). Positive direct ***antiglobulin*** (***Coombs'***) test results may be reported, a reaction that could interfere with ***hematologic studies*** or with ***transfusion cross-matching*** procedures.

INTERACTIONS Drug: TETRACYCLINES may inhibit activity of amoxicillin; **probenecid** prolongs the activity of amoxicillin.

PHARMACOKINETICS Absorption: Rapid and nearly complete absorption. **Peak:** 1–2 h. **Distribution:** Diffuses into most tissues and body fluids, except synovial fluid and CSF (unless meninges are inflamed); crosses placenta; distributed into breast milk in very small amounts. **Metabolism:** Metabolized in liver. **Elimination:** 50%–73% of the amoxicillin and 25%–45% of the clavulanate dose excreted in urine in 2 h. **Half-Life:** Amoxicillin 1–1.3 h, clavulanate 0.78–1.2 h.

NURSING IMPLICATIONS

Assessment & Drug Effects

- Determine previous hypersensitivity reactions to penicillins, cephalosporins, and other allergens prior to therapy.
- Lab tests: Baseline C&S tests prior to initiation of therapy; start drug pending results.
- Monitor for S&S of an urticarial rash (usually occurring within a few days after start of drug) suggestive of a hypersensitivity reaction. If it occurs, look for other signs of hypersensitivity (fever, wheezing, generalized itching, dyspnea), and report to physician immediately.
- Note: Generalized, erythematous, maculopapular rash (ampicillin rash) is not due to hypersensitivity. It is usually mild, but can be severe. Report onset of rash to physician, since hypersensitivity should be ruled out.

Patient & Family Education

- Female patients should report onset of symptoms of *Candidal vaginitis* (e.g., moderate amount of white, cheesy, nonodorous vaginal discharge; vaginal inflammation and itching; vulvar excoriation, inflammation, burning, itching). Therapy may have to be discontinued.
- Note: Use Clinistix or TesTape when monitoring urinary glucose to avoid false readings with diabetes mellitus.
- Do not breast feed while taking this drug without consulting physician.

AMPHETAMINE SULFATE Pr

(am-fet′a-meen)

Racemic Amphetamine Sulfate, Adderall, Adderall XR

Classifications: CENTRAL NERVOUS SYSTEM (CNS) AGENT; CEREBRAL STIMULANT; ANOREXIANT

Pregnancy Category: C

Controlled Substance: Schedule II

AVAILABILITY 5 mg, 10 mg tablets; Adderall 5 mg, 10 mg, 20 mg, 30 mg tablets; 5 mg, 15 mg, 20 mg, 25 mg, 30 mg sustained release capsules

ACTIONS Indirect-acting synthetic sympathomimetic amine with peripheral alpha- and beta-adrenergic activity. Marked stimulant effect on CNS thought to be due to action on cerebral cortex and possibly the Reticular Activating System. Acts indirectly on adrenergic receptors by increasing synaptic release of norepinephrine and dopamine in brain and by blocking reuptake at presynaptic membranes.

THERAPEUTIC EFFECTS CNS stimulation results in increased motor activity, diminished sense of fatigue, alertness, wakefulness, and mood elevation. In hyperkinetic children, it exerts a paradoxic sedative effect by unclear mechanism. Anorexigenic effect thought to result from direct inhibition of hypothalamic appetite center, as well as mood elevation.

USES Narcolepsy, attention deficit disorder in children and adults (hyperkinetic behavioral syndrome, minimal brain dysfunction). Use as short-term adjunct to control exogenous obesity not generally recommended because of its potential for abuse.
UNLABELED USES In combination with other drugs for treatment-resistant depression.

CONTRAINDICATIONS Hypersensitivity to sympathomimetic amines; history of drug abuse; severe agitation; hyperthyroidism; diabetes mellitus; moderate to severe hypertension, advanced arteriosclerosis, angina pectoris or other cardiovascular disorders; Gilles de la Tourette disorder; glaucoma; during or within 14 d after treatment with MAOIs. Safety during pregnancy (category C) or lactation is not established.
CAUTIOUS USE Mild hypertension.

ROUTE & DOSAGE

Narcolepsy
Adult: **PO** 5–60 mg/d divided q4–6h in 2–3 doses
Child: **PO** *>12 y,* 10 mg/d, may increase by 10 mg at weekly intervals; *6–12 y,* 5 mg/d, may increase by 5 mg at weekly intervals

Attention Deficit Disorder
Adult/Adolescent: **PO** 10 mg extended release once daily in a.m.; may increase by 5–10 mg at weekly intervals if needed to max 30 mg/d.
Child: **PO** *6 y,* 5 mg 1–2 times/d, may increase by 5 mg at weekly intervals (max: 40 mg/d); *3–5 y,* 2.5 mg 1–2 times/d, may increase by 2.5 mg at weekly intervals; 10 mg extended release once daily in a.m.; may increase by 5–10 mg at weekly intervals if needed to max of 30 mg/d.

Obesity
Adult: **PO** 5–10 mg 1 h before meals

ADMINISTRATION

Oral
- Give first dose on awakening or early in a.m. when prescribed for narcolepsy.
- Give last dose no later than 6 h before patient retires to avoid insomnia.
- Ensure that sustained release capsules are not crushed or chewed.
- Give drug on an empty stomach 30–60 min before meal to suppress appetite when prescribed for obesity.
- Store at 15°–30° C (59°–86° F) unless otherwise directed.

ADVERSE EFFECTS (≥1%) **Body as a Whole:** Allergy, urticaria, sudden death (reported in children with structural cardiac abnormalities). **CNS:** *Irritability,* psychosis, *restlessness,* nervousness, headache, *insomnia,* weakness, *euphoria,* dysphoria, drowsiness, trembling, hyperactive reflexes. **CV:** *Palpitation,* elevated BP; tachycardia, vasculitis. **Urogenital:** Impotence & change in libido with high doses. **GI:** Dry mouth, anorexia, unusual weight loss, nausea, vomiting, diarrhea, or constipation.

DIAGNOSTIC TEST INTERFERENCE Elevations in ***serum thyroxine (T_4)*** levels with high amphetamine doses.

INTERACTIONS Drug: Acetazolamide, sodium bicarbonate decrease amphetamine elimination; **ammonium chloride, ascorbic acid** increase amphetamine elimination; effects of both amphetamine and BARBITURATE may be antagonized if given together; **furazolidone** may increase BP effects of amphetamines, and interaction may persist for several weeks after furazolidone is discontinued; **guanethidine, guanadryl** antagonize antihypertensive effects; because MAO INHIBITORS, **selegiline** can precipitate hypertensive crisis (fatalities reported), do not administer amphetamines during or within 14 d of these drugs; PHENOTHIAZINES may inhibit mood elevating effects of amphetamines; TRICYCLIC ANTIDEPRESSANTS enhance amphetamine effects through increased **norepinephrine** release; BETA AGONISTS increase cardiovascular adverse effects.

PHARMACOKINETICS Absorption: Rapid. Peak effect: 1–5 h. **Duration:** Up to 10 h. **Distribution:** All tissues, especially CNS. **Metabolism:** Metabolized in liver. **Elimination:** Renal elimination; excreted into breast milk. **Half-Life:** 10–30 h.

NURSING IMPLICATIONS

Assessment & Drug Effects

- Monitor for therapeutic effectiveness. Tolerance to the mood-elevating effects commonly occurs within a few weeks. Drug is usually discontinued when tolerance develops. Generally, tolerance does not occur when used for attention deficit disorder or narcolepsy.
- Monitor for S&S of toxicity in children. Response to this drug is more variable in children than adults; acute toxicity has occurred over a wide range of dosage.
- Monitor for S&S of insomnia or anorexia. Report complaints to physician. Dosage reduction may be required.
- Monitor diabetics closely for loss of glycemic control.
- Monitor growth in children; drug may be discontinued periodically to allow for normal growth.
- Note: Drug's excitatory and euphoric effects are associated with a high abuse potential.

Patient & Family Education

- Keep physician informed of clinical response and persistent or bothersome adverse effects. This drug exerts a stimulating effect that masks fatigue; after exhilaration disappears, fatigue and depression are usually greater than before, and a longer period of rest is needed.
- Report insomnia or undesired weight loss.
- Do not drive or engage in potentially hazardous tasks until response to drug is known.
- Rinse mouth frequently with clear water, especially after eating, to relieve mouth dryness; increase fluid intake, if allowed; chew sugarless gum or sourballs.
- Note: Meticulous oral hygiene is required because decreased saliva encourages demineralization of tooth surfaces and mucosal erosion. Use of a commercially available oral lubricant, such as Moi-Stir or Xero-Lube, can relieve soft tissue problems and reduce the potential of tooth decay.
- Note: Appetite suppression usually lessens within a few weeks and appetite increases; dose increase is not indicated.

- Avoid caffeine-containing beverages because caffeine increases amphetamine effects.
- Note that drug is usually tapered gradually following prolonged administration of high doses. Abrupt withdrawal may result in lethargy, profound depression, or other psychotic manifestations that may persist for several weeks.
- Do not breast feed while taking this drug without consulting physician.

AMPHOTERICIN B (Pr)

(am-foe-ter′i-sin)

Amphocin, Fungizone

AMPHOTERICIN B LIPID-BASED

Abelcet, Amphotec, AmBisome

Classifications: ANTIINFECTIVE; ANTIFUNGAL ANTIBIOTIC

Pregnancy Category: B

AVAILABILITY **Abelcet** 100 mg/ 20 mL suspension for injection **Amphotec** 50 mg, 100 mg powder for injection **AmBisome** 50 mg powder for injection **Fungizone** 50 mg powder for injection; 100 mg/ mL suspension; 3% cream, lotion, ointment

ACTIONS Fungistatic antibiotic produced by *Streptomyces nodosus*. Fungicidal at higher concentrations, depending on sensitivity of fungus.

THERAPEUTIC EFFECTS Exerts antifungal action on both resting and growing cells at least in part by selectively binding to sterols in fungus cell membrane.

USES Used intravenously for a wide spectrum of potentially fatal systemic fungal (mycotic) infections including aspergillosis, blastomycosis, coccidioidomycosis, cryptococcosis, disseminated candidiasis, histoplasmosis, paracoccidioidomycosis, sporotrichosis, and others. Has been used to potentiate antifungal effects of flucytosine (*Ancobon*) and to provide anticandidal prophylaxis in certain susceptible patients receiving immunosuppressive therapy. Used topically for cutaneous and mucocutaneous infections caused by *Candida* (monilia). *Abelcet:* aspergillosis.

UNLABELED USES Treatment of candiduria, fungal endocarditis, meningitis, septicemia; fungal infections of urinary bladder and urinary tract; amebic meningoencephalitis, and paracoccidioidomycosis.

CONTRAINDICATIONS Hypersensitivity to amphotericin.

CAUTIOUS USE Severe bone marrow depression or renal function impairment. Safety during pregnancy (category B) or lactation is not established.

ROUTE & DOSAGE

Systemic Infections [Amphocin, Fungizone]

Adult: **IV Test Dose** 1 mg dissolved in 20 mL of D5W by slow infusion (over 10–30 min) **IV Maintenance Dose** 0.25–0.3 mg/ kg/day infused over 4–6 h, may gradually increase by 0.5–0.75 mg/kg/d up to 1–1.5 mg/kg/d
Child: **IV Test Dose** 0.1 mg/kg up to 1 mg dissolved in 20 mL of D5W by slow infusion (over 10–30 min) **IV Maintenance Dose** 0.4 mg/kg/d infused over 4–6 h, may increase by 0.25 mg/kg/d to target dose of 0.25–1 mg/kg/ d infused over 2–6 h

[Abelcet]

Adult/Child: **IV** 3–5 mg/kg/d infused at 2.5 mg/kg/h

[Amphotec]

Adult/Child: **IV Test Dose** 10 mL (1.6–8.3 mg) of initial dose infused over 10–30 min **IV Maintenance Dose** 3–4 mg/kg/d (max: 7.5 mg/kg/d) infused at 1 mg/kg/h

[AmBisome]

Adult/Child: **IV** 3–5 mg/kg/d infused over 1–2 h

Cryptococcal Meningitis in HIV [AmBisome]

Adult: **IV** 6 mg/kg/d infused over 2 h

Candiduria [Amphocin, Fungizone]

Adult: **Irrigation** 5–50 mg/1000 mL sterile water instilled continuously into the bladder via a 3-way closed drainage catheter system at a rate of 1000 mL/24 h

Oral Candidiasis [Fungizone]

Adult/Child: **PO** 100 mg swish & swallow q.i.d.

Cutaneous Candidiasis [Fungizone]

Adult/Child/Infant: **Topical** apply to lesions 2–4 times/d for 1–4 wks

ADMINISTRATION

Oral

- Instruct patient not to swallow drug immediately, but swish carefully to coat lesions.
- Store according to manufacturer's recommendations.

Topical Application

- Do not cover with plastic wrap, plastic cloth, rubber, or other occlusive dressings. Ask physician to specify when and how lesions are to be washed.
- Discontinue topical treatment promptly if signs of hypersensitivity, irritation, or worsening of lesions occurs.
- Store topical forms in well-closed containers at room temperature, 15°–30° C (59°–86° F), unless otherwise directed.

Intravenous

PREPARE: Each brand of amphotericin is prepared differently according to manufacturer's directions. Refer to specific manufacturer's guidelines for preparation of IV solutions.

ADMINISTER: **Abelcet Intermittent:** Flush existing IV line with D5W before infusion. ▪ Use 5 micron in-line filter. Infuse total daily dose at 2.5 mg/kg/h. ▪ Shake IV bag at least q2h to evenly mix solution. **Amphotec Intermittent:** Do not use an in-line filter. ▪ Infuse total daily dose at 1 mg/kg/h. Infusion time may be shortened but should never be <2 h. Infusion time may also be extended for better tolerance. **AmBisome Intermittent:** Do not use an in-line filter. ▪ Infuse total daily dose over 2 h. Infusion time may be shortened but should never be <1 h. **Fungizone Intermittent:** Use a 1-micron filter. ▪ Infuse total daily dose over 2–6 h. Use longer infusion time for better tolerance. ▪ Alert: Rapid infusion of any amphotericin can cause cardiovascular collapse. If hypotension or arrhythmias develop interrupt infusion and notify physician. ▪ Protect IV solution from light during administration. ▪ Note incompatibilities. When given through an existing IV line, flush before and after with D5W. ▪ Initiate therapy using the most distal vein possible and alternate sites with each dose if possible to reduce the risk of thrombophlebitis. ▪ Check IV site frequently for patency.

INCOMPATIBILITIES **Solution/additive:** Any **saline**-containing solution (precipitate will form), PARENTERAL NUTRITION SOLUTIONS, **calcium chloride, calcium gluconate, cimetidine, edetate calcium disodium, metaraminol, methyldopa, polymyxin, potassium chloride, ranitidine, verapamil**. **Y-site:** AMINOGLYCOSIDES, PENICILLINS, PHENOTHIAZINES, **clindamycin, cotrimoxazole, diphenhydramine, dopamine, dobutamine, heparin** (flush lines with D5W, not NS), **lidocaine, procaine, tetracycline, fluconazole, vitamins, TPN.**

▪ Do not mix Abelcet or Amphotec with any other drugs.

▪ Store according to manufacturer's recommendations for reconstituted and unopened vials.

ADVERSE EFFECTS (≥1%) **Body as a Whole:** Hypersensitivity (pruritus, urticaria, skin rashes, fever, dyspnea, <u>anaphylaxis</u>); *fever, chills*. **CNS:** Headache, sedation, muscle pain, arthralgia, weakness. **CV:** Hypotension, <u>cardiac arrest</u>. **Special Senses:** Ototoxicity with tinnitus, vertigo, loss of hearing. **GI:** nausea, vomiting, diarrhea, epigastric cramps, anorexia, weight loss. **Hematologic:** Anemia, thrombocytopenia. **Metabolic:** *Hypokalemia, hypomagnesemia*. **Urogenital:** <u>Nephrotoxicity</u>, urine with low specific gravity. **Skin:** Dry, erythema, pruritus, burning sensation; allergic contact dermatitis, exacerbation of lesions. **Other:** Pain; arthralgias, thrombophlebitis (IV site), superinfections.

INTERACTIONS Drug: AMINOGLYCOSIDES, **capreomycin, cisplatin, carboplatin, colistin, cyclosporine, mechlorethamine, furosemide, vancomycin** increase the possibility of nephrotoxicity; CORTICOSTEROIDS potentiate hypokalemia; with DIGITALIS GLYCOSIDES, hypokalemia increases the risk of **digitalis** toxicity.

PHARMACOKINETICS Peak: 1–2 h after IV infusion. **Duration:** 20 h. **Distribution:** Minimal amounts enter CNS, eye, bile, pleural, pericardial, synovial, or amniotic fluids; similar plasma and urine concentrations. **Elimination:** Excreted renally; can be detected in blood up to 4 wk and in urine for 4–8 wk after discontinuing therapy. **Half-Life:** 24–48 h.

NURSING IMPLICATIONS

Assessment & Drug Effects

- Lab tests: Baseline C&S tests prior to initiation of therapy; start drug pending results. Baseline and periodic BUN, serum creatinine, creatinine clearance; during therapy periodic CBC, serum electrolytes (especially K^+, Mg^{++}, Na^+, Ca^{++}), and liver function tests.
- Monitor for S&S of local inflammatory reaction or thrombosis at injection site, particularly if extravasation occurs.
- Monitor cardiovascular and respiratory status and observe patient closely for adverse effects during initial IV therapy. If a test dose (1 mg over 20–30 min) is given, monitor vital signs every 30 min for at least 4 h. Febrile reactions (fever, chills, headache, nausea) occur in 20%–90% of patients, usually 1–2 h after beginning infusion, and subside within 4 h after drug is discontinued. The severity of this reaction usually

Common adverse effects in *italic*, life-threatening effects <u>underlined</u>: generic names in **bold**; classifications in SMALL CAPS; ♣ Canadian drug name; ⓟ Prototype drug

decreases with continued therapy. Keep physician informed.

- Monitor I&O and weight. Report immediately oliguria, any change in I&O ratio and pattern, or appearance of urine (e.g., sediment, pink or cloudy urine [hematuria]), abnormal renal function tests, unusual weight gain or loss. Generally, renal damage is reversible if drug is discontinued when first signs of renal dysfunction appear.
- Report to physician and withhold drug, if BUN exceeds 40 mg/dL or serum creatinine rises above 3 mg/dL. Dosage should be reduced or drug discontinued until renal function improves.
- Consult physician about the appearance of mild erythema surrounding topical application to skin lesions. This may be an indication to reduce frequency of topical application.
- Consult physician for guidelines on adequate hydration and adjustment of daily dose as a possible means of avoiding or minimizing nephrotoxicity.
- Report promptly any evidence of hearing loss or complaints of tinnitus, vertigo, or unsteady gait. Tinnitus may not be a complaint in older adults or the very young. Other signs of ototoxicity (i.e., vertigo or hearing loss) are more reliable indicators of ototoxicity in these age groups.

Patient & Family Education

- Notify physician if improvement does not occur within 1–2 wk or if lesions appear to worsen. Nail infections usually require several months or longer to improve.
- Wash towels and clothing that were in contact with affected areas after each treatment.
- Note: Topical cream slightly discolors the skin. Generally, lotion and ointment do not stain skin when rubbed in, but nail lesions may be stained.
- Do not breast feed while taking this drug without consulting physician.

AMPICILLIN (Pr)

(am-pi-sill′in)

Amcill, Ampicin, Novo-Ampicillin ♣, Omnipen, Penbritin ♣, Pfizerpen-A, Polycillin, Principen, SK-Ampicillin, Totacillin

AMPICILLIN SODIUM

Ampicin ♣, Omnipen-N, Penbritin ♣, Polycillin-N, SK-Ampicillin-N, Totacillin-N

Classifications: ANTIINFECTIVE; ANTIBIOTIC; AMINOPENICILLIN

Pregnancy Category: B

AVAILABILITY 250 mg, 500 mg capsules; 125 mg/5 mL, 250 mg/5 mL oral suspension; 125 mg, 250 mg, 500 mg, 1 gm, 2 gm vials

ACTIONS A broad-spectrum semisynthetic, aminopenicillin is highly bactericidal even at low concentrations, but is inactivated by penicillinase (beta-lactamase).

THERAPEUTIC EFFECTS Active against gram-positive microorganisms such as *alpha-* and *beta-Hemolytic streptococci, Diplococcus pneumoniae,* non-penicillinase producing *Staphylococci,* and *Listeria.* Major advantage over penicillin G is enhanced action against most strains of *Enterococci* and several gram-negative strains including *Escherichia coli, Neisseria gonorrhoeae, N. meningitidis, Haemophilus influenzae, Proteus mirabilis, Salmonella* (including typhosa), and *Shigella.* Inactive against *Mycoplasma,* rickettsiae, fungi, and viruses.

USES Infections of GU, respiratory, and GI tracts and skin and soft tissues; also gonococcal infections, bacterial meningitis, otitis media, sinusitis, and septicemia and for prophylaxis of bacterial endocarditis. Used parenterally only for moderately severe to severe infections.

CONTRAINDICATIONS Hypersensitivity to penicillin derivatives; infectious mononucleosis.
CAUTIOUS USE History of severe reactions to cephalosporins; pregnancy (category B) or lactation.

ROUTE & DOSAGE

Systemic Infections
Adult: **PO** 250–500 mg q6h **IV/IM** 250 mg–2 g q6h
Child: **PO** 25–50 mg/kg/d divided q6h **IV/IM** 25–100 mg/kg/d divided q6h
Neonate: **IV/IM** *≤7 d & ≤2000 g,* 50 mg/kg/d divided q12h; *≤7 d & >2000 g,* 75 mg/kg/d divided q8h; *>7 d,* 50–100 mg/kg/d divided q6–12h

Meningitis
Adult/Child: **IV** 150–200 mg/kg/d divided q4–6h
Neonate: **IV/IM** *≤7 d & ≤2000 g,* 100 mg/kg/d divided q12h; *≤7 d & >2000 g,* 150 mg/kg/d divided q8h; *>7 d,* 100–200 mg/kg/d divided q6–12h

Gonorrhea
Adult: **PO** 3.5 g with 1 g probenecid times 1 **IV/IM** 500 mg q8–12h

ADMINISTRATION

Oral
- Give with a full glass of water on an empty stomach (at least 1 h before or 2 h after meals) for maximum absorption. Food hampers rate and extent of oral absorption.

Intramuscular
- Reconstitute each vial by adding the indicated amount of sterile water for injection or bacteriostatic water for injection (1.2 mL to 125 mg; 1 mL to 250 mg; 1.8 mL to 500 mg; 3.5 mL to 1 g; 6.8 mL to 2 g). All reconstituted vials yield 250 mg/mL except the 125 mg vial which yields 125 mg/mL. Administer within 1 h of preparation.
- Withdraw the ordered dose and inject deep IM into a large muscle.

Intravenous

Verify correct IV concentration and rate of infusion with physician for administration to neonates, infants, and children.

PREPARE: **Direct/Intermittent:** Reconstitute each 500 mg or less with at least 5 mL of sterile water for injection. Final concentration must be ≤30 mg/mL; thus may be further diluted in 50 mL or more of NS, D5W, D5/NS, D5W/0.45NS, or RL. ■ Stability of solution varies with diluent and concentration of solution. Solutions in NS are stable for up to 8 h at room temperature; other solutions should be infused within 2–4 h of preparation. Give direct IV within 1 h of preparation. ■ Wear disposable gloves when handling drug repeatedly; contact dermatitis occurs frequently in sensitized individuals.

ADMINISTER: **Direct/Intermittent:** Slowly over at least 15 min. ■ With solutions of 100 mL or more, set rate according to amount of solution, but no faster than direct IV rate. ■ Convulsions may be induced by too rapid administration.

INCOMPATIBILITIES **Solution/additive:** Do not **add to a dextrose** containing solution unless entire dose is given within 1 hour of preparation.

- Store capsules and unopened vials at 15°–30° C (59°–86° F) unless otherwise directed. Keep oral preparations tightly covered.

ADVERSE EFFECTS (≥1%) **Body as a Whole:** Similar to those for penicillin G. Hypersensitivity (pruritus, urticaria, eosinophilia, hemolytic anemia, interstitial nephritis, anaphylactoid reaction); superinfections. **CNS:** Convulsive seizures with high doses. **GI:** *Diarrhea,* nausea, vomiting, pseudomembranous colitis. **Other:** Severe pain (following IM); phlebitis (following IV); **Skin:** *Rash.*

DIAGNOSTIC TEST INTERFERENCE Elevated ***CPK*** levels may result from local skeletal muscle injury following IM injection. ***Urine glucose:*** high urine drug concentrations can result in false-positive test results with ***Clinitest*** or ***Benedict's*** (enzymatic ***glucose oxidase methods,*** e.g., ***Clinistix, Diastix, TesTape,*** are not affected). ***AST*** may be elevated (significance not known).

INTERACTIONS Drug: Allopurinol increases incidence of rash. Effectiveness of the AMINOGLYCOSIDES may be impaired in patients with severe end-stage renal disease. **Chloramphenicol, erythromycin,** and **tetracycline** may reduce bactericidal effects of ampicillin; this interaction is primarily significant when low doses of ampicillin are used. Ampicillin may interfere with the contraceptive action of oral contraceptives **Estrogens.** Female patients should be advised to consider nonhormonal contraception while on antibiotics. **Food:** Food may decrease absorption of ampicillin, so it should be taken 1 h before or 2 h after meals.

PHARMACOKINETICS Absorption: Oral dose is 50% absorbed. Peak effect: 5 min IV, 1 h IM, 2 h PO. **Duration:** 6–8 h. **Distribution:** Most body tissues; high CNS concentrations only with inflamed meninges; crosses the placenta. **Metabolism:** Minimal hepatic metabolism. **Elimination:** 90% excreted in urine; excreted into breast milk. **Half-Life:** 1–1.8 h.

NURSING IMPLICATIONS

Assessment & Drug Effects

- Determine previous hypersensitivity reactions to penicillins, cephalosporins, and other allergens prior to therapy.
- Lab tests: Baseline C&S tests prior to initiation of therapy; start drug pending results. Baseline and periodic assessments of renal, hepatic, and hematologic functions, particularly during prolonged or high-dose therapy.
- Note: Sodium content of drug must be considered in patients on sodium restriction.
- Inspect skin daily and instruct patient to do the same. The appearance of a rash should be carefully evaluated to differentiate a nonallergenic ampicillin rash from a hypersensitivity reaction. Report rash promptly to physician.
- Note: Incidence of ampicillin rash is higher in patients with infectious mononucleosis or other viral infections, *Salmonella* infections, lymphocytic leukemia, or hyperuricemia or in patients taking allopurinol.
- Take medication around the clock; continue taking medica-

tion until it is all gone (usually 10 d) unless otherwise directed by physician or pharmacist.

Patient & Family Education

- Note: Ampicillin rash is believed to be nonallergenic and therefore its appearance is not an absolute contraindication to future therapy.
- Report diarrhea to physician; do not self-medicate. Give a detailed report to the physician regarding onset, duration, character of stools, associated symptoms, temperature and weight loss (if any) to help rule out the possibility of drug-induced, potentially fatal pseudomembranous colitis (see Appendix F).
- Report S&S of superinfection (onset of black, hairy tongue; oral lesions or soreness; rectal or vaginal itching; vaginal discharge; loose, foul-smelling stools; or unusual odor to urine).
- Notify physician if no improvement is noted within a few days after therapy is started.
- Do not breast feed while taking this drug without consulting physician.

AMPICILLIN SODIUM AND SULBACTAM SODIUM

(am-pi-sill'in/sul-bak'tam)

Unasyn

Classifications: ANTIINFECTIVE; ANTIBIOTIC; AMINOPENICILLIN

Prototype: Ampicillin

Pregnancy Category: B

AVAILABILITY 1.5 gm, 3 gm vials

ACTIONS Antibiotic agent with broad spectrum of activity resulting from beta-lactamase inhibition. Sulbactam inhibits beta-lactamases most frequently responsible for transferred drug resistance. Because of this action, a wide range of beta-lactamases found in organisms resistant to penicillins and cephalosporins are inhibited.

THERAPEUTIC EFFECTS Effective against both gram-positive and gram-negative bacteria including those that produce beta-lactamase and nonbeta-lactamase producers. Ampicillin without sulbactam is not effective against beta-lactamase producing strains.

USES Treatment of infections due to susceptible organisms in skin and skin structures (e.g., *Klebsiella pneumoniae, Staphylococcus aureus*) and intraabdominal infections (e.g., *Escherichia coli*) and for gynecologic infections (e.g., *Bacteroides* sp. including *B. fragilis*). Also used for infections caused by ampicillin-susceptible organisms.

CONTRAINDICATIONS Hypersensitivity to penicillins; mononucleosis.

CAUTIOUS USE Hypersensitivity to cephalosporins; pregnancy (category B) or lactation.

ROUTE & DOSAGE

Systemic Infections

Adult/Child: **IV/IM** *≥40 kg,* 1.5 (1 g ampicillin, 0.5 g sulbactam) to 3 g (2 g ampicillin, 1 g sulbactam) q6h (max: 4 g sulbactam/d)
Child: **IV** *≥1 y,* 300 mg/kg/d (200 mg/kg ampicillin and 100 mg/kg sulbactam) divided q6h

ADMINISTRATION

Intramuscular

- Reconstitute solution with sterile water for injection by adding 6.4 mL diluent to a 3 g vial. Each mL contains 250 mg ampicillin and 125 mg sulbactam.

- Give deep IM into a large muscle. Rotate injection sites.

Intravenous

PREPARE: **Direct/Intermittent:** Reconstitute each 1.5 g with 3.2 mL of sterile water for injection to yield 375 mg/mL (250 mg ampicillin/125 mg sulbactam); further dilute with NS, D5W, D5/NS, D5W/0.45NS, or RL to a final concentration within the range of 3–45 mg/mL.
ADMINISTER: **Direct/Intermittent:** Give slowly over at least 15 min. With solutions of 100 mL or more, set rate according to amount of solution but no faster than direct IV rate. ■ Convulsions may be induced by too rapid administration. ■ Use only freshly prepared solution; administer within 1 h after preparation.
INCOMPATIBILITIES **Solution/additive:** Do not add to a **dextrose**-containing solution unless entire dose is given within 1 hour of preparation.

- Store powder for injection at 15°–30° C (59°–86° F) before reconstitution. Storage times and temperatures vary for different concentrations of reconstituted solutions; consult manufacturer's directions.

ADVERSE EFFECTS (≥1%) **Body as a Whole:** Hypersensitivity (rash, itching, anaphylactoid reaction), fatigue, malaise, headache, chills, edema. **GI:** *Diarrhea, nausea,* vomiting, abdominal distention, candidiasis. **Hematologic:** Neutropenia, thrombocytopenia. **Urogenital:** Dysuria. **CNS:** Seizures. **Other:** Local pain at injection site; thrombophlebitis.

INTERACTIONS Drug: Allopurinol increases incidence of rash; effectiveness of the AMINOGLYCOSIDES may be impaired in patients with severe end stage renal disease; **chloramphenicol, erythromycin, tetracycline** may reduce bactericidal effects of ampicillin—this interaction is primarily significant when low doses are used; ampicillin may interfere with the contraceptive action of ORAL CONTRACEPTIVES—female patients should be advised to consider nonhormonal contraception while on antibiotics.

PHARMACOKINETICS Peak: Immediate after IV. **Duration:** 6–8 h. **Distribution:** Most body tissues; high CNS concentrations only with inflamed meninges; crosses placenta; appears in breast milk. **Metabolism:** Minimal hepatic metabolism. **Elimination:** Excreted in urine. **Half-Life:** 1 h.

NURSING IMPLICATIONS

Assessment & Drug Effects

- Determine previous hypersensitivity reactions to penicillins, cephalosporins, and other allergens prior to therapy.
- Lab tests: Baseline C&S tests prior to initiation of therapy; start drug pending results.
- Report promptly unexplained bleeding (e.g., epistaxis, purpura, ecchymoses).
- Monitor patient carefully during the first 30 min after initiation of IV therapy for signs of hypersensitivity and anaphylactoid reaction (see Appendix F). Serious anaphylactoid reactions require immediate use of emergency drugs and airway management.
- Observe for and report symptoms of superinfections (see Appendix F). Withhold drug and notify physician.

- Monitor I&O ratio and pattern. Report dysuria, urine retention, and hematuria.

Patient & Family Education
- Report chills, wheezing, pruritus (itching), respiratory distress, or palpitations to physician immediately.
- Do not breast feed while taking this drug without consulting physician.

AMPRENAVIR

(am-pre'na-vir)
Agenerase
Classifications: ANTIINFECTIVE; ANTIRETROVIRAL AGENT; PROTEASE INHIBITOR
Prototype: Saquinavir
Pregnancy Category: C

AVAILABILITY 50 mg capsules; 15 mg/mL oral solution

ACTIONS Amprenavir inhibits the activity of HIV-1 protease enzyme and thus prevents the cleavage of viral polyproteins essential for the maturation and proliferation of the HIV-1 virus.
THERAPEUTIC EFFECTS The protease inhibitor activity results in the formation of immature, noninfectious viral particles. Amprenavir results in reduction of the viral load (HIV-RNA) in the plasma and an increase in the CD_4 lymphocyte cell count.

USES Treatment of HIV infection in combination with other antiretroviral agents.

CONTRAINDICATIONS Prior sensitivity to amprenavir; pregnancy (category C); lactation, oral solution in children <4 y, infants, neonates; renal failure.

CAUTIOUS USE History of hypersensitivity to other protease inhibitors (e.g., indinavir, ritonavir, saquinavir); hypersensitivity to sulfonamides; hepatic dysfunction; diabetes mellitus; diabetic ketoacidosis, hemophilia A and B; vitamin K deficiencies; anticoagulant therapy, oral contraceptives; coadministration with rifampin or sildenafil; antimicrobial resistance, hypercholesterolemia, hypertriglycerides, hyperglycemia, females, children, hepatic or renal impairment.

ROUTE & DOSAGE

HIV Infection
Adult/Adolescent: **PO** 1200 mg capsules b.i.d.
Child: **PO** *4–12 y or <50 kg,* 20 mg/kg b.i.d. capsules or 15 mg/kg t.i.d. capsules (max: 2400 mg/d); 22.5 mg/kg b.i.d. oral solution or 17 mg/kg t.i.d. oral solution
Hepatic Impairment
Child-Pugh score of 5–8 give 450 mg b.i.d., Child-Pugh score 9–12 give 300 mg b.i.d.

ADMINISTRATION

Oral
- Give without regard to food, BUT not with high fat meal.
- Capsules & oral solution are not interchangeable on mg-for-mg basis.
- Give 1 h before/after antacid.
- Store tablets at 20°–25° C (68°–77° F). Do not refrigerate.

ADVERSE EFFECTS (≥1%) **CNS:** *Oral/perioral paresthesia,* peripheral paresthesia, depression, mood disorders. **GI:** *Nausea, vomiting, diarrhea,* taste disorders, increased triglycerides, hyperglycemia. **Skin:** *Rash,* <u>Stevens-Johnson syndrome</u>.

INTERACTIONS Drug: Administration with **amiodarone, astemizole, bepridil, cisapride, dihydroergotamine, ergotamine, lidocaine, midazolam, quinidine, triazolam,** and TRICYCLIC ANTIDEPRESSANTS may cause life-threatening reactions; **rifampin, rifabutin,** ORAL CONTRACEPTIVES, **phenobarbital, phenytoin, carbamazepine** decrease **amprenavir** concentrations; **amprenavir** may increase **dihydroergotamine, ergotamine sildenafil** concentrations and toxicity; **amprenavir** may decrease **methadone** levels; monitor INR with **warfarin; oral solution** may cause antabuse reaction with **disulfiram, metronidazole. Food:** Decreased absorption with high-fat meal. **Herbal: St. John's wort** may decrease antiretroviral activity.

PHARMACOKINETICS Absorption: Oral solution is less absorbed than capsules. **Peak:** 1–2 h. **Distribution:** 90% bound to plasma proteins. **Metabolism:** Metabolized in liver by CYP3A4. **Elimination:** 14% excreted in urine, 75% excreted in feces as metabolites. **Half-Life:** 7.1–10.6 h.

NURSING IMPLICATIONS

Assessment & Drug Effects

- Monitor for therapeutic effectiveness which is indicated by elevated CD_4 count & decreased HIV RNA copies.
- Monitor for & promptly notify physician of severe skin rash.
- Lab tests: Monitor blood glucose & HbA_{1c}, Hgb & Hct, and lipid profile at periodic intervals.
- Note: Monitor blood levels for coadministered drugs including amiodarone, lidocaine, phenobarbital, phenytoin, quinidine, tricyclic antidepressants; monitor PT and INR with warfarin.

Patient & Family Education

- Follow directions for taking this drug (see ADMINISTRATION).
- Take drug exactly as prescribed at the indicated times. Missed dose: if less than 4 h, wait until the next scheduled dose; otherwise, take immediately.
- Do not take supplemental vitamin E with this drug unless approved by physician.
- Notify physician promptly about skin rash, nausea, vomiting, diarrhea, numbness or tingling around mouth or hands & feet.
- Inform physician of all other prescription/nonprescription drugs being taken. Serious interactions can occur.
- Use alternative barrier contraceptives rather than hormonal contraceptives while taking this drug.
- Note: Redistribution/accumulation of body fat may occur.
- Note: Diabetics may experience loss of glycemic control.
- Do not breast feed while taking this drug.

AMRINONE LACTATE IS NOW INAMRINONE LACTATE

[Note: The generic name amrinone was changed in 2000 to avoid confusion with other drugs.]

AMYL NITRITE

(am′il)

Amyl Nitrite

Classifications: CARDIOVASCULAR AGENT; NITRATE VASODILATOR; ANTIDOTE

Prototype: Nitroglycerin

Pregnancy Category: C

AVAILABILITY 0.3 mL ampules

ACTIONS Short-acting vasodilator and smooth muscle relaxant with actions similar to those of nitroglycerin. Action in treatment of cyanide poisoning based on ability of amyl nitrite to convert hemoglobin to methemoglobin, which forms a nontoxic complex with cyanide ion.

THERAPEUTIC EFFECTS Used for vasodilation of the cardiac vessels and immediate treatment of cyanide poisoning.

USES To relieve pain of renal and gallbladder colic. Also used as an adjunct antidote in the immediate treatment of cyanide poisoning. (Because of adverse effects, unpleasant odor, and expense, infrequently used to treat angina pectoris.)

UNLABELED USES Change intensity of heart murmurs.

CONTRAINDICATIONS Hypersensitivity to nitrites or nitrates; cerebral hemorrhage, head trauma; hypotension; glaucoma; severe anemia; hyperthyroidism; recent MI; acute alcoholism. Safety during pregnancy (category C) and lactation is not established.

ROUTE & DOSAGE

Acute Angina

Adult: **Inhalation** 0.18–0.3 mL prn

Cyanide Poisoning

Adult/Child: **Inhalation** 0.3-mL perle crushed every minute and inhaled for 15–30 s until sodium nitrite infusion is ready

ADMINISTRATION

Inhalation

- Crush ampule between fingers to prepare (amyl nitrite is available in 0.18 mL and 0.3 mL perles, which are thin, friable glass ampules enveloped with woven fabric cover).
- Instruct patient to sit a while immediately after drug is administered.
- Note: Amyl nitrite is volatile and highly flammable; when mixed with air or oxygen, it forms a mixture that can explode if ignited.
- Store at 8°–15° C (46°–59° F), unless otherwise directed. Protect from light.

ADVERSE EFFECTS (≥1%) **Body as a Whole:** Transient flushing, weakness. **CV:** Orthostatic hypotension, palpitation, cardiovascular collapse, tachycardia. **GI:** nausea, vomiting. **Hematologic:** Methemoglobinemia (large doses). **CNS:** *Headache*, dizziness, syncope. **Respiratory:** Respiratory depression.

PHARMACOKINETICS Absorption: Rapidly absorbed from mucous membranes. **Onset:** 10–30 s. **Duration:** 3–5 min.

NURSING IMPLICATIONS

Assessment & Drug Effects

- Monitor for S&S of syncope, due to a sudden drop in systolic BP, which sometimes follows drug inhalation, particularly in older adults.
- Monitor vital signs until stable. Rapid pulse, which usually lasts for a brief period, is an expected response to the fall in BP produced by the drug.
- Chart length of time required for pain to subside after administration of drug.
- Note: Tolerance may develop with repeated use over prolonged periods.

Patient & Family Education

- Note: Drug has a strongly fruity odor.
- Go to the emergency room immediately or consult physician

if no relief from angina is experienced after 3 doses 5 min apart.

- Do not breast feed while taking this drug without consulting physician.

ANAGRELIDE HYDROCHLORIDE

(a-na'gre-lyde)

Agrylin

Classifications: BLOOD FORMERS, COAGULATORS, AND ANTICOAGULANTS; ANTIPLATELET AGENT

Pregnancy Category: C

AVAILABILITY 0.5 mg, 1 mg capsules

ACTIONS Anagrelide action appears to be related to a selective inhibition of platelet production. It inhibits platelet aggregation by affecting several aggregating agents (thrombin and arachidonic acid, ADP, and collagen).

THERAPEUTIC EFFECTS Anagrelide is associated with significant decreases in platelet counts and is thought to prevent early changes in shape of platelets.

USE Essential thrombocythemia.

UNLABELED USE Polycythemia vera.

CONTRAINDICATIONS Safety during pregnancy (category C) or lactation is not established. Hypotension.

CAUTIOUS USE Cardiovascular disease, renal function impairment, hepatic function impairment. Safety and efficacy in patients <16 y are not established.

ROUTE & DOSAGE

Essential Thrombocythemia

Adult: **PO** ≥*16 y*, start with 0.5 mg q.i.d. or 1 mg b.i.d. times 1 wk, may increase by 0.5 mg/d qwk until platelet count is <600,000/mcL (max: 10 mg/d)

ADMINISTRATION

Oral

- Make sure dosage increments do not exceed 0.5 mg/d in any 1 wk.
- Store at 15°–25° C (59°–77° F) in a light-resistant container.

ADVERSE EFFECTS (≥1%) **Body as a Whole:** *Asthenia, pain, edema (general),* paresthesia, back pain, malaise, fever, chills, photosensitivity. **CNS:** Headache, *dizziness,* <u>CVA</u>, syncope, seizures. **CV:** *Palpitations,* chest pain, tachycardia, peripheral edema, CHF, <u>MI, cardiomyopathy, heart block</u>, atrial fibrillation, pericarditis, arrhythmia, hemorrhage. **GI:** *Diarrhea, abdominal pain, nausea,* flatulence, vomiting, dyspepsia, anorexia, pancreatitis, constipation, <u>GI hemorrhage</u>, and ulceration. **Hematologic:** Anemia, thrombocytopenia, ecchymoses, lymphedema. **Respiratory:** *Dyspnea,* pulmonary infiltrates, <u>pulmonary fibrosis</u>, pulmonary hypertension. **Skin:** Rash, urticaria. **Other:** Dysuria.

PHARMACOKINETICS Absorption: 70% absorbed from GI tract. Food reduces bioavailability. **Onset:** 7–14 d at appropriate dose. **Duration:** increased platelet counts were observed 4 d after discontinuing drug. **Metabolism:** Extensively metabolized. **Elimination:** Primarily excreted in urine as metabolites. **Half-Life:** 1.3–1.8 h.

NURSING IMPLICATIONS

Assessment & Drug Effects

- Monitor for therapeutic effectiveness which is indicated by reduction of platelets for at least 4 wk to ≤600,000/mcL or 50% from baseline.

- Monitor for S&S of CHF or myocardial ischemia.
- Monitor for S&S of renal toxicity in patients with renal insufficiency (creatinine ≥2 mg/dL).
- Monitor for S&S of hepatic toxicity in patients with liver functions >1.5 times upper limit of normal.
- Lab tests: Monitor platelet count q2d for first wk, weekly thereafter until maintenance dose reached; closely monitor Hgb, WBC count, liver function tests, and BUN and creatinine while platelet count is being lowered.

Patient & Family Education

- Contact physician if palpitations, fluid retention, breathing difficulty, or any other distressful symptoms develop.
- Avoid excessive exposure to sunlight or UV light.
- Do not breast feed while taking this drug without consulting physician.

ANAKINRA

(an-a-kin'ra)

Kineret

Classifications: IMMUNOMODULATOR; INTERLEUKIN-1 RECEPTOR ANTAGONIST

Pregnancy Category: B

AVAILABILITY 100 mg prefilled syringes

ACTIONS Anakinra is a recombinant human interleukin-1 type-1 receptor antagonist (IL-1R1). It blocks the biologic activity of IL-1 by inhibiting IL-1 from binding to the interleukin receptors that are present in both bone and cartilage as well as other kinds of tissues.

THERAPEUTIC EFFECTS Interleukin-1 is produced in response to inflammation. It mediates various responses of tissues including inflammatory and immunologic responses. Anakinra competes with interleukin-1 (IL-1) by inhibiting it from binding to its receptors in tissues.

USES Treatment of rheumatoid arthritis in patients that have failed other disease modifying antirheumatic drugs (DMARDs). Usually given in combination with another DMARD.

CONTRAINDICATIONS Hypersensitivity to anakinra; E. coli derived products; active infections; live vaccines.

CAUTIOUS USE Pregnancy (category B), lactation; neutropenia, immunosuppressed patients, or patients with frequent, serious infections; concomitant use of tumor necrosis factor blocking agents (TNF), etanercept, or infliximab.

ROUTE & DOSAGE

Rheumatoid Arthritis

Adult: **SC** 100 mg daily

ADMINISTRATION

Subcutaneous

- Do not give anakinra if the patient has an active infection.
- Note that anakinra should not ordinarily be given with tumor necrosis factor (TNF) blocking agents.
- Discard any unused portions as the drug contains no preservative.
- Check expiration date and do not use if expired.
- Store in the refrigerator at 2° to 8° C (36° to 46° F). DO NOT FREEZE OR SHAKE. Protect from light.

ADVERSE EFFECTS (≥1%) **Body as a Whole:** *Bacterial infections (URI,* sinusitis, flu, *other).* **CNS:** Headache. **GI:** Nausea, diarrhea, abdominal pain. **Hematologic:** Decreased neutrophil count, antibody formation. **Other:** *Injection site reactions (erythema, ecchymosis, edema, inflammation, pain).*

INTERACTIONS Drug: Increased risk of infection with live virus vaccine **etanercept, infliximab.** Increase risk of neutropenia as well as infection with **etanercept** and **infliximab.**

PHARMACOKINETICS Absorption: 95% absorbed from SC site. **Peak:** 3–7 h. **Elimination:** Excreted in urine. **Half-Life:** 4–6 h.

NURSING IMPLICATIONS

Assessment & Drug Effects

- Monitor for S&S of infection (e.g., pneumonia or other URI, cellulitis). Withhold drug and notify physician if these appear.
- Lab tests: Monitor absolute neutrophil count (ANC) prior to initiating anakinra, monthly for 3 mo, and q3mo thereafter for 1 y; monitor periodically WBC and platelet counts.
- Monitor closely patients with impaired renal function for S&S of adverse drug reactions.
- Assess for injection site reactions manifested by erythema, ecchymosis, inflammation, and pain.

Patient & Family Education

- Review carefully the "Information for Patients and Caregivers" leaflet for detailed instructions on handling and injecting anakinra.
- Give the injection at approximately the same time every day.
- Administer only 1 dose (the entire contents of 1 prefilled glass syringe) per day. Discard any unused portions as the drug contains no preservative. Do not save unused drug.
- Do not permit vaccination with live vaccines while taking anakinra.
- Withhold drug and notify physician for S&S of upper respiratory, skin, or other infection(s).
- Do not breast feed while taking this drug without consulting physician.

ANASTROZOLE Pr

(a-nas'tro-zole)

Arimidex

Classifications: ANTINEOPLASTIC; HORMONES AND SYNTHETIC SUBSTITUTES; AROMATASE INHIBITOR

Pregnancy Category: D

AVAILABILITY 1 mg tablets

ACTIONS Anastrozole is a potent and selective nonsteroidal aromatase inhibitor that converts estrone to estradiol.

THERAPEUTIC EFFECTS Anastrozole lowers estrogen levels in postmenopausal women by inhibiting adrenally generated androstenedione to estrone and estrone to estradiol. The mechanism occurs in peripheral tissues.

USES Early and advanced breast cancer in postmenopausal women with disease progression following tamoxifen therapy.

CONTRAINDICATIONS Safety during pregnancy (category D) or in children is not established.

CAUTIOUS USE Lactation, severe hepatic disease.

ROUTE & DOSAGE

Breast cancer

Adult: **PO** 1 mg once daily

ADMINISTRATION

Oral

- Give on an empty stomach, 1 h before or 2 h after meals, because food affects extent of absorption.
- Store at 20°–25° C (68°–77° F).

ADVERSE EFFECTS (≥1%) **CNS:** Asthenia, headache, hot flushes, pain, dizziness, depression, paresthesia, malaise, insomnia, confusion, anxiety, nervousness. **CV:** Chest pain, hypertension, thrombophlebitis, edema. **GI:** *Diarrhea,* nausea, vomiting, constipation, abdominal pain, anorexia, dry mouth, increased liver function tests (ALT, AST, GGT). **Respiratory:** Dyspnea, cough, pharyngitis, bronchitis, rhinitis, sinusitis. **Other:** Rash, peripheral edema, pelvic pain, flu-like syndrome.

PHARMACOKINETICS Absorption: Rapidly absorbed from GI tract. **Distribution:** 40% protein bound. **Metabolism:** 85% metabolized in liver to inactive metabolites. **Elimination:** 10% excreted unchanged; 60% as metabolites in urine. **Half-Life:** 50 h.

NURSING IMPLICATIONS

Assessment & Drug Effects

- Lab Tests: Monitor periodically liver enzymes, CBC with differential, alkaline phosphatases, total cholesterol, and lipid profile.
- Assess for hypertension, complications of edema, thrombotic events, and signs of liver toxicity.

Patient & Family Education

- Recognize common adverse effects and seek information on measures to control discomfort.
- Seek medical attention if you experience chest pain, calf pain, or shortness of breath; unexplained loss of appetite or nausea; jaundice.
- Do not breast feed while taking this drug without consulting physician.

ANISINDIONE

(an-i-sin-dye′one)

Miradon

Classifications: BLOOD FORMERS, COAGULATORS & ANTICOAGULANTS; ANTICOAGULANT

Prototype: Warfarin Sodium

Pregnancy Category: X

AVAILABILITY 50 mg tablets

ACTIONS Anisindione inhibits precursor proteins of clotting factors II, VII, IX, and X. Anisindione inhibits formation of the active form of Vitamin K. Therefore, levels of the active form of Vitamin K are depleted.

THERAPEUTIC EFFECTS Reduction of active levels of Vitamin K reduces levels of active clotting factors, and thus produces an anticoagulation effect. The anticoagulant effect inhibits further formation of thrombi. Anisindione does not have a direct thrombolytic effect.

USES Prophylaxis and treatment of venous thrombosis (including in atrial fibrillation) and pulmonary embolism; adjunct in treatment of coronary occlusion.

CONTRAINDICATIONS Pregnancy (category X); labor and delivery; lactation. Hemorrhagic tendencies or blood dyscrasias; recent cerebral hemorrhage; GI ulcer or ulcerative colitis; open wounds.

CAUTIOUS USE Recent surgery of brain, eye, spinal cord, prostate; renal or hepatic disease; severe diabetes; bacterial endocarditis, pericarditis or polyarthritis; diverticulitis or visceral carcinoma; aneurysm, severe or malignant hypertension, eclampsia, or preeclampsia; possible abortion; malnutrition, emaciation, deficiencies of Vitamin C or K; patient noncompliance; elderly females; patients deficient in protein C; congestive heart failure.

ROUTE & DOSAGE

Anticoagulation

Adult: **PO** 300 mg day 1, 200 mg day 2, then 100 mg q.d. Adjust dose to maintain desired PT level (dose range 25–250 mg)

ADMINISTRATION

Oral

- Take at the same time each day.
- Store in a tightly closed container between 15°–30° C (59°–86° F).

ADVERSE EFFECTS (≥1%) **Body as a Whole:** Pyrexia. **GI:** Nausea, vomiting, diarrhea. **Hematologic:** <u>*Hemorrhage*</u>. **Skin:** Dermatitis, urticaria, alopecia.

DIAGNOSTIC TEST INTERFERENCE Anisindione may cause alkaline urine to be red-orange; may enhance ***uric acid*** excretion, cause elevation of ***serum transaminases,*** and may increase ***lactic dehydrogenase*** activity.

INTERACTIONS Drug: In addition to the drugs listed below, many other drugs have been reported to alter the expected response to anisindione; however, clinical importance of these reports has not been substantiated. The addition or withdrawal of any drug to an established drug regimen should be made cautiously, with more frequent **INR** determinations than usual and with careful observation of the patient and dose adjustment as indicated. The following may enhance the anticoagulant effects of anisindione: **Acetohexamide, acetaminophen,** ALKYLATING AGENTS, **allopurinol,** AMINOGLYCOSIDES, **aminosalicylic acid, amiodarone,** ANABOLIC STEROIDS, ANTIBIOTICS (ORAL), ANTIMETABOLITES, ANTIPLATELET DRUGS, **aspirin, asparaginase, capecitabine, celecoxib, chloramphenicol, chlorpropamide, chymotrypsin, cimetidine, clofibrate, co-trimoxazole, danazol, dextran, dextrothyroxine, diazoxide, disulfiram, erythromycin, ethacrynic acid, fluconazole, glucagons, guanethidine,** hepatotoxic drugs, **influenza vaccine, isoniazid, itraconazole, ketoconazole,** MAO INHIBITORS, **meclofenamate, mefenamic acid, methyldopa, methylphenidate, metronidazole, miconazole, mineral oil, nalidixic acid, neomycin (oral),** NONSTEROIDAL ANTI-INFLAMMATORY DRUGS, **plicamycin,** POTASSIUM PRODUCTS, **propoxyphene, propylthiouracil, quinidine, quinine, rofecoxib, salicylates, streptokinase, sulindac,** SULFONAMIDES, SULFONYLUREAS, TETRACYCLINES, THIAZIDES, THYROID DRUGS, **tolbutamide,** TRICYCLIC ANTIDEPRESSANTS, **urokinase, vitamin E, zileuton.** The following may increase or decrease the anticoagulant effects of anisindione: **Alcohol** (acute intoxication may increase, chronic alcoholism may decrease effects), **chloral hydrate,** DIURETIC. The following may decrease the anticoagulant effects of anisindione: **barbiturates, carbamazepine, cholestyramine,** CORTICOSTEROIDS, **corticotropin, ethchlorvynol, glutethimide, griseofulvin,** LAXATIVES, **mercap-**

topurine, ORAL CONTRACEPTIVES, **rifampin, spironolactone, vitamin C, vitamin K. Herbal: Capsicum, celery, chamomile, clove, Devil's claw, Dong quai, Echinacea, fenugreek, feverfew, garlic, ginger, ginkgo, horse chestnut, licorice root, passionflower herb, tumeric, willow bark** may increase risk of bleeding; **ginseng, green tea, St. John's wort** may decrease effectiveness of anisindione.

PHARMACOKINETICS Absorption: Well absorbed. **Peak:** 2–3 d. **Duration:** 1–3 d. **Metabolism:** Metabolized in liver. **Elimination:** Excreted in urine. **Half-Life:** 3–5 d.

NURSING IMPLICATIONS

Assessment & Drug Effects

- Determine PT/INP prior to initiation of therapy and then daily until maintenance dosage is established.
- Obtain a CAREFUL medication history prior to start of therapy and whenever altered responses to therapy require interpretation; extremely IMPORTANT since many drugs interfere with the activity of anticoagulant drugs (see INTERACTIONS).
- Adjust dose to maintain PT at 1.2–1.5 times the control or another parameter set by physician.
- Lab tests: For maintenance dosage, PT/INR determinations at 1–4-wk intervals, or more often, depending on patient's response; periodic Hct, Hgb, platelet count, WBC with differential, urinalyses, stool guaiac, and liver and kidney function tests.
- Monitor closely whenever a new drug is added or removed from the regimen.
- Assess all systems carefully for S&S of hemorrhage.

Patient & Family Education

- Notify physician immediately if you experience any of the following: unusual bleeding or bruising, black or bloody stools, blood in urine, unexplained tiredness or fever, chills or sore throat, or stomach pain.
- Avoid aspirin or other anti-inflammatory pain relievers while taking this drug.
- Do not increase your consumption of foods containing vitamin K, such as liver, green leafy vegetables, broccoli, or cauliflower, without discussing your diet with your doctor.
- Do not breast feed while taking this drug.

ANISTREPLASE (APSAC)

(a-ni'strep-lase)

Eminase

Classifications: BLOOD FORMERS, COAGULATORS, AND ANTICOAGULANTS; THROMBOLYTIC ENZYME

Prototype: Alteplase

Pregnancy Category: C

AVAILABILITY 30 unit vial

ACTIONS A derivative of plasminogen streptokinase activator complex (APSAC). Activation of anistreplase occurs with deacylation of the drug.

THERAPEUTIC EFFECTS The production of plasmin from plasminogen by deacylated anistreplase can take place in the bloodstream or within the thrombus, which is more efficient. Both processes may contribute to thrombolysis.

USES Management of acute MI in adults by lysis of thrombi obstructing coronary arteries and reduction of infarct size. Initiation of treatment occurs immediately after the onset of acute MI.

CONTRAINDICATIONS Active internal bleeding, history of CVA, recent (within 2 mo) intracranial or intraspinal surgery or trauma, intracranial neoplasms, uncontrolled hypertension; severe allergic reactions to either anistreplase or streptokinase. Safety in children not established.

CAUTIOUS USE Pregnancy (category C), lactation, major surgery within preceding 10 d, cerebral vascular disease, recent GI or GU bleeding, recent trauma, hypertension, age >75 y, hemorrhagic ophthalmic conditions, current use of oral anticoagulants.

ROUTE & DOSAGE

Acute MI

Adult: **IV** 30 U IV push over 2–5 min

ADMINISTRATION

Note: Start drug as soon as possible following the onset of clinical symptoms of acute MI.

Intravenous

PREPARE: **Direct:** Dilute each dose with 5 mL sterile water for injection. ■ Slowly add diluent, rolling vial to mix; do not shake. ■ Do not further dilute reconstituted solution. ■ Diluted solution may be clear to pale yellow. ■ Do not administer if particulate matter is present. ■ Discard reconstituted solution after 30 min if not used.

ADMINISTER: **Direct:** Inject over 2–5 min directly into vein or IV line through the most proximal port. ■ During administration, only essential handling or moving of the patient should be done.

ADVERSE EFFECTS (≥1%) **Body as a Whole:** Hypersensitivity (anaphylactic and anaphylactoid reactions in <1% of patients). **CV:** Hemorrhage, *reperfusion arrhythmias, hypotension.*

PHARMACOKINETICS Onset: Immediate. **Peak:** 45 min after end of injection. **Duration:** 4–6 h. **Metabolism:** Metabolized in plasma. **Half-Life:** 105–120 min.

NURSING IMPLICATIONS

Assessment & Drug Effects

- Lab tests: Baseline and periodic aPTT, bleeding time, PT, INR, TT; also draw blood for Hct, Hgb, and platelet counts for baseline values in case of bleeding.
- Monitor vital signs q15min for first 6 h, including BP, pulse, respirations, and temperature. Report promptly bradycardia and allergic reaction.
- Monitor neurological status q30min for 6 h.
- Monitor for bleeding q15min for the first hour of therapy, every 30 min for second to eighth hour, then every 8 h.
- Protect patient from invasive procedures; IM injections are contraindicated. Also avoid potentially traumatic procedures during thrombolytic therapy to prevent bruising.
- Report signs of bleeding: gum bleeding, epistaxis, hematoma, spontaneous ecchymoses, oozing at catheter site, increased pain from internal bleeding. Interrupt infusion until bleeding stops.
- Select radial rather than femoral artery if a blood gas determination is needed because a pressure dressing can more easily be applied to it to control oozing. It may be necessary to apply pressure to puncture sites for as long as 30 min.

- Note: Patient is at risk for post-thrombolytic bleeding for 2–4 d after intracoronary anistreplase treatment. Continue monitoring vital signs until anticoagulant control is attained.

Patient & Family Education
- Report incidents of bleeding to nurse or doctor. Report blood in urine and bloody or tarry stools.
- Continue bed rest during therapy to prevent bleeding.
- Do not breast feed while taking this drug without consulting physician.

APOMORPHINE HYDROCHLORIDE

(a-po-mor'feen)

Apokyn, Apokyn Pen, Uprima

Classifications: CENTRAL NERVOUS SYSTEM AGENT; DOPAMINE RECEPTOR AGONIST; ANTIPARKINSON AGENT

Pregnancy Category: C

AVAILABILITY 10 mg/mL injection

ACTIONS Apomorphine has central dopamine receptor agonist properties. Its mechanism of action in treatment of Parkinson's is unknown, but probably is related to stimulation of centrally located postsynaptic dopamine D2-type receptors.

THERAPEUTIC EFFECTS Diminishes hypomobility associated with "off" episodes ("end-of-dose wearing off" and unpredictable "on/off" episodes) in persons with advanced Parkinson's disease.

USES Rescue of "off" episodes associated with advanced Parkinson's disease.

CONTRAINDICATIONS Concomitant use of drugs of the 5-HT_3 antagonist class (e.g., ondansetron, granisetron, dolasetron, palonosetron, and alosetron); hypersensitivity to the drug or its ingredients (i.e., sodium metabisulfite); benzyl alcohol hypersensitivity; renal failure; QT prolongation; depression, suicidal ideation; decreased alertness, seizures, seizure disorder, unconscious state or coma; pregnancy (category C); lactation.

CAUTIOUS USE Cardiovascular, cerebrovascular, respiratory, renal, or hepatic disease; CNS depression, history of (chronic) depression or suicidal ideation; hypotension; vomiting; bradycardia; hypokalemia and hypomagnesemia; older adult; hypersensitivity to sulfite.

ROUTE & DOSAGE

"Off" Episodes of Parkinson's Disease

Adult: **SC** Start with a test dose where BP can be closely monitored. Escalate test dose no sooner than 2 h after last dose until dose is not tolerated or patient has response. If test dose of 0.2 mL (2 mg) is tolerated and has positive response, continue with 0.2 mL (2 mg); if no response, use test dose of 0.4 mL (4 mg); if tolerated and has a positive response, continue with 0.3 mL (3 mg); if 0.4 mL test dose is not tolerated, try 0.3 mL (3 mg) test dose; if 0.3 mL is tolerated, continue with 0.2 mL (2 mg). May increase by 1 mg every few days, generally should not exceed 0.4 mL (4 mg) as an outpatient. Max dose: 0.6 mL as single injection and max 5 injections/d

ADMINISTRATION

Subcutaneous
- The dosing pen is marked in mL, not mg, increments; a 1 mg dose is equal to 0.1 mL.

- Aspirate to avoid intravascular injection and ensure the injection is SC and not intradermal.
- Rotate SC sites to reduce skin reactions.
- If the patient has not received apomorphine in more than 1 wk, reinstitute it by starting with the initial test dose and titrating to the desired dose.
- Apomorphine SC causes nausea and vomiting; thus the recommendation is to give 300 mg of trimethobenzamide PO t.i.d., starting 3 d before the first injection and continued for at least the first 2 mo of treatment.
- Store at 15°–30° C (59°–86° F).

ADVERSE EFFECTS (≥1%) **Body as a Whole:** Weakness, yawning, tiredness. **CNS:** CNS depression, dizziness, drowsiness, headache, lightheadedness, euphoria, restlessness, tremor, depression, *dyskinesias, hallucinations.* **CV:** Acute circulatory failure, bradycardia, hypertension, orthostatic hypotension, QT prolongation, vasovagal response, syncope. **GI:** *Nausea, vomiting,* hypersalivation, taste perversions. **Metabolic:** Peripheral edema. **Respiratory:** Respiratory depression, tachypnea, cough, pharyngitis, rhinitis. **Skin:** Contact dermatitis, *bruising,* granuloma, pruritus, sweating. **Urogenital:** *Frequent penile erections,* painful erections.

INTERACTIONS Drug: Alosetron, dolasetron, granisetron, ondansetron, palonosetron may cause severe hypotension and unconsciousness; **alfuzosin, amoxapine, bepridil, chloroquine, cisapride, clozapine, cyclobenzaprine, droperidol, flecainide, halofantrine, halothane, levomethadyl,** LOCAL ANESTHETICS, MACROLIDES **(clarithromycin, erythromycin, troleandomycin), maprotiline, mefloquine, methadone, pentamidine,** PHENOTHIAZINES, **probucol, gatifloxacin, gemifloxacin, grepafloxacin, levofloxacin, moxifloxacin, sparfloxacin, tacrolimus,** TRICYCLIC ANTIDEPRESSANTS, **amiodarone, clozapine, disopyramide, dofetilide, dolasetron, haloperidol, ibutilide, mesoridazine, palonosetron, pimozide, procainamide, quinidine, thioridazine, sotalol, ziprasidone** may exacerbate QTc prolongation; may increase CNS depression with other CNS depressants, including TRICYCLIC ANTIDEPRESSANTS, ANXIOLYTICS, SEDATIVES, HYPNOTICS, **dronabinol,** GENERAL ANESTHETICS, **mirtazapine, nefazodone,** OPIATE AGONISTS, **pramipexole, ropinirole,** SKELETAL MUSCLE RELAXANTS, **tramadol, trazodone. Herbal: Kava-kava** may increase the symptoms of Parkinson's disease.

PHARMACOKINETICS Absorption: SC absorption is dependent on site utilized—abdominal injection absorbed faster than thigh; lowering the temperature of the injection site slows absorption. **Onset:** 7–14 min. **Peak:** 40–60 min. **Duration:** Up to 2 h. **Distribution:** 85–90% protein bound. **Metabolism:** Metabolized by glucuronidation, sulfation, and N-demethylation. **Elimination:** Excreted by kidneys. **Half-Life:** 30–60 min.

NURSING IMPLICATIONS

Assessment & Drug Effects

- Periodic ECG, especially in those with known CV disease.
- Withhold drug & notify physician for S&S of torsades de pointes

(i.e., palpitations and syncope), especially in those with bradycardia or suspected hypokalemia or hypomagnesemia.

- Lab tests: Periodic serum electrolytes.
- Monitor closely for orthostatic hypotension, especially when doses are increased, and in patients taking antihypertensive medications and vasodilators (especially nitrates).

Patient & Family Education

- The dosing pen is marked in mL (not mg) increments; a 1 mg dose is equal to 0.1 mL.
- Avoid the use of alcohol while taking this drug.
- Report promptly any of the following: irregular or fast, pounding heartbeat, or palpitations; dizziness, lightheadedness, or fainting; unexplained weakness, tiredness, or sleepiness; confusion, hallucinations, or depression; unusual body movements; vomiting; or prolonged painful erections.
- Do not engage in potentially hazardous activities until reaction to drug is known.
- Do not breast feed while taking this drug.

APRACLONIDINE

(a-pra-clo′ni-deen)

Iopidine

Classifications: EYE PREPARATION; MIOTIC (ANTIGLAUCOMA AGENT)

Prototype: Pilocarpine

Pregnancy Category: C

AVAILABILITY 0.5%, 1% solution

See Appendix A-1.

APREPITANT

(a-pre′pi-tant)

Emend

Classifications: GASTROINTESTINAL AGENT; ANTIEMETIC; SUBSTANCE P NEUROKININ 1 (NK-1) RECEPTOR ANTAGONIST

Pregnancy Category: B

AVAILABILITY 80 mg, 125 mg capsules

ACTIONS Aprepitant is a selective substance P/neurokinin 1 (NK_1) receptor antagonist. Substance P and the NK-1 receptors are present in areas in the brain that control the emetic reflex. Aprepitant crosses the blood–brain barrier and occupies brain NK_1 receptors. Peripheral blockade by NK_1 receptor antagonists at receptors located in the GI is an additional hypothesized mechanism of action.

THERAPEUTIC EFFECTS Aprepitant augments the antiemetic activity of the 5-HT_3-receptor antagonist, ondansetron, and inhibits both the acute and delayed phases of emesis induced by chemotherapy agents.

USES Prevention of acute and delayed nausea and vomiting associated with moderate to severe emetogenic chemotherapy

CONTRAINDICATIONS Hypersensitivity to aprepitant; concurrent use of pimozide, terfenadine, astemizole, or cisapride; children <18 y; lactation.

CAUTIOUS USE Chemotherapeutic agents metabolized through CYP3A4; severe hepatic impairment; severe renal impairment without dialysis; pregnancy (category B).

Common adverse effects in *italic*, life-threatening effects underlined: generic names in **bold**; classifications in SMALL CAPS; ✦ Canadian drug name; Ⓟ Prototype drug

ROUTE & DOSAGE

Chemotherapy-Induced Nausea & Vomiting

Adult: **PO** 125 mg 1 h prior to chemotherapy, then 80 mg qam for the next two days in conjunction with other antiemetics

ADMINISTRATION

Oral

- Ensure that capsule is swallowed whole with a full glass of water. Do not crush or sprinkle the contents of the capsule.
- Give 1 h before start of chemotherapy.
- Store at 20°–25° C (68°–77° F). Keep the desiccant in the original bottle.

ADVERSE EFFECTS (≥1%) **Body as a Whole:** *Fatigue,* asthenia, malaise, dehydration, fever. **CNS:** Dizziness, insomnia, headache, peripheral neuropathy, sensory neuropathy, anxiety, confusion, depression. **GI:** *Constipation, diarrhea, anorexia, nausea, hiccups,* abdominal pain, gastritis, gastroesophageal reflux, abnormal or impaired taste (dysgeusia), dyspepsia, dysphagia, flatulence, hypersalivation, increased taste disturbance, increased AST and ALT. **Hematologic:** Neutropenia, anemia. **Musculoskeletal:** Pain, myalgia. **Respiratory:** Cough, dyspnea, upper or lower respiratory infection, pneumonitis, respiratory insufficiency. **Special Senses:** Tinnitus.

INTERACTIONS Drug: Increased risk of cardiovascular toxicity with **dofetilide, pimozide;** may decrease **warfarin** concentrations and INR; may decrease levels and effectiveness of ORAL CONTRACEPTIVES; **carbamazepine, griseofulvin, modafinil, rifabutin, rifapentine, phenobarbital, primidone** may decrease antiemetic efficacy; may increase levels of **dexamethasone.** Because aprepitant is a substrate of CYP3A4, many additional drug interactions are theoretically possible. **Food: Grapefruit juice** may decrease effectiveness of aprepitant. **Herbal: St. John's wort** may decrease effectiveness of aprepitant.

PHARMACOKINETICS Absorption: 60–65% of oral dose reaches systemic circulation. **Peak:** 4 h. **Duration:** 95% protein bound; readily crosses the blood–brain barrier. **Metabolism:** Metabolized in liver by CYP3A4. **Elimination:** Not renally excreted. **Half-Life:** 9–12 h.

NURSING IMPLICATIONS

Assessment & Drug Effects

- Monitor cardiac status especially with preexisting CV disease or concurrent use of any CYP3A4 substrate drug (e.g., ketoconazole, itraconazole, nefazodone, troleandomycin, clarithromycin).
- Lab tests: Monitor PT/INR 7–10 d after 3-d regimen with concurrent warfarin use; monitor phenytoin level with concurrent use; monitor serum electrolytes, UA, and CBC.

Patient & Family Education

- Report immediately to physician any of the following: skin rash; difficulty breathing or shortness of breath; rapid, slow, or irregular heartbeat; changes in BP; dizziness or confusion; unexplained sharp or severe pain in leg or stomach; rectal bleeding. Inform physician of all other drugs or herbal products you are using. Do not take new drugs (prescription, OTC, herbal) without first consulting physician.

- Use barrier contraception in addition to oral contraceptives while taking drug.
- Do not breast feed while taking this drug.

APROBARBITAL

(a-pro-bar'bi-tol)
Alurate
Classifications: CENTRAL NERVOUS SYSTEM AGENT; ANXIOLYTIC, SEDATIVE-HYPNOTIC; BARBITURATE
Prototype: Secobarbital
Pregnancy Category: D

AVAILABILITY 40 mg/5 mL elixir

ACTIONS Intermediate-acting barbiturate. These agents depress the sensory cortex, decrease motor activity, alter cerebellar function, and produce drowsiness, sedation, and hypnosis. Barbiturates have little analgesic action at subanesthetic doses and may increase the reaction to painful stimuli. All barbiturates exhibit anticonvulsant activity in anesthetic doses.
THERAPEUTIC EFFECTS Barbiturates can produce all levels of CNS mood alteration, from excitation to mild sedation, hypnosis, and deep coma. Barbiturates are respiratory depressants; the degree of respiratory depression is dose dependent. With hypnotic doses, respiratory depression is similar to that which occurs during physiologic sleep.

USES Indicated for routine sedation and as a hypnotic in the short-term treatment of insomnia for up to 2 wk. Barbiturates seem to lose their efficacy for sleep induction and maintenance after this period of time.

CONTRAINDICATIONS Barbiturate hypersensitivity; history of manifest or latent porphyria; impaired liver function; impaired renal function; severe respiratory distress, respiratory disease where dyspnea, obstruction, or cor pulmonale is present; previous addiction to the sedative-hypnotic group; acute or chronic pain. Safety during pregnancy (category D), lactation, or in children is not established.
CAUTIOUS USE Older adults or debilitated patients, presence of fever, hyperthyroidism, diabetes mellitus, severe anemia, debility, severely impaired liver function, pulmonary or cardiac disease, status asthmaticus, shock, uremia, borderline hypoadrenal function.

ROUTE & DOSAGE

Sedative
Adult: **PO** 40 mg t.i.d.
Hypnotic
Adult: **PO** 40–160 mg

ADMINISTRATION

Oral
- Determine if lower initial dose should be used in patient with impaired renal or hepatic function.
- Determine if an increase in dosage is needed for patient on dialysis.
- Note: Not to be used on prolonged basis; demonstrated effectiveness is only 2 wk.
- Store away from heat and direct light in airtight container at 15°–30° C (59°–86° F).

ADVERSE EFFECTS (≥1%) **CNS:** *Somnolence*, agitation, confusion, hyperkinesia, ataxia, vertigo, CNS depression, nightmares, lethargy, *residual sedation (hangover effect)*, paradoxical excitement, nervousness, psychiatric disturbance, hallucinations, insomnia, anxiety, dizziness, thinking abnormalities, delirium and stupor with excessive amounts. **CV:** Bradycardia, circulatory collapse, hypotension, syncope. **GI:** Nausea, vomiting, constipation, diarrhea, epigastric pain. **Hematologic:** Agranulocytosis (rare). **Respiratory:** Hypoventilation, apnea, respiratory depression, laryngospasm, bronchospasm.

DIAGNOSTIC TEST INTERFERENCE

BARBITURATES may cause a false–positive ***phentolamine test*** and decrease serum bilirubin concentrations.

INTERACTIONS Drug: CNS DEPRESSANTS, **alcohol,** SEDATIVES compound CNS depression; MAO INHIBITORS cause excessive CNS depression; ANTICONVULSANTS, **rifampin, phenmetrazine** may decrease effects of aprobarbital. **Herbal: Kava-kava, valerian** may potentiate sedation.

PHARMACOKINETICS Absorption: Well absorbed from GI tract. **Onset:** 45–60 min. **Duration:** 3 h. **Distribution:** Crosses placenta; distributed into breast milk. **Metabolism:** Metabolized in the liver. **Elimination:** Excreted in urine. **Half-Life:** 14–40 h.

NURSING IMPLICATIONS

Assessment & Drug Effects

- Monitor for severe drowsiness, severe confusion, severe weakness, shortness of breath, slow or troubled breathing, slurred speech, staggering gait, and bradycardia.
- Lab tests: Monitor hematologic studies for blood dyscrasia; monitor liver function studies with continuous or prolonged use.
- Monitor older adults for paradoxical response (i.e., irritability, marked excitement, depression, and confusion).
- Monitor phenytoin and barbiturate blood levels frequently if given concurrently because the effect of barbiturates on metabolism is unpredictable.

Patient & Family Education

- Do not increase the dose of the drug without consulting a physician.
- Avoid use of alcohol or other CNS depressants.
- Do not drive or engage in potentially hazardous tasks until response to drug is known.
- Notify physician if any of the following occurs: fever, sore throat, mouth sores, easy bruising or bleeding, nosebleed, or petechiae.
- Do not discontinue use of medication abruptly; physician may want to taper dosage to avoid possibility of withdrawal symptoms.
- Check with physician for suspected psychological or physical dependence.
- Increase vitamin D-fortified foods (e.g., milk products); drug increases vitamin D metabolism, leading to subtherapeutic levels and possible onset of osteomalacia or rickets.
- Do not breast feed while taking this drug without consulting physician.

APROTININ

(a-pro-ti′nin)

Trasylol

Classifications: BLOOD FORMERS, COAGULATORS, AND ANTICOAGULANTS; HEMOSTATIC

Prototype: Aminocaproic acid

Pregnancy Category: B

AVAILABILITY 10,000 KIU/mL injection (one KIU equals 0.14 mg)

ACTIONS Polypeptide of bovine origin that inhibits protease. By interaction with certain proteases, aprotinin has antifibrinolytic effect, hemostatic stabilizing effect, and weak anticoagulant effect.

THERAPEUTIC EFFECTS Aprotinin reduces postoperative bleeding in coronary bypass surgery patients by inhibiting fibrinolytic activity while preserving platelet adhesive function and prolonging postoperative bleeding time.

USES Prophylactically to reduce perioperative blood loss and need for blood transfusions during cardiopulmonary bypass in the course of repeat coronary artery bypass surgery. May also be used in selected cases of primary coronary artery bypass graft surgery where the risk of bleeding is especially high (i.e., impaired hemostasis, coagulopathy).

CONTRAINDICATIONS Hypersensitivity to aprotinin and bovine products.

CAUTIOUS USE Patients with heparinized blood; patients previously treated with aprotinin; pregnancy (category B). Safety and efficacy in children are not established.

ROUTE & DOSAGE

Cardiac Surgery

Adult: **IV Test Dose** 1-mL (10,000 kallikrein inactivator units [KIU]) given at least 10 min prior to loading dose (observe for signs of an allergic reaction) **IV Loading Dose** 2 million KIU over 20–30 min after induction of anesthesia, but prior to sternotomy, add 2 million KIU to the priming fluid of the cardiopulmonary priming pump **IV Maintenance Dose** Constant infusion of 500,000 KIU/h, continue until the patient leaves the OR

ADMINISTRATION

Intravenous

PREPARE: **IV Test Dose/Loading Dose:** Use as supplied (1 mL = 1.4 mg or 10,000 KIU) without further dilution.

ADMINISTER: **IV Test Dose:** Give direct IV push over 1 min. **IV Loading Dose:** Give over 20–30 min. **Continuous:** Follow with infusion at 50 mL/h. Use central venous catheter exclusively for aprotinin.

INCOMPATIBILITIES **Solution/additive:** AMINO ACIDS, CORTICOSTEROIDS, fat emulsion, **heparin,** TETRACYCLINES.

- Store at controlled room temperature.

ADVERSE EFFECTS (≥1%) **Body as a Whole:** Hypersensitivity reactions (rash, urticaria, anaphylaxis). **CV:** Tachycardia. **Hematologic:** Thromboembolism. **Skin:** Rash, urticaria. **Urogenital:** Nephrotoxicity (elevated serum creatinine). **Other:** Bronchospasm.

INTERACTIONS Drug: Heparin results in further prolongation of the whole blood activated clotting time (ACT).

PHARMACOKINETICS Distribution: Rapidly distributes into the extracellular fluid, then accumulates in proximal renal tubular epithelial cells; crosses placenta; distributed into breast milk. **Metabolism:** Metabolized primarily in kidneys to small peptides or amino acids.

Common adverse effects in *italic*, life-threatening effects underlined; generic names in **bold**; classifications in SMALL CAPS; ♣ Canadian drug name; ⊙ Prototype drug

Elimination: Excreted by kidneys. **Half-Life:** Initial 0.7 h, terminal 7 h.

NURSING IMPLICATIONS

Assessment & Drug Effects

- Monitor carefully for S&S of hypersensitivity during administration (see Appendix F). If hypersensitivity occurs, immediately discontinue aprotinin and begin emergency treatment to prevent anaphylaxis.
- Monitor cardiac status and pulmonary function carefully during infusion. Patients with a history of hypersensitivity to any allergens or who have previously received aprotinin are at special risk for hypersensitivity.
- Lab tests: After surgery, monitor aPTT, ACT, and cardiac, pulmonary, renal, and liver functions.

Patient & Family Education

- Do not breast feed while taking this drug without consulting physician.

ARGATROBAN

(ar-ga'tro-ban)

Acova, Novastan

Classifications: BLOOD FORMERS, COAGULATORS, AND ANTICOAGULANTS; THROMBIN INHIBITOR

Prototype: Lepirudin

Pregnancy Category: B

AVAILABILITY 250 mg/2.5 mL vials

ACTIONS Synthetic derivative of arginine, which is a direct thrombin inhibitor. Capable of inhibiting the action of both free and clot-bound thrombin.

THERAPEUTIC EFFECTS Reversibly binds to the thrombin active site, thereby blocking the thrombogenic activity of thrombin.

USES Prophylaxis or treatment of thrombosis in patients with heparin-induced thrombocytopenia (HIT); prophylaxis or treatment of coronary artery thrombosis during percutaneous coronary interventions (PCI) in patients at risk for HIT.

UNLABELED USE Treatment of disseminated intravascular coagulation (DIC).

CONTRAINDICATIONS Hypersensitivity to argatroban; lactation. Any bleeding including intracranial bleeding, GI bleeding, retroperitoneal bleeding.

CAUTIOUS USE Diseased states with increased risk of hemorrhaging; severe hypertension; GI ulcerations, hepatic impairment; pregnancy (category B); spinal anesthesia, stroke, surgery, trauma. Safety and effectiveness in children <18 y are not established.

ROUTE & DOSAGE

Prevention & Treatment of Thrombosis

Adult: **IV** 2 mcg/kg/min, may be adjusted to maintain an aPTT of 1.5–3 times baseline (max: 10 mcg/kg/min)

Hepatic Impairment

Adult: **IV** 0.5 mcg/kg/min, may be adjusted to maintain an aPTT of 1.5–3 times baseline (max: 10 mcg/kg/min)

Prophylaxis or treatment of coronary thrombosis during PCI

Adult: **IV** 350 mcg/kg administered via a large bore IV line over 3–5 min, then 25 mcg/kg/min by continuous infusion, maintain activated clotting time (ACT) 300–450 sec

Disseminated Intravascular Coagulation (DIC)
Adult: **IV** 0.7 mcg/kg/min continuous infusion

ADMINISTRATION

Intravenous

Note: Argatroban is supplied in 100 mg/mL vials which must be diluted 100-fold prior to infusion.

PREPARE: **Continuous:** Dilute each 2.5 mL vial by mixing with 250 mL of D5W, NS, or RL to yield 1 mg/mL. Mix by repeated inversion of the diluent bag for 1 min.
ADMINISTER: **Heparin-Induced Thrombocytopenia (HIT/HITTS): Continuous:** Before administration, discontinue heparin and obtain a baseline aPTT. Give at a rate of 2 mcg/kg/min, or as ordered. Lower initial doses are required with hepatic impairment. Check aPTT 2 h after initiation of therapy. After the initial dose, adjust dose (not to exceed 10 mcg/kg/min) until the steady-state aPTT is 1.5 to 3 times baseline (not to exceed 100 sec). Adjust dose to maintain aPTT at 1.5–3 times baseline, but not >100 sec. Check aPTT 2 h after initiation of therapy to confirm desired therapeutic range. **Percutaneous Coronary Intervention: Continuous:** Start an infusion at 25 mcg/kg/min and give a bolus of 350 mcg/kg, via a large bore IV line, over 3–5 min. Check ACT 5–10 min after the bolus dose. If the ACT is >450 sec, decrease infusion rate to 15 mcg/kg/min. Check ACT q5–10min to maintain an ACT level 300–450 sec.

- Diluted solutions are stable for 24 h at 25° C (77° F) in ambient indoor light. Protect from direct sunlight. Store solutions refrigerated at 2°–8° C (36°–46° F) in the dark.

ADVERSE EFFECTS (≥1%) **Body as a Whole:** Fever, sepsis, pain, allergic reactions (rare). **CV:** Hypotension, <u>cardiac arrest</u>, ventricular tachycardia. **GI:** Diarrhea, nausea, vomiting, coughing, abdominal pain. **Hematologic:** <u>Major GI bleed</u>, *minor GI bleeding, hematuria, decrease Hgb/Hct*, groin bleed, hemoptysis, brachial bleed. **Respiratory:** Dyspnea. **Urogenital:** UTI.

INTERACTIONS Drug: Heparin results in increased bleeding; may prolong PT with **warfarin;** may increase risk of bleeding with THROMBOLYTICS. **Herbal: Feverfew, garlic, ginger, ginkgo** may increase potential for bleeding.

PHARMACOKINETICS Peak: 1–3 h. **Distribution:** Distributes in the extracellular fluid; 54% protein bound. **Metabolism:** Metabolized in liver by CYP3A4/5. **Elimination:** Primarily excreted in bile (78%). **Half-Life:** 39–51 min.

NURSING IMPLICATIONS

Assessment & Drug Effects

- **Heparin-Induced Thrombocytopenia:** Monitor aPTT. Dose adjustment may be needed to reach the target aPTT. Check aPTT 2 h after initiation of therapy. After the initial dose, adjust dose (not to exceed 10 mcg/kg/min), until the steady-state aPTT is 1.5 to 3 times baseline (not to exceed 100 sec).
- Monitor cardiovascular status carefully during therapy.
- Monitor for and report S&S of bleeding: Ecchymosis, epistaxis, GI bleeding, hematuria, hemoptysis.

- Note: Patients with history of GI ulceration, hypertension, recent trauma, or surgery are at increased risk for bleeding.
- Monitor neurologic status and report immediately focal or generalized deficits.
- Lab tests: Baseline and periodic ACT (activated clotting time), thrombin time (TT), platelet count, Hgb & Hct; daily INR when argatroban and warfarin are co-administered; periodic stool test for occult blood; urinalysis.

Patient & Family Education

- Report immediately any of the following to physician: Unexplained back or stomach pain; black, tarry stools; blood in urine, coughing up blood; difficulty breathing; dizziness or fainting spells; heavy menstrual bleeding; nosebleeds; unusual bruising or bleeding at any site.
- Do not breast feed while taking this drug.

ARIPIPRAZOLE

(a-rip′-i-pra-zole)

Abilify

Classifications: CENTRAL NERVOUS SYSTEM (CNS) AGENT; PSYCHOTHERAPEUTIC; ANTIPSYCHOTIC; ATYPICAL

Prototype: Clozapine

Pregnancy Category: C

AVAILABILITY 10 mg, 15 mg, 20 mg, 30 mg tablets

ACTIONS Exhibits high affinity for dopamine D_2 and D_3, serotonin 5-HT_{1A} and 5-HT_{2A} receptors, moderate affinity for dopamine D_4, serotonin 5-HT_{2C} and 5-HT_7, alpha-1 adrenergic and histamine H_1 receptors, and moderate affinity for the serotonin reuptake site. Functions as a partial agonist at the dopamine D_2 and the serotonin 5-H_{1A} receptors, and as an antagonist at serotonin 5-HT_{2A} receptors.

THERAPEUTIC EFFECTS The mechanism of action is unknown. Efficacy of aripiprazole may be mediated through a combination of partial agonist activity at D_2 and 5-HT_{1A} receptors and antagonist activity at 5-HT_{2A} receptors. Actions at other receptors may explain some other clinical effects of aripiprazole (e.g., orthostatic hypotension).

USES Treatment of schizophrenia, bipolar mania.

CONTRAINDICATIONS Hypersensitivity to aripiprazole; lactation; pregnancy (category C).

CAUTIOUS USE History of seizures or conditions that lower seizure threshold (e.g., Alzheimer's dementia); suicidal ideation; brain tumor; dementia; diabetes mellitus; patients with known cardiovascular disease (history of MI or ischemic heart disease, heart failure, or conduction abnormalities), cerebrovascular disease, or conditions that predispose to hypotension (dehydration, hypovolemia, and treatment with antihypertensive medications); dysphagia; ethanol intoxication; hyperglycemia, hypothermia; obesity, elderly, children.

ROUTE & DOSAGE

Schizophrenia

Adult: **PO** 10–15 mg once daily, may increase at 2-wk intervals to max of 30 mg/d if needed

Bipolar Mania

Adult: **PO** 30 mg once daily, may reduce to 15 mg/d

ADMINISTRATION

Oral

- Note that dose should be reduced by 50% with concurrent treatment with ketoconazole, quinidine, fluoxetine, or paroxetine.
- Store at 15°–30° C (59°–86° F).

ADVERSE EFFECTS (≥1%) **Body as a Whole:** *Headache,* asthenia, fever, flu-like symptoms, peripheral edema, chest pain, neck pain, neck rigidity. **CNS:** *Anxiety, insomnia, lightheadedness, somnolence, akathisia*, tremor, extrapyramidal symptoms, depression, nervousness, increased salivation, hostility, suicidal thought, manic reaction, abnormal gait, confusion, cogwheel rigidity. **CV:** Hypertension, tachycardia, hypotension, bradycardia. **GI:** *Nausea, vomiting, constipation,* anorexia. **Hematologic:** Ecchymosis, anemia. **Metabolic:** Weight gain, weight loss, hyperglycemia, diabetes mellitus, increased creatine kinase. **Musculoskeletal:** Muscle cramp. **Respiratory:** Rhinitis, cough. **Skin:** Rash. **Special Senses:** Blurred vision.

INTERACTIONS Drug: Carbamazepine will decrease aripiprazole levels (may need to double aripiprazole dose); **ketoconazole, quinidine, fluoxetine, paroxetine** may increase aripiprazole levels (reduce dose by 1/2); may enhance effects of ANTIHYPERTENSIVE AGENTS.

PHARMACOKINETICS Absorption: Well absorbed, 87% bioavailable. **Peak:** 3–5 h. **Metabolism:** Metabolized in liver by CYP3A4 and 2D6. Major metabolite, dehydroaripiprazole has some activity. **Elimination:** 55% excreted in feces, 25% in urine. **Half-Life:** 75 h (94 h for metabolite).

NURSING IMPLICATIONS

Assessment & Drug Effects

- Monitor diabetics for loss of glycemic control.
- Monitor cardiovascular status. Assess for and report orthostatic hypotension. Take BP supine then in sitting position. Report systolic drop of >15–20 mm Hg. Patients at increased risk are those who are dehydrated, hypovolemic, or receiving concurrent antihypertensive therapy.
- Monitor body temperature in situations likely to elevate core temperature (e.g., exercising strenuously, exposure to extreme heat, receiving drugs with anticholinergic activity, or being subject to dehydration.)
- Monitor for and report signs of tardive dyskinesia.
- Monitor for and immediately report S&S of neuroleptic malignant syndrome (NMS) that include: hyperpyrexia, muscle rigidity, altered mental status, irregular pulse or blood pressure, tachycardia, diaphoresis, and cardiac dysrhythmia. Withhold drug if NMS is suspected.
- Lab tests: Monitor periodically Hct & Hgb. Monitor periodically blood glucose. Monitor for elevated CPK and myoglobinuria if NMS is suspected.

Patient & Family Education

- Carefully monitor blood glucose levels if diabetic.
- Do not drive or engage in other potentially hazardous activities until reaction to drug is known.
- Avoid situations where you are likely to become overheated or dehydrated.
- Notify physician if you become pregnant or intend to become pregnant while taking this drug.
- Do not breast feed while taking this drug.

ASCORBIC ACID (VITAMIN C)

Apo-C ✦, Ascorbicap, Cebid, Cecon, Cenolate, Cemill, C-Span, Cetane, Cevalin, Cevi-Bid, CeVi-Sol ✦, Cevita, Flavorcee, Redoxon ✦, Schiff Effervescent Vitamin C, Vita-C.

ASCORBATE, SODIUM

(a-skor'bate)

Cenolate, Cevita

Classification: VITAMIN
Pregnancy Category: C

AVAILABILITY 25 mg, 50 mg, 100 mg, 250 mg, 500 mg, 1000 mg tablets; 250 mg/mL, 500 mg/mL injection

ACTIONS Water-soluble vitamin essential for synthesis and maintenance of collagen and intercellular ground substance of body tissue cells, blood vessels, cartilage, bones, teeth, skin, and tendons. Unlike most mammals, humans are unable to synthesize ascorbic acid in the body; therefore it must be consumed daily.

THERAPEUTIC EFFECTS Increases protection mechanism of the immune system, thus supporting wound healing. Necessary for wound healing and resistance to infection.

USES Prophylaxis and treatment of scurvy and as a dietary supplement.

UNLABELED USES To acidify urine; to prevent and treat cancer; to treat idiopathic methemoglobinemia; as adjuvant during deferoxamine therapy for iron toxicity; in megadoses will possibly reduce severity and duration of common cold. Widely used as an antioxidant in formulations of parenteral tetracycline and other drugs.

CONTRAINDICATIONS Use of sodium ascorbate in patients on sodium restriction; use of calcium ascorbate in patients receiving digitalis. Safety during pregnancy (category C) or lactation is not established.

CAUTIOUS USE Excessive doses in patients with G6PD deficiency; hemochromatosis, thalassemia, sideroblastic anemia, sickle cell anemia; patients prone to gout or renal calculi.

ROUTE & DOSAGE

Therapeutic

Adult: **PO/IV/IM/SC** 150–500 mg/d in 1–2 doses
Child: **PO/IV/IM/SC** 100–300 mg/d in divided doses

Prophylactic

Adult: **PO/IV/IM/SC** 45–60 mg/d
Child: **PO/IV/IM/SC** 30–60 mg/d

Urinary Acidifier

Adult: **PO/IV/IM/SC** 4–12 g/d in divided doses
Child: **PO/IV/IM/SC** 500 mg q6–8h

ADMINISTRATION

Oral

- Give oral solutions mixed with food.
- Dissolve effervescent tablet in a glass of water immediately before ingestion.

Intramuscular, Subcutaneous

- Open ampules with caution. After prolonged storage, decomposition may occur with release of carbon dioxide and resulting increase in pressure within ampule.
- Be aware that ascorbic acid injection may gradually darken on exposure to light; slight coloration

reportedly does not affect its therapeutic action.

Intravenous

Verify correct IV concentration and rate of infusion for children with physician.

PREPARE: **Direct/Continuous/Intermittent:** Give undiluted or diluted in solutions such as NS, D5W, D5/NS, RL. ▪ Be aware that parenteral vitamin C is incompatible with many drugs. ▪ Consult pharmacist for compatibility information.

ADMINISTER: **Direct:** Give undiluted at a rate of 100 mg or a fraction thereof over 1 min. **Continuous/Intermittent:** Give at ordered rate determined by volume of solution to be infused.

INCOMPATIBILITIES **Solution/additive: Aminophylline, bleomycin, cephapirin, erythromycin, nafcillin, sodium bicarbonate, warfarin**. **Y-site: Cefazolin, doxapram, sodium bicarbonate.**

▪ Store in airtight, light-resistant, nonmetallic containers, away from heat and sunlight, preferably at 15°–30° C (59°–86° F), unless otherwise specified by manufacturer.

ADVERSE EFFECTS (≥1%) **GI:** Nausea, vomiting, heartburn, diarrhea, or abdominal cramps (high doses). **Hematologic:** Acute hemolytic anemia (patients with deficiency of G6PD); sickle cell crisis. **CNS:** Headache or insomnia (high doses). **Urogenital:** Urethritis, dysuria, crystalluria, hyperoxaluria, or hyperuricemia (high doses). **Other:** Mild soreness at injection site; dizziness and temporary faintness with rapid IV administration.

DIAGNOSTIC TEST INTERFERENCE High doses of ascorbic acid can produce false-negative results for ***urine glucose*** with ***glucose oxidase*** methods (e.g., **Clinitest, TesTape, Diastix**); false-positive results with ***copper reduction methods*** (e.g., Benedict's solution, Clinitest); and false increases in ***serum uric acid*** determinations (by ***enzymatic methods***). Interferes with ***urinary steroid*** (17-OHCS) determinations (***by modified Reddy, Jenkins, Thorn procedure***), decreases in ***serum bilirubin,*** and may cause increases in ***serum cholesterol, creatinine,*** and ***uric acid*** (methodologic inferences). May produce false-negative tests for ***occult blood*** in stools if taken within 48–72 h of test.

INTERACTIONS Drug: Large doses may attenuate hypoprothombinemic effects of ORAL ANTICOAGULANTS; SALICYLATES may inhibit ascorbic acid uptake by leukocytes and tissues, and ascorbic acid may decrease elimination of SALICYLATES; chronic high doses of ascorbic acid may diminish the effects of **disulfiram.**

PHARMACOKINETICS Absorption: Readily absorbed PO; however, absorption may be limited with large doses. **Distribution:** Widely distributed to body tissues; crosses placenta; distributed into breast milk. **Metabolism:** Metabolized in liver. **Elimination:** Rapidly excreted from body in urine when plasma level exceeds renal threshold of 1.4 mg/dL.

NURSING IMPLICATIONS

Assessment & Drug Effects

- Lab tests: Periodic Hct & Hgb, serum electrolytes.

- Monitor for S&S of acute hemolytic anemia, sickle cell crisis.

Patient & Family Education

- High doses of vitamin C are not recommended during pregnancy.
- Take large doses of vitamin C in divided amounts because the body uses only what is needed at a particular time and excretes the rest in urine.
- Megadoses can interfere with absorption of vitamin B_{12}.
- Note: Vitamin C increases the absorption of iron when taken at the same time as iron-rich foods.
- Do not breast feed while taking this drug without consulting physician.

ASPARAGINASE

(a-spar'a-gi-nase)

Colaspase, Elspar, Kidrolase A, L-asparaginase

Classifications: ENZYMES; ANTINEOPLASTIC ENZYME

Pregnancy Category: C

AVAILABILITY 10,000 IU vial

ACTIONS A highly toxic drug with a low therapeutic index. Catalyzes hydrolysis of asparagine to aspartic acid and ammonia, thus depleting extracellular supply of an amino acid essential to synthesis of DNA and other nucleoproteins.

THERAPEUTIC EFFECTS Reduced availability of asparagine causes death of tumor cells, since unlike normal cells, tumor cells are unable to synthesize their own supply. Resistance to cytotoxic action develops rapidly; therefore this is not an effective treatment for solid tumors and not recommended for maintenance therapy.

USES Primarily in combination regimens with other antineoplastic agents to treat acute lymphocytic leukemia (ALL).

UNLABELED USES Other leukemias, lymphosarcoma, and (intraarterially) treatment of hypoglycemia due to pancreatic islet cell tumor.

CONTRAINDICATIONS History of/or existing pancreatitis; chickenpox (existing or recent illness or exposure), herpetic infection. Safety during pregnancy (category C) or lactation is not established.

CAUTIOUS USE Liver impairment; diabetes mellitus; infections; history of urate calculi or gout; antineoplastic or radiation therapy.

ROUTE & DOSAGE

Induction Agent

Adult/Child: **IV** 200 IU/kg/d for 28 d, inject over at least 30 min into running IV

ADMINISTRATION

Intravenous

An intradermal skin test is usually performed prior to initial dose and when drug is readministered after an interval of a week or more; allergic reactions are unpredictable.

- Observe test site for at least 1 h for evidence of positive reaction (wheal, erythema). A negative skin test, however, does not preclude possibility of an allergic reaction.
- Administer test dose and IV infusion under constant supervision by clinician experienced in cancer chemotherapy.
- Use only clear solutions.

PREPARE: **Intermittent:** Reconstitute with sterile water or with 0.9% NaCl. ▪ Each 10,000 IU vial is diluted with 5 mL of diluent to yield 2000 IU/mL.

▪ Shake vial well to promote dissolution of powder. Avoid vigorous shaking. Ordinary shaking does not inactivate the enzyme or cause foaming of content.

ADMINISTER: **Intermittent:** Further dilute reconstituted solution with NS or D5W by administration into tubing of an already free flowing infusion of one of these solutions. ▪ Give over a period of not less than 30 min. ▪ Use a 5-mm filter to remove gelatinous fiber-like particles that can develop in solutions on standing.

▪ Store sealed vial of lyophilized powder below 8° C (46° F) unless otherwise directed by manufacturer. Store reconstituted solutions and solutions diluted for IV infusion at 2°–8° C (36°–46° F) for up to 8 h; then discard.

ADVERSE EFFECTS (≥1%) **Body as a Whole:** Hypersensitivity (*Skin rashes, urticaria*, respiratory distress, anaphylaxis), chills, fever, fatal hyperthermia, perspiration, weight loss. **CNS:** Depression, fatigue, lethargy, drowsiness, confusion, agitation, hallucinations, dizziness, Parkinson-like syndrome with tremor and progressive increase in muscle tone. **GI:** *Severe vomiting, nausea,* anorexia, abdominal cramps, diarrhea, acute pancreatitis, liver function abnormalities. **Urogenital:** Uric acid nephropathy, azotemia, proteinuria, renal failure. **Hematologic:** *Reduced clotting factors* (especially V, VII, VIII, IX), *decreased circulating platelets and fibrinogen,* leukopenia. **Metabolic:** Hyperglycemia, glycosuria, polyuria, hypoalbuminemia, hypocalcemia, hyperuricemia. **Other:** Flank pain, infections.

DIAGNOSTIC TEST INTERFERENCE Asparaginase may interfere with ***thyroid function*** tests: decreased total ***serum thyroxine*** and increased ***thyroxine-binding globulin index;*** pretreatment values return within 4 wk after drug is discontinued.

INTERACTIONS Drug: Decreased hypoglycemic effects of SULFONYLUREAS, **insulin;** increased potential for toxicity if asparaginase is given concurrently or immediately before CORTICOSTEROIDS, **vincristine; methotrexate's** antitumor effect blocked if asparaginase is given concurrently or immediately before it.

PHARMACOKINETICS Distribution: Distributed primarily into intravascular space (80%) and lymph; low levels in CSF, pleural and peritoneal fluids. **Metabolism:** Unknown. **Elimination:** Small amounts found in urine. **Half-Life:** 8–30 h.

NURSING IMPLICATIONS

Assessment & Drug Effects

- Have immediately available: Personnel, drugs, and equipment for treating allergic reaction (which may range from urticaria to anaphylactic shock) whenever drug is administered, including skin testing.
- Monitor for S&S and be alert to evidence of hypersensitivity or anaphylactoid reaction (see Appendix F) during drug administration. Anaphylaxis usually occurs within 30–60 min after dose has been given and is more likely with intermittent administrations, particularly at intervals of ≥7 d.

Common adverse effects in *italic*, life-threatening effects underlined: generic names in **bold**; classifications in SMALL CAPS; ♣ Canadian drug name; ⓟ Prototype drug

- Monitor I&O and maintain adequate fluid intake.
- Evaluate CNS function (general behavior, emotional status, level of consciousness, thought content, motor function) before and during therapy.
- Note: Toxicity potential is increased when giving drug immediately before a course of prednisone and vincristine; toxicity appears less when given after these drugs.
- Lab tests: Periodic serum amylase, serum calcium blood glucose, coagulation factors, ammonia and uric acid levels, hepatic and renal function tests, peripheral blood counts, and bone marrow function; liver function tests at least twice weekly during therapy.
- Monitor diabetics for loss of glycemic control.
- Monitor for and report S&S of hyperammonemia: anorexia, vomiting, lethargy, weak pulse, depressed temperature, irritability, asterixis, seizures, coma.
- Anticipate possible prolonged or exaggerated effects of concurrently given drugs or their toxicity because of potential serious hepatic dysfunction that reduces enzymatic detoxification of other drugs. Report incidence promptly.
- Watch for neurotoxic reaction (25% of patients) which usually appears within the first few days of therapy. It is manifested by tiredness and changing levels of consciousness (ranging from confusion to coma).
- Note: Protect from infection during first several days of treatment when circulating lymphoblasts decrease markedly and leukocyte counts may fall below normal. Report promptly S&S of infection: chill, fever, aches, sore throat.
- Report sudden severe abdominal pain with nausea and vomiting, particularly if these symptoms occur after medication is discontinued (may indicate pancreatitis).

Patient & Family Education

- Note: Therapeutic response will most likely be accompanied by some toxicity in all patients; toxicity is reportedly greater in adults than in children.
- Notify physician of continued loss of weight or onset of foot and ankle swelling.
- Notify physician without delay if nausea or vomiting makes it difficult to take all prescribed medication.
- Report onset of unusual bleeding, bruising, petechiae, melena, skin rash or itching, yellowed skin and sclera, joint pain, puffy face, or dyspnea.
- Do not drive or operate equipment that requires alertness and skill. Exercise caution with potentially hazardous activities. These effects can continue several weeks after last dose of the drug.
- Do not breast feed while taking this drug without consulting physician.

ASPIRIN (ACETYLSALICYLIC ACID) Pr

(as'pe-ren)

Alka-Seltzer, A.S.A., Aspergum, Astrin ♣, Bayer, Bayer Children's, Cosprin, Easprin, Ecotrin, Empirin, Entrophen ♣, Halfprin, Measurin, Novasen ♣, St. Joseph Children's, Supasa ♣, Triaphen-10 ♣, ZORprin

Classifications: CENTRAL NERVOUS SYSTEM AGENT; ANALGESIC, SALICYLATE; ANTIPYRETIC

Pregnancy Category: D

AVAILABILITY 81 mg chewable tablets; 325 mg, 500 mg tablets; 81 mg, 165 mg, 325 mg, 500 mg, 650 mg, 975 mg enteric-coated tablets; 650 mg, 800 mg sustained release tablets; 120 mg, 200 mg, 300 mg, 600 mg suppositories

ACTIONS Major actions appear to be associated primarily with inhibiting the formation of prostaglandins involved in the production of inflammation, pain, and fever. **Antiinflammatory action:** Inhibits prostaglandin synthesis. As an antiinflammatory agent, aspirin appears to be involved in enhancing antigen removal and in reducing the spread of inflammation in ground substances. These antiinflammatory actions also contribute to analgesic effects. **Analgesic action:** Principally peripheral with limited action in the CNS, possibly on the hypothalamus; results in relief of mild to moderate pain. **Antipyretic action:** In addition to inhibiting prostaglandin synthesis, aspirin lowers body temperature in fever by indirectly causing centrally mediated peripheral vasodilation and sweating. **Antiplatelet action:** Aspirin (but not other salicylates) powerfully inhibits platelet aggregation. High serum salicylate concentrations can impair hepatic synthesis of blood coagulation factors VII, IX, and X, possibly by inhibiting action of vitamin K.

THERAPEUTIC EFFECTS Reduces inflammation, pain, and fever. Also inhibits platelet aggregation, reducing ability of blood to clot.

USES To relieve pain of low to moderate intensity. Also for various inflammatory conditions, such as acute rheumatic fever, Systemic Lupus, rheumatoid arthritis, osteoarthritis, bursitis, and calcific tendonitis, and to reduce fever in selected febrile conditions. Used to reduce recurrence of TIA due to fibrin platelet emboli and risk of stroke in men; to prevent recurrence of MI; as prophylaxis against MI in men with unstable angina.

UNLABELED USES As prophylactic against thromboembolism; to prevent cataract and progression of diabetic retinopathy; and to control symptoms related to gluten sensitivity.

CONTRAINDICATIONS History of hypersensitivity to salicylates including methyl salicylate (oil of wintergreen); sensitivity to other NSAIDs; patients with "aspirin triad" (aspirin sensitivity, nasal polyps, asthma); chronic rhinitis; chronic urticaria; history of GI ulceration, bleeding, or other problems; hypoprothrombinemia, vitamin K deficiency, hemophilia, or other bleeding disorders; CHF. Do not use aspirin during pregnancy (category D), especially in third trimester; lactation; or in prematures, neonates, or children under 2 y, except under advice and supervision of physician. Do not use in children or teenagers with chickenpox or influenza-like illnesses because of possible association with Reye's syndrome.

CAUTIOUS USE Otic diseases; gout; children with fever accompanied by dehydration; hyperthyroidism; cardiac disease; renal or hepatic impairment; G6PD deficiency; anemia; preoperatively; Hodgkin's disease.

ROUTE & DOSAGE

Mild to Moderate Pain, Fever
Adult: **PO/PR** 350–650 mg q4h (max: 4 g/d)

Child: **PO/PR** 10–15 mg/kg in 4–6 h (max: 3.6 g/d)

Arthritic Conditions

Adult: **PO** 3.6–5.4 g/d in 4–6 divided doses
Child: **PO** 80–100 mg/kg/d in 4–6 divided doses; max 130 mg/kg/d

Thromboembolic Disorders

Adult: **PO** 325–650 mg 1 or 2 times/d

TIA Prophylaxis

Adult: **PO** 650 mg b.i.d.

MI Prophylaxis

Adult: **PO** 80–325 mg/d

ADMINISTRATION

Oral, Suppository

- Give with a full glass of water (240 mL), milk, food, or antacid to minimize gastric irritation.
- Enteric-coated tablets dissolve too quickly if administered with milk and should not be crushed or chewed.
- Store at 15°–30° C (59°–86° F) in airtight container and dry environment unless otherwise directed by manufacturer. Store suppositories in a cool place or refrigerate but do not freeze.

ADVERSE EFFECTS (≥1%) **Body as a Whole:** Hypersensitivity (urticaria, bronchospasm, anaphylactic shock (laryngeal edema). **CNS:** Dizziness, confusion, drowsiness. **Special Senses:** Tinnitus, hearing loss. **GI:** *Nausea,* vomiting, diarrhea, anorexia, *heartburn, stomach pains,* ulceration, occult bleeding, GI bleeding. **Hematologic:** Thrombocytopenia, hemolytic anemia, prolonged bleeding time. **Skin:** Petechiae, easy bruising, rash. **Urogenital:** Impaired renal function. **Other:** Prolonged pregnancy and labor with increased bleeding.

DIAGNOSTIC TEST INTERFERENCE Bleeding time is prolonged 3–8 d (life of exposed platelets) following a single 325-mg (5 grains) dose of aspirin. Large doses of salicylates equivalent to 5 g or more of aspirin per day may cause prolonged ***prothrombin time*** by decreasing prothrombin production; interference with ***pregnancy tests*** (using mouse or rabbit); decreases in ***serum cholesterol, potassium, PBI,*** T_3 and T_4 ***concentrations,*** and an increase in T_3 ***resin uptake. Serum uric acid*** may increase when plasma salicylate levels are below 10 and decrease when above 15 mg/dL using colorimetric methods. ***Urine 5-HIAA:*** aspirin may interfere with tests using fluorescent methods. ***Urine ketones:*** salicylates interfere with Gerhardt test (reaction with ferric chloride produces a reddish color that persists after boiling). ***Urine glucose:*** moderate to large doses of salicylates equivalent to an aspirin dosage ≥2.4 g/d may produce false-negative results with glucose oxidase methods (e.g., Clinistix, TesTape) and false-positive results with copper reduction methods (Benedict's solution, Clinitest). ***Urinary PSP excretion*** may be reduced by salicylates. Salicylates may cause ***urine VMA*** to be falsely elevated (by most tests), or reduced (by Pisano method). Salicylates may interfere with or cause false decreases in plasma theophylline levels using Schack and Waxler method. High plasma salicylate levels may cause abnormalities in ***liver function tests.***

INTERACTIONS Drug: Aminosalicylic acid increases risk of SALICYL-

ATE toxicity. **Ammonium chloride** and other ACIDIFYING AGENTS decrease renal elimination and increase risk of SALICYLATE toxicity. ANTICOAGULANTS increase risk of bleeding. ORAL HYPOGLYCEMIC AGENTS increase hypoglycemic activity with aspirin doses >2 g/d. CARBONIC ANHYDRASE INHIBITORS enhance SALICYLATE toxicity. CORTICOSTEROIDS add to ulcerogenic effects. **Methotrexate** toxicity is increased. Low doses of SALICYLATES may antagonize uricosuric effects of **probenecid** and **sulfinpyrazone**. **Herbal: Feverfew, garlic, ginger, ginkgo** may increase bleeding potential.

PHARMACOKINETICS Absorption: 80%–100% absorbed (depending on formulation), primarily in stomach and upper small intestine. Peak levels: 15 min to 2 h. **Distribution:** Widely distributed in most body tissues; crosses placenta. **Metabolism:** Aspirin is hydrolyzed to salicylate in GI mucosa, plasma, and erythrocytes; salicylate is metabolized in liver. **Elimination:** 50% of dose is eliminated in the urine in 2–4 h (low doses) or 15–30 h (high doses). Excreted into breast milk. **Half-Life:** Aspirin 15–20 min; salicylate 2–18 h (dose dependent).

NURSING IMPLICATIONS

Assessment & Drug Effects

- Monitor for loss of tolerance to aspirin. Previous nonreaction to salicylates does not guarantee future safety. Some individuals develop an acute and specific intolerance to aspirin, although they may have taken it for years without incident. The reaction is nonimmunologic; symptoms usually occur 15 min to 3 h after ingestion: profuse rhinorrhea, erythema, nausea, vomiting, intestinal cramps, diarrhea.
- Monitor for salicylate toxicity. In adults, a sensation of fullness in the ears, tinnitus, and decreased or muffled hearing are the most frequent symptoms associated with chronic salicylate overdosage.
- Monitor children closely because salicylate toxicity is enhanced by the dehydration that frequently accompanies fever or illness. Children tend to manifest salicylate toxicity by hyperventilation, agitation, mental confusion, or other behavioral changes, drowsiness, lethargy, sweating, and constipation.
- Monitor the diabetic child carefully for indicated need of insulin adjustment. Children on high doses of aspirin are particularly prone to develop hypoglycemia (see Appendix F).
- Note: Potential for toxicity is high in older adults and patients with asthma, nasal polyps, perennial vasomotor rhinitis, hay fever, or chronic urticaria.

Patient & Family Education

- Do not give aspirin to children or teenagers with symptoms of varicella (chickenpox) or influenza-like illnesses because of association of aspirin usage with Reye's syndrome.
- Use enteric-coated tablets, extended release tablets, buffered aspirin, or aspirin administered with an antacid to reduce GI disturbances.
- Take aspirin 1–2 d before menses when prescribed for dysmenorrhea. When experiencing heavy menstrual blood loss, take another analgesic, such as acetaminophen, instead of aspirin.
- Discontinue aspirin therapy about 1 wk before surgery to reduce risk of bleeding. Do not use aspi-

rin-containing gum or gargles or chew aspirin products for at least 1 wk following oral surgery.

- Note: Chronic use of high-dose aspirin during the last 3 mo of pregnancy can prolong pregnancy and labor, increase maternal bleeding before and after delivery, and cause weight increase and hemorrhage in the neonate.
- Discontinue aspirin use with onset of ringing or buzzing in the ears, impaired hearing, dizziness, GI discomfort or bleeding, and report to physician.
- Do not use aspirin for self-medication of pain (adults) beyond 5 d without consulting a physician. Do not use aspirin longer than 3 d for fever (adults and children), never for fever over 38.9° C (102° F) in older adults or 39.5° C (103° F) in children and adults under 60 yrs or for recurrent fever without medical direction.
- Consult physician before using aspirin for any fever accompanied by rash, severe headache, stiff neck, marked irritability, or confusion (all possible symptoms of meningitis).
- Avoid alcohol when taking large doses of aspirin.
- Observe and report signs of bleeding (e.g., petechiae, ecchymoses, bleeding gums, bloody or black stools, cloudy or bloody urine).
- Maintain adequate fluid intake when taking repeated doses of aspirin.
- Avoid other medications containing aspirin unless directed by physician, because of danger of overdosing (there are more than 500 OTC aspirin-containing compounds).
- Do not breast feed while taking this drug.

ATAZANAVIR

(a-ta-zan'a-vir)

Reyataz

Classifications: ANTI-INFECTIVE; ANTIVIRAL AGENT; ANTIRETROVIRAL AGENT; PROTEASE INHIBITOR

Prototype: Saquinavir

Pregnancy Category: B

AVAILABILITY 100 mg, 150 mg, 200 mg capsules

ACTIONS Atazanavir is an HIV-1 protease inhibitor that selectively inhibits the replication of HIV. Protease plays a major role in the virus-specific processing of viral Gag and Gag-Pol gene products into key structural proteins and replication enzymes of HIV-1 needed in the replication process of HIV-1 infected cells. Thus, protease is necessary for the production of mature virions.

THERAPEUTIC EFFECTS Protease inhibition renders the virus noninfectious. Because HIV protease inhibitors inhibit the HIV replication cycle after translation and before assembly, they are active in acutely and chronically infected cells. Thus, atazanavir reduces the viral load and increases CD4+ cell count.

USES Treatment of HIV infection in combination with other antiretroviral agents.

CONTRAINDICATIONS Hypersensitivity to atazanavir; severe hepatic insufficiency; lactation; concurrent administration of any of the following: rifampin, irinotecan, midazolam, triazolam, bepridil, dihydroergotamine, ergotamine, ergonovine, methylergonovine, lovastatin, simvastatin, pimozide, indinavir, St. John's wort; lactation; lactase deficiency.

CAUTIOUS USE Moderate hepatic impairment, hepatitis B or C; pregnancy (category B); neonates, infants, children; elderly, females, diabetes mellitus, diabetic ketoacidosis; hemophilia, hepatic disease; hepatitis; jaundice, hypercholesterolemia, hyperglycemia, hypertriglyceridemia; lactic acidosis, pancreatitis, obesity.

ROUTE & DOSAGE

HIV Infection

Adult: **PO** 400 mg once/d with a light meal; reduce dose to 300 mg once/d if giving with efavirenz or ritonavir

Hepatic Impairment

Reduce dose to 300 mg once/d in moderate hepatic insufficiency; not recommended for use in severe hepatic insufficiency

ADMINISTRATION

Oral

- Give with a light meal, not on an empty stomach.
- When coadministered with efavirenz, give atazanavir 300 mg and ritonavir 100 mg with efavirenz 600 mg (all as a single daily dose with food). Atazanavir without ritonavir should not be coadministered with efavirenz.
- When coadministered with didanosine buffered formulations, give atazanavir (with food) 2 h before or 1 h after didanosine.
- Give 2 h before/1 h after antacids or buffered drugs.
- Store at 15°–30° C (59°–86° F).

ADVERSE EFFECTS (≥1%) **Body as a Whole:** *Peripheral neuropathy,* fever, pain, fatigue, allergic reaction, angioedema, asthenia, burning sensation, chest pain, edema, facial atrophy, generalized edema, heat sensitivity, infection, malaise, pallor, peripheral edema, photosensitivity, substernal chest pain, sweating. **CNS:** *Headache,* depression, insomnia, dizziness, abnormal dream, abnormal gait, agitation, amnesia, anxiety, confusion, convulsion, decreased libido, emotional lability, hallucination, hostility, hyperkinesia, hypesthesia, increased reflexes, nervousness, psychosis, sleep disorder, somnolence, suicide attempt, twitch. **CV:** <u>Cardiac arrest</u>, heart block (PR prolongation), hypertension, myocarditis, palpitation, syncope, vasodilatation. **GI:** Hyperbilirubinemia, jaundice, *nausea, vomiting, diarrhea,* abdominal pain, anorexia, aphthous stomatitis, colitis, constipation, dental pain, dyspepsia, enlarged abdomen, esophageal ulcer, esophagitis, flatulence, gastritis, gastroenteritis, gastrointestinal disorder, hepatitis, hepatomegaly, hepatosplenomegaly, increased appetite, liver damage, liver fatty deposit, mouth ulcer, pancreatitis, peptic ulcer. **Endocrine:** Decreased male fertility. **Hematologic:** Ecchymosis, purpura. **Metabolic:** Lipodystrophy syndrome, hypercholesterolemia, hypertriglyceridemia. **Musculoskeletal:** Myalgia, arthralgia. **Respiratory:** Cough, dyspnea, hiccup. **Skin:** *Rash,* alopecia, cellulitis, dermatophytosis, dry skin, eczema, nail disorder, pruritus, seborrhea, urticaria, vesiculobullous rash. **Special Senses:** Otitis, taste perversion, tinnitus. **Urogenital:** Abnormal urine, amenorrhea, crystalluria, gynecomastia, hematuria, impotence, kidney calculus, kidney failure, kidney pain, menstrual disorder, oliguria, pelvic pain, polyuria, proteinuria, urinary frequency, urinary tract infection.

INTERACTIONS Drug: May increase levels and toxicity of **cyclosporine,** systemic **lidocaine, sirolimus, tacrolimus;** increase risk of myopathy and rhabdomyolysis with **atorvastatin, lovastatin, simvastatin;** may increase risk of heart block with **diltiazem;** ANATACIDS, H_2-RECEPTOR ANTAGONISTS, PROTON PUMP INHIBITORS may decrease absorption of atazanavir; **ritonavir** may increase atazanavir levels; may increase toxicity of **irinotecan;** increased risk of prolonged sedations with BENZODIAZEPINES; **indinavir** may increase risk of hyperbilirubinemia; **didanosine, efavirenz, rifampin** may decrease atazanavir levels; **ergotamine, ergonovine dihydroergotamine, bepridil, cisapride, pimozide** may cause serious adverse reactions; may increase risk of hypotension, visual changes, and priapism with **sildenafil, tadalafil, vardenafil. Herbal: St. John's wort** may decrease atazanavir levels.

PHARMACOKINETICS Absorption: 68% absorbed into systemic circulation; taking with food enhances bioavailability. **Peak:** 2–2.5 h. **Metabolism:** Metabolized in liver by CYP3A4. **Elimination:** 70% excreted in feces, 13% excreted in urine. **Half-Life:** 7 h.

NURSING IMPLICATIONS

Assessment & Drug Effects

- Monitor CV status and ECG closely, especially with concurrent treatment with other drugs known to prolong the PR interval.
- Lab tests: Baseline and periodic LFTs; total bilirubin if jaundiced; periodic PT/INR with concurrent warfarin therapy; monitor blood glucose closely, especially if diabetic.

Patient & Family Education

- Do not alter the dose or discontinue therapy without consulting physician.
- Inform physician of all prescription, nonprescription, or herbal meds being used.
- Report promptly any of the following: dizziness or lightheadedness; muscle pain (especially with concurrent statin therapy); severe nausea, vomiting (especially if red or "coffee-ground" in appearance), stomach pain, black tarry stools; yellowing of skin or whites of eyes; skin rash or itchy skin; sore throat, fever, or other S&S of infection; unexplained tiredness or weakness.
- If taking both sildenafil and atazanavir, promptly report any of the following sildenafil-associated adverse effects: hypotension, visual changes, or prolonged penile erection.

ATENOLOL

(a-ten'oh-lole)

Apo-Atenolol ✤, Tenormin

Classifications: AUTONOMIC NERVOUS SYSTEM AGENT; BETA-ADRENERGIC ANTAGONIST (SYMPATHOLYTIC, BLOCKING AGENT); ANTIHYPERTENSIVE AGENT

Prototype: Propranolol

Pregnancy Category: D

AVAILABILITY 25 mg, 50 mg, 100 mg tablets; 5 mg/10 mL vial

ACTIONS In therapeutic doses, atenolol selectively blocks $beta_1$-adrenergic receptors located chiefly in cardiac muscle. With large doses, preferential effect is lost and inhibition of $beta_2$-adrenergic receptors may lead to increased airway resistance, especially in patients with asthma or COPD. Mechanisms for antihypertensive action include central effect leading to decreased sympathetic outflow to periphery, reduction in renin activity with consequent suppression of the renin-angiotensin-aldosterone system, and competitive inhibition of catecholamine binding at beta-adrenergic receptor sites.

THERAPEUTIC EFFECTS Reduces rate and force of cardiac contractions (negative inotropic action); cardiac output is reduced, as well as systolic and diastolic BP. Atenolol decreases peripheral vascular resistance both at rest and with exercise.

USES Management of hypertension as a single agent or concomitantly with other antihypertensive agents, especially a diuretic, and in treatment of stable angina pectoris, MI.

UNLABELED USES Antiarrhythmic, mitral valve prolapse, adjunct in treatment of pheochromocytoma and of thyrotoxicosis; and for vascular headache prophylaxis.

CONTRAINDICATIONS Sinus bradycardia, greater than first-degree AV heart block, uncompensated heart failure, cardiogenic shock, peripheral vascular disease, Raynaud's disease, hypotension; abrupt discontinuation, pulmonary edema. Safety during pregnancy (category D), or lactation is not established.

CAUTIOUS USE Hypertensive patients with CHF controlled by digitalis and diuretics, vasospastic angina (Prinzmetal's angina); asthma, bronchitis, emphysema, and COPD; major depression; diabetes mellitus; impaired renal function, dialysis; myasthenia gravis; pheochromocytoma, hyperthyroidism, thyrotoxicosis; older adults.

ROUTE & DOSAGE

Hypertension, Angina

Adult: **PO** 25–50 mg/d, may increase to 100 mg/d
Child: **PO** 0.8–1.5 mg/kg/d (max: 2 mg/kg/d)

MI

Adult: **PO** 10 min after second IV dose, start 50 mg/d **IV** 5 mg q5min times 2 doses, then switch to PO

ADMINISTRATION

Oral

- Crush tablets, if necessary, before administration and give with fluid of patient's choice.

Intravenous

PREPARE: **Direct:** Use undiluted or diluted in 10–50 mL of NS, D5W, D5/NS, D5/0.45NS, or 0.45NS.

ADMINISTER: **Direct:** Give over 5 min.

- Store in tightly closed, light-resistant container at 15°–30° C (59°–86° F) unless otherwise directed.

ADVERSE EFFECTS (≥1%) **CNS:** Dizziness, vertigo, light-headedness, syncope, fatigue or weakness, lethargy, drowsiness, insomnia, mental changes, depression. **CV:** *Bradycardia, hypotension, CHF,* cold extremities, leg pains, dysrhythmias. **GI:** Nausea, vomiting, diarrhea. **Respiratory:** Pulmonary edema, dyspnea, <u>bronchospasm</u>. **Other:** May mask symptoms of hypoglycemia; decreased sexual ability.

INTERACTIONS Drug: Atropine and other ANTICHOLINERGICS may increase atenolol absorption from GI tract; NSAIDS may decrease hypotensive effects; may mask symptoms of a hypoglycemic reaction induced by **insulin,** SULFONYLUREAS; may increase **lidocaine** levels and toxicity; pharmacologic and toxic effects of both atenolol and **verapamil** are increased. **Prazosin, terazocin** may increase severe hypotensive response to first dose of atenolol.

PHARMACOKINETICS Absorption: 50% of PO dose absorbed. **Peak:** 2–4 h PO; 5 min IV. **Duration:** 24 h. **Distribution:** Does not readily cross blood–brain barrier. **Metabolism:** No hepatic metabolism. **Elimination:** 40%–50% excreted in urine; 50%–60% excreted in feces. **Half-Life:** 6–7 h.

NURSING IMPLICATIONS

Assessment & Drug Effects

- Neonates born to mothers who are receiving atenolol at parturition or breast–feeding may be at risk for hypoglycemia.
- Check apical pulse before giving oral drug, especially in patients receiving digitalis (both drugs slow AV conduction). If below 60 bpm (or other ordered parameter), withhold dose and consult physician.
- Monitor apical pulse, BP, respirations, and peripheral circulation throughout dosage adjustment period. Consult physician for acceptable parameters.

Patient & Family Education

- Adhere rigidly to dose regimen. Sudden discontinuation of drug can exacerbate angina and precipitate tachycardia or MI in patients with coronary artery disease, and thyroid storm in patients with hyperthyroidism.
- Make position changes slowly and in stages, particularly from recumbent to upright posture.
- Do not breast feed while taking this drug without consulting physician.

ATOMOXETINE

(a-to-mox'e-teen)

Strattera

Classifications: CENTRAL NERVOUS SYSTEM (CNS) AGENT; PSYCHOTHERAPEUTIC AGENT; NOREPINEPHRINE REUPTAKE INHIBITOR

Pregnancy Category: C

AVAILABILITY 10 mg, 18 mg, 25 mg, 40 mg, 60 mg capsules

ACTIONS Exact mechanism of action is unknown, but is thought to be related to selective inhibition of the pre-synaptic norepinephrine transporter, resulting in norepinephrine reuptake inhibition.

THERAPEUTIC EFFECTS Improved attentiveness, ability to follow through on tasks with less distraction and forgetfulness, and diminished hyperactivity.

USES Treatment of attention deficit/hyperactivity disorder (ADHD) in adults and children.

CONTRAINDICATIONS Hypersensitive to atomoxetine or any of its constituents; concomitant use or use within 2 wk of MAOIs; narrow angle glaucoma; pregnancy (category C).

CAUTIOUS USE Severe liver injury may progress to liver failure or death in a small percentage of patients. Hypertension, tachycardia, cardiovascular or cerebrovascular disease; any condition that predisposes to hypotension; urinary retention or urinary hesitancy; concomitant use of CYP2D6 inhibitors (e.g., paroxetine, fluoxetine, quinidine), albuterol or other beta-

2 agonists, vasopressor drugs, safety and efficacy in children <6 y and the older adult have not been established; lactation.

ROUTE & DOSAGE

ADHD

Adult: **PO** Start with 40 mg in morning. May increase after 3 days to target dose of 80 mg/d given either once in the morning or divided morning and late afternoon/early evening. May increase to max of 100 mg/d if needed

Child/Adolescent: **PO** *<70 kg,* start with 0.5 mg/kg/d. May increase after 3 d to target dose of 1.2 mg/kg/d. Administer once daily in morning or divide dose and give morning and late afternoon/early evening. Max dose is 1.4 mg/kg or 100 mg, whichever is less. *>70 kg,* the max total daily dose is 100 mg

Hepatic Impairment

Child-Pugh Class B: Initial and target doses should be reduced to 50% of the normal dose

Child-Pugh Class C: Initial dose and target doses should be reduced to 25% of normal

ADMINISTRATION

Oral

- Note that total daily dose in children and adolescents is based on weight. Determine that ordered dose is appropriate for weight prior to administration of drug.
- Note manufacturer recommends dosage adjustments with concomitant administration of strong CYP2D6 inhibitors (e.g., paroxetine, fluoxetine, quinidine). Consult physician.
- Store at 15°–30° C (59°–86° F).

ADVERSE EFFECTS (≥1%) **Body as a Whole:** Flu-like syndrome, flushing, fatigue, fever, rigors. **CNS:** Dizziness, *headache,* somnolence, crying, tearfulness, irritability, mood swings, *insomnia,* depression, tremor, early morning awakenings, paresthesias, abnormal dreams, decreased libido, sleep disorder. **CV:** Increased blood pressure, sinus tachycardia, palpitations. **GI:** *Upper abdominal pain,* constipation, dyspepsia, *vomiting, decreased appetite,* anorexia, dry mouth, diarrhea, flatulence, <u>severe liver injury (rare)</u>. **Endocrine:** Hot flushes. **Metabolic:** Weight loss. **Musculoskeletal:** Arthralgia, myalgia. **Respiratory:** *Cough,* rhinorrhea, nasal congestion, sinusitis. **Skin:** Dermatitis, pruritus, increased sweating. **Special Senses:** Mydriasis. **Urogenital:** Urinary hesitation/retention, dysmenorrhea, ejaculation dysfunction, impotence, delayed onset of menses, irregular menstruation, prostatitis.

INTERACTIONS Drug: Albuterol may potentiate cardiovascular effects of atomoxetine; **fluoxetine, paroxetine, quinidine** may increase atomoxetine levels and toxicity; MAOIS may precipitate a hypertensive crisis; may attenuate effects of ANTIHYPERTENSIVE AGENTS.

PHARMACOKINETICS Absorption: Well absorbed from GI trace. **Peak:** 1–2 h. **Metabolism:** Metabolized in liver by CYP2D6. **Elimination:** Primarily excreted in urine. **Half-Life:** 5.2 h.

NURSING IMPLICATIONS

Assessment & Drug Effects

- Evaluate for continuing therapeutic effectiveness especially with long-term use.

- Monitor cardiovascular status especially with preexisting hypertension.
- Monitor HR and BP at baseline, following a dose increase, and periodically while on therapy.
- Report increased aggression and irritability as these may indicate a need to discontinue the drug.

Patient & Family Education

- Report any of the following to physician: chest pains or palpitations, urinary retention or difficulty initiating voiding urine, appetite loss and weight loss, or insomnia.
- Make position changes slowly if you experience dizziness with arising from a lying or sitting position.
- Do not drive or engage in potentially hazardous activities until reaction to the drug is known.
- Do not breast feed while taking this drug without consulting physician.

ATORVASTATIN CALCIUM

(a-tor-va′sta-tin)

Lipitor

Classifications: CARDIOVASCULAR AGENT; ANTILIPEMIC AGENT; HMG-CoA; REDUCTASE INHIBITOR (STATIN)

Prototype: Lovastatin

Pregnancy Category: X

AVAILABILITY 10 mg, 20 mg, 40 mg tablets

ACTIONS Atorvastatin is an inhibitor of reductase 3-hydroxy-3-methyl-glutaryl coenzyme A (HMG-CoA), which is essential to hepatic production of cholesterol. Lipitor increases the number of hepatic low-density-lipid (LDL) receptors, thus increasing LDL uptake and catabolism of LDL.

THERAPEUTIC EFFECTS Atorvastatin reduces LDL and total triglyceride (TG) production as well as increases the plasma level of high-density lipids (HDL).

USES Adjunct to diet for the reduction of LDL cholesterol and triglycerides in patients with primary hypercholesterolemia and mixed dyslipidemia.

CONTRAINDICATIONS Hypersensitivity to atorvastatin, myopathy, active liver disease, unexplained persistent transaminase elevations, pregnancy (category X), lactation.

CAUTIOUS USE Hypersensitivity to other HMG-CoA reductase inhibitors, history of liver disease, patients who consume substantial quantities of alcohol. Safety and efficacy in children <9 y have not been established.

ROUTE & DOSAGE

Hypercholesterolemia

Adult: **PO** Start with 10–40 mg q.d., may increase up to 80 mg/d

Child/Adolescent: **PO** *10–17 y:* Start with 10 mg q.d., may increase up to 20 mg/d

ADMINISTRATION

Oral

- May be given at any time of day.
- Store at 20°–25° C (68°–77° F).

ADVERSE EFFECTS (≥1%) **Body as a Whole:** Back pain, asthenia, hypersensitivity reaction, myalgia, rhabdomyolysis. **CNS:** Headache. **GI:** Abdominal pain, constipation, diarrhea, dyspepsia, flatulence, increased liver function tests. **Respiratory:** Sinusitis, pharyngitis. **Skin:** Rash.

INTERACTIONS Drug: May increase **digoxin** levels 20%, increases levels of **norethindrone** and **ethinyl estradiol** oral contraceptives; **erythromycin** may increase atorvastatin levels 40%; MACROLIDE ANTIBIOTICS, **cyclosporine, delaviradine, gemfibrozil, niacin, clofibrate,** AZOLE ANTIFUNGALS (**ketoconazole, itraconazole**) may increase risk of rhabdomyolysis; **nelfinavir** may increase atorvastatin levels.

PHARMACOKINETICS Absorption: Rapidly absorbed from GI tract. 30% of active component reaches the systemic circulation. **Onset:** Cholesterol reduction—2 wk. **Peak:** Plasma concentration, 1–2 h; effect 2–4 wk. **Distribution:** ≥98% protein bound. Crosses placenta, distributed into breast milk of animals. **Metabolism:** Metabolized in the liver by CYP3A4 to active metabolites. **Elimination:** Excreted primarily in bile; <2% excreted in urine. **Half-Life:** 14 h; 20–30 h for active metabolites.

NURSING IMPLICATIONS

Assessment & Drug Effects

- Monitor for therapeutic effectiveness which is indicated by reduction in the level of LDL-C.
- Lab tests: Monitor lipid levels within 2–4 wk after initiation of therapy or upon change in dosage; monitor liver functions at 6 and 12 wk after initiation or elevation of dose, and periodically thereafter.
- Assess for muscle pain, tenderness, or weakness; and, if present, monitor CPK level (discontinue drug with marked elevations of CPK or if myopathy is suspected).
- Monitor carefully for digoxin toxicity with concurrent digoxin use.

Patient & Family Education

- Report promptly any of the following: Unexplained muscle pain, tenderness, or weakness, especially with fever or malaise; yellowing of skin or eyes; stomach pain with nausea, vomiting, or loss of appetite; skin rash or hives.
- Do not take drug during pregnancy because it may cause birth defects. Immediately inform physician of a suspected or known pregnancy.
- Inform physician regarding concurrent use of any of the following drugs: erythromycin, niacin, antifungals, or birth control pills.
- Minimize alcohol intake while taking this drug.
- Do not breast feed while taking this drug.

ATOVAQUONE

(a-to′va-quone)

Mepron, Mepron Suspension

Classifications: ANTIINFECTIVE; ANTIPROTOZOAL

Prototype: Metronidazole

Pregnancy Category: C

AVAILABILITY 750 mg/5 mL suspension

ACTIONS Atovaquone is an antiprotozoal with antipneumocystic activity, including *Pneumocystis carinii* and the *Plasmodium* species. Mechanism of action against *P. carinii* is unknown. In the *Plasmodium* species, the site of action is linked to inhibition of the electron transport system in the mitochondria. This results in

Common adverse effects in *italic*, life-threatening effects underlined: generic names in **bold**; classifications in SMALL CAPS; ♣ Canadian drug name; ◉ Prototype drug

the inhibition of nucleic acid and ATP synthesis.

THERAPEUTIC EFFECTS Effective against *Pneumocystis carinii* and the *Plasmodium* species.

USES Second-line oral therapy of mild to moderate *P. carinii* pneumonia (PCP) in immunocompromised patients intolerant of cotrimoxazole.

UNLABELED USES May be effective in the treatment of cerebral toxoplasmosis.

CONTRAINDICATIONS History of potential life-threatening allergies to atovaquone.

CAUTIOUS USE Severe PCP, concurrent pulmonary diseases, older adults, pregnancy (category C), or lactation. Safe use in children is not established.

ROUTE & DOSAGE

Mild to Moderate *Pneumocystis carinii* Pneumonia (PCP)

Adult: **PO** 750 mg (5 mL) suspension b.i.d. for 21 d

ADMINISTRATION

Oral

- Give with meals, because food significantly enhances absorption.
- Store at room temperature 15°–30° C (59°–86° F) unless otherwise directed by the manufacturer.

ADVERSE EFFECTS (≥1%) **Body as a Whole:** *Fever.* **CV:** Hypotension. **CNS:** *Headache, insomnia, dizziness, strange or vivid dreams, anxiety, depression.* **Hematologic:** Anemia, neutropenia. **Metabolic:** Hyponatremia, hypoglycemia. **GI:** *Nausea, diarrhea, vomiting,* abdominal pain, anorexia, dyspepsia, oral candidiasis, oral ulcers. **Skin:** *Rash,* pruritus, erythema multiforme. **Respiratory:** Cough, sinusitis.

DIAGNOSTIC TEST INTERFERENCE May cause increase in **amylase** and other **liver function tests.**

INTERACTIONS Drug: Zidovudine may increase risk of bone marrow toxicity. **Food:** Oral absorption is increased 3- to 4-fold when administered with food, especially with fatty foods.

PHARMACOKINETICS Absorption: Poorly absorbed from GI tract. Absorption is improved when taken with a fatty meal. **Duration:** 6–23 wk after a 3-wk course of therapy. **Distribution:** Penetrates poorly into cerebrospinal fluid; >99.9% protein bound. **Metabolism:** Not metabolized. **Elimination:** >94% excreted in feces over 21 d (enterohepatically cycled). **Half-Life:** 2–3 d.

NURSING IMPLICATIONS

Assessment & Drug Effects

- Assess for therapeutic failure in patients with GI disorders that may limit absorption of drug.
- Lab tests: Monitor CBC with differential, blood glucose, serum sodium, creatinine, BUN, and serum amylase periodically. Report abnormal elevations in these values; drug may need to be discontinued.

Patient & Family Education

- Note: It is necessary to take this drug exactly as prescribed because it is slowly eliminated from the body.
- Do not breast feed while taking this drug without consulting physician.

ATOVAQUONE/PROGUANIL HYDROCHLORIDE

(a-to'va-quone/pro'gua-nil)

Malarone, Malarone Pediatric

Classifications: ANTIINFECTIVE; ANTIPROTOZOAL; ANTIMALARIAL

Prototype: Chloroquine HCl & Metronidazole

Pregnancy Category: C

AVAILABILITY Atovaquone 250 mg/proguanil HCl 100 mg, atovaquone 62.5 mg/proguanil HCl 25 mg tablets

ACTIONS Combination of two antimalarial drugs. Atovaquone inhibits the electron transport system in the mitochondria of the malaria parasite, thus interfering with nucleic acid and ATP synthesis of the parasite. Proguanil interferes with DNA synthesis of the malaria parasite.

THERAPEUTIC EFFECTS Malarone is effective against strains of *Plasmodium* spp. and *P. falciparum*.

USES Prevention and treatment of malaria due to *P. falciparum*, even in chloroquine-resistant areas.

CONTRAINDICATIONS Known hypersensitivity to atovaquone or proguanil; pregnancy (category C); severe malaria.

CAUTIOUS USE Cerebral malaria, complicated malaria, pulmonary edema; renal failure, renal impairment; lactation; older adults; African Americans, Chinese, Japanese; diarrhea, emesis, GI disease; hepatic disease, infection, sunlight (UV) exposure. Use in children weighing <5 kg is not established.

ROUTE & DOSAGE

Prevention of Malaria

Adult: **PO** 1 tablet q.d. with food starting 1–2 d before travel to malarial area and continuing for 7 d after return

Child: **PO** *11–20 kg,* 1 pediatric tablet q.d.; *21–30 kg,* 2 pediatric tablets q.d.; *31–40 kg,* 3 pediatric tablets q.d.; *>40 kg,* 1 adult tablet q.d. with food starting 1–2 d before travel to malarial area and continuing for 7 d after return

Treatment of Malaria

Adult: **PO** 4 tablets as a single daily dose times 3 d

Child: **PO** *5–8 kg,* 2 pediatric tablets; *9–10 kg,* 3 pediatric tablets; *11–20 kg,* 1 adult tablet; *21–30 kg,* 2 adult tablets; *31–40 kg,* 3 adult tablets; *>40 kg,* 4 adult tablets as a single daily dose times 3 d

ADMINISTRATION

Oral

- Give at the same time each day with food or a drink containing milk.
- Give a repeat dose if vomiting occurs within 1 h after dosing.

ADVERSE EFFECTS (≥1%) **Body as a Whole:** Fever, *myalgia*, back pain, asthenia, anorexia. **Digestive:** *Nausea, abdominal pain, diarrhea,* dyspepsia. **CNS:** *Headache*. **Respiratory:** Cough. **Skin:** Pruritus.

INTERACTIONS Drug: Rifampin, rifabutin, tetracycline may decrease serum levels; **metoclopramide** may decrease absorption.

PHARMACOKINETICS Absorption: Atovaquone (A), Poorly absorbed from GI tract, absorption is improved when taken with a fatty meal; **Proguanil (P),** Extensively absorbed. **Duration: A,** 6–23 wk after a 3-wk course of therapy. **Distribution: A,** Penetrates poorly into cerebrospinal fluid; >99.9% protein bound; **P,** 75% protein bound. **Metabolism: A,** Not metabolized; **P,** Metabolized by CYP2C19 to cycloguanil. **Elimination: A,** >94% excreted in feces over 21 d (enterohepatically cycled); **P,** Primarily excreted in urine. **Half-Life: A,** 2–3 d; **P,** 12–21 h.

NURSING IMPLICATIONS

Assessment & Drug Effects

- Lab tests: Monitor AST and ALT periodically, especially with long-term therapy.
- Monitor for S&S of parasitemia in patients receiving tetracycline and in those experiencing diarrhea or vomiting.
- Note: Only use metoclopramide to control vomiting if other antiemetics are not available.

Patient & Family Education

- Take this drug at the same time each day for maximum effectiveness.
- Note: Absorption of this drug may be reduced with diarrhea and vomiting. Consult physician if either of these occurs.
- Do not breast feed while taking this drug without consulting physician.

ATRACURIUM BESYLATE

(a-tra-kyoor'ee-um)

Tracrium

Classifications: AUTONOMIC NERVOUS SYSTEM AGENT; SKELETAL MUSCLE RELAXANT, NONDEPOLARIZING; NEUROMUSCULAR BLOCKER

Prototype: Tubocurarine

Pregnancy Category: C

AVAILABILITY 10 mg/mL injection

ACTIONS Inhibits neuromuscular transmission by binding competitively with acetylcholine to muscle end plate receptors. Lacks analgesic action and has no apparent effect on pain threshold, consciousness, or cerebration. Given in general anesthesia only after unconsciousness has been induced by other drugs.

THERAPEUTIC EFFECTS Synthetic skeletal muscle relaxant pharmacologically similar to tubocurarine that produces shorter duration of neuromuscular blockade, exhibits minimal direct effects on cardiovascular system, and has less histamine-releasing action. Has minimal cumulative tendency with subsequent doses if recovery from the drug begins before dose is repeated.

USES Adjunct for general anesthesia to produce skeletal muscle relaxation during surgery; to facilitate endotracheal intubation. Especially useful for patients with severe renal or hepatic disease, limited cardiac reserve, and in patients with low or atypical pseudocholinesterase levels.

CONTRAINDICATIONS Myasthenia gravis. Safety during pregnancy (category C), lactation, or in children <2 is not established.

CAUTIOUS USE When appreciable histamine release would be hazardous (as in asthma or anaphylactoid reactions, significant cardiovascular disease), neuromuscular disease (e.g., Eaton-Lambert syndrome), carcinomatosis, electrolyte or acid–base imbalances, dehydration, impaired pulmonary function.

ROUTE & DOSAGE

Skeletal Muscle Relaxation

Adult/Child: **IV** ≥2 *y*, 0.4–0.5 mg/kg initial dose, then 0.08–0.1 mg/kg 20–45 min after the first dose if necessary, reduce doses if used with general anesthetics
Child: **IV** *1 mo–2 y*, 0.3–0.4 mg/kg

Mechanical Ventilation

Adult: **IV** 5–9 mcg/kg/min by continuous infusion

ADMINISTRATION

- Verify correct concentration and rate of infusion for infants and children with physician.

Intravenous

PREPARE: **Direct:** Give initial bolus dose undiluted. **Continuous:** Maintenance dose must be diluted with NS, D5W or D5/NS. Do not mix in same syringe or administer through same needle as used for alkaline solutions [incompatible with alkaline solutions (e.g., barbiturates)].

ADMINISTER: **Direct:** Give as bolus dose. **Continuous:** Give infusion.

- Store at 2°–8° C (36°–46° F) to preserve potency unless otherwise directed. Avoid freezing.

ADVERSE EFFECTS (≥1%) **CV:** Bradycardia, tachycardia. **Respiratory:** Respiratory depression. **Other:** Increased salivation, anaphylaxis.

INTERACTIONS Drug: GENERAL ANESTHETICS increase magnitude and duration of neuromuscular blocking action; AMINOGLYCOSIDES, **bacitracin, polymyxin B, clindamycin, lidocaine, parenteral magnesium, quinidine, quinine, trimethaphan, verapamil** increase neuromuscular blockade; DIURETICS may increase or decrease neuromuscular blockade; **lithium** prolongs duration of neuromuscular blockade; NARCOTIC ANALGESICS present possibility of additive respiratory depression; **succinylcholine** increases onset and depth of neuromuscular blockade; **phenytoin** may cause resistance to or reversal of neuromuscular blockade.

PHARMACOKINETICS Onset: 2 min. **Peak:** 3–5 min. **Duration:** 60–70 min. **Distribution:** Well distributed to tissues and extracellular fluids; crosses placenta; distribution into breast milk unknown. **Metabolism:** Rapid nonenzymatic degradation in bloodstream. **Elimination:** 70%–90% excreted in urine in 5–7 h. **Half-Life:** 20 min.

NURSING IMPLICATIONS

Assessment & Drug Effects

- Lab tests: Baseline serum electrolytes, acid–base balance, and renal function as part of preanesthetic assessment.
- Note: Personnel and equipment required for endotracheal intubation, administration of oxygen under positive pressure, artificial respiration, and assisted or controlled ventilation must be immediately available.
- Evaluate degree of neuromuscular blockade and muscle paralysis to avoid risk of overdosage by qualified individual using peripheral nerve stimulator.
- Monitor BP, pulse, and respirations and evaluate patient's recovery from neuromuscular blocking (curare-like) effect as evidenced by ability to breathe naturally or to take deep breaths and cough, keep eyes open, lift

head keeping mouth closed, adequacy of hand-grip strength. Notify physician if recovery is delayed.

- Note: Recovery from neuromuscular blockade usually begins 35–45 min after drug administration and is almost complete in about 1 h. Recovery time may be delayed in patients with cardiovascular disease, edematous states, and in older adults.

ATROPINE SULFATE (Pr)

(a'troe-peen)

Atropair ♣, Atropisol, Isopto Atropine

Classifications: AUTONOMIC NERVOUS SYSTEM AGENT; ANTICHOLINERGIC (PARA-SYMPATHOLYTIC); ANTIMUSCARINIC

Pregnancy Category: C

AVAILABILITY 0.4 mg tablets; 0.05 mg/mL, 0.1 mg/mL, 0.3 mg/mL, 0.4 mg/mL, 0.5 mg/mL, 0.8 mg/mL, 1 mg/mL injection

ACTIONS Acts by selectively blocking all muscarinic responses to acetylcholine (ACh), whether excitatory or inhibitory. Selective depression of CNS relieves rigidity and tremor of Parkinson's syndrome. Antisecretory action (vagolytic effect) suppresses sweating, lacrimation, salivation, and secretions from nose, mouth, pharynx, and bronchi. Blocks vagal impulses to heart with resulting decrease in AV conduction time, increase in heart rate and cardiac output, and shortened PR interval.

THERAPEUTIC EFFECTS Atropine is a potent bronchodilator when bronchoconstriction has been induced by parasympathomimetics. Produces mydriasis (dilation of pupils) and cycloplegia (paralysis of accommodation) by blocking responses of iris sphincter muscle and ciliary muscle of lens to cholinergic stimulation.

USES Adjunct in symptomatic treatment of GI disorders (e.g., peptic ulcer, pylorospasm, GI hypermotility, irritable bowel syndrome) and spastic disorders of biliary tract. Relaxes upper GI tract and colon during hypotonic radiography. *Ophthalmic Use:* To produce mydriasis and cycloplegia before refraction and for treatment of anterior uveitis and iritis. *Preoperative Use:* To suppress salivation, perspiration, and respiratory tract secretions; to reduce incidence of laryngospasm, reflex bradycardia arrhythmia, and hypotension during general anesthesia. *Cardiac Uses:* For sinus bradycardia or asystole during CPR or that is induced by drugs or toxic substances (e.g., pilocarpine, beta-adrenergic blockers, organophosphate pesticides, and *Amanita* mushroom poisoning); for management of selected patients with symptomatic sinus bradycardia and associated hypotension and ventricular irritability; for diagnosis of sinus node dysfunction and in evaluation of coronary artery disease during atrial pacing; for management of chronic symptomatic sinus node dysfunction. *Other Uses:* Oral inhalation for short-term treatment and prevention of bronchospasms associated with asthma, bronchitis, and COPD and as drying agent in upper respiratory infection. Adjunctive therapy for hypermotility of GI tract.

CONTRAINDICATIONS Hypersensitivity to belladonna alkaloids; synechiae; angle-closure glaucoma; parotitis; obstructive uropathy, e.g., bladder neck obstruction caused by prostatic hypertrophy; intestinal atony, paralytic ileus, obstructive diseases of GI tract, severe ulcerative colitis, toxic megacolon; tachycardia secondary to cardiac insufficiency or thyrotoxicosis; acute hemorrhage; myasthenia gravis. Safety during pregnancy (category C) or lactation is not established.

CAUTIOUS USE Myocardial infarction, hypertension, hypotension; coronary artery disease, CHF, tachyarrhythmias; gastric ulcer, GI infections, hiatal hernia with reflux esophagitis; hyperthyroidism; chronic lung disease; hepatic or renal disease; older adults; debilitated patients; children <6 y of age; Down syndrome; autonomic neuropathy, spastic paralysis, brain damage in children; patients exposed to high environmental temperatures; patients with fever.

ROUTE & DOSAGE

Preanesthesia

Adult: **IV/IM/SC** 0.2–1 mg 30–60 min before surgery
Child: **IV/IM/SC** *<5 kg,* 0.02 mg/kg; *>5 kg,* 0.01–0.02 mg/kg 30–60 min before surgery

Arrhythmias

Adult: **IV/IM** 0.5–1 mg q1–2h prn (max: 2 mg)
Child: **IV/IM** 0.01–0.03 mg/kg for 1–2 doses

Organophosphate Antidote

Adult: **IV/IM** 1–2 mg q5–60min until muscarinic signs and symptoms subside (may need up to 50 mg)
Child: **IV/IM** 0.05 mg/kg q10–30 min until muscarinic signs and symptoms subside

COPD

Adult: **Inhalation** 0.025 mg/kg diluted with 3–5 mL saline, via nebulizer 3–4 times daily (max: 2.5 mg/d)
Child: **Inhalation** 0.03–0.05 mg/kg diluted with 3–5 mL saline, via nebulizer 3–4 times daily

Uveitis

Adult/Child: **Ophthalmic** 1–2 drops of solution or small amount of ointment in eye up to t.i.d.

Cycloplegia

Adult: **Ophthalmic** 1 drop of solution or small amount of ointment in eye 1 h before the procedure
Child: **Ophthalmic** 1–2 drops in eye b.i.d. for 1–3 d prior to procedure or a small amount of ointment in conjunctival sac t.i.d. for 1–3 d prior to procedure with last dose applied several hours before the procedure

ADMINISTRATION

Intravenous

PREPARE: **Direct:** Give undiluted or diluted in up to 10 mL of sterile water.

ADMINISTER: **Direct:** Give 1 mg or fraction thereof over 1 min directly into a Y-site.

- Store at room temperature 15°–30° C (59°–86° F) in protected airtight, light-resistant containers unless otherwise directed by manufacturer.

ADVERSE EFFECTS (≥1%) **CNS:** Headache, ataxia, dizziness, excitement, irritability, convulsions, drowsiness, fatigue, weakness; mental depression, confusion, disorientation, hallucinations. **CV:** Hypertension or hypotension, ventricular tachycardia, palpitation, paradoxical bradycardia, AV dissociation, atrial or ventricular fibrillation. **GI:** Dry mouth with thirst, dysphagia, loss of taste; nausea, vomiting, constipation, delayed gastric emptying, antral stasis, paralytic ileus. **Urogenital:** Urinary hesitancy and retention, dysuria, impotence. **Skin:** Flushed, dry skin; anhidrosis, rash, urticaria, contact dermatitis, allergic conjunctivitis, fixed-drug eruption. **Special Senses:** Mydriasis, blurred vision, photophobia, increased intraocular pressure, cycloplegia, eye dryness, local redness.

DIAGNOSTIC TEST INTERFERENCE ***Upper GI series:*** Findings may require qualification because of anticholinergic effects of atropine (reduced gastric motility and delayed gastric emptying). ***PSP excretion test:*** Atropine may decrease urinary excretion of PSP (phenolsulfonphthalein).

INTERACTIONS Drug: Amantadine, ANTIHISTAMINES, TRICYCLIC ANTIDEPRESSANTS, **quinidine, disopyramide, procainamide** add to anticholinergic effects. **Levodopa** effects decreased. **Methotrimeprazine** may precipitate extrapyramidal effects. Antipsychotic effects of PHENOTHIAZINES are decreased due to decreased absorption.

PHARMACOKINETICS Absorption: Well absorbed from all administration sites. Peak effect: 30 min IM, 2–4 min IV, 1–2 h SC, 1.5–4 h inhalation, 30–40 min topical. **Duration:** Inhibition of salivation 4 h; mydriasis 7–14 d. **Distribution:** Distributed in most body tissues; crosses blood–brain barrier and placenta. **Metabolism:** Metabolized in liver. **Elimination:** 77%–94% excreted in urine in 24 h. **Half-Life:** 2–3 h.

NURSING IMPLICATIONS

Assessment & Drug Effects

- Monitor vital signs. HR is a sensitive indicator of patient's response to atropine. Be alert to changes in quality, rate, and rhythm of HR and respiration and to changes in BP and temperature.
- Initial paradoxical bradycardia following IV atropine usually lasts only 1–2 min; it most likely occurs when IV is administered slowly (more than 1 min) or when small doses (less than 0.5 mg) are used. Postural hypotension occurs when patient ambulates too soon after parenteral administration.
- Note: Frequent and continued use of eye preparations, as well as overdosage, can have systemic effects. Some atropine deaths have resulted from systemic absorption following ocular administration in infants and children.
- Monitor I&O, especially in older adults and patients who have had surgery (drug may contribute to urinary retention). Palpate lower abdomen for distention. Have patient void before giving atropine.
- Monitor CNS status. Older adults and debilitated patients sometimes manifest drowsiness or CNS stimulation (excitement, agitation, confusion) with usual doses of drug or other belladonna alkaloids. In addition to dosage adjustment, side rails and supervision of ambulation may be indicated.
- Monitor infants, small children, and older adults for "atropine fever" (hyperpyrexia due to suppression of perspiration and heat loss),

which increases the risk of heatstroke.

- Note: Intraocular tension and depth of anterior chamber should be determined before and during therapy with ophthalmic preparations to avoid glaucoma attacks (ophthalmic solutions and ointments are available in various strengths).
- Patients receiving atropine via inhalation sometimes manifest mild CNS stimulation with doses in excess of 5 mg and mental depression and other mental disturbances with larger doses.

Patient & Family Education

- Follow measures to relieve dry mouth: adequate hydration; small, frequent mouth rinses with tepid water; meticulous mouth and dental hygiene; gum chewing or sucking sugarless sourballs.
- Note: Drug causes drowsiness, sensitivity to light, blurring of near vision, and temporarily impairs ability to judge distance. Avoid driving and other activities requiring visual acuity and mental alertness.
- Discontinue ophthalmic preparations and notify physician if eye pain, conjunctivitis, palpitation, rapid pulse, or dizziness occurs.
- Do not breast feed while taking this drug without consulting physician.

AURANOFIN

(au-rane'eh-fin)

Ridaura

Classifications: GOLD COMPOUND; ANTIINFLAMMATORY; ANTIRHEUMATIC

Prototype: Aurothioglucose

Pregnancy Category: C

AVAILABILITY 3 mg capsules

ACTIONS Strongly lipophilic and almost neutral in solution, properties that may facilitate transport of agent across cell membranes. Action appears to be immunomodulatory: serum immunoglobulin concentrations and rheumatoid factor titers are decreased; and antiinflammatory: gold is taken up by macrophages with resulting inhibition of phagocytosis and lysosomal enzyme release.

THERAPEUTIC EFFECTS Auranofin is immunomodulatory and antiinflammatory.

USES Management of active stage of classic or definite rheumatoid arthritis in adults who do not respond to or tolerate other antiarthritis agents (e.g., NSAIDs, other gold compounds).

UNLABELED USES Juvenile rheumatoid arthritis, active SLE, psoriatic arthritis.

CONTRAINDICATIONS History of gold-induced necrotizing enterocolitis, renal disease, exfoliative dermatitis or bone marrow aplasia; patient who has recently received radiation therapy, history of severe toxicity from previous exposure to gold or other heavy metals. Safety during pregnancy (category C), lactation, or by children is not established.

CAUTIOUS USE Inflammatory bowel disease, rash, liver disease, history of bone marrow depression; older adults; diabetes mellitus, CHF.

ROUTE & DOSAGE

Rheumatoid Arthritis

Adult: **PO** 6 mg/d in 1–2 divided doses, may increase to 6–9 mg/d

in 3 divided doses after 6 mo (max: 9 mg/d)
Child: **PO** Initially 0.1 mg/kg/d, may increase to 0.15 mg/kg/d in 1–2 divided doses (max: 0.2 mg/kg/d)

ADMINISTRATION

Oral

- Give capsule with food or fluid of patient's choice.
- Store at 15°–30° C (59°–86° F); protect from light and moisture.
- Note: Expiration date is 4 y after date of manufacture.

ADVERSE EFFECTS (≥1%) **GI:** *Diarrhea, abdominal cramping* and pain; *nausea,* vomiting, anorexia, dysphagia; *stomatitis,* glossitis, metallic taste; flatulence, constipation, GI bleeding, melena. **Hematologic:** Thrombocytopenia, leukopenia, eosinophilia, agranulocytosis, aplastic anemia. **Urogenital:** Proteinuria, hematuria, renal failure. **Skin:** *Rash, pruritus,* dermatitis, urticaria.

DIAGNOSTIC TEST INTERFERENCE Auranofin may enhance response to a ***tuberculin skin test.***

PHARMACOKINETICS Absorption: 20% absorbed from small intestine. **Peak:** 2 h. **Distribution:** Highest concentrations in kidneys, spleen, lungs, adrenals, and liver; not known if crosses placenta; small amounts distributed into breast milk. **Elimination:** 60% of absorbed gold eliminated in urine, remainder in feces. **Half-Life:** 11–23 d.

NURSING IMPLICATIONS

Assessment & Drug Effects

- Monitor for therapeutic effectiveness which develops slowly and is not usually apparent for 3–4 mo.
- Report any of the following S&S promptly: unexplained bleeding or bruising, metallic taste, sore mouth; pruritus, rash; diarrhea and melena; yellow skin and sclera; unexplained cough or dyspnea.
- Lab tests: Test for signs of possible impending gold toxicity including decreased Hgb; leukocytes <4000/mm^3; granulocytes <1500/mm^3; platelets <150,000/mm^3; proteinuria <500 mg/d. Also urinary protein and hepatic function.
- Note: Drug-induced thrombocytopenia is usually spontaneously reversible several weeks after drug is withdrawn.
- Continue medical surveillance and supportive therapy after drug is discontinued because adverse effects (such as difficulty in breathing, diarrhea and abdominal pain, fatigue, weakness, unexplained bleeding and bruising, metallic taste) may persist for many months.

Patient & Family Education

- Report adverse effects of therapy, especially abdominal cramping and pain; discontinuance of therapy may be necessary.
- Report metallic taste and pruritus with or without rash. These are among earliest symptoms of impending gold toxicity.
- Do not change dosage (dose or dose interval) by omission, increase, or decrease without first consulting physician.
- Use antidiarrheal OTC drug and high-fiber diet for drug-induced diarrhea.
- Avoid exposure to sunlight (especially between 10 a.m. and 4 p.m.) or to artificial ultraviolet light to prevent photosensitivity reaction.

- Rinse mouth with water frequently for symptomatic treatment of mild stomatitis. Avoid commercial mouth rinses; clean teeth with soft tooth brush and gentle brushing to avoid gingival trauma. Floss at least once daily.
- Do not breast feed while taking this drug without consulting physician.

AUROTHIOGLUCOSE (Pr)

(aur-oh-thye-oh-gloo'kose)

Gold thioglucose, Solganal

Classifications: GOLD COMPOUND; ANTIINFLAMMATORY; ANTIRHEUMATIC

Pregnancy Category: C

AVAILABILITY 50 mg/mL injection

ACTIONS Mechanism of antiinflammatory action not clearly understood. Gold uptake by macrophages with subsequent inhibition of migration and phagocytic action, thereby suppressing immune responsiveness, may be principal mechanism.

THERAPEUTIC EFFECTS Major clinical effect is suppression of joint inflammation in early arthritic disease. Has no effect on reparative process, but studies suggest that it may significantly slow or arrest disease progression.

USES Adjunctive treatment of both adult and juvenile active rheumatoid arthritis. Generally used when adequate trial with salicylates or other NSAIDs has not been satisfactory.

UNLABELED USES Psoriatic arthritis, Felty's syndrome, pemphigus, nondisseminated LE.

CONTRAINDICATIONS Gold allergy or history of severe toxicity from previous therapy with gold or other heavy metals; severe debilitation; uncontrolled diabetes mellitus; renal or hepatic insufficiency, history of hepatitis; uncontrolled CHF; marked hypertension; tuberculosis; severe anemia, hemorrhagic diathesis, agranulocytosis or other blood dyscrasias; disseminated LE, Sjögren's syndrome, recent radiation therapy; colitis; urticaria, eczema, history of exfoliative dermatitis. Safety during pregnancy (category C), lactation, or in children <6 y is not established.

CAUTIOUS USE Older adults; history of drug allergy or hypersensitivity; history of blood dyscrasias; history of renal or hepatic disease; compromised cerebral or cardiovascular circulation; presence of skin rash.

ROUTE & DOSAGE

Rheumatoid Arthritis

Adult: **IM** 10 mg 1st wk, 25 mg 2nd and 3rd wk, then 50 mg/wk to a cumulative dose of 1 g **IM Maintenance Dose** with improvement, 25–50 mg q2–3wk, then q3–4wk indefinitely or until adverse effects occur
Child: **IM** *6–12 y*, 0.25–1 mg/kg/wk (max: 25 mg) for 20 wk **IM Maintenance Dose** *6–12 y*, with improvement, 1 mg/kg (max: 25 mg) q2–4wk

ADMINISTRATION

Intramuscular

- Hold vial horizontally and shake vigorously to ensure uniform suspension. Heating vial to body temperature by placing in a warm-water bath facilitates drug withdrawal.
- Give drug by deep IM injection, preferably intragluteally. Use an

18- or 20-gauge, 1 1/2-inch needle (for obese patients a 2-inch needle may be preferable). Patient should be lying down when drug is administered.

- Have patients remain recumbent for 10 min after injection. Observe patient for 20–30 min after injection for hypersensitivity reactions.
- Note: Gold therapy is contraindicated following a severe reaction but may be attempted at reduced initial dosage schedule with careful monitoring after a mild reaction.
- Store at 15°–30° C (59°–86° F) in light-resistant containers unless otherwise directed. Protect from freezing and light.

ADVERSE EFFECTS (≥1%) **Body as a Whole:** Hypersensitivity (Anaphylactic shock, syncope, bradycardia, thickening of tongue, dysphagia, dyspnea), fever. **GI:** Nausea, vomiting, abdominal cramps, anorexia, metallic taste, diarrhea, hepatitis. **Hematologic:** Eosinophilia, agranulocytosis, thrombocytopenia, leukopenia, granulocytopenia, aplastic anemia. **Respiratory:** Pulmonary fibrosis, interstitial pneumonitis. **Skin:** *Pruritus, urticaria, erythema*, "gold dermatitis," fixed-drug eruptions, exfoliative dermatitis with alopecia and nail shedding; gingivitis, glossitis, Stevens-Johnson syndrome, photosensitivity reactions. **Urogenital:** Nephrotic syndrome, proteinuria, hematuria, vaginitis, nephrotic syndrome. **Other:** Immunologic destruction of synovial fluid, exacerbation of arthralgia (temporary), local irritation at injection site.

DIAGNOSTIC TEST INTERFERENCE Low ***PBI*** (by ***chloric acid method***); test interference may persist for several weeks after gold therapy is discontinued.

INTERACTIONS Drug: ANTIMALARIALS, IMMUNOSUPPRESSANTS, **penicillamine, phenylbutazone** increased risk of blood dyscrasias.

PHARMACOKINETICS Absorption: Slowly and irregularly absorbed from IM site. **Peak:** 4–6 h. **Distribution:** Widely distributed, especially to synovial fluid; does not cross blood–brain barrier; crosses placenta. **Metabolism:** Unknown. **Elimination:** 50%–90% of dose ultimately excreted in urine; 10%–50% in feces; excreted into breast milk. **Half-Life:** 3–27 d.

NURSING IMPLICATIONS

Assessment & Drug Effects

- Monitor therapeutic effectiveness which may not be apparent before 6–8 wk of gold therapy.
- Lab tests: Baseline renal and hepatic function tests, CBC, and urinalysis prior to initiation of therapy. Thereafter, perform urinalysis (for protein and sediment) before each injection. Determine CBC (including Hgb, RBC, WBC and differential, platelet counts) before every second injection throughout therapy.
- Withhold drug and notify physician of any of the following: platelet count <100,000/mm^3, or leukocytes <4000/mm^3, granulocytes <1500/mm^3, eosinophils >5%, rapid fall in Hgb value, and presence of proteinuria or hematuria.
- Rule out pregnancy before gold treatment begins. Women of childbearing age should be warned about the potential hazards of becoming pregnant during therapy and counseled about the use of birth control.
- Note: During early treatment, some patients complain of exacerbation of joint pain after injec-

tion. It usually subsides after the first few injections.

- Monitor S&S of beginning gold toxicity. Toxicity generally involves skin and mucous membranes anywhere in body. Inspect skin carefully and examine mouth and throat. Report any of the following promptly: Itching that often precedes dermatitis and eosinophilia, bruising or bleeding, tenderness, metallic taste that frequently precedes sore mouth, tongue, or throat, gray-blue discoloration of skin and mucous membranes, diarrhea or loose stools, indigestion, unexplained malaise; signs of hepatotoxicity (yellow sclerae and skin, clay-colored stools, dark urine, pruritus).
- Note: Rapid improvement in joint pain and mobility also may signify that patient is approaching toxic tissue levels. Interruption of therapy, at least temporarily, may be indicated. Notify physician.

Patient & Family Education

- Review with health care provider and understand the list of possible adverse effects that should be reported. If therapy is interrupted at the onset of gold toxicity, serious reactions can be avoided.
- Note: Adverse reactions are most likely to occur during second and third month of therapy or when cumulative aurothioglucose dose is 300–500 mg. However, they may appear at any time during therapy or several months after treatment has been discontinued.
- Report any unusual color or odor to urine, or change in I&O ratio and pattern.
- Report unusual fatigue or weakness, malaise, chills, fever, sore throat; possible signs of bleeding (e.g., bleeding gums, nosebleeds, dark urine, black stools, petechiae, purpura, easy bruising). Report signs of hepatotoxicity (see Appendix F).
- Avoid contact with anyone who has a cold, recent vaccination, or has been exposed recently to communicable disease.
- Report to physician need to increase the amount of aspirin or other prescribed NSAID for pain as this may indicate diminishing response to gold therapy.
- Minimize exposure to sunlight and artificial ultraviolet light because gray to blue pigmentation may occur on light-exposed skin areas.
- Use careful and thorough oral hygiene. Avoid overuse of mouthwashes, which contain alcohol; these enhance drying and irritation, and can change mouth flora.
- Do not breast feed while taking this drug without consulting physician.

AZACITIDINE

(a-za-ci'ti-deen)

Vidaza

Classifications: ANTINEOPLASTIC AGENT; ANTIMETABOLITE

Prototype: Fluorouracil

Pregnancy Category: D

AVAILABILITY 100 mg powder for injection

ACTIONS Causes changes in DNA in abnormal blood-forming cells in the bone marrow, resulting in restoration of normal function to tumor-suppressor genes that are responsible for regulating cell differentiation and growth.

THERAPEUTIC EFFECTS The cytotoxic effects of azacitidine cause the death of rapidly dividing cancer cells that are no longer responsive to normal growth control mechanisms.

USES Treatment of myelodysplastic syndrome, specifically refractory anemia.

CONTRAINDICATIONS Known hypersensitivity to azacitidine or mannitol; advanced malignant hepatic tumors, myelodysplastic syndrome with hepatic impairment; vaccination; active infection; dental work; intramuscular injections, if platelets <50,000 mm^3; pregnancy (category D), lactation. Safety and efficacy in children have not been established.

CAUTIOUS USE Hypoalbuminemia (<3 g/dL), hepatic disease; bone marrow depression; dental disease; history of varicella zoster or other herpes infections; renal impairment, renal failure; older adults.

ROUTE & DOSAGE

Myelodysplastic Syndrome

Adult: **SC** 75 mg/m^2 once daily for 7 d every 4 wk; may increase to 100 mg/m^2 if no beneficial response is seen after 2 treatment cycles and no toxicity other than nausea and vomiting has occurred

Renal Impairment

If unexplained elevations of BUN or creatinine occur, the next cycle should be delayed until the values return to normal or baseline, and the dose should be reduced by 50% in the next course

ADMINISTRATION

Subcutaneous

- Reconstitute by slowly injecting 4 mL of sterile water for injection into 100 mg vial to yield 25 mg/mL. Invert 2–3 times and gently rotate until a uniform suspension is achieved. The suspension will be cloudy. If not used immediately, see directions for storage.
- Doses greater than 4 mL should be divided equally into 2 syringes and injected into 2 separate sites. Rotate sites for each injection (thigh, abdomen, or upper arm). Give subsequent injections at least 1 in from an old site and never into areas where the site is tender, bruised, red, or hard.
- Storage: Reconstituted suspension may be kept in the vial or syringe. May refrigerate for up to 8 h. Before use, suspension may be kept at room temperature for up to 30 min. Resuspend by inverting the syringe 2–3 times and gently roll between the palms for 30 sec immediately before administration.

ADVERSE EFFECTS (≥1%) **Body as a Whole:** *Fever, fatigue, malaise, weakness, asthenia, limb pain, back pain,* lymphadenopathy, hematoma, night sweats, cellulitis, lethargy. **CNS:** *Dizziness, headache, depression,* syncope. **CV:** *Chest pain,* cardiac murmur, tachycardia, hypotension. **GI:** *Nausea, vomiting, diarrhea, constipation, anorexia, weight loss, abdominal pain,* stomatitis, dyspepsia. **Hematologic:** *Anemia, thrombocytopenia, leukopenia, neutropenia, ecchymosis, febrile neutropenia.* **Metabolic:** *Peripheral edema.* **Musculoskeletal:** *Myalgia, arthralgia,* muscle cramps. **Respiratory:** *Cough, dyspnea, pharyngitis, nasopharyngitis, pneumonia,* wheezing, pleural effusion, rhonchi. **Skin:** *Injection site erythema, injection site reactions, rash, pruritus, sweating,* urticaria. **Urogenital:** Dysuria, urinary tract infection.

INTERACTIONS Drug: ANTICOAGULANTS, NSAIDS, ANTIPLATELET AGENTS may increase risk of bleeding; **filgrastim, sargramostim** may interfere with the efficacy of azacitidine if given within 24 h of azacitidine dose.

PHARMACOKINETICS Peak: 30 min. **Metabolism:** Metabolized in liver. **Elimination:** Excreted by kidneys. **Half-Life:** 4 h.

NURSING IMPLICATIONS

Assessment & Drug Effects

- Monitor for S&S of drug toxicity in those with renal insufficiency.
- Lab tests: Obtain LFTs and serum creatinine before initiation of therapy; monitor CBC with differential before each treatment cycle and prn.
- Withhold drug & notify physician for S&S of hepatic or renal insufficiency; lab values that indicate leukopenia, neutropenia, thrombocytopenia, or hepatic or renal insufficiency; or serum bicarbonate levels less than 20 mEq/L.

Patient & Family Education

- Promptly report S&S of infection or indication of unusual bleeding tendencies (e.g., dark, tarry stools and easy bruising).
- Women should avoid becoming pregnant and men should not father a child while taking this drug.
- Do not breast feed while taking this drug.

AZATADINE MALEATE

(a-za'ta-deen)

Optimine, Trinalin

Classification: ANTIHISTAMINE (H_1-RECEPTOR ANTAGONIST)

Prototype: Diphenhydramine

Pregnancy Category: B

AVAILABILITY 1 mg tablets

ACTIONS Long-acting antihistamine that acts by competitively antagonizing the stimulating effects of histamine at H_1-receptor sites on smooth muscle of blood vessels and respiratory and GI tract.

THERAPEUTIC EFFECTS The effect is to block or reduce intensity of allergic responses associated with histamine release, such as vasodilation, capillary permeability and tissue edema, and itching.

USES Symptomatic relief of hay fever (seasonal allergic rhinitis), perennial (or nonseasonal) allergic rhinitis, and chronic urticaria.

CONTRAINDICATIONS Hypersensitivity to azatadine or to other H_1-receptor antagonists; MAO INHIBITOR therapy. Safety during pregnancy (category B), lactation, or in children <12 y is not established.

CAUTIOUS USE Increased intraocular pressure, narrow-angle glaucoma; pyloroduodenal obstruction, stenosing peptic ulcer; prostatic hypertrophy, bladder neck obstruction; hyperthyroidism; hypertension, cardiovascular disease; convulsive disorders; history of asthma or COPD.

ROUTE & DOSAGE

Allergic Rhinitis

Adult: **PO** 1–2 mg b.i.d.

ADMINISTRATION

Oral

- Give drug with food or milk to minimize GI adverse effects.
- Store at 2°–30° C (36°–86° F) in tightly closed container, unless otherwise directed.

ADVERSE EFFECTS (≥1%) **CNS:** *Drowsiness,* sedation, dizziness, disturbed coordination, fatigue, confusion, euphoria, excitation, nervousness, restlessness, insomnia, tremor, irritability. **CV:** Hypotension, palpitation, tachycardia, extrasystoles. **GI:** *Dry mouth,* epigastric distress, nausea, vomiting, anorexia, diarrhea, or constipation. **Urogenital:** Urinary retention, early menses. **Hematologic:** Hemolytic anemia, thrombocytopenia, agranulocytosis. **Respiratory:** Thickening of bronchial secretions. **Special Senses:** Nasal stuffiness; dryness of nose and throat; tinnitus, blurred vision.

DIAGNOSTIC TEST INTERFERENCE As a general rule, H_1-receptor antagonists are discontinued about 4 d before ***skin testing*** procedures are to be performed since they may produce false-negative results.

INTERACTIONS Drug: Alcohol, CNS DEPRESSANTS add to sedation, drowsiness; MAO INHIBITORS may prolong anticholinergic effects of azatadine; TRICYCLIC ANTIDEPRESSANTS augment anticholinergic effects.

PHARMACOKINETICS Absorption: Readily absorbed from GI tract. **Peak:** 4 h. **Distribution:** Probably crosses blood–brain barrier; crosses placenta; distribution into breast milk unknown. **Metabolism:** Partially metabolized in liver. **Elimination:** 50% excreted in urine in 5 d. **Half-Life:** 9–12 h.

NURSING IMPLICATIONS

Assessment & Drug Effects

- Monitor for sedation, dizziness, hypotension, and confusion which are more common in older adults. Advise patient to report these effects. Reduction in dosage may be indicated.
- Monitor mental status. There may be additive CNS depression with alcohol and other CNS depressants (e.g., sedatives, tranquilizers, sleep medications).

Patient & Family Education

- Do not drive or engage in potentially hazardous activities until response to drug is known. This drug commonly causes drowsiness, sedation, and dizziness.
- Avoid concurrent use of alcohol because of potential for additive CNS depression.
- Avoid prolonged exposure to sunlight or to artificial ultraviolet light. Photosensitivity is a possible adverse effect.
- Relieve dry mouth with frequent rinses with tepid water. Avoid mouthwashes, which contain alcohol that enhances drying.
- Do not breast feed while taking this drug without consulting physician.

AZATHIOPRINE

(ay-za-thye′oh-preen)

Azasan, Imuran

Classification: IMMUNOSUPPRESSANT

Prototype: Cyclosporine

Pregnancy Category: D

AVAILABILITY 50 mg, 75 mg, 100 mg tablets; 100 mg vial

ACTIONS Precise mechanism of immunosuppressant and antiinflammatory actions not determined. Antagonizes purine metabolism and appears to inhibit DNA, RNA, and normal protein synthesis in rapidly growing cells.

THERAPEUTIC EFFECTS Suppresses T cell effects before transplant rejection.

USES Adjunctive agent to prevent rejection of kidney allografts, usu-

ally with other immunosuppressants. Also used in selective adult patients with severe, active rheumatoid arthritis; unresponsive to conventional therapy.
UNLABELED USES SLE, ulcerative colitis, pemphigus, nephrotic syndrome, and other inflammatory and immunologic diseases.

CONTRAINDICATIONS Hypersensitivity to azathioprine or mercaptopurine; clinically active infection, immunization of patient or close family members with live virus vaccines; anuria; pancreatitis; patients receiving alkylating agents (increased risk of neoplasms), concurrent radiation therapy; pregnancy (category D), lactation.
CAUTIOUS USE Impaired kidney and liver function; patients receiving cadaver kidney; myasthenia gravis.

ROUTE & DOSAGE

Renal Transplantation
Adult: **PO** 3–5 mg/kg/d initially, may be able to reduce to 1–3 mg/kg/d **IV** 3–5 mg/kg/d initially, may be able to reduce to 1–3 mg/kg/d

Rheumatoid Arthritis
Adult: **PO** 1 mg/kg/d initially, may be increased by 0.5 mg/kg/d at 4–6 wk intervals if needed up to 2.5 mg/kg/d

Renal Impairment
Cl_{cr} 10–50 mL/min: 75% of usual dose; <10 mL/min: 50% of usual dose

ADMINISTRATION

Oral
- Give oral drug in divided doses (as prescribed) with food or immediately after meals to minimize gastric disturbances.

Intravenous

PREPARE: **Direct/Intermittent:** Reconstitute by adding 10 mL sterile water for injection into vial; swirl until dissolved. May be further diluted with 50 mL NS, D5W, or D5/NS. Reconstituted solution may be stored at room temperature but must be used within 24 h after reconstitution (contains no preservatives).
ADMINISTER: **Direct/Intermittent:** May infuse over 5 min to 8 h. Typical infusion time is 30–60 min or longer. If longer infusion time is ordered, the final volume of the IV solution is increased appropriately. Check with physician.

- Store at 15°–30° C (59°–86° F) in tightly closed, light-resistant containers unless otherwise directed.

ADVERSE EFFECTS (≥1%) **Body as a Whole:** Hypersensitivity (skin eruptions, rash, arthralgia). **GI:** Nausea, vomiting, anorexia, esophagitis, diarrhea, steatorrhea, hepatitis with elevations in bilirubin, alkaline phosphatase, AST, ALT, biliary stasis, toxic hepatitis. **Hematologic:** Bone marrow depression, thrombocytopenia, leukopenia, anemia, agranulocytosis, pancytopenia. **Other:** *Secondary infection (immunosuppression);* dysarthria, alopecia; carcinogenic and teratogenic potential reported.

DIAGNOSTIC TEST INTERFERENCE Azathioprine may decrease plasma and urinary ***uric acid*** in patients with gout.

INTERACTIONS Drug: Allopurinol increases effects and toxicity of azathioprine by reducing metabolism of the active metabolite; **allopurinol** doses should be decreased by one third or one fourth; **tubocurarine** and other NONDEPOLARIZING SKELETAL MUSCLE RELAXANTS may reverse or inhibit neuromuscular blocking effects.

PHARMACOKINETICS Absorption: Readily absorbed from GI tract. **Distribution:** Crosses placenta. **Metabolism:** Extensively metabolized in liver to active metabolite mercaptopurine. **Elimination:** Eliminated in urine. **Half-Life:** 3 h.

NURSING IMPLICATIONS

Assessment & Drug Effects

- Monitor therapeutic effectiveness which usually requires 6–8 wk of therapy for patients with rheumatoid arthritis (improvement in morning stiffness and grip strength). If no improvement has occurred after 12-wk trial period, drug is generally discontinued.
- Lab tests: Perform CBC, including Hgb and platelet counts, prior to and at least weekly during first month of therapy, twice monthly during second and third months, and monthly, or more frequently thereafter, if indicated (e.g., by dosage or therapy changes).
- Monitor for toxicity. Drug has a high toxic potential. Because it may have delayed action, dosage should be reduced or drug withdrawn at the first indication of an abnormally large or persistent decrease in leukocyte or platelet count to avoid irreversible bone marrow depression.
- Monitor vital signs. Report signs of infection.
- Monitor kidney function (urine protein, urine electrolytes, creatinine clearance, serum creatinine, BUN) periodically.
- Monitor I&O ratio; note color, character, and specific gravity of urine. Report an abrupt decrease in urinary output or any change in I&O ratio.
- Monitor liver function (alkaline phosphatase, AST, ALT, serum bilirubin) and repeat at least every 3 mo or more frequently if indicated. If hepatic toxicity (see Appendix F) develops, therapy may have to be withdrawn.
- Monitor for signs of abnormal bleeding (easy bruising, bleeding gums, petechiae, purpura, melena, epistaxis, dark urine [hematuria], hemoptysis, hematemesis). If thrombocytopenia occurs, invasive procedures should be withheld, if possible.
- Use protective isolation for the hospitalized patient to reduce risk of infections.

Patient & Family Education

- Avoid contact with anyone who has a cold or other infection and report signs of impending infection. Exercise scrupulous personal hygiene because infection is a constant hazard of immunosuppressive therapy.
- Practice birth control during therapy and for 4 mo after drug is discontinued. This drug is associated with potential hazards in pregnancy.
- Do not receive/take vaccinations or other immunity-conferring agents during therapy because they may precipitate unusually severe reactions due to the immunosuppressive effects of the drug.
- Do not breast feed while taking this drug without consulting physician.

AZELAIC ACID

(a'ze-laic)

Azelex, Finevin, Finacea

Classifications: SKIN AND MUCOUS MEMBRANE AGENT; ANTIACNE

Prototype: Isotretinoin

Pregnancy Category: B

AVAILABILITY 20% cream; 15% gel

ACTIONS Azelaic acid is a naturally occurring dicarboxylic acid. The antimicrobial action may be attributable to inhibition of the microbial cellular protein synthesis. A normalization of keratinization may also contribute to its clinical effectiveness.

THERAPEUTIC EFFECTS Topical 20% azelaic acid possesses antimicrobial activity against *Propionibacterium acnes* and *Staphylococcus epidermidis.*

USES Mild to moderate inflammatory acne vulgaris, mild to moderate rosacea.

CONTRAINDICATIONS Hypersensitivity to any component in the drug.

CAUTIOUS USE Dark complexion, pregnancy (category B), lactation. Safety and efficacy in children <12 y is not established.

ROUTE & DOSAGE

Acne Vulgaris, Rosacea

Adult/Child: **Topical** >12 y, Apply thin film to clean and dry area b.i.d.

ADMINISTRATION

Topical

- Wash and dry skin thoroughly prior to application of drug.
- Apply by thoroughly massaging a thin film of the cream or gel into the affected area. Avoid occlusive dressing.
- Wash hands before and after application of cream or gel.
- Store at 15°–30° C (59°–86° F).

ADVERSE EFFECTS (≥1%) **Skin:** Pruritus, burning, stinging, tingling, erythema, dryness, rash, peeling, irritation, contact dermatitis, vitiligo depigmentation, hypertrichosis. **Other:** Worsening of asthma.

PHARMACOKINETICS Absorption: Approximately 4% is absorbed through the skin. **Onset:** 4–8 wk. **Distribution:** Distributes into all tissues. **Metabolism:** Partially metabolized by beta oxidation in liver. **Elimination:** Excreted primarily in urine. **Half-Life:** 12 h.

NURSING IMPLICATIONS

Assessment & Drug Effects

- Assess for signs of hypopigmentation and report immediately.
- Monitor for sensitivity or severe irritation, which may warrant drug dosage reduction or discontinuation.

Patient & Family Education

- Learn proper application of cream or gel and avoid contact with eyes or mucous membranes.
- Wash eyes with copious amounts of water if contact with medication occurs.
- Note: Transient pruritus, burning, and stinging are common; however, severe skin irritation or hypopigmentation should be reported.
- Do not breast feed while using this drug without consulting physician.

AZELASTINE HYDROCHLORIDE

(a-ze-las′teen)

Astelin, Optivar

Classifications: ANTIHISTAMINE; H_1-RECEPTOR ANTAGONIST; OCULAR ANTIHISTAMINE

Prototype: Diphenhydramine

Pregnancy Category: C

AVAILABILITY 137 mcg/spray nasal spray; 0.05% ophthalmic solution

ACTIONS First generation antihistamine that is a potent histamine H_1 receptor antagonist.

THERAPEUTIC EFFECTS Effective in the symptomatic treatment of seasonal allergic rhinitis and as a nasal decongestant.

USES Seasonal allergic rhinitis, itching associated with allergic conjunctivitis.

CONTRAINDICATIONS Hypersensitivity to azelastine; concurrent use of CNS depressants; pregnancy (category C), lactation, children <3 y.

CAUTIOUS USE Hepatic or renal disease; children <11 y; asthmatics.

ROUTE & DOSAGE

Allergic Rhinitis

Adult: **Intranasal** 2 sprays per nostril b.i.d.

Child: **Intranasal** *5–11 y,* 1 spray per nostril b.i.d.

Allergic Conjunctivitis

See Appendix A-1.

ADMINISTRATION

Intranasal

- Prime delivery unit before first use (see manufacturer's instructions).
- Instruct patient to clear nasal passages prior to drug installation; then tilt head forward slightly and sniff gently when drug is sprayed into each nostril.
- Store the bottle upright at room temperature, 15°–30° C (59°–86° F).

ADVERSE EFFECTS (≥1%) **Body as a Whole:** Fatigue, dizziness. **GI:** Dry mouth, nausea. **Metabolic:** Weight gain. **CNS:** *Headache, somnolence.* **Respiratory:** Pharyngitis, *rhinitis,* paroxysmal sneezing, *cough,* asthma. **Special Senses:** *Bitter taste,* nasal burning, epistaxis, conjunctivitis.

INTERACTIONS Drug: Alcohol and CNS DEPRESSANTS may cause reduced alertness.

PHARMACOKINETICS Absorption: 40% absorbed from nasal inhalation. **Peak:** 2–3 h. **Metabolism:** Metabolized by CYP450 to active metabolites. **Elimination:** Excreted primarily in feces. **Half-Life:** 22 h.

NURSING IMPLICATIONS

Assessment & Drug Effects

- Monitor level of alertness especially in older adults and with concurrent use of other CNS depressants.

Patient & Family Education

- Follow manufacturer's directions for priming the metered dose spray unit before first use and after storage of >3 d.
- Tilt head forward while instilling spray. Avoid getting spray in eyes.
- Do not drive or engage in potentially hazardous activities until response to drug is known.
- Avoid concurrent use of CNS depressants, such as alcohol, while taking this drug.

- Discard spray unit and dispensing package bottle after 3 mo.
- Do not breast feed while using this drug.

AZITHROMYCIN

(a-zi-thro-mye'sin)
Zithromax
Classifications: ANTIINFECTIVE; MACROLIDE ANTIBIOTIC
Prototype: Erythromycin
Pregnancy Category: B

AVAILABILITY 250 mg, 600 mg tablets; 100 mg/5 mL, 200 mg/5 mL, 1 g/packet oral suspension; 500 mg injection

ACTIONS A macrolide antibiotic that reversibly binds to the 50S ribosomal subunit of susceptible organisms and consequently inhibits protein synthesis.
THERAPEUTIC EFFECTS Effective for treatment of mild to moderate infections caused by pyogenic streptococci, *Streptococcus pneumoniae, Haemophilus influenzae,* and *Staphylococcus aureus.*

USES Pneumonia, lower respiratory tract infections, pharyngitis/tonsillitis, gonorrhea, nongonococcal urethritis, skin and skin structure infections due to susceptible organisms, otitis media, *Mycobacterium avium–intracellulare* complex infections, acute bacterial sinusitis.
UNLABELED USES Bronchitis, *Helicobacter pylori* gastritis.

CONTRAINDICATIONS Hypersensitivity to azithromycin, erythromycin, or any of the macrolide antibiotics.
CAUTIOUS USE Older adults or debilitated persons, hepatic or renal impairment; GI disease; ventricular arrhythmias, QT prolongation; UV exposure; pregnancy (category B), and lactation.

ROUTE & DOSAGE

Bacterial Infections
Adult: **PO** 500 mg on day 1, then 250 mg q24h for 4 more d **IV** 500 mg q.d. times at least 2 d, administer 1 mg/mL over 3 h or 2 mg/mL over 1 h
Child: **PO** ≥6 *mo,* 10 mg/kg on day 1, then 5 mg/kg for 4 more d (max: 250 mg/d)

Acute Bacterial Sinusitis
Adult: **PO** 500 mg once daily × 3 d
Child: **PO** ≥*6 mo,* 10 mg/kg once daily × 3 d

Otitis Media
Child: **PO** >*6 mo,* 30 mg/kg as a single dose or 10 mg/kg once daily (not to exceed 500 mg/d) for 3 days or 10 mg/kg as a single dose on day 1 followed by 5 mg/kg/d on days 2–5.

Gonorrhea
Adult: **PO** 2 g as a single dose

Chancroid
Adult: **PO** 1 g as a single dose
Child: **PO** 20 mg/kg as single dose (max: 1 g)

ADMINISTRATION

Oral
- Give capsule at least 1 h before or 2 h after a meal. Tablets may be taken without regard to food.
- Do not give within 2 h of an aluminum or magnesium-containing antacid.

Intravenous

PREPARE: **Intermittent:** Reconstitute 500-mg vial with 4.8 mL of sterile water for injection and

shake until dissolved. Final concentration is 100 mg/mL. Solution must be further diluted to 1.0 or 2.0 mg/mL by adding 5 mL of the 100-mg/mL solution to 500 mL or 250 mL, respectively, of D5W, D5/NS, 0.45NS, or other compatible solution.
ADMINISTER: **Intermittent:** Administer diluted solution over at least 60 min. Do not give a bolus dose.

- Store drug when diluted as directed for 24 h at or below 30° C (86° F) or for 7 d under 5° C (41° F).

ADVERSE EFFECTS (≥1%) **CNS:** Headache, dizziness. **GI:** Nausea, vomiting, diarrhea, abdominal pain; hepatotoxicity, mild elevations in liver function tests.

DIAGNOSTIC TEST INTERFERENCE Liver function tests: reversible, asymptomatic elevations in ***liver enzymes (AST, ALT, gamma glutamyl transferase, alkaline phosphatase)*** have been reported in some patients treated with azithromycin.

INTERACTIONS Drug: ANTACIDS may decrease peak level of azithromycin; may increase toxicity of **dihydroergotamine, ergotamine. Food:** Food will decrease the amount of azithromycin absorbed by 50%.

PHARMACOKINETICS Absorption: 37% of dose reaches the systemic circulation. **Onset:** 48 h. **Peak:** 2.5–4 h. **Distribution:** Extensively distributed to most tissues including sputum, blister, and vaginal secretions; tissue concentrations are often higher than serum concentrations. **Metabolism:** Metabolized in liver. **Elimination:** 5%–12% of dose is excreted in urine. **Half-Life:** Increases with time after the dose due to slow elimination from tissue sites; ranges from 9.6–40 h.

NURSING IMPLICATIONS

Assessment & Drug Effects

- Monitor for and report loose stools or diarrhea, since pseudomembranous colitis (see Appendix F) must be ruled out.
- Monitor PT and INR closely with concurrent warfarin use.

Patient & Family Education

- Direct sunlight (UV) exposure should be minimized during therapy with drug.
- Take aluminum or magnesium antacids 2 h before or after drug.
- Report onset of loose stools or diarrhea.
- Do not breast feed while taking this drug without consulting physician.

AZTREONAM

(az-tree'oh-nam)
Azactam
Classifications: ANTIINFECTIVE; BETA-LACTAM ANTIBIOTIC
Prototype: Imipenem-Cilastatin
Pregnancy Category: B

AVAILABILITY 500 mg, 1 g, 2 g vials

ACTIONS Differs structurally from other beta-lactam antibiotics (penicillins and cephalosporins) in having a monocyclic rather than a bicyclic nucleus. Acts by inhibiting synthesis of bacterial cell wall, primarily in aerobic, gram-negative bacteria.
THERAPEUTIC EFFECTS Highly resistant to beta-lactamases and does not readily induce their formation. Spectrum of activity limited to aerobic, gram-negative

bacteria. Therapeutically active against *Haemophilus influenzae, Pseudomonas aeruginosa, Neisseria gonorrhoeae,* and against *Enterobacteriaceae* including most strains of *E. coli, Enterobacter, Klebsiella, Proteus, Providencia, Shigella, Salmonella,* and *Serratia.* There appears to be little cross-allergenicity with penicillins and cephalosporins.

USES Gram-negative infections of urinary tract, lower respiratory tract, skin and skin structures; and for intraabdominal and gynecologic infections, septicemia, and as adjunctive therapy for surgical infections. Often used in combination with other antibiotics active against gram-positive and anaerobic bacteria in mixed infections.

CONTRAINDICATIONS Safety during pregnancy (category B), lactation, or in infants and children is not established.

CAUTIOUS USE History of hypersensitivity reaction to penicillin, cephalosporins, or to other drugs; impaired renal or hepatic function.

ROUTE & DOSAGE

Urinary Tract Infection

Adult: **IV/IM** 0.5–1 g q8–12h

Moderate to Severe Infections

Adult: **IV/IM** 1–2 g q6–8h (max: 8 g/24 h)
Neonate: **IV/IM** *≤7 d,* 60–90 mg/kg/d divided q8–12h; *>7 d,* 60–120 mg/kg/d divided q6–12h
Child: **IV/IM** *>1 mo,* 90–120 mg/kg/d divided q6–8h

Cystic Fibrosis

Child: **IV/IM** 50 mg/kg q6–8h (max: 8 g/d)

ADMINISTRATION

Intramuscular

- Reconstitute with at least 3 mL of diluent per gram of drug for IM injection. Immediately and vigorously shake vial to dissolve. Suitable diluents include sterile water for injection; bacteriostatic water for injection (with benzyl alcohol and propyl parabens); NS 0.9% for injection.
- Give IM injections deeply into large muscle mass such as the upper outer quadrant of the gluteus maximus or lateral thigh. Rotate injection sites.

Intravenous

Verify correct IV concentration and rate of infusion/injection with physician before giving to neonates, infants, and children.

PREPARE: **Direct:** Reconstitute a single dose with 6–10 mL of sterile water for injection. ▪ Immediately shake vial until solution is dissolved. ▪ Reconstituted solutions are colorless to light straw yellow and turn slightly pink on standing. **Intermittent:** Each gram of reconstituted aztreonam must be further diluted in at least 50 mL of D5W, NS, or other solution approved by manufacturer to yield a concentration not to exceed 20 mg/mL.

ADMINISTER: **Direct:** Give over 3–5 min. **Intermittent:** Give over 20–60 min through Y-site.

INCOMPATIBILITIES **Solution/additive: Ampicillin, metronidazole, nafcillin.**

ADVERSE EFFECTS (≥1%) **Body as a Whole:** Hypersensitivity (urticaria, eosinophilia, <u>anaphylaxis</u>). **CNS:** Headache, dizziness, confusion, paresthesias, insomnia, seizures. **GI:** Nausea, *diarrhea,* vomiting, elevated liver function tests. **Hematologic:** Eosinophilia. **Special Senses:** Tinnitus, nasal congestion, sneezing, diplopia. **Skin:** Rash, purpura, erythema multiforme, exfoliative dermatitis, diaphoresis; petechiae, pruritus. **Other:** Local reactions (phlebitis, thrombophlebitis (following IV), pain at injection sites), superinfections (gram-positive cocci), vaginal candidiasis.

DIAGNOSTIC TEST INTERFERENCE Aztreonam may cause transient elevations of ***liver function tests,*** increases in ***PT*** and ***PTT,*** minor changes in ***Hgb,*** and positive ***Coombs' test.***

INTERACTIONS Drug: Imipenem-cilastatin, cefoxitin may be antagonistic, **probenecid** slows renal elimination of aztreonam.

PHARMACOKINETICS Peak: 1 h IM. **Distribution:** Widely distributed including synovial and blister fluid, bile, bronchial secretions, prostate, bone, and CSF; crosses placenta; distributed into breast milk in small amounts. **Metabolism:** Not extensively metabolized. **Elimination:** 60%–70% excreted in urine within 24 h. **Half-Life:** 1.6–2.1 h.

NURSING IMPLICATIONS

Assessment & Drug Effects

- Lab tests: Obtain baseline C&S test prior to initiation of therapy. Start drug pending results.
- Baseline and periodic renal function tests, particularly in older adults and in those with history of renal impairment.
- Inspect IV injection sites daily for signs of inflammation. Pain and phlebitis occur in a significant number of patients.

Patient & Family Education

- Determine previous hypersensitivity reactions to penicillins, cephalosporins, and other allergens prior to therapy.
- Monitor for S&S of opportunistic infections (diarrhea, rectal or vaginal itching or discharge, fever, cough) and promptly report onset to physician. Overgrowth of nonsusceptible organisms, particularly *staphylococci, streptococci,* and fungi, is a threat, especially in patients receiving prolonged or repeated therapy.
- Note: IV therapy may cause a change in taste sensation. Report interference with eating.
- Do not breast feed while taking this drug without consulting physician.

BACAMPICILLIN HYDROCHLORIDE

(ba-kam-pi-sill'in)

Penglobe ♣, Spectrobid

Classifications: ANTIINFECTIVE; ANTIBIOTIC; AMINOPENICILLIN

Prototype: Ampicillin

Pregnancy Category: B

AVAILABILITY 400 mg tablets

ACTIONS Acid-stable, penicillinase-sensitive aminopenicillin that is rapidly hydrolyzed to ampicillin in body. Has broad spectrum of antimicrobial activity and exerts antibacterial action by inhibiting bacterial cell wall synthesis. More rapidly and completely absorbed from GI tract than ampicillin is, and serum concentrations attained are higher.

THERAPEUTIC EFFECTS Bacampicillin has a broad spectrum of antimicrobial activity against both gram-positive and gram-negative organisms.

B

USES Infections caused by susceptible microorganisms of upper and lower respiratory tract, urinary tract, skin and skin structures; acute uncomplicated gonorrhea.

CONTRAINDICATIONS Hypersensitivity to penicillins; pregnancy (category B); infectious mononucleosis or other viral diseases; children <25 kg. **CAUTIOUS USE** History of allergy to cephalosporins; lactation.

ROUTE & DOSAGE

Moderate to Severe Infections
Adult: **PO** 400–800 mg q12h
Child: **PO** 12.5–25 mg/kg q12h

Gonorrhea
Adult: **PO** 1.6 g with 1 g probenecid times 1

ADMINISTRATION

Oral
- Note: Tablets may be given without regard to food.
- Do not give concurrently with disulfiram (Antabuse).
- Store in tight container at 15°–30° C (59°–86° F) unless otherwise directed.

ADVERSE EFFECTS (≥1%) **Body as a Whole:** Hypersensitivity (erythematous rash; anaphylaxis). **GI:** *Nausea,* vomiting, anorexia, *diarrhea.* **Hematologic:** Thrombocytopenia, eosinophilia, anemia. **Other:** Superinfections, fixed drug eruption.

DIAGNOSTIC TEST INTERFERENCE High urine bacampicillin concentrations can result in false-positive ***urine glucose determinations with copper sulfate tests*** *(Benedict's, Clinitest, Fehling's);* ***glucose oxidase*** methods *(Clinistix, TesTape)* are not affected. ***Serum ALT*** and ***AST*** may increase.

INTERACTIONS Drug: Allopurinol increases incidence of rash; since ampicillin may interfere with ORAL CONTRACEPTIVE action, female patients should be advised to utilize nonhormonal contraception while on ANTIBIOTICS. **Food:** May decrease absorption of bacampicillin suspension; give 1 h before or 2 h after meals.

PHARMACOKINETICS Absorption: Rapidly and almost completely absorbed; hydrolyzed to ampicillin. **Distribution:** Most body tissues; crosses placenta; appears in breast milk. **Metabolism:** Metabolized in liver. **Elimination:** 75% eliminated as ampicillin in urine within 8 h. **Half-Life:** 0.7–1.1 h.

NURSING IMPLICATIONS

Assessment & Drug Effects
- Determine previous hypersensitivity reactions to penicillins, cephalosporins, and other allergens prior to therapy.
- Lab tests: Baseline C&S tests prior to initiation of therapy; start drug pending results.
- Baseline and periodic checks of renal, hepatic, and hematopoietic status are advised during prolonged therapy, particularly in patients with history of impaired function of these systems, and in premature infants and neonates.

Patient & Family Education
- Report symptoms of an allergic hypersensitivity reaction immediately (see Appendix F).
- Report signs of superinfection (see Appendix F).
- Take all prescribed medicine as prescribed.
- Do not breast feed while taking this drug without consulting physician.

BACITRACIN

(bass-i-tray'sin)

Baciguent, Bacitin

Classifications: ANTIINFECTIVE; ANTIBIOTIC

Pregnancy Category: C

AVAILABILITY 50,000 unit vial; 500 units/g cream

ACTIONS Polypeptide antibiotic derived from cultures of *Bacillus subtilis*. Precise mechanism of action not known. Appears to interfere with function of bacterial cell membrane by inhibiting cell wall synthesis. Spectrum of antibacterial activity similar to that of penicillin. Bactericidal or bacteriostatic depending on concentration and susceptibility of organism.

THERAPEUTIC EFFECTS Active against many gram-positive organisms including *Streptococci, Staphylococci, Pneumococci, Corynebacteria, Clostridia, Neisseria, Haemophilus influenzae,* and *Treponema pallidum*. Also active against *Gonococci* and *Meningococci;* ineffective against most other gram-negative organisms.

USES Parenteral therapy restricted to infants with *Staphylococcal* pneumonia and empyema due to susceptible organisms where adequate laboratory facilities and constant supervision are available. Used topically in treatment of superficial infections of skin.

UNLABELED USES Orally for treatment of antibiotic-associated colitis. Has been used investigationally by various routes (intrathecal, intrapleural, intrasynovial) for serious infections.

CONTRAINDICATIONS Toxic reaction or renal dysfunction associated with bacitracin; impaired renal function; atopic individuals; pregnancy (category C).

CAUTIOUS USE Myasthenia gravis or other neuromuscular disease. Patients allergic to neomycin may be sensitive to bacitracin.

ROUTE & DOSAGE

Systemic Infections

Child: **IM** <2.5 kg up to 900 U/kg/24 h divided q8–12h; >2.5 kg up to 1000 U/kg/24h divided q8–12h

Skin Infections

Adult: **Topical** Apply thin layer of ointment b.i.d., t.i.d., as solution of 250–1000 U/mL in wet dressing

ADMINISTRATION

Intramuscular

- Do not use parenteral bacitracin for longer than 12 d.
- Reconstitute with NS containing 2% procaine hydrochloride (prescribed). Do not reconstitute with diluents containing parabens because solution may precipitate or become cloudy.
- Alternate injection sites since injections are painful.
- Dry bacitracin vials should be stored in refrigerator at 2°–8° C (36°–46° F). Store solution for a maximum of 1 wk if refrigerated. Inactivation occurs at room temperature.

Topical

- Clean affected area prior to application. May be covered with a sterile bandage.
- Store ointments in tightly closed containers at 15°–30° C (59°–86° F) unless otherwise directed.

ADVERSE EFFECTS (≥1%) **GI:** Anorexia, nausea, vomiting, diarrhea,

B

rectal itching and burning. **Hematologic:** Systemic use: Bone marrow depression, blood dyscrasias; eosinophilia. **Body as a Whole:** Hypersensitivity (erythema, anaphylaxis). **Urogenital:** Nephrotoxicity, dose related: Increased BUN, uremia, renal tubular and glomerular necrosis. **Special Senses:** Tinnitus. **Other:** Pain and inflammation at injection site, fever, superinfection, neuromuscular blockade with respiratory depression.

INTERACTIONS Drug: With AMINOGLYCOSIDES, possibility of additive nephrotoxic and neuromuscular blocking effects; with **tubocurarine** and other NONDEPOLARIZING SKELETAL MUSCLE RELAXANTS, possibility of additive neuromuscular blocking effects.

PHARMACOKINETICS Absorption: Poorly absorbed from intact or denuded skin or mucous membranes. **Peak:** 1–2 h IM. **Duration:** 6–8 h. **Distribution:** Widely distributed including peritoneal and ascitic fluids. **Elimination:** Slow renal excretion (10%–40% in 24 h).

NURSING IMPLICATIONS

Assessment & Drug Effects

- Lab tests: Baseline C&S tests prior to initiation of therapy; start drug pending results.
- Determine BUN and nonprotein nitrogen (NPN); examine urine for albumin, casts, and cellular elements, before systemic therapy is started. Monitor renal function daily throughout therapy.
- Watch for signs of local allergic reaction (itching, burning, redness) with topical skin applications. Local reactions have preceded life-threatening anaphylactic episodes.
- Monitor I&O during parenteral therapy. Adequate urinary output is important to reduce possibility of renal toxicity. If fluid intake is inadequate or urinary output decreases, report to physician.
- Inspect urine for turbidity and hematuria, and watch for other S&S of urinary tract dysfunction. Report any changes in urination pattern (e.g., oliguria, urinary frequency, nocturia).
- Note: Prolonged use may result in overgrowth of nonsusceptible organisms, especially *Candida albicans.*

Patient & Family Education

- Report local allergic reactions with topical applications (e.g., itching, burning, redness).

BACLOFEN

(bak'loe-fen)

Lioresal, Lioresal DS

Classifications: AUTONOMIC NERVOUS SYSTEM AGENT; CENTRAL-ACTING SKELETAL MUSCLE RELAXANT

Prototype: Cyclobenzaprine

Pregnancy Category: C

AVAILABILITY 10 mg, 20 mg tablets; 10 mg, 20 mg orally disintegrating tablets; 500 mcg/mL, 2000 mcg/mL ampules

ACTIONS Centrally acting skeletal muscle relaxant. Precise mechanism of action not determined. Depresses monosynaptic and polysynaptic afferent reflex activity at spinal cord level.

THERAPEUTIC EFFECTS Reduces skeletal muscle spasm caused by upper motor neuron lesions.

USES To provide symptomatic relief of painful spasms in multiple sclerosis and in the management of detrusor sphincter dyssynergia in spinal cord injury or disease.

UNLABELED USES Treatment of trigeminal neuralgia and of tardive dystonia associated with antipsychotic medications.

CONTRAINDICATIONS Safety during pregnancy (category C), lactation; coagulopathy, bacteremia, intramuscular or intrathecal administration, subcutaneous administration.

CAUTIOUS USE Impaired renal and hepatic function; bipolar disorder, psychosis, schizophrenia, seizure disorders, seizures, stroke, cerebral palsy, depression, diabetes mellitus, dialysis, head trauma, PKU, epilepsy; thrombocytopenia; psychiatric or brain disorders; older adults, children.

ROUTE & DOSAGE

Muscle Spasm

Adult: **PO** 5 mg t.i.d. may increase by 5 mg/dose q3d prn (max: 80 mg/d)
Child: **PO** *2–7 y:* 10–15 mg/d divided q8h, may increase by 5–15 mg/d q3d (max: 40 mg/d); *≥8 y:* 10–15 mg/d divided q8h, may increase by 5–15 mg/d q3d (max: 60 mg/d)
Adult: **Intrathecal** Prior to infusion pump implantation, initiate trial dose of 50 mcg/mL bolus administered in intrathecal space by barbotage over ≤1 min. Observe patient over next 4–8 h for significant decrease in muscle spasm. If response is less than desired, administer second bolus of 75 mcg/1.5 mL and observe 4–8 h. May repeat in 24 h with a 100 mcg/2-mL bolus if necessary.
Postimplant titration Use screening dose if response lasted >12 h or double screening dose if response lasted <12 h and administer over 24 h. After first 24 h, decrease dose by 10%–30% q24h until desired response achieved. Maintenance doses range from 12–1500 mcg/d, with most patients maintained on 300–800 mcg/d

ADMINISTRATION

Oral

- Give with food or milk to avoid GI distress.

Intrathecal

- Give by direct intrathecal injection (via lumbar puncture or catheter) over at least 1 min or longer.
- Dilute *only* with sterile, preservative free NS injection. Baclofen must be diluted to a concentration of 50 mcg/mL when preparing test doses.
- Intrathecal infusion pump: Do not abruptly discontinue as serious adverse effects may develop.
- Store at 15°–30° C (59°–86° F) in tightly closed container unless otherwise directed.

ADVERSE EFFECTS (≥1%) **CNS:** *Transient drowsiness,* vertigo, dizziness, weakness, fatigue, headache, confusion, insomnia; ataxia, loss of seizure control in epileptic patients; abrupt discontinuation of intrathecal administration may result in high fever, altered mental status, exaggerated rebound spasticity, and muscle rigidity, that in rare cases has advanced to rhabdomyolysis, multiple organ-system failure, and death. **CV:** Hypotension. **Special Senses:** Tinnitus, nasal congestion; blurred vision, mydriasis, nystagmus, diplopia, strabismus, miosis. **GI:** Nausea, constipation, vomiting; mild increases in

B

AST, and alkaline phosphatase, jaundice. **Urogenital:** Urinary frequency.

DIAGNOSTIC TEST INTERFERENCE Possibility of increases in ***blood glucose,*** serum ***alkaline phosphatase,*** and ***AST*** levels.

INTERACTIONS Drug: Alcohol, CNS DEPRESSANTS, MAO INHIBITORS, ANTIHISTAMINES compound CNS depression; baclofen may increase blood **glucose** levels, making it necessary to increase dosage of SULFONYLUREAS, **insulin.**

PHARMACOKINETICS Absorption: Readily absorbed from GI tract. **Peak:** 2–3 h. **Duration:** 8 h. **Distribution:** Minimal amounts cross blood-brain barrier; crosses placenta; distribution into breast milk unknown. **Metabolism:** 15% of dose metabolized in liver. **Elimination:** 70%–85% excreted in urine within 72 h; some elimination in feces. **Half-Life:** 3–4 h.

NURSING IMPLICATIONS

Assessment & Drug Effects

- Supervise ambulation. Initially, the loss of spasticity induced by baclofen may affect patient's ability to stand or walk.
- Lab tests: baseline and periodic BP, weight, blood sugar, hepatic function tests, and urine.
- Monitor for adverse neuropsychiatric or genitourinary symptoms that resemble those of the underlying disease. Assess them carefully and report to the physician.
- Observe carefully for side effects: mental confusion, depression, hallucinations. Older adults are especially sensitive to this drug.
- Monitor patients with epilepsy closely for possible loss of seizure control.

Patient & Family Education

- Note: CNS depressant effects will be additive to other CNS depressants, including alcohol.
- Monitor blood glucose for loss of glycemic control if diabetic.
- Do not drive or engage in other potentially hazardous activities until the response to drug is known.
- Report adverse reactions to physician. Most can be reduced by decreasing dosage. Incidence of CNS symptoms (drowsiness, dizziness, ataxia) are reportedly high in patients >40 y of age.
- Do not self-dose with OTC drugs without physician's approval.
- Do not stop this drug unless directed to do so by physician. Drug withdrawal needs to be accomplished gradually over a period of 2 wk or more. Abrupt withdrawal following prolonged administration may cause anxiety, agitated behavior, auditory and visual hallucinations, severe tachycardia, acute exacerbation of spasticity, and seizures.
- Do not breast feed while taking this drug without consulting physician.

BALSALAZIDE

(bal-sal′a-zide)

Colazal

Classifications: GASTROINTESTINAL AGENT; MUCOUS MEMBRANE AGENT

Prototype: Mesalamine (5-ASA)

Pregnancy Category: B

AVAILABILITY 750 mg capsules

ACTIONS A prodrug of mesalamine that remains intact until it reaches the lumen of the colon. Thought to decrease inflammation of the mucous lining of the colon by blocking cyclooxygenase and inhibiting prostaglandin synthesis in the lining of the colon.

THERAPEUTIC EFFECTS An antiinflammatory agent and a prodrug of 5-ASA.

USES Treatment of mild to moderate active ulcerative colitis.

CONTRAINDICATIONS Prior hypersensitivity to salicylates, balsalazide. **CAUTIOUS USE** Hypersensitivity to mesalamine, sulfasalazine, olsalazine. Allergic response to any medications; hepatic or renal impairment; pregnancy (category B), lactation; pyloric stenosis. Safety and efficacy in children are not established.

ROUTE & DOSAGE

Ulcerative Colitis
Adult: **PO** 2250 mg (3 times 750 mg) t.i.d. for 8–12 wks

ADMINISTRATION

Oral
- Give in a consistent manner with respect to food intake (i.e., either always with or always without food).
- Store at room temperature, preferably between 15°–30° C (59°–86° F).

ADVERSE EFFECTS (≥1%) **Body as a Whole:** Arthralgia, fatigue, fever, pain, back pain. **CNS:** Headache, insomnia. **GI:** Abdominal pain, nausea, diarrhea, vomiting, rectal bleeding, flatulence, dyspepsia, coughing, anorexia. **Respiratory:** Rhinitis, pharyngitis.

INTERACTIONS No clinically significant interactions established.

PHARMACOKINETICS Absorption: Low and variable absorption from the colon. **Distribution:** >99% protein bound. **Metabolism:** Metabolized in colon by bacterial azoreductases to release 5-aminosalicylic acid and 4-aminobenzoyl-beta-alanine. **Elimination:** 25% of metabolites excreted in urine.

NURSING IMPLICATIONS

Assessment & Drug Effects
- Monitor for S&S of myelosuppression in patients also receiving azathioprine.
- Lab tests: Closely monitor CBS with concomitant azathioprine therapy; monitor renal and liver functions when used with other aminosalicylates.

Patient & Family Education
- Report worsening of S&S of colitis to physician (e.g., diarrhea, abdominal pain, fever, rectal bleeding).
- Do not breast feed while taking this drug without consulting physician.

BASILIXIMAB Pr
(bas-i-lix′i-mab)
Simulect
Classifications: IMMUNOSUPPRESSANT; MONOCLONAL ANTIBODY; INTERLEUKIN-2 RECEPTOR ANTIBODY
Pregnancy Category: B

AVAILABILITY 20 mg vials

ACTIONS Immunosuppressant agent that is an interleukin-2 receptor monoclonal antibody produced by recombinant DNA technology. Binds to and blocks interleukin-2R-alpha chain (CD-25 antibodies) on surface of activated T lymphocytes.
THERAPEUTIC EFFECTS Binding to CD-25 antibodies inhibits a critical pathway in the immune response of the lymphocytes involved in allograft rejection.

B

USES Prophylaxis of acute renal transplant rejection.

CONTRAINDICATIONS Hypersensitivity; serious infection or exposure to viral infections (e.g., chickenpox, herpes zoster); lactation.

CAUTIOUS USE History of untoward reactions to dacliximab or other monoclonal antibodies; pregnancy (category B).

ROUTE & DOSAGE

Prophylaxis for Transplant Rejection

Adult: **IV** 20 mg times 2 doses (1st dose 2 h before surgery, 2nd dose 4 d after transplant)
Child: **IV** *2–15 y,* 12 mg/m² (max: 20 mg/dose) times 2 doses (1st dose 2 h before surgery, 2nd dose 4 d after transplant)

ADMINISTRATION

Intravenous

PREPARE: **IV infusion:** Add 5 mL sterile water for injection to a 20 mg vial, rock vial gently to dissolve then further dilute in an infusion bag to a volume of 50 mL of NS or D5W. The resulting solution has a concentration of 2.5 mg/mL. ▪ Invert IV bag to dissolve but do not shake. ▪ Discard if diluted solution is colored or has particulate matter. Use IV solution immediately.

ADMINISTER: Infuse the ordered dose of diluted drug over 20–30 min.

▪ If necessary the diluted solution may be stored at room temperature for 4 h or at 2°–8° C (36°–46° F) for 24 h. Discard after 24 h. ▪ Store undiluted drug at 2°–8° C (36°–46° F).

ADVERSE EFFECTS (≥1%) **Body as a Whole:** Pain, peripheral edema, edema, fever, viral infection, asthenia, arthralgia, acute hypersensitivity reactions with any dose. **CNS:** Headache, tremor, dizziness, insomnia, paresthesias, agitation, depression. **CV:** Hypertension, chest pain, hypotension, arrhythmias. **GI:** Constipation, nausea, diarrhea, abdominal pain, vomiting, dyspepsia, moniliasis, flatulence, GI hemorrhage, melena, esophagitis, erosive stomatitis. **Hematologic:** Anemia, thrombocytopenia, thrombosis, polycythemia. **Respiratory:** Dyspnea, URI, cough, rhinitis, pharyngitis, bronchospasm. **Skin:** Poor wound healing, acne. **Urogenital:** Dysuria, UTI, albuminuria, hematuria, oliguria, frequency, renal tubular necrosis, urinary retention. **Other:** Cataract, conjunctivitis. **Metabolic:** Hyperkalemia, hypokalemia, hyperglycemia, hyperuricemia, hypophosphatemia, hypocalcemia, increased weight, hypercholesterolemia, acidosis.

PHARMACOKINETICS Duration: 36 days. **Distribution:** Binds to interleukin-2R-alpha sites on lymphocytes. **Half-Life:** 7.2 ± 3.2 d in adults, 11.5 ± 6.3 d in children.

NURSING IMPLICATIONS

Assessment & Drug Effects

- Monitor carefully for and immediately report S&S of opportunistic infection or anaphylactoid reaction (see Appendix F).

Patient & Family Education

- Report any distressing adverse effects.
- Avoid vaccination for 2 wk following last dose of drug.
- Do not breast feed while taking this drug.

BCG (BACILLUS CALMETTE-GUÉRIN) VACCINE

(ba-cil'lus cal'met-te guer'in)

Tice, TheraCys

Classifications: VACCINE; ANTINEOPLASTIC; IMMUNOMODULATOR; BIOLOGICAL RESPONSE MODIFIER

Pregnancy Category: C

AVAILABILITY 50 mg, 81 mg, 120 mg powder for suspension

ACTIONS BCG vaccine is an immunization agent for tuberculosis (TB). It is an attenuated strain of the bacillus Calmette and Guérin strain of *Mycobacterium bovis.* BCG vaccine stimulates the reticuloendothelial system (RES) to produce macrophages that do not allow mycobacteria to multiply. BCG live is used intravesically as a biological response modifier for bladder cancer in situ. BCG live is thought to cause a local, chronic inflammatory response involving macrophage and leukocyte infiltration of the bladder. This local inflammatory response leads to destruction of superficial tumor cells.

THERAPEUTIC EFFECTS BCG is active immunotherapy, which stimulates the immune mechanism to reject the tumor. It enhances the cytotoxicity of macrophages.

USES To protect tuberculin skin test-negative infants and children, and groups with an excessive rate of new TB infections; carcinoma in situ of the bladder.

UNLABELED USES Malignant melanoma.

CONTRAINDICATIONS Impaired immune responses, immunosuppressive corticosteroid therapy, asymptomatic carriers with positive HIV serology; fever; UTI; lactation.

CAUTIOUS USE Hypersensitivity to BCG; pregnancy (category C).

ROUTE & DOSAGE

Prevention of Tuberculosis (Tice only)

Adult: **Intradermal** 0.1 mL

Adult/Child: **Percutaneous** *>1 mo,* After reconstitution, 0.2–0.3 mL of vaccine is dropped onto the cleansed surface of the skin and administered using a multiple-puncture disk applied through the vaccine

Child: **Intradermal** *<3 mo,* 0.05 mL; *>3 mo,* 0.1 mL

Child: **Percutaneous** *<1 mo,* reduce adult dose by 1/2 (reconstitute with 2 mL), may need to revaccinate with full dose at 1 y; same as adult

Carcinoma of the Bladder

Adult: **Intravesical** 3 vials of **TheraCys** at 27 mg each (81 mg total) of BCG reconstituted with accompanying diluent 7–14 d after biopsies/transurethral resections once/wk for 6 wk plus one treatment at 3, 6, 12, 18, and 24 mo; 1 vial of **Tice** per intravesical instillation once/wk for 6 wk plus one treatment/mo for 6–12 mo

ADMINISTRATION

WARNING: Do not inject intravenously, subcutaneously, or intradermally.

Percutaneous

- Prepare solution: Add 1 mL sterile water for injection to 1 ampul of vaccine. Draw into syringe and expel back into ampul 3 times to mix.
- Administer drug by dropping 0.2–0.3 mL onto clean surface of

B

skin; then use a sterile multiple-puncture disk to create percutaneous skin punctures.

- Instruct to keep vaccination site dry for 24 h; no dressing is needed.
- Important: Avoid contact with BCG vaccine during preparation and administration.
- Store dry BCG powder, reconstituted vaccine, and diluent refrigerated at 2°–8° C (35°–46° F). Use reconstituted solution within 2 h.

Intravesical Instillation

- **TheraCys:** Dilute 3 vials of **TheraCys** in 50 mL of sterile preservative free NS and instill into bladder slowly by gravity flow via urethral catheter. Patient retains suspension for 2 h and then voids.
- **Tice:** Instill 1 vial of **Tice** intravesically once/wk for 6 wk plus one per mo for 6–12 mo.
- Important: Exercise care, when handling BCG vaccine to avoid contact with the product.

ADVERSE EFFECTS (≥1%) **CNS:** Intravesical administration: *malaise*, dizziness, headache, weakness. **Endocrine:** Hyperpyrexia. **GI:** Abdominal pain, anorexia, constipation, nausea, vomiting, diarrhea; hepatic dysfunction following intratumor injection, granulomatous hepatitis. **Urogenital:** Intravesical administration: bladder spasms, clot retention, decreased bladder capacity, decreased urine flow, *dysuria, hematuria,* incontinence, nocturia, UTI, cystitis, hemorrhagic cystitis, penile pain, prostatism. **Hematologic:** Thrombocytopenia, eosinophilia, *anemia,* leukopenia, <u>disseminated intravascular coagulation</u>. **Respiratory:** Cough (rare), pulmonary granulomas, pulmonary infection. **Skin:** Abscess with recurrent discharge, red papule that scales or ulcerates in about 5–6 wk, dermatomyositis, granulomas at injection site 4–6 wk after inoculation, keloid formation, lupus vulgaris. **Body as a Whole:** Systemic BCG infection, *chills, flu-like syndrome,* <u>anaphylaxis</u> (rare), allergic reactions, lymphadenitis.

DIAGNOSTIC TEST INTERFERENCE Prior BCG vaccination may result in false-positive ***tuberculin skin test (PPD).*** Following BCG vaccination, tuberculin sensitivity may persist for months to years.

INTERACTIONS Drug: Concurrent antimycobacterial therapy (**aminosalicylic acid, capreomycin, cycloserine, ethambutol, ethionamide, isoniazid, pyrazinamide, rifabutin, rifampin, streptomycin**) that inhibits multiplication of BCG bacilli has the potential to antagonize or altogether negate the BCG vaccine-mediated immune response. **Cyclosporine** may reduce the immunologic response to BCG vaccine. ***Cytomegalovirus immune globulin*** and other live vaccines (measles/mumps/rubella, oral polio) may interfere with immune response to BCG. Previous vaccination with or other exposure to BCG may induce variable sensitivity to tuberculin. A greater booster effect following repeat tuberculin testing has been reported in individuals with prior BCG vaccination when compared with individuals without prior vaccination.

PHARMACOKINETICS Not studied.

NURSING IMPLICATIONS

Assessment & Drug Effects

- Monitor for S&S of systemic BCG infection: Fever, chills, severe malaise, or cough.

- Culture blood and urine, if systemic infection is suspected.
- Assess for regional lymph node enlargement and report fistula formation.

Patient & Family Education

- Review potential adverse effects.
- Keep vaccination site clean until local reaction has subsided.
- Do not breast feed until cleared to do so by physician.

BECAPLERMIN

(be-cap′ler-min)

Regranex

Classifications: HORMONES AND SYNTHETIC SUBSTITUTES; GROWTH FACTOR

Pregnancy Category: C

AVAILABILITY 100 mcg/g gel

ACTIONS Recombinant human platelet-derived growth factor B in a topical gel. It induces fibroblast proliferation.

THERAPEUTIC EFFECTS Becaplermin enhances formation of new granulation tissue. It is effective against diabetic neuropathic ulcers that involve subcutaneous or deeper tissue and also have an adequate blood supply.

USES Lower-extremity diabetic neuropathic ulcers.

CONTRAINDICATIONS Hypersensitivity to drug or any component in formulation; neoplasms at site of application; wounds that close by primary intention; lactation.

CAUTIOUS USE Concurrent use of corticosteroids, cancer chemotherapy, or other immunosuppressive agents; ulcer wounds related to arterial or venous insufficiency; thermal, electrical, or radiation burns at wound site; malignancy; pregnancy (category C).

ROUTE & DOSAGE

Diabetic Neuropathic Ulcers

Adult: **Topical** Calculate the length of gel based on ulcer size and apply once/d until healed

ADMINISTRATION

Topical

- Squeeze calculated length of gel onto clean, firm, nonabsorbable surface.
- Apply even layer to ulcer area with clean tongue depressor or cotton swab and cover with saline-moistened dressing. After 12 h, remove dressing, clean ulcer by rinsing with water or saline to remove residual gel, and apply new saline-moistened dressing without becaplermin for next 12 h. Repeat cycle.
- Apply only to ulcers with good blood supply.
- Dosage calculation: Measure greatest length (L) and greatest width (W) of ulcer in inches or centimeters; using 15- or 7.5-g tube multiply ($L \times W$) × 0.6 for dose in inches or ($L \times W$)/4 for dose in cm; using 2-g tube multiply ($L \times W$) × 1.3 for dose in inches or ($L \times W$)/2 for dose in cm.
- Recalculate weekly/biweekly the amount of drug needed.
- Store at 2°–8° C (36°–46° F). Do not freeze and do not use beyond expiration date.

ADVERSE EFFECTS (≥1%) **Skin:** Erythematous rash.

PHARMACOKINETICS Absorption: <3% absorbed into systemic circulation.

NURSING IMPLICATIONS

Assessment & Drug Effects

- Therapeutic effectiveness: 30% decrease in ulcer size after 10 wk or complete healing after 20 wk.

- Monitor for and report appearance of erythematous rash.

Patient & Family Education

- Consult wound care provider who typically recalculates dosage weekly/biweekly.
- Follow directions for application carefully. Gel may be measured out on waxed paper.
- Wash hands prior to application and do not allow tip of tube to contact ulcer or any surface.
- Report worsening ulceration or development of skin rash.
- Do not breast feed while using this drug.

BECLOMETHASONE DIPROPIONATE

(be-kloe-meth'a-sone)

Beclovent, Beconase Nasal Inhaler, QVAR, QVAR Double Strength, Vancenase Nasal Inhaler, Vanceril, Vanceril D, Vancenase AQ

Classifications: HORMONE AND SYNTHETIC SUBSTITUTE; ADRENAL CORTICOSTEROID

Prototype: Hydrocortisone

Pregnancy Category: C

AVAILABILITY 42 mcg, 84 mcg metered dose inhalers; QVAR 40 mcg, 80 mcg inhalers; 42 mcg nasal inhaler; 0.042%, 0.084% nasal spray

See Appendix A-3.

BELLADONNA TINCTURE

(bell-a-don'na)

Classifications: AUTONOMIC NERVOUS SYSTEM AGENT; ANTICHOLINERGIC (PARASYMPATHOLYTIC); ANTIMUSCARINIC, ANTISPASMODIC

Prototype: Atropine

Pregnancy Category: C

AVAILABILITY 27–33 mg/100 mL tincture

ACTIONS Reversibly blocks action of acetylcholine at parasympathetic neuroeffector sites.

THERAPEUTIC EFFECTS Belladonna inhibits smooth muscle contractions and suppresses secretions of secretory glands.

USES Adjunct in treatment of peptic ulcer disease, irritable bowel syndrome, and neurogenic bowel disturbances. Also has been used for dysmenorrhea, nocturnal enuresis, spasms of urinary tract, nausea and vomiting of pregnancy, vertigo, and for symptomatic relief of parkinsonism.

CONTRAINDICATIONS Hypersensitivity to anticholinergic drugs; obstructive uropathy, atony of urinary bladder; esophageal reflux, obstructive disease of GI tract, intestinal atony, paralytic ileus, severe ulcerative colitis, toxic megacolon; myasthenia gravis; narrow-angle glaucoma; unstable cardiovascular status in acute hemorrhages. Safety during pregnancy (category C), lactation, or in children is not established.

CAUTIOUS USE Autonomic neuropathy; heart disease, hypertension; patients >40 y (higher incidence of glaucoma).

ROUTE & DOSAGE

Antispasmodic

Adult: **PO** 0.6–1 mL t.i.d. or q.i.d.
Child: **PO** 0.1 mL/kg/d in 3–4 divided doses (max: 3.5 mL/d)

ADMINISTRATION

Oral

- Administer 30–60 min before meals and at bedtime.

- Space administration of antacid and belladonna preparations at least 2 h apart.
- Store at 15°–30° C (59°–86° F) in tightly covered, light-resistant containers, unless otherwise directed.

ADVERSE EFFECTS (≥1%) **All:** Dose related. **CNS:** Excitement (young children and the older adults), confusion, delirium. **CV:** Rapid heart beat, tachycardia, palpitation. **Special Senses:** Blurred vision, mydriasis, photophobia. **GI:** *Dry mouth, constipation*. **Urogenital:** Urinary retention, urgency.

INTERACTIONS Drug: Amantadine, ANTIHISTAMINES, TRICYCLIC ANTIDEPRESSANTS, **quinidine, disopyramide, procainamide** have additive anticholinergic effects; **levodopa** effects decreased; **methotrimeprazine** may precipitate extrapyramidal effects; antipsychotic effects of PHENOTHIAZINES decreased (decreased absorption).

PHARMACOKINETICS Absorption: Readily absorbed from GI tract. **Onset:** 1–2 h. **Distribution:** Well distributed in body; crosses blood brain barrier. **Elimination:** Excreted unchanged in urine.

NURSING IMPLICATIONS

Assessment & Drug Effects

- Monitor ambulation of older adults or debilitated patients carefully, since drug may cause drowsiness and confusion.
- Monitor I&O and assess for urinary retention.

Patient & Family Education

- Note: Increase in fluid intake and bulk in diet may prevent or relieve constipation. Notify physician if constipation persists.
- Avoid hot baths, saunas, and strenuous work or exercise during hot and humid weather.
- Do not drive or engage in potentially hazardous activities until response to drug is known.
- Practice meticulous oral hygiene. Sugarless gum, lemon drops, and frequent sips of water may help dry mouth.
- Do not breast feed while taking this drug without consulting physician.

BENAZEPRIL HYDROCHLORIDE

(ben-a'ze-pril)
Lotensin
Classifications: CARDIOVASCULAR AGENT; ANGIOTENSIN-CONVERTING ENZYME (ACE) INHIBITOR
Prototype: Captopril
Pregnancy Category: D

AVAILABILITY 5 mg, 10 mg, 20 mg, 40 mg tablets

ACTIONS Lowers blood pressure by specific inhibition of the angiotensin-converting enzyme (ACE) and thus by decreasing angiotensin II (a potent vasoconstrictor) and aldosterone secretion.

THERAPEUTIC EFFECTS Benazepril achieves an antihypertensive effect by suppression of the renin-angiotensin-aldosterone system.

USES Treatment of mild to moderate hypertension.

UNLABELED USES CHF.

CONTRAINDICATIONS Hypersensitivity to benazepril or another ACE inhibitor. Safety during pregnancy (category D), lactation, or in children is not established.

CAUTIOUS USE Renal impairment, renal-artery stenosis; patients with hypovolemia, receiving diuretics, undergoing dialysis; patients in whom excessive hypotension would present a hazard (e.g., cerebrovascular insufficiency); CHF; hepatic impairment; diabetes mellitus.

ROUTE & DOSAGE

Hypertension
Adult: **PO** 10–40 mg/d in 1–2 divided doses

ADMINISTRATION

Oral

- Consult physician about initial dose if patient is also receiving diuretics. Typically an initial dose of 5 mg is used to minimize the risk of hypotension.
- Store at room temperature, but not above 30° C (86° F).

ADVERSE EFFECTS (≥1%) **CV:** Hypotension. **CNS:** *Headache,* dizziness, fatigue, weakness. **Endocrine:** Hyperkalemia (at higher doses). **GI:** Nausea, diarrhea or constipation, gastritis. **Urogenital:** Azotemia, oliguria, renal failure in patients with CHF. **Respiratory:** Cough, rhinitis, bronchitis. **Other:** Back pain.

DIAGNOSTIC TEST INTERFERENCE Elevations in ***serum bilirubin*** have been observed after benazepril administration. Benazepril inhibits ***aldosterone*** secretion, which causes an increase in ***serum potassium.***

INTERACTIONS Drug: POTASSIUM-SPARING DIURETICS may increase the risk of hyperkalemia. Benazepril may increase **lithium** levels, resulting in **lithium** toxicity.

PHARMACOKINETICS Absorption: Readily absorbed from GI tract with 37% reaching the systemic circulation. **Peak:** 2–6 h. **Duration:** 20–24 h. **Distribution:** Small amounts cross the blood-brain barrier; crosses placenta; small amount excreted in breast milk. **Metabolism:** Metabolized in liver to active metabolite, benazeprilat. **Elimination:** Benazeprilat (product of drug) is primarily excreted in urine. **Half-Life:** Benazepril 0.6 h; benazeprilat 22 h.

NURSING IMPLICATIONS

Assessment & Drug Effects

- Assess for hypotension, especially in patients who may be volume depleted (e.g., prolonged diuretic therapy, recent vomiting or diarrhea, salt restriction) or who have CHF.
- Lab tests: Monitor serum potassium levels for hyperkalemia (see Appendix F).

Patient & Family Education

- Do not use salt substitutes unless recommended by physician.
- Report swelling of face, eyes, lips, or tongue or difficulty breathing immediately to physician.
- Do not breast feed while taking this drug without consulting physician.

BENDROFLUMETHIAZIDE

(ben-droe-floo-meth-eye'a-zide)
Naturetin
Classifications: FLUID AND WATER BALANCE AGENT; THIAZIDE DIURETIC
Prototype: Hydrochlorothiazide
Pregnancy Category: C

AVAILABILITY 5 mg, 10 mg tablets

ACTIONS Thiazide diuretic chemically related to the sulfonamides. Similar to hydrochlorothiazide in pharmacologic action.
THERAPEUTIC EFFECTS Bendroflumethiazide decreases blood vol-

ume by increasing excretion of fluid and electrolytes. It has a hypotensive effect.

USES Management of edema associated with CHF, mild hypertension.

UNLABELED USES Lithium-associated diabetes insipidus.

CONTRAINDICATIONS Anuria, hypersensitivity to thiazides, sulfonamides; pregnancy (category C), lactation.

CAUTIOUS USE Renal and hepatic disease; gout; diabetes mellitus.

ROUTE & DOSAGE

Hypertension
Adult: **PO** 2.5–20 mg/d in 1–2 divided doses
Child: **PO** 0.05–0.4 mg/kg/d in 1–2 divided doses

ADMINISTRATION

Oral

- Give drug early in a.m. after patient has eaten to reduce gastric irritation and prevent possibility of interrupted sleep due to diuresis. If 2 daily doses are ordered, administer second dose no later than 3 p.m.
- Store tablets in tightly closed container at 15°–30° C (59°–86° F) unless otherwise specified.

ADVERSE EFFECTS (≥1%) **CV:** Orthostatic hypotension. **Metabolic:** Electrolyte imbalance, hypokalemia, hyperglycemia, impaired glucose tolerance, hyperuricemia. **Musculoskeletal:** Exacerbation of gout.

INTERACTIONS Drug: Cholestyramine, colestipol decrease absorption of the diuretic; **diazoxide** has additive effects; with **digoxin,** the hypokalemia may increase risk of **digitalis** toxicity; increases **lithium** levels and toxicity; may increase blood glucose levels, necessitating adjustment of hypoglycemic therapy (i.e., SULFONYLUREAS), **insulin.**

PHARMACOKINETICS Absorption: Readily absorbed from GI tract. **Onset:** 1–2 h. **Peak:** 6–12 h. **Duration:** 18–24 h. **Elimination:** Excreted unchanged in urine within 24 h.

NURSING IMPLICATIONS

Assessment & Drug Effects

- Monitor BP. Report a sudden fall in BP, which may initiate severe postural hypotension and potentially dangerous perfusion problems of the extremities, especially in older patients. Antihypertensive effects are generally noted in 3–4 d; maximal effects may require 3–4 wk.
- Monitor I&O ratio and pattern, and weight, particularly during first phase of antihypertensive therapy.
- Lab tests: Periodic serum electrolytes. Report hypokalemia promptly.
- Report unexplained onset of joint pain and limitation of motion; may be due to hyperuricemia since thiazides interfere with uric acid excretion, although thiazides rarely precipitate acute gout.
- Monitor diabetics for loss of glycemic control.

Patient & Family Education

- Eat potassium-rich foods such as fruit juices, potatoes, cereals, skim milk, and bananas to prevent onset of hyperuricemia.
- Make position changes slowly and in stages to avoid dizziness or fainting.
- Report joint pain or limited joint movement.

B

- Avoid OTC drugs unless approved by physician.
- Do not breast feed while taking this drug.

BENZALKONIUM CHLORIDE

(benz-al-koe′nee-um)

Benza, Benzalchlor-50, Germicin, Pharmatex ♣, Sabol, Zephiran

Classifications: SKIN AND MUCOUS MEMBRANE AGENT; TOPICAL ANTIINFECTIVE; ANTIBIOTIC

Pregnancy Category: C

AVAILABILITY 17% concentrate, 1:750 solution, 1:750 tincture/tincture spray

ACTIONS Bactericidal or bacteriostatic action (depending on concentration), probably due to inactivation of bacterial enzyme.

THERAPEUTIC EFFECTS Effective against bacteria, some fungi (including yeasts) and certain protozoa (e.g., *Trichomonas vaginalis*). Generally not effective against spore-forming organisms.

USES Antisepsis of intact skin, mucous membranes, superficial injuries, and infected wounds; also for irrigations of the eye and body cavities and for vaginal douching. A component of several contact lens wetting and cushioning solutions, and a preservative for ophthalmic solutions.

CONTRAINDICATIONS Casts, occlusive dressings, anal or vaginal packs, pregnancy (category C), lactation.

CAUTIOUS USE Irrigation of body cavities.

ROUTE & DOSAGE

Minor Wounds or Preoperative Disinfection

Adult: **Topical** 1:750 tincture or spray

Preoperative Disinfection of Denuded Skin and Mucous Membranes

Adult: **Topical** 1:10,000–1:2000 solution

Wet Dressings

Adult: **Topical** 1:5000 solution

Urinary Bladder Irrigation

Adult: **Topical** 1:20,000–1:5000 solution

Urinary Bladder Instillation

Adult: **Topical** 1:40,000–1:20,000 solution

Irrigation of Deep Infected Wounds

Adult: **Topical** 1:20,000–1:3000 solution

Vaginal Irrigation

Adult: **Topical** 1:5000–1:2000 solution

Sterile Storage of Instruments, Thermometers, Ampules

Adult: **Topical** 1:750 solution

ADMINISTRATION

Topical

- Use sterile water for injection as diluent for aqueous solutions to be instilled in wounds or body cavities. For other uses, fresh sterile distilled water is used.
- Do not use tap water (especially hard water) because it may reduce antibacterial potency of benzalkonium chloride.
- Irrigate eyes immediately and repeatedly with water if medication

solution stronger than 1:5000 enters eyes; see a physician promptly.

- Rinse first with water, then with 70% alcohol, before applying benzalkonium for preoperative skin preparation. Avoid pooling or prolonged contact of solution with skin.
- Note: Detergent action is antagonized by pus and other organic matter, and by soap substitutes. If these agents have been used, rinse skin thoroughly with water, dry, and then apply benzalkonium.
- Consult physician about proper dilution of solutions used on denuded skin or inflamed or irritated tissues.
- Store at room temperature, preferably between 15°–30° C (59°–86° F) in airtight container, protected from light.

ADVERSE EFFECTS (≥1%) **Body as a Whole:** Few or no toxic effects in recommended dilutions. **Skin:** Erythema, local burning, hypersensitivity reactions.

PHARMACOKINETICS Not studied.

NURSING IMPLICATIONS

Assessment & Drug Effects

- Monitor wounds carefully. Report increasing signs of infection or lack of healing.

BENZOCAINE

(ben′zoe-caine)

Americaine, Americaine Anesthetic Lubricant, Americaine-Otic, Anbesol, Benzocol, Chigger-Tox, Dermoplast, Foille, Hurricaine, Orabase with Benzocaine, Oracin, Orajel, Rhulicaine, Solarcaine, T-Caine, Unguentine

Classifications: CENTRAL NERVOUS SYSTEM AGENT; LOCAL ANESTHETIC (ESTER TYPE); ANTIPRURITIC
Prototype: Procaine
Pregnancy Category: C

AVAILABILITY 5% spray, cream, ointment; 6% cream; 8% lotion, 20% spray, ointment, gel, liquid

ACTIONS Produces surface anesthesia by inhibiting conduction of nerve impulses from sensory nerve endings. Probable action in certain OTC appetite suppressants is dulling taste for foods. Almost identical to procaine in chemical structure, but has prolonged duration of anesthetic action.

THERAPEUTIC EFFECTS Temporary relief of pain and discomfort.

USES Temporary relief of pain and discomfort in pruritic skin problems, minor burns and sunburn, minor wounds, and insect bites. Otic preparations are used to relieve pain and itching in acute congestive and serous otitis media, swimmer's ear, and otitis externa. Preparations are also available for toothache, minor sore throat pain, canker sores, hemorrhoids, rectal fissures, pruritus ani or vulvae, as male genital desensitizer to slow onset of ejaculation, and for use as anesthetic-lubricant for passage of catheters and endoscopic tubes.

CONTRAINDICATIONS Hypersensitivity to benzocaine or other PABA derivatives (e.g., sunscreen preparations), or to any of the components in the formulation; use of ear preparation in patients with perforated eardrum or ear discharge; applications to large areas; use in children <2 y. Safe use during pregnancy (category C) is not established.

B

CAUTIOUS USE History of drug sensitivity; denuded skin or severely traumatized mucosa; children <6 y.

ROUTE & DOSAGE

Anesthetic
Adult: **Topical** Lowest effective dose
Child: **Topical** Lower strengths

ADMINISTRATION

Topical
- Avoid contact of all preparations with eyes and be careful not to inhale mist when spray form is used.
- Do not use spray near open flame or cautery and do not expose to high temperatures. Hold can at least 12 inches (30 cm) away from affected area when spraying.
- Wash and neutralize chemical burns before benzocaine is applied.
- Clean and dry rectal area before administration of hemorrhoidal preparation. Usually administered morning and evening and after each bowel movement.
- Store at 15°–30° C (59°–86° F) in tight, light-resistant containers unless otherwise specified.

ADVERSE EFFECTS (≥1%) **Body as a Whole:** Low toxicity; sensitization in susceptible individuals; allergic reactions, anaphylaxis. Methemoglobinemia reported in infants.

INTERACTIONS Drug: Benzocaine may antagonize antibacterial activity of SULFONAMIDES.

PHARMACOKINETICS Absorption: Poorly absorbed through intact skin; readily absorbed from mucous membranes. **Peak:** 1 min. **Duration:** 15–30 min. **Metabolism:** Metabolized by plasma cholinesterases and to a lesser extent by hepatic cholinesterases. **Elimination:** Metabolites excreted in urine.

NURSING IMPLICATIONS

Assessment & Drug Effects
- Assess swallowing when used on oral mucosa, as benzocaine may interfere with second (pharyngeal) stage of swallowing; hold food and liquids accordingly.
- Assess for sensitivity. Local anesthetics are potentially sensitizing to susceptible individuals when applied repeatedly or over extensive areas.

Patient & Family Education
- Use specific benzocaine preparation ONLY as prescribed or recommended by manufacturer.
- Discontinue medication if the condition persists, worsens, or if signs of sensitivity, irritation, or infection occur.

BENZONATATE Pr

(ben-zoe′na-tate)

Tessalon

Classification: ANTITUSSIVE
Pregnancy Category: C

AVAILABILITY 100 mg capsules

ACTIONS Nonnarcotic antitussive chemically related to tetracaine. Antitussive activity reported to be somewhat less effective than that of codeine. Does not inhibit respiratory center at recommended doses.

THERAPEUTIC EFFECTS Decreases frequency and intensity of nonproductive cough.

USES Decreases frequency and intensity of nonproductive cough in acute and chronic respiratory conditions. Also used in bronchoscopy, thoracentesis, and other procedures when coughing must be avoided.

CONTRAINDICATIONS Safe use during pregnancy (category C) or lactation is not established.

ROUTE & DOSAGE

Antitussive

Adult: **PO** 100 mg t.i.d. prn up to 600 mg/d
Child: **PO** <10 y, 8 mg/kg/d in 3–6 divided doses

ADMINISTRATION

Oral

- Ensure that soft capsules called perles are swallowed whole.
- Store in airtight containers protected from light.

ADVERSE EFFECTS (≥1%) **Body as a Whole:** Low incidence. **CNS:** Drowsiness, sedation headache, mild dizziness. **GI:** Constipation, nausea. **Skin:** Rash, pruritus.

PHARMACOKINETICS Onset: 15–20 min. **Duration:** 3–8 h.

NURSING IMPLICATIONS

Assessment & Drug Effects

- Auscultate lungs anteriorly and posteriorly at scheduled intervals.
- Observe character and frequency of coughing and volume and quality of sputum. Keep physician informed.

Patient & Family Education

- Do not chew or allow perle to dissolve in mouth; swallow whole. If perle dissolves in mouth, the mouth, tongue, and pharynx will be anesthetized. Also it is unpleasant to taste.
- Do not breast feed while taking this drug without consulting physician.

BENZPHETAMINE HYDROCHLORIDE

(benz-fet′a-meen)

Didrex

Classifications: CENTRAL NERVOUS SYSTEM AGENT; CEREBRAL STIMULANT; ANOREXIANT

Prototype: Amphetamine

Pregnancy Category: X

Controlled Substance: Schedule III

AVAILABILITY 25 mg, 50 mg tablets

ACTIONS Indirect acting sympathomimetic amine with amphetamine-like actions but with fewer side effects than amphetamine.

THERAPEUTIC EFFECTS Anorexiant effect thought to be secondary to stimulation of hypothalamus to release stored catecholamines in the CNS.

USES Short-term adjunct in management of exogenous obesity.

CONTRAINDICATIONS Known hypersensitivity to sympathomimetic amines; angle-closure glaucoma; advanced arteriosclerosis, angina pectoris, severe cardiovascular disease, moderate to severe hypertension; hyperthyroidism, agitated states; history of drug abuse; children <12 y; lactation. Safe use during pregnancy (category X) is not established.

CAUTIOUS USE Diabetes mellitus; older adults; psychosis.

ROUTE & DOSAGE

Obesity

Adult: **PO** 25–50 mg 1–3 times/d

ADMINISTRATION

Oral

- Give as a single daily dose, preferably midmorning or midafternoon, according to patient's eating habits.
- Schedule daily dose no later than 6 h before patient retires to avoid insomnia.
- Store in tight, light-resistant containers at 15°–30° C (59°–86° F) unless otherwise directed.

ADVERSE EFFECTS (≥1%) **CNS:** Euphoria, irritability, hyperactivity, nervousness, *restlessness, insomnia,* tremor, headache, light-headedness, dizziness, depression following stimulant effects. **CV:** *Palpitation,* tachycardia, elevated BP, irregular heart beat. **GI:** Xerostomia, nausea, vomiting, diarrhea or constipation, abdominal cramps. **Chronic Intoxication:** Marked insomnia, irritability, hyperactivity, personality changes, psychosis, severe dermatoses.

INTERACTIONS Drug: Acetazolamide, sodium bicarbonate decrease AMPHETAMINE elimination; **ammonium chloride, ascorbic acid** increase AMPHETAMINE elimination; BARBITURATES may antagonize the effects of both drugs; **furazolidone** may increase BP effects of AMPHETAMINES, and interaction may persist for several weeks after discontinuation of **furazolidone; guanethidine, guanadryl** antagonize antihypertensive effects; because MAO INHIBITORS, **selegiline** can cause hypertensive crisis (fatalities reported); do not administer AMPHETAMINES during or within 14 d of these drugs; PHENOTHIAZINES may inhibit mood-elevating effects of AMPHETAMINES; TRICYCLIC ANTIDEPRESSANTS enhance AMPHETAMINE effects because they increase **norepinephrine** release; BETA AGONISTS increase AMPHETAMINE'S adverse cardiovascular effects.

PHARMACOKINETICS Absorption: Readily absorbed from GI tract. **Duration:** 4 h. **Elimination:** Renal elimination.

NURSING IMPLICATIONS

Assessment & Drug Effects

- Assess for signs of excessive CNS stimulation: insomnia, restlessness, tremor, palpitations. These may indicate need for dosage adjustment.
- Monitor vital signs; report elevated BP, tachycardia, and irregular heart rhythm.
- Monitor diabetics for loss of glycemic control.

Patient & Family Education

- Note: Anorexiant effects are temporary and tolerance may occur; long-term use is not indicated.
- Do not drive or engage in potentially hazardous activities until response to drug is known.
- Do not terminate high dosage therapy abruptly; GI distress, stomach cramps, trembling, unusual tiredness, weakness, and mental depression may result.
- Do not breast feed while taking this drug.

BENZTHIAZIDE

(bens-thye′a-zide)

Aquatag, Exna, Hydrex, Marazide, Proaqua

Classifications: FLUID AND WATER BALANCE AGENT; THIAZIDE DIURETIC; ANTIHYPERTENSIVE

Prototype: Hydrochlorothiazide

Pregnancy Category: D

AVAILABILITY 50 mg tablets

ACTIONS Thiazide diuretic chemically related to sulfonamides. Similar to hydrochlorothiazide. Inhibits renal tubular reabsorption of sodium and chloride, resulting in excretion of sodium and water, accompanied by some loss of bicarbonate and potassium.

THERAPEUTIC EFFECTS Decreases blood volume resulting in a hypotensive effect.

USES Edema and adjunctively with other agents for treatment of mild hypertension.

CONTRAINDICATIONS Hypersensitivity to thiazides or sulfonamides; anuria; pregnancy (category D), lactation.

CAUTIOUS USE History of renal, hepatic, or pancreatic disease; history of gout; diabetes mellitus; hypercalcemia, hypokalemia.

ROUTE & DOSAGE

Edema

Adult: **PO** 25–200 mg/d or q.o.d.
Child: **PO** 1–4 mg/kg/d in 3 divided doses

Hypertension

Adult: **PO** 25–100 mg/d after breakfast, may increase to 200 mg/d in 2–4 divided doses

ADMINISTRATION

Oral

- Give with food or milk to minimize gastric irritation unless otherwise directed by physician.
- Give as a single daily dose to promote diuresis, preferably early in the morning to prevent interrupted sleep.
- Store tablets in tightly closed container at 15°–30° C (59°–86° F) unless otherwise directed.

ADVERSE EFFECTS (≥1%) **Body as a Whole:** Hypersensitivity (dermatitis, photosensitivity, urticaria). **CNS:** Headache, unusual fatigue. **CV:** Irregular heartbeat, vasculitis, orthostatic hypotension, volume depletion. **GI:** Nausea, vomiting, anorexia, constipation, cramps, jaundice. **Metabolic:** Hyperglycemia, hypokalemia; hyperuricemia. **Hematologic:** Rare, thrombocytopenia, agranulocytosis. **Other:** Increased thirst.

DIAGNOSTIC TEST INTERFERENCE

Serum PBI levels may be decreased. Thiazides should be discontinued before ***parathyroid function*** tests because they tend to reduce ***calcium*** excretion.

INTERACTIONS Drug: Cholestyramine, colestipol decrease absorption of the diuretic; **diazoxide** has additive effects; with **digoxin,** hypokalemia may increase risk of **digitalis** toxicity; increases **lithium** levels and toxicity; may increase blood glucose levels, necessitating adjustment of dosage of SULFONYLUREAS, **insulin.**

PHARMACOKINETICS Absorption: Readily absorbed from GI tract. **Onset:** 2 h. **Peak:** 4–6 h. **Duration:** 12–18 h. **Distribution:** Crosses placenta; distributed into breast milk. **Elimination:** Excreted in urine within 24 h.

NURSING IMPLICATIONS

Assessment & Drug Effects

- Assess therapeutic effectiveness. Effects may be noted in 3 or 4 d; maximal effects usually require 3–4 wk.
- Assess patient carefully for signs of hypokalemia, particularly older adults (see Appendix F).

- Lab tests: Baseline and periodic blood counts, serum electrolytes, uric acid, blood sugar, NPN, BUN, and serum creatinine.
- Monitor I&O ratio and pattern.
- Monitor diabetics for loss of glycemic control.

Patient & Family Education

- Eat potassium-rich foods such as fruit juices and bananas to prevent onset of hypokalemia.
- Weigh daily and report sudden weight gain to physician.
- Notify physician if severe nausea, vomiting, or diarrhea occurs in order to prevent dehydration.
- Avoid use of OTC drugs unless approved by physician.
- Notify physician of photosensitivity reaction (like an exaggerated sunburn). Thiazide-related photosensitivity is considered a photoallergy; it occurs 1 1/2–2 wk after initial sun exposure.
- Do not breast feed while taking this drug.

BENZTROPINE MESYLATE

(benz′troe-peen)

Apo-Benztropine ✤, Bensylate ✤, Cogentin, PMS Benztropine ✤

Classifications: AUTONOMIC NERVOUS SYSTEM AGENT; ANTICHOLINERGIC (PARASYMPATHOLYTIC); ANTIPARKINSONISM AGENT

Prototype: Levodopa

Pregnancy Category: C

AVAILABILITY 0.5 mg, 1 mg, 2 mg tablets; 1 mg/mL ampules

ACTIONS Synthetic centrally acting anticholinergic (antimuscarinic) agent. Acts by diminishing excess cholinergic effect associated with dopamine deficiency.

THERAPEUTIC EFFECTS Suppresses tremor and rigidity; does not alleviate tardive dyskinesia.

USES Symptomatic treatment of all forms of parkinsonism (arteriosclerotic, idiopathic, postencephalitic) and to relieve extrapyramidal symptoms associated with neuroleptic drugs, e.g., haloperidol (Haldol), phenothiazines, thiothixene (Navane). Commonly used as supplement with trihexyphenidyl, carbidopa, or levodopa therapy.

CONTRAINDICATIONS Narrow angle glaucoma; myasthenia gravis; obstructive diseases of GU and GI tracts; tendency to tachycardia; tardive dyskinesia, children <3 y. Safety during pregnancy (category C) or lactation is not established.

CAUTIOUS USE Older children, older adults or debilitated patients, patients with poor mental outlook, mental disorders; enlarged prostate; hypertension; history of renal or hepatic disease.

ROUTE & DOSAGE

Parkinsonism

Adult: **PO** 0.5–1 mg/d, may gradually increase as needed up to 6 mg/d

Extrapyramidal Reactions

Adult: **PO** 1–2 mg b.i.d. **IM/IV** 1–2 mg as needed

Child: **PO/IM/IV** *>3 y,* 0.02–0.05 mg/kg, 1–2 times/d

ADMINISTRATION

Oral

- Give immediately after meals or with food to prevent gastric irritation. Tablet can be crushed and sprinkled on or mixed with food.

- Initiate and withdraw drug therapy gradually; effects are cumulative.
- Store in tightly covered, light-resistant container at 15°–30° C (59°–86° F) unless otherwise directed.

Intravenous

IV administration to infants and children: Verify correct IV concentration with physician.

PREPARE: **Direct:** Give undiluted.
ADMINISTER: **Direct:** Give 1 mg or a fraction thereof over 1 min.

ADVERSE EFFECTS (≥1%) **CNS:** *Sedation*, drowsiness, dizziness, paresthesias; agitation, irritability, restlessness, nervousness, insomnia, hallucinations, delirium, mental confusion, toxic psychosis, muscular weakness, ataxia, inability to move certain muscle groups. **CV:** Palpitation, tachycardia, flushing. **Special Senses:** Blurred vision, mydriasis, photophobia. **GI:** Nausea, vomiting, *constipation, dry mouth,* distention, paralytic ileus. **Urogenital:** Dysuria.

INTERACTIONS Drug: Alcohol, CNS DEPRESSANTS have additive sedation and depressant effects; **amantadine,** TRICYCLIC ANTIDEPRESSANTS, MAO INHIBITORS, PHENOTHIAZINES, **procainamide, quinidine** have additive anticholinergic effects and cause confusion, hallucinations, paralyticileus.

PHARMACOKINETICS Onset: 15 min IM/IV; 1 h PO. **Duration:** 6–10 h.

NURSING IMPLICATIONS

Assessment & Drug Effects

- Assess therapeutic effectiveness. Clinical improvement may not be evident for 2–3 d after oral drug is started.
- Monitor I&O ratio and pattern. Advise patient to report difficulty in urination or infrequent voiding. Dosage reduction may be indicated.
- Closely monitor for appearance of S&S of onset of paralytic ileus including intermittent constipation, abdominal pain, diminution of bowel sounds on auscultation, and distension.
- Monitor for and report muscle weakness or inability to move certain muscle groups. Dosage reduction may be needed.
- Supervise ambulation and use bed side rails as necessary.
- Report immediately S&S of CNS depression or stimulation. These usually require interruption of drug therapy.

Patient & Family Education

- Do not drive or engage in potentially hazardous activities until response to drug is known. Seek help walking as necessary.
- Avoid alcohol and other CNS depressants because they may cause additive drowsiness. Do not take OTC cold, cough, or hay fever remedies unless approved by physician.
- Sugarless gum, hard candy, and rinsing mouth with tepid water will help dry mouth.
- Avoid doing manual labor or strenuous exercise in hot weather; diminished sweating may require dose adjustments because of possibility of heat stroke. This condition is most apt to occur in the older adults.
- Do not breast feed while taking this drug without consulting physician.

B

BEPRIDIL HYDROCHLORIDE

(be-pri'dil)

Vascor

Classifications: CARDIOVASCULAR AGENT; CALCIUM CHANNEL BLOCKER

Prototype: Nifedipine

Pregnancy Category: C

AVAILABILITY 200 mg, 300 mg, 400 mg tablets

ACTIONS Selectively blocks calcium ion influx across the cell membrane of cardiac muscle and vascular smooth muscle without changing serum calcium concentrations. Unlike other calcium channel blockers, it also blocks the sodium channel and possibly the potassium channel, resulting in quinidine-like effects.

THERAPEUTIC EFFECTS Bepridil reduces myocardial oxygen use and supply, and relaxes and prevents coronary artery spasm.

USE Chronic stable angina.

CONTRAINDICATIONS Hypersensitivity to bepridil HCl or any other calcium channel blocker, sick sinus syndrome or second or third-degree block, ventricular arrhythmias, hypotension, uncompensated cardiac insufficiency, congenital QT interval prolongation, and with concomitant use of drugs that prolong QT interval; lactation.

CAUTIOUS USE Older adults; CHF, recent MI (≤3 mo); serious hepatic or renal dysfunction; pregnancy (category C).

ROUTE & DOSAGE

Angina

Adult: **PO** start with 200 mg once daily, may be adjusted every 7 d (max: 400 mg/d)

ADMINISTRATION

Oral

- Give with food if nausea occurs.
- Store away from light and moisture in tightly closed containers at 15°–30° C (59°–86° F).

ADVERSE EFFECTS (≥1%) **CNS:** Nervousness, *dizziness,* asthenia, *headache.* **CV:** Negative inotropic effect, proarrhythmic effects (ventricular tachycardia or fibrillation, torsade de pointes), CHF. **GI:** *Nausea, vomiting, diarrhea,* dyspepsia. **Hematologic:** Leukopenia, neutropenia, agranulocytosis (all rare). **Other:** Death has been reported in arrhythmia trials.

INTERACTIONS Drug: Adenosine and BETA BLOCKERS may increase risk of bradycardia. **Amiodarone** may lead to heart block; may increase **digoxin** levels and **digoxin** toxicity. May cause significant hypotension with **fentanyl.** Use with DIURETICS may increase risk of arrhythmias. TRICYCLIC ANTIDEPRESSANTS may exaggerate prolongation of QT interval associated with bepridil. May enhance neuromuscular blockade induced by nondepolarizing agents such as **succinylcholine** and **tubocurarine; warfarin** may increase free bepridil levels.

PHARMACOKINETICS Absorption: Completely absorbed from GI tract; approximately 60% reaches systemic circulation. **Onset:** 60 min. **Peak:** 2–3 h. **Duration:** 24 h. **Distribution:** Distributed into breast milk. **Metabolism:** Metabolized in liver, presumably by hepatic oxidative processes; 17 metabolites have been isolated. **Elimination:** Approximately 65% excreted in urine in 10 d, 23% excreted in feces. **Half-Life:** 42 h.

B

NURSING IMPLICATIONS

Assessment & Drug Effects

- Monitor cardiac status, as bepridil can induce new arrhythmias, including ventricular tachycardia and fibrillation, and CHF
- Monitor closely: Females over age 60 with hypokalemia and sinus bradycardia are at high risk for drug-induced torsade de pointes (a type of ventricular tachycardia).
- Assess safety and need for help with ambulation or other activities (dizziness is a common adverse effect of this drug).
- Monitor common adverse gastrointestinal effects (nausea, vomiting, diarrhea); determine need for intervention.
- Lab tests: Monitor periodically serum transaminase levels, serum electrolytes, WBC with differential, digoxin level when used concurrently.
- Report hypokalemia immediately. The condition should be promptly corrected.
- Monitor diabetics for loss of glycemic control.

Patient & Family Education

- Report ringing in ears to physician.
- Do not breast feed while taking this drug.

BERACTANT (Pr)

(ber-ac'tant)

Survanta

Classification: LUNG SURFACTANT

Pregnancy Category: Not applicable

AVAILABILITY 25 mg/mL suspension

ACTIONS Beractant is a sterile nonpyrogenic pulmonary surfactant. Endogenous pulmonary surfactant lowers surface tension on alveolar surfaces during respiration and stabilizes the alveoli against collapse at resting pressures. Deficiency of surfactant causes respiratory distress syndrome (RDS) in premature infants.

THERAPEUTIC EFFECTS Beractant lowers minimum surface tension and restores pulmonary compliance and oxygenation in premature infants.

USES Prevention and treatment of RDS in premature infants, especially those weighing <1250 g.

UNLABELED USES Infants weighing <600 g or >1750 g; treatment of RDS in adults.

CONTRAINDICATIONS Nosocomial infections.

ROUTE & DOSAGE

Neonate: **Intratracheal** Instill 100 mg/kg (4 mL/kg) birth weight through endotracheal tube, may repeat no more frequently than q6h (max: 4 doses in the first 48 h of life)

ADMINISTRATION

Intratracheal

- Place refrigerated drug at room temperature for at least 20 min or warm in the hand for at least 8 min. Do not use artificial warming methods.
- Give to premature infants weighing less than 1250 g, or who have a surfactant deficiency, preferably within 15 min of birth.
- Give to infants requiring mechanical ventilation and with RDS confirmed by x-ray examination, within 8 h of birth.

B

- Suction infant before administration of beractant.
- Note: Drug color should be white to light brown. If drug has settled, swirl vial gently to suspend.
- Administer using a No. 5 French end-hole catheter inserted into the endotracheal tube.
- Follow specific dosing procedure recommended by the manufacturer. Carefully read and follow exactly accompanying drug administration literature.
- Do not suction for 1 h after drug is administered unless signs of significant airway obstruction occur.
- Unopened vials warmed to room temperature will not lose potency if refrigerated within 8 h of warming. Drug should not be warmed and returned to refrigerator more than once.
- Note: Vials are for single use only. Discard unused drug in opened vials.
- Store unopened vials inside carton to protect from light and refrigerated at 2°–8° C (36°–46° F) until ready to use.

ADVERSE EFFECTS (≥1%) **CV:** *Transient bradycardia.* **Respiratory:** *Oxygen desaturation.* **Other:** Increased probability of posttreatment nosocomial sepsis in surfactant-treated infants was observed in the controlled clinical trials but was not associated with increased mortality.

PHARMACOKINETICS Absorption: Absorbed from the alveolus into lung tissue, where it can be extensively catabolized and reutilized for further phospholipid synthesis and secretion. **Onset:** 0.5–4 h. **Peak:** 2 h. **Duration:** 48–72 h; may need multiple doses to sustain improvement. **Distribution:** Not distributed to the systemic circulation. **Metabolism:** Surfactant is recycled and metabolized exclusively in the lungs. **Elimination:** Recycling may be a dominant metabolic pathway by which surfactant is taken up by type II pneumocytes and reused. **Half-Life:** 20–30 h.

NURSING IMPLICATIONS

Assessment & Drug Effects

- Monitor heart rate, color, chest expansion, facial expressions, oximeter, and endotracheal tube patency and position, during administration. Most adverse effects occur during dosing.
- Monitor frequently with arterial or transcutaneous measurement of systemic oxygen and CO_2.
- Note: Rales and moist breath sounds may occur transiently following drug administration. These do not necessarily indicate a need for suctioning.

BETAMETHASONE

(bay-ta-meth'a-sone)

Betnelan ♣, Celestone

BETAMETHASONE ACETATE AND BETAMETHASONE SODIUM PHOSPHATE

Celestone Soluspan

BETAMETHASONE BENZOATE

Beben ♣, Benisone, Uticort

BETAMETHASONE DIPROPIONATE

Alphatrex, Diprolene, Diprosone, Maxivate

BETAMETHASONE SODIUM PHOSPHATE (PH 8.5)

Betameth, Betnesol ♣, Celestone Phosphate, Celestone S, Cel-U-Jec, Selestoject

BETAMETHASONE VALERATE

Betacort, Betaderm ♣, Betatrex, Beta-Val, Betnovate ♣, Celestoderm ♣, Ectosone Lotion ♣, Luxiq, Metaderm ♣, Novobetamet ♣, Valisone, Valisone Scalp Lotion, Valnac, Psorion cream

Classifications: HORMONE AND SYNTHETIC SUBSTITUTE; ADRENAL CORTICOSTEROID; GLUCOCORTICOID; ANTIINFLAMMATORY

Prototype: Hydrocortisone

Pregnancy Category: C

AVAILABILITY **Betamethasone** 0.6 mg tablets; 0.6 mg/5 mL syrup **Betamethasone Acetate and Betamethasone Sodium** 3 mg acetate, 3 mg sodium phosphate/mL suspension **Betamethasone Benzoate, Betamethasone Dipropionate, and Betamethasone Sodium Phosphate (pH 8.5)** 4 mg/mL injection **Betamethasone Valerate** 0.1% ointment; 0.01%, 0.05%, 0.1% cream; 0.1% lotion; 1.2 mg/g foam

ACTIONS Synthetic, long-acting glucocorticoid with minor mineralocorticoid properties but strong immunosuppressive, antiinflammatory, and metabolic actions.

THERAPEUTIC EFFECTS Relieves antiinflammatory manifestations and is an immunosuppressive agent.

USES Reduces serum calcium in hypercalcemia, suppresses undesirable inflammatory or immune responses, produces temporary remission in nonadrenal disease, and blocks ACTH production in diagnostic tests. Topical use provides relief of inflammatory manifestations of corticosteroid-responsive dermatoses.

UNLABELED USES Prevention of neonatal respiratory distress syndrome (hyaline membrane disease).

CONTRAINDICATIONS In patients with systemic fungal infections. Pregnancy (category C), lactation, vaccines.

CAUTIOUS USE Ocular herpes simplex; concomitant use of aspirin; osteoporosis; diverticulitis, nonspecific ulcerative colitis, abscess or other pyrogenic infection, peptic ulcer disease; hypertension; renal insufficiency; myasthenia gravis.

ROUTE & DOSAGE

Antiinflammatory Agent

Adult: **PO** 0.6–7.2 mg/d **IM/IV** 0.5–9 mg/d as sodium phosphate

Topical See Appendix A-4

Child: **PO** 0.0175–0.25 mg/kg/d or 0.5–0.75 mg/m^2/d divided q6–8h

Child: **IM** 0.0175–0.125 mg/kg/d or 0.5–0.75 mg/m^2/d divided q6–8h

Respiratory Distress Syndrome

Adult: **IM** 2 mL of sodium phosphate to mother once daily 2–3 d before delivery

ADMINISTRATION

Oral

- Give with food or milk to lessen stomach irritation.

Intraarticular, Intramuscular, Intralesional

- Use Celestone Soluspan for intraarticular, IM, and intralesional injection. The preparation is not intended for IV use. Do not mix with diluents containing preservatives (e.g., parabens, phenol).
- Use 1% or 2% lidocaine hydrochloride if prescribed. Withdraw

betamethasone mixture first, then lidocaine; shake syringe briefly.

Intravenous

PREPARE: **Direct:** Give by direct IV undiluted or further diluted in D5W or NS.

ADMINISTER: **Direct:** Give at a rate of 1 dose/min.

INCOMPATIBILITIES **Solution/additive: Amobarbital, ampicillin, bleomycin, colistimethate, dimenhydrinate, doxapram, doxorubicin, ephedrine, heparin, hydralazine, metaraminol, methicillin, nafcillin, pentobarbital, phenobarbital, prochlorperazine, promethazine, secobarbital,** TETRACYCLINE. **Y-site: Ergotamine, phenytoin.**

ADVERSE EFFECTS (≥1%) **Body as a Whole:** Hypersensitivity or <u>anaphylactoid reactions; aggravation or masking of infections</u>; malaise, weight gain, obesity. Most adverse effects are dose and treatment duration dependent. **CNS:** Vertigo, headache, nystagmus, ataxia (rare), increased intracranial pressure with papilledema (usually after discontinuation of medication), mental disturbances, aggravation of preexisting psychiatric conditions, insomnia. **CV:** Hypertension; syncopal episodes, thrombophlebitis, thromboembolism or fat embolism, palpitation, tachycardia, necrotizing angiitis; CHF. **Endocrine:** Suppressed linear growth in children, decreased glucose tolerance; hyperglycemia, manifestations of latent diabetes mellitus; hypocorticism; amenorrhea and other menstrual difficulties. **Special Senses:** Posterior subcapsular cataracts (especially in children), glaucoma, exophthalmos, increased intraocular pressure with optic nerve damage, perforation of the globe, fungal infection of the cornea, decreased or blurred vision. **Metabolic:** Hypocalcemia; *sodium and fluid retention;* hypokalemia and hypokalemic alkalosis; negative nitrogen balance. **GI:** *Nausea,* increased appetite, ulcerative esophagitis, pancreatitis, abdominal distention, peptic ulcer with perforation and hemorrhage, melena; decreased serum concentration of vitamins A and C. **Hematologic:** Thrombocytopenia. **Musculoskeletal:** Osteoporosis, compression fractures, muscle wasting and weakness, tendon rupture, aseptic necrosis of femoral and humeral heads (all resulting from long-term use). **Skin:** Skin thinning and atrophy, *acne, impaired wound healing;* petechiae, ecchymosis, easy bruising; suppression of skin test reaction; hypopigmentation or hyperpigmentation, hirsutism, acneiform eruptions, subcutaneous fat atrophy; allergic dermatitis, urticaria, angioneurotic edema, increased sweating. **Urogenital:** Increased or decreased motility and number of sperm; urinary frequency and urgency, enuresis. **With parenteral therapy, IV site:** Pain, irritation, necrosis, atrophy, sterile abscess; Charcot-like arthropathy following intraarticular use; burning and tingling in perineal area (after IV injection).

DIAGNOSTIC TEST INTERFERENCE May increase serum ***cholesterol, blood glucose,*** serum ***sodium, uric acid*** (in acute leukemia) and ***calcium*** (in bone metastasis). It may decrease serum ***calcium, potassium, PBI, thyroxin (T_4), triiodothyronine (T_3) and reduce thyroid I 131*** uptake. It increases ***urine glucose*** level and ***calcium*** excretion; decreases ***urine***

17-OHCS and ***17-KS*** levels. May produce false-negative results with ***nitroblue tetrazolium test*** for systemic bacterial infection and may suppress reactions to skin tests.

INTERACTIONS Drug: BARBITURATES, **phenytoin, rifampin** may reduce pharmacologic effect of betamethasone by increasing its metabolism.

PHARMACOKINETICS Not studied.

NURSING IMPLICATIONS

Assessment & Drug Effects

- Assess therapeutic effectiveness. Response following intraarticular, intralesional, or intrasynovial administration occurs within a few hours and persists for 1–4 wk. Following IM administration response occurs in 2–3 h and persists for 3–7 d.

Patient & Family Education

- Monitor weight at least weekly.
- Discontinue slowly after systemic use of ≥1 wk. Abrupt withdrawal, especially following high doses or prolonged use, can cause dizziness, nausea, vomiting, fever, muscle and joint pain, weakness.
- Do not breast feed while taking this drug.

BETAXOLOL HYDROCHLORIDE

(be-tax'oh-lol)

Betoptic, Betoptic-S, Kerlone

Classifications: EYE PREPARATION; MIOTIC (ANTIGLAUCOMA AGENT); AUTONOMIC NERVOUS SYSTEM AGENT; BETA-ADRENERGIC BLOCKER

Prototype: Propranolol

Pregnancy Category: C

AVAILABILITY 10 mg, 20 mg tablets; 0.25%, 0.5% ophthalmic solution

ACTIONS Acts as a $beta_1$-selective adrenergic receptor blocking agent, especially in the cardioselective $beta_1$ receptors. Its antihypertensive effect is thought to be due to: (1) decreasing cardiac output, (2) reducing sympathetic nervous system outflow to the periphery resulting in vasodilatation, and (3) suppression of renin activity in the kidney.

THERAPEUTIC EFFECTS All three mechanisms result in its antihypertensive effect.

USES Hypertension. Ocular use for intraocular hypertension, chronic open angle glaucoma (**see Appendix A-1**).

CONTRAINDICATIONS Sinus bradycardia, AV block greater than first degree, cardiogenic shock, glaucoma, angle closure (unless with a miotic). Safety during pregnancy (category C) and in children <18 y is not established.

CAUTIOUS USE Concomitant use of systemic beta-adrenergic blocking agents; history of heart failure; diabetes mellitus; with evidence of airflow obstruction or reactive airway disease; lactation.

ROUTE & DOSAGE

Hypertension

Adult: **PO** 5–10 mg q.d. (max: 20 mg/d in 1–2 divided doses)

ADMINISTRATION

Oral

- Check pulse before administering betaxolol, oral or ophthalmic. If there are extremes (rate or rhythm), withhold medication and call the physician.

B

- Be aware tablet may be crushed before administration and taken with fluid of patient's choice.

ADVERSE EFFECTS (≥1%) **CV:** Bradycardia, hypotension. **CNS:** Depression. **Respiratory:** Increased airway resistance. **Special Senses:** With ophthalmic solution, *mild ocular stinging* and discomfort, tearing.

INTERACTIONS Drug: Reserpine and other CATECHOLAMINE-DEPLETING AGENTS may cause additive hypotensive effects or bradycardia. **Verapamil** may cause additive heart block.

PHARMACOKINETICS Absorption: 90% of PO dose reaches systemic circulation. **Onset:** 0.5–1 h. **Peak:** 2 h. **Duration:** >12 h. **Metabolism:** Metabolized in liver to at least 5 metabolites. **Elimination:** 30%–40% excreted in urine, 50%–60% excreted in bile and feces. **Half-Life:** 3–4 h.

NURSING IMPLICATIONS

Assessment & Drug Effects

- Monitor pulse rate and BP at regular intervals in patients with severe heart disease.
- Monitor therapeutic effectiveness. Some patients develop tolerance during long-term therapy.

Patient & Family Education

- Report unusual pulse rate or significant changes to physician according to parameters provided.
- Adhere to regimen EXACTLY as prescribed. Do not stop drug abruptly; angina may be exacerbated; dosage is reduced over a period of 1–2 wk.
- Report difficulty in breathing promptly to physician. Drug withdrawal may be indicated.
- Do not breast feed while taking this drug without consulting physician.

BETHANECHOL CHLORIDE (Pr)

(be-than'e-kole)

Duvoid, Urabeth, Urecholine

Classifications: AUTONOMIC NERVOUS SYSTEM AGENT; DIRECT-ACTING CHOLINERGIC (PARASYMPATHOMIMETIC) AGENT

Pregnancy Category: C

AVAILABILITY 5 mg, 10 mg, 25 mg, 50 mg tablets; 5 mg/mL injection

ACTIONS Synthetic choline ester with effects similar to those of acetylcholine (ACh). Acts directly on postsynaptic receptors, and since it is not hydrolyzed by cholinesterase, its actions are more prolonged than those of ACh.

THERAPEUTIC EFFECTS Produces muscarinic effects primarily on GI tract and urinary bladder. Increases tone and peristaltic activity of esophagus, stomach, and intestine; contracts detrusor muscle of urinary bladder, usually enough to initiate micturition.

USES Acute postoperative and postpartum nonobstructive (functional) urinary retention, and for neurogenic atony of urinary bladder with retention.

UNLABELED USES In selected cases of adynamic ileus, gastric atony and retention, reflux esophagitis, congenital megacolon, familial dysautonomia; for prevention and treatment of bladder and salivary gland inhibition induced by tricyclic antidepressants, and for prophylaxis and treatment of phenothiazine-induced bladder dysfunction.

CONTRAINDICATIONS COPD; history of or active bronchial asthma; hyperthyroidism; recent urinary bladder surgery, cystitis, bacteriuria, urinary bladder neck or intestinal obstruction, peptic ulcer, recent GI surgery, peritonitis; marked vagotonia, pronounced vasomotor instability, AV conduction defects, severe bradycardia, hypotension or hypertension, coronary artery disease, recent MI; epilepsy, parkinsonism. Safety during pregnancy (category C), lactation, or in children <8 y is not established.

CAUTIOUS USE Urinary retention; bacteriemia.

ROUTE & DOSAGE

Urinary Retention

Adult: **PO** 10–50 mg b.i.d. to q.i.d. (max: 120 mg/d) **SC** 2.5–5 mg t.i.d. or q.i.d. prn
Child: **PO** 0.2 mg/kg or 0.6 mg/m^2 t.i.d.

ADMINISTRATION

Oral

- Give on an empty stomach (1 h before or 2 h after meals) to lessen possibility of nausea and vomiting, unless otherwise advised by physician.
- Determine minimum effective dose: Give 5–10 mg initially and repeat this dose at 1–2 h (max: 50 mg), until a satisfactory response occurs. Alternatively, give 10 mg followed, at 6 h intervals, by 25 mg, then 50 mg, until desired response obtained.

Subcutaneous

- Determine minimum effective dose: Give 2.5 mg initially and repeat this dose at 15–30 min intervals (max: 4 doses), or until a satisfactory response occurs.
- After inserting needle, aspirate carefully before injecting drug to avoid inadvertent entry into a blood vessel.
- DO NOT give by IM or IV; life-threatening symptoms of cholinergic stimulation can occur.
- Overdose management: Atropine sulfate 0.6–1.2 mg for adults administered IM, slow IV, or SC; and 0.01 mg/kg for infants and children repeated every 2 h, if necessary.
- Store at 15°–30° C (59°–86° F), unless otherwise directed.

ADVERSE EFFECTS (≥1%) **Body as a Whole:** Dose-related. Increased sweating, malaise, headache, substernal pain or pressure, hypothermia. **CV:** Hypotension with dizziness, faintness, flushing, orthostatic hypotension (large doses); mild reflex tachycardia, atrial fibrillation (hyperthyroid patients), <u>transient complete heart block</u>. **Special Senses:** Blurred vision, miosis, lacrimation. **GI:** Nausea, vomiting, abdominal cramps, diarrhea, borborygmi, belching, salivation, fecal incontinence (large doses), urge to defecate (or urinate). **Respiratory:** Acute asthmatic attack, dyspnea (large doses).

DIAGNOSTIC TEST INTERFERENCE Bethanechol may cause increases in ***serum amylase*** and ***serum lipase,*** by stimulating pancreatic secretions, and may increase ***AST, serum bilirubin,*** and ***BSP retention*** by causing spasms in sphincter of Oddi.

INTERACTIONS Drug: Ambenonium, neostigmine, other CHOLINESTERASE INHIBITORS compound cholinergic effects and toxicity; **mecamylamine** may cause abdominal symptoms and hypotension; **procainamide, quinidine, atropine, epinephrine** antagonize effects of bethanechol.

PHARMACOKINETICS Absorption: Well absorbed PO. **Onset:** 30 min PO; 5–15 min SC. **Peak:** 60–90 min PO; 15–30 min SC. **Duration:** 1–6 h PO; 2 h SC. **Distribution:** Does not cross blood–brain barrier. **Metabolism:** Unknown. **Elimination:** Unknown.

NURSING IMPLICATIONS

Assessment & Drug Effects

- Monitor BP and pulse. Observe patient for at least 1 h following SC administration. Report early signs of overdosage: Salivation, sweating, flushing, abdominal cramps, nausea.
- Monitor I&O. Observe and record patient's response to bethanechol, and report any failure of the drug to relieve the particular condition for which it was prescribed.
- Monitor respiratory status. Promptly report dyspnea or any other indication of respiratory distress.
- Supervise ambulation as indicated by patient response to drug.

Patient & Family Education

- Make position changes slowly and in stages, particularly from lying down to standing.
- Do not stand still for prolonged periods; sit or lie down at first indication of faintness.
- Do not drive or engage in potentially hazardous activities until response to drug is known.
- Note: Drug may cause blurred vision; take appropriate precautions.
- Do not breast feed while taking this drug without consulting physician.

BEVACIZUMAB

(be-va-ci-zu′mab)

Avastin

Classifications: BIOLOGICAL RESPONSE MODIFIER; MONOCLONAL ANTIBODY

Prototype: Basiliximab

Pregnancy Category: C

AVAILABILITY 25 mg/mL injection

ACTIONS Binds to vascular endothelial growth factor (VEGF) and prevents the interaction of VEGF to its receptors on the surface of endothelial cells. This blocks endothelial cell proliferation and new blood vessel formation in tumor cells.

THERAPEUTIC EFFECTS Believed to cause reduction of microvascularization in the tumor inhibiting the progression of metastatic disease.

USE Metastatic colorectal cancer.

UNLABELED USE Metastatic renal cell cancer.

CONTRAINDICATIONS Pregnancy (category C), lactation; nephrotic syndrome; active bleeding; surgery within 28 d; dental work within 20 d. Safety and effectiveness in children are not established.

CAUTIOUS USE Hypersensitivity to bevacizumab; hypertension, history of arterial thromboembolic, cardiovascular, or cerebrovascular disease.

ROUTE & DOSAGE

Metastatic Colorectal Cancer

Adult: **IV** 5 mg/kg q14d until disease progression

ADMINISTRATION

Intravenous

PREPARE: **IV Infusion:** Withdraw the desired dose of 5 mg/kg and dilute in 100 mL of NS injection. Do not shake and do NOT mix or administer with dextrose solutions. Discard any unused portion.

ADMINISTER: **IV Infusion:** DO NOT administer IV push or bolus. Infuse first dose over 90 min; if well tolerated, infuse second dose over 60 min; if well tolerated, infuse all subsequent doses over 30 min.

INCOMPATIBILITIES **Solution/additive: Dextrose**-containing solutions. **Y-site: Dextrose**-containing solutions.

- Store diluted solution at 2°–8° C (36°–46° F) for up to 8 h. Store vials at 2°–8° C (36°–46° F) and protect from light.

ADVERSE EFFECTS (≥1%) **Body as a Whole:** *Asthenia,* pain, wound dehiscence. **CNS:** Syncope, headache, dizziness, confusion, abnormal gait. **CV:** DVT, *hypertension,* heart failure, intra-abdominal thrombosis. **GI:** Abdominal pain, *diarrhea,* constipation, nausea, vomiting, anorexia, stomatitis, dyspepsia, weight loss, flatulence, dry mouth, colitis, <u>gastrointestinal perforation</u>. **Hematologic:** *Leukopenia, neutropenia,* thrombocytopenia, *thromboembolism.* **Metabolic:** Hypokalemia, hyperbilirubinemia. **Musculoskeletal:** Myalgia. **Respiratory:** Upper respiratory infection, epistaxis, dyspnea, <u>hemoptysis</u>. **Skin:** Exfoliative dermatitis, alopecia. **Special Senses:** Taste disorder, increased tearing. **Urogenital:** *Proteinuria,* urinary frequency/urgency.

INTERACTIONS Drug: None reported.

PHARMACOKINETICS Half-Life: 20 d (11–50 d).

NURSING IMPLICATIONS

Assessment & Drug Effects

- Monitor for S&S of an infusion reaction (hypersensitivity); infusion should be interrupted in all patients with severe infusion reactions and appropriate therapy instituted.
- Monitor BP at least every 2–3 wk; if hypertension develops, monitor more frequently, even after discontinuation of bevacizumab.
- Withhold drug and promptly notify physician for S&S of CHF, hemorrhage (e.g., epistaxis, hemoptysis, or GI bleeding), or unexplained abdominal pain.
- Lab tests: Urinalysis for proteinuria and 24 h urine if protein 2+ or greater.
- Monitor for dizziness, lightheadedness, or loss of balance. Take appropriate safety measures.

Patient & Family Education

- Report any of the following to the physician: bloody or black, tarry stool; changes in patterns of urination; swelling of legs or ankles; increased shortness of breath; severe abdominal pain; change in mental awareness, inability to talk or move one side of the body.
- Women of childbearing age should use effective birth control while receiving bevacizumab.

BEXAROTENE

(bex-a-ro'teen)

Targretin

Classifications: ANTINEOPLASTIC AGENT; SKIN AND MUCOUS MEMBRANE AGENT; RETINOID

Prototype: Isotretinoin

Pregnancy Category: X

B

AVAILABILITY 75 mg capsules; 1% gel

ACTIONS Selectively binds to retinoid X receptors (RXR). Activation of the RXR pathway leads to cell death by interfering with cellular differentiation and proliferation of cells.

THERAPEUTIC EFFECTS Inhibits the growth of tumor cells of squamous (skin) cell origin inducing tumor regression.

USES Treatment of cutaneous manifestations of cutaneous T-cell lymphoma.

CONTRAINDICATIONS Hypersensitivity to bexarotene; pregnancy (X), lactation. Safety and efficacy in children are not established.

CAUTIOUS USE Coronary artery disease; diabetes mellitus; alcoholism, history of pancreatitis, hepatitis; elevated triglycerides, hepatic impairment.

ROUTE & DOSAGE

T-Cell Lymphoma
Adult: **PO** 300 mg/m^2/day as a single dose with a meal, if no response after 8 wks, may increase to 400 mg/m^2/day. Adjust dose downward in 100 mg/m^2/day increments if toxicity occurs **Topical** Apply once q.o.d. times 1 week, increase frequency at weekly intervals to once per day, b.i.d., t.i.d., and q.i.d.

ADMINISTRATION

Oral
- Give drug with or immediately following a meal.
- Do not give oral drug with grapefruit or grapefruit juice.
- Do not initiate therapy in a woman of childbearing age until the possibility of pregnancy has been completely ruled out.

Topical
- Apply a generous coating only to skin lesions; avoid normal skin.
- Do not cover with clothing until gel dries.
- Do not apply more frequently than prescribed.
- Store capsules and gel at 20°–25° C (36°–77° F). Protect from light and avoid high temperatures and humidity after bottle or tube is opened.

ADVERSE EFFECTS (≥1%) **Body as a Whole:** *Headache, asthenia, infection,* chills, fever, flu-like syndrome, back pain, bacterial infection. **CNS:** Insomnia. **CV:** *Peripheral edema.* **GI:** *Abdominal pain, nausea,* diarrhea, vomiting, anorexia. **Endocrine:** *Hyperthyroidism.* **Hematologic:** *Leukopenia,* anemia, hypochromic anemia. **Metabolic:** *Hyperlipidemia, hypercholesterolemia,* increased LDH. **Skin:** *Rash, dry skin,* exfoliative dermatitis, alopecia, photosensitivity.

INTERACTIONS No clinically significant interactions established.

PHARMACOKINETICS **Absorption:** Best absorption with a fat-containing meal. **Peak:** 2 h. **Distribution:** >99% protein bound. **Metabolism:** Metabolized to 4 metabolites by CYP 3A4. **Elimination:** Eliminated primarily in bile. **Half-Life:** 7 h.

NURSING IMPLICATIONS

Assessment & Drug Effects
- Monitor (with oral dose) for S&S of: hypothyroidism, hypertriglyc-

eridemia, hypercholesterolemia, and pancreatitis.

- Lab tests (with oral dose): Baseline blood lipids, then weekly for 2–4 wks, and every 8 wks thereafter; baseline liver function tests, then repeat at 1, 2, 4 wks, and every 8 wks thereafter; baseline WBC and thyroid function tests, then repeat periodically thereafter; periodic serum calcium; for females, pregnancy test q mo throughout therapy.
- Withhold oral drug and notify physician if triglycerides >400 mg/dL or AST, ALT, or bilirubin >3 times upper limit of normal.

Patient & Family Education

- Use effective methods of contraception (both men and women) while taking/using this drug and for at least one month after the last dose of the drug.
- Do not take this drug if you are or could be pregnant.
- Do not take this drug (oral form) if you are also taking gemfibrozil.
- Report immediately any of the following: Swelling in the face, lips, or wheezing; persistent bloating, constipation, diarrhea, vomiting, or stomach pain; persistent headache, severe drowsiness or weakness.
- Limit vitamin A intake to ≤15,000 IU/d while taking this drug (oral form).
- Report changes in vision to the physician. An ophthalmologic evaluation may be needed.
- Limit exposure to sunlight or sun lamps and wear sunscreen.
- Do not use insect repellents that contain the chemical, DEET, while using bexarotene gel.
- Report significant skin irritation.
- Do not breast feed while taking this drug.

BICALUTAMIDE

(bi-ca-lu′ta-mide)

Casodex

Classifications: HORMONES AND SYNTHETIC SUBSTITUTES; ANTIANDROGEN

Prototype: Leuprolide

Pregnancy Category: X

AVAILABILITY 50 mg tablets

ACTIONS Bicalutamide is a nonsteroidal antiandrogen. It inhibits the pharmacologic effects of androgen by binding to the androgen receptors in the target tissue.

THERAPEUTIC EFFECTS Prostatic carcinoma is androgen sensitive; it responds to removal of the source of androgen or treatment that counteracts the effects of androgen.

USES In combination with a luteinizing hormone-releasing hormone (LHRH) analog for advanced prostate cancer.

CONTRAINDICATIONS Hypersensitivity to bicalutamide, pregnancy (category X).

CAUTIOUS USE Moderate to severe hepatic impairment; lactation. Safety and efficacy in children are not established.

ROUTE & DOSAGE

Advanced Prostate Cancer
Adult: **PO** 50 mg once/d

ADMINISTRATION

Oral

- Give drug at the same time each day.
- Start treatment with bicalutamide at the same time as treatment with

B

a luteinizing hormone-releasing hormone (LHRH) analog.
- Store at 15°–30° C (59°–86° F).

ADVERSE EFFECTS (≥1%) **CNS:** Dizziness, paresthesia, insomnia, anxiety, decreased libido, confusion, neuropathy, somnolence, nervousness, headache. **CV:** *Hot flashes,* hypertension, chest pain, CHF. **GI:** *Constipation, nausea, diarrhea,* vomiting, increased liver function tests, abdominal pain, anorexia, dyspepsia, dry mouth, melena. **Urogenital:** Nocturia, hematuria, UTI, impotence, gynecomastia, incontinence, frequency, dysuria, urinary retention, urgency. **Metabolic:** Peripheral edema, hyperglycemia, weight loss, weight gain, gout. **Musculoskeletal:** Myasthenia, arthritis, myalgia, leg cramps, pathologic fractures. **Skin:** Rash, sweating, dry skin, pruritus, alopecia. **Body as a Whole:** Flu syndrome, bone pain, infection, anemia.

INTERACTIONS Drug: May increase effects of ORAL ANTICOAGULANTS.

PHARMACOKINETICS Absorption: Readily absorbed from GI tract. **Metabolism:** Metabolized in liver. **Elimination:** Excreted in urine and feces. **Half-Life:** 5.8 d.

NURSING IMPLICATIONS

Assessment & Drug Effects

- Monitor for S&S of disease progression.
- Lab tests: Periodic PSA levels, CBC, liver functions, renal functions; with concurrent coumadin therapy, closely monitor PT and INR.

Patient & Family Education

- Report jaundice or any other troubling adverse effects immediately.

BIMATOPROST

(bi-mat′o-prost)
Lumigan
Classifications: EYE PREPARATION; PROSTAGLANDIN
Prototype: Latanoprost
Pregnancy Category: C

AVAILABILITY 0.03% solution
See Appendix A-1.

BIPERIDEN HYDROCHLORIDE

(bye-per′i-den)
Akineton

BIPERIDEN LACTATE

Akineton
Classifications: AUTONOMIC NERVOUS SYSTEM AGENT; ANTICHOLINERGIC (PARASYMPATHOLYTIC); ANTIPARKINSONISM AGENT
Prototype: Levodopa
Pregnancy Category: C

AVAILABILITY 2 mg tablets; 5 mg/mL injection

ACTIONS Synthetic tertiary amine, antimuscarinic. In common with other antiparkinsonism drugs has atropine-like (anticholinergic) action. Antiparkinsonism activity is thought to be caused by reducing central excitatory action of acetylcholine on cholinergic receptors in the extrapyramidal system.
THERAPEUTIC EFFECTS This action helps to establish some balance between cholinergic (excitatory) and dopaminergic (inhibitory) activity in the basal ganglia with the result of controlling the effect of extrapyramidal symptoms.

USES Adjunct in all forms of parkinsonism, particularly postencephalitic and idiopathic parkinsonism (appears to be less effective in arteriosclerotic type). Also used to control drug-induced parkinsonism (extrapyramidal symptoms) associated with reserpine and phenothiazine therapy.

CONTRAINDICATIONS Narrow-angle glaucoma; GI or GU obstruction, megacolon; tardive dyskinesia. Safety during pregnancy (category C), lactation, or in children is not established.

CAUTIOUS USE Older adults or debilitated patients; prostatic hypertrophy; glaucoma; cardiac arrhythmias; epilepsy.

ROUTE & DOSAGE

Parkinsonism

Adult: **PO** 2 mg 1–4 times/d **IM/IV** 2 mg injected slowly; may repeat q30min up to 8 mg/24h
Geriatric: **PO** 2 mg 1–2 times/d
Child: **IM/IV** 0.04 mg/kg or 1.2 mg/m^2, may repeat q30min (max: 8 mg/24h)

ADMINISTRATION

Oral

- Give with or after meals to relieve GI disturbances.

Intramuscular

- Give slowly, deep IM into a large muscle.
- Monitor ambulation following IM as incoordination may occur.

Intravenous

PREPARE: **Direct:** Give undiluted.
ADMINISTER: **Direct:** Infuse slowly at a rate of 2 mg or a fraction thereof over 1 min. ▪ Keep patient recumbent when receiving parenteral biperiden and for at least 15 min thereafter. Postural hypotension, disturbances of coordination, and temporary euphoria can occur following IV administration.

- Store in tightly closed, light-resistant containers at 15°–30° C (59°–86° F) unless otherwise directed.

ADVERSE EFFECTS (≥1%) **CNS:** Drowsiness, dizziness, muscle weakness, lack of coordination, disorientation, euphoria, agitation, confusion. **CV:** Mild, transient postural hypotension (following IM), tachycardia. **Special Senses:** *Blurred vision,* photophobia. **GI:** *Dry mouth,* nausea, vomiting, constipation.

INTERACTIONS Drug: Alcohol and other CNS DEPRESSANTS INCREASE SEDATION; **haloperidol,** PHENOTHIAZINES, OPIATES, TRICYCLIC ANTIDEPRESSANTS, **quinidine** increase risk of anticholinergic side effects.

PHARMACOKINETICS Unknown.

NURSING IMPLICATIONS

Assessment & Drug Effects

- Monitor BP and pulse after IV administration. Advise patient to make position changes slowly and in stages, particularly from recumbent to upright position.
- Monitor for and report immediately: Mental confusion, drowsiness, dizziness, agitation, hematuria, and decrease in urinary flow.
- Assess for and report blurred vision.
- Monitor I&O ratio and pattern.
- Note: Biperiden usually reduces muscle rigidity. In patients with severe parkinsonism, tremors may increase as spasticity is relieved.

Patient & Family Education

- Do not drive or engage in potentially hazardous activities until response to drug is known.

B

- Note: Patients on prolonged therapy can develop tolerance; an increase in dosage may be required.
- Do not breast feed while taking this drug without consulting physician.

BISACODYL Pr

(bis-a-koe'dill)

Apo-Bisacodyl ♣, Bisacolax, Bisco-Lax ♣, Dacodyl, Deficol, Dulcolax, Fleet Bisacodyl, Laxit ♣, Theralax

Classifications: GASTROINTESTINAL AGENT; STIMULANT LAXATIVE

Pregnancy Category: C

AVAILABILITY 5 mg tablets; 10 mg suppository

ACTIONS Expands intestinal fluid volume by increasing epithelial permeability.

THERAPEUTIC EFFECTS Induces peristaltic contractions by direct stimulation of sensory nerve endings in the colonic wall.

USES Temporary relief of acute constipation and for evacuation of colon before surgery, proctoscopic, sigmoidoscopic, and radiologic examinations. Also used to cleanse colon before delivery and to relieve constipation in patients with spinal cord damage.

CONTRAINDICATIONS Acute surgical abdomen, nausea, vomiting, abdominal cramps, intestinal obstruction, fecal impaction; use of rectal suppository in presence of anal or rectal fissures, ulcerated hemorrhoids, proctitis.

CAUTIOUS USE Safety during pregnancy (category C), lactation, or in children is not established.

ROUTE & DOSAGE

Laxative

Adult: **PO** 5–15 mg prn (max: 30 mg for special procedures) **PR** 10 mg prn

Child: **PO** ≥6 y, 5–10 mg prn **PR** ≥2 y, 10 mg; <2 y, 5 mg

ADMINISTRATION

Oral

- Give in the evening or before breakfast because of action time required.
- Give enteric coated tablets whole to avoid gastric irritation; do not cut or crush. Patient should not chew tablets. Preferably give with a full glass (240 mL) of water or other liquid.
- Do not give within 1 h of antacids or milk. These substances may cause premature dissolution of enteric coating; early release of drug in stomach may result in gastric irritation and loss of cathartic action.
- Store tablets in tightly closed containers at temperatures not exceeding 30° C (86° F).

Rectal

- Suppository may be inserted at time bowel movement is desired.
- Storage is same as tablets.

ADVERSE EFFECTS (≥1%) Systemic effects not reported. Mild cramping, nausea, diarrhea, fluid and electrolyte disturbances (especially potassium and calcium).

INTERACTIONS Drug: ANTACIDS will cause early dissolution of enteric coated tablets, resulting in abdominal cramping.

PHARMACOKINETICS Absorption: 5%–15% absorbed from GI tract. **Onset:** 6–8 h PO; 15–60 min PR. **Metabolism:** Metabolized in liver.

Elimination: Excreted in urine, bile, and breast milk.

NURSING IMPLICATIONS

Assessment & Drug Effects

- Evaluate periodically patient's need for continued use of drug; bisacodyl usually produces 1 or 2 soft formed stools daily.
- Monitor patients receiving concomitant anticoagulants. Indiscriminate use of laxatives results in decreased absorption of vitamin K.

Patient & Family Education

- Add high-fiber foods slowly to regular diet to avoid gas and diarrhea. Adequate fluid intake includes at least 6–8 glasses/d.
- Do not breast feed while taking this drug without consulting physician.

BISMUTH SUBSALICYLATE

(Bis′muth)

Pepto-Bismol

Classifications: GASTROINTESTINAL AGENT; ANTIDIARRHEAL; SALICYLATE

Prototype: Diphenoxylate with atropine

Pregnancy Category: C

AVAILABILITY 262 mg tablets/caplets; 130 mg/15 mL, 262 mg/15 mL, 524 mg/15 mL liquid

ACTIONS Hydrolyzed in GI tract to salicylate, which is believed to inhibit synthesis of prostaglandins responsible for GI hypermotility and inflammation.

THERAPEUTIC EFFECTS Effectiveness as an antidiarrheal also appears to be due to direct antimicrobial action and to an antisecretory effect on intestinal secretions exposed to toxins particularly of *Escherichia coli* and *Vibrio cholerae.*

USES Prophylaxis and treatment of traveler's diarrhea (turista) and for temporary relief of indigestion.

UNLABELED USES *Helicobacter pylori* associated with peptic ulcer disease.

CONTRAINDICATIONS Hypersensitivity to aspirin or other salicylates; concurrent use with aspirin; use for more than 2 d in presence of high fever or in children <3 y unless prescribed by physician; chicken pox or flu.

CAUTIOUS USE Diabetes and gout; concurrent use with salicylates and anticoagulants; pregnancy (category C), lactation.

ROUTE & DOSAGE

Diarrhea

Adult: **PO** 30 mL or 2 tab q30–60min prn (max: 8 doses/d)
Child: **PO** *3–6 y,* 5 mL or 1/2 tab q30–60min prn (max: 8 doses/d); *6–9 y,* 2/3 tab or 10 mL q30–60 min prn (max: 8 doses/d); *9–12 y,* 15 mL or 1 tab q30–60min prn (max: 8 doses/d)

Traveler's Diarrhea

Adult: **PO** 2–4 tab or 15–30 mL q.i.d. for 3 wk

Peptic Ulcer Disease

Adult: **PO** 2 tablets q.i.d. with 2 additional antibiotics for 10–14 d
Child: **PO** *<10 y,* 15 mL q.i.d. times 6 wk

ADMINISTRATION

Oral

- Ensure chewable tablets are chewed or crushed before being swallowed and followed with at least 8 oz water or other liquid.
- Store at 15°–30° C (59°–86° F) unless otherwise directed.

ADVERSE EFFECTS (≥1%) **GI:** Temporary *darkening of stool* and tongue, metallic taste, bluish gum line; bleeding tendencies. With high doses: fecal impaction. **CNS:** Encephalopathy (disorientation, muscle twitching). **Hematologic:** Bleeding tendency. **Special Senses:** Tinnitus, hearing loss. **Urogenital:** Incontinence.

DIAGNOSTIC TEST INTERFERENCE Because bismuth subsalicylate is radiopaque, it may interfere with ***radiographic studies*** of GI tract.

INTERACTIONS Drug: Bismuth may decrease the absorption of TETRACYCLINES, QUINOLONES **(ciprofloxacin, norfloxacin, ofloxacin).**

PHARMACOKINETICS Absorption: Undergoes chemical dissociation in GI tract to bismuth subcarbonate and sodium salicylate; bismuth is minimally absorbed, but the salicylate is readily absorbed.

NURSING IMPLICATIONS

Assessment & Drug Effects

- Monitor bowel function; note that stools may darken and tongue may appear black. These are temporary effects and will disappear without treatment.
- Lab tests: *H. pylori* breath test when used for peptic ulcers.

Patient & Family Education

- Note: Bismuth contains salicylate. Use caution when taking aspirin and other salicylates. Many OTC medications for colds, fever, and pain contain salicylates.
- Consult physician if diarrhea is accompanied by fever or continues for more than 2 d.
- Note: Temporary grayish black discoloration of tongue and stool may occur.
- Do not breast feed while taking this drug without consulting physician.

BISOPROLOL FUMARATE

(bis-o-pro'lol fum'a-rate)

Zebeta

Classifications: AUTONOMIC NERVOUS SYSTEM AGENT; BETA-ADRENERGIC ANTAGONIST (BLOCKING AGENT); ANTIHYPERTENSIVE

Prototype: Propranolol

Pregnancy Category: C

AVAILABILITY 5 mg, 10 mg tablets

ACTIONS Long-acting cardioselective ($beta_1$) adrenoreceptor blocking agent without membrane-stabilizing activity or intrinsic sympathomimetic activity. To maintain $beta_1$ cardioselectivity, the lowest effective dose is necessary. The mechanism of antihypertensive activity has not been completely established. Bisoprolol decreases heart rate, blood pressure, contractile force, and cardiac workload, which reduces myocardial oxygen consumption and increases blood flow to myocardium.

THERAPEUTIC EFFECTS Bisoprolol has antianginal properties, especially improving exercise tolerance. Factors affecting hypertension may include decreased cardiac output, suppressed renin activity, and decreased sympathetic stimulation from vasomotor centers in the brain.

USE Hypertension.

UNLABELED USE Angina.

CONTRAINDICATIONS History of hypersensitivity to bisoprolol, severe sinus bradycardia, second- and third-degree AV block, overt cardiac failure, cardiogenic shock.

CAUTIOUS USE Asthma or COPD, peripheral vascular disease, diabetes mellitus, hyperthyroidism, renal or hepatic insufficiency, pregnancy (category C), lactation, anesthetic use.

ROUTE & DOSAGE

Hypertension, Angina

Adult: **PO** 2.5–5 mg once daily, may increase to 20 mg/d if necessary

ADMINISTRATION

Oral

- Note: The half life of the drug is increased in those with significant liver dysfunction; usual initial dose is 2.5 mg and may be carefully titrated upward if necessary.
- Discontinue drug gradually over a period of 1–2 wk to avoid rebound, withdrawal angina, or hypertension.
- Store at room temperature, 15°–30° C (59°–86° F).

ADVERSE EFFECTS (≥1%) **CNS:** Dizziness, fatigue, tiredness, vertigo, anxiety, headache, sleep disturbances. **CV:** Bradycardia, orthostatic hypotension, rebound/withdrawal angina or hypertension following abrupt discontinuation, may exacerbate intermittent claudication. **Endocrine:** Increases serum levels of VLDL-C and decreases levels of HDL-C lipoproteins, may cause slight rise in serum potassium. **GI:** Abdominal pain, dyspepsia, nausea, vomiting, constipation, diarrhea. **Respiratory:** Asthma, bronchospasm, cough, dyspnea, pharyngitis, sinusitis. **Skin:** Rash, acne, pruritus, eczema. **Other:** Arthralgia.

INTERACTIONS Drug: Amiodarone may cause significant bradycardia; BETA BLOCKERS may reduce **glucose** tolerance, inhibit **insulin** secretion, alter rate of recovery from hypoglycemia, produce hypertension, reduce peripheral circulation, and suppress hypoglycemic symptoms; **rifampin** decreases bisoprolol blood levels.

PHARMACOKINETICS Absorption: Readily absorbed from GI tract; 82%–94% reaches systemic circulation. **Peak:** Therapeutic effect 2–4 wk. **Duration:** 24 h. **Distribution:** Some CNS penetration. **Metabolism:** 50% metabolized in liver to inactive metabolites. **Elimination:** 50%–60% excreted unchanged in urine. **Half-Life:** 10–12.4 h.

NURSING IMPLICATIONS

Assessment & Drug Effects

- Monitor for therapeutic effectiveness. Time required to achieve optimum antihypertensive effect varies from a few days to several weeks.
- Monitor BP frequently during periods of dose adjustment or drug withdrawal.
- Monitor for activity-induced angina both during therapy and following discontinuation of drug.
- Monitor for and report severe hypotension and bradycardia. Dosage adjustment may be required.
- Monitor for bronchospasms in patients with a history of asthma or COPD.
- Monitor diabetics for loss of glycemic control.
- Lab tests: Periodic CBC, electrolytes, renal function, liver function, lipid profile.

Patient & Family Education

- Report orthostatic hypotension and dizziness to physician.

- Do not discontinue drug abruptly unless specifically instructed to do so.
- Note: Drug-induced nightmares and unpleasant dreams are possible when taking this drug.
- Monitor blood glucose for loss of glycemic control.
- Report cold extremities and development of symptoms of intermittent claudication to physician.
- Do not breast feed while taking this drug without consulting physician.

BITOLTEROL MESYLATE

(bye-tole'ter-ole)

Tornalate

Classifications: AUTONOMIC NERVOUS SYSTEM AGENT; BETA-ADRENERGIC AGONIST (SYMPATHOMIMETIC); BRONCHODILATOR

Prototype: Albuterol

Pregnancy Category: C

AVAILABILITY 0.8% aerosol, 0.2% solution for inhalation

ACTIONS Relaxes bronchial smooth muscle and inhibits the release of mediators of immediate hypersensitivity (e.g., histamine) from lung tissue cells. Cardiovascular effects appear to be similar to or less than those produced by isoproterenol.

THERAPEUTIC EFFECTS Decreases airway resistance and increases vital capacity; bronchodilation is greater and longer in duration than that produced by isoproterenol. Produces prolonged bronchodilation as a beta-adrenergic agent.

USES Prophylaxis and treatment of bronchial asthma and reversible bronchospasm in monotherapy, or concomitantly with theophylline or corticosteroids or both.

CONTRAINDICATIONS Safety during pregnancy (category C), lactation, or in children <12 y is not established.

CAUTIOUS USE Cardiovascular disease, hypertension, hyperthyroidism, diabetes mellitus, convulsive disorders, unusual sensitivity to catecholamines; older patients, psychoneurosis; patient with long standing bronchial asthma, and emphysema with degenerative heart disease.

ROUTE & DOSAGE

Bronchospasm

Adult: **Inhalation** 2 inhalations spaced 1–3 min apart q6–8h (max: 12 inhalations/d)

ADMINISTRATION

Inhalation

- Follow manufacturer's directions for aerosol metered dose inhaler.
- Supervise patient a few times to be certain drug delivery is accomplished.
- Note: Manufacturer recommends bottle containing the drug be removed from the inhaler and plastic mouthpiece be cleansed in warm tap water and thoroughly dried once daily.
- Avoid contacting eyes with bitolterol. If it should happen, flush out with copious amounts of water.
- Note: When an adrenocorticoid inhalation is also being used, administer the two drugs 15 min apart unless otherwise directed by physician. This diminishes the risk of fluorocarbon (propellant) toxicity.
- Store at 15°–30° C (59°–86° F); protect from freezing.

ADVERSE EFFECTS (≥1%) **CNS:** Mild, transient effects include *tremors,* nervousness, headache, dizziness, light-headedness, insomnia; hyperkinesia. **CV:** Palpitations, chest discomfort; tachycardia, flushing, PVCs. **Respiratory:** *Throat irritation,* cough, paradoxical bronchoconstriction, dyspnea, chest tightness. **GI:** Nausea, dyspepsia.

INTERACTIONS Drug: Effects of BETA-ADRENERGIC BLOCKERS (e.g., **propranolol**) and bitolterol may be antagonized.

PHARMACOKINETICS Absorption: Absorption from lungs not fully described. **Onset:** 3–5 min. **Peak:** 0.5–2 h. **Duration:** Up to 8 h. **Distribution:** Not known if it crosses placenta or is distributed into breast milk. **Half-Life:** 3 h.

NURSING IMPLICATIONS

Assessment & Drug Effects

- Keep epinephrine 1:1000 readily available until response to drug is known. Immediate hypersensitivity reactions can occur with this drug (see Appendix F).
- Tremors, a common adverse effect and one due to skeletal muscle stimulation, tend to diminish with continued use of bitolterol. Some find the effect intolerable.
- Note: Overdosage leads to exaggerated adverse effects.

Patient & Family Education

- Do not change dose or dose intervals (i.e., do not omit, increase, or decrease number of inhalations). Notify physician immediately if condition worsens or if there is no response to the usual dose.
- Do not use any other inhaler medication (OTC or leftover medication) without physician approval.
- Do not puncture the canister, use or store it near heat or an open flame, or place it in a fire or incinerator for disposal. Contents of the inhaler are under pressure.
- Do not breast feed while taking this drug without consulting physician.

BIVALIRUDIN

(bi-val′i-ru-den)

Angiomax

Classifications: BLOOD FORMERS, COAGULATORS, AND ANTICOAGULANTS; THROMBIN INHIBITOR

Prototype: Lepirudin

Pregnancy Category: B

AVAILABILITY 250 mg vial

ACTIONS Direct inhibitor of thrombin similar to lepirudin. Capable of inhibiting the action of both free and clot-bound thrombin.

THERAPEUTIC EFFECTS Reversibly binds to the thrombin active site, thereby blocking the thrombogenic activity of thrombin.

USES Used with aspirin as an anticoagulant in patients undergoing PTCA.

CONTRAINDICATIONS Hypersensitivity to bivalirudin; cerebral aneurysm, intracranial hemorrhage; patients with increased risk of bleeding (e.g., recent surgery, trauma, CVA); pregnancy (category B), lactation. Safety and efficacy in children are not established.

CAUTIOUS USE Asthma or allergies; blood dyscrasia or thrombocytopenia; GI ulceration, serious hepatic disease; hypertension, renal impairment.

B

ROUTE & DOSAGE

Anticoagulation

Adult: **IV** 1 mg/kg bolus followed by 2.5 mg/kg/h times 4 h, may continue at 0.2 mg/kg/h up to 20 h if needed

ADMINISTRATION

Intravenous

PREPARE: **Direct/Continuous:** Push (bolus dose) and initial 4-h continuous infusion: Reconstitute each 250 mg vial with 5 mL of sterile water for injection; gently swirl until dissolved. Further dilute each reconstituted vial in 50 mL of D5W or NS to yield 5 mg/mL. **Continuous:** Subsequent infusions are low-rate continuous. Reconstitute each 250 mg vial as above. Further dilute each reconstituted vial in 500 mL of D5W or NS to yield 0.50 mg/mL.

ADMINISTER: **Direct:** Give bolus dose 1 mg/kg (see manufacturer's dosing table) IV push. **Continuous:** Give 2.5 mg/kg/h for 4 h. Subsequent doses, give 0.2 mg/kg/h for up to 20 h as ordered.

- Store reconstituted vials refrigerated at 2°–8° C (35.6°–46.4° F) for up to 24 h. Store diluted concentrations between 0.5 mg/mL and 5 mg/mL at room temperature, 15°–30° C (59°–86° F), for up to 24 h.

ADVERSE EFFECTS (≥1%) **Body as a Whole:** *Back pain,* pain, fever. **CV:** *Hypotension,* hypertension, bradycardia. **GI:** *Nausea,* vomiting, dyspepsia, abdominal pain. **Hematologic:** Bleeding. **CNS:** *Headache,* anxiety, nervousness. **Urogenital:** Urinary retention, pelvic pain. **Other:** Injection site pain.

INTERACTIONS No clinically significant interactions established.

PHARMACOKINETICS Duration: 1 h. **Distribution:** No protein binding. **Metabolism:** Proteolytic cleavage and renal metabolism. **Elimination:** Renal. **Half-Life:** 25 min.

NURSING IMPLICATIONS

Assessment & Drug Effects

- Monitor cardiovascular status carefully during therapy.
- Monitor for and report S&S of bleeding: Ecchymosis, epistaxis, GI bleeding, hematuria, hemoptysis.
- Patients with history of GI ulceration, hypertension, recent trauma or surgery are at increased risk for bleeding.
- Monitor neurologic status and report immediately: focal or generalized deficits.
- Lab tests: Baseline and periodic ACT (activated clotting time), APTT, PT, INR, thrombin time (TT), plasma fibrinopeptide A (especially in unstable angina), platelet count, Hgb and Hct; periodic serum creatinine, stool for occult blood, urinalysis.

Patient & Family Education

- Report any of the following immediately: Unexplained back or stomach pain; black, tarry stools; blood in urine, coughing up blood; difficulty breathing; dizziness or fainting spells; heavy menstrual bleeding; nosebleeds; unusual bruising or bleeding at any site.

BLEOMYCIN SULFATE

(blee-oh-mye'sin)

Blenoxane

Classifications: ANTINEOPLASTIC; ANTIBIOTIC

Prototype: Doxorubicin

Pregnancy Category: D

AVAILABILITY 15 units, 30 units powder for injection

ACTIONS A toxic drug with low therapeutic index; intensely cytotoxic. By unclear mechanism, blocks DNA, RNA, and protein synthesis. A cell cycle-phase nonspecific agent. Widely used in combination with other chemotherapeutic agents because it lacks significant myelosuppressive activity.

THERAPEUTIC EFFECTS This mixture of cytotoxic antibiotics from a strain of *Streptomyces verticillus* has strong affinity for skin and lung tumor cells, in contrast to its low affinity for cells in hematopoietic tissue.

USES As single agent or in combination with other chemotherapeutic agents, as adjunct to surgery and radiation therapy. Squamous cell carcinomas of head, neck, penis, cervix, and vulva; lymphomas (including reticular cell sarcoma, lymphosarcoma, Hodgkin's); testicular carcinoma; malignant pleural effusions.

UNLABELED USES *Mycosis fungoides* and *Verruca vulgaris* (common warts).

CONTRAINDICATIONS History of hypersensitivity or idiosyncrasy to bleomycin; women of childbearing age, pregnancy (category D), lactation.

CAUTIOUS USE Compromised hepatic, renal, or pulmonary function; previous cytotoxic drug or radiation therapy.

ROUTE & DOSAGE

Squamous Cell Carcinoma, Testicular Carcinoma

Adult/Child: **SC, IM, IV** 10–20 U/m² or 0.25–0.5 U/kg 1–2 times/wk (max: 300–400 U)

Lymphomas

Adult/Child: **SC, IM, IV** 10–20 U/m² 1–2 times/wk after a 1–2 U test dose times 2 doses

Hodgkin's Disease, Maintenance

Adult/Child: **SC, IM, IV** 1 U IM or IV/d or 5 U/wk

ADMINISTRATION

Note: Due to risk of anaphylactoid reaction, give lymphoma patients ≤2 U for first two doses. If no reaction, follow regular dosage schedule.

- **Subcutaneous/Intramuscular** Reconstitute with sterile water, NS, or bacteriostatic water by adding 1–5 mL to the 15 U vial or 2–10 mL to the 30 U vial. Amount of diluent is determined by the total volume of solution that will be injected.
- Inject IM deeply into upper outer quadrant of buttock; change sites with each injection.

Intravenous

IV administration to infants and children: Verify correct IV concentration and rate of infusion with physician.

PREPARE: **Intermittent:** Dilute each 15 U with at least 5 mL of sterile water or NS. ■ May be further diluted in 50–100 mL of the chosen diluent. ■ Do not dilute with any solution containing D5W.

ADMINISTER: **Intermittent:** Give each 15 U or fraction thereof over 10 min through Y-tube of free-flowing IV.

INCOMPATIBILITIES **Solution/additive: Aminophylline, ascorbic acid, carbenicillin,** CEPHALOSPORINS, **diazepam, hydrocortisone, methotrexate, mitomycin, nafcillin, penicillin G, terbutaline.**

- Store unopened ampuls at 15°–30° C (59°–86° F) unless otherwise specified by manufacturer.

ADVERSE EFFECTS (≥1%) **Body as a Whole:** Hypersensitivity (anaphylactoid reaction); *mild febrile reaction* **CNS:** Headache, mental confusion. **GI:** Stomatitis, ulcerations of tongue and lips, anorexia, nausea, vomiting, diarrhea, weight loss. **Hematologic:** Thrombocytopenia, leukopenia, (rare). **Respiratory:** Pulmonary toxicity (dose and age-related); interstitial pneumonitis, pneumonia, or fibrosis. **Skin:** Diffuse alopecia (reversible), *hyperpigmentation, pruritic erythema,* vesiculation, acne, thickening of skin and nail beds, *patchy hyperkeratosis*, striae, peeling, bleeding. **Other:** Pain at tumor site; phlebitis; necrosis at injection site.

INTERACTIONS Drug: Other ANTINEOPLASTIC AGENTS increase bone marrow toxicity; decreases effects of **digoxin, phenytoin.**

PHARMACOKINETICS Distribution: Concentrates mainly in skin, lungs, kidneys, lymphocytes, and peritoneum. **Metabolism:** Unknown. **Elimination:** 60%–70% recovered in urine as parent compound. **Half-Life:** 2 h.

NURSING IMPLICATIONS

Assessment & Drug Effects

- Start with a test dose. Monitor patient closely for at least 24 h (vital signs, auscultation of chest, careful observations). If there is no acute reaction (hypotension, hyperpyrexia, chills, confusion, wheezing, cardiopulmonary collapse), start regular dosage schedule. Anaphylactoid reaction can be fatal (see Appendix F). It may occur immediately or several hours after first or second dose, especially in lymphoma patients (10%).
- Therapeutic effectiveness: Favorable response, if any, is expected within 2 wk for treatment of Hodgkin's or testicular tumor, and within 3 wk for squamous cell cancers.
- Monitor vital signs. Febrile reaction (mild chills and fever) is relatively common in patients receiving bleomycin therapy. It usually occurs within the first few hours after administration of a large single dose and lasts about 4–12 h. Reaction tends to become less frequent with continued drug administration, but can recur at any time.
- Monitor for and report any of the following: Unexplained bleeding or bruising; evidence of deterioration of renal function (changed I&O ratio and pattern, decreasing creatinine clearance, weight gain or edema); evidence of pulmonary toxicity (nonproductive cough, chest pain, dyspnea).
- Note: Stomatitis can be a dose-limiting factor because oral ulcerations may interfere with adequate nutrient intake, leading to severe debilitation. Consult physician if an oral local anesthetic is indicated. Apply 10 min before meals to take effect so that patient can eat with less pain.
- Check weight at regular intervals under standard conditions. Weight loss and anorexia may persist a long time after therapy has been discontinued.
- Report symptoms of skin toxicity (hypoesthesia, urticaria, tender swollen hands) promptly. May develop in second or third week of treatment and after 150–200 U of bleomycin have been administered. Therapy may be discontinued.

Patient & Family Education

- Avoid OTC drugs during antineoplastic treatment period unless approved by physician.

B

- Report skin irritation which may not develop for several weeks after therapy begins.
- Hyperpigmentation may occur in areas subject to friction and pressure, skin folds, nail cuticles, scars, and intramuscular sites.
- Do not breast feed while taking this drug.

BORTEZOMIB

(bor-te-zo′mib)

Velcade

Classifications: BIOLOGIC RESPONSE MODIFIER; PROTEOSOME INHIBITOR

Pregnancy Category: D

AVAILABILITY 3.5 mg powder for injection

ACTIONS Bortezomib is a reversible inhibitor of proteasome that is responsible for regulation of protein expression and degradation of damaged or obsolete proteins within the cell; its activity is critical to activation or suppression of cellular functions including the cell cycle, oncogene expression, and apoptosis. Inhibition of breakdown of proteasome proteins has been associated with sensitization of the cell to apoptosis. Malignant cells are much more sensitive to the effects of proteasome inhibition than normal cells.

THERAPEUTIC EFFECTS Proteasome inhibition may reverse some of the changes that allow proliferation of malignant cells and suppress apoptosis (programmed cell death) in malignant cells.

USES Treatment of relapsed or refractory multiple myeloma in patients that have failed two prior therapies.

CONTRAINDICATIONS Hypersensitivity to bortezomib, boron, or mannitol; pregnancy (category D); lactation. Safety and effectiveness in children are not established.

CAUTIOUS USE Peripheral neuropathy; history of syncope, dehydration, hypotension; concurrent antihypertensive drugs; history of allergies, asthma; preexisting electrolyte or acid-base disturbances, especially hypokalemia or hyponatremia; liver disease; myelosuppression, renal impairment; history of peripheral neuropathy or other neurologic disorders; GI toxicities.

ROUTE & DOSAGE

Multiple Myeloma

Adult: **IV** 1.3 mg/m^2 twice weekly for 2 wk (days 1, 4, 8, and 11) followed by a 10-d rest period; at least 72 h should elapse between consecutive doses

ADMINISTRATION

Intravenous

- Wear protective gloves and prevent contact with skin.

PREPARE: **Direct:** Reconstitute 3.6 mg vial with 3.5 mL of NS for injection to yield 1 mg/mL. Discard if not clear and colorless. Give within 8 h of reconstitution.

ADMINISTER: **Direct:** Give as a bolus dose

- Store unopened vials at 15°–30° C (59°–86° F). Protect from light.
- Store reconstituted vials at 15°–30° C (59°–86° F). Give within 8 h of reconstitution. May store up to 3 h in a syringe; however, total storage time must not exceed 8 h when exposed to normal indoor lighting.

B

INCOMPATIBILITIES **Solution/additive:** No data available. Do not recommend mixing or injecting with any other drugs.

ADVERSE EFFECTS (≥1%) **Body as a Whole:** *Asthenia, weakness, fatigue, malaise, fever, dehydration, peripheral neuropathy, rigors, herpes zoster.* **CNS:** *Insomnia, headache, paresthesia, dizziness, anxiety.* **CV:** *Edema, hypotension, orthostatic hypotension.* **GI:** *Nausea, vomiting, diarrhea, anorexia, abdominal pain, constipation, dyspepsia, dysphagia.* **Hematologic:** *Thrombocytopenia, neutropenia, anemia.* **Musculoskeletal:** *Arthralgia, musculoskeletal pain, bone pain, myalgia, back pain, muscle cramps.* **Respiratory:** *Dyspnea, cough, upper respiratory infection.* **Skin:** *Rash, pruritus.* **Special Senses:** *Blurred vision, diplopia.*

INTERACTIONS Drug: Hypoglycemia and hyperglycemia have been reported with ANTIDIABETIC AGENTS; ANTIHYPERTENSIVE AGENTS may exacerbate hypotension; ANTICOAGULANTS, **antithymocyte globulin,** NSAIDS, PLATELET INHIBITORS, **aspirin,** THROMBOLYTIC AGENTS may increase risk of bleeding.

PHARMACOKINETICS Metabolism: Metabolized in the liver primarily by CYP3A4, 2D6, 2C19, 2C9, and 1A2. **Half-Life:** 9–15 h

NURSING IMPLICATIONS

Assessment & Drug Effects

- Monitor for and report S&S of neuropathy (e.g., hyperesthesia, hypoesthesia, paresthesia, discomfort or neuropathic pain).
- Monitor postural vital signs for orthostatic hypotension.
- Monitor I&O and assess for S&S of dehydration or electrolyte imbalance if vomiting and/or diarrhea develop.
- Lab tests: Frequent CBC with platelet count; baseline and periodic LFTs; frequent blood glucose in diabetics.

Patient & Family Education

- Report promptly any of the following: dizziness, light-headedness or fainting spells; numbness, tingling, or other unusual sensations; signs of infection (e.g., fever, chills, cough, sore throat); bruising, pinpoint red spots on the skin; black, tarry stools, nosebleeds, or any other sign of bleeding.
- Do not drive or engage in other hazardous activities until reaction to drug is known.
- Females should use reliable methods of contraception to avoid pregnancy while on this drug.
- Do not breast feed while taking this drug.

BOSENTAN

(bo-sen'tan)

Tracleer

Classifications: CARDIOVASCULAR AGENT; VASODILATOR; ENDOTHELIN RECEPTOR A ANTAGONIST

Pregnancy Category: X

AVAILABILITY 62.5 mg, 125 mg tablets

ACTIONS Bosentan is a potent endothelin A receptor antagonist. Endothelin is a peptide with potent vasoconstrictor activity implicated in the pathogenesis of hypertension, CHF, and renal failure. Bosentan is a potent dilator of pulmonary vascular beds in patients with primary pulmonary hypertension, although it is not selective for pulmonary vasculature alone.

THERAPEUTIC EFFECTS Bosentan vasodilates the pulmonary vasculature thus reducing pulmonary hypertension.

USES Treatment of pulmonary arterial hypertension (PAH).

CONTRAINDICATIONS Hypersensitivity to bosentan; pregnancy (category X), lactation; concomitant administration with cyclosporine or glyburide. Safety and efficacy in pediatric patients have not been established.

CAUTIOUS USE Liver disease or reduces hepatic blood flow; severe hypertension.

ROUTE & DOSAGE

Pulmonary Arterial Hypertension

Adult: **PO** 62.5 mg b.i.d., may titrate up to 125 mg b.i.d.

Hepatic Impairment

If LFTs >3 and ≤5 × upper limit of normal (ULN) reduce dose and monitor LFTs q2wk. If LFTs return to normal may continue treatments. If LFTs >5 and ≤8 × ULN, discontinue and monitor LFTs q2wk. If LFTs return to normal, may restart drug cautiously. If LFTs >8 × ULN, discontinue and do not restart.

ADMINISTRATION

Oral

- Do not administer unless liver function tests have been performed and the patient has been determined to have adequate liver function.
- Give in the morning and evening with or without food.
- Do not administer to anyone also receiving glyburide or cyclosporine.
- Store in a tightly closed container at 15°–30° C (59°–86° F).

ADVERSE EFFECTS (≥1%) **Body as a Whole:** Flushing, lower limb edema, fatigue. **CNS:** *Headache*. **CV:** Hypotension, palpitations, edema. **GI:** *Abnormal AST, ALT*, dyspepsia. **Respiratory:** *Nasopharyngitis*. **Skin:** Pruritus.

INTERACTIONS Drug: MACROLIDE ANTIBIOTICS, **cimetidine, cyclosporine, fluoxetine, ketoconazole** may increase bosentan levels; may decrease concentrations of **simvastatin, tacrolimus; carbamazepine,** ORAL CONTRACEPTIVES, **phenytoin, rifampin** may decrease bosentan levels; **glyburide** may cause increase LFTs and lack of hypoglycemic effects. **Herbal: Ephedra, Ma Huang** may antagonize antihypertensive effects.

PHARMACOKINETICS Absorption: 50% bioavailability. **Peak:** 3–5 h. **Distribution:** 98% protein bound. **Metabolism:** Extensively metabolized by CYP3A4 and CYP2C9 to 3 metabolites, one is active. **Elimination:** Primarily excreted in bile. **Half-Life:** 5 h.

NURSING IMPLICATIONS

Assessment & Drug Effects

- Lab tests: Monitor LFT (ALT, AST, bilirubin) within 3 d of initiating treatment and q2wk thereafter. Use same monitoring schedule following discontinuation and reintroduction of bosentan. Monitor Hgb at periodic intervals.
- Report immediately ALT & AST elevations accompanied by S&S of liver injury (jaundice, nausea, vomiting, fever, abdominal pain, lethargy or fatigue) or bilirubin ≥2 × ULN.

B

- Concurrent drugs: Monitor lipid profile in patients receiving lipid-lowering statin drugs; the dose of the statin drug may need to be adjusted. Monitor PT/INR in patients receiving oral anticoagulants, especially when bosentan is added or withdrawn and periodically during concurrent therapy; adjustments in the anticoagulant may be necessary.

Patient & Family Education

- Use a barrier form of birth control in addition to oral, injected, or implanted contraceptives while taking bosentan.
- Contact physician immediately if you think you are pregnant.
- Do not breast feed while using this drug without consulting physician.
- Do not take glyburide while receiving bosentan. Contact your physician for an alternative drug for control of blood glucose.
- Do not use any OTC medications, vitamins, or herbal supplements without clearance from your physician.
- Notify physician immediately if you experience any of the following: dark-colored urine, pale stools, nausea and vomiting, loss of appetite, stomach pain, yellow skin or eyes, fast or pounding heartbeat, swelling in your ankles or feet.

BOTULINUM TOXIN TYPE A

(bo′tul-i-num)

Botox, BOTOX Cosmetic

Classifications: AUTONOMIC NERVOUS SYSTEM AGENT; SKELETAL MUSCLE RELAXANT; ANTISPASMODIC

Pregnancy Category: C

AVAILABILITY 100 units powder for injection

ACTIONS Botulinum toxin type A blocks neuromuscular transmission by binding to receptor sites on motor nerve terminals, entering the nerve terminals, and inhibiting the release of acetylcholine. This inhibition occurs as the neurotoxin splits a protein molecule integral to the successful docking and releasing of acetylcholine from storage areas located within nerve endings.

THERAPEUTIC EFFECTS When injected intramuscularly at therapeutic doses, botulinum toxin type A produces partial chemical denervation of the muscle resulting in a localized reduction in muscle activity.

USES Treatment of blepharospasm, cervical dystonia, strabismus, glabellar frown wrinkles, severe axillary hyperhidrosis.

UNLABELED USES Treatment of other types of wrinkles, migraine headache, achalasia, focal spasticity associated with cerebral palsy with concurrent equinus gait, spasticity associated with stroke.

CONTRAINDICATIONS Presence of infection at the proposed injection site(s); hypersensitivity to Botox. Patients with dysphagia or respiratory compromise; pregnancy (category C); lactation.

CAUTIOUS USE In individuals with peripheral motor neuropathic diseases (e.g., amyotrophic lateral sclerosis, or motor neuropathy), or neuromuscular junctional disorders (e.g., myasthenia gravis or Lambert-Eaton syndrome); neuromuscular disorders; cardiovascular disease; inflammation at the proposed injection site; weakness in the target muscle(s).

ROUTE & DOSAGE

Blepharospasm
Adult/Child: **Intradermal** *>12 y* 1.25–2.5 U injected at each site, may repeat in 3 mo if needed; cumulative dose should not exceed 200 U in a 30-day period

Cervical Dystonia
Adult/Adolescent: **IM** *>16 y* 198–300 U divided among affected muscles

Frown Wrinkles
Adult: **IM** 25 U divided among affected muscles in 5 step doses, may repeat in 3–4 mo if needed

Other Wrinkles
Adult: **SC** 1–2 U per site

Spasticity
Adult: **IM** 20–50 U per affected site
Child: **IM** *2–18 y* 4 U/kg (max: 200 U per treatment) every 3 mo

Axillary Hyperhydrosis
Adult: **IM** 50 U per site, may repeat in 4 mo

ADMINISTRATION

Intramuscular, Intradermal, Subcutaneous

- Slowly inject required amount of nonpreserved NS (see dilution calculation) into vial. Discard vial if a vacuum does not pull diluent into vial. Gently rotate to mix. Discard if not clear, colorless, and free of particulate matter. Dilution calculation: add 1, 2, 4, or 6 mL of NS to yield, respectively, 10 U/0.1 mL, 5 U/0.1 mL, 2.5 U/0.1 mL, 1.25 U/0.1 mL.
- Note: Injection intervals of BOTOX® Cosmetic should be at least 3 mo apart.
- Store at 2°–8° C (refrigerated). Administer within 4 h of reconstitution.

INCOMPATIBILITIES Do not mix with other solutions/additives.

ADVERSE EFFECTS (≥1%) **Body as a Whole:** Injection site reactions (localized pain, tenderness, bruising), neck pain, flu-like symptoms, hypertonia, asthenia, fever. **CNS:** *Headache,* drowsiness. **GI:** *Dysphagia,* dry mouth, fever, nausea, vomiting. **Hematologic:** Ecchymosis. **Musculoskeletal:** Local muscle weakness, dysarthria. **Respiratory:** Cough, rhinitis, upper respiratory infection. **Special Senses:** *Ptosis,* superficial punctate keratitis, dry eyes, ocular irritation, lacrimation, photophobia, keratitis, diplopia.

INTERACTIONS Drug: AMINOGLYCOSIDES, NEUROMUSCULAR BLOCKING AGENTS may potentiate neuromuscular blockade; **chloroquine** may antagonize blocking effects.

NURSING IMPLICATIONS

Assessment & Drug Effects

- Evaluate for therapeutic effectiveness, maximal at about 1–2 wk (lasting 3–4 mo).

Patient & Family Education

- Inform physician about all prescription, nonprescription, and herbal drugs being taken.
- Report immediately any of the following: difficulty breathing or swallowing, problem with speech; unusual bleeding, bruising, or swelling around injection site.
- Note: Effects of the injection generally last 3–4 mo and then repeat treatments may be given.

B

- Do not breast feed without consulting physician.

BRETYLIUM TOSYLATE

(bre-til′ee-um)

Bretylate ♣, Bretylol

Classifications: CARDIOVASCULAR AGENT; ANTIARRHYTHMIC, CLASS III

Prototype: Amiodarone

Pregnancy Category: C

AVAILABILITY 2 mg/mL, 4 mg/mL, 50 mg/mL injection

ACTIONS Mechanism of action is complex and not fully understood. Suppresses ventricular fibrillation by direct action on the myocardium and ventricular tachycardia by adrenergic blockade. Shortly after administration, norepinephrine is released from adrenergic postganglionic nerve terminals, resulting in a moderate increase in BP, heart rate, and ventricular irritability. Subsequently, (1–2 h) drug-induced release and reuptake of norepinephrine are blocked, leading to a state resembling surgical sympathectomy. Orthostatic hypotension commonly occurs as a result of peripheral adrenergic blockade; some degree of hypotension may occur even while patient is supine. In most patients, tolerance to this effect develops after several days.

THERAPEUTIC EFFECTS Suppresses arrhythmias with a reentry mechanism and decreases dispersion of ectopic foci. PR, QT, and QRS intervals are unchanged. Because onset of desired action is delayed, bretylium is not a first-line antiarrhythmic agent.

USES Short-term prophylaxis and treatment of ventricular fibrillation; life-threatening arrhythmias such as ventricular fibrillation not responsive to conventional therapy [e.g., lidocaine, procainamide, direct current (cardioversion)].

CONTRAINDICATIONS No contraindications for use in life-threatening refractory ventricular arrhythmias. Safety during pregnancy (category C), lactation, or in children is not established.

CAUTIOUS USE Digitalis-induced arrhythmias, patients with fixed cardiac output (e.g., severe aortic stenosis or severe pulmonary hypertension because profound hypotension may result), sinus bradycardia, patients on digitalis maintenance, angina pectoris; impaired renal function.

ROUTE & DOSAGE

Ventricular Fibrillation

Adult: **IV** 5 mg/kg rapid IV injection, may increase to 10 mg/kg and repeat q15–30 min (max: 30 mg/kg/d); may also give by continuous infusion at 1–2 mg/min **IM** 5–10 mg/kg, may repeat in 1–2 h if arrhythmia persists, then 5–10 mg/kg q6–8h for maintenance
Child: **IV** 5 mg/kg, may repeat q10–20min (max: 30 mg/kg) **IM** 2–5 mg/kg as single dose

ADMINISTRATION

Limit use to patients in facilities adequately equipped and staffed for constant monitoring of ECG and BP and for cardiovascular/pulmonary resuscitation and cardioversion.

Intramuscular

- Administer no more than 5 mL in any one IM site.
- Keep a record of injection sites. Injection into same site can cause muscle atrophy, necrosis, and fibrosis.

B

Intravenous

- IV administration to infants and children: Verify correct IV concentration and rate of infusion/injection with physician.

PREPARE: **Direct:** Give undiluted. **Intermittent:** Give diluted in 50 mL or more of NS or D5W.

ADMINISTER: **Direct:** Give undiluted at a rate of 1 dose/15 seconds. **Intermittent:** Give diluted at a rate of 1–2 mg/min.

INCOMPATIBILITIES **Solution/additive: Dobutamine, nitroglycerin, phenytoin. Y-site:** Phenytoin.

- Store at 15°–30° C (59°–86° F) unless otherwise directed.

ADVERSE EFFECTS (≥1%) **CV:** Both supine and postural *hypotension* with dizziness, vertigo, lightheadedness, faintness, syncope, transitory hypertension, bradycardia, increased frequency of PVCs, exacerbation of digitalis-induced arrhythmias. **GI:** ***Nausea, vomiting*** (particularly with rapid IV). **Respiratory:** Respiratory depression.

DIAGNOSTIC TEST INTERFERENCE ***Urinary VMA, epinephrine,*** and ***norepinephrine*** levels may be decreased during bretylium therapy.

INTERACTIONS Drug: Lidocaine, procainamide, quinidine, propranolol may antagonize antiarrhythmic effects and compound hypotension; ANTIHYPERTENSIVE AGENTS will add to hypotensive effects; DIGITALIS GLYCOSIDES may worsen arrhythmias through **digitalis** toxicity.

PHARMACOKINETICS Onset: Minutes after IV; up to 6 h IM. **Peak:** 6–9 h. **Duration:** 6–24 h. **Distribution:** Does not cross blood–brain barrier; not known if crosses placenta or distributed into breast milk. **Metabolism:** Not metabolized. **Elimination:** 70%–80% excreted in urine in 24 h. **Half-Life:** 4–17 h.

NURSING IMPLICATIONS

Assessment & Drug Effects

- Anticipate vomiting. IV administration is associated with a high incidence of nausea and vomiting. These side effects can be minimized by slow administration of drug (≥10 min).
- Establish baseline readings and monitor BP and ECG when drug is administered. Observe for initial transient rise in BP, increased heart rate, PVCs and other arrhythmias, or worsening of existing arrhythmias, which may occur within a few minutes to 1 h after drug administration. Keep physician informed. Initial effect of hypertension is usually followed within 1 h by a fall in supine BP and by orthostatic hypotension.
- Use supine position until patient develops tolerance to hypotensive effect of bretylium (generally in several days). Hypotension can occur in the supine position, particularly in patients with severely compromised cardiac function. It may not readily respond to therapy (e.g., vasopressors, fluids); early reporting is essential.
- Raise or lower head of bed slowly; advise patient to make position changes slowly in order to prevent orthostatic hypotension.
- Monitor I&O, particularly in patients with impaired renal function.

Patient & Family Education

- Make position changes slowly. If allowed to be out of bed, dangle legs for a few minutes before standing, but do not stand still for prolonged periods. Men should sit on toilet to urinate.

- Do not breast feed while taking this drug without consulting physician.

BRIMONIDINE TARTRATE

(bry-mon′i-deen)

Alphagan P

Classifications: EYE PREPARATION; MIOTIC (ANTIGLAUCOMA AGENT)

Prototype: Pilocarpine

Pregnancy Category: B

AVAILABILITY 0.15% solution

See Appendix A-1.

BRINZOLAMIDE

(brin-zol′a-mide)

Azopt

Classifications: EYE PREPARATION; MIOTIC (ANTIGLAUCOMA AGENT); AUTONOMIC NERVOUS SYSTEM AGENT; DIRECT-ACTING CHOLINERGIC (PARASYMPATHOMIMETIC)

Prototype: Pilocarpine, Hydrochloride

Pregnancy Category: C

AVAILABILITY 1% suspension

See Appendix A-1.

BROMOCRIPTINE MESYLATE

(broe-moe-krip′teen)

Parlodel

Classifications: AUTONOMIC NERVOUS SYSTEM AGENT; ERGOT ALKALOID; ANTIPARKINSONISM AGENT

Prototype: Ergotamine

Pregnancy Category: C

AVAILABILITY 2.5 mg tablets; 5 mg capsules

ACTIONS Semisynthetic ergot alkaloid derivative, but devoid of oxytocic activity generally attributed to drugs of this class. Reduces elevated serum prolactin levels in men and women by activating postsynaptic dopaminergic receptors in hypothalamus to stimulate release of prolactin-inhibiting factor and possibly luteinizing hormone release factor.

THERAPEUTIC EFFECTS Restores ovulation and ovarian function in amenorrheic women, thus correcting female infertility secondary to elevated prolactin levels. Activates dopaminergic receptors in neostriatum of CNS, which may explain action in parkinsonism.

USES Short-term management of amenorrhea/galactorrhea or female infertility associated with hyperprolactinemia (when there is no indication of pituitary tumor). Also used as adjunctive to levodopa or levodopa/carbidopa therapy to relieve symptoms of Parkinson's disease and to lower plasma growth hormone in patients with acromegaly.

UNLABELED USES To prevent postpartum lactation, to relieve premenstrual symptoms, to treat hypogonadism and galactorrhea in hyperprolactinemic men; for management of hepatic encephalopathy, Cushing's syndrome, drug-induced neuroleptic malignant syndrome, and cocaine withdrawal.

CONTRAINDICATIONS Hypersensitivity to ergot alkaloids; uncontrolled hypertension; severe ischemic heart disease or peripheral vascular disease; pituitary tumor; normal prolactin levels, lactation. Safe use during pregnancy (category C) or in children <15 y is not established.

CAUTIOUS USE Hepatic and renal dysfunction; history of psychiatric disorder; history of MI with residual arrhythmia.

ROUTE & DOSAGE

Amenorrhea or Galactorrhea, Female Infertility

Adult: **PO** 1.25–2.5 mg/d (max: 2.5 mg 2–3 times/d)

Suppression of Postpartum Lactation

Adult: **PO** 2.5 mg b.i.d. starting at least 4 h after delivery for 14–21 d

Parkinson's Disease

Adult: **PO** 1.25–2.5 mg/d (max: 100 mg/d in divided doses)

Acromegaly

Adult: **PO** 1.25–2.5 mg/d for 3 d, then increase by 1.25–2.5 mg q3–7d until desired effect is achieved, usually 30–60 mg/d in divided doses

ADMINISTRATION

Oral

- Do not begin therapy unless vital signs are stabilized.
- Give with meals, milk, or other food to reduce incidence of GI side effects.
- Have patient in supine position before receiving first dose because dizziness and fainting may occur. For this reason, initial dose is usually prescribed for evening administration.
- Note: Withhold therapy until 4 h after delivery and then begin only if vital signs have stabilized.
- Store in tightly closed, light-resistant containers, preferably at 15°–30° C (59°–86° F) unless otherwise directed.

ADVERSE EFFECTS (≥1%) **Body as a Whole:** Mostly dose related. **CNS:** Headache, dizziness, vertigo, light-headedness, fainting, sedation, nightmares, insomnia, dyskinesia, ataxia; mania, nervousness, anxiety, depression. **CV:** *Orthostatic hypotension,* <u>shock</u>, postpartum hypertension, palpitation, extrasystoles, Raynaud's phenomenon, red, tender, hot, edematous extremities (erythromelalgia), exacerbation of angina, arrhythmias, <u>acute MI</u>. **Special Sense:** Blurred vision, burning sensation in eyes, blepharospasm, diplopia. **GI:** *Nausea,* vomiting, abdominal cramps, epigastric pain, constipation (long-term use) or diarrhea; metallic taste, dry mouth, dysphagia, anorexia, peptic ulcers. **Skin:** Urticaria, rash, mottling, livedo reticularis. **Other:** Fatigue, nasal congestion, asthenia.

INTERACTIONS Drug: Possibility of decreased tolerance to **alcohol;** ANTIHYPERTENSIVE AGENTS add to hypotensive effects; ORAL CONTRACEPTIVES, **estrogen, progestins** may interfere with effect of bromocriptine by causing amenorrhea and galactorrhea; PHENOTHIAZINES, TRICYCLIC ANTIDEPRESSANTS, **methyldopa, reserpine** can cause an increase in **prolactin,** which may interfere with bromocriptine activity.

PHARMACOKINETICS Absorption: Approximately 28% absorbed from GI tract. **Peak:** 1–2 h. **Duration:** 4–8 h. **Metabolism:** Metabolized in liver. **Elimination:** 85% excreted in feces in 5 d; 3%–6% eliminated in urine. **Half-Life:** 50 h.

NURSING IMPLICATIONS

Assessment & Drug Effects

- Monitor vital signs closely during the first few days and periodically throughout therapy.

B

- Lab tests: Periodic CBC, liver functions and renal functions with prolonged therapy.
- Monitor for and report psychotic symptoms and other adverse reactions in Parkinson's patients because larger doses are used.
- Improvement in Parkinson's disease may be noted in 30–90 min following administration of bromocriptine, with maximum effect in 2 h.

Patient & Family Education

- Make position changes slowly and in stages, especially from lying down to standing, and to dangle legs over bed for a few minutes before walking. Lie down immediately if light-headedness or dizziness occurs.
- Do not drive or engage in other potentially hazardous activities until response to drug is known.
- Avoid exposure to cold and report the onset of pallor of fingers or toes.
- Note: Patients taking bromocriptine to suppress postpartum lactation may have temporary rebound breast enlargement and pain following drug withdrawal.
- Note: Restoration of regular menses usually occurs in 6–8 wk. Since fertility may be restored during therapy, advise patients being treated for amenorrhea and galactorrhea to use barrier-type contraceptive measures until normal ovulating cycle is restored. Oral contraceptives are contraindicated.
- Inform physician immediately, if pregnancy occurs during therapy. Bromocriptine should be discontinued without delay.
- Do not breast feed while taking this drug.

BROMPHENIRAMINE MALEATE

(brome-fen-ir'a-meen)

Codimal-A, Conjec-B, Cophene-B, Dehist, Dimetane, Dimetane Extentabs, Nasahist B, Sinusol-B

Classifications: ANTIHISTAMINE; (H_1-RECEPTOR ANTAGONIST)

Prototype: Diphenhydramine

Pregnancy Category: C

AVAILABILITY 10 mg/mL injection; ingredient in many oral combination products containing a decongestant, expectorant, and/or analgesic

ACTIONS Antihistamine similar to diphenhydramine; shares properties of other antihistamines. Has less sedative effect than diphenhydramine. Competes with histamine for H_1-receptor sites on effector cells, thus blocking histamine-mediated responses.

THERAPEUTIC EFFECTS Effective against upper respiratory symptoms and allergic manifestations.

USES Symptomatic treatment of allergic manifestations. Also used in various cough mixtures and antihistamine-decongestant cold formulations.

CONTRAINDICATIONS Hypersensitivity to antihistamines; acute asthma; pregnancy (category C), lactation; newborns.

CAUTIOUS USE Older adults; prostatic hypertrophy; narrow-angle glaucoma; cardiovascular or renal disease; hyperthyroidism.

ROUTE & DOSAGE

Allergy

Adult: **PO** 4–8 mg t.i.d. or q.i.d. or 8–12 mg of sustained release b.i.d. or t.i.d.

SC/IM/IV 5–20 mg q6–12h (max: 40 mg/24 h)
Geriatric: **PO** 4 mg 1–2 times/d
Child: **PO** >6 *y*, 2–4 mg t.i.d. or q.i.d. or 8–12 mg of sustained release b.i.d. (max: 12 mg/24 h); <6 *y*, 0.5 mg/kg in 3–4 divided doses

ADMINISTRATION

Oral

- Give with meals or a snack to prevent gastric irritation.

Subcutaneous/Intramuscular

- Give without further dilution or diluted to a 1:10 ratio with NS.

Intravenous

PREPARE: **Direct:** Give undiluted or diluted with 10 mL D5W or NS.

ADMINISTER: **Direct:** Give IV push slowly over 1 min to a recumbent patient.

INCOMPATIBILITIES **Solution/additive: Radio-contrast media (diatrizoate, iothalamate).**

- Store in tightly covered container at 15°–30° C (59°–86° F) unless otherwise directed. Elixir and parenteral form should be protected from light. Avoid freezing.

ADVERSE EFFECTS (≥1%) **Body as a Whole:** Hypersensitivity reaction (urticaria, increased sweating, agranulocytosis). **CNS:** *Sedation,* drowsiness, dizziness, headache, disturbed coordination. **GI:** Dry mouth, throat, and nose, stomach upset, constipation. **Special Senses:** Ringing or buzzing in ears. **Skin:** Rash, photosensitivity.

DIAGNOSTIC TEST INTERFERENCE May cause false-negative **allergy skin tests.**

INTERACTIONS Drug: Alcohol and other CNS DEPRESSANTS add to sedation.

PHARMACOKINETICS Peak: 3–9 h. **Duration:** Up to 48 h. **Distribution:** Crosses placenta. **Elimination:** 40% excreted in urine within 72 h; 2% in feces. **Half-Life:** 12–34 h.

NURSING IMPLICATIONS

Assessment & Drug Effects

- Drowsiness, sweating, transient hypotension, and syncope may follow IV administration; reaction to drug should be evaluated. Keep physician informed.
- Note: Older adults tend to be particularly susceptible to drug's sedative effect, dizziness, and hypotension. Most symptoms respond to reduction in dosage.
- Lab tests: Periodic CBC in patients receiving long-term therapy.

Patient & Family Education

- Acute hypersensitivity reaction can occur within minutes to hours after drug ingestion. Reaction is manifested by high fever, chills, and possible development of ulcerations of mouth and throat, pneumonia, and prostration. Patient should seek medical attention immediately.
- Follow diligent mouth care. Sugarless gum, lemon drops, or frequent rinses with warm water may relieve dry mouth.
- Do not drive a car or other potentially hazardous activities until response to drug is known.
- Do not take alcoholic beverages or other CNS depressants (e.g., tranquilizers, sedatives, pain or sleeping medicines) without consulting physician.
- Do not breast feed while taking this drug.

B

BUCLIZINE HYDROCHLORIDE

(byoo-cli'zeen)

Bucladin-S Softab

Classifications: ANTIHISTAMINE; ANTIVERTIGO

Prototype: Meclizine

Pregnancy Category: C

AVAILABILITY 50 mg tablets

ACTIONS A piperazine derivative structurally and pharmacologically related to meclizine and cyclizine. Mechanism of action not precisely known but may be related to its central anticholinergic actions. It diminishes vestibular stimulation and depresses labyrinthine function. Action on the medullary chemoreceptive trigger zone (CTZ) may also be involved in its antiemetic effect.

THERAPEUTIC EFFECTS Exhibits antihistaminic, anticholinergic, antivertigo, CNS depressant, and local anesthetic effects.

USES Prevention and treatment of motion sickness and the symptomatic treatment of vertigo.

CONTRAINDICATIONS Hypersensitivity to buclizine hydrochloride, children <2 y, older adults, pregnancy (category C), lactation, Reye's syndrome.

CAUTIOUS USE Patients also receiving other CNS depressants or depressant drugs; angle-closure glaucoma; prostatic hypertrophy; bladder neck obstruction; pyloroduodenal obstruction.

ROUTE & DOSAGE

Motion Sickness

Adult: **PO** 50 mg 30 min before travel, may repeat in 4–6 h if needed

Vertigo

Adult: **PO** 50 mg 1–3 times/d

ADMINISTRATION

Oral

- Give with food, water, or milk to minimize gastric irritation.
- Swallow tablets whole, chewed, or allow to dissolve in mouth without water.
- Store away from heat, light, or moist areas at 15°–30° C (59°–86° F) in a tightly closed container.

ADVERSE EFFECTS (≥1%) **CNS:** *Drowsiness,* headache, jitteriness. **GI:** Dry mouth, nausea.

DIAGNOSTIC TEST INTERFERENCE May interfere with **allergy skin tests.**

INTERACTIONS Drug: Alcohol and other CNS DEPRESSANTS compound CNS depression.

PHARMACOKINETICS Absorption: Readily absorbed from GI tract. **Onset:** 1 h. **Duration:** 4–6 h.

NURSING IMPLICATIONS

Assessment & Drug Effects

- Inquire about history of aspirin allergy. Withhold buclizine if aspirin hypersensitivity is reported.
- Buclizine may mask ototoxic effects of large doses of salicylates.

Patient & Family Education

- Take drug for motion sickness at least 30 min before traveling.
- Do not take more medication than recommended.
- Do not drive or engage in other potentially hazardous tasks until response to drug is known.
- Avoid alcohol and other CNS depressants.
- Do not breast feed while taking this drug.

BUDESONIDE

(bu-des′o-nide)

Entocort EC, Pulmicort Turbuhaler, Rhinocort, Rhinocort Aqua, Rhinocort Turbuhaler

Classifications: HORMONE AND SYNTHETIC SUBSTITUTE; ADRENAL CORTICOSTEROID; GLUCOCORTICOID; MINERALOCORTICOID

Prototype: Hydrocortisone

Pregnancy Category: B for inhaled; C for oral

AVAILABILITY 32 mcg/inhalation; 3 mg capsule

ACTIONS Has potent glucocorticoid and weak mineralocorticoid activity. Its antiinflammatory action on nasal mucosa is unknown.

THERAPEUTIC EFFECTS Glucocorticoids have a wide range of inhibitory activities against multiple cell types (e.g., neutrophils, macrophages) and mediators (e.g., histamine, cytokines) involved in allergic and nonallergic/irritant-mediated inflammation.

USES Treatment of allergic and perennial rhinitis, Crohn's disease; prophylaxis for asthma

CONTRAINDICATIONS Hypersensitivity to budesonide, lactation.

CAUTIOUS USE Concomitant administration of systemic oral steroids; active or quiescent tuberculosis; infections of respiratory tract; in sun-treated fungal, bacterial, or systemic viral infections or ocular herpes simplex; recent nasal septal ulcers; recurrent epistaxis; nasal surgery or trauma; pregnancy (category C for oral; category B for inhaled). Safety and efficacy for children <6 y not established.

ROUTE & DOSAGE

Crohn's Disease

Adult: **PO** 9 mg once/d in a.m. for up to 8 wk, may taper to 6 mg q.d. for 2 wk prior to discontinuing. May repeat 8-wk course for recurring episodes of active Crohn's disease.

Asthma Prophylaxis, Rhinitis
See Appendix A-3.

ADMINISTRATION

Oral

- Ensure that capsules are swallowed whole and not chewed.
- Give only in the morning.
- Patients with moderate to severe liver disease should be monitored for increased signs and/or symptoms of hypercorticism. Reducing the dose of ENTOCORT EC capsules should be considered in these patients
- Store at 25° C (77° F); excursions permitted to 15°–30° C (59°–86° F)

ADVERSE EFFECTS (≥1%) **Body as a Whole:** Arthralgia, fatigue, fever, hyperkinesis, myalgia, asthenia, paresthesia, tremor. **CNS:** Dizziness, emotional lability, facial edema, nervousness, *headache,* agitation, confusion, insomnia, drowsiness. **CV:** Chest pain, hypertension, palpitations, sinus tachycardia. **GI:** Abdominal pain, dyspepsia, gastroenteritis, oral candidiasis, xerostomia, diarrhea, nausea, vomiting, cramps. **Hematologic:** Epistaxis. **Metabolic:** Hypokalemia, weight gain. **Respiratory:** Bronchospasms, *infections,* cough, rhinitis, sinusitis, dyspnea, hoarseness, wheezing. **Skin:** Eczema, pruritus, purpura, rash, alopecia. **Special Senses:** Contact

B

dermatitis, reduced sense of smell, nasal pain. **Urogenital:** Intermenstrual bleeding, dysuria.

INTERACTIONS Drug: Ketoconazole may increase oral budesonide concentrations and toxicity; toxicity may also occur with **anastrozole** (high doses only), **clarithromycin, cyclosporine, danazol, delavirdine, diltiazem, erythromycin, fluconazole, fluoxetine, fluvoxamine, indinavir, isoniazid, INH, itraconazole, mibefradil, nefazodone, nelfinavir, nicardipine, norfloxacin, oxiconazole, quinidine, quinine, ritonavir, saquinavir, troleandomycin, verapamil, and zafirlukast. Food: Grapefruit juice** will significantly increase bioavailability of oral budesonide.

PHARMACOKINETICS Absorption: 20% of nasal inhalation dose, 6–13% of orally inhaled dose, and 9% of oral dose reaches systemic circulation; PO form is absorbed from duodenum at pH >5.5; oral bioavailability increases 2.5 times in hepatic cirrhosis. **Onset:** 8–12 h inhaled, 2 wk oral. **Peak:** 2 wk inhaled, 8 wk oral delayed by high-fat meal. **Distribution:** 90% protein bound. **Metabolism:** 85% of absorbed dose undergoes first pass metabolism to 2 inactive metabolites by CYP 3A4. **Elimination:** 60% excreted in urine, 40% in feces. **Half-Life:** 2–3.6 h

NURSING IMPLICATIONS

Assessment & Drug Effects

- Monitor closely for S&S of hypercorticism if concomitant doses of ketoconazole or other CYP3A4 inhibitors (see Drug Interactions) are being given.
- Monitor patients with moderate to severe liver disease for increased S&S of hypercorticism.
- Lab tests: Periodic serum potassium.

Patient & Family Education

- Notify the physician immediately for any of the following: itching, skin rash, fever, swelling of face and neck, difficulty breathing, or if you develop S&S of infection.
- Do not breast feed while taking this drug.
- Do not drink grapefruit juice or eat grapefruit regularly.
- Avoid people with infections, especially those with chicken pox or measles if you have never had these conditions.

BUMETANIDE

(byoo-met'a-nide)

Bumex

Classifications: FLUID AND WATER BALANCE AGENT; LOOP DIURETIC

Prototype: Furosemide

Pregnancy Category: C

AVAILABILITY 0.5 mg, 1 mg, 2 mg tablets; 0.25 mg/mL injection

ACTIONS Sulfonamide derivative structurally related to furosemide and with similar pharmacologic effects. Diuretic activity is 40 times greater, however, and duration of action is shorter than that of furosemide. Causes both potassium and magnesium wastage.

THERAPEUTIC EFFECTS Inhibits sodium and chloride reabsorption by direct action on proximal ascending limb of the loop of Henle. Also appears to inhibit phosphate and bicarbonate reabsorption. Produces only mild hypotensive effects at usual diuretic doses.

USES Edema associated with CHF; hepatic or renal disease, including nephrotic syndrome. Has been used in management of postoperative and premenstrual edema, edema accompanying disseminated carcinoma, and mild hypertension. May be used concomitantly with a potassium-sparing diuretic.

CONTRAINDICATIONS Hypersensitivity to bumetanide or to other sulfonamides; anuria, markedly elevated BUN; hepatic coma; severe electrolyte deficiency; lactation. Safety during pregnancy (category C) is not established.

CAUTIOUS USE Hepatic cirrhosis, as history of gout; history of hypersensitivity to furosemide.

ROUTE & DOSAGE

Edema

Adult: **PO** 0.5–2 mg once/d, may repeat at 4–5 h intervals if needed (max: 10 mg/d) **IV/IM** 0.5–1 mg over 1–2 min, repeated q2–3h prn (max: 10 mg/d)
Neonate: **PO/IM/IV** 0.01–0.05 mg/kg q24–48h
Infant/Child: **PO/IM/IV** 0.015–0.1 mg/kg q6–24h (max: 10 mg/d)

ADMINISTRATION

Oral

- Give with food or milk to reduce risk of gastrointestinal irritation.
- Administered in the morning as a single dose, either daily or by intermittent schedule. For some patients, diuresis is reportedly more effective when administered in two divided doses, morning and evening.

Intramuscular

- Use undiluted solution for injection.

Intravenous

PREPARE: **Direct/Continuous:** Give direct IV undiluted or diluted for infusion with D5W, NS, RL.
ADMINISTER: **Direct:** Give IV push at a rate of a single dose over 1–2 min. **Continuous:** Use diluted solution and give at prescribed rate.
INCOMPATIBILITIES **Solution/additive: Dobutamine.**

Diluted infusion should be used within 24 h after preparation.

- Store in tight, light-resistant container at 15°–30° C (59°–86° F) unless otherwise directed.

ADVERSE EFFECTS (≥1%) **Body as a Whole:** Sweating, hyperventilation, glycosuria. **CNS:** Dizziness, headache, weakness, fatigue. **CV:** Hypotension, ECG changes, chest pain, *hypovolemia*. **GI:** Nausea, vomiting, abdominal or stomach pain, GI distress, diarrhea, dry mouth. **Metabolic:** *Hypokalemia*, hyponatremia, hyperuricemia, hyperglycemia; *hypomagnesemia;* decreased calcium, chloride. **Musculoskeletal:** Muscle cramps, muscle pain, stiffness or tenderness; arthritic pain. **Special Senses:** Ear discomfort, ringing or buzzing in ears, impaired hearing.

INTERACTIONS Drug: AMINOGLYCOSIDES, **cisplatin** increase risk of ototoxicity; bumetanide increases risk of hypokalemia-induced **digoxin** toxicity; NONSTEROIDAL ANTIINFLAMMATORY DRUGS (NSAID) may attenuate diuretic and hypotensive response; **probenecid** may antagonize diuretic activity; bumetanide may decrease renal elimination of **lithium.**

PHARMACOKINETICS Absorption: Readily absorbed from GI tract. **Onset:** 30–60 min PO; 40 min IV.

B

Peak: 0.5–2 h. **Duration:** 4–6 h. **Distribution:** Distributed into breast milk. **Metabolism:** Partially metabolized in liver. **Elimination:** 80% excreted in urine in 48 h, 10%–20% excreted in feces. **Half-Life:** 60–90 min.

NURSING IMPLICATIONS

Assessment & Drug Effects

- Monitor I&O and report onset of oliguria or other changes in I&O ratio and pattern promptly.
- Monitor weight, BP, and pulse rate. Assess for hypovolemia by taking BP and pulse rate while patient is lying, sitting, and standing. Older adults are particularly at risk for hypovolemia with resulting thrombi and emboli.
- Lab tests: Serum electrolytes, blood studies, liver and kidney function tests, uric acid (particularly patients with history of gout), and blood glucose. Determine values initially and at regular intervals; measurements are especially important in patients receiving prolonged treatment, high doses, or who are on sodium restriction.
- Monitor for S&S of hypomagnesemia and hypokalemia (see Appendix F) especially in those receiving digitalis or who have CHF, hepatic cirrhosis, ascites, diarrhea, or potassium-depleting nephropathy.
- Monitor patients with hepatic disease carefully for fluid and electrolyte imbalances which can precipitate encephalopathy (inappropriate behavior, altered mood, impaired judgment, confusion, drowsiness, coma).
- Question patient about hearing difficulty or ear discomfort. Patients at risk of ototoxic effects include those receiving the drug IV, especially at high doses, those with severely impaired renal function, and those receiving other potentially ototoxic or nephrotoxic drugs (see Appendix F).
- Monitor diabetics for loss of glycemic control.

Patient & Family Education

- Report symptoms of electrolyte imbalance to physician promptly (e.g., weakness, dizziness, fatigue, faintness, confusion, muscle cramps, headache, paresthesias).
- Eat potassium-rich foods such as fruit juices, potatoes, cereals, skim milk, and bananas while taking bumetanide.
- Report S&S of ototoxicity promptly to physician (see Appendix F).
- Monitor blood glucose for loss of glycemic control if diabetic.
- Do not breast feed while taking this drug.

BUPIVACAINE HYDROCHLORIDE

(byoo-piv′a-kane)

Marcaine, Sensorcaine

Classifications: CENTRAL NERVOUS SYSTEM AGENT; LOCAL ANESTHETIC (AMIDE-TYPE)

Prototype: Procaine

Pregnancy Category: C

AVAILABILITY 0.25%, 0.5%, 0.75% injection

ACTIONS Anesthetic of the amide type. Decreases sodium flux into nerve cell, inhibiting initial depolarization, and prevents propagation and conduction of the nerve impulse. Progression of anesthesia, related to diameter, myelination, and conduction velocity of affected fibers is manifested clinically as sequential loss of nerve function. May stimulate or depress the CNS or do both.

THERAPEUTIC EFFECTS Primary depressant effect is in medulla and higher centers affecting patient's reaction to pain, temperature, and touch, as well as proprioception and skeletal muscle tone.

USES Infiltration anesthesia; peripheral, sympathetic nerve, and epidural (including caudal) block anesthesia; 0.75% bupivacaine solution in dextrose is used for spinal anesthesia.

CONTRAINDICATIONS Known sensitivity to bupivacaine, local anesthetics, other amide-type anesthetics. Parabens, or metabisulfites; acidosis; heart block; severe hemorrhage; hypotension and shock; hypertension, cerebrospinal diseases; obstetrical paracervical anesthesia or spinal anesthesia in septicemia; topical or IV regional anesthesia; intercurrent use with chloroprocaine; history of malignant hyperthermia. Safety during pregnancy (category C) other than during labor, lactation, or children <12 y is not established.

CAUTIOUS USE Older adults or debilitated patients; hepatic or renal disease; known drug allergies and sensitivities; dysrhythmias; children >12 y; obstetrical delivery.

ROUTE & DOSAGE

Infiltration Anesthesia

Adult: **IM Local infiltration, sympathetic block** 0.25% solution; **Lumbar epidural** 0.25%, 0.5%, 0.75% solutions; **Caudal block, peripheral nerve block** 0.25%, 0.5% solutions; **Retrobulbar block** 0.75% solution
Child: **IM** 1–3.7 mg/kg

ADMINISTRATION

Intramuscular

- Inject slowly with frequent aspirations to avoid intravascular injection.

Intrathecal

- Do not use preparations containing preservatives for epidural or spinal anesthesia.
- Do not use multiple-dose vial for lumbar or caudal epidural block.
- Store ampuls at 15°–30° C (59°–86° F); protect from freezing. Solutions with epinephrine should be protected from light.

INCOMPATIBILITIES **Solution/additive: Sodium bicarbonate**

ADVERSE EFFECTS (≥1%) **Body as a Whole:** Hypersensitivity [cutaneous lesions, urticaria, sneezing, diaphoresis, syncope, hyperthermia, angioneurotic edema <u>(including laryngeal edema), anaphylaxis, anaphylactoid reaction</u>]. **CNS:** Nervousness, unusual anxiety, excitement, dizziness, drowsiness, tremors, convulsions, unconsciousness, <u>respiratory arrest</u>. **Special Senses:** Pupillary constriction; blurred or double vision; tinnitus. **GI:** Nausea, vomiting. **Other:** Inflammation or sepsis at injection site, chills, pupillary constriction. **Associated with Epidural Anesthesia, Body as a Whole:** Total spinal block, persistent analgesia, paresthesia. **Urogenital:** Urinary retention, fecal incontinence, loss of perineal sensation and sexual function. **Other:** Slowing of labor, increased incidence of forceps delivery, cranial nerve palsies (with inadvertent intrathecal injection).

INTERACTIONS Drug: CNS DEPRESSANTS augment CNS depression; with **isoproterenol, ergonovine** there is persistent hypertension and a risk of CVA if bupivacaine used with **epinephrine.** MAO INHIBITORS, TRICYCLIC ANTIDEPRESSANTS, PHENOTHIAZINES cause severe or prolonged hypotension or hypertension if bupivacaine used with **epinephrine.**

PHARMACOKINETICS Onset: 4–17 min for epidural, caudal, peripheral, or sympathetic block; within 1 min for spinal block. **Duration:** 3–5 h for epidural, caudal, peripheral, or sympathetic block; 1.25–2.5 h for spinal block. **Distribution:** Crosses placenta. **Metabolism:** Metabolized in liver. **Elimination:** 6% excreted unchanged in urine. **Half-Life:** 1.5–5.5 h in adults, 8.1 h in neonates.

NURSING IMPLICATIONS

Assessment & Drug Effects

- Monitor for signs of inadvertent intravascular injection, which can produce a transient "epinephrine response" (increased heart rate or systolic BP or both, circumoral pallor, palpitations, nervousness) within 45 seconds in the unsedated patient and an increase by 20 bpm or more in heart rate for at least 15 seconds in sedated patient.
- Vasoconstrictor-containing solution should be administered cautiously, if at all, to areas with end arteries (e.g., digits, penis) or to areas that have a compromised blood supply; ischemia and gangrene can result. Inspect areas for evidence of reduced perfusion because of vasospasm: pale, cold, sensitive skin.
- Note: Systemic reactions (toxicity) are more apt to occur in children or older adults and may develop rapidly or be delayed for as long as 30 min after administration.
- Monitor for toxicity: CNS stimulation (unusual anxiety, excitement, restlessness) usually occurs first, followed by CNS depression (drowsiness, unconsciousness, respiratory arrest). However, because stimulation is apt to be transient or absent, drowsiness may be the first sign in some patients (especially children and older adults).
- Monitor BP and fetal heart rate continuously during labor because maternal hypotension may accompany regional anesthesia. Place mother on left side with legs elevated.
- Monitor cardiac and respiratory status continuously in patients receiving retrobulbar and dental blocks.

Patient & Family Education

- After spinal anesthesia, sensation to lower extremities may not return for 2.5–3.5 h.

BUPRENORPHINE HYDROCHLORIDE

(byoo-pre-nor′feen)

Buprenex, Subutex

BUPRENORPHINE HYDROCHLORIDE/NALOXONE HYDROCHLORIDE DIHYDRATE

Suboxone

Classifications: CENTRAL NERVOUS SYSTEM AGENT; ANALGESIC; NARCOTIC (OPIATE) AGONIST-ANTAGONIST
Prototype: Pentazocine
Pregnancy Category: C
Controlled Substance: Schedule III

AVAILABILITY 0.324 mg/mL injection; 2 mg, 8 mg sublingual tablets; 2 mg buprenorphine/0.5 mg naloxone, 8 mg buprenorphine/2 mg naloxone sublingual tablets

ACTIONS Opiate agonist-antagonist with agonist activity approximately 30 times that of morphine and antagonist activity equal to or up to 3 times greater than that of naloxone. Respiratory depression occurs infrequently, probably due to drug's opiate antagonist activity. Psychologic and limited physical dependence develops infrequently; tolerance to drug rarely develops.

THERAPEUTIC EFFECTS Dose-related analgesia results from a high affinity of buprenorphine for mu-opioid receptors and an antagonist at the kappa-opiate receptors in the CNS. Naloxone is an antagonist at the mu-opioid receptor.

USES *Injectable* used principally for moderate to severe postoperative pain. Also for pain associated with cancer and trigeminal neuralgia, accidental trauma, ureteral calculi, MI. *Sublingual tablets* used for treatment of opioid dependence.

UNLABELED USES *Injectable* to reverse fentanyl-induced anesthesia. *Sublingual tablets* may be used to ease cocaine withdrawal.

CONTRAINDICATIONS Known hypersensitivity to buprenorphine (both drug forms) or hypersensitivity to naloxone (Suboxone). Safety during pregnancy (category C), lactation, or in children <13 y is not established.

CAUTIOUS USE Patient with history of opiate use; compromised respiratory function (e.g., chronic obstructive pulmonary disease (COPD), cor pulmonale, decreased respiratory reserve, hypoxia, hypercapnia, or preexisting respiratory depression); concomitant use of other respiratory depressants; hypothyroidism, myxedema, Addison's disease; severe renal or hepatic impairment; geriatric or debilitated patients; acute alcoholism, delirium tremens; prostatic hypertrophy, urethral stricture; comatose patient; patients with CNS depression, head injury, or intracranial lesion; biliary tract dysfunction.

ROUTE & DOSAGE

Postoperative Pain

Adult: **IV/IM** 0.3 mg q6h up to 0.6 mg q4h or 25–50 mcg/h by IV infusion
Geriatric: **IV/IM** give 1/2 adult dose
Child: **IV/IM** 2–12 y 2–6 mcg/kg q4–6h prn

Opioid Dependence/Cocaine Withdrawal

Adult: **SL** Initiate with 8 mg q.d. Subutex on day 1 at least 4 h after last opioid dose, 16 mg q.d. Subutex on day 2, then switch to Suboxone for maintenance therapy at the same buprenorphine dose as day 2 (e.g., 16 mg q.d.). Adjust dose daily until opiate withdrawal effects are suppressed. Maintenance dose range 4 mg–24 mg/d buprenorphine

ADMINISTRATION

Sublingual

- Place SUBONONE and SUBUTEX tablets under tongue until dissolved. For doses requiring more than two tablets, place all tablets at once under tongue, or if patient cannot accommodate all tablets, place two tablets at a time under tongue.
- Instruct to hold the tablets under tongue until dissolved; advise not to swallow.

Intramuscular

- Give undiluted, deep IM into a large muscle.

B

Intravenous

PREPARE: **Direct:** Give undiluted. Do not use if discolored or contains particulate matter.

ADMINISTER: **Direct:** Give slowly at a rate of 0.3 mg over 2 min to a patient in a recumbent position.

- Store at 15°–30° C (59°–86° F); avoid freezing.

ADVERSE EFFECTS (≥1%) **CNS:** *Sedation, drowsiness,* dizziness, vertigo, *headache,* amnesia, euphoria, asthenia, *insomnia, pain* (when used for withdrawal), *withdrawal symptoms.* **CV:** Hypotension, vasodilation. **Special Senses:** Miosis. **GI:** *Nausea,* vomiting, diarrhea, *constipation.* **Respiratory:** Respiratory depression, hyperventilation. **Skin:** Pruritus, injection site reactions, *sweating.*

INTERACTIONS Drug: Alcohol, OPIATES, other CNS DEPRESSANTS, BENZODIAZEPINES augment CNS depression; **diazepam** may cause respiratory or cardiovascular collapse; AZOLE ANTIFUNGALS (e.g., **fluconazole**), MACROLIDE ANTIBIOTICS (e.g., **erythromycin**), and PROTEASE INHIBITORS (e.g., **saquinavir**) may increase buprenorphine levels.

PHARMACOKINETICS Absorption: Widely variable sublingual absorption. **Onset:** 10–30 min IM/IV. **Peak:** 1 h IM/IV; 2–6 h SL. **Duration:** 6–10 h. **Metabolism:** Metabolized extensively in liver by CYP3A4 to active metabolite norbuprenorphine. **Elimination:** 70% eliminated in feces and 30% in urine in 7 d. **Half-Life:** 2.2 h IM/IV; 37 h SL.

NURSING IMPLICATIONS

Assessment & Drug Effects

- Monitor respiratory status during therapy. Buprenorphine-induced respiratory depression is about equal to that produced by 10 mg morphine, but onset is slower, and if it occurs, it lasts longer.
- Note: Respiratory depression in the healthy adult plateaus or may even decrease in severity with doses more than 1.2 mg because of antagonist activity of the drug.
- Use lower dosing of buprenorphine with a concurrent NSAID or other nonnarcotic analgesic due to additive analgesic effect.
- Monitor I&O ratio and pattern during buprenorphine therapy; urinary retention is a potential adverse effect.
- Lab tests: Baseline liver function, renal function, alkaline phosphatase, and PSA.
- Supervise ambulation; drowsiness occurs in 66% of patients taking this drug.

Patient & Family Education

- Do not drive or engage in other potentially hazardous activities until response to drug is known.
- Do not use alcohol or other CNS depressing drugs without consulting physician. An additive effect exists between buprenorphine hydrochloride and other CNS depressants including alcohol.
- Do not breast feed while taking this drug without consulting physician.

BUPROPION HYDROCHLORIDE

(byoo-pro′pi-on)

Wellbutrin, Wellbutrin SR, Wellbutrin XL, Zyban

Classifications: CENTRAL NERVOUS SYSTEM (CNS) AGENT; ANTIDEPRESSANT

Pregnancy Category: B

AVAILABILITY 75 mg, 100 mg tablets; 100 mg, 150 mg, 200 mg sustained-release tablets; 150 mg, 300 mg extended-release tablets

ACTIONS The neurochemical mechanism of bupropion is unknown. It does not inhibit monoamine oxidase. Compared to tricyclic antidepressants (TCA), it is a weak blocker of neural uptake of serotonin and norepinephrine.

THERAPEUTIC EFFECTS Its antidepressive effect is related to CNS stimulant effects.

USES Indicated for mental depression; since it has been associated with increased risk of seizures, it is not the agent of first choice; adjunct for smoking cessation.

UNLABELED USES Cyclic mood disorders, schizoaffective disorders.

CONTRAINDICATIONS Hypersensitivity to bupropion; history of seizure disorder; current or prior diagnosis of bulimia or anorexia nervosa; concurrent administration of an MAO inhibitor; head trauma; CNS tumor; recent MI; abrupt discontinuation, anorexia nervosa, bulimia nervosa, children <18 y; lactation.

CAUTIOUS USE Renal or hepatic function impairment; drug abuse or dependence; pregnancy (category B); cardiac disease, MI, hepatic disease, biliary cirrhosis; hypertension, bipolar disorder, mania, psychosis, diabetes mellitus, older adults, ethanol intoxication, suicidal ideation, tics, Tourette's syndrome.

ROUTE & DOSAGE

Depression

Adult: **PO** 75–100 mg t.i.d., start with 75 mg t.i.d., or 100 mg SR b.i.d., or 150 mg XL q.d., and increase dose q3d to 300 mg/d; doses >450 mg/d are associated with an increased risk of adverse reactions including seizures

Geriatric: **PO** 50–100 mg/d, may increase by 50–100 mg q3–4d (max: 150 mg/dose)

Smoking Cessation

Adult: **PO** Start with 150 mg once daily × 3 d, then increase to 150 mg b.i.d. (max: 300 mg/d) for 7–12 wk

ADMINISTRATION

Oral

- Give with meals to decrease incidence of nausea and vomiting.
- Ensure that sustained-release tablets are not chewed or crushed. They must be swallowed whole.
- Note: Increases in dosage should not exceed 100 mg/d over a 3-d period. Greater increments increase the seizure potential.
- Store away from heat, direct light, and moisture.

ADVERSE EFFECTS (≥1%) **Body as a Whole:** Weight loss, weight gain. **CNS:** Seizures. The risk of seizure appears to be strongly associated with dose (especially >450 mg/d) and may be increased by predisposing factors (e.g., head trauma, CNS tumor) or a history of prior seizure; *agitation, insomnia, dry mouth, blurred vision, headache, dizziness, tremor.* **GI:** *Nausea, vomiting, constipation.* **CV:** Tachycardia. **Skin:** Rash.

INTERACTIONS Drug: May increase metabolism of **carbamazepine, cimetidine, phenytoin, phenobarbital,** decreasing their effect; may increase incidence of adverse effects of **levodopa,** MAO INHIBITORS.

PHARMACOKINETICS Absorption: Readily absorbed from GI tract.

B

Onset: 3–4 wk. **Peak:** 1–3 h. **Metabolism:** Metabolized in liver (including first pass metabolism) to active metabolites. **Elimination:** 80% excreted in urine as inactive metabolites **Half-Life:** 8–24 h.

NURSING IMPLICATIONS

Assessment & Drug Effects

- Monitor for therapeutic effectiveness. The full antidepressant effect of drug may not be realized for 4 or more weeks.
- Close observation for worsening of depression or suicidal tendencies.
- Use extreme caution when administering drug to patient with history of seizures, cranial trauma, or other factors predisposing to seizures; during sudden and large increments in dose, seizure potential is increased.
- Report significant restlessness, agitation, anxiety, and insomnia. Symptoms may require treatment or discontinuation of drug.
- Monitor for and report delusions, hallucinations, psychotic episodes, confusion, and paranoia.
- Lab tests: Monitor hepatic and renal function tests while patient is taking this drug.

Patient & Family Education

- Take drug at the same times each day.
- Monitor your weight at least weekly. Report significant changes in weight (+/–5 lb) to physician.
- Minimize or avoid alcohol because it increases the risk of seizures.
- Do not drive or engage in potentially hazardous activities until response to drug is known because judgment or motor and cognitive skills may be impaired.
- Do not abruptly discontinue drug. Gradual dosage reduction may be necessary to prevent adverse effects.
- Do not take any OTC drugs without consulting physician.
- Do not breast feed while taking this drug.

BUSPIRONE HYDROCHLORIDE

(byoo-spye′rone)

BuSpar

Classifications: CENTRAL NERVOUS SYSTEM AGENT; ANXIOLYTIC

Prototype: Lorazepam

Pregnancy Category: B

AVAILABILITY 5 mg, 10 mg, 15 mg tablets

ACTIONS First generation agent in a new class of anxiolytics. Has chemical and pharmacologic properties unrelated to those of the benzodiazepines or other psychotherapeutic agents. Action is unclear, but appears to be focused mainly on the brain D_2-dopamine receptors. It has agonist effects on presynaptic dopamine receptors and also a high affinity for serotonin ($5\text{-}HT_{1A}$) receptors. Unlike other anxiolytics, it seems to cause less clinically significant impairment of cognitive and motor performance and produces minimal if any interaction with other CNS depressants, including alcohol.

THERAPEUTIC EFFECTS Antianxiety effect is due to its serotonin reuptake inhibition and agonist effects on dopamine receptors of the brain.

USES Management of anxiety disorders and for short-term treatment of generalized anxiety.

UNLABELED USES Adjuvant for nicotine withdrawal.

CONTRAINDICATIONS Concomitant use of alcohol and buspirone. Safety during pregnancy (category B), labor and delivery, lactation, or in children <18 y is not established.
CAUTIOUS USE Moderate to severe renal or hepatic impairment.

ROUTE & DOSAGE

Anxiety
Adult: **PO** 7.5–15 mg/d in divided doses, may increase by 5 mg/d q2–3d as needed (max: 60 mg/d)
Geriatric: **PO** 5 mg b.i.d., may increase to max 60 mg/d

ADMINISTRATION

Oral
- Give with food to decrease nausea.
- Give 8 h before or after drinking grapefruit juice.
- Store at 15°–30° C (59°–86° F) in tightly closed container unless otherwise directed.

ADVERSE EFFECTS (≥1%) **CNS:** Numbness, paresthesia, tremors, *dizziness, headache,* nervousness, *drowsiness,* light-headedness, dream disturbances, decreased concentration, excitement, mood changes. **CV:** Tachycardia, palpitation. **Special Senses:** Blurred vision. **GI:** *Nausea,* vomiting, dry mouth, abdominal/gastric distress, diarrhea, constipation. **Urogenital:** Urinary frequency, hesitancy. **Musculoskeletal:** Arthralgias. **Respiratory:** Hyperventilation, shortness of breath. **Skin:** Rash, edema, pruritus, flushing, easy bruising, hair loss, dry skin. **Other:** Fatigue, weakness.

DIAGNOSTIC TEST INTERFERENCE Buspirone may increase serum concentrations of ***hepatic aminotransferases (ALT, AST).***

INTERACTIONS Drug: May cause hypertension with MAO INHIBITORS, **trazodone,** possible increase in liver transaminases; increased **haloperidol** serum levels.

PHARMACOKINETICS Absorption: Readily absorbed from GI tract but undergoes first pass metabolism. **Onset:** 5–7 d. **Peak:** 1 h. **Metabolism:** Metabolized in liver. **Elimination:** 30%–63% excreted in urine as metabolites within 24 h. **Half-Life:** 2–4 h.

NURSING IMPLICATIONS

Assessment & Drug Effects
- Monitor for therapeutic effectiveness. Desired response may begin within 7–10 d; however, optimal results take 3–4 wk. Reinforce the importance of continuing treatment to patient.
- Benzodiazepines or sedative-hypnotic drugs are withdrawn gradually before buspirone therapy is started. Observe patient for rebound symptoms, which may occur over varying time periods during first phase of treatment.
- Note: Buspirone may displace digoxin from its serum binding, increasing the potential for toxic serum levels of digoxin. If the two drugs must be given concomitantly, monitor cardiovascular parameters (BP, pulse) until dosage has been stabilized.
- Monitor for and report dystonia, motor restlessness, and involuntary repetitious movement of facial or cervical muscle.
- Observe for and report swollen ankles, decreased urinary output, changes in voiding pattern, jaundice, itching, nausea, or vomiting.

Patient & Family Education
- Take exactly as prescribed: Specifically, do not omit, skip, in-

crease or decrease doses without advice of the physician.

- Report any of the following immediately: Involuntary, repetitive movements of face or neck; weakness, nervousness, nightmares, headache, or blurred vision; depression or thoughts of suicide.
- Do not use OTC drugs without advice of the physician while taking buspirone.
- Note: Adverse effects subside during continued therapy with or without dosage adjustment. Do not discontinue therapy.
- Do not drive or engage in other potentially hazardous activities until response to drug is known.
- Alert physician if you become pregnant; buspirone must be discontinued during pregnancy.
- Discuss limits of alcohol intake with physician; cautious use is generally advised.
- Note: It is important to understand the planned schedule for changes in doses and intervals to ensure low incidence of withdrawal or rebound symptoms when therapy is discontinued.
- Do not breast feed while taking this drug without consulting physician.

BUSULFAN

(byoo-sul'fan)

Busulfex, Myleran

Classifications: ANTINEOPLASTIC; ALKYLATING AGENT

Prototype: Cyclophosphamide

Pregnancy Category: D

AVAILABILITY 2 mg tablets; 6 mg/mL injection

ACTIONS Potent cytotoxic alkylating agent that may be mutagenic and carcinogenic. Cell cycle nonspecific. Reduces total granulocyte mass but has little effect on lymphocytes and platelets except in large doses. May cause widespread epithelial cellular dysplasia severe enough to make it difficult to interpret exfoliative cytologic examinations from lung, breast, bladder, and uterine cervix.

THERAPEUTIC EFFECTS Causes cell death by acting predominantly on slowly proliferating stem cells by inducing cross linkage in DNA, thus blocking replication. Acquired resistance may develop, probably due to intracellular inactivation of busulfan.

USES Palliative treatment of chronic myelogenous (myeloid, granulocytic, myelocytic) leukemia for patients no longer responsive to radiation therapy or to previously tried antineoplastics. Does not appreciably extend survival time.

UNLABELED USES Polycythemia vera, severe thrombocytosis, as adjunct in treatment of myelofibrosis, allogenic bone transplantation in patients with acute nonlymphocytic leukemia.

CONTRAINDICATIONS Therapy-resistant chronic lymphocytic leukemia; lymphoblastic crisis of chronic myelogenous leukemia; bone marrow depression, immunizations (patient and household members), chickenpox (including recent exposure), herpetic infections. Safety during pregnancy (category D) or lactation is not established.

CAUTIOUS USE Men and women in childbearing years; history of gout or urate renal stones; prior irradiation or chemotherapy.

ROUTE & DOSAGE

Chronic Myelogenous Leukemia

Adult: **PO** 4–8 mg/d until maximal clinical and hematologic improvement, may use 1–4 mg/d if remission is shorter than 3 mo

Child: **PO** 0.06–0.12 mg/kg/d or 1.8–4.6 mg/m²

ADMINISTRATION

Oral

- Give at same time each day.
- Give on an empty stomach to minimize nausea and vomiting.
- Store in tightly capped, light-resistant container at 15°–30° C (59°–86° F), unless otherwise specified.

ADVERSE EFFECTS (≥1%) **Hematologic:** Major toxic effects are related to <u>bone marrow failure; agranulocytosis</u> (rare), pancytopenia, thrombocytopenia, leukopenia, *anemia*. **Urogenital:** Flank pain, renal calculi, uric acid nephropathy, <u>acute renal failure</u>, gynecomastia, testicular atrophy, azoospermia, impotence, sterility in males, ovarian suppression, menstrual changes, amenorrhea (potentially irreversible), menopausal symptoms. **Respiratory:** Irreversible <u>pulmonary fibrosis</u> ("busulfan lung"). **Skin:** Alopecia, hyperpigmentation. **Other:** Endocardial fibrosis, dizziness, cholestatic jaundice, infections.

DIAGNOSTIC TEST INTERFERENCE

Busulfan may decrease ***urinary 17-OHCS*** excretion, and may increase ***blood and urine uric acid*** levels. Drug-induced cellular dysplasia may interfere with interpretation of ***cytologic studies.***

INTERACTIONS Drug: Probenecid, sulfinpyrazone may increase **uric acid** levels.

PHARMACOKINETICS Absorption: Readily absorbed from GI tract. **Peak:** 4 h. **Duration:** 4 h. **Metabolism:** Metabolized in liver. **Elimination:** 10%–50% excreted in urine within 48 h.

NURSING IMPLICATIONS

Assessment & Drug Effects

- Monitor for therapeutic effectiveness: Normal leukocyte count is usually achieved in about 2 mo.
- Monitor the following: Vital signs, weight, I&O ratio and pattern. Urge patient to increase fluid intake to 10–12 [8 oz] glasses daily (if allowed) to assure adequate urinary output.
- Monitor for and report symptoms suggestive of superinfection (see Appendix F), particularly when patient develops leukopenia.
- Lab test: Baseline Hgb, Hct, WBC with differential, platelet count, liver function, kidney function, serum uric acid; repeat at least weekly.
- Avoid invasive procedures during periods of platelet count depression.

Patient & Family Education

- Report to physician any of the following: Easy bruising or bleeding, cloudy or pink urine, dark or black stools; sore mouth or throat, unusual fatigue, blurred vision, flank or joint pain, swelling of lower legs and feet; yellowing white of eye, dark urine, light-colored stools, abdominal discomfort, or itching (hepatotoxicity).
- Use contraceptive measures during busulfan therapy and for at least 3 mo after drug is withdrawn.

B

- Do not breast feed while taking this drug without consulting physician.

BUTABARBITAL SODIUM

(byoo-ta-bar'bi-tal)

Barbased, Butalan, Butisol Sodium, Sarisol No. 2

Classifications: CENTRAL NERVOUS SYSTEM AGENT; BARBITURATE; ANXIOLYTIC; SEDATIVE-HYPNOTIC

Prototype: Phenobarbital

Pregnancy Category: C

Controlled Substance: Schedule III

AVAILABILITY 15 mg, 30 mg, 50 mg, 100 mg tablets; 30 mg/5 mL elixir

ACTIONS Intermediate-acting barbiturate, similar to phenobarbital. Appears to act at thalamus level, where it interferes with transmission of impulses to the cerebral cortex.

THERAPEUTIC EFFECTS Preoperative sedative agent that also is an effective antianxiety agent.

USES Hypnotic in short-term treatment of simple insomnia, as sedative for relief of anxiety, and to provide sedation preoperatively.

CONTRAINDICATIONS Porphyria; uncontrolled pain; severe respiratory disease; history of addiction; pregnancy (category C), lactation.

CAUTIOUS USE Severe renal or hepatic impairment; acute abdominal conditions; older adults or debilitated patients. Safe use in children <12 is not established.

ROUTE & DOSAGE

Daytime Sedation

Adult: **PO** 15–30 mg t.i.d. or q.i.d.

Child: **PO** 7.5–30 mg t.i.d.

Preoperative Sedation

Adult: **PO** 50–100 mg 60–90 min before surgery

Child: **PO** 2–6 mg/kg in 3 equally divided doses (max: 100 mg)

Hypnotic

Adult: **PO** 50–100 mg h.s.

ADMINISTRATION

Oral

- Schedule slow withdrawal following long-term use to avoid precipitating withdrawal symptoms.
- Store in tightly covered containers, preferably at 15°–30° C (59°–86° F), unless otherwise directed.

ADVERSE EFFECTS (≥1%) **CNS:** Drowsiness, ***residual sedation*** ("hangover"), headache. **GI:** Nausea, vomiting, constipation, diarrhea. **Skin:** Urticaria, skin rash. **Musculoskeletal:** Muscle or joint pain.

INTERACTIONS Drug: Alcohol and other CNS DEPRESSANTS add to CNS and respiratory depression; butabarbital increases the metabolism of ORAL ANTICOAGULANTS, BETA BLOCKERS, CORTICOSTEROIDS, **doxycycline, griseofulvin, quinidine,** THEOPHYLLINES, ORAL CONTRACEPTIVES, decreasing their effectiveness. **Herbal: Kava-kava, valerian** may potentiate sedation.

PHARMACOKINETICS Absorption: Readily absorbed from GI tract. **Onset:** 40–60 min. **Peak:** 3–4 h. **Duration:** 6–8 h. **Distribution:** Crosses placenta; distributed into breast milk. **Metabolism:** Metabolized in liver. **Elimination:** Excreted in urine primarily as metabolites. **Half-Life:** Average 100 h.

NURSING IMPLICATIONS

Assessment & Drug Effects

- Assess for adverse effects. Older adults and debilitated patients sometimes manifest excitement, confusion, or depression. Children also may react with paradoxical excitement. Side rails may be advisable. Report these reactions to physician.

Patient & Family Education

- Do not drive or engage in other potentially hazardous activities until response to drug is known.
- Do not drink alcoholic beverages while taking this drug. Other CNS depressants may produce additive drowsiness; do not take without approval of physician.
- Note: Prolonged use is not recommended because tolerance to drug occurs in about 14 d.
- Do not breast feed while taking this drug.

BUTENAFINE HYDROCHLORIDE

(bu-ten′a-feen)

Mentax

Classifications: ANTIINFECTIVE; ANTIFUNGAL ANTIBIOTIC

Prototype: Fluconazole

Pregnancy Category: B

AVAILABILITY 1% cream

ACTIONS Exerts antifungal action by inhibiting sterol synthesis, which may enhance susceptibility of the fungal membrane to damage by butenafine.

THERAPEUTIC EFFECTS Antifungal effectiveness against interdigital *tinea pedis* (athlete's foot), *tinea corporis* (ringworm), and *tinea cruris* (jock itch).

USES Treatment of tinea pedis, tinea corporis, and tinea cruris due to *Epidermophyton floccosum, Trichophyton mentagrophytes, Trichophyton rubrum.*

CONTRAINDICATIONS Hypersensitivity to butenafine.

CAUTIOUS USE Hypersensitivity to naftifine or tolnaftate; pregnancy (category B); lactation. Safety and efficacy in children <12 y are not established.

ROUTE & DOSAGE

Tinea Pedis

Adult/Child: **Topical** >*12 y,* Apply to affected area and surrounding skin b.i.d. times 7 d or q.d. times 4 wk

Tinea Corporis, Tinea Cruris

Adult/Child: **Topical** >*12 y,* Apply to affected area and surrounding skin once daily

ADMINISTRATION

Topical

- Apply sufficient cream to cover affected skin and surrounding areas.
- Do not use occlusive dressing unless specifically directed to do so.
- Store at 5°–30° C (41°–86° F).

ADVERSE EFFECTS (≥1%) **Skin:** Burning/stinging at application site, contact dermatitis, erythema, irritation, itching.

NURSING IMPLICATIONS

Assessment & Drug Effects

- Note: 2–4 wk of therapy are usually required for effective treatment.

Patient & Family Education

- Discontinue medication and notify physician if irritation or sensitivity develops.

- Avoid contact with mucous membranes.
- Wash hands thoroughly before and after application of cream.
- Do not breast feed while taking this drug without consulting physician.

BUTOCONAZOLE NITRATE

(byoo-toe-koe′na-zole)

Femstat 3, Femstat-One

Classifications: ANTIINFECTIVE; ANTIFUNGAL ANTIBIOTIC

Prototype: Fluconazole

Pregnancy Category: C

AVAILABILITY 2% cream

ACTIONS Imidazole derivative with antifungal activity. Alters fungal cell membrane permeability, permitting loss of phosphorous compounds, potassium, and other essential intracellular constituents with consequent loss of ability to replicate. Action takes place primarily on medicated infected surface tissues.

THERAPEUTIC EFFECTS Has fungicidal effect against *Candida, Trichophyton, Microsporum,* and *Epidermophyton* as well as some gram-positive bacteria.

USES Local treatment of vulvovaginal candidiasis.

CONTRAINDICATIONS First trimester of pregnancy (category C). Safety during lactation or in children is not established.

CAUTIOUS USE Second and third trimester of pregnancy.

ROUTE & DOSAGE

Vulvovaginal Candidiasis

Adult: **Topical** 1 applicator full intravaginally h.s. for 3 d, may be extended another 3 d if needed; *Pregnant women,* **Topical** 1 applicator full intravaginally h.s. for 6 d

ADMINISTRATION

Topical Intravaginal

- Continue treatment even during menstruation.
- Store medication at 15°–30° C (59°–86° F); avoid extreme temperature and freezing.

ADVERSE EFFECTS (≥1%) **Urogenital:** Vulvar or vaginal burning, vulvar itching, discharge, soreness, swelling; urinary frequency and burning. **Skin:** Itching of fingers. **CNS:** Headache.

PHARMACOKINETICS Absorption: Small amount absorbed systemically from intravaginal administration. **Distribution:** Crosses placenta in animals. **Metabolism:** Metabolized in liver. **Elimination:** Excreted in equal amounts in urine and feces within 4–7 d. **Half-Life:** 21–24 h.

NURSING IMPLICATIONS

Assessment & Drug Effects

- Monitor for therapeutic effectiveness. Candidiasis in nonpregnant women is usually controlled in 3 d.

Patient & Family Education

- Take medication exactly as prescribed; do not increase or decrease dosage or discontinue or extend treatment period. Contact physician if symptoms (vaginal burning, discharge, or itching) persist; drug may be discontinued if acute irritation occurs.
- Patient's sexual partner should wear a condom during intercourse.
- Do not breast feed while taking this drug without consulting physician.

BUTORPHANOL TARTRATE

(byoo-tor'fa-nole)

Stadol, Stadol NS

Classifications: CENTRAL NERVOUS SYSTEM AGENT; ANALGESIC; NARCOTIC (OPIATE) AGONIST-ANTAGONIST

Prototype: Pentazocine

Pregnancy Category: C

Controlled Substance: Schedule IV

AVAILABILITY 1 mg/mL, 2 mg/mL injection; 10 mg/mL spray

ACTIONS Synthetic, centrally acting analgesic with mixed narcotic agonist and antagonist actions. Acts as agonist on one type of opioid receptor and as a competitive antagonist at others. Site of analgesic action believed to be subcortical, possibly in the limbic system. On a weight basis, analgesic potency appears to be about 5 times that of morphine, 40 times that of meperidine, and 15–30 times that of pentazocine. Narcotic antagonist potential is approximately 30 times that of pentazocine and 1/40 that of naloxone. Respiratory depression does not increase appreciably with higher doses, as it does with morphine, but duration of action increases. Like pentazocine, analgesic doses may increase pulmonary arterial pressure and cardiac work load.

THERAPEUTIC EFFECTS Analgesic that relieves moderate to severe pain with apparently low potential for dependence.

USES Relief of moderate to severe pain, preoperative or preanesthetic sedation and analgesia, obstetrical analgesia during labor, cancer pain, renal colic, burns.

UNLABELED USES Musculoskeletal and postepisiotomy pain.

CONTRAINDICATIONS Narcotic-dependent patients. Safety during pregnancy prior to labor (category C), lactation, or in children <8 y is not established.

CAUTIOUS USE History of drug abuse or dependence; emotionally unstable individuals; head injury, increased intracranial pressure; acute MI, ventricular dysfunction, coronary insufficiency, hypertension; patients undergoing biliary tract surgery; respiratory depression, bronchial asthma, obstructive respiratory disease; and renal or hepatic dysfunction.

ROUTE & DOSAGE

Pain Relief

Adult: **IM** 1–4 mg q3–4h as needed (max: 4 mg/dose) **IV** 0.5–2 mg q3–4h as needed
Geriatric: **IM/IV** 0.5–2 mg q6–8h **Intranasal** 1 mg (1 spray) in one nostril, may repeat in 90 s, then may repeat these 2 doses q3–4h prn

ADMINISTRATION

Intranasal

- Give 1 spray into one nostril only. One spray provides a 1 mg dose.

Intramuscular

- Do not give more than 4 mg in a single IM dose.
- Give preoperative IM injection 60–90 min before surgery.

Intravenous

PREPARE: **Direct:** Give undiluted.
ADMINISTER: **Direct:** Give at a rate of 2 mg over 3–5 min.
INCOMPATIBILITIES **Solution/additive: Dimenhydrinate, pentobarbital. Y-site:** Pentobarbital.

- Store at 15°–30° C (59°–86° F) unless otherwise directed. Protect from light.

C

ADVERSE EFFECTS (≥1%) **CNS:** Drowsiness, *sedation,* headache, vertigo, dizziness, floating feeling, weakness, lethargy, confusion, light-headedness, insomnia, nervousness, respiratory depression. **CV:** Palpitation, bradycardia. **GI:** Nausea. **Skin:** Clammy skin, tingling sensation, flushing and warmth, cyanosis of extremities, diaphoresis, sensitivity to cold, urticaria, pruritus. **Genitourinary:** Difficulty in urinating, biliary spasm.

INTERACTIONS Drug: Alcohol and other CNS DEPRESSANTS augment CNS and respiratory depression.

PHARMACOKINETICS Onset: 10–30 min IM; 1 min IV. **Peak:** 0.5–1 h IM; 4–5 min IV. **Duration:** 3–4 h IM; 2–4 h IV. **Distribution:** Crosses placenta; distributed into breast milk. **Metabolism:** Metabolized in liver in inactive metabolites. **Elimination:** Excreted primarily in urine. **Half-Life:** 3–4 h.

NURSING IMPLICATIONS

Assessment & Drug Effects

- Monitor for respiratory depression. Do not administer drug if respiratory rate is <12 breaths/min.
- Monitor vital signs. Report marked changes in BP or bradycardia.
- Note: If used during labor or delivery, observe neonate for signs of respiratory depression.
- Note: Drug can induce acute withdrawal symptoms in opiate-dependent patients.
- Schedule gradual withdrawal following chronic administration. Abrupt withdrawal may produce vomiting, loss of appetite, restlessness, abdominal cramps, increase in BP and temperature, mydriasis, faintness. Withdrawal symptoms peak 48 h after discontinuation of drug.

Patient & Family Education

- Lie down to control drug-induced nausea.
- Do not take alcohol or other CNS depressants with this drug without consulting physician because of possible additive effects.
- Do not drive or engage in other potentially hazardous activities until response to drug is known.
- Do not breast feed while taking this drug without consulting physician.

CABERGOLINE

(ka-ber′go-leen)

Dostinex

Classifications: AUTONOMIC NERVOUS SYSTEM AGENT; ERGOT ALKALOID

Prototype: Ergotamine

Pregnancy Category: B

AVAILABILITY 0.5 mg tablets

ACTIONS Cabergoline is a synthetic ergot derivative, long-acting dopamine receptor agonist with a high affinity for D_2 receptors.

THERAPEUTIC EFFECTS Cabergoline inhibits both puerperal lactation and pathologic hyperprolactinemia.

USES Treatment of hyperprolactinemia (idiopathic or secondary to pituitary adenomas).

UNLABELED USES Treatment of Parkinson's disease.

CONTRAINDICATIONS Uncontrolled hypertension and hypersensitivity to ergot derivatives; pregnancy (category B), pregnancy-induced hypertension, lactation.

C

CAUTIOUS USE Hepatic function impairment. Safety and efficacy in pediatric patients are unknown.

ROUTE & DOSAGE

Hyperprolactinemia

Adult: **PO** Start with 0.25 mg 2 times/wk, may increase by 0.25 mg 2 times/wk to a max of 1 mg 2 times/wk

Parkinson's Disease

Adult: **PO** Start with 0.5 mg q.d., may increase up to 2.5 mg q.d. (max 5 mg/d)

ADMINISTRATION

Oral

- Give on same days each week.

ADVERSE EFFECTS (≥1%) **Body as a Whole:** Asthenia, fatigue, hot flashes. **CV:** Postural hypotension. **GI:** *Nausea, constipation,* abdominal pain, dyspepsia, vomiting, dry mouth, diarrhea, flatulence. **Endocrine:** Breast pain, dysmenorrhea. **CNS:** *Headache, dizziness,* paresthesia, somnolence, depression, nervousness.

INTERACTIONS Drug: Cabergoline should not be used concurrently with PHENOTHIAZINES, BUTYROPHENONES, THIOXANTHINES, and **metoclopramide** to avoid decreased therapeutic effects of both drugs.

PHARMACOKINETICS Absorption: Rapidly absorbed from GI tract, undergoes first-pass metabolism. **Peak:** 2–3 h. **Distribution:** 40–42% protein bound. Crosses placenta, will interfere with ability to lactate. **Metabolism:** Extensively metabolized. **Elimination:** Approximately 22% excreted in urine, 60% in feces. **Half-Life:** 63–69 h.

NURSING IMPLICATIONS

Assessment & Drug Effects

- Lab tests: Monitor serum prolactin levels to assess response to each dosing level.
- Monitor for hypotension, especially when given with other drugs known to lower BP.

Patient & Family Education

- Discontinue this drug once physician advises that serum prolactin level has been maintained for 6 mo.
- Do not breast feed while taking this drug.

CAFFEINE (Pr)

(kaf-een')

Caffedrine, Dexitac, NoDoz, Quick Pep, S-250, Tirend, Vivarin

CAFFEINE AND SODIUM BENZOATE

CITRATED CAFFEINE

Cafcit

Classifications: CENTRAL NERVOUS SYSTEM AGENT; RESPIRATORY AND CEREBRAL STIMULANT; XANTHINE

Pregnancy Category: C

AVAILABILITY 100 mg, 150 mg, 200 mg tablets; 250 mg/mL solution; 20 mg/mL caffeine citrate injection

ACTIONS Chief action is thought to be related to inhibition of the enzyme phosphodiesterase, which results in higher concentrations of cyclic AMP. Releases epinephrine and norepinephrine from adrenal medulla, producing CNS stimulation. Small doses improve psychic and sensory awareness and reduce

C

drowsiness and fatigue by stimulating cerebral cortex. Higher doses stimulate medullary, respiratory, vasomotor, and vagal centers. Produces smooth muscle relaxation (especially bronchi) and dilation of coronary, pulmonary, and systemic blood vessels by direct action on vascular musculature. Mild diuretic action may result from increase in renal blood flow and glomerular filtration rate and decrease in renal tubular reabsorption of sodium and water. Increases contractile force of heart and cardiac output by direct stimulation of myocardium. Also stimulates secretion of gastric acid and digestive enzymes.

THERAPEUTIC EFFECTS Effective in managing neonatal apnea, and as an adjuvant for pain control in headaches and following dural puncture. Relief of headache is perhaps due to mild cerebral vasoconstriction action and increased vascular tone. It acts as a bronchodilator in asthma and may improve psychomotor performance through CNS stimulation.

USES Orally as a mild CNS stimulant to aid in staying awake and restoring mental alertness, and as an adjunct in narcotic and nonnarcotic analgesia. Used parenterally as an emergency stimulant in acute circulatory failure, as a diuretic, and to relieve spinal puncture headache.

UNLABELED USES Topical treatment of atopic dermatitis; neonatal apnea.

CONTRAINDICATIONS Acute MI, symptomatic cardiac arrhythmias, palpitations; peptic ulcer; insomnia, panic attacks. Safe use during pregnancy (category C), in lactation, and in children not established.

CAUTIOUS USE Diabetes mellitus; hiatal hernia; hypertension with heart disease.

ROUTE & DOSAGE

Mental Stimulant

Adult: **PO** 100–200 mg q3–4h prn

Circulatory Stimulant

Adult: **IM** 200–500 mg prn

Spinal Puncture Headaches

Adult: **IV** 500 mg over 1 h, may repeat times 1 dose

Neonatal Apnea

Neonate: **PO/IV** 20–30 mg/kg caffeine citrate as a loading dose, followed by a maintenance dose 5 mg/kg citrate 24 h later of once daily up to max 10–12 d

ADMINISTRATION

Oral

- Give sustained-release oral preparations not less than 6 h before bedtime.
- Ensure that timed-release form of drug is not chewed or crushed. It must be swallowed whole.

Intramuscular

- Give deep IM into a large muscle.

Intravenous

- Note: IV route reserved for emergency situations only.

PREPARE: **Direct:** Give undiluted.

ADMINISTER: **Direct:** Emergency situations: IV push at a rate of 250 mg or fraction thereof over 1 min. With neonates use caffeine without sodium benzoate and check with physician regarding preferred rate.

ADVERSE EFFECTS (≥1%) **CV:** Tingling of face, flushing, palpitation, tachycardia or bradycardia, ventricular ectopic beats. **GI:** Nausea, vomiting; epigastric discomfort, gastric irritation (oral form), diarrhea, hematemesis, kernicterus (neonates). **CNS:** *Nervousness, insomnia,* restlessness, irritability, confusion, agitation, fasciculations, delirium, twitching, tremors, clonic convulsions. **Respiratory:** Tachypnea. **Special Senses:** Scintillating scotomas, tinnitus. **Urogenital:** Increased urination, diuresis.

DIAGNOSTIC TEST INTERFERENCE Caffeine reportedly may interfere with diagnosis of pheochromocytoma or neuroblastoma by increasing urinary excretion of ***catecholamines, VMA,*** and ***5-HIAA*** and may cause false positive increases in ***serum urate*** (by ***Bittner method***).

INTERACTIONS Drug: Increases effects of **cimetidine;** increases cardiovascular stimulating effects of BETA-ADRENERGIC AGONISTS; possibly increases **theophylline** toxicity.

PHARMACOKINETICS Absorption: Rapidly absorbed. **Peak:** 15–45 min. **Distribution:** Widely distributed throughout body; crosses blood-brain barrier and placenta. **Metabolism:** Metabolized in liver. **Elimination:** Excreted in urine as metabolites; excreted in breast milk in small amounts. **Half-Life:** 3–5 h in adults, 36–144 h in neonates.

NURSING IMPLICATIONS

Assessment & Drug Effects

- Monitor vital signs closely as large doses may cause intensification rather than reversal of severe drug-induced depressions.
- Observe children closely following administration as they are more susceptible than adults to the CNS effects of caffeine.
- Lab tests: Monitor blood glucose and HbA_{1c} levels in diabetics.

Patient & Family Education

- Caffeine in large amounts may impair glucose tolerance in diabetics.
- Do not consume large amounts of caffeine as headache, dizziness, anxiety, irritability, nervousness, and muscle tension may result from excessive use, as well as from abrupt withdrawal of coffee (or oral caffeine). Withdrawal symptoms usually occur 12–18 h following last coffee intake.

CALCIFEDIOL

(kal-si-fe-dye'ole)

Calderol

Classifications: HORMONE AND SYNTHETIC SUBSTITUTE; VITAMIN D ANALOG

Prototype: Calcitriol

Pregnancy Category: C

AVAILABILITY 20 mcg, 50 mcg capsules

ACTIONS Vitamin D analog and major transport form of cholecalciferol (D_3) Vitamin D analog is fat soluble. Because it is activated in the body and has regulatory effects, it is considered a hormone. Primary action leads to regulation of serum calcium, which is affected also by the activity of other vitamin D analogs (e.g., ergocalciferol), parathyroid hormone, and calcitonin. Pharmacologic effects of calcifediol are related to its intrinsic vitamin D activity as well as to the properties of active metabolites (e.g., calcitriol), which result from renal metabolism.

THERAPEUTIC EFFECTS Helps to maintain serum calcium in patients undergoing chronic renal dialysis and effective in renal osteodystrophy and promotes healing in hepatic osteomalacia.

USES Management of metabolic bone disease and hypocalcemia associated with chronic renal failure in patients undergoing renal dialysis.
UNLABELED USES Osteopenia caused by prolonged glucocorticoid therapy and osteomalacia secondary to hepatic disease.

CONTRAINDICATIONS Hypersensitivity to vitamin D, vitamin D toxicity, hypercalcemia. Safe use of doses in excess of RDA during pregnancy (category C), lactation, and children not established.
CAUTIOUS USE Patients receiving digitalis glycosides.

ROUTE & DOSAGE

Metabolic Bone Disease in Patients With Chronic Renal Failure
Adult: **PO** Initially 300–350 mcg/wk administered on a daily or alternate day schedule, may increase at 4-wk intervals if necessary; patients with normal calcium may only need 20 mcg q.o.d. (usual range 50–100 mcg/d or 100–200 mcg q.o.d.)

ADMINISTRATION

Oral
- Since calcitriol is a metabolite of vitamin D_3, all sources of vitamin D are usually withheld during therapy or at least must be considered when calculating dosage.

ADVERSE EFFECTS (≥1%) **Body as a Whole:** Muscle or bone pain, idiosyncratic reaction (headache, nausea, vomiting, diarrhea, fever). **GI:** Anorexia, nausea, vomiting, dry mouth, thirst, constipation, diarrhea, abdominal cramps, metallic taste. **Metabolic:** Vitamin D intoxication, hypercalcemia, polyuria, hypercalciuria, hyperphosphatemia. **CNS:** Lethargy, headache, weakness, vertigo.

INTERACTIONS Drug: THIAZIDE DIURETICS may cause hypercalcemia; may precipitate digitalis arrhythmias with **digoxin.**

PHARMACOKINETICS Absorption: Readily absorbed from small intestines. **Peak:** 4 h. **Duration:** 15–20 d. **Distribution:** Stored chiefly in liver and fat deposits. **Metabolism:** Activated in kidneys. **Elimination:** Excreted primarily in bile and feces. **Half-Life:** 12–22 d.

NURSING IMPLICATIONS

Assessment & Drug Effects
- Lab tests: Determine baseline and periodic values for serum calcium, phosphorus, magnesium, and alkaline phosphatase. Monitor serum calcium whenever dosage adjustments are made. Measure urinary calcium and phosphorus levels q24h.
- Effectiveness of therapy depends on an adequate daily intake of calcium. Since dietary calcium and phosphate are difficult to control, the physician may prescribe a calcium supplement as needed.
- Monitor for manifestations of hypercalcemia (see Appendix F). If hypercalcemia occurs, discontinue calcifediol until serum calcium returns to normal (9–10.6 mg/dL).
- Report a fall in serum alkaline phosphatase as this usually signals the onset of hypercalcemia.

Patient & Family Education
- Do not take this drug if experiencing S&S of hypercalcemia (see Appendix F), and report immediately to physician.
- Consult physician before taking an OTC medication. Calcium, phosphate, or magnesium-containing

laxatives and antacids, mineral oil, and vitamin D preparations may increase adverse effects of calcifediol and therefore should be avoided.

- Note: Patients undergoing dialysis may require aluminum carbonate or hydroxide gels to bind intestinal phosphate and thus lower serum phosphate levels.
- Do not breast feed while taking this drug.

CALCIPOTRIENE

(cal-ci′po-tri-een)
Dovonex

Classifications: SKIN AND MUCOUS MEMBRANE AGENT; VITAMIN D ANALOG
Prototype: Calcitriol
Pregnancy Category: C

AVAILABILITY 0.005% ointment and cream

ACTIONS Calcipotriene is a synthetic vitamin D_3 analog for the treatment of moderate plaque psoriasis. The scaly red patches of psoriasis are caused by abnormal growth and production of skin cells known as keratinocytes.

THERAPEUTIC EFFECTS Calcipotriene controls psoriasis by inhibiting proliferation of keratinocytes, reducing the number of polymorphonuclear leukocytes (PMNs) in the skin cells, and decreasing the number of epithelial cells.

USE Treatment of moderate plaque psoriasis.

CONTRAINDICATIONS Hypersensitivity to calcipotriene, hypercalcemia or vitamin D toxicity.

CAUTIOUS USE Dermatoses other than psoriasis; patients >65 y old; pregnancy (category C), lactation. Safety and efficacy in children not established.

ROUTE & DOSAGE

Adult: **Topical** Apply a thin layer to affected area once or twice daily

ADMINISTRATION

Topical

- A thin layer should be applied to the affected skin and rubbed in gently and completely.
- Calcipotriene should not be applied to the face.
- Wash hands before and after application of medication.

ADVERSE EFFECTS (≥1%) **Skin:** Facial dermatitis, burning, stinging, erythema, folliculitis, mild transient itching.

INTERACTIONS No clinically significant interactions established.

PHARMACOKINETICS Absorption: Approximately 6% absorbed systemically. **Onset:** 1 wk. **Peak:** 8 wk. **Duration:** 4 wk. **Metabolism:** Recycled via liver. **Elimination:** Excreted in bile.

NURSING IMPLICATIONS

Assessment & Drug Effects

- Observe reductions in scaling, erythema, and lesion thickness indicating a positive therapeutic response.
- Significant reduction in psoriatic lesions usually occurs following 1 wk of treatment. Marked improvement is generally noted by the 8th wk of treatment.
- Lab tests: Monitor periodically serum calcium, phosphate, and calcitriol levels, during long-term therapy.

C

Patient & Family Education

- Treatment with calcipotriene may be indefinite, as reappearance of psoriatic lesions is common following discontinuation of the drug.
- Adverse effects may include burning and stinging with drug application; these are usually transient.
- Do not mix calcipotriene with any other topical medicine.
- Report appearance of facial dermatitis (erythema and scaling around mouth and nose).
- Do not breast feed while taking this drug without consulting physician.

CALCITONIN (HUMAN)

(kal-si-toe′nin)

Cibacalcin

CALCITONIN (SALMON)

Calcimar, Miacalcin

Classifications: HORMONES AND SYNTHETIC SUBSTITUTES; BONE METABOLISM REGULATOR

Prototype: Etidronate

Pregnancy Category: C

AVAILABILITY 200 IU/mL injection; 200 IU/spray

ACTIONS Calcitonin human and calcitonin salmon are synthetic polypeptides. Pharmacologic actions are the same, but calcitonin salmon is considerably more potent and has a longer duration of action. Antibody formation occurs commonly with calcitonin salmon and only rarely with calcitonin human. Calcitonin opposes the effects of parathyroid hormone on bone and kidneys, reduces serum calcium by binding to a specific receptor site on osteoclast cell membrane, and alters transmembrane passage of calcium and phosphorus. Promotes renal excretion of calcium and phosphorus and causes transient sodium and water loss.

THERAPEUTIC EFFECTS Effective in osteoporosis due to inhibition of bone resorption. Effective in symptomatic hypercalcemia by rapidly lowering of serum calcium.

USES Symptomatic Paget's disease of bone (osteitis deformans), postmenopausal osteoporosis. Orphan drug approval (calcitonin human): short-term adjunctive treatment of severe hypercalcemic emergencies.

UNLABELED USES Diagnosis and management of medullary carcinoma of thyroid; treatment of osteogenesis imperfecta.

CONTRAINDICATIONS Hypersensitivity to fish proteins or to synthetic calcitonin; history of allergy. Safe use in children, pregnancy (category C), and lactation not established.

CAUTIOUS USE Renal impairment; osteoporosis; pernicious anemia; Zollinger-Ellison syndrome.

ROUTE & DOSAGE

Paget's Disease

Adult: **SC** Human 0.5 mg/d *or* 2–3 times/wk *or* 0.25 mg/d up to 0.5 mg b.i.d. **SC/IM** Salmon 100 IU/d, may decrease to 50–100 IU/d or q.o.d.

Hypercalcemia

Adult: **SC/IM** Salmon 4 IU/kg q12h, may increase to 8 U/kg q6h if needed

Postmenopausal Osteoporosis
Adult: **SC/IM** Salmon 100 IU/d **Intranasal** Miacalcin 1 spray (200 IU) daily, alternate nostrils

ADMINISTRATION

Allergy Test Dose
- An allergy skin test is usually done prior to initiation of therapy. The appearance of more than mild erythema or wheal 15 min after intracutaneous injection indicates that the drug should not be given.

Intranasal
- Activate the pump prior to first use; hold bottle upright and depress white side arms 6 times.
- The nasal spray is administered in one nostril daily; alternate nostrils.

Subcutaneous
- Calcitonin human is administered only by SC injection; calcitonin salmon may be administered by SC or IM injection.

Intramuscular
- Use IM route when the volume to be injected is >2 mL.
- Rotate injection sites.
- Store calcitonin (human) at 25° C (77° F) or less, protected from light, unless otherwise specified by manufacturer.
- Store calcitonin (salmon) in refrigerator, preferably at 2°–8° C (36°–46° F) unless otherwise directed.

ADVERSE EFFECTS (≥1%) **Body as a Whole:** Headache, eye pain, feverish sensation, hypersensitivity reactions, <u>anaphylaxis</u>. Reported for calcitonin human only: Urinary frequency, chills, chest pressure, weakness, paresthesias, tender palms and soles, dizziness, nasal congestion, shortness of breath. **GI:** *Transient nausea,* vomiting, anorexia, unusual taste sensation, abdominal pain, diarrhea. **Skin:** Inflammatory reactions at injection site, flushing of face or hands, pruritus of ear lobes, edema of feet, skin rashes. **Urogenital:** Nocturia, diuresis, abnormal urine sediment.

INTERACTIONS Drug: may decrease serum **lithium** levels.

PHARMACOKINETICS (salmon calcitonin). **Onset:** 15 min. **Peak:** 4 h. **Duration:** 8–24 h. **Distribution:** Does not cross placenta; distribution into breast milk unknown. **Metabolism:** Metabolized in kidneys. **Elimination:** Excreted in urine. **Half-Life:** 1.25 h (1 h for human calcitonin).

NURSING IMPLICATIONS

Assessment & Drug Effects
- Have on hand epinephrine 1:1000, antihistamines, and oxygen in the event of a reaction. Also have readily available parenteral calcium, particularly during early therapy. Hypocalcemic tetany is a theoretical possibility.
- Examine urine specimens periodically for sediment with long-term therapy.
- Lab tests: Monitor for hypocalcemia (see Signs & Symptoms, Appendix F). Theoretically, calcitonin can lead to hypocalcemic tetany. Latent tetany may be demonstrated by Chvostek's or Trousseau's signs and by serum calcium values: 7–8 mg/dL (latent tetany); below 7 mg/dL (manifest tetany).
- Examine nasal passages prior to treatment with the nasal spray and anytime nasal irritation occurs.
- Nasal ulceration or heavy bleeding are indications for drug discontinuation.

C

Patient & Family Education

- Use the SC route for self-administration.
- Watch for redness, warmth or swelling at injection site and report to physician, as these may indicate an inflammatory reaction. The transient flushing that commonly occurs following injection of calcitonin, particularly during early therapy, may be minimized by administrating the drug at bedtime. Consult physician.
- Maintain your drug regimen even though symptoms have been ameliorated to prevent early relapses.
- Ensure that you feel comfortable using the nasal pump properly. Notify physician if significant nasal irritation occurs.
- Consult physician before using OTC preparations. Some supervitamins, hematinics, and antacids contain calcium and vitamin D (vitamin may antagonize calcitonin effects).

CALCITRIOL (Pr)

(kal-si-trye′ole)

Calcijex, Rocaltrol

Classifications: HORMONES AND SYNTHETIC SUBSTITUTES; VITAMIN D ANALOG

Pregnancy Category: C

AVAILABILITY 0.25 mcg, 0.5 mcg tablets; 1 mcg/mL oral solution; 1 mcg/mL, 2 mcg/mL injection

ACTIONS Synthetic form of an active metabolite of ergocalciferol (vitamin D_2). In the liver, cholecalciferol (vitamin D_3) and ergocalciferol (vitamin D_2) are enzymatically metabolized to calcifediol, an activated form of vitamin D_3. Calcifediol is biodegraded in the kidney to calcitriol, the most potent form of vitamin D_3. Patients with nonfunctioning kidneys are unable to synthesize sufficient calcitriol and therefore must receive it pharmacologically.

THERAPEUTIC EFFECTS By promoting intestinal absorption and renal retention of calcium, calcitriol elevates serum calcium levels, decreases elevated blood levels of phosphate and parathyroid hormone, and decreases subperiosteal bone resorption and mineralization defects in some patients.

USES Management of hypocalcemia in patients undergoing chronic renal dialysis and in patients with hypoparathyroidism or pseudohypoparathyroidism.

UNLABELED USES Selected patients with vitamin D-dependent rickets, familial hypophosphatemia (vitamin D-resistant rickets); management of hypocalcemia in premature infants.

CONTRAINDICATIONS Hypercalcemia or vitamin D toxicity; pregnancy (category C), lactation. Safe use in children not established.

CAUTIOUS USE Hyperphosphatemia, patients receiving digitalis glycosides.

ROUTE & DOSAGE

Hypocalcemia

Adult: **PO** 0.25 mcg/d, may be increased by 0.25 mcg/d q4–8wk for dialysis patients or q2–4wk for hypoparathyroid patients if necessary. **IV** 0.5 mcg 3 times/wk at the end of dialysis, may need up to 3 mcg 3 times/wk

Child: **PO** On hemodialysis: 0.25–2 mcg/d. **IV** 0.01–0.05 mcg/kg 3 times/wk
Renal failure without dialysis: **PO** 0.014–0.041 mcg/kg/d

ADMINISTRATION

Oral

- Oral dose can be taken either with food or milk or on an empty stomach. Discuss with physician.
- When given for hypoparathyroidism, the dose is given in the morning.
- Capsules should be protected from heat, light, and moisture. Store in tightly closed container.

Intravenous

PREPARE: **Direct:** Give undiluted.
ADMINISTER: **Direct:** Give IV push over 30–60 s.

ADVERSE EFFECTS (≥1%) **Body as a Whole:** Muscle or bone pain. **CV:** Palpitation. **GI:** Anorexia, nausea, vomiting, dry mouth, thirst, constipation, abdominal cramps, metallic taste. **Metabolic:** Vitamin D intoxication, hypercalcemia, hypercalciuria, hyperphosphatemia. **CNS:** Headache, weakness. **Special Senses:** Blurred vision, photophobia. **Urogenital:** Increased urination.

INTERACTIONS Drug: THIAZIDE DIURETICS may cause hypercalcemia; calcifediol-induced hypercalcemia may precipitate digitalis arrhythmias in patients receiving DIGITALIS GLYCOSIDES.

PHARMACOKINETICS Absorption: Readily absorbed from GI tract. **Onset:** 2–6 h. **Peak:** 10–12 h. **Duration:** 3–5 d. **Metabolism:** Metabolized in liver. **Elimination:** Excreted mainly in feces. **Half-Life:** 3–6 h.

NURSING IMPLICATIONS

Assessment & Drug Effects

- Lab tests: Determine baseline and periodic levels of serum calcium, phosphorus, magnesium, alkaline phosphatase, creatinine; measure urinary calcium and phosphorus levels q24h.
- Effectiveness of therapy depends on an adequate daily intake of calcium and phosphate. The physician may prescribe a calcium supplement on an as-needed basis.
- Monitor for hypercalcemia (see Signs & Symptoms, Appendix F). During dosage adjustment period, monitor serum calcium levels particularly twice weekly to avoid hypercalcemia.
- If hypercalcemia develops, withhold calcitriol and calcium supplements and notify physician. Drugs may be reinitiated when serum calcium returns to normal.

Patient & Family Education

- Discontinue the drug if experiencing any symptoms of hypercalcemia (see Appendix F) and contact physician.
- Do not use any other source of vitamin D during therapy, since calcitriol is the most potent form of vitamin D_3. This will avoid the possibility of hypercalcemia.
- Consult physician before taking an OTC medication. (Many products contain calcium, vitamin D, phosphates, or magnesium, which can increase adverse effects of calcitriol.)
- Maintain an adequate daily fluid intake unless you have kidney problems, in which case consult your physician about fluids.
- Do not breast feed while taking this drug.

C

CALCIUM CARBONATE
Apo-Cal ✦, BioCal, Calcite-500, Calsan ✦, Cal-Sup, Caltrate ✦, Chooz, Dicarbosil, Equilet, Mallamint, Mega-Cal, Nu-Cal, Os-Cal, Oystercal, Titralac, Tums

CALCIUM ACETATE
PhosLo

CALCIUM CITRATE
Citracal

CALCIUM PHOSPHATE TRIBASIC (TRICALCIUM PHOSPHATE)
Posture

Classifications: FLUID AND ELECTROLYTIC BALANCE AGENT; REPLACEMENT SOLUTION; ANTACID
Prototype: Calcium gluconate
Pregnancy Category: C for calcium acetate; other salts not rated

AVAILABILITY **Calcium carbonate:** 125 mg, 250 mg, 650 mg, 750 mg, 1.25 g, 1.5 g tablets **Calcium acetate:** 667 mg tablets **Calcium citrate:** 950 mg, 2376 mg tablets **Calcium phosphate tribasic:** 1565.2 mg tablets

ACTIONS Rapid-acting antacid with high neutralizing capacity and relatively prolonged duration of action. Decreases gastric acidity, thereby inhibiting proteolytic action of pepsin on gastric mucosa. Also increases lower esophageal sphincter tone. Although classified as a nonsystemic antacid, a slight to moderate alkalosis usually develops with prolonged therapy. Acid rebound, which may follow even low doses, is thought to be caused by release of gastrin triggered by action of calcium in small intestines.

THERAPEUTIC EFFECTS Effectively relieves symptoms of acid indigestion and useful as a calcium supplement.

USES Relief of transient symptoms of hyperacidity as in acid indigestion, heartburn, peptic esophagitis, and hiatal hernia. Also used as calcium supplement when calcium intake may be inadequate and in treatment of mild calcium deficiency states. Control of hyperphosphatemia in chronic renal failure (calcium acetate).
UNLABELED USES For treatment of hyperphosphatemia in patients with chronic renal failure and to lower BP in selected patients with hypertension.

CONTRAINDICATIONS Hypercalcemia and hypercalciuria (e.g., hyperparathyroidism, vitamin D overdosage, decalcifying tumors, bone metastases), calcium loss due to immobilization, severe renal disease, renal calculi, GI hemorrhage or obstruction, dehydration, hypochloremic alkalosis, ventricular fibrillation, cardiac disease, pregnancy (category C).
CAUTIOUS USE Decreased bowel motility (e.g., with anticholinergics, antidiarrheals, antispasmodics), the older adult, lactation.

ROUTE & DOSAGE

All doses are in terms of *elemental calcium:* 1 g calcium carbonate = 400 mg (20 mEq, 40%) elemental calcium; 1 g calcium acetate = 250 mg (12.6 mEq, 25%) elemental calcium; 1 g calcium citrate = 210 mg (12 mEq, 21%) elemental calcium; 1g tricalcium phosphate = 390 mg (19.3 mEq, 39%) elemental calcium

Supplement for Osteoporosis
Adult: **PO** 1–2 g b.i.d. or t.i.d.
Antacid
Adult: **PO** 0.5–2 g 4–6 times/d
Hyperphosphatemia
Adult: **PO** calcium acetate 2–4 tablets with each meal

ADMINISTRATION

Oral

- When used as antacid, give 1 h after meals and at bedtime. When used as calcium supplement, give 1–1 1/2 h after meals, unless otherwise directed by physician.
- Chewable tablet should be chewed well before swallowing or allowed to dissolve completely in mouth, followed with water. Powder form may be mixed with water.
- Ensure that sustained-release form of drug is not chewed or crushed. It must be swallowed whole.

ADVERSE EFFECTS (≥1%) **GI:** *Constipation* or laxative effect, acid rebound, nausea, eructation, *flatulence,* vomiting, fecal concretions. **Metabolic:** Hypercalcemia with alkalosis, metastatic calcinosis, hypercalciuria, hypomagnesemia, hypophosphatemia (when phosphate intake is low). **CNS:** Mood and mental changes. **Urogenital:** Polyuria, renal calculi.

INTERACTIONS Drug: May enhance inotropic and toxic effects of **digoxin; magnesium** may compete for GI absorption; decreases absorption of TETRACYCLINES, QUINOLONES **(ciprofloxacin).**

PHARMACOKINETICS Absorption: Approximately 1/3 of dose absorbed from small intestine. **Distribution:** Crosses placenta. **Elimination:** Primarily excreted in feces; small amounts excreted in urine, pancreatic juice, saliva, breast milk.

NURSING IMPLICATIONS

Assessment & Drug Effects

- Note number and consistency of stools. If constipation is a problem, physician may prescribe alternate or combination therapy with a magnesium antacid or advise patient to take a laxative or stool softener as necessary.
- Lab tests: Determine serum and urine calcium weekly in patients receiving prolonged therapy and in patients with renal dysfunction.
- Record amelioration of symptoms of hypocalcemia (see Signs & Symptoms, Appendix F).
- Observe for S&S of hypercalcemia in patients receiving frequent or high doses, or who have impaired renal function (see Appendix F).

Patient & Family Education

- Do not continue this medication beyond 1–2 wk, since it may cause acid rebound, which generally occurs after repeated use for 1 or 2 wk and leads to chronic use. It is potentially dangerous to self-medicate. Do not take antacids longer than 2 wk without medical supervision.
- Avoid taking calcium carbonate with cereals or other foods high in oxalates. Oxalates combine with calcium carbonate to form insoluble, nonabsorbable compounds.
- Do not use calcium carbonate repeatedly with foods high in vitamin D (such as milk) or sodium bicarbonate, as it may cause milk-alkali syndrome: hypercalcemia, distaste for food, headache, confusion, nausea, vomiting, abdominal pain, metabolic alkalosis,

C

hypercalciuria, polyuria, soft tissue calcification (calcinosis), hyperphosphatemia and renal insufficiency. Predisposing factors include renal dysfunction, dehydration, electrolyte imbalance, and hypertension.

- Do not breast feed while taking this drug without consulting physician.

CALCIUM CHLORIDE

Calciject, Calcitrans, Solucalcine

Classifications: FLUID AND ELECTROLYTIC BALANCE AGENT; REPLACEMENT SOLUTION

Prototype: Calcium gluconate

Pregnancy Category: C

AVAILABILITY 10% injection

ACTIONS Actions similar to those of calcium gluconate. Ionizes more readily and thus is more potent than calcium gluconate and more irritating to tissues. Provides excess chloride ions that promote acidosis and temporary (1–2 d) diuresis secondary to excretion of sodium.

THERAPEUTIC EFFECTS Rapidly and effectively restores serum calcium levels in acute hypocalcemia of various origins and an effective cardiac stabilizer under conditions of hyperkalemia or resuscitation.

USES Treatment of cardiac resuscitation when epinephrine fails to improve myocardial contractions; for treatment of acute hypocalcemia (as in tetany due to parathyroid deficiency, vitamin D deficiency, alkalosis, insect bites or stings, and during exchange transfusions), for treatment of hypermagnesemia, and for cardiac disturbances of hyperkalemia.

CONTRAINDICATIONS Ventricular fibrillation, hypercalcemia, digitalis toxicity, injection into myocardium or other tissue; pregnancy (category C).

CAUTIOUS USE Digitalized patients; sarcoidosis, renal insufficiency, history of renal stone formation; cor pulmonale, respiratory acidosis, respiratory failure; lactation.

ROUTE & DOSAGE

All doses are in terms of *elemental calcium:* 1 g calcium chloride = 272 mg (13.6 mEq) elemental calcium

Hypocalcemia

Adult: **IV** 0.5–1 g (7–14 mEq) at 1–3 d intervals as determined by patient response and serum calcium levels
Child: **IV** 25 mg/kg (1–7 mEq) administered slowly
Neonate: **IV** <1 mEq/d

Hypocalcemic Tetany

Adult: **IV** 4.5–16 mEq prn
Child: **IV** 0.5–0.7 mEq/kg t.i.d. or q.i.d.
Neonate: **IV** 2.4 mEq/kg/d in divided doses

CPR

Adult: **IV** 2.7–3.7 mEq × 1
Child: **IV** 20 mg/kg, may repeat in 10 min

ADMINISTRATION

Intravenous

- IV administration to neonates, infants, and children: Verify correct IV concentration and rate of infusion with physician.

PREPARE: **Direct:** May be given undiluted or diluted (preferred) with an equal volume of NS for injection. Solution should be warmed to body temperature before administration.

ADMINISTER: **Direct:** Give at 0.5–1 mL/min or more slowly if irritation develops. Avoid rapid administration. Use a small-bore needle and inject into a large vein to minimize venous irritation and undesirable reactions

INCOMPATIBILITIES **Solution/additive: Amphotericin B, chlopheniramine, dobutamine. Y-site: Amphotericin B cholesteryl complex, propofol, sodium bicarbonate**

ADVERSE EFFECTS (≥1%) **Body as a Whole:** Tingling sensation. With rapid IV, sensations of heat waves (peripheral vasodilation), fainting, **CV:** (With rapid infusion) hypotension, bradycardia, cardiac arrhythmias, <u>cardiac arrest</u>. **Skin:** Pain and burning at IV site, severe venous thrombosis, necrosis and sloughing (with extravasation).

INTERACTIONS Drug: May enhance inotropic and toxic effects of **digoxin;** antagonizes the effects of **verapamil** and possibly other CALCIUM CHANNEL BLOCKERS.

PHARMACOKINETICS Distribution: Crosses placenta. **Elimination:** Primarily excreted in feces; small amounts excreted in urine, pancreatic juice, saliva, and breast milk.

NURSING IMPLICATIONS

Assessment & Drug Effects

- Monitor ECG and BP and observe patient closely during administration. IV injection may be accompanied by cutaneous burning sensation and peripheral vasodilation, with moderate fall in BP.
- Advise ambulatory patient to remain in bed for 15–30 min or more depending on response following injection.
- Observe digitalized patients closely since an increase in serum calcium increases risk of digitalis toxicity.
- Lab tests: Determine serum pH, calcium, and other electrolytes frequently as guides to dosage adjustments.

Patient & Family Education

- Remain in bed for 15–30 min or more following injection and depending on response.
- Symptoms of mild hypercalcemia, such as loss of appetite, nausea, vomiting, or constipation may occur. If hypercalcemia becomes severe, call health care provider if feeling confused or extremely excited.
- Do not use other calcium supplements or eat foods high in calcium, like milk, cheese, yogurt, eggs, meats, and some cereals, during therapy.
- Do not breast feed while taking this drug without consulting physician.

CALCIUM GLUCEPTATE

(gloo-sep'tate)

Calcium Glucoheptonate, Glucalcium, Calcitrans

Classifications: FLUID AND ELECTROLYTIC BALANCE AGENT; REPLACEMENT SOLUTION

Prototype: Calcium gluconate

Pregnancy Category: C

AVAILABILITY 1.1 g/5 mL injection

ACTIONS Calcium is an essential element for regulating the excitation threshold of nerves and muscles, blood clotting mechanisms, cardiac function, maintenance of renal function, and body skeleton and teeth. Also plays a role in regulating neurotransmitters and hormones, and functional integrity of cell membranes and capillaries. Calcium gluceptate acts like digitalis on the heart, increasing cardiac muscle tone and force of systolic contractions (positive inotropic effect).

THERAPEUTIC EFFECTS Preferred for use when IM administration is required as in neonatal tetany. Rapidly and effectively restores serum calcium levels in acute hypocalcemia of various origins and an effective cardiac stabilizer under conditions of hyperkalemia or resuscitation.

USES To correct hypocalcemia and following each 100 mL of exchange transfusion in newborns.

CONTRAINDICATIONS Ventricular fibrillation, hypercalcemia, digitalis toxicity, injection into myocardium or other tissue; pregnancy (category C).

CAUTIOUS USE Digitalized patients; sarcoidosis, renal insufficiency, history of renal stone formation; cor pulmonale, respiratory acidosis, respiratory failure; lactation.

ROUTE & DOSAGE

All doses are in terms of *elemental calcium:* 1 g calcium gluceptate = 82 mg (4.1 mEq) elemental calcium

Hypocalcemia

Adult: **IV** 1.1–4.4 g/d. **IM** 0.5–1.1 g.d. in 2–5 mL (220 mg/mL)
Child: **IV** 200–500 mg/kg/d divided q6h. **IM** 0.5–1.1 g/d in 2–5 mL (220 mg/mL)

Exchange Transfusions with Citrated Blood

Neonate: **IV** 0.5 mL after each 100 mL of blood exchanged

ADMINISTRATION

Intramuscular

- IM injection may produce mild local reactions. Generally, this route is used only in adults when IV administration is not feasible.
- Recommended IM site for adults is the upper outer quadrant of the buttock and in infants (if prescribed) the midlateral thigh.

Intravenous

PREPARE: **Direct:** May be given undiluted. Solution should be warmed to body temperature before administration.

ADMINISTER: **Direct:** Give at a rate not to exceed 1 mL/min or more slowly if irritation develops. Avoid rapid administration.

- Patient may complain of a transient tingling sensation and metallic taste following IV administration.

ADVERSE EFFECTS (≥1%) **Body as a Whole:** Tingling sensation. With rapid IV, sensations of heat waves (peripheral vasodilation), fainting, **CV:** (With rapid infusion) hypotension, bradycardia, cardiac arrhythmias, <u>cardiac arrest</u>, **Skin:** Pain and burning at IV site, severe venous thrombosis, necrosis and sloughing (with extravasation).

INTERACTIONS Drug: May enhance inotropic and toxic effects of **digoxin;** antagonizes the effects of **verapamil** and possibly other CALCIUM CHANNEL BLOCKERS.

PHARMACOKINETICS Duration: 2–3 h IV; 1–4 h IM. **Distribution:** Crosses placenta. **Elimination:** Primarily excreted in feces; small amounts excreted in urine, pancreatic juice, saliva, and breast milk.

NURSING IMPLICATIONS

See calcium gluconate for additional **NURSING IMPLICATIONS.**

CALCIUM GLUCONATE Pr

(gloo'koe-nate)

Kalcinate

Classifications: FLUID AND ELECTROLYTIC AND WATER BALANCE AGENT; REPLACEMENT SOLUTION

Pregnancy Category: B

AVAILABILITY 500 mg, 650 mg, 975 mg, 1 gm tablets; 10% injection

ACTIONS Calcium is an essential element for regulating the excitation threshold of nerves and muscles, for blood clotting mechanisms, cardiac function (rhythm, tonicity, contractility), maintenance of renal function, for body skeleton and teeth. Also plays a role in regulating storage and release of neurotransmitters and hormones; regulating amino acid uptake and absorption of vitamin B_{12}, gastrin secretion, and in maintaining structural and functional integrity of cell membranes and capillaries. Calcium gluconate acts like digitalis on the heart, increasing cardiac muscle tone and force of systolic contractions (positive inotropic effect).

THERAPEUTIC EFFECTS Rapidly and effectively restores serum calcium levels in acute hypocalcemia of various origins and effective cardiac stabilizer under conditions of hyperkalemia or resuscitation.

USES Negative calcium balance (as in neonatal tetany, hypoparathyroidism, vitamin D deficiency, alkalosis). Also to overcome cardiac toxicity of hyperkalemia, for cardiopulmonary resuscitation, to prevent hypocalcemia during transfusion of citrated blood. Also as antidote for magnesium sulfate, for acute symptoms of lead colic, to decrease capillary permeability in sensitivity reactions, and to relieve muscle cramps from insect bites or stings. Oral calcium may be used to maintain normal calcium balance during pregnancy, lactation, and childhood growth and to prevent primary osteoporosis. Also in osteoporosis, osteomalacia, chronic hypoparathyroidism, rickets, and as adjunct in treatment of myasthenia gravis and Eaton-Lambert syndrome.

UNLABELED USES To antagonize aminoglycoside-induced neuromuscular blockage, and as "calcium challenge" to diagnose Zollinger-Ellison syndrome and medullary thyroid carcinoma.

CONTRAINDICATIONS Ventricular fibrillation, metastatic bone disease, injection into myocardium; administration by SC or IM routes; renal calculi, hypercalcemia, predisposition to hypercalcemia (hyperparathyroidism, certain malignancies); pregnancy (category B).

CAUTIOUS USE Digitalized patients, renal or cardiac insufficiency, sarcoidosis, history of lithiasis, immobilized patients; lactation.

ROUTE & DOSAGE

All doses are in terms of *elemental calcium:* 1 g calcium gluconate = 90 mg (4.5 mEq, 9.3%) elemental calcium

Supplement for Osteoporosis

Adult: **PO** 1–2 g b.i.d. to q.i.d. **IV** 7 mEq q 1–3d

Child: **PO** 45–65 mg/kg/d in divided doses. **IV** 1–7 mEq q1–3d

C

Neonate: **PO** 50–130 mg/kg/d (max: 1 g). **IV** mEq q1–3d

Hypocalcemic Tetany

Adult: **IV** 4.5–16 mEq prn
Child: **IV** 0.5–0.7 mEq/kg t.i.d. or q.i.d.
Neonate: **IV** 2.4 mEq/kg/d in divided doses

CPR

Adult: **IV** 2.3–3.7 mEq x 1

Hyperkalemia with Cardiac Toxicity

Adult: **IV** 2.25–14 mEq q 1–2 min

Exchange Transfusions with Citrated Blood

Adult: **IV** 1.35 mEq for each 100 mL of blood
Neonate: **IV** 0.45 mEq for each 100 mL of blood

ADMINISTRATION

Oral

- Ensure that chewable tablets are chewed or crushed before being swallowed with a liquid.
- Give with meals to enhance absorption.

Intravenous

PREPARE: **Direct:** May be given undiluted **Intermittent/Continuous:** May be diluted in 1000 mL of NS.

ADMINISTER: **Direct:** Give direct IV at a rate of 0.5 mL or a fraction thereof over 1 min. Do not exceed 2 mL/min. **Intermittent/Continuous:** Give slowly, not to exceed 200 mg/min, through a small-bore needle into a large vein to avoid possibility of extravasation and resultant necrosis. With children, scalp veins should be avoided. Avoid rapid infusion. High concentrations of calcium suddenly reaching the heart can cause fatal cardiac arrest.

INCOMPATIBILITIES **Solution/additive: Amphotericin B, cefamandole, dobutamine, methylprednisolone, metoclopramide. Y-site: Amphotericin B cholesteryl complex, fluconazole, indomethacin.**

- Injection should be stopped if patient complains of any discomfort. ■ Patient should be advised to remain in bed for 15–30 min or more following injection, depending on response.

ADVERSE EFFECTS (≥1%) **Body as a Whole:** Tingling sensation. With rapid IV, sensations of heat waves (peripheral vasodilation), fainting. **GI:** PO preparation: Constipation, increased gastric acid secretion. **CV:** (With rapid infusion) hypotension, bradycardia, cardiac arrhythmias, <u>cardiac arrest</u>, **Skin:** Pain and burning at IV site, severe venous thrombosis, necrosis and sloughing (with extravasation).

DIAGNOSTIC TEST INTERFERENCE IV calcium may cause false decreases in ***serum and urine magnesium*** (by ***Titan yellow method***) and transient elevations of ***plasma 11-OHCS*** levels by ***Glenn-Nelson technique.*** Values usually return to control levels after 60 min; ***urinary steroid values (17-OHCS)*** may be decreased.

INTERACTIONS Drug: May enhance inotropic and toxic effects of **digoxin; magnesium** may compete for GI absorption; decreases absorption of TETRACYCLINES, QUINOLONES (**ciprofloxacin**); antagonizes the effects of **verapamil** and possibly other CALCIUM CHANNEL BLOCKERS (IV administration).

PHARMACOKINETICS Absorption: Approximately 1/3 of dose absorbed from small intestine. **Onset:** Immediately after IV. **Distribution:** Crosses placenta. **Elimination:** Primarily excreted in feces; small amounts excreted in urine, pancreatic juice, saliva, and breast milk.

NURSING IMPLICATIONS

Assessment & Drug Effects

- Assess for cutaneous burning sensations and peripheral vasodilation, with moderate fall in BP, during direct IV injection.
- Monitor ECG during IV administration to detect evidence of hypercalcemia: decreased QT interval associated with inverted T wave.
- Observe IV site closely. Extravasation may result in tissue irritation and necrosis.
- Monitor for hypocalcemia and hypercalcemia (see Signs & Symptoms, Appendix F).
- Lab tests: Determine levels of calcium and phosphorus (tend to vary inversely) and magnesium frequently, during sustained therapy. Deficiencies in other ions, particularly magnesium, frequently coexist with calcium ion depletion.

Patient & Family Education

- Report S&S of hypercalcemia (see Appendix F) promptly to your care provider.
- Milk and milk products are the best sources of calcium (and phosphorus). Other good sources include dark green vegetables, soy beans, tofu, and canned fish with bones.
- Calcium absorption can be inhibited by zinc-rich foods: nuts, seeds, sprouts, legumes, soy products (tofu).
- Check with physician before self-medicating with a calcium supplement.
- Do not breast feed while taking this drug without consulting physician.

C

CALCIUM LACTATE

(lak'tate)

Cal-Lac, Calcimax, Calcium Unison, Ridactate

Classifications: FLUID AND ELECTROLYTIC BALANCE AGENT; REPLACEMENT SOLUTION

Prototype: Calcium gluconate

Pregnancy Category: B

AVAILABILITY 325 mg, 650 mg tablets

ACTIONS Oral calcium preparation reportedly well tolerated. Calcium is an essential element for regulating the excitation threshold of nerves and muscles, for blood clotting mechanisms, cardiac function, maintenance of renal function, for body skeleton and teeth. Also plays a role in regulating storage and release of neurotransmitters and hormones, and in maintaining structural and functional integrity of cell membranes and capillaries. It increases cardiac muscle tone and force of systolic contractions (positive inotropic effect).

THERAPEUTIC EFFECTS Rapidly and effectively restores serum calcium levels in mild hypocalcemia of various origins and effective for calcium maintenance therapy.

USES Mild hypocalcemia and maintenance calcium therapy.

CONTRAINDICATIONS Ventricular fibrillation, metastatic bone disease, injection into myocardium; administration by SC or IM routes; renal cal-

C

culi, hypercalcemia, predisposition to hypercalcemia (hyperparathyroidism, certain malignancies); pregnancy (category B).

CAUTIOUS USE Digitalized patients, renal or cardiac insufficiency, sarcoidosis, history of lithiasis, immobilized patients; lactation.

ROUTE & DOSAGE

All doses are in terms of *elemental calcium:* 1 g calcium lactate = 130 mg (6.5 mEq, 13%) elemental calcium

Supplement for Mild Hypocalcemia

Adult: **PO** 325 mg–1.3 g t.i.d. with meals
Child: **PO** 500 mg/kg/d in divided doses

ADMINISTRATION

Oral

- Tablets or powder can be dissolved in hot water (if patient unable to swallow whole), then add cool water to make palatable.
- Calcium lactate may be administered with lactose (amount prescribed) to increase solubility.

ADVERSE EFFECTS (≥1%) **GI:** *Constipation* or laxative effect, acid rebound, nausea, eructation, *flatulence,* vomiting, fecal concretions. **Metabolic:** Hypercalcemia with alkalosis, metastatic calcinosis, hypercalciuria, hypomagnesemia, hypophosphatemia (when phosphate intake is low). **CNS:** Mood and mental changes, **Urogenital:** Polyuria, renal calculi.

INTERACTIONS Drug: May enhance inotropic and toxic effects of **digoxin; magnesium** may compete for GI absorption; decreases absorption of TETRACYCLINES, QUINOLONES (**ciprofloxacin**).

PHARMACOKINETICS Absorption: Approximately 1/3 of dose absorbed from small intestine. **Distribution:** Crosses placenta. **Elimination:** Primarily excreted in feces; small amounts excreted in urine, pancreatic juice, saliva, and breast milk.

NURSING IMPLICATIONS

Assessment & Drug Effects

- Monitor for hypercalcemia (see Signs & Symptoms, Appendix F).
- Lab tests: Check serum calcium levels periodically. Hypercalcemia can occur during prolonged administration particularly if patient is also taking vitamin D.
- Monitor increases in serum calcium in digitalized patients as this increases risk of digitalis toxicity.

Patient & Family Education

- Confer with physician regarding need for vitamin D supplementation.
- Calcium absorption can be inhibited by zinc-rich foods such as nuts, sprouts, legumes, and soy products.
- Do not breast feed while taking this drug without consulting physician.

CALCIUM POLYCARBOPHIL

(pol-ee-kar'boe-fil)

FiberCon, Mitrolan

Classifications: GASTROINTESTINAL AGENT; BULK LAXATIVE; ANTIDIARRHEAL

Prototype: Psyllium hydrophilic muciloid

Pregnancy Category: C

AVAILABILITY 500 mg, 625 mg, tablets

C

ACTIONS Hydrophilic, bulk-producing laxative that restores normal moisture level and bulk content of intestinal tract. In constipation, retains free water in intestinal lumen, thereby indirectly opposing dehydrating forces of the bowel; in diarrhea, when intestinal mucosa is incapable of absorbing fluid, drug absorbs fecal fluid to form a gel. In both conditions, peristalsis is encouraged and a well-formed stool is produced.

THERAPEUTIC EFFECTS Relieves constipation or diarrhea associated with bowel disorders and acute nonspecific diarrhea.

USES Constipation or diarrhea associated with diverticulitis or irritable bowel syndrome; acute nonspecific diarrhea.

CONTRAINDICATIONS GI obstruction; children <6 y.

CAUTIOUS USE Pregnancy (category C); lactation.

ROUTE & DOSAGE

Constipation or Diarrhea
Adult: **PO** 1 g q.i.d. as needed (max: 6 g/24 h)
Child: **PO** *6–12 y,* 500 mg 1–3 times/d (max: 3 g/24 h); *<6 y,* 500 mg 1–2 times/d (max: 1.5 g/24 h)

ADMINISTRATION

Oral

- Administer with at least 180–240 mL (6–8 oz) water or other fluid of patient's choice when used as a laxative and with at least 60–90 mL (2–3 oz) of fluid when used as an antidiarrheal. Chewed tablets should not be swallowed dry.
- If diarrhea is severe, dose can be repeated every half hour up to maximum daily dose.

ADVERSE EFFECTS (≥1%) **GI:** *Flatulence,* abdominal fullness, intestinal obstruction; laxative dependence (long-term use).

PHARMACOKINETICS Absorption: Calcium polycarbophil is not absorbed from the intestine. Bowel movement usually occurs within 12–72 hrs. **Elimination:** Excreted in feces.

NURSING IMPLICATIONS

Assessment & Drug Effects

- Evaluate effectiveness of medication. If it is ineffective as an antidiarrheal, report to physician.
- Report rectal bleeding, very dark stools, or abdominal pain promptly.

Patient & Family Education

- You will likely have a bowel movement within 12–72 h.
- This is an OTC product. Take this drug exactly as ordered. Do not increase the dose if response is inadequate. Consult physician. Do not use other laxatives while you are taking calcium polycarbophil.
- Do not breast feed while taking this drug without consulting physician.

CALFACTANT

(cal-fac'tant)
Infasurf
Classification: LUNG SURFACTANT
Prototype: Beractant
Pregnancy Category: Not applicable

AVAILABILITY 35 mg/mL suspension

ACTIONS Pulmonary surfactant. Lowers the surface tension on alveolar surfaces during respiration and stabilizes the alveoli against

C

collapse at resting pressure. Deficiency of surfactant causes respiratory disease syndrome (RDS) in premature infants.

THERAPEUTIC EFFECTS Effectively relieves and prevents RDS in neonates.

USES Prevention and treatment of RDS in infants at high risk for RDS.

CONTRAINDICATIONS Nosocomial infections.

ROUTE & DOSAGE

Prevention & Treatment of RDS

Infant: **Intratracheal** 3 mL/kg of birth weight administered through an endotracheal tube q12h times 3 doses

ADMINISTRATION

Intratracheal

- Swirl vial to disperse suspension; do not dilute and DO NOT SHAKE. Withdraw with 20-gauge or larger needle. Avoid excess foaming. Instill into the endotracheal tube, preferably within 30 min of birth.
- Stop administration of calfactant if reflux into endotracheal tube occurs as indicated by cyanosis, bradycardia, or other signs of airway obstruction.

ADVERSE EFFECTS (≥1%) **CV:** *Bradycardia.* **Respiratory:** *Cyanosis, airway obstruction, reflux of surfactant* into endotracheal tube.

INTERACTIONS Drug: No clinically significant interactions established.

PHARMACOKINETICS Absorption: Absorbs rapidly to air; liquid interface of lung surface. No other human pharmacokinetic information available.

NURSING IMPLICATIONS

Assessment & Drug Effects

- Monitor closely during and after administration; adjustments in oxygen therapy and ventilator pressures are usually needed.

Patient & Family Education

- This drug will help baby to breathe properly and support normal respiratory function.

CANDESARTAN CILEXETIL

(can-de-sar′tan ci-lex′e-til)

Atacand

Classifications: CARDIOVASCULAR AGENT; ANGIOTENSIN II RECEPTOR ANTAGONIST

Prototype: Losartan

Pregnancy Category: C (first trimester); D (second and third trimesters)

AVAILABILITY 4 mg, 8 mg, 16 mg, 32 mg tablets

ACTIONS Angiotensin II receptor (type AT_1) antagonist. Angiotensin II is a potent vasoconstrictor and primary vasoactive hormone of the renin–angiotensin–aldosterone system. Candesartan selectively blocks binding of angiotensin II to the AT_1 receptors found in many tissues (e.g., vascular smooth muscle, adrenal glands).

THERAPEUTIC EFFECTS This results in blocking the vasoconstricting and the aldosterone-secreting effects of angiotensin II, resulting in an antihypertensive effect. Effectively lowers BP from hypertensive to normotensive range.

USE Hypertension.

CONTRAINDICATIONS Known sensitivity to candesartan or any other angiotensin II (AT_1) receptor antagonist (e.g., losartan, valsartan); primary hyperaldosteronism; bilateral renal artery stenosis; pregnancy (category C, first trimester; category D, second and third trimesters); lactation.

CAUTIOUS USE Concurrent administration with high-dose diuretics, potassium-sparing diuretics, or potassium salt substitutes; unilateral renal artery stenosis; aortic or mitral valve stenosis; hypertrophic cardiomyopathy; CHF; diabetes; lactation; significant renal failure.

ROUTE & DOSAGE

Hypertension

Adult: **PO** Start at 16 mg q.d. (range 8–32 mg divided once or twice daily)

ADMINISTRATION

Oral

- Volume depletion should be corrected prior to initiation of therapy to prevent hypotension.
- Dose is individualized and may be given once or twice daily. The daily dose may be titrated up to 32 mg; larger doses are not likely to provide additional benefit.

ADVERSE EFFECTS (≥1%) **Body as a Whole:** Fatigue, peripheral edema, back pain, arthralgia. **CV:** Chest pain. **GI:** Nausea, abdominal pain, diarrhea, vomiting. **CNS:** Headache, dizziness. **Respiratory:** Cough, sinusitis, upper respiratory infection, pharyngitis, rhinitis. **Urogenital:** Albuminuria.

PHARMACOKINETICS Absorption: Rapidly absorbed from GI tract; activated by ester hydrolysis during absorption; 15% reaches systemic circulation. **Peak:** Serum concentration, 3–4 h; therapeutic effect, 2–4 wk. **Duration:** 24 h. **Distribution:** >99% protein bound; crosses placenta; distributed into breast milk. **Metabolism:** Minimally metabolized in liver. **Elimination:** Excreted primarily unchanged in bile (67%) and urine (33%). **Half-Life:** 9 h.

NURSING IMPLICATIONS

Assessment & Drug Effects

- Monitor BP as therapeutic effectiveness is indicated by decreases in systolic and diastolic BP within 2 wk with maximal effect at 4–6 wk.
- Monitor for transient hypotension in volume/salt-depleted patients; if hypotension occurs, place in supine position and notify physician.
- Monitor BP periodically; trough readings, just prior to the next scheduled dose, should be made when possible.
- Lab tests: Periodically monitor BUN and creatinine, serum potassium, liver enzymes, and CBC with differential.

Patient & Family Education

- Inform your physician immediately if you become pregnant.
- You may not notice maximum pressure-lowering effect for 6 wk.
- Report episodes of dizziness especially when making position changes.
- Do not breast feed while taking this drug.

CAPECITABINE

(cap-e-si′ta-been)

Xeloda

Classifications: ANTINEOPLASTIC; ANTIMETABOLITE

Prototype: Fluorouracil (5-FU)

Pregnancy Category: D

AVAILABILITY 150 mg, 500 mg tablets

ACTIONS Pyrimidine antagonist and cell cycle-specific antimetabolite. Prodrug of 5-FU. Blocks actions of enzymes essential to normal DNA and RNA synthesis. May become incorporated into RNA molecules thereby interfering with RNA and protein synthesis.

THERAPEUTIC EFFECTS Reduces or stabilizes tumor size in metastatic breast cancer.

USES Metastatic breast cancer refractory to other treatments, colorectal cancer, adjuvant therapy for colon cancer after surgery.

CONTRAINDICATIONS Hypersensitivity to capecitabine, doxifluridine, 5-FU; myelosuppression; dihydropyrimidine dehydrogenase (DPD) deficiency; females of childbearing age; active infection; jaundice; severe renal failure or impairment; pregnancy (category D); lactation, children <18 y.

CAUTIOUS USE Mild to moderate renal or hepatic dysfunction; bacterial or viral infection; coronary artery disease, angina, cardiac arrhythmias; history of varicella zoster or other herpes infections; older adults.

ROUTE & DOSAGE

Breast Cancer, Colorectal Cancer

Adult: **PO** 2500 $mg/m^2/d$ in 2 divided doses times 2 wk, then 1 wk off. Repeat

Renal Impairment

Cl_{cr} 30–50 mL/min reduce dose by 25%, <30 mL/min do not use

ADMINISTRATION

Oral

- Morning and evening doses (about 12 h apart) should be given within 30 min of the end of a meal. Water is the preferred liquid for taking this drug.

ADVERSE EFFECTS (≥1%) **Body as a Whole:** *Fatigue,* pyrexia, pain, myalgia. **CV:** Edema. **GI:** *Severe diarrhea, nausea, vomiting, stomatitis,* abdominal pain, constipation, dyspepsia, *anorexia*. **Hematologic:** *Neutropenia, thrombocytopenia, anemia, lymphopenia*. **Metabolic:** Dehydration, hyperbilirubinemia. **CNS:** Paresthesias, headache, dizziness, insomnia. **Skin:** Hand-and-foot syndrome, *dermatitis,* nail disorder. **Special Senses:** Eye irritation.

INTERACTIONS Drug: Leucovorin increases concentration and toxicity of **5-FU,** altered coagulation and/or bleeding reported with **warfarin.**

PHARMACOKINETICS Absorption: Absorption significantly reduced by food. **Peak:** 1.5–2 h. **Distribution:** Approx 35% protein bound. **Metabolism:** Extensively metabolized to 5-FU. **Elimination:** Excreted in urine. **Half-Life:** 45 min.

NURSING IMPLICATIONS

Assessment & Drug Effects

- Lab tests: Monitor periodically CBC with differential and liver functions including bilirubin, transaminases, alkaline phosphatase.
- Monitor carefully for S&S of grade 2 or greater toxicity: diarrhea >4 BMs/day or at night; vomiting >1 time/24 h; significant loss of appetite or anorexia; stomatitis; hand-and-foot syndrome (pain, swelling, erythema, desquamation, blistering); temperature = 100.5° F; and S&S of infection.
- Withhold drug and immediately report S&S of grade 2 or greater toxicity.
- Monitor for dehydration and replace fluids as needed.

- Monitor carefully patients with coronary artery disease for S&S of cardiotoxicity (e.g., increasing angina).

Patient & Family Education

- Report immediately significant nausea, loss of appetite, diarrhea, soreness of tongue, fever of 100.5° F or more, or signs of infection. Review patient drug package insert carefully for more detail.
- Inform physician immediately if you become pregnant.
- Do not breast feed while taking this drug.

CAPREOMYCIN SULFATE

(kap-ree-oh-mye'sin)

Capastat Sulfate

Classifications: ANTIINFECTIVE; ANTITUBERCULOSIS AGENT

Prototype: Isoniazid

Pregnancy Category: C

AVAILABILITY 1 gm powder for injection

ACTIONS Polypeptide antibiotic derived from *Streptomyces capreolus*. Action mechanism not clear. Cross-resistance between capreomycin and both kanamycin and neomycin has been reported. Bacterial resistance can develop rapidly when used alone.

THERAPEUTIC EFFECTS Bacteriostatic against human strains of *Mycobacterium tuberculosis* and other species of *Mycobacterium*. Effective second-line antimycobacterial in conjunction with other antitubercular drugs.

USES Only in conjunction with other appropriate antitubercular drugs in treatment of pulmonary tuberculosis when bactericidal agents, e.g., isoniazid and rifampin, cannot be tolerated or when causative organism has become resistant.

CONTRAINDICATIONS Pregnancy (category C), in lactation. Safe use in infants and children not established.

CAUTIOUS USE Renal insufficiency (extreme caution); acoustic nerve impairment; history of allergies (especially to drugs); preexisting liver disease; myasthenia gravis; parkinsonism.

ROUTE & DOSAGE

Tuberculosis

Adult: **IM** 1 g/d (not to exceed 20 mg/kg/d) for 60–120 d, then 1 g 2–3 times/wk. See prescribing information for dose adjustments for renal insufficiency

ADMINISTRATION

Intramuscular

- Reconstitute by adding 2 mL of NS injection or sterile water for injection to each 1 g vial. Allow 2–3 min for drug to dissolve completely.
- Make IM injections deep into large muscle mass. Superficial injections are more painful and are associated with sterile abscess. Rotate injection sites.
- Solution may become pale straw color and darken with time, but this does not indicate loss of potency.
- After reconstitution, solution may be stored 48 h at room temperature and up to 14 d under refrigeration unless otherwise directed.

ADVERSE EFFECTS (≥1%) **Skin:** Urticaria, maculopapular rash, photosensitivity. **Hematologic:** Leukocytosis, leukopenia, *eosinophilia*. **CNS:** Neuromuscular blockage (large doses: skeletal muscle weakness, respiratory depression or arrest). **Urogenital:** Nephrotoxicity (long-term therapy), tubular necrosis. **Special Senses:** *Ototoxicity,* eighth nerve (auditory and vestibular) damage. **Metabolic:** Hypokalemia, and other electrolyte imbalances; **Other:** impaired hepatic function (decreased BSP excretion); IM site reactions: pain, induration, excessive bleeding, sterile abscesses.

DIAGNOSTIC TEST INTERFERENCE ***BSP*** and ***PSP*** excretion tests may be decreased.

INTERACTIONS Drug: Increased risk of nephrotoxicity and ototoxicity with AMINOGLYCOSIDES, **amphotericin B, colistin, polymyxin B, cisplatin, vancomycin.**

PHARMACOKINETICS Peak: 1–2 h. **Distribution:** Does not cross blood–brain barrier; crosses placenta; distribution into breast milk unknown. **Elimination:** 52% excreted in urine unchanged in 12 h; small amount excreted in bile. **Half-Life:** 4–6 h.

NURSING IMPLICATIONS

Assessment & Drug Effects

- Observe injection sites for signs of excessive bleeding and inflammation.
- Lab tests: Perform the following as guidelines for therapy before drug is started and at regular intervals during therapy: appropriate bacterial sensitivity tests; CBC; SMA-12 screening weekly; weekly renal function studies (BUN, NPN, creatinine clearance, sediment); liver function tests (periodically); serum potassium levels (monthly).
- Reduce dosage of capreomycin in patients with impaired renal function, as it is cumulative. Follow renal function tests closely.
- Monitor I&O rates and pattern: Report immediately any change in output or I&O ratio, any unusual appearance of urine, or elevation of BUN above 30 mg/dL. (Normal BUN: 10–20 mg/dL.)
- Evaluate hearing and balance by audiometric measurements (twice weekly or weekly) and tests of vestibular function (periodically).

Patient & Family Education

- Report any change in hearing or disturbance of balance. These effects are sometimes reversible if drug is withdrawn promptly when first symptoms appear.
- Ensure that you know about adverse reactions and what to do about them. Report immediately the appearance of any unusual symptom, regardless of how vague it may seem.
- Do not breast feed while taking this drug.

CAPSAICIN

(cap-say′i-sin)

Axsain, Capsaicin, Capsin, Capsacin-P, Dolorac, Zostrix, Zostrix-HP

Classifications: SKIN AND MUCOUS MEMBRANE AGENT; TOPICAL ANALGESIC

AVAILABILITY 0.025%, 0.075% lotion; 0.025%, 0.075%, 0.25% cream; 0.025%, 0.05% gel

ACTIONS Capsaicin is an alkaloid derived from plants and is the active ingredient in hot peppers. It is used as a topical analgesic. Capsaicin's precise mechanism is not fully understood. Substance P is thought to act as a principal neurotransmitter of pain sensations from the peripheral neurons to the CNS.

THERAPEUTIC EFFECTS It is thought that the drug renders skin and joints insensitive to pain by preventing the reaccumulation of substance P in peripheral sensory neurons. Thus capsaicin is an effective peripheral analgesic.

USES Temporary relief of pain from arthritis, neuralgias, diabetic neuropathy, and herpes zoster.

UNLABELED USES Phantom limb pain, psoriasis, intractable pruritus.

CONTRAINDICATIONS Hypersensitivity to capsaicin or any ingredient in the cream.

CAUTIOUS USE Patients on ACE inhibitors. Safety and efficacy in children <2 y have not been established.

ROUTE & DOSAGE

Analgesia

Adult: **Topical** Apply to affected area not more than 3–4 times/d
Child ≥2 y: **Topical** Apply to affected area not more than 3–4 times/d

ADMINISTRATION

Topical

- Apply to affected areas only and avoid contact with eyes or broken or irritated skin.
- If applied with bare hand, wash immediately following application. An applicator or gloved hand may be used to apply cream.
- Avoid tight bandages over areas of application of the cream.

ADVERSE EFFECTS (≥1%) **CNS:** Concentration >1%: neurotoxicity, hyperalgesia. **Skin:** *Burning, stinging, redness,* itching. **Other:** Cough.

INTERACTIONS Drug: May increase incidence of cough with ACE INHIBITORS.

PHARMACOKINETICS Onset: Postherpetic neuralgia: 2–6 wk.

NURSING IMPLICATIONS

Assessment & Drug Effects

- Monitor for significant pain relief, which may require 4–6 wk of application three or four times daily.
- Monitor for and report signs of skin breakdown as these generally indicate need for drug discontinuation.

Patient & Family Education

- Report local discomfort at site of application if discomfort is distressing or persists beyond the first 3–4 d of use.
- Use caution in handling contact lenses following application of cream. Wash hands thoroughly before touching lenses.
- Notify physician if symptoms do not improve or condition worsens within 14–28 d.
- Apply frequently three or four times daily to maximize therapeutic effectiveness.

CAPTOPRIL (Pr)

(kap'toe-pril)

Capoten

Classifications: CARDIOVASCULAR AGENT; ANGIOTENSIN-CONVERTING ENZYME (ACE) INHIBITOR; ANTIHYPERTENSIVE AGENT

Pregnancy Category: D

AVAILABILITY 12.5 mg, 25 mg, 50 mg, 100 mg tablets

ACTIONS Lowers blood pressure by specific inhibition of the angiotensin-converting enzyme (ACE). This interrupts conversion sequences initiated by renin that lead to formation of angiotensin II, a potent endogenous vasoconstrictor. ACE inhibition alters hemodynamics without compensatory reflex tachycardia or changes in cardiac output (except in patients with CHF). Peripheral vascular resistance is lowered by vasodilation. Inhibition of ACE also leads to decreased circulating aldosterone. Reduced circulating aldosterone is associated with a potassium-sparing effect. In heart failure, captopril administration is followed by a fall in CVP and pulmonary wedge pressure; hypotensive action appears to be unrelated to plasma renin levels.

THERAPEUTIC EFFECTS Effective in stepped protocol management of hypertension to convert to normotensive range, and in congestive heart failure with resulting decreases in dyspnea and improved exercise tolerance.

USES Hypertension; in conjunction with digitalis and diuretics in CHF, diabetic nephropathy.

UNLABELED USE Idiopathic edema.

CONTRAINDICATIONS Angioedema, hypersensitivity to captopril or ACE inhibitors; hypotension; pregnancy (category D), lactation.

CAUTIOUS USE Impaired renal function, patient with solitary kidney; collagen-vascular diseases (scleroderma, SLE); patients receiving IMMUNOSUPPRESSANTS or other drugs that cause leukopenia or agranulocytosis; autoimmune disease, bone marrow suppression, coronary or cerebrovascular disease; cardiomyopathy, aortic stenosis; severe salt/volume depletion; heart failure, renal artery stenosis, renal disease, renal failure, renal impairment; hyperkalemia, children, elderly.

ROUTE & DOSAGE

Hypertension

Adult: **PO** 6.25–25 mg t.i.d., may increase to 50 mg t.i.d. (max: 450 mg/d)
Child: **PO** 0.3–12.5 mg/kg q12–24h, may titrate up to max of 6 mg/kg/d in 2–4 divided doses
Infant: **PO** 0.15–0.3 mg/kg, may titrate up to 6 mg/kg/d in 1–4 divided doses
Neonate: **PO** 0.05–0.1 mg/kg q8–24 h, may titrate up to 0.5 mg/kg q6–24 h
Premature infant: **PO** 0.01 mg/kg q8–12h

Congestive Heart Failure

Adult: **PO** 6.25–12.5 mg t.i.d., may increase to 50 mg t.i.d. (max: 450 mg/d)

ADMINISTRATION

Oral

- Give Captopril 1 h before meals. Food reduces absorption by 30–40%.
- Store in light-resistant containers at no more than 30° C (86° F) unless otherwise directed.

ADVERSE EFFECTS (≥1%) **Body as a Whole:** Hypersensitivity reactions, serum sickness-like reaction, arthralgia, skin eruptions. **CV:** Slight increase in heart rate, first dose hypotension, dizziness, fainting. **GI:** Altered taste sensation (loss of taste perception, persistent salt or metallic taste); weight loss, intestinal angioedema. **Hematologic:** Hyperkalemia, neutropenia, agranulocytosis (rare). **Respiratory:** *cough*. **Skin:** *Maculopapular rash,* urticaria, pruritus, angioedema, photosensitivity. **Urogenital:** Azotemia, impaired renal function, nephrotic syndrome, membranous glomerulonephritis. **Other:** Positive antinuclear antibody (ANA) titers.

DIAGNOSTIC TEST INTERFERENCE In some patients, elevated ***urine protein levels*** may persist even after captopril has been discontinued. Possibility of transient elevations of ***BUN*** and ***serum creatinine,*** slight increase in ***serum potassium,*** and ***serum prolactin,*** increases in ***liver enzymes,*** and false-positive ***urine acetone*** (using ***sodium nitroprusside reagent***). Captopril may decrease ***fasting blood sugar*** in the nondiabetic and cause hypoglycemia in the diabetic patient controlled with antidiabetic drug therapy.

INTERACTIONS Drug: NITRATES, DIURETICS, and ANTIHYPERTENSIVES enhance hypotensive effects. **Aspirin** and other NSAIDS may antagonize hypotensive effects. POTASSIUM-SPARING DIURETICS **(spironolactone, amiloride)** increase potassium levels. **Probenecid** decreases elimination and increases effects. **Food:** Food decreases absorption; take 30–60 min before meals.

PHARMACOKINETICS Absorption: 60–75% absorbed; food may decrease absorption 25–40%. **Onset:** 15 min. **Peak:** 1–2 h. **Duration:** 6–12 h. **Distribution:** Distributed to all tissues except CNS; crosses placenta. **Metabolism:** Some liver metabolism. **Elimination:** Excreted primarily in urine; excreted in breast milk.

NURSING IMPLICATIONS

Assessment & Drug Effects

- Monitor BP closely following the first dose. A sudden exaggerated hypotensive response may occur within 1–3 h of first dose, especially in those with high BP or on a diuretic and restricted salt intake.
- Advise bed rest and BP monitoring for the first 3 h after the initial dose.
- Monitor therapeutic effectiveness. At least 2 wk of therapy may be required before full therapeutic effects are achieved.
- Lab tests: Establish baseline urinary protein levels before initiation of therapy and check at monthly intervals for the first 8 mo of treatment and then periodically thereafter. Perform WBC and differential counts before therapy is begun and at approximately 2-wk intervals for the first 3 mo of therapy and then periodically thereafter.

Patient & Family Education

- Report to physician without delay the onset of unexplained fever, unusual fatigue, sore mouth or throat, easy bruising or bleeding (pathognomonic of agranulocytosis).
- Mild skin eruptions are most likely to appear during the first 4 wk of therapy and may be accompanied by fever and eosinophilia.
- Consult physician promptly if vomiting or diarrhea occur.
- Report darkening or crumbling of nailbeds (reversible with dosage reduction).
- Taste impairment occurs in 5–10% of patients and generally reverses in 2–3 mo even with continued therapy.
- Use OTC medications only with approval of the physician. Inform surgeon or dentist that captopril is being taken. Alert diabetic patient that captopril may produce hypoglycemia. Monitor blood glucose and HbA_{1c} closely during first few weeks of therapy.

- Do not breast feed while taking this drug.

CARBACHOL INTRAOCULAR

(kar'ba-kole)

Miostat

CARBACHOL TOPICAL

Isopto Carbachol

Classifications: EYE, EAR, NOSE AND THROAT PREPARATION; MIOTIC; AUTONOMIC NERVOUS SYSTEM AGENT; DIRECT-ACTING CHOLINERGIC (PARASYMPATHOMIMETIC)

Prototype: Pilocarpine

Pregnancy Category: C

AVAILABILITY 0.75%, 1.5%, 2.25%, 3% solution

See Appendix A-1.

CARBAMAZEPINE (Pr)

(kar-ba-maz'e-peen)

Apo-Carbamazepine ♣, Carbatrol, Epitol, Mazepine ♣, PMS-Carbamazepine ♣, Tegretol, Tegretol XR, Teril

Classifications: CENTRAL NERVOUS SYSTEM AGENT; ANTICONVULSANT; TRICYCLIC

Pregnancy Category: D

AVAILABILITY 100 mg chewable tablets; 200 mg tablets; 100 mg, 200 mg, 400 mg sustained-release tablets; 200 mg, 300 mg sustained-release capsules; 100 mg/5 mL suspension

ACTIONS Structurally related to tricyclic antidepressants (TCAs) but lacks antidepressant properties. Anticonvulsant actions appear qualitatively similar to those of phenytoin. Like phenytoin, provides relief in trigeminal neuralgia by reducing synaptic transmission within trigeminal nucleus. Also has sedative, anticholinergic, antidepressant, and muscle relaxant (by inhibition of neuromuscular transmission) effects and slight analgesic actions.

THERAPEUTIC EFFECTS Effective anticonvulsant for a range of seizure disorders and as an adjuvant reduces depressive signs and symptoms and stabilizes mood. It is effective for pain and other symptoms associated with neurologic disorders.

USES Alone or concomitantly with other anticonvulsants in treatment of grand mal and psychomotor or temporal lobe epilepsy and mixed seizures in patients who have not responded satisfactorily to other agents. Also used for symptomatic treatment of trigeminal (tic douloureux) and glossopharyngeal neuralgias and for pain and paroxysmal symptoms associated with multiple sclerosis and other neurologic disorders.

UNLABELED USES Certain psychiatric disorders including prophylaxis and treatment of manic-depressive illness, treatment of schizoaffective illness, resistant schizophrenia, dyscontrol syndrome; for management of alcohol withdrawal, rage outbursts, and for antidiuretic effect in diabetes insipidus.

CONTRAINDICATIONS Hypersensitivity to carbamazepine and to TCAs; history of myelosuppression or hematologic reaction to other drugs; increased IOP; SLE; cardiac, hepatic, or renal disease; coronary artery disease; hypertension; pregnancy (category D), lactation. Safe use in children <6 mo not established.

CAUTIOUS USE The older adult; history of cardiac disease.

ROUTE & DOSAGE

Epilepsy

Adult: **PO** 200 mg b.i.d., gradually increased to 800–1200 mg/d in 3–4 divided doses. Tegretol XR dosed b.i.d.
Child: **PO** *<6 y:* 10–20 mg/kg/d, may gradually increase weekly, recommended max 35 mg/kg/d in 3–4 divided doses; *6–12 y:* 100 mg b.i.d., gradually increased to 400–800 mg/d in 3–4 divided doses (max: 1 g/d); *<6 y:* 20–30 mg/kg/d in 3–4 divided doses

Trigeminal Neuralgia

Adult: **PO** 100 mg b.i.d., gradually increased by 100 mg increments q12h until relief; usual dose 200–800 mg/d in 3–4 divided doses (max: 1.2 g/d). Tegretol XR dosed b.i.d.

ADMINISTRATION

Oral

- Do not administer within 14 d of patient receiving a MAO inhibitor.
- Give with a meal to increase absorption.
- Ensure that chewable tablets are chewed or crushed before being swallowed with a liquid.
- Ensure that sustained-release form of drug is not chewed or crushed. It must be swallowed whole.
- Do not administer carbamazepine suspension simultaneously with other liquid medications: a precipitate may form in the stomach.

ADVERSE EFFECTS (≥1%) **Body as a Whole:** Myalgia, arthralgia, leg cramps, carbamazepine-induced SLE. **CV:** Edema, syncope, arrhythmias, heart block. **GI:** Nausea, vomiting, anorexia, abdominal pain, diarrhea, constipation, dry mouth and pharynx, abnormal liver function tests, hepatitis, cholestatic and hepatocellular jaundice, pancreatitis. **Endocrine:** Hypothyroidism, SIADH. **Hematologic:** Aplastic anemia, *leukopenia* (transient), leukocytosis, agranulocytosis, eosinophilia, thrombocytopenia. **CNS:** Dizziness, vertigo, drowsiness, disturbances of coordination, ataxia, confusion, headache, fatigue, listlessness, speech difficulty, development of minor motor seizures, hyperreflexia, akathisia, involuntary movements, tremors, visual hallucinations, activation of latent psychosis, aggression; agitation, respiratory depression. **Skin:** Skin rashes, urticaria, petechiae, erythema multiforme, Stevens-Johnson syndrome, photosensitivity reactions, altered skin pigmentation, exfoliative dermatitis, alopecia. **Special Senses:** Abnormal hearing acuity, scotomas, conjunctivitis, blurred vision, transient diplopia, oculomotor disturbances, oscillopsia, nystagmus. **Urogenital:** Urinary frequency or retention, oliguria, impotence.

DIAGNOSTIC TEST INTERFERENCE False-negative ***pregnancy test*** results with tests involving ***human chorionic gonadotropin.***

INTERACTIONS Drug: Serum concentrations of other ANTICONVULSANTS may decrease because of increased metabolism; **verapamil, erythromycin, ketoconazole, nefazadone** may increase carbamazepine levels; decreases hypoprothrombinemic effects of ORAL ANTICOAGULANTS; increases metabolism of ESTROGENS, thus decreasing effectiveness of ORAL CONTRACEP-

TIVES. **Herbal: Ginkgo** may decrease anticonvulsant effectiveness.

PHARMACOKINETICS Absorption: Slowly absorbed from GI tract. **Peak:** 2–8 h. **Distribution:** Widely distributed; high concentrations in CSF; crosses placenta; distributed into breast milk. **Metabolism:** Metabolized in liver; can induce liver microsomal enzymes. **Elimination:** Excreted in urine and feces. **Half-Life:** 14–16 h (decreases with long-term use).

NURSING IMPLICATIONS

Assessment & Drug Effects

- Lab tests: Baseline and periodic CBCs including platelets, reticulocytes, serum electrolytes and serum iron, liver function tests, BUN, and complete urinalysis.
- At least 3 mo into therapy, it is recommended that physician attempt dosage reduction or termination of drug therapy, if possible, in patients with trigeminal neuralgia. Some patients develop tolerance to the effects of carbamazepine.
- Monitor for the following reactions, which commonly occur during early therapy: drowsiness, dizziness, light-headedness, ataxia, gastric upset. If these symptoms do not subside within a few days, dosage adjustments may be indicated.
- Withhold drug and notify physician if any of the following signs of myelosuppression occur: RBC <4 million/mm^3, Hct <32%, Hgb <11 g/dL, WBC <4000/mm^3, platelet count <100,000/mm^3, reticulocyte count <20,000/mm^3, serum iron >150 mg/dL.
- Monitor for toxicity, which can develop when serum concentrations are even slightly above the therapeutic range.
- Monitor I&O ratio and vital signs during period of dosage adjustment. Report oliguria, signs of fluid retention, changes in I&O ratio, and changes in BP or pulse patterns.
- Cardiac syncope may resemble epileptic seizures. Therefore, it is recommended that patients who experience an apparent increase in frequency of seizures or a change in their character should be checked by continuous ECG monitoring for 24 h.
- Doses higher than 600 mg/d may precipitate arrhythmias in patients with heart disease.
- Confusion and agitation may be aggravated in the older adult; therefore, side rails and supervision of ambulation may be indicated.

Patient & Family Education

- Discontinue drug and notify physician immediately if early signs of toxicity or a possible hematologic problem appear, (e.g., anorexia, fever, sore throat or mouth, malaise, unusual fatigue, tendency to bruise or bleed, petechiae, ecchymoses, bleeding gums, nose bleeds).
- Avoid hazardous tasks requiring mental alertness and physical coordination until reaction to drug is known, since dizziness, drowsiness, and ataxia are common adverse effects.
- Remain under close medical supervision throughout therapy.
- Avoid excessive sunlight, as photosensitivity reactions have been reported. Apply a sunscreen (if allowed) with SPF of 12 or above.
- Carbamazepine may cause breakthrough bleeding and may also

affect the reliability of oral contraceptives.

- Be aware that abrupt withdrawal of any anticonvulsant drug may precipitate seizures or even status epilepticus.
- Do not breast feed while taking this drug.

CARBENICILLIN INDANYL SODIUM

(kar-ben-i-sill'in)

Geocillin, Geopen Oral ♣

Classifications: ANTIINFECTIVE; ANTIBIOTIC; ANTIPSEUDOMONAL PENICILLIN

Prototype: Mezlocillin

Pregnancy Category: B

AVAILABILITY 382 mg tablets

ACTIONS Broad-spectrum, semisynthetic penicillin and acid stable ester of carbenicillin prepared for oral use. Rapidly hydrolyzed to carbenicillin in body.

THERAPEUTIC EFFECTS Like carbenicillin disodium, it is bactericidal and penicillinase sensitive and has similar antimicrobial activity but achieves lower blood concentrations than parent compound. Reduces the discomfort of prostatitis and effective in reducing symptoms of urinary tract infections.

USES Mainly in the treatment of prostatitis and acute and chronic infections of upper and lower urinary tract caused by susceptible strains of *Escherichia coli, Enterobacter, Enterococcus, Proteus,* and *Pseudomonas species.*

CONTRAINDICATIONS Hypersensitivity to penicillins; pregnancy (category B). Safe use in children not established.

CAUTIOUS USE History of or suspected atopy or allergies; history of allergy to cephalosporins; lactation; impaired renal and hepatic function; patients on sodium restriction.

ROUTE & DOSAGE

Urinary Tract Infections

Adult: **PO** 382–764 mg q6h for 10 d, continue for 2–4 wk for prostatitis

ADMINISTRATION

Oral

- Give with a full glass (240 mL) of water on an empty stomach (either 1 h before or 2 h after meals) to attain maximum therapeutic drug levels in urine. Consult physician.
- Protect tablets from moisture.

ADVERSE EFFECTS (≥1%) **Body as a Whole:** Hypersensitivity (Rash, fever, urticaria, eosinophilia, pruritus, anaphylaxis), superinfections, especially of vagina. **GI:** *Nausea,* vomiting, heartburn; *diarrhea,* abdominal cramps, flatulence, unpleasant aftertaste, dry mouth. **Hematologic:** Neutropenia, leukopenia, thrombocytopenia, hemolytic anemia, increased AST.

PHARMACOKINETICS Absorption: Incompletely absorbed from GI tract. **Peak:** 0.5–1 h. **Distribution:** Very low systemic concentrations; crosses placenta; distributed into breast milk. **Elimination:** 80–99% excreted unchanged in urine within 24 h. **Half-Life:** 67 min.

NURSING IMPLICATIONS

Assessment & Drug Effects

- Lab tests: Perform culture and sensitivity tests prior to and at regular intervals throughout therapy. Therapy may be initiated pending test results. Evaluate renal, hepatic, and hematopoietic systems at regular intervals during prolonged therapy. Patients with creatinine clearance of less than 10 mL/min (normal: 105–130 mL/min) will not attain therapeutic urine levels.
- Inquire carefully concerning patient's previous exposure and sensitivity to penicillin and cephalosporins and other allergic reactions of any kind before treatment is initiated.
- Note that drug-induced nausea, unpleasant aftertaste and smell, dry mouth, and furry tongue may be so objectionable as to necessitate drug withdrawal. Report to physician if symptoms persist.
- Monitor I&O rates and pattern: Check with physician regarding optimum daily fluid intake. Report any change in quality or quantity of urine or in I&O ratio.
- Observe patient for signs of electrolyte imbalance. Each 1 g of drug contains approximately 1 mEq of sodium.

Patient & Family Education

- Take this medication with a full glass of water on an empty stomach.
- Take medication around the clock, do not miss any doses, and continue taking medication until it is all gone unless otherwise directed by physician.
- Do not breast feed while taking this drug without consulting physician.

CARBIDOPA-LEVODOPA

(kar-bi-doe′pa)

Sinemet, Sinemet-CR, Parcopa

CARBIDOPA

Lodosyn

Classifications: AUTONOMIC NERVOUS SYSTEM AGENT; ANTICHOLINERGIC (PARASYMPATHOLYTIC); ANTI-PARKINSONISM AGENT

Prototype: Levodopa

Pregnancy Category: C

AVAILABILITY **Carbidopa:** 25 mg tablet **Carbidopa/Levodopa:** 10 mg/100 mg, 25 mg/100 mg, 25 mg/250 mg tablets; 25 mg/100 mg, 50 mg/200 mg sustained-release tablets and orally disintegrating tablets

ACTIONS When levodopa is given alone, large doses must be administered. Carbidopa prevents peripheral metabolism (decarboxylation) of levodopa and thereby makes more levodopa available for transport to the brain. Carbidopa does not cross blood-brain barrier and therefore does not affect metabolism of levodopa within the brain. Carbidopa also prevents the inhibitory effect of pyridoxine (vitamin B_6) on levodopa.

THERAPEUTIC EFFECTS Effective in management of symptoms of Parkinson's disease and parkinsonism of secondary origin and improving life expectancy and quality of life.

USES Symptomatic treatment of idiopathic Parkinson's disease (paralysis agitans), postencephalitic parkinsonism, and parkinsonism following carbon dioxide and manganese intoxication. Carbidopa is available alone from manufacturer, on request by physician, for use with levodopa when separate titration of each agent is indicated, and for investigational purposes.

CONTRAINDICATIONS Hypersensitivity to carbidopa or levodopa; narrow-angle glaucoma; history of or suspected melanoma. Safe use in women of childbearing potential, during pregnancy (category C), in lactation, and in children <18 y not established.

CAUTIOUS USE Cardiovascular, hepatic, pulmonary, or renal disorders; urinary retention; history of peptic ulcer; psychiatric states; endocrine disease; chronic wide-angle glaucoma; seizure disorders.

ROUTE & DOSAGE

Parkinson's Disease in Patients Not Currently Receiving Levodopa

Adult: **PO** 1 tablet containing 10 mg carbidopa/100 mg levodopa *or* 25 mg carbidopa/100 mg levodopa t.i.d., increased by 1 tablet q.d. or q.o.d. up to 6 tablets/d

Patients Receiving Levodopa

Adult: **PO** 1 tablet of the 25/250 mixture t.i.d. or q.i.d., adjusted by 1/2–1 tablet as needed up to 8 tablets/d (start at 20–25% of initial dose of levodopa)

ADMINISTRATION

Oral

- Ensure that sustained-release form of drug (Sinemet CR) is not chewed or crushed. It may be broken in half but otherwise swallowed whole.
- Give consistently with respect to food. High protein meals may interfere with absorption of levodopa.
- When patient has been taking levodopa alone, carbidopa-levodopa is usually initiated with a morning dose after patient has been without levodopa for at least 8 h.
- Store in tight, light-resistant containers.

ADVERSE EFFECTS (≥1%) **Body as a Whole:** Hoarseness, unusual breathing patterns, neuroleptic malignant syndrome. **CV:** Orthostatic hypotension, irregular heart beat, palpitation, arrhythmias, phlebitis, edema. **GI:** Nausea, anorexia, dry mouth, bruxism, vomiting, excess salivation. **Hematologic:** Hemolytic and nonhemolytic anemia, thrombocytopenia, agranulocytosis. **Metabolic:** Abnormal liver function tests, abnormal BUN. **CNS:** *Involuntary movements (dyskinetic, dystonic, choreiform),* ataxia, muscle twitching, increase in hand tremor, numbness, headache, dizziness, euphoria, fatigue, confusion, insomnia, nightmares, mental disturbances, anxiety, depression with suicidal tendencies, delirium, seizures. **Skin:** Body odor, skin rash, dark sweat, loss of hair. **Special Senses:** Blepharospasm, mydriasis, miosis, blurred vision, diplopia, oculogyric crisis. **Urogenital:** Dark urine, priapism, urinary frequency, retention, incontinence.

DIAGNOSTIC TEST INTERFERENCE **Urine glucose:** false-negative tests may result with use of ***glucose oxidase methods*** (e.g., ***Clinistix, TesTape***) and false-positive results with ***copper reduction methods*** (e.g., ***Benedict's, Clinitest***), especially in patients receiving large doses. It is reported that ***Clinistix*** and ***TesTape*** may be used if reading is taken at margin of wet and dry tape. There is also the possibility of false-positive tests for ***uri-***

C

nary ketones by ***dipstick tests,*** e.g., ***Acetest*** (equivocal), ***Ketostix, Labstix;*** false elevation of ***serum*** and ***urinary uric acid*** levels by ***colorimetric methods*** (***not*** with ***uricase***); and interference with ***urine PKU test*** results.

INTERACTIONS Drug: MAO INHIBITORS may precipitate hypertensive crisis; TRICYCLIC ANTIDEPRESSANTS potentiate postural hypotension; PHENOTHIAZINES, **haloperidol** may antagonize effects of levodopa; ANTICHOLINERGIC AGENTS may enhance levodopa effects but can exacerbate involuntary movements; **methyldopa, guanethidine** increase hypotensive and CNS effects; **phenytoin, papaverine** may interfere with levodopa effects.

PHARMACOKINETICS Absorption: 40–70% of carbidopa absorbed after PO dose; carbidopa may enhance absorption of levodopa. **Distribution:** Widely distributed in most body tissues except CNS; crosses placenta; excreted in breast milk. **Elimination:** Excreted in urine. **Half-Life:** 2 h.

NURSING IMPLICATIONS

Assessment & Drug Effects

- Make accurate observations and report promptly adverse reactions and therapeutic effects. Rate of dosage increase is determined primarily by patient's tolerance and response to levodopa.
- Monitor vital signs, particularly during period of dosage adjustment. Report alterations in BP, pulse, and respiratory rate and rhythm.
- Monitor all patients closely for behavior changes. Patients in depression should be closely observed for suicidal tendencies.
- Monitor for changes in intraocular pressure in patients with chronic wide-angle glaucoma.
- Monitor patients with diabetes carefully for alterations in diabetes control. Frequent monitoring of blood sugar is advised.
- Lab tests: Periodic blood glucose, hepatic and renal function tests, CBC with differential, Hgb and Hct.
- Report promptly abnormal involuntary movement such as facial grimacing, exaggerated chewing, protrusion of tongue, rhythmic opening and closing of mouth, bobbing of head, jerky arm and leg movements, and exaggerated respiration.
- Assess for "on-off" phenomenon: sudden, unpredictable loss of drug effectiveness ("off" effect), which lasts 1 min–1 h. This is followed by an equally abrupt return of function ("on" effect). Sometimes symptoms can be controlled by increasing number of doses per day.
- Monitor therapeutic effects. Some patients manifest increase in bradykinesia ("leg freezing" or slow body movement). The patient is unable to start walking and frequently falls. Reduction of dosage may be indicated in these patients.
- Patients who require more frequent drug administration are most likely to manifest gradual return of parkinsonian symptoms toward the end of a dose period.

Patient & Family Education

- Follow physician's directions regarding continuation or discontinuation of levodopa. Both adverse reactions and therapeutic effects occur more rapidly with carbidopa-levodopa combination than with levodopa alone.
- Make positional changes slowly and in stages, particularly from recumbent to upright position, dan-

gle your legs a few minutes before standing, and walk in place before ambulating, as some patients experience weakness, dizziness, and faintness. Tolerance to this effect usually develops within a few months of therapy. Support stockings may help. Consult physician.

- Report muscle twitching and spasmodic winking promptly, as these may be early signs of overdosage.
- You may notice elevation of mood and sense of well-being before any objective improvement. Resume activities gradually and observe safety precautions to avoid injury.
- Maintain your prescribed drug regimen. Abrupt withdrawal can lead to parkinsonian crisis with return of marked muscle rigidity, akinesia, tremor, hyperpyrexia, mental changes.
- Avoid driving or other hazardous activities until reaction to drug is determined.
- Levodopa may cause urine to darken on standing and may also cause sweat to be dark-colored. This effect is not clinically significant.
- Wear medical identification. Inform all health care providers that you are taking carbidopa-levodopa.
- Do not breast feed while taking this drug.

CARBOPLATIN

(car-bo-pla'tin)

Paraplatin

Classifications: ANTINEOPLASTIC; ALKYLATING AGENT

Prototype: Cyclophosphamide

Pregnancy Category: D

AVAILABILITY 50 mg, 150 mg, 450 mg vials

ACTIONS Carboplatin is a platinum compound that is a chemotherapeutic agent. It produces interstrand DNA cross-linkages, thus interfering with DNA, RNA, and protein synthesis. Carboplatin is cell-cycle nonspecific, i.e., effective throughout the entire cell life cycle.

THERAPEUTIC EFFECTS Full or partial activity against a variety of cancers resulting in reduction or stabilization of tumor size and useful in patients with impaired renal function, patients unable to accommodate high-volume hydration, or patients at high risk for neurotoxicity and/or ototoxicity.

USES Monotherapy or combination therapy for ovarian cancer.

UNLABELED USES Combination therapy for breast, cervical, colon, endometrial, head and neck, and lung cancer; leukemia, lymphoma, and melanoma.

CONTRAINDICATIONS History of severe reactions to carboplatin or other platinum compounds, severe bone marrow depression; significant bleeding; impaired renal function; pregnancy (category D), and lactation.

CAUTIOUS USE Use with other nephrotoxic drugs.

ROUTE & DOSAGE

Ovarian Cancer

Adult: **IV** 360 mg/m^2 once q4wk. May be repeated when neutrophil count is at least 2000 mm^3 and platelet count is at least 100,000 mm^3. If neutrophil and platelet counts are lower, dose of carboplatin should be reduced by 50–75% of initial dose. Alternatively, 400 mg/m^2 as a 24-h infusion for 2 consecutive d can be used

C

Head and Neck and Small Cell Lung Cancer
Adult: **IV** 300–400 mg/m^2 q4wk
Child: **IV** Up to 560 mg/m^2 once q4wk or up to 175 mg/m^2 q2wk. Other dosage regimens have been used for specific dosing protocols

Important Note
Aluminum reacts with carboplatin to form an inactive precipitate; therefore, intravenous infusion sets and needles containing aluminum should not be used

ADMINISTRATION

Intravenous

PREPARE: **IV Infusion:** Do not use needles or IV sets containing aluminum. Immediately before use, reconstitute with either sterile water for injection or D5W or NS as follows: 50-mg vial plus 5 mL diluent; 150-mg vial plus 15 mL diluent; 450-mg vial plus 45 mL diluent. All dilutions yield 10 mg/mL. May be further diluted to 0.5 mg/mL with D5W or NS.
ADMINISTER: **IV Infusion:** Give IV solution over 15 min or longer, depending on total amount of solution and patient tolerance. Lengthening duration of administration may decrease nausea and vomiting.
INCOMPATIBILITIES **Solution/additive: Sodium bicarbonate, fluorouracil, mesna. Y-site: Amphotericin B cholesteryl complex.**

■ Premedication with a parenteral antiemetic 1/2 h before and on a scheduled basis thereafter is normally used. ■ Do not repeat doses until the neutrophil count is at least 2000/mm^3 and platelet count at least 100,000/mm^3.

■ Protect from light. Reconstituted solutions are stable for 8 h at room temperature; discard solutions 8 h after dilution.

ADVERSE EFFECTS (≥1%) **Body as a Whole:** Hypersensitivity reactions. **GI:** *Mild to moderate nausea and vomiting,* anorexia, hypogeusia, dysgeusia, mucositis, diarrhea, constipation, elevated liver enzymes. **Hematologic:** *Thrombocytopenia, leukopenia, neutropenia, anemia.* **Metabolic:** *Mild hyponatremia, hypomagnesemia, hypocalcemia, and hypokalemia.* **CNS:** Peripheral neuropathy. **Skin:** Rash, alopecia. **Special Senses:** Tinnitus. **Urogenital:** Nephrotoxicity.

DIAGNOSTIC TEST INTERFERENCE Decreased ***calcium levels;*** mild increases in ***liver function tests;*** decreased levels of ***magnesium, potassium,*** and ***sodium.***

INTERACTIONS Drug: AMINOGLYCOSIDES may increase the risk of ototoxicity and nephrotoxicity. May decrease **phenytoin** levels.

PHARMACOKINETICS Onset: 8 wk (2 cycles). **Duration:** 2–16 mo. **Distribution:** Highest concentration is seen in the liver, lung, kidney, skin, and tumors. Not bound to plasma proteins. **Metabolism:** Hydrolyzed in the serum. **Elimination:** Primarily eliminated by the kidneys; 60–80% excreted in urine within 24 h. **Half-Life:** 3 h.

NURSING IMPLICATIONS

Assessment & Drug Effects

- Monitor closely during first 15 min of infusion, since allergic reactions have occurred within minutes of carboplatin administration.
- Lab tests: Baseline and periodic CBC with differential, platelet

count, Hgb and Hct. Monitor periodically kidney function with creatinine clearance tests and serum electrolytes.

- Monitor results of peripheral blood counts. Median nadir occurs at day 21. Leukopenia, neutropenia, and thrombocytopenia are dose related and may produce dose-limiting toxicity.
- Monitor for peripheral neuropathy (e.g., paresthesias), ototoxicity, and visual disturbances.
- Monitor serum electrolyte studies, because carboplatin has been associated with decreases in sodium, potassium, calcium, and magnesium. Special precautions may be warranted for patients on diuretic therapy.

Patient & Family Education

- Learn about the range of potential adverse effects. Strategies for nausea prevention should receive special attention.
- During therapy you are at risk for infection and hemorrhagic complications related to bone marrow suppression. Avoid unnecessary exposure to crowds or infected persons during the nadir period.
- Report paresthesias (numbness, tingling), visual disturbances, or symptoms of ototoxicity (hearing loss and/or tinnitus).
- Do not breast feed while taking this drug.

CARBOPROST TROMETHAMINE

(kar'boe-prost)
Hemabate
Classifications: PROSTAGLANDIN; ABORTIFACIENT
Prototype: Dinosprostone
Pregnancy Category: D

AVAILABILITY 250 mcg/mL injection

ACTIONS Synthetic analog of naturally occurring prostaglandin F_2 alpha with longer duration of biologic activity. Stimulates myometrial contractions of gravid uterus; contractions are qualitatively similar to those occurring at term labor. Mean time to abortion 16 h; mean dose required 2.6 mL. Length of time to abortion and total dose of carboprost required decrease with greater parity but increase with greater gestational age. Can be employed as abortifacient even if membranes are ruptured.

THERAPEUTIC EFFECTS Effectively stimulates uterine contraction and is used to induce abortion over a wide range of gestational age. Useful in treatment of postpartum hemorrhage due to uterine atony unresponsive to usual measures.

USES To induce abortion between 13th and 20th week of pregnancy, as calculated from first day of last menstrual period. Also for refractory postpartum bleeding.

UNLABELED USES To reduce blood loss secondary to uterine atony; to induce labor in intrauterine fetal death and hydatidiform mole.

CONTRAINDICATIONS Acute pelvic inflammatory disease; active cardiac, pulmonary, renal, or hepatic disease; pregnancy (category D); lactation.

CAUTIOUS USE History of asthma; adrenal disease; anemia; hypotension; hypertension; diabetes mellitus; epilepsy; history of uterine surgery; cervical stenosis; fibroids.

ROUTE & DOSAGE

Abortion, Postpartum Bleeding
Adult: **IM** Initial: 250 mcg (1 mL) repeated at 1 1/2–3 1/2-h inter

C

vals if indicated by uterine response. Dosage may be increased to 500 mcg (2 mL) if uterine contractility is inadequate after several doses of 250 mcg (1 mL), not to exceed total dose of 12 mg or continuous administration for more than 2 d

ADMINISTRATION

- Because nausea and diarrhea occur in about 60% of patients, an antiemetic and an antidiarrheal agent may be prescribed before and during carboprost administration.
- Give deep IM into a large muscle. Aspirate carefully before injecting drug to avoid inadvertent entry into blood vessel which can result in bronchospasm, tetanic contractions, and shock. Do not use same site for subsequent doses.
- Store drug in refrigerator at 2°–4° C (36°–39° F) unless otherwise specified.

ADVERSE EFFECTS (≥1%) **Body as a Whole:** Fever, flushing, chills, cough, headache, pain (muscles, joints, lower abdomen, eyes), hiccups, breast tenderness. **GI:** *Nausea,* diarrhea, vomiting.

PHARMACOKINETICS Peak: After IM injection, time to peak in plasma is 30–90 mins. **Elimination:** Renal within 24 hrs.

NURSING IMPLICATIONS

Assessment & Drug Effects

- Monitor uterine contractions and observe and report excessive vaginal bleeding and cramping pain. Save all clots and tissue for physician inspection and laboratory analysis.
- Check vital signs at regular intervals. Carboprost-induced febrile reaction occurs in more than 10% of patients and must be differentiated from endometritis, which occurs around third day after abortion.

Patient & Family Education

- Report promptly onset of bleeding, foul-smelling discharge, abdominal pain, or fever.
- Since ovulation may reoccur as early as 2 wk post-abortion, you may wish to consider appropriate contraception.
- Do not breast feed while taking this drug.

CARISOPRODOL

(kar-eye-soe-proe′dole)

Rela, Soma

Classifications: AUTONOMIC NERVOUS SYSTEM AGENT; SKELETAL MUSCLE RELAXANT: CENTRAL-ACTING

Prototype: Cyclobenzaprine

Pregnancy Category: C

AVAILABILITY 350 mg tablets

ACTIONS Propanediol derivative carbamate with central depressant action pharmacologically related to meprobamate. Precise action mechanism of CNS depression is not clear. Skeletal muscle relaxant effect, unlike that of neuromuscular blocking agents, appears to be due to sedative action. Voluntary motor function is not lost, but there may be slight reduction in muscle tone leading to relief of pain and discomfort of muscle spasm.

THERAPEUTIC EFFECTS Effective spasmolytic and reduces pain associated with acute musculoskeletal disorders.

USES Skeletal muscle spasm, stiffness, and pain in a variety of musculoskeletal disorders and to relieve spasticity and rigidity in cerebral palsy.

CONTRAINDICATIONS Hypersensitivity to carisoprodol and related compounds (e.g., meprobamate, tybamate); acute intermittent porphyria; children <5 y; pregnancy (category C), lactation.
CAUTIOUS USE Impaired liver or kidney function, addiction-prone individuals.

ROUTE & DOSAGE

Muscle Spasm
Adult: **PO** 350 mg t.i.d.
Child: **PO** >5 y, 25 mg/kg/d in 4 divided doses

ADMINISTRATION

Oral
- Give with food, as needed, to reduce GI symptoms. Last dose should be taken at bedtime.
- Store in tightly closed container.

ADVERSE EFFECTS (≥1%) **Body as a Whole:** Eosinophilia, asthma, fever, anaphylactic shock. **CV:** Tachycardia, postural hypotension, facial flushing. **GI:** Nausea, vomiting, hiccups. **CNS:** *Drowsiness, dizziness,* vertigo, ataxia, tremor, headache, irritability, depressive reactions, syncope, insomnia. **Skin:** Skin rash, erythema multiforme, pruritus.

INTERACTIONS Drug: Alcohol, CNS DEPRESSANTS potentiate CNS effects.

PHARMACOKINETICS Onset: 30 min. **Duration:** 4–6 h. **Distribution:** Crosses placenta. **Metabolism:** Metabolized in liver. **Elimination:** Excreted by kidneys; excreted in breast milk (2–4 times the plasma concentrations). **Half-Life:** 8 h.

NURSING IMPLICATIONS

Assessment & Drug Effects
- Monitor for allergic or idiosyncratic reactions that generally occur from the first to the fourth dose in patients taking the drug for the first time. Symptoms usually subside after several hours; they are treated by supportive and symptomatic measures.

Patient & Family Education
- Avoid driving and other potentially hazardous activities until response to the drug has been evaluated. Drowsiness is a common side effect and may require reduction in dosage.
- Report to physician if symptoms of dizziness and faintness persist. Symptoms may be controlled by making position changes slowly and in stages.
- Do not take alcohol or other CNS depressants (effects may be additive) unless otherwise directed by physician.
- Discontinue drug and notify physician if skin rash, diplopia, dizziness, or other unusual signs or symptoms appear.
- Do not breast feed while taking this drug.

CARMUSTINE

(kar-mus'teen)
BCNU, BiCNU, Gliadel
Classifications: ANTINEOPLASTIC; ALKYLATING AGENT
Prototype: Cyclophosphamide
Pregnancy Category: D

AVAILABILITY 100 mg injection; 7.7 mg wafer

ACTIONS Highly lipid-soluble nitrosourea derivative with cell-cycle-nonspecific activity against

C

rapidly proliferating cell populations. Produces cross-linkage of DNA strands, thereby blocking DNA, RNA, and protein synthesis. Major toxic effect is bone marrow suppression.

THERAPEUTIC EFFECTS Drug metabolites thought to be responsible for antineoplastic activities. Full or partial activity against a variety of cancers resulting in reduction or stabilization of tumor size and increased survival rates.

USES As single agent or in combination with other antineoplastics in treatment of Hodgkin's disease and other lymphomas, melanoma, primary and metastatic tumors of brain, and GI tract malignancies.

UNLABELED USES Treatment of carcinomas of breast and lungs, Ewing's sarcoma, Burkitt's tumor, malignant melanoma, and topically for mycosis fungoides.

CONTRAINDICATIONS History of pulmonary function impairment; recent illness with or exposure to chickenpox or herpes zoster; infection, decreased circulating platelets, leukocytes, or erythrocytes; pregnancy (category D), lactation.

CAUTIOUS USE Hepatic and renal insufficiency; patient with previous cytotoxic medication, or radiation therapy.

ROUTE & DOSAGE

Previously Untreated Patients—Carcinoma

Adult: **IV** 150–200 mg/m^2 q6wk in one dose *or* given over 2 d

Child: **IV** 200–250 mg/m^2 q4–6wk as single dose. Doses adjusted based on hematologic parameters

Mycosis Fungoides

Adult: **Topical** 0.05–0.4% solution in 30% alcohol to paint entire body (60 mLs) or ointment 1–2 times/d for 6–8 wk (10 mg/d) (must be specially compounded)

ADMINISTRATION

Note: When administering IV to infants and children, verify correct IV concentration and rate of infusion with physician.

Intravenous

PREPARE: **IV Infusion:** Wear disposable gloves; contact of drug with skin can cause burning, dermatitis, and hyperpigmentation. Add supplied diluent to the 100 mg vial. Further dilute with 27 mL of sterile water for injection to yield a concentration of 3.3 mg/mL. Each dose is then added to 100–500 mL of D5W or NS. If possible avoid using PVC IV tubing and bags.

ADMINISTER: **IV Infusion:** Infuse a single dose over at least 1 h. Slow infusion over 1–2 h and adequate dilution will reduce pain of administration. Avoid starting infusion into dorsum of hand, wrist, or the antecubital veins; extravasation in these areas can damage underlying tendons and nerves leading to loss of mobility of entire limb.

INCOMPATIBILITIES **Solution/additive: Sodium bicarbonate. Y-site: Allopurinol.**

- Frequently check rate of flow and blood return; palpate injection site for extravasation. If there is any question about patency, line should be restarted.

- Reconstituted solutions of carmustine are clear and colorless and may be stored at 2°–8° C

(36°–46° F) for 24 h protected from light. ▪ Store unopened vials at 2°–8° C (36°–46° F), protected from light, unless otherwise directed by manufacturer. ▪ Signs of decomposition of carmustine in unopened vial: liquefaction and appearance of oil film at bottom of vial. Discard drug in this condition.

ADVERSE EFFECTS (≥1%) **Hematologic:** Delayed myelosuppression (dose-related); thrombocytopenia. **CNS:** Dizziness, ataxia. **Respiratory:** Pulmonary infiltration or fibrosis. **Skin:** Skin flushing and burning pain at injection site, hyperpigmentation of skin (from contact). **Special Senses:** (with high doses) Eye infarctions, retinal hemorrhage, suffusion of conjunctiva. **GI:** Stomatitis, *nausea, vomiting*.

INTERACTIONS Drug: Cimetidine may potentiate neutropenia and thrombocytopenia.

PHARMACOKINETICS Distribution: Readily crosses blood–brain barrier; CSF concentrations 15–70% of plasma concentrations. **Metabolism:** Rapidly metabolized; metabolic fate not completely known. **Elimination:** 60–70% excreted in urine in 96 h; 6% excreted through lungs, 1% in feces; excreted in breast milk.

NURSING IMPLICATIONS

Assessment & Drug Effects

- Monitor for nausea and vomiting (dose related), which may occur within 2 h after drug administration and persist for up to 6 h. Prior administration of an antiemetic may help to decrease or prevent these adverse effects.
- Lab tests: Baseline CBC with differential and platelet count, repeat blood studies following infusion at weekly intervals for at least 6 wk. Baseline and periodic tests of hepatic and renal function.
- Platelet nadir usually occurs within 4–5 wk, and leukocyte nadir within 5–6 wk after therapy is terminated. Thrombocytopenia may be more severe than leukopenia; anemia is less severe.
- Check temperature daily. Avoid use of rectal thermometer to prevent injury to mucosa. An elevation of 0.6° F or more above usual temperature warrants reporting.
- Report symptoms of lung toxicity (cough, shortness of breath, fever) to the physician immediately.
- Be alert to signs of hepatic toxicity (jaundice, dark urine, pruritus, light-colored stools) and renal insufficiency (dysuria, oliguria, hematuria, swelling of lower legs and feet).

Patient & Family Education

- Report burning sensation immediately, as carmustine can cause burning discomfort even in the absence of extravasation. Infusion will be discontinued and restarted in another site. Ice application over the area may decrease the discomfort.
- Intense flushing of skin may occur during IV infusion. This usually disappears in 2–4 h.
- You will be highly susceptible to infection and to hemorrhagic disorders. Be alert to hazardous periods that occur 4–6 wk after a dose of carmustine. If possible, avoid invasive procedures (e.g., IM injections, enemas, rectal temperatures) during this period.
- Report promptly the onset of sore throat, weakness, fever, chills, infection of any kind, or abnormal bleeding (ecchymosis, petechiae, epistaxis, bleeding gums, hematemesis, melena).

C

■ Do not breast feed while taking this drug.

CARTEOLOL HYDROCHLORIDE

(car'tee-oh-lole)

Cartrol, Ocupress

Classifications: AUTONOMIC NERVOUS SYSTEM AGENT; BETA-ADRENERGIC ANTAGONIST (BLOCKING AGENT, SYMPATHOLYTIC); ANTIHYPERTENSIVE

Prototype: Propranolol

Pregnancy Category: C

AVAILABILITY 2.5 mg, 5 mg tablets; 1% solution

ACTIONS Carteolol is a beta-adrenergic blocking agent (antagonist) that competes for available beta receptor sites. It inhibits both $beta_1$ receptors (chiefly in cardiac muscle) and $beta_2$ receptors (chiefly in the bronchial and vascular musculature). It decreases standing and supine hypertension.

THERAPEUTIC EFFECTS Effective antihypertensive agent by reducing BP to normotensive range and useful in mananging some angina, dysrhythmias, and CHF by decreasing myocardial oxygen demand and lowering cardiac work load.

USES For hypertension, either alone or in combination with other drugs, particularly a thiazide diuretic (not indicated for hypertensive crisis); chronic open-angle glaucoma.

UNLABELED USES To reduce the frequency of anginal attacks.

CONTRAINDICATIONS Sinus bradycardia, greater than first-degree heart block, cardiogenic shock, CHF secondary to tachycardia treatable with beta-blockers, overt cardiac failure, hypersensitivity to beta-blocking agents, persistent severe bradycardia, bronchial asthma or bronchospasm, and severe COPD; pregnancy (category C).

CAUTIOUS USE CHF patients treated with digitalis and diuretics, peripheral vascular disease; diabetes, hypoglycemia, thyrotoxicosis; lactation.

ROUTE & DOSAGE

Hypertension

Adult: **PO** 2.5 mg once/d, may increase to 5–10 mg if needed (max: 10 mg/d)

Open-Angle Glaucoma

Adult: **Ophthalmic** 1 drop in affected eye b.i.d.

ADMINISTRATION

Oral

- Consult physician if patient's creatinine clearance is below normal. Dosage adjustment may be needed.
- Administer capsule or tablet whole. Do not crush or break and instruct patient not to chew before swallowing.
- Store away from heat, light, or moisture.

ADVERSE EFFECTS (≥1%) **Body as a Whole:** Rash, muscle cramps, bronchospasm. **CV:** Increased angina, hypotension, CHF, bradycardia. **GI:** Abdominal pain, diarrhea, nausea. **Endocrine:** Hyperglycemia. **CNS:** *Headache, dizziness,* drowsiness, insomnia, anxiety, tremor, paresthesia, weakness.

INTERACTIONS Drug: DIURETICS and other HYPOTENSIVE AGENTS increase hypotensive effect; carteolol and **albuterol, metoproterenol, terbutaline, pirbuterol** are mutually antagonistic; NSAIDS may blunt hypotensive effect; decreases hypoglycemic effect of **glyburide;** may increase bradycardia and sinus arrest with **amiodarone.**

PHARMACOKINETICS Absorption: Readily absorbed from GI tract; 85% reaches systemic circulation. **Peak:** 1–3 h. **Duration:** 24–48 h. **Distribution:** Crosses placenta; distributed into breast milk. **Metabolism:** Metabolized in liver to active metabolite. **Elimination:** Excreted primarily in urine. **Half-Life:** 4–6 h.

NURSING IMPLICATIONS

Assessment & Drug Effects

- Assess heart rate prior to administration. If pulse is less than 50 bpm, withhold drug and notify physician.
- Monitor BP and pulse frequently during period of adjustment and periodically throughout therapy.
- If hypotension (systolic BP <90 mm Hg) occurs, discontinue the drug and carefully assess the hemodynamic status of the patient.
- Monitor daily weight and assess for evidence of fluid overload since drug may precipitate CHF (see Signs & Symptoms, Appendix F).
- Monitor mental status. Mental depression may be increased by use of this drug.
- Assess respiratory status closely if the patient has history of bronchitis or emphysema, assess for respiratory difficulty.
- Monitor diabetic for loss of diabetic control. Drug may prevent the appearance of early S&S of acute hypoglycemia (see Appendix F).
- Drug may reduce tolerance to cold temperatures in older adults or in those who have circulatory problems.

Patient & Family Education

- Report the first sign or symptom of impending CHF (see Signs & Symptoms, Appendix F) or unexplained respiratory symptoms.
- Do not discontinue medication abruptly, since sudden withdrawal may precipitate or exacerbate angina.
- Do not use any OTC products such as nasal decongestants and cold preparations without consultation.
- Report slow pulse rate, confusion or depression, dizziness or lightheadedness, skin rash, fever, sore throat, or unusual bleeding or bruising.
- Be cautious while driving or performing other hazardous activities until response to drug is known.
- Continue to take this medication as instructed by your physician no matter how well you feel.
- Take your BP at least twice a week and report significant changes.
- Take your pulse before and after taking the medication. If it is much slower than normal rate (or less than 50 bpm), check with your physician.
- Do not breast feed while taking this drug without consulting physician.

CARVEDILOL

(car-ve-di'lol)

Coreg, Kredex ♣

Classifications: AUTONOMIC NERVOUS SYSTEM AGENT; ALPHA- AND BETA-ADRENERGIC ANTAGONIST; ANTIHYPERTENSIVE

Prototype: Propanolol HCl

Pregnancy Category: C

AVAILABILITY 3.125 mg, 6.25 mg, 12.5 mg, 25 mg tablets

ACTIONS Adrenergic receptor blocking agent that combines selective alpha activity and nonselective beta-adrenergic blocking actions. Both activities contribute to blood pressure reduction. Peripheral vasodilatation and, therefore, decreased peripheral resistance results from $alpha_1$-blocking activity of Coreg. It is 3–5 times more potent than labetalol in lowering blood pressure.

THERAPEUTIC EFFECTS An effective antihypertensive agent reducing BP to normotensive range and useful in managing some angina, dysrhythmias, and CHF by decreasing myocardial oxygen demand and lowering cardiac work load.

USES Management of essential hypertension, CHF, in conjunction with other heart failure medications.

CONTRAINDICATIONS Patients with class IV decompensated cardiac failure, bronchial asthma, or related bronchospastic conditions (e.g., chronic bronchitis and emphysema), second- and third-degree AV block, cardiogenic shock or severe bradycardia; pregnancy (category C), lactation.

CAUTIOUS USE Patients on MAOI agents, diabetes, hypoglycemia; patients at high risk for anaphylactic reaction, peripheral vascular disease, hepatic impairment. Safety and efficacy in patients <18 y of age have not been established.

ROUTE & DOSAGE

CHF

Adult: **PO** Start with 3.125 mg b.i.d. times 2 wk, may double dose q2wk as tolerated up to 25 mg b.i.d. if <85 kg *or* 50 mg b.i.d. if >85 kg

Hypertension

Adult: **PO** Start with 6.25 mg b.i.d., may increase by 6.25 mg b.i.d. to max of 50 mg/d

ADMINISTRATION

Oral

- Give with food to slow absorption and minimize risk of orthostatic hypotension.
- Dose increments should be made at 7- to 14-day intervals.

ADVERSE EFFECTS (≥1%) **Body as a Whole:** Increased sweating, fatigue, chest pain, pain, arthralgia. **CV:** Bradycardia, hypotension, syncope, hypertension, AV block, angina. **GI:** Diarrhea, nausea, abdominal pain, vomiting. **Respiratory:** Sinusitis, bronchitis. **Hematologic:** Thrombocytopenia, **Metabolic:** Hyperglycemia, weight increase, gout. **CNS:** *Dizziness,* headache, paresthesias.

INTERACTIONS Drug: Rifampin significantly decreases **carvedilol** levels; **cimetidine** may increase **carvedilol** levels; **clonidine, reserpine,** MAO INHIBITORS may cause hypotension or bradycardia; **carvedilol** may increase **digoxin** levels and may enhance hypoglycemic effects of **insulin** and ORAL HYPOGLYCEMIC AGENTS.

PHARMACOKINETICS Absorption: Rapidly absorbed from GI tract, 25–35% reaches the systemic circulation. **Peak:** Antihypertensive effect 7–14 d. **Distribution:** >98% protein bound. **Metabolism:** Metabolized in the liver by CYP2D6 and CYP2C9 enzymes. **Elimination:** Primarily eliminated via the bile through the feces. **Half-Life:** 7–10 h.

C

NURSING IMPLICATIONS

Assessment & Drug Effects

- Monitor for therapeutic effectiveness which is indicated by lessening of S&S of CHF and improved BP control.
- Lab tests: Monitor liver function tests periodically; at first sign of hepatic toxicity (see Appendix F) stop drug and notify physician.
- Monitor for worsening of symptoms in patients with PVD.
- Monitor digoxin levels with concurrent use; plasma digoxin concentration may increase.

Patient & Family Education

- Do not abruptly discontinue taking this drug.
- You may experience dizziness or faintness, as a risk of orthostatic hypotension.
- Do not engage in hazardous activities while experiencing dizziness.
- If you have diabetes, the drug may increase effects of hypoglycemic drugs and mask S&S of hypoglycemia.
- Do not breast feed while taking this drug.

CASCARA SAGRADA

(kas-kar'a)

Cascara Sagrada Aromatic Fluid-extract, Cascara Sagrada Fluidextract

Classifications: GASTROINTESTINAL AGENT; STIMULANT, LAXATIVE

Prototype: Bisacodyl

Pregnancy Category: C

AVAILABILITY 325 mg tablets; liquid

ACTIONS Anthraquinone derivative obtained from bark of buckhorn tree (*Rhamnus purshiana*). Acts principally in large intestine by stimulating propulsive movements of colon through direct chemical irritation. Casanthrol, which is present in a variety of OTC mixtures, is a derivative of cascara sagrada.

THERAPEUTIC EFFECTS Effective laxative with results in 6–12 hrs. Useful in conditions where straining at stool is to be avoided.

USES Temporary relief of constipation and to prevent straining at stool in various disease conditions. Sometimes used with milk of magnesia.

CONTRAINDICATIONS Abdominal pain, fecal impaction; GI bleeding, ulcerations; appendicitis, gastroenteritis, intestinal obstruction, CHF; pregnancy (category C).

CAUTIOUS USE Lactation; renal impairment; diabetic patients; rectal bleeding; concomitant laxative use.

ROUTE & DOSAGE

Laxative

Adult: **PO** Tablet: 325–1000 mg/d; fluid extract: 0.5–1.5 mL/d; aromatic fluid extract: 2–6 mL/d
Child: **PO** *2–12 y:* 1/2 of adult dose; *<2 y:* 1/4 of adult dose
Infant: **PO** Aromatic fluid extract: 1.25 mL/d as single dose

ADMINISTRATION

Oral

- Administer with a full glass of water on an empty stomach for best results. Results may be delayed somewhat by food.
- Store in tightly covered, light-resistant containers, unless otherwise directed by manufacturer.

ADVERSE EFFECTS (≥1%) **GI:** Anorexia, nausea, gripping, abnormally loose stools, constipation

C

rebound, melanosis of colon. **Metabolic:** Hypokalemia, impaired glucose tolerance, calcium deficiency, **Urogenital:** Discoloration of urine.

DIAGNOSTIC TEST INTERFERENCE Possibility of interference with ***PSP excretion test*** because of urine discoloration.

INTERACTIONS Drug: Decreased effect of ORAL ANTICOAGULANTS.

PHARMACOKINETICS Absorption: Minimal absorption from GI tract. **Onset:** 6–12 h. **Metabolism:** Metabolized in liver. **Elimination:** Eliminated in feces and urine; excreted in breast milk.

NURSING IMPLICATIONS

Assessment & Drug Effects

- Monitor electrolyte balance if significant diarrhea occurs, especially with frail older adults.
- Monitor restoration of normal bowel function.

Patient & Family Education

- A single dose taken before retiring usually results in evacuation of soft stool 6–12 h later.
- Frequent or prolonged use of irritant cathartics disrupts normal reflex activity of colon and rectum and can lead to drug dependence for evacuation.
- See bisacodyl for additional information.

CASPOFUNGIN ACETATE

(cas-po-fung'in)

Cancidas

Classifications: ANTIINFECTIVE; ANTIBIOTIC; ANTIFUNGAL

Prototype: Amphotericin B

Pregnancy Category: C

AVAILABILITY 50 mg, 70 mg vials

ACTIONS Inhibits synthesis of an essential component of the cell wall of many filamentous fungi.

THERAPEUTIC EFFECTS Interferes with reproduction and growth of susceptible fungi.

USES Treatment of invasive *Aspergillosis* in patients refractory to other antifungal therapies; empiric therapy for presumed fungal infection in febrile neutropenic patients.

UNLABELED USES Other fungal infections due to *Candida sp.*

CONTRAINDICATIONS Hypersensitivity to caspofungin acetate.

CAUTIOUS USE Concomitant use of cyclosporine; impaired liver function; jaundice, hepatic disease, lactation. Safety and efficacy in children are not established.

ROUTE & DOSAGE

Aspergillosis Infections

Adult: **IV Loading Dose** 70 mg infused over 1 h on day 1 **IV Maintenance Dose** 50 mg infused over 1 h q.d. times approximately 30 d depending on infection

ADMINISTRATION

Note: Dosage reductions are recommended with moderate hepatic insufficiency (35 mg/d maintenance dose), and concomitant use with cyclosporine is not recommended.

Intravenous

PREPARE: **IV Loading Dose:** For 70 mg dose—When using one 70 mg vial, bring refrigerated vial to room temperature, then add 10.5 mL NS to vial and mix gently to dissolve. Transfer 10 mL reconstituted solution to a 250 mL NS IV solution. When using two 50 mg vials, bring refrigerated vials to room temperature then add 10.5 mL NS to each vial and mix gently to dissolve. Transfer a total of 14 mL reconstituted solution to a 250 mL NS IV solution. **IV Maintenance Dose:** For 50 mg dose—Bring refrigerated 50 mg vial to room temperature then add 10.5 mL NS to vial and mix gently to dissolve. Transfer 10 mL reconstituted solution to a 250 mL NS IV solution (or 100 mL if reduced volume is medically necessary). For 35 mg dose—Reconstitute the 50 mg vial as for the 50 mg infusion, however, transfer only 7 mL of reconstituted solution to a 250 mL NS IV solution (or 100 mL if reduced volume is medically necessary).

ADMINISTER: **IV Loading & Maintenance Doses:** Give slowly over at least 1 h. Do NOT mix with or add to dextrose infusions.

INCOMPATIBILITIES **Solution/additive: Dextrose**-containing solutions. Do not mix or co-infuse with other medications.

- Store unopened vials at 2°–4° C (34°–46° F). Store IV solution for 24 h at ≤25° C (≤77° F).

ADVERSE EFFECTS (≥1%) **Body as a Whole:** Flushing, edema, facial edema, myalgia, back pain, asthenia, fatigue, *fever,* chills, flu-like symptoms, malaise, pain, warm sensation, <u>anaphylaxis</u>. **CNS:** Headache, insomnia, paresthesia, tremor. **CV:** *Phlebitis/thrombophlebitis from infusion,* tachycardia, vasculitis. **GI:** Nausea, vomiting, abdominal pain, anorexia, diarrhea, *increased AST, ALT.* **Hematologic:** Eosinophilia, anemia, neutropenia, thrombocytopenia, increased prothrombin time. **Metabolic:** Hypokalemia. **Respiratory:** Tachypnea. **Skin:** Erythema, induration, pruritus, rash, sweating.

INTERACTIONS Drug: May decrease **tacrolimus** levels; **cyclosporine** increased caspofungin levels; **carbamazepine, dexamethasone, efavirenz, nelfinavir, nevirapine, phenytoin, rifampin** may decrease caspofungin levels.

PHARMACOKINETICS Distribution: Extensively distributes into tissues. **Metabolism:** Slowly hydrolyzed in plasma. **Elimination:** Equally excreted in urine and feces. **Half-Life:** Initial 9–11 h, 40–50 h after distribution to tissues.

NURSING IMPLICATIONS

Assessment & Drug Effects

- Monitor for S&S of respiratory distress; interrupt or withhold drug and notify physician immediately.
- Monitor for S&S of hypersensitivity, phlebitis or thrombophlebitis.
- Lab tests: Baseline and periodic ALT/AST, CBC with differential, platelet count, PT, urinalysis, serum albumin, serum alkaline phosphatase, serum potassium, and serum creatinine.

Patient & Family Education

- Report any of the following to a health care provider: Shortness of breath, facial swelling, itching, or an unusual sense of warmth.
- Do not breast feed while taking this drug without consulting physician.

CEFACLOR

(sef'a-klor)

Ceclor, Ceclor CD

Classifications: ANTIINFECTIVE; ANTIBIOTIC; SECOND-GENERATION CEPHALOSPORIN

Prototype: Cefonicid sodium

Pregnancy Category: B

AVAILABILITY 250 mg, 500 mg tablets; 375 mg, 500 mg sustained-release tablets; 125 mg/5 mL, 187 mg/5 mL, 250 mg/5 mL, 375 mg/5 mL suspension

ACTIONS Semisynthetic, second-generation oral cephalosporin antibiotic similar to cefonicid. Possibly more active than other oral cephalosporins against gram-negative bacilli, especially beta-lactamase-producing *Haemophilus influenzae*, including ampicillin-resistant strains. Also active against *Escherichia coli, Proteus mirabilis, Klebsiella sp* and certain gram-positive strains, e.g., *Streptococcus pneumoniae, S. pyogenes,* and *Staphylococcus aureus*. Preferentially binds to one or more of the penicillin-binding proteins (PBPs) located on cell walls of susceptible organisms. This inhibits third and final stage of bacterial cell wall synthesis, thus killing the bacterium.

THERAPEUTIC EFFECTS Effective in treating acute otitis media and acute sinusitis where the causative agent is resistant to other antibiotics. Useful in treating gonorrhea, respiratory and urinary tract infections. Partial cross-allergenicity between penicillins and cephalosporins has been reported.

USES Treatment of otitis media and infections of upper and lower respiratory tract, urinary tract, and skin and skin structures caused by ampicillin-resistant *H. influenzae;* acute uncomplicated UTI.

CONTRAINDICATIONS Hypersensitivity to cephalosporins and related antibiotics; pregnancy (category B), lactation. Safe use in infants <1 mo not established.

CAUTIOUS USE History of sensitivity to penicillins or other drug allergies; markedly impaired renal function.

ROUTE & DOSAGE

Mild to Moderate Infections
Adult: **PO** 250–500 mg q8h, or Ceclor CD 250–500 mg/q12h
Child >1 mo: **PO** 20–40 mg/kg/d divided q8h (max: 2 g/d)

ADMINISTRATION

Oral

- Give sustained-release tablets with food to enhance absorption. Food does not affect absorption of capsules.
- Ensure that sustained-release tablets are not chewed or crushed. They must be swallowed whole.
- After stock oral suspension is prepared, it should be kept refrigerated. Expiration date should appear on label. Discard unused portion after 14 d. Shake well before pouring.
- Store pulvules in tightly closed container unless otherwise directed.

ADVERSE EFFECTS (≥1%) **Body as a Whole:** Serum sickness-like reaction, eosinophilia, joint pain or swelling, fever, superinfections. **GI:** *Diarrhea,* nausea, vomiting, anorexia, <u>pseudomembranous colitis</u> (rare). **Skin:** Urticaria, pruritus, morbilliform eruptions.

DIAGNOSTIC TEST INTERFERENCE Cefaclor may produce positive ***direct Coombs' test,*** which can complicate ***cross-matching procedures*** and ***hematologic studies.*** False-positive ***urine glucose*** determinations may result with use of ***copper sulfate reduction methods,*** e.g., ***Clinitest*** or ***Benedict's reagent,*** but not with ***glucose oxidase*** (enzymatic) ***tests*** such as ***Clinistix, Diastix, Tes-Tape.***

INTERACTIONS Drug: Probenecid decreases renal excretion of cefaclor.

PHARMACOKINETICS Absorption: Well absorbed; acid stable. **Peak:** 30–60 min. **Elimination:** 60% of dose eliminated renally in 8 h; crosses placenta; excreted in breast milk. **Half-Life:** 0.5–1 h.

NURSING IMPLICATIONS

Assessment & Drug Effects

- Determine previous hypersensitivity to cephalosporins, penicillins, and other drug allergies before therapy is initiated.
- Lab tests: Perform culture and sensitivity tests prior to and periodically during therapy.
- Diarrhea, the most frequent adverse effect, may be due to a pharmacologic effect or to associated change in intestinal flora. If it persists, interruption of therapy may be necessary.
- Monitor for manifestations of drug hypersensitivity (see Appendix F). Discontinue drug and promptly report them if they appear.
- Monitor for manifestations of superinfection (see Appendix F). Promptly report their appearance.

Patient & Family Education

- Report promptly any signs or symptoms of superinfection (see Appendix F).
- Yogurt or buttermilk (if allowed) may serve as a prophylactic against intestinal superinfections by helping to maintain normal intestinal flora.
- Take your medication for the full course of therapy as directed by physician.
- Do not breast feed while taking this drug.

CEFADROXIL

(sef-a-drox'ill)

Duricef, Ultracef

Classifications: ANTIINFECTIVE; ANTIBIOTIC; FIRST-GENERATION CEPHALOSPORIN

Prototype: Cefazolin

Pregnancy Category: B

AVAILABILITY 500 mg capsules; 1 g tablets; 125 mg/5 mL, 250 mg/5 mL, 500 mg/5 mL suspension

ACTIONS Semisynthetic, first-generation cephalosporin antibiotic with antibacterial spectrum similar to that of cefazolin. Bactericidal action (similar to that of penicillins): drug penetrates bacterial cell wall, resists beta-lactamases and inactivates enzymes essential to cell wall synthesis. At equivalent doses, reportedly attains greater concentrations in serum and urine than other oral cephalosporins.

THERAPEUTIC EFFECTS Active against organisms that liberate cephalosporinase and penicillinase (beta-lactamases). According to clinical and laboratory evidence, partial cross-allergenicity exists between penicillins and cephalosporins. Effective in reducing signs and symptoms of urinary tract infections, bone and joint infections, skin and soft tissue infections, and pharyngitis.

USES Primarily in treatment of urinary tract infections caused by *Escherichia coli, Proteus mirabilis,* and *Klebsiella sp;* infections of skin and skin structures caused by *Staphylococci* and *Streptococci;* and for treatment of *Group A beta-Hemolytic Streptococcal* pharyngitis and tonsillitis.

CONTRAINDICATIONS Hypersensitivity to cephalosporins and related antibiotics; pregnancy (category B), lactation.

CAUTIOUS USE Sensitivity to penicillins or other drug allergies; impaired renal function, history of colitis.

ROUTE & DOSAGE

Uncomplicated Urinary Tract Infection

Adult: **PO** 1–2 g/d in 1–2 divided doses
Child: **PO** 30 mg/kg/d in 2 divided doses

Skin and Skin Structure Infections, Streptococcal Pharyngitis, or Tonsillitis

Adult: **PO** 1 g/d in 1–2 divided doses
Child: **PO** 30 mg/kg/d in 2 divided doses

Adjustment for Renal Impairment

Cl_{cr} <25 mL/min
Adult: **PO** 1 g q24h
Child: **PO** 15 mg/kg q24h

ADMINISTRATION

Oral

- Give with food or milk to reduce nausea. If nausea persists, termination of therapy may be necessary.
- Follow directions for mixing oral suspension found on drug label. Reconstituted solution contains 125 mg or 250 mg cefadroxil per 5 mL suspension.
- Shake suspension well before use; discard after 14 d.
- Store in tight container unless otherwise directed. Oral suspensions are stable for 14 d under refrigeration at 2°–8° C (36°–46° F). Avoid freezing. Note expiration date on label.

ADVERSE EFFECTS (≥1%) **Body as a Whole:** Hypersensitivity [Rash, swollen eyelids (angioedema)], pruritus, chills), superinfections. **GI:** Nausea, *diarrhea,* vomiting, heartburn, gastritis, bloating, abdominal cramps.

DIAGNOSTIC TEST INTERFERENCE False-positive ***urine glucose*** determinations using ***copper sulfate reduction reagents,*** such as ***Clinitest*** or ***Benedict's reagent,*** but not with ***glucose oxidase tests,*** e.g., ***Clinistix, Diastix, TesTape. Cefadroxil-induced positive direct Coombs' test*** may interfere with ***cross-matching procedures*** and ***hematologic studies.***

INTERACTIONS Drug: Probenecid decreases renal excretion of cefadroxil.

PHARMACOKINETICS Absorption: Acid stable; rapidly absorbed from GI tract. **Peak:** 1 h. **Elimination:** 90% excreted unchanged in urine within 8 h; bacterial inhibitory levels persist 20–22 h; crosses placenta; excreted in breast milk. **Half-Life:** 1–12 h.

NURSING IMPLICATIONS

Assessment & Drug Effects

- Determine previous hypersensitivity to cephalosporins, penicillins, and other drug allergies, before therapy is initiated.
- Lab tests: Perform culture and sensitivity testing prior to and periodically during therapy.
- Lab tests: Perform baseline and periodic renal function studies in patients with renal function impairment, and monitor I&O ratio and pattern.
- Monitor for manifestations of drug hypersensitivity (see Signs & Symptoms, Appendix F). Discontinue drug and promptly report them if they appear.
- Monitor for manifestations of superinfection (see Signs & Symptoms, Appendix F). Promptly report their appearance.

Patient & Family Education

- Report promptly the onset of rash, urticaria, pruritus, or fever,

as the possibility of an allergic reaction is high, if you are allergic to penicillin.
- Take medication for the full course of therapy as directed by your physician.
- Report promptly S&S of superinfections (see Appendix F).
- Do not breast feed while taking this drug.

CEFAMANDOLE NAFATE

(sef-a-man′dole)

Mandol

Classifications: ANTIINFECTIVE; ANTIBIOTIC; SECOND-GENERATION CEPHALOSPORIN

Prototype: Cefonicid sodium

Pregnancy Category: B

AVAILABILITY 1 g, 2 g injection

ACTIONS Semisynthetic, second-generation cephalosporin antibiotic similar to other drugs of this class. Preferentially binds to one or more of the penicillin-binding proteins (PBP) located on cell walls of susceptible organisms. This inhibits third and final stage of bacterial wall synthesis, thus killing the bacterium.

THERAPEUTIC EFFECTS Usually active against organisms susceptible to first generation cephalosporins. In addition, it is active against the anaerobes *Clostridium sp, Peptococcus sp, Fusobacterium sp;* and against some strains of *Providencia sp, Enterobacter, Serratia, Proteus, E. coli,* and *Klebsiella* resistant to first generation cephalosporins. Inactive against *Enterococci,* methicillin-resistant *Staphylococci* (MRSA), *Listeria monocytogenes* and *Pseudomonas.* Partial cross-allergenicity between penicillins and cephalosporins has been reported. Effective treatment for bone and joint infections, lower respiratory tract infections, peritonitis, urinary tract infections and surgical prophylaxis.

USES Serious infections of respiratory, genitourinary, and biliary tracts, skin and soft tissue, bones and joints, and in septicemia and peritonitis (caused by *E. coli* and other coliform microbes); also perioperative prophylaxis to reduce infections in patient undergoing potentially contaminated procedure.

CONTRAINDICATIONS Hypersensitivity to cephalosporins and related antibiotics; pregnancy (category B), lactation. Safe use in children between 1 and 6 mo not established.

CAUTIOUS USE History of sensitivity to penicillins or other drug allergies; renal function impairment; history of GI disease, particularly colitis.

ROUTE & DOSAGE

Moderate to Severe Infections

Adult: **IV/IM** 500 mg–1 g q4–8h, up to 2 g q4h

Child: **IV/IM** 50–100 mg/kg/d in 3–6 divided doses, up to 150 mg/kg/d (not to exceed adult doses)

Surgical Prophylaxis

Adult: **IV/IM** 1–2 g 30–60 min before surgery, then q6h for 24 h

Child: **IV/IM** 50–100 mg/kg 30–60 min before surgery, then q6h for 24 h

ADMINISTRATION

Intramuscular
- To each gram of cefamandole add 3 mL of sterile water for injection or bacteriostatic water for injection, or NS, or D5W. Resulting solution contains 285 mg/mL. Administer IM deep into a large muscle mass such as gluteus maximus or lateral thigh.

Intravenous

PREPARE: **Direct:** Reconstitute each gram with 10 mL sterile water for injection, D5W, or NS. **Intermittent/Continuous:** May be further diluted in 100–1000 mL of D5W or NS.

ADMINISTER: **Direct:** Give slowly over 3–5 min. **Intermittent/Continuous:** The rate of infusion is determined by the amount of solution and status of patient.

INCOMPATIBILITIES **Solution/additive: Ringer's lactate, calcium gluconate, calcium gluceptate, cimetidine,** AMINOGLYCOSIDES, **metronidazole, magnesium, ranitidine. Y-site:** AMINOGLYCOSIDES, **amiodarone, hetastarch.**

- Prolonged exposure to light causes cefamandole powder to discolor. Once reconstituted, cefamandole is no longer light sensitive. Solutions appear light yellow to amber. Do not use if otherwise colored or if a precipitate is present.
- After reconstitution, cefamandole may liberate CO_2. Do not store medication in syringes, as pressure build-up from CO_2 may force plunger out of barrel.

- Protect from light. Reconstituted drug remains stable at room temperature for 24 h and when refrigerated at 5° C (41° F), for 96 h.

ADVERSE EFFECTS (≥1%) **Body as a Whole:** Drug fever, eosinophilia, pain, redness and induration, sterile abscess at injection site, superinfections. **GI:** Abdominal cramps, *diarrhea,* <u>pseudomembranous colitis</u>. **Hematologic:** Hypoprothrombinemia (vitamin K deficiency). **Skin:** Rash, urticaria.

DIAGNOSTIC TEST INTERFERENCE False-positive ***urine glucose*** determinations using ***copper sulfate reduction methods,*** e.g., ***Clinitest*** or ***Benedict's reagent,*** but not with ***glucose oxidase*** (enzymatic) ***tests*** such as ***Clinistix, Diastix, Tes-Tape.*** Cefamandole-induced positive ***direct Coombs' test*** may interfere with ***cross-matching procedures*** and ***hematologic studies.***

INTERACTIONS Drug: Probenecid decreases renal elimination of cefamandole; **alcohol** causes disulfiram reaction.

PHARMACOKINETICS Peak: 0.5–2 h after IM; 10 min after IV. **Distribution:** Poor CNS penetration even with inflamed meninges; extensive enterohepatic circulation; high concentrations in bile. **Metabolism:** Rapidly hydrolyzed in plasma to active metabolite. **Elimination:** 68–85% excreted unchanged in urine in 6–8 h. **Half-Life:** 30–120 min.

NURSING IMPLICATIONS

Assessment & Drug Effects

- Determine previous hypersensitivity to cephalosporins, penicillins, and other drugs prior to initiating therapy.
- Lab tests: Perform culture and sensitivity testing prior to and periodically during therapy. Cefamandole therapy may be instituted pending test results. Baseline and periodic studies of renal function and PT determinations should be performed.
- Monitor I&O rates and pattern: Particularly important in patients with impaired renal function, patients >50 y, or patients who are receiving high doses.
- Antibiotic-associated pseudomembranous enterocolitis (life-threatening) is a superinfection caused by *Clostridia difficile* and may occur in 4–9 d or as long as 6 wk after cefamandole is discontinued (see Signs & Symptoms, Appendix F). Most likely to occur in the chroni-

cally ill or debilitated older adult patient, especially if undergoing abdominal surgery or if in an ICU.

Patient & Family Education

- Check for fever if you have diarrhea and report fever and diarrhea to your physician.
- If you experience any signs or symptoms of hypersensitivity (see Appendix F), discontinue your drug and consult with your physician.
- Avoid use of alcohol during and for 48–72 h after taking cefamandole. A drug-induced disulfiram-like reaction (see Appendix F) may follow alcohol intake.
- Report promptly any signs or symptoms of superinfection (see Appendix F). Superinfections may occur, particularly during prolonged use of cephalosporins.
- Yogurt or buttermilk, 120 mL (4 oz) of either (if allowed), may serve as a prophylactic against intestinal superinfection by helping to maintain normal intestinal flora.
- Do not breast feed while taking this drug.

CEFAZOLIN SODIUM (Pr)

(sef-a′zoe-lin)

Ancef, Kefzol, Zolicef

Classifications: ANTIINFECTIVE; ANTIBIOTIC; FIRST-GENERATION CEPHALOSPORIN

Pregnancy Category: B

AVAILABILITY 250 mg, 500 mg, 1 g, injection

ACTIONS Semisynthetic, first-generation derivative of cephalosporin C; antibiotic activity similar to that of cefazolin. Activity against gram-negative organisms is limited. Bactericidal action: preferentially binds to one or more of the penicillin-binding proteins (PBP) located on cell walls of susceptible organisms. This inhibits third and final stage of bacterial cell wall synthesis, thus killing the bacterium.

THERAPEUTIC EFFECTS Effective treatment for bone and joint infections, biliary tract infections, enocarditis prophylaxis and treatment, respiratory tract and genital tract infections, septicemia and skin infections, and surgical prophylaxis.

USES Severe infections of urinary and biliary tracts, skin, soft tissue, and bone, and for bacteremia and endocarditis caused by susceptible organisms; also perioperative prophylaxis in patients undergoing procedures associated with high risk of infection, e.g., open heart surgery.

CONTRAINDICATIONS Hypersensitivity to any cephalosporin and related antibiotics; pregnancy (category B), lactation.

CAUTIOUS USE History of penicillin sensitivity, impaired renal function, patients on sodium restriction.

ROUTE & DOSAGE

Moderate to Severe Infections

Adult: **IV/IM** 250 mg–2 g q8h, up to 2 g q4h (max: 12 g/d)
Child: **IV/IM** 25–100 mg/kg/d in 3–4 divided doses, up to 100 mg/kg/d (not to exceed adult doses)
Neonate: **IV** = 7 d: 40 mg/kg/d divided q12h; >7 d: 40–60 mg/kg/d divided q8–12h

Adjustment for Renal Impairment

Cl_{cr} <35 mL/min: dose q12h

Surgical Prophylaxis

Adult: **IV/IM** 1–2 g 30–60 min before surgery, then q8h for 24 h
Child: **IV/IM** 25–50 mg/kg 30–60 min before surgery, then q8h for 24 h

C

ADMINISTRATION

Intramuscular

- Preparation of IM solution: Reconstitute with sterile water for injection, bacteriostatic water for injection, or 0.9% sodium chloride injection. Reconstituted solutions are stable for 24 hr at room temperature and for 96 hr refrigerated.
- IM injections should be made deep into large muscle mass. Pain on injection is usually minimal. Rotate injection sites.

Intravenous

- IV administration to neonates, infants, and children: Verify correct IV concentration and rate of infusion with physician.

PREPARE: **Direct:** Dilute each 1 g with 10 mL of sterile water for injection. **Intermittent:** Further dilute with 50–100 mL of NS or D5W.

ADMINISTER: **Direct/Intermittent:** Infuse 1 g over 5 min or longer as determined by the amount of solution. The risk of IV site reactions may be reduced by proper dilution of IV solution, use of small bore IV needle in a large vein, and by rotating injection sites.

INCOMPATIBILITIES **Solution/additive:** AMINOGLYCOSIDES, **ascorbic acid, atracurium, bleomycin, cimetidine, hydromorphone, lidocaine, ranididine, vitamin B complex with C. Y-site: Amiodarone,** AMINOGLYCOSIDES, **amphotericin B cholesteryl complex, idarubicin, pentamidine, vinorelbine.**

ADVERSE EFFECTS (≥1%) **Body as a Whole:** Anaphylaxis, fever, eosinophilia, superinfections, seizure (high doses in patients with renal insufficiency). **GI:** *Diarrhea,* anorexia, abdominal cramps. **Skin:** Maculopapular rash, urticaria.

DIAGNOSTIC TEST INTERFERENCE Because of cefazolin effect on the ***direct Coombs' test,*** transfusion ***cross-matching procedures*** and ***hematologic studies*** may be complicated. False-positive ***urine glucose*** determinations are possible with use of ***copper sulfate tests*** (e.g., ***Clinitest*** or ***Benedict's reagent***) but not with ***glucose oxidase tests*** such as ***TesTape, Diastix,*** or ***Clinistix.***

INTERACTIONS Drug: Probenecid decreases renal elimination of cefazolin.

PHARMACOKINETICS Peak: 1–2 h after IM; 5 min after IV. **Distribution:** Poor CNS penetration even with inflamed meninges; high concentrations in bile and in diseased bone; crosses placenta. **Elimination:** 70% excreted unchanged in urine in 6 h; small amount excreted in breast milk. **Half-Life:** 90–130 min.

NURSING IMPLICATIONS

Assessment & Drug Effects

- Determine history of hypersensitivity to cephalosporins, penicillins, and other drugs, before therapy is initiated.
- Lab tests: Perform culture and sensitivity testing prior to and during therapy. Therapy may be initiated pending results.
- Monitor I&O rates and pattern: Be alert to changes in BUN, serum creatinine.
- If patient has had a reaction to penicillin, be alert to signs of hypersensitivity with use of cefazolin. Cross-allergenicity between cephalosporins and penicillin has been reported. Prompt attention should be given to onset of signs of hypersensitivity (see Appendix F).
- Promptly report the onset of diarrhea, which may or may not be

dose related. It is seen especially in patients with history of drug-related GI disturbances. Pseudomembranous colitis, a potentially life-threatening condition, starts with diarrhea.

Patient & Family Education

- Report promptly any signs or symptoms of superinfection (see Appendix F).
- Report signs of hemostatic defects: ecchymoses, petechiae, nosebleed.
- Do not breast feed while taking this drug.

CEFDINIR

(cef'di-nir)

Omnicef

Classifications: ANTIINFECTIVE; THIRD-GENERATION CEPHALOSPORIN

Prototype: Cefotaxime Sodium

Pregnancy Category: B

AVAILABILITY 300 mg capsules; 125 mg/5 mL suspension

ACTIONS Broad-spectrum semisynthetic third-generation cephalosporin antibiotic. Generally active against a wide variety of gram-positive and gram-negative bacteria.

THERAPEUTIC EFFECTS Effective against most *Enterobacteriaceae* and *Pseudomonas,* and most strains of *Staphylococci* and *Streptococci* including methicillin-resistant *strains* (MRSA). Effectively treats pneumonia, acute and chronic bronchitis, otitis media, sinusitis, vaginitis, and skin infections reducing or eliminating signs and symptoms of infection.

USES Community-acquired pneumonia, acute exacerbations of chronic bronchitis, acute maxillary sinusitis, pharyngitis, tonsillitis, uncomplicated skin infections, bacterial otitis media.

CONTRAINDICATIONS Hypersensitivity to cefdinir and other cephalosporins; pregnancy (category B).

CAUTIOUS USE Hypersensitivity to penicillins, penicillin derivatives; renal impairment; ulcerative colitis or antibiotic-induced colitis; bleeding disorders; lactation; GI disorders; liver or kidney disease. Safety and efficacy in neonates and infants <6 mo old not established.

ROUTE & DOSAGE

Community-Acquired Pneumonia, Skin Infections

Adult: **PO** 300 mg q12h times 10 d
Child 6 mo–12 y: **PO** 7 mg/kg q12h times 10 d

Chronic Bronchitis, Maxillary Sinusitis, Pharyngitis, Tonsillitis

Adult: **PO** 600 mg q24h or 300 mg q12h times 10 d
Child 6 mo–12 y: **PO** 14 mg/kg q24h or 7 mg/kg q12h times 10 d

ADMINISTRATION

Oral

- Do not give within 2 h of aluminum- or magnesium-containing antacids or iron supplements.
- Reconstitute oral suspension to 125 mg/mL by adding water (38-mL to 60-mL bottle or 63-mL to 100-mL bottle). Shake well before each use.
- Consult physician for dosage adjustment if creatinine clearance <30 mL/min and for patients on hemodialysis.
- Store in tightly closed container. Discard after 10 days.

ADVERSE EFFECTS (≥1%) **GI:** *Diarrhea,* nausea, abdominal pain. **Metabolic:** Increased GGT, increased urine protein, hematuria. **CNS:** Headache. **Skin:** Rash, cuta-

C

neous moniliasis. **Urogenital:** Vaginal moniliasis, vaginitis.

DIAGNOSTIC TEST INTERFERENCE False positive for ***ketones*** or ***glucose*** in urine using ***nitroprusside*** or ***Clinitest.***

INTERACTIONS Drug: ANTACIDS should be taken at least 2 h before or after cefdinir; **probenecid** prolongs cefdinir elimination; **iron** decreases absorption.

PHARMACOKINETICS Absorption: 16–25% bioavailability. **Peak:** 2–4 h. **Distribution:** 60–70% protein bound; penetrates sinus tissue, blister fluid, lung tissue, middle ear fluid. **Metabolism:** Not metabolized. **Elimination:** Excreted in urine. **Half-Life:** 1.6 h.

NURSING IMPLICATIONS

Assessment & Drug Effects

- Determine previous hypersensitivity to cephalosporins, penicillins, and other drug allergies before therapy is initiated.
- Carefully monitor for and immediately report S&S of: hypersensitivity, superinfection, or pseudomembranous colitis (see Appendix F).
- Discontinue drug and notify physician if seizures associated with drug therapy occur.

Patient & Family Education

- Allow a minimum of 2 h between cefdinir and antacids containing aluminum or magnesium, or drugs containing iron.
- Immediately contact physician if a rash, diarrhea, or new infection (e.g., yeast infection) develops.
- Drug may cause false positive for urine ketones or glucose. Consult package insert.
- Do not breast feed while taking this drug without consulting physician.

CEFDITOREN PIVOXIL

(cef-ditor′en)
Spectracef
Classifications: ANTIINFECTIVE; ANTIBIOTIC; CEPHALOSPORIN; THIRD GENERATION
Prototype: Cefotaxime Sodium
Pregnancy Category: B

ACTIONS Semi-synthetic cephalosporin with antibacterial activity against both aerobic gram-positive and aerobic gram-negative bacteria. Bactericidal activity results from the inhibition of cell wall synthesis through an affinity for penicillin-binding proteins (PBPs). Stable in the presence of a variety of bacterial beta-lactamase enzymes, including penicillinases and some cephalosporinases.

THERAPEUTIC EFFECTS Resolution of bronchitis, pharyngitis, tonsillitis, or uncomplicated skin infections caused by susceptible bacteria including most strains of: *Staphylococcus aureus* (except MRSA), *Streptococcus pneumonia, Streptococcus pyogenes, Haemophilus influenzae, Haemophilus parainfluenzae,* and *Moraxella catarrhalis.*

USES Acute exacerbation of bacterial chronic bronchitis, pharyngitis, tonsillitis, uncomplicated skin and skin-structure infections.

CONTRAINDICATIONS Known allergy to cephalosporins or any of the components of cefditoren; carnitine deficiency; milk protein hypersensitivity; lactation.

CAUTIOUS USE History of hypersensitivity to penicillin or other drugs; renal or hepatic impairment; poor nutritional status; concurrent anticoagulant therapy. Safety and efficacy in children <12 y are not established.

ROUTE & DOSAGE

Chronic Bronchitis

Adult: **PO** 400 mg b.i.d. times 10 d

Pharyngitis, Tonsillitis, Skin Infections

Adult: **PO** 200 mg b.i.d. times 10 d

Renal Impairment

Cl_{cr} 30–49 mL/min: 200 mg b.i.d.; <30 mL/min: 200 mg q.d.

ADMINISTRATION

Oral

- Give with food to enhance absorption.
- Do not give within 2 h of an antacid or H_2-receptor antagonist (such as cimetidine).
- Verify dose for patients with renal insufficiency. Manufacturer recommends doses not to exceed 200 mg b.i.d. for patients with creatinine clearance of 30–49 mL/min and doses not to exceed 200 mg q.d. for patients with creatinine clearance of <30 mL/min.
- Store at 15°–30° C (58°–86° F). Protect from light and moisture.

ADVERSE EFFECTS (≥1%) **GI:** *Diarrhea,* nausea, abdominal pain, dyspepsia, vomiting. **Hematologic:** Anemia, leukocytosis. **CNS:** Headache. **Urogenital:** Vaginal moniliasis, hematuria.

INTERACTIONS Drug: ANTACIDS, H_2-RECEPTOR ANTAGONISTS may decrease absorption; **probenecid** will decrease elimination.

PHARMACOKINETICS Absorption: 14% reaches systemic circulation. **Distribution:** 88% protein bound, distributes into blister fluid, tonsils. **Metabolism:** Minimal metabolism. **Elimination:** Primarily excreted in urine. **Half-Life:** 1.6 h.

NURSING IMPLICATIONS

Assessment & Drug Effects

- Obtain history of hypersensitivity to cephalosporins, penicillins, and other drug allergies.
- Lab tests: Baseline C&S tests recommended prior to and periodically during therapy. Initiate drug pending results. Baseline and periodic studies of kidney function; frequent PT determinations in patients at risk for increased prothrombin time; as indicated, Hct & Hgb, CBC with differential, urinalysis, serum electrolytes, and liver enzymes.
- Monitor for manifestations of drug hypersensitivity (see Appendix F). Withhold drug and report promptly to physician if they appear.
- Monitor for and report promptly manifestations of superinfection (see Appendix F), especially diarrhea. Diarrhea may indicate a change in intestinal flora and development of enterocolitis. If it persists, interruption of therapy may be necessary.
- Monitor for and report immediately signs of seizure activity or loss of seizure control.

Patient & Family Education

- Do not take within 2 h of antacids or other drugs used to reduce stomach acids.
- Discontinue drug and report to physician signs of an allergic reaction (e.g., rash, urticaria, pruritus, fever).
- Report promptly S&S of superinfection (see Appendix F), especially unexplained diarrhea. Antibiotic-associated colitis is a superinfection that may occur in 4–9 d or as long as 6 wk after drug is discontinued.
- Use daily yogurt or buttermilk (if allowed) as a prophylactic against intestinal superinfections.
- Do not breast feed while taking this drug.

C

CEFEPIME HYDROCHLORIDE

(cef'e-peem)

Maxipime

Classifications: ANTIINFECTIVE; ANTIBIOTIC; FOURTH-GENERATION CEPHALOSPORIN

Prototype: Cefotaxime sodium

Pregnancy Category: B

AVAILABILITY 500 mg, 1 g, 2 g vials

ACTIONS Cefepime, considered to be a fourth-generation cephalosporin antibiotic, is similar to third-generation cephalosporins with respect to broad gram-negative coverage; however, cefepime has broader gram-positive coverage than third-generation cephalosporins. It is highly resistant to hydrolysis by most beta-lactamase bacteria. Cefepime preferentially binds to one or more of the penicillin-binding proteins (PBPs) located on cell walls of susceptible organisms. This inhibits the third and final stage of bacterial cell wall synthesis, thus killing the bacteria (bactericidal).

THERAPEUTIC EFFECTS Effectively treats pneumonia, skin and soft tissue infections, febrile neutropenia, respiratory tract, intra-abdominal infections, and urinary tract infections by reducing or eliminating signs and symptoms of infection.

USES Uncomplicated and complicated UTI, skin and skin structure infections, pneumonia caused by susceptible organisms (*Escherichia coli, Klebsiella pneumoniae, Proteus mirabilis, Staphylococcus aureus* [methicillin-sensitive], *Streptococcus pyogenes, Streptococcus pneumoniae, Pseudomonas aeruginosa, Enterobacter sp*). Empiric monotherapy for febrile neutropenic patients.

CONTRAINDICATIONS Hypersensitivity to cefepime, other cephalosporins, penicillins, or other beta-lactam antibiotics.

CAUTIOUS USE Patients with history of GI disease, particularly colitis, renal insufficiency; pregnancy (category B), lactation. Safety and efficacy of cefepime in children <12 y not known.

ROUTE & DOSAGE

Mild to Moderate Infections

Adult: **IV/IM** 0.5–1g q12h times 7–10 d

Moderate to Severe Infections

Adult: **IV** 1–2g q12h times 10 d

Febrile Neutropenia

Adult: **IV** 2 g q8h for 7 d or until resolution of neutropenia

Adjustment for Renal Impairment

Cl_{cr} 30–60 mL/min: dose q24h; 11–29 mL/min: give 50% of normal dose q24h; <10 mL/min: 250–500 mg q24h

ADMINISTRATION

Intramuscular

- Reconstitute 500-mg vial and 1-g vial, respectively, with 1.3 or 2.4 mL of one of the following: Sterile Water for Injection, 0.9% NaCl Injection, Bacteriostatic Water for Injection with Parabens or benzyl alcohol, or other compatible solution.

Intravenous

PREPARE: **Intermittent:** Dilute with 50–100 mL of one of the following: NS, D5W, D5/NS or other compatible solution.

ADMINISTER: **Intermittent:** Infuse over 30 min; with Y-type administration set, discontinue other compatible solutions while infusing cefepime.

***INCOMPATIBILITIES* Solution/additive:** AMINOGLYCOSIDES, **ampicillin, aminophylline, metronidazole.**: **Y-site: Acyclovir, amphotericin B, amphotericin B cholesteryl complex, chlordiazepoxide, chlorpromazine, cimetidine, ciproxfloxacin, cisplatin, dacarbazine, daunorubicin, diazepam, diphenhydramine, dobutamine, dopamine, doxorubicin, droperidol, enalaprilat, etoposide, famotidine, filgrastim, floxuridine, ganciclovir, haloperidol, hydroxyzine, idarubicin, ifosfamide, magnesium sulfate, mannitol, mechlorethamine, meperidine, metoclopramide, mitomycin, mitoxantrone, morphine, nalbuphine, ofloxacin, ondansetron, plicamycin, prochlorperazine, promethazine, streptozocin, vancomycin, vinblastine, vincristine.**

- Store reconstituted solution at 20°–25° C (68°–77° F) for 24 h or in refrigerator at 2°–8° C (36°–46° F) for 7 days. Protect from light.

ADVERSE EFFECTS (≥1%) **Body as a Whole:** Eosinophilia. **GI:** Antibiotic-associated colitis, diarrhea, nausea, oral moniliasis, vomiting, elevated liver function tests (ALT, AST). **CNS:** Headache, fever. **Skin:** Phlebitis, pain, inflammation, rash, pruritus, urticaria, **Urogenital:** Vaginitis.

DIAGNOSTIC TEST INTERFERENCE Positive ***Coombs' test*** without hemolysis. May cause false-positive ***urine glucose test*** with ***Clinitest.***

INTERACTIONS Drug: AMINOGLYCOSIDES may increase risk of nephrotoxicity and have additive/synergistic effects. May decrease efficacy of ORAL CONTRACEPTIVES. **Probenecid** may increase levels.

PHARMACOKINETICS Absorption: Well absorbed after IM administration; serum levels significantly lower than after equivalent IV dose. **Distribution:** 20% protein bound, widely distributed, may cross inflamed meninges; crosses placenta, secreted into breast milk. **Metabolism:** Metabolized in liver. **Elimination:** Excreted in urine. **Half-Life:** 2 h.

NURSING IMPLICATIONS

Assessment & Drug Effects

- Determine history of hypersensitivity reactions to cephalosporins, penicillins, or other drugs before therapy is initiated.
- Lab tests: Perform culture and sensitivity tests before initiation of therapy. Dosage may be started pending test results.
- Monitor for S&S of hypersensitivity (see Appendix F). Report their appearance promptly and discontinue drug.
- Monitor for S&S of superinfection or pseudomembranous colitis (see Appendix F); immediately report either to physician.
- With concurrent high-dose aminoglycoside therapy, closely monitor for nephrotoxicity and ototoxicity.

Patient & Family Education

- Promptly report any S&S of hypersensitivity, superinfection, and pseudomembranous colitis.
- Do not breast feed while taking this drug without consulting physician.

C

CEFIXIME

(ce-fix'ime)
Suprax
Classifications: ANTIINFECTIVE; ANTIBIOTIC; THIRD-GENERATION CEPHALOSPORIN
Prototype: Cefotaxime sodium
Pregnancy Category: B

AVAILABILITY 200 mg, 400 mg tablets; 100 mg/5 mL suspension

ACTIONS A third-generation cephalosporin that is highly stable in the presence of beta-lactamases (penicillinases and cephalosporinases) and therefore has excellent activity against a wide range of gram-negative bacteria. It is bactericidal against susceptible bacteria. Cephalosporins inhibit mucopeptide synthesis in the bacterial cell wall.
THERAPEUTIC EFFECTS Effectively treats respiratory tract, urinary tract infection, otitis media and gonorrhea, reducing or eliminating signs and symptoms of infection.

USES Effective against *Streptococcus pyogenes, Streptococcus pneumoniae,* and gram-negative bacilli, including *Haemophilus influenzae, Branhamella catarrhalis,* and *Neisseria gonorrhoeae*. Little activity against *Staphylococci,* and no activity against *Pseudomonas aeruginosa;* also uncomplicated UTI, otitis media, pharyngitis, tonsillitis, and bronchitis.

CONTRAINDICATIONS Patients with known allergy to the cephalosporin group of antibiotics.
CAUTIOUS USE Allergy to penicillin, history of colitis, renal insufficiency, pregnancy (category B), lactation. Safety and effectiveness in infants <6 mo have not been established.

ROUTE & DOSAGE

Infection
Adult: **PO** 400 mg/d in 1–2 divided doses
Child: **PO** 8 mg/kg/d in 1–2 divided doses

ADMINISTRATION

Oral
- Do not substitute tablets for liquid in treatment of otitis media because of lack of bioequivalence.
- After reconstitution, suspension may be kept for 14 d at room temperature or refrigerated. Store away from heat and light. Keep tightly closed and shake well before using.

ADVERSE EFFECTS (≥1%) **GI:** *Diarrhea,* loose stools, nausea, vomiting, dyspepsia, flatulence. **CNS:** Drug fever, headache, dizziness. **Skin:** Rash, pruritus, **Urogenital:** Vaginitis, genital pruritus.

INTERACTIONS Drug: AMINOGLYCOSIDES may increase risk of nephrotoxicity and have additive/synergistic effects. May decrease efficacy of ORAL CONTRACEPTIVES. **Probenecid** may increase levels.

PHARMACOKINETICS Absorption: 40–50% absorbed from GI tract. **Peak:** 2–6 h. **Distribution:** Distributed into breast milk. **Elimination:** 50% excreted in urine, 50% in bile. **Half-Life:** 3–4 h.

NURSING IMPLICATIONS

Assessment & Drug Effects
- Determine previous hypersensitivity reactions to cephalosporins, penicillins, and history of other allergies, particularly to drugs prior to initiation of therapy.
- Lab tests: Perform culture and sensitivity tests prior to initiation

of therapy and periodically during therapy. Therapy may be implemented pending test results.

- Discontinue if seizures associated with the drug therapy occur.
- Monitor for superinfections (see Appendix F) caused by overgrowth of nonsusceptible organisms, particularly during prolonged use.
- Monitor I&O rates and pattern: Nephrotoxicity occurs more frequently in patients >50 y, with impaired renal function, in the debilitated, and in patients receiving high doses or other nephrotoxic drugs.
- Carefully monitor anyone with a history of allergies, especially to drugs. Report manifestations of hypersensitivity (see Appendix F).
- Promptly report loose stools or diarrhea, which may indicate pseudomembranous colitis (see Appendix F). Discontinuation of drug may be necessary.

Patient & Family Education

- Report loose stools or diarrhea during drug therapy and for several weeks after. Older adult patients are especially susceptible to pseudomembranous colitis.
- Take this antibiotic for the full course of treatment.
- Do not miss any doses and take the doses at evenly spaced times, day and night.
- Do not breast feed while taking this drug without consulting physician.

CEFMETAZOLE

(sef-met'a-zol)

Zefazone

Classifications: ANTIINFECTIVE; ANTIBIOTIC; THIRD-GENERATION CEPHALOSPORIN

Prototype: Cefotaxime sodium

Pregnancy Category: B

AVAILABILITY 1 g, 2 g injection

ACTIONS Cefmetazole is a synthetic cephalosporin antibiotic. Its bactericidal action results from inhibition of cell wall synthesis.

THERAPEUTIC EFFECTS Active against a wide range of gram-positive and gram-negative aerobic and anaerobic bacteria. Effectively treats abdominal and respiratory tract infections, pelvic inflammatory disease, urinary tract infections, skin and soft tissue infections and used for surgical prophylaxis, reducing or eliminating signs and symptoms of infection.

USES UTI infections caused by *Escherichia coli,* lower respiratory tract infections, namely pneumonia and bronchitis caused by *Streptococcus pneumoniae, Staphylococcus aureus, E. coli, Haemophilus influenzae.* In addition, it is effective against *Staphylococcus epidermidis, Streptococcus pyogenes, Streptococcus agalactiae, Proteus vulgaris,* and *Bacteroides fragilis;* preoperative prophylaxis of cesarean section, hysterectomy, cholecystectomy, and colorectal surgery.

CONTRAINDICATIONS Patients with known allergy to cefmetazole or to any other cephalosporin antibiotic.

CAUTIOUS USE Allergy to penicillin, history of colitis, renal insufficiency, pregnancy (category B), lactation.

ROUTE & DOSAGE

Systemic Infections

Adult: **IV** 1–2 g q6–12h

Surgical Prophylaxis

Adult: **IV** 1–2 g 30–90 min before surgery; then q8h for 2 more doses

Adjustment for Renal Impairment

Cl_{cr} <30 mL/min: 1–2 g q24h

C

ADMINISTRATION

Intravenous

PREPARE: **Direct/Intermittent:** Reconstitute with sterile water for injection, bacteriostatic water for injection, or NS. Dilute 1 g with 3.7 mL to yield 250 mg/mL or with 10 mL to yield 100 mg/mL. Dilute 2 g with 7 mL to yield 250 mg/mL or with 15 mL to yield 125 mg/mL. Solution may be further diluted to concentrations ranging from 1–20 mg/mL by adding it to D5W, NS, or RL.

ADMINISTER: **Direct/Intermittent:** Drug can be given direct IV over 3–5 min (for surgical prophylaxis only) or infused over 10–60 min.

INCOMPATIBILITIES **Solution/additive:** AMINOGLYCOSIDES. **Y-site:** AMINOGLYCOSIDES.

- Observe IV sites for evidence of inflammatory reaction. Risk of phlebitis may be reduced by use of a small needle in a large vein.
- Potency is retained for 24 h after reconstitution at room temperature, 7 d under refrigeration, and for 6 wk if frozen. Store away from heat, light, and moisture; do not refreeze.

ADVERSE EFFECTS (≥1%) **Body as a Whole:** Hypersensitivity reactions. **GI:** *Diarrhea,* loose stools, nausea, vomiting, dyspepsia, flatulence. **CNS:** Drug fever, headache, dizziness. **Skin:** Rash, pruritus. **Urogenital:** Vaginitis, genital pruritus.

INTERACTIONS Drug: Probenecid decreases renal elimination of cefmetazole.

PHARMACOKINETICS Elimination: Excreted unchanged in urine. **Half-Life:** 1.2 h.

NURSING IMPLICATIONS

Assessment & Drug Effects

- Determine previous hypersensitivity to cephalosporins, penicillins, and history of other allergies, particularly to drugs, before therapy is initiated.
- Lab tests: Perform culture and sensitivity tests before initiation of therapy and periodically during therapy. Therapy may be implemented pending test results. Monitor PT in patients with renal or hepatic disease or those receiving a long course of antibiotic therapy.
- Assess for S&S of superinfections (see Appendix F) caused by overgrowth of nonsusceptible organisms, particularly with prolonged use.
- Promptly report loose stools or diarrhea because of risk of pseudomembranous colitis (see Appendix F). Older adults are especially susceptible. Drug may be discontinued.

Patient & Family Education

- Report onset of loose stools or diarrhea even for several weeks after drug is discontinued.
- Do not ingest alcohol within 24 h of drug as this may cause a disulfiram-like reaction (see Appendix F).
- Do not breast feed while taking this drug without consulting physician.

CEFONICID SODIUM (Pr)

(se-fon′i-sid)

Monocid

Classifications: ANTIINFECTIVE; BETA-LACTAM ANTIBIOTIC; SECOND-GENERATION CEPHALOSPORIN

Pregnancy Category: B

AVAILABILITY 1 g injection

ACTIONS Semisynthetic, second-generation cephalosporin antibiotic with drug structure characterized by a beta-lactam ring (like the penicillin structure); generally resistant to hydrolysis by beta-lactamases. Preferentially binds to one or more of the penicillin-binding proteins (PBP) located on cell walls of susceptible organisms. This inhibits third and final stage of bacterial wall synthesis, thus killing the bacterium. Second generation cephalosporins are usually active against the organisms susceptible to first generation cephalosporins.

THERAPEUTIC EFFECTS Active against *Haemophilus influenzae, Providencia sp, Clostridium sp, Peptococcus sp,* and against some strains of *Citrobacter, Enterobacter, Serratia, Neisseria, Proteus, Escherichia coli,* and *Klebsiella* that are resistant to first generation cephalosporins. Second generation agents are generally inactive against *Enterococci,* methicillin-resistant *Staphylococci* (MRSA), *Acinetobacter, Listeria monocytogenes,* and *Pseudomonas.* Active against a wide range of gram-positive and gram-negative aerobic and anaerobic bacteria. Effectively treats bone and joint infections, gonorrhea, lower respiratory tract infections, urinary tract infections, septicemia, skin and soft tissue infections and used for surgical prophylaxis, reducing or eliminating signs and symptoms of infection.

USES Moderate to severe infections such as septicemia, infections of lower respiratory tract, bones and joints, skin and skin structures, and urinary tract (UTI). Also used for perioperative prophylaxis.

UNLABELED USE Uncomplicated gonorrhea.

CONTRAINDICATIONS Hypersensitivity to cephalosporins and related antibiotics; severely impaired renal or hepatic function; pregnancy (category B). Safe use in children not established.

CAUTIOUS USE Lactation; patient with history of delayed-type reaction to penicillins or other drugs; GI disease, especially colitis.

ROUTE & DOSAGE

Moderate to Severe Infections

Adult: **IV/IM** 1 g q24h, up to 2 g/24 h

Surgical Prophylaxis

Adult: **IV/IM** 1 g 60 min before surgery

ADMINISTRATION

- Note: When cefonicid is given for prophylaxis during cesarean section, it is administered only after umbilical cord has been clamped.

Intramuscular

- Reconstitute with sterile water for injection. Add 2 mL of diluent to 500 mg of drug to yield 220 mg/mL; add 2.5 mL diluent to 1 g of drug to yield 325 mg 1 mL. Shake well to assure complete dissolution of drug. After reconstitution, inspect for particulate matter; if present, discard solution.
- IM injections should be made deeply into large muscle mass. Pain and discomfort at IM site occurs commonly. If dose is 2 g, give 1/2 dose in a different large muscle mass. Rotate injection sites.

Intravenous

PREPARE: **Direct:** Reconstitute as for IM injection. **Intermittent:** Further dilute reconstituted cefonicid in 50–100 mL D5W, NS, RL, or other compatible diluent.

ADMINISTER: **Direct:** Give a single dose slowly over 3–5 min.

C

May give directly or through IV tubing of a compatible parenteral fluid. **Intermittent:** Give a single dose over 30 min.
INCOMPATIBILITIES **Solution/additive:** AMINOGLYCOSIDES. **Y-site:** AMINOGLYCOSIDES.

- Examine IV site daily for evidence of inflammation.
- After reconstitution or dilution, solutions are stable for 24 h at room temperature or 72 h if refrigerated 5° C (41° F). Slight yellowing does not indicate loss of potency.

ADVERSE EFFECTS (≥1%) **Body as a Whole:** Hypersensitivity, fever, rash, pruritus, erythema, myalgia, anaphylactoid reaction, pain with IM injection; burning sensation, phlebitis (IV administration), flu-like syndrome, superinfections (by *Candida, Pseudomonas, Enterobacter sp*). **GI:** Nausea, vomiting, *diarrhea*, pseudomembranous enterocolitis. **Hematologic:** Neutropenia (rare).

DIAGNOSTIC TEST INTERFERENCE A false-positive reaction for ***urine glucose*** may occur with ***copper sulfate reduction reagents,*** e.g., ***Benedict's*** or ***Clinitest; tests*** based ***on glucose oxidase reactions*** are apparently not affected, e.g., ***TesTape, Clinistix, Diastix.***

INTERACTIONS Drug: Probenecid decreases renal elimination.

PHARMACOKINETICS Peak: 1 h after IM; 5 min after IV. **Distribution:** Poor CNS penetration even with inflamed meninges; crosses placenta. **Metabolism:** Not metabolized. **Elimination:** 90–99% excreted unchanged in urine within 24 h; small amount excreted in breast milk. **Half-Life:** 3.5–5.8 h.

NURSING IMPLICATIONS

Assessment & Drug Effects

- Determine history of hypersensitivity to cephalosporins, penicillins, or other drugs before therapy begins.
- Lab tests: Perform culture and sensitivity tests before and periodically during therapy, if indicated. Therapy may be initiated before test results are available. Perform periodic hematologic studies including PT/INR and PTT and evaluations of renal and hepatic functions in patients receiving high doses and during prolonged therapy.
- Monitor I&O rates and pattern: Particularly important in patients with impaired renal function, patients >50 y, or who are receiving high doses.
- Monitor temperature. Report temperature alterations and the onset of flu-like symptoms (chills, malaise).
- Monitor for superinfections caused by overgrowth of nonsusceptible organisms, particularly during prolonged use of cephalosporins.
- Antibiotic-associated pseudomembranous enterocolitis is a life-threatening superinfection caused by *Clostridium difficile;* may occur in 4–9 d or as long as 6 wk after cefonicid is discontinued. Most apt to occur in the chronically ill or debilitated older adult patient, especially if undergoing abdominal surgery or if in an intensive care unit.
- Check for fever if diarrhea occurs. Report diarrhea and fever promptly.

Patient & Family Education

- Superinfections caused by overgrowth of nonsusceptible organisms may occur, particularly during prolonged use of cephalosporins. Report early S&S (see Appendix F) promptly.

- Report loose stools or diarrhea.
- Yogurt or buttermilk, 120 mL (4 oz) of either (if allowed), may serve as a prophylactic against intestinal superinfection by helping to maintain normal intestinal flora.
- Do not breast feed while taking this drug without consulting physician.

CEFOPERAZONE SODIUM

(sef-oh-per'a-zone)

Cefobid

Classifications: ANTIINFECTIVE; ANTIBIOTIC; THIRD-GENERATION CEPHALOSPORIN

Prototype: Cefotaxime sodium

Pregnancy Category: B

AVAILABILITY 1 g, 2 g injection

ACTIONS Semisynthetic third-generation cephalosporin antibiotic. Preferentially binds to one or more of the penicillin-binding proteins (PBP) located on cell walls of susceptible organisms. This inhibits third and final stage of bacterial cell wall synthesis, thus killing the bacterium. Spectrum of activity is similar to that of cefotaxime.

THERAPEUTIC EFFECTS Generally active against a wide variety of gram-negative bacteria, including some strains of *Pseudomonas aeruginosa*. Also active against some organisms resistant to first and second generation cephalosporins and currently available aminoglycoside antibiotics and penicillins: e.g., *Escherichia coli, Klebsiella pneumoniae,* and *Serratia marcescens*. Other susceptible organisms include *Proteus mirabilis, Salmonella, Shigella, Haemophilus influenzae, Neisseria gonorrhoeae,* groups A and B *Streptococci, Staphylococcus aureus,* and some strains of *Pseudomonas* sp. Cefoperazone inhibits some strains of *Clostridium,* but *C. difficle* is resistant to the drug, as is *Listeria monocytogenes*. It has a broad antibacterial spectrum, including gram-positive bacteria and *Pseudomonas aeruginosa*. Effectively treats biliary tract infections, gynecologic infections and gonorrhea, intra-abdominal and soft tissue infections, respiratory tract infections, urinary tract infections, skin infections, septicemia, and surgical infections, reducing or eliminating signs and symptoms of infection.

USES Infections of skin and skin structures, urinary tract, respiratory tract; peritonitis and other intra-abdominal infections, pelvic inflammatory disease, endometritis and other infections of the female genital tract; bacterial septicemia.

UNLABELED USE Children <12 y.

CONTRAINDICATIONS Hypersensitivity to cephalosporins and related beta-lactam antibiotics; pregnancy (category B).

CAUTIOUS USE History of hypersensitivity to penicillins, history of allergy, particularly to drugs; hepatic disease, history of colitis or other GI disease, history of bleeding disorders; lactation.

ROUTE & DOSAGE

Moderate to Severe Infections

Adult: **IV/IM** 1–2 g q12h; 16 g/d in 2–4 divided doses

Child <12 y: **IV/IM** 100–150 mg/kg/d divided q8–12h (max: 12 g/d)

ADMINISTRATION

Intramuscular

- To prepare IM injections, appropriate diluents include sterile water for injection, bacteriostatic water for injection, and 0.5% lidocaine. See package insert for reconstitution procedure.

- Reconstitute for IM: Dilute each 1 g with 5 mL sterile water. Shake vigorously to dissolve. If concentrations of ≥250 mg/mL are needed for IM injection, 2% lidocaine should be added. See manufacturer's directions.

Intravenous

- IV administration to infants and children: Verify correct IV concentration and rate of infusion with physician.
- Rapid, direct (bolus) IV injections are not recommended.

PREPARE: **Intermittent:** Dilute each 1 g with 5 mL sterile water. Shake vigorously to dissolve, then dilute in 50–100 mL of D5W or NS. **Continuous: Further** dilute in 500–1000 mL of the selected IV solution.

ADMINISTER: **Intermittent:** Give over 15–30 min. **Continuous:** Give 500–1000 mL over 6–24 h.

INCOMPATIBILITIES **Solution/additive:** AMINOGLYCOSIDES, doxapram. **Y-site:** AMINOGLYCOSIDES, **amifostine, amphotericin B cholesteryl complex, cisatracurium, diltiazem, doxorubicin liposome, filgrastim, gemcitabine, hetastarch, labetalol, meperidine, ondansetron, pentamidine, perphenazine, promethazine, sargramostim, vinorelbine.**

- Protect sterile powder and piggyback units from light and store at or below 25° C (77° F). Reconstituted solutions may be stored in original containers for 24 h at 15°–25° C (59°–77° F); for 5 d under refrigeration at 5° C (41° F) or less, or for at least 3 wk in freezer.

ADVERSE EFFECTS (≥1%) **Body as a Whole:** Fever, eosinophilia, phlebitis (IV site), transient pain (IM site), superinfections. **GI:** Abdominal cramps, bloating, loose stools or *diarrhea,* pseudomembranous colitis, elevated liver function tests (AST, ALT, alkaline phosphatase). **Hematologic:** Abnormal PT/INR and PTT; hypoprothrombinemia. **Skin:** Skin rash, urticaria, pruritus. **Urogenital:** Transient increases in serum creatinine and BUN, oliguria.

DIAGNOSTIC TEST INTERFERENCE Cefoperazone can cause positive ***direct Coombs' test,*** which may result in interferences with ***hematologic studies*** and ***cross-matching*** procedures. False-positive results for ***urine glucose*** using ***copper sulfate tests (Benedict's, Clinitest),*** but not with ***glucose enzymatic tests,*** e.g., ***Clinistix, TesTape, Diastix.*** Also causes ***prolonged prothrombin*** twice during therapy.

INTERACTIONS Drug: Probenecid decreases renal elimination of cefoperazone; **alcohol** produces disulfiram reaction.

PHARMACOKINETICS Peak: 1–2 h after IM; 15–20 min after IV. **Distribution:** Low CNS penetration except with inflamed meninges; highest concentrations in bile; crosses placenta. **Elimination:** 70–75% excreted unchanged in bile in 6–12 h, small amount excreted in breast milk. **Half-Life:** 2 h.

NURSING IMPLICATIONS

Assessment & Drug Effects

- Determine hypersensitivity to cephalosporins, penicillins, and other drug allergies before therapy begins.

- Lab tests: Perform culture and sensitivity studies before initiation of therapy and during therapy, as indicated. Therapy may begin pending test results. Perform PTT and PT/INR before and during therapy.
- Observe for and question patient about signs of hemostatic defects: wound bleeding (e.g., surgical patient), nose bleeds, bleeding gums, bloody sputum, hematuria. Hypoprothrombinemia and vitamin K deficiency are possible complications of therapy and can result in significant blood loss in some patients. Patients at risk are those with poor nutritional states, malabsorption problems, patients on hyperalimentation regimens, and alcoholism. Vitamin K supplements may be prescribed for these patients, if indicated.
- Report the onset of loose stools or diarrhea. Most patients respond to replacement of fluids, electrolytes, and proteins. Discontinuation of drug may be required for some patients.
- Monitor cefoperazone serum levels (at steady state: 150 mg/mL) in patients with hepatic disease or biliary obstruction who are receiving over 4 g/d, patients with both hepatic and renal disease receiving over 1–2 g/d, and patients with renal impairment on high dose therapy.

Patient & Family Education

- Do not ingest alcohol within 72 h after drug administration as this will cause a disulfiram-like reaction (see Signs & Symptoms, Appendix F). Effects generally appear within 15–30 min after alcohol is taken and disappear spontaneously 1–2 h later.
- Report promptly any signs or symptoms of superinfection (see Appendix F).
- Do not breast feed while taking this drug without consulting physician.

CEFOTAXIME SODIUM (Pr)

(sef-oh-taks′eem)

Claforan

Classifications: ANTIINFECTIVE; BETA-LACTAM ANTIBIOTIC; THIRD-GENERATION CEPHALOSPORIN

Pregnancy Category: B

AVAILABILITY 500 mg, 1 g, 2 g injection

ACTIONS Broad-spectrum semisynthetic third-generation cephalosporin antibiotic. Preferentially binds to one or more of the penicillin-binding proteins (PBP) located on cell walls of susceptible organisms. This inhibits third and final stage of bacterial cell wall synthesis, thus killing the bacterium.

THERAPEUTIC EFFECTS Generally active against a wide variety of gram-negative bacteria including most of the *Enterobacteriaceae*. Also active against some organisms resistant to first and second generation cephalosporins and currently available aminoglycoside antibiotics and penicillins, e.g., *Escherichia coli, Klebsiella pneumoniae,* and *Serratia marcescens*. Other susceptible organisms: *Bacteroides fragilis, Morganella morganii, Proteus mirabilis, Salmonella, Shigella, Hemophilus influenzae, Neisseria gonorrhoeae,* groups A and B *Streptococci, Staphylococcus aureus, Bacteroides, Eubacterium, Peptostreptococcus,* and *Peptococcus*. Inhibits some strains of *Clostridium*, but *C. difficile* is resistant to the drug, as is *Listeria monocytogenes*. It is the drug of choice in the treatment of gram-negative adult bacillary meningitis, neonatal and

C

childhood meningitis, and *Enterobacteriaceae*. Effectively treats bone and joint infections, CNS infections, gynecologic infections and gonorrhea, lower respiratory tract infections, intra-abdominal infections, skin and urinary tract infections, and is used for surgical prophylaxis to reduce or eliminate infection.

USES Serious infections of lower respiratory tract, skin and skin structures, bones and joints, CNS (including meningitis and ventriculitis), gynecologic and GU tract infections, including uncomplicated gonococcal infections caused by penicillinase-producing *Neisseria gonorrhoeae* (PPNG). Also used to treat bacteremia or septicemia, intra-abdominal infections, and for perioperative prophylaxis.

UNLABELED USES Currently recommended by CDC for treatment of disseminated gonococcal infections (gonococcal arthritis-dermatitis syndrome) and as drug of choice for gonococcal ophthalmia caused by PPNG in adults, children, and neonates.

CONTRAINDICATIONS Hypersensitivity to cephalosporins and other beta-lactam antibiotics; pregnancy (category B).

CAUTIOUS USE History of type I hypersensitivity reactions to penicillin; history of allergy to other beta-lactam; antibiotics; renal impairment; history of colitis or other GI disease; lactation.

ROUTE & DOSAGE

Moderate to Severe Infections

Adult: **IV/IM** 1–2 g q8–12h, up to 2 g q4h (max 12 g/d)
Child: **IV/IM** *≤1wk:* 50 mg/kg q12h; *1–4 wk:* 50 mg/kg q8h; *1 mo–12 y:* 100–200 mg/kg/d divided q4–8h

Surgical Prophylaxis

Adult: **IV/IM** 1 g 30–90 min before surgery

ADMINISTRATION

Intramuscular

- Add 3 mL sterile water for injection or bacteriostatic water for injection to vial containing 1 g drug, providing a solution of approximately 300 mg cefotaxime/mL.
- Administer IM injection deeply into large muscle mass (e.g., upper outer quadrant of gluteus maximus). Aspirate to avoid inadvertent injection into blood vessel. If IM dose is 2 g, divide dose and administer into 2 different sites.
- Risk of phlebitis may be reduced by use of a small needle in a large vein.

Intravenous

- IV administration to infants and children: Verify correct IV concentration and rate of infusion with physician.
- Do not admix cefotaxime with sodium bicarbonate or any fluid with a pH >7.5.

PREPARE: **Direct:** Add 10 mL diluent to vial with 1 or 2 g drug providing a solution containing 95 or 180 mg/mL, respectively. **Intermittent:** To 1 or 2 g drug add 50 or 100 mL D5W, NS, D5/NS, D5/.45% NaCl, RL, or other compatible diluent. **Continuous:** Dilute in 500–1000 mL compatible IV solution.

ADMINISTER: **Direct:** Give over 3–5 min. **Intermittent:** Give over 20–30 min, preferably via butterfly or scalp vein-type needles. **Continuous:** Infuse over 6–24 h.

INCOMPATIBILITIES **Solution/additive:** AMINOGLYCOSIDES, **aminophylline, doxapram, sodium bicarbonate, vancomycin. Y-site: Allopurinol,** AMINOGLYCOSIDES, **aminophylline, doxapram, filgrastim, fluconazole, gemcitabine, hetastarch, sodium bicarbonate; pentamidine, vancomycin.**

- Protect from excessive light. Reconstituted solutions may be stored in original containers for 24 h at room temperature; for 10 days under refrigeration at 5° C (41° F) or less; or for at least 13 wk in frozen state.

ADVERSE EFFECTS (≥1%) **Body as a Whole:** Fever, nocturnal perspiration, inflammatory reaction at IV site, phlebitis, thrombophlebitis; pain, induration, and tenderness at IM site, superinfections. **GI:** Nausea, vomiting, *diarrhea,* abdominal pain, colitis, <u>pseudomembranous colitis</u>, anorexia. **Metabolic:** Transient increases in serum AST, ALT, LDH, bilirubin, alkaline phosphatase concentrations. **Skin:** Rash, pruritus.

DIAGNOSTIC TEST INTERFERENCE May cause falsely elevated ***serum*** or ***urine creatinine*** values ***(Jaffe reaction)***. False-positive reactions for ***urine glucose*** have not been reported using ***copper sulfate reduction methods,*** e.g., ***Benedict's, Clinitest:*** however, since it has occurred with other cephalosporins, it may be advisable to use ***glucose oxidase tests (Clinistix, TesTape, Diastix).*** Positive ***direct antiglobulin (Coombs') test*** results may interfere with ***hematologic studies*** and ***cross-matching*** procedures.

INTERACTIONS Drug: Probenecid decreases renal elimination; **alcohol** produces disulfiram reaction.

PHARMACOKINETICS Peak: 30 min after IM; 5 min after IV. **Distribution:** CNS penetration except with inflamed meninges; also penetrates aqueous humor, ascitic and prostatic fluids; crosses placenta. **Metabolism:** Partially metabolized in liver to active metabolites. **Elimination:** 50–60% excreted unchanged in urine in 24 h; small amount excreted in breast milk. **Half-Life:** 1 h.

NURSING IMPLICATIONS

Assessment & Drug Effects

- Determine previous hypersensitivity reactions to cephalosporins and penicillins, and history of other allergies, particularly to drugs, before therapy is initiated.
- Lab tests: Perform culture and sensitivity tests before initiation of therapy and periodically during therapy if indicated. Therapy may be instituted pending test results. Serum creatinine, creatinine clearance, BUN should be evaluated at regular intervals during therapy and for several months after drug has been discontinued. Perform periodic hematologic studies (including PT and PTT) and evaluation of hepatic functions with high doses or prolonged therapy.
- Monitor I&O rates and patterns: Report change in I&O in patients with impaired renal function or with chronic UTI or who are receiving high dosages or an aminoglycoside concomitantly.
- Superinfection due to overgrowth of nonsusceptible organisms may occur, particularly with prolonged therapy.
- Report onset of diarrhea promptly. Check for fever. If diarrhea is mild, discontinuation of cefotaxime may be sufficient.

C

- If diarrhea is severe, suspect antibiotic-associated pseudomembranous colitis, a life-threatening superinfection (may occur in 4–9 d or as long as 6 wk after cephalosporin therapy is discontinued). Chronically ill or debilitated older adult patients undergoing abdominal surgery or those in an intensive care unit are most vulnerable.

Patient & Family Education

- Report any early signs or symptoms of superinfection promptly. Superinfections caused by overgrowth of nonsusceptible organisms may occur, particularly during prolonged use.
- Yogurt or buttermilk, 120 mL (4 oz) of either (if allowed), may serve as a prophylactic against intestinal superinfection by helping to maintain normal intestinal flora.
- Report loose stools or diarrhea.
- Do not breast feed while taking this drug without consulting physician.

CEFOTETAN DISODIUM

(sef'oh-tee-tan)
Cefotan
Classifications: ANTIINFECTIVE; ANTIBIOTIC; THIRD-GENERATION CEPHALOSPORIN
Prototype: Cefotaxime sodium
Pregnancy Category: B

AVAILABILITY 1 g, 2 g injection

ACTIONS Semisynthetic beta-lactam antibiotic, classified as a third-generation cephalosporin. Preferentially binds to one or more of the penicillin-binding proteins (PBP) located on cell walls of susceptible organisms. This inhibits third and final stage of bacterial cell wall synthesis, thus killing the bacterium. Generally less active against susceptible *Staphylococci* than first generation cephalosporins are but has broad spectrum of activity against gram-negative bacteria when compared to first and second generation cephalosporins.

THERAPEUTIC EFFECTS Spectrum of activity is like that of cefotaxime including *Escherichia coli, Klebsiella sp, Enterobacter sp, Proteus sp, Streptococcus pneumoniae, Staphylococcus aureus,* penicillinase- and nonpenicillinase-producing *Haemophilus influenzae, Salmonella, Shigella, Neisseria gonorrhoeae,* and many anaerobes. Generally inactive against *Pseudomonas aeruginosa*. It is active against the *Enterobacteriaceae* and anaerobes, and shows moderate activity against gram-positive organisms. Effectively treats bone and joint infections, gynecologic and intra-abdominal infections, lower respiratory tract infections, skin infections, urinary tract infections, and is used for surgical prophylaxis, reducing or eliminating infection.

USES Infections caused by susceptible organisms in urinary tract, lower respiratory tract, skin and skin structures, bones and joints, gynecologic tract; also intra-abdominal infections, bacteremia, and perioperative prophylaxis.

CONTRAINDICATIONS Hypersensitivity to cephalosporins and related beta-lactam antibiotics; pregnancy (category B).
CAUTIOUS USE Lactation.

ROUTE & DOSAGE

Moderate to Severe Infections
Adult: **IV/IM** 1–2 g q12h
Child: **IV/IM** 40–80 mg/kg/d divided q12h (max: 6 g/d)

Surgical Prophylaxis
Adult: **IV/IM** 1–2 g 30–60 min before surgery

ADMINISTRATION

Intramuscular

- For IM reconstitution (follow manufacturer's directions for selection of diluent), add 2 mL diluent to 1 g vial; withdraw approximately 2.4 mL to yield 375 mg drug/mL.
- For IM administration, inject well into body of large muscle such as upper outer quadrant of buttock (gluteus maximus).

Intravenous

- IV administration to infants and children: Verify correct IV concentration and rate of infusion with physician.

PREPARE: **Direct:** Dilute each 1 g with 10 mL of sterile water for injection. **Intermittent:** Following reconstitution, dilute each 1 g with 50–100 mL of D5W or NS.

ADMINISTER: **Direct:** Give over 3–5 min. **Intermittent:** Give a single dose over 30 min. For IV infusion, solution may be given for longer period of time through tubing system through which other IV solutions are being given.

INCOMPATIBILITIES **Solution/additive:** AMINOGLYCOSIDES, **doxapram,** HEPARIN, **promethazine,** TETRACYCLINES. **Y-site:** AMINOGLYCOSIDES, **promethazine, vancomycin, vinorelbine.**

- Protect sterile powder from light; store at 22° C (71.6° F) or less; remains stable 24 mo after date of manufacture. May darken with age, but potency is unaffected. Reconstituted solutions: stable for 24 h at 25° C (77° F); 96 h when refrigerated at 5° C (41° F); or at least 1 wk when frozen at –20° C (–4° F).

ADVERSE EFFECTS (≥1%) **Body as a Whole:** Fever, chills, injection site pain, inflammation, disulfiram-like reaction. **GI:** Nausea, vomiting, *diarrhea,* abdominal pain, antibiotic-associated colitis. **Hematologic:** Thrombocytopenia, prolongation of bleeding time or prothrombin time. **Skin:** Rash, pruritus.

DIAGNOSTIC TEST INTERFERENCE May cause falsely elevated ***serum*** or ***urine creatinine*** values ***(Jaffe reaction).*** False-positive reactions for ***urine glucose*** have not been reported using ***copper sulfate reduction methods,*** e.g., ***Benedict's, Clinitest;*** however, since it has occurred with other cephalosporins, it may be advisable to use ***glucose oxidase tests (Clinistix, TesTape, Diastix).*** Positive ***direct antiglobulin (Coombs') test*** results may interfere with ***hematologic studies*** and ***cross-matching*** procedures.

INTERACTIONS Drug: Probenecid decreases renal elimination of cefotetan; **alcohol** produces disulfiram reaction.

PHARMACOKINETICS Peak: 1.5–3 h after IM. **Distribution:** Poor CNS penetration; widely distributed to body tissues and fluids, including bile, sputum, prostatic and peritoneal fluids; crosses placenta. **Elimination:** 51–81% excreted unchanged in urine; 20% excreted in bile; small amount excreted in breast milk. **Half-Life:** 180–270 min.

NURSING IMPLICATIONS

Assessment & Drug Effects

- Determine history of hypersensitivity to cephalosporins and penicillins, and other drug allergies, before therapy begins.
- Lab tests: Perform culture and sensitivity studies before initiation of therapy and during therapy, as in-

C

dicated. Therapy may begin pending test results. Perform periodic hematologic studies (including PT/INR and PTT) and evaluation of renal function, especially if cefotetan dose is high or if therapy is prolonged in order to recognize symptoms of nephrotoxicity and ototoxicity (see Appendix F).

- Report onset of loose stools or diarrhea. If diarrhea is severe, suspect pseudomembranous colitis (see Appendix F) caused by *Clostridium difficile*. Check temperature. Report fever and severe diarrhea to physician; drug should be discontinued.

Patient & Family Education

- Report promptly S&S of superinfection (see Appendix F).
- Report loose stools or diarrhea.
- Do not breast feed while taking this drug without consulting physician.

CEFOXITIN SODIUM

(se-fox′i-tin)

Mefoxin

Classifications: ANTIINFECTIVE; ANTIBIOTIC; SECOND-GENERATION CEPHALOSPORIN

Prototype: Cefonicid sodium

Pregnancy Category: B

AVAILABILITY 1 g, 2 g injection

ACTIONS Semisynthetic, broad-spectrum beta-lactam antibiotic derivative of cephamycin C (produced by *Streptomyces lactamdurans*). Classified as second generation cephalosporin; structurally and pharmacologically related to cephalosporins and penicillins. Antimicrobial spectrum of activity resembles that of cefonicid. Considerably less active than most cephalosporins against *Staphylococci*. Preferentially binds to one or more of the penicillin-binding proteins (PBP) located on cell walls of susceptible organisms.

THERAPEUTIC EFFECTS It shows enhanced activity against a wide variety of gram-negative organisms and is effective for mixed aerobic-anaerobic infections. Effectively treats gynecologic, bone and joint and intra-abdominal infections, gonorrhea, skin and urinary tract infections, and is used for surgical prophylaxis, reducing or eliminating infection.

USES Infections caused by susceptible organisms in the lower respiratory tract, urinary tract, skin and skin structures, bones and joints; also intra-abdominal endocarditis, gynecological infections, septicemia, uncomplicated gonorrhea, and perioperative prophylaxis in prosthetic arthroplasty or cardiovascular surgery. May be cephalosporin of choice for mixed aerobic-anaerobic infections (e.g., *Bacteroides fragilis*).

CONTRAINDICATIONS Hypersensitivity to cephalosporins and related antibiotics; pregnancy (category B), lactation. Safe use in children <3 mo not established.

CAUTIOUS USE History of sensitivity to penicillin or other allergies, particularly to drugs; impaired renal function.

ROUTE & DOSAGE

Moderate to Severe Infections

Adult: **IV/IM** 1–2 g q6–8h, up to 12 g/d
Child >3 mo:: **IV/IM** 80–160 mg/kg/d in 4–6 divided doses (max: 12 g/d)
Neonate: **IV/IM** 90–100 mg/kg/d divided q8h

Surgical Prophylaxis

Adult: **IV/IM** 2 g 30–60 min before surgery, then 2 g q6h for 24 h
Child: **IV/IM** 30–40 mg/kg 30–60 min before surgery, then 2 g q6h for 24 h

Uncomplicated Gonorrhea

Adult: **IV/IM** 2 g given concurrently with 1 g probenecid PO

ADMINISTRATION

Intramuscular

- Reconstitute each 1 g with 2 mL sterile water for injection or 0.5 or 1% lidocaine hydrochloride (without epinephrine), used to reduce discomfort of IM injection. After reconstitution for IM use, shake vial and allow solution to stand until it becomes clear.
- Administer IM injections deep into large muscle mass such as upper outer quadrant of gluteus maximus. Aspirate before injecting drug. Rotate injection sites.

Intravenous

- IV administration to neonates, infants and children: Verify correct IV concentration and rate of infusion/injection with physician.

PREPARE: **Direct:** Dilute each 1 g with 10 mL sterile water, D5W, or NS. **Intermittent:** Following reconstitution, dilute 1–2 g in 50–100 mL of D5W or NS.

ADMINISTER: **Direct:** Give over 3–5 min. **Intermittent:** Give over 15 min.

INCOMPATIBILITIES **Solution/additive:** AMINOGLYCOSIDES, **ranitidine. Y-site:** AMINOGLYCOSIDES, **filgrastim, hetastarch, pentamidine, vancomycin.**

- Reconstituted solution may become discolored (usually light yellow to amber) if exposed to high temperatures; however, potency is not affected. Solution may be cloudy immediately after reconstitution; let stand and it will clear.
- After reconstitution, solution is stable for 24 h at 25° C (77° F); 7 d when refrigerated at 4° C (39° F), or 30 wk when frozen at –20° C (–4° F).

ADVERSE EFFECTS (≥1%) **Body as a Whole:** Drug fever, eosinophilia, superinfections, local reactions: pain, tenderness, and induration (IM site), thrombophlebitis (IV site). **GI:** *Diarrhea,* <u>pseudomembranous colitis</u>. **Skin:** Rash, <u>exfoliative dermatitis</u>, pruritus, urticaria. **Urogenital:** nephrotoxicity, interstitial nephritis.

DIAGNOSTIC TEST INTERFERENCE Cefoxitin causes false-positive (black-brown or green-brown color) ***urine glucose*** reaction with ***copper reduction reagents*** such as ***Benedict's*** or ***Clinitest,*** but not with ***enzymatic glucose oxidase reagents (Clinistix, Tes-Tape)***. With high doses, falsely elevated ***serum and urine creatinine*** (with ***Jaffee reaction***) reported. False-positive ***direct Coombs' test*** (may interfere with ***cross-matching procedures*** and ***hematologic studies***) has also been reported.

INTERACTIONS Drug: Probenecid decreases renal elimination of cefoxitin.

PHARMACOKINETICS Peak: 20–30 min after IM; 5 min after IV. **Distribution:** Poor CNS penetration even with inflamed meninges; widely distributed in body tissues including pleural, synovial, and ascitic fluid and bile; crosses placenta. **Elimination:** 85% excreted unchanged in urine in 6 h, small amount excreted in breast milk. **Half-Life:** 45–60 min.

NURSING IMPLICATIONS

Assessment & Drug Effects

- Determine previous hypersensitivity to cephalosporins, penicillins, and other drug allergies before therapy is initiated.
- Lab tests: Perform culture and sensitivity testing prior to and periodically during therapy. Periodic renal function tests.
- Inspect injection sites regularly. Report evidence of inflammation and patient's complaint of pain.
- Monitor I&O rates and pattern: Nephrotoxicity occurs most frequently in patients >50 y, in patients with impaired renal function, the debilitated, and in patients receiving high doses or other nephrotoxic drugs.
- Be alert to S&S of superinfections (see Appendix F). This condition is most apt to occur in older adult patients, especially when drug has been used for prolonged period.
- Report onset of diarrhea (may be dose related). If severe, pseudomembranous colitis (see Signs & Symptoms, Appendix F) must be ruled out. Older adult patients are especially susceptible.

Patient & Family Education

- Report promptly S&S of superinfection (see Appendix F).
- Report watery or bloody loose stools or severe diarrhea.
- Report severe vomiting or stomach pain.
- Report infusion site swelling, pain, or redness.
- Do not breast feed while taking this drug.

CEFPODOXIME

(cef-po-dox'eem)

Vantin

Classifications: ANTIINFECTIVE; ANTIBIOTIC; THIRD-GENERATION CEPHALOSPORIN

Prototype: Cefotaxime sodium

Pregnancy Category: B

AVAILABILITY 100 mg, 200 mg tablets; 50 mg/5 mL, 100 mg/5 mL suspension

ACTIONS Semisynthetic cephalosporin antibiotic with antibacterial activity resembling that of other third-generation cephalosporins. Stable in the presence of beta-lactamases. Highly active against gram-negative bacteria.

THERAPEUTIC EFFECTS It is effective against most common pathogens causing upper and lower respiratory infections. Effectively treats gonorrhea, otitis media, upper and lower respiratory infections, and skin and urinary tract infections, reducing or eliminating infection.

USES Gonorrhea, otitis media, lower and upper respiratory tract infections, urinary tract infections.

UNLABELED USES Skin and soft tissue infections.

CONTRAINDICATIONS Hypersensitivity to cephalosporins and other beta-lactam antibiotics; pregnancy (category B).

CAUTIOUS USE Renal impairment, history of type I hypersensitivity reactions to penicillins; history of colitis or other GI disease; lactation.

ROUTE & DOSAGE

Respiratory Tract, Skin, and Soft Tissue Infections

Adult: **PO** 200 mg q12h for 10 d

Child: **PO** 10 mg/kg/d divided q12h

Urinary Tract Infections

Adult: **PO** 100 mg q12h

Gonorrhea

Adult: **PO** 200 mg as single dose

Otitis Media

Child 5 mo–12 y: **PO** 10 mg/kg/d divided q12–24h

ADMINISTRATION

Oral

- Give with food to enhance absorption.
- Give 1 h before or 2 h after an antacid.
- Consult physician regarding patients with renal impairment (i.e., creatinine clearance less than 30 mL/min); dosage intervals should be every 12 h.
- Patients on hemodialysis should be given usual dose 3 times weekly after hemodialysis.
- Preparation of suspension: To either the 50 mg/5 mL strength or the 100 mg/5 mL strength, add 25 mL of distilled water, then shake vigorously for 15 seconds. Next, to the 50 mg/5 mL strength add 33 mL, or to the 100 mg/5 mL strength add 32 mL, of distilled water, and shake for at least 3 minutes.
- Store suspension for up to 14 d in a refrigerator (2°–8° C/36°–46° F). Shake well before using.

ADVERSE EFFECTS (≥1%) **Body as a Whole:** Eye itching, cough, epistaxis, fever, decreased appetite, malaise. **GI:** Diarrhea, nausea, vomiting, abdominal pain, soft stools, flatulance, pseudomembranous colitis (rare). **CNS:** rare: Headache, asthenia, dizziness, fatigue, anxiety, insomnia, flushing, nightmares, weakness. **Urogenital:** Vaginal candidiasis. **Skin:** Urticaria, rash, scaling, peeling.

INTERACTIONS Drug: ANTACIDS, **ranitidine** may decrease absorption. **Food:** Food may increase the absorption.

PHARMACOKINETICS Absorption: 40–50% absorbed from GI tract increased with food. **Onset:** Therapeutic effect in 3 d. **Distribution:** Distributes well into inflammatory, pulmonary, and pleural fluid, and tonsils. Some distribution into prostate. 40% bound to plasma proteins. Distributed into breast milk. **Elimination:** 80% excreted in urine. **Half-Life:** 2–3 h.

NURSING IMPLICATIONS

Assessment & Drug Effects

- Determine history of hypersensitivity reactions to cephalosporins and penicillins, and history of allergies, particularly to drugs, before therapy is initiated.
- Lab tests: Perform culture and sensitivity tests before initiation of therapy and periodically during therapy, if indicated. Therapy may be instituted pending test results.
- Report onset of loose stools or diarrhea. Although pseudomembranous enterocolitis (see Appendix F) rarely occurs, this potentially life-threatening complication should be ruled out as the cause of diarrhea during and after antibiotic therapy.
- Monitor for manifestations of hypersensitivity (see Appendix F). Discontinue drug and report S&S of hypersensitivity promptly.
- Monitor I&O rates and pattern: Especially important with high doses; report any significant changes.

Patient & Family Education

- Report any signs or symptoms of hypersensitivity immediately.

C

- Report loose stools, or diarrhea, especially if containing blood, mucus, or pus.
- Complete the full course of drug therapy even if symptoms improve.
- Do not breast feed while taking this drug without consulting physician.

CEFPROZIL

(cef′pro-zil)
Cefzil
Classifications: ANTIINFECTIVE; ANTIBIOTIC; SECOND-GENERATION CEPHALOSPORIN
Prototype: Cefonicid sodium
Pregnancy Category: B

AVAILABILITY 250 mg, 500 mg tablets; 125 mg/5 mL, 250 mg/5 mL suspension

ACTIONS Semisynthetic, second-generation cephalosporin antibiotic with drug structure characterized by a beta-lactam ring; generally resistant to hydrolysis by beta-lactamases. Preferentially binds to proteins in cell walls of susceptible organisms, thus killing the bacteria. Also active against organisms susceptible to first generation cephalosporin.

THERAPEUTIC EFFECTS Active against *Streptococcus pyogenes, Streptococcus pneumoniae, Haemophilus influenzae, Moraxella catarrhalis*, and *Staphylococcus aureus*. Effectively treats upper and lower respiratory tract infections, otitis media and sinusitis, and skin infections, eliminating or reducing infection.

USES Upper and lower respiratory tract infections, otitis media, skin infections.

CONTRAINDICATIONS Hypersensitivity to cephalosporin and related antibiotics; severely impaired renal or hepatic function; pregnancy (category B).

CAUTIOUS USE Lactation; patients with delayed reaction to penicillin or other drugs; GI disease, especially colitis.

ROUTE & DOSAGE

Mild to Moderate Infections
Adult: **PO** 250–500 mg q12–24h for 10–14 d
Child >6 mo: **PO** 15 mg/kg q12h

ADMINISTRATION

Oral

- Drug may be given without regard to meals.
- Consult physician for patients with impaired renal function. Dose is reduced by 50% when creatinine clearance is 0–30 mL/min.
- Administer after hemodialysis since drug is partially removed by dialysis.
- After reconstitution, oral suspension is refrigerated. Discard unused portion after 14 days.

ADVERSE EFFECTS (≥1%) **Body as a Whole:** Hypersensitivity reactions, superinfections. **GI:** Nausea, vomiting, diarrhea, abdominal pain. **Hematologic:** Eosinophilia. **CNS:** Headache. **Skin:** Rash, diaper rash. **Urogenital:** Genital pruritus, vaginal candidiasis.

DIAGNOSTIC TEST INTERFERENCE May cause a positive ***direct Coombs' test;*** false-negative results in the ferricyanide assay for ***blood glucose***; false-positive reactions for ***urine glucose*** with ***copper reduction tests*** such as ***Benedict's*** or ***Fehling's solution*** or ***Clinitest tablets;*** increased ***partial thromboplastin time,*** indicating thrombocytosis, eosinophilia; minor elevations in ***serum alanine aminotransferase (ALT), aspartate aminotransferase (AST),*** and ***bilirubin.***

INTERACTIONS Drug: Probenecid prolongs the elimination of cefprozil.

PHARMACOKINETICS Absorption: Readily absorbed from GI tract. **Peak:** 1–2 h. **Distribution:** Distributes into blister fluid at 50% of the serum level. **Elimination:** Primarily excreted by the kidneys. **Half-Life:** 1–2 h.

NURSING IMPLICATIONS

Assessment & Drug Effects

- Determine previous hypersensitivity to cephalosporins or penicillins before treatment.
- Withhold drug and notify physician if hypersensitivity occurs (e.g., rash, urticaria).
- Lab tests: Perform culture and sensitivity tests before and periodically during therapy. Therapy may be initiated while results are pending.
- Monitor for and report diarrhea, as pseudomembranous colitis is a potential adverse effect.
- Monitor for and report signs of superinfection (see Appendix F).
- When given concurrently with other cephalosporins or aminoglycosides, monitor for signs of nephrotoxicity.

Patient & Family Education

- Complete the prescribed course of therapy, even if symptom free.
- Report rash or other signs of hypersensitivity immediately.
- Report signs of superinfection (see Appendix F).
- Report loose stools and diarrhea even after completion of drug therapy.
- Do not breast feed while taking this drug without consulting physician.

CEFTAZIDIME

(sef′tay-zi-deem)

Fortaz, Tazicef, Tazidime

Classifications: ANTIINFECTIVE; ANTIBIOTIC; THIRD-GENERATION CEPHALOSPORIN

Prototype: Cefotaxime sodium

Pregnancy Category: B

AVAILABILITY 500 mg, 1 g, 2 g injection

ACTIONS Semisynthetic, third-generation broad-spectrum cephalosporin antibiotic similar to cefotaxime but more active against *Pseudomonas aeruginosa* and less active against *Staphylococci* and *Bacteroides fragilis.* Preferentially binds to one or more of the penicillin-binding proteins (PBP) located on cell walls of susceptible microbes; this inhibits third and final stage of bacterial cell wall synthesis, leading to cell death of the bacterium.

THERAPEUTIC EFFECTS Most strains of gonococci, meningococci, and *Haemophilus influenzae* are highly susceptible to ceftazidime; *Listeria monocytogenes* organisms are resistant. Emergence of resistance during treatment has been reported. May be used concomitantly with other antibiotics (e.g., aminoglycosides, vancomycin, clindamycin). It is effective against *Pseudomonas, Serratia* and the *Enterobacteriaceae.* Effectively treats bone and joint infections, gynecologic and gram negative infections, meningitis, intra-abdominal infections, septicemia, and respiratory tract, urinary tract, and skin and soft tissue infections, by reducing or eliminating the infection.

USES To treat infections of lower respiratory tract, skin and skin structures, urinary tract, bones and joints; also used to treat bacteremia, gynecological, intra-abdominal and CNS infections (including meningitis).

UNLABELED USE Surgical prophylaxis.

CONTRAINDICATIONS Hypersensitivity to cephalosporins and related beta-lactam antibiotics; pregnancy (category B).

CAUTIOUS USE Lactation.

ROUTE & DOSAGE

Moderate to Severe Infections

Adult: **IV/IM** 1–2 g q8–12h, up to 2 g q6h
Geriatric: **IV/IM** 1–2 g q12h
Child: **IV/IM** *<4 wk,* 30 mg/kg q12h; *1 mo–12 y,* 30–50 mg/kg/d in 3 divided doses (max: 6 g/d)

ADMINISTRATION

Intramuscular

- Reconstitute by adding 3 mL sterile water or bacteriostatic water for injection or 0.5% or 1% lidocaine HCl injection to 1 g vial to yield 280 mg/mL.
- Inject into large muscle mass (e.g., upper outer quadrant of gluteus maximus or lateral part of thigh).

Intravenous

PREPARE: **Direct:** Add 10 mL of sterile water for injection to 1 g to yield 280 mg/mL. **Intermittent:** Further dilute with 50–100 mL of D5W, NS, or RL.

ADMINISTER: **Direct:** Give over 3–5 min. **Intermittent:** Give over 30–60 min. If given through a Y-type set, discontinue other solutions during infusion of ceftazidime.

INCOMPATIBILITIES **Solution/additive:** AMINOGLYCOSIDES, **aminophylline, ranidine. Y-site:** AMINOGLYCOSIDES, **amphotericin B cholesteryl complex, amsacrine, doxorubicin liposome, fluconazole, idarubicin, midazolam, pentamidine, sargramostim, vancomycin, warfarin.**

- Protect sterile powder from light. Reconstituted solution is stable 7 d when refrigerated at 4°–5° C (39°–41° F); for 18–24 h when stored at 15°–30° C (59°–86° F).

ADVERSE EFFECTS (≥1%) **Body as a Whole:** Fever, phlebitis, pain or inflammation at injection site, superinfections. **GI:** Nausea, vomiting, *diarrhea,* abdominal pain, metallic taste, drug-associated <u>pseudomembranous colitis</u>. **Skin:** Pruritus, rash, urticaria. **Urogenital:** Vaginitis, candidiasis.

DIAGNOSTIC TEST INTERFERENCE False-positive reactions for ***urine glucose*** have been reported using ***copper sulfate*** (e.g., ***Benedict's solution, Clinitest***). ***Glucose oxidase tests (Clinistix, TesTape)*** are unaffected. May cause positive ***direct antiglobulin (Coombs') test*** results, which can interfere with ***hematologic studies*** and ***transfusion cross-matching procedures.***

INTERACTIONS Drug: Probenecid decreases renal elimination of ceftazidine.

PHARMACOKINETICS Peak: 1 h after IM or IV. **Distribution:** CNS penetration with inflamed meninges;

also penetrates bone, gallbladder, bile, endometrium, heart, skin, and ascitic and pleural fluids; crosses placenta. **Metabolism:** Not metabolized. **Elimination:** 80–90% excreted unchanged in urine in 24 h; small amount excreted in breast milk. **Half-Life:** 25–60 min.

NURSING IMPLICATIONS

Assessment & Drug Effects

- Determine history of hypersensitivity to cephalosporins and penicillins, and other drug allergies, before therapy begins.
- Lab tests: Perform culture and sensitivity studies before initiation of therapy and during therapy as indicated. Therapy may begin pending test results.
- If administered concomitantly with another antibiotic, monitor renal function and report if symptoms of dysfunction appear (e.g., changes in I&O ratio and pattern, dysuria).
- Be alert to onset of rash, itching, and dyspnea. Check patient's temperature. If it is elevated, suspect onset of hypersensitivity reaction (see Signs & Symptoms, Appendix F).
- Monitor for superinfection. (See Signs & Symptoms, Appendix F).
- If diarrhea occurs and is severe, suspect pseudomembranous colitis (caused by *Clostridium difficile*). Check temperature: Report fever and severe diarrhea to physician; drug should be discontinued.

Patient & Family Education

- Report loose stools or diarrhea promptly.
- Report any signs or symptoms of superinfection promptly (see Appendix F).
- Do not breast feed while taking this drug without consulting physician.

CEFTIBUTEN

(sef-ti-bu′ten)

Cedax

Classifications: ANTIINFECTIVE; BETA-LACTAM ANTIBIOTIC; THIRD-GENERATION CEPHALOSPORIN

Prototype: Cefotaxime sodium

Pregnancy Category: B

AVAILABILITY 400 mg capsules; 90 mg/5 mL, 180 mg/5 mL suspension

ACTIONS Ceftibuten is a broad-spectrum, third-generation beta-lactam antibiotic. Preferentially binds to one or more of the penicillin-binding proteins located in the cell wall of susceptible organisms. This inhibits third and final stage of bacterial cell wall synthesis, thus killing the bacterium. It is highly resistant to hydrolysis by most beta-lactamase bacteria.

THERAPEUTIC EFFECTS It has antibacterial activity against both gram-negative and gram-positive bacteria, including *Haemophilus influenzae* (beta-lactamase-producing strains also), *Streptococcus pneumoniae,* and *Streptococcus pyogenes.* Effectively treats bronchitis, otitis media, pharyngitis, and urinary tract infections, reducing or eliminating infection.

USES Acute bacterial exacerbations of chronic bronchitis caused by *H. influenzae, Moraxella catarrhalis,* or *S. pneumoniae;* acute bacterial otitis media caused by *H. influenzae, M. catarrhalis,* or *S. pyogenes;* pharyngitis or tonsillitis caused by *S. pyogenes.*

CONTRAINDICATIONS Hypersensitivity to ceftibuten or cephalosporins.

CAUTIOUS USE Renal dysfunction, penicillin hypersensitivity, history of colitis or diabetes, pregnancy (category B), lactation. Safety and efficacy in infants <6 mo not established.

ROUTE & DOSAGE

Mild to Moderate Infections

Adult: **PO** 400 mg once daily for 10 d

Renal Insufficiency

Cl_{cr} 30–49: 200 mg q24h; Cl_{cr} <30: 100 mg q24h
Child (6 mo–12 y): **PO** 9 mg/kg once daily (max 400 mg) for 10 d

Renal Impairment

Cl_{cr} 30–49 mL/min: 4.5 mg/kg q24h; <30 mL/min: 2.25 mg/kg q24h

ADMINISTRATION

Oral

- Give oral suspension 1 h before or 2 h after a meal.
- Children weighing more than 45 kg may receive maximum daily dose.
- Hemodialysis patients should receive drug at the end of dialysis.
- Store capsules at 2°–25° C (36°–77° F); keep container tightly closed. Reconstituted oral suspension is stable for 14 d under refrigeration at 2°–8° C (36°–46° F).

ADVERSE EFFECTS (≥1%) **Body as a Whole:** Dyspnea, dysuria, fatigue, vaginitis, moniliasis, urticaria, pruritus, rash, paresthesia, taste perversion. **GI:** Nausea, vomiting, diarrhea, dyspepsia, abdominal pain, anorexia, constipation, dry mouth, eructation, flatulence. **CNS:** Headache, dizziness, nasal congestion, somnolence.

INTERACTIONS Drug: AMINOGLYCOSIDES may increase risk of nephrotoxicity and have additive/synergistic effects. May decrease efficacy of ORAL CONTRACEPTIVES. **Probenecid** may increase levels.

PHARMACOKINETICS Absorption: Rapidly absorbed from GI tract. **Peak:** Approx 2–3 h. **Distribution:** Bronchial mucosa levels are approx 37% of plasma levels, middle ear levels approx 50% of plasma levels. **Elimination:** Excreted primarily in urine. **Half-Life:** 1.5–2.5 h.

NURSING IMPLICATIONS

Assessment & Drug Effects

- Determine history of hypersensitivity reactions to cephalosporins, penicillins, or other drugs, before therapy is initiated. Monitor for S&S of hypersensitivity (see Appendix F); report their appearance promptly and discontinue drug.
- Lab tests: Perform culture and sensitivity tests before initiation of therapy. Dosage may be started pending test results.
- Monitor for S&S of superinfection or pseudomembranous colitis (see Appendix F); immediately report either to physician.
- Closely monitor patients with renal impairment; if seizures develop, discontinue drug and notify physician.

Patient & Family Education

- If on dialysis treatment, take this drug after dialysis.
- Report any S&S of hypersensitivity, superinfection, and pseudomembranous colitis promptly.
- Do not breast feed while taking this drug without consulting physician.

CEFTIZOXIME SODIUM

(sef-ti-zox′eem)

Cefizox

Classifications: ANTIINFECTIVE; ANTIBIOTIC; THIRD-GENERATION CEPHALOSPORIN

Prototype: Cefotaxime sodium

Pregnancy Category: B

AVAILABILITY 500 mg, 1 g, 2 g injection

ACTIONS Semisynthetic third-generation cephalosporin antibiotic. Preferentially binds to one or more of the penicillin-binding proteins (PBP) located on cell walls of susceptible organisms. This inhibits third and final stage of bacterial cell wall synthesis, thus killing the bacterium. Spectrum of activity similar to that of cefotaxime. Generally resistant to inactivation by beta-lactamases that act principally as cephalosporinases and penicillinases.

THERAPEUTIC EFFECTS *Clostridium difficile,* enterococci including *Streptococcus faecalis,* and most strains of *Listeria monocytogenes* are resistant to ceftizoxime. Incompatible with the aminoglycoside antibiotics. Evidence of partial cross-allergenicity among cephalosporins and other beta-lactamase antibiotics has been reported. It is used for gram-negative bacillary meningitis and drug-resistant *Enterobacteriaceae.* Effectively treats endocarditis, bone and joint infections, gonorrhea and gynecologic infections including PID, *E. coli* infections, *Haemophilus influenzae* infections, intra-abdominal infections, meningitis, osteomyelitis, lower respiratory tract infections, *Serratia sp.* infections, septicemia and skin infections, urinary tract infections, and is used for surgical prophylaxis, reducing or eliminating infection.

USES Infections caused by susceptible organisms in lower respiratory tract, skin and skin structures, urinary tract, bones and joints; also used to treat intra-abdominal infections, pelvic inflammatory disease, uncomplicated gonorrhea, meningitis *(Haemophilus influenzae, Streptococcus pneumoniae),* and for surgical prophylaxis.

UNLABELED USES Meningitis caused by *Neisseria meningitidis* and *Escherichia coli.*

CONTRAINDICATIONS Hypersensitivity to cephalosporins and other beta-lactam antibiotics; pregnancy (category B).

CAUTIOUS USE Lactation.

ROUTE & DOSAGE

Moderate to Severe Infections
Adult: **IV/IM** 1–2 g q8–12h, up to 2 g q4h
Child: **IV/IM** ≥6 mo, 50 mg/kg q6–8h, up to 200 mg/kg/d

ADMINISTRATION

Intramuscular

- Reconstitute as follows with sterile water for injection: add 1.5 mL to 500 mg to yield 280 mg/mL; add 3 mL to 1 g or 6 mL to 2 g to yield 270 mg/mL.
- Give deep IM into a large muscle. Give no more than 1 g into a single injection site.

Intravenous

PREPARE: **Direct:** Reconstitute each 1 g with 10 mL sterile water. Shake well. **Intermittent:** Further dilute in 50–100 mL D5W, NS, D5/NS, D5/.45% NaCl, RL, or other compatible IV solution.
ADMINISTER: **Direct:** Give over 3–5 min. **Intermittent:** Give over 30 min.
INCOMPATIBILITIES **Solution/additive:** AMINOGLYCOSIDES. **Y-site:** AMINOGLYCOSIDES, **filgrastim.**

- Protect from light. Consult manufacturer's directions concerning storage of reconstituted solutions.

C

ADVERSE EFFECTS (≥1%) **Body as a Whole:** Fever, phlebitis, vaginitis, pain and induration at injection site, paresthesia. **GI:** Nausea, vomiting, diarrhea, pseudomembranous colitis. **Skin:** Rash, pruritus.

DIAGNOSTIC TEST INTERFERENCE Ceftizoxime causes false-positive ***direct Coombs' test*** (may interfere with ***cross-matching procedures*** and ***hematologic studies).***

INTERACTIONS Drug: Probenecid decreases renal elimination of ceftizoxime.

PHARMACOKINETICS Peak: 1 h after IM or IV. **Distribution:** Crosses placenta. **Metabolism:** Not metabolized. **Elimination:** 80–90% excreted unchanged in urine in 24 h; small amount excreted in breast milk. **Half-Life:** 25–60 min.

NURSING IMPLICATIONS

Assessment & Drug Effects

- Determine history of hypersensitivity reactions to cephalosporins, penicillin, or other drugs before therapy is instituted. Report to physician history of allergy, particularly to drugs.
- Lab tests: Perform culture and sensitivity tests before initiation of therapy and periodically during therapy if indicated. Therapy may be instituted pending test results.
- Be alert to symptoms of hypersensitivity reaction (see Appendix F). Serious reactions may require emergency measures.

Patient & Family Education

- Report loose stools or diarrhea promptly.
- Report any signs or symptoms of hypersensitivity (see Appendix F) promptly.
- Do not breast feed while taking this drug without consulting physician.

CEFTRIAXONE SODIUM

(sef-try-ax'one)

Rocephin

Classifications: ANTIINFECTIVE; ANTIBIOTIC; THIRD-GENERATION CEPHALOSPORIN

Prototype: Cefotaxime sodium

Pregnancy Category: B

AVAILABILITY 250 mg, 500 mg, 1 g, 2 g injection

ACTIONS Semisynthetic third-generation cephalosporin antibiotic. Preferentially binds to one or more of the penicillin-binding proteins (PBP) located on cell walls of susceptible organisms. This inhibits third and final stage of bacterial cell wall synthesis, thus killing the bacterium.

THERAPEUTIC EFFECTS Spectrum of activity similar to that of cefotaxime including most *Enterobacteriaceae,* most gram-positive aerobic cocci, *Neisseria meningitidis,* and most strains of penicillinase-producing and nonpenicillinase-producing *Neisseria gonorrhoeae.* Has some activity against *Treponema pallidum* but none against most strains of *Clostridia.* Effectively treats bone and joint infections, gonorrhea and intra-abdominal infections, meningitis and lower respiratory tract infections, otitis media, pelvic inflammatory disease, *Proteus* infections, septicemia, skin and soft tissue infections, urinary tract infections, and is used for surgical prophylaxis, reducing or eliminating infection.

USES Infections caused by susceptible organisms in lower respiratory tract, skin and skin structures, urinary tract, bones and joints; also intra-abdominal infections, pelvic inflammatory disease, uncomplicated gonorrhea, meningitis, and surgical prophylaxis.

CONTRAINDICATIONS Hypersensitivity to cephalosporins and related antibiotics; pregnancy (category B). **CAUTIOUS USE** Lactation.

ROUTE & DOSAGE

Moderate to Severe Infections

Adult: **IV/IM** 1–2 g q12–24h (max: 4 g/d)
Child: **IV/IM** 50–75 mg/kg/d in 2 divided doses (max: 2 g/d)

Meningitis

Adult: **IV/IM** 2 g q12h
Child: **IV/IM** 75 mg/kg loading dose, then 100 mg/kg/d in 2 divided doses (max: 4 g/d)

Surgical Prophylaxis

Adult: **IV/IM** 1 g 30–120 min before surgery

Uncomplicated Gonorrhea

Adult: **IM** 250 mg as single dose
Child: **IM** 125 mg as single dose

ADMINISTRATION

Intramuscular

- Reconstitute the 1 g or 2 g vial by adding 2.1 mL or 4.2 mL, respectively, of sterile water for injection. Yields 3.50 mg/mL. See manufacturer's directions for other dilutions.
- Give deep IM into a large muscle.

Intravenous

- IV administration to infants and children: Verify correct IV concentration and rate of infusion with physician.

PREPARE: **Intermittent:** Reconstitute each 250 mg with 2.4 mL of sterile water, D5W, NS, or D5/NS to yield 100 mg/mL. Further dilute with 50–100 mL of the selected IV solution.

ADMINISTER: **Intermittent:** Give over 30 min.

INCOMPATIBILITIES **Solution/additive:** AMINOGLYCOSIDES, **aminophylline, clindamycin, lidocaine, metronidazole, theophylline. Y-site:** AMINOGLYCOSIDES, **amphotericin B cholesteryl complex, amsacrine, fluconazole, filgrastim, labetalol, pentamidine, vancomycin, vinorelbine.**

- Protect sterile powder from light. Store at 15°–25° C (59°–77° F). Reconstituted solutions: diluent, concentration of solutions are determinants of stability. See manufacturer's instructions for storage.

ADVERSE EFFECTS (≥1%) **Body as a Whole:** Pruritus, fever, chills, pain, induration at IM injection site; phlebitis (IV site). **GI:** *Diarrhea,* abdominal cramps, pseudomembranous colitis, biliary sludge. **Urogenital:** Genital pruritus; moniliasis.

DIAGNOSTIC TEST INTERFERENCE Causes prolonged ***PT/INR*** during therapy.

INTERACTIONS Drug: Probenecid decreases renal elimination of ceftriaxone; **alcohol** produces disulfiram reaction.

PHARMACOKINETICS Peak: 1.5–4 h after IM; immediately after IV infusion. **Distribution:** Widely distributed in body tissues and fluids; good CNS penetration, especially with inflamed meninges; crosses placenta. **Metabolism:** Not metabolized. **Elimination:** 33–65% excreted unchanged in urine; also excreted in bile; small amount excreted in breast milk. **Half-Life:** 5–10 h.

C

NURSING IMPLICATIONS

Assessment & Drug Effects

- Determine history of hypersensitivity reactions to cephalosporins and penicillins and history of other allergies, particularly to drugs, before therapy is initiated.
- Lab tests: Perform culture and sensitivity tests before initiation of therapy and periodically during therapy. Dosage may be started pending test results. Periodic coagulation studies (PT and INR) should be done.
- Inspect injection sites for induration and inflammation. Rotate sites. Note IV injection sites for signs of phlebitis (redness, swelling, pain).
- Monitor for manifestations of hypersensitivity (see Signs & Symptoms, Appendix F). Report their appearance promptly and discontinue drug.
- Watch for and report signs: petechiae, ecchymotic areas, epistaxis, or any unexplained bleeding. Ceftriaxone appears to alter vitamin K-producing gut bacteria; therefore, hypoprothrombinemic bleeding may occur.
- Check for fever if diarrhea occurs: Report both promptly. The incidence of antibiotic-produced pseudomembranous colitis (see Appendix F) is higher than with most cephalosporins. Most vulnerable patients: chronically ill or debilitated older adult patients undergoing abdominal surgery.

Patient & Family Education

- Report any signs of bleeding.
- Report loose stools or diarrhea promptly.
- Do not breast feed while taking this drug without consulting physician.

CEFUROXIME SODIUM

(se-fyoor-ox′eem)

Kefurox, Zinacef

CEFUROXIME AXETIL

Ceftin

Classifications: ANTIINFECTIVE; ANTIBIOTIC; SECOND-GENERATION CEPHALOSPORIN

Prototype: Cefonicid sodium

Pregnancy Category: B

AVAILABILITY 125 mg, 250 mg, 500 mg tablets; 125 mg/5 mL, 250 mg/5 mL suspension; 750 mg, 1.5 g injection

ACTIONS Semisynthetic second-generation cephalosporin antibiotic with structure similar to that of the penicillins. Resistance against beta-lactamase-producing strains exceeds that of first generation cephalosporins. Antimicrobial spectrum of activity resembles that of cefonicid. Preferentially binds to one or more of the penicillin-binding proteins (PBP) located on cell walls of susceptible organisms. This inhibits third and final stage of bacterial cell wall synthesis, thus killing the bacterium. Partial cross-allergenicity between other beta-lactam antibiotics and cephalosporins has been reported.

THERAPEUTIC EFFECTS It is effective for the treatment of penicillinase-producing *Neisseria gonorrhoea* (PPNG). Effectively treats bone and joint infections, bronchitis, meningitis, gonorrhea, otitis media, pharyngitis/tonsillitis, sinusitis, lower respiratory tract infections, skin and soft tissue infections, urinary tract infections, and is used for surgical prophylaxis, reducing or eliminating infection.

USES Infections caused by susceptible organisms in the lower respiratory tract, urinary tract, skin, and skin structures; also used for treatment of meningitis, gonorrhea, and otitis media and for perioperative prophylaxis (e.g., open-heart surgery), early Lyme disease.

CONTRAINDICATIONS Hypersensitivity to cephalosporins and related antibiotics; pregnancy (category B), lactation.

CAUTIOUS USE History of allergy, particularly to drugs; penicillin sensitivity; renal insufficiency; history of colitis or other GI disease; potent diuretics.

ROUTE & DOSAGE

Moderate to Severe Infections

Adult: **PO** 250–500 mg q12h. **IV/IM** 750 mg–1.5 g q6–8h
Child (3 mo–12 y): **PO** 10–15 mg/kg (125–250 mg) q12h. **IV/IM** 75–100 mg/kg/d divided q8h (max 6 g/d)
Neonate: **IM/IV** 20–100 mg/kg/d divided q12h

Bacterial Meningitis

Adult: **IV/IM** 3 g q8h
Child: **IV/IM** 200–240 mg/kg/d divided q6–8h; reduced to 100 mg/kg/d upon improvement

Surgical Prophylaxis

Adult: **IV/IM** 1.5 g 30–60 min before surgery, then 750 mg q8h for 24 h
Child: **IV/IM** Same as for adult

ADMINISTRATION

Oral

- Cefuroxime tablets and oral suspension are not substitutable on a mg-for-mg basis.
- The oral suspension is for infants and children 3 mo to 12 y. Each teaspoon (5 mL) contains the equivalent of 125 mg cefuroxime. Shake oral suspension well before each use.

Intramuscular

- Shake IM suspension gently before administration. IM injections should be made deeply into large muscle mass. Rotate injection sites.

Intravenous

- IV administration to neonates, infants and children: Verify correct IV concentration and rate of infusion/injection with physician.

PREPARE: **Direct:** Dilute each 750 mg with 9 mL sterile water, D5W, or NS. **Intermittent:** Further dilute in 50–100 mL of compatible solution. **Continuous:** May be added to 1000 mL of IV compatible solution.

ADMINISTER: **Direct:** Give slowly over 3–5 min. **Intermittent:** Give over 30 min. **Continuous:** Give over 6–24 h.

INCOMPATIBILITIES **Solution/additive:** AMINOGLYCOSIDES, **doxapram, ranitidine, sodium bicarbonate. Y-site:** AMINOGLYCOSIDES, **filgrastim, fluconazole, midazolam, sodium bicarbonate, vancomycin, vinorelbine.**

- Cefuroxime powder and solutions of the drug may range in color from light yellow to amber without adversely affecting product potency.

- Store powder protected from light unless otherwise directed. After reconstitution, store suspension at 2°–30° C (36°–86° F). Discard after 10 d.

ADVERSE EFFECTS (≥1%) **Body as a Whole:** Thrombophlebitis (IV site); pain, burning, cellulitis (IM site); superinfections, positive Coombs' test. **GI:** *Diarrhea,* nausea, antibiotic-associated colitis. **Skin:** Rash, pruritus, urticaria. **Urogenital:** Increased se-

C

rum creatinine and BUN, decreased creatinine clearance.

DIAGNOSTIC TEST INTERFERENCE Cefuroxime causes false-positive (black-brown or green-brown color) ***urine glucose*** reaction with ***copper reduction reagents,*** e.g., ***Benedict's*** or ***Clinitest,*** but not with ***enzymatic glucose oxidase reagents,*** e.g., ***Clinistix, TesTape.*** False-positive ***direct Coombs' test*** (may interfere with ***cross-matching procedures*** and ***hematologic studies***) has been reported.

INTERACTIONS Drug: Probenecid decreases renal elimination of cefuroxime, thus prolonging its action.

PHARMACOKINETICS Absorption: Axetil salt well absorbed from GI tract; hydrolyzed to active drug in GI mucosa. **Peak:** PO 2 h; IM 30 min. **Distribution:** Widely distributed in body tissues and fluids; adequate CNS penetration with inflamed meninges; crosses placenta. **Elimination:** 66–100% excreted in urine in 24 h; excreted in breast milk. **Half-Life:** 1–2 h.

NURSING IMPLICATIONS

Assessment & Drug Effects

- Determine history of hypersensitivity reactions to cephalosporins, penicillins, and history of allergies, particularly to drugs, before therapy is initiated.
- Lab tests: Perform culture and sensitivity tests before initiation of therapy and periodically during therapy if indicated. Therapy may be instituted pending test results. Monitor periodically BUN and creatinine clearance.
- Inspect IM and IV injection sites frequently for signs of phlebitis.
- Report onset of loose stools or diarrhea. Although pseudomembranous colitis (see Signs & Symptoms, Appendix F) rarely occurs, this potentially life-threatening complication should be ruled out as the cause of diarrhea during and after antibiotic therapy.
- Monitor for manifestations of hypersensitivity (see Appendix F). Discontinue drug and report their appearance promptly.
- Monitor I&O rates and pattern: Especially important in severely ill patients receiving high doses. Report any significant changes.

Patient & Family Education

- Report loose stools or diarrhea promptly.
- Report any signs or symptoms of hypersensitivity (see Appendix F).
- Do not breast feed while taking this drug.

CELECOXIB Pr

(cel-e-cox'ib)

Celebrex

Classification: CENTRAL NERVOUS SYSTEM AGENT, ANALGESIC, NSAID, CYCLOOXYGENASE-2 INHIBITOR, ANTIPYRETIC

Pregnancy Category: C first and second trimesters; D third trimester

AVAILABILITY 100 mg, 200 mg, 400 mg capsules

ACTIONS NSAID that exhibits antiinflammatory, analgesic, and antipyretic activities. Unlike ibuprofen, inhibits prostaglandin synthesis by inhibiting cyclooxygenase-2 (COX-2), but does not inhibit cyclooxygenase-1 (COX-1).

THERAPEUTIC EFFECTS Reduces or eliminates the pain of rheumatoid and osteoarthritis.

USES Relief of S&S of osteoarthritis and rheumatoid arthritis. Treatment of acute pain and primary dysmenorrhea. Reduction of polyp formation in Familial Adenomatous Polyposis (FAP)

CONTRAINDICATIONS Severe hepatic impairment; hypersensitivity to celecoxib; asthmatic patients with aspirin triad; advanced renal disease; concurrent use of diuretics and ACE inhibitors; anemia; pregnancy (category D) in third trimester; lactation.
CAUTIOUS USE Patients who are P450 2C9 poor metabolizers; patients who weigh <50 kg; moderate hepatic impairment; renal insufficiency; aspirin use; prior history of GI bleeding or peptic ulcer disease; asthmatics; pregnancy (category C) in first and second trimesters, and (category D) in third trimester; elevated liver function tests; heart failure; kidney disease; hypertension; fluid retention.

ROUTE & DOSAGE

Arthritis

Adult: **PO** 100–200 mg b.i.d. or 200 mg q.d.

Acute Pain, Dysmenorrhea

Adult: **PO** 400 mg 1st dose, then 200 mg same day if needed, then 200 mg b.i.d. prn

FAP

Adult: **PO** 400 mg b.i.d.

ADMINISTRATION

Oral

- Give 2 h before/after magnesium or aluminum-containing antacids.
- Store in tightly closed container and protect from light.

ADVERSE EFFECTS (≥1%) **Body as a Whole:** Back pain, peripheral edema. **GI:** Abdominal pain, diarrhea, dyspepsia, flatulence, nausea. **CNS:** Dizziness, headache, insomnia. **Respiratory:** Pharyngitis, rhinitis, sinusitis, URI. **Skin:** Rash.

INTERACTIONS Drug: May diminish effectiveness of ACE INHIBITORS; **fluconazole** increases celecoxib concentrations; may increase **lithium** concentrations; may increase INR in older patients on **warfarin.**

PHARMACOKINETICS Peak: 3 h. **Distribution:** 97% protein bound; crosses placenta. **Metabolism:** Metabolized in liver by cytochrome P450 2C9 enzymes. **Elimination:** Excreted primarily in feces (57%), 27% excreted in urine. **Half-Life:** 11.2 h.

NURSING IMPLICATIONS

Assessment & Drug Effects

- Therapeutic effectiveness is indicated by relief of joint pain.
- Lab tests: Periodically monitor Hct and Hgb, liver functions, BUN and creatinine, and serum electrolytes.
- Monitor closely lithium levels when the two drugs are given concurrently.
- Monitor closely PT/INR when used concurrently with warfarin.
- Monitor for fluid retention and edema especially in those with a history of hypertension or CHF.

Patient & Family Education

- Avoid using celecoxib during the third trimester of pregnancy.
- Promptly report any of the following: unexplained weight gain, edema, skin rash.
- Stop taking celecoxib and promptly report to physician if any of the following occurs: S&S of liver dysfunction including nausea, fatigue, lethargy, itching, jaundice, abdominal pain, and flulike symptoms; S&S of GI ulceration including black, tarry stools and upper GI distress.
- Do not breast feed while taking this drug.

C

CELLULOSE SODIUM PHOSPHATE (CSP)

Calcibind

Classifications: RESIN EXCHANGE AGENT, CATION; ANTILITHIC

Pregnancy Category: C

AVAILABILITY 2.5 g/packet; 300 g bottle

ACTIONS When taken with meals, releases sodium in exchange for bivalent cations (e.g., dietary and secreted calcium and magnesium) in intestines to form a nonabsorbable complex. Binding of these bivalent ions renders them unavailable for complexing with oxalate; thus formation of renal calculi is inhibited. Does not generally cause significant alterations in serum phosphate or calcium in most patients. Serum magnesium is predictably reduced, however, and therefore supplementation is necessary.

THERAPEUTIC EFFECTS It binds dietary and secreted calcium, interfering with its absorption in the gut, effectively lowering urinary calcium excretion and causing fecal excretion of calcium. Effectively treats nephrolithiasis by lowering calcium absorption in patients with Type I absorptive hypercalciuria.

USES Adjunct to dietary restriction to reduce renal calculi formation in absorptive hypercalciuria type I with recurrent calcium oxalate and calcium phosphate nephrolithiasis.

UNLABELED USES Adjunct in treatment of hypercalcemia (e.g., associated with parathyroid carcinoma or sarcoidosis) and in management of calcinosis cutis.

CONTRAINDICATIONS Bone disease, hypocalcemia, hypomagnesemia, hyperoxaluria; primary and secondary hyperparathyroidism, including renal hypercalciuria; high fasting urinary calcium or hypophosphatemia; conditions associated with high skeletal mobilization of calcium; pregnancy (category C), lactation. Safe use in children <16 y not established.

CAUTIOUS USE Sodium restriction, CHF, ascites, nephrotic syndrome.

ROUTE & DOSAGE

Urinary Calcium Exceeding 300 mg/d

Adult: **PO** Initial: 5 g t.i.d. with each meal, decrease to 5 g with the main meal and 2.5 g with the other 2 meals when urinary calcium is <150 mg/d

ADMINISTRATION

Oral

- Powder can be mixed with full glass (240 mL) of water, soft drink, or fruit juice and taken with meals. CSP is not palatable.
- Oral magnesium supplement (e.g., magnesium gluconate) should be administered to prevent hypomagnesemia. It can be given at any time as long as it is at least 1 h before or after CSP to avoid binding of magnesium.
- Doses of oral magnesium supplement depend on dose of CSP. Patients receiving 15 g/d of CSP should take 1.5 g magnesium gluconate before breakfast and again at bedtime (separately from CSP). Patients taking 10 g/d of CSP should take 1 g magnesium gluconate twice a day.
- Store in tightly closed container protected from moisture, unless otherwise directed.

ADVERSE EFFECTS (≥1%) **Body as a Whole:** Acute arthritis, arthralgia, hyperparathyroid bone disease. **GI:** Loose stools, diarrhea, GI discomfort, dyspepsia, anorexia, nausea, vomiting. **Metabolic:** Hypomagnesemia, hypomagnesuria, hyperoxaluria, symptoms related to electrolyte imbalances, or depletion of trace elements copper, zinc, and iron.

INTERACTIONS Drug: CALCIUM SUPPLEMENTS counteract calcium-lowering effects of CSP; CSP also binds **magnesium,** decreasing its absorption—Separate administration by at least 1 h; THIAZIDE DIURETICS may have additive effects; **ascorbic acid** is metabolized to oxalate and can counteract oxalate-lowering effects of CSP.

PHARMACOKINETICS Absorption: Not absorbed from GI tract. **Metabolism:** Partially hydrolyzed in intestines, causing release of phosphorous ions, which are absorbed by the intestines. **Elimination:** Nonabsorbable complex of calcium and cellulose phosphate excreted in feces along with unchanged resin.

NURSING IMPLICATIONS

Assessment & Drug Effects

- Monitor I&O rates and pattern: Fluid intake should be encouraged to maintain a urinary output of at least 2 L/d (approximately 240 mL/h while awake).
- Lab tests: Evaluate serum parathyroid hormone (PTH) levels at least once between first 2 wk–3 mo of therapy, and then every 3–6 mo during therapy. Serum and urinary calcium and oxalate, serum magnesium, copper, iron, and zinc, and CBC should be monitored every 3–6 mo throughout therapy.
- Monitor urinary calcium levels. A reduction of less than 30 mg/5 g in urinary calcium in patients on moderate calcium and sodium restriction indicates treatment failure. Drug is usually discontinued.
- Discontinuation of therapy is also indicated in patients on moderate oxalate restriction with urinary oxalate levels in excess of 55 mg/d. A rise in serum PTH above normal also points to the need to adjust dosage or stop the drug.
- To increase therapeutic effectiveness of CSP, dietary restriction of sodium, calcium, oxalate, and ascorbic acid is essential. Collaborate with physician and dietitian.
- With long-term use, monitor for manifestations of hypomagnesemia (see Signs & Symptoms, Appendix F).

Patient & Family Education

- Take this drug with meals or at least within 30 min of a meal, otherwise it will not be effective.
- Report S&S of hypomagnesemia (see Appendix F) if you are on long term therapy.
- Do not breast feed while taking this drug.

CEPHALEXIN

(sef-a-lex'in)

Cefanex, Ceporex_A, Keflet, Keflex, Keftab, Novolexin_A

Classifications: ANTIINFECTIVE; ANTIBIOTIC; FIRST-GENERATION CEPHALOSPORIN

Prototype: Cefazolin

Pregnancy Category: B

AVAILABILITY 250 mg, 500 mg capsules; 250 mg, 500 mg, 1 g tablets; 125 mg/5 mL, 250 mg/5 mL suspension

C

ACTIONS Semisynthetic derivative of cephalosporin C. Broad-spectrum, first-generation cephalosporin antibiotic with antiinfective activity similar to that of cefazolin but reportedly less potent. Preferentially binds to one or more of the penicillin-binding proteins (PBP) located on cell walls of susceptible organisms. This inhibits third and final stage of bacterial cell wall synthesis, thus killing the bacterium. Ineffective against many gram-negative or anaerobic organisms. Cross-allergenicity between cephalosporins and penicillins has been reported.

THERAPEUTIC EFFECTS It is active against many gram-positive aerobic cocci and much less active against gram-negative bacteria. Effectively treats osteomyelitis, otitis media, streptococcal pharyngitis, prostate and respiratory infections, skin and urinary tract infections, eliminating or reducing infection.

USES To treat infections caused by susceptible pathogens in respiratory and urinary tracts, middle ear, skin, soft tissue, and bone.

CONTRAINDICATIONS Hypersensitivity to cephalosporins and related antibiotics; pregnancy (category B), lactation. Safe use in infants <1 mo not established.

CAUTIOUS USE History of hypersensitivity to penicillin or other drug allergy; severely impaired renal function.

ROUTE & DOSAGE

Mild to Moderate Infection
Adult: **PO** 250–500 mg q6h
Child: **PO** 25–100 mg/kg/d in 4 divided doses

Skin and Skin Structure Infections
Adult: **PO** 500 mg q12h

Otitis Media
Child: **PO** 75–100 mg/kg/d in 4 divided doses

ADMINISTRATION

Oral

- Cephalexin oral suspension should be refrigerated; discard unused portions 14 d after preparation. Label should indicate expiration date. Keep tightly covered. Shake suspension well before pouring.

ADVERSE EFFECTS (≥1%) **Body as a Whole:** Angioedema, anaphylaxis, superinfections. **GI:** *Diarrhea* (generally mild), nausea, vomiting, anorexia, abdominal pain. **CNS:** Dizziness, headache, fatigue. **Skin:** Rash, urticaria.

DIAGNOSTIC TEST INTERFERENCE False-positive ***urine glucose*** determinations using ***copper sulfate reagents,*** e.g., ***Clinitest, Benedict's reagent,*** but not with ***glucose oxidase (enzymatic) tests,*** e.g., ***Tes-Tape, Diastix, Clinistix.*** Positive ***direct Coombs' test*** may complicate transfusion ***cross-matching procedures*** and ***hematologic studies.***

INTERACTIONS Drug: Probenecid decreases renal elimination of cephalexin.

PHARMACOKINETICS Absorption: rapidly absorbed from GI tract; stable in stomach acid. **Peak:** 1 h. **Distribution:** Widely distributed in body fluids with highest concentration in kidney; crosses placenta. **Elimination:** 80–100% eliminated unchanged in urine in 8 h; excreted in breast milk. **Half-Life:** 38–70 min.

C

NURSING IMPLICATIONS

Assessment & Drug Effects

- Determine history of hypersensitivity reactions to cephalosporins and penicillin and history of other drug allergies before therapy is initiated.
- Lab tests: Evaluate renal and hepatic function periodically in patients receiving prolonged therapy.
- Monitor for manifestations of hypersensitivity (see Signs & Symptoms, Appendix F). Discontinue drug and report their appearance promptly.

Patient & Family Education

- Take medication for the full course of therapy as directed by physician.
- Keep physician informed if adverse reactions appear.
- Be alert to S&S of superinfections (see Appendix F). These symptoms should be reported promptly and appropriate therapy instituted.
- Do not breast feed while taking this drug.

CEPHAPIRIN SODIUM

(sef-a-pye′rin)

Cefadyl

Classifications: ANTIINFECTIVE; ANTIBIOTIC; FIRST-GENERATION CEPHALOSPORIN

Prototype: Cefazolin

Pregnancy Category: B

AVAILABILITY 1 g injection

ACTIONS Semisynthetic, first-generation, broad-spectrum cephalosporin antibiotic similar to cefazolin. Reported to cause less tissue irritation and to be less nephrotoxic than cefazolin. Preferentially binds to one or more of the penicillin-binding proteins (PBP) located on cell walls of susceptible organisms. This inhibits third and final stage of bacterial cell wall synthesis, thus killing the bacterium. Cross-allergenicity between cephalosporins and penicillins has been reported.

THERAPEUTIC EFFECTS Effectively treats osteomyelitis, respiratory tract infections, skin infections, urinary tract infections, *Streptococcal* infections, infective endocarditis, septicemia, and is used for preoperative prophylaxis, reducing or eliminating infection.

USES Serious infections of respiratory and urinary tracts, skin and soft tissue, and for osteomyelitis, septicemia, and endocarditis caused by susceptible pathogens, e.g., group A *beta-hemolytic Streptococci,* penicillinase- and nonpenicillinase-producing *Staphylococcus aureus, Streptococcus pneumoniae, viridans streptococci, Haemophilus influenzae, Escherichia coli, Proteus mirabilis,* and *Klebsiella sp;* also to prevent postoperative infection when infection at operative site is a risk.

CONTRAINDICATIONS Hypersensitivity to cephalosporins and related antibiotics; pregnancy (category B), lactation. Safe use in children <3 mo not established.

CAUTIOUS USE History of sensitivity to penicillins and other allergies, particularly to drugs; sodium restriction, impaired renal function.

ROUTE & DOSAGE

Mild to Moderate Infection

Adult: **IM/IV** 500 mg–1 g q4–6h up to 12 g/d
Child: **IM/IV** 40–80 mg/kg/d in 4 divided doses

C

Perioperative Prophylaxis
Adult: **IM/IV** 1–2 g 30–60 min before surgery, 1–2 g during surgery, then 1–2 g q6h for 24 h
Adjustment for Renal Impairment
Cl_{cr} <5 mg/dL: **IM/IV** 7.5–15 mg/kg q12h

ADMINISTRATION

Intramuscular

- Reconstitute the 500 mg and 1 g vials with 1 or 2 mL sterile water for injection or bacteriostatic water for injection, respectively. Resulting solutions will contain 500 mg of cephapirin per 1.2 mL.
- IM injections should be made deep into large muscle mass. Rotate injection sites.

Intravenous

PREPARE: **Direct:** Reconstitute 1 g or 2 g vial with at least 10 mL bacteriostatic water for injection, D5W, or NS. **Intermittent:** Further dilute with 50–100 mL of D5W or NS.
ADMINISTER: **Direct:** Give over 5 min. **Intermittent:** Give over 30 min.
INCOMPATIBILITIES **Solution/additive:** AMINOGLYCOSIDES, **aminophylline, ascorbic acid, epinephrine, norepinephrine, mannitol, phenytoin,** TETRACYCLINES, **thiopental. Y-site:** AMINOGLYCOSIDES, TETRACYCLINES, **thiopental, phenytoin.**

- After reconstitution, depending on diluent and amount used, solutions retain potency for 12–48 h at room temperature or for 10 d if refrigerated at 4° C. See package insert for specific information. ■ Solutions may become slightly yellow, but this does not affect potency.

ADVERSE EFFECTS (≥1%) **Body as a Whole:** Rash, urticaria, drug fever, eosinophilia, serum sickness-like reactions, anaphylaxis. **GI:** Nausea, vomiting, *diarrhea,* abdominal cramps. **Other:** Needle site reactions (infrequent).

DIAGNOSTIC TEST INTERFERENCE False-positive ***urine glucose*** determinations, using ***copper sulfate reduction methods,*** e.g., ***Clinitest*** or ***Benedict's reagent,*** but not with ***glucose oxidase (enzymatic) tests,*** e.g., ***Clinistix, Diastix, Tes-Tape.*** Positive ***Coombs' test*** may **complicate** ***cross-matching procedures*** and ***hematologic studies.***

INTERACTIONS Drug: Probenecid decreases renal elimination of cephapirin.

PHARMACOKINETICS Peak: 30 min after IM; 5 min after IV. **Distribution:** Widely distributed in body fluids with highest concentration in kidney; crosses placenta. **Metabolism:** Partially metabolized in liver and kidneys. **Elimination:** 60–85% eliminated unchanged in urine in 6 h; excreted in breast milk. **Half-Life:** 36–54 min.

NURSING IMPLICATIONS

Assessment & Drug Effects

- Determine history of previous hypersensitivity to cephalosporins, penicillins, and other allergies, particularly to drugs, before therapy begins.
- Lab tests: Perform culture and sensitivity testing before treatment is begun. Therapy may be initiated before results are obtained. Monitor periodically renal function.
- Advise patient to report changes in I&O ratio and pattern or evidence of blood or pus in urine.

- Monitor for manifestations of hypersensitivity (see Signs & Symptoms, Appendix F). Discontinue drug and report their appearance promptly.

Patient & Family Education

- Report promptly any signs or symptoms of superinfections (see Appendix F).
- Report S&S of hypersensitivity (see Appendix F).
- Do not breast feed while taking this drug.

CEPHRADINE

(sef'ra-deen)

Anspor, Velosef

Classifications: ANTIINFECTIVE; ANTIBIOTIC; FIRST-GENERATION CEPHALOSPORIN

Prototype: Cefazolin

Pregnancy Category: B

AVAILABILITY 250 mg, 500 mg capsules; 125 mg/5 mL, 250 mg/5 mL suspension; 250 mg, 500 mg, 1 g, 2 g injection

ACTIONS Semisynthetic acid-stable, first generation, broad-spectrum cephalosporin similar to cefazolin. Preferentially binds to one or more of the penicillin-binding proteins (PBP) located on cell walls of susceptible organisms. This inhibits third and final stage of bacterial cell wall synthesis, thus killing the bacterium. Cross-allergenicity between cephalosporins and penicillins has been reported.

THERAPEUTIC EFFECTS It is active against many gram-positive aerobic cocci and much less active against gram-negative bacteria. Effectively treats bone infections, otitis media, respiratory tract infections, septicemia and skin infections, and urinary tract infections, reducing or eliminating infection.

USES Serious infections of respiratory and urinary tracts, skin and soft tissues, and for otitis media caused by susceptible pathogens; for perioperative prophylaxis, in cesarean section (intraoperative and postoperative); in septicemia (due to *Streptococcus pneumoniae, Staphylococcus aureus, Proteus mirabilis,* and *Escherichia coli*). Also used to treat urinary tract infections due to *Klebsiella sp* and enterococci *(Streptococcus faecalis)*.

CONTRAINDICATIONS Hypersensitivity to cephalosporins and related antibiotics; pregnancy (category B), lactation. Safe use in children <9 mo not established.

CAUTIOUS USE History of penicillin or other allergies, particularly to drugs; impaired renal function, sodium restriction (parenteral cephradine).

ROUTE & DOSAGE

Mild to Moderate Infection

Adult: **PO** 250–500 mg q6h or 500 mg–1 g q12h up to 4 g/d. **IM/IV** 2–4 g/d in 4 divided doses (max: 8 g/d)
Child: **PO** 25–50 mg/kg/d in 2–4 divided doses up to 4 g/d. **IM/IV** 50–100 mg/kg/d in 4 divided doses up to 8 g/d

Perioperative Prophylaxis

Adult: **PO** 1 g 30–60 min before surgery; 1 g during surgery; then 1 g q4–6h for 24 h

ADMINISTRATION

Oral

- Oral cephradine may be given without regard to meals (acid stable); however, the presence of food may delay absorption.

Intramuscular

- Inject deep into large muscle mass, such as gluteus maximus or lateral aspect of thigh, to minimize pain and induration of IM site.

Intravenous

***PREPARE:* Direct:** Dilute each 500 mg with 5 mL sterile water for injection. **Intermittent:** Further dilute in 10–20 mL of D5W or NS. Do not mix with RL.

***ADMINISTER:* Direct:** Give over 3–5 min. **Intermittent:** Give over 30–60 min.

***INCOMPATIBILITIES* Solution/additive:** AMINOGLYCOSIDES, TPN SOLUTIONS, other ANTIBIOTICS. **Y-site:** AMINOGLYCOSIDES, TPN SOLUTIONS, other ANTIBIOTICS.

The risk of thrombophlebitis may be reduced by proper dilution of IV fluid, use of small IV needles and large veins, and by alternating injection sites.

- Oral suspension may be stored at room temperature up to 7 d or in refrigerator for up to 14 d. - After reconstitution, IM or IV solutions should be used within 2 h if kept at room temperature or 24 h if refrigerated. - Protect from concentrated light or direct sunlight.

ADVERSE EFFECTS (≥1%) **Body as a Whole:** Joint pains, eosinophilia, tightness in chest, pain, induration and tissue sloughing (IM injection site); thrombophlebitis (IV site); paresthesias, superinfections. **GI:** *Diarrhea* or loose stools, abdominal pain, heartburn. **CNS:** Dizziness. **Skin:** Urticaria, rash, pruritus.

DIAGNOSTIC TEST INTERFERENCE Cephradine causes false-positive (black-brown or green-brown color) ***urine glucose*** reaction with ***copper reduction reagents,*** (e.g., as ***Benedict's*** or ***Clinitest***), but not with ***enzymatic glucose oxidase reagents,*** e.g., ***Clinistix, TesTape.*** False-positive ***direct Coombs' test*** (may interfere with ***cross-matching procedures*** and ***hematologic studies***) has also been reported.

INTERACTIONS Drug: Probenecid decreases renal elimination of cephradine.

PHARMACOKINETICS Absorption: Well absorbed from GI tract. **Peak:** 1 h after PO; 1–2 h after IM; 5 min after IV. **Distribution:** Widely distributed in body fluids, with highest concentration in kidney; crosses placenta. **Elimination:** 80–90% eliminated unchanged in urine in 6 h; excreted in breast milk. **Half-Life:** 1–2 h.

NURSING IMPLICATIONS

Assessment & Drug Effects

- Determine history of previous hypersensitivity to cephalosporins, penicillins, and other drug allergies before therapy is initiated.
- Inspect IV insertion site frequently for thrombophlebitis (see Signs & Symptoms, Appendix F).
- Lab tests: Perform culture and sensitivity tests and renal function studies before and periodically during drug therapy.
- Consult physician if patient's creatinine clearance is below normal. Recommended dosage schedule in patients with reduced renal function is lowered based on creatinine clearance determinations and severity of infection.
- Pseudomembranous enterocolitis, a potentially life-threatening superinfection caused by *Clostridium difficile,* may occur during or after cephalosporin therapy. If di-

C

arrhea occurs, check for fever. Report diarrhea and fever promptly.
- Monitor for signs of superinfection (see Appendix F). Report their appearance promptly.

Patient & Family Education
- Take this medication for the full course of therapy as directed by your physician. Therapy is usually continued for at least 48–72 h after you become asymptomatic.
- Superinfections caused by overgrowth of nonsusceptible organisms may occur. Report early S&S (see Appendix F) promptly.
- Report loose stools or diarrhea promptly.
- Do not breast feed while taking this drug.

CETIRIZINE

(ce-tir'i-zeen)

Reactine ♣, Zyrtec

Classifications: ANTIHISTAMINE; H_1-RECEPTOR ANTAGONIST; NON-SEDATING

Prototype: Loratidine

Pregnancy Category: B

AVAILABILITY 5 mg, 10 mg tablets; 5 mg, 10 mg chewable tablets; 5 mg/5 mL syrup

ACTIONS Cetirizine is a potent H_1-receptor antagonist and thus an antihistamine without significant anticholinergic or CNS activity. Low lipophilicity combined with its H_1-receptor selectivity probably accounts for its relative lack of anticholinergic and sedative properties.

THERAPEUTIC EFFECTS Effectively treats allergic rhinitis, and chronic urticaria by eliminating or reducing the local and systemic effects of histamine release.

USES Seasonal and perennial allergic rhinitis and chronic idiopathic urticaria.

CONTRAINDICATIONS Hypersensitivity to H_1-receptor antihistamines; lactation, children <2 y.

CAUTIOUS USE Moderate to severe renal impairment, pregnancy (category B), children.

ROUTE & DOSAGE

Allergic Rhinitis

Adult: **PO** 5–10 mg once/d

Child: **PO** *2–5 y:* 2.5 mg q.d. (max: 5 mg/d); *≥6 y:* 5–10 mg q.d.

Chronic Urticaria

Adult: **PO** 10 mg q.d. or b.i.d.

ADMINISTRATION

Oral
- Consult physician about dosage if significant adverse effects appear. As elimination half-life is prolonged in the older adult, dosage adjustments may be warranted.

ADVERSE EFFECTS (≥1%) **GI:** Constipation, diarrhea, dry mouth. **CNS:** *Drowsiness, sedation, headache,* depression.

INTERACTIONS Drug: Theophylline may decrease cetirizine clearance leading to toxicity.

PHARMACOKINETICS Absorption: Readily absorbed from GI tract. **Peak:** 1 h. **Distribution:** 93% protein bound; minimal CNS concentrations. **Metabolism:** minimal. **Elimination:** 60% excreted unchanged in urine within 24 h, 5% excreted in feces. **Half-Life:** 7.4 h.

NURSING IMPLICATIONS

Assessment & Drug Effects
- Monitor for drug interactions. As the drug is highly protein

C

bound, the potential for interactions with other protein-bound drugs exists.

- Monitor for sedation, especially the older adult.

Patient & Family Education

- Do not use in combination with OTC antihistamines.
- Do not engage in driving or other hazardous activities, before experiencing your responses to the drug.
- Do not breast feed while taking this drug without consulting physician.

CETRORELIX

(ce-tro-re'lix)

Cetrotide

Classifications: HORMONES & SYNTHETIC SUBSTITUTES; GONADOTROPIN-RELEASING HORMONE ANTAGONIST

Pregnancy Category: X

AVAILABILITY 0.25 mg, 3 mg injection

ACTIONS Centrotide is a luteinizing hormone-releasing hormone (LHRH) antagonist.

THERAPEUTIC EFFECTS It prevents premature LH surges in patients undergoing controlled ovarian hyperstimulation for assisted reproduction.

USES Treatment of infertility as part of an assisted reproduction program.

CONTRAINDICATIONS Hypersensitivity to cetrorelix, extrinsic peptide hormones, mannitol, gonadotropin-releasing hormone analogs; pregnancy (category X); known or suspected pregnancy; lactation.

CAUTIOUS USE Hepatic insufficiency.

ROUTE & DOSAGE

Infertility

Adult: **SC** 0.25 mg/d during the early to mid follicular phase of the cycle (stimulation day 5 or 6) following the initiation of FSH or 3 mg as a single dose is administered when the serum estradiol level is indicative of an appropriate stimulation response, usually on FSH stimulation day 7 (range day 5–9). If HCG has not been administered within 4 d after the injection of 3 mg, then 0.25 mg should be administered once daily until the day of HCG administration

ADMINISTRATION

Subcutaneous

- Reconstitute the 0.25 or 3 mL vial with 1 or 3 mL, respectively, of sterile water for injection.
- Inject into lower abdominal wall following reconstitution. Rotate injection sites.
- Store the 3 mg dose at room temperature, 15°–30° C (59°–86° F). Store the 0.25 mg dose in the refrigerator.

ADVERSE EFFECTS (≥1%) **CNS:** Headache. **GI:** Nausea, vomiting, abdominal pain. **Endocrine:** Hot flashes. **Skin:** Pruritus at injection site. **Urogenital:** Ovarian enlargement, ovarian hyperstimulation syndrome, pelvic pain.

INTERACTIONS Drug: Cimetidine, methyldopa, metoclopramide, reserpine, PHENOTHIAZINES may interfere with fertility efforts. **Herbal: Black cohosh, DHEA** may antagonize fertility efforts.

PHARMACOKINETICS Absorption: 85% absorbed from SC injection site.

Peak: 1–2 h. **Metabolism:** Metabolized by peptidases. **Elimination:** 2–4% excreted in urine, 5–10% excreted in bile. **Half-Life:** 62 h after single dose, 20 h after multiple doses.

NURSING IMPLICATIONS

Assessment & Drug Effects

- Lab test: Monitor routine blood chemistries.
- Monitor weight and report development of edema and/or shortness of breath.

Patient & Family Education

- Contact physician immediately for any of the following: Abdominal or stomach pain, persistent or severe nausea, vomiting or diarrhea; decreased urination; pelvic pain; moderate to severe bloating, rapid weight gain; shortness of breath; swelling of lower legs.
- Understand that hot flashes are a common side effect of this drug.
- Do not breast feed while using this drug without consulting physician.

CETUXIMAB

(ce-tux′i-mab)

Erbitux

Classifications: BIOLOGIC RESPONSE MODIFIER; MONOCLONAL ANTIBODY

Prototype: Basiliximab

Pregnancy Category: C

AVAILABILITY 100 mg/50 mL injection

ACTIONS Cetuximab is a recombinant, monoclonal antibody that binds specifically to the epidermal growth factor receptor (EGFR, HER1, c-ErbB-1) on both normal and tumor cells. Binding to the EGFR results in inhibition of cell growth, induction of apoptosis, and decreased vascular endothelial growth factor production.

THERAPEUTIC EFFECTS Overexpression of EGFR is detected in many human cancers, including those of the colon and rectum. Cetuximab inhibits the growth and survival of tumor cells that overexpress the EGFR.

USES Treatment of EGFR-expressing metastatic colorectal cancer in combination with irinotecan in patients who are refractory to irinotecan-based chemotherapy or as monotherapy in patients who are intolerant to irinotecan-based chemotherapy.

CONTRAINDICATIONS Pregnancy (category C), lactation within 60 d of using cetuximab. Safety and efficacy in children have not been established.

CAUTIOUS USE Infusion reaction, especially with first time users; history of hypersensitivity to murine proteins or cetuximab; pulmonary disease, pulmonary fibrosis; UV exposure, radiation therapy.

ROUTE & DOSAGE

Colorectal Cancer

Adult: **IV** Start with 400 mg/m^2 over 2 h; continue with 250 mg/m^2 over 1 h weekly

ADMINISTRATION

Intravenous

- Administer with full resuscitation equipment available and under the supervision of a physician experienced with chemotherapy.
- Premedication with an H_1-receptor antagonist (e.g., di-

phenhydramine 50 mg IV) is recommended.

- Monitor for an infusion reaction for at least 1 h following completion of infusion.

PREPARE: **IV Infusion:** Do not shake or further dilute vial. Do not mix with other medication. Inject cetuximab solution into a sterile, evacuated container or bag (i.e., glass, polyolefin, ethylene vinyl acetate, DEHP plasticized PVC, or PVC); repeat until needed dose has been added to container, using a new needle for each vial. Attach to infusion set with a low-protein-binding 0.22-micron filter and prime line with cetuximab. May also administer by syringe and syringe pump; use a new needle and filter for each vial.

ADMINISTER: **IV Infusion:** Do NOT administer a bolus dose. Give IV infusion via an infusion pump or syringe pump at ≤5 mL/min; piggyback into the patient's IV line. ▪ Flush line with NS after infusion. ▪ Note: Slow infusion rate by 50% if a prior, mild infusion reaction occurred.

INCOMPATIBILITIES **Solution/additive:** Do not mix with other additives. **Y-site:** No data available.

- Store unopened vials at 2°–8° C (36°–46° F). Note: Vials may contain a small amount of easily visible, white particles.
- Cetuximab in IV bag is stable for up to 12 h refrigerated and up to 8 h at 20°–25° C (68°–77° F).

ADVERSE EFFECTS (≥1%) **Body as a Whole:** Infusion reactions (allergic reaction, anaphylactoid reaction, fever, chills, dyspnea, bronchospasm stridor, hoarseness, urticaria, hypotension), *fever,* sepsis, *asthenia, malaise,* pain, infection. **CNS:** *Headache,* insomnia, depression. **GI:** *Nausea, vomiting diarrhea, abdominal pain, constipation,* stomatitis, dyspepsia. **Hematologic:** Leukopenia, anemia. **Metabolic:** Weight loss, peripheral edema, dehydration. **Respiratory:** Pulmonary embolism, <u>pulmonary fibrosis (rare)</u>, *dyspnea,* cough. **Skin:** *Rash,* alopecia, pruritus. **Urogenital:** Kidney failure.

INTERACTIONS Drug: None reported.

PHARMACOKINETICS Half-Life: 114 h (75–188 h).

NURSING IMPLICATIONS

Assessment & Drug Effects

- Withhold drug and notify physician for S&S of an infusion reaction: chills, fever, bronchospasm, stridor, hoarseness, urticaria, and/or hypotension. Institute supportive measure immediately if a severe reaction occurs.
- Monitor pulmonary status and report onset of acute or worsening pulmonary symptoms.
- Lab tests: Periodic CBC with differential, Hct and Hgb.

Patient & Family Education

- Report immediately: especially difficulty breathing, wheezing, shortness of breath, hives, faintness and/or dizziness anytime during IV infusion.
- Report promptly any of the following: eye inflammation, mouth sores, skin rash, redness, or severe dry skin.
- Wear sunscreen and a hat and limit sun exposure while being treated with this drug.
- Do not breast feed while taking this drug.

CEVIMELINE HYDROCHLORIDE (Pr)

(cev-i-may'leen)

Evoxac

Classifications: AUTONOMIC NERVOUS SYSTEM AGENT; CHOLINERGIC (PARASYMPATHOMIMETIC)

Pregnancy Category: C

AVAILABILITY 30 mg capsules

ACTIONS Cholinergic agent that binds to muscarinic receptors.

THERAPEUTIC EFFECTS Increases secretion of exocrine glands, such as salivary and sweat glands. It relieves severe dry mouth.

USES Treatment of dry mouth in patients with Sjögren's Syndrome.

CONTRAINDICATIONS Hypersensitivity to cevimeline; uncontrolled asthma; acute iritis; narrow-angle glaucoma; lactation.

CAUTIOUS USE Controlled asthma; chronic bronchitis, COPD; myocardial infarction; history of nephrolithiasis or cholelithiasis; pregnancy (category C); older adults. Safety and effectiveness in children are not established.

ROUTE & DOSAGE

Dry Mouth

Adult: **PO** 30 mg t.i.d.

ADMINISTRATION

Oral

- Give without regard to food.
- Store refrigerated at 2°–8° C (35.6°–46.4° F) with occasional fluctuations between 15°–30° C (59°–86° F).

ADVERSE EFFECTS (≥1%) **Body as a Whole:** *Excessive sweating, headache,* back pain, dizziness, fatigue, pain, hot flushes, rigors, tremor, hypertonia, myalgia, fever, eye pain, ear ache, flu-like symptoms. **CNS:** Insomnia, anxiety, vertigo, depression, hyporeflexia. **CV:** Peripheral edema, chest pain. **GI:** *Nausea, diarrhea,* excessive salivation, dyspepsia, abdominal pain, coughing, vomiting, constipation, anorexia, dry mouth, hiccup. **Respiratory:** *Rhinitis, sinusitis, upper respiratory tract infection,* pharyngitis, bronchitis. **Skin:** Rash, conjunctivitis, pruritus. **Special Senses:** Abnormal vision. **Urogenital:** Urinary tract infection.

INTERACTIONS Drug: BETA-ADRENERGIC AGONISTS may cause conduction disturbances; PARASYMPATHOMIMETIC DRUGS may have additive effects.

PHARMACOKINETICS Absorption: Rapidly absorbed. **Peak:** 1.5–2 h. **Distribution:** <20% protein bound. **Metabolism:** Metabolized in liver by CYP 2D6 and 3A3/4. **Elimination:** Excreted primarily in urine. **Half-Life:** 5 h.

NURSING IMPLICATIONS

Assessment & Drug Effects

- Monitor for S&S of increased airway resistance, especially in patient with asthma, bronchitis, emphysema, or COPD.
- Monitor cardiac status, especially in those with known cardiac disease or dysfunction.
- Monitor fluid status, especially in those at risk for dehydration.
- Lab tests: Routine blood chemistry during long-term therapy.
- Report S&S of excess cholinergic activity (e.g., diaphoresis, frequent urge to urinate, nausea and/or diarrhea).

Patient & Family Education

- Do not drive or engage in potentially hazardous activities until response to drug is known.

- Consult physician if confusion, dizziness, or faintness occur.
- Report diminished night vision or depth perception.
- Drink fluids liberally (2000–3000 mL/d) in the event of excessive sweating when it occurs.
- Do not breast feed while taking this drug.

CHARCOAL, ACTIVATED (LIQUID ANTIDOTE)

Actidose, CharcoAid, Charcocaps, Charcodote, Insta-Char

Classifications: ANTIDOTE; ADSORBENT

Pregnancy Category: C

AVAILABILITY 208 mg/mL, 15g, 30 g, 50 mg liquid/suspension

ACTIONS Residue from destructive distillation of organic materials treated to reduce particle size, which increases surface area and adsorptive power. Activated charcoal (carbon) is a chemically inert, odorless, tasteless, fine black powder with wide spectrum of adsorptive activity. Acts by binding (adsorbing) toxic substances, thereby inhibiting their GI absorption, enterohepatic circulation, and thus bioavailability.

THERAPEUTIC EFFECTS Recent studies indicate that administration by "gastric dialysis" (repetitive doses) effectively increases clearance of drugs already absorbed into the systemic circulation. Action appears to result from increased rate of drug diffusion from plasma into GI tract where it is adsorbed by activated charcoal. Effectively adsorbs toxins in the gut preventing their systemic absorption and impact.

USES General purpose emergency antidote in the treatment of poisonings by most drugs and chemicals, e.g., acetaminophen, aspirin, atropine, barbiturates, digitalis glycosides, phenytoin, propoxyphene, strychnine, tricyclic antidepressants, among many others. Gastric dialysis (repetitive doses) in uremia to adsorb various waste products from GI tract; severe acute poisoning. Has been used to adsorb intestinal gases in treatment of dyspepsia, flatulence, and distension (value in these conditions not established). Sometimes used topically as a deodorant for foul-smelling wounds and ulcers.

CONTRAINDICATIONS Reportedly not effective for poisonings by cyanide, mineral acids, caustic alkalis, organic solvents, iron, ethanol, methanol.

CAUTIOUS USE Pregnancy (category C); lactation.

ROUTE & DOSAGE

Acute Poisonings

Adult: **PO** 30–100 g in at least 180–240 mL (6–8 oz) of water or 1 g/kg

Child 1–12 y: **PO** 1–2 g/kg or 15–30 g in at least 6–8 oz of water

Infant <1 y: **PO** 1 g/kg

Gastric Dialysis

Adult: **PO** 20–40 g q6h for 1 or 2 d

GI Disturbances

Adult: **PO** 520–975 mg p.c. up to 5 g/d

ADMINISTRATION

Oral

- Activated charcoal tablets or capsules are less adsorptive and thus less effective than powder or liquid form; therefore, they are not recommended in treatment of acute poisoning.

- Drug is most effective when administered as soon as possible after acute poisoning (preferably within 30 min).
- In an emergency, dose may be approximated by stirring sufficient activated charcoal into tap water to make a slurry the consistency of soup (about 20–30 g in at least 240 mL of water).
- Activated charcoal can be swallowed or given through a nasogastric tube. If administered too rapidly, patient may vomit.
- If necessary, palatability may be improved by adding a small amount of concentrated fruit juice or chocolate powder to the slurry. Reportedly, these agents do not appreciably alter adsorptive activity.
- To prevent adsorption of gases from the air, store in tightly covered container.

ADVERSE EFFECTS (≥1%) **GI:** Vomiting (rapid ingestion of high doses), constipation, diarrhea (from sorbitol).

INTERACTIONS Drug: May decrease absorption of all other oral medications—administer at least 2 h apart.

PHARMACOKINETICS Absorption: Not absorbed. **Elimination:** Excreted in feces.

NURSING IMPLICATIONS

Assessment & Drug Effects

- Record appearance, color, consistency, frequency, and relative amount of stools. Inform patient that activated charcoal will color feces black.

Patient & Family Education

- Do not breast feed while taking this drug without consulting physician.

CHLORAL HYDRATE

(klor′al hye′drate)

Aquachloral Supprettes, Noctec, Novochlorhydrate ♣

Classifications: CENTRAL NERVOUS SYSTEM AGENT; ANXIOLYTIC, SEDATIVE-HYPNOTIC

Prototype: Secobarbital

Pregnancy Category: C

Controlled Substance: Schedule IV

AVAILABILITY 500 mg capsules; 250 mg/5 mL, 500 mg/5 mL syrup; 324 mg, 500 mg, 648 mg suppositories

ACTIONS Produces "physiologic sleep" by mild cerebral depression with little effect on respirations or BP and little or no hangover.

THERAPEUTIC EFFECTS Chloral hydrate is a sedative-hypnotic which does not affect sleep physiology (e.g., REM sleep) in low doses. Has little or no analgesic action.

USES Short-term management of insomnia, for general sedation (especially in the young and the older adult), for sedation before and after surgery, to reduce anxiety associated with drug withdrawal, and alone or with paraldehyde to prevent or suppress alcohol withdrawal symptoms.

CONTRAINDICATIONS Known hypersensitivity to chloral hydrate or chloral derivatives; severe hepatic, renal, or cardiac disease; rectal dosage form in patients with proctitis; oral use in patients with esophagitis, gastritis, gastric or duodenal ulcers; pregnancy (category C), lactation.

CAUTIOUS USE History of intermittent porphyria, asthma, history of or proneness to drug dependence, depression, suicidal tendencies.

C

ROUTE & DOSAGE

Sedative

Adult: **PO/PR** 250 mg t.i.d. p.c.
Child: **PO/PR** 25–50 mg/kg/d divided q6–8h (max: 500 mg/dose)

Hypnotic

Adult: **PO/PR** 500 mg–1 g 15–30 min before h.s. or 30 min before surgery
Geriatric: **PO/PR** 250 mg h.s.
Child: **PO/PR** 50 mg/kg 15–30 min before h.s. or 30 min before surgery (max: 1 g)

EEG Premedication

Child: **PO/PR** 20–25 mg/kg 30–60 min prior to procedure

ADMINISTRATION

Oral

- Dilute liquid preparations in chilled fluids to minimize unpleasant taste.
- Watch to see that drug is not cheeked and hoarded.

Rectal

- Moisten suppository with a water-based lubricant, such as K-Y jelly, prior to insertion.
- Solutions are preserved in tightly covered, light-resistant containers.

ADVERSE EFFECTS (≥1%) **Body as a Whole:** Angioedema, eosinophilia, breath odor, leukopenia, ketonuria, renal and hepatic damage, sudden death. **CV:** Arrhythmias, cardiac arrest. **GI:** *Nausea, vomiting, diarrhea,* severe gastritis. **CNS:** Dizziness, motor incoordination, headache. **Skin:** Purpura, urticaria, erythematous rash, eczema, erythema multiforme, fixed drug eruptions. **Special Senses:** Conjunctivitis.

DIAGNOSTIC TEST INTERFERENCE False-positive results for ***urine glucose*** with ***Benedict's solutions,*** and possibly with ***Clinitest*** but not with ***glucose oxidase methods*** (e.g., ***Clinistix, Diastix, TesTape***). Possible interference with fluorometric test for ***urine catecholamines*** (if chloral hydrate is administered within 48 h of test) and ***urinary 17-OHCS*** determinations (by modification of ***Reddy, Jenkins, Thorn procedure***).

INTERACTIONS Drug: Alcohol, BARBITURATES, **paraldehyde,** other CNS DEPRESSANTS potentiate CNS depression; tachycardia may also occur with **alcohol**; increases anticoagulant effect of ORAL ANTICOAGULANTS; **furosemide** IV can produce flushing, diaphoresis, BP changes.

PHARMACOKINETICS Absorption: Readily absorbed from oral or rectal administration. **Onset:** 30–60 min. **Peak:** 1–3 h. **Duration:** 4–8 h. **Distribution:** Well distributed to all tissues; 70–80% protein bound; crosses placenta. **Metabolism:** Metabolized in liver to the active metabolite trichloroethanol. **Elimination:** Excreted primarily by kidneys, with a small amount excreted in feces via bile. **Half-Life:** 8–11 h.

NURSING IMPLICATIONS

Assessment & Drug Effects

- Chloral hydrate is not intended for relief of pain. When used in the presence of pain, it may cause excitement and delirium.
- Do not discontinue abruptly following prolonged use. Sudden withdrawal from dependent patients may produce delirium, mania, or convulsions.
- Monitor for S&S of allergic skin reactions, which may occur within

several hours or as long as 10 d after drug administration.
- Evaluate patient's response to chloral hydrate and continued need for the drug.

Patient & Family Education
- Do not ambulate without assistance until response to drug is known.
- Avoid concomitant use of alcoholic beverages.
- Avoid driving and other potentially hazardous activities while under the influence of chloral hydrate.
- Do not breast feed while taking this drug.

CHLORAMBUCIL

(klor-am′byoo-sil)
Leukeran
Classifications: ANTINEOPLASTIC; ALKYLATING AGENT
Prototype: Cyclophosphamide
Pregnancy Category: D

AVAILABILITY 2 mg tablets

ACTIONS Potent aromatic derivative of the alkylating agent nitrogen mustard which is slowest acting and least toxic of the nitrogen mustards. A cell-cycle nonspecific drug (kills both resting and dividing cells), it causes cytotoxic cross linkage in DNA, thus preventing synthesis of DNA, RNA, and proteins. Myelosuppression in therapeutic doses is moderate and rapidly reversible.
THERAPEUTIC EFFECTS Lymphocytic effect is marked, thus it is effective in treatment of various lymphomas.

USES As single agent or in combination with other antineoplastics in treatment of chronic lymphocytic leukemia, malignant lymphomas including lymphosarcoma, Hodgkin's disease, and giant follicular lymphoma, and in treatment of carcinoma of the ovary, breast, and testes.
UNLABELED USES Nonneoplastic conditions: vasculitis complicating rheumatoid arthritis, autoimmune hemolytic anemias associated with cold agglutinins, lupus glomerulonephritis, idiopathic nephrotic syndrome, polycythemia vera, macroglobulinemia.

CONTRAINDICATIONS Hypersensitivity to chlorambucil or to other alkylating agents; administration within 4 wk of a full course of radiation or chemotherapy; full dosage if bone marrow is infiltrated with lymphomatous tissue or is hypoplastic; smallpox and other vaccines; pregnancy (category D), lactation.
CAUTIOUS USE Excessive or prolonged dosage, pneumococcus vaccination, history of seizures or head trauma.

ROUTE & DOSAGE

Malignant Diseases (Lymphomas, Hodgkin's Disease, etc.)
Adult: **PO** 0.1–0.2 mg/kg/d (usual dose 4–10 mg/d)
Child: **PO** 0.1–0.2 mg/kg/d in single or divided doses

ADMINISTRATION
Oral
- Control nausea and vomiting by giving entire daily dose at one time, 1 h before breakfast or 2 h after evening meal, or at bedtime. Consult physician.
- With confirmation of bone marrow depression (low platelet and neutrophil counts or peripheral

C

lymphocytosis), it is recommended that dosage not exceed 0.1 mg/kg.

- Store in tightly closed, light-resistant container.

ADVERSE EFFECTS (≥1%) **Body as a Whole:** Drug fever, skin rashes, papilledema, alopecia, peripheral neuropathy, sterile cystitis, pulmonary complications, seizures (high doses). **GI:** Low incidence of gastric discomfort, hepatotoxicity. **Hematologic:** Bone marrow depression: *leukopenia,* thrombocytopenia, anemia. **Metabolic:** Sterility, hyperuricemia.

INTERACTIONS Drug: May have to adjust dose of **allopurinol, colchicine** because of chlorambucil-associated hyperuricemia.

PHARMACOKINETICS Absorption: Rapidly and completely absorbed from GI tract. **Peak:** 1 h. **Distribution:** Extensively bound to plasma and tissue proteins; crosses placenta. **Metabolism:** Extensively metabolized in liver. **Elimination:** 60% eliminated in urine as metabolites within 24 h. **Half-Life:** 1.5–2.5 h.

NURSING IMPLICATIONS

Assessment & Drug Effects

- Lab tests: CBC, Hgb, total and differential leukocyte counts, and serum uric acid initially and at least once weekly during treatment.
- Leukopenia usually develops after the third week of treatment; it may continue for up to 10 d after last dose, then rapidly return to normal.
- Avoid or reduce to minimum injections and other invasive procedures (e.g., rectal temperatures, enemas) when platelet count is low because of danger of bleeding.
- Monitor for S&S of skin rashes, which are rare, but appear to show a consistent pattern: pustular eruption on mouth, chin, cheeks; urticarial erythema on trunk that spreads to legs. The rash occurs early in treatment period and lasts about 10 d after last dose.

Patient & Family Education

- Keep appointments with physician. During treatment it is dangerous to go longer than 2 wk without a clinical examination and blood studies.
- Notify physician if the following symptoms occur: unusual bleeding or bruising, sores on lips or in mouth; flank, stomach, or joint pain; fever, chills, or other signs of infection, sore throat, cough, dyspnea.
- Report immediately the onset of cutaneous reaction.
- Drink at least 10–12 glasses (240 mL [8 oz] each) of fluid per day, if not contraindicated, and report to physician if urine output decreases below normal amounts.
- Report to physician immediately if pregnant, as there is a potential hazard to the fetus.
- Do not breast feed while taking this drug.

CHLORAMPHENICOL

(klor-am-fen′i-kole)

Chlorofair, Chloromycetin, Chloroptic, Chloroptic S.O.P., Fenicol, Isopto Fenicol, Novochlorocap ✦, Ophthochlor, Pentamycetin ✦

CHLORAMPHENICOL SODIUM SUCCINATE

Chloromycetin Sodium Succinate

Classifications: ANTIINFECTIVE; ANTIBIOTIC

Pregnancy Category: C

AVAILABILITY 250 mg capsules; 100 mg/mL injection; 5 mg/mL ophth solution; 10 mg/g ointment; 0.5% otic solution

ACTIONS Synthetic broad-spectrum antibiotic formerly derived from *Streptomyces venezuelae.* Principally bacteriostatic but may be bactericidal in certain species (e.g., *Haemophilus influenzae*) or when given in higher concentrations. Believed to act by binding to the 50S ribosome of bacteria and thus interfering with protein synthesis.

THERAPEUTIC EFFECTS Effective against a wide variety of gram-negative and gram-positive bacteria and most anaerobic microorganisms.

USES Severe infections when other antibiotics are ineffective or are contraindicated. Particularly effective against *Salmonella typhi* and other *Salmonella* sp, *Streptococcus pneumoniae, Neisseria,* meningeal infections caused by *H. influenzae,* and infections involving *Bacteroides fragilis* and other anaerobic organisms, *Rickettsia rickettsii* (cause of Rocky Mountain spotted fever) and other rickettsiae, the lymphogranuloma-psittacosis group *(Chlamydia),* and *Mycoplasma.* Also used in cystic fibrosis antiinfective regimens and topically for infections of skin, eyes, and external auditory canal.

CONTRAINDICATIONS History of hypersensitivity or toxic reaction to chloramphenicol; treatment of minor infections, prophylactic use; typhoid carrier state, history or family history of drug-induced bone marrow depression, concomitant therapy with drugs that produce bone marrow depression; pregnancy (category C); lactation.

CAUTIOUS USE Impaired hepatic or renal function, premature and full-term infants, children; intermittent porphyria; patients with G6PD deficiency; patient or family history of drug-induced bone marrow depression.

ROUTE & DOSAGE

Serious Infections

Adult: **PO/IV** 50 mg/kg/d in 4 divided doses. **Topical** 1–2 drops of ophthalmic solution q3–6h or small strip of ophthalmic ointment in lower conjunctival sac q3–6h or 2–3 drops of otic solution in ear t.i.d.

Neonate: **IV** 25–50 mg/kg/d divided q12–24h

Infant/Child: **PO/IV** 50–75 mg/kg/d divided q6h (max: 4 g/d)

Meningitis

Adult: **IV** 75–100 mg/kg/d divided q6h

Child: **IV** Same as for adult

ADMINISTRATION

Oral

- Give preferably with a full glass of water on an empty stomach, at least 1 h before or 2 h after a meal, to achieve optimum blood levels.

Ophthalmic

- Apply light pressure to lacrimal duct after instillation for 1–2 min to prevent drainage into nasopharynx and systemic absorption. This is an extremely important step to decrease absorption. Several cases of aplastic anemia have been associated with use of ophthalmic preparations.

Intravenous

- IV administration to neonates, infants, children: Verify correct IV concentration and rate of infusion with physician.

PREPARE: **Direct:** Dilute each 1 g with 10 mL of sterile water or D5W. **Intermittent:** Further dilute in 50–100 mL of D5W. **Continuous:** Dilute with additional D5W for a longer infusion time.
ADMINISTER: **Direct:** Give slowly over a period of at least 1 min. **Intermittent:** Give over 30–60 min. **Continuous:** Infuse over 4–6 h.
INCOMPATIBILITIES **Solutions/additives: Chlorpromazine, glycopyrrolate, metoclopramide, polymyxin B, prochlorperazine, promethazine,** TETRACYCLINES, **vancomycin. Y-site: Fluconazole.**

- Solution for infusion may form crystals or a second layer when stored at low temperatures. Solution can be clarified by shaking vial. Do not use cloudy solutions.
- Store topical ophthalmic, otic, and skin preparations, PO forms, and unopened ampuls at room temperature and protected from light unless otherwise directed by manufacturer.

ADVERSE EFFECTS (≥1%) **Body as a Whole:** Hypersensitivity, angioedema, dyspnea, fever, anaphylaxis, superinfections, Gray syndrome. **GI:** Nausea, vomiting, diarrhea, perianal irritation, enterocolitis, glossitis, stomatitis, unpleasant taste, xerostomia. **Hematologic:** Bone marrow depression (dose-related and reversible): reticulocytosis, leukopenia, granulocytopenia, thrombocytopenia, increased plasma iron, reduced Hgb, hypoplastic anemia, hypoprothrombinemia. Non-dose-related and irreversible pancytopenia, agranulocytosis, aplastic anemia, paroxysmal nocturnal hemoglobinuria, leukemia. **CNS:** Neurotoxicity: headache, mental depression, confusion, delirium, digital paresthesias, peripheral neuritis. **Skin:** Urticaria, contact dermatitis, maculopapular and vesicular rashes, fixed-drug eruptions. **Special Senses:** Visual disturbances, optic neuritis, optic nerve atrophy, contact conjunctivitis.

DIAGNOSTIC TEST INTERFERENCE Possibility of false-positive results for ***urine glucose*** by ***copper reduction methods*** (e.g., ***Benedict's solution, Clinitest***). Chloramphenicol may interfere with ***17-OHCS*** (urinary steroid) determinations (modification of ***Reddy, Jenkins, Thorn procedure*** not affected), with ***urobilinogen excretion,*** and with responses to ***tetanus toxoid*** and possibly other active immunizing agents.

INTERACTIONS Drug: The metabolism of **chlorpropamide, dicumarol, phenytoin, tolbutamide** may be decreased, prolonging their activity. **Phenobarbital** decreases chloramphenicol levels. The response to **iron** preparations, **folic acid,** and **vitamin B_{12}** may be delayed.

PHARMACOKINETICS Absorption: Rapidly absorbed from GI tract. **Peak:** PO: 1–3 h; IV: 1 h. **Distribution:** Widely distributed to most body tissues including saliva and ascitic, pleural and synovial fluid; concentrates in liver and kidneys; penetrates CNS; crosses placenta. **Metabolism:** Primarily inactivated in liver. **Elimination:** Much longer in neonates; metabolite and free drug excreted in urine; excreted in breast milk. **Half-Life:** 1.5–4.1 h.

NURSING IMPLICATIONS

Assessment & Drug Effects

- Lab tests: Perform bacterial culture and susceptibility tests prior to first dose and periodically thereafter. Baseline CBC, platelets, serum iron, and reticulocyte cell counts before initiation of therapy, at 48 h intervals during therapy, and periodically. Monitor chloramphenicol blood levels weekly or more frequently with hepatic dysfunction and in patients receiving therapy for longer than 2 wk. Desired concentrations: peak 10–20 mg/mL; through 5–10 mg/mL.

- Monitor blood studies. Chloramphenicol should be discontinued upon appearance of leukopenia, reticulocytopenia, thrombocytopenia, or anemia.
- Non-dose-related irreversible bone marrow depression may appear weeks or months after drug therapy is terminated. The potential for this side effect is greatest in patients with impaired hepatic or renal function, infants, children, and premenopausal women.
- Observe the patient closely, because blood studies are not always reliable predictors of irreversible bone marrow depression.
- Check temperature at least q4h. Usually chloramphenicol is discontinued if temperature remains normal for 48 h.
- Monitor I&O ratio or pattern: Report any appreciable change.
- More frequent determinations of serum glucose are recommended in patients receiving oral antidiabetic agents.
- Monitor for S&S of Gray syndrome, which has occurred 2–9 d after initiation of high dose chloramphenicol therapy in premature infants and neonates and in children ≤2 y. Report early signs: abdominal distention, failure to feed, pallor, changes in vital signs. Early detection and prompt termination of therapy can interrupt a potentially fatal course.

Patient & Family Education

- A bitter taste may occur 15–20 s after IV injection; it usually lasts only 2–3 min.
- Report immediately sore throat, fever, fatigue, petechiae, nose bleeds, bleeding gums, or other unusual bleeding or bruising, or any other suspicious sign of symptom. Drug therapy should be discontinued if abnormal bleeding occurs.
- Watch for S&S of superinfection (see Appendix F).
- Follow dosage and duration of therapy as prescribed by physician.
- Avoid prolonged or frequent intermittent use of topical preparations because systemic absorption and toxicity can occur.
- Withhold medication and check with physician immediately if signs of hypersensitivity reaction (see Appendix F), irritation, superinfection, or other adverse reactions appear.
- Do not breast feed while taking this drug.

CHLORDIAZEPOXIDE HYDROCHLORIDE

(klor-dye-az-e-pox'ide)

Libritabs, Librium, Lipoxide, Medilium ✤, Novopoxide ✤, Sereen, Solium ✤

Classifications: CENTRAL NERVOUS SYSTEM AGENT; ANXIOLYTIC; SEDATIVE-HYPNOTIC; BENZODIAZEPINE

Prototype: Lorazepam

Pregnancy Category: D

Controlled Substance: Schedule IV

AVAILABILITY 5 mg, 10 mg, 25 mg capsules; 10 mg, 25 mg tablets; 100 mg/amp injection

C

ACTIONS Benzodiazepine derivative. Acts on the limbic, thalamic, and hypothalamic areas of the CNS. Has long-acting hypnotic properties. Causes mild suppression of REM sleep and of deeper phases, particularly stage 4, while increasing total sleep time.

THERAPEUTIC EFFECTS Produces mild anxiolytic (reduces anxiety), sedative, anticonvulsant, and skeletal muscle relaxant effects.

USES Relief of various anxiety and tension states, preoperative apprehension and anxiety, and for management of alcohol withdrawal.

UNLABELED USE Essential, familial, and senile action tremors.

CONTRAINDICATIONS Hypersensitivity to chlordiazepoxide and other benzodiazepines; narrow angle glaucoma, prostatic hypertrophy, shock, comatose states, primary depressive disorder or psychoses, pregnancy (category D), lactation, oral use in children <6 y, parenteral use in children <12 y, acute alcohol intoxication.

CAUTIOUS USE Anxiety states associated with impending depression, history of impaired hepatic or renal function; addiction-prone individuals, blood dyscrasias; in the older adult, debilitated patients, children; hyperkinesis, COPD.

ROUTE & DOSAGE

Mild Anxiety, Preoperative Anxiety

Adult: **PO** 5–10 mg t.i.d. or q.i.d. **IM/IV** 50–100 mg 1 h before surgery
Geriatric: **PO** 5 mg b.i.d. to q.i.d.
Child: **PO** 5 mg b.i.d. to q.i.d.; may be increased to 10 mg t.i.d.

Severe Anxiety and Tension

Adult: **PO** 20–25 mg t.i.d. or q.i.d. **IM/IV** 50–100 mg, then 25–50 mg t.i.d. or q.i.d.

Alcohol Withdrawal Syndrome

Adult: **PO** 50–100 mg prn up to 300 mg/d. **IM/IV** 50–100 mg, may repeat in 2–3 h if necessary

ADMINISTRATION

Oral

- Give with or immediately after meals or with milk to reduce GI distress. If an antacid is prescribed, it should be taken at least 1 h before or after chlordiazepoxide to prevent delay in drug absorption.
- Supervise drug ingestion to prevent "cheeking" pills, a maneuver that leads to hoarding or omission of drug.

Intramuscular

- Prepare parenteral solution immediately before use; discard unused portion. Drug is unstable in light and when in solution.
- Use special diluent provided by manufacturer to make the IM solution. Add diluent carefully to avoid bubble formation; gently agitate until solution is clear. Resulting solution: 50 mg/mL. Discard diluent if it is not clear.

Intravenous

PREPARE: **Direct:** Dilute each 100 mg ampul of dry powder with 5 mL sterile water for injection or NS. Agitate gently until dissolved. DO NOT use supplied diluent which is for IM injection only.

ADMINISTER: **Direct:** Give at a rate of 100 mg or a fraction thereof over at least 1 min.

INCOMPATIBILITIES **Y-site: Cefepime.**

- Store in tight, light-resistant containers at room temperature unless otherwise specified by manufacturer. The special diluent supplied by manufacturer for IM preparation should be kept refrigerated, preferably at 2°–8° C (36°–46° F) until ready for use.

ADVERSE EFFECTS (≥1%) **Body as a Whole:** Edema, pain in injection site, jaundice, hiccups, respiratory depression. **CV:** Orthostatic hypotension, tachycardia, changes in ECG patterns seen with rapid IV administration. **GI:** Nausea, dry mouth, vomiting, constipation, increased appetite. **CNS:** *Drowsiness,* dizziness, *lethargy,* changes in EEG pattern; vivid dreams, nightmares, headache, vertigo, syncope, tinnitus, confusion, hallucinations, paradoxic rage, depression, delirium, ataxia. **Skin:** Photosensitivity, skin rash. **Urogenital:** Urinary frequency.

DIAGNOSTIC TEST INTERFERENCE Chlordiazepoxide increases ***serum bilirubin, AST*** and ***ALT;*** decreases ***radioactive iodine uptake;*** and may falsely increase readings for ***urinary 17-OHCS*** (modified ***Glenn-Nelson*** technique).

INTERACTIONS Drug: Alcohol, CNS DEPRESSANTS, ANTICONVULSANTS potentiate CNS depression; **cimetidine** increases **chlordiazepoxide** plasma levels, thus increasing toxicity; may decrease antiparkinson effects of **levodopa;** may increase **phenytoin** levels; smoking decreases sedative and antianxiety effects. **Herbal: Kava-kava, valerian** may potentiate sedation.

PHARMACOKINETICS Absorption: Well absorbed from GI tract; slow erratic absorption from IM. **Peak:** 1–4 h PO; 15–30 min IM; 3–30 min IV. **Distribution:** Widely distributed throughout body; crosses placenta. **Metabolism:** Metabolized in liver to long-acting active metabolite. **Elimination:** Slowly excreted in urine (may last several days); excreted in breast milk. **Half-Life:** 5–30 h.

NURSING IMPLICATIONS

Assessment & Drug Effects

- Monitor for S&S of orthostatic hypotension and tachycardia, which occur more frequently with parenteral administration. Patient should stay recumbent 2–3 h after IM or IV injection; observe closely and monitor vital signs.
- Check BP and pulse before giving benzodiazepine in early part of therapy. If blood pressure falls 20 mm Hg or more or if pulse rate is above 120 bpm, delay medication and consult physician.
- Lab tests: Periodic blood cell counts and liver function tests are recommended during prolonged therapy.
- Monitor for S&S of agranulocytosis: sore throat or mouth, upper respiratory infection, fever, and malaise. Total and differential WBC counts should be ordered immediately, and protective isolation instituted.
- Monitor I&O until drug dosage is stabilized. Report changes in I&O ratio and dysuria to physician. Cumulative (overdosage) effects can result in renal dysfunction. Older adults are especially vulnerable.
- Monitor for S&S of paradoxic reactions—excitement, stimulation, disturbed sleep patterns, acute rage—which may occur during first few weeks of therapy in psychiatric patients and in hyperactive and aggressive children receiving chlordiazepoxide. Withhold drug and report to physician.
- Assess patient's sleep pattern. If dreams or nightmares interfere with rest, notify physician. A

change in the dosing schedule, dose, or an alternate drug may be prescribed.

- Supervision of ambulation especially with older adults & debilitated patients.
- Observe for signs of developing physical or psychologic dependency such as requests for change in drug regimen (dose and dose interval), diminishing favorable response (e.g., disturbed sleep pattern, increase in psychomotor activity), withdrawal symptoms. Investigate the symptoms of ataxia, vertigo, slurred speech; the patient may be taking more than the prescribed dose.
- Abrupt discontinuation of drug in patients receiving high doses for long periods (≥4 mo) has precipitated withdrawal symptoms, but not for at least 5–7 d because of slow elimination.

Patient & Family Education

- Take drug specifically as prescribed: do not skip, increase, or decrease doses, change intervals, or terminate therapy without physician's advice and do not lend or offer any of drug to another person.
- Do not take OTC drugs unless prescribed.
- Long-term use of this drug may cause xerostomia. Good oral hygiene can alleviate the discomfort.
- Avoid activities requiring mental alertness until reaction to the drug has been evaluated.
- Avoid drinking alcoholic beverages. When combined with chlordiazepoxide, effects of both are potentiated.
- If pregnant during therapy or intending to become pregnant, communicate with physician about continuing therapy.
- Avoid excessive sunlight. Photosensitivity has been reported. Use sun screen lotion (SPF 12 or above) if allowed.
- Do not breast feed while taking this drug.

CHLOROPROCAINE HYDROCHLORIDE

(klor-oh-proe′kane)

Nesacaine, Nesacaine-CE ♣

Classifications: CENTRAL NERVOUS SYSTEM AGENT; LOCAL ANESTHETIC (ESTER-TYPE)

Prototype: Procaine

Pregnancy Category: C

AVAILABILITY 1%, 2%, 3% injection

ACTIONS Short-acting ester-type local anesthetic similar to procaine. Decreases sodium influx into nerve cells, thus preventing initial depolarization, propagation, and conduction of the nerve impulse.

THERAPEUTIC EFFECTS Produces anesthetic effect, but not used for spinal, topical, or IV regional anesthesia.

USES Infiltration anesthesia and for peripheral, sympathetic, and epidural (including caudal) block anesthesia.

CONTRAINDICATIONS Known sensitivity to ester-type anesthetics, bisulfites, parabens (preservative) or PABA; intercurrent use of bupivacaine; pregnancy (category C), lactation. Safe use children <12 y not established.

CAUTIOUS USE Cardiac function impairment; history of drug hypersensitivity; debilitated, older adult, or acutely ill patients; dysrhythmias.

ROUTE & DOSAGE

Infiltration and Nerve Block
Adult: 1–2% solution: max of 800 mg without epinephrine, 1 g with epinephrine

Caudal and Epidural Block (Without Preservatives)
Adult: 2–3% solution: max of 800 mg without epinephrine, 1 g with epinephrine

ADMINISTRATION

Caudal/Epidural

- A test dose (3 mL of 3% solution or 5 mL of 2% solution) may be given before epidural use to check for intravascular or subarachnoid injection. Signs of intravascular injection: "epinephrine response" (tachycardia, circumoral pallor, palpitations, nervousness). Signs of subarachnoid injection: motor paralysis and extensive sensory anesthesia.
- If patient is moved with potential displacement of epidural catheter, test dose is repeated. At least 5 min should elapse between each test dose. Total dose for anesthesia is administered in fractional doses.
- Nesacaine formulation incorporates parabens (preservative) and sodium bisulfite; Nesacaine-CE is preservative-free but incorporates sodium bisulfite. Both parabens and bisulfites may initiate an allergic reaction in some individuals. Determine patient's sensitivity before administration of drug.
- Chloroprocaine is incompatible with alkali hydroxides and their carbonates: soaps, iodine, iodides, silver salts. Avoid use of any of these agents for skin or mucous membrane disinfection before chloroprocaine administration.
- Do not administer solution that is colored. Discard partially used solutions that are preservative-free.
- Store vials at 15°–30° C (59°–86° F); protect from freezing and from direct light.

ADVERSE EFFECTS (≥1%) **Body as a Whole:** *Sneezing*, anaphylactoid reactions. **CV:** Myocardial depression, hypotension, arrhythmias, bradycardia, cardiac arrest. **GI:** Nausea, vomiting. **CNS:** Anxiety, nervousness, tremors, sedation, circumoral paresthesia, convulsions followed by drowsiness, respiratory arrest. **Skin:** Cutaneous lesions of delayed onset; urticaria. **Special Senses:** Blurred or double vision, tinnitus. **Other:** With caudal or epidural anesthesia: urinary retention, fecal or urinary incontinence, slowing of labor and increased incidence of forceps delivery, headache, backache, edema, status asthmaticus.

INTERACTIONS Drug: May antagonize effects of SULFONAMIDES; increased risk of hypotension with MAO INHIBITORS, ANTIHYPERTENSIVE AGENTS.

PHARMACOKINETICS Onset: 6–12 min. **Duration:** 30–60 min without epinephrine; 60–90 min with epinephrine. **Metabolism:** Hydrolyzed by plasma pseudocholinesterases. **Elimination:** Excreted by kidneys.

NURSING IMPLICATIONS

Assessment & Drug Effects

- Monitor vital signs throughout period of drug use.
- Have immediately available resuscitation equipment, oxygen, resuscitative drugs, and vasopressors when chloroprocaine is in use.

Patient & Family Education

- Report urinary retention or urinary or fecal incontinence.

CHLOROQUINE HYDROCHLORIDE (Pr)

(klor'oh-kwin)

Aralen Hydrochloride

CHLOROQUINE PHOSPHATE

Aralen Phosphate

Classifications: ANTIINFECTIVE; ANTIMALARIAL

Pregnancy Category: C

AVAILABILITY **Hydrochloride:** 250 mg, 500 mg tablets; 5 mg, 50 mg/mL ampule **Phosphate:** 250 mg, 500 mg tablets

ACTIONS Antimalarial activity is believed to be based on its ability to form complexes with DNA of parasite, thereby inhibiting replication and transcription to RNA and nucleic acid synthesis. Highly active against asexual erythrocytic forms of the four species of *Plasmodium: P. vivax, P. malariae, P. ovale,* and most strains of *P. falciparum*. Action mechanism is unknown.

THERAPEUTIC EFFECTS Acts as a suppressive agent in patient with *P. vivax* or *P. malariae* malaria; terminates acute attacks and increases intervals between treatment and relapse of malaria. Abolishes the acute attack of *P. falciparum* malaria but does not prevent the infection. Chloroquine-resistant strains have been reported. Also acts as a tissue amebicide, has antiinflammatory, antihistamine, and antiserotonic properties.

USES Suppression and treatment of malaria caused by *P. malariae, P. ovale, P. vivax,* and susceptible forms of *P. falciparum,* and in the treatment of extraintestinal amebiasis. Concomitant therapy with primaquine is necessary for radical cure of *P. vivax* and *P. malariae* malarias.

UNLABELED USES Discoid and systemic lupus erythematosus, porphyria cutanea tarda, solar urticaria, polymorphous light eruptions, and in rheumatoid arthritis (as second-line therapy).

CONTRAINDICATIONS Hypersensitivity to 4-aminoquinolines, psoriasis; porphyria, renal disease, 4-aminoquinoline-induced retinal or visual field changes; long-term therapy in children; pregnancy (category C), lactation. Safe use in women of childbearing potential not established.

CAUTIOUS USE Impaired hepatic function, alcoholism, eczema, patients with G6PD deficiency, infants and children, hematologic, GI, and neurologic disorders.

ROUTE & DOSAGE

Doses are expressed in terms of chloroquine base: 500 mg tablet = 300 mg base; 50 mg injection = 40 mg base

Acute Malaria

Adult: **PO** 600 mg base followed by 300 mg base at 6, 24, and 48 h. **IM** 200 mg base q6h prn, not to exceed 800 mg base/24 h

Child: **PO** 10 mg base/kg, then 5 mg base/kg at 6, 24, and 48 h. **IM** 5 mg base/kg q12h

Malaria Suppression

Adult: **PO** 300 mg base the same day each week starting 2 wk before exposure and continuing for 4–6 wk after leaving the area of exposure (max: 300 mg base/wk)

Child: **PO** 5 mg base/kg the same day each week starting 2 wk before exposure and continuing for 4–6 wk after leaving the area of exposure (max 300 mg base/wk)

Extraintestinal Amebiasis

Adult: **PO** 600 mg base/d for 2 d, then 300 mg base/d for 2–3 wk
Child: **PO** 10 mg base/kg/d for 2–3 wk

Rheumatoid Arthritis, SLE

Adult: **PO** 150 mg base/d with evening meal

ADMINISTRATION

Oral

- Give immediately before or after meals to minimize GI distress.
- Monitor child's dose closely. Children are extremely susceptible to overdosage.

Intramuscular

- IM administration should generally be reserved for those who cannot take the oral form.
- Give undiluted, deep IM into a large muscle.
- Store tablets in tightly closed container; store tablets and ampules preferably between 15°–30° C (59°–86° F), unless otherwise directed by manufacturer.

ADVERSE EFFECTS (≥1%) **Body as a Whole:** Slight weight loss, myalgia, lymphedema of upper limbs. **CV:** Hypotension; ECG changes. **GI:** *Diarrhea,* abdominal cramps, *nausea,* vomiting, anorexia. **Hematologic:** Hemolytic anemia in patients with G6PD deficiency. **CNS:** Mild transient headache, fatigue, irritability, confusion, nightmares, skeletal muscle weakness, paresthesias, reduced reflexes, vertigo. **Skin:** Bleaching of scalp, eyebrows, body hair, and freckles, pruritus, patchy alopecia (reversible). **Special Senses:** (usually reversible): Blurred vision, disturbances of accommodation, night blindness, scotomas, visual field defects, photophobia, corneal edema, opacity or deposits, ototoxicity (rare).

INTERACTIONS Drug: Aluminum- and **magnesium-**containing ANTACIDS and LAXATIVES decrease chloroquine absorption, so separate administration by at least 4 h; chloroquine may interfere with response to **rabies vaccine.**

PHARMACOKINETICS Absorption: Rapidly and almost completely absorbed. **Peak:** 1–2 h. **Distribution:** Widely distributed; concentrates in lungs, liver, erythrocytes, eyes, skin, and kidneys; crosses placenta. **Metabolism:** Partially metabolized in liver to active metabolites. **Elimination:** Eliminated in urine; excreted in breast milk. **Half-Life:** 70–120 h.

NURSING IMPLICATIONS

Assessment & Drug Effects

- Lab tests: CBC and ECG are advised before initiation of therapy and periodically thereafter in patients on long-term therapy. A test for G6PD deficiency is recommended for American blacks and individuals of Mediterranean ancestry before therapy.
- Monitor for changes in vision. Retinopathy (generally irreversible) can be progressive even after termination of therapy. Patient may be asymptomatic or complain of night blindness, scotomas, visual field changes, blurred vision, or difficulty in focusing. Chloroquine should be discontinued immediately.
- Question patients on long-term therapy regularly about skeletal muscle weakness. Periodic tests

should be made of muscle strength and deep tendon reflexes. Positive signs are indications to terminate therapy.

Patient & Family Education

- Report promptly visual or hearing disturbances, muscle weakness, or loss of balance, symptoms of blood dyscrasia (fever, sore mouth or throat, unexplained fatigue, easy bruising or bleeding).
- Use of dark glasses in sunlight or bright light may provide comfort (because of photophobia) and reduce risk of ocular damage.
- Avoid driving or other potentially hazardous activities until reaction to drug is known.
- May cause rusty yellow or brown discoloration of urine.
- Do not breast feed while taking this drug.

CHLOROTHIAZIDE

(klor-oh-thye'a-zide)

Diachlor, Diuril, SK-Chlorothiazide

CHLOROTHIAZIDE SODIUM

Sodium Diuril

Classifications: ELECTROLYTE & WATER BALANCE AGENT; THIAZIDE DIURETIC; ANTIHYPERTENSIVE

Prototype: Hydrochlorothiazide

Pregnancy Category: C

AVAILABILITY 250 mg, 500 mg tablets; 250 mg/5 mL suspension; 500 mg injection

ACTIONS Thiazide diuretic chemically related to sulfonamides. Primary action is production of diuresis by direct action on the distal convoluted tubules. Inhibits reabsorption of sodium, potassium, and chloride ions. Promotes renal excretion of sodium (and water), bicarbonate, and potassium; decreases renal calcium excretion and supports uric acid excretion.

THERAPEUTIC EFFECTS Antihypertensive mechanism is unclear but correlates with contraction of extracellular and intravascular fluid volumes and direct vasodilatory effect on vascular wall. This initially reduces cardiac output with subsequent decrease in peripheral resistance through autoregulatory mechanisms.

USES Adjunctively to manage edema associated with CHF, hepatic cirrhosis, renal dysfunction, corticosteroid, or estrogen therapy. Used alone as step 1 agent in stepped-care approach, or in combination with other agents for treatment of hypertension.

UNLABELED USES To reduce polyuria of central and nephrogenic diabetes insipidus, to prevent calcium-containing renal stones, and to treat renal tubular acidosis.

CONTRAINDICATIONS Hypersensitivity to thiazide or sulfonamides; anuria; hypokalemia; pregnancy (category C).

CAUTIOUS USE History of sulfa allergy; impaired renal or hepatic function or gout; lactation; hypercalcemia, diabetes mellitus, older adult or debilitated patients, pancreatitis, sympathectomy, jaundiced children.

ROUTE & DOSAGE

Hypertension, Edema

Adult: **PO** 250 mg–1 g/d in 1–2 divided doses **IV** 250 mg–1 g/d in 1–2 divided doses

Geriatric: **PO** 500 mg qd or 1 g 3 times/wk

Edema

Child: **PO** *<6 mo:* 20–40 mg/kg/d in 1–2 divided doses; *>6 mo:* 20 mg/kg/d in 2 divided doses **IV** *<6 mo:* 2–4 mg/kg/d in 2 divided doses; *>6 mo:* 4 mg/kg/d

ADMINISTRATION

Oral

- Give with or after food to prevent gastric irritation. Extent of absorption appears to be increased by taking it with food.
- Schedule daily doses to avoid nocturia and interrupted sleep.

Intravenous

Reserve for emergency or when patient unable to take oral medication. IV administration to infants and children: Verify correct IV concentration and rate of infusion with physician.

PREPARE: **Intermittent:** Reconstitute the 500 mg vial with at least 18 mL sterile water for injection. May be further diluted with D5W or NS.

ADMINISTER: **Intermittent:** Give at a rate of 0.5 gram over 5 min.

INCOMPATIBILITIES **Solution/additive: Amikacin, chlorpromazine, hydralazine, insulin, levorphanol, morphine, norepinephrine, polymyxin B, procaine, prochlorperazine, promazine, promethazine, streptomycin, triflupromazine, vancomycin.**

- Thiazide preparations are extremely irritating to the tissues, and great care must be taken to avoid extravasation. If infiltration occurs, stop medication, remove needle, and apply ice if area is small.

- Store tablets, PO solutions, and parenteral dosage forms at 15°–30° C (59°–86° F) unless otherwise directed by manufacturer. Unused reconstituted IV solutions may be stored at room temperature up to 24 h. Use only clear solutions.

ADVERSE EFFECTS (≥1%) **Body as a Whole:** Fever, respiratory distress, <u>anaphylactic reaction</u>. **CV:** Irregular heart beat, weak pulse, orthostatic hypotension. **GI:** Vomiting, acute pancreatitis, diarrhea. **Hematologic:** <u>Agranulocytosis</u> (rare), <u>aplastic anemia</u> (rare), asymptomatic hyperuricemia, hyperglycemia, glycosuria, SIADH secretion. **Metabolic:** *Hypokalemia,* hypercalcemia, hyponatremia, hypochloremic alkalosis, elevated cholesterol and triglyceride levels. **CNS:** Unusual fatigue, dizziness, mental changes, vertigo, headache. **Skin:** Urticaria, photosensitivity, skin rash.

DIAGNOSTIC TEST INTERFERENCE Chlorothiazide (thiazides) may cause: marked increases in ***serum amylase*** values, decrease in ***PBI*** determinations; increase in excretion of ***PSP***; increase in ***BSP retention***; false-negative ***phentolamine*** and ***tyramine*** tests; interference with ***urine steroid*** determinations, and possibly the ***histamine test*** for pheochromocytoma. Thiazides should be discontinued at least 3 d before ***bentiromide test*** (thiazides can invalidate test) and before ***parathyroid function tests*** because they tend to decrease calcium excretion.

INTERACTIONS Drug: Amphotericin B, CORTICOSTEROIDS increase hypokalemic effects of chlorothiazide; the hypoglycemic effects of SULFONYLUREAS and **insulin** may be antagonized; **cholestyramine, colestipol** decrease thiazide absorption; intensifies hypoglycemic and hypotensive effects of **diazoxide**; increased potassium and magnesium loss may cause **digoxin** toxicity; decreases **lithium** excretion, increasing its toxicity; increases risk of NSAID-induced renal failure and may attenuate diuresis.

PHARMACOKINETICS Absorption: Incompletely absorbed PO. **Onset:** 2 h PO; 15 min IV. **Peak:** 3–6 h PO; 30 min IV. **Duration:** 6–12 h PO; 2 h IV. **Distribution:** Distributed throughout extracellular tissue; concentrates in kidney; crosses placenta. **Metabolism:** Does not appear to be metabolized. **Elimination:** Excreted in urine and breast milk. **Half-Life:** 45–120 min.

NURSING IMPLICATIONS

Assessment & Drug Effects

- Monitor for therapeutic effect. Antihypertensive action of a thiazide diuretic requires several days before effects are observed; usually optimum therapeutic effect is not established for 3–4 wk.
- Lab tests: Baseline and periodic determinations are indicated for blood count, serum electrolytes, CO_2, BUN, creatinine, uric acid, and blood glucose.
- Monitor for hyperglycemia. Thiazide therapy can cause hyperglycemia (see Appendix F) and glycosuria in diabetic and diabetic-prone individuals. Dosage adjustment of hypoglycemic drugs may be required.
- Monitor patients with gout. Asymptomatic hyperuricemia can be produced because of interference with uric acid excretion.
- Establish baseline weight before initiation of therapy. Weigh patient at the same time each a.m. under standard conditions. A gain of more than 1 kg (2.2) within 2 or 3 d and a gradual weight gain over the week's period is reportable. Tell patient to report signs of edema (hands, ankles, pretibial areas).
- Monitor BP closely during early drug therapy.
- Inspect skin and mucous membranes daily for evidence of petechiae in patients receiving large doses and those on prolonged therapy.
- Monitor I&O rates and patterns: Excessive diuresis or oliguria may cause electrolyte imbalance and necessitate prompt dosage adjustment.
- Monitor patients on digitalis therapy for S&S of hypokalemia (see Appendix G). Even moderate reduction in serum potassium can precipitate digitalis intoxication in these patients.

Patient & Family Education

- Urination will occur in greater amounts and with more frequency than usual, and there will be an unusual sense of tiredness. With continued therapy, diuretic action decreases; hypotensive effects usually are maintained, and sense of tiredness diminishes.
- If orthostatic hypotension is a troublesome symptom (and it may be, especially in the older adult), consult physician for measures that will help tolerate the effect and to prevent falling.
- Report to physician any illness accompanied by prolonged vomiting or diarrhea.
- Avoid drinking large quantities of coffee or other caffeine drinks. Caffeine is a CNS stimulant with diuretic effects.
- Report S&S of hypokalemia, hypercalcemia, or hyperglycemia (see Appendix F).

- Hypokalemia may be prevented if the daily diet contains potassium-rich foods. Eat a banana and drink at least 6 oz orange juice every day. Collaborate with dietitian and physician.
- Report photosensitivity reaction to physician if it occurs. Thiazide-related photosensitivity is considered a photoallergy (radiation changes drug structure and makes it allergenic for some individuals). It occurs 1 1/2–2 wk after initial sun exposure.
- Do not breast feed while taking this drug without consulting physician.

CHLORPHENIRAMINE MALEATE

(klor-fen-eer′a-meen)

Aller-Chlor, Chlo-Amine, Chlorate, Chlor-Pro, Chlorspan, Chlortab, Chlor-Trimeton, Chlor-Tripolon ♣, Novopheniram ♣, Pfeiffer Allergy, Phenetron, Telachlor, Teldrin, Trymegan

Classification: ANTIHISTAMINE (H_1-RECEPTOR ANTAGONIST)

Prototype: Diphenhydramine

Pregnancy Category: B first and second trimester; category D in third trimester

AVAILABILITY 2 mg, 4 mg tablets; 8 mg, 12 mg sustained-release tablets; 2 mg/5 mL syrup

ACTIONS Antihistamine that competes with histamine for H_1-receptor sites on effector cells, thus it prevents histamine action that promotes capillary permeability and edema formation and constrictive action on respiratory, gastrointestinal, and vascular smooth muscles. It generally produces less drowsiness than other antihistamines, but adverse effects involving CNS stimulation may be more common.

THERAPEUTIC EFFECTS Has effective antihistamine reaction resulting in decreasing allergic symptomatology.

USES Symptomatic relief of various uncomplicated allergic conditions; to prevent transfusion and drug reactions in susceptible patients, and as adjunct to epinephrine and other standard measures in anaphylactic reactions.

CONTRAINDICATIONS Hypersensitivity to antihistamines of similar structure; lower respiratory tract symptoms, narrow-angle glaucoma, obstructive prostatic hypertrophy or other bladder neck obstruction, GI obstruction or stenosis; pregnancy [(category B in first and second trimester) and (category D in third trimester)], lactation; premature and newborn infants; during or within 14 days of MAO INHIBITOR therapy.

CAUTIOUS USE Convulsive disorders, increased intraocular pressure, hyperthyroidism, cardiovascular disease, hypertension, diabetes mellitus, history of bronchial asthma, older adult patients, patients with G6PD deficiency.

ROUTE & DOSAGE

Symptomatic Allergy Relief

Adult: **PO** 2–4 mg t.i.d. or q.i.d. *or* 8–12 mg b.i.d. or t.i.d., max 24 mg/d

Geriatric: **PO** 4 mg q.d. or b.i.d. *or* 8 mg sustained-release h.s.

Child: **PO** *6–12 y:* 2 mg q4–6h (max: 12 mg/d); *2–6 y:* 1 mg q4–6h

Allergic Reactions to Blood

Adult: **SC/IV/IM** 10–20 mg (max: 40 mg/d)

C

ADMINISTRATION

Oral

- Give on an empty stomach for fastest response.
- Sustained-release tablets should be swallowed whole and not crushed or chewed.
- Ensure that chewable tablets are chewed or crushed before being swallowed with a liquid.

Subcutaneous/Intramuscular/Intravenous

- The 100 mg/mL preparation is intended for IM or SC use only. It should not be administered IV because it contains preservatives. The 10 mg/mL injection can be given IV, IM, or SC. It contains no preservatives.

Intravenous

PREPARE: **Direct:** Give undiluted.
ADMINISTER: **Direct:** Give 10 mg or fraction thereof over at least 1 min.

- If patient manifests any reaction after parenteral administration, drug should be discontinued. (Exception: Patient may experience transitory stinging sensation that rarely lasts longer than a few minutes.)

- Store preferably between 15° and 30° C (59° and 86° F) unless otherwise directed by manufacturer. Syrup and injection forms should be protected from light to prevent discoloration.

ADVERSE EFFECTS (≥1%) **Body as a Whole:** Sensation of chest tightness. **CV:** Palpitation, tachycardia, mild hypotension or hypertension. **GI:** Epigastric distress, anorexia, nausea, vomiting, constipation, or diarrhea. **CNS:** *Drowsiness,* sedation, headache, dizziness, vertigo, fatigue, disturbed coordination, tremors, euphoria, nervousness, restlessness, insomnia. **Special Senses:** *Dryness of mouth,* nose, and throat, tinnitus, vertigo, acute labyrinthitis, thickened bronchial secretions, blurred vision, diplopia. **Urogenital:** Urinary frequency or retention, dysuria.

DIAGNOSTIC TEST INTERFERENCE Antihistamines should be discontinued 4 d before ***skin testing*** procedures for allergy because they may obscure otherwise positive reactions.

INTERACTIONS Drug: Alcohol (ethanol) and other CNS DEPRESSANTS produce additive sedation and CNS depression.

PHARMACOKINETICS Absorption: Well absorbed from GI tract; about 45% of dose reaches systemic circulation intact. **Onset:** Within 6 h. **Peak:** 2–6 h. **Distribution:** Highest concentrations in lung, heart, kidney, brain, small intestine, and spleen. **Half-Life:** 12–43 h.

NURSING IMPLICATIONS

Assessment & Drug Effects

- Monitor for CNS depression and sedation, especially when chlorpheniramine is given in combination with other CNS depressants.
- Monitor BP in hypertensive patients since chlorpheniramine may elevate BP.

Patient & Family Education

- Avoid driving a car and other potentially hazardous activities until drug response has been determined.
- Avoid or minimize alcohol intake. Antihistamines have additive effects with alcohol.
- Report any of the following: tinnitus or palpitations.

- Consult physician before taking additional OTC drugs for allergy relief.
- Do not breast feed while taking this drug.

CHLORPROMAZINE Pr

(klor-proe'ma-zeen)

CHLORPROMAZINE HYDROCHLORIDE

Chlorpromanyl ♣, Largactil ♣, Novochlorpromazine ♣, Ormazine, Promapar, Promaz, Sonazine, Thorazine, Thor-Prom

Classifications: CENTRAL NERVOUS SYSTEM AGENT; PSYCHOTHERAPEUTIC; ANTIPSYCHOTIC; PHENOTHIAZINE; ANTIEMETIC

Pregnancy Category: C

AVAILABILITY 10 mg, 25 mg, 50 mg, 100 mg, 200 mg tablets; 30 mg, 75 mg, 150 mg sustained-release capsules; 10 mg/5 mL syrup; 30 mg/mL, 100 mg/mL oral concentrate; 25 mg, 100 mg suppositories; 25 mg/mL injection

ACTIONS Phenothiazine derivative with actions at all levels of CNS with a mechanism that produces strong antipsychotic effects. Actions on hypothalamus and reticular formation produce strong sedation, hypotension, and depressed temperature regulation. Has strong alpha-adrenergic blocking action and weak anticholinergic effects. Directly depresses the heart; may increase coronary blood flow. Exerts quinidine-like antiarrhythmic action. Antiemetic effect due to suppression of the chemoreceptor trigger zone (CTZ). Inhibitory effect on dopamine reuptake may be the basis for moderate extrapyramidal symptoms. Antipsychotic drugs are sometimes called neuroleptics because they tend to reduce initiative and interest in the environment, decrease displays of emotions or affect, suppress spontaneous movements and complex behavior, and decrease psychotic symptoms. Spinal reflexes and unconditioned nociceptive-avoidance behaviors remain intact.

THERAPEUTIC EFFECTS Mechanism that produces strong antipsychotic effects is unclear, but thought to be related to blockade of postsynaptic dopamine receptors in the brain. Also has antiemetic effects due to its action on the CTZ.

USES To control manic phase of manic-depressive illness, for symptomatic management of psychotic disorders, including schizophrenia, in management of severe nausea and vomiting, to control excessive anxiety and agitation before surgery, and for treatment of severe behavior problems in children, e.g., attention deficit disorder. Also used for treatment of acute intermittent porphyria, intractable hiccups, and as adjunct in treatment of tetanus.

CONTRAINDICATIONS Hypersensitivity to phenothiazine derivatives; withdrawal states from alcohol; comatose states, brain damage, bone marrow depression, Reye's syndrome; children <6 mo; pregnancy (category C), lactation.

CAUTIOUS USE Agitated states accompanied by depression, seizure disorders, respiratory impairment due to infection or COPD; glaucoma, diabetes, hypertensive disease, peptic ulcer, prostatic hypertrophy; thyroid, cardiovascular, and hepatic disorders; patients exposed to extreme heat or organophosphate insecticides; previously detected breast cancer.

ROUTE & DOSAGE

Psychotic Disorders, Agitation

Adult: **PO** 25–100 mg t.i.d. or q.i.d., may need up to 1000 mg/d. **IM/IV** 25–50 mg up to 600 mg q4–6h
Child: **PO** *>6 mo,* 0.55 mg/kg q4–6h prn up to 500 mg/d **PR** *>6 mo,* 1.1 mg/kg q6–8h **IM/IV** *>6 mo,* 0.55 mg/kg q6–8h

Nausea and Vomiting

Adult: **PO** 10–25 mg q4–6h prn. **PR** 50–100 mg q6–8h **IM/IV** 25–50 mg q3–4h prn
Child: **PO** *>6 mo,* 0.55 mg/kg q4–6h prn up to 500 mg/d. **PR** *>6 mo,* 1.1 mg/kg q6–8h **IM/IV** *>6 mo,* 0.55 mg/kg q6–8h

Dementia

Geriatric: **PO** Initial 10–25 mg 1–2 times/d, may increase q4–7d by 10–25 mg/d (max: 800 mg/d)

Intractable Hiccups

Adult: **PO/IM/IV** 25–50 mg t.i.d. or q.i.d.

ADMINISTRATION

Oral

- Give with food or a full glass of fluid to minimize GI distress.
- Ensure that oral drug is swallowed and not hoarded. Suicide attempt is a constant possibility in depressed patients, particularly when they are improving.
- Mix chlorpromazine concentrate just before administration in at least 1/2 glass juice, milk, water, coffee, tea, carbonated beverage, or with semisolid food.
- Ensure that sustained-release form of drug is not chewed or crushed. It must be swallowed whole.

Intramuscular/Intravenous

- Avoid parenteral drug contact with skin, eyes, and clothing because of its potential for causing contact dermatitis.
- Keep patient recumbent for at least 1/2 h after parenteral administration. Observe closely. Report hypotensive reactions.

Intramuscular

- Inject IM preparations slowly and deep into upper outer quadrant of buttock. Avoid SC injection; it may cause tissue irritation and nodule formation. If irritation is a problem, consult physician about diluting medication with normal saline or 2% procaine. Rotate injection sites.

Intravenous

PREPARE: **Direct:** Dilute 25 mg with 24 mL of NS to yield 1 mg/mL. **Continuous:** May be further diluted in up to 1000 mL of NS.

ADMINISTER: **Direct:** Administer 1 mg or fraction thereof over 1 min for adults and over 2 min for children. **Continuous:** Give slowly at a rate not to exceed 1 mg/min.

INCOMPATIBILITIES **Solution/additive: Aminophylline, amphotericin B, ampicillin, chloramphenicol, chlorothiazide, cimetidine, dimenhydrinate, furosemide, heparin, methohexital, penicillin G, pentobarbital, phenobarbital, thiopental. Y-site: Allopurinol, amifostine, aminophylline, amphotericin B; cholesteryl complex, aztreonam, cefe- pime, chloramphenicol, chlorothiazide, etoposide, fludarabine, melphalan, methotrexate, paclitaxel, piperacillin/tazobactam, remifentanil, sargramostim.**

- Lemon yellow color of parenteral preparation does not alter potency; if otherwise colored or markedly discolored, solution should be discarded.
- All forms are stored preferably between 15°–30° C (59°–86° F) protected from light, unless otherwise specified by the manufacturer. Avoid freezing.

ADVERSE EFFECTS (≥1%) **Body as a Whole:** Idiopathic edema, muscle necrosis (following IM), SLE-like syndrome, sudden unexplained death. **CV:** Orthostatic hypotension, palpitation, tachycardia, ECG changes (usually reversible): prolonged QT and PR intervals, blunting of T waves, ST depression. **GI:** Dry mouth; constipation, adynamic ileus, cholestatic jaundice, aggravation of peptic ulcer, dyspepsia, increased appetite. **Hematologic:** Agranulocytosis, thrombocytopenic purpura, pancytopenia (rare). **Metabolic:** Weight gain, hypoglycemia, hyperglycemia, glycosuria (high doses), enlargement of parotid glands. **CNS:** *Sedation, drowsiness,* dizziness, restlessness, neuroleptic malignant syndrome, tardive dyskinesias, tumor, syncope, headache, weakness, insomnia, reduced REM sleep, bizarre dreams, cerebral edema, convulsive seizures, hypothermia, inability to sweat, depressed cough reflex, *extrapyramidal symptoms,* EEG changes. **Respiratory:** Laryngospasm. **Skin:** Fixed-drug eruption, urticaria, reduced perspiration, contact dermatitis, exfoliative dermatitis, photosensitivity, eczema, anaphylactoid reactions, hypersensitivity vasculitis; hirsutism (long-term therapy). **Special Senses:** Blurred vision, lenticular opacities, mydriasis, photophobia. **Urogenital:** Anovulation, infertility, pseudopregnancy, menstrual irregularity, gynecomastia, galactorrhea, priapism, inhibition of ejaculation, reduced libido, urinary retention and frequency.

DIAGNOSTIC TEST INTERFERENCE Chlorpromazine (phenothiazines) may increase ***cephalin flocculation,*** and possibly other ***liver function tests***; also may increase ***PBI.*** False-positive result may occur for ***amylase, 5-hydroxyindole acetic acid, porphobilinogens, urobilinogen (Ehrlich's reagent),*** and ***urine bilirubin (Bili-Labstix).*** False-positive or false-negative ***pregnancy test*** results possibly caused by a metabolite of phenothiazines, which discolors urine depending on test used.

INTERACTIONS Drug: Alcohol, CNS DEPRESSANTS increase CNS depression; ANTACIDS, ANTIDIARRHEALS decrease absorption—space administration 2 h before or after administration of chlorpromazine; **phenobarbital** increases metabolism of phenothiazine; GENERAL ANESTHETICS increase excitation and hypotension; antagonizes antihypertensive action of **guanethidine**; **phenylpropanolamine** poses possibility of sudden death; TRICYCLIC ANTIDEPRESSANTS intensify hypotensive and anticholinergic effects; ANTICONVULSANTS decrease seizure threshold—may need to increase anticonvulsant dose. **Herbal: Kava-kava** increased risk and severity of dystonic reaction.

PHARMACOKINETICS Absorption: Rapid absorption with considerable first pass metabolism in liver; rapid absorption after IM. **Onset:** 30–60 min. **Peak:** 2–4 h PO; 15–20 min IM. **Duration:** 4–6 h. **Distribu-**

tion: Widely distributed; accumulates in brain; crosses placenta. **Metabolism:** Metabolized in liver. **Elimination:** Excreted in urine as metabolites; excreted in breast milk. **Half-Life:** Biphasic 2 and 30 h.

NURSING IMPLICATIONS

Assessment & Drug Effects

- Establish baseline BP (in standing and recumbent positions), and pulse, before initiating treatment.
- Monitor BP frequently. Hypotensive reactions, dizziness, and sedation are common during early therapy, particularly in patients on high doses and in the older adult receiving parenteral doses. Patients usually develop tolerance to these adverse effects; however, lower doses or longer intervals between doses may be required.
- Lab tests: Periodic CBC with differential, liver function tests, urinalysis, and blood glucose.
- Monitor cardiac status with baseline ECG in patients with preexisting cardiovascular disease.
- Be alert for signs of neuroleptic malignant syndrome (see Appendix G). Report immediately.
- Observe and record smoking since it increases metabolism of phenothiazines, resulting in shortened half-life and more rapid clearance of drug. Higher dosage in smokers may be required. Advise patient to stop or at least reduce smoking, if possible.
- Monitor I&O ratio and pattern: Urinary retention due to mental depression and compromised renal function may occur. If serum creatinine becomes elevated, therapy should be discontinued.
- Monitor for antiemetic effect of chlorpromazine, which may obscure signs of overdosage of other drugs or other causes of nausea and vomiting.
- Be alert to complaints of diminished visual acuity, reduced night vision, photophobia, and a perceived brownish discoloration of objects. Patient may be more comfortable with dark glasses.
- Monitor diabetics or prediabetics on long-term, high-dose therapy for reduced glucose tolerance and loss of diabetes control.
- Ocular examinations, and EEG (in patients >50 y) are recommended before and periodically during prolonged therapy.

Patient & Family Education

- Take medication as prescribed and keep appointments for follow-up evaluation of dosage regimen. Improvement may not be experienced until 7 or 8 wk into therapy.
- Do not alter dosing regimen, and do not give the drug to another person.
- May cause pink to red-brown discoloration of urine.
- Wear protective clothing and sunscreen lotion with SPF above 12 when outdoors, even on dark days. Photosensitivity associated with chlorpromazine therapy is a phototoxic reaction. Severity of response depends on amount of exposure and drug dose. Exposed skin areas have appearance of an exaggerated sunburn. If reaction occurs, report to physician.
- Practice meticulous oral hygiene. Oral candidiasis occurs frequently in patients receiving phenothiazines.
- Report extrapyramidal symptoms that occur most often in patients on high dosage, the pediatric patient with severe de-

hydration and acute infection, the older adult, and women.

- Avoid driving a car or undertaking activities requiring precision and mental alertness until drug response is known.
- Do not abruptly stop this drug. Abrupt withdrawal of drug or deliberate dose skipping, especially after prolonged therapy with large doses, can cause onset of extrapyramidal symptoms (see Appendix F) and severe GI disturbances. When drug is to be discontinued, dosage must be tapered off gradually over a period of several weeks.
- Do not breast feed while taking this drug.

CHLORPROPAMIDE

(klor-proe′pa-mide)

Apo-Chlorpropamide ✦, Chloronase, Diabinese, Glucamide, Novopropamide ✦

Classifications: HORMONE AND SYNTHETIC SUBSTITUTE; ANTIDIABETIC SULFONYLUREA

Prototype: Glyburide

Pregnancy Category: C

AVAILABILITY 100 mg, 250 mg tablets

ACTIONS Longest-acting first-generation sulfonylurea compound, structurally and pharmacologically related to tolbutamide. Although a sulfonamide derivative, it has no antiinfective activity. Lowers blood glucose by stimulating beta cells in pancreas to synthesize and release endogenous insulin. May potentiate available antidiuretic hormone (ADH) secretion, a property not shared by other sulfonylureas.

THERAPEUTIC EFFECTS Antidiabetic effect is due to the ability of the drug to stimulate the beta cells of the pancreas to manufacture and release insulin. Therapeutic effectiveness is indicated by HbA_{1c} levels >7%.

USES Mild to moderately severe, stable non-insulin-dependent diabetes mellitus (type 2) in patients who cannot be controlled by diet alone and who do not have complications of diabetes.

UNLABELED USE Neurogenic diabetes insipidus.

CONTRAINDICATIONS Known hypersensitivity to sulfonylureas and to sulfonamides; diabetes complicated by severe infection; acidosis; severe renal, hepatic, or thyroid insufficiency. Safe use during pregnancy (category C), in nursing mothers, and in children not established.

CAUTIOUS USE Older adult patients, Addison's disease, CHF, and hepatic porphyria.

ROUTE & DOSAGE

Antidiabetic

Adult: **PO** Initial: 100–250 mg/d with breakfast, adjust by 50–125 mg/d q3–5d until glycemic control is achieved, up to 750 mg/d

Antidiuretic

Adult: **PO** 100–250 mg/d, may adjust q2–3d up to 500 mg/d

ADMINISTRATION

Oral

- Give as a single morning dose with breakfast. To reduce GI adverse effects, drug may be prescribed as 2 or 3 doses and taken with meals.
- Store below 40° C (104° F), preferably at 15°–30° C (59°–86° F)

C

in a tightly closed container, unless otherwise directed.

ADVERSE EFFECTS (≥1%) **Body as a Whole:** Flushing, photosensitivity, alcohol intolerance. **GI:** GI distress, anorexia, nausea, diarrhea, constipation, cholestatic jaundice. **Hematologic:** Leukopenia, thrombocytopenia, agranulocytosis. **Metabolic:** Hypoglycemia, antidiuretic effect (SIADH), dilutional hyponatremia, water intoxication. **CNS:** Drowsiness, muscle cramps, weakness, paresthesias. **Skin:** Rash, pruritus.

INTERACTIONS Drug: Adverse effects of ORAL ANTICOAGULANTS, **phenytoin,** SALICYLATES, NSAIDS may be increased along with those of chlorpropamide; THIAZIDE DIURETICS may increase blood sugar; **alcohol** produces disulfiram reaction; **probenecid,** MAO INHIBITORS may increase hypoglycemic effects. **Herbal: Garlic, ginseng** may increase hypoglycemic effects.

PHARMACOKINETICS Absorption: Readily absorbed from GI tract. **Onset:** 1 h. **Peak:** 3–6 h. **Distribution:** Highly protein bound; distributed into breast milk. **Metabolism:** Metabolized in liver. **Elimination:** 80–90% excreted in urine in 96 h. **Half-Life:** 36 h.

NURSING IMPLICATIONS

Assessment & Drug Effects

- Monitor therapeutic effectiveness: Indicated by HbA_{1c} levels >7%.
- Monitor blood and urine glucose to determine effectiveness of glycemic control.
- Lab tests: Periodic fasting and postprandial blood glucose; HbA_{1c} every 3 mo; baseline and periodic hematologic and hepatic studies are advisable, particularly in patients receiving high doses. A CBC should be performed if symptoms of anemia appear.
- Report dizziness, shortness of breath, malaise, fatigue.
- Monitor for S&S of hypoglycemia (see Appendix F).
- Monitor I&O ratio and pattern: Infrequently, chlorpropamide produces an antidiuretic effect, with resulting severe hyponatremia, edema, and water intoxication. If fluid intake far exceeds output and edema develops (weight gain), report to the physician.

Patient & Family Education

- Report hypoglycemic episodes to physician. Because chlorpropamide has a long half-life, hypoglycemia can be severe, although onset is not as fast or as dramatic as with use of insulin.
- Report any of the following immediately to physician: skin eruptions, malaise, fever, or photosensitivity. Immediately report these symptoms to physician. A change to another hypoglycemic agent may be indicated.
- Do not self-dose with OTC drugs unless approved or prescribed by the physician.
- Do not breast feed while using this drug.

CHLORTHALIDONE

(klor-thal′ i-done)

Hygroton, Hylidone, Novothalidone ♣, Thalitone, Uridon ♣

Classifications: ELECTROLYTE & WATER BALANCE AGENT; THIAZIDE DIURETIC

Prototype: Hydrochlorothiazide

Pregnancy Category: B

AVAILABILITY 15 mg, 25 mg, 50 mg, 100 mg tablets

ACTIONS Sulfonamide derivative. Differs chemically from thiazides but shares similar actions. Increases excretion of sodium and chloride by inhibiting their reabsorption in the cortical diluting segment of the ascending loop of Henle. Reportedly, in some patients, it causes elevations in total cholesterol, LDL cholesterol, and triglycerides.

THERAPEUTIC EFFECTS Antihypertensive effect is correlated to the decrease in extracellular and intracellular volumes. Decreased volume results in reduced cardiac output with subsequent decrease in peripheral resistance.

USES Edema associated with CHF, renal decompensation, hepatic cirrhosis, corticosteroid and estrogen therapy; as sole agent or with other antihypertensives to treat hypertension.

CONTRAINDICATIONS Hypersensitivity to sulfonamide derivatives; anuria, hypokalemia; pregnancy (category B), lactation. Safe use in children not established.

CAUTIOUS USE History of renal and hepatic disease, gout, SLE, diabetes mellitus.

ROUTE & DOSAGE

Hypertension

Adult: **PO** 12.5–25 mg/d, may be increased to 100 mg/d if needed

Child: **PO** 2 mg/kg 3 times/wk

Edema

Adult: **PO** 50–100 mg/d, may be increased to 200 mg/d if needed

ADMINISTRATION

Oral

- Administer as single dose in a.m. to reduce potential for interrupted sleep because of diuresis.
- Consult physician when chlorthalidone is used as a diuretic; an intermittent dose schedule may reduce incidence of adverse reactions.
- Store tablets in tightly closed container at 15°–30° C (59°–86° F) unless otherwise advised.

ADVERSE EFFECTS (≥1%) **CV:** Orthostatic hypotension. **GI:** Anorexia, nausea, vomiting, diarrhea, constipation, cramping, jaundice. **Hematologic:** Agranulocytosis, thrombocytopenia, aplastic anemia. **CNS:** Dizziness, vertigo, paresthesias, headache. **Metabolic:** *Hypokalemia,* hyponatremia, hypochloremia, hypercalcemia, glycosuria, hyperglycemia, exacerbation of gout. **Skin:** Rash, urticaria, photosensitivity, vasculitis. **Urogenital:** Impotence.

INTERACTIONS Drug: Increased risk of **digoxin** toxicity because of hypokalemia; CORTICOSTEROIDS, **amphotericin B** increases hypokalemia; decreases **lithium** elimination; may antagonize the hypoglycemic effects of SULFONYLUREAS; NSAIDS may attenuate diuretic effects; **cholestyramine** decreases thiazide absorption.

PHARMACOKINETICS Absorption: Readily absorbed from GI tract. **Onset:** 2 h. **Peak:** 3–6 h. **Duration:** 24–72 h. **Distribution:** Crosses placenta; appears in breast milk. **Elimination:** 30–60% excreted in urine in 24 h. **Half-Life:** 54 h.

NURSING IMPLICATIONS

Assessment & Drug Effects

- Establish baseline BP measurements and check at regular inter-

C

vals during period of dosage adjustment when chlorthalidone is used for hypertension.

- Be alert to signs of hypokalemia (see Appendix F). Older adult patients are more sensitive to adverse effects of drug-induced diuresis because of age-related changes in the cardiovascular and renal systems.
- Lab tests: Baseline and periodic: serum electrolytes (particularly K, Mg, Ca), serum uric acid, creatinine, BUN, and uric acid and blood glucose (especially in patients with diabetes).
- Monitor lithium and digoxin levels closely when either of these drugs is used concurrently.

Patient & Family Education

- Maintain adequate potassium intake, monitor weight, and make a daily estimate of I&O ratio.
- Do not breast feed while taking this drug.

CHLORZOXAZONE

(klor-zox'a-zone)

Paraflex, Parafon Forte

Classifications: AUTONOMIC NERVOUS SYSTEM AGENT; CENTRALLY ACTING SKELETAL MUSCLE RELAXANT

Prototype: Cyclobenzaprine

Pregnancy Category: C

AVAILABILITY 250 mg, 500 mg tablets

ACTIONS Centrally acting skeletal muscle relaxant. Acts indirectly by depressing nerve transmission through polysynaptic pathways in spinal cord, subcortical centers, and brainstem; also possibly has a sedative effect.

THERAPEUTIC EFFECTS Effectively controls muscle spasms and pain associated with musculoskeletal conditions. Not effective for spastic or dyskinetic CNS disorders, e.g., cerebral palsy.

USE Symptomatic treatment of muscle spasm and pain associated with various musculoskeletal conditions.

CONTRAINDICATIONS Impaired liver function; pregnancy (category C), lactation.

CAUTIOUS USE Patients with known allergies or history of drug allergies; history of liver disease; older adult patients.

ROUTE & DOSAGE

Skeletal Muscle Relaxant

Adult: **PO** 250–500 mg t.i.d. or q.i.d. (max: 3 g/d)
Child: **PO** 20 mg/kg/d in 3–4 divided doses

ADMINISTRATION

Oral

- Give with food or meals to prevent gastric distress. If necessary, tablet may be crushed and mixed with food or liquid, e.g., milk, fruit juice.
- Store in tight container at 15°–30° C (59°–86° F) unless otherwise directed.

ADVERSE EFFECTS (≥1%) **GI:** Anorexia, heartburn, nausea, vomiting, constipation, diarrhea, abdominal pain, hepatotoxicity: jaundice, liver damage. **CNS:** *Drowsiness, dizziness,* light-headedness, headache, malaise, overstimulation. **Skin:** Erythema, rash, pruritus, urticaria, petechiae, ecchymoses.

INTERACTIONS Drug: Alcohol, CNS DEPRESSANTS add to CNS depression.

PHARMACOKINETICS Absorption: Readily absorbed from GI tract. **Onset:** 1 h. **Peak:** 1–4 h. **Duration:** 3–4 h. **Distribution:** Not known if crosses placenta or distributed into breast milk. **Metabolism:** Metabolized in liver. **Elimination:** Excreted in urine. **Half-Life:** 66 min.

NURSING IMPLICATIONS

Assessment & Drug Effects

- Monitor ambulation during early drug therapy; some patients may require supervision.
- Lab tests: Periodic liver function tests are advised in patients receiving long-term therapy even if sporadic.
- Note: Since chlorzoxazone metabolite may discolor urine, dark urine cannot be a reliable sign of a hepatotoxic reaction.

Patient & Family Education

- Avoid activities requiring mental alertness, judgment, and physical coordination until reaction to drug is known, since sedation, drowsiness, and dizziness may occur.
- Drug may discolor urine orange to purplish red, but this is of no clinical significance.
- Discontinue drug and notify physician if signs of hypersensitivity (see Appendix F) or of liver dysfunction appear (abdominal discomfort, yellow sclerae or skin, pruritus, malaise, nausea, vomiting).
- Check with physician before taking an OTC depressant (e.g., antihistamine, sedative, alcohol) since effects may be additive.
- Do not breast feed while using this drug.

CHOLESTYRAMINE RESIN (Pr)

(koe-less-tear'a-meen)

LoCHOLEST, Questran, Questran Light, Prevalite

Classifications: CARDIOVASCULAR AGENT; ANTILIPEMIC; BILE ACID SEQUESTRANT

Pregnancy Category: C

AVAILABILITY 4 g powder for suspension; 1 g tablet

ACTIONS Anion-exchange resin used for its cholesterol-lowering effect. Adsorbs and combines with intestinal bile acids in exchange for chloride ions to form an insoluble, nonabsorbable complex that is excreted in the feces. As a result, bile salts are continually (but not entirely) prevented from reentry into the enterohepatic circulation, thus, increasing fecal loss of bile acids. This leads to lowered serum total cholesterol by decreasing low-density lipoprotein (LDL) cholesterol.

THERAPEUTIC EFFECTS The resin anion-exchange agent increases fecal loss of bile acids which leads to lowered serum total cholesterol by decreasing (LDL) cholesterol, and reducing bile acid deposit in dermal tissues (decreasing pruritus). Serum triglyceride levels may increase or remain unchanged.

USES As adjunct to diet therapy in management of patients with primary hypercholesterolemia (type IIa hyperlipidemia) with a significant risk of atherosclerotic heart disease and MI; for relief of pruritus secondary to partial biliary stasis.

UNLABELED USES To control diarrhea caused by excess bile acids in colon; for hyperoxaluria.

C

CONTRAINDICATIONS Complete biliary obstruction, hypersensitivity to bile acid sequestrants; pregnancy (category C), lactation. Safe use in children ≤6 y not established.

CAUTIOUS USE Bleeding disorders; hemorrhoids; impaired GI function, peptic ulcer, malabsorption states (e.g., steatorrhea); phenylketonuria (Questran Light only).

ROUTE & DOSAGE

Hypercholesterolemia

Adult: **PO** 4 g b.i.d. to q.i.d. a.c. and h.s., may need up to 24 g/d
Child: **PO** 240 mg/kg/d in 3 divided doses

Hyperlipoproteinemia

Adult: **PO** 4–8 g b.i.d. to q.i.d. a.c. and h.s. (≤32 g/d)

Pruritus

Adult: **PO** 4 g b.i.d. to q.i.d. a.c. and h.s. (≤16 g/d)

ADMINISTRATION

Oral

- Place contents of one packet or one level scoopful on surface of at least 120 to 180 mL (4–6 oz) of water or other preferred liquid. Permit drug to hydrate by standing without stirring 1–2 min, twirling glass occasionally, then stir until suspension is uniform. Rinse glass with small amount of liquid and have patient drink remainder to ensure entire dose is taken. Administer before meals.
- Always dissolve cholestyramine powder before administration; it is irritating to mucous membranes and may cause esophageal impaction if administered dry.
- Store in tightly closed container at 15°–30° C (59°–86° F) unless otherwise specified.

ADVERSE EFFECTS (≥1%) **GI:** *Constipation,* fecal impaction, hemorrhoids, abdominal pain and distension, flatulence, bloating sensation, belching, nausea, vomiting, heartburn, anorexia, diarrhea, steatorrhea. **Endocrine:** Increased libido. **Metabolic:** Weight loss or gain, iron, calcium, vitamin A, D, and K deficiencies (from poor absorption); hypoprothrombinemia, hyperchloremic acidosis, decreased erythrocyte folate levels. **Skin:** Rash, irritations of skin, tongue, and perianal areas. **Special Senses:** Arcus juvenilis, uveitis.

DIAGNOSTIC TEST INTERFERENCE Cholestyramine therapy may be accompanied by increased ***serum AST, phosphorus, chloride,*** and ***alkaline phosphatase*** levels; decreased ***serum calcium, sodium,*** and ***potassium*** levels.

INTERACTIONS Drug: Decreases the absorption of ORAL ANTICOAGULANTS, **digoxin,** TETRACYCLINES, **penicillins, phenobarbital,** THYROID HORMONES, THIAZIDE DIURETICS, IRON SALTS, FAT-SOLUBLE VITAMINS (A, D, E, K) from the GI tract—administer cholestyramine 4 h before or 2 h after these drugs.

PHARMACOKINETICS Absorption: Not absorbed from GI tract. **Elimination:** Excreted in feces as insoluble complex.

NURSING IMPLICATIONS

Assessment & Drug Effects

- Monitor therapeutic effect. Serum cholesterol levels are reduced within 24–48 h after treatment starts and may continue to decline for a year. After withdrawal of cholestyramine, cholesterol levels usually return to baseline level in about 2 to 4 wk.

- Be alert to early symptoms of hypoprothrombinemia (petechiae, ecchymoses, abnormal bleeding from mucous membranes, tarry stools) and report their occurrence promptly. Long-term use of cholestyramine resin can increase bleeding tendency.
- Preexisting constipation may be worsened in the older adult, women, and in those taking >24 g/d.
- Consult physician regarding supplemental vitamins A and D and folic acid that may be required by patient on long-term therapy.
- Lab tests: Periodic CBC, platelet count, serum electrolytes, and lipid profile.

Patient & Family Education

- Report constipation immediately to physician. High-bulk diet with adequate fluid intake is an essential adjunct to cholestyramine treatment and generally resolves the problems of constipation and bloating sensation.
- Do not omit doses. Sudden withdrawal can promote uninhibited absorption of other drugs taken concomitantly, leading to toxicity or overdosage.
- GI adverse effects usually subside after the first month of drug therapy.
- The following symptoms may be drug-induced and should be reported promptly: severe gastric distress with nausea and vomiting, unusual weight loss, black stools, severe hemorrhoids (GI bleeding), sudden back pain.
- Do not breast feed while using this drug.

CHOLINE MAGNESIUM TRISALICYLATE

(cho'leen mag-ne'si-um tri-sal'i-ci-late)

Trilisate

Classifications: CENTRAL NERVOUS SYSTEM AGENT; ANALGESIC, SALICYLATE; ANTIPYRETIC

Prototype: Aspirin

Pregnancy Category: C

AVAILABILITY 500 mg, 750 mg, 1000 mg tablets; 500 mg/5 mL liquid

ACTIONS Trilisate is a nonsteroidal, antiinflammatory preparation combining choline salicylate and magnesium salicylate. Mode of action is by inhibiting prostaglandin synthesis.

THERAPEUTIC EFFECTS Trilisate has antiinflammatory, analgesic, and antipyretic action. Platelet aggregation is not affected.

USES Osteoarthritis, rheumatoid arthritis, and other arthrides. Preferable to aspirin for patients with GI bleeding.

CONTRAINDICATIONS Hypersensitivity to nonacetylated salicylates; children <6 y; children and teenagers with chickenpox, influenza, or flu symptoms because of the potential for Reye's syndrome; pregnancy (category C); contraindicated in late pregnancy, near term, or in labor and delivery.

CAUTIOUS USE Chronic renal and hepatic failure, peptic ulcer; patients on coumadin or heparin; lactation; older adults.

ROUTE & DOSAGE

Arthritis

Adult: **PO** 1.5–2.5 g/d in 1–3 divided doses (max: 4.5 g/d)

Mild to Moderate Pain, Fever
Adult: **PO** 2–3 g/d in 2 divided doses
Child: **PO** 30–60 mg/kg/d in 3–4 divided doses

ADMINISTRATION

Oral
- Give with food to reduce gastric upset. Do not give with antacids.
- Store at 59°–86° F (15°–30° C).

ADVERSE EFFECTS (≥1%) **GI:** Vomiting, diarrhea. **CNS:** Headache, vertigo, confusion, drowsiness. **Special Senses:** Tinnitus.

INTERACTIONS Drug: Aminosalicylic acid increases risk of salicylate toxicity; **ammonium chloride** and other **acidifying agents** decrease its renal elimination, increasing risk of salicylate toxicity; ANTICOAGULANTS increase risk of bleeding; CARBONIC ANHYDRASE INHIBITORS enhance salicylate toxicity; CORTICOSTEROIDS compound ulcerogenic effects; increases **methotrexate** toxicity; low doses of salicylates may antagonize uricosuric effects of **probenecid, sulfinpyrazone.**

PHARMACOKINETICS Absorption: Readily absorbed from small intestine. **Onset:** 30 min. **Peak:** 1–3 h. **Metabolism:** Metabolized in liver. **Elimination:** Excreted in urine. **Half-Life:** 2–3 h.

NURSING IMPLICATIONS

Assessment & Drug Effects
- As with other NSAIDS, the antipyretic and antiinflammatory effects may mask usual S&S of infection or other diseases.
- Assess for GI discomfort; nausea, gastric irritation, indigestion, diarrhea, and constipation are frequent complaints.
- Monitor for S&S of bleeding. Closely monitor PT if used concurrently with warfarin.

Patient & Family Education
- Avoid taking aspirin, NSAIDS, or acetaminophen concurrently with drug.
- Avoid dangerous activities until reaction to drug is determined, due to possible CNS effects (e.g., vertigo, drowsiness).
- Report tinnitus or persistent gastric irritation and epigastric pain.
- Report any unexplained bruising or bleeding to physician.
- Hypoglycemic effects may be enhanced for those with type 2 diabetes taking an oral hypoglycemic agent (OHA).
- Do not give to children or teenagers with chickenpox, influenza, or flu symptoms because of association with Reye's syndrome.
- Do not breast feed without consulting physician.

CHOLINE SALICYLATE
(koe'leen)
Arthropan
Classifications: CENTRAL NERVOUS SYSTEM AGENT; ANALGESIC, SALICYLATE; ANTIPYRETIC
Prototype: Aspirin
Pregnancy Category: C

AVAILABILITY 870 mg/5 mL liquid

ACTIONS Choline salt of salicylic acid available commercially as a liquid preparation which is a nonsteroidal antiinflammatory agent. Mode of action is by inhibiting prostaglandin synthesis.

THERAPEUTIC EFFECTS Reported to be less potent than aspirin as an analgesic, antiinflammatory, and antipyretic, and produces less gastric irritation and bleeding. Unlike aspirin, believed to have no appreciable effect on platelet function.

USES Analgesic and antiinflammatory in rheumatoid arthritis, rheumatic fever, osteoarthritis, and other conditions for which oral salicylates are usually recommended. May be indicated for patients who have difficulty swallowing tablets or capsules or as an alternative preparation for patients who show gastric intolerance to aspirin or who should avoid sodium-containing salicylates.

CONTRAINDICATIONS Salicylate hypersensitivity; children <12 y; children and teenagers with chickenpox, influenza, or flu symptoms because of the potential for Reye's syndrome; pregnancy (category C); contraindicated in late pregnancy, near term, or in labor and delivery.

CAUTIOUS USE Chronic renal and hepatic failure, peptic ulcer; patients on coumadin or heparin; lactation; older adults.

ROUTE & DOSAGE

Analgesic, Antipyretic

Adult: **PO** 435–870 mg (2.5–5 mL) q4h

Child: **PO** *2–11 y:* 2 g (115 mL)/m^2 in 4–6 divided doses

Arthritis

Adult: **PO** 4.8–7.2 g (28–41 mL)/d in 4–6 divided doses

Child: **PO** 107–134 mg (0.6–0.8 mL)/kg/d in 4–6 divided doses

ADMINISTRATION

Oral

- May be mixed with or followed by fruit juice, a carbonated beverage, or water. Do not administer with an antacid.
- If patient requires an antacid, administer choline salicylate before meals and the antacid 2 h after meals.
- Store in tightly capped container at temperature between 15° and 30° C (59° and 86° F). Protect from freezing.

ADVERSE EFFECTS (≥1%) **GI:** *Nausea,* vomiting, hepatotoxicity. **CNS:** Dizziness, sweating, mental confusion, hyperventilation. **Special Senses:** Tinnitus, deafness.

DIAGNOSTIC TEST INTERFERENCE As for aspirin with the exception of ***5-HIAA*** which is not affected by choline salicylate.

INTERACTIONS Drug: Aminosalicylate increases risk of salicylate toxicity; increases risk of bleeding with ORAL ANTICOAGULANTS; SULFONYLUREAS pose increased risk of hypoglycemia with large doses of salicylates; CARBONIC ANHYDRASE INHIBITORS cause metabolic acidosis that may increase salicylate toxicity; CORTICOSTEROIDS add to ulcerogenic effects; may increase **methotrexate** levels; small doses of salicylates may blunt uricosuric effects of **probenecid, sulfinpyrazone.**

PHARMACOKINETICS Absorption: Readily absorbed from GI tract. **Peak:** 10–30 min. **Distribution:** Widely distributed in most body tissues; crosses placenta; distributed in breast milk. **Elimination:** Excreted in urine. **Half-Life:** 2–3 h.

NURSING IMPLICATIONS

Assessment & Drug Effects

- Monitor effectiveness of drug in relieving pain in arthritic joints.
- Assess for signs of bleeding, especially in patients on anticoagulant therapy.

C

Patient & Family Education

- Report any of the following to physician: tinnitus, persistent gastric irritation, epigastric pain, unexplained bruising or bleeding.
- This drug is available OTC. Do not exceed recommended dosage and keep medicine out of the reach of children.
- Avoid concurrent use of other drugs containing aspirin or salicylates unless otherwise advised by physician.
- Do not breast feed without consulting physician.

CHORIONIC GONADOTROPIN

(go-nad'oh-troe-pin)

Antuitrin, A.P.L., Chorex, Chorigon, Choron 10, Corgonject-5, Follutein, Glukor, Gonic, HCG, Pregnyl, Profasi HP

Classification: HORMONE & SYNTHETIC SUBSTITUTE

Pregnancy Category: X

AVAILABILITY 5,000 units, 10,000 units, 20,000 units vials

ACTIONS Human chorionic gonadotropin (HCG) is a polypeptide hormone produced by the placenta and extracted from urine during first trimester of pregnancy. Actions nearly identical to those of pituitary luteinizing hormone (LH). Promotes production of gonadal steroid hormones by stimulating interstitial cells of the testes to produce androgen, and the corpus luteum of the ovary to produce progesterone.

THERAPEUTIC EFFECTS Administration of HCG to women of childbearing age with normal functioning ovaries causes maturation of the ovarian follicle and triggers ovulation. When given during normal pregnancy, it maintains corpus luteum after LH decreases, supports continuing secretion of estrogen and progesterone, and prevents ovulation.

USES Prepubertal cryptorchidism not due to anatomic obstruction and male hypogonadism secondary to pituitary deficiency. Also used in conjunction with menotropins to induce ovulation and pregnancy in infertile women in whom the cause of anovulation is secondary; ovulation usually occurs within 18 h. To stimulate spermatogenesis in males with hypogonadism.

UNLABELED USES Corpus luteum dysfunction.

CONTRAINDICATIONS Known hypersensitivity to HCG, hypogonadism of testicular origin, hypertrophy or tumor of pituitary, prostatic carcinoma or other androgen-dependent neoplasms, precocious puberty; children <4 y; pregnancy (category X).

CAUTIOUS USE Epilepsy, migraine, asthma, cardiac or renal disease; lactation.

ROUTE & DOSAGE

Prepubertal Cryptorchidism

Child: **IM** 4000 units 3 times/wk for 3 wk, *or* 5000 U q.o.d. for 4 doses, *or* 500–1000 U 3 times/wk for 4–6 wk

Hypogonadotropic Hypogonadism

Adult: **IM** 500–1000 U 3 times/wk for 3 wk, then 2 times/wk for 3 wk *or* 4000 U 3 times/wk for 6–9 mo followed by 2000 U 3 times/wk for 3 mo

Stimulation of Spermatogenesis

Adult: **IM** 5000 U 3 times/wk until normal testosterone levels are achieved (4–6 mo), then 2000 U 2 times/wk with menotropins for 4 mo

Induction of Ovulation

Adult: **IM** 500–1000 U 1 d following last dose of menotropins

ADMINISTRATION

- Reconstitute only with diluent supplied by manufacturer.
- Following reconstitution solution is stable for 30–90 d, depending on manufacturer, when refrigerated; thereafter potency decreases.
- Store powder for injection at 15°–30° C (59°–86° F) unless otherwise directed.

ADVERSE EFFECTS (≥1%) **Body as a Whole:** Edema, pain at injection site, arterial thromboembolism. **Endocrine:** Gynecomastia, precocious puberty, increased urinary steroid excretion, ectopic pregnancy (incidence low). When used with menotropins (human menopausal gonadotropin): Ovarian hyperstimulation (ascites with or without pain, pleural effusion, ruptured ovarian cysts with resultant hemoperitoneum, multiple births). **CNS:** Headache, irritability, restlessness, depression, fatigue.

DIAGNOSTIC TEST INTERFERENCE ***Pregnancy tests:*** possibility of false results.

INTERACTIONS Drug: No clinically significant drug interactions established. **Herbal: Black cohosh** may antagonize fertility effects.

PHARMACOKINETICS Onset: 2 h. **Peak:** 6 h. **Distribution:** Testes in males, ovaries in females. **Elimination:** 10–12% excreted in urine within 24 h. **Half-Life:** 23 h.

NURSING IMPLICATIONS

Assessment & Drug Effects

- Assess prepubescent males for development of secondary sex characteristics.
- Assess females for and report excessive menstrual bleeding, irregular menstrual cycles, and abdominal/pelvic distention or pain.

Patient & Family Education

- Treatment for prepubertal cryptorchidism is usually started between 4 and 9 y. HCG can help predict whether orchidopexy will be needed in the future.
- When used for treatment of infertility, timing of coitus is important. Daily intercourse is encouraged from day before HCG is given until ovulation occurs.
- Report promptly onset of abdominal pain and distension (ovarian hyperstimulation syndrome).
- Report to physician if the following appear: axillary, facial, pubic hair; penile growth; acne; deepening of voice. Induction of androgen secretion by HCG may induce precocious puberty in patient treated for cryptorchidism.
- Observe for signs of fluid retention. A weight chart should be maintained for a biweekly record. Report to physician if weight gain is associated with edema.
- Report vaginal bleeding during treatment of corpus luteum deficiency; drug will be discontinued.
- Do not breast feed without consulting physician.

C

CICLOPIROX OLAMINE

(sye-kloe-peer'ox)
Loprox, Penlac Nail Lacquer
Classifications: ANTIINFECTIVE; ANTIFUNGAL ANTIBIOTIC
Prototype: Fluconazole
Pregnancy Category: B

AVAILABILITY 1% cream, ointment; 8% nail lacquer; 1% shampoo

ACTIONS Synthetic broad-spectrum antifungal agent with activity against pathogenic fungi. Inhibits transport of amino acids within fungal cell, thereby interfering with synthesis of fungal protein, RNA, and DNA.

THERAPEUTIC EFFECTS Effective against the following organisms: dermatophytes, yeasts, and *Malassezia furfur,* some species of *Mycoplasma* and *Trichomonas vaginalis,* and certain strains of gram-positive and gram-negative bacteria.

USES Topically for treatment of tinea cruris and tinea corporis (ringworm) due to *Trichophyton rubrum, Trichophyton mentagrophytes, Epidermophyton floccosum,* and *Microsporum canis,* and for tinea (pityriasis) versicolor due to *Malassezia furfur;* also cutaneous candidiasis (moniliasis) caused by *Candida albicans.* Nail lacquer indicated for onychomycosis of fingernails and toenails due to *Trichophyton rubrum;* seborrheic dermatitis of the scalp.

CONTRAINDICATIONS Hypersensitivity to ciclopirox olamine or to any component in the formulation; pregnancy (category B). Safe use in children <10 y not established.

CAUTIOUS USE Lactation; type 1 diabetic patient.

ROUTE & DOSAGE

Tinea

Adult: **Topical** Massage cream into affected area and surrounding skin twice daily, morning and evening.

Onychomycosis

Adult: **Topical** Paint affected nail(s) under the surface of the nail and on the nail bed once daily at bedtime (at least 8 h before washing). After 7 d, remove lacquer with alcohol and remove or trim away unattached nail. Continue times 48 wk

Seborrheic Dermatitis

Adult: **Topical** Wet hair and apply approximately 1 tsp (5 mL) to the scalp (may use up to 10 mL for long hair), leave on scalp for 3 min, then rinse. Repeat treatment twice/wk × 4 wk, with a min 3 d between applications.

ADMINISTRATION

- Wash hands thoroughly before and after treatments.
- Consult with physician about specific procedure for cleansing the skin before medication is applied. Regardless of method used, dry skin thoroughly before drug application.
- Avoid occlusive dressing, wrapping, or clothing over site where cream is applied.
- Store at 15°–30° C (59°–86° F) unless otherwise directed.

ADVERSE EFFECTS (≥1%) **Skin:** Irritation, pruritus, burning, worsening of clinical condition.

INTERACTIONS Drug: No clinically significant interactions established.

PHARMACOKINETICS Absorption: 1.3% absorbed through intact skin. **Distribution:** Distributed to epidermis, corium (dermis), including hair and hair follicles and sebaceous glands; not known if crosses placenta or is distributed into breast milk. **Elimination:** Excreted primarily by kidneys. **Half-Life:** 1.7 h.

NURSING IMPLICATIONS

Assessment & Drug Effects

- Monitor for therapeutic effectiveness. Tinea versicolor generally responds to drug treatment in about 2 wk. Tinea pedis ("athlete's foot"), tinea corporis (ringworm), tinea cruris ("jock itch"), and candidiasis (moniliasis) require about 4 wk of therapy.

Patient & Family Education

- Use medication for the prescribed time even though symptoms improve.
- Report skin irritation or other possible signs of sensitization. A reaction suggestive of sensitization warrants drug discontinuation.
- Do not use occlusive dressings or wrappings.
- Avoid contact of drug in or near the eyes.
- Wear light clothing and footwear that will allow ventilation. Loose-fitting cotton underwear or socks are preferred.
- Do not breast feed without consulting physician.

CIDOFOVIR

(cye-do′fo-ver)

Vistide

Classifications: ANTIINFECTIVE; ANTIVIRAL

Prototype: Acyclovir

Pregnancy Category: C

AVAILABILITY 75 mg/mL injection

ACTIONS Cidofovir, a nucleotide analog, suppresses cytomegalovirus (CMV) replication by inhibiting CMV DNA polymerase.

THERAPEUTIC EFFECTS Cidofovir reduces the rate of viral DNA synthesis of CMV. Cidofovir is limited for use in treating CMV retinitis in patients with AIDS.

USES Treatment of CMV retinitis in patients with AIDS.

CONTRAINDICATIONS Hypersensitivity to cidofovir, history of severe hypersensitivity to probenecid or other sulfa-containing medications, lactation; childbearing women and men without barrier contraception; pregnancy (category C); severe renal dysfunction. Safety and effectiveness in children not established.

CAUTIOUS USE Renal function impairment, history of diabetes, myelosuppression, previous hypersensitivity to other nucleoside analogs; older adults.

ROUTE & DOSAGE

CMV Retinitis: Induction

Adult: **IV** 5 mg/kg once weekly for 2 wk. Also give 2 g probenecid 3 h prior to infusion and 1 g 8 h after infusion (4 g total)

CMV Retinitis: Maintenance

Adult: **IV** 5 mg/kg once every 2 wk. Also give 2 g probenecid 3 h prior to infusion and 1 g 8 h after infusion (4 g total)

Renal Impairment

Cl_{cr} 41–55 mL/min: 2 mg/kg; 30–40: 1.5 mg/kg; 20–29 mL/min: 1 mg/kg; <20 mL/min: 0.5 mg/kg

C

ADMINISTRATION

- Pretreatment: Prehydrate with IV of 1 L NS infused over 1–2 h immediately before cidofovir infusion. If able to tolerate fluid load, infuse second liter over 1–3 h starting at beginning (or end) of cidofovir infusion.

Intravenous

PREPARE: **IV Infusion:** Dilute the calculated dose in 100 mL of NS.
ADMINISTER: **IV Infusion:** Give over 1 h at constant rate.

- Do not coadminister with other agents with significant nephrotoxic potential.

- Store vials at 20°–25° C (68°–77° F); may store diluted IV solution at 2°–8° C (36°–46° F) for up to 24 h.

ADVERSE EFFECTS (≥1%) **Body as a Whole:** Infection, allergic reactions. **GI:** Nausea, vomiting, diarrhea. **Metabolic:** Metabolic acidosis. **Hematologic:** Neutropenia. **CNS:** *Fever, headache,* asthenia. **Respiratory:** Dyspnea, pneumonia. **Special Senses:** Ocular hypotony. **Urogenital:** *Nephrotoxicity, proteinuria.*

INTERACTIONS Drug: AMINOGLYCOSIDES, **amphotericin B, foscarnet, pentamidine** can increase risk of nephrotoxicity.

PHARMACOKINETICS Duration: Probenecid increases serum levels and area under concentration–time curve. **Elimination:** 80–100% recovered in urine, probenecid delays urinary excretion.

NURSING IMPLICATIONS

Assessment & Drug Effects

- Evaluate concurrent medications. Nephrotoxic drugs are usually discontinued 7 d prior to starting cidofovir.
- Lab tests: Baseline and periodic serum creatinine, urine protein; periodic and WBC count with differential prior to each dose. Dose adjustments or discontinuation may be required.
- In patients with proteinuria, administer IV hydration and repeat test.
- Periodically monitor visual acuity and intraocular pressure.
- Monitor for S&S of hypersensitivity (see Appendix F). Report their appearance promptly.

Patient & Family Education

- Those taking zidovudine should discontinue or decrease dose to 50% on days of cidofovir administration.
- Initiate or continue regular ophthalmologic exams.
- Be alert to potential adverse reactions caused by probenecid (e.g., headache, nausea, vomiting, hypersensitivity reactions) and cidofovir.
- Closely monitor renal function.
- Women: Use effective contraception during and 1 mo after treatment.
- Men: Use barrier contraception during and 3 mo after treatment.
- Do not breast feed while taking this drug.

CILOSTAZOL

(sil-os′tah-zol)

Pletal

Classifications: CARDIOVASCULAR AGENT; COAGULATOR; VASODILATOR; ANTIPLATELET AGENT; PHOSPHODIESTERASE INHIBITOR

Pregnancy Category: C

AVAILABILITY 50 mg, 100 mg tablets

ACTIONS Inhibition of an isoenzyme which results in vasodilatation and inhibition of platelet aggregation induced by collagen or arachidonic acid.

THERAPEUTIC EFFECTS Increases the skin temperature of the extremities and improves claudication. Effectiveness is indicated by increased ability to walk further without claudication.

USES Intermittent claudication.

CONTRAINDICATIONS Congestive heart failure of any severity; hypersensitivity to cilostazol; pregnancy (category C), lactation.

CAUTIOUS USE Safety and efficacy in children <18 y are not established.

ROUTE & DOSAGE

Intermittent Claudication

Adult: **PO** 100 mg b.i.d. 0.5 h before or 2 h after meals, may need to reduce to 50 mg b.i.d. with concomitant ketoconazole, itraconazole, erythromycin, diltiazem or omeprazole

ADMINISTRATION

Oral

- Give at least 1/2 h before or 2 h after a meal. Do not give with grapefruit juice.
- Store at 20°–25° C (68°–77° F).

ADVERSE EFFECTS (≥1%) **Body as a Whole:** Back pain, *headache,* infection, myalgia. **CNS:** Dizziness, vertigo. **CV:** Palpitations, tachycardia. **GI:** Abdominal pain, *abnormal stools, diarrhea,* dyspepsia, flatulence, nausea. **Respiratory:** Cough, pharyngitis, rhinitis.

INTERACTIONS Drug: Diltiazem, erythromycin, fluconazole, fluvoxamine, fluoxetine, ketoconazole, itraconazole, MACROLIDE ANTIBIOTICS, **miconazole, nefazodone, omeprazole, sertraline** may increase **cilostazol** levels. **Food:** Grapefruit juice may decrease absorption.

PHARMACOKINETICS Absorption: Well absorbed from GI tract. **Onset:** 2–4 wks. **Distribution:** 95%–98% protein bound. Smoking may decrease serum levels. May be excreted in breast milk. **Metabolism:** Metabolized by CYP3A4 to active metabolites. **Elimination:** Metabolites primarily excreted in urine. **Half-Life:** 1–13 hr.

NURSING IMPLICATIONS

Assessment & Drug Effects

- Monitor therapeutic effectiveness indicated by ability to walk farther without leg pain.
- Monitor for S&S of CHF. Do not give cilostazol to patients with preexisting CHF.

Patient & Family Education

- Avoid grapefruit or grapefruit juice while taking cilostazol.
- Allow 2–12 wk for therapeutic response.
- Do not breast feed while taking this drug.

CIMETIDINE (Pr)

(sye-met'i-deen)

Novocimetine ♣, Peptol ♣, Tagamet, Tagamet HB

Classifications: GASTROINTESTINAL AGENT; ANTISECRETORY (H_2-RECEPTOR ANTAGONIST)

Pregnancy Category: B

AVAILABILITY 100 mg, 200 mg, 400 mg, 800 mg tablets; 300 mg/5 mL liquid; 150 mg/mL injection

ACTIONS Enzyme inhibitor structurally similar to histamine. Be-

C

longs to the antihistamine group with high selectivity for histamine H_2-receptors on parietal cells of the stomach (minimal effect on H_1-receptors). By reversible competitive inhibition of histamine at the H_2-receptor sites, it suppresses all phases of daytime and nocturnal basal gastric acid secretion in the stomach. Indirectly reduces pepsin secretion; it is not a cholinergic. Has no effect on lower esophageal sphincter pressure, gastric motility or emptying, biliary or pancreatic secretion.

THERAPEUTIC EFFECTS Cimetidine blocks the H_2-receptor on the parietal cells of the stomach, thus decreasing gastric acid secretion, raises the pH of the stomach and, thereby, reduces pepsin secretion.

USES Short-term treatment of active duodenal ulcer and prevention of ulcer recurrence (at reduced dosage) after it is healed. Also used for short-term treatment of active benign gastric ulcer, pathologic hypersecretory conditions such as Zollinger-Ellison syndrome, and heartburn.

UNLABELED USES Prophylaxis of stress-induced ulcers, upper GI bleeding, and aspiration pneumonitis; gastroesophageal reflux; chronic urticaria; acetaminophen toxicity.

CONTRAINDICATIONS Known hypersensitivity to cimetidine or other H_2 receptor antagonists; lactation, pregnancy (category B). Safe use in children <16 y not established.

CAUTIOUS USE Older adults or critically ill patients; impaired renal or hepatic function; organic brain syndrome; gastric ulcers; immunocompromised patients.

ROUTE & DOSAGE

Duodenal Ulcer

Adult: **PO** 300 mg q.i.d. *or* 400 mg b.i.d. *or* 800 mg h.s. **IM/IV** 300 mg q6–8h
Child: **PO/IM/IV** 20–40 mg/kg/d in 4 divided doses
Neonate: **PO/IM/IV** 5–10 mg/kg/d divided q8–12h
Infant: **PO/IM/IV** 10–20 mg/kg/d divided q6–12h

Duodenal Ulcer, Maintenance Therapy

Adult: **PO** 400 mg h.s.

Gastric Ulcer

Adult: **PO** 300 mg q.i.d. with meals and h.s. **IM/IV** 300 mg q6–8h

Heartburn

Adult: **PO** 200 mg 2–4 times/d

Pathologic Hypersecretory Disease

Adult: **PO** 300 mg q.i.d. with meals and h.s., may increase up to 2400 mg/d **IM/IV** 300 mg q6–8h, may increase up to 2400 mg/d

Adjustment for Renal Impairment

Cl_{cr} 20–40 mL/min: dose q8h; Cl_{cr} <20 mL/min: dose q12h

ADMINISTRATION

Oral

- Give 1 h before or 2 h after an antacid.

Intravenous

- IV administration to neonates, infants and children: Verify correct IV concentration and rate of infusion/injection with physician.

PREPARE: **Direct:** Dilute 300 mg in 18 mL D5W or NS to yield

300 mg/20 mL. **Intermittent:** Dilute 300 mg in 50 mL D5W or NS. **Continuous:** Further dilute in up to 1000 mL of selected IV solution.

ADMINISTER: **Direct:** Give 300 mg or fraction thereof over at least 5 min. **Intermittent:** Give over 15–20 min. **Continuous:** Give a loading dose of 150 mg at the intermittent infusion rate; then give continuous infusion equally spaced over 24 h.

INCOMPATIBILITIES **Solution/additive: Amphotericin B, atropine, cefamandole, cefazolin, chlorpromazine, pentobarbital, secobarbital. Y-site: Allopurinol, amphotericin B cholesteryl complex, amsacrine, cefepime, indomethacin, warfarin.**

- Parenteral solutions are stable for 48 h at room temperature when added to commonly used IV solutions for dilution. Follow manufacturer's directions. - Store all forms of cimetidine at 15°–30° C (59°–86° F) protected from light unless otherwise directed by manufacturer.

ADVERSE EFFECTS (≥1%) **Body as a Whole:** Fever. **CV (rare):** Cardiac arrhythmias and cardiac arrest after rapid IV bolus dose. **GI:** Mild transient diarrhea; severe diarrhea, constipation, abdominal discomfort. **Hematologic:** Increased prothrombin time; neutropenia (rare), thrombocytopenia (rare), aplastic anemia. **Metabolic:** Slight increase in serum uric acid, BUN, creatinine; transient pain at IM site; hypospermia. **Musculoskeletal:** Exacerbation of joint symptoms in patients with preexisting arthritis. **CNS:** Drowsiness, dizziness, lightheadedness, depression, headache, reversible confusional states, paranoid psychosis. **Skin:** Rash, Stevens-Johnson syndrome, reversible alopecia. **Urogenital:** Gynecomastia and breast soreness, galactorrhea, reversible impotence.

DIAGNOSTIC TEST INTERFERENCE Cimetidine may cause false-positive ***Hemoccult test for gastric bleeding*** if test is performed within 15 min of oral cimetidine administration.

INTERACTIONS Drug: Cimetidine decreases the hepatic metabolism of **warfarin, phenobarbital, phenytoin, diazepam, propranolol, lidocaine, theophylline,** thus increasing their activity and toxicity; ANTACIDS may decrease absorption of cimetidine.

PHARMACOKINETICS Absorption: 70% of oral dose absorbed from GI tract. **Peak:** 1–1.5 h. **Distribution:** Widely distributed; crosses blood–brain barrier and placenta. **Metabolism:** Metabolized in liver. **Elimination:** Most of drug excreted in urine in 24 h; excreted in breast milk. **Half-Life:** 2 h.

NURSING IMPLICATIONS

Assessment & Drug Effects

- Ulcer healing may occur within the first 2 wk of therapy but generally requires at least 4 wk in most patients. Short-term (i.e., 8 wk) therapy of active duodenal ulcer does not prevent ulcer recurrence when drug is discontinued.
- Monitor pulse of patient during first few days of drug regimen. Bradycardia after PO as well as IV administration should be reported. Pulse usually returns to normal within 24 h after drug discontinuation.
- Monitor I&O ratio and pattern: Particularly in the older adult, se-

verely ill, and in patients with impaired renal function.

- Report loss of bowel sounds, absence of bowel movement or flatus, vomiting, crampy pain, abdominal distention. Adynamic ileus has been reported in patients receiving cimetidine to prevent and treat stress ulcers.
- Lab tests: Periodic evaluations of blood count and renal and hepatic function are advised during therapy.
- Be alert to onset of confusional states, particularly in the older adult or severely ill patient. Symptoms occur within 2–3 d after first dose. Report immediately: drug should be withdrawn. Symptoms usually resolve within 3–4 d after therapy is discontinued.
- Check BP and report an elevation to the physician, if patient complains of severe headache.
- Cimetidine impairs absorption of protein-bound vitamin B_{12}; therefore patient who takes cimetidine in divided doses to continuously suppress acid gastric secretion is at risk for vitamin B_{12} deficiency (no risk for patient who takes drug at bedtime to suppress nocturnal acid production).

Patient & Family Education

- Cimetidine must be taken exactly as prescribed. Sudden discontinuation of therapy reportedly has caused perforation of chronic peptic ulcer.
- Seek advice about self-medication with any OTC drug.
- Report breast tenderness or enlargement. Mild bilateral gynecomastia and breast soreness may occur after ≥1 mo of therapy. It may disappear spontaneously or remain throughout therapy.
- Report recurrence of gastric pain or bleeding (black, tarry stools or "coffee ground" vomitus) immediately, and notify physician if diarrhea continues more than 1 d.
- Avoid driving and other potentially hazardous activities until reaction to drug is known.
- Duodenal or gastric ulcer is a chronic, recurrent condition that requires long-term maintenance drug therapy.
- Maintenance therapy at reduced dosage after healing of active duodenal ulcer appears to limit recurrence, particularly if patient undertakes other antiulcer therapeutic measures: no smoking, life-style that promotes reduced stress.
- Do not breast feed while taking this drug.

CINACALCET HYDROCHLORIDE

(sin-a′ca-let)

Sensipar

Classifications: HORMONES & SYNTHETIC SUBSTITUTES; PARATHYROID AGENT; CALCIUM RECEPTOR AGONIST

Pregnancy Category: C

AVAILABILITY 30 mg, 60 mg, 90 mg tablets

ACTIONS Directly lowers parathyroid hormone (PTH) levels by increasing the sensitivity of calcium-sensing receptors on the parathyroid gland to extracellular calcium. The reduction in PTH causes decreased calcium and phosphate adsorption from bone, and thus decreased serum calcium and phosphate levels. The drug is a calcium receptor agonist, also known as a calcimimetic agent.

THERAPEUTIC EFFECTS Lowers PTH production; this also decreases rate of bone turnover and bone fibrosis in chronic renal failure discase (CRFD).

USES Treatment of secondary hyperparathyroidism in patients with chronic kidney disease on dialysis; hypercalcemia in patients with parathyroid cancer.

CONTRAINDICATIONS Hypersensitivity to cinacalcet; pregnancy (category C), lactation, children <18 y.

CAUTIOUS USE Moderate and severe hepatic impairment, hypocalcemia, history of seizures.

ROUTE & DOSAGE

Secondary Hyperparathyroidism

Adult: **PO** Start with 30 mg once daily; may increase q2–4wk until target iPTH of 150–300 pg/mL (max: 300 mg/d)

Parathyroid Cancer

Adult: **PO** 30 mg twice daily; titrate q2–4wk as 60 mg b.i.d., 90 mg b.i.d., then 90 mg 3–4 times daily as needed to normalize calcium concentrations

ADMINISTRATION

Oral

- Give with food or shortly after a meal.
- Tablets should be swallowed whole and not divided, crushed, or chewed.
- Store at 15°–30° C (59°–86° F).

ADVERSE EFFECTS (≥1%) **Body as a Whole:** Dizziness, asthenia, noncardiac chest pain, dialysis access infection. **CV:** Hypertension. **GI:** *Nausea, vomiting, diarrhea,* anorexia. **Metabolic:** Hypocalcemia. **Musculoskeletal:** *Myalgia,* adynamic bone disease (renal osteodystrophy).

INTERACTIONS Drug: May increase **amoxapine, atomoxetine, carvedilol, metoprolol, propranolol, timolol, encainide, flecainide, mexiletine, propafenone, clozapine, codeine, cyclobenzaprine, fenfluramine, dexfenfluramine, dextromethorphan, donepezil, fluoxetine, haloperidol, hydrocodone, maprotiline, meperidine, methadone, methamphetamine, morphine, oxycodone, paroxetine, perphenazine, risperidone, thioridazine** (use may be contraindicated with cinacalcet), **tramadol, trazodone**, tricyclic antidepressants, **venlafaxine, zolpidem** levels; cinacalcet levels may be increased by strong CYP3A4 inhibitors such as **fluconazole, itraconazole, ketoconazole, miconazole, voriconazole, clarithromycin, erythromycin, dalfopristin; quinupristin, troleandomycin, verapamil, diltiazem, amiodarone, aprepitant, fluvoxamine, nefazodone, zafirlukast, zileuton. Food: Grapefruit juice** may increase cinacalcet levels.

PHARMACOKINETICS Peak: 2–6 h. **Distribution:** 93–97% protein bound. **Metabolism:** Metabolized in liver by CYP3A4. **Elimination:** 80% excreted by kidneys, 15% excreted in feces. **Half-Life:** 30–40 h.

NURSING IMPLICATIONS

Assessment & Drug Effects

- Monitor for S&S of hypocalcemia (e.g., paresthesias, myalgias, cramping, tetany, convulsions).
- Withhold drug and notify physician for serum calcium <7.5 mg/dL or symptoms of hypocalcemia. Drug should not be resumed until serum calcium levels reach 8.0 mg/dL, and/or symptoms of hypocalcemia resolve.

C

- Lab tests: Serum calcium and phosphorus within 1 wk after and iPTH 1–4 wk after initiation of drug or dose adjustment; thereafter, monthly serum calcium and phosphorus (more often with a history of a seizure disorder), and iPTH every 1–3 mo.
- Closely monitor iPTH and serum calcium with concurrent administration of a strong CYP3A4 (e.g., ketoconazole, erythromycin, itraconazole).

Patient & Family Education

- Report promptly any of the following: seizure or convulsion; muscle spasms or cramping of the abdomen, back, legs, face; burning, numbness, pricking, tickling, or tingling of the face, lips, tongue, hands, or feet; changes in mental status.
- Do not breast feed while taking this drug without consulting physician.

CINOXACIN

(sin-ox′a-sin)
Cinobac
Classifications: URINARY TRACT ANTIINFECTIVE; QUINOLONE ANTIBIOTIC
Prototype: Trimethoprim
Pregnancy Category: B

AVAILABILITY 250 mg, 500 mg capsules

ACTIONS Synthetic bactericidal agent with properties similar to those of nalidixic acid but with fewer adverse effects. Acts intracellularly to inhibit bacterial DNA replication and protein synthesis.

THERAPEUTIC EFFECTS Effective against a wide variety of gram-negative pathogens, particularly most strains of *Escherichia coli, Klebsiella* and *Enterobacter* species, *Proteus mirabilis,* and *Proteus vulgaris.* Not active against *Staphylococci, Enterococci,* or *Pseudomonas.*

USE Initial and recurrent UTIs in adults caused by susceptible microorganisms.

CONTRAINDICATIONS Hypersensitivity to cinoxacin or to other quinolones; anuria; dehydration; pregnancy (category B), lactation. Safe use in prepubertal children or children <18 y not established.

CAUTIOUS USE Impaired renal or hepatic function; known CNS disorders, i.e. seizures, tremors, confusion; severe cerebral atherosclerosis.

ROUTE & DOSAGE

UTI
Adult: **PO** 1 g/d in 2–4 divided doses

ADMINISTRATION

Oral

- Give the drug at evenly spaced intervals throughout 24 h so that urinary drug concentration is maintained and therapeutic effectiveness enhanced.

ADVERSE EFFECTS (≥1%) **Body as a Whole:** Edema, swelling of extremities, arthropathy. **CNS:** *Headache, dizziness,* insomnia, tingling sensations, agitation, anxiety. **Skin:** Urticaria, pruritus, rash. **Special Senses:** Tinnitus, photophobia, blurred vision. **GI:** *Nausea,* vomiting, anorexia, constipation, rectal itching, metallic taste, sore gums, abdominal cramps, diarrhea.

DIAGNOSTIC TEST INTERFERENCE May cause false positive on ***opiate screening tests.***

INTERACTIONS Drug: Probenecid decreases renal elimination of cinoxacin.

PHARMACOKINETICS Absorption: Readily absorbed from GI tract. **Peak:** 2–3 h. **Duration:** 12 h. **Distribution:** Concentrates in renal and prostatic tissues; crosses placenta; distribution into breast milk unknown. **Elimination:** 97% excreted in urine within 24 h. **Half-Life:** 1.5 h.

NURSING IMPLICATIONS

Assessment & Drug Effects

- Lab tests: Culture and sensitivity tests should be performed before start of therapy and during therapy if response is not satisfactory.
- Monitor ambulation since dizziness is a possible side effect, especially with the older adult and debilitated, may be warranted.

Patient & Family Education

- Take drug for the full course of therapy as prescribed.
- Report to physician if symptoms do not improve within a few days or if they become worse.
- Avoid driving and other potentially hazardous tasks until reaction to drug is known.
- Report to physician if tinnitus develops.
- Do not breast feed while taking this drug.

CIPROFLOXACIN HYDROCHLORIDE (Pr)

(ci-pro-flox'a-cin)

Cipro, Cipro IV, Cipro XR

CIPROFLOXACIN OPHTHALMIC

Ciloxan

Classifications: ANTIINFECTIVE; QUINOLONE ANTIBIOTIC

Pregnancy Category: C

AVAILABILITY 100 mg, 250 mg, 500 mg, 750 mg tablets; 500 mg extended-release tablets; 50 mg/mL, 100 mg/mL suspension; 200 mg, 400 mg injection; 3.5 mg/mL ophth solution

ACTIONS Synthetic quinolone that is a broad spectrum bactericidal agent. Inhibits DNA-gyrase, an enzyme necessary for bacterial DNA replication and some aspects of transcription, repair, recombination, and transposition.

THERAPEUTIC EFFECTS Effective against many gram-positive and gram-negative organisms including *Citrobacter diversus, Enterobacter cloacae, Enterobacter aerogenes, Escherichia coli, Haemophilus influenzae, Klebsiella pneumoniae, Neisseria gonorrhoeae, Proteus mirabalis, Proteus vulgaris, Pseudomonas aeruginosa, Serratia marcescens, Staphylococcus aureus, Streptococcus pyogenes, Shigella,* and *Salmonella*. Less active against gram-positive than gram-negative bacteria, although active against many gram-positive aerobic bacteria, including penicillinase-producing, non-penicillinase-producing, and methicillin-resistant *Staphylococci.* However, many strains of *Streptococci* are relatively resistant to the drug. Inactive against most anaerobic bacteria. Resistant to some strains of methicillin-resistant *Staphylococcus aureus* (MRSA).

USES UTIs, lower respiratory tract infections, skin and skin structure infections, bone and joint infections, GI infection or infectious diarrhea, chronic bacterial prostatitis, nosocomial pneumonia, acute sinusitis. Post-exposure prophylaxis for anthrax. **Ophthalmic:** Corneal ulcers, bacterial

C

conjunctivitis caused by *Staphylococci, Streptococci,* and *P. aeruginosa*.

CONTRAINDICATIONS Known hypersensitivity to ciprofloxacin or other quinolones, syphilis, viral infection; tendon inflammation or tendon pain; pregnant women (category C), lactation.

CAUTIOUS USE Known or suspected CNS disorders (i.e., severe cerebral arteriosclerosis or seizure disorders); myasthenia gravis; myocardial ischemia, atrial fibrillation, QT elongation, CHF; GI disease, colitis; CVA; uncorrected hypokalemia; patients receiving theophylline derivatives or caffeine, severe renal impairment and crystalluria during ciprofloxacin therapy, and patients on coumarin therapy; children.

ROUTE & DOSAGE

Uncomplicated UTI

Adult: **PO** 250 mg q12h or 500 mg XR q.d. × 3 d. **IV** 200 mg q12h, infused over 60 min

Complicated UTI

Adult: **PO** 1000 mg XR q.d. × 7–14 d. **IV** 400 mg q12h, infused over 60 min

Acute Sinusitis

Adult: **PO** 500 mg b.i.d. × 10 d

Moderate to Severe Systemic Infection

Adult: **PO** 500–750 mg q12h **IV** 200–400 mg q12h, infused over 60 min

Renal Impairment

Cl_{cr} 30–50 mL/min: **PO** 250–500 mg q12h, **IV** no change in dose; <30 mL/min: **PO** 250–500 mg q18h, **IV** 200–400 mg q18–24h

Bacterial Conjunctivitis

Adult: **Ophthalmic** 1–2 drops in conjunctival sac q2h while awake for 2 d, then 1–2 drops q4h while awake for the next 5 d **Ointment** 1/2-inch ribbon into conjunctival sac t.i.d. times 2 d, then b.i.d. times 5 d

Corneal Ulcers

Adult: **Ophthalmic** 2 drops q15min for 6 h, 2 drops q30min for the next 18 h, then 2 drops q1h for 24 h, then 2 drops q4h for 14 d

ADMINISTRATION

- For patients with renal impairment, oral and IV doses are lowered according to creatinine clearance.

Oral

- Do not give an antacid within 4 h of the oral ciprofloxacin dose.

Intravenous

PREPARE: **Intermittent:** Dilute in NS or D5W to a final concentration of 0.5–2 mg/mL. Typical dilutions are 200 mg in 100–250 mL and 400 mg in 250–500 mL.
ADMINISTER: **Intermittent:** Give slowly over 60 min. Avoid rapid infusion and use of a small vein.
INCOMPATIBILITIES **Solution/additive: Aminophylline, clindamycin, heparin. Y-site: Aminophylline, ampicillin, ampicillin/sulbactam, cefepime, dexamethasone, furosemide, heparin, hydrocortisone, phenytoin, propofol, sodium bicarbonate, theophylline, warfarin.**

- Discontinue other IV infusion while infusing ciprofloxacin or infuse through another site.
- Reconstituted IV solution is stable for 14 d refrigerated.

ADVERSE EFFECTS (≥1%) **GI:** Nausea, vomiting, diarrhea, cramps, gas, pseudomembranous colitis. **Metabolic:** Transient increases in liver transaminases, alkaline phosphatase, lactic dehydrogenase, and eosinophilia count. **Musculoskeletal:** Tendon rupture. **CNS:** Headache, vertigo, malaise, peripheral neuropathy, seizures (especially with rapid IV infusion). **Skin:** Rash, phlebitis, pain, burning, pruritus, and erythema at infusion site. **Special Senses:** *Local burning and discomfort, crystalline precipitate on superficial portion of cornea,* lid margin crusting, scales, foreign body sensation, itching, and conjunctival hyperemia.

DIAGNOSTIC TEST INTERFERENCE Ciprofloxacin does not interfere with ***urinary glucose*** determinations using ***cupric sulfate solution*** or with ***glucose oxidase tests;*** may cause false positive on ***opiate screening tests.***

INTERACTIONS Drug: May increase **theophylline** levels 15–30%; ANTACIDS, **sulcralfate, iron** decrease absorption of ciprofloxacin; may increase PT for patients on **warfarin.**

PHARMACOKINETICS Absorption: 60–80% absorbed from GI tract. **Ophthalmic:** Minimal absorption through cornea or conjuctiva. **Onset:** Topical 0.5–2 h. **Duration:** Topical 12 h. **Peak:** 1–2 h. **Distribution:** Widely distributed including prostate, lung, and bone; crosses placenta; distributed into breast milk. **Elimination:** Excreted primarily in urine with some biliary excretion. **Half-Life:** 3.5–4 h.

NURSING IMPLICATIONS

Assessment & Drug Effects

- Report tendon inflammation or pain. Cipro needs to be discontinued.
- Lab tests: Culture and sensitivity tests should be done prior to initial dose. Treatment may be implemented pending results.
- Monitor urine pH; it should be less than 6.8, especially in the older adult and patients receiving high dosages of ciprofloxacin, to reduce the risk of crystalluria.
- Monitor I&O ratio and patterns: Patients should be well hydrated; assess for S&S of crystalluria.
- Monitor plasma theophylline concentrations, since drug may interfere with half-life.
- Administration with theophylline derivatives or caffeine can cause CNS stimulation.
- Assess for S&S of GI irritation (e.g., nausea, diarrhea, vomiting, abdominal discomfort) in clients receiving high dosages and in older adults.
- Monitor PT and INR in patients receiving coumarin therapy.
- Assess for S&S of superinfections (see Appendix F).

Patient & Family Education

- Immediately report tendon inflammation or pain. Cipro should be discontinued.
- Fluid intake of 2–3 L/d is advised, if not contraindicated.
- Report sudden, unexplained joint pain.
- Restrict caffeine due to the following effects (e.g., nervousness, insomnia, anxiety, tachycardia).
- Report possible toxicity. If taking theophylline derivatives, there is potential for adverse effects.
- Report nausea, diarrhea, vomiting, and abdominal pain or discomfort.

C

- Use caution with hazardous activities until reaction to drug is known. Drug may cause lightheadedness.
- Do not breast feed while taking this drug.

CISATRACURIUM BESYLATE

(cis-a-tra-kyoo-ri'um)

Nimbex

Classifications: AUTONOMIC NERVOUS SYSTEM AGENT; SKELETAL MUSCLE RELAXANT, NONDEPOLARIZING

Prototype: Tubocurarine chloride

Pregnancy Category: B

AVAILABILITY 2 mg/mL, 10 mg/mL injection

ACTIONS Cisatracurium is a neuromuscular blocking agent with intermediate onset and duration of action compared with similar agents. It binds competitively to cholinergic receptors on motor endplate of neurons, antagonizing the action of acetylcholine.

THERAPEUTIC EFFECTS Antagonism of acetylcholine blocks neuromuscular transmission of nerve impulses. This action can be reversed or antagonized by acetylcholinesterase inhibitors (e.g., neostigmine).

USES Adjunct to general anesthesia to facilitate tracheal intubation and provide skeletal muscle relaxation during surgery or mechanical ventilation.

CONTRAINDICATIONS Hypersensitivity to cisatracurium or other related agents; rapid-sequence endotracheal intubation. Not studied in children <2 y.

CAUTIOUS USE History of hemiparesis, electrolyte imbalances, burn patients, neuromuscular diseases (e.g., myasthenia gravis), older adults, renal function impairment, pregnancy (category B), lactation.

ROUTE & DOSAGE

Intubation

Adult: **IV** 0.15 or 0.20 mg/kg
Child ≥2 y: **IV** 0.1 mg/kg over 5–10 sec

Maintenance

Adult: **IV** 0.03 mg/kg q20min prn *or* 1–2 mcg/kg/min
Child ≥2 y: **IV** 1–2 mcg/kg/min

Mechanical Ventilation in ICU

Adult: **IV** 3 mcg/kg/min (can range from 0.5 to 10.2 mcg/kg/min)

ADMINISTRATION

- Administer carefully adjusted, individualized doses using a peripheral nerve stimulator to evaluate neuromuscular function.
- Give only by or under supervision of expert clinician familiar with the drug's actions and potential complications.
- Have immediately available personnel and facilities for resuscitation and life support and an antagonist of cisatracurium.
- Refer to manufacturer's guidelines for preparation and administration. Note that 10-mL multiple-dose vials contain benzyl alcohol and should not be used with neonates.

Intravenous

PREPARE: **Direct:** Give undiluted. **IV Infusion:** Dilute 10 mg in 95 mL or 40 mg in 80 mL of compatible IV fluid to prepare 0.1 mg/mL or 0.4 mg/mL, respectively, IV solution. Compatible IV fluids include D5W, NS, D5/NS, D5/RL. **ICU IV Infusion:** Dilute the contents of the 200 mg vial (i.e., 10 mg/mL) in 1000 mL or 500 mL of compatible IV fluid to prepare 0.2 mg/mL or 0.4 g/mL, respectively, IV solutions.

ADMINISTER: **Direct:** Give a single dose over 5–10 sec. **IV Infusion:** Adjust the rate based on patient's weight.

INCOMPATIBILITIES **Solution/additive:** **Ketorolac, propofol, sodium bicarbonate.** **Y-site:** **Amphotericin B, amphotericin B cholesteryl complex, cefoperazone, cefuroxime, diazepam, sodium bicarbonate.**

- Refrigerate vials at 2°–8° C (36°–46° F). Protect from light. Diluted solutions may be stored refrigerated or at room temperature for 24 h.

ADVERSE EFFECTS (≥1%) **CV:** Bradycardia, hypotension, flushing. **Respiratory:** Bronchospasm. **Skin:** Rash.

PHARMACOKINETICS **Onset:** Varies with dose from 1.5 to 3.3 min (higher the dose, faster the onset). **Peak:** Varies with dose from 1.5 to 3.3 min (higher the dose, faster to peak). **Duration:** Varies with dose from 46 to 121 min (higher dose, longer recovery time). **Metabolism:** Undergoes Hoffman elimination (pH- and temperature-dependent degradation) and hydrolysis by plasma esterases. **Elimination:** Excreted in urine. **Half-Life:** 22 min.

NURSING IMPLICATIONS

Assessment & Drug Effects

- Perform neuromuscular monitoring only on nonparetic limbs.
- Time-to-maximum neuromuscular block is ≈1 min slower in the older adult.
- Monitor for bradycardia, hypotension, and bronchospasms; monitor ICU patients for spontaneous seizures.
- Antagonists should not be given when complete neuromuscular block is present.

CISPLATIN (cis-DDP, cis-PLATINUM II)

(sis′pla-tin)

Abiplatin ♦, Platinol

Classifications: ANTINEOPLASTIC; ALKYLATING AGENT

Prototype: Cyclophosphamide

Pregnancy Category: D

AVAILABILITY 1 mg/mL injection

ACTIONS A heavy metal complex with platinum as central atom surrounded by 2 chloride atoms and 2 ammonia molecules in the cis chemical position. Biochemical properties similar to those of bifunctional alkylating agents. Produces interstrand and intrastrand cross linkage in DNA of rapidly dividing cells, thus preventing DNA, RNA, and protein synthesis.

THERAPEUTIC EFFECTS Cell cycle-nonspecific, i.e., effective throughout the entire cell life cycle. Carcinogenicity has not been fully studied, but other compounds with similar action mechanisms and mutogenicity have been studied.

USES Established combination therapy (cisplatin, vinblastine, bleomycin) in patient with metastatic testicular tumors and with doxorubicin for metastatic ovarian tumors following appropriate surgical or radiation therapy.

UNLABELED USES Carcinoma of endometrium, bladder, head, and neck.

CONTRAINDICATIONS History of hypersensitivity to cisplatin or

C

other platinum-containing compounds; impaired renal function; myelosuppression; impaired hearing; history of gout and urate renal stones; hypomagnesia; concurrent administration with loop diuretics; Raynard syndrome; pregnancy (category D), lactation. Safe use in children not established.

CAUTIOUS USE Previous cytotoxic drug or radiation therapy with other ototoxic and nephrotoxic drugs; hyperuricemia. Electrolyte imbalances, hepatic impairment; history of circulatory disorders.

ROUTE & DOSAGE

Testicular Neoplasms

Adult: **IV** 20 mg/m²/d for 5 d q3–4wk for 3 courses

Ovarian Neoplasms

Adult: **IV** *Combination therapy:* 50 mg/m² once q3–4wk; *Single agent:* 100 mg/m² once q3–4wk

ADMINISTRATION

- Administered only under supervision of a qualified physician experienced in the use of antineoplastics.
- Usually a parenteral antiemetic agent is administered 1/2 h before cisplatin therapy is instituted and given on a scheduled basis throughout day and night as long as necessary.
- Before the initial dose is given, hydration is started with 1–2 L IV infusion fluid to reduce risk of nephrotoxicity and ototoxicity.

Intravenous

PREPARE: **IV Infusion:** Use disposable gloves when preparing cisplatin solutions. If drug accidentally contacts skin or mucosa, wash immediately and thoroughly with soap and water. Do not use any equipment containing aluminum. Withdraw required dose and dilute in 2 L D5W 5% dextrose in 1/2 or 1/3 normal saline containing 37.5 g mannitol.

ADMINISTER: **IV Infusion:** Give 2 L over 6–8 h

INCOMPATIBILITIES **Solution/additive: 5% dextrose, fluorouracil, mesna, metoclopramide, sodium bicarbonate, thiotepa. Y-site: Amifostine, amphotericin B, cholesteryl, cefepime, piperacillin/tazobactam, thiotepa, TPN.**

- Hydration and forced diuresis are continued for at least 24 h after drug administration to ensure adequate urinary output.
- Store at 15°–30° C (59°–86° F). Do not refrigerate. Protect from light. Once vial is opened, solution is stable for 28 d protected from light or 7 d in fluorescent light.

ADVERSE EFFECTS (≥1%) **Body as a Whole:** <u>Anaphylactic-like reactions.</u> **CV:** Cardiac abnormalities. **GI:** *Marked nausea, vomiting,* anorexia, stomatitis, xerostomia, diarrhea, constipation. **Hematologic:** Myelosuppression (25–30% patients): leukopenia, thrombocytopenia; hemolytic anemia, hemolysis. **Metabolic:** Hypocalcemia, *hypomagnesemia,* hyperuricemia, elevated AST, SIADH. **CNS:** Seizures, headache; peripheral neuropathies (may be irreversible): paresthesia, unsteady gait, clumsiness of hands and feet, exacerbation of neuropathy with exercise, loss of taste. **Special Senses:** Ototoxicity (may be irreversible): tinnitus, hearing loss, deafness, vertigo, blurred vision, changes in ability to see colors (optic neuritis, papilledema). **Urogenital:** Nephrotoxicity.

INTERACTIONS Drug: AMINOGLYCOSIDES, **amphotericin B, vancomycin,** other **nephrotoxic drugs** increase nephrotoxicity and acute renal failure—try to separate by at least 1–2 wk; AMINOGLYCOSIDES, **furosemide** increase risk of ototoxicity.

PHARMACOKINETICS Peak: Immediately after end of infusion. **Distribution:** Widely distributed in body fluids and tissues; concentrated in kidneys, liver, and prostate; accumulated in tissues. **Metabolism:** Not completely known. **Elimination:** 15–50% of dose excreted in urine within 24–48 h. **Half-Life:** 73–290 h.

NURSING IMPLICATIONS

Assessment & Drug Effects

- Obtain baseline ECG and cardiac monitoring during induction therapy because of possible myocarditis or focal irritability.
- Lab tests: The following tests should be done *before* initiating every course of therapy and repeated each week during treatment period: serum uric acid, serum creatinine, BUN, urinary creatinine clearance. CBC and platelet counts are done weekly for 2 wk after each course of treatment. Monitor periodically serum electrolytes and liver function tests.
- A repeat course of therapy should not be given until (1) serum creatinine is below 1.5 mg/dL; (2) BUN is below 25 mg/dL; (3) platelets ≥100,000/mm^3; (4) WBC ≥4000/mm^3; (5) audiometric test is within normal limits.
- Monitor urine output and specific gravity for 4 consecutive hours before treatment and for 24 h after therapy. Report if output is less than 100 mL/h or if specific gravity is more than 1.030. A urine output of less than 75 mL/h necessitates medical intervention to avert a renal emergency.
- Audiometric testing should be performed before the first dose and before each subsequent dose. Ototoxicity (reported in 31% of patients) may occur after a single dose of 50 mg/m^2. Children who receive repeated doses are especially susceptible.
- Monitor for anaphylactoid reactions (particularly in patient previously exposed to cisplatin), which may occur within minutes of drug administration.
- Monitor closely for dose-related adverse reactions. Drug action is cumulative; therefore severity of most adverse effects increases with repeated doses.
- Nephrotoxicity (reported in 28–36% of patients receiving a single dose of 50 mg/m^2) usually occurs within 2 wk after drug administration and becomes more severe and prolonged with repeated courses of cisplatin.
- Suspect ototoxicity if patient manifests tinnitus or difficulty hearing in the high frequency range.
- Intractable nausea and vomiting severe enough to warrant discontinuation of drug usually begin 1–4 h after treatment and may last 24 h or persist for up to 1 wk after treatment is ended.
- Monitor and report abnormal electrolyte levels: sodium >145 or <135 mEq/L, and potassium >5 or <3.5 mEq/L.
- Monitor results of blood studies. The nadirs in platelet and leukocyte counts occur between day

18 and 23 (range: 7.5–45) with most patients recovering in 13–62 d. A decrease in Hgb (more than 2 g/dL) occurs at approximately the same time and with the same frequency.

- Check BP, mental status, pupils, and fundi every hour during therapy. Hydration and mannitol may increase the danger of elevated intracranial pressure (ICP).
- Neurologic examinations at regular intervals should include tests of muscle strength, Romberg, vibratory and position sense, tests of sensation.
- Monitor and report abnormal bowel elimination pattern. Constipation and the possibility of fecal impaction may be caused by neurotoxicity; diarrhea is a possible response to GI irritation.
- Inspect oral membranes for xerostomia (white patches and ulcerations) and tongue for signs of fungal overgrowth (black, furry appearance).
- Institute infection precautions promptly if a temperature increase of 0.6° F over the previous reading is noted.
- Weigh the patient under standard conditions every day. A gradual ascending weight profile occurring over a period of several days should be reported.

Patient & Family Education

- Continue maintenance of adequate hydration (at least 3000 mL/24 h oral fluid if physician agrees) and report promptly: reduced urinary output, flank pain, anorexia, nausea, vomiting, dry mucosae, itching skin, urine odor on breath, fluid retention, and weight gain.
- Avoid rapid changes in position to minimize risk of dizziness or falling.
- Tingling, numbness, and tremors of extremities, loss of position sense and taste, and constipation are early signs of neurotoxicity. Report their occurrence promptly to prevent irreversibility. Pain with heel walking and difficulty in getting out of bed or chair are late indicators of nerve damage.
- Report tinnitus or any hearing impairment.
- Report promptly evidence of unexplained bleeding and easy bruising.
- Report unusual fatigue, fever, sore mouth and throat, abnormal body discharges.
- Do not breast feed while taking this drug.

CITALOPRAM HYDROBROMIDE

(cit-a-lo′pram)

Celexa

Classifications: CENTRAL NERVOUS SYSTEM (CNS) AGENT; PSYCHOTHERAPEUTIC AGENT; SELECTIVE SEROTONIN-REUPTAKE INHIBITOR (SSRI)

Prototype: Fluoxetine

Pregnancy Category: C

AVAILABILITY 20 mg, 40 mg tablets; 10 mg/5 mL oral solution

ACTIONS Selective serotonin reuptake inhibitor (SSRI) in the CNS. Antidepressant effect is presumed to be linked to its inhibition of CNS presynaptic neuronal uptake of serotonin which results in antidepressant activity. Does not produce any sympathomimetic response or anticholinergic activity.

THERAPEUTIC EFFECTS Does not inhibit MAOIs. Selective serotonin reuptake inhibition mechanism results in the antidepressant activity of citalopram.

USE Depression.

CONTRAINDICATIONS Hypersensitivity to citalopram; concurrent use of MAOIs or use within 14 d of discontinuing MAOIs; pregnancy (category C); volume depleted; lactation; children <18 y.

CAUTIOUS USE Hypersensitivity to other SSRIs; renal or hepatic insufficiency; older adults; concurrent use of diuretics, dehydration, renal impairment or renal failure, cardiovascular disease (e.g., dysrhythmias, conduction defects, myocardial ischemia); history of seizure disorders or suicidal tendencies; ECT treatments.

ROUTE & DOSAGE

Depression

Adult: **PO** Start at 20 mg q.d., may increase to 40 mg q.d. if needed
Geriatric: **PO** 20 mg q.d.

ADMINISTRATION

Oral

- Do not begin this drug within 14 d of stopping an MAOI.
- Reduced doses are advised for the older adult and those with hepatic or renal impairment.
- Dose increments should be separated by at least 1 wk.
- Store at 15°–30° C (59°–86° F) in tightly closed container and protect from light.

ADVERSE EFFECTS (≥1%) **Body as a Whole:** Asthenia, fatigue, fever, arthralgia, myalgia. **CV:** Tachycardia, postural hypotension, hypotension. **GI:** *Nausea,* vomiting, diarrhea, dyspepsia, abdominal pain, *dry mouth,* anorexia, flatulence. **CNS :** Dizziness, *insomnia, somnolence,* agitation, tremor, anxiety, paresthesia, migraine. **Respiratory:** URI, rhinitis, sinusitis. **Skin:** Increased sweating. **Urogenital:** Dysmenorrhea, decreased libido, ejaculation disorder, impotence.

INTERACTIONS Drug: Combination with MAOIS could result in hypertensive crisis, hyperthermia, rigidity, myoclonus, autonomic instability; **cimetidine** may increase citalopram levels; **linezolid** may cause serotonin syndrome. **Herbal: St. John's wort** may cause serotonin syndrome.

PHARMACOKINETICS Absorption: Rapidly absorbed from GI tract; approximately 80% reaches systemic circulation. **Peak:** Steady-state serum concentrations in 1 wk; peak blood levels at 4 h. **Distribution:** 80% protein bound; crosses placenta; distributed into breast milk. **Metabolism:** Metabolized in liver by cytochrome P450 3A4 and cytochrome P450 2C9 enzymes. **Elimination:** 20% excreted in urine, 80% in bile. **Half-Life:** 35 h.

NURSING IMPLICATIONS

Assessment & Drug Effects

- Watch closely for worsening of depression or emergence of suicidal ideations.
- Monitor for therapeutic effectiveness: Indicated by elevation of mood; 1–4 wk may be needed before improvement is noted.
- Lab tests: Monitor periodically hepatic functions, CBC, serum sodium, and lithium levels when the two drugs are given concurrently.
- Monitor periodically HR and BP, and carefully monitor complete cardiac status in person with known or suspected cardiac disease.
- Monitor closely older adult patients for adverse effects especially with doses >20 mg/d.

C

Patient & Family Education

- Do not engage in hazardous activities until reaction to this drug is known.
- Avoid using alcohol while taking citalopram.
- Inform physician of commonly used OTC drugs as there is potential for drug interactions.
- Report distressing adverse effects including any changes in sexual functioning or response.
- Periodic ophthalmology exams are advised with long-term treatment.
- Do not breast feed while taking this drug.

CLADRIBINE

(cla′dri-been)
Leustatin
Classification: ANTINEOPLASTIC
Pregnancy Category: D

AVAILABILITY 1 mg/mL injection

ACTIONS Cladribine is a synthetic antineoplastic agent with selective toxicity toward certain normal and malignant lymphocytes and monocytes. It accumulates intracellularly, preventing repair of single-stranded DNA breaks and ultimately interfering with cellular metabolism and DNA synthesis.
THERAPEUTIC EFFECTS Cladribine is cytotoxic to both actively dividing and quiescent lymphocytes and monocytes, inhibiting both DNA synthesis and repair.

USE Treatment of hairy cell leukemia.
UNLABELED USES Advanced cutaneous T-cell lymphomas, chronic lymphocytic leukemia, non-Hodgkin's lymphomas, acute myeloid leukemia, autoimmune hemolytic anemia, mycosis fungoides.

CONTRAINDICATIONS Hypersensitivity to cladribine; pregnancy (category D).
CAUTIOUS USE Hepatic or renal impairment. Safety and efficacy in children not established.

ROUTE & DOSAGE

Hairy Cell Leukemia
Adult: **IV** 0.09 mg/kg/d by 7 d continuous infusion

Chronic Lymphocytic Leukemia
Adult: **IV** 0.1 mg/kg/d by 7 d continuous infusion *or* 0.028–0.14 mg/kg/d as 2 h infusion for 5 consecutive d

ADMINISTRATION

- Solutions for cladribine should not be mixed with any other IV drugs or additives, nor administered through an IV line used for other drugs or solutions.
- Use disposable gloves and protective clothing when handling the drug.
- Wash immediately if skin contact occurs.

Intravenous

PREPARE: **IV Infusion (single daily dose):** IV infusion (7-day dose): The calculated dose of cladribine is injected into an infusion reservoir using a 0.22 micron filter. An amount of bacteriostatic NS is added through a 0.22 micron filter to bring the total to 100 mL. (Note: reservoir usually prepared by the pharmacist.)
ADMINISTER: **IV Infusion (single daily dose):** Distribute evenly over ordered time (i.e., 2 h or 24 h). **IV infusion (7-day dose):** Give through a central line and control by a pump device (e.g., Deltec pump) to deliver 100 mL evenly over 7 d.

INCOMPATIBILITIES **Solution/additive:** Do not mix with any other diluents or drugs.

▪ Diluted solutions of cladribine may be stored refrigerated for up to 8 h prior to administration. ▪ Store unopened vials in refrigerator (2°–8° C/36°–46° F), and protect from light.

ADVERSE EFFECTS (≥1%) **CNS:** Headache, dizziness. **GI:** Nausea, diarrhea. **Hematologic:** *Myelosuppression (neutropenia), anemia,* thrombocytopenia. **Metabolic:** *Fever.* **CNS:** Headache, dizziness. **Urogenital:** Elevated serum creatinine.

INTERACTIONS Drug: Additive risk of bleeding with ANTICOAGULANTS, NSAIDS, PLATELET INHIBITORS, SALICYLATES.

PHARMACOKINETICS Onset: Therapeutic effect 10 d to 4 mo. **Duration:** 7–25+ mo. **Distribution:** Crosses placenta; distributed into breast milk. **Metabolism:** In malignant leukocytes, cladribine is phosphorylated to form its monophosphate and triphosphate forms, presumably its active forms, which are subsequently incorporated into cellular DNA. **Half-Life:** Initial 35 min, terminal 6.7 h.

NURSING IMPLICATIONS

Assessment & Drug Effects

- Monitor vital signs during and after drug infusion. Fever (>100° F) is common during the 5th to 7th day in patients with hairy cell leukemia, and severe fever (>104° F) may develop within the first month of therapy.
- Lab tests: Frequent hematologic studies; periodic serum creatinine and liver function tests.
- Closely monitor hematologic status; myelosuppression is common during the first month after starting therapy.
- Monitor for and report S&S of infection. Note that within the first month, fever may occur in the absence of infection.
- With high doses of cladribine, monitor for neurologic toxicity (paraparesis/quadriparesis) and acute nephrotoxicity.

Patient & Family Education

- Be fully informed regarding adverse responses to the drug.
- Understand the need for close follow-up during and after treatment with the drug.

CLARITHROMYCIN

(clar′i-thro-my-sin)

Biaxin Filmtabs, Biaxin XL

Classifications: ANTIINFECTIVE; MACROLIDE ANTIBIOTIC

Prototype: Erythromycin

Pregnancy Category: C

AVAILABILITY 250 mg, 500 mg tablets; 500 mg sustained-release tablets; 125 mg/5 mL, 250 mg/5 mL suspension

ACTIONS A semisynthetic macrolide antibiotic that binds to the 50S ribosomal subunit of susceptible bacterial organisms and thus inhibits protein synthesis of the bacteria.

THERAPEUTIC EFFECTS It is active against both aerobic and anaerobic gram-positive and gram-negative organisms including *Streptococcus pyogenes, Streptococcus pneumoniae, Haemophilus influenzae, Moraxella catarrhalis, Mycoplasma pneumoniae,* and *Staphylococcus aureus.*

USES Treatment of upper respiratory, lower respiratory infections;

C

acute maxillary sinusitis; otitis media; and skin and soft tissue infections caused by clinically significant aerobic and anaerobic gram-negative and gram-positive organisms, including *S. aureus, H. influenzae, S. pneumoniae, M. catarrhalis, S. pyogenes, M. pneumoniae.* Prevention and treatment of *Mycobacterium avium complex* (MAC) infections in patients with HIV. Used in combination for *H. pylori.*

CONTRAINDICATIONS Hypersensitivity to clarithromycin, erythromycin, or any other macrolide antibiotics; patients receiving cisapride, astemizole or pimozide; suspected or potential bacteremias; acute porphyria; severe hepatic or biliary disease; pregnancy (category C). Safety and efficacy in children <6 y not established.
CAUTIOUS USE Renal impairment, older adults, and lactation.

ROUTE & DOSAGE

Mild to Moderate Infections

Adult: **PO** 250–500 mg b.i.d. or 500 mg XL q.d. for 10–14 d
Child: **PO** 7.5 mg/kg q12h

Mycobacterial Infections

Adult: **PO** 500 mg q12h
Child: **PO** 7.5 mg/kg q12h

***H. pylori* Infections**

Adult: **PO** 500 mg b.i.d. to t.i.d.

Renal Impairment

Cl_{cr} <30 mL/min, decrease dose by 1/2 or double the dosing interval

ADMINISTRATION

Oral

- Ensure that sustained-release form of drug is not chewed or crushed. It must be swallowed whole.
- Shake suspension well before use.
- Store at 15°–30° C (59°–86° F).

ADVERSE EFFECTS (≥1%) **GI:** Diarrhea, abdominal discomfort, nausea, abnormal taste, dyspepsia. **Hematologic:** Eosinophilia. **CNS:** Headache. **Skin:** Rash, urticaria.

DIAGNOSTIC TEST INTERFERENCE May increase serum AST and ALT levels.

INTERACTIONS Drug: May increase **theophylline** levels; drugs known to interact with **erythromycin** (i.e., **digoxin, carbamazepine, triazolam, warfarin, ergotamine, dihydroergotamine**) should be monitored carefully for increased levels and toxicity; **pimozide** may increase risk of arrhythmias.

PHARMACOKINETICS Absorption: Readily absorbed from GI tract; 50% reaches the systemic circulation. **Peak:** 2–4 h. **Distribution:** Widely distributes into most body tissue (excluding CNS); high pulmonary tissue concentrations. **Metabolism:** Partially metabolized in the liver; active 14-OH metabolite acts synergistically with the parent compound against *H. influenzae.* **Elimination:** 20% excreted unchanged in urine; 10–15% of 14-OH metabolite excreted in urine. **Half-Life:** 3–5 h.

NURSING IMPLICATIONS

Assessment & Drug Effects

- Inquire about previous hypersensitivity to other macrolides (e.g., erythromycin) before treatment.
- Withhold drug and notify physician, if hypersensitivity occurs (e.g., rash, urticaria).

- Monitor for and report loose stools or diarrhea, since pseudomembranous colitis must be ruled out.
- When clarithromycin is given concurrently with anticoagulants, digoxin, or theophylline, blood levels of these drugs may be elevated. Monitor appropriate serum levels and assess for S&S of drug toxicity.

Patient & Family Education

- Complete prescribed course of therapy.
- Report rash or other signs of hypersensitivity immediately.
- Report loose stools or diarrhea even after completion of drug therapy.
- Do not breast feed without consulting physician.

CLEMASTINE FUMARATE

(klem'as-teen)

Tavist, Tavist-1

Classification: ANTIHISTAMINE (H_1-RECEPTOR ANTAGONIST)

Prototype: Diphenhydramine

Pregnancy Category: B

AVAILABILITY 1.34 mg, 2.68 mg tablets; 0.67 mg/5 mL syrup

ACTIONS An antihistamine (H_1-receptor antagonist) which competes for H_1 receptor sites on effector cells, thus blocking histamine release. Has greater selectivity for preripheral H_1 receptors and, consequently, it produces little sedation. Has prominent antipruritic activity and low incidence of unpleasant adverse effects.

THERAPEUTIC EFFECTS Effective in controlling various allergic reactions, e.g. nasal congestion, sneezing, itching.

USES Symptomatic relief of allergic rhinitis (sneezing, rhinorrhea, pruritus) and mild uncomplicated allergic skin manifestations such as urticaria and angioedema.

CONTRAINDICATIONS Hypersensitivity to clemastine or to other antihistamines of similar chemical structure; lower respiratory tract symptoms, including acute asthma; concomitant MAO INHIBITOR therapy. Safe use in children <6 y not established. Pregnancy (category B), lactation.

CAUTIOUS USE History of bronchial asthma, increased intraocular pressure, GI or GU obstruction, hyperthyroidism, cardiovascular disease, hypertension, older adults.

ROUTE & DOSAGE

Allergic Rhinitis

Adult: **PO** 1.34 mg b.i.d., may increase up to 8.04 mg/d
Child: **PO** *>6 y:* 0.67 mg b.i.d., may increase up to 4.02 mg/d; *<6 y:* 0.335–0.67 mg/kg/d in 2 divided doses (max: 1.34 mg/d)

Allergic Urticaria

Adult: **PO** 2.68 mg b.i.d. or t.i.d., may increase up to 8.04 mg/d
Child: **PO** 1.34 mg b.i.d., may increase up to 4.02 mg/d

ADMINISTRATION

Oral

- Drug may be administered with food, water, or milk to reduce possibility of gastric irritation.
- Older adult patients usually require less than average adult dose.
- Store at 15°–30° C (59°–86° F) unless otherwise directed.

ADVERSE EFFECTS (≥1%) **Body as a Whole:** Anaphylaxis, excess perspiration, chills. **CV:** Hypotension, palpitation, tachycardia, extrasystoles. **GI:** *Dry mouth,* epigastric distress, anorexia, nausea, vomiting, diarrhea, constipation. **Hematologic:** Hemolytic anemia, thrombocytopenia, agranulocytosis. **CNS:** Sedation, *transient drowsiness,* dry nose and throat, headache, dizziness, weakness, fatigue, disturbed coordination; confusion, restlessness, nervousness, hysteria, convulsions, tremors, irritability, euphoria, insomnia, paresthesias, neuritis. **Respiratory:** Dry nose and throat, thickening of bronchial secretions, tightness of chest, wheezing, nasal stuffiness. **Skin:** Urticaria, rash, photosensitivity. **Special Senses:** Vertigo, tinnitus, acute labyrinthitis, blurred vision, diplopia. **Urogenital:** Difficult urination, urinary retention, early menses.

INTERACTIONS Drug: Alcohol and other CNS DEPRESSANTS increase sedation; MAO INHIBITORS may prolong and intensify anticholinergic effects.

PHARMACOKINETICS Absorption: Readily absorbed from GI tract. **Peak:** 5–7 h. **Duration:** 10–12 h. **Distribution:** Distributed into breast milk. **Metabolism:** Metabolized in liver. **Elimination:** Excreted chiefly in urine.

NURSING IMPLICATIONS

Assessment & Drug Effects

- Monitor for drowsiness, poor coordination, or dizziness, especially in the older adult or debilitated. Supervision of ambulation may be warranted.
- Assess for symptomatic relief with use of the medication.
- Lab tests: Periodic hematological studies with long-term use.

Patient & Family Education

- Check with physician before taking alcohol or other CNS depressants, since effects may be additive.
- Clemastine may cause lethargy and drowsiness; therefore, necessary safety precautions should be taken.
- Older adults should make position changes slowly and in stages, particularly from recumbent to upright posture, as dizziness and hypotension occur more frequently than in younger patients.
- Avoid driving and other potentially hazardous activities until response to the drug has been established.
- Frequent sips of water or sugarless hard candy to relieve dry mouth.
- Do not breast feed while taking this drug.

CLINDAMYCIN HYDROCHLORIDE (Pr)

(klin-da-mye′sin)

Cleocin, Dalacin C ♣

CLINDAMYCIN PALMITATE HYDROCHLORIDE

Cleocin Pediatric

CLINDAMYCIN PHOSPHATE

Cleocin Phosphate, Cleocin T, Dalacin C, Cleocin Vaginal Ovules or Cream

Classifications: ANTIINFECTIVE; ANTIBIOTIC

Pregnancy Category: B

AVAILABILITY 75 mg, 150 mg, 300 mg capsules; 75 mg/5 mL oral suspension; 150 mg/mL injection; 2% vaginal cream; 100 mg suppositories; 10 mg gel, lotion

ACTIONS Semisynthetic derivative of lincomycin with which it shares neuromuscular blocking properties and other actions. Reported to have a greater degree of antibacterial activity in vitro, better absorption, and lower incidence of GI adverse effects than lincomycin. Suppresses protein synthesis by binding to 50 S subunits of bacterial ribosomes, and therefore inhibits other antibiotics (e.g., erythromycin) that act at this site.

THERAPEUTIC EFFECTS Particularly effective against susceptible strains of anaerobic streptococci, *Bacteroides* (especially *B. fragilis*), *Fusobacterium, Actinomyces israelii, Peptococcus,* and *Clostridium sp.* Also effective against aerobic gram-positive cocci, including *Staphylococcus aureus, Staphylococcus epidermidis,* Streptococci (except *S. faecalis*), and *Pneumococci.*

USES Serious infections when less toxic alternatives are inappropriate. Topical applications are used in treatment of acne vulgaris. Vaginal applications are used in treatment of bacterial vaginosis in nonpregnant women.

UNLABELED USES In combination with pyrimethamine for toxoplasmosis in patients with AIDS.

CONTRAINDICATIONS History of hypersensitivity to clindamycin or lincomycin; history of regional enteritis, ulcerative colitis, or antibiotic-associated colitis. Pregnancy (category B), lactation. Not recommended for infants <1 mo.

CAUTIOUS USE History of GI disease, renal or hepatic disease; atopic individuals (history of eczema, asthma, hay fever); older patients >60 y.

ROUTE & DOSAGE

Moderate to Severe Infections

Adult: **PO** 150–450 mg q6h **IM/IV** 300–900 mg q6–8h (max: 2700 mg/d)
Child: **PO** 10–30 mg/kg/d q6–8h. **IM/IV** 25–40 mg/kg/d q6–8h
Neonate: **IM/IV** = 7 d: 10–15 mg/kg/d divided q8–12h; >7 d: 10–20 mg/kg/d divided q6–12h

Acne Vulgaris

Adult: **Topical** Apply to affected areas b.i.d.

Bacterial Vaginosis

Adult: **Topical** Insert 1 suppository intravaginally at bedtime times 3 d, or insert 1 applicator full of cream intravaginally at bedtime times 7 d

ADMINISTRATION

- Determine history of any previous sensitivities to drugs or other allergens prior to administration.

Oral

- Administer clindamycin capsules with a full (240 mL [8 oz]) glass of water to prevent esophagitis.
- Note expiration date of oral solution; retains potency for 14 d at room temperature. Do not refrigerate, as chilling causes thickening and thus makes pouring it difficult.

Intramuscular

- Deep IM injection is recommended. Rotate injection sites and observe daily for evidence of inflammatory reaction. Single IM doses should not exceed 600 mg.

Intravenous

- IV administration to neonates, infants, and children: Verify correct IV concentration and rate of infusion with physician.

PREPARE: **Intermittent:** Each 18 mg must be diluted with at least 1 mL of D5W, NS, D5/.45% NaCl, or other compatible solution. Final concentration should never exceed 18 mg/mL.

C

ADMINISTER: **Intermittent:** Never give a bolus dose. Do not give >1200 mg in a single 1-h infusion. Infusion rate should not exceed 30 mg/min.
INCOMPATIBILITIES **Solution/additive: Aminophylline, ceftriaxone, ciprofloxacin, fluconazole, ranitidine, tobramycin. Y-site: Allopurinol, filgrastim, fluconazole, idarubicin.**

- Store in tight containers at 15°–30° C (59°–86° F) unless otherwise directed.

ADVERSE EFFECTS (≥1%) **Body as a Whole:** Fever, serum sickness, sensitization, swelling of face (following topical use), generalized myalgia, superinfections, proctitis, vaginitis, pain, induration, sterile abscess (following IM injections); thrombophlebitis (IV infusion). **CV:** Hypotension (following IM), cardiac arrest (rapid IV). **GI:** *Diarrhea,* abdominal pain, flatulence, bloating, *nausea, vomiting,* pseudomembranous colitis; esophageal irritation, loss of taste, medicinal taste (high IV doses), jaundice, abnormal liver function tests. **Hematologic:** Leukopenia, eosinophilia, agranulocytosis, thrombocytopenia. **Skin:** *Skin rashes,* urticaria, pruritus, dryness, contact dermatitis, gram-negative folliculitis, irritation, oily skin.

DIAGNOSTIC TEST INTERFERENCE Clindamycin may cause increases in ***serum alkaline phosphatase, bilirubin, creatine phosphokinase (CPK)*** from muscle irritation following IM injection; ***AST, ALT.***

INTERACTIONS Drug: Chloramphenicol, erythromycin possibly are mutually antagonistic to clindamycin; neuromuscular blocking action enhanced by NEUROMUSCULAR BLOCKING AGENTS **(atracurium, tubocurarine, pancuronium).**

PHARMACOKINETICS Absorption: Approximately 90% absorbed from GI tract; 10% of topical application is absorbed through skin. **Peak:** 45–60 min PO; 3 h IM. **Duration:** 6 h PO; 8–12 h IM. **Distribution:** Widely distributed except for CNS; crosses placenta; distributed into breast milk. **Metabolism:** Metabolized in liver. **Elimination:** Excreted in urine and feces. **Half-Life:** 2–3 h.

NURSING IMPLICATIONS

Assessment & Drug Effects

- Lab tests: Culture and susceptibility testing should be performed initially and periodically during therapy. Periodic CBC with differential and platelet count.
- Monitor BP and pulse in patients receiving drug parenterally. Hypotension has occurred following IM injection. Advise patient to remain recumbent following drug administration until BP has stabilized.
- Severe diarrhea and colitis, including pseudomembranous colitis, have been associated with oral (highest incidence), parenteral, and topical clindamycin. Report immediately the onset of watery diarrhea, with or without fever; passage of tarry or bloody stools, pus, intestinal tissue, or mucus; abdominal cramps, or ileus. Symptoms may appear within a few days to 2 wk after therapy is begun or up to several weeks following cessation of therapy.
- Closely observe older adult and bedridden patients, as they are at a higher risk of developing severe colitis.
- Be alert to signs of superinfection (see Appendix F).

- Be alert for signs of anaphylactoid reactions (see Appendix F), that require immediate attention.

Patient & Family Education

- Take drug for the full course of therapy as prescribed.
- Report loose stools or diarrhea promptly.
- Stop drug therapy if significant diarrhea develops (more than 5 loose stools daily) and notify physician.
- Do not self-medicate with antidiarrheal preparations. Antiperistaltic agents may prolong and worsen diarrhea by delaying removal of toxins from colon.
- If using topical preparation for acne, discontinue other acne preparations unless otherwise directed by physician. Keep medication away from eyes.
- Since 10% absorption of topical medication is possible, report the onset of systemic reactions to physician.
- Do not breast feed while taking this drug.

CLIOQUINOL (IODOCHLORHYDROXYQUIN)

(klee-oh-kwee′nole)

Torofor, Vioform

Classifications: ANTIINFECTIVE; ANTIBIOTIC; ANTIFUNGAL

Prototype: Fluconazole

Pregnancy Category: C

AVAILABILITY 3% cream, ointment

ACTIONS Halogenated hydroxyquinoline with broad spectrum topical antiinfective.

THERAPEUTIC EFFECTS It is both antifungal and antibacterial in activity. Available OTC.

USES Topically for treatment of inflamed cutaneous conditions such as eczema, athlete's foot, and other fungal conditions.

CONTRAINDICATIONS Hypersensitivity to chloroxine, iodine, or iodine-containing preparations; tuberculosis; vaccinia, varicella, or other viral skin conditions; severe renal disease; hepatic damage; thyroid disorder; pregnancy (category C), lactation.

ROUTE & DOSAGE

Inflamed Cutaneous Conditions

Adult: **Topical** Apply thin layer to affected area b.i.d. or t.i.d. for 1 wk only

ADMINISTRATION

Topical

- Wash area to be treated with soap and water and dry thoroughly before each application. Consult physician.
- Do not apply an occlusive dressing without a physician's order.
- Preserve in tightly covered, light-resistant containers at 15°–30° C (59°–86° F) unless otherwise directed.

ADVERSE EFFECTS (≥1%) **Body as a Whole:** Iodism, hypersensitivity reaction, slight enlargement of thyroid gland, hair loss, subacute myeloptic neuropathy. **Hematologic:** Agranulocytosis. **Skin:** Local burning, irritation, redness, swelling, itching, rash, staining of hair and skin.

DIAGNOSTIC TEST INTERFERENCE Possibility of elevated ***PBI,*** decreased ***iodine 131 thyroidal uptake,*** and elevation of ***butanol-extractable iodine (BEI).*** False-positive ***ferric chloride test*** for ***phenylketonuria (PKU)*** may re-

C

sult if clioquinol is present on diaper or in urine.

PHARMACOKINETICS Absorption: Minimally absorbed through intact skin. **Elimination:** Some is rapidly excreted in urine; the rest may persist in body 1 mo or more.

NURSING IMPLICATIONS

Assessment & Drug Effects

- Monitor for signs of skin irritation. Notify physician if they appear. Drug may be discontinued.
- Monitor for signs of systemic absorption such as thyroid enlargement and hair loss. Notify physician if they occur. Drug may be discontinued.

Patient & Family Education

- Avoid contact of drug in or around eyes. Drug may stain fabric, skin, or hair yellow on contact.
- Clioquinol should be discontinued if skin irritation, rash, or other signs of sensitivity or systemic absorption develop. Report to physician.
- Treatment is usually continued 4 wk for athlete's foot or ringworm and 2 wk for jock itch.
- Notify physician if there is no improvement within 1–2 wk. Apply the drug as directed and only for the period of time prescribed.
- Do not breast feed while taking this drug.

CLOBETASOL PROPIONATE

(cloe-bay'ta-sol)

Clobex, Dermovate, Temovate, Embeline gel; Olux Foam

Classifications: SKIN AND MUCOUS MEMBRANE AGENT; ANTIINFLAMMATORY; CORTICOSTEROID

Prototype: Hydrocortisone

Pregnancy Category: C

AVAILABILITY 0.05% ointment, cream, gel, scalp lotion, foam

See Appendix A-4.

CLOCORTOLONE PIVALATE

(kloe-kor'toe-lone)

Cloderm

Classifications: SKIN AND MUCOUS MEMBRANE AGENT; ANTIINFLAMMATORY; STEROID

Prototype: Hydrocortisone

Pregnancy Category: C

AVAILABILITY 0.1% cream

See Appendix A-4.

CLOFAZIMINE

(kloe-fa'zi-meen)

Lamprene

Classifications: ANTIINFECTIVE; ANTILEPROSY AGENT

Prototype: Dapsone

Pregnancy Category: C

AVAILABILITY 50 mg capsules

ACTIONS Exerts a slow bactericidal effect on *Mycobacterium leprae* (Hansen's bacillus). Binds preferentially to DNA of all mycobacteria and inhibits their growth. Its antiinflammatory action (precise mechanism unknown) controls erythema nodosum leprosum reactions. Bacterial killing is not detectable in biopsy tissue from leprosy patient until 50 d after start of therapy.

THERAPEUTIC EFFECTS Exerts a slow bactericidal effect on *Mycobacterium leprae* (Hansen's bacillus) and has antiinflammatory activity. Clofazimine is not effective against all forms of leprosy. Does not show cross-resistance with rifampin or dapsone. Has no clinically useful activity against microorganisms other than mycobacteria.

USES Chiefly in multiinfective therapy of multibacillary leprosy (with dapsone, rifampin, ethionamide) to prevent development of drug resistance. Also in lepromatous leprosy, including dapsone-resistant lepromatous leprosy and leprosy complicated by erythema nodosum leprosum (lepra) reaction.

UNLABELED USE *Mycobacterium avium-intracellulare complex* infections in patients with AIDS.

CONTRAINDICATIONS Pregnancy (category C), lactation, children <12 y.

CAUTIOUS USE Patients with GI problems.

ROUTE & DOSAGE

Dapsone-resistant Leprosy

Adult: **PO** 100 mg/d in combination with 1 or more antileprosy drugs for 3 y, then 100 mg/d as monotherapy

Child: **PO** 1 mg/kg/d in combination with dapsone and rifampin

Erythema Nodosum Leprosum

Adult: **PO** 100–300 mg/d for up to 3 mo; taper dose to 100 mg/d as soon as possible

Mycobacterium avium-intracellulare

Adult: **PO** 100 mg 1–3 times/d

Child: **PO** 1–2 mg/kg/d (max: 100 mg/d)

ADMINISTRATION

Oral

- Drug should be taken with meals or milk to reduce gastric irritation.
- Doses of more than 100 mg/d are given for as short a period of time as possible and should be administered under close medical supervision.
- Store capsules at 15°–30° C (59°–86° F); protect from moisture.

ADVERSE EFFECTS (≥1%) **GI:** *Abdominal/epigastric pain* (dose-related), *nausea, vomiting, diarrhea,* bowel obstruction, hepatitis, jaundice, enlarged liver. **Hematologic:** Eosinophilia. **Metabolic:** Hypokalemia; elevated albumin, serum bilirubin, and AST. **CNS:** Drowsiness, fatigue, headache, giddiness, dizziness, neuralgia, taste disorder. **Skin:** *Pink-brown skin discoloration, ichthyosis, dryness,* rash, pruritus, phototoxicity, erythema nodosum leprosum (lepra) reaction. **Special Senses:** *Conjunctival and corneal discoloration,* dryness, burning, itching, irritation.

INTERACTIONS Drug: Isoniazid may decrease clofazimine concentrations in skin. **Food:** Food will increase absorption.

PHARMACOKINETICS Absorption: Slowly absorbed from GI tract; approximately 50% absorbed. **Peak:** 4–12 h. **Distribution:** Distributed predominantly to fatty tissues and reticuloendothelial system; crosses placenta; distributed into breast milk. **Elimination:** Primarily eliminated in feces through bile. **Half-Life:** 70 d.

NURSING IMPLICATIONS

Assessment & Drug Effects

- Assess for serious adverse effects (e.g., pain in bones and joints, GI bleeding, diminished vision). Reactions are usually reversible but may require months or years to diminish.

- Lab tests: Periodic WBC with differential, serum electrolytes, serum albumin, and liver function tests.
- Drug-induced reddish-brown discoloration of skin, cornea, conjunctiva, and body fluids (including tears, sweat, sputum, urine, and feces) occurs in 75–90% of patients within a few weeks of treatment. Skin discoloration may take months or years to disappear after drug is discontinued.
- Monitor for the onset of tender, erythematous nodules with lymphadenopathy, joint swelling, epistaxis, iritis which suggests a type 2 leprosy reactional state. Dosage may be increased to 200 mg/d. After reactive episode is controlled, dosage is tapered to 100 mg/d as soon as possible. Patient should remain under medical surveillance during the episode.

Patient & Family Education

- Adhere strictly to established drug regimen. No drug dosage should be omitted, increased, or decreased without advice of physician.
- Report promptly bone and joint pain; GI bleeding, colicky abdominal pain, nausea, vomiting, diarrhea; diminished vision.
- Minimize use of soap, avoid applying it directly to dry skin, and thoroughly rinse it off.
- When dizziness, drowsiness, or visual impairment adverse effects are experienced, do not drive or work with hazardous equipment. These symptoms are generally dose related. Discuss with physician.
- Do not breast feed while taking this drug.

CLOFIBRATE (Pr)

(kloe-fy′brate)

Atromid-S, Claripex ♣, Novofibrate ♣

Classifications: CARDIOVASCULAR DRUG; ANTILIPEMIC; FIBRATE

Pregnancy Category: C

AVAILABILITY 500 mg capsules

ACTIONS Structurally related to gemfibrozil. Reduces very low density lipoproteins (VLDL) to a greater extent than it reduces low density lipoproteins (LDL). Mechanism of action is unclear; it appears to inhibit cholesterol biosynthesis prior to transfer of triglycerides from liver to serum. Interferes with binding of free fatty acids to albumin and increases fecal excretion of neutral sterols. It affects the mobilization of cholesterol from tissue. Reduces platelet adhesiveness and increases release of ADH from posterior pituitary.

THERAPEUTIC EFFECTS Reduces very low density lipoproteins (VLDL) to a greater extent than it reduces low density lipoproteins (LDL).

USES Adjunct for treatment of severe primary (type III) hyperlipidemia.

UNLABELED USE Management of diabetes insipidus.

CONTRAINDICATIONS Impaired renal or hepatic function, primary biliary cirrhosis; pregnancy (category C), lactation. Safe use in children <14 y not established.

CAUTIOUS USE History of jaundice or hepatic disease; gallstones; peptic ulcer; hypothyroidism; cardiovascular disease.

ROUTE & DOSAGE

Hyperlipidemia
Adult: **PO** 2 g/d in 2–4 divided doses
Diabetes Insipidus
Adult: **PO** 1.5–2 g/d in 2–4 divided doses

ADMINISTRATION

Oral
- If gastric distress is a problem, administer drug with meals.
- Preserve in closed, light-resistant containers at 15°–30° C (59°–86° F) unless otherwise directed.

ADVERSE EFFECTS (≥1%) **CV:** Increase or decrease in angina, CHF, arrhythmias. **GI:** *Nausea,* vomiting, loose stools, diarrhea, flatulence, abdominal distress, gastritis, stomatitis, cholelithiasis. **Hematologic:** Neutropenia, leukopenia, anemia, eosinophilia, agranulocytosis, potentiation of anticoagulant effect. **Metabolic:** Elevated AST and ALT. **Musculoskeletal:** Flu-like symptoms. **CNS:** Drowsiness, dizziness, headache. **Skin:** Swelling and phlebitis at xanthoma sites, skin rash, allergy, urticaria, pruritus. **Urogenital:** Renal insufficiency, impotence, decreased libido.

DIAGNOSTIC TEST INTERFERENCE Clofibrate therapy may lead to increased ***BSP*** retention, ***thymol*** turbidity; increased ***serum creatine phosphokinase (CPK); proteinuria,*** parodoxical increase in ***LDL*** or ***cholesterol*** levels (if there is a large decrease in VLDL level). Lower fasting ***blood glucose*** and ***serum insulin*** levels in patients with diabetes mellitus.

INTERACTIONS Drug: ORAL ANTICOAGULANTS increase hypoprothrombinemia and increase risk of bleeding; **probenecid** increases effects of clofibrate; SULFONYLUREAS increase hypoglycemic effects.

PHARMACOKINETICS Absorption: Readily absorbed from GI tract. **Peak:** 4–6 h. **Distribution:** Distributed to extracellular space; crosses placenta; distribution into breast milk unknown. **Metabolism:** Hydrolyzed in plasma to clofibric acid, which is further metabolized in liver. **Elimination:** Excreted in urine. **Half-Life:** 12–35 h.

NURSING IMPLICATIONS

Assessment & Drug Effects
- Lab tests: Baseline and periodic lipid profile; periodic liver function tests, CBC, renal function tests, and determinations of plasma and urine steroid levels, serum electrolyte levels, and blood glucose.
- Therapeutic response generally occurs during the first or second month of therapy. Rebound may occur in second or third month, followed by a further decrease, and may also occur with sudden withdrawal of drug.
- Clofibrate therapy for increased serum cholesterol and triglycerides is generally withdrawn after 3 mo if the response is not adequate.

Patient & Family Education
- Report flu-like symptoms (malaise, muscle soreness, aching, weakness) promptly to physician. Other reportable conditions include leukopenia, pulmonary edema, and renal insufficiency (see Appendix F) and gastric pain, nausea, and vomiting.

C

- Women of childbearing years should be on birth control regimen. If pregnancy is desired, clofibrate therapy should be discontinued at least 2 mo before conception.
- Do not self-dose with OTC drugs without the approval of physician.
- Do not breast feed while taking this drug.

CLOMIPHENE CITRATE

(kloe′mi-feen)

Clomid, Milophene, Serophene

Classifications: HORMONES AND SYNTHETIC SUBSTITUTES; OVULATION STIMULANT; ANTIESTROGENIC

Pregnancy Category: X

AVAILABILITY 50 mg tablets

ACTIONS Oral nonsteroidal estrogen agonist or antagonist. Induces ovulation in selected anovulatory women. Lacks androgenic, antiandrogenic, or progestational effects and does not appear to effect pituitary-adrenal or pituitary-thyroid functions. May act by binding to hypothalamic estrogen receptors, decreasing their numbers, and by inhibiting receptor replenishment.

THERAPEUTIC EFFECTS Inhibition of receptor replenishment results in a false hypoestrogenic state which stimulates pituitary release of luteinizing hormone (LH), follicle-stimulating hormone (FSH), and gonadotropins, leading to ovarian stimulation. Normal ovulatory function does not usually resume after treatment or after pregnancy.

USES Infertility in appropriately selected women desiring pregnancy whose partners are fertile and potent.

UNLABELED USES Male infertility, menstrual abnormalities, gynecomastia, fibrocystic breast disease, regulation of cycles in patients using rhythm method of contraception, endometrial hyperplasia, persistent lactation.

CONTRAINDICATIONS Pregnancy (category X); lactation; neoplastic lesions, ovarian cyst; hepatic disease or dysfunction; abnormal uterine bleeding; visual abnormalities; mental depression; thrombophlebitis.

CAUTIOUS USE Polycystic ovarian enlargement, pelvic discomfort, sensitivity to pituitary gonadotropins.

ROUTE & DOSAGE

Infertility

Adult: **PO First course:** 50 mg/d for 5 d; start on 5th day of cycle following start of spontaneous or induced bleeding (with progestin) or at any time in the patient who has had no recent uterine bleeding
Second course if ovulation: repeat first course until conception or for 3 cycles
Second course if no ovulation: 100 mg/d for 5 d as above (max: 100 mg/d)

ADMINISTRATION

Oral

- Pretreatment with estrogen is indicated for the patient who has been hypoestrogenic for a long time. Estrogen therapy is stopped immediately before clomiphene therapy begins.
- Each course of therapy should start on or about the 5th cycle day once ovulation has been established.
- Store at 15°–30° C (59°–86° F) in tightly capped, light-resistant container.

ADVERSE EFFECTS (≥1%) **Body as a Whole:** *Vasomotor flushes,* breast discomfort, abdominal pain, heavy menses, exacerbation of endometriosis; mental depression, headache, fatigue, insomnia, dizziness, vertigo. **GI:** Nausea, vomiting, increased appetite with weight gain, constipation, bloating. **Endocrine:** Spontaneous abortion, multiple ovulations, ovarian failure, *ovarian hyperstimulation syndrome, enlarged ovaries with multiple follicular cysts.* **Special Senses:** Transient blurring, diplopia, scotomas, photophobia, floaters, prolonged after-images. **Urogenital:** Urinary frequency, polyuria.

DIAGNOSTIC TEST INTERFERENCE Clomiphene may increase BSP retention; ***plasma transcortin, thyroxine*** and ***sex hormone binding globulin*** levels. Also increases ***follicle-stimulating*** and ***luteinizing hormone*** secretion in most patients.

INTERACTIONS Drug: No clinically significant drug interactions established. **Herbal: Black cohosh** may antagonize infertility treatments.

PHARMACOKINETICS Absorption: Readily absorbed from GI tract. **Metabolism:** Metabolized in liver. **Elimination:** Excreted primarily in feces in 5 d; the remainder is excreted slowly from enterohepatic pool or is stored in body fat for later release. **Half-Life:** 5 d.

NURSING IMPLICATIONS

Assessment & Drug Effects

- Monitor for abnormal bleeding. If it occurs, full diagnostic measures are crucial. Report it immediately.
- Monitor for visual disturbances. Their occurrence indicates the need for a complete ophthalmologic evaluation. Drug will be stopped until symptoms subside.
- If clomiphene is continued more than 1 y, patient should have an ophthalmologic examination at regular intervals.
- Pelvic pain indicates the need for immediate pelvic examination for diagnostic purposes.

Patient & Family Education

- Take the medicine at same time every day to maintain drug levels and prevent forgetting a dose.
- Missed dose: Take drug as soon as possible. If not remembered until time for next dose, double the dose, then resume regular dosing schedule. If more than one dose is missed, check with physician.
- Incidence of multiple births during clomiphene use is reportedly increased to 6 times normal and appears to increase with dose increases.
- Patient who is going to respond usually ovulates 4–10 d after last day of treatment.
- Report these symptoms: hot flushes resembling those associated with menopause; nausea, vomiting, headache. Appropriate drug therapy may be prescribed. Symptoms disappear after clomiphene is discontinued.
- Reported promptly yellowing of eyes, light-colored stools, yellow, itchy skin, and fever symptomatic of jaundice.
- Stop taking clomiphene if pregnancy is suspected. Contact physician for a confirmatory examination.
- Because of the possibility of light-headedness, dizziness, and visual disturbances, do not perform hazardous tasks requiring skill and coordination in an environment with variable lighting.

C

- Report promptly excessive weight gain, signs of edema, bloating, decreased urinary output.
- Do not breast feed while taking this drug.

CLOMIPRAMINE HYDROCHLORIDE

(clo-mi'pra-meen)

Anafranil

Classifications: CENTRAL NERVOUS SYSTEM AGENT; PSYCHOTHERAPEUTIC; TRICYCLIC ANTIDEPRESSANT

Prototype: Imipramine

Pregnancy Category: C

AVAILABILITY 25 mg, 50 mg, 75 mg capsules

ACTIONS Inhibits the reuptake of norepinephrine and serotonin at the presynaptic neuron. Elevates serum levels of these two amines.

THERAPEUTIC EFFECTS The basis of its antidepressant effects is thought to be due to the elevated serum levels of norepinephrine and serotonin. Exhibits anticholinergic, antihistaminic, hypotensive, sedative, mild analgesic, and peripheral vasodilator effects.

USES Obsessive-compulsive disorder (OCD).

UNLABELED USES Panic disorder, anxiety, agoraphobia.

CONTRAINDICATIONS Hypersensitivity to other tricyclic compounds; acute recovery period after MI, children <10 y, pregnancy (category C), lactation.

CAUTIOUS USE History of convulsive disorders, prostatic hypertrophy, urinary retention, cardiovascular, hepatic, GI, or blood disorders.

ROUTE & DOSAGE

Obsessive-compulsive Disorder

Adult: **PO** 75–300 mg/d in divided doses

Child: **PO** *10–18 y:* 100–200 mg/d in divided doses, start at 50 mg/d

Depression

Adult: **PO** 50–150 mg/d in single or divided doses

ADMINISTRATION

Oral

- Give in divided doses with meals to reduce GI adverse effects.
- Following titration to the full dose, drug may be given as a single dose at bedtime to reduce daytime sedation.
- Store at 15°–30° C (59°–86° F).

ADVERSE EFFECTS (≥1%) **Body as a Whole:** Diaphoresis. **CV:** Hypotension, tachycardia. **GI:** Constipation, *dry mouth*. **Endocrine:** Galactorrhea, hyperprolactinemia, amenorrhea, *weight gain*. **Hematologic:** Leukopenia, agranulocytosis, thrombocytopenia, anemia. **CNS:** Mania, *tremor,* dizziness, hyperthermia, neuroleptic malignant syndrome, seizures (especially with abrupt withdrawal). **Urogenital:** Delayed ejaculation, anorgasmia.

DIAGNOSTIC TEST INTERFERENCE Clomipramine appears to elevate serum ***prolactin*** levels. ***Serum AST and ALT*** are elevated. Serum levels of ***triiodothyronine (T_3) and free triiodothyronine (FT_3)*** have been significantly reduced from baseline. ***Thyroxine-binding globulin (TBG)*** levels were increased from baseline, whereas ***thyroxine (T_4), free thyroxine***

(FT_4), and reverse *T_3* were unchanged.

INTERACTIONS Drug: MAO INHIBITORS may precipitate hyperpyrexic crisis, tachycardia, or seizures; ANTIHYPERTENSIVE AGENTS potentiate orthostatic hypotension; CNS DEPRESSANTS, **alcohol** add to CNS depression; **norepinephrine** and other SYMPATHOMIMETICS may increase cardiac toxicity; **cimetidine** decreases hepatic metabolism, thus increasing imipramine levels; **methylphenidate** inhibits metabolism of **imipramine** and thus may increase its toxicity. **Herbal: Ginkgo** may decrease seizure threshold; **St. John's wort** may cause serotonin syndrome.

PHARMACOKINETICS Absorption: Rapidly absorbed from GI tract; 20–78% reaches systemic circulation. **Onset:** Depression: approx 2 wk; OCD: approx 4–10 wk. **Peak:** 2–6 h. **Distribution:** Widely distributed including the CSF; crosses placenta. **Metabolism:** Extensive first-pass metabolism in the liver; active metabolite is desmethylclomipramine. **Elimination:** 50–60% excreted in urine, 24–32% in feces. **Half-Life:** 20–30 h.

NURSING IMPLICATIONS

Assessment & Drug Effects

- Monitor for seizures, especially in those with predisposing factors such as alcoholism, brain injury, or concurrent therapy with other drugs that lower seizure threshold.
- Lab tests: Periodic CBC with differential, platelet count, and Hct and Hgb. Monitor liver functions, especially with long-term therapy.
- Monitor for and report signs of neuroleptic malignant syndrome (see Appendix F).
- Monitor for sedation and vertigo, especially at the beginning of therapy and following dosage increases. Supervision of ambulation may be indicated.
- Notify physician of fever and complaints of sore throat since these may indicated need to rule out adverse hematologic changes.

Patient & Family Education

- Do not take nonprescribed drugs or discontinue therapy without consent of physician. Abrupt discontinuation may cause nausea, headache, malaise, or seizures.
- Men should understand that the drug may cause impotence or ejaculation failure. Advise them to report this problem to physician.
- Report promptly a sore throat accompanied by fever.
- Use caution with ambulation until response to drug is known.
- Moderate alcohol intake since it may potentiate adverse drug effects.
- Do not breast feed while taking this drug.

CLONAZEPAM

(kloe-na'zi-pam)

Klonopin, Klonopin Wafers, Rivotril ♣

Classifications: CENTRAL NERVOUS SYSTEM AGENT; ANTICONVULSANT; BENZODIAZEPINE

Prototype: Diazepam

Pregnancy Category: C

Controlled Substance: Schedule IV

AVAILABILITY 0.5 mg, 1 mg, 2 mg tablets; 0.125 mg, 0.25 mg, 0.5 mg, 1 mg, and 2 mg orally disintegrating wafers

ACTIONS BENZODIAZEPINE derivative with strong anticonvulsant ac-

C

tivity and several other pharmacologic properties characteristic of the drug class.
THERAPEUTIC EFFECTS Suppresses spike and wave discharge in absence seizures (petit mal) and decreases amplitude, frequency, duration, and spread of discharge in minor motor seizures.

USES Alone or with other drugs in absence, myoclonic, and akinetic seizures, Lennox-Gastaut syndrome, absence seizures refractory to succinimides or valproic acid, and for infantile spasms and restless legs.
UNLABELED USES Panic disorder, complex partial seizure pattern, and generalized tonic-clonic convulsions.

CONTRAINDICATIONS Hypersensitivity to benzodiazepines; liver disease; acute narrow-angle glaucoma; pregnancy (category C), lactation.
CAUTIOUS USE Renal disease; COPD; drug-controlled open-angle glaucoma; addiction-prone individuals; children (because of unknown consequences of long-term use on growth and development); patient with mixed seizure disorders.

ROUTE & DOSAGE

Seizures

Adult: **PO** 1.5 mg/d in 3 divided doses, increased by 0.5–1 mg q3d until seizures are controlled or until intolerable adverse effects (max recommended dose: 20 mg/d)
Child: **PO** *<10 y,* 0.01–0.03 mg/kg/d (not to exceed 0.05 mg/kg/d) in 3 divided doses; may increase by 0.25–0.5 mg q3d until seizures are controlled or until intolerable adverse effects (max recommended dose: 0.2 mg/kg/d)

Panic Disorders

Adult: **PO** 1–2 mg/d in divided doses (max: 4 mg/d)

ADMINISTRATION

Oral

- Give largest dose at bedtime if daily dose cannot be equally divided.
- Place wafer form on tongue to dissolve.
- If clonazepam is to replace a different anticonvulsant, verify whether or not the prior drug should be gradually tapered.
- Store in tightly closed container protected from light at 15°–30° C (59°–86° F) unless otherwise specified.

ADVERSE EFFECTS (≥1%) **CV:** Palpitations. **GI:** Dry mouth, sore gums, anorexia, coated tongue, increased salivation, increased appetite, nausea, constipation, diarrhea. **Hematologic** Anemia, leukopenia, thrombocytopenia, eosinophilia. **CNS:** *Drowsiness, sedation, ataxia,* insomnia, aphonia, choreiform movements, coma, dysarthria, "glassy-eyed" appearance, headache, hemiparesis, hypotonia, slurred speech, tremor, vertigo, confusion, depression, hallucinations, aggressive behavior problems, hysteria, suicide attempt. **Respiratory:** Chest congestion, respiratory depression, rhinorrhea, dyspnea, hypersecretion in upper respiratory passages. **Skin:** Hirsutism, hair loss, skin rash, ankle and facial edema. **Special Senses:** Diplopia, nystagmus, abnormal eye movements. **Urogenital:** Increased libido, dysuria, enuresis, nocturia, urinary retention.

DIAGNOSTIC TEST INTERFERENCE Clonazepam causes transient elevations of ***serum transaminase*** and ***alkaline phosphatase.***

INTERACTIONS Drug: Alcohol and other CNS DEPRESSANTS increase sedation and CNS depression; may increase **phenytoin** levels. **Herbal: Kava-kava, valerian** may potentiate sedation.

PHARMACOKINETICS Absorption: Readily absorbed from GI tract. **Onset:** 60 min. **Peak:** 1–2 h. **Duration:** Up to 12 h in adults; 6–8 h in children. **Distribution:** Crosses placenta; distributed into breast milk. **Metabolism:** Metabolized in liver. **Elimination:** Excreted in urine primarily as metabolites. **Half-Life:** 18–40 h.

NURSING IMPLICATIONS

Assessment & Drug Effects

- Monitor I&O ratio and patterns: Excess accumulation of metabolites due to impaired excretion leads to toxicity.
- Assess carefully for signs of overdosage or drug interaction, i.e., increased depressant adverse effects, if multiple anticonvulsants are being given.
- Lab tests: Periodic liver function tests, platelet counts, blood counts, and renal function tests.
- Watch patient to see that he or she does not cheek the tablet. Both psychological and physical dependence may occur in the patient on long-term, high-dose therapy. Limit availability of large amounts of drug in the addiction-prone individual.
- Monitor for S&S of overdose, including somnolence, confusion, irritability, sweating, muscle and abdominal cramps, diminished reflexes, coma.

Patient & Family Education

- Report loss of seizure control promptly. Anticonvulsant activity is often lost after 3 mo of therapy; dosage adjustment may reestablish efficacy.
- Do not abruptly discontinue this drug. Abrupt withdrawal can precipitate seizures. Other withdrawal symptoms include convulsion, tremor, abdominal and muscle cramps, vomiting, sweating.
- Take drug as prescribed and do not alter dosing regimen without consulting physician.
- Do not self-medicate with OTC drugs before consulting the physician.
- Do not drive a car or engage in other activities requiring mental alertness and physical coordination until reaction to the drug is known. Drowsiness occurs in approximately 50% of patients.
- Carry identification (e.g., Medic Alert) bearing information about medication in use and the diagnosis.
- Do not breast feed while taking this drug.

CLONIDINE HYDROCHLORIDE

(kloe′ni-deen)

Catapres, Catapres-TTS, Dixaril ♦, Duraclon

Classifications: CARDIOVASCULAR AGENT; CENTRAL-ACTING ANTIHYPERTENSIVE; ANALGESIC

Prototype: Methyldopa

Pregnancy Category: C

AVAILABILITY 0.1 mg, 0.2 mg, 0.3 mg tablets; 0.1 mg/24 h, 0.2 mg/24 h; 0.3 mg/24 h transdermal patch; 100 mcg/mL, 500 mcg/mL injection

ACTIONS Centrally acting antiadrenergic derivative. Stimulates $alpha_2$-adrenergic receptors in CNS to inhibit sympathetic vasomotor centers. Central actions reduce plasma concentrations of norepinephrine.

It decreases systolic and diastolic BP and heart rate. Orthostatic effects tend to be mild and occur infrequently. Also inhibits renin release from kidneys.

THERAPEUTIC EFFECTS Decreases systolic and diastolic BP and heart rate. Orthostatic effects tend to be mild and occur infrequently. Reportedly minimizes or eliminates many of the common clinical S&S associated with withdrawal of heroin, methadone, or other opiates.

USES Step 2 drug in stepped-care approach to treatment of hypertension, either alone or with diuretic or other antihypertensive agents. Epidural administration as adjunct therapy for severe pain.

UNLABELED USES Prophylaxis for migraine; treatment of dysmenorrhea, menopausal flushing, diarrhea, paroxysmal localized hyperhidroses; alcohol, smoking, opiate, and benzodiazepine withdrawal; in the clonidine suppression test for diagnosis of pheochromocytoma; Gilles de la Tourette syndrome; attention deficit disorder with hyperactivity (ADDH) in children.

CONTRAINDICATIONS Pregnancy (category C), lactation. Use of clonidine patch in polyarteritis nodosa, scleroderma, SLE.

CAUTIOUS USE Severe coronary insufficiency, recent MI, sinus node dysfunction, cerebrovascular disease; chronic renal failure; Raynaud's disease, thromboangiitis obliterans; history of mental depression.

ROUTE & DOSAGE

Hypertension

Adult: **PO** 0.1 mg b.i.d. or t.i.d., may increase by 0.1–0.2 mg/d until desired response is achieved (max: 2.4 mg/d) **Transdermal** 0.1 mg patch once q7d, may increase by 0.1 mg q1–2 wk
Geriatric: **PO** Start with 0.1 mg once daily
Child: **PO** 5–10 mcg/kg/d divided q8–12h, may increase to 5–25 mcg/kg/d divided q6h (max: 0.9 mg/d)

Severe Pain

Adult: **Epidural** start infusion at 30 mcg/h and titrate to response. Use rates >40 mcg/h with caution
Child: **Epidural** start infusion at 0.5 mcg/kg/h and titrate to response

ADDH

Child: **PO** 5 mcg/kg/d in 4 divided doses (average dose, 0.15–0.2 mg/d) **Transdermal** 0.2–0.3 mg/d q5–7d

ADMINISTRATION

- Give last PO dose immediately before patient retires to ensure overnight BP control and to minimize daytime drowsiness.
- Oral dosage is increased gradually over a period of weeks so as not to lower BP abruptly (especially important in the older adult). Follow-up visits should be scheduled every 2–4 wk until BP stabilizes, then every 2–4 mo.
- Apply transdermal patch to dry skin, free of hair and rash. Avoid irritated, abraded, or scarred skin. Recommended areas for applying transdermal patch are upper outer arm and anterior chest. Less drug is absorbed from thighs. Rotate application sites and keep a record.
- During change from PO clonidine to transdermal system, PO clonidine should be maintained for at least 24 h after patch is applied. Consult physician.

- Do not abruptly discontinue drug. It should be withdrawn over a period of 2–4 d. Abrupt withdrawal resembles sympathetic stimulation and may result in restlessness and headache 2–3 h after a missed dose and a hypertensive crisis within 8–18 h.
- Store in tightly closed container at 15°–30° C (59°–86° F) unless otherwise directed.

ADVERSE EFFECTS (≥1%) **CV:** *Hypotension (epidural),* postural hypotension (mild), peripheral edema, ECG changes, tachycardia, bradycardia, flushing, rapid increase in BP with abrupt withdrawal. **GI:** *Dry mouth, constipation,* abdominal pain, pseudo-obstruction of large bowel, altered taste, nausea, vomiting, hepatitis, hyperbilirubinemia, weight gain (sodium retention). **CNS:** *Drowsiness, sedation,* dizziness, headache, fatigue, weakness, sluggishness, dyspnea, vivid dreams, nightmares, insomnia, behavior changes, agitation, hallucination, nervousness, restlessness, anxiety, mental depression. **Skin:** Rash, pruritus, thinning of hair, exacerbation of psoriasis; with transdermal patch: hyperpigmentation, recurrent herpes simplex, skin irritation, contact dermatitis, mild erythema. **Special Senses:** Dry eyes. **Urogenital:** Impotence, loss of libido.

DIAGNOSTIC TEST INTERFERENCE Possibility of decreased urinary excretion of ***aldosterone, catecholamines,*** and ***VMA*** (however, sudden withdrawal of clonidine may cause increases in these values); transient increases in ***blood glucose;*** weakly positive ***direct antiglobulin (Coombs') tests.***

INTERACTIONS Drug: Alcohol and other CNS DEPRESSANTS add to CNS depression; TRICYCLIC ANTIDEPRESSANTS may reduce antihypertensive effects. OPIATE ANALGESICS increase hypotension with epidural clonidine. Increased risk of bradycardia or AV block when epidural clonidine is used with **digoxin,** CALCIUM CHANNEL BLOCKERS, or BETA-BLOCKERS.

PHARMACOKINETICS Absorption: Readily absorbed from GI tract. **Onset:** 30–60 min PO; 1–3 d transdermal. **Peak:** 2–4 h PO; 2–3 d transdermal. **Duration:** 8 h PO; 7 d transdermal. **Distribution:** Widely distributed; crosses blood–brain barrier; not known if crosses placenta or distributed into breast milk. **Metabolism:** Metabolized in liver. **Elimination:** 80% excreted in urine, 20% in feces. **Half-Life:** 6–20 h.

NURSING IMPLICATIONS

Assessment & Drug Effects

- Monitor BR closely. Determine positional changes (supine, sitting, standing).
- With epidural administration, frequently monitor BP and HR. Hypotension is a common side effect that may require intervention.
- Monitor BP closely whenever a drug is added to or withdrawn from therapeutic regimen.
- Monitor I&O during period of dosage adjustment. Report change in I&O ratio or change in voiding pattern.
- Determine weight daily. Patients not receiving a concomitant diuretic agent may gain weight, particularly during first 3 or 4 d of therapy, because of marked sodium and water retention.
- Supervise closely patients with history of mental depression, as they may be subject to further depressive episodes.

Patient & Family Education

- Although postural hypotension occurs infrequently, make position changes slowly, and in stages, particularly from recumbent to upright position, and dangle and move legs a few minutes before standing. Lie down immediately if faintness or dizziness occurs.
- Avoid potentially hazardous activities until reaction to drug has been determined due to possible sedative effects.
- Do not omit doses or stop the drug without consulting the physician.
- Do not take OTC medications, alcohol, or other CNS depressants without prior discussion with physician.
- Examine site when transdermal patch is removed and report to physician if erythema, rash, irritation, or hyperpigmentation occurs.
- If transdermal patch loosens, tape it in place with adhesive. The patch should never be cut or trimmed.
- Do not breast feed while taking this drug.

CLOPIDOGREL BISULFATE

(clo-pi'do-grel)
Plavix
Classifications: BLOOD FORMERS, COAGULATORS, AND ANTICOAGULANTS; ANTIPLATELET AGENT
Prototype: Ticlopidine
Pregnancy Category: B

AVAILABILITY 75 mg tablets

ACTIONS Inhibits platelet aggregation by selectively preventing the binding of adenosine diphosphate to its platelet receptor. It is an analog of ticlopidine. The drug's effect on the adenosine diphosphate receptor of a platelet is irreversible.

THERAPEUTIC EFFECTS Consequently, clopidrogrel prolongs bleeding time.

USES Secondary prevention of MI, stroke, and vascular death in patients with recent MI, stroke, unstable angina or established peripheral arterial disease.

UNLABELED USE Reduction of restenosis after stent placement.

CONTRAINDICATIONS Hypersensitivity to clopidogrel; intracranial hemorrhage, peptic ulcer, or any other active pathologic bleeding; pregnancy (category B). Discontinue clopidogrel 7 days before surgery and during lactation. Safety and efficacy not established in children.

CAUTIOUS USE Concurrent use with drugs that might induce gastrointestinal bleeding; GI bleeding; hepatic impairment (moderate to severe); patients at risk for increased bleeding.

ROUTE & DOSAGE

Secondary Prevention
Adult: **PO** 75 mg q.d.

ADMINISTRATION

Oral

- Do not administer to persons with active pathologic bleeding.
- Discontinue drug 7 d prior to surgery.
- Store at 15°–30° C (59°–86° F) in tightly closed container and protect from light.

ADVERSE EFFECTS (≥1%) **Body as a Whole:** Flu-like syndrome, fatigue, pain, arthralgia, back pain. **CV:** Chest pain, edema, hypertension. **GI:** Abdominal pain, dyspepsia, diarrhea, nausea, hypercholesterolemia. **Hematologic:** Thrombotic thrombocytopenic purpura, epistaxis. **CNS:** Headache, dizziness, depression. **Respiratory:** URI, dyspnea, rhinitis, bronchitis, cough. **Skin:** Rash, pruritus.

INTERACTIONS Drug: NSAIDS may increase risk of bleeding events. **Herbal: Feverfew, garlic, ginger, ginkgo** may increase risk of bleeding.

PHARMACOKINETICS Absorption: Rapidly absorbed from GI tract. **Onset:** 2 h; reaches steady state in 3–7 d. **Distribution:** 94–98% protein bound. **Metabolism:** Rapidly hydrolyzed in plasma to active metabolite. **Elimination:** 50% excreted in urine and 50% in feces. **Half-Life:** 8 h.

NURSING IMPLICATIONS

Assessment & Drug Effects

- Carefully monitor for and immediately report S&S of GI bleeding, especially when coadministered with NSAIDS, aspirin, heparin, or warfarin.
- Lab tests: Periodic platelet count and lipid profile.
- Evaluate patients with unexplained fever or infection for myelotoxicity.

Patient & Family Education

- Report promptly any unusual bleeding (e.g., black, tarry stools).
- Avoid chronic aspirin or NSAID use unless approved by physician.
- Do not breast feed while taking this drug.

CLORAZEPATE DIPOTASSIUM

(klor-az′e-pate)

Novoclopate ✦, Tranxene, Tranxene-SD

Classifications: CENTRAL NERVOUS SYSTEM AGENT; ANXIOLYTIC; SEDATIVE-HYPNOTIC; ANTICONVULSANT; BENZODIAZEPINE

Prototype: Lorazepam

Pregnancy Category: D

Controlled Substance: Schedule IV

AVAILABILITY 3.75 mg, 7.5 mg, 15 mg capsules and tablets; 11.25 mg, 22.5 mg long acting tablets

ACTIONS Anxiolytic qualitatively similar to lorazepam. It has depressant effects on the CNS, thus controlling anxiety associated with stress.

THERAPEUTIC EFFECTS Effective in controlling anxiety and withdrawal symptoms of alcohol.

USES Management of anxiety disorders, short-term relief of anxiety symptoms, as adjunct in management of partial seizures, and symptomatic relief of acute alcohol withdrawal.

CONTRAINDICATIONS Hypersensitivity to clorazepate and other benzodiazepines; acute narrow-angle glaucoma; depressive neuroses, psychotic reactions, drug abusers. Safe use during pregnancy (category D), lactation, and in children <9 y not established.

CAUTIOUS USE Older adults; debilitated patients; hepatic disease; kidney disease.

ROUTE & DOSAGE

Anxiety

Adult: **PO** 15 mg/d h.s., may increase to 15–60 mg/d in divided doses (max: 60 mg/d)

C

Acute Alcohol Withdrawal

Adult: **PO** 30 mg followed by 30–60 mg in divided doses (max: 90 mg/d), taper by 15 mg/d over 4 d to 7.5–15 mg/d until patient is stable

Partial Seizures

Adult: **PO** 7.5 mg t.i.d.
Child: 9–12 y: **PO** 3.75–7.5 mg b.i.d., may increase by no more than 3.75 mg/wk (max: 60 mg/d)

ADMINISTRATION

Oral

- Give with food to minimize gastric distress. Give antacid no less than 1 h before or 1 h after drug ingestion.
- Ensure that sustained-release form of drug is not chewed or crushed. It must be swallowed whole.
- Taper drug dose gradually over several days when drug is to be discontinued. Abrupt termination may lead to memory impairment, severe GI symptoms, muscle pain, restlessness, irritability, fatigue, insomnia.
- Store in light-resistant container at 15°–30° C (59°–86° F) unless otherwise specified.

ADVERSE EFFECTS (≥1%) **Body as a Whole:** Allergic reactions. **CV:** Hypotension. **GI:** GI disturbances, abnormal liver function tests, xerostomia. **Hematologic:** Decreased Hct, blood dyscrasias. **CNS:** *Drowsiness,* ataxia, dizziness, headache, paradoxical excitement, mental confusion, insomnia. **Special Senses:** diplopia, blurred vision.

INTERACTIONS Drug: Alcohol and other CNS DEPRESSANTS compound CNS depression; clorazepate increases effects of **cimetidine, disulfiram,** causing excessive sedation. **Herbal: Ginkgo** may decrease anticonvulsant effectiveness.

PHARMACOKINETICS Absorption: Decarboxylated in stomach; absorbed as active metabolite, desmethyldiazepam. **Peak:** 1 h. **Duration:** 24 h. **Distribution:** Crosses placenta; distributed into breast milk. **Metabolism:** Metabolized in liver to oxazepam. **Elimination:** Excreted primarily in urine. **Half-Life:** 30–200 h.

NURSING IMPLICATIONS

Assessment & Drug Effects

- Drowsiness, a common side effect, is more likely to occur at initiation of therapy and with dose increments on successive days.
- Lab tests: Periodic blood counts and tests of liver and kidney function should be performed throughout therapy.
- Monitor patient with history of cardiovascular disease in early therapy for drug-induced responses. If systolic BP drops more than 20 mm Hg or if there is a sudden increase in pulse rate, withhold drug and notify physician.

Patient & Family Education

- Take drug as prescribed and do not change dose or abruptly stop taking the drug without physician's approval.
- Do not self-dose with OTC drugs (cold remedies, sleep medications, antacids) without consulting physician.
- Avoid driving and other potentially hazardous activities until reaction to drug is known.
- Do not use alcohol and other CNS depressants while on clorazepate therapy.

- If a woman becomes pregnant during therapy or intends to become pregnant, communicate with physician about the desirability of discontinuing the drug.
- Do not breast feed while taking this drug.

CLOTRIMAZOLE

(kloe-trim'a-zole)

Canesten ♣, Gyne-Lotrimin, Gyne-Lotrimin-3, Lotrimin, Mycelex, Mycelex-G

Classifications: ANTIINFECTIVE; ANTIBIOTIC; ANTIFUNGAL

Prototype: Fluconazole

Pregnancy Category: B (topical) C (oral)

AVAILABILITY 1% cream, solution, lotion; 10 mg troches; 100 mg, 200 mg, 500 mg vaginal tablets; 1% vaginal cream

ACTIONS Has broad-spectrum fungicidal activity. Acts by altering fungal cell membrane permeability, permitting loss of phosphorous compounds, potassium, and other essential intracellular constituents with consequent loss of ability to replicate.

THERAPEUTIC EFFECTS Active against *Trichophyton rubrum, Trichophyton mentagrophytes, Epidermophyton floccosum, Microsporum canis, Malassezia furfur,* and *Candida sp,* including *Candida albicans*. Natural or acquired fungal resistance to clotrimazole is rare.

USES Dermal infections including tinea pedis, tinea cruris, tinea corporis, tinea versicolor; also vulvovaginal and oropharyngeal candidiasis.

UNLABELED USE Trichomoniasis.

CONTRAINDICATIONS Ophthalmic uses; systemic mycoses. Safe use during pregnancy (category C for oral troches, category B for topical preparations), lactation, and in children <3 y not established.

CAUTIOUS USE Hepatic impairment.

ROUTE & DOSAGE

Dermal Infections

Adult: **Topical** Apply small amount onto affected areas b.i.d. a.m. and p.m.

Vulvovaginal Infections

Adult: **Intravaginal** Insert 1 applicator full or one 100 mg vaginal tablet into vagina at bedtime for 7 d, or one 500 mg vaginal tablet at bedtime for 1 dose

Oropharyngeal Candidiasis

Adult/Child: **PO** 1 troche (lozenge) 5 times/d q3h for 14 d

ADMINISTRATION

- Instruct patient taking the oral lozenge to allow it to dissolve slowly in mouth over 15–30 min for maximum effectiveness.
- Apply skin cream and solution preparations sparingly. Protect hands with latex gloves when applying medication.
- Avoid contact of clotrimazole preparations with the eyes.
- Do not use occlusive dressings unless directed by physician to do so.
- Consult physician about skin cleansing procedure before applying medication. Regardless of procedure used, dry skin thoroughly.
- Store cream and solution formulations at 15°–30° C (59°–86° F); do not store troches or vaginal tablets above 35° C (95° F) unless otherwise directed.

C

ADVERSE EFFECTS (≥1%) **GI:** Abnormal liver function tests; occasional nausea and vomiting (with oral troche). **Skin:** Stinging, erythema, edema, vesication, desquamation, pruritus, urticaria, skin fissures. **Urogenital:** Mild burning sensation, lower abdominal cramps, bloating, cystitis, urethritis, mild urinary frequency, vulval erythema and itching, pain and vaginal soreness during intercourse.

INTERACTIONS Drug: Intravaginal preparations may inactivate SPERMICIDES.

PHARMACOKINETICS Absorption: Minimal systemic absorption; minimally absorbed topically. **Peak:** High saliva concentrations <3 h; high vaginal concentrations in 8–24 h. **Metabolism:** Metabolized in liver. **Elimination:** Eliminated as metabolite in bile.

NURSING IMPLICATIONS

Assessment & Drug Effects

- Evaluate effectiveness of treatment. Report any signs of skin irritation with dermal preparations.
- Anticipate signs of clinical improvement within the first week of drug use.

Patient & Family Education

- Use clotrimazole as directed and for the length of time prescribed by physician.
- Generally, clinical improvement is apparent during first week of therapy. Report to physician if condition worsens or if signs of irritation or sensitivity develop, or if no improvement is noted after 4 wk of therapy.
- If receiving the drug vaginally, your sexual partner may experience burning and irritation of penis or urethritis; refrain from sexual intercourse during therapy or have sexual partner wear a condom.
- Do not breast feed while taking this drug.

CLOXACILLIN, SODIUM

(klox-a-sill'in)

Apo-Cloxi ✦, Cloxapen, Cloxilean, Novocloxin ✦, Orbenin, Tegopen

Classifications: ANTIINFECTIVE; ANTIBIOTIC, NATURAL PENICILLIN; BETA-LACTAM

Prototype: Penicillin G

Pregnancy Category: B

AVAILABILITY 250 mg, 500 mg capsules; 125 mg/5 mL oral suspension

ACTIONS Semisynthetic, acid-stable, penicillinase-resistant, isoxazolyl penicillin. Effective against most gram-positive bacteria.

THERAPEUTIC EFFECTS In common with other isoxazolyl penicillins (dicloxacillin, oxacillin), highly active against most penicillinase-producing staphylococci, less potent than penicillin G against penicillin-sensitive microorganisms, and generally ineffective against gram-negative bacteria and methicillin-resistant staphylococci (MRSA).

USES Primarily in infections caused by penicillinase-producing staphylococci and penicillin-resistant staphylococci. May be used to initiate therapy in suspected staphylococcal infections pending culture and susceptibility test results. As with other penicillins, serum concentrations are enhanced by concurrent use of probenecid.

CONTRAINDICATIONS Sensitivity to penicillins; pregnancy (category

B), lactation. Safe use in neonates not established.

CAUTIOUS USE History of or suspected atopy or allergy (asthma, eczema, hives, hay fever), renal or hepatic function impairment, history of allergy to cephalosporins.

ROUTE & DOSAGE

Mild to Moderate Infections
Adult: **PO** 250–500 mg q6h
Child: **PO** <20 kg: 12.5–25 mg/kg q6h (max: 4 g/d)

ADMINISTRATION

Oral

- Give on an empty stomach (at least 1 h before or 2 h after meals) unless otherwise advised by physician. Food reduces rate and extent of drug absorption.
- After reconstitution PO solution retains potency for 14 d if refrigerated (shake well before pouring).
- Unless otherwise advised, store capsules at 15°–30° C (59°–86° F).

ADVERSE EFFECTS (≥1%) **Body as a Whole:** Wheezing, sneezing, chills, drug fever, anaphylaxis, superinfections. **GI:** *Nausea,* vomiting, flatulence, *diarrhea.* **Hematologic:** Eosinophilia, leukopenia, agranulocytosis. **Metabolic:** Elevated AST, ALT; jaundice (possibly of allergic etiology). **Skin:** Pruritus, urticaria, rash.

INTERACTIONS Drug: Probenecid decreases cloxacillin elimination.

PHARMACOKINETICS Absorption: 37–60% absorbed from GI tract. **Peak:** 0.5–2 h. **Duration:** 4–6 h. **Distribution:** Distributed throughout body with highest concentrations in liver, kidney, spleen, bone, bile, and pleural fluid; low CSF penetration; crosses placenta; distributed into breast milk. **Metabolism:** Metabolized in liver. **Elimination:** Excreted primarily in urine with some elimination through bile. **Half-Life:** 30–60 min.

NURSING IMPLICATIONS

Assessment & Drug Effects

- Determine previous exposure and sensitivity to penicillins and cephalosporins and other allergic reactions of any kind before treatment is initiated.
- Monitor for S&S of anaphylactoid reaction (see Appendix G) or other signs or symptoms of hypersensitivity reaction (see Appendix F) as with other penicillins.
- Lab tests: Periodic assessments of renal, hepatic, and hematopoietic function are advised in patients on long-term therapy.

Patient & Family Education

- Take medication around the clock, do not miss a dose, and continue taking the medication until it is finished.
- Report to physician the onset of hypersensitivity reaction (see Appendix F) and superinfections.
- Check with physician if GI adverse effects (nausea, vomiting, diarrhea) appear.
- Do not breast feed while taking this drug.

CLOZAPINE (Pr)

(clo′za-pin)

Clozaril, Fazaclo

Classifications: CENTRAL NERVOUS SYSTEM (CNS) AGENT; PSYCHOTHERAPEUTIC AGENT; ANTIPSYCHOTIC; ATYPICAL

Prototype: Clozapine

Pregnancy Category: B

C

AVAILABILITY 25 mg, 100 mg tablets and orally disintegrating tablets

ACTIONS Mechanism is not defined. Interferes with binding of dopamine to D_1 and D_2 receptors in the limbic region of brain. It binds primarily to nondopaminergic sites (e.g., alpha-adrenergic, serotonergic, and cholinergic receptors).

THERAPEUTIC EFFECTS Utilized for treatment of schizophrenia uncontrolled by other agents.

USE Indicated only in the management of severely ill schizophrenic patients who have failed to respond to other neuroleptic agents.

CONTRAINDICATIONS Severe CNS depression, blood dyscrasia, history of bone marrow depression; patients with myeloproliferative disorders, uncontrolled epilepsy; clozapine-induced agranulocytosis, severe granulocytosis, chemotherapy, coma, leukemia, leukopenia, neutropenia, myocarditis, concurrent administration of benzodiazepines or other psychotropic drugs; renal failure, dialysis, hepatitis, jaundice; infants, lactation.

CAUTIOUS USE Arrhythmias, GI disorders, narrow-angle glaucoma, hepatic and renal impairment, prostatic hypertrophy, history of seizures; patients with cardiovascular and/or pulmonary disease; cerebrovascular disease, cardiac arrhythmias, tachycardia, dehydration, neurological disease, tardive dyskinesia, previous history of agranulocytosis; surgery, glaucoma, infection, pregnancy (category B); older adults. Safety and efficacy in children have not been established.

ROUTE & DOSAGE

Schizophrenia
Adult: **PO** *>16 y:* Initiate at 25–50 mg/d and titrate to a target dose of 350–450 mg/d in 3 divided doses at 2 wk intervals, further increases can be made if necessary, max of 900 mg/d

ADMINISTRATION

Oral
- Drug is usually withdrawn gradually over 1–2 wk if therapy must be discontinued.
- Store the drug away from heat or light.

ADVERSE EFFECTS (≥1%) **CV:** Orthostatic hypotension, *tachycardia,* ECG changes, increased risk of myocarditis especially during first month of therapy, pericarditis, pericardial effusion, cardiomyopathy, heart failure, MI, mitral insufficiency. **GI:** Nausea, dry mouth, constipation, hypersalivation. **Hematologic:** Agranulocytosis. **CNS:** Seizures, *transient fever,* sedation, neuroleptic malignant syndrome (rare), dystonic reactions (rare). **Metabolic:** Hyperglycemia, diabetes mellitus. **Urogenital:** Urinary retention.

INTERACTIONS Drug: Alcohol and other CNS DEPRESSANTS compound depressant effects; ANTICHOLINERGIC AGENTS potentiate anticholinergic effects; ANTIHYPERTENSIVE AGENTS may potentiate hypotension.

PHARMACOKINETICS Absorption: Readily absorbed from GI tract. **Onset:** 2–4 wk. **Peak:** 2.5 h. **Distribution:** Possibly distributed into breast milk. **Metabolism:** Metabolized in liver. **Elimination:** 50% excreted in urine, 30% in feces. **Half-Life:** 8–12 h.

NURSING IMPLICATIONS

Assessment & Drug Effects

- Lab tests: Baseline WBC and differential count must be made before initial treatment, every week for first 6 mo, then every 2 wk for next 6 mo, and for 4 wk after the drug is discontinued. Periodically monitor blood glucose.
- Monitor diabetics for loss of glycemic control.
- Monitor for seizure activity; seizure potential increases at the higher dose level.
- Closely monitor for recurrence of psychotic symptoms if the drug is being discontinued.
- Monitor cardiovascular status, especially during the first month of therapy. Report promptly S&S of CHF and other potential cardiac problems.
- Monitor for development of tachycardia or hypotension, which may pose a serious risk for patients with compromised cardiovascular function.
- Monitor daily temperature and report fever. Transient elevation above 38° C (100.4° F), with peak incidence during first 3 wk of drug therapy, may occur.

Patient & Family Education

- Carefully monitor blood glucose levels if diabetic.
- Do not engage in any hazardous activity until response to the drug is known. Drowsiness and sedation are common adverse effects.
- Due to the risk of agranulocytosis (see Appendix F) it is important to comply with blood test regimen. Report flulike symptoms, fever, sore throat, lethargy, malaise, or other signs of infection.
- Rise slowly to avoid orthostatic hypotension.
- Report immediately any of the following: unexplained fatigue, especially with activity; shortness of breath, sudden weight gain or edema of the lower extremities.
- Take drug exactly as ordered.
- Do not use OTC drugs or alcohol without permission of physician.
- Do not breast feed while taking clozapine.

COCAINE

(koe-kane′)

COCAINE HYDROCHLORIDE

Classifications: CENTRAL NERVOUS SYSTEM AGENT; ANESTHETIC, LOCAL
Prototype: Procaine
Pregnancy Category: C
Controlled Substance: Schedule II

AVAILABILITY 4%, 10% topical solution

ACTIONS Alkaloid obtained from leaves of *Erythroxylon coca*. Topical application blocks nerve conduction and produces surface anesthesia accompanied by local vasoconstriction. Exerts adrenergic effect by potentiating action of endogenous (and injected) epinephrine and norepinephrine, possibly by inhibiting reuptake of catecholamines into sympathetic nerve terminals.

THERAPEUTIC EFFECTS Systemic absorption produces descending CNS stimulation, with intense, short-lived euphoria accompanied by indifference to pain or hunger and with illusions of great strength, endurance, and mental capacity, all the basis for drug abuse.

USES Surface anesthesia of ear, nose, throat, rectum, and vagina. Ophthalmic use largely abandoned because of its tendency to cause corneal sloughing. Sometimes used as ingredient in Brompton's cocktail.

CONTRAINDICATIONS Hypersensitivity to local anesthetics; sepsis in region of proposed application; pregnancy (category C), lactation. **CAUTIOUS USE** History of drug sensitivities, history of drug abuse.

ROUTE & DOSAGE

Surface Anesthesia

Adult: **Topical** 1–10% solution (use >4% solution with caution), max single dose of 1 mg/kg

ADMINISTRATION

Topical

- Exercise caution to ensure that drug is taken as prescribed.
- Preserve in tightly closed, light-resistant containers.

ADVERSE EFFECTS (≥1%) **Body as a Whole:** Formication ("cocaine bugs"), hypersensitivity reactions. **CV:** Tachycardia, ventricular fibrillation, MI, angina pectoris. **GI:** Nausea, vomiting, anorexia, abdominal pain. **CNS:** *CNS stimulation* and CNS depression (respiratory and circulatory failure). **Respiratory:** pneumonia, lung damage (chronic cocaine smoking). **Special Senses:** Runny nose, perforated nasal septum; clouding, pitting, and ulceration of cornea.

INTERACTIONS Drug: Epinephrine entails risk of severe hypertension and arrhythmias; MAO INHIBITORS potentiate pharmacologic effects of cocaine.

PHARMACOKINETICS Absorption: Readily absorbed from mucous membranes; absorption limited by vasoconstriction. **Onset:** 1 min. **Peak:** 15–120 min. **Duration:** 30 min–2 h. **Distribution:** Crosses placenta; distributed into breast milk. **Metabolism:** Hydrolyzed in serum. **Elimination:** Excreted in urine; detectable for up to 30 h. **Half-Life:** 1–2.5 h.

NURSING IMPLICATIONS

Assessment & Drug Effects

- When used for anesthesia of throat, cocaine causes temporary paralysis of cilia of respiratory tract cells, reducing protection against aspiration. It also may interfere with pharyngeal stage of swallowing. Give nothing by mouth until sensation returns.
- Monitor cardiovascular status, especially in patients with known cardiac disease. Report promptly cardiac arrhythmias.

Patient & Family Education

- Promptly report angina or chest pain or respiratory distress.
- Do not breast feed while taking this drug.

CODEINE

(koe′deen)

CODEINE PHOSPHATE

Paveral ♣

CODEINE SULFATE

Classifications: CENTRAL NERVOUS SYSTEM AGENT; NARCOTIC (OPIATE) AGONIST ANALGESIC; ANTITUSSIVE
Prototype: Morphine
Pregnancy Category: C
Controlled Substance: Schedule II

AVAILABILITY 15 mg, 30 mg, 60 mg tablets; 15 mg/5 mL oral solution; 30 mg, 60 mg injection

ACTIONS Opium derivative similar to morphine. In equianalgesic doses, parenteral codeine produces degree of respiratory depression similar to that of morphine. In contrast to morphine, orally administered codeine is about 60% as potent as the parenteral form. Histamine-releasing action appears to be more potent than that of morphine and may result in hypotension, flushing, and rarely bronchoconstriction.

THERAPEUTIC EFFECTS Analgesic potency is about one-sixth that of morphine; antitussive activity is also a little less than that of morphine.

USES Symptomatic relief of mild to moderately severe pain when control cannot be obtained by nonnarcotic analgesics and to suppress hyperactive or nonproductive cough.

CONTRAINDICATIONS Hypersensitivity to codeine or other morphine derivatives; acute asthma, COPD; increased intracranial pressure, head injury, acute alcoholism, hepatic or renal dysfunction, hypothyroidism. Pregnancy (category C), lactation. Safe use in neonates not established.

CAUTIOUS USE Prostatic hypertrophy, debilitated patients, very young and very old patients; history of drug abuse.

ROUTE & DOSAGE

Analgesic

Adult: **PO/IM/SC** 15–60 mg q.i.d.
Child: **PO/IM/SC** 0.5–1 mg/kg q4–6h prn (max: 60 mg/dose)

Antitussive

Adult: **PO** 10–20 mg q4–6h prn (max: 120 mg/24h)
Child: **PO** *6–12 y:* 5–10 mg q4–6h (max: 60 mg/24 h); *2–6 y:* 2.5–5 mg q4–6h (max: 30 mg/24 h)

ADMINISTRATION

Oral

- Administer PO codeine with milk or other food to reduce possibility of GI distress.

Subcutaneous/Intramuscular

- Give parenterally to achieve greatest effectiveness. An oral dose is about 60% as effective as an equal parenteral dose.
- Preserve in tight, light-resistant containers at 15°–30° C (59°–86° F) unless otherwise directed.

ADVERSE EFFECTS (≥1%) **Body as a Whole:** Shortness of breath, anaphylactoid reaction. **CV:** Palpitation, hypotension, orthostatic hypotension, bradycardia, tachycardia, circulatory collapse. **GI:** *Nausea,* vomiting, *constipation.* **CNS:** *Dizziness,* light-headedness, *drowsiness,* sedation, lethargy, euphoria, agitation; restlessness, exhilaration, convulsions, narcosis, respiratory depression. **Skin:** Diffuse erythema, rash, urticaria, *pruritus,* excessive perspiration, facial flushing, fixed-drug eruption. **Special Senses:** Miosis. **Urogenital:** Urinary retention.

INTERACTIONS Drug: Alcohol and other CNS DEPRESSANTS augment CNS depressant effects. **Herbal: St. John's wort** may cause increase sedation.

PHARMACOKINETICS Absorption: Readily absorbed from GI tract. **Onset:** 15–30 min. **Peak:** 1–1.5 h. **Duration:** 4–6 h. **Distribution:** Crosses placenta; distributed into breast milk. **Metabolism:** Metabolized in liver. **Elimination:** Excreted in urine. **Half-Life:** 2.5–4 h.

C

NURSING IMPLICATIONS

Assessment & Drug Effects

- Record relief of pain and duration of analgesia.
- Evaluate effectiveness as cough suppressant. Treatment of cough is directed toward decreasing frequency and intensity of cough without abolishing cough reflex, need to remove bronchial secretions.
- Although codeine has less abuse liability than morphine, dependence is a major unwanted effect.
- Supervision of ambulation and use other safety precautions as warranted since drug may cause dizziness and light-headedness.
- Monitor for nausea, a common side effect. Report nausea accompanied by vomiting. Change to another analgesic may be warranted.

Patient & Family Education

- Make position changes slowly and in stages particularly from recumbent to upright posture. Lie down immediately if light-headedness or dizziness occurs.
- Lie down when feeling nauseated and to notify physician if this symptom persists. Nausea appears to be aggravated by ambulation.
- Avoid driving and other potentially hazardous activities until reaction to drug is known. Codeine may impair ability to perform tasks requiring mental alertness and therefore to.
- Do not take alcohol or other CNS depressants unless approved by physician.
- Hyperactive cough may be lessened by avoiding irritants such as smoking, dust, fumes, and other air pollutants. Humidification of ambient air may provide some relief.
- Do not breast feed while taking this drug.

COLCHICINE Pr

(kol'chi-seen)

Novocolchine ♣

Classification: ANTIGOUT AGENT

Pregnancy Category: C

AVAILABILITY 0.5 mg, 0.6 mg tablets; 0.5 mg/mL injection

ACTIONS Alkaloid of the plant *Colchicum autumnale* with antimitotic and indirect antiinflammatory properties.

THERAPEUTIC EFFECTS Inhibition of inflammation and reduction of pain and swelling which occurs in gouty arthritis. Colchicine is nonanalgesic and nonuricosuric. Tolerance to colchicine does not develop.

USES Prophylactically for recurrent gouty arthritis and for acute gout, either as single agent or in combination with a uricosuric such as probenecid, allopurinol, or sulfinpyrazone.

UNLABELED USES Sarcoid arthritis, chondrocalcinosis (pseudogout), arthritis associated with erythema nodosum, leukemia, adenocarcinoma, acute calcific tendonitis, familial Mediterranean fever, multiple sclerosis, primary biliary cirrhosis, mycosis fungoides, and in experimental studies of normal and abnormal cell division.

CONTRAINDICATIONS Blood dyscrasias; severe GI, renal, hepatic, or cardiac disease; use of IV colchicine in patients with both renal and hepatic dysfunction. Severe local irritation can result from SC or IM use. Pregnancy (category C), safe use in children not established.

CAUTIOUS USE Older adult and debilitated patients, lactation, early manifestations of GI, renal, hepatic, or cardiac disease.

C

ROUTE & DOSAGE

Acute Gouty Attack

Adult: **PO** 0.5–1.2 mg followed by 0.5–0.6 mg q1–2h until pain relief or intolerable GI symptoms (max: 4 mg/attack). **IV** 2 mg followed by 0.5 mg q6h until relief or intolerable GI symptoms (max: 4 mg/attack)

Prophylaxis

Adult: **PO** 0.5 or 0.6 mg every night or every other night as needed (up to 1.8 mg/d may be needed for severe cases). **IV** 0.5–1 mg 1–2 times/d

Surgical Patients

Adult: **PO** 0.5 or 0.6 mg t.i.d. starting 3 d before surgery and continuing for 3 d after surgery

Renal Impairment

Cl_{cr} 10–50 mL/min: prolonged use is not recommended. Cl_{cr} <10 mL/min: reduce recommended dose by 50%

ADMINISTRATION

Oral

- Administer oral drug with milk or food to reduce possibility of GI upset.

Intravenous

PREPARE: **Direct/Intermittent:** Dilute a single dose with NS without a bacteriostatic agent. Discard turbid solutions.

ADMINISTER: **Direct/Intermittent:** Give over 2–5 min by direct IV or into tubing of free-flowing IV with compatible fluid (not compatible with dextrose solutions).

- Care must be taken to prevent extravasation of IV colchicine because severe tissue irritation including nerve damage can result.

- Preserve in tight, light-resistant containers preferably between 15°–30° C (59°–86° F), unless otherwise directed by manufacturer.

ADVERSE EFFECTS (≥1%) **GI:** *Nausea, vomiting, diarrhea, abdominal pain,* anorexia, hemorrhagic gastroenteritis, steatorrhea, hepatotoxicity, pancreatitis. **Hematologic:** Neutropenia, bone marrow depression, thrombocytopenia, agranulocytosis, aplastic anemia. **CNS:** Mental confusion, peripheral neuritis, syndrome of muscle weakness (accompanied by elevated serum creatine kinase). **Skin:** Severe irritation and tissue damage if IV administration leaks around injection site. **Urogenital:** Azotemia, proteinuria, hematuria, oliguria.

DIAGNOSTIC TEST INTERFERENCE Possible interference with ***urinary steroid (17-OHCS)*** determinations when done by modifications of ***Reddy, Jenkins, Thorn procedure.*** False-positive ***urine tests for RBCs and Hgb*** reported.

INTERACTIONS Drug: May decrease intestinal absorption of vitamin B_{12}.

PHARMACOKINETICS Absorption: Rapidly absorbed from GI tract. **Peak:** 0.5–2 h; may have multiple peaks because of enterohepatic cycling. **Distribution:** Widely distributed; concentrates in leukocytes, kidney, liver, spleen, and intestinal tract. **Metabolism:** Partially metabolized in liver. **Elimination:** Primarily excreted in feces; 10–20% excreted in urine in 24 h.

NURSING IMPLICATIONS

Assessment & Drug Effects

- Lab tests: Baseline and periodic determinations of serum uric acid and creatinine are advised, as well as CBC, including Hgb, platelet count, serum electrolytes, and urinalysis.

- Monitor for dose-related adverse effects; they are most likely to occur during the initial course of treatment.
- Monitor for early signs of colchicine toxicity including weakness, abdominal discomfort, anorexia, nausea, vomiting, and diarrhea, regardless of administration route. Report to physician. To avoid more serious toxicity, drug should be discontinued promptly until symptoms subside.
- Monitor I&O ratio and pattern (during acute gouty attack): High fluid intake promotes excretion and reduces danger of crystal formation in kidneys and ureters.
- Keep physician informed of patient's progress. Drug should be stopped when pain of acute gout is relieved. Therapeutic response: articular pain and swelling generally subside within 8–12 h and usually disappear in 24–72 h after PO therapy, and 6–12 h after IV administration.

Patient & Family Education

- If taking colchicine at home, withhold drug and report to the physician the onset of GI symptoms or signs of bone marrow depression (nausea, sore throat, bleeding gums, sore mouth, fever, fatigue, malaise, unusual bleeding or bruising).
- Keep colchicine on hand at all times to start therapy or increase dosage, as prescribed by physician, at the first suggestion of an acute attack.
- Physician may prescribe sodium bicarbonate, or sodium or potassium citrate, to maintain alkaline urine and thus prevent formation of urate stones.
- Avoid fermented beverages such as beer, ale, and wine as they may precipitate gouty attack. The physician may allow distilled alcoholic beverages in moderation.
- Do not breast feed without consulting physician.

COLESEVELAM HYDROCHLORIDE

(co-less′e-ve-lam)

Welchol

Classifications: CARDIOVASCULAR AGENT; ANTILIPEMIC; BILE ACID SEQUESTRANT

Prototype: Cholestyramine Resin

Pregnancy Category: B

AVAILABILITY 625 mg tablets

ACTIONS Anion exchange resin used for its cholesterol-lowering effect. Binds with bile salts in the intestinal tract to form an insoluble complex that is excreted in the feces, thus reducing circulating cholesterol and increasing serum LDL removal rate. Serum triglyceride levels may increase slightly.

THERAPEUTIC EFFECTS Decreases serum LDL and total cholesterol level. Removes bile salts from the intestine.

USES Adjunctive therapy to diet and exercise for reduction of elevated LDL cholesterol alone or in combination with an HMG-CoA reductase inhibitor (statin).

CONTRAINDICATIONS Hypersensitivity to colesevelam; complete biliary obstruction; bowel obstruction; children <2 y of age.

CAUTIOUS USE Preexisting GI disorders or bowel disease, primary biliary cirrhosis, partial biliary obstruction, biliary atresia; hypertriglyceridemia; older adults, pregnancy (category B), lactation; malabsorption states; bleeding disorders.

ROUTE & DOSAGE

Hypercholesterolemia, Monotherapy
Adult: **PO** 3 tablets b.i.d. with meals or 6 tablets q.d. with a meal, may be increased to 7 tablets/d

Hypercholesterolemia, Combination Therapy
Adult: **PO** 4–6 tablets/d with meals or 6 tablets q.d. with a meal

ADMINISTRATION

Oral

- Give with meals (mandatory) and adequate liquid (e.g., 8 oz).
- Store at 15°–30° C (59°–86° F) with occasional fluctuations to 40° C (90° F); protect from moisture.

ADVERSE EFFECTS (≥1%) **Body as a Whole:** Infection, pain, flu-like syndrome, asthenia, myalgia. **CNS:** Headache. **GI:** Abdominal pain, *flatulence, constipation,* diarrhea, nausea, dyspepsia. **Respiratory:** Sinusitis, rhinitis, cough, pharyngitis.

INTERACTIONS Drug: May decrease absorption of **verapamil.**

PHARMACOKINETICS Absorption: Not absorbed. **Metabolism:** Not metabolized. **Elimination:** Excreted in feces.

NURSING IMPLICATIONS

Assessment & Drug Effects

- Lab tests: Monitor total cholesterol, LDL-C, HDL-C, and triglycerides periodically.
- Withhold drug and notify physician for triglycerides >300 mg/dL.

Patient & Family Education

- Report S&S of GI distress (see Appendix F), especially constipation.
- Do not breast feed while taking this drug without consulting physician.

COLESTIPOL HYDROCHLORIDE

(koe-les'ti-pole)
Cholestabyl ♣, Colestid, Lestid ♣
Classifications: CARDIOVASCULAR DRUG; ANTILIPEMIC; BILE ACID SEQUESTRANT
Prototype: Cholestyramine
Pregnancy Category: C

AVAILABILITY 1 g tablets; 5 g powder for suspension

ACTIONS Insoluble chloride salt of a basic anion exchange resin with high molecular weight, which adsorbs and combines with intestinal bile acids in exchange for chloride ions to form an insoluble, nonabsorbable complex that is excreted in the feces.

THERAPEUTIC EFFECTS Binds with bile acids in intestinal tract to form an insoluble complex that is excreted in the feces, thus reducing circulating cholesterol and increasing serum LDL removal rate. Serum triglycerides are not affected or are minimally increased.

USES Pruritus associated with partial biliary obstruction; also as adjunct to diet therapy of patient with primary hypercholesterolemia (type IIa hyperlipoproteinemia) or with coronary artery disease unresponsive to diet or other measures alone.

UNLABELED USES Digitoxin overdose and hyperoxaluria and to control postoperative diarrhea caused by excess bile acids in colon.

CONTRAINDICATIONS Complete biliary obstruction, hypersensitivity to bile acid sequestrants; pregnancy (category C), lactation. Safe use in children not established.

CAUTIOUS USE Hemorrhoids; bleeding disorders; malabsorption states; the older adult.

ROUTE & DOSAGE

Hypercholesterolemia

Adult: **PO** 15–30 g/d in 2–4 doses a.c. and h.s., or 1–2 tabs 1–2 times/d

Digitalis Toxicity

Adult: **PO** 10 g followed by 5 g q6–8h as needed

ADMINISTRATION

Oral

- Give 30 min before a meal when ordered a.c.
- Ensure that tablets are not chewed or crushed. They must be swallowed whole.
- Always mix granule form with liquids, juices, soups, cereals, or pulpy fruits. Add powder to at least 90 mL fluid. When carbonated drink is used, slowly stir in a large glass because excess foaming may occur. Rinse glass with small amount extra fluid to be sure all the drug is taken.
- Drugs given concomitantly should be scheduled at least 1 h before or 4 h after ingestion of colestipol to reduce interference with their absorption (see drug interactions).
- Store at 15°–30° C (59°–86° F) in tightly closed container unless otherwise instructed.

ADVERSE EFFECTS (≥1%) **Body as a Whole:** Joint and muscle pain, arthritis, shortness of breath. **GI:** *Constipation,* abdominal pain or distention, belching, flatulence, nausea, vomiting, diarrhea. **Metabolic:** Transient increases in liver enzyme tests, serum phosphorus and chloride; decreases in serum sodium and potassium. **Skin:** Dermatitis, urticaria.

INTERACTIONS Drug: Because it decreases the absorption from the GI tract of ORAL ANTICOAGULANTS, **digoxin,** TETRACYCLINES, PENICILLINS, **phenobarbital,** THYROID HORMONES, THIAZIDE DIURETICS, IRON SALTS, FAT-SOLUBLE VITAMINS (A, D, E, K), administer cholestyramine 4 h before or 2 h after these drugs.

PHARMACOKINETICS Absorption: Not absorbed from GI tract. **Elimination:** Excreted in feces as insoluble complex.

NURSING IMPLICATIONS

Assessment & Drug Effects

- Watch for changes in bowel elimination pattern. Constipation should not be allowed to persist without medical attention.
- Lab test: Monitor serum sodium and potassium levels. Monitor for and report S&S of hyponatremia and hypokalemia (see Appendix F).

Patient & Family Education

- Do not change the times for taking each drug, nor omit or increase doses. Any change in established regimens should be approved by the physician. It is important to keep to established regimens for colestipol and other drugs.
- If receiving prolonged therapy, report unusual bleeding (vitamin K deficiency). Colestipol

prevents absorption of FAT-SOLUBLE VITAMINS (A, D, E, K).

- Do not use OTC drugs unless physician has given approval.
- Check with physician regarding permitted amount of alcohol intake.
- Do not breast feed while taking this drug.

COLFOSCERIL PALMITATE

(col-fos′ce-ril)

Exosurf Neonatal

Classification: LUNG SURFACTANT

Prototype: Beractant

Pregnancy Category: Not applicable

AVAILABILITY 108 mg powder for injection

ACTIONS Synthetic lung surfactant. Endogenous pulmonary surfactant lowers surface tension on alveolar surfaces during respiration and stabilizes the alveoli against collapse at resting pressures.

THERAPEUTIC EFFECTS Deficiency of surfactant causes respiratory distress syndrome (RDS) in premature infants. Colfosceril lowers minimum surface tension on alveolar surfaces and restores pulmonary compliance and oxygenation in premature infants.

USES Prophylactic treatment of infants with birth weights <1350 g who are at risk of developing RDS. Prophylactic therapy of infants with birth weights >1350 g who show evidence of pulmonary immaturity.

UNLABELED USES Rescue treatment of infants with established RDS; RDS in adults.

CONTRAINDICATIONS Infants who have major congenital abnormalities or who are suspected of having congenital infections.

ROUTE & DOSAGE

Prophylaxis

Infant: **Intratracheal** 3 doses of 5 mL/kg are recommended, with the first dose being given as soon as possible after birth and repeat doses 12 and 24 h later to infants who remain on mechanical ventilation

Rescue Therapy

Infant: **Intratracheal** 2 doses of 5 mL/kg are recommended, the first dose being initiated as soon as the diagnosis of RDS is confirmed and the second 12 h later in infants remaining on mechanical ventilation

ADMINISTRATION

Intratracheal

- Reconstitute immediately before use if possible. Use only supplied diluent for reconstitution.
- Reconstitute as follows: (1) withdraw diluent with 18–19-gauge needle attached to 10–12-mL syringe; (2) inject into vial by allowing vacuum to draw diluent in; (3) do not withdraw needle and aspirate as much of solution as possible back into syringe; (4) maintain vacuum and quickly release plunger. Repeat steps 3 and 4 three or four times to ensure adequate mixing.
- Reconstituted drug is a milky white suspension. Gently shake if needed to resuspend it.
- Withdraw entire ordered dose into syringe while maintaining vacuum in vial.
- Before administration of drug, ensure that endotracheal tube tip is in the trachea.

C

- Before administration of drug, the infant should be suctioned. If possible, avoid suctioning for 2 h after drug administration.
- Drug is administered without interrupting mechanical ventilation. Use side port on the endotracheal tube adaptor.
- Administer dose in halves, each half over 1–2 min. Give first half dose with head in midline position; then turn head and torso to the right. Wait 30 s; then return to midline position for second half dose. Give each dose in short bursts timed with inspiration. After second half dose, turn head and torso to left for 30 s; then return to midline.
- Slow or stop drug administration and adjust ventilator rate or FIO_2 if any of the following occur: heart rate decreases, infant becomes dusky or agitated, or O_2 saturation drops.
- Store at 15°–30° C (59°–86° F) in a dry place. Reconstituted solution is stable for 12 h.

INCOMPATIBILITIES **Solution/additive:** Do not mix any antibiotics with surfactant; this may inactivate surfactant.

ADVERSE EFFECTS (≥1%) **CV:** Bradycardia, tachycardia. **Respiratory:** Decreased oxygen saturation, mucous plugging, apnea, pulmonary hemorrhage.

INTERACTIONS Drug: No clinically significant interactions established.

PHARMACOKINETICS Absorption: Absorbed from the alveolus into lung tissue, **Duration:** at least 7 d. **Distribution:** Distributes uniformly to all lobes of the lung, distal airways, and alveolar spaces; **Metabolism:** recycled and metabolized exclusively in the lungs. **Half-Life:** 20–36 h.

NURSING IMPLICATIONS

Assessment & Drug Effects

- During administration of drug, continuous ECG and transcutaneous monitoring are required. Also monitor chest expansion and facial expression.
- Monitor pulmonary function during administration. Rapid changes may require immediate adjustment of peak inspiratory pressure, ventilator rate, or FIO_2.
- Monitor continuously for 30 min following administration. Frequent arterial blood gas sampling is required to prevent hyperoxia and hypocarbia.

COLISTIMETHATE SODIUM

(koe-lis-ti-meth'ate)

Coly-Mycin M

Classifications: URINARY TRACT ANTIINFECTIVE; ANTIBIOTIC

Prototype: Trimethoprim

Pregnancy Category: B

AVAILABILITY 150 mg injection

ACTIONS Polymyxin antibiotic and parenteral form of colistin. Similar to polymyxin B in structure and actions but about one-third to one-fifth as potent. Antibacterial activity and overall toxicity are less, but nephrotoxic potential is almost identical with that of polymyxin B. Believed to act by affecting phospholipid component in bacterial cytoplasmic membranes with resulting damage and leakage of essential intracellular components.

THERAPEUTIC EFFECTS Bactericidal against most gram-negative organisms including *Pseudomonas aeruginosa, Escherichia coli, Enterobacter aerogenes, Haemophilus sp, Klebsiella pneumoniae, Brucella, Salmonella, Shigella, Bordetella, Pas-*

teurella, and *Vibrio.* Not effective against *Proteus* or *Neisseria* species. Complete cross-resistance and cross-sensitivity to polymyxin B reported but not to broad-spectrum antibiotics.

USES Particularly for severe, acute and chronic UTIs caused by susceptible strains of gram-negative organisms resistant to other antibiotics. Has been used with carbenicillin for *Pseudomonas* sepsis in children with acute leukopenia.

CONTRAINDICATIONS Hypersensitivity to polypeptide antibiotics; concomitant use of drugs that potentiate neuromuscular blocking effect (aminoglycoside antibiotics, other polymyxins, anticholinesterases, curariform muscle relaxants, ether, sodium citrate); nephrotoxic and ototoxic drugs; pregnancy (category B).
CAUTIOUS USE Impaired renal function; myasthenia gravis; older adult patients, infants; lactation.

ROUTE & DOSAGE

Urinary Tract Infections

Adult/Child: **IM/IV** 2.5–5 mg/kg/d divided in 2–4 doses, max of 5 mg/kg/d

Renal Impairment

Cl_{cr} 1.3–1.5 mg/dL: 2.5–3.8 mg/kg/d in 2 divided doses; 1.6–2.5 mg/dL: 2.5 mg/kg/d in a single dose or 2 divided doses; 2.6–4 mg/dL: 1.5 mg/kg q36h

ADMINISTRATION

Intramuscular

- Reconstitute each 150-mg vial with 2 mL of sterile water for injection to yield a concentration of 75 mg/mL. Swirl vial gently during reconstitution to avoid bubble formation. IM injection should be made deep into upper outer quadrant of buttock. Patients commonly experience pain at injection site. Rotate sites.

Intravenous

PREPARE: **Direct/Intermittent:** Prepare first half of total daily dose as directed for IM then further dilute with 20 mL sterile water for injection. Prepare second half of total daily dose by diluting further in 50 mL or more of D5W, NS, D5/NS, RL or other compatible solution. IV infusion solution should be freshly prepared and used within 24 h.

ADMINISTER: **Direct/Intermittent:** First half of total daily dose: Give slowly over 3–5 min. Second half of total daily dose: Starting 1–2 h after the first half dose has been given, infuse the second half dose over the next 22–23 h.

INCOMPATIBILITIES **Solution/additive: Carbenicillin, cephalothin, erythromycin, hydrocortisone, kanamycin.**

- Reconstituted solution may be stored in refrigerator at 2°–8° C (36°–46° F) or at controlled room temperature of 15°–30° C (59°–86° F). Use within 7 d. Store unopened vials at controlled room temperature.

ADVERSE EFFECTS (≥1%) **Body as a Whole:** Drug fever, pain at IM site. **GI:** GI disturbances. **CNS:** Circumoral, lingual, and peripheral paresthesias; visual and speech disturbances, neuromuscular blockade (generalized muscle weakness, dyspnea, respiratory depression or paralysis), seizures, psychosis. **Respiratory:** Respiratory arrest after IM injection. **Skin:** Pruritus, urticaria, dermatoses. **Special Senses:** Ototoxicity. **Urogenital:** Nephrotoxicity.

C

INTERACTIONS Drug: Tubocurarine, pancuronium, atracurium, AMINOGLYCOSIDES may compound and prolong respiratory depression; AMINOGLYCOSIDES, **amphotericin B, vancomycin** augment nephrotoxicity.

PHARMACOKINETICS Peak: 1–2 h IM. **Duration:** 8–12 h. **Distribution:** Widely distributed in most tissues except CNS; crosses placenta; distributed into breast milk in low concentrations. **Metabolism:** Metabolized in liver. **Elimination:** 66–75% excreted in urine within 24h. **Half-Life:** 2–3 h.

NURSING IMPLICATIONS

Assessment & Drug Effects

- Lab tests: Culture and susceptibility tests should be performed initially and periodically during therapy to determine responsiveness of causative organisms. Baseline renal function tests should be performed prior to therapy; frequent monitoring of renal function and urine drug levels is advisable during therapy. Impaired renal function increases the possibility of nephrotoxicity, apnea, and neuromuscular blockade.
- Report restlessness or dyspnea promptly. Respiratory arrest has been reported after IM administration.
- Monitor I&O ratio and patterns: Decrease in urine output or change in I&O ratio and rising BUN, serum creatinine, and serum drug levels (without dosage increase) are indications of renal toxicity. If they occur, withhold drug and report to physician.
- Close monitoring of older adult patients and infants is essential. They are particularly prone to renal toxicity because they tend to have inadequate renal reserves.
- Be alert to neurologic symptoms: changes in speech and hearing, visual changes, drowsiness, dizziness, ataxia, and transient paresthesias, and keep physician informed.
- Monitor closely postoperative patients who have received curariform muscle relaxants, ether, or sodium citrate for signs of neuromuscular blockade (delayed recovery, muscle weakness, depressed respiration).

Patient & Family Education

- Avoid operating a vehicle or other potentially hazardous activities while on drug therapy because of the possibility of transient neurologic disturbances.
- Do not breast feed without consulting the physician.

CORTICOTROPIN

(kor-ti-koe-troe′pin)
ACTH, Acthar

CORTICOTROPIN REPOSITORY

ACTH Gel, Acthron, Cortigel, Cortrophin-Gel, Cotropic Gel, H.P. Acthar Gel

Classifications: HORMONE AND SYNTHETIC SUBSTITUTE; ADRENAL CORTICOSTEROID
Prototype: Prednisone
Pregnancy Category: C

AVAILABILITY 25 unit, 40 unit vials for injection; **Repository:** 40 units/mL, 80 units/mL

ACTIONS Adrenocorticotropic hormone (ACTH) extracted from pituitary of domestic animals (usually pigs). Stimulates functioning adrenal cortex to produce and secrete corticosterone, cortisol (hydrocortisone), several weak androgens, and limited amounts of aldosterone.

THERAPEUTIC EFFECTS Therapeutic effects appear more rapidly than do those of prednisone. Suppresses further release of corticotropin by negative feedback mechanism. Chronic administration of exogenous corticosteroids decreases ACTH store and causes structural changes in pituitary. Lack of ACTH stimulation can lead to adrenal cortex atrophy.

USES Diagnostic test of adrenocortical function and adjunctively to treat adrenal insufficiency secondary to inadequate corticotropin secretion. Effective in treatment of adrenocorticoid-responsive diseases, such as multiple sclerosis, but adrenocorticoid therapy is preferred.

CONTRAINDICATIONS Ocular herpes simplex; recent surgery; CHF; scleroderma; osteoporosis; systemic fungoid infections; hypertension; sensitivity to porcine proteins; conditions accompanied by primary adrenocortical insufficiency or hyperfunction; pregnancy (category C), lactation.
CAUTIOUS USE Patients with latent tuberculosis or those reacting to tuberculin; hypothyroiditis, impaired hepatic function.

ROUTE & DOSAGE

Diagnostic Test
Adult: **IV** 10–25 U in 500 mL D5W infused over 8 h

Therapeutic
Adult: **IM/SC** 40–80 U/d, dose and frequency individualized; **Repository** 40–80 U q24–72h
Child: **IM/IV/SC** 1.6 U/kg/d divided q6–8h; **Repository** 0.8 U/kg/d divided q12h

Acute Multiple Sclerosis
Adult: **IM/SC** 80–120 U/d for 2–3 wk; **Repository** 80–120 U/d for 2–3 wk

ADMINISTRATION

Subcutaneous/Intramuscular
- Dosage is individualized. Changes in dosage regimen are gradual and only after full drug effects have become apparent.
- Corticotropin repository is only for SC and IM use. Do not use IV.
- Shake corticotropin zinc hydroxide bottle well before injecting drug deep into gluteal muscle.
- Give deep IM into a large muscle.

Intravenous
- IV administration to infants and children: Verify correct IV concentration and rate of infusion with physician.

PREPARE: **Continuous:** Use only the vial labeled for IV use. Dilute powder with 2 mL sterile water or NS for injection; desired dose is withdrawn from vial and further diluted with 500 mL of D5W.
ADMINISTER: **Continuous:** Give over 8 h.
INCOMPATIBILITIES **Solution/additive: Aminophylline, sodium bicarbonate.**

- Administration of the hormone at high dosage levels is tapered rather than withdrawn suddenly. A 2–5 d period of adrenocortical hypofunction follows discontinuation of corticotropin.

- Storage: Corticotropin for injection (reconstituted solution) is stable for 24 h or 7 d, depending on product, when stored at 2°–8° C (36°–46° F). Store corticotropin repository at 2°–15° C (36°–59° F). Store corticotropin zinc hydroxide at 15°–30° C (59°–86° F).

ADVERSE EFFECTS (≥1%) **Body as a Whole:** Loss of muscle mass, hypersensitivity, activation of latent tuberculosis, vertebral compression fracture. **GI:** Nausea, vomiting, abdominal distention, peptic ulcer with perforation and hemorrhage. **Endocrine:** Hirsutism, amenorrhea, osteoporosis, cushingoid state, activation of latent diabetes mellitus. **Metabolic:** Sodium and water retention; potassium and calcium loss, negative nitrogen balance, hyperglycemia. **CNS:** Euphoria, insomnia, headache, convulsions, papilledema, mood swings, depression. **Skin:** Acne, impaired wound healing, fragile skin, petechiae, ecchymosis. **Special Senses:** Cataract, glaucoma.

INTERACTIONS Drug: Aspirin, NSAIDS increase potential for hypoprothrombinemia; BARBITURATES, **phenytoin, rifampin** decrease effects of corticotropin; ESTROGENS may increase corticotropin binding and effects; **amphotericin B,** THIAZIDE AND LOOP DIURETICS increase potassium loss.

PHARMACOKINETICS Absorption: Readily absorbed from IM site. **Onset:** 6 h. **Duration:** 2–4 h IV/IM; 12–24 h repository. **Distribution:** concentrated in many tissues; not known if crosses placenta or distributed into breast milk. **Metabolism:** metabolized in liver. **Elimination:** Excreted in urine. **Half-Life:** <20 min.

NURSING IMPLICATIONS

Assessment & Drug Effects

- Before giving corticotropin to patient with suspected sensitivity to porcine proteins, hypersensitivity skin testing should be performed.
- Observe patient closely for 15 min for hypersensitivity reactions during IV administration or immediately after SC or IM injections (urticaria, pruritus, dizziness, nausea, vomiting, anaphylactic shock). Epinephrine 1:1000 should be readily available for emergency treatment.
- Prolonged use of corticotropin increases risk of hypersensitivity reaction (see Appendix F).
- Adrenal response to corticotropin is measured against a baseline plasma cortisol level 1 h before the 8 h test. Another plasma level is determined after at least 1 h of the infusion.
- Corticotropin may suppress S&S of chronic disease.
- New infections can appear during treatment. Because of decreased resistance and inability to localize the infection, it may be severe. Report immediately.
- Monitor carefully growth and development of a child receiving this drug.

Patient & Family Education

- Corticotropin administration increases requirements for insulin and oral antidiabetic agents. If you have diabetes mellitus, monitor blood glucose closely until response to the drug is stabilized.
- Monitor weight and report a steady gain, especially if accompanied by edema. Also promptly report headache, muscle weakness, abdominal pain.
- Do not self-medicate with OTC drugs without consulting physician.
- Eye examinations should be done before initiation of expected long-term therapy and periodically during treatment. Report to physician if blurred vision occurs.
- Dietary salt restriction and potassium supplementation may be necessary to minimize edema

caused by overstimulation of the adrenal cortex by corticotropin.

- Do not receive live vaccine immunizations while receiving corticotropin.
- Do not breast feed while taking this drug.

CORTISONE ACETATE

(kor'ti-sone)

Cortistan, Cortone

Classifications: HORMONES AND SYNTHETIC SUBSTITUTES; SYNTHETIC ADRENAL CORTICOSTEROID; GLUCOCORTICOID

Prototype: Prednisone

Pregnancy Category: D

AVAILABILITY 5 mg, 10 mg, 25 mg tablets; 50 mg/mL injection

ACTIONS Short-acting synthetic steroid with prominent glucocorticoid activity and mineralocorticoid effects approximately equal to those of prednisone (cortisol). Because therapeutic activity of cortisone results from its conversion in body to cortisol, its effects simulate those of hydrocortisone. Metabolic effects include promotion of protein, carbohydrate, and fat metabolism and interference with linear growth in children.

THERAPEUTIC EFFECTS Mineralocorticoid actions include promotion of sodium retention and potassium excretion. May foster development of osteoporosis. Has antiinflammatory and immunosuppressive actions.

USES Replacement therapy for primary or secondary adrenocortical insufficiency and inflammatory and allergic disorders.

CONTRAINDICATIONS Hypersensitivity to glucocorticoids; psychoses; viral or bacterial diseases of skin; Cushing's syndrome, immunologic procedures; pregnancy (category D), lactation. Safe use in children not established.

CAUTIOUS USE Diabetes mellitus; hypertension, CHF; active or arrested tuberculosis; active or latent peptic ulcer.

ROUTE & DOSAGE

Replacement or Inflammatory Disorders

Adult: **PO/IM** 20–300 mg/d in 1 or more divided doses, try to reduce periodically by 10–25 mg/d to lowest effective dose

Child: **PO** 2.5–10 mg/kg/d divided q6–8h; **IM** 1–5 mg/kg/d divided q12–24h

ADMINISTRATION

Oral

- Administer cortisone (usually in a.m.) with food or fluid of patient's choice to reduce gastric irritation.
- Sodium chloride and a mineralocorticoid are usually given with cortisone as part of replacement therapy.

Intramuscular

- Parenteral cortisone is a suspension (25 mg/mL) and therefore should not be used IV. Shake bottle well before withdrawing dose.
- Give deep IM into a large muscle.
- Drug must be gradually tapered rather than withdrawn abruptly.
- Store at 15°–30° C (59°–86° F) in tightly closed container unless otherwise directed by manufacturer. Protect from heat and freezing.

ADVERSE EFFECTS (≥1%) **CV:** CHF, hypertension, *edema.* **GI:** *Nausea,* peptic ulcer, pancreatitis. **Endocrine:** Hyperglycemia. **Hematologic:** Thrombocytopenia. **Musculoskele-**

C

tal: *Compression fracture,* osteoporosis, muscle weakness. **CNS:** Euphoria, insomnia, vertigo, nystagmus. **Skin:** Impaired wound healing, petechiae, ecchymosis, acne. **Special Senses:** *Cataracts,* glaucoma, blurred vision.

INTERACTIONS Drug: BARBITURATES, **phenytoin, rifampin** decrease effects of cortisone.

PHARMACOKINETICS Absorption: Readily absorbed from GI tract. **Onset:** Rapid PO; 24–48 h IM. **Peak:** 2 h PO; 24–48 h IM. **Duration:** 1.25–1.5 d. **Distribution:** Concentrated in many tissues; crosses placenta; distributed into breast milk. **Metabolism:** Metabolized in liver. **Elimination:** Excreted in urine. **Half-Life:** 0.5 h; HPA suppression: 8–12 h.

NURSING IMPLICATIONS

Assessment & Drug Effects

- Monitor for S&S of Cushing's syndrome (see Appendix F), especially in patients on long-term therapy.
- Lab tests: Periodic blood glucose and CBC with platelet count.
- Cortisone may mask some signs of infection, and new infections may appear.
- Be alert to clinical indications of infection: malaise, anorexia, depression, and evidence of delayed healing. (Classic signs of inflammation are suppressed by cortisone.)
- Report ecchymotic areas, unexplained bleeding, and easy bruising.

Patient & Family Education

- Take drug exactly as prescribed. Do not alter dose intervals or stop therapy abruptly.
- Monitor weight and report a steady gain especially if it is accompanied by signs of fluid retention (e.g., edema of ankles or hands).
- Report changes in visual acuity, including blurring, promptly.
- Inform physician or dentist that cortisone is being taken. Carry identification card or jewelry that states drug being taken and physician's name.
- Do not breast feed while taking this drug.

COSYNTROPIN

(koe-sin-troe′pin)

Cortrosyn

Classification: DIAGNOSTIC AGENT

Prototype: Prednisone

Pregnancy Category: C

AVAILABILITY 0.25 mg injection

ACTIONS Synthetic polypeptide resembling corticotropin (ACTH) in relation to the first 24 of the 39 amino acids in naturally occurring ACTH. Has less immunologic activity and is associated with less risk of sensitivity than corticotropin.

THERAPEUTIC EFFECTS In patient with normal adrenocortical function, stimulates adrenal cortex to secrete corticosterone, cortisol (hydrocortisone), several weak androgenic substances, and limited amounts of aldosterone.

USES Diagnostic tool to differentiate primary adrenal from secondary (pituitary) adrenocortical insufficiency.

UNLABELED USE In patients with normal adrenocortical function for the long-term treatment of chronic inflammatory or degenerative disorders responsive to glucocorticoids.

CONTRAINDICATIONS History of allergic disorders; scleroderma, osteoporosis; systemic fungal infections, ocular herpes simplex; recent surgery; history of or presence of peptic ulcer; CHF; hypertension; adrenocortical insufficiency and adrenocortical hyperfunction; pregnancy (category C), lactation; immunizations, tuberculosis, infections.

CAUTIOUS USE Multiple sclerosis, acute gouty arthritis, mental disturbances, diabetes, abscess, pyrogenic infections, diverticulitis, renal insufficiency, myasthenia gravis, children.

ROUTE & DOSAGE

Rapid Screening Test
Adult/Child: >2 y: **IM/IV** 0.25 mg injected over 2 min
Child: <2 y: **IM** 0.125 mg injected over 2 min; **IV** 0.125 mg at 0.04 mg/h over 6 h
Neonate: **IM/IV** 0.015 mg/kg

ADMINISTRATION

Intramuscular

- Reconstitute cosyntropin powder by adding 1.1 mL NS (diluent provided by manufacturer) to vial labeled 0.25 mg to provide solution containing 0.25 mg/mL.
- Inject deep IM into a large muscle.

Intravenous

- IV administration to neonates, infants and children: Verify correct IV concentration and rate of infusion/injection with physician.

PREPARE: **Direct:** Reconstitute as for IM. **IV Infusion:** Further dilute in 250–500 mL of D5W or NS.

ADMINISTER: **Direct:** Give over 2 min. **IV Infusion:** Give at an approximate rate of 40 mcg/h over 4–6 h.

- Reconstituted solutions remain stable 24 h at room temperature or 21 d at 2°–8° C. ▪ Cosyntropin should not be added to blood or to plasma infusions.

ADVERSE EFFECTS (≥1%) **Body as a Whole:** Mild fever. **GI:** chronic pancreatitis. **Skin:** Pruritus.

DIAGNOSTIC TEST INTERFERENCE **Cortisone, hydrocortisone, estrogen, spironolactone** elevated ***bilirubin***, and presence of ***free Hgb*** in plasma may interfere with ***plasma cortisol*** determinations.

INTERACTIONS Drug: Cortisone, hydrocortisone can exhibit abnormally high baseline values of cortisol and a decreased response to cosyntropin test.

PHARMACOKINETICS Absorption: Plasma cortisol levels double in 15–30 min. **Peak:** 1 h. **Duration:** 2–4 h. **Distribution:** Unknown; does not cross placenta. **Metabolism:** Unknown.

NURSING IMPLICATIONS

Assessment & Drug Effects

- Normal 17-KS levels in men are 10–25 mg/24 h; in women <50 y, 5–15 mg/24 h; and in women >50 y, 4–8 mg/24 h.
- Normal 17-OHCS levels in men are 5–12 mg/24 h; in women, 3–10 mg/24 h; in children 8–12 y, <4.5 mg/24 h; in younger children, 1.5 mg/24 h. Levels may be slightly higher in obese or muscular individuals.

CROMOLYN SODIUM ℗

(kroe′moe-lin)

Disodium Cromoglycate, Crolom, DSCG, Fivent ♣, Intal, Nasalcrom, Opticrom, Rynacrom ♣, Vistacrom ♣, Gastrocrom

Classification: MAST CELL STABILIZER
Pregnancy Category: B

AVAILABILITY 20 mg/2 mL solution for nebulization; 800 mcg spray; 40 mg/mL nasal solution; 4% ophth solution; 100 mg/5 mL oral concentrate ampules

ACTIONS Synthetic asthma-prophylactic agent with unique action. Inhibits release of bronchoconstrictors—histamine and SRS-A (slow-reacting substance of anaphylaxis) from sensitized pulmonary mast cells, thereby suppressing an allergic response. Has no intrinsic bronchodilator, antihistaminic, or vasoconstrictor properties, thus only of value when taken prophylactically.

THERAPEUTIC EFFECTS Particularly effective for IgE-mediated or "extrinsic asthma" precipitated by exposure to specific allergen, e.g., pollens, dust, animal dander by inhibiting the release of bronchoconstrictor substances.

USES Primarily for prophylaxis of mild to moderate seasonal and perennial bronchial asthma and allergic rhinitis. Also used for prevention of exercise-related bronchospasm, prevention of acute bronchospasm induced by known pollutants or antigens, and for prevention and treatment of allergic rhinitis. Orally for systemic mastocytosis. **Ophthalmic use:** Allergic ocular disorders, conjunctivitis, vernal keratoconjunctivitis.

UNLABELED USE Orally for prophylaxis of GI and systemic reactions to food allergy.

CONTRAINDICATIONS Use of aerosol (because of fluorocarbon propellants) in patients with coronary artery disease or history of arrhythmias; dyspnea, acute asthma, status asthmaticus; patients unable to coordinate actions or follow instructions, pregnancy (category B), lactation. Safe use in children <6 y not determined; use of capsule not recommended for children.

CAUTIOUS USE Renal or hepatic dysfunction.

ROUTE & DOSAGE

Allergies

Adult: **Inhalation** Metered dose inhaler or capsule: 1 spray or 1 capsule inhaled q.i.d.; nasal solution: 1 spray in each nostril 3–6 times/d at regular intervals
Child: **Inhalation** *>6 y:* Metered dose inhaler or capsule: same as for adult; *>6 y:* nasal solution: same as for adult

Conjunctivitis see Appendix A-1

Mastocytosis

Adult: **PO** 2 ampules q.i.d. 30 min a.c. and h.s.
Child: **PO** *2–12 y:* 1 ampule q.i.d. 30 min a.c. and h.s.

ADMINISTRATION

- Patients should receive detailed instructions for loading and administering the spinhaler or nasalmatic device. See manufacturer's instructions. Therapeutic effect is dependent on proper inhalation technique.
- Advise patient to clear as much mucus as possible before inhalation treatments.
- Instruct patient to exhale as completely as possible before placing inhaler mouthpiece between lips, tilt head backward and inhale rapidly and deeply with steady, even breaths. Remove inhaler from mouth, hold breath for a few seconds, then exhale into the air. Repeat until entire dose is taken.
- Caution patient not to exhale into inhaler because moisture from breath will interfere with its

proper operation. Also inform patient that capsule is intended for inhalation only and is ineffective if swallowed.

- Protect cromolyn from moisture and heat. Store in tightly closed, light-resistant container at 15°–30° C (59°–86° F) unless otherwise directed.

ADVERSE EFFECTS (≥1%) **Body as a Whole:** Peripheral eosinophilia, angioedema, bronchospasm, anaphylaxis (rare). **GI:** Swelling of parotid glands, dry mouth, slightly bitter after-taste, *nausea,* vomiting, esophagitis. **CNS:** Headache, dizziness, peripheral neuritis. **Skin:** Erythema, urticaria, rash, contact dermatitis. **Special Senses:** *Sneezing, nasal stinging and burning,* dryness and *irritation of throat and trachea; cough;* nasal congestion, itchy, puffy eyes, lacrimation, *transient ocular burning, stinging.*

INTERACTIONS Drug: No clinically significant interactions established.

PHARMACOKINETICS Absorption: Approximately 8% of dose absorbed from lungs. **Onset:** 1 wk with regular use. **Peak:** 15 min. **Duration:** 4–6 h; may last as long as 2–3 wk. **Elimination:** Excreted in bile and urine in equal amounts. **Half-Life:** 80 min.

NURSING IMPLICATIONS

Assessment & Drug Effects

- Withhold drug and notify physician if any of the following occur; angioedema or bronchospasm.
- Monitor for exacerbation of asthmatic symptoms including breathlessness and cough that may occur in patients receiving cromolyn during corticosteroid withdrawal.
- For patients with asthma, therapeutic effects may be noted within a few days but generally not until after 1–2 wk of therapy.

Patient & Family Education

- Throat irritation, cough, and hoarseness can be minimized by gargling with water, drinking a few swallows of water, or by sucking on a lozenge after each treatment.
- Talk to your physician about what to do in the event of an acute asthmatic attack. Cromolyn is of no value in acute asthma.
- Cromolyn does not eliminate the continued need for therapy with bronchodilators, expectorants, antibiotics, or corticosteroids, but the amount and frequency of use of these medications may be appreciably reduced.
- Report any unusual signs or symptoms. Hypersensitivity reactions (see Signs & Symptoms, Appendix F) can be severe and life-threatening. Drug should be discontinued if an allergic reaction occurs.
- Treatment with cromolyn 15 min before doing protracted exercises reportedly blunts the effects of vigorous exercise as well as cold air.
- Ophthalmic use: Do not wear soft contact lenses during therapy with ophthalmic drug. They may be worn within a few hours after therapy is discontinued.
- Learn the proper technique for instillation of ophthalmic drops.
- Do not breast feed while taking this drug.

CROTAMITON

(kroe-tam′i-tonn)

Eurax

Classifications: SKIN AND MUCOUS MEMBRANE AGENT; SCABICIDE; ANTIPRURITIC

Prototype: Lindane

Pregnancy Category: C

C

AVAILABILITY 10% cream, lotion

ACTIONS Scabicidal and antipruritic agent. Available in an emollient-lotion base or in a vanishing cream.

THERAPEUTIC EFFECTS By unknown mechanisms, drug eradicates *Sarcoptes scabiei* and effectively relieves itching.

USES Treatment of scabies and for symptomatic treatment of pruritus.

CONTRAINDICATIONS Application to acutely inflamed skin, raw or weeping surfaces, eyes, or mouth; history of previous sensitivity to crotamiton; pregnancy (category C).

ROUTE & DOSAGE

Scabies
Adult/Child: **Topical** Apply a thin layer of cream from neck to toes; apply a second layer 24 h later. Bathe 48 h after last application to remove drug

ADMINISTRATION

Topical
- Shake container well before use of solution.
- The skin must be thoroughly dry before applying medication.
- If drug accidentally contacts eyes, thoroughly flush out medication with water.
- Pruritus treatment: massage medication gently into affected areas until it is completely absorbed. Repeat as needed (usually effective for 6–10 h).
- Store in tightly closed containers at 15°–30° C (59°–86° F). Do not freeze.

ADVERSE EFFECTS (≥1%) **Skin:** Skin irritation (particularly with prolonged use), rash, erythema, sensation of warmth, allergic sensitization.

INTERACTIONS Drug: No clinically significant interactions established.

NURSING IMPLICATIONS

Assessment & Drug Effects
- Monitor for and report significant skin irritation or allergic sensitization.

Patient & Family Education
- Review package insert before treatment begins.
- Discontinue medication and report to physician if irritation or sensitization develops.

CYANOCOBALAMIN

(sye-an-oh-koe-bal'a-min)

Anacobin ♣, Bedoz ♣, Betalin 12, Cobex, Crystamine, Crysti-12, Cyanabin, Cyanoject, Kaybovite, Nascobal Redisol, Rubesol, Rubion ♣, Rubramin PC

Classifications: HORMONE AND SYNTHETIC SUBSTITUTE; VITAMIN B_{12}

Pregnancy Category: A; C (parenteral)

AVAILABILITY 25 mcg, 50 mcg, 100 mcg, 250 mcg tablets; 400 mcg/unit, 500 mcg/0.1 mL nasal gel

ACTIONS Vitamin B_{12} is a cobalt-containing B complex vitamin produced by *Streptomyces griseus*. Essential for normal growth, cell reproduction, maturation of RBCs, nucleoprotein synthesis, maintenance of nervous system (myelin synthesis), and believed to be involved in protein and carbohydrate metabolism. Also acts as coenzyme in various biologic reactions. Vitamin B_{12} deficiency results in megaloblastic anemia, dysfunction of spinal cord with paralysis, GI lesions.

THERAPEUTIC EFFECTS Therapeutically effective for treatment of vitamin B_{12} deficiency and pernicious anemia.

USES Vitamin B_{12} deficiency due to malabsorption syndrome as in pernicious (Addison's) anemia, sprue; GI pathology, dysfunction, or surgery; fish tapeworm infestation, and gluten enteropathy. Also used in B_{12} deficiency caused by increased physiologic requirements or inadequate dietary intake, and in vitamin B_{12} absorption (Schilling) test.

UNLABELED USE To prevent and treat toxicity associated with sodium nitroprusside.

CONTRAINDICATIONS History of sensitivity to vitamin B_{12}, other cobalamins, or cobalt; early Leber's disease (hereditary optic nerve atrophy), indiscriminate use in folic acid deficiency. Safe use during pregnancy [category A, category C (parenteral)], lactation, and in children not established.

CAUTIOUS USE Heart disease, anemia, pulmonary disease.

ROUTE & DOSAGE

Vitamin B_{12} Deficiency

Adult: **IM/Deep SC** 30 mcg/d for 5–10 d, then 100–200 mcg/mo
Child: **IM/Deep SC** 100 mcg doses to a total of 1–5 mg over 2 wk, then 60 mcg/mo

Pernicious Anemia

Adult: **IM/Deep SC** 100–1000 mcg/d for 2–3 wk, then 100–1000 mcg q2–4wk **Intranasal** one pump of gel in one nostril once weekly
Child: **IM** 30–50 mcg/d times 2 wk to total of 1000 mcg, then 100 mcg/mo
Infant: **IM** 1000 mcg/d times at least 2 wk, then 50 mcg/mo

Diagnosis of Megaloblastic Anemia

Adult: **IM/Deep SC** 1 mcg/d for 10 d while maintaining a low folate and vitamin B_{12} diet

Schilling Test

Adult: **IM/Deep SC** 1000 mcg times 1 dose

Nutritional Supplement

Adult: **PO** 1–25 mcg/d
Child: **PO** *<1 y:* 0.3 mcg/d; *≥1 y:* 1 mcg/d

ADMINISTRATION

Oral

- PO preparations may be mixed with fruit juices. However, administer promptly since ascorbic acid affects the stability of vitamin B_{12}.
- Administration of oral vitamin B_{12} with meals increases its absorption.

Subcutaneous/Intramuscular

- Give deep SC by slightly tenting the skin at the injection site.
- IM may be given into any normal IM injection site.
- Preserved in light-resistant containers at room temperature preferably at 15°–30° C (59°–86° F) unless otherwise directed by manufacturer.

ADVERSE EFFECTS (≥1%) **Body as a Whole:** Feeling of swelling of body, anaphylactic shock, sudden death. **CV:** Peripheral vascular thrombosis, pulmonary edema, CHF. **GI:** Mild transient diarrhea. **Hematologic:** Unmasking of polycythemia vera (with correction of vitamin B_{12} deficiency). **Metabolic:** Hypokalemia. **Skin:** Itching, rash, flushing. **Special Senses:** Severe optic nerve atrophy (patients with Leber's disease).

DIAGNOSTIC TEST INTERFERENCE Most antibiotics, methotrexate, and pyrimethamine may produce invalid diagnostic ***blood assays for vitamin B_{12}***. Possibility of false-positive test for ***intrinsic factor antibodies.***

INTERACTIONS Drug: Alcohol, aminosalicylic acid, neomycin, colchicine may decrease absorption of oral cyanocobalamin; **chloramphenicol** may interfere with therapeutic response to cyanocobalamin.

PHARMACOKINETICS Absorption: Intestinal absorption requires presence of intrinsic factor in terminal ileum. **Distribution:** Widely distributed; principally stored in liver, kidneys, and adrenals; crosses placenta, excreted in breast milk. **Metabolism:** Converted in tissues to active co-enzymes; enterohepatically cycled. **Elimination:** 50–95% of doses ≥100 mcg are excreted in urine in 48 h. **Half-Life:** 6 d (400 d in liver).

NURSING IMPLICATIONS

Assessment & Drug Effects

- Lab tests: Before initiation of therapy, reticulocyte and erythrocyte counts, Hgb, Hct, vitamin B_{12}, and serum folate levels should be determined; then repeated between 5 and 7 d after start of therapy and at regular intervals during therapy. Monitor potassium levels during the first 48 h. Conversion to normal erythropoiesis increases erythrocyte potassium requirement and can result in severe hypokalemia and sudden death.
- Obtain a careful history of sensitivities. Sensitization to cyanocobalamin can take as long as 8 y to develop.
- Monitor vital signs in patients with cardiac disease and in those receiving parenteral cyanocobalamin, and be alert to symptoms of pulmonary edema, which generally occur early in therapy.
- Therapeutic response to drug therapy is usually dramatic, occurring within 48 h. Effectiveness is measured by laboratory values and improvement in manifestations of vitamin B_{12} deficiency.
- Characteristically, reticulocyte concentration rises in 3–4 d, peaks in 5–8 d, and then gradually declines as erythrocyte count and Hgb rise to normal levels (in 4–6 wk).
- Obtain a complete diet and drug history and inquire into alcohol drinking patterns for all patients receiving cyanocobalamin to identify and correct poor habits.

Patient & Family Education

- Notify physician of any intercurrent disease or infection. Increased dosage may be required.
- To prevent irreversible neurologic damage resulting from pernicious anemia, drug therapy must be continued throughout life.
- Rich food sources of B_{12} are nutrient-added breakfast cereals, vitamin B_{12}-fortified soy milk, organ meats, clams, oysters, egg yolk, crab, salmon, sardines, muscle meat, milk, and dairy products.
- Do not breast feed while taking this drug.

C

CYCLIZINE HYDROCHLORIDE

(sye'kli-zeen)

Marezine, Marzine ♦

CYCLIZINE LACTATE

Marezine Lactate, Marzine

Classifications: ANTIHISTAMINE (H_1-RECEPTOR ANTAGONIST); ANTI-VERTIGO AGENT; ANTIEMETIC

Prototype: Meclizine

Pregnancy Category: B

AVAILABILITY 50 mg tablets; 50 mg/mL injection

ACTIONS Piperazine antihistamine (H_1-receptor blocking agent) structurally and pharmacologically related to other cyclizine compounds (e.g., buclizine, hydroxyzine, meclizine). In common with these agents, it exhibits CNS depression and anticholinergic, antispasmodic, local anesthetic, and antihistaminic activity. Mechanism of action is not known.

THERAPEUTIC EFFECTS Has prominent depressant action on labyrinthine excitability and on conduction in vestibular-cerebellar pathways, thus producing marked antimotion and antiemetic effects.

USES Chiefly for prevention and treatment of motion sickness and postoperative nausea and vomiting.

CONTRAINDICATIONS Pregnancy (category B), lactation, children <6 y.

CAUTIOUS USE Narrow-angle glaucoma; prostatic hypertrophy; obstructive disease of GU or GI tracts; postoperative patients.

ROUTE & DOSAGE

Motion Sickness

Adult: **PO** 50 mg 30 min before travel, then q4–6h prn (max: 200 mg/d). **IM** 50 mg q4–6h prn

Child: **PO** *6–12 y,* 25 mg q4–6h prn (max 75 mg/d). **IM** *6–12y,* 1 mg/kg t.i.d. prn (max: 75 mg/d)

Postoperative Vomiting

Adult: **IM** 50 mg 15–30 min before end of operation, may repeat q4–6h (t.i.d.) prn during first few days after surgery

ADMINISTRATION

Oral

- Give dose 30 min prior to any activity likely to cause motion sickness.

Intramuscular

- Aspirate needle carefully before injecting IM. Anaphylactic reactions following inadvertent IV injection have been reported.
- For prophylaxis of postoperative nausea and vomiting, drug usually prescribed with preoperative medication or is administered 20–30 min before expected termination of surgery.
- Store tablets in tight, light-resistant container at 15°–30° C (59°–86° F) unless otherwise directed. Store parenteral form in a cold place at 5°–10° C (41°–50° F). When parenteral solution is stored at room temperature for prolonged periods, it may become slightly yellow, but this does not indicate loss of potency.

ADVERSE EFFECTS (≥1%) **CV:** Hypotension, palpitation, tachycardia. **GI:** Anorexia, nausea, vomiting, diarrhea, or constipation, cholestatic jaundice. **CNS:** *Drowsiness,* excitement, euphoria, auditory and visual hallucinations, hyperexcitability alternating with

C

drowsiness, convulsions, respiratory paralysis (rare). **Skin:** Urticaria, rash. **Special Senses:** *Dry mouth,* nose, and throat; blurred vision, diplopia; tinnitus. **Other:** Pain at IM injection site.

DIAGNOSTIC TEST INTERFERENCE Because cyclizine is an antihistamine, inform patient that ***skin testing*** procedures should not be scheduled for about 4 d after drug is discontinued or false-negative reactions may result.

INTERACTIONS **Drug: Alcohol,** BARBITURATES, CNS DEPRESSANTS (e.g., HYPNOTICS, SEDATIVES, and ANXIOLYTICS) may compound effects of cyclizine.

PHARMACOKINETICS **Onset:** Rapid. **Duration:** 4–6 h. **Metabolism:** Unknown.

NURSING IMPLICATIONS

Assessment & Drug Effects

- Monitor post-operative patient's vital signs closely, as cyclizine can cause hypotension.
- Monitor for and report signs of CNS stimulation (e.g., hyperexcitability, euphoria). Dose reduction or discontinuation of drug may be indicated.

Patient & Family Education

- Take cyclizine with food or a glass of milk or water to minimize GI irritation.
- Do not drive a car or engage in other potentially hazardous activities until reaction to the drug is known. Adverse effects include drowsiness and dizziness.
- Alcohol, barbiturates, narcotic analgesic, and other CNS depressants may compound sedative action.
- Do not breast feed while taking this drug.

CYCLOBENZAPRINE HYDROCHLORIDE (Pr)

(sye-kloe-ben′za-preen)

Cycoflex, Flexeril

Classifications: AUTONOMIC NERVOUS SYSTEM AGENT; SKELETAL MUSCLE RELAXANT, CENTRAL ACTING

Pregnancy Category: B

AVAILABILITY 5 mg, 10 mg tablets

ACTIONS Structurally and pharmacologically related to tricyclic antidepressants. Relieves skeletal muscle spasm of local origin without interfering with muscle function. Believed to act primarily within CNS at brain stem; some action at spinal cord level is also probable. Depresses tonic somatic motor activity, although both gamma and alpha motor neurons are affected.

THERAPEUTIC EFFECTS In common with other tricyclic compounds, it increases circulating norepinephrine by blocking its synaptic reuptake, thus producing its antidepressant effect. Also has sedative effects and potent central and peripheral anticholinergic activity.

USES Short-term adjunct to rest and physical therapy for relief of muscle spasm associated with acute musculoskeletal conditions. Not effective in treatment of spasticity associated with cerebral palsy or cerebral or cord disease.

CONTRAINDICATIONS Acute recovery phase of MI, patients with cardiac arrhythmias, heart block or conduction disturbances, CHF, hyperthyroidism. Use for periods longer than 2 or 3 wk not recommended by manufacturer. Pregnancy (category B), lactation. Safe use in children <15 y not established.

C

CAUTIOUS USE Patients receiving anticholinergic medications; prostatic hypertrophy, history of urinary retention, angle-closure glaucoma; increased IOP, seizures; cardiovascular disease; hepatic impairment; older adults, debilitated patients; history of psychiatric illness.

ROUTE & DOSAGE

Muscle Spasm
Adult: **PO** 5–10 mg t.i.d. (max: 60 mg/d)
Geriatric: Start with 5 mg
Mild Hepatic Impairment
Start with 5 mg
Moderate to Severe Hepatic Impairment
not recommended

ADMINISTRATION

Oral

- Do not administer drug if patient is receiving an MAO INHIBITOR (e.g., furazolidone, isocarboxazid, pargyline, tranylcypromine).
- Cyclobenzaprine is intended for short-term (2 or 3 wk) use.
- Store in tightly closed container, preferably at 15°–30° C (59°–86° F) unless otherwise directed by manufacturer.

ADVERSE EFFECTS (≥1%) **Body as a Whole:** Edema of tongue and face, sweating, myalgia, hepatitis, alopecia. Shares toxic potential of tricyclic antidepressants. **CV:** Tachycardia, syncope, palpitation, vasodilation, chest pain, orthostatic hypotension, dyspnea; with high doses, possibility of severe arrhythmias. **GI:** *Dry mouth,* indigestion, unpleasant taste, coated tongue, tongue discoloration, vomiting, anorexia, abdominal pain, flatulence, diarrhea, paralytic ileus. **CNS:** *Drowsiness, dizziness,* weakness, fatigue, asthenia, paresthesias, tremors, muscle twitching, insomnia, euphoria, disorientation, mania, ataxia. **Skin:** Pruritus, urticaria, skin rash. **Urogenital:** Increased or decreased libido, impotence.

INTERACTIONS Drug: Alcohol, BARBITURATES, other CNS DEPRESSANTS enhance CNS depression; potentiates anticholinergic effects of **phenothiazine** and other ANTICHOLINERGICS; MAO INHIBITORS may precipitate hypertensive crisis—use with extreme caution.

PHARMACOKINETICS Absorption: Well absorbed from GI tract with some first-pass elimination in liver. **Onset:** 1 h. **Peak:** 3–8 h. **Duration:** 12–24 h. **Distribution:** Highly protein bound (93%). **Metabolism:** Metabolized in liver to inactive metabolites. **Elimination:** Slowly excreted in urine with some elimination in feces; may be excreted in breast milk. **Half-Life:** 1–3 d.

NURSING IMPLICATIONS

Assessment & Drug Effects

- Supervision of ambulation may be indicated, especially in the older adult because of risk of drowsiness and dizziness.
- Withhold drug and notify physician if signs of hypersensitivity, e.g., pruritus, urticaria, rash, appear.

Patient & Family Education

- Avoid driving and other potentially hazardous activities until reaction to drug is known. Adverse effects include drowsiness and dizziness.
- Avoid alcohol and other CNS DEPRESSANTS (unless otherwise directed by physician) because cyclobenzaprine enhances their effects.

C

- Dry mouth may be relieved by increasing total fluid intake (if not contraindicated).
- Keep physician informed of therapeutic effectiveness. Spasmolytic effect usually begins within 1 or 2 d and may be manifested by lessening of pain and tenderness, increase in range of motion, and ability to perform ADL.
- Do not breast feed while taking this drug.

CYCLOPENTOLATE HYDROCHLORIDE (Pr)

(sye-kloe-pen'toe-late)

Ak-Pentolate, Cyclogyl, Pentalair

Classifications: EYE PREPARATION; CYCLOPLEGIC; MYDRIATIC

Pregnancy Category: C

AVAILABILITY 0.5%, 1%, 2% ophth solution

ACTIONS Tertiary amine antimuscarinic compound with systemic side effects and CNS toxicity, similar to those of atropine. Acts by blocking response of iris sphincter muscle, and muscle of accommodation in the ciliary body to cholinergic stimulation.

THERAPEUTIC EFFECTS This results in dilation and paralysis of accommodation of the eyes. It binds to melanin in pupil; thus highly pigmented eyes may be less responsive to cycloplegic and mydriatic actions of the drug.

USES Induction of cycloplegia or mydriasis for ophthalmic diagnostic procedures.

CONTRAINDICATIONS Narrow angle glaucoma, excessively increased intraocular pressure; pregnancy (category C), lactation.

CAUTIOUS USE Elderly patients, brain damage (in children), Down's syndrome, spastic paralysis in children, blue-eyed individuals.

ROUTE & DOSAGE

Cycloplegia or Mydriasis

Adult: **Topical** 1 drop of 1% solution in eye 40–50 min before procedure, followed by 1 drop in 5 min; may need 2% solution in patients with darkly pigmented eyes.

Child: **Topical** 1 drop of 0.5–1% solution in eye 40–50 min before procedure, followed by 1 drop in 5 min; may need 2% solution in patients with darkly pigmented eyes.

ADMINISTRATION

Topical

- Clarify with physician which strength (1% or 2%) should be used.
- Ask patient to remove soft contact lenses prior to installation of drops.

ADVERSE EFFECTS (≥1%) **Body as a Whole:** Flushing, fever. **CNS:** Drowsiness dysarthria, disorientation, ataxia, hallucinations, hyperkinesis, psychosis, seizures. **CV:** Sinus tachycardia, hypotension. **GI:** Dry mouth, abdominal distention in infants. **Skin:** Rash, contact urticaria. **Special Senses:** Burning, stinging, transient increases in intraocular pressure, irritation, punctate keratitis, blurred vision, hyperemia, synechiae, conjunctivitis, photophobia. **Urogenital:** Urinary retention.

INTERACTIONS Drug: May interfere with the ocular antihypertensive effects of **carbachol, pilocarpine, physostigmine.**

PHARMACOKINETICS Peak: 15–60 min. **Duration:** 24 h.

NURSING IMPLICATIONS

Assessment & Drug Effects

- Monitor cardiac status especially with preexisting heart disease.

Patient & Family Education

- Do not touch the dropper to any surface, including your skin or eyes.
- Exercise caution when driving or engaging in other potentially hazardous activities as cyclopentolate ophthalmic may cause blurred vision. If you experience blurred vision, avoid these activities.
- Protect your eyes when in bright light. Cyclopentolate ophthalmic may cause increased light sensitivity.
- Do not wear soft contact lenses when the eye drops are being inserted.
- Report immediately any of the following: difficulty breathing, swelling of your lips, tongue, face or hives; palpitations; and unusual behavior.
- Do not breast feed while using this drug.

CYCLOPHOSPHAMIDE Pr

(sye-kloe-foss′fa-mide)

Cytoxan, Neosar, Procytox ♣

Classifications: ANTINEOPLASTIC; ALKYLATING AGENT

Pregnancy Category: C

AVAILABILITY 25 mg, 50 mg tablets; 100 mg, 200 mg, 500 mg, 1 g, 2 g vials

ACTIONS Cell-cycle-nonspecific alkylating agent chemically related to the nitrogen mustards. Action mechanism unknown but thought to be the result of cross-linkage of DNA strands, thereby blocking synthesis of DNA, RNA, and protein. Associated with increased risk of secondary malignancies that may be detected several years after cyclophosphamide has been discontinued.

THERAPEUTIC EFFECTS Has pronounced immunosuppressive activity and is a highly toxic drug; thus therapeutic effects are usually accompanied by some evidence of toxicity.

USES As single agent or in combination with other chemotherapeutic agents in treatment of malignant lymphoma, multiple myeloma, leukemias, mycosis fungoides (advanced disease), neuroblastoma, adenocarcinoma of ovary, carcinoma of breast, or malignant neoplasms of lung.

UNLABELED USES To prevent rejection in homotransplantation; to treat severe rheumatoid arthritis, multiple sclerosis, systemic lupus erythematosus, Wegener's granulomatosis, nephrotic syndrome.

CONTRAINDICATIONS Men and women in childbearing years; serious infections (including chickenpox, herpes zoster); live virus vaccines; myelosuppression; pregnancy (category C), lactation.

CAUTIOUS USE History of radiation or cytotoxic drug therapy; hepatic and renal impairment, recent history of steroid therapy; bone marrow infiltration with tumor cells; history of urate calculi and gout; patients with leukopenia, thrombocytopenia.

ROUTE & DOSAGE

Neoplasm

Adult: **PO initial:** 1–5 mg/kg/d; **Maintenance:** 1–5 mg/kg q7–10d. **IV Initial:** 40–50 mg/kg in divided doses over 2–5 d up to 100 mg/kg; **Maintenance:** 10–

C

15 mg/kg q7–10d *or* 3–5 mg twice weekly
Child: **PO initial:** 2–8 mg/kg or 60–250 mg/m^2; **Maintenance:** 2–5 mg/kg *or* 50–150 mg/m^2 twice weekly. **IV Initial:** 2–8 mg/kg *or* 60–250 mg/m^2

Rheumatoid Arthritis

Adult/Child: **PO** 1.5–2.5 mg/kg/d in combination with other agents **IV** 0.5–1 g/m^2 monthly times 6 mo then q 2–3 mo in combination with other agents

ADMINISTRATION

Oral

- Administer PO drug on empty stomach. If nausea and vomiting are severe, however, it may be taken with food. An antiemetic medication may be prescribed to be given before the drug.
- Store cyclophosphamide PO solution in refrigerator at 2°–8° C (36°–46° F), and use within 14 d.

Intravenous

PREPARE: **Direct:** Add 5 mL sterile water for injection or bacteriostatic water for injection (paraben-preserved only) to each 100 mg and shake gently to dissolve. **Intermittent:** May be further diluted with 100–250 mL D5W, NS, D5/NS, RL, or other compatible solution.

ADMINISTER: **Direct/Intermittent:** Give each 100 mg or fraction thereof over 10–15 min.

INCOMPATIBILITIES **Y-site: Amphotericin B, cholesteryl complex.**

- Store at temperature between 2° and 30° C (36° and 86° F) unless otherwise recommended by the manufacturer.

ADVERSE EFFECTS (≥1%) **Body as a Whole:** Transient dizziness, fatigue, facial flushing, diaphoresis, drug fever, anaphylaxis, secondary neoplasia. **GI:** *Nausea, vomiting,* mucositis, *anorexia,* hepatotoxicity, diarrhea. **Hematologic:** Leukopenia, *neutropenia,* acute myeloid leukemia, anemia, thrombophlebitis, interference with normal healing. **Metabolic:** Severe hyperkalemia, SIADH, hyponatremia, weight gain (but without edema) or weight loss, hyperuricemia. **Respiratory:** Pulmonary emboli and edema, pneumonitis, interstitial pulmonary fibrosis. **Skin:** *Alopecia* (reversible), transverse ridging of nails, pigmentation of nail beds and skin (reversible), nonspecific dermatitis, toxic epidermal necrolysis, Stevens-Johnson syndrome. **Urogenital:** Sterile hemorrhagic and nonhemorrhagic cystitis, bladder fibrosis, nephrotoxicity.

DIAGNOSTIC TEST INTERFERENCE Cyclophosphamide suppresses positive reactions to ***Candida, mumps, trichophytons,*** and ***tuberculin PPD skin tests. Papanicolaou (PAP)*** smear may be falsely positive.

INTERACTIONS Drug: Succinylcholine, prolonged neuromuscular blocking activity; **doxorubicin** may increase cardiac toxicity.

PHARMACOKINETICS Absorption: Readily absorbed from GI tract. **Peak:** 1 h PO. **Distribution:** Widely distributed, including brain, breast milk; crosses placenta. **Metabolism:** Metabolized in liver. **Elimination:** Excreted in urine as active metabolites and unchanged drug. **Half-Life:** 4–6 h.

NURSING IMPLICATIONS

Assessment & Drug Effects

- Lab tests: Total and differential leukocyte count, platelet count, and Hct are determined initially and at least 2 times per week during maintenance period. Baseline and periodic determinations of liver and kidney function and serum electrolytes also should be made. Microscopic urine examinations are recommended after large IV doses.

- Thrombocytopenia is rare, but if it occurs (count of 100,000/mm^3 or lower), assess for signs of unexplained bleeding or easy bruising. If platelet count indicates thrombocytopenia ($\leq$100,000/mm^3), drug will be discontinued.
- Marked leukopenia is the most serious side effect. It can be fatal. Nadir may occur in 2–8 d after first dose but may be as late as 1 mo after a series of several daily doses. Leukopenia usually reverses 7–10 d after therapy is discontinued.
- During severe leukopenic period, protect patient from infection and trauma and from visitors and medical personnel who have colds or other infections.
- Report onset of unexplained chills, sore throat, tachycardia. Monitor temperature carefully and report an elevation immediately. The development of fever in a neutropenic patient (granulocyte count <1000) is a medical emergency because sepsis can develop quickly in these patients.
- Observe and report character of wound drainage. During period of neutropenia, purulent drainage may become serosanguineous because there are not enough WBC to create pus. Because of suppressed immune mechanisms, wound healing may be prolonged or incomplete.
- Monitor I&O ratio and patterns: Since the drug is a chemical irritant, PO and IV fluid intake is generally increased to help prevent renal irritation and hemorrhagic cystitis. Have patient void frequently, especially after each dose and just before retiring to bed.
- Watch for symptoms of water intoxication or dilutional hyponatremia; patients are usually well hydrated as part of the therapy.
- Promptly report hematuria or dysuria. Drug schedule is usually interrupted and fluids are forced.
- Record body weight at least twice weekly (basis for dose determination). Alert physician to sudden change or slow, steady weight gain or loss over a period of time that appears inconsistent with caloric intake.
- Diarrhea may signal onset of hyperkalemia, particularly if accompanied by colicky pain, nausea, bradycardia, and skeletal muscle weakness. These symptoms warrant prompt reporting to physician.
- Monitor for hyperuricemia, which occurs commonly during early treatment period in patients with leukemias or lymphoma. Report edema of lower legs and feet; joint, flank, or stomach pain.
- Protect patient from potential sources of infection. Cyclophosphamide makes the patient particularly susceptible to varicella-zoster infections (chickenpox, herpes zoster).
- Report any sign of overgrowth with opportunistic organisms, especially in patient receiving corticosteroids or who has recently been on steroid therapy.
- Report fever, dyspnea, and nonproductive cough. Pulmonary toxicity is not common, but the already debilitated patient is particularly susceptible.

Patient & Family Education

- Adhere to dosage regimen and do not omit, increase, decrease, or delay doses. If for any reason drug cannot be taken, notify physician.

- Alopecia occurs in about 33% of patients on cyclophosphamide therapy. Hair loss may be noted 3 wk after therapy begins; regrowth (often differs in texture and color) usually starts 5–6 wk after drug is withdrawn and may occur while on maintenance doses.
- Use adequate means of contraception during and for at least 4 mo after termination of drug treatment. Breast-feeding should be discontinued before cyclophosphamide therapy is initiated.
- Amenorrhea may last up to 1 y after cessation of therapy in 10–30% of women.
- Do not breast feed while taking this drug.

CYCLOSERINE

(sye-kloe-ser'een)

Seromycin

Classifications: ANTIINFECTIVE; ANTITUBERCULOSIS AGENT

Prototype: Isoniazid

Pregnancy Category: C

AVAILABILITY 250 mg capsules

ACTIONS Broad-spectrum antiinfective derived from strains of *Streptomyces orchidaceus* or *S. garyphalus;* also produced synthetically. Structural analog of the amino acid D-alanine. Inhibits cell wall synthesis in susceptible strains. Bacteriostatic or bactericidal depending on concentration and susceptibility of organism.

THERAPEUTIC EFFECTS Effective against gram-positive and gram-negative bacteria and in *Mycobacterium tuberculosis* by competitively interfering with the incorporation of D-alanine into the bacterial cell wall.

USES In conjunction with other tuberculostatic drugs in treatment of active pulmonary and extrapulmonary tuberculosis when primary agents isoniazid, rifampin, ethambutol, streptomycin have failed. Also used in treatment of acute UTI caused by *Enterobacter sp.* and *Escherichia coli* that are unresponsive to conventional treatment.

UNLABELED USE Treatment of tuberculosis meningitis and nocardiosis.

CONTRAINDICATIONS Epilepsy; depression, severe anxiety, history of psychoses; severe renal insufficiency; chronic alcoholism; pregnancy (category C), lactation. Safe use in children not established.

CAUTIOUS USE Renal impairment, anemia.

ROUTE & DOSAGE

Tuberculosis

Adult: **PO** 250 mg q12h for 2 wk, may increase to 500 mg q12h (max: 1 g/d)

Urinary Tract Infection

Adult: **PO** 250 mg q12h for 2 wk

ADMINISTRATION

Oral

- Pyridoxine 200–300 mg/d may be ordered concurrently to prevent neurotoxic effects of cycloserine.
- Store in tightly closed container at 15°–30° C (59°–86° F) unless otherwise directed.

ADVERSE EFFECTS (≥1%) **CV:** Arrhythmias, CHF. **Hematologic:** Vitamin B_{12} and folic acid deficiency, megaloblastic or sideroblastic anemia. **CNS:** *Drowsiness,* anxiety, *headache,* tremors, myoclonic jerking, convulsions, vertigo, visual disturbances, speech difficulties (dysarthria), lethargy, depression, disorientation with loss of memory, confusion, nervousness, psychoses, tic episodes, character changes, hyperirritability, aggression, hyperreflexia, peripheral neuropathy, paresthesias, paresis, dyskinesias. **Skin:** Dermatitis, photosensitivity. **Special Senses:** Eye pain (optic neuritis), photophobia.

INTERACTIONS Drug: Alcohol increases risk of seizures; **ethionamide, isoniazid** potentiate neurotoxic effects; may inhibit **phenytoin** metabolism, increasing its toxicity.

PHARMACOKINETICS Absorption: 70–90% absorbed from GI tract. **Peak:** 3–4 h. **Distribution:** Distributed to lung, ascitic, pleural and synovial fluids, and CSF; crosses placenta; distributed into breast milk. **Metabolism:** Not metabolized. **Elimination:** 60–70% excreted in urine within 72 h; small amount in feces. **Half-Life:** 10 h.

NURSING IMPLICATIONS

Assessment & Drug Effects

- Lab tests: Culture and susceptibility tests should be performed before initiation of therapy and periodically thereafter to detect possible bacterial resistance. Monitor plasma drug levels weekly and hematologic, renal, and hepatic function at regular intervals.
- Maintenance of blood-drug level below 30 mg/mL considerably reduces incidence of neurotoxicity. Possibility of neurotoxicity increases when dose is 500 mg or more or when renal clearance is inadequate.
- Observe patient carefully for signs of hypersensitivity and neurologic effects. Neurotoxicity generally appears within first 2 wk of therapy and disappears after drug is discontinued.
- Drug should be withheld and physician notified or dosage reduced if symptoms of CNS toxicity or hypersensitivity reaction (see Appendix F) develop.

Patient & Family Education

- Take cycloserine after meals to prevent GI irritation.
- Notify physician immediately of the onset of skin rash and early signs of CNS toxicity (see Appendix F).
- Avoid potentially hazardous tasks such as driving until reaction to cycloserine has been determined.
- Take drug precisely as prescribed and to keep follow-up appointments. Continuous therapy may extend into months or years.
- Do not breast feed while taking this drug.

CYCLOSPORINE Pr

(sye'kloe-spor-een)

Gengraf, Neoral, Sandimmune, Restasis

Classification: IMMUNOSUPPRESSANT

Pregnancy Category: C

AVAILABILITY Sandimmune: 25 mg, 50 mg, 100 mg capsules; 100 mg/mL oral solution **Gengraf, Neoral:** (microemulsion) 25 mg, 100 mg capsules; 100 mg/mL oral solution; 50 mg/mL injection **Restasis:** 0.05% ophthalmic emulsion

ACTIONS Immunosuppressant agent derived from extract of a soil fungus. Action in reducing transplant rejection appears to be due to selective and reversible inhibition of helper T-lymphocytes (which normally stimulate antibody production).

THERAPEUTIC EFFECTS This creates an imbalance in favor of suppressor T-lymphocytes (which inhibit antibody production); thus immune response is subdued. Unlike other immunosuppressive agents, it does not cause clinically significant bone marrow suppression.

USES In conjunction with adrenal corticosteroids to prevent organ rejection after kidney, liver, and heart transplants (allografts). Has had limited use in pancreas, bone marrow, and heart/lung transplantations. Also used for treatment of chronic transplant rejection in patients previously treated with other immunosuppressants; rheumatoid arthritis, severe psoriasis. Ophthalmic emulsion for the treatment of keratoconjunctivitis sicca.

UNLABELED USES Sjögren's syndrome, to prevent rejection of heart-lung and pancreatic transplants, ulcerative colitis.

CONTRAINDICATIONS Hypersensitivity to cyclosporine or to ingredients in commercially available formulations, e.g., Cremophor (polyoxyl 35 castor oil); recent contact with or bout of chickenpox, herpes zoster; administration of live virus vaccines to patient or family members; RA patients with abnormal renal function, uncontrolled hypertension, or malignancies; ocular infection, pregnancy (category C), lactation.

CAUTIOUS USE Renal, hepatic, pancreatic, or bowel dysfunction; biliary tract disease, jaundice, hyperkalemia; electrolyte imbalance, hyperuricemia, hypertension; infection; radiation therapy, older adults, encephalopathy, females of childbearing age, fungal or viral infection, gout, herpes infection, lymphoma, neoplastic disease, malabsorption problems (e.g., liver transplant patients).

ROUTE & DOSAGE

Prevention of Organ Rejection

Adult: **PO** 14–18 mg/kg beginning 4–12 h before transplantation and continued for 1–2 wk after surgery, then gradual reduction by 5%/wk, max dose of microemulsion, 10 mg/kg/d; **Maintenance:** 5–10 mg/kg/d. **IV** 5–6 mg/kg beginning 4–12 h before transplantation and continued after surgery until patient can take oral

Child: **PO** Same as for adult. **IV** Same as for adult

Rheumatoid Arthritis (Neoral)

Adult: **PO** 2.5 mg/kg/d divided into 2 doses. May increase by 0.5–0.75 mg/kg/d q4wk to a max of 4 mg/kg/d

Severe Psoriasis (Neoral)

Adult: **PO** 1.25 mg/kg b.i.d. If significant improvement has not occurred after 4 wk, may increase dose by 0.5 mg/kg/d every 2 wk to max of 4 mg/kg/d

Keratoconjunctivitis sicca

Adult: **Ophthalmic** 1 drop in affected eye(s) twice daily approximately 12 h apart

ADMINISTRATION

Oral

- Do not dilute oral solution with grapefruit juice. Dilute with orange or apple juice, stir well, then administer immediately.

- Neoral (microemulsion) and Sandimmune are not bioequivalent and cannot be used interchangeably without physician supervision.

Intravenous

PREPARE: **IV Infusion:** Dilute each 1 mL immediately before administration in 20–100 mL of D5W or NS.
ADMINISTER: **IV Infusion:** Give by slow infusion over approximately 2–6 h. Rapid IV can result in nephrotoxicity.
INCOMPATIBILITIES **Solution/additive: Magnesium Sulfate. Y-site: Amphotericin B cholesteryl complex, TPN.**

- Store preferably at 15°–30° C (59°–86° F) in well-closed containers. Do not refrigerate. Protect ampuls from light.

ADVERSE EFFECTS (≥1%) **Body as a Whole:** Lymphoma, gynecomastia, chest pain, leg cramps, edema, fever, chills, weight loss, increased risk of skin malignancies in psoriasis patients previously treated with methotrexate, psoralens, or UV light therapy. **CV:** *Hypertension,* MI (rare). **GI:** Gingival hyperplasia, diarrhea, nausea, *vomiting,* abdominal discomfort, anorexia, gastritis, constipation. **Hematologic:** Leukopenia, anemia, thrombocytopenia, *hypermagnesemia, hyperkalemia,* hyperuricemia, *decreased serum bicarbonate,* hyperglycemia. **CNS:** *Tremor,* convulsions, headache, paresthesias, hyperesthesia, flushing, night sweats, insomnia, visual hallucinations, confusion, anxiety, flat affect, depression, lethargy, weakness, paraparesis, ataxia, amnesia. **Skin:** *Hirsutism,* acne, oily skin, flushing. **Special Senses:** Sinusitis, tinnitus, hearing loss, sore throat. **Urogenital:** Urinary retention, frequency, *nephrotoxicity (oliguria).*

DIAGNOSTIC TEST INTERFERENCE ***Hyperlipidemia*** and abnormalities in ***electrophoresis*** reported; believed to be due to polyoxyl 35 castor oil (Cremophor) in IV cyclosporine.

INTERACTIONS Drug: AMINOGLYCOSIDES, **danazol, diltiazem, doxycycline, erythromycin, ketoconazole, methylprednisolone, metoclopramide, nicardipine,** NSAIDS, **prednisolone, verapamil** may increase cyclosporine levels; **carbamazepine, isoniazid, octreotide, phenobarbital, phenytoin, rifampin** may decrease cyclosporine levels; **acyclovir,** AMINOGLYCOSIDES, **amphotericin B, cimetidine, erythromycin, ketoconazole, melphalan, ranitidine, cotrimoxazole, trimethoprim** may increase risk of nephrotoxicity; POTASSIUM-SPARING DIURETICS, ACE INHIBITORS **(captopril, enalapril)** may potentiate hyperkalemia. **Herbal: St. John's wort** may decrease cyclosporine levels.

PHARMACOKINETICS Absorption: Variably and incompletely absorbed (30%). Microemulsion formulation (Neoral) has less variability in absorption and may produce significantly higher serum levels compared with the standard formulation. **Peak:** 3–4 h. **Distribution:** Widely distributed; 33–47% distributed to plasma; 41–50% to RBCs; crosses placenta; distributed into breast milk. **Metabolism:** Extensively metabolized in liver, including significant first pass metabolism; considerable enterohepatic circulation. **Elimination:** Primarily eliminated in bile and feces; 6% excreted in urine. **Half-Life:** 19–27 h.

NURSING IMPLICATIONS

Assessment & Drug Effects

- Observe patients receiving the drug parenterally for at least 30 min continuously after start of IV infusion, and at frequent intervals thereafter to detect allergic or other adverse reactions.
- Hypersensitivity reactions have been associated with Cremophor emulsifying agent in the parenteral formulation but not with the PO solution, which does not contain this ingredient.
- Monitor I&O ratio and pattern: Nephrotoxicity has been reported in about one third of transplant patients. It has occurred in mild forms as late as 2–3 mo after transplantation. In severe form, it can be irreversible, and therefore early recognition is critical.
- Monitor vital signs. Be alert to indicators of local or systemic infection that can be fungal, viral, or bacterial. Also report significant rise in BP.
- Lab tests: Baseline and periodic tests are advised for (1) renal function (BUN, serum creatinine), (2) liver function (AST, ALT, serum amylase, bilirubin, and alkaline phosphatase), and (3) serum potassium.
- Lab tests: In psoriasis patients, CBC, BUN, uric acid, potassium, lipids, and magnesium should be monitored biweekly during first 3 mo.
- Periodic tests should be made of neurologic function. Neurotoxic effects generally occur over 13–195 days after initiation of cyclosporine therapy. Signs and symptoms are reportedly fully reversible with dosage reduction or discontinuation of drug.
- Monitor blood or plasma drug concentrations at regular intervals, particularly in patients receiving the drug orally for prolonged periods, as drug absorption is erratic.

Patient & Family Education

- Use the specially calibrated pipette provided to measure dose.
- Take medication with meals to reduce nausea or GI irritation.
- Enhance palatability of oral solution by mixing it with milk, chocolate milk, or orange juice, preferably at room temperature. Mix in a glass rather than a plastic container. Stir well, drink immediately, and rinse glass with small quantity of diluent to assure getting entire dose.
- Take medication at same time each day to maintain therapeutic blood levels.
- Keep scheduled follow-up appointments.
- If possible, see a dentist before start of cyclosporine treatment, and practice good oral hygiene. Inspect mouth daily for white patches, sores, swollen gums.
- Hirsutism is reversible with discontinuation of drug.
- Do not breast feed while taking this drug.

CYPROHEPTADINE HYDROCHLORIDE

(si-proe-hep′ta-deen)

Periactin, Vimicon ♣

Classifications: ANTIHISTAMINE, H_1-RECEPTOR ANTAGONIST; ANTIPRURITIC

Prototype: Diphenhydramine

Pregnancy Category: B

AVAILABILITY 4 mg tablets

ACTIONS Potent piperidine antihistamine with pharmacologic actions similar to those of azatadine. Acts by competing with histamine for H_1-receptor sites on effector cells, thus preventing histamine-mediated responses.

THERAPEUTIC EFFECTS Produces mild central depression and moderate anticholinergic effects; lacks antiemetic action. Has significant antipruritic, local anesthetic, and antiserotonin activity.

USES Symptomatic relief of various allergic conditions, including hay fever, vasomotor rhinitis, allergic conjunctivitis, urticaria caused by cold sensitivity, and pruritus of allergic dermatoses. Effective in treatment of anaphylactoid reactions as adjunct to epinephrine and other standard measures after acute symptoms have been controlled.

UNLABELED USES Cushing's disease, carcinoid syndrome, vascular headaches, appetite stimulant.

CONTRAINDICATIONS Hypersensitivity to cyproheptadine or other H_1-receptor antagonist antihistamines; acute asthma attack. Safe use during pregnancy (category B), lactation, and in children <2 y not established.

CAUTIOUS USE Older adult and debilitated patients; patients predisposed to urinary retention; glaucoma; asthma; hyperthyroidism; cardiovascular disease, hypertension; GI or GU tract obstruction.

ROUTE & DOSAGE

Allergies

Adult: **PO** 4 mg t.i.d. or q.i.d. (4–20 mg/d), max 0.5 mg/kg/d
Geriatric: **PO** Start with 4 mg b.i.d.
Child: **PO** 0.25 mg/kg/d in 3–4 divided doses (max: 12 mg/d for *2–6 y*, 16 mg/d for *6–12 y*)

ADMINISTRATION

Oral

- GI adverse effects may be minimized by administering drug with food or milk.
- Store in tightly covered container at 15°–30° C (59°–86° F) unless otherwise directed.

ADVERSE EFFECTS (≥1%) **GI:** *Dry mouth,* nausea, vomiting, epigastric distress, appetite stimulation, weight gain, transient decrease in fasting blood sugar level, increased serum amylase level, cholestatic jaundice. **CNS:** *Drowsiness,* dizziness, faintness, headache, tremulousness, fatigue, disturbed coordination. **Respiratory:** Thickened bronchial secretions. **Skin:** Skin rash. **Special Senses:** Dry nose and throat. **Urogenital:** Urinary frequency, retention, and difficult urination.

DIAGNOSTIC TEST INTERFERENCE As a general rule, antihistamines are discontinued about 4 d before ***skin testing procedures*** are to be performed because they may produce false-negative results.

INTERACTIONS Drug: Alcohol and CNS DEPRESSANTS add to CNS depression; TRICYCLIC ANTIDEPRESSANTS and other ANTICHOLINERGICS have additive anticholinergic effects; may inhibit pressor effects of **epinephrine.**

PHARMACOKINETICS Absorption: Readily absorbed from GI tract. **Duration:** 6–9 h. **Distribution:** Distribution into breast milk not known. **Metabolism:** Metabolized in liver. **Elimination:** Excreted in urine.

C

NURSING IMPLICATIONS

Assessment & Drug Effects

- Monitor level of alertness. In some patients, the sedative effect disappears spontaneously after 3–4 d of drug administration.
- Since drug may cause dizziness, supervision of ambulation and other safety precautions may be warranted.

Patient & Family Education

- Avoid activities requiring mental alertness and physical coordination, such as driving a car, until reaction to the drug is known.
- Drug causes sedation, dizziness, and hypotension in older adults. Report these symptoms. Children are more apt to manifest CNS stimulation, e.g., confusion, agitation, tremors, hallucinations. Reduction in dosage may be indicated.
- Cyproheptadine may increase and prolong the effects of alcohol, barbiturates, narcotic analgesics, anxiolytics, and other CNS depressants.
- Monitor weight and keep physician informed of any significant weight gain.
- Maintain sufficient fluid intake to help to relieve dry mouth and also reduce risk of cholestatic jaundice.
- Do not breast feed while taking this drug.

CYTARABINE

(sye-tare'a-been)

ARA-C, Cytosar-U, Cytosine Arabinoside, DepoCyt, Tarabine

Classifications: ANTINEOPLASTIC; ANTIMETABOLITE; IMMUNOSUPPRESSANT

Prototype: Fluorouracil

Pregnancy Category: D

AVAILABILITY 10 mg/mL liposomal, 20 mg/mL, 100 mg, 500 mg, 1g, 2 g injection

ACTIONS Pyrimidine analog with cell phase specificity affecting rapidly dividing cells in S phase (DNA synthesis). In certain conditions prevents development of cell from G_1 to S phase. Interferes with DNA and RNA synthesis.

THERAPEUTIC EFFECTS Antineoplastic agent which has strong myelosuppressant activity. Immunosuppressant properties are exhibited by obliterated cell-mediated immune responses, such as delayed hypersensitivity skin reactions.

USES To induce and maintain remission in acute myelocytic leukemia, acute lymphocytic leukemia, and meningeal leukemia and for treatment of lymphomas. Used in combination with other antineoplastics in established chemotherapeutic protocols.

CONTRAINDICATIONS History of drug-induced myelosuppression; immunization procedures; pregnancy (category D) particularly during first trimester, lactation. Safe use in infants not established.

CAUTIOUS USE Impaired renal or hepatic function, gout, drug-induced myelosuppression.

ROUTE & DOSAGE

Leukemias

Adult/Child: **IV** 200 mg/m² by continuous infusion over 24 h **SC** 1 mg/kg 1–2 times/wk
Intrathecal 5–75 mg once q4d or once/d for 4 d

ADMINISTRATION

Intrathecal

- For intrathecal injection, reconstitute with an isotonic, buffered diluent without preservatives. Follow manufacturer's recommendations.

Intravenous

PREPARE: **Direct:** Reconstitute with bacteriostatic water for injection (without benzyl alcohol for neonates) as follows: add 5 mL to the 100-mg vial to yield 20 mg/mL; add 10 mL to the 500 mg vial to yield 50 mg/mL. **IV Infusion:** May be further diluted with 100 mL or more of D5W or NS.

ADMINISTER: **Direct:** Give at a rate of 100 mg or a fraction thereof over 3 min. IV Infusion: Give over 30 min or longer depending on the total volume of IV solution to be infused.

INCOMPATIBILITIES **Solution/additive: Fluorouracil, gentamicin, heparin, insulin, nafcillin, oxacillin, penicillin G. Y-site: Allopurinol, ganciclovir, TPN.**

- Store cytarabine in refrigerator until reconstituted. Reconstituted solutions may be stored at 15°–30° C (59°–86° F) for 48 h. Discard solutions with a slight haze.

ADVERSE EFFECTS (≥1%) **Body as a Whole:** Weight loss, sore throat, fever, thrombophlebitis and pain at injection site; pericarditis, bleeding (any site), pneumonia. Potentially carcinogenic and mutagenic. **GI:** *Nausea, vomiting,* diarrhea, stomatitis, oral or anal inflammation or ulceration, esophagitis, anorexia, <u>hemorrhage</u>, hepatotoxicity, jaundice. **Hematologic:** *Leukopenia, thrombocytopenia,* anemia, megaloblastosis, myelosuppression (reversible); transient hyperuricemia. **CNS:** Headache, <u>neurotoxicity</u>; peripheral neuropathy, brachial plexus neuropathy, personality change, neuritis, vertigo, lethargy, somnolence, confusion. **Skin:** Rash, erythema, freckling, cellulitis, skin ulcerations, pruritus, urticaria, bulla formation, desquamation. **Special Senses:** Conjunctivitis, keratitis, photophobia. **Urogenital:** Renal dysfunction, urinary retention.

INTERACTIONS Drug: GI toxicity may decrease **digoxin** absorption; decreases AMINOGLYCOSIDES activity against *Klebsiella pneumoniae.*

PHARMACOKINETICS Peak: 20–60 min SC. **Distribution:** Crosses blood-brain barrier in moderate amounts; crosses placenta. **Metabolism:** Metabolized primarily in liver. **Elimination:** 80% excreted in urine in 24 h. **Half-Life:** 1–3 h.

NURSING IMPLICATIONS

Assessment & Drug Effects

- Inspect patient's mouth before the administration of each dose. Toxicity necessitating dosage alterations almost always occurs. Report adverse reactions immediately.
- Lab tests: Hct and platelet counts and total and differential leukocyte counts should be evaluated daily during initial therapy. Serum uric acid and hepatic function tests should be performed at regular intervals throughout treatment period.
- Hyperuricemia due to rapid destruction of neoplastic cells may accompany cytarabine therapy. A regimen that includes a uricosuric agent such as allopurinol, urine alkalinization, and adequate hydration may be started. To reduce potential for urate stone formation, fluids are forced in excess of 2 L, if tolerated. Consult physician.
- Monitor I&O ratio and pattern.
- Monitor body temperature. Be alert to the most subtle signs of

C

infection, especially low-grade fever, and report promptly.

- When platelet count falls below 50,000/mm^3 and polymorphonuclear leukocytes to below 1000/mm^3, therapy may be suspended. WBC nadir is usually reached in 5–7 d after therapy has been stopped. Therapy is restarted with appearance of bone marrow recovery and when preceding cell counts are reached.
- Provide good oral hygiene to diminish adverse effects and chance of superinfection. Stomatitis and cheilosis usually appear 5–10 d into the therapy.

Patient & Family Education

- Report promptly protracted vomiting or signs of nephrotoxicity (see Appendix F).
- Flu-like syndrome occurs usually within 6–12 wk after drug administration and may recur with successive therapy. Report chills, fever, achy joints and muscles.
- Report any S&S of superinfection (see Appendix F).
- Do not breast feed while taking this drug.

CYTOMEGALOVIRUS IMMUNE GLOBULIN (CMVIG, CMV-IVIG)

(cy-to-meg'a-lo-vi-rus)

CytoGam

Classifications: IMMUNOMODULATOR; ANTIVIRAL

Prototype: Interferon Alfa-2a

Pregnancy Category: C

AVAILABILITY 50 mg/mL injection

ACTIONS Cytomegalovirus immune globulin (CMVIG) is a preparation of immunoglobulin G (IgG) antibodies derived from a large number of healthy donors with high concentrations of antibodies directed against cytomegalovirus (CMV).

THERAPEUTIC EFFECTS The CMV antibodies attenuate or reduce the incidence of serious CMV disease, such as CMV-associated pneumonia, CMV-associated hepatitis, and concomitant fungi and parasitic superinfections.

USES Attenuation of primary cytomegalovirus (CMV) disease associated with kidney transplantation.

UNLABELED USE Prevention of CMV disease in other organ transplants (especially heart) when the recipient is seronegative for CMV and the donor is seropositive.

CONTRAINDICATIONS History of previous severe reactions associated with CMVIG or other human immunoglobulin preparations, selective immunoglobulin A (IgA) deficiency; lactation.

CAUTIOUS USE Myelosuppression, cardiac disease, pregnancy (category C).

ROUTE & DOSAGE

Prevention of CMV Disease

Adult: **IV** 150 mg/kg within 72 h of transplantation, then 100 mg/kg 2, 4, 6, and 8 wk posttransplant, then 50 mg/kg 12 and 16 wk posttransplant

ADMINISTRATION

Intravenous

- CMVIG should be administered through a separate IV line using an infusion pump. See manufacturer's directions if this is not possible.

PREPARE: **IV Infusion:** Use a double ended transfer needle or large syringe to reconstitute with 50 mL sterile water. Gently rotate vial to dissolve; do not shake. Allow 30 min to dissolve powder. Reconstituted solution contains 50 mg/mL. Must be completely infused within 12 h since solution contains no preservative.

ADMINISTER: **IV Infusion:** Use a constant infusion pump and give at rate of 15, 30, 60 mg/kg/h over first 30 min, second 30 min, third 30 min, respectively. Monitor closely during and after each rate change. If flushing, nausea, back pain, fever, or chills develops, slow or temporarily discontinue infusion. If BP begins to decrease, stop infusion and institute emergency measures. **Infusion of subsequent IV doses:** The intervals for increasing the dose from 15 to 30 to 60 mg may be shortened from 30 to 15 min. Never infuse more than 75 mL/h CMVIG.

- Reconstituted solution should be started within 6 h and completed within 12 h of preparation. Discard solution if cloudy.

ADVERSE EFFECTS (≥1%) **Body as a Whole:** Muscle aches, back pain, <u>anaphylaxis</u> (rare), fever and chills during infusion. **CV:** Hypotension, palpitations. **GI:** Nausea, vomiting, metallic taste. **CNS:** Headache, anxiety. **Respiratory:** Shortness of breath, wheezing. **Skin:** Flushing.

INTERACTIONS Drug: May interfere with the immune response to LIVE VIRUS VACCINES **(BCG, measles/mumps/rubella, live polio),** defer vaccination with live viral vaccines for approximately 3 mo after administration of CMVIG; revaccination may be necessary if these vaccines were given shortly after CMVIG.

NURSING IMPLICATIONS

Assessment & Drug Effects

- Monitor vital signs preinfusion, before increases in infusion rate, periodically during infusion, and postinfusion.
- Notify physician immediately if any of the following occur: flushing, nausea, back pain, fall in BP, other signs of anaphylaxis.
- Emergency drugs should be available for treatment of acute anaphylactic reactions.
- Monitor for CMV-associated syndromes (e.g., leukopenia, thrombocytopenia, hepatitis, pneumonia) and for superinfections.

Patient & Family Education

- Familiarize yourself with potential adverse effects and know which to report to physician.
- Defer vaccination with live viral vaccines for 3 mo after administration of CMVIG.
- Do not breast feed while taking this drug.

DACARBAZINE

(da-kar'ba-zeen)

DTIC, DTIC-Dome, Imidazole Carboxamide

Classifications: ANTINEOPLASTIC; ALKYLATING AGENT

Prototype: Cyclophosphamide

Pregnancy Category: C

AVAILABILITY 10 mg/mL injection

ACTIONS Cytotoxic agent with alkylating properties, which is cell-cycle nonspecific. Interferes with purine metabolism and with RNA and protein synthesis in rapidly proliferating cells.

THERAPEUTIC EFFECTS Has minimal immunosuppressive activity; reportedly carcinogenic, mutagenic, and teratogenic.

D

USES As single agent or in combination with other antineoplastics in treatment of metastatic malignant melanoma, refractory Hodgkin's disease, various sarcomas, and neuroblastoma.

UNLABELED USES Soft tissue metastatic sarcoma and malignant glucagonoma.

CONTRAINDICATIONS Hypersensitivity to dacarbazine; lactation. Safe use during pregnancy (category C) is not established.

ROUTE & DOSAGE

Neoplasms

Adult: **IV** 2–4.5 mg/kg/d for 10 d repeated at 4-wk intervals or 250 $mg/m^2/d$ for 5 d repeated at 3-wk intervals

Child: **IV** 200–470 $mg/m^2/d$ over 5 d q21–28d

ADMINISTRATION

Intravenous

IV administration to infants and children: Verify correct IV concentration and rate of infusion with physician.

- Wear gloves when handling this drug. If solution gets into the eyes, wash them with soap and water immediately, then irrigate with water or isotonic saline.

PREPARE: **Direct:** Reconstitute drug with sterile water for injection to make a solution containing 10 mg/mL dacarbazine (pH 3.0–4.0) by adding 9.9 mL to 100 mg or 19.8 mL to 200 mg. **IV Infusion:** Dilute further in 50 mL of D5W or NS.

ADMINISTER: **Direct:** Give by direct IV over 1 min. **IV Infusion:** Infuse IV over 30 min. If possible, avoid using antecubital vein or veins on dorsum of hand or wrist where extravasation could lead to loss of mobility of entire limb. Avoid veins in extremity with compromised venous or lymphatic drainage and veins near joint spaces.

INCOMPATIBILITIES **Solution/additive: Heparin.**

- Administer dacarbazine only to patients under close supervision because close observation and frequent laboratory studies are required during and after therapy.
- IV extravasation: Monitor injection site frequently (instruct patient to do so, if able). Give prompt attention to patient's complaint of swelling, stinging, and burning sensation around injection site. Extravasation can occur painlessly and without visual signs. Danger areas for extravasation are dorsum of hand or ankle (especially if peripheral arteriosclerosis is present), joint spaces, and previously irradiated areas. If extravasation is suspected, infusion should be stopped immediately and restarted in another vein. Report to the physician. Prompt institution of local treatment is IMPERATIVE.
- Store reconstituted solution up to 72 h at 4° C (39° F) or at room temperature 15°–30° C; (59°–86° F) for up to 8 h. Store diluted reconstituted solution for 24 h at 4° C (39° F) or at room temperature for up to 8 h. Protect from light.

ADVERSE EFFECTS (≥1%) **Body as a Whole:** Hypersensitivity (erythematosus, urticarial rashes, hepatotoxicity, photosensitivity); facial paresthesia and flushing, flu-like syndrome, myalgia, malaise, anaphylaxis. **CNS:** Confusion, headache, seizures, blurred vision. **GI:** *Anorexia, nausea, vomiting*. **Hematologic:** Severe leukopenia and thrombocytopenia, mild anemia. **Skin:** Alopecia. **Other:** *Pain along injected vein*.

PHARMACOKINETICS Distribution: Localizes primarily in liver. **Metabolism:** Extensively metabolized in liver. **Elimination:** 35%–50% excreted in urine in 6 h. **Half-Life:** 5 h.

NURSING IMPLICATIONS

Assessment & Drug Effects

- Monitor IV site carefully for extravasation; if suspected, discontinue IV immediately and notify physician.
- Note: Skin damage by dacarbazine can lead to deep necrosis requiring surgical debridement, skin grafting, and even amputation. Older adults, the very young, comatose, and debilitated patients are especially at risk. Other risk factors include establishing an IV line in a vein previously punctured several times and the use of nonplastic catheters.
- Lab tests: Monitor for hematopoietic toxicity that usually appears about 4 wk after first dose. Generally, a leukocyte count of <3000/mm^3 and a platelet count of <100,000/mm^3 require suspension or cessation of therapy.
- Avoid, if possible, all tests and treatments during platelet nadir requiring needle punctures (e.g., IM). Observe carefully and report evidence of unexplained bleeding.
- Monitor for severe nausea and vomiting (>90% of patients) that begin within 1 h after drug administration and may last for as long as 12 h.
- Check patient's mouth for ulcerative stomatitis prior to the administration of each dose.
- Monitor I&O ratio and pattern and daily temperature. Renal impairment extends the half-life and increases danger of toxicity. Report symptoms of renal dysfunction and even a slight elevation of temperature.

Patient & Family Education

- Learn about all potential adverse drug effects.
- Report flu-like syndrome that may occur during or even a week after treatment is terminated and last 7–21 d. Symptoms frequently recur with successive treatments.
- Avoid prolonged exposure to sunlight or to ultraviolet light during treatment period and for at least 2 wk after last dose. Protect exposed skin with sunscreen lotion (SPF 15) and avoid exposure in midday.
- Report promptly the onset of blurred vision or paresthesia.
- Do not breast feed while taking this drug.

DACLIZUMAB

(dac'li-zu-mab)

Zenapax

Classifications: IMMUNOSUPPRESSANT; MONOCLONAL ANTIBODY; INTERLEUKIN-2 RECEPTOR ANTAGONIST

Prototype: Basiliximab

Pregnancy Category: C

AVAILABILITY 25 mg/5 mL injection

ACTIONS Immunosuppressant IgG-1 monoclonal antibody produced by recombinant DNA technology. Binds to interleukin-2 (IL-2) receptor complex of lymphocytes.

THERAPEUTIC EFFECTS Therefore, daclizumab inhibits IL-2–mediated activation of lymphocytes which is the major pathway for cellular immune rejection of allografts.

USES Prophylaxis of acute organ rejection in renal transplant.

CONTRAINDICATIONS Hypersensitivity to daclizumab; murine protein hypersensitivity, pregnancy (category C), lactation.
CAUTIOUS USE Moderate-to-severe renal impairment; allergies, asthma, or history of allergic responses to medications; fungal or herpes infection, lymphoma, neoplastic disease, vaccination, varicella, viral infection.

ROUTE & DOSAGE

Renal Transplant
Adult/Child: **IV** *>11 mo,* 1 mg/kg. Start first dose no more than 24 h prior to transplant, then repeat q14d for 4 more doses

ADMINISTRATION

Intravenous

PREPARE: **IV Infusion:** Add calculated amount of drug (based on patient's body weight) to 50 mL of NS. Invert infusion bag to dissolve, but do not shake. Discard if diluted solution is colored or has particulate matter.
ADMINISTER: **IV Infusion:** Infuse diluted drug over 15 min.

- Use diluted solution immediately or store at room temperature for 4 h or at 2°–8° C (36°–46° F) for 24 h. Discard after 24 h.
- Store unopened vials at 2°–8° C (36°–46° F) and protect from light.

ADVERSE EFFECTS (≥1%) **Body as a Whole:** Edema (general and in extremities), pain, fever, fatigue, shivering, generalized weakness, arthralgia, myalgia, hypersensitivity reactions. **CNS:** Tremor, headache, dizziness, insomnia, anxiety, depression. **CV:** Chest pain, hypertension, hypotension, tachycardia, thrombosis, bleeding. **GI:** Constipation, nausea, diarrhea, vomiting, abdominal pain, dyspepsia, abdominal distention, epigastric pain, flatulence, gastritis, hemorrhoids. **Urogenital:** Oliguria, dysuria, renal tubular necrosis, hydronephrosis, urinary tract bleeding, renal insufficiency. **Respiratory:** Dyspnea, pulmonary edema; cough, atelectasis, congestion, pharyngitis, rhinitis, hypoxia, rales, abnormal breath sounds, pleural effusion. **Skin:** Impaired wound healing, acne, pruritus, hirsutism, rash, night sweats. **Other:** Diabetes mellitus, dehydration, blurred vision.

INTERACTIONS Drug: Mycophenolate, cyclosporine may increase mortality.

PHARMACOKINETICS Duration: 120 d. **Half-Life:** 20 d (11–38 d).

NURSING IMPLICATIONS

Assessment & Drug Effects
- Monitor carefully for and immediately report S&S of opportunistic infection or anaphylactoid reaction (see Appendix F).

Patient & Family Education
- Use effective contraception before beginning daclizumab therapy, during therapy, and for 4 mo after completion of therapy.
- Avoid vaccinations during daclizumab therapy.
- Do not breast feed while taking this drug.

DACTINOMYCIN

(dak-ti-noe-mye′sin)
Actinomycin-D, Cosmegen
Classifications: ANTINEOPLASTIC; ANTIBIOTIC
Prototype: Doxorubicin
Pregnancy Category: C

AVAILABILITY 0.5 mg injection

ACTIONS Potent cytotoxic antibiotic derived from mixture of actinomycins produced by *Streptomyces parvulus.* Toxic properties preclude its use as antibiotic. Complexes with DNA, thereby inhibiting DNA, RNA, and protein synthesis. Causes delayed myelosuppression. Potentiates effects of x-ray therapy; the converse also appears likely.
THERAPEUTIC EFFECTS Drug has antineoplastic properties that result from inhibiting DNA and RNA synthesis.

USES As single agent or in combination with other antineoplastics or radiation to treat Wilms' tumor, rhabdomyosarcoma, carcinoma of testes and uterus, Ewing's sarcoma, and sarcoma botryoides.
UNLABELED USES Malignant melanoma, trophoblastic tumors, Kaposi's sarcoma, osteogenic sarcoma, among others.

CONTRAINDICATIONS Chickenpox, herpes zoster, and other viral infections; pregnancy (category C), lactation, infants <6 mo.
CAUTIOUS USE Previous therapy with antineoplastics or radiation within 3–6 wk, bone marrow depression; infections; history of gout; impairment of kidney or liver function; obesity.

ROUTE & DOSAGE

Neoplasms

Adult: **IV** 500 mcg/d for 5 d max., may repeat at 2–4 wk intervals if tolerated (if patient is obese or edematous, give 400–600 mcg/m^2/d to relate dosage to lean body mass) monitor for symptoms of toxicity from overdosage
Child: **IV** 15 mcg/kg/d (max: 500 mcg) for 5 d or 2.5 mg/m^2 over 7 d, may repeat at 2–4 wk intervals if tolerated

Isolation Perfusion

Adult: **IV** 50 mcg/kg for lower extremity or pelvis; 35 mcg/kg for upper extremity

ADMINISTRATION

Intravenous

Use gloves and eye shield when preparing solution. If skin is contaminated, rinse with running water for 10 min; then rinse with buffered phosphate solution. If solution gets into the eyes, wash with water immediately; then irrigate with water or isotonic saline for 10 min.

PREPARE: **Direct:** Reconstitute 0.5 mg vial by adding 1.1 mL sterile water (without preservative) for injection; the resulting solution will contain approximately 0.5 mg/mL. **IV Infusion:** Further dilute in 50 mL of D5W or NS for infusion.

ADMINISTER: **Direct:** Use two-needle technique for direct IV: Withdraw calculated dose from vial with one needle, change to new needle to give directly into vein without using an infusion. Give over 2–3 min. Or give directly into an infusing solutions of D5W or NS, or into tubing or side arm of a running IV infusion. **IV Infusion:** Give diluted solution as a single dose over 15–30 min.

- Store drug at 15°–30° C (59°–86° F) unless otherwise directed. Protect from heat and light.

ADVERSE EFFECTS (≥1%) **GI:** *Nausea, vomiting,* anorexia, abdominal pain, diarrhea, proctitis, GI ulceration, *stomatitis,* cheilitis, glossitis, dysphagia, hepatitis. **Hematologic:** Anemia (including aplastic anemia), agranulocytosis, *leukopenia, thrombocytopenia,* pancytopenia, reticulopenia. **Skin:** Acne, desquamation, hyperpigmentation and reactivation of erythema especially over previously irradiated areas, *alopecia* (reversible). **Other:** Malaise, fatigue, lethargy, fever, myalgia, anaphylaxis, gonadal suppression, hypocalcemia, hyperuricemia, thrombophlebitis; *necrosis, sloughing, and contractures at site of extravasation;* hepatitis, hepatomegaly.

INTERACTIONS Drug: Elevated **uric acid** level produced by dactinomycin may necessitate dose adjustment of ANTIGOUT AGENTS; effects of both dactinomycin and other MYELOSUPPRESSANTS are potentiated; effects of both **radiation** and dactinomycin are potentiated, and dactinomycin may reactivate erythema from previous radiation therapy; **vitamin K** effects (antihemorrhagic) decreased, leading to prolonged clotting time and potential hemorrhage.

PHARMACOKINETICS Distribution: Concentrated in liver, spleen, kidneys, and bone marrow; does not cross blood–brain barrier; crosses placenta; distribution into breast milk not known. **Elimination:** 50% excreted unchanged in bile and 10% in urine; only 30% excreted in urine over 9 d. **Half-Life:** 36 h.

NURSING IMPLICATIONS

Assessment & Drug Effects

- Observe injection site frequently; if extravasation occurs, stop infusion immediately. Restart infusion in another vein. Report to physician. Institute prompt local treatment to prevent thrombophlebitis and necrosis.
- Monitor for severe toxic effects that occur with high frequency. Effects usually appear 2–4 d after a course of therapy is stopped and may reach maximal severity 1–2 wk following discontinuation of therapy.
- Use antiemetic drugs to control nausea and vomiting, which often occur a few hours after drug administration. Vomiting may be severe enough to require intermittent therapy. Observe patient daily for signs of drug toxicity.
- Lab tests: Frequent renal, hepatic, and bone marrow function tests are advised. Perform WBC counts daily, and platelet counts every 3 d to detect hematopoietic depression.
- Monitor temperature and inspect oral membranes daily for stomatitis.
- Monitor for stomatitis, diarrhea, and severe hematopoietic depression. These may require prompt interruption of therapy until drug toxicity subsides.
- Report onset of unexplained bleeding, jaundice, and wheezing. Also, be alert to signs of agranulocytosis (see Appendix F). Report to physician. Antibiotic therapy, protective isolation, and discontinuation of the antineoplastic are indicated.

- Observe and report symptoms of hyperuricemia (see Appendix F). Urge patient to increase fluid intake up to 3000 mL/d if allowed.

Patient & Family Education

- Note: Infertility is a possible, irreversible adverse effect of this drug.
- Learn preventative measures to minimize nausea and vomiting.
- Note: Alopecia (hair loss) is an anticipated reversible adverse effect of this drug. Seek appropriate supportive guidance.
- Do not breast feed while taking this drug.

DALTEPARIN SODIUM

(dal-tep-a′rin)

Fragmin

Classification: BLOOD FORMERS, COAGULATORS, AND ANTICOAGULANTS

Prototype: Enoxaparin

Pregnancy Category: B

AVAILABILITY 2500 IU/0.2 mL, 5000 IU/0.2 mL, 10,000 IU/0.2 mL injection

See Appendix A-2.

DANAZOL

(da′na-zole)

Cyclomen ♣, Danocrine

Classifications: HORMONES AND SYNTHETIC SUBSTITUTES; ANDROGEN/ ANABOLIC STEROID

Prototype: Testosterone

Pregnancy Category: C

AVAILABILITY 50 mg, 100 mg, 200 mg capsules

ACTIONS Synthetic androgen steroid; derivative of testosterone with dose-related mild androgenic effects but no estrogenic or progestational activity.

THERAPEUTIC EFFECTS Suppresses pituitary output of FSH and LH, resulting in anovulation and associated amenorrhea. Interrupts progress and pain of endometriosis by causing atrophy and involution of both normal and ectopic endometrial tissue.

USES Palliative treatment of endometriosis when alternative hormonal therapy is ineffective, contraindicated, or intolerable. Also used to treat fibrocystic breast disease and hereditary angioedema.

UNLABELED USES To treat precocious puberty, gynecomastia, menorrhagia, premenstrual syndrome (PMS), chronic immune thrombocytopenic purpura (ITP), autoimmune hemolytic anemia, hemophilia A and B.

CONTRAINDICATIONS Pregnancy (category C), lactation; children; undiagnosed abnormal genital bleeding; impaired renal, cardiac, or hepatic function.

CAUTIOUS USE Migraine headache, epilepsy.

ROUTE & DOSAGE

Endometriosis

Adult: **PO** 400 mg b.i.d. for 3–6 mo, start during menstruation or if pregnancy test is negative, may extended to 9 mo if necessary. Do not repeat regimen

Fibrocystic Breast Disease

Adult: **PO** 100–400 mg in 2 divided doses, start during menstruation or if pregnancy test is negative

Hereditary Angioedema

Adult: **PO** 200 mg b.i.d. or t.i.d., may decrease by 50% at intervals of 1–3 mo or longer, start during menstruation or if pregnancy test is negative

ADMINISTRATION

Oral

- Start therapy during menstruation, or after a negative pregnancy test.
- Store capsules at 15°–30° C (59°–86° F) in tightly closed container.

ADVERSE EFFECTS (≥1%) **Body as a Whole:** Hypersensitivity (skin rashes, nasal congestion). **Endocrine:** Androgenic effects (acne, mild hirsutism, deepening of voice, oily skin and hair, hair loss, edema, weight gain, pitch breaks, voice weakness, decrease in breast size); hypoestrogenic effects (*hot flashes;* sweating; emotional lability; nervousness; vaginitis with itching, drying, burning, or bleeding; *amenorrhea, irregular menstrual patterns);* impairment in glucose tolerance. **CNS:** Dizziness, sleep disorders, fatigue, tremor, irritability. **Special Senses:** Conjunctival edema. **CV:** Elevated BP. **GI:** Gastroenteritis, hepatic damage (rare), increased LDL, decreased HDL. **Urogenital:** Decreased libido. **Musculoskeletal:** Joint lock-up, joint swelling.

INTERACTIONS Herbal: Echinacea possibility of increased hepatotoxicity.

PHARMACOKINETICS Elimination: other pharmacokinetic information is not known. **Half-Life:** 4.5 h.

NURSING IMPLICATIONS

Assessment & Drug Effects

- Routine breast examinations should be carried out during therapy. Carcinoma of the breast should be ruled out prior to start of therapy for fibrocystic breast disease. Advise patient to report to physician if any nodule enlarges or becomes tender or hard during therapy.
- Because danazol may cause fluid retention, patients with cardiac or renal dysfunction, epilepsy, or migraine should be observed closely during therapy, as these problems could worsen. Monitor weight.
- Drug-induced edema may compress the median nerve, producing symptoms of carpal tunnel syndrome. If patient complains of wrist pain that worsens at night, paresthesias in radial palmar aspect of the hand and fingers, consult physician.
- Lab tests: Baseline and periodic liver function tests should be performed in all patients. Patients with diabetes (or history of) should have blood glucose tests.

Patient & Family Education

- Note: Pain and discomfort are usually relieved in 2 or 3 mo; the nodularity in 4–6 mo. Menses may be regular or irregular in pattern during therapy.
- Note: Drug-induced amenorrhea is reversible. Ovulation and cyclic bleeding usually return within 60–90 d after therapeutic regimen is discontinued as well as the potential for conception.
- Use a nonhormonal contraceptive during treatment because ovulation may not be suppressed until 6–8 wk after therapy is begun. If pregnancy occurs while taking this drug, discontinue danzol. Continue discussing the question of continuing the pregnancy considered.
- Report voice changes promptly. Stop drug to avoid permanent damage to voice. Virilizing adverse effects may persist even after drug therapy is terminated.
- Do not breast feed while taking this drug.

DANTROLENE SODIUM

(dan'troe-leen)

Dantrium

Classifications: AUTONOMIC NERVOUS SYSTEM AGENT; CENTRAL-ACTING SKELETAL MUSCLE RELAXANT

Prototype: Cyclobenzaprine

Pregnancy Category: C

AVAILABILITY 25 mg, 50 mg, 100 mg capsules; 20 mg vial

ACTIONS Hydantoin derivative, structurally related to phenytoin, with peripheral skeletal muscle relaxant action. Directly relaxes the spastic muscle by interfering with calcium ion release from sarcoplasmic reticulum. Clinical doses produce about a 50% decrease in contractility of skeletal muscles but no effect on smooth or cardiac muscles.

THERAPEUTIC EFFECTS Relief of spasticity may be accompanied by muscle weakness sufficient to affect overall functional capacity of the patient.

USES Orally for the symptomatic treatment of skeletal muscle spasms secondary to spinal cord injury, stroke, cerebral palsy, multiple sclerosis. Used intravenously for the management of malignant hyperthermia. Oral dantrolene has been used prophylactically (2 or 3 d before anesthesia) for patients with a history of malignant hyperthermia or with a family history of the disorder.

UNLABELED USES Neuroleptic malignant syndrome, exercise–induced muscle pain, and flexor spasms.

CONTRAINDICATIONS Active hepatic disease; when spasticity is necessary to sustain upright posture and balance in locomotion or to maintain increased body function; spasticity due to rheumatic disorders. Safe use during pregnancy (category C), lactation, or in children <5 y is not established.

CAUTIOUS USE Impaired cardiac or pulmonary function, patients >35 y, especially women.

ROUTE & DOSAGE

Relief of Spasticity

Adult: **PO** 25 mg once/d, increase to 25 mg b.i.d. to q.i.d., may increase q4–7d up to 100 mg b.i.d. to q.i.d.
Child: **PO** 0.5 mg/kg b.i.d., increase to 0.5 mg/kg t.i.d. or q.i.d., may increase by 0.5 mg/kg up to 3 mg/kg b.i.d. to q.i.d. (max: 100 mg q.i.d.)

Malignant Hyperthermia

Adult/Child: **IV** 1 mg/kg rapid direct IV push repeated prn up to a total of 10 mg/kg **PO** May be necessary to continue orally with 1–2 mg/kg q.i.d. for 1–3 d to prevent recurrence

ADMINISTRATION

Oral

- Prepare oral suspension for a single dose, when necessary, by emptying contents of capsule(s) into fruit juice or other liquid. Shake suspension well before pouring. Avoid contamination, keep refrigerated, and use within several days, since it will not contain a preservative.

Intravenous

PREPARE: **Direct:** Dilute each 20 mg with 60 mL sterile water without preservatives. Shake until clear.

ADMINISTER: **Direct:** Give by rapid direct IV push. Avoid extravasation; solution has a high pH and therefore is extremely irritating to tissue. Ensure IV patency prior to IV push.

- Store capsules in tightly closed, light-resistant container. Contents of vial (for IV use) must be protected from direct light and used within 6 h after reconstitution, since it does not contain a preservative. Store both PO and parenteral forms at 15°–30° C (59°–86° F) unless otherwise directed.

ADVERSE EFFECTS (≥1%) **Body as a Whole:** Hypersensitivity (pruritus, urticaria, eczematoid skin eruption, photosensitivity, eosinophilic pleural effusion). **CNS:** Drowsiness, *muscle weakness,* dizziness, lightheadedness, unusual fatigue, speech disturbances, headache, confusion, nervousness, mental depression, insomnia, euphoria, seizures. **CV:** Tachycardia, erratic BP. **Special Senses:** Blurred vision, diplopia, photophobia. **GI:** *Diarrhea,* constipation, nausea, vomiting, anorexia, swallowing difficulty, alterations of taste, gastric irritation, abdominal cramps, GI bleeding; hepatitis, jaundice, hepatomegaly, <u>hepatic necrosis</u> (all related to prolonged use of high doses). **Urogenital:** Crystalluria with pain or burning with urination, urinary frequency, urinary retention, nocturia, enuresis, difficult erection.

INTERACTIONS Drug: Alcohol and other CNS DEPRESSANTS compound CNS depression; **estrogens** increase risk of hepatotoxicity in women >35 y; **verapamil** and other CALCIUM CHANNEL BLOCKERS increase risk of ventricular fibrillation and cardiovascular collapse with IV dantrolene.

PHARMACOKINETICS Absorption: About 35% slowly and incompletely absorbed from GI tract. **Peak:** 5 h. **Distribution:** Crosses placenta. **Metabolism:** Metabolized in liver. **Elimination:** excreted in urine chiefly as metabolites. **Half-Life:** 8.7 h.

NURSING IMPLICATIONS

Assessment & Drug Effects

- Monitor for therapeutic effectiveness. Improvement may not be apparent until 1 wk or more of drug therapy.
- Monitor vital signs during IV infusion. Also monitor ECG, CVP, and serum potassium.
- Supervise ambulation until patient's reaction to drug is known. Relief of spasticity may be accompanied by some loss of strength.
- Note: Most common adverse effects are generally transient, lasting up to 14 d after initiation of therapy. Keep physician informed.
- Monitor patients with impaired cardiac or pulmonary function closely for cardiovascular or respiratory symptoms such as tachycardia, BP changes, feeling of suffocation.
- Monitor for and report symptoms of allergy and allergic pleural effusion: Shortness of breath, pleuritic pain, dry cough.
- Alert physician if improvement is not evident within 45 d. Drug may be discontinued because of the possibility of hepatotoxicity (see Appendix F).
- Lab tests: Perform baseline and regularly scheduled hepatic function tests (alkaline phosphatase, AST, ALT, total bilirubin), blood cell counts, and renal function tests.
- Monitor bowel function. Persistent diarrhea may necessitate drug withdrawal. Severe constipation with abdominal distention and signs of intestinal obstruction have been reported.

Patient & Family Education

- Report promptly the onset of jaundice: yellow skin or sclerae; dark urine, clay-colored stools, itching, abdominal discomfort. Hepatotoxicity frequently occurs between 3rd and 12th mo of therapy.
- Do not drive or engage in other potentially hazardous activities until response to drug is known.
- Do not use OTC medications, alcoholic beverages, or other CNS depressants unless otherwise advised by physician. Liver toxicity occurs more commonly when other drugs are taken concurrently.
- Do not breast feed while taking this drug without consulting physician.

DAPSONE (Pr)

(dap′sone)

Avlosulfon ✤, DDS

Classifications: ANTIINFECTIVE; ANTILEPROSY (SULFONE) AGENT

Pregnancy Category: C

AVAILABILITY 25 mg, 100 mg tablets

ACTIONS Sulfone derivative chemically related to sulfonamides, with bacteriostatic and bactericidal activity similar to that group. Interferes with bacterial cell growth by competitive inhibition of folic acid synthesis by susceptible organisms.

THERAPEUTIC EFFECTS Spectrum of activity includes *Mycobacterium leprae* (Hansen's bacillus), *Mycobacterium tuberculosis,* and limited activity against *Pneumocystis carinii* and *Plasmodium*. Drug is effective against dapsone-sensitive multibacillary (borderline, borderline lepromatous, or lepromatous) leprosy, and dapsone-sensitive paucibacillary (indeterminate, tuberculoid, or borderline tuberculoid) leprosy. Resistant strains of initially susceptible *M. leprae* develop slowly in a stepwise fashion over periods of 5–24 y.

USES Drug of choice for treatment of all forms of leprosy (unless organism is shown to be dapsone resistant). Used in dapsone-sensitive multibacillary leprosy (with clofazimine and rifampin) and in dapsone-sensitive paucibacillary leprosy (with rifampin, clofazimine, or ethionamide). Also used prophylactically in contacts of patients with all forms of leprosy except tuberculoid and indeterminate leprosy. Used for treatment of dermatitis herpetiformis.

UNLABELED USES Chemoprophylaxis of malaria (with pyrimethamine), systemic and discoid lupus erythematosus, pemphigus vulgaris, dermatosis (especially those associated with bullous eruptions, mucocutaneous lesions, inflammation or pustules); rheumatoid arthritis, allergic vasculitis; treatment of initial episodes of *P. carinii* pneumonia (with trimethoprim) in limited number of adults with AIDS.

CONTRAINDICATIONS Hypersensitivity to sulfones or its derivatives; advanced renal amyloidosis, anemia, methemoglobin reductase deficiency. Safe use during pregnancy (category C) or lactation is not established.

CAUTIOUS USE Chronic renal, hepatic, pulmonary, or cardiovascular disease, refractory anemias, albuminuria, G6PD deficiency.

ROUTE & DOSAGE

Tuberculoid and Indeterminate-type Leprosy

Adult: **PO** 100 mg/d (with 6 mo of rifampin 600 mg/d) for a minimum of 3 y

D

Lepromatous and Borderline Lepromatous Leprosy

Adult: **PO** 100 mg/d for ≥10 y
Child: **PO** 1–2 mg/kg/d once daily in combination therapy (max: 100 mg/d)

Dermatitis Herpetiformis

Adult: **PO** 50 mg/d, may be increased to 300 mg/d if necessary (max: 500 mg/d)

Prophylaxis for Close Contacts of Patient with Multibacillary Leprosy

Adult: **PO** 50 mg/d
Child: **PO** *<6 mo,* 6 mg 3 times/wk; *6–23 mo,* 12 mg 3 times/wk; *2–5 y,* 25 mg 3 times/wk; *6–12 y,* 25 mg/d

***P. carinii* Pneumonia Prophylaxis**

Adult: **PO** 50 mg b.i.d. or 100 mg q.d.
Child: **PO** 2 mg/kg once daily (max: 100 mg/d)

ADMINISTRATION

Oral

- Give with food to reduce possibility of GI distress.
- Store in tightly covered, light-resistant containers at 15°–30° C (59°–86° F). Drug discoloration apparently does not indicate a chemical change.

ADVERSE EFFECTS (≥1%) **Body as a Whole:** Hypersensitivity (cutaneous reactions); erythema multiforme, exfoliative dermatitis, toxic epidermal necrolysis [rare], allergic rhinitis, urticaria, fever, infectious mononucleosis-like syndrome. **CNS:** Headache, nervousness, insomnia, vertigo; paresthesia, *muscle weakness.* **CV:** Tachycardia. **GI:** Anorexia, nausea, vomiting, abdominal pain; toxic hepatitis, cholestatic jaundice (reversible with discontinuation of drug therapy); increased ALT, AST, LDH; hyperbilirubinemia. **Hematologic:** In patient with or without G6PD deficiency; *dose-related hemolysis,* Heinz body formation, *methemoglobinemia with cyanosis,* hemolytic anemia; aplastic anemia (rare), agranulocytosis. **Skin:** Drug-induced lupus erythematosus, phototoxicity. **Special Senses:** Blurred vision, tinnitus. **Other:** Male infertility; sulfone syndrome (fever, malaise, exfoliative dermatitis, hepatic necrosis with jaundice, lymphadenopathy, methemoglobinemia, anemia).

INTERACTIONS Drug: Activated charcoal decreases dapsone absorption and enterohepatic circulation; **pyrimethamine, trimethoprim** increase risk of adverse hematologic reactions; **rifampin** decreases dapsone levels 7–10 fold.

PHARMACOKINETICS Absorption: Rapidly and nearly completely absorbed from GI tract. **Peak:** 2–8 h. **Distribution:** Distributed to all body tissues; high concentrations in kidney, liver, muscle, and skin; crosses placenta; distributed into breast milk. **Metabolism:** Metabolized in liver. **Elimination:** 70%–85% excreted in urine; remainder excreted in feces; traces of drug may be found in body for 3 wk after discontinuation of repeated doses. **Half-Life:** 20–30 h.

NURSING IMPLICATIONS

Assessment & Drug Effects

- Monitor for therapeutic effectiveness that may not appear for leprosy until after 3–6 mo of therapy. Skin lesions respond well; recovery from nerve involvement is usually limited.
- Lab tests: Perform baseline then weekly CBC during the first

month of therapy, at monthly intervals for at least 6 mo, and semiannually thereafter.
- Determine periodic dapsone blood levels.
- Perform liver function tests in patients who complain of malaise, fever, chills, anorexia, nausea, vomiting, and have jaundice. Dapsone therapy is usually suspended until etiology is identified.
- Monitor severity of anemia. Nearly all patients demonstrate hemolysis. Manufacturer states that Hgb level is generally decreased by 1–2 g/dL; reticulocytes increase by 2%–12%; RBC life span is shortened; and methemoglobinemia occurs in most patients receiving dapsone.
- Monitor temperature during first few weeks of therapy. If fever is frequent or severe, leprosy reactional state should be ruled out. Reduction of or interruption of therapy may be sufficient for improvement.
- Report cyanotic appearance or mucous membranes with brownish hue to physician as possible methemoglobinemia.

Patient & Family Education
- Report symptoms of leprosy that do not improve within 3 mo or get worse to physician.
- Report the appearance of a rash with bullous lesions around elbows and other joints promptly. Drug-induced or worsening skin lesions require withdrawal of dapsone.
- Report symptoms of peripheral neuropathy with motor loss (muscle weakness) promptly.
- Do not breast feed while taking this drug without consulting physician.

DAPTOMYCIN

(dap-to-my'sin)
Cubicin
Classifications: ANTI-INFECTIVE; ANTIBIOTIC; LIPOPEPTIDE
Pregnancy Category: B

AVAILABILITY 250 mg, 500 mg vial

ACTIONS Daptomycin is cyclic lipopeptide antibiotic. It binds to bacterial membranes of gram-positive bacteria causing rapid depolarization of the membrane potential leading to inhibition of protein, DNA, and RNA synthesis and bacterial cell death. Lipopeptides are bactericidal against gram-positive bacteria.
THERAPEUTIC EFFECTS Daptomycin is effective against a broad spectrum of gram-positive organisms, including both susceptible and resistant strains of *S. aureus*.

USES Complicated skin and skin structure infections.

CONTRAINDICATIONS GI disease, pseudomembranous colitis; myopathy, peripheral neuropathy; rhabdomyolysis; infants, children, elderly, lactation.
CAUTIOUS USE Severe renal or hepatic impairment, end-stage renal impairment; pregnancy (category B).

ROUTE & DOSAGE

Skin Infections
Adult: **IV** 4 mg/kg q24h × 7–14 d
Renal Impairment
Cl_{cr} <30 mL/min: 4 mg/kg q48h

ADMINISTRATION

Intravenous

PREPARE: **IV Infusion:** Reconstitute the 250 mg vial or the 500

D

mg vial with 5 mL or 10 mL, respectively, of NS to yield 50 mg/mL. Further dilute the 50 mg/mL solution in 50-100 mL of NS or RL.
ADMINISTER: **IV Infusion:** Infuse over 30 min; if same IV line is used for infusion of other drugs, flush line before/after with NS or RL.
INCOMPATIBILITIES **Solution/additive:** Little data available, thus additives or other medications should not be added or infused simultaneously through the same intravenous line.

- Store unopened vials in 2°–8° C (36°–46° F). Avoid excessive heat. May store reconstituted, single-use vials or IV solution for 12 h at room temperature or 48 h if refrigerated.

ADVERSE EFFECTS (≥1%) **Body as a Whole:** Injection site reactions, fever, fungal infections. **CNS:** Headache, insomnia, dizziness. **CV:** Hypotension, hypertension. **GI:** Constipation, nausea, vomiting, diarrhea, abnormal liver function tests. **Hematologic:** Anemia. **Metabolic:** Elevated CPK. **Musculoskeletal:** Limb pain, arthralgia. **Respiratory:** Dyspnea. **Skin:** Rash, pruritus. **Urogenital:** UTIs, renal failure.

INTERACTIONS Drug: Potential increased risk of myopathy with STATINS.

PHARMACOKINETICS Metabolism: Site of metabolism not determined. **Elimination:** Primarily renal. **Half-Life:** 8 h.

NURSING IMPLICATIONS

Assessment & Drug Effects

- Monitor for and report: muscle pain or weakness, especially with concurrent therapy with HMG-CoA reductase inhibitors (statin drugs); S&S of peripheral neuropathy, superinfection such as candidiasis.
- Lab tests: Perform C&S before treatment is begun; baseline renal function tests; weekly CPK levels; PT/INR during first few days of daptomycin therapy with concurrent warfarin use; daily blood glucose monitoring in diabetics; serum electrolytes if S&S of hypokalemia or hypomagnesemia (see Appendix F) appear.
- Withhold drug and notify physician if S&S of myopathy develop with CPK elevation >1000 U/L (~5 × ULN), or if CPK level is ≥10 × ULN.

Patient & Family Education

- Report any of the following to the physician: muscle pain, weakness or unusual tiredness; numbness or tingling; difficulty breathing or shortness of breath; severe diarrhea or vomiting; skin rash or itching.
- Do not breast feed without consulting the physician.

DARBEPOETIN ALFA

(dar-be-po-e'tin)
ARANESP
Classifications: BLOOD FORMERS, COAGULATORS AND ANTICOAGULANTS; HEMATOPOIETIC GROWTH FACTOR
Prototype: Epoetin alfa
Pregnancy Category: C

AVAILABILITY 25 mcg/mL, 40 mcg/mL, 60 mcg/mL, 100 mcg/mL vials; 300 mcg/0.6 mL syringe

ACTIONS Darbepoetin is an erythropoiesis-stimulating protein closely related to erythropoietin. Erythropoietin is a primary growth factor for erythroid development. It is produced naturally in the kidney in response to hypoxia, and stimulates red blood cell production in the bone marrow.

THERAPEUTIC EFFECTS Production of endogenous erythropoietin is impaired in patients with chronic renal failure (CRF) resulting in anemia. Darbepoetin stimulates erythropoiesis by the same mechanism as endogenous erythropoietin.

USES Treatment of anemia in patients with chronic renal failure or chemotherapy-associated anemia.

CONTRAINDICATIONS Patients with uncontrolled hypertension; hypersensitivity to darbepoetin, pregnancy (category C).

CAUTIOUS USE Controlled hypertension, elevated hemoglobin, folic acid or vitamin B_{12} deficiencies, infections, inflammatory or malignant processes, osteofibrosis, occult blood loss, hemolysis, severe aluminum toxicity, bone marrow fibrosis, chronic renal failure patients not on dialysis, lactation, hematologic diseases.

ROUTE & DOSAGE

Anemia

Adult: **IV/SC** Initially, 0.45 mcg/kg once/wk. Reduce dose by 25% if there is a rapid increase (i.e., more than 1 g/dl in any 2-wk period) in Hgb or if the Hgb is increasing and approaching 12 g/dl. If the Hgb does not increase by 1 g/dl after 4 wk of therapy and iron stores are adequate, increase the dose by 25%. Maintenance dose is 0.26–0.65 mcg/kg once/wk

Converting epoetin alfa to darbepoetin

Adults: **IV/SC** Estimate the starting dose of darbepoetin alfa based on the total weekly dose of epoetin alfa at the time of conversion. If the patient was receiving epoetin alfa 2–3 times/wk, administer darbepoetin alfa once per week; if the patient was receiving epoetin alfa once per week, administer darbepoetin alfa once every 2 wks. The route of administration (i.e., SC or IV) should be maintained. Note: The following darbepoetin alfa dosage recommendations are estimates based on total amount of epoetin alfa administered per week. Because of individual variability, titrate doses to maintain the target Hgb.

Epoetin alfa <2500 Units/week: Initial darbepoetin alfa dose 6.25 mcg/wk

Epoetin alfa 2500–4999 Units/week: Initial darbepoetin alfa dose 12.5 mcg/wk

Epoetin alfa 5000–10,999 Units/week: Initial darbepoetin alfa dose 25 mcg/wk

Epoetin alfa 11,000–17,999 Units/week: Initial darbepoetin alfa dose 40 mcg/wk

Epoetin alfa 18,000–33,999 Units/week: Initial darbepoetin alfa dose 60 mcg/wk

Epoetin alfa 34,000–89,999 Units/week: Initial darbepoetin alfa dose 100 mcg/wk

Epoetin alfa ≥90,000 Units/week: Initial darbepoetin alfa dose 200 mcg/wk

ADMINISTRATION

All Routes

- Correct deficiencies of folic acid or vitamin B_{12} prior to initiation of therapy.

Subcutaneous

- Do not shake solution. Shaking may denature the darbepoetin, rendering it biologically inactive.

D

- Inspect solution for particulate matter prior to use. Do not use if solution is discolored or if it contains particulate matter.
- Use only one dose per vial, and do not reenter vial.
- Do not give with any other drug solution.

Intravenous

PREPARE: **Direct:** Withdraw the desired dose and give undiluted. Discard the unused portion.
ADMINISTER: **Direct:** Give direct IV as a bolus dose over 1 min.

- Discard any unused portion of the vial. It contains no preservatives.

- Store at 2°–8° C (36°–46° F). Do not freeze or shake. Protect from light.

ADVERSE EFFECTS (≥1%) **Body as a Whole:** Injection site pain, *peripheral edema,* fatigue, fever, death, chest pain, fluid overload, access infection, access hemorrhage, flu-like symptoms, asthenia, *infection.* **CNS:** *Headache,* dizziness. **CV:** *Hypertension, hypotension, arrhythmias,* cardiac arrest, angina, chest pain, vascular access thrombosis, CHF. **GI:** *Nausea, vomiting, diarrhea,* constipation. **Musculoskeletal:** *Myalgia, arthralgia,* limb pain, back pain. **Respiratory:** *Upper respiratory infection, dyspnea, cough,* bronchitis. **Skin:** Pruritus.

INTERACTIONS Drug: No clinically significant reactions reported to date.

PHARMACOKINETICS Absorption: 37% absorbed from SC site. **Peak:** 24–72 h SC. **Distribution:** Distribution confined primarily to intravascular space. **Elimination:** 10% excreted in urine. **Half-Life:** 21 h IV, 49 h SC.

NURSING IMPLICATIONS

Assessment & Drug Effects

- Control BP adequately prior to initiation of therapy and closely monitor and control during therapy. Report immediately S&S of CHF, cardiac arrhythmias, or sepsis. Note that hypertension is an adverse effect that must be controlled.
- Notify physician of a rapid rise in Hgb as dosage will need to be reduced because of risk of serious hypertension. Note that BP may rise during early therapy as Hgb increases.
- Monitor for premonitory neurological symptoms (i.e., aura, and report their appearance promptly). The potential for seizures exists during periods of rapid Hgb increase (e.g., >1.0 g/dl in any 2-wk period).
- Monitor closely and report immediately S&S of thrombotic events (e.g., MI, CVA, TIA), especially for patients with CRF.
- Lab tests: At baseline and periodically thereafter, evaluate iron stores, including transferrin and serum ferritin; Hgb twice weekly until stabilized and maintenance dose is established, then weekly for at least 4 wk, and at regular intervals thereafter; CBC with differential and platelet count at regular interval; periodic BUN, creatinine, serum phosphorus, and serum potassium.

Patient & Family Education

- Adhere closely to antihypertensive drug regimen and dietary restrictions.
- Monitor BP as directed by physician.
- Do not drive or engage in other potentially hazardous activity during the first 90 d of therapy because of possible seizure activity.
- Report any of the following to the physician: chest pain, difficulty

breathing, shortness of breath, severe or persistent headache, fever, muscle aches and pains, or nausea.
- Do not breast feed while taking this drug without consulting physician.

DAUNORUBICIN HYDROCHLORIDE

(daw-noe-roo'bi-sin)
Cerubidine

DAUNORUBICIN CITRATED LIPOSOMAL

DaunoXome
Classifications: ANTINEOPLASTIC; ANTIBIOTIC
Prototype: Doxorubicin HCl
Pregnancy Category: D

AVAILABILITY **Daunorubicin HCl** 10 mg, 20 mg, 50 mg, 100 mg, 150 mg lyophilized vials; 2 mg/mL injection; **Daunorubicin Citrated Liposomal** 2 mg/mL (equivalent to 50 mg daunorubicin base) injection

ACTIONS Cytotoxic and antimitotic glycoside antibiotic; cell-cycle specific for S-phase of cell division. Toxic properties preclude its use as an antibiotic. Mechanism of action unclear but may be due to rapid intercalating of DNA molecule resulting in inhibition of DNA, RNA, and protein synthesis.
THERAPEUTIC EFFECTS A potent bone marrow suppressant with immunosuppressive properties as well as antineoplastic properties. It interferes with DNA and RNA synthesis. Induces cardiac toxicity and may be mutagenic and carcinogenic (development of secondary carcinomas).

USES To induce remission in acute nonlymphocytic leukemia (myelogenous, monocytic, erythroid) in adults.
UNLABELED USES Solid tumors of childhood and non-Hodgkin's lymphoma.

CONTRAINDICATIONS Severe myelosuppression; immunizations (patient, family), and preexisting cardiac disease unless risk-benefit is evaluated; lactation; uncontrolled systemic infection. Safe use during pregnancy (category D) is not established.
CAUTIOUS USE History of gout, urate calculi, hepatic or renal function impairment; older adult patients with inadequate bone reserve due to age or previous cytotoxic drug therapy, tumor cell infiltration of bone marrow, patient who has received potentially cardiotoxic drugs or related antineoplastics.

ROUTE & DOSAGE

Neoplasms
Adult: **IV** As a single agent, 30–60 mg/m^2/d for 3–5 d q3–4wk (max: total cumulative dose 500–600 mg/m^2); As combination therapy, 30–45 mg/m^2/d on days 1, 2, 3 of first course and days 1 and 2 of subsequent courses.
Child: **IV** As combination therapy, *≥2 y,* 25–45 mg/m^2; *<2 y,* calculated on body weight (mg/kg) rather than body surface area

Kaposi's Sarcoma (DaunoXome)
Adult: **IV** 40 mg/m^2 over 1 h, repeat q2wk (for serum bilirubin >3 mg/dL or S_{cr} >3 mg/dL, administer half normal dose)

ADMINISTRATION

Intravenous
Use gloves during preparation for infusion to prevent skin contact

with this drug. If contact occurs, decontaminate skin with copious amounts of water with soap.

PREPARE: **Direct:** Reconstitute 20 mg vial with 4 mL sterile water for injection. The concentration of the solution will be 5 mg/mL. ▪ Withdraw dose into syringe containing 10–15 mL normal saline. **IV Infusion:** Dilute further in 100 mL NS as required.

ADMINISTER: **Direct:** Inject over approximately 3 min into the tubing or side arm of a rapidly flowing IV infusion of D5W or NS. **Infusion:** Give a single dose over 30 min.

Specific to DaunoXome

PREPARE: **IV Infusion:** Each vial of DaunoXome contains the equivalent of 50 mg daunorubicin base. Dilute with enough D5W to produce a concentration of 1 mg/1mL.

ADMINISTER: **IV Infusion:** Give DaunoXome over 60 min. Do not use a filter with DaunoXome.

INCOMPATIBILITIES **Solution/additive: Dexamethasone, Heparin.**

▪ Avoid extravasation because it can cause severe tissue necrosis.

▪ Store reconstituted solution at room temperature (15°–30° C; 59°–86° F) for 24 h and under refrigeration at 2°–8° C (36°–46° F) for 48 h. Protect from light.

ADVERSE EFFECTS (≥1%) **Body as a Whole:** Fever. **CNS:** Amnesia, anxiety, ataxia, confusion, hallucinations, emotional lability, tremors. **CV:** Pericarditis, myocarditis, arrhythmias, peripheral edema, CHF, hypertension, tachycardia. **GI:** *Acute nausea and vomiting* (mild), anorexia, *stomatitis,* mucositis, diarrhea (occasionally) hemorrhage. **Urogenital:** Dysuria, nocturia, polyuria, dry skin. **Hematologic:** *Bone marrow depression thrombocytopenia, leukopenia,* anemia, **Skin:** Generalized *alopecia* (reversible), transverse pigmentation of nails, severe cellulitis or tissue necrosis at site of drug extravasation. **Endocrine:** Hyperuricemia, gonadal suppression.

PHARMACOKINETICS Distribution: Highest concentrations in spleen, kidneys, liver, lungs, and heart; does not cross blood–brain barrier; crosses placenta; distribution into breast milk not known. **Metabolism:** Metabolized in liver to active metabolite. **Elimination:** 25% excreted in urine, 40% in bile. **Half-Life:** 18.5–26.7 h.

NURSING IMPLICATIONS

Assessment & Drug Effects

- Monitor for therapeutic effectiveness. A profound suppression of bone marrow is required to induce a complete remission. Nadirs for thrombocytes and leukocytes are usually reached in 10–14 d.
- Monitor serum bilirubin; drug dose needs to be reduced when bilirubin is >1.2 mg/dL.
- Lab tests: Perform Hct, platelet count, total and differential leukocyte count, serum uric acid, chest x-ray, and cardiac, hepatic, and renal function tests prior to and periodically during therapy.
- Monitor BP, temperature, pulse, and respiratory function during treatment.
- Monitor for S&S of acute CHF. It can occur suddenly, especially when total dosage exceeds 550 mg/m^2, or in patients with compromised heart function because of previous radiation therapy to heart area.

- Report immediately: Breathlessness, orthopnea, change in pulse and BP parameters. Early clinical diagnosis of drug-induced CHF is essential for successful treatment.
- Report promptly S&S of superinfections including elevation of temperature, chills, upper respiratory tract infection, tachycardia, overgrowth with opportunistic organisms because myelosuppression imposes risk of superimposed infection (see Appendix F).
- Protect patient from contact with persons with infections. The most hazardous period is during nadirs of thrombocytes and leukocytes.
- Control nausea and vomiting (usually mild) by antiemetic therapy.
- Inspect oral membranes daily. Mucositis may occur 3–7 d after drug is administered.

Patient & Family Education

- Note: Loss of hair is probable; recovery is usual in 6–10 wk.
- Use barrier contraceptives during treatment because this drug is teratogic. Tell your physician immediately if you become pregnant during therapy.
- Note: A transient effect of the drug is to turn urine red on the day of infusion.
- Do not breast feed while taking this drug.

DEFEROXAMINE MESYLATE

(de-fer-ox'a-meen)

Desferal

Classifications: CHELATING AGENT; ANTIDOTE

Pregnancy Category: C

AVAILABILITY 500 mg vials

ACTIONS Chelating agent isolated from *Streptomyces pilosus* with specific affinity for ferric ion and low affinity for calcium.

THERAPEUTIC EFFECTS Binds ferric ions to form a stable water-soluble chelate readily excreted by kidneys. Main effect is removal of iron from ferritin, hemosiderin, and transferrin.

USES Adjunct in treatment of acute iron intoxication. Has been used in management of hemochromatosis and hemosiderosis secondary to increased iron storage as from multiple transfusions used in treatment of congenital anemias, e.g., thalassemia (Cooley's or Mediterranean anemia), sickle cell anemia, and other chronic anemias.

UNLABELED USES To promote aluminum excretion in aluminum-associated dialysis encephalopathy and aluminum accumulation in bones of patients in renal failure.

CONTRAINDICATIONS Severe renal disease, anuria, pyelonephritis; pregnancy (category C), and children <3 y of age.

CAUTIOUS USE History of pyelonephritis; lactation.

ROUTE & DOSAGE

Acute Iron Intoxication

Adult: **IM/IV** 1 g followed by 500 mg at 4 h intervals for 2 doses, subsequent doses of 500 mg q4–12h may be given if necessary (max: 6 g/24 h), infuse at ≤15 mg/kg/h
Child: **IM/IV** 20 mg/kg followed by 10 mg/kg at 4 h intervals for 2 doses, subsequent doses of 10 mg/kg q4–12h may be given if necessary (max: 6 g/24 h), infuse at ≤15 mg/kg/h

Chronic Iron Overload

Adult/Child: **IM** 500 mg–1 g/d
IV 2 g with each unit of blood transfused, infuse at ≤15 mg/kg/h

SC 1–2 g/d (20–40 mg/kg/d) infused over 8–24 h (*Child,* max: 6 g/d or 2 g/dose)

D

ADMINISTRATION

Subcutaneous/Intramuscular

- Reconstitute by adding 2 mL sterile water for injection to 500-mg vial to yield 250 mg/mL. Dissolve drug completely before it is withdrawn from vial.
- Administer SC dose over 8–24 h using portable minipump devices.
- Use IM route for all patients not in shock; preferred route for acute intoxication.

Intravenous

For infants and children: Verify correct IV concentration and rate with physician.

PREPARE: **IV Infusion:** Reconstitute by adding 5 mL sterile water for injection to 500-mg vial to yield 100 mg/mL. ▪ After drug is completely dissolved, withdraw prescribed amount from vial and add to NS, D5W, or RL solution.

ADMINISTER: **IV Infusion:** Give initial 1000 mg dose at a rate not to exceed 15 mg/kg/h. ▪ Give subsequent 500 mg doses at a rate of 125 mg/h.

- Do not infuse IV rapidly; such infusion is associated with the occurrence of more adverse effects.

- Store at room temperature 15°–30° C (59°–86° F) for not longer than 1 wk. Protect from light.

ADVERSE EFFECTS (≥1%) **Body as a Whole:** Hypersensitivity (generalized itching, cutaneous wheal formation, rash, fever, <u>anaphylactoid reaction</u>). **CV:** Hypotension, tachycardia. **Special Senses:** Decreased hearing; blurred vision, decreased visual acuity and visual fields, color vision abnormalities, night blindness, retinal pigmentary degeneration. **GI:** Abdominal discomfort, diarrhea. **Urogenital:** Dysuria, exacerbation of pyelonephritis, orange-rose discoloration of urine. **Other:** *Pain and induration at injection site.*

PHARMACOKINETICS Distribution: Widely distributed in body tissues. **Metabolism:** Forms nontoxic complex with iron. **Elimination:** Excreted primarily in urine; some excreted in feces.

NURSING IMPLICATIONS

Assessment & Drug Effects

- Lab tests: Perform baseline kidney function tests prior to drug administration.
- Monitor injection site. If pain and induration occur, move infusion to another site.
- Monitor I&O ratio and pattern. Report any change. Observe stools for blood (iron intoxication frequently causes necrosis of GI tract).
- Note: Periodic ophthalmoscopic (slit lamp) examinations and audiometry are advised for patients on prolonged or high-dose therapy for chronic iron overload.

Patient & Family Education

- Deferoxamine chelate makes urine turn a reddish color.
- Report blurred vision or any other visual abnormality.
- Do not breast feed while taking this drug without consulting physician.

DELAVIRDINE MESYLATE

(del-a-vir′deen)

Rescriptor

Classifications: ANTIINFECTIVE; ANTIVIRAL; NONNUCLEOSIDE REVERSE TRANSCRIPTASE INHIBITOR

Prototype: Nevirapine

Pregnancy Category: C

AVAILABILITY 100 mg tablets

ACTIONS Nonnucleoside reverse transcriptase inhibitor (NNRTI) of HIV-1 binds directly to reverse transcriptase (RT) and blocks RNA- and DNA-dependent DNA polymerase activities.

THERAPEUTIC EFFECTS Thus, it prevents replication of the HIV-1 virus. HIV-2 RT and human DNA polymerases such as polymerases alpha, gamma, and delta are not inhibited by delavirdine. Resistant strains appear rapidly.

USES Treatment of HIV infection in combination with other antiretroviral agents.

CONTRAINDICATIONS Hypersensitivity to delavirdine; lactation.

CAUTIOUS USE Impaired liver function, pregnancy (category C). Safety and efficiency in children ≤16 y have not been established.

ROUTE & DOSAGE

HIV Infection
Adult: **PO** 400 mg t.i.d.
Child: **PO** ≤*16 y*, 400 mg t.i.d.

ADMINISTRATION

Oral

- Disperse in water by adding a single dose to at least 3 oz of water, let stand for a few minutes, then stir to create a uniform suspension just prior to administration.
- Give drug to patients with achlorhydria with an acid beverage such as orange or cranberry juice.
- Store at 20°–25° C (68°–77° F) and protect from high humidity in a tightly closed container.

ADVERSE EFFECTS (≥1%) **Body as a Whole:** Headache, fatigue, allergic reaction, chills, edema, arthralgia. **CNS:** Abnormal coordination, agitation, amnesia, anxiety, confusion, dizziness. **CV:** Chest pain, bradycardia, palpitations, postural hypotension, tachycardia. **GI:** Nausea, vomiting, diarrhea, increased LFTs, abdominal cramps, anorexia, aphthous stomatitis. **Hematologic:** Neutropenia. **Respiratory:** Bronchitis, cough, dyspnea. **Skin:** *Rash,* pruritus.

INTERACTIONS Drug: ANTACIDS, H_2-RECEPTOR ANTAGONISTS decrease absorption; **didanosine** and **delavirdine** should be taken 1 h apart to avoid decreased delavirdine levels; **clarithromycin, fluoxetine, ketoconazole** may increase delavirdine levels; **carbamazepine, phenobarbital, phenytoin, rifabutin, rifampin** may decrease delavirdine levels; delavirdine may increase levels of **clarithromycin, astemizole, indinavir, saquinavir, dapsone, rifabutin, alprazolam, midazolam, triazolam,** DIHYDROPYRIDINE, CALCIUM CHANNEL BLOCKERS (e.g., **nifedipine, nicardipine**, etc.), **cisapride, quinidine, warfarin. Herbal: St. John's wort** may decrease antiretroviral activity.

PHARMACOKINETICS Absorption: Rapidly absorbed from GI tract, 80% reaches systemic circulation. **Peak:** 1 h. **Distribution:** 98% protein bound. **Metabolism:** Metabolized in the liver by the CYP3A enzymes. **Elimination:** Approximately 51% excreted in urine, 44% in feces. **Half-Life:** 2–11 h.

NURSING IMPLICATIONS

Assessment & Drug Effects

- Therapeutic effectiveness: Indicated by decreased viral load.
- Monitor for and immediately report appearance of a rash, generally

within 1–3 wk of starting therapy; rash is usually diffuse, maculopapular, erythematous, and pruritic.

Patient & Family Education

- Take this drug exactly as prescribed. Missed doses increase risk of drug resistance.
- Do not take antacids and delavirdine at the same time; separate by at least 1 h.
- Report all prescription and nonprescription drugs used to physician because of multiple drug interactions.
- Discontinue medication and notify physician if rash is accompanied by any of the following: Fever, blistering, oral lesions, conjunctivitis, swelling, muscle or joint pain.
- Do not breast feed while taking this drug.

DEMECARIUM BROMIDE

(dem-e-kare′ee-um)

Humorsol

Classifications: EYE PREPARATION; MIOTIC (ANTIGLAUCOMA); AUTONOMIC NERVOUS SYSTEM AGENT; CHOLINERGIC; CHOLINESTERASE INHIBITOR

Prototype: Pilocarpine HCl

Pregnancy Category: C

AVAILABILITY 0.125%, 0.25% ophthalmic solution

See Appendix A-1.

DEMECLOCYCLINE HYDROCHLORIDE

(dem-e-kloe-sye′kleen)

Declomycin

Classifications: ANTIINFECTIVE; ANTIBIOTIC; TETRACYCLINE

Prototype: Tetracycline

Pregnancy Category: D

AVAILABILITY 150 mg capsules; 150 mg, 300 mg tablets

ACTIONS Broad-spectrum, tetracycline antibiotic isolated from mutant strain of *Streptomyces aureofaciens*. Similar to tetracycline but is absorbed more readily, excreted much more slowly.

THERAPEUTIC EFFECTS Drug has longer duration of effective blood levels than tetracycline; therefore intervals between doses can be longer. Primarily bacteriostatic in action.

USES Similar to those of tetracycline.

UNLABELED USES Treatment of chronic SIADH (Syndrome of Inappropriate [excessive] Antidiuretic Hormone) secretion.

CONTRAINDICATIONS Hypersensitivity to any of the tetracyclines; cirrhosis, common bile duct obstruction; period of tooth development [last half of pregnancy (category D), lactation, children <8 y (causes permanent yellow discoloration of teeth, enamel hypoplasia, and retarded bone growth)].

CAUTIOUS USE Impaired renal or hepatic function; nephrogenic diabetes insipidus; use of capsule or tablet formulations in patients with esophageal compression or obstruction.

ROUTE & DOSAGE

Antiinfective

Adult: **PO** 150 mg q6h or 300 mg q12h (max: 2.4 g/d)
Child: **PO** *>8 y*, 8–12 mg/kg/d divided q8–12h

Gonorrhea

Adult: **PO** 600 mg followed by 300 mg q12h for 4 d

SIADH
Adult: **PO** 600–1200 mg/d in 3–4 divided doses

ADMINISTRATION

Oral

- Give not less than 1 h before or 2 h after meals. Foods rich in iron (e.g., red meat or dark green vegetables) or calcium (e.g., milk products) impair absorption.
- Concomitant therapy: Do not give antacids with tetracyclines.
- Check expiration date before giving drug. Renal damage and death have resulted from use of outdated tetracyclines.
- Request physician order to give with light meal if gastric distress is a problem. Absorption may be reduced; keep meal dairy free.
- Store in tight, light-resistant containers, preferably at 15°–30° C (59°–86° F) unless otherwise directed. Tetracyclines form toxic products when outdated or exposed to light, heat, or humidity.

ADVERSE EFFECTS (≥1%) **Body as a Whole:** Hypersensitivity (*photosensitivity,* pericarditis, anaphylaxis [rare]). **GI:** *Nausea,* vomiting, *diarrhea,* esophageal irritation or ulceration, enterocolitis, abdominal cramps, anorexia. **Urogenital:** Diabetes insipidus, azotemia, hyperphosphatemia. **Skin:** Pruritus, erythematous eruptions, exfoliative dermatitis.

DIAGNOSTIC TEST INTERFERENCE Like other tetracyclines, demeclocycline may cause false increases in ***urine catecholamines*** (**fluorometric** methods); false decreases in ***urine urobilinogen;*** and false-negative ***urine glucose*** with **glucose oxidase** methods (e.g., **Clinistix, TesTape**).

INTERACTIONS Drug: ANTACIDS, IRON PREPARATION, **calcium, magnesium, zinc, kaolin-pectin, sodium bicarbonate** can significantly decrease demeclocycline absorption; effects of **desmopressin** and demeclocycline antagonized; increases **digoxin** absorption, increasing risk of **digoxin** toxicity; **methoxyflurane** increases risk of renal failure. **Food:** Dairy products significantly decrease demeclocycline absorption; food may decrease drug absorption also.

PHARMACOKINETICS Absorption: 60%–80% absorbed from GI tract. **Peak:** 3–4 h. **Distribution:** Concentrated in liver; crosses placenta; distributed into breast milk. **Metabolism:** Metabolized in liver; enterohepatic circulation. **Elimination:** 40%–50% excreted in urine and 31% in feces in 48 h. **Half-Life:** 10–17 h.

NURSING IMPLICATIONS

Assessment & Drug Effects

- Lab tests: C&S prior to initial therapy and periodically during prolonged therapy. With prolonged therapy, add periodic evaluations of serum drug levels, electrolytes, and renal, hepatic, and hematopoietic systems.
- Monitor I&O ratio and pattern and record weights in patients with impaired kidney or liver function, or on prolonged or high dose therapy. Some patients develop diabetes insipidus-like syndrome (SIADH).

Patient & Family Education

- Do not use antacids while taking this drug.
- Take drug on an empty stomach to enhance absorption. Because esophageal irritation and ulceration have been reported, take

D

each dose with a full glass (240 mL) of water; remain upright for at least 90 s after taking medication; and avoid taking drug within 1 h of lying down or bedtime.

- Notify physician if gastric distress is a problem; a snack or light meal free of dairy products may be added to the regimen.
- Report symptoms of superinfections; this is VERY important (see Appendix F).
- Demeclocycline-induced phototoxic reaction can be unusually severe. Avoid sunlight as much as possible and use sunscreen.
- Do not breast feed while taking this drug.

DENILEUKIN DIFTITOX

(den-i-leu′kin dif′ti-tox)

Ontak

Classifications: ANTINEOPLASTIC; INTERLEUKIN-2 (IL-2) INHIBITOR; IMMUNOMODULATOR

Pregnancy Category: C

AVAILABILITY 300 mcg/2 mL vial

ACTIONS A recombinant DNA cytotoxic protein which is an interleukin-2 receptor-specific protein that acts as an antineoplastic agent against malignant cells that express the CD25 component of the interleukin-2 (IL-2) receptor on the cell surface.

THERAPEUTIC EFFECTS Effectiveness is indicated by reduced tumor burden. Interacts with high affinity to CD25 IL-2 receptors on the cell surface in certain leukemias and lymphomas, thus inhibiting cellular protein synthesis and resulting in cell death in malignant tumors.

USES Persistent or recurrent T-cell lymphoma.

CONTRAINDICATIONS Hypersensitivity to denileukin, diphtheria toxin, or interleukin-2; pregnancy (category C), lactation.

CAUTIOUS USE Cardiovascular disease; hepatic and renal impairment, preexisting lower of serum albumin levels, serum albumin levels below 3 grams/dL. Safety and efficacy in children <18 y are unknown.

ROUTE & DOSAGE

T-Cell Lymphoma

Adult: **IV** 9 or 18 mcg/kg/day infused over at least 15 min daily for 5 d every 21 d

ADMINISTRATION

Intravenous

PREPARE: **IV Infusion:** Bring vials to room temperature (solution will be clear when room temperature is reached). Swirl to mix, but do not shake. Use only plastic syringe and plastic IV bag. Withdraw the calculated dose and inject it into an empty IV bag. Add NO MORE THAN 9 mL sterile saline without preservative to IV bag for each 1 mL of drug. Use within 6 h of preparation.

ADMINISTER: **IV Infusion:** Infuse over at least 15 minutes without an in-line filter. Stop infusion and notify physician if S&S of hypersensitivity occur.

INCOMPATIBILITIES **Solution/additive:** Do not physically mix with any other drug.

ADVERSE EFFECTS (≥1%) **Body as a Whole:** *Chills, fever, asthenia, infection, pain, headache, chest pain,* flu-like syndrome; injection site reaction; *acute hypersensitivity reaction (hypotension, back pain, dysp-*

nea, vasodilation, rash, chest pain or tightness, tachycardia, dysphagia, syncope, *anaphylaxis),* myalgia, arthralgia. **CNS:** *Dizziness, paresthesia, nervousness,* confusion, insomnia. **CV:** *Vascular leak syndrome (hypotension, edema, hypoalbuminemia); hypotension, vasodilation, tachycardia,* thrombotic events, hypertension, arrhythmia. **GI:** *Nausea, vomiting, anorexia, diarrhea,* constipation, dyspepsia, dysphagia. **Hematologic:** *Anemia,* thrombocytopenia, leukopenia. **Metabolic:** *Hypoalbuminemia; transaminase increase; edema; hypocalcemia; weight loss;* dehydration; hypokalemia. **Respiratory:** *Dyspnea, cough, pharyngitis, rhinitis,* lung disorder. **Skin:** *Rash, pruritus, sweating.* **Urogenital:** *Hematuria, albuminuria, pyuria, increased creatinine.*

INTERACTIONS: No clinically significant interactions established.

PHARMACOKINETICS Distribution: Primarily distributed to liver and kidneys. **Metabolism:** Metabolized by proteolytic degradation. **Half-Life:** 70–80 min.

NURSING IMPLICATIONS

Assessment & Drug Effects

- Monitor and notify physician immediately for S&S of hypersensitivity or anaphylaxis that occur during/within 24 h of infusion.
- Monitor and notify physician immediately for S&S of flu-like syndrome that occur within several hours to days following infusion.
- Monitor outpatients for weight gain, developing edema, or declining blood pressure. Notify physician immediately for S&S of vascular leak syndrome (e.g., edema PLUS hypotension or hypoalbuminemia) that may occur within 2 wk of infusion.
- Lab tests: Baseline and weekly CBC with differential, platelet count, blood chemistry panel (including serum electrolytes, serum albumin, renal and liver functions).

Patient & Family Education

- Report S&S of infection promptly to physician.
- Check weight daily and report rapid weight gain or swelling of extremities promptly.
- Report bothersome adverse effects or S&S of infection or flu-like symptoms (e.g., fever, nausea, vomiting, diarrhea, rash).
- Do not breast feed while taking this drug.

DESIPRAMINE HYDROCHLORIDE

(dess-ip′ra-meen)

Norpramin, Pertofrane

Classifications: CENTRAL NERVOUS SYSTEM AGENT; PSYCHOTHERAPEUTIC; TRICYCLIC ANTIDEPRESSANT

Prototype: Imipramine

Pregnancy Category: C

AVAILABILITY 10 mg, 25 mg, 50 mg, 75 mg, 100 mg, 150 mg tablets

ACTIONS Dibenzoxazepine tricyclic antidepressant (TCA) and secondary amine. Desipramine is the active metabolite of imipramine and has similar pharmacologic actions. Unlike imipramine, onset of action is more rapid, and it has lower potential for producing sedative and anticholinergic effects and orthostatic hypotension.

THERAPEUTIC EFFECTS In common with other TCAs, antidepressant activity appears to be related to inhibition of reuptake of norepinephrine and serotonin in the CNS. Restoration of the levels of these neurotransmitters is a proposed mechanism of antidepressant action.

D

USES Endogenous depression and various depression syndromes.

UNLABELED USES Attention deficit disorder in children >6 y and adolescents; to prevent depression in cocaine withdrawal.

CONTRAINDICATIONS Hypersensitivity to tricyclic compounds; recent MI. Safe use during pregnancy (category C), lactation, or in children <12 y is not established.

CAUTIOUS USE Urinary retention, prostatic hypertrophy; narrow-angle glaucoma; epilepsy; alcoholism; adolescents, older adults; thyroid; cardiovascular, renal, and hepatic disease; suicidal tendency; ECT; elective surgery.

ROUTE & DOSAGE

Antidepressant

Adult: **PO** 75–100 mg/d at bedtime or in divided doses, may gradually increase to 150–300 mg/d (use lower doses in older adult patients)
Adolescent: **PO** 25–50 mg/d (max: 100 mg/d) in divided doses
Child: **PO** *6–12 y,* 1–3 mg/kg/d in divided doses (max: 5 mg/kg/d)

ADMINISTRATION

Oral

- Give drug with or immediately after food to reduce possibility of gastric irritation.
- Give maintenance dose at bedtime to minimize daytime sedation.
- Store drug in tightly closed container at 15°–30° C (59°–86° F) unless otherwise specified.

ADVERSE EFFECTS (≥1%) **Body as a Whole:** Hypersensitivity (rash, urticaria, photosensitivity). **CNS:** *Drowsiness,* dizziness, weakness, fatigue, headache, insomnia, confusional states, depressive reaction, paresthesias, ataxia. **CV:** *Postural hypotension,* hypotension, palpitation, tachycardia, ECG changes, flushing, heart block. **Special Senses:** Tinnitus, parotid swelling; blurred vision, disturbances in accommodation, mydriasis, increased IOP. **GI:** *Dry mouth, constipation,* bad taste, diarrhea, nausea. **Urogenital:** *Urinary retention,* frequency, delayed micturition, nocturia; impaired sexual function, galactorrhea. **Hematologic:** Bone marrow depression and agranulocytosis (rare). **Other:** Sweating, craving for sweets, weight gain or loss, SIADH secretion, hyperpyrexia, eosinophilic pneumonia.

INTERACTIONS Drug: May somewhat decrease response TO ANTIHYPERTENSIVES; CNS DEPRESSANTS, **alcohol,** HYPNOTICS, BARBITURATES, SEDATIVES potentiate CNS depression; may increase hypoprothombinemic effect of ORAL ANTICOAGULANTS; **ethchlorvynol** may cause transient delirium; **levodopa,** SYMPATHOMIMETICS (e.g., **epinephrine, norepinephrine**) pose possibility of sympathetic hyperactivity with hypertension and hyperpyrexia; MAO INHIBITORS pose possibility of severe reactions, toxic psychosis, cardiovascular instability; **methylphenidate** increases plasma TCA levels; THYROID AGENTS may increase possibility of arrhythmias; **cimetidine** may increase plasma TCA levels. **Herbal: Ginkgo** may decrease seizure threshold; **St. John's wort** may cause **serotonin** syndrome.

PHARMACOKINETICS Absorption: Rapidly absorbed from GI tract and injection sites. **Peak:** 4–6 h. **Distribution:** Crosses placenta. **Metabolism:** Metabolized in liver.

Elimination: Primarily excreted in urine. **Half-Life:** 7–60 h.

NURSING IMPLICATIONS

Assessment & Drug Effects

- Monitor for therapeutic effectiveness: Usually not realized until after at least 2 wk of therapy.
- Monitor BP and pulse rate during early phase of therapy, particularly in older adult, debilitated, or cardiovascular patients. If BP rises or falls more than 20 mm Hg or if there is a sudden increase in pulse rate or change in rhythm, withhold drug and inform physician.
- Note: Drowsiness, dizziness, and orthostatic hypotension are signs of impending toxicity in patient on long-term, high dosage therapy. Prolonged QT or QRS intervals indicate possible toxicity. Report to physician.
- Observe patient with history of glaucoma. Report symptoms that may signal acute attack: Severe headache, eye pain, dilated pupils, halos of light, nausea, vomiting.
- Monitor bowel elimination pattern and I&O ratio. Severe constipation and urinary retention are potential problems of TCA therapy.
- Note: Norpramin tablets may contain tartrazine, which can cause allergic-type reactions including bronchial asthma in susceptible individuals. Such individuals are frequently also sensitive to aspirin.

Patient & Family Education

- Make all position changes slowly and in stages, particularly from recumbent to standing position.
- Do not drive or engage in other potentially hazardous activities until reaction to drug is known.
- Take medication exactly as prescribed; do not change dose or dose intervals.
- Note: Patients who receive high doses for prolonged periods may experience withdrawal symptoms including headache, nausea, musculoskeletal pain, and weakness if drug is discontinued abruptly.
- Do not take OTC drugs unless physician has approved their use.
- Stop, or at least limit, smoking because it may increase the metabolism of desipramine, thereby diminishing its therapeutic action.
- Do not breast feed while taking this drug without consulting physician.

DESLORATADINE

(des-lor-a-ta′deen)

Clarinex

Classifications: ANTIHISTAMINE, NON-SEDATING; H_1-RECEPTOR ANTAGONIST

Prototype: Loratadine

Pregnancy Category: C

AVAILABILITY 5 mg tablets; 0.5 mg/mL syrup

ACTIONS A long-acting, nonsedating antihistamine with selective H_1 receptor antagonist properties. The drug reduces human mast cell release of the inflammatory cytokines. Therefore, it also exhibits antiallergic effects.

THERAPEUTIC EFFECTS It is more potent than loratadine or terfenadine as an antagonist at H_1 receptors. Desloratadine is effective in controlling allergic rhinitis and inhibiting histamine-induced wheals and flare (hives).

USES Treatment of seasonal or perennial allergic rhinitis and idiopathic urticaria.

CONTRAINDICATIONS Hypersensitivity to desloratadine or loratadine; neonates; pregnancy (category C); lactation.

D

CAUTIOUS USE Renal and hepatic insufficiencies; bladder neck obstruction or urinary retention; prostatic hypertrophy; glaucoma. Safety and efficacy in children <12 y not known.

ROUTE & DOSAGE

Allergic Rhinitis, Idiopathic Urticaria

Adult: **PO** 5 mg q.d.

Renal Impairment

Adult: **PO** Cl_{cr} <50 mL/min: 5 mg every other day

Hepatic Impairment

Adult: **PO** 5 mg every other day

ADMINISTRATION

Oral

- Note that drug should be given q.o.d. to patients with significant renal or hepatic impairment.
- Store between 2°–25° C (36°–77° F).

ADVERSE EFFECTS (≥1%) **Body as a Whole:** Pharyngitis, fatigue, flu-like symptoms, myalgia. **CNS:** Somnolence, dizziness. **GI:** Dry mouth, nausea, dry throat. **Urogenital:** Dysmenorrhea.

INTERACTIONS Drug: No clinically significant interactions established.

PHARMACOKINETICS Absorption: Well absorbed. **Peak:** 3 h. **Distribution:** 85–89% protein bound. **Metabolism:** Extensively metabolized in liver to 3-hydroxydesloratadine, an active metabolite. **Elimination:** Excreted equally in urine and feces. **Half-Life:** 27 h.

NURSING IMPLICATIONS

Assessment & Drug Effects

- Assess carefully for and report distressing or dangerous S&S that occur after initiation of the drug. A variety of adverse effects, although not common, are possible. Some are an indication to discontinue the drug.
- Monitor cardiovascular status and report significant changes in BP and palpitations or tachycardia.
- Lab tests: Monitor periodically renal and liver function tests.
- Concurrent drugs: Monitor ECG when used in combination with any other drug that can increase blood level of desloratidine in patients with preexisting cardiac disease.

Patient & Family Education

- Drug may cause significant drowsiness in older adult patients and those with liver or kidney impairment.
- Note: Concurrent use of alcohol and other CNS depressants may have an additive effect.
- Do not take this drug more often than every other day if you have renal impairment.
- Do not breast feed while taking this drug without consulting physician.

DESMOPRESSIN ACETATE

(des-moe-pres′sin)

DDAVP, Stimate

Classifications: HORMONES AND SYNTHETIC SUBSTITUTES; PITUITARY (ANTIDIURETIC) HORMONE

Prototype: Vasopressin

Pregnancy Category: B

AVAILABILITY 0.1 mg, 0.2 mg tablets; 0.1 mg/mL, 1.5 mg/mL nasal solution; 4 mcg/mL, 15 mcg/mL injection

ACTIONS Synthetic analog of the natural human posterior pituitary (antidiuretic) hormone, arginine vasopressin. Has more specific and longer duration of action than antidiuretic hormone and lower incidence of allergic reactions. Also, oxytocic and vasopressor actions are not apparent at therapeutic dosages. Unlike vasopressin, it does not stimulate release of adrenocorticotropic hormone nor does it increase plasma cortisol, growth hormone, prolactin, or luteinizing hormone levels.

THERAPEUTIC EFFECTS Reduces urine volume and osmolality in patients with central diabetes insipidus by increasing reabsorption of water by kidney collecting tubules. Produces a dose-related increase in factor VIII (antihemophilic factor) and von Willebrand's factor.

USES To control and prevent symptoms and complications of central (neurohypophyseal) diabetes insipidus, and to relieve temporary polyuria and polydipsia associated with trauma or surgery in the pituitary region.

UNLABELED USES To increase factor VIII activity in selected patients with mild to moderate hemophilia A and in type I von Willebrand's disease or uremia, and to control enuresis in children.

CONTRAINDICATIONS Nephrogenic diabetes insipidus, type II B von Willebrand's disease. Safe use during pregnancy (category B) or lactation is not established.

CAUTIOUS USE Coronary artery insufficiency, hypertensive cardiovascular disease.

ROUTE & DOSAGE

Diabetes Insipidus

Adult: **Intranasal** 0.1–0.4 mL (10–40 mcg) in 1–3 divided doses **IV/SC** 2–4 mcg in 2 divided doses **PO** 0.2–0.4 mg/d

Child: **Intranasal** 3 *mo–12 y,* 0.05–0.3 mL in 1–2 divided doses **IV/SC** 0.3 mcg/kg infused over 15–30 min **PO** 0.05 mg titrated to response

Enuresis

Adult/Child: **Intranasal** 5–40 mcg h.s.

Child: **PO** ≥6 *y,* 0.2 mg h.s., may titrate up to 0.6 mg h.s.

Von Willebrand's Disease

Adult/Child: **IV/SC** >*3 mo,* 0.3 mcg/kg 30 min preop, may repeat in 48 h if needed

ADMINISTRATION

Oral

- Note that 0.2 mg PO is equivalent to 10 mcg (0.1 mL) intranasal.

Intranasal

- Follow manufacturer's instructions for proper technique with nasal spray.
- Give initial dose in the evening, and observe antidiuretic effect. Dose is increased each evening until uninterrupted sleep is obtained. If daily urine volume is more than 2 L after nocturia is controlled, morning dose is started and adjusted daily until urine volume does not exceed 1.5–2 L/24 h.

Intravenous

PREPARE: **Direct:** Give undiluted for diabetes insipidus. **IV Infusion:** Dilute 0.3 mcg/kg in 10 mL of NS (children ≤10 kg) or 50 mL of NS (children >10 kg and adults) for von Willebrand's disease (type I).

ADMINISTER: **Direct:** Give direct IV over 30 s for diabetes insipidus. **IV Infusion:** Give over 15–30 min for von Willebrand's disease (type I).

D

▪ Store parenteral and nasal solution in refrigerator preferably at 4° C (39.2° F) unless otherwise directed. Avoid freezing. ▪ Nasal spray can be stored at room temperature. ▪ Discard solutions that are discolored or contain particulate matter.

ADVERSE EFFECTS (≥1%) **All:** Dose related. **CNS:** Transient headache, drowsiness, listlessness. **Special Senses:** Nasal congestion, rhinitis, nasal irritation. **GI:** Nausea, heartburn, mild abdominal cramps. **Other:** Vulval pain, shortness of breath, slight rise in BP, facial flushing, pain and swelling at injection site.

INTERACTIONS Drug: Demeclocycline, lithium, other VASOPRESSORS may decrease antidiuretic response; **carbamazepine, chlorpropamide, clofibrate** may prolong antidiuretic response.

PHARMACOKINETICS Absorption: 10%–20% absorbed through nasal mucosa. **Onset:** 15–60 min. **Peak:** 1–5 h. **Duration:** 5–21 h. **Distribution:** Small amount crosses blood–brain barrier; distributed into breast milk. **Half-Life:** 76 min.

NURSING IMPLICATIONS

Assessment & Drug Effects

- Monitor I&O ratio and pattern (intervals). Fluid intake must be carefully controlled, particularly in older adults and the very young to avoid water retention and sodium depletion.
- Weigh patient daily and observe for edema. Severe water retention may require reduction in dosage and use of a diuretic.
- Monitor BP during dosage-regulating period and whenever drug is administered parenterally.
- Monitor urine and plasma osmolality. An increase in urine osmolality and a decrease in plasma osmolality indicate effectiveness of treatment in diabetes insipidus.

Patient & Family Education

- Report upper respiratory tract infection or nasal congestion.
- Follow manufacturer's instructions for insertion to ensure delivery of drug high into nasal cavity and not down throat. A flexible calibrated plastic tube is provided.
- Do not breast feed while taking this drug without consulting physician.

DESONIDE

(dess′oh-nide)

DesOwen, Tridesilon

Classifications: SKIN AND MUCOUS MEMBRANE; ANTIINFLAMMATORY; STEROID

Prototype: Hydrocortisone

Pregnancy Category: C

AVAILABILITY 0.05% ointment, cream, lotion

See Appendix A-4.

DESOXIMETASONE

(des-ox-i-met′a-sone)

Topicort, Topicort-LP

Classifications: SKIN AND MUCOUS MEMBRANE; ANTIINFLAMMATORY; STEROID

Prototype: Hydrocortisone

Pregnancy Category: C

AVAILABILITY 0.25% ointment; 0.25%, 0.05% cream; 0.05% gel

See Appendix A-4.

D

DEXAMETHASONE

(dex-a-meth'a-sone)

Aeroseb-Dex, Decaderm, Decadron, Decaspray, Deronil ♣, Dexameth, Dexamethasone Intensol, Dexasone, Dexone, Hexadrol, Maxidex, Mymethasone, Oradexon ♣

DEXAMETHASONE ACETATE

Dalalone D. P., Dalalone-LA, Decadron-LA, Decaject-LA, Dexacen LA-8, Dexasone-LA, Dexo-LA, Dexon LA, Dexone LA, Solurex-LA

DEXAMETHASONE SODIUM PHOSPHATE

AK-Dex, Alba Dex, Dalalone, Decadrol, Decadron Phosphate, Decaject, Dex-4, Dexacen-4, Dexasone, Dexon, Dexone, Hexadrol Phosphate, Maxidex Ophthalmic, Savacort-D, Solurex

Classifications: HORMONES AND SYNTHETIC SUBSTITUTES, ADRENAL CORTICOSTEROID; GLUCOCORTICOID; STEROID

Prototype: Prednisone

Pregnancy Category: C

AVAILABILITY **Dexamethasone** 0.25 mg, 0.5 mg, 0.75 mg, 1 mg, 1.5 mg, 2 mg, 4 mg, 6 mg tablets; 0.5 mg/5 mL, 0.5 mg/0.5 mg oral solution; 0.01%, 0.04% topical aerosol; **Dexamethasone Acetate** 8 mg/mL, 16 mg/mL injection suspension; **Dexamethasone Sodium Phosphate** 4 mg/mL, 10 mg/mL, 20 mg/mL, 24 mg/mL injection; 0.1% cream; 0.1% ophthalmic solution, suspension; 0.05% ophthalmic ointment

ACTIONS Long-acting synthetic adrenocorticoid with intense anti-inflammatory (glucocorticoid) activity and minimal mineralocorticoid activity. ***Antiinflammatory action:*** Prevents accumulation of inflammatory cells at sites of infection; inhibits phagocytosis, lysosomal enzyme release, and synthesis of selected chemical mediators of inflammation; reduces capillary dilation and permeability. ***Immunosuppression:*** Not clearly understood, but may be due to prevention or suppression of delayed hypersensitivity immune reaction.

THERAPEUTIC EFFECTS Drug has antiinflammatory and immunosuppression properties.

USES Adrenal insufficiency concomitantly with a mineralocorticoid; inflammatory conditions, allergic states, collagen diseases, hematologic disorders, cerebral edema, and addisonian shock. Also palliative treatment of neoplastic disease, as adjunctive short-term therapy in acute rheumatic disorders and GI diseases, and as a diagnostic test for Cushing's syndrome and for differential diagnosis of adrenal hyperplasia and adrenal adenoma.

UNLABELED USES As an antiemetic in cancer chemotherapy; as a diagnostic test for endogenous depression; and to prevent hyaline membrane disease in premature infants.

CONTRAINDICATIONS Systemic fungal infection, acute infections, active or resting tuberculosis, vaccinia, varicella, administration of live virus vaccines (to patient, family members), latent or active amebiasis. ***Ophthalmic use:*** Primary open-angle glaucoma, eye infections, superficial ocular herpes simplex, keratitis and tuberculosis of eye. Safe use during pregnancy (category C), lactation, or in children is not established.

D

CAUTIOUS USE Stromal herpes simplex, keratitis, GI ulceration, renal disease, diabetes mellitus, hypothyroidism, myasthenia gravis, CHF, cirrhosis, psychic disorders, seizures.

ROUTE & DOSAGE

Allergies, Inflammation, Neoplasias

Adult: **PO** 0.25–4 mg b.i.d. to q.i.d. **IM** 8–16 mg q1–3 wk or 0.8–1.6 mg intralesional q1–3 wk
Child: **PO/IV/IM** 0.08–0.3 mg/kg/d divided q6–12h

Cerebral Edema

Adult: **IV** 10 mg followed by 4 mg q4h, reduce dose after 2–4 d then taper over 5–7 d
Child: **PO/IV/IM** 1–2 mg/kg loading dose, then 1–1.5 mg/kg/d divided q4–6h (max: 16 mg/d)

Shock

Adult: **IV** 1–6 mg/kg as a single dose or 40 mg repeated q2–6h if needed

Dexamethasone Suppression Test

Adult: **PO** 0.5 mg q6h for 48 h

Inflammation

Adult/Child: **Ophthalmic/Topical/Inhalation/Intranasal See Appendix A.**

ADMINISTRATION

Oral

- Give the once-daily dose in the A.M. with food or liquid of patient's choice.
- Taper dosage over a period of time before discontinuing because adrenal suppression can occur with prolonged use.
- Do not store or expose aerosol to temperature above 48.9°C (120°F); do not puncture or discard into a fire or an incinerator.

Intramuscular

- Give IM injection deep into a large muscle mass (e.g., gluteus maximus). Avoid SC injection: Atrophy and sterile abscesses may occur.
- Use repository form, dexamethasone acetate, for IM or local injection only. The white suspension settles on standing; mild shaking will resuspend drug.

Intravenous

PREPARE: **Direct:** Give undiluted. **Intermittent:** Dilute in D5W or NS for infusion.

ADMINISTER: **Direct:** Give direct IV push over 30 sec or less. **Intermittent:** Set rate as prescribed or according to amount of solution to infuse.

INCOMPATIBILITIES **Solution/additive: Daunorubicin, doxorubicin, doxapram, glycopyrrolate, metaraminol, vancomycin.**

- Store at 15°–30° C (59°–86° F) unless otherwise directed.

ADVERSE EFFECTS (≥1%) **Aerosol therapy:** *Nasal irritation,* dryness, epistaxis, rebound congestion, bronchial asthma, anosomia, perforation of nasal septum. ***Systemic Absorption*—CNS:** Euphoria, insomnia, convulsions, increased ICP, vertigo, headache, psychic disturbances. **CV:** CHF, hypertension, *edema*. **Endocrine:** Menstrual irregularities, *hyperglycemia;* cushingoid state; growth suppression in children; hirsutism. **Special Senses:** *Posterior subcapsular cataract,* increased IOP, glaucoma, exophthalmos. **GI:** Peptic ulcer with possible perforation, abdominal distension, nausea, increased appetite, heartburn, dyspepsia, pancreatitis, bowel perforation, *oral candidiasis.* **Musculoskeletal:** Muscle weakness, loss of muscle mass, vertebral compression fracture, pathologic fracture of long bones, tendon rupture. **Skin:** Acne, *impaired wound healing,* petechiae, ecchymoses, diaphoresis, allergic dermatitis, hypo- or hyperpigmentation, SC and cutaneous atrophy, burning and tingling in perineal area (following IV injection).

DIAGNOSTIC TEST INTERFERENCE ***Dexamethasone suppression test for endogenous depression:*** false-positive results may be caused by **alcohol, glutethimide, meprobamate;** false-negative results may be caused by high doses of benzodiazepines (e.g., **chlordiazepoxide** and **cyproheptadine**), long-term glucocorticoid treatment, **indomethacin, ephedrine,** estrogens or hepatic enzyme-inducing agents **(phenytoin)** may also cause false-positive results in ***test for Cushing's syndrome.***

INTERACTIONS Drug: BARBITURATES, **phenytoin, rifampin** increase steroid metabolism—dosage of dexamethasone may need to be increased; **amphotericin B,** DIURETICS compound potassium loss; **ambenonium, neostigmine, pyridostigmine** may cause severe muscle weakness in patients with myasthenia gravis; may inhibit antibody response to VACCINES, TOXOIDS.

PHARMACOKINETICS Absorption: Readily absorbed from GI tract. **Onset:** Rapid onset. **Peak:** 1–2 h PO; 8 h IM. **Duration:** 2.75 d PO; 6 d IM; 1–3 wk intralesional, intraarticular. **Distribution:** Crosses placenta; distributed into breast milk. **Elimination:** Hypothalamus-pituitary axis suppression: 36–54 h. **Half-Life:** 3–4.5 h.

NURSING IMPLICATIONS

Assessment & Drug Effects

- Monitor and report S&S of Cushing's syndrome (see Appendix F) or other systemic adverse effects.
- Monitor neonates born to a mother who has been receiving a corticosteroid during pregnancy for symptoms of hypoadrenocorticism.
- Monitor for S&S of a hypersensitivity reaction (see Appendix F). The acetate and sodium phosphate formulations may contain bisulfites, parabens, or both; these inactive ingredients are allergenic to some individuals.

Patient & Family Education

- Take drug exactly as prescribed.
- Report lack of response to medication or malaise, orthostatic hypotension, muscular weakness and pain, nausea, vomiting, anorexia, hypoglycemic reactions (see Appendix F), or mental depression to physician. These symptoms may signal hypoadrenocorticism.
- Report changes in appearance and easy bruising to physician. These symptoms may signal hyperadrenocorticism.
- Note: Hiccups that occur for several hours following each dose may be a complication of high-dose oral dexamethasone.
- Keep appointments for check-ups; make sure electrolytes and BP are evaluated during therapy at regular intervals.
- Add potassium-rich foods to diet; report signs of hypokalemia (see Appendix F). Concomitant potassium-depleting diuretic can enhance dexamethasone-induced potassium loss.
- Note: Dexamethasone dose regimen may need to be altered dur-

ing stress (e.g., surgery, infections, emotional stress, illness, acute bronchial attacks, trauma). Consult physician if change in living or working environment is anticipated.

- Discontinue drug gradually under the guidance of the physician.
- Note: It is important to prevent exposure to infection, trauma, and sudden changes in environmental factors, as much as possible, because drug is an immunosuppressor.
- Do not breast feed while taking this drug without consulting physician.

DEXCHLORPHENIRAMINE MALEATE

(dex-klor-fen-eer'a-meen)

Dexchlor, Poladex T. D., Polaramine, Polargen

Classification: ANTIHISTAMINE (H_1-RECEPTOR ANTAGONIST)

Prototype: Diphenhydramine

Pregnancy Category: B

AVAILABILITY 2 mg tablets; 4 mg, 6 mg sustained release tablets; 2 mg/5 mL syrup

ACTIONS Competes for H_1 receptor sites on cells thus blocking histamine release.

THERAPEUTIC EFFECTS H_1-receptor antagonist and alkyl amine antihistamine. In common with other antihistamines, has anticholinergic properties and produces mild to moderate drowsiness and sedation.

USES Perennial and seasonal allergic rhinitis, other manifestations of allergy, and vasomotor rhinitis. Also as adjunct to epinephrine in treatment of anaphylactic reactions.

CONTRAINDICATIONS Hypersensitivity to antihistamines of similar class; acute asthmatic attack, lower respiratory tract symptoms, newborns, premature infants. Safe use during pregnancy (category B) or lactation is not established.

CAUTIOUS USE Increased intraocular pressure; prostatic hypertrophy; hyperthyroidism; renal and cardiovascular disease; older adults.

ROUTE & DOSAGE

Allergic Rhinitis

Adult: **PO** 2 mg q4–6h or 4–6 mg of repeat-action tablets h.s. or q8–10h during the day

Child: **PO** *2–5 y,* 0.5 mg q4–6h (max: 3 mg/24 h); *6–11 y,* 1 mg q4–6h (max: 6 mg/24 h) or 4 mg of repeat-action tablets h.s.

ADMINISTRATION

Oral

- Ensure that sustained release form of drug is not chewed or crushed. It must be swallowed whole.
- Give regular tablet whole or crushed and taken with fluid or mixed with food.
- Give medication with food, water, or milk to lessen GI distress.
- Store at 15°–30° C (59°–86° F) unless otherwise directed.

ADVERSE EFFECTS (≥1%) **CNS:** *Drowsiness*, dizziness, weakness, headache, excitation, neuritis, disturbed coordination, insomnia, euphoria, paresthesias. **Special Senses:** Vertigo, tinnitus, acute labyrinthitis; blurred vision. **CV:** Palpitation, tachycardia, hypotension, extrasystoles. **GI:** Nausea, vomiting, anorexia, *dry mouth,* constipation, diarrhea. **Urogenital:** Difficulty in urinating, *urinary retention,* urinary frequency, early menses. **Hematologic:** Agranulocytosis (rare), hemolytic or hypoplastic anemia. **Skin:** Skin eruptions, photosensitivity.

DIAGNOSTIC TEST INTERFERENCE In common with other antihistamines, dexchlorpheniramine may interfere with ***skin tests for allergy;*** discontinue dexchlorpheniramine at least 72 h before tests.

INTERACTIONS Drug: Alcohol and other CNS DEPRESSANTS, MAO INHIBITORS compound CNS depression.

PHARMACOKINETICS Absorption: Readily absorbed from GI tract. **Onset:** 15–30 min. **Peak:** 3 h. **Distribution:** Small amounts distributed into breast milk. **Metabolism:** Metabolized in liver. **Elimination:** Excreted in urine within 24 h.

NURSING IMPLICATIONS

Assessment & Drug Effects

- Supervise ambulation and take safety precautions, especially with older adult patients.
- Monitor I&O and assess for difficulty voiding (e.g., frequency or retention).

Patient & Family Education

- Swallow timed or sustained release tablet whole. Do not break, crush, or chew.
- Do not drive or engage in other potentially hazardous activities until reaction to drug is known.
- Ask physician about the use of alcohol, tranquilizers, sedatives, or other CNS depressants because the effects of dexchlorpheniramine will be additive.
- Discontinue dexchlorpheniramine about 4 d before skin tests for allergies, since it can make test results inaccurate.
- Do not breast feed while taking this drug without consulting physician.

DEXMEDETOMIDINE HYDROCHLORIDE

(dex-med-e-to′mi-deen)

Precedex

Classifications: AUTONOMIC NERVOUS SYSTEM AGENT; ALPHA$_2$-ADRENERGIC AGONIST (SYMPATHOMIMETIC); SEDATIVE-HYPNOTIC

Prototype: Methoxamine HCl

Pregnancy Category: C

AVAILABILITY 100 mcg/mL in 2 mL ampule or vial

ACTIONS A selective alpha$_2$-adrenergic agonist with sedative properties. Dexmedetomidine stimulates alpha$_2$-adrenergic receptors in the CNS (primarily in the medulla oblongata) causing inhibition of the sympathetic vasomotor center of the brain.

THERAPEUTIC EFFECTS Sedative properties utilized in intubating patients and for initially maintaining them on a mechanical ventilator. Hemodynamic responses of the heart affected by alpha$_2$ receptors are better controlled with dexmedetomidine than with other related drugs (e.g., midazolam).

USES Sedation of initially intubated or mechanically ventilated patients.

CONTRAINDICATIONS Hypersensitivity to dexmedetomidine; labor and delivery, including cesarean section.

CAUTIOUS USE Patients with arrhythmias or cardiovascular disease; renal or hepatic insufficiency; signs of light anesthesia; pregnancy (category C), lactation; older adults >65 y. Safety and efficacy in children <18 y are unknown.

D

ROUTE & DOSAGE

Sedation

Adult: **IV** Start with 1 mcg/kg infused over 10 min, then continue with infusion of 0.2–0.7 mcg/kg/hr for up to 24 h, may need to decrease dosage in patients with renal or hepatic impairment

ADMINISTRATION

Intravenous

PREPARE: **Continuous:** Withdraw 2 mL of dexmedetomidine and add to 48 mL of 0.9% NaCl injection. Shake gently to mix.

ADMINISTER: **Continuous:** Administer using a controlled infusion device. A loading dose of 1 mcg/kg is infused over 10 min followed by the ordered maintenance dose. Do NOT use administration set containing natural rubber. Do NOT infuse longer than 24 h.

- Store at 15°–30° C (59°–86° F).

ADVERSE EFFECTS (≥1%) **Body as a Whole:** Pain, infection. **CV:** *Hypotension,* bradycardia, atrial fibrillation. **GI:** *Nausea,* thirst. **Respiratory:** Hypoxia, pleural effusion, pulmonary edema. **Hematologic:** Anemia, leukocytosis. **Urogenital:** Oliguria.

INTERACTIONS Drug: BARBITURATES, BENZODIAZEPINES, GENERAL ANESTHETICS, OPIATE AGONISTS, ANXIOLYTICS, SEDATIVES/HYPNOTICS, **ethanol,** TRICYCLIC ANTIDEPRESSANTS, **tramadol,** PHENOTHIAZINES, SKELETAL MUSCLE RELAXANTS, **azatadine, brompheniramine, carbinoxamine, chlorpheniramine, clemastine, cyproheptadine, dexchlorpheniramine, dimenhydrinate, diphenhydramine, doxylamine, hydroxyzine, methdilazine, phenindamine, promethazine, tripelennamine** enhance CNS depression possibly prolong recovery from anesthesia.

PHARMACOKINETICS Distribution: Half-life 6 min. **Metabolism:** Extensively metabolized in the liver (CYP 2A6). **Elimination:** Primarily excreted in urine. **Half-Life:** 2 h.

NURSING IMPLICATIONS

Assessment & Drug Effects

- Monitor for hypertension during loading dose; reduction of loading dose may be required.
- Monitor cardiovascular status continuously; notify physician immediately if hypotension or bradycardia occur.

DEXMETHYLPHENIDATE

(dex-meth-ill-fen′i-date)

Focalin

Classifications: CENTRAL NERVOUS SYSTEM AGENT; CEREBRAL STIMULANT

Prototype: Amphetamine

Pregnancy Category: C

Controlled Substance: Schedule II

AVAILABILITY 2.5 mg, 5 mg, 10 mg tablets

ACTIONS Thought to block the reuptake of norepinephrine and dopamine into the presynaptic neurons and, thereby, increasing release of these substances into the synapse. The mode of action in controlling the symptoms of Attention Deficit Hyperactivity Disorder (ADHD) by Focalin is not fully understood.

THERAPEUTIC EFFECTS Focalin is used for control of ADHD syndrome in conjunction with other measures (psychological, educational, and social). The use of stimulants is contraindicated in patients who exhibit ADHD symptoms secondary to environmental factors, and/or other primary psychiatric disorders, including psychosis.

USES Attention deficit hyperactivity disorder (ADHD).

CONTRAINDICATIONS Hypersensitivity to dexmethylphenidate or methylphenidate; severe agitation, anxiety, or tension; glaucoma; motor tics other than Tourette's syndrome; concurrent MAOI therapy; children <6 y; seizures; pregnancy (category C).

CAUTIOUS USE Moderate to severe hepatic insufficiency; Tourette's syndrome; depression; emotional instability; alcoholism or drug dependence; history of seizure disorders; psychotic symptomatology; hypertension or other cardiovascular disease; hyperthyroidism; lactation.

ROUTE & DOSAGE

Attention Deficit Hyperactivity Disorder

Adult/Child: **PO** >6 y 2.5 mg b.i.d., may increase by 2.5 mg–5 mg/d at weekly intervals to max of 20 mg/d. If converting from methylphenidate, start with 1/2 of methylphenidate dose

ADMINISTRATION

Oral

- Do not administer with or within 14 d following discontinuation of a MAO inhibitor.
- Give b.i.d. doses at least 4 h apart.
- Store at 15°–30° C (59°–86° F).

ADVERSE EFFECTS (≥1%) **Body as a Whole:** Fever, allergic reactions. **CNS:** Dizziness, insomnia, nervousness, tics, abnormal thinking, hallucinations, emotional lability, CNS overstimulation or sympathomimetic effects (angina, anxiety, agitation, biting, blurred vision, delirium, diaphoresis, flushing or pallor, hallucinations, hyperthermia, labile blood pressure and heart rate (hypotension or hypertension), mydriasis, palpitations, paranoia, purposeless movements, psychosis, sinus tachycardia, tachypnea, or tremor). **CV:** Hypertension, tachycardia. **GI:** *Abdominal pain,* decreased appetite, nausea, vomiting.

INTERACTIONS Drug: Additive stimulant effects with other STIMULANTS (including **amphetamine, caffeine**); increased vasopressor effects with **dopamine, epinephrine, norepinephrine, phenylpropanolamine, pseudoephedrine;** MAO INHIBITORS may cause hypertensive crisis; antagonizes hypotensive effects of **guanethidine, bretylium;** may inhibit metabolism and increase serum levels of **fosphenytoin, phenytoin, phenobarbital, and primidone, warfarin,** TRICYCLIC ANTIDEPRESSANTS.

PHARMACOKINETICS Absorption: well absorbed. **Peak:** 1–1.5 h. **Metabolism:** De-esterified in liver. No interaction with CYP450 system. **Elimination:** Primarily excreted in urine. **Half-Life:** 2.2 h.

NURSING IMPLICATIONS

Assessment & Drug Effects

- Withhold drug and notify physician if patient has a seizure. Monitor closely for loss of seizure control with a prior history of seizures.
- Monitor BP in all patients receiving this drug. Monitor cardiac status and report palpitations or other signs of arrhythmias.

D

- Monitor for potential abuse and dependence on this drug. Careful supervision is needed during drug withdrawal since severe depression may occur.
- Lab tests: Periodic CBC, differential, platelet counts, and LFTs during prolonged therapy.
- Concurrent drugs: Monitor patients on BP-lowering drugs for loss of BP control. Monitor plasma levels of oral anticoagulants and anticonvulsants; doses of these drugs may need to be decreased.

Patient & Family Education

- Withhold drug and report immediately any of the following signs of overdose: vomiting, agitation, tremors, muscle twitching, convulsions, confusion, hallucinations, delirium, sweating, flushing, headache, or high temperature.
- Note that drug is usually discontinued if improvement is not observed after appropriate dosage adjustment over 1 mo.
- Do not breast feed while taking this drug without consulting physician.

DEXPANTHENOL (PANTOTHENIC ACID)

(dex-pan'the-nole)

Dexol, Ilopan, Panthoderm

Classifications: AUTONOMIC NERVOUS SYSTEM AGENT; CHOLINERGIC, DIRECT ACTING

Prototype: Bethanechol

Pregnancy Category: C

AVAILABILITY 250 mg/mL injection

ACTIONS Analog of the coenzyme vitamin pantothenic acid, to which it is readily converted. A member of the B-complex group and precursor of coenzyme A, which is essential to normal epithelial function and biosynthesis of fatty acids, amino acids, and acetylcholine.

THERAPEUTIC EFFECTS Increases GI peristalsis and intestinal tone by stimulating acetylcholine. Topical application reportedly relieves itching and may aid healing of skin lesions by stimulating epithelialization and granulation.

USES Prevention or treatment of postoperative abdominal distention, intestinal atony, and paralytic ileus. Topically to relieve itching and to promote healing in minor skin lesions.

CONTRAINDICATIONS Hemophilia; ileus due to mechanical obstruction. Safe use during pregnancy (category C), lactation, or in children is not established.

CAUTIOUS USE Hypokalemia.

ROUTE & DOSAGE

Postoperative Abdominal Distension, Intestinal Atony, Paralytic Ileus

Adult: **IM** 250–500 mg, repeat in 2 h, then repeat q4–12h prn **IV** 500 mg by slow IV infusion
Child: **IM** 11–12.5 mg/kg, repeat in 2 h, then repeat q4–12h prn

Itching

Adult: **Topical** Apply to affected area 1–2 times/d

ADMINISTRATION

Topical

- Do not administer within 1 h of succinylcholine.

Intramuscular

- Give deep IM into a large muscle.

Intravenous

PREPARE: **IV infusion:** Dilute in at least 500 mL of D5W or RL.
ADMINISTER: **IV infusion:** Infuse slowly over 3–6 h.

- Store at 15°–30° C (59°–86° F); protect from freezing and excessive heat.

ADVERSE EFFECTS (≥1%) **All:** Generally well tolerated.

INTERACTIONS Drug: Prolongs muscle relaxation effects of **succinylcholine.**

PHARMACOKINETICS Absorption: Readily absorbed from IM site. **Distribution:** Highest concentration in liver, adrenals, heart, and kidneys; small amount distributed into breast milk. **Metabolism:** Rapidly converted to pantothenic acid, the active moiety. **Elimination:** 70% excreted in urine, 30% in feces.

NURSING IMPLICATIONS

Assessment & Drug Effects

- Monitor for therapeutic effectiveness: May not see results in patients with hypokalemia until potassium imbalance is corrected.
- Observe for and report bleeding tendency. Dexpanthenol may prolong bleeding time in some patients.
- Report immediately any evidence of a hypersensitivity reaction (see Appendix F); drug should be discontinued.

Patient & Family Education

- Report abdominal cramping or diarrhea to physician.
- Do not breast feed while taking this drug without consulting physician.

DEXRAZOXANE

(dex-ra-zox'ane)

Zinecard

Classifications: CHELATING AGENT; CARDIOPROTECTIVE FOR DOXORUBICIN

Pregnancy Category: C

AVAILABILITY 250 mg, 500 mg vials for injection

ACTIONS Drug is a derivative of EDTA that readily penetrates cell membranes. The mechanism by which dexrazoxane exerts its cardioprotective activity is not fully understood.

THERAPEUTIC EFFECTS Dexrazoxane is converted intracellularly to a chelating agent that interferes with iron-mediated free radical generation thought to be partially responsible for one form of cardiomyopathy.

USES Reduction of the incidence and severity of cardiomyopathy associated with doxorubicin in women with metastatic breast cancer who have received a cumulative doxorubicin dose of 300 mg/m^2.

CONTRAINDICATIONS Chemotherapy regimens that do not contain anthracycline, lactation.

CAUTIOUS USE Myelosuppression, pregnancy (category C). Safety and efficacy in children have not been established.

ROUTE & DOSAGE

Cardiomyopathy

Adult: **IV** 10 parts dexrazoxane to 1 part doxorubicin or 500 mg/m^2 for every 50 mg/m^2 of doxorubicin, repeated q3wk

ADMINISTRATION

Intravenous

Wear gloves when handling dexrazoxane. Immediately wash with soap and water if drug contacts skin or mucosa.

- Doxorubicin dose MUST be started within 30 min of beginning dexrazoxane.

D

PREPARE: **Direct:** Reconstitute by adding 25 or 50 mL of 0.167 M sodium lactate injection (provided by manufacturer) to the 250- or 500-mg vial, respectively, to produce a 10-mg/mL solution. **IV Infusion:** Further dilute with NS or D5W in an IV bag to a concentration of 1.3–5.0 mg/mL for infusion.

ADMINISTER: **Direct:** Give slow IV push. **IV Infusion:** Give over 10 min.

- Store reconstituted solutions for 6 h at 15°–30° C (59°–86° F).

ADVERSE EFFECTS (≥1%) **All:** Adverse effects of dexrazoxane are difficult to distinguish from those of the chemotherapeutic agents. Pain at injection site, leukopenia, granulocytopenia, and thrombocytopenia appear to occur more frequently with the addition of dexrazoxane than with placebo.

PHARMACOKINETICS Distribution: Not bound to plasma proteins. **Metabolism:** Metabolized in liver. **Elimination:** 42% excreted in urine. **Half-Life:** 2–2.5 h.

NURSING IMPLICATIONS

Assessment & Drug Effects

- Monitor cardiac function. Drug does not eliminate risk of doxorubicin cardiotoxicity.
- Lab tests: Monitor hepatic, renal, and hematopoietic status throughout course of therapy.
- Note: Adverse effects are likely due to concurrent cytotoxic drugs rather than dexrazoxane.

Patient & Family Education

- Report any of the following to physician: Worsening shortness of breath, swelling extremities, or chest pains.
- Do not breast feed while taking this drug.

DEXTRAN 40

(dex'tran)

Gentran 40, Hyskon, 10% LMD, Rheomacrodex

Classifications: BLOOD DERIVATIVE; PLASMA VOLUME EXPANDER; REPLACEMENT SOLUTION

Prototype: Albumin

Pregnancy Category: C

AVAILABILITY 10% solution in D5W or NS

ACTIONS Low-molecular-weight polysaccharide. As a hypertonic colloidal solution, produces immediate and short-lived expansion of plasma volume by increasing colloidal osmotic pressure and drawing fluid from interstitial to intravascular space. Reduces possibility of deep venous thrombosis and pulmonary embolism, primarily by inhibiting venous stasis and platelet adhesiveness.

THERAPEUTIC EFFECTS Cardiovascular response to volume expansion includes increased BP, pulse pressure, CVP, cardiac output, venous return to heart, and urinary output.

USES Adjunctively to expand plasma volume and provide fluid replacement in treatment of shock or impending shock caused by hemorrhage, burns, surgery, or other trauma. Also used in prophylaxis and therapy of venous thrombosis and pulmonary embolism. Used as priming fluid or as additive to other primers during extracorporeal circulation.

CONTRAINDICATIONS Hypersensitivity to dextrans, renal failure, hypervolemic conditions, severe CHF, thrombocytopenia, significant anemia, hypofibrinogenemia or other marked hemostatic defects including those caused by drugs, (e.g., heparin, warfarin); pregnancy (category C), lactation.

CAUTIOUS USE Active hemorrhage; severe dehydration; chronic liver disease; impaired renal function; patients susceptible to pulmonary edema or CHF.

ROUTE & DOSAGE

Shock

Adult: **IV** 500 mL administered rapidly (over 15–30 min), additional doses may be given more slowly up to 20 mL/kg in the first 24 h (doses up to 10 mL/kg/d may be given for an additional 4 d if needed)
Child: **IV** Total dose ≤20 mL/kg in first 24 h and ≤10 mL/kg/d (max: 5 d total)

Prophylaxis for Thromboembolic Complications

Adult: **IV** 500–1000 mL (10 mL/kg) on the day of operation followed by 500 mL/d for 2–3 d, may continue with 500 mL q2–3d for up to 2 wk if necessary

Priming for Extracorporeal Circulation

Adult: **IV** 10–20 mL/kg added to perfusion circuit

ADMINISTRATION

Intravenous

If blood is to be administered, draw a cross-match specimen before dextran infusion.

PREPARE: **IV Infusion:** Use only if seal is intact, vacuum is detectable, and solution is absolutely clear.

ADMINISTER: **IV Infusion:** Specific flow rate should be prescribed by physician. For emergency treatment of shock in adults give first 500 mL rapidly (e.g., 20–40 mL/min); give remaining portion of the daily dose over 8–24 h or at the rate prescribed.

- Store at a constant temperature, preferably 25° C (77° F). Once opened, discard unused portion because dextran contains no preservative.

ADVERSE EFFECTS (≥1%) **Body as a Whole:** Hypersensitivity (mild to generalized urticaria, pruritus, anaphylactic shock (rare), angioedema, dyspnea). **Other:** Renal tubular vacuolization (osmotic nephrosis), stasis, and blocking; oliguria, renal failure; increased AST and ALT, interference with platelet function, prolonged bleeding and coagulation times.

DIAGNOSTIC TEST INTERFERENCE When blood samples are drawn for study, notify laboratory that patient has received dextran. ***Blood glucose:*** false increases (utilizing ***ortho-toluidine methods*** or ***sulfuric*** or ***acetic acid*** hydrolysis). ***Urinary protein:*** false increases (utilizing ***Lowry method***). ***Bilirubin assays:*** false increases when alcohol is used. ***Total protein assays:*** false increases using ***biuret reagent. Rh testing, blood typing*** and ***cross-matching*** procedures: dextran may interfere with results (by inducing rouleaux formation) when ***proteolytic enzyme techniques*** are used (***saline agglutination*** and ***indirect antiglobulin methods*** reportedly not affected).

PHARMACOKINETICS Onset: Volume expansion within minutes of infusion. **Duration:** 12 h. **Metabolism:** Degraded to glucose and metabolized to CO_2 and water over a period of a few weeks. **Elimination:** 75% excreted in urine within 24 h; small amount excreted in feces.

D

NURSING IMPLICATIONS

Assessment & Drug Effects

- Evaluate patient's state of hydration before dextran therapy begins. Administration to severely dehydrated patients can result in renal failure.
- Lab tests: Baseline Hct prior to and after initiation of dextran (dextran usually lowers Hct). Notify physician if Hct is depressed below 30% by volume.
- Monitor vital signs and observe patient closely for at least the first 30 min of infusion. Hypersensitivity reaction is most likely to occur during the first few minutes of administration. Terminate therapy at the first sign of a hypersensitivity reaction (see Appendix F).
- Monitor CVP as an estimate of blood volume status and a guide for determining dosage. Normal CVP: 5–10 cm H_2O.
- Observe for S&S of circulatory overload (see Appendix F).
- Note: When sodium restriction is indicated, know that 500 mL of dextran 40 in 0.9% normal saline contains 77 mEq of both sodium and chloride.
- Monitor I&O ratio and check urine specific gravity at regular intervals. Low urine specific gravity may signify failure of renal dextran clearance and is an indication to discontinue therapy.
- Report oliguria, anuria, or lack of improvement in urinary output (dextran usually causes an increase in urinary output). Discontinue dextran at first sign of renal dysfunction.
- High doses are associated with transient prolongation of bleeding time and interference with normal blood coagulation.

Patient & Family Education

- Report immediately S&S of bleeding: easy bruising, blood in urine or dark tarry stool.
- Do not breast feed while taking this drug.

DEXTRAN 70

(dex'tran)
Macrodex

DEXTRAN 75

Gentran 75

Classifications: BLOOD FORMER AND COAGULANT; PLASMA VOLUME EXPANDER; REPLACEMENT SOLUTION
Prototype: Albumin
Pregnancy Category: C

AVAILABILITY 6% solution in D5W or NS

ACTIONS High-molecular-weight polysaccharides. Dextran 70 has an average molecular weight of 70,000; that of dextran 75 is 75,000. Colloidal properties approximate those of serum albumin.

THERAPEUTIC EFFECTS Cardiovascular response to volume expansion includes increased BP, pulse pressure, CVP, cardiac output, venous return to heart, and urinary output.

USES Primarily for emergency treatment of hypovolemic shock or impending shock caused by hemorrhage, burns, surgery, or other trauma. Intended for emergency treatment only when whole blood or blood products are not available or when haste precludes cross-matching of blood.

UNLABELED USES Nephrosis, toxemia of pregnancy, and prophylaxis of deep-vein thrombosis.

CONTRAINDICATIONS Known hypersensitivity to dextrans; severe bleeding disorders; severe CHF; severe renal failure; pregnancy (category C), lactation.
CAUTIOUS USE Impaired renal function, pulmonary edema, CHF, pathological GI disorders.

ROUTE & DOSAGE

Shock
Adult: **IV** 500 mL administered rapidly (over 15–30 min), additional doses may be given more slowly up to 20 mL/kg in the first 24 h (doses up to 10 mL/kg/d may be given for an additional 4 d if needed)

ADMINISTRATION

Intravenous

PREPARE: **IV Infusion:** Use only if seal is intact, vacuum is detectable, and solution is absolutely clear.
ADMINISTER: **IV Infusion:** Specific flow rate should be prescribed by physician. For emergency treatment of shock, rate of administration for first 500 mL may be 20–40 mL/min; thereafter, unless patient is hypovolemic, rate should not exceed 4 mL/min.

- Store at a constant temperature, preferably 25° C (77° F).

ADVERSE EFFECTS (≥1%) **All:** *Allergic reactions,* urticaria, wheezing, mild hypotension, nausea, vomiting, fever, arthralgia, severe anaphylactoid reaction.

PHARMACOKINETICS Onset: Volume expansion within minutes of infusion. **Duration:** 12 h. **Metabolism:** Degraded to glucose and metabolized to carbon dioxide and water over a period of a few weeks. **Elimination:** 75% excreted in urine within 24 h; small amount excreted in feces.

NURSING IMPLICATIONS

Assessment & Drug Effects
- Observe closely for S&S of anaphylaxis (see Appendix F) especially during first 30 min of infusion. Severe reactions have resulted in fatalities.
- Note: Bleeding time may be temporarily prolonged in patients receiving more than 1000 mL of dextran 70 or 75.
- Monitor I&O ratio and pattern. Monitor vital signs frequently as warranted by condition of patient.

Patient & Family Education
- Report immediately S&S of bleeding to physician: Easy bruising, blood in urine, or dark tarry stool.
- Do not breast feed while taking this drug.

DEXTROAMPHETAMINE SULFATE

(dex-troe-am-fet'a-meen)
Dexampex, Dexedrine, Oxydess II ✤, Spancap No. 1
Classifications: CENTRAL NERVOUS SYSTEM AGENT; RESPIRATORY AND CEREBRAL STIMULANT; AMPHETAMINE; ANOREXIANT
Prototype: Amphetamine
Pregnancy Category: C
Controlled Substance: Schedule II

AVAILABILITY 5 mg, 10 mg tablets; 5 mg, 10 mg, 15 mg sustained release capsules

ACTIONS Dextrorotatory isomer of amphetamine. Anorexigenic action is thought to result from CNS stimulation and possibly from loss of acuity of smell and taste.

THERAPEUTIC EFFECTS On a weight basis, has less pronounced effect on cardiovascular and peripheral nervous systems and is a more potent appetite suppressant than amphetamine. CNS stimulating effect approximately twice that of racemic amphetamine. In hyperkinetic children, amphetamines reduce motor restlessness by an unknown mechanism.

USES Adjunct in short-term treatment of exogenous obesity, narcolepsy, and attention deficit disorder with hyperactivity in children (also called minimal brain dysfunction or hyperkinetic syndrome).

UNLABELED USES Adjunct in epilepsy to control ataxia and drowsiness induced by barbiturates; to combat sedative effects of trimethadione in absence seizures.

CONTRAINDICATIONS Hypersensitivity to sympathomimetic amines, glaucoma, agitated states, psychoses (especially in children), advanced arteriosclerosis, symptomatic heart disease, moderate to severe hypertension, hyperthyroidism, history of drug abuse, during or within 14 d of MAO inhibitor therapy, as anorexiant in children <12 y, for attention deficit disorder in children <3 y, lactation.

CAUTIOUS USE Pregnancy (category C). Safety and efficacy in children <3 y have not been established.

ROUTE & DOSAGE

Narcolepsy

Adult: **PO** 5–20 mg 1–3 times/d at 4–6 h intervals

Child: **PO** *6–12 y,* 5 mg/d, may increase by 5 mg at weekly intervals; *>12 y,* 10 mg/d, may increase by 10 mg at weekly intervals

Attention Deficit Disorder

Child: **PO** *3–5 y,* 2.5 mg 1–2 times/d, may increase by 2.5 mg at weekly intervals; *≥6 y,* 5 mg 1–2 times/d, may increase by 5 mg at weekly intervals (max: 40 mg/d)

Obesity

Adult: **PO** 5–10 mg 1–3 times/d or 10–15 mg of sustained release once/d 30–60 min a.c.

ADMINISTRATION

Oral

- Ensure that sustained release capsule is not chewed or crushed. It MUST be swallowed whole.
- Give 30–60 min before meals for treatment of obesity. Give long-acting form in the morning.
- Give last dose no later than 6 h before patient retires (10–14 h before bedtime for sustained release form) to avoid insomnia.
- Store in tightly closed containers at 15°–30° C (59°–86° F) unless otherwise directed.

ADVERSE EFFECTS (≥1%) **CNS:** Nervousness, *restlessness,* hyperactivity, *insomnia,* euphoria, dizziness, headache; ***with prolonged use***—severe depression, psychotic reactions. **CV:** Palpitation, tachycardia, elevated BP. **GI:** Dry mouth, unpleasant taste, anorexia, weight loss, diarrhea, constipation, abdominal pain. **Other:** Impotence, changes in libido, unusual fatigue, increased intraocular pressure, marked dystonia of head, neck, and extremities; sweating.

D

DIAGNOSTIC TEST INTERFERENCE Dextroamphetamine may cause significant elevations in ***plasma corticosteroids*** (evening levels are highest) and increases in ***urinary epinephrine*** excretion (during first 3 h after drug administration).

INTERACTIONS Drug: Acetazolamide, sodium bicarbonate decrease dextroamphetamine elimination; **ammonium chloride, ascorbic acid** increase dextroamphetamine elimination; effects of both BARBITURATES and dextroamphetamine may be antagonized; **furazolidone** may increase BP effects of AMPHETAMINES—interaction may persist for several weeks after discontinuing **furazolidone;** antagonizes antihypertensive effects of **guanethidine, guanadrel;** MAO INHIBITORS, **selegiline** can cause—hypertensive crisis (fatalities reported)—do not administer AMPHETAMINES during or within 14 d of these drugs; PHENOTHIAZINES may inhibit mood elevating effects of AMPHETAMINES; TRICYCLIC ANTIDEPRESSANTS enhance dextroamphetamine effects because of increased **norepinephrine** release; BETA-ADRENERGIC AGONISTS increase cardiovascular adverse effects.

PHARMACOKINETICS Absorption: Rapid. **Peak:** 1–5 h. **Duration:** Up to 10 h. **Distribution:** All tissues especially the CNS. **Metabolism:** Metabolized in liver. **Elimination:** Renal elimination; excreted in breast milk. **Half-Life:** 10–30 h.

NURSING IMPLICATIONS

Assessment & Drug Effects

- Monitor growth rate closely in children.
- Interrupt therapy or reduce dosage periodically to assess effectiveness in behavior disorders.
- Note: Tolerance to anorexiant effects may develop after a few weeks, however, tolerance does not appear to develop when dextroamphetamine is used to treat narcolepsy.

Patient & Family Education

- Swallow sustained release capsule whole with a liquid; do not chew or crush.
- Do not drive or engage in other potentially hazardous activities until response to drug is known.
- Taper drug gradually following long-term use to avoid extreme fatigue, mental depression, and prolonged sleep pattern.
- Do not breast feed while taking this drug.

DEXTROMETHORPHAN HYDROBROMIDE

(dex-troe-meth-or′fan)

Balminil DM ✦, Benylin DM, Cremacoat 1, Delsym, DM Cough, Hold, Koffex ✦, Mediquell, Neo-DM ✦, Ornex DM ✦, Pedia Care, Pertussin 8 Hour Cough Formula, Robidex ✦, Robitussin DM, Romilar CF, Romilar Children's Cough, Sedatuss ✦, Sucrets Cough Control

Classification: ANTITUSSIVE

Prototype: Benzonatate

Pregnancy Category: C

AVAILABILITY 30 mg capsules; 2.5 mg, 5 mg, 7.5 mg, 15 mg lozenges; 10 mg/15 mL, 3.5 mg/5 mL, 7.5 mg/5 mL, 15 mg/5 mL liquid; 15 mg/15 mL, 10 mg/5 mL syrup

ACTIONS Nonnarcotic derivative of levorphanol. Chemically related to morphine but without central hypnotic or analgesic effect or capacity to cause tolerance or addiction. Antitussive activity comparable to that of codeine but is less likely than codeine to cause constipation, drowsiness, or GI disturbances.

THERAPEUTIC EFFECTS Controls cough spasms by depressing cough center in medulla. Temporarily relieves coughing spasm.

USES Temporary relief of cough spasms in nonproductive coughs due to colds, pertussis, and influenza.

CONTRAINDICATIONS Children <2 y, asthma, productive cough, persistent or chronic cough; hepatic function impairment; pregnancy (category C).

CAUTIOUS USE Chronic pulmonary disease; enlarged prostate; patients on MAO INHIBITORS.

ROUTE & DOSAGE

Cough

Adult: **PO** 10–20 mg q4h or 30 mg q6–8h (max: 120 mg/d) or 60 mg of sustained action liquid b.i.d.

Child: **PO** *2–6 y,* 2.5–5 mg q4h or 7.5 mg q6–8h (max: 30 mg/d) or 15 mg sustained action liquid b.i.d.; *6–12 y,* 5–10 mg q4h or 15 mg q6–8h (max: 60 mg/d) or 30 mg sustained action liquid b.i.d.

ADMINISTRATION

Oral

- Do not give lozenges to children <6 y.
- Ensure that extended release form of drug is not chewed or crushed. It MUST be swallowed whole.
- Note: Although soothing local effect of the syrup may be enhanced if given undiluted, depression of cough center depends only on systemic absorption of drug.

ADVERSE EFFECTS (≥1%) **CNS:** Dizziness, drowsiness, CNS depression with very large doses; excitability, especially in children. **GI:** GI upset, constipation, abdominal discomfort.

INTERACTIONS Drug: High risk of excitation, hypotension, and hyperpyrexia with MAO INHIBITORS.

PHARMACOKINETICS Absorption: Readily absorbed from GI tract. **Onset:** 15–30 min. **Duration:** 3–6 h. **Metabolism:** Metabolized in liver. **Elimination:** Excreted in urine.

NURSING IMPLICATIONS

Assessment & Drug Effects

- Monitor for dizziness and drowsiness, especially when concurrent therapy with CNS depressant is used.

Patient & Family Education

- Avoid irritants such as smoking, dust, fumes, and other air pollutants to lessen unnecessary cough. Humidify ambient air to provide some relief.
- Note: Treatment aims to decrease the frequency and intensity of cough without completely eliminating protective cough reflex.
- While dextromethorphan is available OTC, any cough persisting longer than 1 wk–10 d needs to be medically diagnosed.

DEXTROTHYROXINE SODIUM

(dex-troe-thye-rox'een)

Choloxin

Classifications: CARDIOVASCULAR DRUG; ANTILIPEMIC; LIPID-LOWERING AGENT

Pregnancy Category: C

AVAILABILITY 2 mg, 4 mg tablets

ACTIONS Sodium salt and dextrorotatory isomer of thyroxine. Reduces serum cholesterol and LDL levels in hyperlipidemia; triglycerides and beta-lipoproteins may also be lowered from previously elevated levels, but effect is variable.

THERAPEUTIC EFFECTS By an unclear mechanism, liver is stimulated to increase catabolism and excretion of cholesterol and its degradation products via the biliary route into feces. Greatest decrease in serum cholesterol occurs in patients with highest baseline concentrations, with maximum therapeutic effects in 1 or 2 mo.

USES Adjunct to other medications in the treatment of primary hypercholesterolemia (type IIa hyperlipidemia), particularly euthyroid patients with significant risk but no evidence of coronary artery disease.

CONTRAINDICATIONS Euthyroids with one or more of the following: known organic heart disease including angina pectoris, arrhythmias, decompensated or borderline compensated cardiac states; history of MI or CHF; rheumatic heart disease; hypertension; advanced liver or kidney disease; history of iodism; pregnancy (category C), lactation; 2 wk prior to elective surgery.

CAUTIOUS USE Hypothyroid patients with concomitant coronary artery disease; women of childbearing age with familial hypercholesterolemia; diabetes mellitus; liver and kidney impairment; children, older adults.

ROUTE & DOSAGE

Euthyroid Hyperlipidemia

Adult: **PO** 1–2 mg/d, increased by 1 or 2 mg every month if needed (max: 8 mg/d)

Child: **PO** 0.05 mg/kg/d, increased by not more than 0.05 mg/kg every month if needed (max: 4 mg/d)

ADMINISTRATION

Oral

- Give at any time without respect to meals.
- Store medication in light- and moisture-proof container at 15°–30° C (59°–86° F) unless otherwise specified.

ADVERSE EFFECTS (≥1%) **All:** Mainly due to increased metabolism. **CNS:** Insomnia, nervousness, dizziness, psychic changes, paresthesias. **CV:** Angina pectoris, palpitation, cardiac arrhythmia, ECG evidence of ischemic myocardial changes, increase in heart size; MI (relationship not conclusive), worsening of peripheral vascular disease. **Special Senses:** Tinnitus, hoarseness; visual disturbances, exophthalmos, retinopathy, lid lag. **GI:** Nausea, constipation, diarrhea, bitter taste, weight loss. **Other:** Acneiform rash, pruritus, coryza, conjunctivitis, stomatitis, brassy taste, laryngitis, bronchitis.

INTERACTIONS Drug: Cholestyramine, colestipol decrease absorption of dextrothyroxine; compounds thyroid effects of other THYROID PREPARATIONS; increases risk of hypoprothrombinemia associated with **warfarin; digoxin** may enhance myocardial stimulation; may increase blood **glucose**, requiring adjustment of **insulin** and SULFONYLUREAS.

PHARMACOKINETICS Absorption: About 25% absorbed from GI tract. **Distribution:** Crosses placenta; distribution into breast milk not known. **Metabolism:** Metabolized in liver. **Elimination:** Excreted in urine and feces. **Half-Life:** 18 h.

NURSING IMPLICATIONS

Assessment & Drug Effects

- Monitor for therapeutic effectiveness. Initial decrease in cholesterol levels may not occur until 2 wk–1 mo after initiation of therapy. Maximum decrease usually occurs during second or third month of therapy.
- Lab test: Determine & evaluate serum lipids initially and at periodic intervals during therapy. Patient should follow a normal diet for several days prior to the test.
- Observe patients with cardiac disease closely, particularly during early therapy, and at frequent intervals throughout the treatment period.
- Note: Hypothyroid patients with organic heart disease have a high incidence of adverse effects.
- Report immediately new signs and symptoms of cardiac disease or increased decompensation in the borderline compensated patient. Dose adjustment may be indicated.
- Concomitant drugs: Carefully monitor coagulation studies with warfarin.
- Monitor diabetics for loss of glycemic control.

Patient & Family Education

- Note: Serum lipids generally return to pretreatment levels within 6 wk–3 mo after drug is withdrawn.
- Report chest pain, palpitations, sweating, diarrhea, headache, or skin rash to physician.
- Report to physician immediately any of the following: Acne-type rash, itching, conjunctivitis, inflamed mouth, significant nasal discharge, brassy taste, laryngitis, or bronchitis.
- Do not take OTC medications without physician's approval.
- Inform physician or dentist in an emergency situation that you are taking dextrothyroxine before any surgery is performed.
- Do not breast feed while taking this drug.

DEZOCINE

(de′zo-ceen)

Dalgan

Classifications: CENTRAL NERVOUS SYSTEM AGENT; NARCOTIC (OPIATE) AGONIST-ANTAGONIST; ANALGESIC

Prototype: Pentazocine

Pregnancy Category: C

Controlled Substance: Schedule IV

AVAILABILITY 5 mg/mL, 10 mg/mL, 15 mg/mL injection

ACTIONS Dezocine is an agonist–antagonist opioid. Because of its narcotic antagonist activity, dezocine may precipitate withdrawal symptoms in individuals with opiate dependence. Causes less respiratory depression and hypotension than morphine and no bronchoconstrictive or histamine-releasing activity following its administration.

THERAPEUTIC EFFECTS It is comparable to morphine in analgesic potency, onset, and duration of action in the relief of postoperative pain.

USES Management of pain when the use of an opioid is appropriate.

CONTRAINDICATIONS Hypersensitivity to dezocine or structurally related drugs, concurrent use of CNS depressants; children <18 y; lactation.

CAUTIOUS USE COPD, chronic bronchitis, emphysema, head injury, increased intracranial pressure, pregnancy (category C).

ROUTE & DOSAGE

Adult: **IV** 2.5–10 mg (usually 5 mg) q2–4h **IM** 5–20 mg (usually 10 mg), may repeat q3–6h (max: 20 mg single dose; max: 120 mg/d)

ADMINISTRATION

- Do not administer to anyone with a known sulfite allergy.

Intramuscular

- Note: 20 mg is the maximum single IM dose; 120 mg is the maximum daily IM dose.
- Doses should be reduced for older adult patients and those with renal or hepatic insufficiency.

Intravenous

PREPARE: **Direct:** Give undiluted. ***ADMINISTER:*** **Direct:** Give by direct IV over 30–60 s.

- Store at room temperature, 15°–30° C (59°–86° F), and protect from light. Do not use if precipitate is visible.

ADVERSE EFFECTS (≥1%) **CNS:** Headache, dizziness, anxiety, euphoria, dysphoria, sedation. **CV:** Bradycardia, hypotension. **GI:** *Nausea, vomiting.* **Respiratory:** Respiratory depression. **Other:** Miosis, pruritus, mild itching, drug dependence.

INTERACTIONS Drug: BARBITURATES, other OPIATES, INHALATION GENERAL ANESTHETICS, and other CNS DEPRESSANTS may enhance the cardiovascular and CNS effects; MONOAMINE OXIDASE INHIBITORS should be avoided; increased respiratory depression when used with other OPIOIDS.

PHARMACOKINETICS Absorption: Completely absorbed from IM site. **Onset:** 15–30 min. **Peak:** 10–90 min IM. **Duration:** 4–6 h. **Metabolism:** Metabolized in liver. **Elimination:** Excreted in urine. **Half-Life:** 2.6 h.

NURSING IMPLICATIONS

Assessment & Drug Effects

- Assess for pain relief; onset occurs within 15–30 min, with peak effect at 60 min. Effective analgesia usually lasts 4–6 h.
- Monitor for respiratory depression (especially with preexisting pulmonary disease), changes in BP and heart rate (especially hypotension and bradycardia), and excess CNS depression.
- Supervise ambulation; drug may cause dizziness.

Patient & Family Education

- Use caution with position changes and walking; drug may cause hypotension and dizziness.
- Do not drive or engage in other hazardous activities until response to drug is known.
- Report adverse drug effects. A dosage reduction or change of drug may be warranted.
- Do not breast feed while taking this drug.

DIAZEPAM Pr

(dye-az'e-pam)

Apo-Diazepam ♣, Diastat, Diazemuls ♣, E-Pam ♣, Meval ♣, Novodipam ♣, Valium, Valrelease, Vivol ♣

DIAZEPAM EMULSIFIED

Dizac

Classifications: CENTRAL NERVOUS SYSTEM AGENT; BENZODIAZEPINE ANTICONVULSANT; ANXIOLYTIC

Pregnancy Category: D

Controlled Substance: Schedule IV

D

AVAILABILITY 2 mg, 5 mg, 10 mg tablets; 1 mg/mL, 5 mg/mL, 5 mg/5 mL oral solution; 5 mg/mL injection; 2.5 mg, 5 mg, 10 mg, 15 mg, 20 mg rectal gel

ACTIONS Psychotherapeutic agent related to chlordiazepoxide; reportedly superior in antianxiety and anticonvulsant activity, with somewhat shorter duration of action. Like chlordiazepoxide, it appears to act at both limbic and subcortical levels of CNS.

THERAPEUTIC EFFECTS Shortens REM and stage 4 sleep but increases total sleep time. Antianxiety and anticonvulsant agent.

USES Drug of choice for status epilepticus. Management of anxiety disorders, for short-term relief of anxiety symptoms, to allay anxiety and tension prior to surgery, cardioversion and endoscopic procedures, as an amnesic, and treatment for restless legs. Also used to alleviate acute withdrawal symptoms of alcoholism, voiding problems in older adults, and adjunctively for relief of skeletal muscle spasm associated with cerebral palsy, paraplegia, athetosis, stiff-man syndrome, tetanus.

CONTRAINDICATIONS ***Injectable form:*** Shock, coma, acute alcohol intoxication, depressed vital signs, obstetrical patients, infants <30 d of age. ***Tablet form:*** Infants <6 mo of age, acute narrow-angle glaucoma, untreated open-angle glaucoma; during or within 14 d of MAO inhibitor therapy. Safe use during pregnancy (category D) and lactation is not established.

CAUTIOUS USE Epilepsy, psychoses, mental depression; myasthenia gravis; impaired hepatic or renal function; drug abuse, addiction-prone individuals. Injectable diazepam used with extreme caution in older adults, the very ill, and patients with COPD.

ROUTE & DOSAGE

Status Epilepticus

Adult: **IV/IM** 5–10 mg, repeat if needed at 10–15 min intervals up to 30 mg, then repeat if needed q2–4h
Child: **IV/IM** *<5 y,* 0.2–0.5 mg slowly q2–5min up to 5 mg; *>5 y,* 1 mg slowly q2–5min up to 10 mg, repeat if needed q2–4 h

Anxiety, Muscle Spasm, Convulsions, Alcohol Withdrawal

Adult: **PO** 2–10 mg b.i.d. to q.i.d. or 15–30 mg/d sustained release **IV/IM** 2–10 mg, repeat if needed in 3–4 h
Geriatric: **PO** 1–2 mg 1–2 times/d (max: 10 mg/d)
Child: **PO** *>6 mo,* 1–2.5 mg b.i.d. or t.i.d.

ADMINISTRATION

Note: Dizac emulsion is administered by IV only.

Oral

- Ensure that sustained release form is not chewed or crushed. It MUST be swallowed whole. Give other tablets crushed with fluid or mixed with food if necessary.
- Supervise oral ingestion to ensure drug is swallowed.
- Avoid abrupt discontinuation of diazepam. Taper doses to termination.

Intramuscular

- Give deep into large muscle mass. Inject slowly. Rotate injection sites.
- Do NOT give emulsion form (Dizac) as IM or SC. It is for IV use only.

Intravenous

PREPARE: **Direct:** Do not dilute or mix with any other drug.

ADMINISTER: **Direct:** Give direct IV by injecting drug slowly, taking at least 1 min for each 5 mg (1 mL) given to adults and taking at least 3 min to inject 0.25 mg/kg body weight of children. ▪ If injection cannot be made directly into vein, inject slowly through infusion tubing as close as possible to vein insertion. ▪ The emulsion form is incompatible with PVC infusion sets. ▪ Avoid small veins and take extreme care to avoid intraarterial administration or extravasation.

INCOMPATIBILITIES **Solution/additive: Bleomycin, benzquinamide, dobutamine, doxapram, doxorubicin, fluorouracil, glycopyrrolate, heparin, nalbuphone, sufentanil.** Emulsion also incompatible with **morphine. Y-site: Furosemide, heparin, potassium chloride, vitamin B complex with C.** Emulsion also incompatible with **morphine.** Do not mix emulsion with any other drugs. Do not administer through **polyvinyl chloride (PVC)** infusion sets.

▪ Store in tight, light-resistant containers at 15°–30° C (59°–86° F), unless otherwise specified by manufacturer. Store Dizac emulsion at 2°–8° C (36°–46° F). Do not freeze.

ADVERSE EFFECTS (≥1%) **Body as a Whole:** Throat and chest pain. **CNS:** *Drowsiness,* fatigue, ataxia, confusion, paradoxic rage, dizziness, vertigo, amnesia, vivid dreams, headache, slurred speech, tremor; EEG changes, tardive dyskinesia. **CV:** Hypotension, tachycardia, edema, <u>cardiovascular collapse.</u> **Special Senses:** Blurred vision, diplopia, nystagmus. **GI:** Xerostomia, nausea, constipation, hepatic dysfunction. **Urogenital:** Incontinence, urinary retention, gynecomastia (prolonged use), menstrual irregularities, ovulation failure. **Respiratory:** Hiccups, coughing, <u>laryngospasm</u>. **Other:** Pain, venous thrombosis, phlebitis at injection site.

INTERACTIONS Drug: Alcohol, CNS DEPRESSANTS, ANTICONVULSANTS potentiate CNS depression; **cimetidine** increases diazepam plasma levels, increases toxicity; may decrease antiparkinson effects of **levodopa;** may increase **phenytoin** levels; smoking decreases sedative and antianxiety effects. **Herbal: Kava kava, valerian** may potentiate sedation.

PHARMACOKINETICS Absorption: Readily absorbed from GI tract; erratic IM absorption. **Onset:** 30–60 min PO; 15–30 min IM; 1–5 min IV. **Peak:** 1–2 h PO. **Duration:** 15 min–1 h IV; up to 3 h PO. **Distribution:** Crosses blood–brain barrier and placenta; distributed into breast milk. **Metabolism:** Metabolized in liver to active metabolites. **Elimination:** Excreted primarily in urine. **Half-Life:** 20–50 h.

NURSING IMPLICATIONS

Assessment & Drug Effects

- Monitor for adverse reactions. Most are dose related. Physician will rely on accurate observation and reports of patient response to the drug to determine lowest effective maintenance dose.
- Monitor for therapeutic effectiveness. Maximum effect may require 1–2 wk; patient tolerance to therapeutic effects may develop after 4 wk of treatment.
- Observe necessary preventive precautions for suicidal tendencies

that may be present in anxiety states accompanied by depression.

- Observe patient closely and monitor vital signs when diazepam is given parenterally; hypotension, muscular weakness, tachycardia, and respiratory depression may occur.
- Lab tests: Periodic CBC and liver function tests during prolonged therapy.
- Supervise ambulation. Adverse reactions such as drowsiness and ataxia are more likely to occur in older adults and debilitated or those receiving larger doses. Dosage adjustment may be necessary.
- Monitor I&O ratio, including urinary and bowel elimination.
- Note: Smoking increases metabolism of diazepam; lowering clinical effectiveness. Heavy smokers may need a higher dose than the nonsmoker.
- Note: Psychic and physical dependence may occur in patients on long-term high dosage therapy, in those with histories of alcohol or drug addiction, or in those who self-medicate.

Patient & Family Education

- Avoid alcohol and other CNS depressants during therapy unless otherwise advised by physician. Concomitant use of these agents can cause severe drowsiness, respiratory depression, and apnea.
- Do not drive or engage in other potentially hazardous activities or those requiring mental precision until reaction to drug is known.
- Tell physician if you become or intend to become pregnant during therapy; drug may need to be discontinued.
- Take drug as prescribed; do not change dose or dose intervals.
- Check with physician before taking any OTC drugs.
- Do not breast feed while taking this drug without consulting physician.

DIAZOXIDE

(dye-az-ox'ide)

Hyperstat I. V., Proglycem

Classifications: CARDIOVASCULAR AGENT; ANTIHYPERTENSIVE; VASODILATOR; SULFONYLUREA

Prototype: Hydralazine

Pregnancy Category: C

AVAILABILITY 50 mg capsules; 50 mg/mL suspension; 15 mg/mL injection

ACTIONS Rapid-acting thiazide nondiuretic hypotensive and hyperglycemic agent. In contrast to thiazide diuretics, causes sodium and water retention and decreases urinary output, probably because it increases proximal tubular reabsorption of sodium and decreases glomerular filtration rate. Hypotensive effect may be accompanied by marked reflex increase in heart rate, cardiac output, and stroke volume; thus cerebral and coronary blood flow are usually maintained.

THERAPEUTIC EFFECTS Reduces peripheral vascular resistance and BP by direct vasodilatory effect on peripheral arteriolar smooth muscles, perhaps by direct competition for calcium receptor sites.

USES Intravenously for emergency lowering of BP in hospitalized patients with malignant hypertension, particularly when associated with renal impairment. Not effective in pheochromocytoma. Commonly used with a diuretic such as furosemide (Lasix) to counteract diazoxide-induced sodium and water retention. Orally in treatment of various diagnosed hypoglycemic states due to hyperinsulinism when other medical treatment or surgical management has been unsuccessful or is not feasible.

CONTRAINDICATIONS Hypersensitivity to diazoxide or to other thiazides; cerebral bleeding, eclampsia; aortic coarctation; AV shunt, significant coronary artery disease. Safe use during pregnancy (category C) or lactation is not established. Use of oral diazoxide for functional hypoglycemia or in presence of increased bilirubin in newborns.
CAUTIOUS USE Diabetes mellitus; impaired cerebral or cardiac circulation; impaired renal function; patients taking corticosteroids or estrogen–progestogen combinations; hyperuricemia, history of gout, uremia.

ROUTE & DOSAGE

Severe Hypertension
Adult/Child: **IV** 1–3 mg/kg up to 150 mg, repeat at 5–15 min intervals if necessary
Hypoglycemia
Adult/Child: **PO** 3–8 mg/kg/d divided q8–12h
Neonate/Infant: **PO** 8–15 mg/kg/d divided q8–12h

ADMINISTRATION

Intravenous

Note: Give any prescribed diuretic 30–60 min prior to IV diazoxide. Keep patient recumbent 8–10 h because of possible additive hypotensive effect.

PREPARE: **Direct:** Give undiluted.
ADMINISTER: **Direct:** Give IV by rapid direct injection over 10–30 s. Keep patient recumbent while receiving IV and for at least 30 min following administration.

- Check IV injection site frequently. Solution is strongly alkaline. Extravasation of medication into tissues can cause severe inflammatory reaction. Administer drug by peripheral vein ONLY.

- Do not give darkened solutions. Store capsules, oral suspension, and injectables at 2°–30° C (36°–86° F) unless otherwise directed. Protect from light, heat, and freezing.

ADVERSE EFFECTS (≥1%) **CNS:** Headache, weakness, malaise, *dizziness,* polyneuritis, sleepiness, insomnia, euphoria, anxiety, extrapyramidal signs. **CV:** Palpitations, atrial and ventricular arrhythmias, flushing, shock; *orthostatic hypotension,* CHF, transient hypertension. **Special Senses:** Tinnitus, momentary hearing loss; blurred vision, transient cataracts, subconjunctival hemorrhage, ring scotoma, diplopia, lacrimation, papilledema. **GI:** *Nausea, vomiting,* abdominal discomfort, diarrhea, constipation, ileus, anorexia, transient loss of taste, impaired hepatic function. **Hematologic:** Transient neutropenia, eosinophilia, decreased Hgb/Hct, decreased IgG. **Body as a Whole:** Hypersensitivity (rash, fever, leukopenia); chest and back pain, muscle cramps. **Urogenital:** Decreased urinary output, nephrotic syndrome (reversible), hematuria, increased nocturia, proteinuria, azotemia; inhibition of labor. **Skin:** Pruritus, flushing, monilial dermatitis, herpes, hirsutism; loss of scalp hair, sweating, sensation of warmth, burning, or itching. **Endocrine:** Advance in bone age (children), *hyperglycemia, sodium and water retention, edema,* hyperuricemia, glycosuria, enlargement of breast lump, galactorrhea; decreased immunoglobulinemia, hirsutism.

DIAGNOSTIC TEST INTERFERENCE Diazoxide can cause false-negative response to ***glucagon.***

INTERACTIONS Drug: SULFONYLUREAS antagonize effects; THIAZIDE DIURETICS may intensify hyperglycemia and antihypertensive effects; **phenytoin** increases risk of hyperglycemia, and diazoxide may increase **phenytoin** metabolism, causing loss of seizure control.

PHARMACOKINETICS Onset: 30–60 s IV; 1 h PO. **Peak:** 5 min IV. **Duration:** 2–12 or more h IV; 8 h PO. **Distribution:** Crosses blood–brain barrier and placenta. **Metabolism:** Partially metabolized in the liver. **Elimination:** Excreted in urine. **Half-Life:** 21–45 h.

NURSING IMPLICATIONS

Assessment & Drug Effects

- Monitor for therapeutic effectiveness. Discontinue if not effective in 2 or 3 wk.
- Lab tests: Initial blood glucose, serum electrolytes, and CBC and at regular intervals in patients receiving multiple doses.
- Monitor BP q5min for the first 15–30 min or until stabilized, then hourly for balance of drug effect.
- Notify physician immediately if BP continues to fall 30 min or more after IV drug administration. Cause other than drug effect is probable.
- Monitor pulse: Tachycardia has occurred immediately following IV; palpitation and bradycardia have also been reported.
- Report promptly any change in I&O ratio.
- Observe patient closely for S&S of CHF (see Appendix F).
- Monitor diabetics carefully for loss of glycemic control.
- Evaluate serum electrolyte levels at regular intervals, particularly in patients with impaired renal function; hypokalemia potentiates hyperglycemic effect of diazoxide.
- Note: In contrast to IV diazoxide, oral administration usually does not produce marked effects on BP. However, do make periodic measurements of BP and vital signs.
- Monitor S&S for up to 7 d for both oral and parenteral forms; essential because of long half-life of diazoxide.

Patient & Family Education

- Note: Drug may cause hyperglycemia and glycosuria in diabetic and diabetic-prone individuals. Closely monitor blood and urine glucose; report any abnormalities to physician.
- Report palpitations, chest pain, dizziness, fainting, or severe headache.
- Note: Lanugo-type hirsutism occurs frequently, commonly in children and women. It is reversible with discontinuation of drug.
- Do not breast feed while taking this drug without consulting physician.

DIBUCAINE

(dye′byoo-kane)
Nupercainal
Classifications: CENTRAL NERVOUS SYSTEM AGENT; ANESTHETIC, LOCAL (AMIDE-TYPE)
Prototype: Procaine
Pregnancy Category: C

AVAILABILITY 1% ointment; 0.5% cream

ACTIONS Long-acting anesthetic of the amide type and reportedly one of the most potent and most toxic. Appears to inhibit initiation and

conduction of nerve impulses by reducing permeability of nerve cell membrane to sodium ions.
THERAPEUTIC EFFECTS Relief of pain and itching due to inhibiting conduction of nerve impulses.

USES Fast, temporary relief of pain and itching due to hemorrhoids and other anorectal disorders, nonpoisonous insect bites, sunburn, minor burns, cuts, and scratches.

CONTRAINDICATIONS Hypersensitivity to amide-type anesthetics, pregnancy (category C), children <1 y.
CAUTIOUS USE Lactation, children <12 y.

ROUTE & DOSAGE

Itching Due to Insect Bites or Hemorrhoids

Adult: **Topical** Apply skin cream or ointment to affected area as needed (max: 1 oz [28 g]/24 h); insert rectal ointment morning and evening and after each bowel movement
Child: **Topical** Apply skin cream or ointment to affected area as needed (max: 1/4 oz [7 g]/24 h)

ADMINISTRATION

Topical

- Apply cream preparation after bathing or swimming (water soluble).
- Store at 15°–30° C (59°–86° F) in tight, light-resistant containers.

ADVERSE EFFECTS (≥1%) **Skin:** Irritation, contact dermatitis; rectal bleeding (suppository).

PHARMACOKINETICS Absorption: Poorly absorbed from intact skin; readily absorbed from mucous membranes or abraded skin. **Onset:** 15 min. **Duration:** 2–4 h.

NURSING IMPLICATIONS

Patient & Family Education

- Use OTC preparations as directed. Always review package instructions.
- Discontinue if irritation or rectal bleeding (following use of rectal preparations) develops and consult physician.
- Hemorrhoids can be caused or worsened by constipation, excessive straining at stool, excessive standing, sitting, and coughing.
- Physician may prescribe sitz baths 3–4 times/d to reduce the swelling and pain of hemorrhoids.
- Note: Medication is intended for temporary relief of mild to moderate itching or pain. Seek medical advice for continuing discomfort, pain, bleeding, or sensation of rectal pressure.
- Do not breast feed while taking this drug without consulting physician.

DICHLORPHENAMIDE

(dye-klor-fen'a-mide)
Daranide, Oratrol
Classifications: EYE PREPARATION; CARBONIC ANHYDRASE INHIBITOR; ANTIGLAUCOMA
Prototype: Acetazolamide
Pregnancy Category: C

AVAILABILITY 50 mg tablets

ACTIONS Nonbacteriostatic sulfonamide derivative similar to acetazolamide except that chloride excretion is increased, and thus potential for significant metabolic acidosis is less.
THERAPEUTIC EFFECTS Lowers IOP by decreasing production of aqueous humor.

D

USES Adjunctive treatment of open-angle glaucoma and preoperatively in narrow-angle glaucoma when delay of surgery is desired to lower IOP. Commonly used in conjunction with a miotic; an osmotic agent may also be used to enhance reduction of IOP in acute angle-closure glaucoma.

CONTRAINDICATIONS Hypersensitivity to sulfonamides and sulfonamide derivative diuretics; depressed sodium and potassium levels, severe pulmonary obstruction, marked kidney or liver dysfunction, hyperchloremic acidosis, adrenocortical insufficiency, long-term use in noncongestive angle-closure glaucoma. Safe use during pregnancy (category C) or lactation is not established.
CAUTIOUS USE Respiratory acidosis, reduced respiratory capacity, diabetes mellitus.

ROUTE & DOSAGE

Glaucoma
Adult: **PO** 100–200 mg followed by 100 mg q12h until desired response is obtained **PO Maintenance Dose:** 25–50 mg 1–3 times/d

ADMINISTRATION

Oral
- Take drug with meals to reduce gastric irritation.
- Store at room temperature.

ADVERSE EFFECTS (≥1%) **CNS:** Paresthesia, sedation, drowsiness, fatigue, dizziness, ataxia. **GI:** Anorexia, nausea, vomiting, metallic taste, diarrhea, abdominal discomfort. **Hematologic:** Leukopenia, agranulocytosis, thrombocytopenia, hemolytic anemia. **Urogenital:** Urinary frequency, crystalluria, renal calculi. **Skin:** Urticaria, pruritus, rash. **Other:** Weight loss, fever, glycosuria, asymptomatic hyperuricemia.

INTERACTIONS Drug: Renal excretion of AMPHETAMINES, **ephedrine, flecainide, quinidine, procainamide,** TRICYCLIC ANTIDEPRESSANTS may be decreased, thereby enhancing or prolonging their effects; increases renal excretion of **lithium;** excretion of **phenobarbital** may be increased; **amphotericin B,** CORTICOSTEROIDS may increase **potassium** loss; dichlorphenamide-induced hypokalemia may predispose patients taking DIGITALIS GLYCOSIDES to **digitalis** toxicity; patients on high doses of SALICYLATES are at higher risk for SALICYLATE toxicity.

PHARMACOKINETICS Absorption: Well absorbed from GI tract. **Onset:** 0.5–1 h. **Peak:** 2–4 h. **Duration:** 6–12 h.

NURSING IMPLICATIONS

Assessment & Drug Effects
- Supervise ambulation since drug may cause dizziness and ataxia; other safety precautions may be warranted.
- Monitor for hematologic reactions common to sulfonamides. Obtain baseline CBC and platelet counts before initiating therapy and at regular intervals.

Patient & Family Education
- Increase fluid intake to a high level to reduce risk of renal calculi. Consult physician.
- Report to physician the onset of sore throat, fever, unusual bleeding or bruising, tremors, flank or loin pain, skin rash.
- Do not drive or engage in other potentially hazardous activities until reaction to drug is known.

- Do not breast feed while taking this drug without consulting physician.

DICLOFENAC SODIUM

(di-klo′fen-ak)

Voltaren, Voltaren-XR, Solaraze

DICLOFENAC POTASSIUM

Cataflam

Classifications: CENTRAL NERVOUS SYSTEM AGENT; ANALGESIC, ANTIPYRETIC; NSAID

Prototype: Ibuprofen

Pregnancy Category: B

AVAILABILITY **Diclofenac Sodium** 25 mg, 50 mg, 75 mg tablets; 100 mg sustained release tablets; 0.1% ophthalmic solution; 3% gel **Diclofenac Potassium** 50 mg tablets

ACTIONS Although its exact mechanism of action has not been fully elucidated, it appears to be a potent inhibitor of cyclooxygenase, thereby decreasing the synthesis of prostaglandins.

THERAPEUTIC EFFECTS Nonsteroidal antiinflammatory drug (NSAID) with analgesic and antipyretic activity.

USES Analgesic and antipyretic effects in symptomatic treatment of rheumatoid arthritis, osteoarthritis, and ankylosing spondylitis. Also acute gout; juvenile rheumatoid arthritis; various rheumatic conditions including bursitis, myalgia, sciatica, and tendinitis; acute soft tissue injuries including sprains and strains; dysmenorrhea; headache, migraine, and dental, minor surgical, and postpartum pain; and renal or biliary colic. **Ophthalmic:** Cataract surgery; photophobia associated with refractive surgery. **Topical:** Treatment of actinic keratosis.

CONTRAINDICATIONS Hypersensitivity to diclofenac, patients in whom asthma, urticaria, angioedema, bronchospasm, severe rhinitis, shock, or other sensitivity reaction is precipitated by aspirin or other NSAIDS, pregnancy (category B), lactation.

CAUTIOUS USE Geriatric patients and children; patients receiving anticoagulant therapy; history of GI disease; GU tract problems such as dysuria, cystitis, hematuria, nephritis, nephrotic syndrome, patients who must restrict their sodium intake; impaired hepatic function; SLE; heart failure; hypertension.

ROUTE & DOSAGE

Rheumatoid Arthritis

Adult: **PO** 150–200 mg/d in 3–4 divided doses
Child: **PO** 25 mg b.i.d. or t.i.d.

Osteoarthritis

Adult: **PO** 100–150 mg/d in 3–4 divided doses 100 mg sustained release q.d.

Ankylosing Spondylitis

Adult: **PO** 25 mg q.i.d. and 25 mg h.s.

Cataract Surgery

Adult: **Ophthalmic** 1 drop of 0.1% solution in affected eye q.i.d. beginning 24 h after surgery and continuing for 2 wk

Actinic Keratosis

Adult: **Topical** Apply to affected area b.i.d. for 60–90 d

ADMINISTRATION

Oral

- Ensure that sustained release or enteric coated forms of drug are

D

not chewed or crushed. MUST be swallowed whole.

- Give on an empty stomach, 1 h before or after a meal; absorption is delayed markedly by food. Minimize gastric irritation by administering it with a full glass of milk or water.
- Schedule administration 30 min before physical therapy or planned exercise to keep discomfort at a minimum.
- Discontinue therapy about 1 wk before surgery to reduce risk of bleeding.
- Use with caution in anyone who must restrict sodium intake.
- Store at 15°–30° C (59°–86° F) away from heat and direct light.

ADVERSE EFFECTS (≥1%) **CNS:** Dizziness, headache, drowsiness. **Special Senses:** Tinnitus. **Skin:** Rash, pruritus. **GI:** *Dyspepsia,* nausea, vomiting, abdominal pain, cramps, constipation, diarrhea, indigestion, abdominal distension, flatulence, peptic ulcer; liver enzymes, transaminases increased, liver test abnormalities. **CV:** Fluid retention, hypertension, CHF. **Respiratory:** Asthma. **Body as a Whole:** Back, leg, or joint pain. **Endocrine:** Hyperglycemia. **Hematologic:** Prolonged bleeding time; inhibits platelet aggregation.

DIAGNOSTIC TEST INTERFERENCE Liver function test values may be increased. Liver function test abnormalities may return to normal despite continued use; however, if significant abnormalities occur, clinical signs and symptoms consistent with liver disease develop, or systemic manifestations such as eosinophilia or rash occur, the medication should be discontinued. Serum uric acid concentrations may be decreased because of increased renal clearance.

INTERACTIONS Drug: Increases **cyclosporine**-induced nephrotoxicity; increases **methotrexate** levels (increases toxicity); may decrease BP-lowering effects of DIURETICS; may increase levels and toxicity of **lithium;** may increase **digoxin** levels. **Herbal: Feverfew, garlic, ginger, ginkgo** may increase risk of bleeding.

PHARMACOKINETICS Absorption: Readily absorbed from GI tract; 50%–60% reaches systemic circulation. **Peak:** 2–3 h. **Distribution:** Widely distributed including synovial fluid and into breast milk. **Metabolism:** Extensively metabolized in liver. **Elimination:** 50%–70% excreted in urine, 30%–35% in feces. **Half-Life:** 1.2–2 h.

NURSING IMPLICATIONS

Assessment & Drug Effects

- Monitor for therapeutic effectiveness. Up to 3 wks may be needed for beneficial effects with rheumatoid arthritis or osteoarthritis.
- Lab tests: Periodic liver function, serum uric acid concentrations Hct, PT/INR, and blood glucose.
- Observe and report signs of bleeding (e.g., petechiae, ecchymoses, bleeding gums, bloody or black stools, cloudy or bloody urine).
- Monitor BP for hypertension and blood sugar for hyperglycemia.
- Monitor diabetics closely for loss of diabetic control.
- Monitor for increased serum sodium and potassium in patients receiving potassium-sparing diuretics.
- Monitor weight and report gains greater than 1 kg (2 lb)/24 h.
- Monitor for signs and symptoms of GI irritation and ulceration.

Patient & Family Education

Oral Form

- Do not lie down for 15–30 min after taking medicine to decrease esophageal irritation.
- Discontinue use with onset of ringing or buzzing in the ears, impaired hearing, dizziness, GI discomfort, or bleeding and notify physician.
- Do not take aspirin or other OTC analgesics without permission of the physician.
- Avoid alcohol or other CNS depressants.
- Do not drive or engage in other potentially hazardous activities until reaction to drug is known.
- Note: Diabetics need to monitor blood glucose carefully for loss of glycemic control.
- Do not breast feed while taking this drug.

DICLOXACILLIN SODIUM

(dye-klox-a-sill′in)

Dycill, Dynapen, Pathocil

Classifications: ANTIINFECTIVE; ANTIBIOTIC; SEMISYNTHETIC PENICILLIN

Prototype: Penicillin G potassium

Pregnancy Category: B

AVAILABILITY 125 mg, 250 mg, 500 mg capsules; 62.5 mg/5 mL suspension

ACTIONS Semisynthetic, acid-stable, penicillinase-resistant isoxazolyl penicillin. Action is bactericidal. Inhibits biosynthesis of bacterial cell wall during stage of active multiplication.

THERAPEUTIC EFFECTS Reportedly the most active of the isoxazolyl penicillins (cloxacillin, oxacillin) against penicillinase-producing *Staphylococci*. Generally ineffective against methicillin-resistant *Staphylococci* and gram-negative bacteria.

USES Primarily in systemic infections caused by penicillinase-producing *Staphylococci* and penicillin-resistant *Staphylococci*.

CONTRAINDICATIONS Hypersensitivity to penicillins. Safe use during pregnancy (category B) or in neonates is not established.

CAUTIOUS USE History of or suspected atopy or allergy (asthma, eczema, hives, hay fever); history of hypersensitivity to cephalosporins; lactation; renal or hepatic impairment.

ROUTE & DOSAGE

Mild to Moderate Infections

Adult: **PO** 125–500 mg q6h

Child: **PO** <40 kg, 12.5–25 mg/kg q6h (max: 4 g/d)

ADMINISTRATION

Oral

- Give on an empty stomach at least 1 h before or 2 h after meals. Food reduces drug absorption.
- Reconstitute powder for oral suspension by shaking container to loosen powder. Add water according to label starting with half of the amount, then shake vigorously. Add remaining half and shake again vigorously. Shake well before each use.
- Store reconstituted oral suspensions for 7 d at room temperature (15°–30° C; 59°–86° F) or 14 d under refrigeration at 2°–8° C (36°–46° F). Date and label container. Store capsules at room temperature in tight containers unless otherwise directed.

ADVERSE EFFECTS (≥1%) **Body as a Whole:** Hypersensitivity (pruritus, urticaria, rash, wheezing, sneezing, anaphylaxis; eosinophilia). **GI:** Nausea, vomiting, flatulence, *diarrhea*, abdominal pain. **Other:** Transient elevations of ALT, superinfections.

INTERACTIONS Drug: Probenecid decreases dicloxacillin elimination.

PHARMACOKINETICS Absorption: 35%–76% absorbed from GI tract. **Peak:** 0.5–2 h. **Duration:** 4–6 h. **Distribution:** Distributed throughout body with highest concentrations in liver and kidney; low CSF penetration; crosses placenta; distributed into breast milk. **Metabolism:** Metabolized in liver. **Elimination:** Excreted primarily in urine with some elimination through bile. **Half-Life:** 30–60 min.

NURSING IMPLICATIONS

Assessment & Drug Effects

- Note: Take care to establish previous exposure and sensitivity to penicillins and cephalosporins as well as other allergic reactions of any kind before initiating therapy.
- Obtain C&S prior to initiation of therapy to determine susceptibility of causative organism. Therapy may begin pending test results.
- Lab tests: Baseline blood cultures, WBC, and differential counts and at least weekly for patients on prolonged therapy. Periodic ALT and AST determinations, urinalysis, BUN, and creatinine are also advised for these patients.

Patient & Family Education

- Take medication around the clock. Do not miss a dose and continue taking medication until it is all gone, unless otherwise directed by physician.
- Check with physician if GI side effects appear.
- Watch for and report the signs of hypersensitivity reactions and superinfections (see Appendix F).
- Do not breast feed while taking this drug without consulting physician.

DICUMAROL

(dye-koo′ma-role)
Bishydroxycoumarin
Classification: BLOOD FORMERS, COAGULATORS, AND ORAL ANTICOAGULANTS
Prototype: Warfarin
Pregnancy Category: D

AVAILABILITY 25 mg tablets

ACTIONS Long-acting coumarin derivative.
THERAPEUTIC EFFECTS Interferes with blood clotting by depressing hepatic synthesis of vitamin K-dependent coagulation factors: II, VII, IX, X.

USES Prophylaxis and treatment of DVT.

CONTRAINDICATIONS Hemorrhagic tendencies: hemophilia, thrombocytopenia, leukemia; open wounds or ulcers; renal or hepatic impairment, vitamin C or K deficiency; severe hypertension; subacute bacterial endocarditis; visceral carcinoma. Safe use during pregnancy (category D), lactation, or in children is not established.
CAUTIOUS USE Active tuberculosis, major surgery, indwelling catheters.

ROUTE & DOSAGE

Anticoagulant
Adult: **PO** 200–300 mg on day 1, then 25–200 mg/d based on PT time

ADMINISTRATION

Oral

- Give with food to enhance drug absorption. Frequent dosage adjustment may be necessary during first 1–2 wk of therapy because drug absorption is so variable.
- Give consistently with respect to time of day.
- Store in tightly closed container at 15°–30° C (59°–86° F) unless otherwise directed.

ADVERSE EFFECTS (≥1%) **GI:** Diarrhea, flatulence, nausea, vomiting, anorexia, abdominal cramping. **Urogenital:** Hematuria, priapism. **Hematologic:** Leukopenia, agranulocytosis, hemorrhage. **Skin:** Unusual hair loss, urticaria, dermatitis. **Other:** Hypersensitivity, fever.

INTERACTIONS Drug: See **warfarin.**

PHARMACOKINETICS Absorption: Slowly and incompletely absorbed from GI tract. **Peak:** 1–4 d. **Duration:** 2–10 d. **Distribution:** Crosses placenta; distributed into breast milk. **Metabolism:** Metabolized in liver. **Elimination:** 70%–85% excreted in urine, 15%–30% in feces. **Half-Life:** 1–2 d.

NURSING IMPLICATIONS

Assessment & Drug Effects

- Lab tests: Check PT and INR daily during period of dosage adjustment; obtain dose order following results. Check PT and INR in patient on controlled maintenance dose semiweekly, weekly for 3–4 wk, then at 1- to 4-wk intervals, depending on stability of patient's response.
- Draw blood for PT and INR at least 5 h after an IV bolus dose of heparin or 24 h following a full therapeutic SC heparin dose. Continuous IV infusion or low doses of heparin SC usually do not cause a significant increase in PT; therefore, blood can be drawn at any time.

Patient & Family Education

- Inform physician of any other medication being taken, including OTC drugs.
- Do not add or discontinue any medication without approval of physician or pharmacist.
- Report immediately to physician any unexplained bleeding, easy bruising, or prolonged bleeding time.
- Tell all doctors and dentists before care that you are on anticoagulant therapy.
- Avoid unusual changes in vitamin intake, diet, or life-style without consulting physician. Also notify physician of any changes in health status. Illness may increase anticoagulant requirement.
- Do not breast feed while taking this drug without consulting physician.

DICYCLOMINE HYDROCHLORIDE

(dye-sye′kloe-meen)

Antispas, A-spas, Bentyl, Bentylol ♣, Byclomine, Dibent, Di-Cyclonex, Dilomine, DiSpaz, Formulex ♣, Lominex ♣, Neoquess, Nospaz, Or-Tyl, Protylol ♣, Spasmoban ♣, Spasmoject, Viscerol ♣

Classifications: AUTONOMIC NERVOUS SYSTEM AGENT; ANTICHOLINERGIC (PARASYMPATHOLYTIC); ANTISPASMODIC

Prototype: Atropine

Pregnancy Category: B

AVAILABILITY 10 mg, 20 mg capsules; 20 mg tablets; 10 mg/5 mL syrup; 10 mg/mL injection

ACTIONS Synthetic tertiary amine with antispasmodic properties.
THERAPEUTIC EFFECTS Relieves smooth muscle spasm in GI and biliary tracts, uterus, and ureters by nonspecific direct relaxant action.

USES Adjunctively in treatment of functional bowel disorders/irritable bowel syndrome.
UNLABELED USES Acute enterocolitis, peptic ulcer, and infant colic.

CONTRAINDICATIONS Hypersensitivity to anticholinergic drugs; obstructive diseases of GU and GI tracts, paralytic ileus, intestinal atony, biliary tract disease; unstable cardiovascular status; severe ulcerative colitis, toxic megacolon; myasthenia gravis; infants <6 mo. Safe use during pregnancy (category B), lactation, or in children is not established.
CAUTIOUS USE Glaucoma; prostatic hypertrophy; autonomic neuropathy; ulcerative colitis; hyperthyroidism; coronary heart disease, CHF, arrhythmias, hypertension; hepatic or renal disease; hiatal hernia associated with esophageal reflux.

ROUTE & DOSAGE

Irritable Bowel Disorders
Adult: **PO** 20–40 mg q.i.d. **IM** 20 mg q.i.d.
Child: **PO** 10 mg t.i.d. or q.i.d. (max: 40 mg/d)
Infant: **PO** 5 mg t.i.d. or q.i.d.

ADMINISTRATION

Oral
- Give 30 min before meals and at bedtime.

Intramuscular
- Give deep IM into a large muscle. Do NOT give IV.
- Store below 30° C (86° F) unless otherwise directed.

ADVERSE EFFECTS (≥1%) **All:** Dose related. **Body as a Whole:** Allergic reactions; curare-like effect (cyanosis, apnea, respiratory arrest); decreased sweating; suppression of lactation; urticaria. **CNS:** Lightheadedness, drowsiness, headache, insomnia, brief euphoria, fever, restlessness, irritability, coma, seizures. **CV:** Fluctuations in heart rate, palpitation, tachycardia. **GI:** *Dry mouth,* nausea, *constipation,* paralytic ileus, vomiting, diminished sense of taste, bloated feeling. **Urogenital:** Urinary hesitancy, *urinary retention,* impotence. **Special Senses:** Blurred vision.

PHARMACOKINETICS Absorption: Readily absorbed from GI tract. **Onset:** 1–2 h. **Duration:** 4 h. **Metabolism:** Metabolized in liver. **Elimination:** 80% excreted in urine, 10% in feces. **Half-Life:** 9–10 h.

NURSING IMPLICATIONS

Assessment & Drug Effects
- Monitor for adverse effects especially in infants. Treatment of infant colic with dicyclomine includes some risk, especially in infants <2 mo of age. Doubling the usual dose of 5 mg can produce serious toxic effects. Infants <6 wk have developed respiratory symptoms as well as seizures, fluctuations in heart rate, weakness, and coma within minutes after taking syrup formulation. Symptoms generally last 20–30 min and are believed to be due to local irritation.
- Monitor I&O to assess for urinary retention.

- If drug produces drowsiness and light-headedness, supervision of ambulation and other safety precautions are warranted.

Patient & Family Education

- Exercise caution in hot weather. Dicyclomine may increase risk of heatstroke by decreasing sweating, especially in older adults.
- Do not drive or engage in other potentially hazardous activities until reaction to drug is known.
- Report changes in urine volume, voiding pattern.
- Do not breast feed while taking this drug without consulting physician.

DIDANOSINE (DDI)

(di-dan'o-sine)

Videx, Videx EC

Classifications: ANTIINFECTIVE; ANTIRETROVIRAL AGENT; NUCLEOSIDE REVERSE TRANSCRIPTASE INHIBITOR

Prototype: Zidovudine

Pregnancy Category: B

AVAILABILITY 25 mg, 50 mg, 100 mg, 150 mg, 200 mg tablets; 125 mg, 200 mg, 250 mg, 400 mg delayed release capsules; 100 mg, 167 mg, 250 mg, 2 g, 4 g powder for oral solution

ACTIONS DDI interferes with the HIV RNA-dependent DNA polymerase (reverse transcriptase), thus preventing replication of the virus.

THERAPEUTIC EFFECTS Synthetic purine nucleotide that inhibits replication of HIV.

USES Advanced HIV infection in patients who are intolerant to zidovudine (AZT) or who demonstrate significant clinical or immunological deterioration during zidovudine therapy.

CONTRAINDICATIONS Hypersensitivity to any of the components in the formulation, pregnancy (category B), lactation.

CAUTIOUS USE Individuals with peripheral vascular disease, history of neuropathy, chronic pancreatitis, renal impairment, or any liver impairment.

ROUTE & DOSAGE

HIV Infection

Adult: **PO** *<60 kg,* tablets, 250 mg q.d. or 125 mg b.i.d. (take 2 tablets at each dose to ensure adequate buffering); *<60 kg,* powder, 167 mg b.i.d.; *≥60 kg,* tablets, 400 mg q.d. or 200 mg b.i.d.; *≥60 kg,* powder, 250 mg b.i.d.
Child: **PO** 120 mg/m^2 b.i.d., *<1 y,* give a 1-tablet dose; *>1 y,* give a 2-tablet dose

ADMINISTRATION

Oral

- Give drug on an empty stomach. Food should not be consumed within 15–30 min of drug administration.
- Give with water. Do NOT give with fruit juice or any other acid-containing liquid.
- Chewable tablets must be thoroughly chewed or crushed and dispersed in at least 30 mL (1 oz) of water and immediately swallowed.
- Mix powder for oral solution (buffered) with at least 120 mL (4 oz) of water, stir until dissolved (requires 2–3 min), and immediately swallowed.
- Note: Powder for oral solution (pediatric) is prepared by pharmacist to yield a concentration of 10 mg/mL. Shake solution thoroughly before administration.

D

- Dosage reduction may be indicated in those with renal or hepatic impairment.
- Store reconstituted liquid in a tightly closed container in refrigerator for up to 30 d.

ADVERSE EFFECTS (≥1%) **CV:** Palpitations, thrombophlebitis, arrhythmias, *vasodilation*. **CNS:** *Headache, dizziness, nervousness, insomnia, peripheral neuropathy,* lethargy, poor coordination, seizures. **Special Senses:** Retinal depigmentation, photophobia, blurred vision, optic neuritis, diplopia, blindness. **GI:** *Abdominal pain, nausea, vomiting, diarrhea,* constipation, stomatitis, dry mouth, pancreatitis, increased liver enzymes. **Hematologic:** Increased WBC, neutrophil, lymphocyte, and platelet counts; increased Hgb, thrombocytopenia, ecchymosis, hemorrhage, petechiae. **Metabolic:** Hypocalcemia, hypokalemia, hypomagnesemia, hyperuricemia (asymptomatic), *hypertriglyceridemia*. **Musculoskeletal:** Muscle atrophy, myalgia, arthritis, decreased strength. **Respiratory:** *Asthma, cough, dyspnea, epistaxis, rhinitis, rhinorrhea,* hypoventilation, pharyngitis, rhonchi or rales, sinusitis, congestion. **Skin:** Rash, impetigo, eczema, *pruritus, sweating,* erythema.

INTERACTIONS Drug: ALUMINUM- and MAGNESIUM-CONTAINING ANTACIDS may increase the aluminum- and magnesium-associated adverse effects of tablets. The effectiveness of **dapsone** in prophylaxis of *Pneumocystis carinii* pneumonia may be reduced by concomitant didanosine. May cause additive neuropathy with **zalcitabine** (ddC). **Food:** Absorption is significantly decreased by food. Take on an empty stomach.

PHARMACOKINETICS Absorption: Rapidly absorbed from GI tract when administered to fasting patient with antacids; 23%–40% reaches systemic circulation. **Peak:** 0.6–1 h. **Distribution:** Distributed primarily to body water; 21% reaches CSF; crosses placenta. **Elimination:** 36% excreted in urine. **Half-Life:** 0.8–1.5 h.

NURSING IMPLICATIONS

Assessment & Drug Effects

- Monitor for S&S of pancreatitis (e.g., abdominal pain, nausea, vomiting, elevated serum amylase). Report immediately to physician and withhold drug until ruled out.
- Monitor for S&S of peripheral neuropathy (e.g., numbness, tingling, burning, pain in hands or feet). Report to physician; dose reduction may be indicated.
- Monitor patients with renal impairment for drug toxicity and hypermagnesemia manifested by muscle weakness and confusion.

Patient & Family Education

- Report immediately to physician any of the following: Abdominal pain, nausea, or vomiting.
- Do not breast feed while taking this drug.

DIETHYLPROPION HYDROCHLORIDE Pr

(dye-eth-il-proe′pee-on)

Nobesine ♣, Propion, Ten-Tab, Tenuate, Tenuate Dospan, Tepanil

Classifications: GASTROINTESTINAL AGENT; ANOREXIANT

Pregnancy Category: B

Controlled Substance: Schedule IV

Common adverse effects in *italic*, life-threatening effects underlined: generic names in **bold**; classifications in SMALL CAPS; ♣ Canadian drug name; Pr Prototype drug

AVAILABILITY 25 mg tablets; 75 mg sustained release tablets

ACTIONS Sympathomimetic amine and amphetamine congener. Has lower incidence of amphetamine-type adverse effects but reportedly is less effective as an appetite suppressant. Anorexigenic action probably secondary to direct (CNS) stimulation of appetite control center in hypothalamus and limbic regions. Also produces mild psychic stimulation and vasopressor effects.

THERAPEUTIC EFFECTS Suppresses appetite as a result of drug action on CNS appetite control center.

USES Used solely in management of exogenous obesity as short-term (a few weeks) adjunct in a regimen of weight reduction based on caloric restriction.

CONTRAINDICATIONS Known hypersensitivity or idiosyncrasy to sympathomimetic amines; severe hypertension, advanced arteriosclerosis; hyperthyroidism; glaucoma; agitated states, history of drug abuse. Safe use during pregnancy (category B) or in children <12 y is not established.

CAUTIOUS USE Hypertension, arrhythmias, symptomatic cardiovascular disease; epilepsy; diabetes mellitus; lactation.

ROUTE & DOSAGE

Obesity

Adult: **PO** 25 mg t.i.d. 30–60 min a.c. or 75 mg sustained release q.d. midmorning

ADMINISTRATION

Oral

- Give on an empty stomach, 1/2–1 h before meals.
- Note: Additional dose sometimes prescribed in midevening to control nighttime hunger. Rarely causes insomnia except in high doses.
- Titrate dosage carefully in patients with diabetes.
- Store between 15°–30° C (59°–86° F) in well-closed container unless otherwise specified.

ADVERSE EFFECTS (≥1%) **Body as a Whole:** Hypersensitivity (urticaria, rash, erythema); muscle pain, dyspnea, hair loss, blurred vision, severe dermatoses (chronic intoxication), increased sweating. **CNS:** Mild euphoria, restlessness, *nervousness,* dizziness, headache, irritability, hyperactivity, insomnia, drowsiness, mood changes, lethargy, increase in convulsive episodes in patients with epilepsy. **CV:** Palpitation, tachycardia, precordial pain, rise in BP. **GI:** Nausea, vomiting, diarrhea, constipation, dry mouth, unpleasant taste. **Urogenital:** Impotence, changes in libido, gynecomastia, menstrual irregularities; polyuria, dysuria.

INTERACTIONS Drug: Acetazolamide, sodium bicarbonate decrease diethylpropion elimination; **ammonium chloride, ascorbic acid** increase diethylpropion elimination; a BARBITURATE and diethylpropion taken together may antagonize the effects of both drugs; **furazolidone** may increase blood pressure effects of AMPHETAMINES, and interaction may persist for several weeks after discontinuation of **furazolidone; guanethidine, guanadryl** antagonize antihypertensive effects; MAO INHIBITORS, **selegiline** can cause hypertensive crisis (fatalities reported)—AMPHETAMINES should not be administered at the same time as or within 14 days of these drugs; PHENOTHIAZINES may inhibit mood elevating effects of AMPHETAMINES; TRICYCLIC ANTIDEPRESSANTS enhance AMPHETAMINES' effects by increasing **norepinephrine** release; BETA AGONISTS increase cardiovascular adverse effects.

PHARMACOKINETICS Absorption: Readily absorbed from GI tract. **Duration:** 4 h, regular tablets; 10–14 h, sustained release. **Elimination:** Excreted in urine. **Half-Life:** 4–6 h.

NURSING IMPLICATIONS

Assessment & Drug Effects

- Observe patients with epilepsy closely for reduction in seizure control.
- Anorexigenic effect seldom lasts more than a few weeks. Discontinue if tolerance develops.
- Note: Varying degrees of psychologic and rarely physical dependence can occur.

Patient & Family Education

- Swallow sustained release tablets whole; do NOT chew.
- Do not drive or engage in other potentially hazardous activities until reaction to drug is known.
- Do not breast feed while taking this drug without consulting physician.

DIETHYLSTILBESTROL (DES)

(dye-eth-il-stil-bess'trole)

Stilbestrol

DIETHYLSTILBESTROL DIPHOSPHATE

Honval ✦, Stilphostrol

Classifications: HORMONES AND SYNTHETIC SUBSTITUTES; ESTROGEN; ANTINEOPLASTIC

Prototype: Estradiol

Pregnancy Category: X

AVAILABILITY 50 mg tablets; 0.25 mg/5 mL injection

ACTIONS Potent nonsteroidal synthetic estrogen compound with strong teratogenic potential: may cause vaginal or cervical cancer in offspring if mother is treated with diethylstilbestrol (DES) during pregnancy. Interferes with release of FSH and LH with resultant inhibition of lactation, ovulation, and androgen secretion.

THERAPEUTIC EFFECTS Changes the hormonal environment essential for the survival of tumor cells by competing for their androgen or estrogen receptors.

USES Estrogen deficiency states, including female hypogonadism or castration, primary ovarian failure, menopausal symptoms, atrophic vaginitis, kraurosis vulvae, and for palliative treatment of advanced metastatic carcinoma of the breast in selected men and postmenopausal women and advanced inoperable carcinoma of prostate.

UNLABELED USES Emergency postcoital contraceptive (a morning after pill).

CONTRAINDICATIONS Use for birth control (except emergency postcoital contraception); malignancies or precarcinomatous lesions (vagina, vulva, or breasts); pregnancy (category X); blood clotting disorders; hepatic dysfunction; undiagnosed vaginal bleeding; long-term use during menopause; lactation.

CAUTIOUS USE Hypertension; migraine; diabetes mellitus; asthma.

ROUTE & DOSAGE

Carcinoma Palliation

Adult: **PO** 15 mg/d for breast cancer; 1–3 mg/d, may increase in advanced cases for prostate cancer

Postcoital Contraception

Adult: **PO** 25 mg b.i.d. for 5 d, must start within 72 h after coitus

Prostate Carcinoma

Adult: **PO** 50 mg t.i.d., may increase to 200 mg or more t.i.d. depending on tolerance of patient
IV 0.5 g followed by 1 g/d for 5 or more days, then may reduce to 0.25–0.5 g 1–2 times/wk

ADMINISTRATION

Oral

- Swallow enteric-coated tablets whole.

Intravenous

PREPARE: **Intermittent:** Dilute a single dose in 300 mL NS or D5W.

ADMINISTER: **Intermittent:** Give slowly (1–2 mL/min) during first 10–15 min and then adjust flow rate to permit remainder of solution to be given over a period of 1 h. Patient should be lying down during infusion to reduce incidence of dizziness.

- Store reconstituted solution at room temperature if protected from direct light for 5 d. Do not use if a precipitate or cloudiness is present.
- Store tablets and ampuls at 15°–30° C (59°–86° F) in a tightly closed container. Protect from light and freezing.

ADVERSE EFFECTS (≥1%) **CV:** Thromboembolic disorders, hypertension, edema, MI. **CNS:** Headache, dizziness, chronic depression. **Special Senses:** Intolerance to contact lenses, worsening of myopia. **GI:** *Nausea,* vomiting, diarrhea, anorexia, constipation, cramps, bloating, cholestatic jaundice. **Metabolic:** Reduced carbohydrate tolerance, hypercalcemia, folic acid deficiency. **Urogenital:** Gynecomastia, mastodynia, breast secretions, breakthrough bleeding, changes in menstrual flow, dysmenorrhea, amenorrhea, vaginal candidiasis, changes in libido. **Skin:** Melasma (discoloration), erythema multiforme or nodosum, loss of scalp hair, hirsutism. **Other:** Weight changes, leg cramps.

INTERACTIONS Drug: Rifampin may increase DES metabolism; may antagonize anticoagulant effects of **warfarin**.

PHARMACOKINETICS Absorption: Readily absorbed from GI tract. **Metabolism:** Metabolized in liver. **Elimination:** Excreted in urine and feces.

NURSING IMPLICATIONS

Assessment & Drug Effects

- Monitor for nausea and vomiting which are common in the menopausal group of patients receiving ≥1 mg/d and relatively uncommon in men and nonpregnant women even when doses are 3–5 mg/d.
- Note: Severe nausea and vomiting with contraceptive doses can lead to noncompliance. An antiemetic may be required.
- Monitor for S&S of deep vein thrombosis or thrombophlebitis (see Appendix F); risk of blood clot formation is high.

Patient & Family Education

- Report the onset of vaginal bleeding or any other unusual signs if uterus is intact because of the risk for endometrial cancer.
- Note: Women should have breasts and pelvic organs examined prior to treatment and at intervals throughout therapy. Learn self-

examination of breasts. Keep check-up appointments.

- Take pregnancy test prior to therapy with DES. Know teratogenic potential of this drug.
- Drug-induced loss of libido and development of feminine characteristics in males disappear with termination of therapy.
- Do not breast feed while taking this drug.

DIFLORASONE DIACETATE

(dye-flor'a-sone)

Florone, Florone E, Maxiflor, Psorcon

Classifications: SKIN AND MUCOUS MEMBRANE AGENT; ANTIINFLAMMATORY; STEROID

Prototype: Hydrocortisone

Pregnancy Category: C

AVAILABILITY 0.05% cream, ointment

See Appendix A-4.

DIFLUNISAL

(dye-floo'ni-sal)

Dolobid

Classifications: CENTRAL NERVOUS SYSTEM AGENT; ANALGESIC; NSAID

Prototype: Ibuprofen

Pregnancy Category: C

AVAILABILITY 250 mg, 500 mg tablets

ACTIONS A long-acting nonsteroidal antiinflammatory drug (NSAID) unlike aspirin, in which, inhibition of platelet function and effect on bleeding time are dose related and reversible, lasting only about 24 h after drug is discontinued. Is a nonnarcotic analgesic agent. Exerts mild antipyretic effect; therefore it is not used clinically for this purpose. Has some uricosuric activity at usual dosages.

THERAPEUTIC EFFECTS This NSAID has peripheral analgesic properties by inhibition of prostaglandin synthesis. It is more potent than aspirin and acetaminophen in equianalgesic doses and has longer duration of effect.

USES Acute and long-term relief of mild to moderate pain and symptomatic treatment of osteoarthritis and rheumatoid arthritis.

CONTRAINDICATIONS Patients in whom aspirin or other NSAIDS precipitate an acute asthmatic attack (bronchospasm), urticaria, angioedema, severe rhinitis, or shock; active peptic ulcer, GI bleeding. Safe use during pregnancy (category C), lactation, or children <12 y is not established. Use during third trimester of pregnancy specifically contraindicated because NSAIDS are known to cause premature closure of ductus arteriosus in fetus.

CAUTIOUS USE History of upper GI disease; impaired renal or hepatic function; compromised cardiac function, and other conditions associated with fluid retention; patients receiving diuretics; geriatric patients; hypertension; patients who may be adversely affected by prolonged bleeding time.

ROUTE & DOSAGE

Pain Relief

Adult: **PO** 1000 mg followed by 500 mg q8–12h

Arthritis

Adult: **PO** 500–1000 mg/d in 2 divided doses (max: 1500 mg/d)

ADMINISTRATION

Oral

- Give with water, milk, or food to reduce GI irritation. Food causes slight reduction in absorption rate, but does not affect total amount absorbed.
- Store at 15°–30° C (59°–86° F) in tightly closed containers unless otherwise directed.

ADVERSE EFFECTS (≥1%) **Body as a Whole:** Hypersensitivity syndrome (fever, chills, rash, eosinophilia, changes in renal and hepatic function, anaphylactic reactions with bronchospasm). **CNS:** Headache, drowsiness, insomnia, dizziness, vertigo, light-headedness, fatigue, weakness, nervousness, confusion, disorientation. **CV:** Palpitation, tachycardia, *peripheral edema*. **Special Senses:** Tinnitus, hearing loss; blurred vision, reduced visual acuity, changes in color vision, scotomas, corneal deposits, retinal disturbances. **GI:** *Nausea,* GI pain, flatulence, GI bleeding, peptic ulcer, anorexia, eructation, cholestatic jaundice. **Urogenital:** Hematuria, proteinuria, interstitial nephritis, renal failure. **Hematologic:** Prolonged PT, anemia, decreased serum uric acid, transient elevations of liver function tests. **Skin:** Rash, toxic epidermal necrolysis, exfoliative dermatitis, urticaria. **Other:** Weight gain, hyperventilation, dyspnea, photosensitivity.

DIAGNOSTIC TEST INTERFERENCE Diflunisal can lower ***serum uric acid*** concentrations by as much as 1.4 mg/dL and increased renal clearance of uric acid.

INTERACTIONS Drug: ANTACIDS decrease diflunisal absorption; **aspirin** and other NSAIDS increase risk of GI bleeding; increases risk of **warfarin**-induced hypoprothrombinemia; increases **methotrexate** levels and toxicity.

PHARMACOKINETICS Absorption: Readily absorbed from GI tract. **Onset:** 1 h. **Peak:** 2–3 h. **Duration:** 12 h. **Distribution:** Probably crosses placenta; distributed into breast milk. **Metabolism:** Metabolized in liver. **Elimination:** Excreted in urine. **Half-Life:** 8–12 h.

NURSING IMPLICATIONS

Assessment & Drug Effects

- Monitor for therapeutic effectiveness: Full antiinflammatory effect for arthritis may not occur until 8 d to several weeks into therapy.
- Discontinue if patient presents signs of hepatic toxicity (see Appendix F).
- Note: Although the antipyretic effect is mild, chronic or high doses may mask fever in some patients.

Patient & Family Education

- Swallow tablet whole; do not crush or chew.
- Take drug as prescribed. Doubling the dosage can produce greater than doubling of drug accumulation, particularly in patients receiving repetitive doses.
- Report onset of visual or auditory problems immediately to physician.
- Be aware of I&O ratio and pattern and check for and report peripheral edema and unusual weight gain.
- Report promptly to physician the onset of melena, hematemesis, or severe stomach pain.
- Do not drive or engage in other potentially hazardous activities until reaction to drug is known.
- Do not breast feed while taking this drug without consulting physician.

D

DIGOXIN (Pr)

(di-jox'in)

Lanoxicaps, Lanoxin

Classifications: CARDIOVASCULAR AGENT; CARDIAC GLYCOSIDE; ANTIARRHYTHMIC

Pregnancy Category: A

AVAILABILITY 0.05 mg, 0.1 mg, 0.2 mg capsules; 0.125 mg, 0.25 mg, 0.5 mg tablets; 0.05 mg/mL elixir; 0.25 mg/mL, 0.1 mg/mL injection

ACTIONS Widely used cardiac glycoside of *Digitalis lanata*. Acts by increasing the force and velocity of myocardial systolic contraction (positive inotropic effect). It also decreases conduction velocity through the atrioventricular node. Action is more prompt and less prolonged than that of digitalis and digitoxin.

THERAPEUTIC EFFECTS Increases the contractility of the heart muscle (positive inotropic effect).

USES Rapid digitalization and for maintenance therapy in CHF, atrial fibrillation, atrial flutter, paroxysmal atrial tachycardia.

CONTRAINDICATIONS Digitalis hypersensitivity, ventricular fibrillation, ventricular tachycardia unless due to CHF. Full digitalizing dose not given if patient has received digoxin during previous week or if slowly excreted cardiotonic glycoside has been given during previous 2 wk.

CAUTIOUS USE Renal insufficiency, hypokalemia, advanced heart disease, acute MI, incomplete AV block, cor pulmonale; hypothyroidism; lung disease; pregnancy (category A), lactation, premature and immature infants, children, older adults, or debilitated patients.

ROUTE & DOSAGE

Digitalizing Dose

Adult: **PO** 10–15 mcg/kg (1 mg) in divided doses over 24–48 h
IV 10–15 mcg/kg (1 mg) in divided doses over 24 h
Child: **PO/IV** <2 *y*, 40–60 mcg/kg; *2–10 y*, 20–40 mcg/kg; >*10 y*, 10–15 mcg/kg (1.5–2 mg)
Neonate: **PO/IV** 30–50 mcg/kg
Premature neonate: **PO/IV** 20 mcg/kg

Maintenance Dose

Adult: **PO/IV** 0.1–0.375 mg/d
Child: **PO/IV** <*2 y*, 7.5–9 mcg/kg/d; *2–10 y*, 6–7.5 mcg/kg/d; >*10 y*, 0.125–0.25 mg/d
Neonate: 6–7.5 mcg/kg/d
Premature neonate: 3.75 mcg/kg/d

ADMINISTRATION

Oral

- Give without regard to food. Administration after food may slightly delay rate of absorption, but total amount absorbed is not affected.
- Crush and mix with fluid or food if patient cannot swallow it whole.

Intravenous

PREPARE: **Direct:** Give undiluted or diluted in 4 mL of sterile water, D5W, or NS (less diluent may cause precipitation).

ADMINISTER: **Direct:** Give each dose over at least 5 min.

INCOMPATIBILITIES **Solution/additive: Dobutamine, doxapram.**

- Monitor IV site frequently. Infiltration of parenteral drug into subcutaneous tissue can cause local irritation and sloughing.

- Store tablets, elixir, and injection solution at 25° C (77° F) or at 15°–30° C (59°–86° F).

ADVERSE EFFECTS (≥1%) **CNS:** Fatigue, muscle weakness, headache, facial neuralgia, mental depression, paresthesias, hallucinations, confusion, drowsiness, agitation, dizziness. **CV:** Arrhythmias, hypotension, AV block. **Special Senses:** Visual disturbances. **GI:** Anorexia, *nausea*, vomiting, diarrhea. **Other:** Diaphoresis, recurrent malaise, dysphagia.

INTERACTIONS Drug: ANTACIDS, **cholestyramine, colestipol** decrease digoxin absorption; DIURETICS, CORTICOSTEROIDS, **amphotericin B,** LAXATIVES, **sodium polystyrene sulfonate** may cause hypokalemia, increasing the risk of digoxin toxicity; **calcium IV** may increase risk of arrhythmias if administered together with digoxin; **quinidine, verapamil, amiodarone, flecainide** significantly increase digoxin levels, and digoxin dose should be decreased by 50%; **erythromycin** may increase digoxin levels; **succinylcholine** may potentiate arrhythmogenic effects; **nefazodone** may increase digoxin levels. **Herbal: Ginseng** increase digoxin toxicity; **ma huang, ephedra** may induce arrhythmias.

PHARMACOKINETICS Absorption: 70% PO tablets; 90% PO liquid and capsules. **Onset:** 1–2 h PO; 5–30 min IV. **Peak:** 6–8 h PO; 1–5 h IV. **Duration:** 3–4 d in fully digitalized patient. **Distribution:** Widely distributed; tissue levels significantly higher than plasma levels; crosses placenta. **Metabolism:** Approximately 14% in liver. **Elimination:** 80%–90% excreted by kidneys; may appear in breast milk. **Half-Life:** 34–44 h.

NURSING IMPLICATIONS

Assessment & Drug Effects

- Be familiar with patient's baseline data (e.g., quality of peripheral pulses, blood pressure, clinical symptoms, serum electrolytes, creatinine clearance) as a foundation for making assessments.
- Lab tests: Baseline and periodic serum digoxin, potassium, magnesium, and calcium. Notify physician of abnormal values. Draw blood samples for determining plasma digoxin levels at least 6 h after daily dose and preferably just before next scheduled daily dose. Therapeutic range of serum digoxin is 0.8–2 ng/mL; toxic levels are >2 ng/mL.
- Take apical pulse for 1 full min noting rate, rhythm, and quality before administering. If changes are noted, withhold digoxin, take rhythm strip if patient is on ECG monitor, notify physician promptly.
- Withhold medication and notify physician if apical pulse falls below ordered parameters (e.g., >50 or 60/min in adults and >60 or 70/min in children).
- Monitor for S&S of drug toxicity: In children, cardiac arrhythmias are usually reliable signs of early toxicity. Early indicators in adults (anorexia, nausea, vomiting, diarrhea, visual disturbances) are rarely initial signs in children.
- Monitor I&O ratio during digitalization, particularly in patients with impaired renal function. Also monitor for edema daily and auscultate chest for rales.
- Monitor serum digoxin levels closely during concurrent antibiotic–digoxin therapy, which can precipitate toxicity because of altered intestinal flora.
- Observe patients closely when being transferred from one preparation (tablet, elixir, or parenteral) to another; when tablet is replaced by elixir potential for toxicity increases since ≥30% of drug is absorbed.

D

Patient & Family Education

- Report to physician if pulse falls below 60 or rises above 110 or if you detect skipped beats or other changes in rhythm, when digoxin is prescribed for atrial fibrillation.
- Suspect toxicity and report to physician if any of the following occur: Anorexia, nausea, vomiting, diarrhea, or visual disturbances.
- Weigh each day under standard conditions. Report weight gain >1 kg (2 lb)/d.
- Take digoxin PRECISELY as prescribed, do not skip or double a dose or change dose intervals, and take it at same time each day.
- Do not to take OTC medications, especially those for coughs, colds, allergy, GI upset, or obesity, without prior approval of physician.
- Continue with brand originally prescribed unless otherwise directed by physician.
- Do not breast feed while taking this drug without consulting physician.

DIGOXIN IMMUNE FAB (OVINE)

(di-jox′in)

Digibind, DigiFab

Classification: ANTIDOTE

Pregnancy Category: C

AVAILABILITY 38 mg, 40 mg vial

ACTIONS Purified fragments of antibodies specific for digoxin (but also effective for digitoxin) produced in sheep immunized with digoxin–albumin conjugate. Use of fragments of antidigoxin antibodies (Fab) instead of whole antibody molecules permits more extensive and faster distribution to serum and toxic cellular sites.

THERAPEUTIC EFFECTS FAB acts by selectively complexing with circulating digoxin or digitoxin, thereby preventing drug from binding at receptor sites; the complex is then eliminated in urine.

USES Treatment of potentially life-threatening digoxin or digitoxin intoxication in carefully selected patients.

CONTRAINDICATIONS Hypersensitivity to sheep products; renal or cardiac failure. Safe use during pregnancy (category C) or lactation is not established.

CAUTIOUS USE Prior treatment with sheep antibodies or ovine Fab fragments; history of allergies; impaired renal function.

ROUTE & DOSAGE

Serious Digoxin Toxicity Secondary to Overdose

Adult/Child: **IV** Dosages vary according to amount of digoxin to be neutralized; dosages are based on total body load or steady state serum digoxin concentrations (see package insert); some patients may require a second dose after several hours

ADMINISTRATION

Intravenous

PREPARE: **Direct:** Reconstitute by dissolving 38 mg (1 vial) in 4 mL of sterile water for injection; mix gently (solution will contain 9.5 mg/mL). **IV Infusion:** Dilute further with any volume of NS compatible with cardiac status.

ADMINISTER: **Direct:** Give undiluted bolus only if cardiac arrest is imminent. **IV Infusion:** Give IV infusion over 30 min, preferably through a 0.22-micron membrane filter. ■ For administration to infants: Reconstitute for direct IV and administer with a tuberculin syringe. For small doses (e.g., 2 mg or less), dilute the reconstituted 40 mg vial with 36 mL of NS to yield 1 mg/mL. Closely monitor for fluid overload.

- Use reconstituted solutions promptly or refrigerated at 2°–8° C (36°–46° F) for up to 4 h.

ADVERSE EFFECTS (≥1%) Adverse reactions associated with use of digoxin immune Fab are related primarily to the effects of **digitalis** withdrawal on the heart (see Nursing Implications). Allergic reactions have been reported rarely. Hypokalemia.

DIAGNOSTIC TEST INTERFERENCE Digoxin immune Fab may interfere with ***serum digoxin*** determinations by immunoassay tests.

INTERACTIONS Drug: Not established.

PHARMACOKINETICS Onset: <1 min after IV administration. **Elimination:** Excreted in urine over 5–7 d. **Half-Life:** 14–20 h.

NURSING IMPLICATIONS

Assessment & Drug Effects

- Perform skin testing for allergy prior to administration of immune Fab, particularly in patients with history of allergy or who have had previous therapy with immune Fab.
- Keep emergency equipment and drugs immediately available before skin testing is done or first dose is given and until patient is out of danger.
- Monitor for therapeutic effectiveness: Reflected in improvement in cardiac rhythm abnormalities, mental orientation and other neurologic symptoms, and GI and visual disturbances. S&S of reversal of digitalis toxicity occurs in 15–60 min in adults and usually within minutes in children.
- Baseline and frequent vital signs and EGG during administration.
- Lab tests: Baseline and periodic serum potassium and serum digoxin; serum digoxin or digitoxin concentration (this measurement will not be accurate for at least 5–7 d after therapy begins because of test interference by immune Fab).
- Note: Serum potassium is particularly critical during first several hours following administration of immune Fab. Monitor closely.
- Monitor closely: Cardiac status may deteriorate as inotropic action of digitalis is withdrawn by action of immune Fab. CHF, arrhythmias, increase in heart rate, and hypokalemia can occur.
- Make sure serum digoxin levels and ECG readings are obtained for at least 2–3 wk.

Patient & Family Education

- Do not breast feed while taking this drug without consulting physician.

DIHYDROERGOTAMINE MESYLATE

(dye-hye-droe-er-got'a-meen)

D.H.E. 45, Migranal

Classifications: AUTONOMIC NERVOUS SYSTEM AGENT; ALPHA-ADRENERGIC ANTAGONIST; ERGOT ALKALOID

Prototype: Ergotamine

Pregnancy Category: X

AVAILABILITY 4 mg/mL nasal spray; 1 mg/mL injection

D

ACTIONS Alpha-adrenergic blocking agent and dihydrogenated ergot alkaloid with direct constricting effect on smooth muscle of peripheral and cranial blood vessels. Maintains elevated levels of circulating norepinephrine (vasoconstrictor action) by inhibiting its reuptake. Vasoconstrictor action is more prominent on capacitance vessels (veins, venules) than on resistance vessels (arteries, arterioles).

THERAPEUTIC EFFECTS Reduces rate of serotonin-induced platelet aggregation. Has somewhat weaker vasoconstrictor action than ergotamine but greater adrenergic blocking activity.

USES To prevent or abort vascular headache (e.g., migraine or histaminic cephalalgia) when rapid control is desired or other routes are not feasible. With low-dose heparin therapy to prevent postoperative deep-vein thrombosis and pulmonary embolism.

UNLABELED USES To treat postural hypotension.

CONTRAINDICATIONS History of hypersensitivity to ergot preparations; peripheral vascular disease, coronary heart disease, hypertension; peptic ulcer; impaired hepatic or renal function; sepsis. Safe use during pregnancy (category X), lactation, or in children is not established.

ROUTE & DOSAGE

Migraine Headache

Adult: **IV/IM/SC** 1 mg, may be repeated at 1 h intervals to a total of 3 mg IM or 2 mg IV/SC (max: 6 mg/wk) **Intranasal** 1 spray (0.5 mg) in each nostril, may repeat with additional spray in 15 min if no relief (max: 4 sprays per attack); wait 6–8 h before treating another attack (max: 8 sprays per 24 h, 24 sprays/wk)

ADMINISTRATION

Intranasal

- Give at first warning of migraine headache.
- Optimum results: Titrate the doses required to bring relief for several headaches to determine the minimal effective dose. Use the established dose for subsequent attacks.

Intramuscular/Subcutaneous

- Withdraw IM or SC dose directly from ampule. Do not dilute.
- Note: Onset of action is about 20 min; when rapid relief is required, the IV route is prescribed.

Intravenous

PREPARE: **Direct:** Give undiluted.
ADMINISTER: **Direct:** Give at a rate of 1 mg/60 sec.

- Store at 15°–30° C (59°–86° F) unless otherwise directed. ▪ Protect ampoules from heat and light; do not freeze. ▪ Discard ampoule if solution appears discolored.

ADVERSE EFFECTS (≥1%) **CV:** Vasospasm: coldness, numbness and tingling in fingers and toes, muscle pains and weakness of legs, precordial distress and pain, transient tachycardia or bradycardia, hypertension (large doses). **GI:** *Nausea, vomiting.* **Body as a Whole:** Dizziness, dysphoria, *localized edema and itching;* ergotism (excessive doses).

INTERACTIONS Drug: BETA BLOCKERS, **erythromycin** increase peripheral vasoconstriction with risk of ischemia; increased **ergotamine** toxicity with drugs that inhibit CYP3A4 (e.g., PROTEASE INHIBITORS, **amprenavir, ritonavir, nelfina-**

vir, indinavir, saquinavir), MACROLIDE ANTIBIOTICS **(erythromycin, azithromycin, clarithromycin)**, AZOLE ANTIFUNGALS **(ketoconazole, itraconazole, fluconazole, clotrimazole), nefazodone, fluoxetine, fluvoxamine. Food: Grapefruit juice** may increase toxicity.

PHARMACOKINETICS Onset: 15–30 min IM; <5 min IV. **Duration:** 3– 4 h. **Distribution:** Probably distributed into breast milk. **Metabolism:** Metabolized in liver. **Elimination:** Excreted primarily in urine; some excreted in feces. **Half-Life:** 21–32 h.

NURSING IMPLICATIONS

Assessment & Drug Effects

- Monitor cardiac status, especially when large doses are given.
- Monitor for and report numbness and tingling of fingers and toes, extremity weakness, muscle pain, or intermittent claudication.

Patient & Family Education

- Take at first warning of migraine headache.
- Lie down in a quiet, darkened room for several hours after drug administration for best results.
- Report immediately if any of the following S&S develop: Chest pain, nausea, vomiting, change in heartbeat, numbness, tingling, pain or weakness of extremities, edema, or itching.
- Do not breast feed while taking this drug without consulting physician.

DIHYDROTACHYSTEROL

(dye-hye-droe-tak-iss′ter-ole)

DHT, DHT Intensol, Hytakerol

Classifications: VITAMIN D; REGULATOR, SERUM CALCIUM

Pregnancy Category: A

AVAILABILITY 0.125 mg, 0.2 mg, 0.4 mg tablets; 0.2 mg/mL oral solution; 0.125 mg capsules

ACTIONS Oil-soluble reduction product of ergocalciferol (vitamin D_2) with pharmacologic actions similar to those of both ergocalciferol and parathyroid hormone. In comparison with ergocalciferol, dihydrotachysterol promotes less intestinal absorption of calcium but almost equal phosphate diuresis.

THERAPEUTIC EFFECTS Acts like parathyroid hormone in ability to raise serum calcium concentrations rapidly; also reported to increase intestinal absorption of sodium, potassium, and magnesium.

USES Hypocalcemia associated with hypoparathyroidism, both postoperative and idiopathic, and in pseudohypoparathyroidism. Also for prophylaxis of hypocalcemic tetany following thyroid surgery.

UNLABELED USES Vitamin D-resistant rickets (familial hypophosphatemia), osteoporosis, and renal osteodystrophy.

CONTRAINDICATIONS Sensitivity to vitamin D; hypercalcemia and hypocalcemia associated with renal insufficiency and hyperphosphatemia; renal stones, hypervitaminosis D. Safe use during pregnancy (category A), lactation, or in children in amounts exceeding RDA is not established.

ROUTE & DOSAGE

Hypoparathyroidism, Pseudohypoparathyroidism

Adult: **PO** 0.75–2.5 mg/d for several days, then 0.2–1 mg/d (may need 1.5 mg/d)
Child: **PO** 1–5 mg/d for 4 d then 0.5–1.5 mg/d

D

Neonate: **PO** 0.05–0.1 mg/d

Thyroidectomy-induced Hypocalcemia

Adult: **PO** 0.25 mg/d

Renal Osteodystrophy

Adult: **PO** 0.1–0.6 mg/d
Child: **PO** 0.1–0.5 mg/d

ADMINISTRATION

Oral

- Withhold drug if signs and symptoms of hypercalcemia appear (see Appendix F) and report to physician.
- Store in tightly closed, light-resistant containers at 15°–30° C (59°–86° F) unless otherwise directed.

ADVERSE EFFECTS (≥1%) **CNS:** Drowsiness, headache, weakness, vertigo, ataxia, atonia, mental depression. **Endocrine:** Hypercalcemia. **GI:** Anorexia, nausea, vomiting, metallic taste, dry mouth, thirst, diarrhea, constipation, abdominal pain. **Urogenital:** Nocturia, polyuria, renal calculi. **Special Senses:** Tinnitus.

INTERACTIONS Drug: Not established.

PHARMACOKINETICS Absorption: Readily absorbed from small intestines. **Peak:** 2 wk. **Duration:** 2 wk. **Distribution:** Distributed in breast milk. **Metabolism:** Metabolized in liver to active metabolite. **Elimination:** Excreted primarily in bile and feces.

NURSING IMPLICATIONS

Assessment & Drug Effects

- Lab tests: serum and urinary calcium levels at least weekly during first month of therapy until they are stabilized, then monthly thereafter.
- Supplement with 10–15 g of oral calcium lactate or gluconate daily; adequate calcium intake is necessary for clinical response to therapy.
- Restrict dietary phosphate or administer calcium carbonate supplements with meals, or both, to bind intestinal phosphates and improve calcium balance in patients with hyperphosphatemia.
- Monitor hypoparathyroid patients receiving thiazide diuretics closely; they are prone to develop hypercalcemia.

Patient & Family Education

- Learn S&S of hypercalcemia (see Appendix F).
- Do not breast feed while taking this drug without consulting physician.

DILTIAZEM

(dil-tye′a-zem)

Cardizem, Cardizem CD, Cardizem LA, Cardizem SR, Cardizem Lyo-Ject, Cartia XT, Dilacor XR, Tiamate, Tiazac, Taztia XT

DILTIAZEM IV

Cardizem IV

Classifications: CARDIOVASCULAR AGENT; CALCIUM CHANNEL BLOCKING AGENT; ANTIHYPERTENSIVE

Prototype: Verapamil

Pregnancy Category: C

AVAILABILITY 30 mg, 60 mg, 90 mg, 120 mg tablets; 120 mg, 180 mg, 240 mg sustained-release tablets; 60 mg, 90 mg, 120 mg, 180 mg, 240 mg, 300 mg, 360 mg sustained-release capsules; 120 mg, 180 mg, 240 mg, 300 mg, 360 mg, 420 mg extended-release tablets; 25 mg, 50 mg vials

ACTIONS Slow channel blocker with pharmacologic actions similar to those of verapamil. Inhibits calcium ion influx through slow channels into cell of myocardial and arterial smooth muscle (both coronary and peripheral blood vessels). As a result, intracellular calcium remains at subthreshold levels insufficient to stimulate cell excitation and contraction. Slows SA and AV node conduction (antiarrhythmic effect) without affecting normal arterial action potential or intraventricular conduction.

THERAPEUTIC EFFECTS Dilates coronary arteries and arterioles and inhibits coronary artery spasm; thus myocardial oxygen delivery is increased (antianginal effect). By vasodilation of peripheral arterioles, drug decreases total peripheral vascular resistance and reduces arterial BP at rest (antihypertensive effect).

USES Vasospastic angina (Prinzmetal's variant or at rest angina), chronic stable (classic effort-associated) angina, essential hypertension. *IV form:* Atrial fibrillation, atrial flutter, supraventricular tachycardia.

UNLABELED USES Prevention of reinfarction in non-Q-wave MI.

CONTRAINDICATIONS Known hypersensitivity to drug; sick sinus syndrome (unless pacemaker is in place and functioning); second- or third-degree AV block; severe hypotension (systolic <90 mm Hg or diastolic <60 mm Hg); patients undergoing intracranial surgery; bleeding aneurysms. Safe use during pregnancy (category C), lactation, or in children is not established.

CAUTIOUS USE CHF (especially if patient is also receiving beta blocker), conduction abnormalities; renal or hepatic impairment; older adults.

ROUTE & DOSAGE

Angina

Adult: **PO** 30 mg q.i.d., may increase q1–2d as required (usual range: 180–360 mg/d in divided doses)

Hypertension

Adult: **PO** 60–120 mg sustained-release b.i.d. (usual range: 240–360 mg/d) or 120–540 mg of CD or LA once daily

Atrial Fibrillation

Adult: **IV** 0.25 mg/kg IV bolus over 2 min, if inadequate response, may repeat in 15 min with 0.35 mg/kg, followed by a continuous infusion of 5–10 mg/h (max: 15 mg/h for 24 h)

ADMINISTRATION

Oral

- Do not crush sustained-release capsules or tablets. They must be swallowed whole.
- Withhold if systolic BP is <90 mm Hg or diastolic is <60 mm Hg.
- Give before meals and at bedtime.
- Store at 15°–30° C (59°–86° F).

Intravenous

PREPARE: **Direct:** Give undiluted. **Continuous:** For IV infusion, add to a volume of D5W, NS, or D5/0.45% NaCl that can be administered in 24 h or less.

ADMINISTER: **Direct:** Give as a bolus dose over 2 min. A second bolus may be given after 15 min. **Continuous:** Give at a rate 5–15 mg/h. Infusion duration longer than 24 h and infusion rate >15 mg/h are not recommended.

INCOMPATIBILITIES **Solution/additive: Furosemide. Y-site: Furosemide.**

D

ADVERSE EFFECTS (≥1%) **CNS:** *Headache,* fatigue, dizziness, asthenia, drowsiness, nervousness, insomnia, confusion, tremor, gait abnormality. **CV:** Edema, arrhythmias, angina, second- or third-degree AV block, bradycardia, CHF, flushing, hypotension, syncope, palpitations. **GI:** Nausea, constipation, anorexia, vomiting, diarrhea, impaired taste, weight increase. **Skin:** Rash.

INTERACTIONS Drug: BETA BLOCKERS, **digoxin** may have additive effects on av node conduction prolongation; may increase **digoxin** or **quinidine** levels; **cimetidine** may increase diltiazem levels, thus increasing effects; may increase **cyclosporine** levels.

PHARMACOKINETICS Absorption: Approximately 80% absorbed from GI tract, with 40% reaching systemic circulation. **Peak:** 2–3 h; 6–11 h sustained release; 11–18 h Cardizem LA. **Distribution:** Distributed into breast milk. **Metabolism:** Metabolized in liver. **Elimination:** Excreted primarily in urine with some elimination in feces. **Half-Life:** Oral 3.5–9 h, IV 2 h.

NURSING IMPLICATIONS

Assessment & Drug Effects

- Check BP and ECG before initiation of therapy and monitor particularly during dosage adjustment period.
- Lab tests: Do baseline and periodic liver and renal function tests.
- Monitor for and report S&S of CHF.
- Monitor for headache. An analgesic may be required.
- Supervise ambulation as indicated.

Patient & Family Education

- Make position changes slowly and in stages; light-headedness and dizziness (hypotension) are possible.
- Do not drive or engage in other potentially hazardous activities until reaction to drug is known.
- Keep follow-up appointments and physician informed.
- Do not breast feed while taking this drug without consulting physician.

DIMENHYDRINATE

(dye-men-hye′dri-nate)

Apo-Dimenhydrinate ♣, Calm-X, Dimenhydrinate Injection, Dimentabs, Dinate, Dommanate, Dramanate, Dramamine, Dramilin, Dramocen, Dramoject, Dymenate, Gravol ♣, Hydrate, Marmine, Motion-Aid, Nauseatol ♣, Novodimenate ♣, PMS Dimenhydrinate ♣, Travamine ♣, Travel Aid, Travel Eze, Wehamine

Classifications: ANTIHISTAMINE (H_1-RECEPTOR ANTAGONIST); ANTIEMETIC; ANTIVERTIGO AGENT

Prototype: Diphenhydramine

Pregnancy Category: B

AVAILABILITY 50 mg tablets; 50 mg/mL injection; 15.62 mg/5 mL, 12.5 mg/4 mL, 12.5 mg/5 mL liquid

ACTIONS H_1-receptor antagonist and salt of diphenhydramine, with which it shares similar properties.

THERAPEUTIC EFFECTS Precise mode of antinauseant action not known, but thought to involve ability to inhibit cholinergic stimulation in vestibular and associated neural pathways.

USES Chiefly in prevention and treatment of motion sickness. Also has been used in management of vertigo, nausea, and vomiting associated with radiation sickness, labyrinthitis, Ménière's syndrome, stapedectomy, anesthesia, and various medications.

CONTRAINDICATIONS Narrow-angle glaucoma, prostatic hypertrophy. Safe use during pregnancy (category B), lactation, or in children <2 y is not established.
CAUTIOUS USE Convulsive disorders.

ROUTE & DOSAGE

Motion Sickness

Adult: **PO** 50–100 mg q4–6h (max: 400 mg/24h) **IV/IM** 50 mg as needed
Child: **PO** *2–6 y,* up to 25 mg q6–8h (max: 75 mg/24h); *6–12 y,* 25–50 mg q6–8h (max:150 mg/24h) **IV/IM** *2–6 y,* 1.25 mg/kg q.i.d. up to 300 mg/d; *6–12 y,* 1.25 mg/kg q.i.d. up to 300 mg/d

ADMINISTRATION

Note: Give 30–60 min before treatment, then repeat 90 min after treatment, and again in 3 h to prevent radiation sickness.

Intramuscular
- Give undiluted and inject deep IM into a large muscle.

Intravenous

PREPARE: **Direct:** Dilute each 50 mg in 10 mL of NS.
ADMINISTER: **Direct:** Give each 50 mg or fraction thereof over 2 min.
INCOMPATIBILITIES **Solution/additive: Aminophylline, amobarbital, butorphanol, chlorpromazine, glycopyrrolate, hydroxyzine, midazolam, pentobarbital, prochlorperazine, promazine, promethazine, thiopental.**

- Store preferably at 15°–30° C (59°–86° F), unless otherwise directed by manufacturer. ▪ Examine parenteral preparation for particulate matter and discoloration. Do not use unless absolutely clear.

ADVERSE EFFECTS (≥1%) **CNS:** *Drowsiness,* headache, incoordination, dizziness, blurred vision, nervousness, restlessness, *insomnia (especially children).* **CV:** Hypotension, palpitation. **GI:** Dry mouth, nose, throat; anorexia, constipation or diarrhea. **Urogenital:** Urinary frequency, dysuria.

DIAGNOSTIC TEST INTERFERENCE ***Skin testing*** procedures should not be performed within 72 h after use of an antihistamine.

INTERACTIONS Drug: Alcohol and other CNS DEPRESSANTS enhance CNS depression, drowsiness; TRICYCLIC ANTIDEPRESSANTS compound anticholinergic effects.

PHARMACOKINETICS Absorption: Readily absorbed from GI tract. **Onset:** 15–30 min PO; immediate IV; 20–30 min IM. **Duration:** 3–6 h. **Distribution:** Distributed into breast milk. **Elimination:** Excreted in urine.

NURSING IMPLICATIONS

Assessment & Drug Effects
- Use side rails and supervise ambulation; drug produces high incidence of drowsiness.
- Note: Tolerance to CNS depressant effects usually occurs after a few days of drug therapy; some decrease in antiemetic action may result with prolonged use.
- Monitor for dizziness, nausea, and vomiting; these may indicate drug toxicity.

Patient & Family Education

- Do not drive or engage in other potentially hazardous activities until response to drug is known.
- Take 30 min before departure to prevent motion sickness; repeat before meals and upon retiring.
- Do not breast feed while taking this drug without consulting physician.

DIMERCAPROL

(dye-mer-kap'role)

BAL in Oil, British Anti-Lewisite

Classifications: CHELATING AGENT; ANTIDOTE

Pregnancy Category: D

AVAILABILITY 100 mg/mL injection

ACTIONS Dithiol compound that combines with ions of various heavy metals to form relatively stable, nontoxic, soluble complexes called chelates, which can be excreted; inhibition of enzymes by toxic metals is thus prevented. May also reactivate affected enzymes but is most effective when administered prior to enzyme damage.

THERAPEUTIC EFFECTS Neutralizes the effects of various heavy metals.

USES Acute poisoning by arsenic, gold, and mercury; as adjunct to edetate calcium disodium (EDTA) in treatment of lead encephalopathy.

UNLABELED USES Chromium dermatitis; ocular and dermatologic manifestations of arsenic poisoning, as adjunct to penicillamine to increase rate of copper excretion in Wilson's disease, and for poisoning with antimony, bismuth, chromium, copper, nickel, tungsten, zinc.

CONTRAINDICATIONS Hepatic insufficiency (with exception of postarsenical jaundice); severe renal insufficiency; poisoning due to cadmium, iron, selenium, or uranium; pregnancy (category D), lactation.

CAUTIOUS USE Hypertension, patients with G6PD deficiency.

ROUTE & DOSAGE

Arsenic or Gold Poisoning

Adult/Child: **IM** 2.5–3 mg/kg q4h for first 2 d, then q.i.d. on third day, then b.i.d. for 10 d

Mercury Poisoning

Adult/Child: **IM** 5 mg/kg initially, followed by 2.5 mg/kg 1–2 times/d for 10 d

Acute Lead Encephalopathy

Adult/Child: **IM** 4 mg/kg initially, then 3–4 mg/kg q4h with EDTA for 2–7 d depending on response

ADMINISTRATION

Intramuscular

- Initiate therapy ASAP (within 1–2 h) after ingestion of the poison because irreversible tissue damage occurs quickly, particularly in mercury poisoning.
- Give by deep IM injection only. Local pain, gluteal abscess, and skin sensitization possible. Rotate injection sites and observe daily.
- Determine if a local anesthetic may be given with the injection to decrease injection site pain.
- Handle with caution; contact of drug with skin may produce erythema, edema, dermatitis.
- Note: Presence of sediment in ampul reportedly does not indicate drug deterioration.

ADVERSE EFFECTS (≥1%) **CNS:** Headache, anxiety, muscle pain or weakness, restlessness, paresthesias, tremors, *convulsions,* shock.

D

CV: *Elevated BP,* tachycardia. **Special Senses:** Rhinorrhea; burning sensation, feeling of pain and constriction in throat. **GI:** Nausea, *vomiting;* burning sensation in lips and mouth, halitosis, salivation; abdominal pain, metabolic acidosis. **Urogenital:** Burning sensation in penis, renal damage. **Other:** Pains in chest or hands, pain and sterile abscess at injection site, sweating, reduction in polymorphonuclear leukocytes, dental pain.

DIAGNOSTIC TEST INTERFERENCE ***I^{131} thyroid uptake*** values may be decreased if test is done during or immediately following dimercaprol therapy.

INTERACTIONS Drug: Iron, cadmium, selenium, uranium form toxic complexes with dimercaprol.

PHARMACOKINETICS Peak: 30–60 min. **Distribution:** Distributed mainly in intracellular spaces, including brain; highest concentrations in liver and kidneys. **Elimination:** Completely excreted in urine and bile within 4 h. **Half-Life:** Short.

NURSING IMPLICATIONS

Assessment & Drug Effects

- Monitor vital signs. Elevations of systolic and diastolic BPs accompanied by tachycardia frequently occur within a few minutes following injection and may remain elevated up to 2 h.
- Note: Fever occurs in approximately 30% of children receiving treatment and may persist throughout therapy.
- Monitor I&O. Drug is potentially nephrotoxic. Report oliguria or change in I&O ratio to physician.
- Keep urine alkaline to reduce possibility of renal damage during elimination of dimercaprol chelate.
- Check urine daily for albumin, blood, casts, and pH. Blood and urinary levels of the metal serve as guides for dosage adjustments.
- Minor adverse reactions generally reach maximum 15–20 min after drug administration and subside in 30–90 min. Ephedrine or an antihistamine is sometimes administered to prevent symptoms.

Patient & Family Education

- Drink as much fluid as the physician will permit.
- Do not breast feed while taking this drug without consulting physician.

DIMETHYL SULFOXIDE

(dye-meth'il sul-fox'ide)

DMSO, Rimso-50

Classifications: SKIN AND MUCOUS MEMBRANE AGENT; ANTIINFLAMMATORY; LOCAL

Pregnancy Category: C

AVAILABILITY 50% solution

ACTIONS Mechanism of action not known.

THERAPEUTIC EFFECTS Reported effects include antiinflammatory effects, membrane penetration, collagen dissolution, vasodilation, muscle relaxation, diuresis, weak bacteriostatic and antifungal actions, initiation of histamine release at administration site, cholinesterase inhibition.

USES Symptomatic treatment of interstitial cystitis.

UNLABELED USES Topical treatment of a variety of musculoskeletal disorders, arthritis, scleroderma, tendinitis, breast and prostate malignancies, retinitis pigmentosa, herpesvirus infections, head and spinal cord injuries, shock, and as a carrier to en-

D

hance penetration and absorption of other drugs. Also used to protect living cells and tissues during cold storage (cryo-protection). Widely used as an industrial solvent and in veterinary medicine for treatment of musculoskeletal injuries.

CONTRAINDICATIONS Safe use during pregnancy (category C), lactation, or in children is not established.
CAUTIOUS USE Hepatic or renal dysfunction.

ROUTE & DOSAGE

Interstitial Cystitis

Adult: **Instillation** 50 mL of 50% solution instilled slowly into urinary bladder and retained for 15 min; may repeat q2wk until maximum relief obtained, then increase intervals between treatments

ADMINISTRATION

Instillation

- Apply analgesic lubricant such as lidocaine jelly to urethra to facilitate insertion of catheter.
- Instruct patient to retain instillation for 15 min and then expel it by spontaneous voiding.
- Note: Discomfort associated with instillation usually lessens with repeated administration. Physician may prescribe an oral analgesic or suppository containing belladonna and an opiate prior to instillation to reduce bladder spasm.
- Store at 15°–30° C (59°–86° F) unless otherwise directed. Protect from strong light. Avoid contact with plastics.

ADVERSE EFFECTS (≥1%) **Special Senses:** Transient disturbances in color vision, photophobia. **GI:** Nausea, diarrhea. Hypersensitivity: Local or generalized rash, erythema, pruritus, urticaria, swelling of face, dyspnea (<u>anaphylactoid reaction</u>). **Other:** Nasal congestion, headache, sedation, drowsiness. **Following instillation:** *Garlic-like odor on breath and skin; garlic-like taste;* discomfort during administration; transient cystitis. **Following topical application:** Vesicle formation.

INTERACTIONS Drug: Decreases effectiveness of **sulindac,** possibly causing severe peripheral neuropathy.

PHARMACOKINETICS Absorption: Readily absorbed systemically. **Peak:** 4–8 h. **Distribution:** Widely distributed in tissues and body fluids; penetrates blood–brain barrier; distributed into breast milk. **Metabolism:** Metabolized to dimethyl sulfide (garlic breath) and dimethyl sulfone. **Elimination:** Dimethyl sulfide excreted through lungs and skin; dimethyl sulfone may remain in serum >2 wk and is excreted in urine and feces.

NURSING IMPLICATIONS

Assessment & Drug Effects

- Lab tests: Do CBC and liver and renal function tests initially and at 6-mo intervals.
- Do complete eye evaluation including slit-lamp examination prior to and at regular intervals during therapy.

Patient & Family Education

- Note: Garlic-like taste may be experienced within minutes after drug instillation and may last for several hours. Garlic-like odor on breath and skin may last as long as 72 h.
- Do not use OTC topical medications without consulting physician.
- Do not breast feed while taking this drug without consulting physician.

DINOPROSTONE (PGE2, PROSTAGLANDIN E2) (Pr)

(dye-noe-prost′one)

Cervidil, Prostin E2, Prepidil

Classifications: HORMONES AND SYNTHETIC SUBSTITUTES; PROSTAGLANDIN; OXYTOCIC

Pregnancy Category: C

AVAILABILITY 20 mg suppository; **Prepidil** 0.5 mg gel; **Cervidil** 10 mg vaginal insert

ACTIONS Synthetically prepared member of the prostaglandin E_2 series that appears to act directly on myometrium and on gastrointestinal, bronchial, and vascular smooth muscle. Stimulation of gravid uterus in early weeks of gestation is more potent than that of oxytocin.

THERAPEUTIC EFFECTS Contractions are qualitatively similar to those that occur during term labor. Has high success rate when used as abortifacient before twentieth week and for stimulation of labor in cases of intrauterine fetal death.

USES To terminate pregnancy from twelfth week through second trimester as calculated from first day of last regular menstrual period; to evacuate uterine contents in management of missed abortion or intrauterine fetal death up to 28 wk gestational age; to manage benign hydatidiform mole; cervical ripening prior to labor induction.

CONTRAINDICATIONS Acute pelvic inflammatory disease, history of pelvic surgery, uterine fibroids, cervical stenosis, active cardiac, pulmonary, renal, or hepatic disease, pregnancy (category C).

CAUTIOUS USE History of hypertension, hypotension, asthma, epilepsy, anemia, diabetes mellitus; jaundice, history of hepatic, renal, or cardiovascular disease; cervicitis, acute vaginitis, infected endocervical lesion.

ROUTE & DOSAGE

Induction of Labor

Adult: **Endocervical** Place *Prepidil* 0.5 mg endocervically, may repeat q6h (max: of 1.5 mg); Place *Cervidil* insert 10-mg transversely in the posterior fornix of the vagina, remove on onset of active labor or 12 h after insertion

Evacuation of Uterus

Adult: **Intravaginal** Insert suppository high in vagina, repeat q2–5 h until abortion occurs or membranes rupture (max: total dose 240 mg)

ADMINISTRATION

Endocervical & Intravaginal

- Antiemetic and antidiarrheal medication may be prescribed to be given before dinoprostone to minimize GI side effects.
- Place vaginal insert in the vagina immediately after removal from the foil package. Do NOT use without retrieval system.
- Keep patient in supine position for 10 min after administration of suppository to prevent expulsion and enhance absorption.
- Store suppositories in freezer at temperature not exceeding –20° C (–4° F) unless otherwise specified.

ADVERSE EFFECTS (≥1%) **CNS:** Headache, tremor, tension. **CV:** Transient hypotension, flushing, cardiac arrhythmias. **GI:** *Nausea, vomiting, diarrhea*. **Urogenital:** Vaginal pain, endometritis, uterine rupture. **Respiratory:** Dyspnea, cough, hiccups. **Body as a Whole:** Chills, *fever,* dehydration, diaphoresis, rash.

D

INTERACTIONS Drug: OXYTOCICS used with extreme caution.

PHARMACOKINETICS Absorption: Slowly absorbed from vagina; Cervidil insert releases approximately 0.3 mg/h. **Onset:** 10 min. **Duration:** 2–3 h. **Distribution:** Widely distributed in body. **Metabolism:** Rapidly metabolized in lungs, kidneys, spleen, and other tissues. **Elimination:** Excreted mainly in urine; some excreted in feces.

NURSING IMPLICATIONS

Assessment & Drug Effects

- Observe patient carefully, after insertion of the drug. Rupture of the membranes is not a contraindication to drug, but be aware that profuse bleeding may result in expulsion of the suppository. Report wheezing, chest pain, dyspnea, and significant changes in BP and pulse to the physician.
- Monitor uterine contractions and observe for and report excessive vaginal bleeding and cramping pain. Keep pad count. Save all clots and tissues for physician inspection and laboratory analysis.
- Abortion usually occurs within 30 h. When used in conjunction with oxytocin, time may be shortened to 12–14 h.
- Monitor vital signs. Fever is a physiologic response of the hypothalamus to use of dinoprostone and occurs within 15–45 min after insertion of suppository. Temperature returns to normal within 2–6 h after discontinuation of medication.

Patient & Family Education

- Continue taking your temperature (late afternoon) for a few days after discharge. Contact physician with onset of fever, bleeding, abdominal cramps, abnormal or foul-smelling vaginal discharge.
- Avoid douches, tampons, intercourse, and tub baths for at least 2 wk. Clarify with physician.
- Note: Dinoprostone may exacerbate joint pain and limitation due to its effect on the inflammatory process.

DIPHENHYDRAMINE HYDROCHLORIDE (Pr)

(dye-fen-hye′dra-meen)

Allerdryl ♣, Banophen, Belix, Ben-Allergin, Bena-D, Benadryl, Benadryl Dye-Free, Benahist, Benoject, Benylin, Compoz, Diahist, Dihydrex, Diphen, Diphenacen-50, Fenylhist, Hyrexin, Insomnal, Nordryl, Nytol with DPH, Sleep-Eze 3, Sominex Formula 2, Tusstat, Twilite, Valdrene, Wehdryl

Classifications: ANTIHISTAMINE; H_1-RECEPTOR ANTAGONIST

Pregnancy Category: C

AVAILABILITY 25 mg, 50 mg capsules, tablets; 6.25 mg/5 mL, 12.5 mg/5 mL syrup; 50 mg/mL injection

ACTIONS H_1-receptor antagonist and antihistamine with significant anticholinergic activity. High incidence of drowsiness, but GI side effects are minor. Effects in parkinsonism and drug-induced extrapyramidal symptoms are apparently related to its ability to suppress central cholinergic activity and to prolong action of dopamine by inhibiting its reuptake and storage.

THERAPEUTIC EFFECTS Competes for H_1-receptor sites on effector cells, thus blocking histamine release.

USES Temporary symptomatic relief of various allergic conditions and to treat or prevent motion sickness, vertigo, and reactions to blood or plasma in susceptible patients. Also used in anaphylaxis as adjunct to epinephrine and other standard measures after acute symptoms have been controlled; in treatment of parkinsonism and drug-induced extrapyramidal reactions; as a non-narcotic cough suppressant; as a sedative-hypnotic; and for treatment of intractable insomnia.

CONTRAINDICATIONS Hypersensitivity to antihistamines of similar structure; lower respiratory tract symptoms (including acute asthma); narrow-angle glaucoma; prostatic hypertrophy, bladder neck obstruction; GI obstruction or stenosis; pregnancy (category C), lactation, premature neonates, and neonates; use as nighttime sleep aid in children <12 y.

CAUTIOUS USE History of asthma; convulsive disorders; increased IOP; hyperthyroidism; hypertension, cardiovascular disease; diabetes mellitus; older adults, infants, and young children.

ROUTE & DOSAGE

Allergy Symptoms, Antiparkinsonism, Motion Sickness, Nighttime Sedation

Adult: **PO** 25–50 mg t.i.d. or q.i.d. (max: 300 mg/d) **IV/IM** 10–50 mg q4–6h (max: 400 mg/d)
Child: **PO/IV/IM** *2–6 y,* 6.25 mg q4–6h (max: 300 mg/24 h); *6–12 y,* 12.5–25 mg q4–6h (max: 300 mg/24 h)

Nonproductive Cough

Adult: **PO** 25 mg q4–6h (max: 100 mg/d)
Child: **PO** *2–6 y,* 6.25 mg q4–6h (max: 25 mg/24 h); *6–12 y,* 12.5 mg q4–6h (max: 50 mg/24 h)

ADMINISTRATION

Oral

- Give with food or milk to lessen GI adverse effects.
- For motion sickness: Give the first dose 30 min before exposure to motion; give remaining doses before meals and at bedtime.

Intramuscular

- Give IM injection deep into large muscle mass; alternate injection sites. Avoid perivascular or SC injections because of its irritating effects.
- Note: Hypersensitivity reactions (including anaphylactic shock) are more likely to occur with parenteral than PO administration.

Intravenous

PREPARE: **Direct:** Give undiluted.
ADMINISTER: **Direct:** Give at a rate of 25 mg or a fraction thereof over 1 min.
INCOMPATIBILITIES **Y-site: Furosemide.**

- Store in tightly covered containers at 15°–30° C (59°–86° F) unless otherwise directed by manufacturer. Keep injection and elixir formulations in light-resistant containers.

ADVERSE EFFECTS (≥1%) **CNS:** *Drowsiness,* dizziness, headache, fatigue, disturbed coordination, tingling, heaviness and weakness of hands, tremors, euphoria, nervousness, restlessness, insomnia; confusion; (especially in children): excitement, fever. **CV:** Palpitation, *tachycardia,* mild hypotension or hypertension, <u>cardiovascular collapse</u>. **Special Senses:** Tinnitus, vertigo, dry nose, throat, nasal stuffiness; blurred vision, diplopia, photosensitivity, dry eyes. **GI:** *Dry mouth,* nausea, epigastric distress, anorexia, vomiting, constipation, or diarrhea. **Urogenital:** Urinary frequency or retention, dysuria. **Body as a Whole:** Hypersensitivity (skin rash, urticaria, photosensitivity, anaphylactic shock). **Respiratory:** Thickened bronchial secretions, wheezing, sensation of chest tightness.

DIAGNOSTIC TEST INTERFERENCE In common with other antihistamines, diphenhydramine should be discontinued 4 d prior to ***skin testing*** procedures for allergy because it may obscure otherwise positive reactions.

INTERACTIONS Drug: Alcohol and other CNS DEPRESSANTS, MAO INHIBITORS compound CNS depression.

PHARMACOKINETICS Absorption: Readily absorbed from GI tract but only 40%–60% reaches systemic circulation. **Onset:** 15–30 min. **Peak:** 1–4 h. **Duration:** 4–7 h. **Distribution:** Crosses placenta; distributed into breast milk. **Metabolism:** Metabolized in liver; some degradation in lung and kidney. **Elimination:** Mostly excreted in urine within 24 h.

NURSING IMPLICATIONS

Assessment & Drug Effects

- Monitor cardiovascular status especially with pre-existing cardiovascular disease.
- Monitor for adverse effects especially in children and the older adult.
- Supervise ambulation and use side-rails as necessary. Drowsiness is most prominent during the first few days of therapy and often disappears with continued therapy. Older adults are especially likely to manifest dizziness, sedation, and hypotension.

Patient & Family Education

- Do not use alcohol and other CNS depressants because of the possible additive CNS depressant effects with concurrent use.
- Do not drive or engage in other potentially hazardous activities until the response to drug is known.
- Increase fluid intake, if not contraindicated; drug has an atropine-like drying effect (thickens bronchial secretions) that may make expectoration difficult.
- Do not breast feed while taking this drug.

DIPHENOXYLATE HYDROCHLORIDE WITH ATROPINE SULFATE (Pr)

(dye-fen-ox′i-late)

Diphenatol, Lofene, Lomanate, Lomotil, Lonox, Lo-Trol, Low-Quel, Nor-Mil

Classifications: GASTROINTESTINAL AGENT; ANTIDIARRHEAL

Pregnancy Category: C

Controlled Substance: Schedule V

AVAILABILITY 2.5 mg tablets; 2.5 mg/5 mL liquid

ACTIONS Diphenoxylate is a synthetic narcotic structurally related to meperidine. Commercially available only with atropine sulfate, added in subtherapeutic doses to discourage deliberate overdosage.

THERAPEUTIC EFFECTS Has little or no analgesic activity or risk of dependence, except in high doses. Inhibits mucosal receptors responsible for peristaltic reflex, thereby reducing GI motility.

USES Adjunct in symptomatic management of diarrhea.

CONTRAINDICATIONS Hypersensitivity to diphenoxylate or atropine; severe dehydration or electrolyte imbalance, advanced liver disease, obstructive jaundice, diarrhea caused by pseudomembranous enterocolitis associated with use of broad-spectrum antibiotics; diarrhea associated with organisms that penetrate intestinal mucosa; diarrhea induced by poisons until toxic material is eliminated from GI tract; glaucoma; children <2 y of age. Safe use during pregnancy (category C) or lactation is not established.

CAUTIOUS USE Advanced hepatic disease, abnormal liver function tests; renal function impairment, patients receiving addicting drugs, addiction-prone individuals or those whose history suggests drug abuse; ulcerative colitis; young children (particularly patients with Down syndrome).

ROUTE & DOSAGE

Diarrhea

Adult: **PO** 1–2 tablets or 1–2 teaspoons full (5 mL) 3–4 times/d (each tablet or 5 mL contains 2.5 mg diphenoxylate HCl and 0.025 mg atropine sulfate)
Child: **PO** *2–12 y,* 0.3–0.4 mg/kg/d of liquid in divided doses

ADMINISTRATION

Oral

- Crush tablet if necessary and give with fluid of patient's choice.
- Reduce dosage as soon as initial control of symptoms occurs.
- Withhold drug in presence of severe dehydration or electrolyte imbalance until appropriate corrective therapy has been initiated.
- Note: Treatment is generally continued for 24–36 h before it is considered ineffective.
- Store in tightly covered, light-resistant container, preferably 15°–30° C (59°–86° F), unless otherwise directed by manufacturer.

ADVERSE EFFECTS (≥1%) **Body as a Whole:** Hypersensitivity (pruritus, angioneurotic edema, giant urticaria, rash). **CNS:** Headache, sedation, drowsiness, dizziness, lethargy, numbness of extremities; restlessness, euphoria, mental depression, weakness, general malaise. **CV:** Flushing, palpitation, tachycardia. **Special Senses:** Nystagmus, mydriasis, blurred vision, miosis (toxicity). **GI:** Nausea, vomiting, anorexia, dry mouth, abdominal discomfort or distension, paralytic ileus, toxic megacolon. **Other:** Urinary retention, swelling of gums.

INTERACTIONS Drug: MAO INHIBITORS may precipitate hypertensive crisis; **alcohol** and other CNS DEPRESSANTS may enhance CNS effects; also see **atropine.**

PHARMACOKINETICS Absorption: Readily absorbed from GI tract. **Onset:** 45–60 min. **Peak:** 2 h. **Duration:** 3–4 h. **Distribution:** Distributed into breast milk. **Metabolism:** Rapidly metabolized to active and inactive metabolites in liver. **Elimination:** Excreted slowly through bile into feces; small amount excreted in urine. **Half-Life:** 4.4 h.

NURSING IMPLICATIONS

Assessment & Drug Effects

- Assess GI function; report abdominal distention and signs of decreased peristalsis.
- Monitor for S&S of dehydration (see Appendix F). It is essential to monitor young children closely; dehydration occurs more rapidly in this age group and may influence variability of response to diphenoxylate and predispose patient to delayed toxic effects.

D

- Monitor frequency and consistency of stools.

Patient & Family Education

- Take medication only as directed by physician.
- Notify physician if diarrhea persists or if fever, bloody stools, palpitation, or other adverse reactions occur.
- Do not drive or engage in other potentially hazardous activities until response to drug is known.
- Do not breast feed while taking this drug without consulting physician.

DIPIVEFRIN HYDROCHLORIDE

(dye-pi've-frin)

Propine

Classifications: EYE PREPARATION; MYDRIATIC; AUTONOMIC NERVOUS SYSTEM AGENT; ADRENERGIC AGONIST (SYMPATHOMIMETIC)

Prototype: Pilocarpine

Pregnancy Category: B

AVAILABILITY 0.1% solution

See Appendix A-1.

DIPYRIDAMOLE

(dye-peer-id'a-mole)

Apo-Dipyridamole ♣, Persantine, Pyridamole, IV Persantine

Classifications: BLOOD FORMERS, COAGULATORS, AND ANTICOAGULANTS; ANTIPLATELET AGENT

Prototype: Ticlopidine

Pregnancy Category: C

AVAILABILITY 25 mg, 50 mg, 75 mg tablets; 10 mg injection

ACTIONS Nonnitrate coronary vasodilator with many properties similar to those of papaverine.

THERAPEUTIC EFFECTS Increases coronary blood flow by selectively dilating coronary arteries, thereby increasing myocardial oxygen supply. Exhibits mild inotropic action. Also has antiplatelet activity.

USES To prevent postoperative thromboembolic complications associated with prosthetic heart valves and as adjunct for thallium stress testing.

UNLABELED USES To reduce rate of reinfarction following MI; to prevent TIAs (transient ischemic attacks) and coronary bypass graft occlusion.

CONTRAINDICATIONS Pregnancy (category C), lactation.

CAUTIOUS USE Hypotension, anticoagulant therapy.

ROUTE & DOSAGE

Prevention of Thromboembolism in Cardiac Valve Replacement

Adult: **PO** 75–100 mg q.i.d.
Child: **PO** 1–2 mg t.i.d.

Thromboembolic Disorders

Adult: **PO** 150–400 mg/d in divided doses

Thallium Stress Test

Adult: **IV** 0.142 mg/kg/min for 4 min

ADMINISTRATION

Oral

- Give on an empty stomach at least 1 h before or 2 h after meals, with a full glass of water. Physician may prescribe with food if gastric distress persists.

Intravenous

PREPARE: **Direct:** Dilute to at least a 1:2 ratio with 0.45%

NaCl, NS, or D5W to yield a final volume of 20–50 mL.

ADMINISTER: **Direct:** Give a single dose over 4 min (0.142 mg kg/min).

- Store in tightly closed container at 15°–30° C (59°–86° F) unless otherwise directed. Protect injection from direct light.

ADVERSE EFFECTS (≥1%) Usually dose related, minimal, and transient. **CNS:** Headache, dizziness, faintness, syncope, weakness. **CV:** Peripheral vasodilation, flushing. **GI:** Nausea, vomiting, diarrhea, abdominal distress. **Skin:** Skin rash, pruritus.

PHARMACOKINETICS Absorption: Readily absorbed from GI tract. **Peak:** 45–150 min. **Distribution:** Small amount crosses placenta. **Metabolism:** Metabolized in liver. **Elimination:** Mainly excreted in feces. **Half-Life:** 10–12 h.

NURSING IMPLICATIONS

Assessment & Drug Effects

- Monitor therapeutic effectiveness. Clinical response may not be evident before second or third month of continuous therapy. Effects include reduced frequency or elimination of anginal episodes, improved exercise tolerance, reduced requirement for nitrates.

Patient & Family Education

- Notify physician of any adverse effects.
- Make all position changes slowly and in stages, especially from recumbent to upright posture, if postural hypotension or dizziness is a problem.
- Do not breast feed while taking this drug without consulting physician.

DIRITHROMYCIN

(dir-ith-roe-my'sin)

Dynabac

Classifications: ANTIINFECTIVE; MACROLIDE ANTIBIOTIC

Prototype: Erythromycin

Pregnancy Category: C

AVAILABILITY 250 mg enteric tablets

ACTIONS Dirithromycin is an analog of erythromycin. It binds reversibly to the 235 component of the 50-S ribosomal subunit of the bacteria, thus inhibiting RNA-dependent protein synthesis in bacterial cells.

THERAPEUTIC EFFECTS It is more active against gram-positive organisms than gram-negative organisms, including *Legionella, Helicobacter pylori,* and *Chlamydia trachomatis.* It is not effective against *Pseudomonas* or methicillin-resistant *Staphylococcus aureus (MRSA), S. epidermidis, Listeria monocytogenes, Legionella pneumophila, Haemophilus influenzae,* or *Neisseria gonorrhoeae.*

USES Acute bacterial exacerbations of chronic bronchitis, community-acquired pneumonia, pharyngitis/tonsillitis, uncomplicated skin/skin structure infections due to susceptible bacteria.

CONTRAINDICATIONS Known hypersensitivity to dirithromycin, erythromycin, or any other macrolide antibiotic; known or suspected bacteremias.

CAUTIOUS USE Concurrent administration of terfenadine, hepatic impairment, pregnancy (category C). Safety and effectiveness in lactation or children <2 y are not established.

D

ROUTE & DOSAGE

Bacterial Infections
Adult/Child: **PO** 500 mg once/d

ADMINISTRATION

Oral
- Give with food or within 1 h of eating.
- Do not cut, crush, or chew tablets.
- Store at 15°–30° C (59°–86° F).

ADVERSE EFFECTS (≥1%) **CNS:** Headache, dizziness, asthenia. **CV:** Chest pain. **GI:** *Abdominal pain, nausea, diarrhea, vomiting, dyspepsia, flatulence;* elevated liver function tests (ALT, AST, GGT). **Skin:** Rash, urticaria. **Respiratory:** Dyspnea, asthma-like symptoms, rhinitis, pharyngitis, increased coughing.

INTERACTIONS Drug: May increase **theophylline** levels. May increase risk of arrhythmias with **terfenadine.**

PHARMACOKINETICS Absorption: Readily absorbed from GI tract; 60%–90% hydrolyzed to active metabolite, erythromycylamine, within 35 min. **Peak:** 1.5 h. **Distribution:** High tissue concentrations of active metabolite; slowly released back into the circulation. **Metabolism:** Rapidly converted to active metabolite, erythromycylamine, in absorption and distribution phases. **Elimination:** 81%–97% excreted in bile and feces. **Half-Life:** 20–50 h.

NURSING IMPLICATIONS

Assessment & Drug Effects
- Take history of previous hypersensitivity to other macrolides (e.g., erythromycin) prior to initiation of therapy.
- Withhold drug and notify physician if signs and symptoms of hypersensitivity occur (see Appendix F).
- Monitor liver and renal function in patients with mild liver or renal impairment.
- Monitor for S&S of superinfection (see Appendix F).
- Monitor theophylline levels if given concurrently with dirithromycin.
- Note: Dirithromycin may increase the blood level of theophylline, necessitating theophylline dosage adjustment.

Patient & Family Education
- Take tablets whole and within 1 h of meals.
- Monitor for and report S&S of superinfection or pseudomembranous enterocolitis (see Appendix F).
- Report any worsening of signs and symptoms of infection.
- Do not breast feed while taking this drug without consulting physician.

DISOPYRAMIDE PHOSPHATE

(dye-soe-peer'a-mide)

Napamide, Norpace, Norpace CR, Rythmodan ♣, Rythmodan-LA ♣

Classifications: CARDIOVASCULAR AGENT; ANTIARRHYTHMIC, CLASS IA
Prototype: Procainamide
Pregnancy Category: C

AVAILABILITY 100 mg, 150 mg regular and sustained release capsules

ACTIONS Class IA antiarrhythmic agent with pharmacologic actions similar to those of quinidine and procainamide, although chemically unrelated. Disopyramide shortens sinus node recovery time and increases atrial and ventricular effective refractory period but has minimal effect on refractoriness and conduction time of AV node or on conduction time of His-Purkinje system or QRS duration.

THERAPEUTIC EFFECTS Acts as myocardial depressant by reducing rate of spontaneous diastolic depolarization in pacemaker cells, thereby suppressing ectopic focal activity.

USES To suppress and prevent recurrence of premature ventricular contractions (unifocal, multifocal, paired) and ventricular tachycardia not severe enough to require cardioversion.

UNLABELED USES In combination with other antiarrhythmic drugs to treat or prevent serious refractory arrhythmias. To convert atrial fibrillation, atrial flutter, and paroxysmal atrial tachycardia to normal sinus rhythm.

CONTRAINDICATIONS Cardiogenic shock, preexisting 2nd or 3rd degree AV block (if no pacemaker is present); uncompensated or inadequately compensated CHF, hypotension (unless secondary to cardiac arrhythmia), hypokalemia. Safe use during pregnancy (category C), lactation, or in children is not established.

CAUTIOUS USE Sick sinus syndrome (bradycardia-tachycardia); Wolff-Parkinson-White (WPW) syndrome or bundle branch block, myocarditis or other cardiomyopathy, underlying cardiac conduction abnormalities; hepatic or renal impairment; urinary tract disease (especially prostatic hypertrophy); myasthenia gravis; narrow-angle glaucoma, family history of glaucoma.

ROUTE & DOSAGE

Arrhythmias

Adult: **PO** *<50 kg,* 100 mg q6h or 200 mg sustained release q12h; *>50 kg,* 100–200 mg q6h or 300 mg sustained release capsule q12h

Child: **PO** *<1 y,* 10–30 mg/kg/d in divided doses q6h; *1–4 y,* 10–20 mg/kg/d in divided doses q6h; *4–12 y,* 10–15 mg/kg/d in divided doses q6h; *12–18 y,* 6–15 mg/kg/d in divided doses q6h

ADMINISTRATION

Oral

- Start drug 6–12 h after last quinidine dose and 3–6 h after last procainamide dose for patients who have been receiving either quinidine or procainamide.
- Give sustained release capsules whole.
- Do not use sustained release capsules in loading doses when rapid control is required or in patients with creatinine clearance of ≤40 mL/min.
- Start sustained release capsules 6 h after last dose of conventional capsule if change in drug form is made.
- Store at 15°–30° C (59°–86° F) unless otherwise directed.

ADVERSE EFFECTS (≥1%) **Body as a Whole:** Hypersensitivity (pruritus, urticaria, rash, photosensitivity, laryngospasm). **CNS:** Dizziness, headache, fatigue, muscle weakness, convulsions, paresthesias, nervousness, acute psychosis, peripheral neuropathy. **CV:** *Hypotension,* chest pain, edema, dyspnea, syncope, bradycardia, tachycardia; worsening of CHF or cardiac arrhythmia; cardiogenic shock, heart block; edema with weight gain. **Special Senses:** *Blurred vision,* dry eyes, increased IOP, precipitation of acute angle-closure glaucoma. **GI:** *Dry mouth, constipation,* epigastric or abdominal pain, cholestatic jaundice. **Urogenital:** *Hesitancy* and *retention,* urinary frequency, urgency, renal insufficiency. **Other:** Dry nose and throat, drying of bronchial secretions, initiation of uterine contractions (pregnant patient); muscle aches, precipitation of myasthenia gravis, agranulocytosis (rare), thrombocytopenia.

INTERACTIONS Drug: ANTICHOLINERGIC DRUGS (e.g., TRICYCLIC ANTIDEPRESSANTS, ANTIHISTAMINES) compound anticholinergic effects; other ANTIARRHYTHMICS compound toxicities; **phenytoin, rifampin** may increase disopyramide metabolism and decrease levels; may increase **warfarin**-induced hypoprothrombinemia.

PHARMACOKINETICS Absorption: Readily absorbed from GI tract; 60%–83% reaches systemic circulation. **Onset:** 30 min–3.5 h. **Peak:** 1–2 h. **Duration:** 1.5–8.5 h. **Distribution:** Distributed in extracellular fluid; crosses placenta; distributed into breast milk. **Metabolism:** Metabolized in liver. **Elimination:** 80% excreted in urine, 10% in feces. **Half-Life:** 4–10 h.

NURSING IMPLICATIONS

Assessment & Drug Effects

- Check apical pulse before administering drug. Withhold drug and notify physician if pulse rate is slower than 60 bpm, faster than 120 bpm, or if there is any unusual change in rate, rhythm, or quality.
- Monitor ECG closely. The following signs are indications for drug withdrawal: Prolongation of QT interval and worsening of arrhythmia interval, QRS widening (>25%).
- Monitor for rapid weight gain or other signs of fluid retention.
- Lab tests: Baseline and periodic hepatic and renal function tests, blood glucose, and serum potassium. Correct hypokalemia or other imbalances before initiation of therapy.
- Monitor BP closely in all patients during periods of dosage adjustment and in those receiving high dosages.
- Monitor I&O, particularly in older adults and patients with impaired renal function or prostatic hypertrophy. Persistent urinary hesitancy or retention may necessitate lower dosage or discontinuation of drug.
- Report S&S of hyperkalemia (see Appendix F); it enhances drug's toxic effects.
- Measure IOP before treatment begins in patients with a family history of glaucoma.
- Monitor for S&S of CHF.
- Discontinue promptly if S&S of agranulocytosis, peripheral neuritis, or jaundice appear (see Appendix F).

Patient & Family Education

- Take drug precisely as prescribed to maintain regularity of heartbeat. Do not skip or stop medication or change dose without consulting physician.
- Weigh daily under standard conditions and check ankles for edema. Report to physician a weekly weight gain of ≥1–2 kg (2–4 lb).
- Make position changes slowly, particularly when getting up from lying down because of the possibility of hypotension; dangle legs for a few minutes before walking, and do not stand still for prolonged periods. If you feel

light-headed, lie down or sit down.
- Do not take OTC medications unless approved by physician.
- Avoid exposure to sunlight or ultraviolet light; drug may cause photosensitivity.
- Do not drive or engage in other potentially hazardous activities until response to drug is known.
- Do not drink alcoholic beverages while taking disopyramide.
- Do not breast feed while taking this drug without consulting physician.

DISULFIRAM

(dye-sul′fi-ram)

Antabuse, Cronetal, Ro-sulfiram

Classifications: ENZYME INHIBITOR; ANTIALCOHOL AGENT

Pregnancy Category: X

AVAILABILITY 250 mg, 500 mg tablets

ACTIONS Acts as a deterrent to alcohol ingestion by inhibiting the enzyme acetaldehyde dehydrogenase, which normally metabolizes alcohol in the body.

THERAPEUTIC EFFECTS When a small amount of alcohol is ingested, a complex of highly unpleasant symptoms known as the disulfiram reaction occurs, which serves as a deterrent to further drinking.

USES Adjunct in treatment of the patient with chronic alcoholism who sincerely wants to maintain sobriety.

CONTRAINDICATIONS Severe myocardial disease; psychoses; pregnancy (category X), lactation; patients who have recently ingested alcohol, metronidazole, paraldehyde; multiple drug dependence.

CAUTIOUS USE Diabetes mellitus; epilepsy; hypothyroidism; coronary artery disease, cerebral damage; chronic and acute nephritis; hepatic cirrhosis or insufficiency; abnormal EEG.

ROUTE & DOSAGE

Alcoholism

Adult: **PO** 500 mg/d for 1–2 wk, then 125–500 mg/d (max: 500 mg/d)

ADMINISTRATION

Oral
- Give daily dose in the morning when the resolve not to drink may be strongest.
- Give at bedtime to minimize sedative effect of the drug. Decrease in dose may also reduce sedative effect.
- Make sure patient has abstained from alcohol and alcohol-containing preparations for at least 12 h and preferably 48 h before initiating therapy.
- Determine compliance periodically. Maintenance therapy may be required for months or even years.
- Store at 15°–30° C (59°–86° F) unless otherwise directed. Protect tablets from light.

ADVERSE EFFECTS (≥1%) **Reaction with alcohol ingestion:** Flushing of face, chest, arms, pulsating headache, nausea, violent vomiting, thirst, sweating, marked uneasiness, confusion, weakness, vertigo, blurred vision, pruritic skin rash, hyperventilation, abnormal gait, slurred speech, disorientation, confusion, personality changes, bizarre behavior, psychoses, tachycardia, palpitation, chest pain, hypotension to shock level arrhythmias, acute congestive fail-

D

ure. **Severe reactions:** Marked respiratory depression, unconsciousness, convulsions, sudden death. **Body as a Whole:** Hypersensitivity (allergic or acneiform dermatitis; urticaria, fixed-drug eruption). **CNS:** Drowsiness, fatigue, restlessness, headache, tremor, psychoses (usually with high doses), polyneuritis, peripheral neuropathy, optic neuritis. **GI:** Mild GI disturbances, garlic-like or metallic taste, hepatotoxicity, hypersensitivity hepatitis.

DIAGNOSTIC TEST INTERFERENCE Disulfiram can reduce ***uptake of*** I^{131}; or decreases ***PBI*** test results (rare).

INTERACTIONS Drug: Alcohol (including in liquid OTC drugs, **IV nitroglycerin, IV cotrimoxazole**), **metronidazole, paraldehyde** will produce disulfiram reaction; **isoniazid** can produce neurological symptoms; may increase blood levels and toxicity of **warfarin, paraldehyde,** BARBITURATES, **phenytoin.**

PHARMACOKINETICS Absorption: Readily absorbed from GI tract. **Onset:** Up to 12 h. **Duration:** Up to 2 wk. **Distribution:** Initially deposited in fat. **Metabolism:** Metabolized slowly in liver. **Elimination:** 5%–20% excreted in feces; 20% remains in body for 1–2 wk; some may be excreted in breath as carbon disulfide.

NURSING IMPLICATIONS

Assessment & Drug Effects

- Do a complete physical examination and careful drug history prior to initiation of therapy.
- Lab tests: Baseline and follow-up transaminase studies every 10–14 d to detect hepatic dysfunction, and perform CBC and sequential multiple analysis (SMA-12) tests every 6 mo.
- Note: Disulfiram reaction occurs within 5–10 min following ingestion of alcohol and may last 30 min to several hours. Intensity of reaction varies with each individual, but is generally proportional to the amount of alcohol ingested.
- Treat patient with severe disulfiram reaction as though in shock. Monitor potassium levels, especially if patient has diabetes mellitus.

Patient & Family Education

- Understand fully the possible dangers if alcohol is ingested during disulfiram treatment before consenting to therapy.
- Report promptly to physician the onset of nausea with right upper quadrant pain or discomfort, itching, jaundiced sclerae or skin, dark urine, clay-colored stools. Withhold drug pending liver function tests.
- Note: Ingestion of even small amounts of alcohol or use of external applications that contain alcohol may be sufficient to produce a reaction. Read all labels and avoid use of anything containing alcohol.
- Prolonged administration of disulfiram does not produce tolerance; the longer the therapy, the higher the sensitivity to alcohol.
- Alcohol sensitivity may last as long as 2 wk after disulfiram has been discontinued.
- Note: Adverse effects of drug are often experienced during first 2 wk of therapy; symptoms usually disappear with continued therapy or with dose reduction.
- Carry an identification card stating you are on disulfiram therapy and describing the symptoms of disulfiram reaction. Also provide the name of the physician or institution to contact in an emergency.

- Do not drive or engage in other potentially hazardous activities until response to drug is known.
- Do not breast feed while taking this drug.

DOBUTAMINE HYDROCHLORIDE

(doe-byoo'ta-meen)

Dobutrex

Classifications: AUTONOMIC NERVOUS SYSTEM AGENT; BETA-ADRENERGIC AGONIST; CATECHOLAMINE

Prototype: Isoproterenol

Pregnancy Category: C

AVAILABILITY 12.5 mg/mL injection

ACTIONS Produces inotropic effect by acting on beta receptors and primarily on myocardial alpha-adrenergic receptors. Increases cardiac output and decreases pulmonary wedge pressure and total systemic vascular resistance with comparatively little or no effect on BP. Also increases conduction through AV node. Has lower potential for precipitating arrhythmias than dopamine.

THERAPEUTIC EFFECTS In CHF or cardiogenic shock, increase in cardiac output enhances renal perfusion and increases renal output and renal sodium excretion.

USES Inotropic support in short-term treatment of adults with cardiac decompensation due to depressed myocardial contractility (cardiogenic shock) resulting from either organic heart disease or from cardiac surgery.

UNLABELED USES To augment cardiovascular function in children undergoing cardiac catheterization, stress thallium testing.

CONTRAINDICATIONS History of hypersensitivity to other sympathomimetic amines, ventricular tachycardia, idiopathic hypertrophic subaortic stenosis. Safe use during pregnancy (category C), lactation, children, or following acute MI is not established.

CAUTIOUS USE Preexisting hypertension, atrial fibrillation.

ROUTE & DOSAGE

Cardiac Decompensation

Adult/Child: **IV** 2.5–10 mcg/kg/min (max: 40 mcg/kg/min), has been given for up to 72 h without decrease in effectiveness

ADMINISTRATION

Intravenous

PREPARE: **Continuous:** Reconstitute by adding 10 mL sterile water for injection or D5W to 250-mg vial; if not completely dissolved, add an additional 10 mL of diluent. ▪ Further dilute to a volume of at least 50 mL with D5W, NS, LR, D5/LR, or sodium lactate injection. ▪ Use IV solutions within 24 h.

ADMINISTER: **Continuous:** Rate of infusion is determined by body weight and controlled by an infusion pump (preferred) or a microdrip IV infusion set.
▪ IV infusion rate and duration of therapy are determined by heart rate, blood pressure, ectopic activity, urine output, and whenever possible, by measurements of cardiac output and central venous or pulmonary wedge pressures.

INCOMPATIBILITIES **Solution/additive: Sodium bicarbonate, aminophylline, bretylium, bumetanide, calcium chloride, calcium gluconate, diazepam, doxapram, digoxin, epinephrine, furosemide, heparin,**

insulin, magnesium sulfate, phenytoin, potassium chloride, potassium phosphate. Y-site: Acyclovir, aminophylline, sodium bicarbonate.

- Refrigerate reconstituted solution at 2°–15° C (36°–59° F) for 48 h or store for 6 h at room temperature.

ADVERSE EFFECTS (≥1%) **All:** Generally dose related. **CNS:** Headache, tremors, paresthesias, mild leg cramps, nervousness, fatigue (with overdosage). **CV:** *Increased heart rate and BP,* premature ventricular beats, palpitation, *anginal pain.* **GI:** Nausea, vomiting. **Other:** Nonspecific chest pain, shortness of breath.

INTERACTIONS Drug: GENERAL ANESTHETICS (especially **cyclopropane** and **halothane**) may sensitize myocardium to effects of CATECHOLAMINES such as dobutamine and lead to serious arrhythmias—used with extreme caution; BETA-ADRENERGIC BLOCKING AGENTS, e.g., **metoprolol, propranolol,** may make dobutamine ineffective in increasing cardiac output, but total peripheral resistance may increase—concomitant use generally avoided; MAO INHIBITORS, TRICYCLIC ANTIDEPRESSANTS potentiate pressor effects—use with extreme caution.

PHARMACOKINETICS Onset: 2–10 min. **Peak:** 10–20 min. **Metabolism:** Metabolized in liver and other tissues by COMT. **Elimination:** Excreted in urine. **Half-Life:** 2 min.

NURSING IMPLICATIONS

Assessment & Drug Effects

- Correct hypovolemia by administration of appropriate volume expanders prior to initiation of therapy.
- Monitor therapeutic effectiveness. At any given dosage level, drug takes 10–20 min to produce peak effects.
- Monitor ECG and BP continuously during administration.
- Note: Marked increases in blood pressure (systolic pressure is the most likely to be affected) and heart rate, or the appearance of arrhythmias or other adverse cardiac effects are usually reversed promptly by reduction in dosage.
- Observe patients with preexisting hypertension closely for exaggerated pressor response.
- Note: Tolerance has been observed with continuous or prolonged infusions; adverse reactions are no different than those seen with shorter infusions.
- Monitor I&O ratio and pattern. Urine output and sodium excretion generally increase because of improved cardiac output and renal perfusion.

Patient & Family Education

- Report anginal pain to physician promptly.
- Do not breast feed while taking this drug without consulting physician.

DOCETAXEL

(doc-e-tax′el)

Taxotere

Classifications: ANTINEOPLASTIC AGENT; TAXANE AGENT

Prototype: Paclitaxel

Pregnancy Category: D

AVAILABILITY 20 mg, 80 mg injection

ACTIONS Docetaxel is a semisynthetic analog of paclitaxel. Potential advantages over paclitaxel are greater antitumor activity and lower toxicity potential. Docetaxel, like paclitaxel, binds to the microtubule network essential for interphase and mitosis of the cell cycle.

THERAPEUTIC EFFECTS Docetaxel stabilizes the microtubules involved in cell division and prevents their normal functioning, which results in inhibiting mitosis in cells.

USES Metastatic breast cancer, metastatic prostate cancer.

CONTRAINDICATIONS Hypersensitivity to docetaxel or other drugs formulated with polysorbate 80, paclitaxel, neutrophil count <1500 cells/mm^3, biliary tract disease, hepatic disease, jaundice, neutropenia, intramuscular injections, thrombocytopenia, lactation, pregnancy (category D), acute infection.

CAUTIOUS USE Bone marrow suppression, bone marrow transplant patients, CHF, ascites, peripheral edema, pleural effusion, radiation therapy, pulmonary disorders, acute bronchospasm; cardiac tamponade, dental disease, dental work, herpes infection, hypotension, infection. Safety and effectiveness in children not established.

ROUTE & DOSAGE

Breast Cancer

Adult: **IV** 60–100 mg/m^2 once every 3 wk (premedicate patients with dexamethasone 8 mg b.i.d. × 5 d, starting 1 d prior to docetaxel)

Prostate Cancer

Adult: **IV** 75 mg/m^2 over 1 h every 21 d plus prednisone (5 mg PO twice daily) for 10 cycles (premedicate patients with dexamethasone 8 mg q12h, 3h, and 1h prior to starting docetaxel infusion)

ADMINISTRATION

Note: If drug contacts skin during preparation, wash immediately with soap and water.

Intravenous

PREPARE: **IV Infusion:** Bring vials to room temperature for 5 min; add provided diluent, gently rotate for 15 s; let stand until surface foam dissipates. ▪ Inject required amount of diluted solution into a 250-mL, or larger, bag of NS or D5W; the final concentration should not exceed 0.9 mg/mL. ▪ Use glass or polypropylene bottles or polypropylene or polyolefin plastic bags and administer through polyethylene-lined administration sets. Do not use PVC administration sets or containers. ▪ Mix completely by manual rotation. ▪ Use within 4 h (including the 1 h infusion time).

ADMINISTER: **IV Infusion:** Give at a constant rate over 1 h. Administer ONLY after premedication with corticosteroids to prevent hypersensitivity.

▪ Reduce dose by 25% following severe neutropenia (<500 cells/mm^3) for 7 d or longer for febrile neutropenia, severe cutaneous reactions, or severe peripheral neuropathy.

▪ Refrigerate vials at 2°–8° C (36°–46° F). Protect from light. Do not store in PVC bags. Store diluted solutions in refrigerator or at room temperature for 8 h.

ADVERSE EFFECTS (≥1%) **CNS:** Paresthesia, pain, burning sensation, weakness, confusion. **CV:** Hypotension, *fluid retention (peripheral edema, weight gain),* pleural effusion. **GI:** *Nausea, vomiting, diarrhea, stomatitis,* abdominal pain; increased liver function tests (AST or

D

ALT). **Hematologic:** *Neutropenia, leukopenia, thrombocytopenia, anemia*, febrile neutropenia. **Skin:** Rash, localized eruptions, desquamation, *alopecia*, nail changes (hyper/hypopigmentation, onycholysis). **Body as a Whole:** *Hypersensitivity reactions*, infusion site reactions (hyperpigmentation, inflammation, redness, dryness, phlebitis, extravasation).

INTERACTIONS Drug: Possibility of interacting with other drugs metabolized by the cytochrome P4503A system **(cyclosporine, erythromycin, ketoconazole, terfenadine, troleandomycin).**

PHARMACOKINETICS Distribution: 97% protein bound. **Metabolism:** Metabolized in liver by cytochrome P4503A isoenzymes. **Elimination:** 80% eliminated in feces, 20% renally excreted. **Half-Life:** 11.1 h.

NURSING IMPLICATIONS

Assessment & Drug Effects

- Lab tests: Monitor bilirubin, AST or ALT, and alkaline phosphatase prior to each drug cycle. Generally, do not give to patients with elevations of bilirubin or with significant elevations of transaminases concurrent with elevations of alkaline phosphatase. Monitor frequently CBCs with differential. Withhold drug if platelets <100,000 or neutrophils <1500 cells/mm^3.
- Monitor for S&S of hypersensitivity (see Appendix F), which may develop within a few minutes of initiation of infusion. It is usually not necessary to discontinue infusion for minor reactions (i.e., flushing or local skin reaction).
- Assess throughout therapy and report cardiovascular dysfunction, respiratory distress; fluid retention; development of neurosensory symptoms; severe, cutaneous eruptions on feet, hands, arms, face, or thorax; and S&S of infection.

Patient & Family Education

- Learn common adverse effects and measures to control or minimize them when possible. Report immediately any distressing adverse effects.
- Note: It is extremely important to comply with corticosteroid therapy and monitoring of lab values.
- Avoid pregnancy during therapy.
- Do not breast feed while taking this drug.

DOCOSANOL

(doc′os-a-nol)
Abreva
Classifications: ANTIINFECTIVE; ANTIVIRAL-LIKE
Pregnancy Category: C

AVAILABILITY 10% cream

ACTIONS Precise mechanism of action is not fully understood; however, current evidence suggests that 1-docosanol inhibits viral replication by interfering with the early intracellular events surrounding viral entry into target cells. It is possible that interaction between the highly lipophilic compound and components of target cell membranes renders such target cells less susceptible to viral fusion or entry.

THERAPEUTIC EFFECTS Believed to exert its anti-viral effect by inhibiting fusion of the HSV (herpes virus) envelope with the human cell plasma membrane, therefore making it difficult for the virus to enter the cell and replicate. Thus docosanol-treated cells resist infection by the herpes virus.

USES Treatment of herpes simplex infections of the face and lips (i.e., cold sores).

CONTRAINDICATIONS Hypersensitivity to docosanol or any of the inactive ingredients in the ointment.
CAUTIOUS USE Safety and efficacy in children are not established.

ROUTE & DOSAGE

Herpes Simplex Infections
Adult: **Topical** Apply to lesions 5 times/day for up to 10 d, starting at onset of symptoms

ADMINISTRATION

Topical
- Apply cream only to the affected areas using a gloved finger. Rub in gently but completely.
- Do not apply near or in the eyes.
- Avoid application to the mucous membranes inside of the mouth.
- Store at 20°–25° C (68°–77° F).

ADVERSE EFFECTS (≥1%) **CNS:** Headache. **Skin:** Skin irritation, burning.

INTERACTIONS Drug: No clinically significant interactions established.

PHARMACOKINETICS Not studied.

NURSING IMPLICATIONS
Assessment & Drug Effects
- Monitor severity and extent of infection.
- Notify physician if improvement is not seen within 10 days of initiating treatment

Patient & Family Education
- Wash hands before and after applying cream.
- Do not share this cream with any other individual as this may spread the herpes virus.
- Report to physician if your condition worsens or does not improve within 10 days of beginning treatment.
- Report to the emergency room or contact a poison control center immediately if a significant amount of cream is swallowed.

DOCUSATE CALCIUM (DIOCTYL CALCIUM SULFOSUCCINATE) (Pr)

(dok'yoo-sate)
DCS, PMS-Docusate Calcium, Pro-Cal-Sof, Surfak

DOCUSATE POTASSIUM

Dialose, Diocto-K, Kasof

DOCUSATE SODIUM

Colace, Colace Enema, Dio-Sul, Disonate, DGSS, D-S-S, Duosol, Lax-gel, Laxinate 100, Modane Soft, Pro-Sof, Regulax ♣, Regutol, Therevac-Plus, Therevac-SB
Classifications: GASTROINTESTINAL AGENT; STOOL SOFTENER
Pregnancy Category: C

AVAILABILITY Docusate Calcium 50 mg, 240 mg capsules **Docusate Potassium** 100 mg tablets; 240 mg capsules **Docusate Sodium** 100 mg tablets; 50 mg, 100 mg, 240 mg, 250 mg capsules; 50 mg/15 mL 60 mg/15 mL, 150 mg/15 mL syrup

ACTIONS Anionic surface-active agent with emulsifying and wetting properties.
THERAPEUTIC EFFECTS Detergent action lowers surface tension, permitting water and fats to penetrate and soften stools for easier passage.

USES Prophylactically in patients who should avoid straining during defecation and for treatment of constipation associated with hard, dry stools (e.g., following anorectal surgery, MI).

CONTRAINDICATIONS Atonic constipation, nausea, vomiting, abdominal pain, fecal impaction, structural anomalies of colon and rectum, intestinal obstruction or perforation; use of docusate sodium in patients on sodium restriction; use of docusate potassium in patients with renal dysfunction; concomitant use of mineral oil; pregnancy (category C).
CAUTIOUS USE History of CHF, edema, diabetes melitus.

ROUTE & DOSAGE

Stool Softener

Adult: **PO** 50–500 mg/d **PR** 50–100 mg added to enema fluid
Child: **PO** *<3 y,* 10–40 mg/d; *3–6 y,* 20–60 mg/d; *6–12 y,* 40–120 mg/d

ADMINISTRATION

Oral

- Give with a full glass of water if allowed.
- Store syrup formulations in tight, light-resistant containers at 15°–30° C (59°–86° F) unless directed otherwise.

Rectal

- Microenema: Insert full length of nozzle (half length for children) into the rectum. Squeeze entire contents of tube and remove completely before releasing grip on tube.
- Store in tightly covered containers.

ADVERSE EFFECTS (≥1%) **GI:** Occasional mild abdominal cramps, *diarrhea,* nausea, bitter taste. **Other:** Throat irritation (liquid preparation), rash.

INTERACTIONS Drug: Docusate will increase systemic absorption of **mineral oil.**

PHARMACOKINETICS Not studied.

NURSING IMPLICATIONS

Assessment & Drug Effects

- Withhold drug if diarrhea develops and notify physician.
- Therapeutic effectiveness: Usually apparent 1–3 d after first dose.

Patient & Family Education

- Take sufficient liquid with each dose and increase fluid intake during the day, if allowed. Oral liquid (NOT syrup) may be administered in milk, fruit juice, or infant formula to mask bitter taste.
- Do not take concomitantly with mineral oil.
- Do not take for prolonged periods in lieu of proper dietary management or treatment of underlying causes of constipation.

DOFETILIDE

(do-fe-ti′lyde)
Tikosyn
Classifications: CARDIOVASCULAR AGENT; ANTIARRHYTHMIC, CLASS III; POTASSIUM CHANNEL BLOCKER
Prototype: Amiodarone HCl
Pregnancy Category: C

AVAILABILITY 125 mcg, 250 mcg, 500 mcg capsules

ACTIONS Class III antiarrhythmic agent that prolongs the cardiac action potential by blocking the potassium channels and thus one or more of the potassium currents.
THERAPEUTIC EFFECTS Effectiveness indicated by correction of cardiac arrhythmias. Action results in suppression of arrhythmias dependent upon re-entry of potassium ions. It also prolongs the atrial and ventricular refractory period.

USES Symptomatic atrial fibrillation and flutter.

CONTRAINDICATIONS Baseline QT/QT_C interval of >420 milliseconds; ventricular arrhythmias; hypersensitivity to dofetilide; concurrent administration with verapamil, cimetidine, trimethoprim, ketoconazole; lactation.

CAUTIOUS USE Atrioventricular block, bradycardia, CHF, electrolyte imbalances (e.g., hypokalemia, hypomagnesia, etc.); concurrent administration of potassium depleting diuretics, hepatic or renal impairment; history of moderate QT_C interval prolongation; moderate to severe hypertension; recent MI or unstable angina; vascular heart disease; pregnancy (category C); older adults. Safety and efficacy in children <18 y are unknown.

ROUTE & DOSAGE

Atrial Fibrillation/Flutter

Adult: **PO** Based on creatinine clearance (Cl_{cr}) and QT_c interval, if QT_c increases by >15% from baseline or is >500 msec 2–3 h after initial dose. Decrease subsequent doses by 50%

Renal Impairment

Cl_{cr} >60 mL/min: 500 mcg b.i.d.; 40–60 mL/min: 250 mcg b.i.d.; 20–39 mL/min: 125 mcg b.i.d.

ADMINISTRATION

Oral

- Do not give dofetilide if QT/QT_c interval >420 milliseconds (or >500 milliseconds with ventricular conduction abnormalities).
- Individualize doses on creatinine clearance; QT_c interval is used if HR <60 bpm.
- Administer only with continuous ECG monitoring.
- Do not initiate therapy until 3 mo after withdrawal of previous antiarrhythmic therapy.
- Do not initiate therapy until 3 mo after amiodarone has been withdrawn or plasma level is <0.3 mcg/mL.
- Store at 15°–30° C (59°–86° F); protect from moisture and humidity.

ADVERSE EFFECTS (≥1%) **Body as a Whole:** Flu-like syndrome, back pain. **CNS:** *Headache,* dizziness, insomnia. **CV:** <u>Torsade de pointes arrhythmia,</u> <u>*ventricular arrhythmias,*</u> AV block, *chest pain.* **GI:** Nausea, diarrhea, abdominal pain. **Respiratory:** Respiratory infection, dyspnea. **Skin:** Rash.

INTERACTIONS Drug: Dofetilide levels increased by **verapamil, cimetidine, trimethoprim, ketoconazole, prochlorperazine, megestrol;** do not give with drugs known to increase the QT_c interval such as **cisapride, bepridil,** PHENOTHIAZINE, TRICYCLIC ANTIDEPRESSANTS, ORAL MACROLIDES, other ANTIARRHYTHMICS.

PHARMACOKINETICS Absorption: >90% bioavailable. **Peak:** 2–3 h. **Distribution:** 60%–70% protein bound. **Metabolism:** Metabolized in liver. **Elimination:** Primarily excreted unchanged in urine. **Half-Life:** 10 h.

NURSING IMPLICATIONS

Assessment & Drug Effects

- Monitor ECG continuously during first 3 mo of therapy; then periodically.
- Do not discharge patient until 12 h after conversion to normal sinus rhythm.
- Lab tests: Baseline and periodic serum electrolytes (including magnesium), periodic CBC, and routine blood chemistry. Serum potassium must be within normal limits prior to and throughout therapy with dofetilide.

D

- Notify physician immediately of electrolyte imbalances, especially hypokalemia and hypomagnesemia.

Patient & Family Education

- Report immediately conditions that cause potassium loss (e.g., prolonged vomiting, diarrhea, excessive sweating).
- Do NOT take concurrently cimetidine, verapamil, ketoconazole, trimethoprim.
- Do not breast feed while taking this drug.

DOLASETRON MESYLATE

(dol-a-se′tron)

Anzemet

Classifications: GASTROINTESTINAL AGENT; ANTIEMETIC; 5-HT_3 ANTAGONIST

Prototype: Ondansetron

Pregnancy Category: B

AVAILABILITY 50 mg, 100 mg tablets; 20 mg/mL injection

ACTIONS Dolasetron is a selective serotonin (5-HT_3) receptor antagonist used for control of nausea and vomiting associated with cancer chemotherapy. Serotonin receptors affected by dolasetron are located in the chemoreceptor trigger zone (CTZ) of the brain and peripherally on the vagal nerve terminal. Serotonin, released from the cells of the small intestine, activate 5-HT_3 receptors located on vagal efferent, neurons, thus initiating the vomiting reflex. Dolasetron causes ECG changes lasting from 6 to 24 h.

THERAPEUTIC EFFECTS This selective serotonin (5-HT_3) receptor antagonist has antiemetic properties that help patients on chemotherapy.

USES Prevention of nausea and vomiting from emetogenic chemotherapy, prevention and treatment of postoperative nausea and vomiting.

CONTRAINDICATIONS Hypersensitivity to dolasetron.

CAUTIOUS USE Patients who have or may develop prolongation of cardiac conduction intervals, particularly QT_c (i.e., patients with hypokalemia, hypomagnesia, diuretics, congenital QT syndrome; patients taking antiarrhythmic drugs and high-dose anthracycline therapy, etc.), pregnancy (category B), and lactation. Safety and efficacy in children <2 y are not established.

ROUTE & DOSAGE

Prevention of Chemotherapy-induced Nausea and Vomiting

Adult: **IV** 1.8 mg/kg or 100 mg administered over 30 s, 30 min prior to chemotherapy **PO** 100 mg 1 h prior to chemotherapy
Child: **IV** >2 *y,* 1.8 mg/kg or 100 mg administered over 30 s, 30 min prior to chemotherapy **PO** >2 *y,* 1.8 mg/kg up to 100 mg 1 h before chemotherapy

Pre/Postoperative Nausea and Vomiting

Adult: **IV** 12.5 mg 15 min before cessation of anesthesia or when post-op nausea and vomiting occurs **PO** 100 mg within 2 h prior to surgery
Child: **IV** >2 *y,* 0.35 mg/kg up to 12.5 mg 15 min before cessation of anesthesia or when post-op nausea and vomiting occurs **PO** >2 *y,* 1.2 mg/kg up to 100 mg starting 2 h prior to surgery (may also mix IV formulation in apple or apple-grape juice and administer orally)

ADMINISTRATION

Oral

- Give dissolved in apple or apple-grape juice 1 h before chemotherapy.
- Give within 2 h before surgery, when used for post-op nausea.

Intravenous

PREPARE: **Direct:** Give undiluted. **IV Infusion:** Dilute in 50 mL of any of the following: NS, D5W, D5/0.45% NaCl, LR.

ADMINISTER: **Direct:** Inject undiluted drug over 30 s. **IV Infusion:** Infuse diluted drug over 15 min.

- Store at 20°–25° C (66°–77° F) and protect from light. ▪ Diluted IV solution may be stored refrigerated up to 48 h.

ADVERSE EFFECTS (≥1%) **Body as a Whole:** Fever, fatigue, pain, chills or shivering. **CNS:** *Headache,* dizziness, drowsiness. **CV:** Hypertension. **GI:** *Diarrhea,* increased LFTs, abdominal pain. **Genitourinary:** Urinary retention.

PHARMACOKINETICS Absorption: Rapidly absorbed from GI tract, converted to hydrodolasetron, the active metabolite. **Peak:** 0.6 h IV, 1 h PO. **Distribution:** Crosses placenta, distributed into breast milk. **Metabolism:** Metabolized to hydrodolasetron by carbonyl reductase. Hydrodolasetron is metabolized in the liver by CYP2D6. **Elimination:** Primarily excreted in urine as unchanged hydrodolasetron. **Half-Life:** 10 min dolasetron, 7.3 h hydrodolasetron.

NURSING IMPLICATIONS

Assessment & Drug Effects

- Therapeutic effectiveness: Prevention of nausea and vomiting.
- Determine serum electrolytes before initiating drug. Hypokalemia and hypomagnesemia should be correct before initiating therapy.
- Monitor closely cardiac status especially with vomiting, excess diuresis, or other conditions that may result in electrolyte imbalances.
- Monitor ECG, especially in those taking concurrent antiarrhythmic or other drugs that may cause QT prolongation.
- Monitor for and report signs of bleeding (e.g., hematuria, epistaxis, purpura, hematoma).
- Lab tests: With prolonged therapy, periodically monitor liver functions, PTT, CBC with platelet count, and alkaline phosphatase.

Patient & Family Education

- Headache requiring analgesic for relief is a common adverse effect.
- Do not breast feed while taking this drug without consulting physician.

D

DONEPEZIL HYDROCHLORIDE (Pr)

(don-e′pe-zil)

Aricept, Aricept ODT

Classifications: AUTONOMIC NERVOUS SYSTEM AGENT; CHOLINERGIC (PARASYMPATHOMIMETIC) AGENT; CHOLINESTERASE INHIBITOR; CHOLINERGIC, CENTRAL ACTING

Pregnancy Category: C

AVAILABILITY 5 mg, 10 mg tablets and orally disintegrating tablets

ACTIONS In early stages of Alzheimer's disease, pathologic changes in neurons result in deficiency of acetylcholine.

THERAPEUTIC EFFECTS Aricept, a cholesterase inhibitor, presumably elevates acetylcholine concentration in the cerebral cortex by slowing degradation of acetylcholine released by remaining intact neurons.

USES Mild to moderate dementia of Alzheimer's type.

CONTRAINDICATIONS Hypersensitivity to donepezil or tracine; pregnancy (category C), lactation; children; GI bleeding, jaundice.

CAUTIOUS USE Anesthesia, sick sinus rhythm, AV block, bradycardia, cardiac arrhythmias, cardiac disease, hypotension; hyperthyroidism, history of ulcers, abnormal liver function; patients with asthma or obstructive pulmonary disease, history of seizures, seizures, urinary tract obstruction, intestinal obstruction; diarrhea, emesis, GI disease, renal failure, renal impairment, surgery.

ROUTE & DOSAGE

Alzheimer's Disease

Adult: **PO** 5–10 mg h.s.

ADMINISTRATION

Oral

- Give at h.s. just prior to going to bed.
- Increase dosage to 10 mg ONLY after 4–6 wk of therapy with the 5-mg dose.
- Store at 15°–30° C (59°–86° F).

ADVERSE EFFECTS (≥1%) **Body as a Whole:** *Headache,* fatigue. **CNS:** *Insomnia,* dizziness, depression, tremor, irritability, vertigo, ataxia. **CV:** Syncope, hypertension, atrial fibrillation, hot flashes, hypotension. **GI:** *Nausea, diarrhea, vomiting, muscle cramps, anorexia,* GI bleeding, bloating, fecal incontinence, epigastric pain. **Respiratory:** Dyspnea. **Skin:** Pruritus, sweating, urticaria. **Other:** Ecchymoses, muscle cramps, dehydration, blurred vision, urinary incontinence, nocturia.

INTERACTIONS Drug: Ketoconazole, quinidine may inhibit donepezil metabolism; **carbamazepine, dexamethasone, phenobarbital, phenytoin, rifampin** may increase donepezil elimination; donepezil may interfere with the action of ANTICHOLINERGIC AGENTS.

PHARMACOKINETICS Absorption: Rapidly absorbed from GI tract. **Peak plasma concentration:** 3–4 h. **Distribution:** 96% protein bound. **Metabolism:** Metabolized in the liver by CYP2D6 and CYP3A4 to at least 2 active metabolites. **Elimination:** Primarily excreted in urine. **Half-Life:** 70 h.

NURSING IMPLICATIONS

Assessment & Drug Effects

- Monitor therapeutic effectiveness: Improvement as noted on the Alzheimer's Disease Assessment Scale.
- Monitor closely for S&S of GI ulceration and bleeding, especially with concurrent use of NSAIDS.
- Monitor carefully patients with a history of asthma or obstructive pulmonary disease.
- Monitor cardiovascular status; drug may have vagotonic effect on the heart, causing bradycardia, especially in presence of conduction abnormalities.

Patient & Family Education

- Exercise caution. Fainting episodes related to slowing the heart rate may occur.
- Report immediately to physician any S&S of GI ulceration or bleeding (e.g., "coffee-grounds" emesis, tarry stools, epigastric pain).

DOPAMINE HYDROCHLORIDE

(doe′pa-meen)

Dopastat, Intropin, Revimine ♣

Classifications: AUTONOMIC NERVOUS SYSTEM AGENT; ALPHA- AND BETA-ADRENERGIC AGONIST (SYMPATHOMIMETIC)

Prototype: Epinephrine

Pregnancy Category: C

AVAILABILITY 40 mg/mL, 80 mg/mL, 160 mg/mL injection

ACTIONS Naturally occurring neurotransmitter and immediate precursor of norepinephrine. Major cardiovascular effects produced by direct action on alpha- and beta-adrenergic receptors and on specific dopaminergic receptors in mesenteric and renal vascular beds.

THERAPEUTIC EFFECTS Positive inotropic effect on myocardium increases cardiac output with increase in systolic and pulse pressure and little or no effect on diastolic pressure. Improves circulation to renal vascular bed by decreasing renal vascular resistance with resulting increase in glomerular filtration rate and urinary output.

USES To correct hemodynamic imbalance in shock syndrome due to MI (cardiogenic shock), trauma, endotoxic septicemia (septic shock), open heart surgery, and CHF.

UNLABELED USES Acute renal failure; cirrhosis; hepatorenal syndrome; barbiturate intoxication.

CONTRAINDICATIONS Pheochromocytoma; tachyarrhythmias or ventricular fibrillation. Safe use during pregnancy (category C), lactation, or children is not established.

CAUTIOUS USE Patients with history of occlusive vascular disease (e.g., Buerger's or Raynaud's disease); cold injury; diabetic endarteritis, arterial embolism.

ROUTE & DOSAGE

Shock

Adult/Child: **IV** 2–5 mcg/kg/min increased gradually up to 20–50 mcg/kg/min if necessary

Renal Failure

Adult: **IV** 2–5 mcg/kg/min

ADMINISTRATION

Intravenous

PREPARE: **Continuous:** Dilute just prior to administration. ▪ Dilute each ampule in one of the following: D5W, D5/NS, D5/LR, D5/0.45% NaCl, NS. ▪ Dilute 200 mg ampule in 250 mL, 500 mL, or 1000 mL IV solution to yield 800 mcg/mL, 400 mcg/mL, or 200 mcg/mL, respectively. Dilute 400 mg ampule in 250 mL, 500 mL, or 1000 mL IV solution to yield 1600 mcg/mL, 800 mcg/mL or 400 mcg/mL, respectively. ▪ Dilute 800 mg ampule in 250 mL, 500 mL, or 1000 mL IV solution to yield 3200 mcg/mL, 1600 mcg/mL or 800 mcg/mL, respectively. ▪ Consult package information for other dilutions.

ADMINISTER: **Continuous:** Infusion rate is based on body weight. ▪ Infusion rate and guidelines for adjusting rate relative changes in blood pressure are prescribed by physician. ▪ Microdrip and other reliable metering device should be used for accuracy of flow rate.

INCOMPATIBILITIES **Solution/additive: Sodium bicarbonate, aminophylline, amphotericin B, ampicillin, cephalothin, penicillin G. Y-site: Acyclovir,**

D

aminophylline, amphotericin B, sodium bicarbonate.

▪ Correct hypovolemia, if possible, with either whole blood or plasma before initiation of dopamine therapy. ▪ Monitor infusion continuously for free flow, and take care to avoid extravasation, which can result in tissue sloughing and gangrene. Use a large vein of the antecubital fossa. ▪ Antidote for extravasation: Stop infusion promptly and remove needle. Immediately infiltrate the ischemic area with 5–10 mg phentolamine mesylate in 10–15 mL of NS, using syringe and fine needle. ▪ Protect dopamine from light. Discolored solutions should not be used.

▪ Store reconstituted solution for 24 h at 2°–15° C (36°–59° F) or 6 h at room temperature 15°–30° C.

ADVERSE EFFECTS (≥1%) **CV:** *Hypotension,* ectopic beats, *tachycardia,* anginal pain, palpitation, vasoconstriction (indicated by disproportionate rise in diastolic pressure), cold extremities; less frequent: aberrant conduction, bradycardia, widening of QRS complex, elevated blood pressure. **GI:** Nausea, vomiting. **CNS:** Headache. **Skin:** Necrosis, tissue sloughing with extravasation, gangrene, piloerection. **Other:** Azotemia, dyspnea, dilated pupils (high doses).

DIAGNOSTIC TEST INTERFERENCE Dopamine may modify test response when histamine is used as a control for ***intradermal skin tests.***

INTERACTIONS Drug: MAO INHIBITORS, ERGOT ALKALOIDS, **furazolidine** increase alpha-adrenergic effects (headache, hyperpyrexia, hypertension); **guanethidine, phenytoin** may decrease dopamine action; BETA BLOCKERS antagonize cardiac effects; ALPHA BLOCKERS antagonize peripheral vasoconstriction; **halothane, cyclopropane** increase risk of hypertension and ventricular arrhythmias.

PHARMACOKINETICS Onset: <5 min. **Duration:** <10 min. **Distribution:** Widely distributed; does not cross blood–brain barrier. **Metabolism:** Inactive in the liver, kidney, and plasma by monoamine oxidase and COMT. **Elimination:** Excreted in urine. **Half-Life:** 2 min.

NURSING IMPLICATIONS

Assessment & Drug Effects

- Monitor blood pressure, pulse, peripheral pulses, and urinary output at intervals prescribed by physician. Precise measurements are essential for accurate titration of dosage.
- Report the following indicators promptly to physician for use in decreasing or temporarily suspending dose: Reduced urine flow rate in absence of hypotension; ascending tachycardia; dysrhythmias; disproportionate rise in diastolic pressure (marked decrease in pulse pressure); signs of peripheral ischemia (pallor, cyanosis, mottling, coldness, complaints of tenderness, pain, numbness, or burning sensation).
- Monitor therapeutic effectiveness. In addition to improvement in vital signs and urine flow, other indices of adequate dosage and perfusion of vital organs include loss of pallor, increase in toe temperature, adequacy of nail bed capillary filling, and reversal of confusion or comatose state.

DORNASE ALFA

(dor'naze)
Pulmozyme
Classifications: ANTITUSSIVE, EXPECTORANT, AND MUCOLYTIC AGENTS; MUCOLYTIC
Prototype: Acetylcysteine
Pregnancy Category: B

AVAILABILITY 1 mg/mL solution for inhalation

ACTIONS Dornase is a solution of recombinant human deoxyribonuclease (DNAse), an enzyme that selectively cleaves DNA. In cystic fibrosis (CF) patients, viscous, purulent secretions in the airway reduce pulmonary function and lead to exacerbations of infection. Purulent pulmonary secretions contain very high concentrations of DNA released by degenerating leukocytes that are present in response to infection.
THERAPEUTIC EFFECTS Dornase hydrolyzes the DNA in sputum of CF patients and reduces sputum viscosity. Use of dornase significantly reduces number of upper respiratory infections acquired by patients with CF.

USES In combination with standard therapies to reduce the frequency of respiratory infections in patients with CF and to improve pulmonary function.

CONTRAINDICATIONS Hypersensitivity to dornase.
CAUTIOUS USE Pregnancy (category B), lactation. Safety and efficacy in children <5 y of age is not known.

ROUTE & DOSAGE

Cystic Fibrosis
Adult/Child: **Inhalation** >*3 mo,* 2.5 mg (1 ampule) inhaled once daily using a recommended nebulizer, may increase to twice daily (do not mix with other agents in nebulizer)

ADMINISTRATION

Inhalation
- Do not dilute or mix with any other drugs or solutions in the nebulizer.
- Use only with nebulizer systems recommended by the drug manufacturer.
- Do not shake ampuls; do not use ampuls that have been at room temperature longer than 24 h or have become cloudy or discolored.
- Store refrigerated at 2°–8° C (36°–46° F) in protective foil pouch.

ADVERSE EFFECTS (≥1%) **Respiratory:** Hoarseness, sore throat, voice alterations, pharyngitis, laryngitis, cough, rhinitis. **Other:** Conjunctivitis, chest pain, rash.

PHARMACOKINETICS Absorption: Minimal systemic absorption. **Onset:** 3–8 d. **Duration:** Benefit lasts up to 4 d after discontinuing treatment.

NURSING IMPLICATIONS

Assessment & Drug Effects
- Monitor for improvement in dyspnea and sputum clearance.
- Monitor for S&S of hypersensitivity (see Appendix F). Patients with a history of hypersensitivity to bovine pancreatic dornase are at high risk.
- Monitor for adverse effects; rarely, dosage adjustments may be required.

Patient & Family Education
- Report rash, hives, itching, or other S&S of hypersensitivity to physician immediately.

- Know potential adverse effects and report those that are bothersome or do not disappear.
- Take a missed dose as soon as possible; if it is almost time for the next dose, skip the missed dose.
- Do not breast feed while taking this drug without consulting physician.

DORZOLAMIDE HYDROCHLORIDE

(dor-zol′a-mide)

Trusopt

Classifications: EYE PREPARATION; CARBONIC ANHYDRASE INHIBITOR

Prototype: Acetazolamide

Pregnancy Category: C

AVAILABILITY 2% ophthalmic solution

ACTIONS Dorzolamide is a sulfonamide and inhibits carbonic anhydrase in the eye, thus reducing the rate of aqueous humor formation with subsequent lowering of IOP. Elevated IOP is a major risk factor in the pathogenesis of optic nerve damage and visual field loss due to glaucoma.

THERAPEUTIC EFFECTS Lowers IOP in glaucoma or ocular hypertension.

USES Elevated intraocular pressure in patients with ocular hypertension or open-angle glaucoma.

CONTRAINDICATIONS Previous hypersensitivity to dorzolamide; pregnancy (category C).

CAUTIOUS USE History of hypersensitivity to other carbonic anhydrase inhibitors, sulfonamides, or thiazide diuretics; ocular infection or inflammation; recent ocular surgery; moderate-to-severe renal or hepatic insufficiency; angle-closure glaucoma; concomitant use of oral carbonic anhydrase inhibitors; older adults, corneal abrasion.

ROUTE & DOSAGE

Glaucoma, Ocular Hypertension

Adult/Child: **Ophthalmic** 1 drop in affected eye t.i.d.

ADMINISTRATION

Instillation

- Apply gentle pressure to lacrimal sac during and immediately following drug instillation for about 1 min to lessen degree of systemic absorption.
- Administer at least 10 min apart, if another ophthalmic drug is being used concurrently.
- Store at 15°–30° C (59°–86° F).

ADVERSE EFFECTS (≥1%) **CNS:** Headache. **GI:** Bitter taste, nausea. **Special Senses:** *Transient burning or stinging, transient blurred vision,* superficial punctate keratitis, tearing, dryness, photophobia, ocular allergic reaction. **Skin:** Rash.

PHARMACOKINETICS Absorption: Some systemic absorption from topical instillation. **Onset:** 2 h. **Duration:** 8–12 h. **Distribution:** Distributes into red blood cells. **Elimination:** Excreted in urine. **Half-Life:** RBC elimination about 4 mo.

NURSING IMPLICATIONS

Assessment & Drug Effects

- Inquire about previous hypersensitivity to sulfonamides prior to therapy.
- Withhold drug and notify physician if S&S of local or systemic hypersensitivity occur (see Appendix F).
- Withhold the drug and notify the physician if ocular irritation occurs.

- Lab tests: Monitor CBC, serum electrolytes, and renal and liver function tests periodically with long-term therapy.

Patient & Family Education

- Learn proper technique for applying eyedrops.
- Do not allow tip of drug dipenser to come in contact with the eye.
- Discontinue drug and report to physician: ocular irritation, infection, or S&S of systemic hypersensitivity occur (see Appendix F).

DOXACURIUM CHLORIDE

(dox′a-cur-i-um)

Nuromax

Classifications: AUTONOMIC NERVOUS SYSTEM AGENT; SKELETAL MUSCLE RELAXANT, NONDEPOLARIZING AGENT

Prototype: Tubocurarine

Pregnancy Category: C

AVAILABILITY 1 mg/mL injection

ACTIONS Long-acting neuromuscular blocking agent. Binds competitively to cholinergic receptors on the motor end-plate, thus resulting in a block of neuromuscular transmission. Most patients require a pharmacologic reversal prior to full spontaneous recovery from a neuromuscular block using an anticholinesterase.

THERAPEUTIC EFFECTS Produces skeletal muscle relaxation during surgery.

USES Skeletal muscle relaxation during surgery after induction with general anesthesia.

UNLABELED USES Facilitates endotracheal intubation.

CONTRAINDICATIONS Hypersensitivity to doxacurium, pregnancy (category C), or children <2 years of age

CAUTIOUS USE Neuromuscular diseases (e.g., myasthenia gravis); burn patients; acid–base or serum electrolyte imbalances; newborn infants, older adults, lactation.

ROUTE & DOSAGE

Intubation or Induction

Adult: **IV** 0.05 mg/kg administered as rapid bolus injection over 5–10 s. Use lower doses in older adults or patients with renal or hepatic dysfunction

Child: **IV** *2–12 y,* 0.03–0.05 mg/kg with halothane general anesthesia

Maintenance with General Anesthesia

Adult/Child: **IV** *2–12 y,* same dose as adult, but may have to give more frequently; 0.0005–0.01 mg/kg q60–100min administered as rapid bolus injection over 5–10 s (dosing interval adjusted for each individual patient; use lower dosage in patients with renal or hepatic dysfunction)

ADMINISTRATION

Intravenous

PREPARE: **Direct:** Dilute each 1 mL (1 mg) with 10 mL of D5W, NS, D5/NS, LR, or D5/LR to yield 0.1 mg/mL.

ADMINISTER: **Direct:** Give IV push over 5–10 s.

Individualize doses according to age, body size, and presence of kidney, liver, and neuromuscular diseases. ■ Note: Doxacurium contains benzyl alcohol, which has been associated with fatal complications in newborns.
■ Doxacurium should be adminis-

tered under the supervision of expert clinicians. ▪ See manufacturer's guidelines for dilution, compatibility, and administration.

▪ Store undiluted at room temperature 15°–25° C (41°–77° F). Do not freeze. Diluted drug may be stored in polypropylene syringes for up to 24 h at 5°–25° C (41°–77° F).

ADVERSE EFFECTS (≥1%) **CV:** Bradycardia, hypotension, cutaneous flushing, histamine release.

INTERACTIONS Drug: VOLATILE ANESTHETICS **(isoflurane, enflurane, halothane)** potentiate the effects of doxacurium, requiring a reduced dose of doxacurium. Certain ANTIBIOTICS, including the AMINOGLYCOSIDES, **capreomycin, tetracycline, bacitracin, polymyxins, lincomycin, clindamycin,** and **colistin,** increase the neuromuscular blocking effect of doxacurium. **Carbamazepine** or **phenytoin** may increase the onset and decrease the duration of neuromuscular blockade. **Lithium, magnesium, procainamide,** or **quinidine** may enhance neuromuscular blockade.

PHARMACOKINETICS Onset: 5–10 min. **Peak:** 10 min. **Duration:** 60–160 min depending on dose. **Distribution:** 30% protein bound. **Metabolism:** Minimal to no hepatic metabolism. **Elimination:** 40%–50% excreted in urine within 12 h. some excretion in bile. **Half-Life:** 1.5 h.

NURSING IMPLICATIONS

Assessment & Drug Effects

- Monitor for evidence of prolonged neuromuscular block which may range from skeletal muscle weakness to prolonged paralysis with respiratory insufficiency and apnea.
- Monitor for full recovery of skeletal muscle function. Support ventilation until full recovery occurs.
- Note: Duration of neuromuscular block may be longer in persons >60 years old and in obese patients whose doses have not been adjusted according to ideal body weight.
- Monitor accordingly, knowing that drugs used to antagonize doxacurium may wear off before the effects of doxacurium.

DOXAPRAM HYDROCHLORIDE

(dox'a-pram)
Dopram
Classifications: CENTRAL NERVOUS SYSTEM AGENT; CEREBRAL STIMULANT
Prototype: Caffeine
Pregnancy Category: B

AVAILABILITY 20 mg/mL injection

ACTIONS Short-acting analeptic capable of stimulating all levels of the cerebrospinal axis. Has minor effect on cortex. Respiratory stimulation by direct medullary action or possibly by indirect activation of peripheral chemoreceptors increases tidal volume and slightly increases respiratory rate.
THERAPEUTIC EFFECTS Decreases Pco_2 and increases Po_2 by increasing alveolar ventilation; may elevate BP and pulse rate by stimulation of brain stem vasomotor area.

USES Short-term adjunctive therapy to alleviate postanesthesia and drug-induced respiratory depression and to hasten arousal and return of pharyngeal and laryngeal reflexes. Also as a temporary measure (approximately 2 h) in hospitalized patients with COPD associated with acute respiratory insufficiency as an aid to prevent elevation of $Paco_2$ during administration of oxygen. (Not used with mechanical ventilation.)

UNLABELED USES Neonatal apnea refractory to xanthine therapy.

CONTRAINDICATIONS Epilepsy and other convulsive disorders; of ventilatory mechanism due to muscle paresis, pulmonary fibrosis, flail chest, pneumothorax, airway obstruction, extreme dyspnea, or acute bronchial asthma; severe hypertension, coronary artery disease, uncompensated heart failure, CVA. Safe use during pregnancy (category B), lactation, or in children <12 y is not established.

CAUTIOUS USE History of bronchial asthma, COPD; cardiac disease, severe tachycardia, arrhythmias, hypertension; hyperthyroidism; pheochromocytoma; head injury, cerebral edema, increased intracranial pressure; peptic ulcer, patients undergoing gastric surgery; acute agitation.

ROUTE & DOSAGE

Postanesthesia

Adult: **IV** 0.5–1 mg/kg single injection not to exceed 1.5 mg/kg or 2 mg/kg total dose when repeated at 5 min intervals or 1–3 mg/min infusion (max: 4 mg/kg or 300 mg, not to exceed 3 g/d)

Drug-Induced CNS Depression

Adult: **IV** 1–2 mg/kg repeat in 5 min, then q1–2h until patient awakens (if relapse occurs, resume q1–2h injections (max: total dose 3 g), if no response after priming dose, may give 1–3 mg/min for up to 2 h until patient awakens)

Chronic Obstructive Pulmonary Disease

Adult: **IV** 1–2 mg/min for a max of 2 h (max: rate 3 mg/min)

Neonatal Apnea

Neonate: **IV** 2.5–3 mg/kg followed by 1 mg/kg/h (titrate to max: 2.5 mg/kg/h)

D

ADMINISTRATION

- IV administration to neonates: Verify correct IV concentration and rate of infusion with physician. Generally do not use in newborns because doxapram contains benzyl alcohol.
- Ensure adequacy of airway and oxygenation before initiation of doxapram therapy.

Intravenous

PREPARE: **Direct:** Give undiluted. **IV Infusion:** Dilute 250 mg (12.5 mL) in 250 mL of D5W or NS.

ADMINISTER: **Direct:** Give undiluted over 5 min. **IV Infusion:** Give at a rate of 1–3 mg/min, depending on patient response. Never exceed 3 mg/min.

INCOMPATIBILITIES **Solution/additive: Aminophylline, ascorbic acid,** CEPHALOSPORINS, **carbenicillin, dexamethasone, diazepam, digoxin, dobutamine, folic acid, furosemide, hydrocortisone, ketamine, methylprednisolone, minocycline, thiopental, ticarcillin.**

- Store at 15°–30° C (59°–86° F) unless otherwise directed.

ADVERSE EFFECTS (≥1%) **CNS:** Dizziness, sneezing, apprehension, confusion, *involuntary movements,* hyperactivity, paresthesias; feeling of warmth and burning, especially of genitalia and perineum; flushing, sweating, hyperpyrexia, headache, pilomotor erection, pruritus, muscle tremor, rigidity, convulsions, *increased deep-tendon reflexes,* bilateral Babinski sign, *carpopedal spasm,* pupillary dilation, mild delayed narcosis. **CV:** *Mild to moderate increase in BP, sinus tachycardia,* bradycardia, extrasystoles, lowered T waves, PVCs, chest pains, tightness in chest. **GI:** Nausea, vomiting, diarrhea, salivation, sour taste. **Urogenital:** Urinary retention, frequency, incontinence. **Respiratory:** Dyspnea, tachypnea, cough, <u>laryngospasm, bronchospasm</u>, hiccups, rebound hypoventilation, hypocapnia with tetany. **Other:** Local skin irritation, thrombophlebitis with extravasation; decreased Hgb, Hct, and RBC count; elevated BUN; albuminuria.

INTERACTIONS Drug: MAO INHIBITORS, SYMPATHOMIMETIC AGENTS add to pressor effects.

PHARMACOKINETICS Onset: 20–40 s. **Peak:** 1–2 min. **Duration:** 5–12 min. **Metabolism:** Rapidly metabolized. **Elimination:** Excreted in urine as metabolites.

NURSING IMPLICATIONS

Assessment & Drug Effects

- Monitor IV site frequently. Extravasation or use of same IV site for prolonged periods can cause thrombophlebitis (see Appendix F) or tissue irritation.
- Monitor carefully and observe accurately: BP, pulse, deep tendon reflexes, airway, and arterial blood gases. All are essential guides for determining minimum effective dosage and preventing overdosage. Make baseline determinations for comparison.
- Lab tests: Draw arterial Po_2 and Pco_2 and O_2 saturation prior to both initiation of doxapram infusion and oxygen administration in patients with COPD, and then at least every 30 min during infusion. Infusion should not be administered for longer than 2 h.
- Discontinue doxapram if arterial blood gases show evidence of deterioration and when mechanical ventilation is initiated.
- Observe patient continuously during therapy and maintain vigilance until patient is fully alert (usually about 1 h) and protective pharyngeal and laryngeal reflexes are completely restored.
- Notify physician immediately of any adverse effects. Be alert for early signs of toxicity: Tachycardia, muscle tremor, spasticity, hyperactive reflexes.
- Note: A mild to moderate increase in BP commonly occurs.
- Discontinue if sudden hypotension or dyspnea develops.

DOXAZOSIN MESYLATE

(dox-a'zo-sin)

Cardura

Classifications: AUTONOMIC NERVOUS SYSTEM AGENT; ALPHA-ADRENERGIC ANTAGONIST (SYMPATHOLYTIC, ADRENERGIC BLOCKING AGENT)

Prototype: Prazosin

Pregnancy Category: B

AVAILABILITY 1 mg, 2 mg, 4 mg, 8 mg tablets

ACTIONS By selective competitive inhibition of $alpha_1$-adrenoreceptors, it produces vasodilation in both resistance (arterioles) and capacitance (veins) vessels with the result that both peripheral vascular resistance and blood pressure are reduced.

THERAPEUTIC EFFECTS Lowers blood pressure in supine or standing individuals with most pronounced effect on diastolic pressure.

USES Mild to moderate hypertension, benign prostatic hypertrophy.

UNLABELED USE CHF.

CONTRAINDICATIONS Hypersensitivity to doxazosin, prazosin, and terazosin; hypotension, syncope. Safe use during pregnancy (category B) or in children is not established.

CAUTIOUS USE Hepatic impairment or disease; renal disease, impairment, or failure; lactation.

ROUTE & DOSAGE

Hypertension

Adult: **PO** Start with 1 mg h.s. and titrate up to maximum of 16 mg/d in 1–2 divided doses

Geriatric: **PO** Start with 0.5 mg h.s.

ADMINISTRATION

Oral

- Give initial dose at bedtime to minimize problems with postural hypotension and syncope.
- Individualize maintenance dose according to the standing BP response.
- Store at 15°–30° C (59°–86° F).

ADVERSE EFFECTS (≥1%) **CV:** *Orthostatic hypotension,* edema. **CNS:** Vertigo, *headache,* dizziness, somnolence, fatigue, nervousness, anxiety. **GI:** Nausea, abdominal pain. **Hematologic:** Leukopenia. **Skin:** Pruritus, eczema.

PHARMACOKINETICS Absorption: Readily absorbed from GI tract; 62%–69% of dose reaches systemic circulation. **Peak:** 2–6 h. **Duration:** Up to 24 h. **Distribution:** Highly protein bound (98%–99%). **Metabolism:** Approximately 35% of dose is metabolized in liver. **Elimination:** 9% excreted in urine, 63% in feces. **Half-Life:** 9–12 h.

NURSING IMPLICATIONS

Assessment & Drug Effects

- Monitor BP with patient lying down and standing; doses above 4 mg increase the risk of postural hypotension.
- Monitor BP 2–6 h after initial dose or any dose increase. This is when postural hypotension is most likely to occur.

Patient & Family Education

- Do not drive or engage in other potentially hazardous activities for 12–24 h after the first dose or an increase in dosage or when medication is restarted after an interruption in dosage.
- Use caution when rising from a sitting or supine position in order to avoid orthostatic hypotension and syncope; make position and directional changes slowly and in stages.
- Report to the physician episodes of dizziness or palpitations. These will require a dosage adjustment.
- Do not breast feed while taking this drug.

DOXEPIN HYDROCHLORIDE

(dox′e-pin)

Adapin, Sinequan, Triadapin ✦, Zonalon

Classifications: CENTRAL NERVOUS SYSTEM AGENT; PSYCHOTHERAPEUTIC; TRICYCLIC ANTIDEPRESSANT

Prototype: Imipramine

Pregnancy Category: C

AVAILABILITY 10 mg, 25 mg, 50 mg, 75 mg, 100 mg, 150 mg capsules; 10 mg/mL oral concentrate

ACTIONS Dibenzoxepin is a tricyclic antidepressant (TCA). Reportedly one of the most sedating of the TCAs. Inhibits serotonin reuptake from the synaptic gap; also inhibits norepinephrine reuptake to a moderate degree.

THERAPEUTIC EFFECTS Restores the level of these neurotransmitters (serotonin and norepinephrine) as the proposed mechanism of antidepressant action.

USES Psychoneurotic anxiety or depressive reactions; mixed symptoms of anxiety and depression; anxiety or depression associated with alcoholism; organic disease; psychotic depressive disorders; topical for treatment of pruritus.
UNLABELED USES Peptic ulcer disease, neuralgia.

CONTRAINDICATIONS Prior sensitivity to any TCA; during acute recovery phase following MI; glaucoma; prostatic hypertrophy; tendency for urinary retention; concurrent use of MAO inhibitors. Safe use during pregnancy (category C), lactation, or in children <12 y is not established.
CAUTIOUS USE Patients receiving Electroconvulsive Therapy, patients with suicidal tendency; renal, cardiovascular or hepatic dysfunction.

ROUTE & DOSAGE

Antidepressant
Adult: **PO** 30–150 mg/d h.s. or in divided doses, may gradually increase to 300 mg/d (use lower doses in older adult patients)
Geriatric: **PO** 10–25 mg h.s., may gradually increase to 75 mg/d
Child: **PO** 1–3 mg/kg/d in single or divided doses

Pruritus
Adult: **Topical** apply a thin film q.i.d. with at least 3–4 h between applications, may use up to 8 d

ADMINISTRATION

Oral
- Give oral concentrate diluted with approximately 120 mL water, milk, or fruit juice.
- Empty capsule and swallow contents with fluid or mix with food as necessary if it cannot be swallowed whole.
- Inform physician if daytime sedation is pronounced. Entire daily dose (up to 150 mg) may be prescribed for bedtime administration.

Topical
- Apply a thin film to affected areas; allow 3–4 h between applications.
- Store all forms at 15°–30° C (59°–86° F) in tightly closed, light-resistant container.

ADVERSE EFFECTS (≥1%) **All:** Anticholinergic. **CNS:** *Drowsiness,* dizziness, weakness, fatigue, headache, hypomania, confusion, tremors, paresthesias. **CV:** *Orthostatic hypotension,* palpitation, hypertension, tachycardia, ECG changes. **Special Senses:** Mydriasis, blurred vision, photophobia. **GI:** *Dry-mouth,* sour or metallic taste, epigastric distress, constipation. **Urogenital:** Urinary retention, delayed micturition, urinary frequency. **Other:** Increased perspiration, tinnitus, weight gain, photosensitivity reaction, skin rash, agranulocytosis, *burning or stinging at application site,* edema.

INTERACTIONS Drug: May decrease some antihypertensive response to ANTIHYPERTENSIVES; CNS DEPRESSANTS, **alcohol,** HYPNOTICS, BARBITURATES, SEDATIVES potentiate CNS depression; may increase hypoprothrombinemic effect of ORAL ANTICOAGULANTS; **ethchlorvynol** may cause transient delirium; **levodopa,** SYMPATHOMIMETICS (e.g., **epinephrine, norepinephrine**) introduce possibility of sympathetic hyperactivity with hypertension and hyperpyrexia; MAO INHIBITORS introduce possibility of severe reactions, toxic psychosis, cardiovascular instability; **methylphenidate** increases plasma TCA levels; THYROID AGENTS may increase possibility of arrhythmias; **cimetidine** may increase plasma TCA levels. **Herbal: Ginkgo** may decrease seizure threshold; **St. John's wort** may cause **serotonin** syndrome.

PHARMACOKINETICS Absorption: Rapidly absorbed from GI sites through intact skin. **Peak:** 2 h. **Distribution:** Crosses placenta; distributed into breast milk. **Metabolism:** Metabolized in liver. **Elimination:** Primarily excreted in urine. **Half-Life:** 6–8 h.

NURSING IMPLICATIONS

Assessment & Drug Effects

- Monitor use of other CNS depressants, including alcohol. Danger of overdosage or suicide attempt is increased when patient uses excessive amounts of alcohol.
- Be alert to changes in voiding and evaluate patient for constipation and abdominal distention; drug has moderate to strong anticholinergic effects.

Patient & Family Education

- Maintain established dosage regimen and avoid change of intervals, doubling, reducing, or skipping doses.
- Consult physician about safe amount of alcohol, if any, that can be taken. The actions of both alcohol and doxepin are potentiated when used together and for up to 2 wk after doxepin is discontinued.
- Do not drive or engage in other potentially hazardous activities until response to drug is known.
- Do not breast feed while taking this drug without consulting physician.

DOXERCALCIFEROL

(dox-er-kal'si-fe-rol)

Hectorol

Classifications: HORMONES AND SYNTHETIC SUBSTITUTES; VITAMIN D ANALOG

Prototype: Calcitriol

Pregnancy Category: B

AVAILABILITY 0.5 mcg, 2.5 mcg capsule; 2 mcg/mL injection

ACTIONS Vitamin D_2 analog that is activated by the liver. Regulates the blood calcium levels.

THERAPEUTIC EFFECTS Activated Vitamin D is needed for absorption of dietary calcium in the intestine, and the parathyroid hormone (PTH) which mobilizes calcium from the bone tissue.

USES Reduction of elevated iPTH in secondary hyperparathyroidism in patients undergoing chronic renal dialysis; secondary hyperparathyroidism in chronic kidney disease not on dialysis.

CONTRAINDICATIONS Hypersensitivity to doxercalciferol or other Vitamin D analogs; recent hypercalcemia, recent hyperphosphatemia, hypervitaminosis D; lactation.

CAUTIOUS USE Renal or hepatic insufficiency; renal osteodystrophy with hyperphosphatemia, prolonged hypercalcemia; pregnancy (category B). Safety and efficacy in children are not established.

ROUTE & DOSAGE

Secondary Hyperparathyroidism

Adult: **PO** 10 mcg 3 times per wk at dialysis, adjust dose as needed to lower iPTH into the range of 150–300 pg/mL by increasing the dose in 2.5 mcg increments every 8 wks (max: 60 mcg/wk) **IV** 4 mcg 3 times/wk at end of dialysis (max: 18 mcg/wk)

D

ADMINISTRATION

Oral

- Give at time of dialysis.
- Withhold drug and notify physician if any of the following occurs: iPTH <100 pg/mL, hypercalcemia, hyperphosphatemia, or product of serum calcium times serum phosphorus >70.
- Use beyond 16 wk is not recommended.
- Store at 20°–25° C (66°–77° F); excursions to 15°–30° C (59°–86° F) are permitted.

Intravenous

PREPARE: **Direct:** No dilution is needed. ▪ Withdraw appropriate dose from ampule using a filter needle. ▪ Change needles before injecting as an IV bolus. Discard any unused portion.

ADMINISTER: **Direct:** Give a bolus injection at the end of dialysis sessions.

- Store at 15°–20° C (59°–77° F).

ADVERSE EFFECTS (≥1%) **Body as a Whole:** Abscess, *headache, malaise,* arthralgia. **CNS:** *Dizziness,* sleep disorder. **CV:** Bradycardia, *edema.* **GI:** Anorexia, constipation, dyspepsia, *nausea, vomiting.* **Respiratory:** *Dyspnea.* **Skin:** Pruritus. **Other:** Weight gain.

INTERACTIONS Drug: Cholestyramine, mineral oil may decrease absorption; MAGNESIUM-CONTAINING ANTACIDS may cause hypermagnesemia; other VIT D ANALOGS may increase toxicity and hypercalcemia.

PHARMACOKINETICS Absorption: Absorbed from GI tract and is activated in the liver. **Peak:** 11–12 h. **Metabolism:** Activated by CYP 27 to form 1alpha, 25-$(OH)_2D_2$ (major metabolite) and 1alpha, 24-dihydroxyvitamin D_2 (minor metabolite). **Half-Life:** 32–37 h.

NURSING IMPLICATIONS

Assessment & Drug Effects

- Lab tests: Baseline and periodic iPTH, serum calcium, serum phosphorus. Monitor levels weekly during dose titration.
- Monitor for S&S of hypercalcemia (see Appendix F).

Patient & Family Education

- Do not take antacids without consulting the physician.
- Notify the physician if you become pregnant while taking this drug.
- Do not use mineral oil on the days doxercalciferol is taken. Mineral oil may decrease absorption of drug.
- Do not take nonprescription drugs containing magnesium while taking doxercalciferol.
- Report S&S of hypercalcemia immediately: Bone or muscle pain, dry mouth with metallic taste, rhinorrhea, itching, photophobia, conjunctivitis, frequent urination, anorexia and weight loss.
- Do not breast feed while taking this drug.

DOXORUBICIN HYDROCHLORIDE (Pr)

(dox-oh-roo′bi-sin)

Adriamycin, Rubex

DOXORUBICIN LIPOSOME

Doxil

Classifications: ANTINEOPLASTIC; ANTIBIOTIC

Pregnancy Category: D

AVAILABILITY 10 mg, 20 mg, 50 mg, 100 mg, 150 mg powder for injection; 2 mg/mL injection; 20 mg liposomal injection

ACTIONS Cytotoxic antibiotic with wide spectrum of antitumor activity and strong immunosuppressive properties. Intercalates with preformed DNA residues, blocking effective DNA and RNA transcription. A potent radiosensitizer capable of enhancing radiation reactions. No clinical cross-resistance to standard antineoplastics; therefore, it may be especially effective in patients with less advanced disease.
THERAPEUTIC EFFECTS Highly destructive to rapidly proliferating cells and slowly developing carcinomas; selectively toxic to cardiac tissue.

USES To produce regression in neoplastic conditions, including acute lymphoblastic and myeloblastic leukemias, Wilms' tumor, neuroblastoma, soft tissue and bone sarcomas, breast and ovary carcinomas, lymphomas, bronchogenic carcinoma. Generally used in combined modalities with surgery, radiation, and immunotherapy. Effective pretreatment to sensitize superficial tumors to local radiation therapy. Kaposi's sarcoma (Doxil).
UNLABELED USES Multiple myeloma.

CONTRAINDICATIONS Myelosuppression, impaired cardiac function, obstructive jaundice, previous treatment with complete cumulative doses of doxorubicin or daunorubicin; lactation. Safe use during pregnancy (category D) is not established.
CAUTIOUS USE Impaired hepatic or renal function; patients who have received cyclophosphamide or pelvic irradiation or radiotherapy to areas surrounding heart; history of atopic dermatitis.

ROUTE & DOSAGE

Neoplasm
Adult: **IV** 60–75 mg/m^2 as single dose at 21 d intervals or 30 mg/m^2 on each of 3 consecutive days repeated every 4 wk (max: total cumulative dose 500–550 mg/m^2)
Child: **IV** 35–75 mg/m^2 as single dose, repeat at 21-d interval, or 20–30 mg/m^2 once weekly

Kaposi's Sarcoma
Adult: **IV Doxil** 20 mg/m^2 every 3 wk. Infuse over 30 min (do not use in-line filters)

ADMINISTRATION

Intravenous

IV administration to infants and children: Verify correct IV concentration and rate of infusion with physician. ▪ Wear gloves and use caution when preparing drug solution. If powder or solution contacts skin or mucosa, wash copiously with soap and water. ▪ Exposure to doxorubicin during the first trimester of pregnancy can result in losing the fetus.

PREPARE: **Direct:** Dilute the powder with NS to yield a final concentration of 2 mg/mL. Bacteriostatic diluents are not recommended.
ADMINISTER: **Direct:** Administer slowly into y-site of freely running IV infusion of NS or D5W. Tubing should be attached to a butterfly needle inserted into a large vein. Usually infused over 3–5 min. Rate will be specifically ordered.

D

INCOMPATIBILITIES **Solution/additive: Aminophylline, cephalothin, dexamethasone, diazepam, fluorouracil, furosemide, hydrocortisone, heparin, vinblastine. Y-site: Furosemide, heparin,** TPN.

▪ Facial flushing and local red streaking along the vein may occur if drug is administered too rapidly. ▪ Avoid using antecubital vein or veins on dorsum of hand or wrist, if possible, where extravasation could damage underlying tendons and nerves. Also avoid veins in extremity with compromised venous or lymphatic drainage.

▪ Store reconstituted solution for 24 h at room temperature; refrigerated at 4°–10° C (39°–50° F) for 48 h. Protect from sunlight; discard unused solution.

ADVERSE EFFECTS (≥1%) **Body as a Whole:** Hypersensitivity (red flare around injection site, erythema, skin rash, pruritus, angioedema, urticaria, eosinophilia, fever, chills, anaphylactoid reaction). **CV:** Serious, irreversible myocardial toxicity with delayed CHF, ventricular arrhythmias, acute left ventricular failure, hypertension, hypotension. **GI:** *Stomatitis,* esophagitis with ulcerations; nausea, vomiting, anorexia, inanition, diarrhea. **Hematologic:** *Severe myelosuppression* (60–85% of patients); *leukopenia (principally granulocytes),* thrombocytopenia, anemia. **Skin:** Hyperpigmentation of nail beds, tongue, and buccal mucosa (especially in blacks); *complete alopecia* (reversible), hyperpigmentation of dermal creases (especially in children), rash, *recall phenomenon (skin reaction due to prior radiotherapy).* **Other:** Lacrimation, drowsiness, fever, facial flush with too rapid IV infusion rate, microscopic hematuria, hyperuricemia. *With extravasation: severe cellulitis, vesication, tissue necrosis,* lymphangitis, phlebosclerosis.

INTERACTIONS Drug: BARBITURATES may decrease pharmacologic effects of doxorubicin by increasing its hepatic metabolism—increase in doxorubicin dosage may be needed; **streptozocin** (Zanosar) may prolong doxorubicin half-life—dosage reduction of doxorubicin may be indicated.

PHARMACOKINETICS Distribution: Widely distributed; does not cross blood–brain barrier; crosses placenta; distribution into breast milk not known. **Metabolism:** Metabolized in liver to active metabolite. **Elimination:** Excreted primarily in bile. **Half-Life:** 16.7–31.7 h.

NURSING IMPLICATIONS

Assessment & Drug Effects

- Stop infusion, remove IV needle, and notify physician promptly if patient complains of stinging or burning sensation at the injection site.
- Monitor any area of extravasation closely for 3–4 wk. If ulceration begins (usually 1–4 wk after extravasation), a plastic surgeon should be consulted.
- Begin a flow chart to establish baseline data. Include temperature, pulse, respiration, BP, body weight, laboratory values, and I&O ratio and pattern.
- Lab tests: Baseline and periodic hepatic function, renal function, CBC with differential throughout therapy.
- Note: The nadir of leukopenia (an expected 1000/mm^3) typically occurs 10–14 d after single

dose, with recovery occurring within 21 d.

- Evaluate cardiac function (ECG) prior to initiation of therapy, at regular intervals, and at end of therapy.
- Be alert to and report early signs of cardiotoxicity (see Appendix F). Acute life-threatening arrhythmias may occur within a few hours of drug administration.
- Report promptly objective signs of hepatic dysfunction (jaundice, dark urine, pruritus) or kidney dysfunction (altered I&O ratio and pattern, local discomfort with voiding).
- Promote fastidious oral hygiene, especially before and after meals. Stomatitis, generally maximal in second week of therapy, frequently begins with a burning sensation accompanied by erythema of oral mucosa that may progress to ulceration and dysphagia in 2 or 3 d.
- Report signs of superinfection (see Appendix F) promptly; these may result from antibiotic therapy during leukopenic period.
- Avoid rectal medications and use of rectal thermometer; rectal trauma is associated with bloody diarrhea resulting from an antiblastic effect on rapidly growing intestinal mucosal cells.

Patient & Family Education

- Note: Complete loss of hair (reversible) is an expected adverse effect. It may also involve eyelashes and eyebrows, beard and mustache, pubic and axillary hair. Regrowth of hair usually begins 2–3 mo after drug is discontinued.
- Drug turns urine red for 1–2 d after administration.
- Keep hands away from eyes to prevent conjunctivitis. Increased tearing for 5–10 d after a single dose is possible.
- Do not breast feed while taking this drug.

D

DOXYCYCLINE HYCLATE

(dox-i-sye′kleen)

Adoxa, Apo-Doxy ✤, Doryx, Doxy, Doxy-Caps, Doxychel, Doxycin ✤, Doxy-Lemmon, Monodox, Novodoxylin ✤, SK-Doxycycline, Vibramycin, Vibra-Tabs, Vivox

Classifications: ANTIINFECTIVE; ANTIBIOTIC; TETRACYCLINE

Prototype: Tetracycline

Pregnancy Category: D

AVAILABILITY 50 mg, 75 mg, 100 mg capsules, tablets; 200 mg injection

ACTIONS Semisynthetic broad-spectrum tetracycline antibiotic derived from oxytetracycline. More completely absorbed with effective blood levels maintained for longer periods and excreted more slowly than most other tetracyclines. Thus it requires smaller and less frequent dosing.

THERAPEUTIC EFFECTS Primarily bacteriostatic in effect. Similar in use to tetracycline (e.g., effective against *chlamydial* and *mycoplasmal* infections; gonorrhea, syphilis, rickettsia).

USES Similar to those of tetracycline, e.g., chlamydial and mycoplasmal infections; gonorrhea, syphilis in penicillin-allergic patients; rickettsial diseases; acute exacerbations of chronic bronchitis.

UNLABELED USES Treatment of acute PID, leptospirosis, prophylaxis for rape victims, suppression and chemoprophylaxis of chloroquine-resistant *Plasmodium falciparum* malaria, short-term prophylaxis and treatment of travelers' diarrhea caused by enterotoxigenic strains of *Escherichia coli*. Intrapleural administration for malignant pleural effusions.

CONTRAINDICATIONS Sensitivity to any of the tetracyclines; use during period of tooth development including last half of pregnancy (category D), lactation, infants, and children <8 y (causes permanent yellow discoloration of teeth, enamel hypoplasia, and retardation of bone growth).
CAUTIOUS USE Alcoholism.

ROUTE & DOSAGE

Antiinfective
Adult: **PO/IV** 100 mg q12h on day 1, then 100 mg/d as single dose (max: 100 mg q12h)
Child: **PO/IV** *>8 y,* 4.4 mg/kg in 1–2 doses on day 1, then 2.2–4.4 mg/kg/d in 1–2 divided doses

Gonorrhea
Adult: **PO** 200 mg immediately, followed by 100 mg h.s., then 100 mg b.i.d. for 3 d

Primary and Secondary Syphilis
Adult: **PO** 300 mg/d in divided doses for at least 10 d

Travelers' Diarrhea
Adult: **PO** 100 mg/d during risk period (up to 2 wk) beginning day 1 of travel

Acne
Adult: **PO** 100 mg q12h on day 1, then 100 mg q.d.
Child: **PO** *>8 y and >45 kg,* 100 mg q12h on day 1, then 100 mg q.d.; *>8 y and <45 kg,* 2.2 mg/kg q12h day 1 then 2.2 mg/kg/q.d.

ADMINISTRATION

Oral
- Check expiration date. Degradation products of tetracycline are toxic to the kidneys.
- Give with food or a full glass of milk to minimize nausea without significantly affecting bioavailability of drug (UNLIKE MOST TETRACYCLINES).
- Consult physician about ordering the oral suspension for patients who are bedridden or have difficulty swallowing.

Intravenous

PREPARE: **Intermittent/Continuous:** Reconstitute by adding 10 mL sterile water for injection, or D5W, NS, LR, D5/LR, or other diluent recommended by manufacturer, to each 100 mg of drug. ▪ Further dilute with 100–1000 mL (per 100 mg of drug) of compatible infusion solution to produce concentrations ranging from 0.1 to 1 mg/mL.

ADMINISTER: **Intermittent/Continuous:** IV infusion rate will usually be prescribed by physician. ▪ Duration of infusion varies with dose but is usually 1–4 h. ▪ Recommended minimum infusion time for 100 mg of 0.5 mg/mL solution is 1 h. Infusion should be completed within 12 h of dilution. ▪ When diluted with LR or D5/LR, infusion must be completed within 6 h to ensure adequate stability. ▪ Protect all solutions from direct sunlight during infusion.

- Store oral and parenteral forms (prior to reconstitution) in tightly covered, light-resistant containers at 15°–30° C (59°–86° F) unless otherwise directed. ▪ Refrigerate reconstituted solutions for up to 72 h. After this time, infusion must be completed within 12 h.

ADVERSE EFFECTS (≥1%) **Special Senses:** Interference with color vision. **GI:** Anorexia, *nausea,* vomiting, diarrhea, enterocolitis; esophageal irritation (oral capsule and tablet). **Skin:** Rashes, photosensitivity reaction. **Other:** Thrombophlebitis (IV use), superinfections.

DIAGNOSTIC TEST INTERFERENCE Like other ***tetracyclines,*** doxycycline may cause false increases in ***urinary catecholamines*** (fluorometric methods); false decreases in ***urinary urobilinogen;*** false-negative ***urine glucose*** with ***glucose oxidase methods*** (e.g., ***Clinistix, TesTape***); parenteral doxycycline (containing ascorbic acid) may cause false-positive determinations using ***Benedict's reagent*** or ***Clinitest.***

INTERACTIONS Drug: ANTACIDS, **iron** preparation, **calcium, magnesium, zinc, kaolin-pectin, sodium bicarbonate** can significantly decrease absorption; effects of both doxycycline and **desmopressin** antagonized; increases **digoxin** absorption, thus increasing risk of **digoxin** toxicity; **methoxyflurane** increases risk of renal failure.

PHARMACOKINETICS Absorption: Completely absorbed from GI tract. **Peak:** 1.5–4 h. **Distribution:** Penetrates eye, prostate, and CSF; crosses placenta; distributed into breast milk. **Metabolism:** Not metabolized. **Elimination:** 20%–30% excreted in urine and 20%–40% in feces in 48 h. **Half-Life:** 14–24 h.

NURSING IMPLICATIONS

Assessment & Drug Effects

- Report sudden onset of painful or difficult swallowing promptly to physician. Doxycycline (capsule and tablet forms) is associated with a comparatively high incidence of esophagitis, especially in patients >40 y.
- Report evidence of superinfections (see Appendix F).

Patient & Family Education

- Take capsule or tablet forms with a full glass (240 mL) of water to ensure passage into stomach and prevent esophageal ulceration. Avoid taking capsule or tablet within 1 h of lying down or retiring.
- Avoid exposure to direct sunlight and ultraviolet light during and for 4 or 5 d after therapy is terminated to reduce risk of phototoxic reaction. Phototoxic reaction appears like an exaggerated sunburn. Sunscreens provide little protection.
- Do not breast feed while taking this drug.

D

DRONABINOL

(droe-nab′i-nol)

Marinol, THC

Classifications: CENTRAL NERVOUS SYSTEM AGENT; ANTIEMETIC; CANNABINOID

Pregnancy Category: B

Controlled Substance: Schedule III

AVAILABILITY 2.5 mg, 5 mg, 10 mg capsules

ACTIONS Synthetic derivative of tetrahydrocannabinol (THC), the principal psychoactive constituent of marijuana *(Cannabis sativa).* Mechanism unclear: Inhibits vomiting through control mechanism in the medulla oblongata, producing potent antiemetic effect; nontherapeutic actions are exactly like those of marijuana. Has complex CNS effect that necessitates close supervision of the patient during drug use. Decreases REM sleep; effect on BP is unpredictable; oral temperature may be decreased, and heart rate may be increased. Risk of drug abuse is high.

THERAPEUTIC EFFECTS Drug produces potent antiemetic effect and is used to treat chemotherapy-induced nausea and vomiting.

USES To treat chemotherapy-induced nausea and vomiting in cancer patients who fail to respond to conventional antiemetic therapy. Appetite stimulant for AIDS patients.

UNLABELED USES Glaucoma.

CONTRAINDICATIONS Nausea and vomiting caused by other than chemotherapeutic agents; hypersensitivity to dronabinol or sesame oil; use during pregnancy (category B) only if clearly necessary; lactation.

CAUTIOUS USE First exposure, especially in the older adult or cardiac patient; hypertension, cardiovascular disorders; epilepsy; psychiatric illness, patient receiving other psychoactive drugs; severe hepatic dysfunction.

ROUTE & DOSAGE

Chemotherapy-induced Nausea

Adult/Child: **PO** 5 mg/m^2 1–3 h before administration of chemotherapy, then q2–4h after chemotherapy for a total of 4–6 doses, dose may be increased by 2.5 mg/m^2 (max: of 15 mg/m^2 if necessary)

Appetite Stimulant

Adult: **PO** 2.5 mg b.i.d., before lunch and dinner

ADMINISTRATION

Oral

- Do not repeat dose following a reaction until patient's mental state has returned to normal and the circumstances have been evaluated.
- Store at 8°–15° C (46°–59° F).

ADVERSE EFFECTS (≥1%) **CNS:** *Drowsiness,* psychologic high, dizziness, anxiety, confusion, euphoria, sensory or perceptual difficulties, impaired coordination, depression, irritability, headache, ataxia, memory lapse, paresthesias, paranoia, depersonalization, disorientation, tinnitus, nightmares, speech difficulty, facial flush, diaphoresis. **CV:** Tachycardia, orthostatic hypotension, hypertension, syncope. **GI:** Dry mouth, diarrhea, fecal incontinence. **Other:** Muscular pains.

INTERACTIONS Drug: Alcohol and other CNS DEPRESSANTS may exaggerate psychoactive effects of dronabinol; TRICYCLIC ANTIDEPRESSANTS, **atropine** may cause tachycardia.

PHARMACOKINETICS Absorption: Rapidly absorbed from GI tract, with bioavailability of 10%–20%. **Peak:** 2–3 h. **Distribution:** Fat soluble; distributed to many organs; distributed into breast milk. **Metabolism:** Metabolized in liver; extensive first-pass metabolism. **Elimination:** Excreted principally in bile; 50% excreted in feces within 72 h; 10%–15% excreted in urine. **Half-Life:** 25–36 h.

NURSING IMPLICATIONS

Assessment & Drug Effects

- Monitor patients with hypertension or heart disease for BP and cardiac status.
- Response to dronabinol is varied, and previous uneventful use does not guarantee that adverse reactions will not occur. Effects of drug may persist an unpredictably long time (days). Extended use at therapeutic dosage may cause accumulation of toxic amounts of dronabinol and its metabolites.
- Watch for disturbing psychiatric symptoms if dose is increased:

Altered mental state, loss of coordination, evidence of a psychologic high (easy laughing, elation and heightened awareness), or depression.

- Note: Abrupt withdrawal is associated with symptoms (within 12 h) of irritability, insomnia, restlessness. Peak intensity occurs at about 24 h: Hot flashes, diaphoresis, rhinorrhea, watery diarrhea, hiccups, anorexia. Usually, syndrome is over in 96 h.

Patient & Family Education

- Do not drive or engage in other potentially hazardous activities that require alertness and judgment because of high incidence of dizziness and drowsiness.
- Understand potential (reversible) for drug-induced mood or behavior changes that may occur during dronabinol use.
- Do not ingest alcohol during period of systemic dronabinol effect. Effect on blood ethanol levels is complex and unpredictable.
- Do not breast feed while taking this drug.

DROPERIDOL

(droe-per'i-dole)

Inapsine

Classifications: CENTRAL NERVOUS SYSTEM AGENT; BUTYROPHENONE; ANTIEMETIC

Prototype: Haloperidol

Pregnancy Category: C

AVAILABILITY 2.5 mg/mL injection

ACTIONS Butyrophenone derivative structurally and pharmacologically related to haloperidol. Antagonizes emetic effects of morphine-like analgesics and other drugs that act on chemoreceptor trigger zone. Mild alpha-adrenergic blocking activity and direct vasodilator effect may cause hypotension. Acts primarily at subcortical level to produce sedation.

THERAPEUTIC EFFECTS Sedative property reduces anxiety and motor activity without necessarily inducing sleep; patient remains responsive. Potentiates other CNS depressants. Also has antiemetic properties.

USES To produce tranquilizing effect and to reduce nausea and vomiting during surgical and diagnostic procedures. Also for premedication, during induction, and as adjunct in maintenance of general or regional anesthesia. Principally used in fixed combination with the potent narcotic analgesic fentanyl (Innovar) to produce neuroleptanalgesia (quiescence, reduced motor activity, and indifference to pain and environmental stimuli) to permit carrying out a variety of diagnostic and minor surgical procedures.

UNLABELED USES IV antiemetic in cancer chemotherapy.

CONTRAINDICATIONS Known intolerance to droperidol. Safe use during pregnancy (category C), lactation, or in children <2 y is not established.

CAUTIOUS USE Older adult, debilitated, and other poor-risk patients; Parkinson's disease; hypotension; liver, kidney, cardiac disease; cardiac bradyarrhythmias.

ROUTE & DOSAGE

Premedication

Adult: **IV/IM** 2.5–10 mg 30–60 min preoperatively

Child: **IV/IM** *2–12 y,* 0.088–0.165 mg/kg 30–60 min preoperatively

D

Maintenance of General Anesthesia

Adult: **IV/IM** *Induction*, 0.22–0.275 mg/kg; *Maintenance*, 1.25–2.5 mg
Child: **IV/IM** *2–12 y*, 0.088–0.165 mg/kg

ADMINISTRATION

Intramuscular

- Give deep IM into a large muscle.

Intravenous

IV administration to infants and children: Verify correct rate of IV injection with physician.

PREPARE: **Direct:** Give undiluted.

ADMINISTER: **Direct:** Give at a rate of 10 mg or fraction thereof over 30–60 s.

INCOMPATIBILITIES **Solution/additive: Fluorouracil, furosemide, heparin, leucovorin, methotrexate, pentobarbital. Y-site: Fluorouracil, furosemide, heparin, leucovorin, methotrexate, nafcillin.**

- Store at 15°–30° C (59°–86° F), unless otherwise directed by manufacturer. Protect from light.

ADVERSE EFFECTS (≥1%) **CNS:** *Postoperative drowsiness, extrapyramidal symptoms:* dystonia, akathisia, oculogyric crisis; dizziness, restlessness, anxiety, hallucinations, mental depression. **CV:** *Hypotension, tachycardia,* irregular heartbeats *(prolonged QTc interval even at low doses)*. **Other:** Chills, shivering, laryngospasm, bronchospasm.

PHARMACOKINETICS Onset: 3–10 min. **Peak:** 30 min. **Duration:** 2–4 h; may persist up to 12 h. **Distribution:** Crosses placenta. **Metabolism:** Metabolized in liver. **Elimination:** Excreted in urine and feces.

NURSING IMPLICATIONS

Assessment & Drug Effects

- Monitor ECG throughout therapy. Report immediately prolongation of QTc interval.
- Monitor vital signs closely. Hypotension and tachycardia are common adverse effects.
- Exercise care in moving medicated patients because of possibility of severe orthostatic hypotension. Avoid abrupt changes in position.
- Observe patients for signs of impending respiratory depression carefully when receiving a concurrent narcotic analgesic carefully.
- Note: EEG patterns are slow to return to normal during the postoperative period.
- Observe carefully and report promptly to physician early signs of acute dystonia: Facial grimacing, restlessness, tremors, torticollis, oculogyric crisis. Extrapyramidal symptoms may occur within 24–48 h postoperatively.
- Note: Droperidol may aggravate symptoms of acute depression.

Patient & Family Education

- Do not breast feed while taking this drug without consulting physician.

DROTRECOGIN ALFA (ACTIVATED)

(dro-tree′co-gin)

Xigris

Classifications: IMMUNOMODULATOR; RECOMBINANT HUMAN ACTIVATED PROTEIN C

Pregnancy Category: C

AVAILABILITY 5 mg, 20 mg vials

ACTIONS Drotrecogin alfa is a recombinant form of Human Activated Protein C. Protein C deficiencies are found in most septic patients and result in a higher mortality rate. Activated Protein C exerts antithrombotic and anticoagulant effects by inhibiting clotting Factor Va and VIIIa. Activated Protein C may exert an antiinflammatory effect by inhibiting human tumor necrosis factor (TNF) produced by monocytes, and by limiting the thrombin-induced inflammatory responses of the endothelial lining of the vasculature.

THERAPEUTIC EFFECTS Drotrecogin alfa possesses anticoagulant, profibrinolytic and antiinflammatory properties.

USES Reduction in mortality in patients with severe sepsis and evidence of organ dysfunction.

CONTRAINDICATIONS Prior hypersensitivity to drotrecogin alfa; chronic severe hepatic disease; active internal bleeding or trauma; recent hemorrhagic stroke (within 3 months); invasive surgery or invasive procedures; recent intracranial or intraspinal surgery, or severe head trauma (within 2 mo); intracranial neoplasm, lesion, aneurysm, or herniation; presence of an epidural catheter; pregnancy (category C), lactation.

CAUTIOUS USE Immunosuppression; increased risk of bleeding, hypercoagulability; concurrent use of anticoagulants, or aspirin; children <18; recent ischemic stroke, or intracranial aneurysm.

ROUTE & DOSAGE

Sepsis

Adult: **IV** 24 mcg/kg/h continuous infusion for 96 h

ADMINISTRATION

Intravenous

PREPARE: **Continuous:** Prepare immediately prior to use. Reconstitute 5 mg or 20 mg vials with 2.5 mL or 10 mL, respectively, of sterile water for injection to yield approximate concentration of 2 mg/mL. Slowly add sterile water to vial, avoid inverting or shaking vial, gently swirl until powder is completely dissolved. Slowly withdraw calculated dose from vial, add to infusion bag of NS by directing stream to side of bag to minimize agitation, then gently invert to mix. Final concentration should be 100–200 mcg/mL. Do not transport infusion bag between locations attached to mechanical pump. Note: When using a syringe pump, solution is typically diluted to a final concentration of 100–1000 mcg/mL.

ADMINISTER: **Continuous:** Give over 96 h. Dose adjustment based on clinical or laboratory parameters is not recommended. IV must be completed within 12 h after solution is prepared.

INCOMPATIBILITIES **Solution/additive:** Do not mix with any other drugs. **Y-site:** Do not infuse with any other drugs.

- Storage: Reconstituted vial may be held at 15°–30° C (59°–86° F), but must be used within 3 h of preparation.

ADVERSE EFFECTS (≥1%) **Hematologic:** *Bleeding* (including intracranial).

DIAGNOSTIC TEST INTERFERENCE May affect the ***APTT assay.*** This interference may result in an apparent factor concentration that is lower than the true concentration.

INTERACTIONS Drug: ANTICOAGULANTS, NSAIDS, ANTIPLATELET AGENTS may increase risk of bleeding.

PHARMACOKINETICS Absorption: Steady state reached in 2 h. **Dura-**

tion: Serum levels undetectable 2 h after end of infusion. **Half-Life:** 1.6 h.

NURSING IMPLICATIONS

Assessment & Drug Effects

- Monitor closely for S&S of hemorrhage. Stop infusion immediately should clinically important bleeding occur. There is no antidote for drotrecogin alfa.
- Discontinue drotrecogin alfa 2 h prior to invasive procedures with an inherent risk of bleeding. Reinitiation may be reconsidered 12 h after major invasive procedure or immediately after uncomplicated less invasive procedures.
- Lab tests: Monitor closely PT; APTT is not a reliable indication of coagulation.

DULOXETINE HYDROCHLORIDE

(du-lox′e-teen)

Cymbalta

Classifications: CENTRAL NERVOUS SYSTEM AGENT; PSYCHOTHERAPEUTIC AGENT; ANTIDEPRESSANT; SEROTONIN NOREPINEPHRINE REUPTAKE INHIBITOR (SNRI)

Prototype: Venlafaxine

Pregnancy Category: C

AVAILABILITY 20 mg, 30 mg, 60 mg capsules

ACTIONS Exact mechanism of action in controlling depression or pain is unknown. As a selective serotonin and norepinephrine reuptake inhibitor (SSNRI), duloxetine causes potentiation of serotonergic and noradrenergic activity in the CNS.

THERAPEUTIC EFFECTS Antidepressant effect is presumed to be due to its dual inhibition of CNS presynaptic neuronal uptake of serotonin and norepinephrine, thus increasing the serum levels of both substances.

USES Treatment of major depression, diabetic peripheral neuropathy.

UNLABELED USES Stress urinary incontinence.

CONTRAINDICATIONS MAOI therapy; uncontrolled narrow-angle glaucoma; abrupt discontinuation; pregnancy (category C), lactation. Safety and efficacy in children <18 y not established.

CAUTIOUS USE Anorexia nervosa, history of mania, history of suicidal ideation; cardiac or hepatic disease; renal impairment or renal failure; hypertension.

ROUTE & DOSAGE

Depression

Adult: **PO** 40–60 mg/d in one or two divided doses

Diabetic Neuropathy

Adult: **PO** 40–60 mg/d in one or two divided doses

ADMINISTRATION

Oral

- Do not initiate therapy within 14 d of the last dose of an MAOI.
- Must be swallowed whole. Do not cut, chew, or crush. Do not sprinkle on food or mix with liquids.
- Store at 15°–30° C (59°–86° F).

ADVERSE EFFECTS (≥1%) **Body as a Whole:** Fatigue, hot flashes. **CNS:** Dizziness, somnolence, tremor, *insomnia.* **GI:** *Nausea, dry mouth, constipation,* diarrhea, vomiting. **Metabolic:** Decreased appetite, weight loss. **Skin:** Increased sweating. **Special Senses:** Blurred vision. **Urogenital:** Decreased libido, abnormal orgasm, erectile dysfunction, ejaculatory dysfunction.

INTERACTIONS Drug: Alcohol may result in increased liver function tests; MAOIS may result in hyperthermia, rigidity, mental status changes, myoclonus, autonomic instability, features resembling neuroleptic malignant syndrome; **cimetidine, fluoxetine, fluvoxamine, paroxetine, quinidine,** QUINOLONES may increase levels and half-life of duloxetine; may increase levels and toxicity of **thioridazine,** TRICYCLIC ANTIDEPRESSANTS. **Amphetamine, dextroamphetamine, buspirone, cocaine, dexfenfluramine, fenfluramine, lithium, phentermine, sibutramine, nefazodone,** SSRIS, TRIPTANS, **tramadol, trazodone** may cause serotonin syndrome. **Herbal: St. John's Wort, tryptophan** may cause serotonin syndrome.

PHARMACOKINETICS Peak: 6 h. **Metabolism:** Metabolized in the liver by CYP2D6 and CYP1A2. **Elimination:** 70% excreted in urine, 20% excreted in feces. **Half-Life:** 12 h (8–17 h).

NURSING IMPLICATIONS

Assessment & Drug Effects

- Ensure that a complete list of all concurrent medications is obtained.
- Monitor for S&S of numerous drug-drug interactions (see Interaction section).
- Monitor closely for and report suicide ideation, especially when drug is initiated or dosage changed.
- Report emergence of any of the following: anxiety, agitation, panic attacks, insomnia, irritability, hostility, psychomotor restlessness, hypomania, and mania.
- Monitor BP, especially in those being treated for hypertension.

Patient & Family Education

- The beneficial effects of this drug may not be felt for approximately 4 wk.
- Report any of the following: suicidal ideation (especially early in treatment or when dosage is changed), palpitations, anxiety, hyperactivity, agitation, panic attacks, insomnia, irritability, hostility, restlessness.
- Do not abruptly discontinue taking this drug. Notify physician if side effects are bothersome.
- Avoid or minimize use of alcohol while taking this drug.
- Do not self-treat for coughs, colds, or allergies. Consult physician.
- Do not breast feed while taking this drug.

DUTASTERIDE

(du-tas'ter-ide)

Avodart

Classifications: HORMONES & SYNTHETIC SUBSTITUTES; ANTIANDROGEN; 5-ALPHA REDUCTASE INHIBITOR

Prototype: Finasteride

Pregnancy Category: X

AVAILABILITY 0.5 mg capsules

ACTIONS Specific inhibitor of the steroid 5-alpha-reductase, an enzyme necessary to convert testosterone into the potent androgen 5-alpha-dihydrotestosterone (DHT) in the prostate gland.

THERAPEUTIC EFFECTS Decreases the production of testosterone in the prostate gland.

USES Treatment of benign prostatic hypertrophy (BPH).

UNLABELED USES Treatment of male pattern baldness.

CONTRAINDICATIONS Hypersensitivity to dutasteride or finasteride;

pregnancy (category X), lactation, and children.
CAUTIOUS USE Hepatic impairment, obstructive uropathy.

D

ROUTE & DOSAGE

BPH
Adult: **PO** 0.5 mg once daily
Male Pattern Baldness
Adult: **PO** 0.25–0.5 mg once daily

ADMINISTRATION

Oral
- Do not handle capsules if you are or may become pregnant because of the potential for absorption of dutasteride and the subsequent risk to a developing male fetus.
- Do not open or crush capsules. They must be swallowed whole.
- Store at 15°–30° C (59°–86° F).

ADVERSE EFFECTS (≥1%) **Endocrine:** Gynecomastia. **Urogenital:** Ejaculation dysfunction, impotence, decreased libido.

INTERACTIONS Drug: Diltiazem, verapamil may decrease clearance of dutasteride. **Herbal:** May see exaggerated effects with **Saw Palmetto.**

PHARMACOKINETICS Absorption: Rapidly absorbed. 60% bioavailability. **Peak:** 2–3 h. **Distribution:** 99% protein bound. **Metabolism:** Metabolized in liver by CYP3A4 to one active and 2 inactive metabolites. **Elimination:** Primarily excreted in feces. **Half-Life:** 5 weeks.

NURSING IMPLICATIONS

Assessment & Drug Effects
- Monitor voiding patterns, assessing for ease of starting a stream, frequency, and urgency.
- Lab tests: Monitor baseline PSA and again at 3–6 mo to establish new baseline to use to assess potentially cancer-related changes in PSA. After 6 mo of treatment, obtained PSA values should be doubled for comparison with normal values in untreated men.

Patient & Family Education
- Do not donate blood until at least 6 mo following last dose to prevent administration of dutasteride to a pregnant female transfusion recipient.
- Ejaculate volume might be decreased during treatment but this does not seem to interfere with normal sexual function.
- Note that the incidence of most drug-related sexual adverse events (impotence, decreased libido, and ejaculation disorder) typically decrease with duration of treatment.

DYCLONINE HYDROCHLORIDE

(dye-kloe-neen)
Dyclone
Classifications: CENTRAL NERVOUS SYSTEM AGENT; ANESTHETIC, LOCAL (MUCOSAL); ANTIPRURITIC
Prototype: Procaine
Pregnancy Category: C

AVAILABILITY 0.5% solution

ACTIONS Synthetic local topical anesthetic agent. Unrelated to amide derivatives.
THERAPEUTIC EFFECTS Produces local anesthesia by blocking impulses at peripheral nerve endings in skin and mucous membranes.

USES Topical anesthesia of mucous membranes preparatory for endoscopic examinations and gynecologic and proctologic procedures. Also to suppress gag reflex, to relieve pain of minor burns or trauma, and to alleviate itching of pruritus ani or vulvae.

UNLABELED USES To provide relief from discomfort of fever blisters.

CONTRAINDICATIONS Cystoscopic procedures following IV pyelography (because contrast media containing iodine may precipitate and interfere with visualization); applications to extensive areas or to bleeding surfaces. Safe use during pregnancy (category C) is not established.

CAUTIOUS USE Debilitated or older adult patients, children, lactation, patients with drug sensitivities or family history of allergies; severe trauma or sepsis in region of application.

ROUTE & DOSAGE

Topical Anesthesia

Adult: **Topical** Apply 0.5–1% solution by swabbing, gargling, spray, instillation, wet compress, or rinse

Before Urologic Endoscopy

Adult: **Topical** Instill 30–60 mL of 0.5–1% solution into urethra and retain 5–10 min before procedure

ADMINISTRATION

Topical

- Use to relieve pain of esophageal lesions; 5–15 mL of 0.5% dyclonine solution may be swallowed as prescribed.
- Avoid contact with eyes or eyelids. Also avoid applications to large areas.
- Store at 15°–30° C (59°–86° F) in tight, light-resistant container unless otherwise directed.

ADVERSE EFFECTS (≥1%) **Body as a Whole:** Systemic absorption (nervousness, dizziness, drowsiness, excitement or depression, tremors, *seizures*, blurred vision). **CV:** Hypotension, bradycardia, cardiac or respiratory arrest. **Skin:** Urticaria, edema, contact dermatitis (local): burning, tenderness, swelling, irritation, urethritis.

DIAGNOSTIC TEST INTERFERENCE Dyclonine may interfere with visualization in cystoscopic procedures by causing precipitation of iodine in ***contrast media.***

PHARMACOKINETICS Absorption: Absorbed through skin and mucous membranes. **Onset:** 2–10 min. **Duration:** Up to 1 h.

NURSING IMPLICATIONS

Assessment & Drug Effects

- Do not give patient anything by mouth within 60 min (until return of gag reflex) following drug administration. Drug may interfere with second stage of swallowing when applied orally.
- Test gag reflex by gently stroking soft palate with a cotton swab (while holding tongue down with a depressor). If patient does not gag or swallow, give nothing by mouth. Suctioning secretions as necessary to prevent aspiration.
- Note: A sip of clear water should be the first thing swallowed when gag reflex returns.

Patient & Family Education

- Understand suppression of gag reflex and appropriate safety CAUTIOUS USE.
- Do not breast feed while taking this drug without consulting physician.

D

DYPHYLLINE

(dye'fi-lin)

Dilor, Dyflex, Dyline-GG, Lufyllin, Neothylline, Protophylline ♣, Thylline

Classifications: BRONCHODILATOR; RESPIRATORY SMOOTH MUSCLE RELAXANT; XANTHINE

Prototype: Theophylline

Pregnancy Category: C

AVAILABILITY 200 mg, 400 mg tablets; 100 mg/15 mL, 160 mg/15 mL elixir; 250 mg/mL injection

ACTIONS Xanthine and derivative of theophylline with which it shares similar pharmacologic effects: bronchodilation, myocardial stimulation, vasodilation, diuresis, and smooth muscle relaxation. Unlike other xanthines, dyphylline is not metabolized to theophylline in body; therefore serum theophylline levels are not useful.

THERAPEUTIC EFFECTS Drug has bronchodilator effects.

USES Acute bronchial asthma and reversible bronchospasm associated with chronic bronchitis and emphysema.

CONTRAINDICATIONS Hypersensitivity to xanthine compounds; apnea in newborns. Safe use during pregnancy (category C) or lactation is not established.

CAUTIOUS USE Severe cardiac disease, hypertension, acute myocardial injury; renal or hepatic dysfunction; glaucoma; hyperthyroidism; peptic ulcer; in the older adults or children; concomitant administration of other xanthine formulations or other CNS-stimulating drugs.

ROUTE & DOSAGE

Asthma

Adult: **PO** 200–800 mg q6h up to 15 mg/kg q.i.d. **IM** 250–500 mg q6h (max: 15 mg/kg q.i.d.)
Child: **PO/IM** ≥6 y, 4.4–6.6 mg/kg/d in divided doses

ADMINISTRATION

Oral

- Give oral preparation with a full glass of water on an empty stomach (e.g., 1 h before or 2 h after meals) to enhance absorption. However, administration after meals may help to relieve gastric discomfort.
- Exercise care in the amount of elixir given to children because it has a high alcohol content (18%–20%).

Intramuscular

- Aspirate carefully before injecting and inject slowly. Give deep IM into a large muscle.
- Do not use parenteral form if a precipitate is present.
- Store at 15°–30° C (59°–86° F) unless otherwise directed. Protect dyphylline injection from light.

ADVERSE EFFECTS (≥1%) **CNS:** Headache, irritability, restlessness, dizziness, insomnia, light-headedness, muscle twitching, <u>convulsions</u>. **CV:** Palpitation, *tachycardia,* extrasystoles, flushing, hypotension. **GI:** *Nausea,* vomiting, diarrhea, anorexia, epigastric distress. **Respiratory:** Tachypnea. **Other:** Albuminuria, fever, dehydration.

INTERACTIONS Drug: BETA BLOCKERS may antagonize bronchodilating effects of dyphylline; **halothane** increases risk of cardiac arrhythmias; **probenecid** may decrease dyphylline elimination.

PHARMACOKINETICS Absorption: Readily absorbed from GI tract. **Peak:** 1 h. **Metabolism:** Metabolized in liver (but not to theophylline). **Elimination:** Excreted in urine. **Half-Life:** 2 h.

NURSING IMPLICATIONS

Assessment & Drug Effects

- Lab tests; Baseline and periodic pulmonary function tests to assess therapeutic effectiveness.
- Monitor therapeutic effectiveness; usually occurs at a blood level of at least 12 mcg/mL.
- Note: Toxic dyphylline plasma levels, although rare with normal dosage, are a risk in patients with a diminished capacity for dyphylline clearance, e.g., those with CHF or hepatic impairment or who are >55 y or <1 y of age.

Patient & Family Education

- Take medication consistently with or without food at the same time each day.
- Notify physician of adverse effects: Nausea, vomiting, insomnia, jitteriness, headache, rash, severe GI pain, restlessness, convulsions, or irregular heartbeat.
- Avoid alcohol and also large amounts of coffee and other xanthine-containing beverages (e.g., tea, cocoa, cola) during therapy.
- Consult physician before taking OTC preparations. Many OTC drugs for coughs, colds, and allergies contain ephedrine or other sympathomimetics and xanthines (e.g., caffeine, theophylline, aminophylline).
- Do not breast feed while taking this drug without consulting physician.

ECHOTHIOPHATE IODIDE

(ek-oh-thye′oh-fate)

Phospholine Iodide

Classifications: EYE PREPARATION; MIOTIC (ANTIGLAUCOMA AGENT)

Prototype: Pilocarpine HCl

Pregnancy Category: C

AVAILABILITY 1.5 mg, 3 mg, 6.25 mg, 12.5 mg powder for reconstitution

See Appendix A-1.

ECONAZOLE NITRATE

(e-kone′a-zole)

Ecostatin ♣, Spectazole

Classifications: ANTIINFECTIVE; ANTIBIOTIC; ANTIFUNGAL

Prototype: Fluconazole

Pregnancy Category: C

AVAILABILITY 1% cream

ACTIONS Synthetic imidazole derivative with broad antifungal spectrum of activity similar to that of miconazole. Exerts fungistatic action but may be fungicidal for certain microorganisms.

THERAPEUTIC EFFECTS Active against dermatophytes (including *Trichophyton mentagrophytes, T. rubrum, T. tonsurans, Epidermophyton floccosum, Microsporum audouini, M. canis*), yeasts [e.g., *Candida albicans, Pityrosporum obiculare (tinea versicolor)*], and many other genera of fungi. Also appears to be active against some gram-positive bacteria (e.g., *Staphylococcus aureus, Streptococcus pyogenes, Corynebacterium diphtheriae*). Clinical improvement occurs within the first 1–2 wk of therapy.

USES Topically for treatment of *tinea pedis* (athlete's foot or ringworm of foot), *tinea cruris* ("jock itch" or ringworm of groin), *tinea corporis* (ringworm of body), *tinea versicolor*, and *cutaneous candidiasis* (moniliasis).

UNLABELED USES Has been used for topical treatment of erythrasma and with corticosteroids for fungal or bacterial dermatoses associated with inflammation.

CONTRAINDICATIONS Safety during pregnancy (category C) or lactation is not established.

ROUTE & DOSAGE

Tinea Cruris, Tinea Corporis, Tinea Pedis, Cutaneous Candidiasis

Adult/Child: **Topical** Apply sufficient amount to affected areas twice daily, morning and evening

Tinea Versicolor

Adult: **Topical** Apply sufficient amount to affected areas once daily

ADMINISTRATION

Topical

- Cleanse skin with soap and water and dry thoroughly before applying medication (unless otherwise directed by physician). Wash hands thoroughly before and after treatments.
- Do not use occlusive dressings unless prescribed by physician.
- Store at less than 30° C (86° F) unless otherwise directed.

ADVERSE EFFECTS (≥1%) **Skin:** Burning, stinging sensation, pruritus, erythema.

INTERACTIONS Drug: No clinically significant interactions established.

PHARMACOKINETICS Absorption: Minimal percutaneous absorption through intact skin; increased absorption from denuded skin. **Peak:** 0.5–5 h. **Elimination:** <1% of applied dose is eliminated in urine and feces.

NURSING IMPLICATIONS

Patient & Family Education

- Use medication for the prescribed time even if symptoms improve and report to physician skin reactions suggestive of irritation or sensitization.
- Notify physician if full course of therapy does not result in improvement. Diagnosis should be reevaluated.
- Do not to apply the topical cream in or near the eyes or intravaginally.
- Do not breast feed while using this drug without consulting physician.

EDETATE CALCIUM DISODIUM

(ed′e-tate)

Calcium Disodium Versenate, Calcium EDTA

Classification: CHELATING AGENT

Pregnancy Category: C

AVAILABILITY 200 mg/mL injection

ACTIONS Chelating agent that combines with divalent and trivalent metals to form stable, nonionizing soluble complexes that can be readily excreted by kidneys. Action is dependent on ability of heavy metal to displace the less strongly bound calcium in the drug molecule.

THERAPEUTIC EFFECTS Chelating agent that binds with heavy metals such as lead to form a soluble complex which can be excreted through the kidney, thereby ridding the body of the poisonous substance.

USES Principally as adjunct in treatment of acute and chronic lead poisoning (plumbism). Generally used in combination with dimercaprol (BAL) in treatment of lead encephalopathy or when blood lead level exceeds 100 mcg/dL. Also used to diagnose suspected lead poisoning.
UNLABELED USES Treatment of poisoning from other heavy metals such as chromium, manganese, nickel, zinc, and possibly vanadium; removal of radioactive and nuclear fission products such as plutonium, yttrium, uranium. Not effective in poisoning from arsenic, gold, or mercury.

CONTRAINDICATIONS Severe kidney disease, anuria; IV use in patients with lead encephalopathy not generally recommended (because of possible increase in intracranial pressure); pregnancy (category C).
CAUTIOUS USE Kidney dysfunction; active tubercular lesions; history of gout; lactation.

ROUTE & DOSAGE

Diagnosis of Lead Poisoning

Adult: **IV/IM** 500 mg/m^2 (max: 1 g) over 1 h, then collect urine for 24 h (if mcg lead:mg EDTA ratio in urine is >1, the test is positive)
Child: **IM** 50 mg/kg (max: 1 g), then collect urine for 6–8 h, (if mcg lead:mg EDTA ratio in urine is >0.5, the test is positive)

Treatment of Lead Poisoning

Adult/Child: **IV** 1–1.5 g/m^2/d infused over 8–24 h for up to 5 d
IM 1–1.5 g/m^2/d divided q8–12 h

Lead Nephropathy/Renal Impairment

Adult: **IV** Serum creatinine <2 mg/dL 1 g/m^2/d, 2–3 mg/dL 500 mg/m^2/d, 3.1–4 mg/dL 400 mg/m^2 q48h, >4 mg/dL 500 mg/m^2 once/wk. Infuse over 8–24 h for 5 d, may repeat monthly until lead excretion is reduced toward normal

ADMINISTRATION

Note: Calcium disodium edetate can produce potentially fatal effects when higher than recommended doses are used or when it is continued after toxic effects appear.

Intramuscular

- IM route preferred for symptomatic children and recommended for patients with incipient or overt lead-induced encephalopathy.
- Add Procaine HCl to minimize pain at injection site (usually 1 mL of procaine 1% to each 1 mL of concentrated drug). Consult physician.
- Use separate injections sites when dimercaprol (BAL) and Calcium EDTA are given concurrently.

Intravenous

PREPARE: **IV Infusion:** Dilute the 5 mL ampule with 250–500 mL of NS or D5W.
ADMINISTER: **IV Infusion:** Warning: Rapid IV infusion may be LETHAL by suddenly increasing intracranial pressure in patients who already have cerebral edema. Manufacturer recommends total daily dose over 8–12 h. Some clinicians recommend infusing over 1–2 h. Consult physician for specific rate.
INCOMPATIBILITIES **Solution/additive: Amphotericin B, hydralazine, Ringer's Lactate.**

ADVERSE EFFECTS (≥1%) **CV:** Hypotension, thrombophlebitis. **GI:** Anorexia, nausea, vomiting, diar-

E

rhea, abdominal cramps, cheilosis. **Hematologic:** Transient bone marrow depression, depletion of blood metals. **Urogenital:** Nephrotoxicity (renal tubular necrosis), proteinuria, hematuria. **Body as a Whole:** *Febrile reaction* (excessive thirst, fever, chills, severe myalgia, arthralgia, GI distress), *histamine-like reactions* (flushing, throbbing headache, sweating, sneezing, nasal congestion, lacrimation, postural hypotension, tachycardia).

DIAGNOSTIC TEST INTERFERENCE Edetate calcium disodium may decrease ***serum cholesterol, plasma lipid*** levels (if elevated), and ***serum potassium*** values. ***Glycosuria*** may occur with toxic doses.

INTERACTIONS Drug: No clinically significant interactions established.

PHARMACOKINETICS Absorption: Well absorbed IM. **Onset:** 1 h. **Peak:** Peak chelation 24–48 h. **Distribution:** Distributed to extracellular fluid; does not enter CSF. **Metabolism:** Not metabolized. **Elimination:** Chelated lead excreted in urine; 50% excreted in 1 h. **Half-Life:** 20–60 min IV, 90 min IM.

NURSING IMPLICATIONS

Assessment & Drug Effects

- Determine adequacy of urinary output prior to therapy. This may be done by administering IV fluids before giving first dose.
- Increase fluid intake to enhance urinary excretion of chelates. Avoid excess fluid intake, however, in patients with lead encephalopathy because of the danger of further increasing intracranial pressure. Consult physician regarding allowable intake.
- Monitor I&O. Since drug is excreted almost exclusively via kidneys, toxicity may develop if output is inadequate. Stop therapy if urine flow is markedly diminished or absent. Report any change in output or I&O ratio to physician.
- Lab tests: Obtain serum creatinine, calcium, and phosphorus before and during each course of therapy. Monitor baseline and frequent BUN levels and ECG during therapy. With prolonged therapy determine periodic determinations of blood trace element metals (e.g., copper, zinc, magnesium).
- Be alert for occurrence of febrile reaction that may appear 4–8 h after drug infusion (see ADVERSE EFFECTS).

Patient & Family Education

- Do not breast feed while taking this drug without consulting physician.

EDROPHONIUM CHLORIDE

(ed-roe-foe′nee-um)

Enlon, Reversol, Tensilon

Classifications: AUTONOMIC NERVOUS SYSTEM AGENT; CHOLINERGIC (PARASYMPATHOMIMETIC) CHOLINESTERASE INHIBITOR

Prototype: Neostigmine

Pregnancy Category: C

AVAILABILITY 10 mg/mL injection

ACTIONS Indirect-acting cholinesterase inhibitor similar to neostigmine that is rapidly reversible. Acts as antidote to curariform drugs by displacing them from muscle cell receptor sites, thus permitting resumption of normal transmission of neuromuscular impulses. Like neostigmine, it prolongs skeletal muscle relaxant action of succinylcholine chloride and decamethonium bromide.

THERAPEUTIC EFFECTS Acts as antidote to curariform drugs by displacing them from muscle cell receptor sites, thus permitting resumption of normal transmission of neuromuscular impulses.

USES Differential diagnosis and as adjunct in evaluation of treatment requirements of myasthenia gravis, for differentiating myasthenic from cholinergic crisis, and to reverse neuromuscular blockade produced by overdosage of nondepolarizing skeletal muscle relaxants, e.g., tubocurarine, gallamine. Not recommended for maintenance therapy in myasthenia gravis because of its short duration of action.

UNLABELED USES To terminate paroxysmal atrial tachycardia, as an aid in diagnosing supraventricular tachyarrhythmias, and to evaluate function of demand pacemakers.

CONTRAINDICATIONS Hypersensitivity to anticholinesterase agents; intestinal and urinary obstruction. Safety during pregnancy (category C) or lactation is not established.

CAUTIOUS USE Bronchial asthma; cardiac arrhythmias; patients receiving digitalis.

ROUTE & DOSAGE

Edrophonium Test for Myasthenia Gravis

Adult: **IV** Prepare 10 mg in a syringe; inject 2 mg over 15–30 s, if no reaction after 45 s, inject the remaining 8 mg, may repeat test after 30 min **IM** Inject 10 mg, if cholinergic reaction occurs, retest after 30 min with 2 mg to rule out false-negative reaction

Child: **IV** *≤34 kg,* 1 mg, if no response after 45 s, dose may be titrated up to 5 mg **IM** 2 mg **IV** *>34 kg,* 2 mg, if no response after 45 s, dose may be titrated up to 10 mg **IM** 5 mg

Infant: **IM** 0.5–1 mg

Evaluation of Myasthenia Treatment

Adult: **IV** 1–2 mg administered 1 h after last PO dose of anticholinesterase medication

Curare Antagonist

Adult: **IV** 10 mg administered over 30–45 s, may repeat q5–10 min as needed up to 40 mg

ADMINISTRATION

Note: Have antidote (atropine sulfate) immediately available and facilities for endotracheal intubation, tracheostomy, suction, assisted respiration, and cardiac monitoring for treatment of cholinergic reaction.

Intravenous

PREPARE: **Direct:** May be given undiluted.

ADMINISTER: **Direct:** USE for diagnosis of MG—Inject 2 mg (adult & child >34 kg) or 1 mg (child ≤34 kg) over 15–30 s; if no reaction after 45 s, inject additional 8 mg (adult) or titrate up to a total of 8 mg additional (child >34 kg) or titrate in 1 mg increments up to a total of 4 mg additional (child ≤34 kg), may repeat test after 30 min. If cholinergic reaction (increased muscle weakness) is obtained after initial 1 or 2 mg, discontinue test and give atropine IV (as ordered).

- Note: Some clinicians recommend giving a 1–2 mg test dose of edrophonium to older adult patients, to those with history of heart disease or who take digitalis, and possibly to all patients.

E

ADVERSE EFFECTS (≥1%) **Body as a Whole:** Severe adverse effects uncommon with usual doses. **CNS:** Weakness, muscle cramps, dysphoria, fasciculations, incoordination, dysarthria, dysphagia, convulsions, respiratory paralysis. **CV:** Bradycardia, irregular pulse, hypotension, pulmonary edema. **Special Senses:** Miosis, blurred vision, diplopia, lacrimation. **GI:** Diarrhea, abdominal cramps, nausea, vomiting, excessive salivation. **Respiratory:** Increased bronchial secretions, bronchospasm, laryngospasm, pulmonary edema. **Other:** Excessive sweating, urinary frequency, incontinence.

INTERACTIONS Drug: Procainamide, quinidine may antagonize the effects of edrophonium; DIGITALIS GLYCOSIDES increase the sensitivity of the heart to edrophonium; **succinylcholine, decamethonium** may prolong neuromuscular blockade.

PHARMACOKINETICS Onset: 30–60 s IV; 2–10 min IM. **Duration:** 5–10 min IV; 5–30 min IM.

NURSING IMPLICATIONS

Assessment & Drug Effects

- Monitor vital signs. Observe for signs of respiratory distress. Patients >50 y are particularly likely to develop bradycardia, hypotension, and cardiac arrest.
- Edrophonium test for myasthenia gravis: All cholinesterase inhibitors (anticholinesterases) should be discontinued for at least 8 h before test. Positive response to edrophonium test consists of brief improvement in muscle strength unaccompanied by lingual or skeletal muscle fasciculations.
- Evaluation of myasthenic treatment: *Myasthenic response* (immediate subjective improvement with increased muscle strength, absence of fasciculations; generally indicates that patient requires larger dose of anticholinesterase agent or longer-acting drug); *Cholinergic response* muscarinic adverse effects (lacrimation, diaphoresis, salivation, abdominal cramps, diarrhea, nausea, vomiting; accompanied by decrease in muscle strength; usually indicates over-treatment with cholinesterase inhibitor); *Adequate response* (no change in muscle strength; fasciculations may be present or absent; minimal cholinergic adverse effects (observed in patients at or near optimal dosage level).

Patient & Family Education

- Do not breast feed while taking this drug without consulting physician.

EFALIZUMAB

(e-fal-i-zoo′-mab)
Raptiva
Classifications: BIOLOGIC RESPONSE MODIFIER; MONOCLONAL ANTIBODY
Prototype: Basiliximab
Pregnancy Category: C

AVAILABILITY 125 mg vial

ACTIONS An anti-CD11a antibody that targets this receptor subunit on the surface of T-lymphocytes; inhibits binding of T-cells to endothelial cells, prevents migration of T-cells out of the blood stream into the skin, and prevents activation of T-cells. Lymphocyte activation and movement to skin play a key role in the pathophysiology of chronic plaque psoriasis.

THERAPEUTIC EFFECTS Prevents activation of T-cells and their migration out of the circulatory system to sites of inflammation, thus slowing processes that result in plaque psoriasis.

USES Treatment of moderate to severe plaque psoriasis.

CONTRAINDICATIONS Hypersensitivity to efalizumab; severe infection or exposure to viral infections (e.g., chicken pox, herpes zoster), live vaccines; pregnancy (category C); lactation.
CAUTIOUS USE History of untoward reactions to other monoclonal antibodies.

ROUTE & DOSAGE

Plaque Psoriasis
Adult: **SC** 0.7 mg/kg first dose, then 1 mg/kg (max: 200 mg) once weekly

ADMINISTRATION

Subcutaneous

- Note: A reduced initial dose is used to prevent first dose reaction including headache, fever, nausea, and vomiting.
- Reconstitute immediately before use. Inject 1.3 mL of the supplied diluent (using prefilled syringe with sterile water for injection) slowly into vial. Swirl gently to dissolve but DO NOT SHAKE; dissolves in >5 min. Should be clear to pale yellow and free of particulates.
- Replace needle on syringe used for reconstitution with a new needle. Insert needle into vial keeping needle below the level of the liquid; withdraw the required dose.
- Inject SC into thigh, abdomen, buttocks, or upper arm. Rotate sites.
- If reconstituted vial is not used immediately, store at room temperature but use within 8 h.
- Store powder vials at 2°–8° C (36°–46° F). Protect from light.

ADVERSE EFFECTS (≥1%) **Body as a Whole:** First dose reaction (headache, fever, nausea, vomiting, myalgia), increased risk of *infection* or reactivation of latent infection, *chills,* pain, myalgia, flu syndrome, asthenia, hypersensitivity reactions, peripheral edema. **CNS:** *Headache.* **GI:** *Nausea.* **Hematologic:** Thrombocytopenia. **Musculoskeletal:** Arthralgia. **Skin:** Worsening of psoriasis, acne, urticaria.

INTERACTIONS Drug: Do not administer live or live-attenuated VACCINES; increased risk of immunosuppression with other IMMUNOSUPPRESSANTS.

PHARMACOKINETICS Absorption: 50% absorbed from SC site. **Peak:** Steady-state levels reached in 4 wk. **Elimination:** Drug eliminated approximately 25 d after last steady-state dose.

NURSING IMPLICATIONS

Assessment & Drug Effects

- Monitor for S&S of infection. Withhold drug and notify physician if infection is suspected.
- Lab tests: Periodic platelet counts.

Patient & Family Education

- Seek immediate medical attention for bleeding from gums, bruising, petechiae (numerous small red spots on skin), or S&S of an infection (fever, abscess, sore throat with breathing difficulty, etc.), or worsening of psoriasis.
- Do not accept a live virus vaccine without consulting physician.
- Notify physician immediately if you become pregnant while taking this drug, or within 6 wk of last dose of drug.
- Do not breast feed while taking this drug without consulting physician.

E

EFAVIRENZ

(e-fa′vi-renz)

Sustiva

Classifications: ANTIINFECTIVE; ANTIVIRAL AGENT; NONNUCLEOSIDE REVERSE TRANSCRIPTASE INHIBITOR (NNRTI)

Prototype: Nevirapine

Pregnancy Category: C

AVAILABILITY 50 mg, 100 mg, 200 mg capsules; 300 mg, 600 mg tablets

ACTIONS Nonnucleoside reverse transcriptase inhibitor (NNRTI) of HIV-1. Binds directly to reverse transcriptase and blocks RNA polymerase activities.

THERAPEUTIC EFFECTS Prevents replication of the HIV-1 virus. HIV-2 reverse transcriptase and DNA polymerases alpha, beta, gamma, and delta are not inhibited by efavirenz. Resistant strains appear rapidly. Effectiveness indicated by reduction in viral load (plasma HIV RNA).

USES HIV-1 infection in combination with other antiretroviral agents.

CONTRAINDICATIONS Hypersensitivity to efavirenz; pregnancy (category C), lactation.

CAUTIOUS USE Liver disease, alcoholism, hepatitis, hypertriglyceridemia, hypercholesterolemia, substance abuse, antimicrobial resistance, bipolar disorder, depression, suicidal ideation, exfoliative dermatitis; females of childbearing age, CNS disorders. Safety and efficacy in children <3 y old or who weigh <13 kg (29 lb) are not known.

ROUTE & DOSAGE

HIV Infection

Adult: **PO** 600 mg q.d.
Child: **PO** *≥3 y, 10–15 kg,* 200 mg q.d.; *15–20 kg,* 250 mg q.d.; *20–25 kg,* 300 mg q.d.; *25–32.5 kg,* 350 mg q.d.; *32.5–40 kg,* 400 mg q.d.; *>40 kg,* 600 mg q.d.

ADMINISTRATION

Oral

- Use bedtime dosing to increase tolerability of CNS adverse effects.
- Give exactly as ordered. Do not skip a dose or discontinue therapy without consulting the physician.
- Do not give efavirenz following a high fat meal.
- Store at 15°–30° C (59°–86° F) in a tightly closed container and protect from light.

ADVERSE EFFECTS (≥1%) **Body as a Whole:** Fatigue, fever. **CNS:** Dizziness, headache, hypoesthesia, impaired concentration, insomnia, abnormal dreams, somnolence, depression, nervousness, adverse psychiatric experiences. **CV:** Hypercholesterolemia. **GI:** *Nausea,* vomiting, *diarrhea,* dyspepsia, abdominal pain, flatulence, anorexia, increased liver function tests (ALT, AST). **Respiratory:** Cough. **Skin:** *Rash* (erythematous rash, pruritus, *maculopapular rash,* <u>erythema multiforme, Stevens–Johnson syndrome, toxic epidermal necrolysis</u>), increased sweating. **Urogenital:** Renal calculus, hematuria.

DIAGNOSTIC TEST INTERFERENCE False-positive urine tests for **marijuana.**

INTERACTIONS Drug: Decreased concentrations of **clarithromycin, indinavir, nelfinavir, saquinavir, voriconazole;** increased concentrations of **ritonavir, azithromycin, ethinyl estradiol.** Efavirenz levels are increased by **ritonavir, fluconazole** and decreased by **saquinavir, rifampin.** Additional drugs not recommended for administration with efavirenz include **astemizole, midazolam, triazolam, cisapride,**

ERGOT DERIVATIVES, **warfarin.** **Herbal: St. John's wort** may decrease antiretroviral activity.

PHARMACOKINETICS Peak: 5 h; steady-state 6–10 d. **Distribution:** 99% protein bound. **Metabolism:** Metabolized in liver by cytochrome P450 3A4 and 2B6; can induce (increase) its own metabolism. **Elimination:** 14%–34% excreted in urine, 16%–61% excreted in feces. **Half-Life:** 52–76 h after single dose, 40–55 h after multiple doses.

NURSING IMPLICATIONS

Assessment & Drug Effects

- Monitor GI status and evaluate ability to maintain a normal diet.
- Lab tests: Periodic liver functions and lipid profile.

Patient & Family Education

- Contact physician promptly if any of the following occurs: skin rash, delusions, inappropriate behavior, thoughts of suicide.
- Use or add barrier contraception if using hormonal contraceptive.
- Notify physician immediately if you become pregnant.
- Do not drive or engage in potentially hazardous activities until response to the drug is known. Dizziness, impaired concentration, and drowsiness usually improve with continued therapy.
- Do not breast feed while taking this drug.

EFLORNITHINE HYDROCHLORIDE

(e-flor'ni-theen)

Vaniqa

Classifications: SKIN AND MUCOUS MEMBRANE AGENT; DERMATOLOGICAL AGENT

Pregnancy Category: C

AVAILABILITY 13.9% cream

ACTIONS Inhibits enzyme activity in the skin that is required for hair growth.

THERAPEUTIC EFFECTS Results in retarding the rate of hair growth.

USES Reduction of unwanted facial hair in women.

CONTRAINDICATIONS Hypersensitivity to eflornithine or its components; lactation, children <12 y.

CAUTIOUS USE Pregnancy (category C).

ROUTE & DOSAGE

Hair Removal

Adult: **Topical** Apply thin layer to affected areas of the face and adjacent involved areas under the chin and rub in thoroughly b.i.d. at least 8 h apart

ADMINISTRATION

Topical

- Apply thin layer to affected skin areas on face and under chin and rub in thoroughly.
- Do not wash treated areas for at least 4 h after application.
- Store at 15°–30° C (59°–86° F).

ADVERSE EFFECTS (≥1%) **Body as a Whole:** Facial edema. **CNS:** Dizziness. **GI:** Dyspepsia, anorexia. **Skin:** *Acne, pseudofolliculitis barbae,* stinging, burning, pruritus, erythema, tingling, irritation, rash, alopecia, folliculitis, ingrown hair.

INTERACTIONS No clinically significant interactions established.

PHARMACOKINETICS Absorption: <1% absorbed through intact skin. **Metabolism:** Not metabolized. **Elimination:** Excreted primarily in urine. **Half-Life:** 8 h.

E

NURSING IMPLICATIONS

Assessment & Drug Effects

- Monitor for and report skin irritation.
- Note: Drug slows growth of facial hair, but is not a depilatory.

Patient & Family Education

- Note: Effect of drug is usually not apparent for 4–8 wks.
- Reduce frequency of drug application to once daily if skin irritation occurs. If irritation continues, contact physician.
- Do not breast feed while using this drug.

ELETRIPTAN HYDROBROMIDE

(e-le-trip'tan)
Relpax
Classifications: AUTONOMIC NERVOUS SYSTEM AGENT; 5-HT_1 SEROTONIN AGONIST
Prototype: Sumatriptan
Pregnancy Category: C

AVAILABILITY 20 mg, 40 mg tablets

ACTIONS Eletriptan is a potent agonist at central serotonin 5-HT_{1B}, 5-HT_{1D}, and 5-HT_{1F} receptors, and has modest affinity for 5-HT_{1A}, 5-HT_{1E}, 5-HT_{2B}, and 5-HT_7 receptors. Eletriptan stimulates presynaptic 5-HT_{1D} receptors inhibiting dural vasodilation and agonizes vascular 5-HT_{1B} receptors causing vasoconstriction of intracranial extracerebral vessels.
THERAPEUTIC EFFECTS Inhibits dural vasodilation and inflammation, and causes vasoconstriction of painfully dilated intracranial extracerebral vessels, thus relieving the migraine headache. Also relieves photophobia, phonophobia, and nausea and vomiting associated with migraine attacks.

USES Treatment of acute migraine attacks with or without aura.

CONTRAINDICATIONS Hypersensitivity to eletriptan; CVA or TIA; within 24 hours of administering of another ergotamine; pregnancy (category C), lactation within 24 hours after dose; children <18 y; severe hepatic insufficiency; hemiplegic or basilar migraine; ischemic heart disease; peripheral vascular disease; uncontrolled hypertension.
CAUTIOUS USE Hypotension in the elderly; lactation; mild to moderate hepatic impairment; ischemic or vasospastic coronary artery disease; diabetes, obesity, smoking, high cholesterol; history of coronary artery disease; men over 40 years of age; postmenopausal women. Use within 72 h of potent CYP3A4 metabolizing drugs.

ROUTE & DOSAGE

Acute Migraine
Adult: **PO** 20 mg or 40 mg at onset of migraine (max: 40 mg/dose and 80 mg/day), may repeat dose in 2 h if partial response
Geriatric: Use not recommended

Hepatic Impairment
Use not recommended in severe hepatic impairment

ADMINISTRATION

Oral

- Give one tablet as soon as the migraine begins.
- May give 2nd tablet if headache improves but returns after 2 h.
- If 1st tablet is ineffective, do not give a 2nd without consulting physician.
- Do not give within 72 h of potent CYP3A4 inhibitors (see INTERACTIONS).

- Store at 15°–30° C (59°–86° F). Protect from light and moisture

ADVERSE EFFECTS (≥1%) **Body as a Whole:** *Asthenia,* paresthesia, flushing, back pain, chills. **CNS:** Dizziness, drowsiness, headache, somnolence, hypertonia, hypesthesia. **CV:** Chest tightness/pressure, palpitation, hypertension. The following are rare, usually seen in patients with cardiovascular disease risk factors: Coronary vasospasm, transient myocardial ischemia, MI, ventricular tachycardia, atrial fibrillation, ventricular fibrillation. **GI:** Abdominal pain, dyspepsia, dysphagia, nausea, vomiting, dry mouth. **Respiratory:** Pharyngitis. **Skin:** Sweating.

INTERACTIONS Drug: Drugs that inhibit CYP3A4 may increase eletriptan levels and toxicity, do not administer eletriptan within 72 h of AZOLE ANTIFUNGALS (especially **itraconazole, ketoconazole, voriconazole**), **amiodarone, cimetidine, dalfopristin, quinupristin, diltiazem, metronidazole, nicardipine, norfloxacin, quinine, verapamil, zafirlukast, zileuton,** MACROLIDE ANTIBIOTICS, NONNUCLEOTIDE REVERSE TRANSCRIPTASE INHIBITORS, PROTEASE INHIBITORS, SELECTIVE SEROTONIN REUPTAKE INHIBITORS, **sibutramine;** ERGOT ALKALOIDS may prolong vasospastic adverse reactions (do not use within 24 h of ergot-containing drugs); do not administer within 24 h of other 5-HT_1 AGONISTS (may cause increased adverse effects). **Food: Grapefruit juice** may increase eletriptan levels and toxicity. **Herbal: Gingko, ginseng, echinacea, St. John's wort** may increase triptan toxicity.

PHARMACOKINETICS Absorption: Rapidly absorbed, 50% reaches systemic circulation. **Onset:** 1–2 h. **Peak:** 1.5 h. **Distribution:** 85% protein bound. **Metabolism:** Metabolized in liver by CYP3A4. **Elimination:** 90% cleared by nonrenal routes, 9% eliminated in urine. **Half-Life:** 4–5 h.

NURSING IMPLICATIONS

Assessment & Drug Effects

- Monitor CV status carefully following first dose in patients at risk for coronary artery disease (e.g., history of hypertension, postmenopausal women, men >40 y, persons with known CAD risk factors) or who have coronary artery vasospasms.
- Report immediately chest pain, tightness in chest or throat that is severe or does not quickly resolve following a dose of eletriptan.
- Monitor therapeutic effectiveness. Pain relief is usually achieved within 1 h.

Patient & Family Education

- Note: If first dose is ineffective, do not take a second dose as it will not work for the same attack.
- Inform physician of all prescription, nonprescription, and herbal drugs you are taking. Do not add additional drugs without informing physician as many drugs interact with eletriptan.
- Report promptly any of the following: headache more severe than usual, migraine; dizziness, faintness, blurred vision; chest, neck, or throat pain; irregular heart beat, palpitations; shortness of breath, wheezing, difficulty breathing; tingling, pain, or numbness in the face, hands, or feet; seizures; severe stomach pain, cramping, or bloody diarrhea.
- Do not drive or engage in any potentially hazardous task until reaction to drug is known.
- Do not breast feed without consulting physician.

E

EMEDASTINE DIFUMARATE

(em-e-das'teen di-foom'a-rate)
Emadine
Classifications: EYE, EAR, NOSE AND THROAT (EENT) PREPARATION; ANTIHISTAMINE; OCULAR
Prototype: Levocabastine
Pregnancy Category: C

AVAILABILITY 0.05% solution

See Appendix A-1.

EMLA (EUTECTIC MIXTURE OF LIDOCAINE AND PRILOCAINE)

EMLA cream
Classifications: CENTRAL NERVOUS SYSTEM AGENT; LOCAL ANESTHETIC
Prototype: Procaine
Pregnancy Category: B

AVAILABILITY 2.5% lidocaine/2.5% prilocaine cream

ACTIONS EMLA cream is a mixture of lidocaine and prilocaine. The mixture forms a liquid at room temperature. Concentration of anesthetic in liquid versus an emulsifier is 80% versus 20%.
THERAPEUTIC EFFECTS EMLA is a topical analgesic.

USES Topical anesthetic on normal intact skin for local anesthesia.
UNLABELED USES Topical anesthetic prior to leg ulcer debridement; treatment of postherpetic neuralgia.

CONTRAINDICATIONS Patients with known sensitivity to local anesthetics; patients with congenital or idiopathy methemoglobinemia.
CAUTIOUS USE Acutely ill, debilitated, or older adult patients; severe liver disease; pregnancy (category B), lactation; children <7 years of age.

ROUTE & DOSAGE

Topical Anesthetic
Adult/Child: **Topical** *>1 mo,* Apply 2.5 g of cream (1/2 of 5-g tube) over 20–25 cm^2 of skin, cover with occlusive dressing and wait at least 1 h, then remove dressing and wipe off cream, cleanse area with an antiseptic solution and prepare patient for the procedure

ADMINISTRATION

Topical
- Apply a thick layer to skin (approximately 1/2 of 5-g tube per 20–25 cm^2 or 2 × 2 in) at site of procedure. Apply an occlusive dressing. Do not spread out cream. Seal edges of dressing well to avoid leakage.
- Apply EMLA cream 1 h before routine procedure and 2 h before painful procedure.
- Remove EMLA cream prior to skin puncture and clean area with an aseptic solution.
- Store at room temperature 15°–30° C (59°–86° F).

ADVERSE EFFECTS (≥1%) **Hematologic:** Methemoglobinemia, especially in infants, small children, and patients with G6PD deficiency. **Skin:** *Blanching and redness,* itching, heat sensation. **Body as a Whole:** Edema, soreness, aching, numbness, heaviness. **Other:** The adverse effects of lidocaine could occur with large doses or if there is significant systemic absorption.

INTERACTIONS Drug: May cause additive toxicity with CLASS I ANTIARRHYTHMICS; may increase risk of developing methemoglobin when used with **acetaminophen, chlo-**

roquine, dapsone, fosphenytoin, NITRATES and NITRITES, **nitric oxide, nitrofurantoin, nitroprusside, pamaquine, phenobarbital, phenytoin, primaquine, quinine,** or SULFONAMIDES.

PHARMACOKINETICS Absorption: Penetrates intact skin. **Onset:** 15–60 min. **Peak:** 2–3 h. **Duration:** 1–2 h after removal of cream. **Distribution:** Crosses blood–brain barrier and placenta, distributed into breast milk. **Metabolism:** Metabolized in liver. **Elimination:** 98% of absorbed dose is excreted in urine. **Half-Life:** 60–150 min.

NURSING IMPLICATIONS

Assessment & Drug Effects

- Monitor for local skin reactions including erythema, edema, itching, abnormal temperature sensations, and rash. These reactions are very common and usually disappear in 1–2 h.
- Note: Patients taking Class 1 antiarrhythmic drugs may experience toxic effects on the cardiovascular system. EMLA should be used with caution in these patients.
- Wash immediately with water or saline if contact with the eye occurs; protect the eye until sensation returns.

Patient & Family Education

- Skin analgesia lasts for 1 h following removal of the occlusive dressing. Analgesia may be accompanied by temporary loss of all sensation in the treated skin. Advise caution until sensation returns.
- Do not breast feed while using this drug without consulting physician.

EMTRICITABINE

(em-tri′ci-ta-been)
Emtriva
Classifications: ANTI-INFECTIVE; ANTIRETROVIRAL; NUCLEOSIDE REVERSE TRANSCRIPTASE INHIBITOR (NRTI)
Prototype: Zidovudine
Pregnancy Category: B

AVAILABILITY 200 mg capsules

ACTIONS Emtricitabine is a synthetic nucleoside analogue with inhibitory activity against HIV. It inhibits HIV-1 reverse transcriptase (RT), both by competing with the natural DNA nucleoside and by incorporation into viral DNA, which terminates the formation of the viral DNA chain.
THERAPEUTIC EFFECTS The viral load is decreased as measured by an increase in CD4 leukocyte count and suppression of viral RNA.

USES Treatment of HIV in combination with other antiretroviral agents
UNLABELED USES Treatment of chronic hepatitis B in HIV-positive patients

CONTRAINDICATIONS Safety and efficacy in children and elderly are not established; lactation.
CAUTIOUS USE Renal impairment, and with end-stage renal disease; pregnancy (category B).

ROUTE & DOSAGE

HIV
Adult: **PO** 200 mg once/d

Renal Impairment
Cl_{cr} 30–49 mL/min: 200 mg q48h; 15–29 mL/min: 200 mg q72h; <15 mL/min: 200 mg q96h

ADMINISTRATION

Oral

- Give at the same time daily.
- Store between 15°–30° C (59°–86° F) in a tightly closed container.

E

ADVERSE EFFECTS (≥1%) **Body as a Whole:** Asthenia, neuropathy, peripheral neuritis. **CNS:** *Headache,* depression, dizziness, insomnia. **GI:** *Diarrhea, nausea,* dyspepsia, abdominal pain, hepatomegaly. **Metabolic:** Lactic acidosis. **Musculoskeletal:** Arthralgia, myalgia, paresthesias. **Respiratory:** Cough, rhinitis. **Skin:** *Rash,* hyperpigmentation of palms and soles of feet.

INTERACTIONS None yet reported.

PHARMACOKINETICS Absorption: 93% reaches systemic circulation. **Peak:** 1–2 h. **Distribution:** 4% protein bound. **Metabolism:** Metabolized in liver. **Elimination:** Urine. **Half-Life:** 10 h (active metabolite has intracellular half-life of 39 h).

NURSING IMPLICATIONS

Assessment & Drug Effects

- Note: Persons with a detectable viral load to be switched from lamivudine to emtricitabine should have genotypic testing to determine whether the M184 mutation is present.
- Monitor closely for S&S of lactic acidosis, especially in persons with known risk factors such as female gender, obesity, alcoholism, or hepatic disease.
- Withhold drug and notify physician if S&S suggestive of lactic acidosis or hepatotoxicity occur.
- Lab tests: Baseline renal function tests; frequent LFTs and serum electrolytes during the last trimester of pregnancy; complete blood chemistry if lactic acidosis is suspected; and periodic lipid profile.

Patient & Family Education

- Inform physician, prior to taking this drug, if you have used lamivudine and developed resistance to it.
- Report any of the following to the physician: difficulty breathing, shortness of breath, fast or irregular heartbeat; weight gain with fullness around waist and/or face; vomiting or diarrhea; unexplained muscle aches, pains, weakness, or fatigue; yellow eyes or skin.
- Avoid alcoholic drinks while taking this drug.
- Do not self-treat nausea, vomiting, or stomach pain. Contact physician for guidance.
- Do not breast feed while taking this drug.

ENALAPRIL MALEATE

(e-nal'a-pril)

Vasotec

ENALAPRILAT

Vasotec I.V.

Classifications: CARDIOVASCULAR AGENT; ANGIOTENSIN-CONVERTING ENZYME (ACE) INHIBITOR; ANTIHYPERTENSIVE

Prototype: Captopril

Pregnancy Category: D

AVAILABILITY 2.5 mg, 5 mg, 10 mg, 20 mg tablets; 1.25 mg/mL injection; 1 mg/mL suspension

ACTIONS Angiotensin-converting enzyme (ACE) inhibitor. ACE catalyzes the conversion of angiotensin I to angiotensin II, a vasoconstrictor substance. Therefore, inhibition of ACE decreases angiotensin II levels, which decreases vasopressor activity and aldosterone secretion. Both actions achieve an antihypertensive effect by suppression of the renin–angiotensin–aldosterone sys-

tem. ACE inhibitors also reduce peripheral arterial resistance (afterload), pulmonary capillary wedge pressure (PCWP), a measure of preload, pulmonary vascular resistance, and improve cardiac output as well as exercise tolerance.
THERAPEUTIC EFFECTS Antihypertensive effect related to suppression of the renin-angiotensin-aldosterone system causes vasodilation and, therefore, lower blood pressure. Improvement in cardiac output results in increased exercise tolerance.

USES Management of mild to moderate hypertension as monotherapy or with a diuretic. Malignant, refractory, accelerated, and renovascular hypertension (except in bilateral renal artery stenosis or renal artery stenosis in a solitary kidney), CHF.
UNLABELED USES Hypertension or renal crisis in scleroderma.

CONTRAINDICATIONS Hypersensitivity to enalapril or captopril. There has been evidence of fetotoxicity and kidney damage in newborns exposed to ACE inhibitors during pregnancy (category D). Safety during lactation or in children is not established.
CAUTIOUS USE Renal impairment, renal artery stenosis; patients with hypovolemia, receiving diuretics, undergoing dialysis; patients in whom excessive hypotension would present a hazard (e.g., cerebrovascular insufficiency); CHF; hepatic impairment; diabetes mellitus.

ROUTE & DOSAGE

Hypertension

Adult: **PO** 5 mg/d, may increase to 10–40 mg/d in 1–2 divided doses **IV** 1.25 q6h, may give up to 5 mg q6h in hypertensive emergencies
Neonate: **PO** 0.1 mg/kg q24h **IV** 5–10 mcg/kg q8–24h
Child: **PO** 0.08 mg/kg/d in 1–2 divided doses, may increase (max: 5 mg/kg/d) **IV** 5–10 mcg/kg q8–24h

Congestive Heart Failure

Adult: **PO** 2.5 mg 1–2 times/d, may increase up to 5–20 mg/d in 1–2 divided doses (max: 40 mg/d)

ADMINISTRATION

Oral

- Discontinue diuretics, if possible, for 2–3 d prior to initial oral dose to reduce incidence of hypotension. If the diuretic cannot be discontinued, give an initial dose of 2.5 mg. Keep patient under medical supervision for at least 2 h and until BP has stabilized for at least an additional hour.
- Give with food or drink of patient's choice.
- Protect from heat and light. Expiration date: 30 mo following date of manufacture if stored at <30° C.
- Conversion from IV to oral therapy: Recommended initial dose is 5 mg once a day with a creatinine clearance of (Cl_{cr}) >30 mL/min, and 2.5 mg once daily with a Cl_{cr} <30 mL/min.
- Store tablets at 30° C (86° F); protect from heat and light.

Intravenous

Note: Verify correct IV concentration and rate of infusion/injection with physician for neonates, infants, children.

PREPARE: **Direct:** Give undiluted. **Intermittent:** Dilute in 50 mL of D5W, NS, D5/NS, D5/LR.
ADMINISTER: **Direct/Intermittent:** Give direct IV slowly over at least 5 min through a port of a

free flowing infusion of D5W or NS or as an infusion over 5 min. ***INCOMPATIBILITIES*** **Y-site: amphotericin B, amphotericin B cholesteryl, cefepime, phenytoin.**

E

ADVERSE EFFECTS (≥1%) **CNS:** *Headache, dizziness,* fatigue, nervousness, paresthesias, asthenia, insomnia, somnolence. **CV:** *Hypotension including postural hypotension;* syncope, palpitations, chest pain. **GI:** Diarrhea, nausea, abdominal pain, loss of taste, dyspepsia. **Hematologic:** Decreased Hgb and Hct. **Urogenital:** Acute kidney failure, deterioration in kidney function. **Skin:** Pruritus with and without *rash,* angioedema, erythema. **Metabolic:** Hyperkalemia. **Respiratory:** Cough.

INTERACTIONS Drug: Indomethacin and other NSAIDS may decrease antihypertensive activity; POTASSIUM SUPPLEMENTS, POTASSIUM-SPARING DIURETICS may cause hyperkalemia; may increase **lithium** levels and toxicity.

PHARMACOKINETICS Absorption: 70% absorbed from GI tract. **Onset:** 1 h PO; 15 min IV. **Peak:** 4–8 h PO; 4 h IV. **Duration:** 12–24 h PO; 6 h IV. **Distribution:** Limited amount crosses blood–brain barrier; crosses placenta. **Metabolism:** Oral dose undergoes first-pass metabolism in liver to active form, enalaprilat. **Elimination:** 60% excreted in urine, 33% in feces within 24 h. **Half-Life:** 2 h.

NURSING IMPLICATIONS

Assessment & Drug Effects

- Monitor for therapeutic effectiveness. Peak effects after the first IV dose may not occur for up to 4 h; peak effects of subsequent doses may exceed those of the first.
- Maintain bedrest and monitor BP for the first 3 h after the initial IV dose. First-dose phenomenon (i.e., a sudden exaggerated hypotensive response) may occur within 1–3 h of first IV dose, especially in the patient with very high blood pressure or one on a diuretic and controlled salt intake regimen. An IV infusion of normal saline for volume expansion may be ordered to counteract the hypotensive response. This initial response is not an indicator to stop therapy.
- Monitor BP for first several days of therapy. If antihypertensive effect is diminished before 24 h, the total dose may be given as 2 divided doses.
- Report transient hypotension with lightheadedness. Older adults are particularly sensitive to drug-induced hypotension. Supervise ambulation until BP has stabilized.
- Lab tests: Monitor serum potassium and be alert to symptoms of hyperkalemia (K^+ >5.7 mEq/L). Patients who have diabetes, impaired kidney function, or CHF are at risk of developing hyperkalemia during enalapril treatment. Monitor kidney function closely during first few weeks of therapy.

Patient & Family Education

- Full antihypertensive effect may not be experienced until several weeks after enalapril therapy starts.
- When drug is discontinued due to severe hypotension, the hypotensive effect may persist a week or longer after termination because of long duration of drug action.
- Do not follow a low-sodium diet (e.g., low-sodium foods or low-sodium milk) without approval from physician.
- Avoid use of salt substitute (principal ingredient: potassium salt) and potassium supplements be-

cause of the potential for hyperkalemia.

- Notify physician of a persistent nonproductive cough, especially at night, accompanied by nasal congestion.
- Report to physician promptly if swelling of face, eyelids, tongue, lips, or extremities occurs. Angioedema is a rare adverse effect and, if accompanied by laryngeal edema, may be fatal.
- Do not drive or engage in other potentially hazardous activities until response to drug is known.
- Do not breast feed while taking this drug without consulting physician.

ENFUVIRTIDE

(en-fu-vir'tide)

Fuzeon

Classifications: ANTIVIRAL; ANTIRETROVIRAL; FUSION INHIBITOR

Pregnancy Category: B

AVAILABILITY 90 mg/mL injection

ACTIONS Enfuvirtide interferes with entry of HIV-1 into host cells by inhibiting fusion of the virus and cell membranes. For HIV-1 to enter and infect a human cell, the viral surface glycoprotein gp120 must bind to the host CD4+ cell. Then, the viral glycoprotein gp41 undergoes a change in shape facilitating the fusion of viral membranes with the cell. Enfuvirtide binds to viral envelope glycoprotein and prevents the change in shape required for membrane fusion and viral entry into target cells.

THERAPEUTIC EFFECTS Prevents entry of the HIV-1 virus into host cells.

USES Treatment of advanced HIV disease with evidence of resistance to other therapies.

CONTRAINDICATIONS Hypersensitivity to enfuvirtide or any of its components; lactation.

CAUTIOUS USE Pregnancy (category B); renal and hepatic impairment; renal clearance of <35 mL/min; bacterial pneumonia, low initial CD4 count, past history of lung disease, high initial viral load, IV drug use. Safety and efficacy have not been established in children <6 y.

ROUTE & DOSAGE

Advanced HIV Disease

Adult/Adolescent: **SC** *≥16 y or ≥42.6 kg,* 90 mg b.i.d.

Child/Adolescent: **SC** *6–16 y or <42.6 kg,* 2 mg/kg (up to 90 mg) b.i.d.

ADMINISTRATION

Subcutaneous

- Reconstitute by adding 1.1 mL sterile water for injection into vial. Mix by gently tapping vial for 10 sec, then gently rolling in palms of hands. Ensure that no drug is remaining on vial wall. Allow vial to stand until powder completely dissolves (up to 45 min). Solution should be clear, colorless, and without bubbles or particulate matter.
- Bring refrigerated reconstituted solution to room temperature before injection. Ensure that powder is fully dissolved and solution is clear, colorless, and without bubbles or particulate matter.
- Inject into upper arm, abdomen, or anterior thigh.
- Rotate injection sites and inject in an area with no current injection site reaction.
- Store unreconstituted vials at 15°–30° C (59°–86° F) or refriger-

ated at 2°–6° C (3°–46° F); do not freeze.

ADVERSE EFFECTS (≥1%) **Body as a Whole:** *Injection site reactions (pain, induration, erythema, nodules, cysts, pruritus, ecchymoses),* infection at injection site, *fatigue,* hypersensitivity reactions, Guillain-Barre syndrome, asthenia, herpes simplex infections, influenza, lymphadenopathy, myalgia, peripheral neuropathy. **CNS:** Anxiety, depression, *insomnia.* **GI:** *Diarrhea, nausea,* abdominal pain, anorexia, constipation, dysgeusia, pancreatitis, weight loss. **Hematologic:** Eosinophilia, anemia. **Metabolic:** Increased amylase, increased lipase, increased ALT and AST, hypertriglyceridemia. **Respiratory:** Bacterial pneumonia, acute respiratory distress syndrome, cough, sinusitis. **Skin:** Pruritus, skin papilloma. **Special Senses:** Conjunctivitis. **Urogenital:** Glomerulonephritis.

INTERACTIONS None yet reported.

PHARMACOKINETICS Absorption: 84.3% absorbed from SC site. **Peak:** Average 4–8 h. **Distribution:** 92% protein bound. **Metabolism:** Catabolized into constituent amino acids. **Half-Life:** 4 h.

NURSING IMPLICATIONS

Assessment & Drug Effects

- Inspect SC sites for S&S of site reactions (e.g., itching, swelling, redness, pain, tenderness, or hardened skin) that usually last for <7 d postinjection.
- Monitor closely for S&S of pneumonia, especially with low initial CD4 count, high initial viral load, IV drug use, smoking, or prior history of lung disease.
- Lab tests: Periodic LFTs, serum lipase and amylase, lipid profile, and CBC with differential.

Patient & Family Education

- Report promptly S&S of infection at SC injection sites: increased heat, redness, pain, or oozing.
- Report promptly S&S of pneumonia: cough with fever, rapid breathing, shortness of breath.
- Do not breast feed while taking this drug.

ENOXACIN

(e-nox'a-sin)

Penetrex

Classifications: ANTIINFECTIVE; ANTIBIOTIC; QUINOLONE

Prototype: Ciprofloxacin

Pregnancy Category: X

AVAILABILITY 200 mg, 400 mg tablets

ACTIONS Synthetic quinolone broad-spectrum antibiotic. Inhibits DNA-gyrase, an enzyme necessary for bacterial DNA replication and some aspects of transcription, repair, recombination, and transposition.

THERAPEUTIC EFFECTS Effective against *Neisseria gonorrhoeae, Escherichia coli, Staphylococcus epidermidis, Staphylococcus saprophyticus, Klebsiella pneumoniae, Proteus mirabilis, Pseudomonas aeruginosa,* and *Enterobacter cloacae.*

USES Uncomplicated urethral or cervical gonorrhea and uncomplicated and complicated urinary tract infections due to susceptible organisms.

UNLABELED USES Ear, nose, and throat infections, lower respiratory tract infections, and skin infections.

CONTRAINDICATIONS Known hypersensitivity to enoxacin, ciprofloxacin, or other quinolones; pregnant women (category X), lactation, and children.

CAUTIOUS USE Severe renal impairment and known or suspected CNS disorders.

ROUTE & DOSAGE

Urinary Tract Infections
Adult: **PO** 200–400 mg q12h for 7–14 d
Uncomplicated Gonorrhea
Adult: **PO** 400 mg single dose
Renal Impairment
CL_{cr} ≤30 mL/min: Reduce dose by 50%

ADMINISTRATION

Oral
- Give 1 h before or 2 h after meals.
- Keep patient well hydrated.
- Lower dose for patients with renal impairment according to Cl_{cr}.

ADVERSE EFFECTS (≥1%) **CNS:** Headache, hallucinations, seizures. **GI:** Nausea, vomiting, gastric pain. **Skin:** Rash, photosensitivity.

DIAGNOSTIC TEST INTERFERENCE May cause false positive on ***opiate screening tests.***

INTERACTIONS Drug: Ranitidine may decrease enoxacin levels by 40% when given 2 h before enoxacin. Enoxacin decreases **theophylline** clearance by at least 50%, thus increasing theophylline levels and toxicity. ALUMINUM- AND MAGNESIUM-CONTAINING ANTACIDS may decrease the absorption of enoxacin.

PHARMACOKINETICS Absorption: Readily absorbed from GI tract; 90% of dose reaches systemic circulation. **Peak:** Serum, 1–2 h; urine, 2.5–7 h. **Distribution:** Widely distributed including blister fluid, middle ear fluid, and prostatic tissue; crosses placenta; distributed into breast milk. **Metabolism:** 15%–20% of dose metabolized in liver. **Elimination:** 26%–72% excreted in urine within 72 h. **Half-Life:** 3–6 h.

NURSING IMPLICATIONS

Assessment & Drug Effects
- Lab tests: Determine C&S prior to initial dose. Treatment may be started pending results.
- Discontinue the drug immediately and notify physician for hypersensitivity reaction, including skin rash or other allergic response; may occur after just one dose.
- Monitor for increased digoxin level and possible toxicity with concurrent digoxin administration.
- Monitor patients with seizure disorders carefully, since enoxacin may lower the seizure threshold.

Patient Education
- Discontinue drug and notify physician promptly at first sign of an allergic response.
- Restrict caffeine intake; enoxacin may reduce rate of caffeine clearance, producing insomnia, nervousness, tachycardia.
- Phototoxicity may occur with excessive exposure to sunlight.
- Do not breast feed while taking this drug.

ENOXAPARIN Pr

(e-nox'a-pa-rin)
Lovenox
Classifications: BLOOD FORMERS, COAGULATORS, AND ANTICOAGULANTS; LOW MOLECULAR WEIGHT HEPARIN
Pregnancy Category: B

AVAILABILITY 30 mg/0.3 mL, 40 mg/0.4 mL, 60 mg/0.6 mL, 80 mg/0.8 mL, 100 mg/1 mL injection

E

ACTIONS Low molecular weight heparin with antithrombotic properties. Does not affect PT. Does affect thrombin time (TT) and activated thromboplastin time (aPTT) up to 1.8 times the control value.

THERAPEUTIC EFFECTS Antithrombotic properties are due to its antifactor Xa and antithrombin (antifactor IIa) in the coagulation activities. An effective anticoagulation agent; used for prophylactic treatment as an antithrombotic agent following certain types of surgery.

USES Prevention of deep vein thrombosis (DVT) after hip, knee, or abdominal surgery, treatment of DVT and pulmonary embolism, management of acute coronary syndrome.

CONTRAINDICATIONS Patients with active major bleeding, GI bleeding, hemophilia, heparin hypersensitivity, heparin-induced thrombocytopenia (HIT), thrombocytopenia associated with an antiplatelet antibody in the presence of enoxaparin, bleeding disorders, idiopathic thrombocytopenia purpura (ITP), hypersensitivity to enoxaparin; porcine protein hypersensitivity, neonates.

CAUTIOUS USE Uncontrolled arterial hypertension, recent history of GI disease, benzyl alcohol hypersensitivity, conditions or surgery with increased risk of bleeding, hepatic disease, hypertension, coagulopathy, thrombolytic therapy, thrombocytopenia, dental disease, dental work, diabetic retinopathy, dialysis, diverticulitis, inflammatory bowel disease, intramuscular injections, lumbar puncture, menstruation, obesity, peptic ulcer disease, older adults, endocarditis, renal disease, renal impairment, spinal anesthesia, stroke, surgery, pregnancy (category B), lactation. Safety and effectiveness in children are not established.

ROUTE & DOSAGE

Prevention of DVT after Hip or Knee Surgery

Adult: **SC** 30 mg b.i.d. for 10–14 d starting 12–24 h post-surgery

Prevention of DVT after Abdominal Surgery

Adult: **SC** 40 mg q.d. starting 2 h before surgery and continuing for 7–10 d (max: 12 d)

Treatment of DVT and Pulmonary Embolus

Adult: **SC** 1 mg/kg q12h or 1.5 mg/kg/d; monitor anti-Xa activity to determine appropriate dose

Acute Coronary Syndrome

Adult: **SC** 1 mg/kg q12h for 2–8 d, give concurrently with aspirin 100–325 mg/d

Adjustment for Renal Impairment

Cl_{cr} <30 mL/min: 30 mg or 1 mg/kg q24h

ADMINISTRATION

Subcutaneous

- Use a TB syringe or prefilled syringe to ensure accurate dosage.
- Do not expel the air bubble from the 30 or 40 mg prefilled syringe before injection.
- Place patient in a supine position for injection of the drug.
- Alternate injections between the left and right anterolateral abdominal wall.
- Hold the skin fold between the thumb and forefinger and insert the whole length of the needle into the skin fold. Hold skin fold throughout the injection. Do not rub site post injection.
- Store at 15°–30° C (59°–86° F).

ADVERSE EFFECTS (≥1%) **Body as a Whole:** Allergic reactions (rash, urticaria), fever, angioedema arthralgia, pain and inflammation at injection site, peripheral edema, arthralgia, fever. **Digestive:** Abnormal liver function tests. **Hematologic:** *Hemorrhage,* thrombocytopenia, ecchymoses, anemia. **Respiratory:** Dyspnea. **Skin:** Rash, pruritus.

INTERACTIONS Drug: Aspirin, NSAIDS, **warfarin** can increase risk of hemorrhage. **Herbal: Garlic, ginger, ginkgo, feverfew, horse chestnut** may increase risk of bleeding.

PHARMACOKINETICS Absorption: 91% absorbed from SC injection site. **Peak:** 3 h. **Duration:** 4.6 h. **Distribution:** Appears to accumulate in liver, kidneys, and spleen. Does not cross placenta. **Elimination:** Primarily excreted in urine. **Half-Life:** 4.6 h.

NURSING IMPLICATIONS

Assessment & Drug Effects

- Lab tests: Baseline coagulation studies; periodic CBC, platelet count, urine and stool for occult blood.
- Monitor platelet count closely. Withhold drug and notify physician if platelet count less than 100,000/mm^3.
- Monitor closely patients with renal insufficiency and older adults who are at higher risk for thrombocytopenia.
- Monitor for and report immediately any sign or symptom of unexplained bleeding.

Patient & Family Education

- Report to physician promptly signs of unexplained bleeding such as: pink, red, or dark brown urine; red or dark brown vomitus; bleeding gums or bloody sputum; dark, tarry stools.
- Do not take any OTC drugs without first consulting physician.
- Do not breast feed while taking this drug without consulting physician.

ENTACAPONE

(en-ta'ca-pone)

Comtan

Classifications: AUTONOMIC NERVOUS SYSTEM AGENT; CATECHOLAMINE O-METHYLTRANSFERASE (COMT) INHIBITOR; ANTIPARKINSONISM AGENT

Prototype: Tolcapone

Pregnancy Category: C

AVAILABILITY 200 mg tablets

ACTIONS Selective inhibitor of catecholamine O-methyltransferase (COMT). COMT is responsible for metabolizing levodopa to an intermediate compound 3-O-methyldopa, a chemical which interferes with the availability of levodopa to the brain.

THERAPEUTIC EFFECTS Taken with levodopa, it decreases the formation of 3-O-methyldopa, thus increasing the duration of the motor response of the brain to levodopa in Parkinson's disease. Indicated by diminished Parkinson's manifestations.

USES Adjunct to levodopa/carbidopa to treat Parkinson's disease.

CONTRAINDICATIONS Hypersensitivity to entacapone; concurrent MAO inhibitors; pregnancy (category D), lactation.

CAUTIOUS USE Hepatic impairment; biliary obstruction; concomitant administration with CNS depressants; lactation; drugs metabolized by COMT (e.g., isoproterenol, epinephrine, etc.); history of hypotension or syncope.

E

ROUTE & DOSAGE

Parkinson's Disease
Adult: **PO** 200 mg administered with each dose of levodopa/carbidopa up to 8 times/d

ADMINISTRATION

Oral

- Give simultaneously with each levodopa/carbidopa dose.
- Must be tapered if discontinued. Never discontinue abruptly.
- Do not administer to patients receiving nonselective MAO inhibitors.
- Store at 15°–30° C (59°–86° F).

ADVERSE EFFECTS (≥1%) **Body as a Whole:** Back pain, fatigue, asthenia. **CNS:** *Dyskinesia, hyperkinesia,* hypokinesia, dizziness, anxiety, somnolence, agitation. **GI:** Taste perversion, *nausea, diarrhea,* abdominal pain, constipation, vomiting, dry mouth, dyspepsia, flatulence, gastritis. **Respiratory:** Dyspnea. **Skin:** Increased sweating. **Other:** *Urine discoloration,* purpura.

INTERACTIONS Drug: Extreme caution must be used if administered with a nonselective MAOI; **bitolterol, dobutamine, dopamine, epinephrine, isoetharine, isoproterenol, methyldopa, norepinephrine** may increase heart rates, possibly cause arrhythmias, excessive changes in BP.

PHARMACOKINETICS Absorption: Rapidly absorbed, 35% bioavailable. **Peak:** 1 h. **Distribution:** Highly protein bound. **Metabolism:** Extensively metabolized in plasma and erythrocytes. **Elimination:** Primarily excreted in feces. **Half-Life:** 2.4 h (terminal).

NURSING IMPLICATIONS

Assessment & Drug Effects

- Monitor carefully for hyperpyrexia, confusion, or emergence of Parkinson's S&S during drug withdrawal.
- Monitor for orthostatic hypotension & worsening of dyskinesia or hyperkinesia.
- Lab tests: Hgb and serum ferritin levels with prolonged therapy.

Patient & Family Education

- Take with levodopa/carbidopa; not effective alone.
- Do not discontinue abruptly; gradually reduce dosage.
- Exercise caution when rising from a sitting or lying position because faintness/dizziness can occur.
- Exercise caution with hazardous activities until reaction to the drug is known.
- Harmless brownish-orange discoloration of urine is possible.
- Report unusual adverse effects (e.g., hallucinations/unexplained diarrhea).
- Do not breast feed while taking this drug.

EPHEDRINE HYDROCHLORIDE

(e-fed'rin)
Efedron

EPHEDRINE SULFATE

Ectasule, Ephedsol, Vatronol

Classifications: AUTONOMIC NERVOUS SYSTEM AGENT; ALPHA- AND BETA-ADRENERGIC AGONIST (SYMPATHOMIMETIC); BRONCHODILATOR
Prototype: Epinephrine HCl
Pregnancy Category: C

AVAILABILITY 25 mg capsules; 50 mg/mL injection; 0.25% nasal spray; 1% nasal gel

ACTIONS Both indirect- and direct-acting sympathomimetic amine. Thought to act indirectly by releasing tissue stores of norepinephrine and directly by stimulation of alpha-, $beta_1$-, and $beta_2$-adrenergic receptors.

THERAPEUTIC EFFECTS Like epinephrine, contracts dilated arterioles of nasal mucosa, thus reducing engorgement and edema and facilitating ventilation and drainage. Local application to eye produces mydriasis without loss of light reflexes or accommodation or change in intraocular pressure (IOP).

USES Temporary relief of congestion of hay fever, allergic rhinitis, and sinusitis; and in treatment and prophylaxis of mild cases of acute asthma and in patients with chronic asthma requiring continuing treatment. Also has been used for its CNS stimulant actions in treatment of narcolepsy, to improve respiration in narcotic and barbiturate poisoning, to combat hypotensive states, especially those associated with spinal anesthesia; in management of enuresis or impaired bladder control; as adjunct in treatment of myasthenia gravis; as mydriatic; to relieve dysmenorrhea; and for temporary support of ventricular rate in Adams-Stokes syndrome; for peripheral edema secondary to type I diabetic neuropathy.

CONTRAINDICATIONS History of hypersensitivity to ephedrine or other sympathomimetics; narrow-angle glaucoma; pregnancy (category C), lactation.

CAUTIOUS USE Exercise extreme caution if used at all in hypertension, arteriosclerosis, angina pectoris, coronary insufficiency, chronic heart disease; diabetes mellitus; hyperthyroidism; prostatic hypertrophy.

ROUTE & DOSAGE

Bronchodilator, Nasal Decongestant

Adult: **PO** 25–50 mg q3–4h prn (max: 150 mg/24 h) **IM/IV/SC** 12.5–25 mg
Child: **PO** >2 *y,* 2–3 mg/kg/d in 4–6 divided doses; *6–12 y,* 6.25–12.5 mg q4h (max: 75 mg/24 h)

Hypotension

Adult: **PO** 25 mg 1–4 times/d (max: 150 mg/24 h) **IM/SC/IV** 10–50 mg IM/SC or 10–25 mg slow IV, may repeat in 5–10 min if necessary (max: 150 mg/24 h)
Child: **PO/IM/SC/IV** 3 mg/kg/d in 4–6 divided doses (max: 75 mg/24 h)

Myasthenia Gravis

Adult: **PO** 25 mg t.i.d. or q.i.d.

Enuresis

Adult: **PO** 25 mg h.s.

Urinary Incontinence

Geriatric: **PO** 25–50 mg q6h.

Nasal Decongestant

Adult: **Intranasal** 2–4 drops or a small amount of jelly in each nostril no more than q.i.d. for 3–4 consecutive days

ADMINISTRATION

Oral

- Administer last dose a few hours before bedtime, if possible, to minimize insomnia.
- Store at 15°–30° C (59°–86° F) in tightly closed, light-resistant containers unless otherwise directed by the manufacturer.

Intranasal

- Have patient clear nose before instilling drops. Instruct patient to blow gently with both nostrils open. Generally, nose drops are instilled with head in lateral, head-low position to avoid entry of drug into throat. Check with physician.

Intravenous

***PREPARE:* Direct:** Give undiluted.
***ADMINISTER:* Direct:** Direct IV at a rate of 10 mg or fraction thereof over 30–60 seconds.
***INCOMPATIBILITIES* Solution/additive: Hydrocortisone, pentobarbital, phenobarbital, secobarbital, thiopental. Y-site: thiopental**

- Store in tightly closed, light-resistant containers. Do not use liquid formulation unless it is absolutely clear.

ADVERSE EFFECTS (≥1%) **CNS:** Headache, insomnia, *nervousness,* anxiety, tremulousness, giddiness. **CV:** Palpitation, tachycardia, precordial pain, cardiac arrhythmias. **GU:** Difficult or painful urination, acute urinary retention (especially older men with prostatism). **GI:** Nausea, vomiting, anorexia. **Body as a Whole:** Sweating, thirst, overdosage: euphoria, confusion, delirium, convulsions, pyrexia, hypertension, rebound hypotension, respiratory difficulty. **Skin:** Fixed-drug eruption. Topical use: *Burning, stinging,* dryness of nasal mucosa, sneezing, rebound congestion.

DIAGNOSTIC TEST INTERFERENCE Ephedrine is generally withdrawn at least 12 h before ***sensitivity tests*** are made to prevent false-positive reactions.

INTERACTIONS Drug: MAO INHIBITORS, TRICYCLIC ANTIDEPRESSANTS, **furazolidone, guanethidine** may increase alpha-adrenergic effects (headache, hyperpyrexia, hypertension); **sodium bicarbonate** decreases renal elimination of ephedrine, increasing its CNS effects; **epinephrine, norepinephrine** compound sympathomimetic effects; effects of ALPHA AND BETA BLOCKERS and ephedrine antagonized.

PHARMACOKINETICS Absorption: Readily absorbed from GI tract. **Peak:** 15 min–1 h. **Duration:** Bronchodilation 2–4 h; cardiac & pressor effects up to 4 h PO and 1 h IV. **Distribution:** Widely distributed; crosses blood–brain barrier and placenta; distributed into breast milk. **Metabolism:** Small amounts metabolized in liver. **Elimination:** Excreted in urine. **Half-Life:** 3–6 h.

NURSING IMPLICATIONS

Assessment & Drug Effects

- Supervise continuously patients receiving ephedrine IV. Take baseline BP and other vital signs. Check BP repeatedly during first 5 min, then q3–5min until stabilized.
- Monitor I&O ratio and pattern, especially in older male patients. Encourage patient to void before taking medication (see ADVERSE EFFECTS).
- Monitor for systemic effects of nose drops that can occur because of excessive dosage from rapid absorption of drug solution through nasal mucosa. This is most likely to occur in older adults.

Patient & Family Education

- Note: Ephedrine is a commonly abused drug. Learn adverse effects and dangers; take medication ONLY as prescribed.
- Do not take OTC medications for coughs, colds, allergies, or asthma unless approved by physician. Ephedrine is a common ingredient in these preparations.
- Do not breast feed while taking this drug without consulting physician.

EPINASTINE HYDROCHLORIDE

(e-pi-nas'teen)
Elestat
Classifications: EYE, EAR, NOSE & THROAT (EENT) PREPARATIONS; ANTIHISTAMINE, OCULAR
Prototype: Levocabastine HCl
Pregnancy Category: C

AVAILABILITY 0.05% ophthalmic solution

See Appendix A-1.

EPINEPHRINE ℗

(ep-i-ne'frin)
Bronkaid Mist, Epi-E-Zpen, Epinephrine Pediatric, EpiPen Auto-Injector, Primatene Mist Suspension

EPINEPHRINE BITARTRATE

AsthmaHaler, Bronkaid Mist Suspension, Bronitin Mist Suspension, Epitrate, Medihaler-Epi, Primatene Mist Suspension

EPINEPHRINE HYDROCHLORIDE

Adrenalin Chloride, Bronkaid Mistometer, Dysne-Inhal, Epifrin, Glaucon, SusPhrine ♣

EPINEPHRINE, RACEMIC

AsthmaNefrin, Dey-Dose Epinephrine, microNefrin, Vaponefrin ♣

EPINEPHRYL BORATE

(ep-i-ne'frill bor'ate)
Epinal, Eppy/N
Classifications: AUTONOMIC NERVOUS SYSTEM AGENT; ALPHA- AND BETA-ADRENERGIC AGONIST; BRONCHODILATOR
Pregnancy Category: C

AVAILABILITY 1:100, 1:1000, 2.25% solution for inhalation; 0.35 mg, 0.2 mg spray; 1:1000, 1:2000, 1:10,000, 1:100,000 injection; 1:200 suspension; 0.1%, 0.5%, 1%, 2% ophthalmic solution; 0.1% nasal solution

ACTIONS Naturally occurring catecholamine obtained from animal adrenal glands; also prepared synthetically. Acts directly on both alpha and beta receptors; the most potent activator of alpha receptors. Strengthens myocardial contraction; increases systolic but may decrease diastolic blood pressure; increases cardiac rate and cardiac output.

THERAPEUTIC EFFECTS Constricts bronchial arterioles and inhibits histamine release, thus reducing congestion and edema and increasing tidal volume and vital capacity. Relaxes uterine smooth musculature and inhibits uterine contractions. Imitates all actions of sympathetic nervous system except those on arteries of the face and sweat glands.

USES Temporary relief of bronchospasm, acute asthmatic attack, mucosal congestion, hypersensitivity and anaphylactic reactions, syncope due to heart block or carotid sinus hypersensitivity, and to restore cardiac rhythm in cardiac arrest. Ophthalmic preparation is used in management of simple (open-angle) glaucoma, generally as an adjunct to topical miotics and oral carbonic anhydrase inhibitors; also used as ophthalmic decongestant. Relaxes myometrium and inhibits uterine contractions; prolongs action and delays systemic absorption of local and intraspinal anesthetics. Used topically to control superficial bleeding.

CONTRAINDICATIONS Hypersensitivity to sympathomimetic amines; narrow-angle glaucoma; hemorrhagic, traumatic, or cardiogenic shock; cardiac dilatation, cerebral arteriosclerosis, coronary insufficiency, arrhythmias, organic heart or brain disease; during second stage of labor; for local anesthesia of fingers, toes, ears, nose, genitalia. Safety during pregnancy (category C) or lactation is not established.

CAUTIOUS USE Older adult or debilitated patients; prostatic hypertrophy; hypertension; diabetes mellitus; hyperthyroidism; Parkinson's disease; tuberculosis; psychoneurosis; in patients with long-standing bronchial asthma and emphysema with degenerative heart disease; in children <6 y of age.

ROUTE & DOSAGE

Anaphylaxis

Adult: **SC** 0.1–0.5 mL of 1:1000 q10–15min prn **IV** 0.1–0.25 mL of 1:1000 q10–15min
Child: **SC** 0.01 mL/kg of, 1:1000 q10–15min prn **IV** 0.01 mL/kg of 1:1000 q10–15min
Neonate: **IV Intratracheal** 0.01–0.03 mg/kg (0.1–0.3 mL/kg of 1:10,000) q3–5min prn

Cardiac Arrest

Adult: **IV** 0.1–1 mg (1–10 mL of 1:10,000) q5min as needed **Intracardiac** 0.1–1 mg
Child: **IV** 0.01 mg/kg (0.1 mL/kg of 1:10,000) q5min as needed **Intracardiac** 0.05–0.1 mg/kg

Asthma

Adult: **SC** 0.1–0.5 mL of 1:1000 q20min–4h **Inhalation** 1 inhalation q4h prn
Child: **SC** 0.01 mL/kg of 1:1000 q20min–4h **Inhalation** 1 inhalation q4h prn

Glaucoma

Adult/Child: **Instillation** 1–2 drops 0.25%–2% solution 1/d or b.i.d.

Ocular Mydriasis

See Appendix A-1

Nasal Hemostasis

Adult/Child: **Instillation** 1–2 drops 0.1% ophthalmic or 0.1% nasal solution

Topical Hemostatic

Adult/Child: **Topical** 1:50,000–1:1000 applied topically or 1:500,000–1:50,000 mixed with a local anesthetic

ADMINISTRATION

Inhalation

- Have patient in an upright position when aerosol preparation is used. The reclining position can result in overdosage by producing large droplets instead of fine spray.
- Instruct patient to rinse mouth and throat with water immediately after inhalation to avoid swallowing residual drug (may cause epigastric pain and systemic effects from the propellant in the aerosol preparation) and to prevent dryness of oropharyngeal membranes.
- Do not give isoproterenol concurrently with epinephrine. Allow 4-h interval to elapse before a change is made from one drug to the other.

Instillation

- Instill nose drops with head in lateral, head-low position to prevent entry of drug into throat.
- Instruct patient to rinse nose dropper or spray tip with hot water after each use to prevent contamination of solution with nasal secretions.

Ophthalmic

- Remove soft contact lenses before instilling eye drops.
- Instruct patient to apply gentle finger pressure against nasolacrimal duct immediately after drug is instilled for at least 1 or 2 min following instillation to prevent excessive systemic absorption.
- When separate solutions of epinephrine and a topical miotic are used, the miotic should be instilled 2–10 min prior to epinephrine because of the conjunctival sac's limited capacity.

Subcutaneous

- Use tuberculin syringe to ensure greater accuracy in measurement of parenteral doses.
- Protect epinephrine injection from exposure to light at all times. Do not remove ampul or vial from carton until ready to use.
- Shake vial or ampul thoroughly to disperse particles before withdrawing epinephrine suspension into syringe; then inject promptly.
- Aspirate carefully before injecting epinephrine. Inadvertent IV injection of usual SC doses can result in sudden hypertension and possibly cerebral hemorrhage.
- Rotate injection sites and observe for signs of blanching. Vascular constriction from repeated injections may cause tissue necrosis.

Intravenous

Note: Verify correct rate of IV injection to neonates, infants, children with physician.

- Note: 1:1000 solution contains 1 mg/1 mL. 1:10,000 solution contains 0.1 mg/1 mL.

PREPARE: **Direct:** Dilute each 1 mg of 1:1000 solution with 10 mL of NS to yield 1:10,000 solution. **IV Infusion:** Further dilute in 250–500 mL of D5W.

ADMINISTER: **Direct:** Give each 1 mg over 1 min or longer; may give more rapidly in cardiac arrest. **IV Infusion:** 1–10 mcg/min titrated according to patient's condition.

INCOMPATIBILITIES **Solution/additive: Aminophylline, cephapirin, hyaluronidase, mephentermine, sodium bicarbonate, warfarin. Y-site: Ampicillin, thiopental, sodium bicarbonate.**

ADVERSE EFFECTS (≥1%) **Special Senses:** *Nasal burning or stinging,* dryness of nasal mucosa, sneezing, rebound congestion. *Transient stinging or burning of eyes,* lacrimation, browache, headache, rebound conjunctival hyperemia, allergy, iritis; with prolonged use: melanin-like deposits on lids, conjunctiva, and cornea; corneal edema; loss of lashes (reversible); maculopathy with central scotoma in aphakic patients (reversible). **Body as a Whole:** *Nervousness,* restlessness, sleeplessness, fear, anxiety, *tremors,* severe headache, cerebrovascular accident, weakness, dizziness, syncope, pallor, sweating, dyspnea. **Digestive:** Nausea, vomiting. **Cardiovascular:** Precordial pain, *palpitations,* hypertension, <u>MI</u>, tachyarrhythmias including <u>ventricular fibrillation</u>. **Respiratory:** Bronchial and <u>pulmonary edema</u>. **Urogenital:** Urinary retention. **Skin:** Tissue necrosis with repeated injections. **Metabolic:** Metabolic acidoses, elevated serum lactic acid, transient elevations of blood glucose. **Nervous System:** Altered state of perception and thought, psychosis.

INTERACTIONS Drug: May increase hypotension in circulatory collapse or hypotension caused by PHENOTHI-

E

AZINES, **oxytocin, entacapone.** Additive toxicities with other SYMPATHOMIMETICS **(albuterol, dobutamine, dopamine, isoproterenol, metaproterenol, norepinephrine, phenylephrine, phenylpropanolamine, pseudoephedrine, ritodrine, salmeterol, terbutaline),** MAO INHIBITORS, TRICYCLIC ANTIDEPRESSANTS. ALPHA- AND BETA-ADRENERGIC BLOCKING AGENTS (e.g., **ergotamine, propranolol**) antagonize effects of epinephrine. GENERAL ANESTHETICS increase cardiac irritability.

PHARMACOKINETICS Absorption: Inactivated in GI tract. **Onset:** 3–5 min, 1 h on conjunctiva. **Peak:** 20 min, 4–8 h on conjunctiva. **Duration:** 12–24 h topically. **Distribution:** Widely distributed; does not cross blood–brain barrier; crosses placenta. **Metabolism:** Metabolized in tissue and liver by monoamine oxidase (MAO) and catecholamine-methyltransferase (COMT). **Elimination:** Small amount excreted unchanged in urine; excreted in breast milk.

NURSING IMPLICATIONS

Assessment & Drug Effects

- Monitor BP, pulse, respirations, and urinary output and observe patient closely following IV administration. Epinephrine may widen pulse pressure. If disturbances in cardiac rhythm occur, withhold epinephrine and notify physician immediately.
- Keep physician informed of any changes in intake-output ratio.
- Use cardiac monitor with patients receiving epinephrine IV. Have full crash cart immediately available.
- Check BP repeatedly when epinephrine is administered IV during first 5 min, then q3–5min until stabilized.
- Advise patient to report to physician if symptoms are not relieved in 20 min or if they become worse following inhalation.
- Advise patient to report bronchial irritation, nervousness, or sleeplessness. Dosage should be reduced.
- Monitor blood glucose & HbA1c for loss of glycemic control if diabetic.

Patient & Family Education

- Be aware intranasal application may sting slightly.
- Administer ophthalmic drug at bedtime or following prescribed miotic to minimize mydriasis, with blurred vision and sensitivity to light (possible in some patients being treated for glaucoma).
- Transitory stinging may follow initial ophthalmic administration and that headache and browache occur frequently at first but usually subside with continued use. Notify physician if symptoms persist.
- Discontinue epinephrine eye drops and consult a physician if signs of hypersensitivity develop (edema of lids, itching, discharge, crusting eyelids).
- Learn how to administer epinephrine subcutaneously. Keep medication and equipment available for home emergency. Confer with physician.
- Note: Inhalation epinephrine reduces bronchial secretions and thus may make mucous plugs more difficult to dislodge.
- Report tolerance to physician; may occur with repeated or prolonged use. Continued use of epinephrine in the presence of tolerance can be dangerous.
- Take medication only as prescribed and immediately notify physician of onset of systemic effects of epinephrine.

- Discard discolored or precipitated solutions.
- Do not breast feed while taking this drug without consulting physician.

EPIRUBICIN HYDROCHLORIDE

(e-pi-roo'bi-sin)

Ellence

Classifications: ANTINEOPLASTIC; ANTIBIOTIC

Prototype: Doxorubicin HCl

Pregnancy Category: D

AVAILABILITY 50 mg/25 mL, 200 mg/100 mL vials

ACTIONS Cytotoxic antibiotic with wide spectrum of antitumor activity and strong immunosuppressive properties. Intercalates with preformed DNA residues, blocking effective DNA and RNA transcription.

THERAPEUTIC EFFECTS Highly destructive to rapidly proliferating cells. Utilized effectively in the treatment of breast carcinomas. Indicated by tumor regression.

USES Adjunctive therapy for axillary node-positive breast cancer.

CONTRAINDICATIONS Hypersensitivity to epirubicin and other related drugs; marked myelosuppression, impaired cardiac function; previous treatment with maximum doses of epirubicin, doxorubicin, or daunorubicin; pregnancy (category D), lactation.

CAUTIOUS USE Arrhythmias; liver dysfunction; severe renal insufficiency.

ROUTE & DOSAGE

Breast Cancer

Adult: **IV** 100–120 mg/m^2 infused over 3–5 min on day 1 of a 3–4 wk cycle or 50–60 mg/m^2 on day 1 and 8 of a 3–4 wk cycle

ADMINISTRATION

Intravenous

Note: Pregnant women should NOT prepare or administer this drug. Wear protective goggles, gowns and disposable gloves and masks when handling this drug. Discard ALL equipment used in preparation of this drug in high-risk, waste-disposal bags for incineration. Treat accidental contact with skin or eyes by rinsing with copious amounts of water followed by prompt medical attention.

Note: Reduce dosages when serum creatinine >5 mg/dL or AST 2–4 times the upper limit of normal.

PREPARE: **IV Infusion:** Epirubicin is manufactured as a preservative-free ready-to-use solution. The contents of a vial must be used within 25 h of first penetrating the rubber stopper. Discard unused solution.

ADMINISTER: **IV Infusion:** Measure ordered dose and inject into a port of a freely flowing IV solution of D5W or NS over 3–5 min. DO NOT give by direct IV push into a vein. Avoid IV sites that enter small veins or repeated injections into the same vein. Monitor IV site closely for S&S of extravasation and if suspected, notify physician immediately.

INCOMPATIBILITIES **Solution/additive:** ALKALINE SOLUTIONS (including **sodium bicarbonate**), **fluorouracil, ifosfamide, heparin, fluorouracil.**

- Store between 2°–8° C (36°–46° F). Protect from light.

E

ADVERSE EFFECTS (≥1%) **Body as a Whole:** *Lethargy,* fever. **CV:** Asymptomatic decrease in LVEF, CHF. **GI:** *Nausea, vomiting, mucositis, diarrhea,* anorexia. **Hematologic:** Leukopenia, neutropenia, anemia, thrombocytopenia, AML. **Skin:** *Alopecia, injection site reaction,* rash, itching, skin changes. **Other:** *Amenorrhea, hot flashes, infection, conjunctivitis/keratitis.*

INTERACTIONS Drug: Cimetidine increases epirubicin levels; concomitant use with cardioactive drugs (e.g., CALCIUM CHANNEL BLOCKERS).

PHARMACOKINETICS Distribution: Widely distributed, 77% protein bound, concentrated in red blood cells. **Metabolism:** Extensively metabolized in liver, blood and other organs. Clearance is reduced in patients with hepatic impairment. **Elimination:** Primarily excreted in bile, some urinary excretion; clearance decreases in older adult female patients. **Half-Life:** 33 h.

NURSING IMPLICATIONS

Assessment & Drug Effects

- Withhold drug and notify physician of any of the following: neutrophil count <1500 cells/mm^3, recent MI, suspicion of severe myocardial insufficiency.
- Obtain baseline and periodic (before each cycle of therapy) cardiac evaluation: left ventricular ejection fraction, ECG and ECHO (tests are recommended especially in the presence of risk factors of cardiac toxicity).
- Monitor cardiac status closely throughout therapy as the risk of developing severe CHF increases rapidly when cumulative doses approach 900 mg/m^2. Report significant ECG changes immediately. Report immediately S&S of the following: tachycardia, gallop rhythm, pleural effusion, pulmonary edema, dependent edema, ascites, or hepatomegaly.
- Lab tests: Baseline and periodic (before each cycle of therapy), CBC with differential, platelet count, serum total bilirubin, AST, serum creatinine.

Patient & Family Education

- Review all literature regarding the adverse effects of epirubicin therapy carefully.
- Report any of the following to physician immediately: Pain at the site of IV infusion, chest pain, palpitations, shortness of breath or difficulty breathing, sudden weight gain, swelling of hands, feet or legs, or any unexplained bleeding.
- Be aware that your urine may turn red for 1–2 d after receiving this drug. This change is expected and harmless.
- Do not take OTC cimetidine or any other OTC drug without consulting physician.
- Use effective means of contraception (both men and women) while on epirubicin therapy.
- Do not breast feed while taking this drug.

EPLERENONE (Pr)

(e-ple're-none)

Inspra

Classifications: ELECTROLYE & WATER BALANCE AGENT; SELECTIVE ALDOSTERONE RECEPTOR ANTAGONIST

Pregnancy Category: B

AVAILABILITY 25 mg, 50 mg, 100 mg tablets

ACTIONS Binds to mineralocorticoid receptors and blocks the binding of aldosterone, a component of the renin-angiotensin-

aldosterone-system (RAAS). Thus eplerenone blocks the primary effect of aldosterone which is sodium reabsorption.
THERAPEUTIC EFFECTS Lowers blood pressure by inhibiting sodium and water retention thus reducing total plasma volume.

USES Treatment of hypertension, alone or with other antihypertensive agents. Adjunctive therapy for post MI heart failure.

CONTRAINDICATIONS Serum potassium >5.5 meq/L; type 2 diabetes with microalbuminuria; serum creatinine >2.0 mg/dL in males or >1.8 mg/dL in females; creatinine clearance <50 mL/min; concomitant treatment with potassium supplements or potassium-sparing diuretics (amiloride, spironolactone, or triamterene), or strong inhibitors of CYP450 3A4 (e.g., ketoconazole, itraconazole).
CAUTIOUS USE Hepatic impairment; concomitant use of another mineralocorticoid receptor blocker and ACE inhibitors or angiotensin II antagonists; concomitant treatment with moderate inhibitors of CYP450 3A4 (e.g., fluconazole, erythromycin, verapamil, saquinavir); pregnancy (category B); lactation; safety and efficacy in pediatric patients are not established.

ROUTE & DOSAGE

Hypertension
Adult: **PO** 50 mg once daily, may be increased to 50 mg b.i.d. or 100 mg q.d., if inadequate response after 4 wk

ADMINISTRATION

Oral
- Do not administer in combination with potassium supplements or potassium-sparing diuretics.
- Manufacturer recommends dosage reduction to 25 mg once daily with concurrent administration of erythromycin, saquinavir, verapamil, or fluconazole.
- Store at 15°–30° C (59°–86° F).

ADVERSE EFFECTS (≥1%) **Body as a Whole:** Fatigue, flu-like syndrome. **CNS:** Headache, dizziness. **CV:** Angina, MI. **GI:** Diarrhea, abdominal pain. **Endocrine:** Gynecomastia. **Metabolic:** *Hyperkalemia*, increased GGT, hypercholesterolemia, hypertriglyceridemia, decreased sodium levels. **Respiratory:** Cough. **Urogenital:** Albuminuria, abnormal vaginal bleeding.

INTERACTIONS Drug: ACE INHIBITORS, ANGIOTENSIN II RECEPTOR BLOCKERS, AZOLE ANTIFUNGALS (e.g., **fluconazole, itraconazole, ketoconazole), erythromycin, saquinavir, verapamil** may increase risk of hyperkalemia. **Food: Potassium**-containing SALT SUBSTITUTES may increase risk of hyperkalemia.

PHARMACOKINETICS Absorption: Rapidly absorbed. **Peak:** 1.5 h. **Distribution:** 50% protein bound, primarily to alpha1-acid glycoproteins. **Metabolism:** Metabolized in liver by CYP3A4. **Elimination:** 32% excreted in feces, 67% excreted in urine. **Half-Life:** 4–6 h.

NURSING IMPLICATIONS

Assessment & Drug Effects
- Monitor cardiovascular status with frequent BP determinations. Note that BP lowering usually occurs within 2 wk with maximal antihypertensive effects achieved within 4 wk.

E

- Lab tests: Monitor baseline and periodic serum potassium, serum sodium, renal function tests, lipid profile, and LFTs. Monitor type 2 diabetics for microalbuminuria.
- Concurrent drugs: Monitor serum potassium levels more frequently when patient also receiving an ACE inhibitor or an angiontensin II receptor antagonist. Monitor frequently for lithium toxicity with concurrent use.
- Withhold drug and notify physician for any of the following: serum potassium >5.5 mEq/L, serum creatinine >2.0 mg/dL in males or >1.8 mg/dL in females, creatinine clearance <50 mL/min, microalbuminuria in type 2 diabetics.

Patient & Family Education

- Do not use potassium supplements, salt substitutes containing potassium, or contraindicated drugs (e.g., ketoconazole, itraconazole) without consulting physician.
- Do not use OTC nonsteroidal anti-inflammatory drugs without consulting physician.
- Do not breast feed without consulting physician.

EPOETIN ALFA (HUMAN RECOMBINANT ERYTHROPOIETIN) Pr

(e-po-e-tin)

Epogen, Eprex ♣, Procrit

Classifications: BLOOD FORMERS, COAGULATORS, AND ANTICOAGULANTS; HEMATOPOIETIC GROWTH FACTOR

Pregnancy Category: C

AVAILABILITY 2000 units/mL, 3000 units/mL, 4000 units/mL, 10,000 units/mL, 20,000 units/mL

ACTIONS Glycoprotein that stimulates RBC production. Hypoxia and anemia generally increase the production of erythropoietin.

THERAPEUTIC EFFECTS Produced in the kidney and stimulates bone marrow production of RBCs (erythropoiesis).

USES Elevates the hematocrit of patients with anemia secondary to chronic kidney failure (CRF); patients may or may not be on dialysis; other anemias related to malignancies and AIDS. Autologous blood donations for anticipated transfusions. Reduces need for blood in anemic surgical patients.

CONTRAINDICATIONS Uncontrolled hypertension and known hypersensitivity to mammalian cell–derived products and albumin (human).

CAUTIOUS USE Pregnancy (category C) or lactation. Safety and effectiveness in children are not established.

ROUTE & DOSAGE

Anemia

Adult: **SC/IV** 3–500 U/kg/dose 3 times/wk, usually start with 50–100 U/kg/dose until target Hct range of 30%–33% (max: 36%) is reached, Hct should not increase by more than 4 points in any 2-wk period, rapid increase in Hct increases the risk of serious adverse reactions (hypertension, seizures), may increase dose if Hct has not increased 5–6 points after 8 wk of therapy, reduce dose after target range is reached or the Hct increases by >4 points in any 2-wk period, dose usually increased or decreased by 25 U/kg increments

Child: **SC** 150 U/kg/dose 3 times/wk initially, when Hct increased to 35%, decrease dose by 25 U/kg/dose until Hct reaches 40%

ADMINISTRATION

Subcutaneous

- Do not shake solution. Shaking may denature the glycoprotein, rendering it biologically inactive.
- Inspect solution for particulate matter prior to use. Do not use if solution is discolored or if it contains particulate matter.
- Use only one dose per vial, and do not reenter vial.
- Do not give with any other drug solution.

Intravenous

PREPARE: **Direct:** Give undiluted.
ADMINISTER: **Direct:** Give direct IV as a bolus dose over 1 min.

- Discard any unused portion of the vial. It contains no preservatives.
- Store at 2°–8° C (36°–46° F). Do not freeze or shake.

ADVERSE EFFECTS (≥1%) **CNS:** Seizures, *headache*. **CV:** *Hypertension*. **GI:** Nausea, diarrhea. **Hematologic:** *Iron deficiency,* thrombocytosis, *clotting of AV fistula*. **Other:** Sweating, bone pain, arthralgias.

INTERACTIONS Drug: No clinically significant interactions established.

PHARMACOKINETICS Onset: 7–14 d. **Metabolism:** Metabolized in serum. **Elimination:** Minimal recovery in urine. **Half-Life:** 4–13 h.

NURSING IMPLICATIONS

Assessment & Drug Effects

- Control BP adequately prior to initiation of therapy and closely monitor and control during therapy. Hypertension is an adverse effect that must be controlled.
- Be aware that BP may rise during early therapy as the Hct increases. Notify physician of a rapid rise in Hct (>4 points in 2 wk). Dosage will need to be reduced because of risk of serious hypertension.
- Monitor for hypertensive encephalopathy in patients with CRF during period of increasing Hct.
- Monitor for premonitory neurological symptoms (i.e., aura, and report their appearance promptly). The potential for seizures exists during periods of rapid Hct increase (>4 points in 2 wk).
- Monitor closely for thrombotic events (e.g., MI, CVA, TIA), especially for patients with CRF.
- Lab tests: Baseline transferrin and serum ferritin. Monitor aPTT & INR closely. Patients may require additional heparin during dialysis to prevent clotting of the vascular access or artificial kidney. Determine Hct twice weekly until it is stabilized in the target range (30%–33%) and the maintenance dose of epoetin alfa has been determined; then monitor at regular intervals. Perform CBC with differential and platelet count regularly. Monitor BUN, creatinine, phosphorus, and potassium regularly.

Patient & Family Education

- Important to comply with antihypertensive medication and dietary restrictions.
- Do not drive or engage in other potentially hazardous activity during the first 90 d of therapy because of possible seizure activity.
- Note: As Hct increases, there is an improved sense of well-being and quality of life. It is important to continue compliance with dietary and dialysis prescriptions.
- Understand that headache is a common adverse effect. Report if

severe or persistent, may indicate developing hypertension.

- Keep all follow-up appointments.
- Do not breast feed while taking this drug without consulting physician.

E

EPOPROSTENOL SODIUM

(e-po-pros'te-nol)

Flolan

Classifications: PROSTAGLANDIN; ANTIHYPERTENSIVE; ANTIPLATELET AGENT

Prototype: Dinoprostone

Pregnancy Category: B

AVAILABILITY 0.5 mg, 1.5 mg powder for injection

ACTIONS Naturally occurring prostaglandin. Reduces right and left ventricular afterload, increases cardiac output, and increases stroke volume through its vasodilation effect. May also decrease pulmonary vascular resistance and mean systemic arterial pressure, depending on the dose.

THERAPEUTIC EFFECTS Potent vasodilator of pulmonary and systemic arterial vascular beds and an inhibitor of platelet aggregation.

USES Long-term treatment of primary pulmonary hypertension in NYHA Class III and IV patients.

CONTRAINDICATIONS Chronic use with CHF patients, hypersensitivity to epoprostenol or related compounds.

CAUTIOUS USE Older adults, pregnancy (category B), lactation. Safety and efficacy in children are not established.

ROUTE & DOSAGE

Primary Pulmonary Hypertension

Adult: **IV** *Acute dose,* Initiate with 2 ng/kg/min, increase by 2 ng/kg/min q15 min until dose-limiting effects occur (e.g., nausea, vomiting, headache, hypotension, flushing); *Chronic administration,* Start infusion at 4 ng/kg/min less than the maximum tolerated infusion; if maximum tolerated infusion is ≤5 ng/kg/min, start maintenance infusion at 50% of maximum tolerated dose

ADMINISTRATION

Note: Anticoagulation therapy is generally initiated along with epoprostenol.

Intravenous

PREPARE: **Continuous:** Must be reconstituted using sterile diluent for epoprostenol; must not be mixed with any other medications or solution prior to or during administration. To make 100 mL of 3000 ng/mL, add 5 mL of diluent to one 0.5 mg vial; withdraw 3 mL and add to enough diluent to make a total of 100 mL. To make 100 mL of 5000 ng/mL, add 5 mL of diluent to one 0.5 mg vial; withdraw contents of vial and add to enough diluent to make a total of 100 mL. To make 100 mL of 10,000 ng/mL, add 5 mL of diluent to each of two 0.5 mg vials; withdraw contents of each vial and add to enough diluent to make a total of 100 mL. To make 100 mL of 15,000 ng/mL, add 5 mL of diluent to a 1.5 mg vial; withdraw contents of vial and add to enough diluent to make a total of 100 mL.

ADMINISTER: **Continuous:** Give at ordered rate using an infusion control device. Avoid abrupt infusion interruption or large dosage reduction.

INCOMPATIBILITIES **Solution/additive:** Do not mix or infuse with any other drugs.

- Store unopened vials at 15°–25° C (59°–77° F). Protect from light. See manufacturer's directions for stability or storage of reconstituted solutions.

ADVERSE EFFECTS (≥1%) **CNS:** *Chills, fever, flu-like syndrome, dizziness,* syncope, *headache*, anxiety*/nervousness,* hyperesthesia, paresthesia, dizziness*. **CV:** *Tachycardia*, hypotension*, flushing*, chest pain*,* bradycardia*. **GI:** *Diarrhea, nausea*, vomiting*,* abdominal pain*. **Musculoskeletal:** *Jaw pain, myalgia, nonspecific musculoskeletal pain*.* **Respiratory:** Dyspnea*. ***Dose-limiting effects.**

INTERACTIONS Drug: Hypotension if administered with other vasodilators or antihypertensives.

PHARMACOKINETICS Peak: Approximately 15 min. **Metabolism:** Rapidly hydrolyzed at neutral pH in blood; also subject to enzyme degradation. **Elimination:** 82% eliminated in urine. **Half-Life:** Approximately 6 min.

NURSING IMPLICATIONS

Assessment & Drug Effects

- Assess carefully for development of pulmonary edema during dose ranging.
- Monitor respiratory and cardiovascular status frequently during entire period of chronic use of epoprostenol.
- Monitor for and report recurrence or worsening of symptoms associated with primary pulmonary hypertension (e.g., dyspnea, dizziness, exercise intolerance) or adverse effects of drug; dosage adjustments may be needed.

Patient & Family Education

- Learn correct techniques for storage, reconstitution, and administration of drug, and maintenance of catheter site (see ADMINISTRATION).
- Notify physician immediately of S&S of worsening primary pulmonary hypertension, adverse drug reactions, and S&S of infection at catheter site or sepsis.
- Do not breast feed while taking this drug without consulting physician.

EPROSARTAN MESYLATE

(e-pro-sar'tan)

Teveten

Classifications: CARDIOVASCULAR AGENT; ANGIOTENSIN II RECEPTOR ANTAGONIST; ANTIHYPERTENSIVE

Prototype: Losartan potassium

Pregnancy Category: C (first trimester); D (second and third trimester)

AVAILABILITY 400 mg, 600 mg tablets

ACTIONS Angiotensin II receptor (type AT_1) antagonist. Angiotensin II is a potent vasoconstrictor and primary vasoactive hormone of the renin-angiotensin-aldosterone system.

THERAPEUTIC EFFECTS Selectively blocks the binding of angiotensin II to the AT_1 receptors found in many tissues. This blocks the vasoconstricting and aldosterone-secreting effects of angiotensin II, thus resulting in an antihypertensive effect. This is indicated by decreases in systolic and diastolic BP.

USES Treatment of hypertension.

CONTRAINDICATIONS Hypersensitivity to eprosartan, losartan or other angiotensin II receptor antagonists; pregnancy [(category C) first trimester, and (category D) second and third trimesters], lactation.

E

CAUTIOUS USE Angioedema, aortic or mitral value stenosis, coronary artery disease, cardiomyopathy, hypotension, CHF; biliary obstruction; older adults; hepatic dysfunction, renal artery stenosis, renal impairment.

ROUTE & DOSAGE

Hypertension

Adult: **PO** 600 mg q.d. or 400 mg q.d. to b.i.d. (max: 800 mg/d)

ADMINISTRATION

Oral

- Correct volume depletion prior to therapy to prevent hypotension.
- Store at 15°–30° C (59°–86° F); protect from moisture and direct light.

ADVERSE EFFECTS (≥1%) **Body as a Whole:** Viral infection, fatigue, arthralgia. **CNS:** Depression. **GI:** Abdominal pain, hypertriglyceridemia. **Respiratory:** Upper respiratory infection, rhinitis, pharyngitis, cough.

PHARMACOKINETICS Absorption: Only 13% of oral dose reaches systemic circulation. **Peak:** 1–2 h. **Metabolism:** Minimal metabolism. **Elimination:** 61% excreted in feces and 37% in urine. **Half-Life:** 5–9 h.

NURSING IMPLICATIONS

Assessment & Drug Effects

- Monitor BP periodically; do trough readings just before scheduled dose when possible.
- Monitor for S&S of angioedema (may occur within 30 min or as long as 30 d after initial dose).
- Lab tests: Monitor liver function, BUN & creatinine, serum potassium, CBC with differential periodically.

Patient & Family Education

- Inform physician immediately of pregnancy.
- Report episodes of dizziness especially associated with position changes.
- Report swelling of lips, tongue, face, or feeling of obstruction in neck immediately.
- Do not breast feed while taking this drug.

EPTIFIBATIDE

(ep-ti-fib′a-tide)

Integrilin

Classifications: CARDIOVASCULAR AGENT; ANTITHROMBOTIC AGENT; ANTIPLATELET ANTIBODY; GLYCOPROTEIN IIB/IIIA INHIBITOR

Prototype: Abciximab

Pregnancy Category: B

AVAILABILITY 0.75 mg/mL, 2 mg/mL injection

ACTIONS Binds to the glycoprotein IIb/IIIa (GPIIb/IIIa) receptor sites of platelets.

THERAPEUTIC EFFECTS Inhibits platelet aggregation by preventing fibrinogen, von Willebrand's factor, and other molecules from adhering to GPIIb/IIIa receptor sites on platelets.

USES Treatment of acute coronary syndromes (unstable angina, non-Q-wave MI) and patients undergoing percutaneous coronary interventions (PCIs).

CONTRAINDICATIONS Hypersensitivity to eptifibatide; active bleeding; GI or GU bleeding within 6 weeks; thrombocytopenia; recent major surgery or trauma; intracranial neoplasm, intracranial bleeding within 6 mo; concurrent administration of another GPIIb/

IIIa receptor inhibitor (e.g., abciximab); renal dialysis; severe hypertension (systolic blood pressure >200 mm Hg or diastolic blood pressure >110 mm Hg), aneurysm.
CAUTIOUS USE Hypersensitivity to related compounds (e.g., abciximab, tirofiban, lamifiban); concurrent administration of other anticoagulants; pregnancy (category B), lactation. Safety and effectiveness in children are not established.

ROUTE & DOSAGE

Acute Coronary Syndromes (ACS)

Adult: **IV** 180 mcg/kg initial bolus followed by 2 mcg/kg/min until hospital discharge or up to 72 h

PCI in Patients with ACS

Adult: **IV** 180 mcg/kg initial bolus followed by 0.5 mcg/kg/min for 20–24 h after end of procedure

PCI in Patients without ACS

Adult: **IV** 135 mcg/kg initial bolus followed by 0.5 mcg/kg/min for 20–24 h after end of procedure

ADMINISTRATION

Note: Review contraindications to administration prior to giving this drug.

Intravenous

PREPARE: **Direct:** Give undiluted.
ADMINISTER: **Direct:** Give bolus doses IV push over 1–2. **Continuous:** Start continuous infusion immediately following bolus dose. Give undiluted directly from the 100-mL vial (at a rate based on patient's weight) using a vented infusion set. May be given in the same IV line with NS or D5/NS (either solution may contain up to 60 mEq KCl).

- Store unopened vials at 2°–8° C (36°–46° F) and protect from light. Discard any unused portion in opened vial.

ADVERSE EFFECTS (≥1%) **CNS:** Intracranial bleed (rare). **GI:** GI bleeding. **Hematologic:** *Bleeding* (major bleeding 4.4%–11%), anemia, thrombocytopenia.

INTERACTIONS Drug: ORAL ANTICOAGULANTS, NSAIDS, **dipyridamole, ticlopidine, dextran** may increase risk of bleeding.

PHARMACOKINETICS Duration: 6–8 h after stopping infusion. **Distribution:** 25% protein bound. **Metabolism:** Minimally metabolized. **Elimination:** 50% excreted in urine. **Half-Life:** 2.5 h.

NURSING IMPLICATIONS

Assessment & Drug Effects

- Lab tests: Prior to infusion determine PT/aPTT & INR, ACT for those undergoing percutaneous coronary intervention (PCI); Hct or Hgb; platelet count; and serum creatinine.
- Lab tests: Monitor aPTT & INR (target aPPT, 50–70 s); during PCI (target ACT, 300–350 s).
- Minimize all vascular and other trauma during treatment. When obtaining IV access, avoid using a noncompressible site such as the subclavian vein.
- Monitor carefully for and immediately report S&S of bleeding (e.g., femoral artery access site bleeding, intracerebral hemorrhage, GI bleeding).
- Immediately stop infusion of eptifibatide and heparin if bleeding at the arterial access site cannot be controlled by pressure.
- Achieve hemostasis at the arterial access site by standard compres-

sion for a minimum of 4 h prior to hospital discharge following discontinuation of eptifibatide and heparin.

E

ERGOCALCIFEROL

(er-goe-kal-si'fe-role)

Activated Ergosterol, Calciferol, Deltalin, Drisdol, D-ViSol, Ostoforte ✦, Radiostol ✦, Radiostol Forte ✦, Vitamin D_2

Classifications: HORMONES AND SYNTHETIC SUBSTITUTES; VITAMIN D ANALOG

Prototype: Calcitriol

Pregnancy Category: C

AVAILABILITY 8000 IU/mL oral liquid; 50,000 units capsules, tablets; 500,000 IU/mL injection

ACTIONS The name Vitamin D encompasses two related fat-soluble substances (sterols) that occur in nature or are synthetically prepared. Vitamin D acts like a hormone in that it is distributed through the circulation and plays a major regulatory role.

THERAPEUTIC EFFECTS Maintains normal blood calcium and phosphate ion levels by enhancing their intestinal absorption and by promoting mobilization of calcium from bone and renal tubular resorption of phosphate.

USES Familial hypophosphatemia (vitamin D-resistant rickets), osteomalacia (adult rickets), anticonvulsant-induced rickets and osteomalacia, osteoporosis, renal osteodystrophy, hypocalcemia associated with hypoparathyroidism; prophylaxis and treatment of nutritional rickets. Also hypophosphatemia in Fanconi's syndrome.

UNLABELED USES With varying clinical results in lupus vulgaris, psoriasis, and rheumatoid arthritis.

CONTRAINDICATIONS Hypersensitivity to vitamin D, hypervitaminosis D, hypercalcemia, hyperphosphatemia, renal osteodystrophy with hyperphosphatemia, malabsorption syndrome, decreased kidney function. Safe use of amounts in excess of 400 IU (10 mcg) daily during pregnancy (category C) is not established.

CAUTIOUS USE Coronary disease; lactation; arteriosclerosis (especially in older adults); history of kidney stones.

ROUTE & DOSAGE

Nutritional Rickets, Osteomalacia

Adult: **PO/IM** 25–125 mcg/d for 6–12 wk, may need up to 7.5 mg/d in patients with malabsorption

Child: **PO/IM** 50–125 mcg/d, may need up to 250–625 mcg/d in patients with malabsorption

Vitamin D–Dependent Rickets

Adult: **PO/IM** 250 mcg–1.5 mg/d, may need up to 12.5 mg/d (prolonged therapy with >2.5 mg/d increases risk of toxicity)

Child: **PO/IM** 75–125 mcg/d, may need up to 1.5 mg/d

Hypoparathyroidism, Pseudohypoparathyroidism

Adult: **PO/IM** 625 mcg–5 mg/d, may need up to 10 mg/d (prolonged therapy with >2.5 mg/d increases risk of toxicity)

Child: **PO/IM** 1.25–5 mg/d, (prolonged therapy with >2.5 mg/d increases risk of toxicity)

ADMINISTRATION

Note: 40 U = 1 mcg. Reduce dosage, once symptoms of vitamin D deficiency are relieved, to prevent hypercalcemia.

Intramuscular

- Give injection deeply, preferably into gluteus maximus and inject slowly. Aspirate carefully. Rotate injection sites.
- Preserve in tightly covered, light-resistant containers. Drug decomposes when exposed to light and air.

ADVERSE EFFECTS (≥1%) **Body as a Whole:** Fatigue, weakness, vertigo, tinnitus, ataxia, muscle and joint pain, hypotonia (infants), exanthema, rhinorrhea; pruritus; mild acidosis. **Nervous System:** Headache, drowsiness, convulsions. **Digestive:** Metallic taste, dry mouth, anorexia, nausea, vomiting, diarrhea, constipation, abdominal cramps. **Hematologic:** Anemia. **Musculoskeletal:** Calcification of soft tissues (kidneys, blood vessels, myocardium, lungs, skin). **Urogenital:** Nephrotoxicity (polyuria, hyposthenuria, polydipsia, nocturia, casts, albuminuria, hematuria), kidney failure. **Cardiovascular:** Hypertension, cardiac arrhythmias. **Special Senses:** Conjunctivitis (calcific); photophobia. **Metabolic:** Osteoporosis (adults); weight loss, chronic hypervitaminosis D in children (mental and physical retardation, suppression of linear growth).

DIAGNOSTIC TEST INTERFERENCE Vitamin D may cause false increase in ***serum cholesterol*** measurements (***Zlatkis-Zak reaction***).

INTERACTIONS Drug: Cholestyramine, colestipol, mineral oil may decrease absorption of vitamin D.

PHARMACOKINETICS Absorption: Readily absorbed from GI tract. **Peak activity:** After 4 wk. **Duration:** 2 mo or more. **Distribution:** Most of drug first appears in lymph, then concentrates in liver; stored chiefly in liver and to a lesser extent in skin, brain, spleen, and bones. **Metabolism:** Metabolized in liver and kidney to active metabolites. **Elimination:** About 50% of oral dose excreted in bile; may be stored in tissues for months. **Half-Life:** 12–24 h.

NURSING IMPLICATIONS

Assessment & Drug Effects

- Monitor closely patients receiving therapeutic doses of vitamin D must remain under close medical supervision.
- Lab tests: When high therapeutic doses are used, progress is followed by frequent determinations (q2wk or more often) of serum calcium, phosphorus, magnesium, alkaline phosphatase, BUN, and determinations of urine calcium, casts, albumin, and RBC. Blood calcium concentration is generally kept between 9 and 10 mg/dL.
- Monitor for hypercalcemia; in patients with osteomalacia a decrease in serum alkaline phosphatase may signal the onset of hypercalcemia.

Patient & Family Education

- Avoid magnesium-containing antacids and laxatives with chronic kidney failure when receiving vitamin D preparations since vitamin D increases the risk of magnesium intoxication than other patients.
- Do not use OTC medications unless approved by physician.
- Do not breast feed while taking this drug without consulting physician.

E

ERGOLOID MESYLATE

(er'goe-loid mess'i-late)

Gerimal, Hydergine, Hydroloid G, Niloric

Classifications: AUTONOMIC NERVOUS SYSTEM AGENT; ALPHA-ADRENERGIC ANTAGONIST (BLOCKING AGENT, SYMPATHOLYTIC); ERGOT ALKALOID

Prototype: Ergotamine tartrate

Pregnancy Category: C

AVAILABILITY 0.5 mg, 1 mg sublingual tablets; 0.5 mg, 1 mg tablets; 1 mg capsules; 1 mg/mL oral liquid

ACTIONS Combination of three hydrogenated derivatives of ergot alkaloids. Produces peripheral vasodilation primarily by central action and may cause slight reduction in BP and heart rate.

THERAPEUTIC EFFECTS Reportedly relieves symptoms of cerebral arteriosclerosis, possibly by increasing cerebral metabolism with consequent increase in blood flow. Improvement may not be apparent until after 3–4 wk of therapy.

USES Senile dementia of Alzheimer type.

CONTRAINDICATIONS Acute or chronic psychosis; hypersensitivity to ergoloid. Safety during pregnancy (category C), lactation, or in children is not established.

CAUTIOUS USE Acute intermittent porphyria.

ROUTE & DOSAGE

Senile Dementia of Alzheimer Type

Adult: **PO** 1 mg t.i.d.; doses up to 4.5–12 mg/d have been used

ADMINISTRATION

Sublingual

- Instruct patient to allow sublingual (SL) tablet to dissolve under tongue and not to drink, eat, or smoke while tablet is in place. Do not crush SL tablets.
- Store in tightly closed container.

ADVERSE EFFECTS (≥1%) **Body as a Whole:** Mostly dose related. **CV:** Orthostatic hypotension, dizziness or light-headedness, flushing, sinus bradycardia. **Special Senses:** Blurred vision, nasal stuffiness, increased nasopharyngeal secretions. **GI:** Sublingual irritation, anorexia, stomach cramps, transient nausea and vomiting, heartburn. **Skin:** Skin rash. **CNS:** Drowsiness, headache. **Other:** Precipitation of acute intermittent porphyria.

INTERACTIONS Drug: No clinically significant interactions established.

PHARMACOKINETICS Absorption: Incompletely absorbed from GI tract; approximately 50% reaches systemic circulation. **Peak:** 1.5–3 h. **Metabolism:** Undergoes rapid first-pass metabolism in liver. **Elimination:** Primarily excreted in feces. **Half-Life:** 2–12 h.

NURSING IMPLICATIONS

Assessment & Drug Effects

- Establish baseline values of BP and pulse; check at regular intervals throughout therapy.
- Report to physician sinus bradycardia (40 bpm); has been reported in patients receiving 1.5 mg doses. Pulse rate usually returns to normal within 2 d after drug is discontinued.
- Withdraw drug permanently if marked bradycardia or hypotension occurs.

Patient & Family Education

- Make position changes slowly, particularly from recumbent to upright posture, and move ankles and feet for a few minutes before walking.
- Do not breast feed while taking this drug without consulting physician.

ERGOTAMINE TARTRATE Pr

(er-got'a-meen)

Ergomar, Ergostat

Classifications: AUTONOMIC NERVOUS SYSTEM AGENT; ALPHA-ADRENERGIC ANTAGONIST (SYMPATHOLYTIC); ERGOT ALKALOID

Pregnancy Category: X

AVAILABILITY 2 mg sublingual tablets

ACTIONS Natural amino acid alkaloid of ergot. Alpha-adrenergic blocking agent with direct stimulating action on cranial and peripheral vascular smooth muscles and depressant effect on central vasomotor centers. Ergotamine activity can damage vascular endothelium by unknown mechanism, with subsequent occlusion, thrombosis, and gangrene.

THERAPEUTIC EFFECTS In vascular headache, exerts vasoconstrictive action on previously dilated cerebral vessels, reduces amplitude of arterial pulsations, and antagonizes effects of serotonin.

USES As single agent or in combination with caffeine to prevent or abort migraine, cluster headache (histamine cephalalgia), and other vascular headaches. Not recommended for migraine prophylaxis because of the possibility of adverse effects.

CONTRAINDICATIONS Hypersensitivity to ergotamine; sepsis, obliterative vascular disease, thromboembolic disease, prolonged use of excessive dosage, liver and kidney disease, severe pruritus, marked arteriosclerosis, history of MI, coronary artery disease, hypertension; infectious states, anemia, malnutrition; pregnancy (category X), use in children.

CAUTIOUS USE Lactation, older adult patients.

ROUTE & DOSAGE

Vascular Headaches

Adult: **SL** 1–2 mg followed by 1–2 mg q30min until headache abates or until max of 6 mg/24h or 10 mg/wk

ADMINISTRATION

Sublingual

- Instruct patient to allow sublingual (SL) tablet to dissolve under tongue and not to drink, eat, or smoke while tablet is in place. Do not crush SL tablets.

ADVERSE EFFECTS (≥1%) **Body as a Whole:** Paresthesias*; pain (spasms) of facial muscles*, tongue*, limbs*, and lumbar region with difficulty in walking*; muscle pains*, *weakness**, numbness*, coldness and cyanosis of digits (Raynaud's phenomenon)*. **Nervous System:** Delirium*; convulsive seizures*; confusion*; depression; drowsiness; **Digestive:** *Nausea*; vomiting**; diarrhea*; abdominal pain*; unquenchable thirst*; partial necrosis of tongue, disagreeable aftertaste. **Cardiovascular:** Rapid, weak, or irregular pulse*; intermittent claudication*, complete absence of medium- and large-vessel pulsations in extremities; precordial distress and pain; angina pectoris, transient bradycardia or tachycardia; elevated or lowered BP. **Skin:** Itching* and cold skin*; gangrene of nose, digits, ears*. **Urogenital:** Kidney failure. ***Symptoms of ergotism.**

INTERACTIONS Drug: With high doses of BETA-ADRENERGIC BLOCKERS, SYMPATHOMIMETICS, possibility of additive vasoconstrictor effects; **erythromycin, troleandomycin** may cause severe peripheral vasospasm. **Eletriptan, naratriptan, rizatriptan, sumatriptan, or zolmitriptan** may increase risk of coronary ischemia, separate drugs by 24 h; AZOLE ANTIFUNGALS (**ketoconazole, itraconazole, fluconazole, clotrimazole**), **nefazodone, fluoxetine, fluvoxamine,** amprenavir, **delavirdine, efavirenz, indinavir, nelfinavir, ritonavir, and saquinavir,** may inhibit ergot metabolism and increase toxicity; **sibutramine, dexfenfluramine, nefazodone, fluvoxamine** may increase risk of serotonin syndrome. **Food:** Grapefruit juice may increase toxicity.

PHARMACOKINETICS Absorption: Variable absorption orally. **Peak:** 0.5–3 h. **Distribution:** Crosses blood–brain barrier. **Metabolism:** Extensive first-pass metabolism in liver. **Elimination:** 96% eliminated in feces; excreted in breast milk. **Half-Life:** 2.7 h initial phase, 21 h terminal phase.

NURSING IMPLICATIONS

Assessment & Drug Effects

- Monitor adverse GI effects. Nausea and vomiting are adverse reactions that occur in about 10% of patients after they take ergotamine. Patient may need an antiemetic. Consult with physician.
- Monitor patients with PVD carefully for development of peripheral ischemia.
- Monitor long-term effectiveness. Patients receiving high ergotamine doses for prolonged periods may experience increased frequency of headaches, fatigue, and depression. Discontinuation of the drug in these patients results in severe withdrawal headache that may last a few days.
- Overdose symptoms: Nausea, vomiting, weakness and pain in legs, numbness and tingling in fingers and toes, tachycardia or bradycardia, hypertension or hypotension, and localized edema.

Patient & Family Education

- Begin drug therapy as soon after onset of migraine attack as possible, preferably during migraine prodrome (scintillating scotomas, visual field defects, nausea, paresthesias usually on side opposite to that of the migraine).
- Notify physician if migraine attacks occur more frequently or are not relieved.
- Lie down in a quiet, dark room for 2–3 h after drug administration.
- Report claudication, muscle pain or weakness of extremities, cold or numb digits, irregular heartbeat, nausea, or vomiting. Carefully protect extremities from exposure to cold temperatures; provide warmth, but not heat, to ischemic areas.
- Do NOT increase dosage without consulting physician; overdosage is the chief cause of adverse effects from the drug.
- Do not breast feed while taking this drug without consulting physician.

ERLOTINIB

(er-lo′ti-nib)

Tarceva

Classifications: ANTINEOPLASTIC AGENTS; EPIDERMAL GROWTH FACTOR RECEPTOR INHIBITOR

Prototype: Gefitinib

Pregnancy Category: D

AVAILABILITY 25 mg, 100 mg, 150 mg tablets

ACTIONS Erlotinib is a human epidermal growth factor receptor type 1 (HER1/EGFR) inhibitor. Antitumor action of erlotinib is believed to be due to inhibition of EGFR present on the cell surface of both normal and cancer cells.
THERAPEUTIC EFFECTS Inhibition of EGFR in cancer cells diminishes their capacity for cell proliferation, cell survival, and decreases metastases.

USES Treatment of patients with locally advanced or metastatic non–small cell lung cancer (NSCLC) after failure of at least one prior chemotherapy regimen.
UNLABELED USES Pancreatic cancer.

CONTRAINDICATIONS Hypersensitivity to erlotinib; pregnancy (category D); lactation.
CAUTIOUS USE Hepatic dysfunction, interstitial pulmonary disease (interstitial pneumonia, pneumonitis, alveolitis); myelosuppression; ocular toxicities (corneal ulcer, eye pain). Concurrent use of ketoconazole and other strong CYP3A4 inhibitors (e.g., atazanavir, clarithromycin, indinavir, itraconazole, nefazodone, nelfinavir, ritonavir, saquinavir, telithromycin, troleandomycin, and voriconazole).

ROUTE & DOSAGE

Metastatic Non–Small Cell Lung Cancer

Adult: **PO** 150 mg once daily at least 1 h before or 2 h after meals

ADMINISTRATION

Oral
- Give at least 1 h before or 2 h after eating.
- Store at 15–30° C (59–86° F). Keep container tightly closed. Protect from light.

ADVERSE EFFECTS (≥1%) **Body as a Whole:** Infection. **GI:** *Diarrhea,* anorexia, *fatigue,* nausea, vomiting, stomatitis, abdominal pain. **Metabolic:** Increased LFTs. **Respiratory:** *Dyspnea,* cough, <u>interstitial lung disease (sometimes fatal)</u>. **Skin:** *Acneiform rash,* pruritus, dry skin. **Special Senses:** Conjunctivitis, dry eyes.

INTERACTIONS Drug: Atazanavir, clarithromycin, indinavir, itraconazole, ketoconazole, nefazodone, nelfinavir, ritonavir, saquinavir, telithromycin, troleandomycin, voriconazole may increase erlotinib levels and toxicity; **rifampin, rifabutin, rifapentine, phenytoin, carbamazepine, phenobarbital** may decrease erlotinib levels. **Herbal: St. John's wort** may decrease erlotinib levels.

PHARMACOKINETICS Absorption: 60% absorbed orally; food can increase to 100%. **Peak:** 4 h. **Metabolism:** Metabolized in liver by CYP3A4. **Elimination:** Primarily excreted in feces (83%). **Half-Life:** 36.2 h.

NURSING IMPLICATIONS

Assessment & Drug Effects
- Monitor closely changes in pulmonary function.
- Withhold drug and notify physician for acute onset of new or progressive pulmonary symptoms (e.g., dyspnea, cough, or fever) or significant changes in liver functions as indicated by elevated transaminases, bilirubin, and alkaline phosphatase.
- Lab tests: periodic LFTs.

E

Patient & Family Education

- Report promptly any of the following: severe or persistent diarrhea, nausea, anorexia, or vomiting; onset or worsening of unexplained shortness of breath or cough; eye irritation.
- Monitor closely PT/INR values with concurrent warfarin therapy.
- Women should use effective means to avoid pregnancy while taking this drug.
- Do not breast feed while taking this drug without consulting physician.

ERTAPENEM SODIUM

(er-ta-pen'em)
Invanz
Classifications: ANTIINFECTIVE; BETA-LACTAM ANTIBIOTIC
Prototype: Imepenem-Cilastatin
Pregnancy Category: B

AVAILABILITY 1 g vial

ACTIONS Broad-spectrum carbapenem antibiotic that inhibits the cell wall synthesis of gram-positive and gram-negative bacteria by its strong affinity for penicillin-binding proteins (PBPs) of the bacterial cell wall.
THERAPEUTIC EFFECTS Effective against both gram-positive and gram-negative bacteria. Highly resistant to most bacterial beta-lactamases. Effective against most *Enterobacteriaceae, Pseudomonas aeruginosa*, and *Acinetobacter spp*. It is poorly effective against *Enterococci* bacteria, particularly vancomycin-resistant strains (VRSA).

USES Complicated intraabdominal infections, complicated skin and skin structure infections, community-acquired pneumonia, complicated UTI (including pyelonephritis), and acute pelvic infections due to susceptible bacteria.

CONTRAINDICATIONS Hypersensitivity to ertapenem; hypersensitivity to amide-type local anesthetics such as lidocaine; hypersensitivity to meropenem or imipenem; previous anaphylactic reaction to beta-lactams.
CAUTIOUS USE Renal impairment; history of CNS disorders; history of seizures; hypersensitivity to other beta-lactam antibiotics (penicillins, cephalosporins); pregnancy (category B); hypersensitivity to other allergens; meningitis; lactation (bottle feed during, and for 5 d after therapy ends).

ROUTE & DOSAGE

Community Acquired Pneumonia; Complicated UTI
Adult: **IV/IM** 1 g q.d. × 10–14 d May switch to appropriate PO antibiotic after 3 d if responding
Intraabdominal Infection
Adult: **IV/IM** 1 g q.d. × 5–14 d
Skin and Skin Structure Infections
Adult: **IV/IM** 1 g q.d. × 7–14 d
Acute Pelvic Infections
Adult: **IV/IM** 1 g q.d. × 3–10 d
Renal Impairment (all indications)
Cl_{cr} <30 mL/min, reduce dose to 500 mg q.d.

ADMINISTRATION

Intramuscular

- Reconstitute 1 g vial with 3.2 mL of 1.0% lidocaine HCI injection (without epinephrine). Shake vial thoroughly to form solution. Use immediately.
- Inject deep IM into a large muscle mass (such as the gluteal muscles or lateral part of the thigh).

- The reconstituted IM solution should be used within 1 h after preparation. Note: DO NOT use this solution for IV administration.

Intravenous

PREPARE: **Intermittent:** Reconstitute 1 g vial with 10 mL of sterile water for injection, NS, or bacteriostatic water for injection. Shake well to dissolve and immediately transfer contents to 50 mL of NS injection solution.

ADMINISTER: **Intermittent:** Infuse over 30 min. Note: Infusion should be completed within 6 h of reconstitution.

INCOMPATIBILITIES **Solution/additive: Dextrose. Y-site:** Do not mix or infuse with any other drugs.

- Store lyophilized powder above 25° C (77° F). May store reconstituted solution for 6 h at room temperature (not greater than 25° C/77° F) or for 24 h under refrigeration. Use within 4 h of removal from refrigeration. Do not freeze.

ADVERSE EFFECTS (≥1%) **Body as a Whole:** Phlebitis or thrombosis at injection site, asthenia, fatigue, <u>death</u>, fever, leg pain. **CNS:** Anxiety, altered mental status, dizziness, headache, insomnia. **CV:** Chest pain, hypertension, hypotension, tachycardia, edema. **GI:** Abdominal pain, *diarrhea*, acid regurgitation, constipation, dyspepsia, nausea, vomiting, increased AST and ALT. **Respiratory:** Cough, dyspnea, pharyngitis, rales/rhonchi, and respiratory distress. **Skin:** Erythema, pruritus, rash. **Urogenital:** Vaginitis.

INTERACTIONS Drug: Probenecid decreases renal excretion.

PHARMACOKINETICS Absorption: 90% absorbed from IM site. **Peak:** 2.3 h. **Distribution:** 95% protein bound, distributes into breast milk, may cross placenta. **Metabolism:** Hydrolysis of beta-lactam ring. **Elimination:** 80% excreted in urine, 10% in feces. **Half-Life:** 4.5 h.

NURSING IMPLICATIONS

Assessment & Drug Effects

- Lab tests: Perform C&S tests prior to therapy. Monitor periodically liver and kidney function.
- Determine history of hypersensitivity reactions to other beta-lactams, cephalosporins, penicillins, or other drugs.
- Discontinue drug and immediately report S&S of hypersensitivity (see Appendix F).
- Report S&S of superinfection or pseudomembranous colitis (see Appendix F).
- Monitor for seizures especially in older adults and those with renal insufficiency.
- Lab tests: Monitor AST, ALT, alkaline phosphatase, CBC, platelet count, and routine blood chemistry during prolonged therapy.

Patient & Family Education

- Learn S&S of hypersensitivity, superinfection, and pseudomembranous colitis (see Appendix F); report any of these to physician promptly.
- Do not breast feed during and for at least 5 d following termination of therapy.

ERYTHROMYCIN Pr

(er-ith-roe-mye′sin)

Akne-Mycin Ery-Tab, Apo-Erythro Base ♣, A/T/S, E-Mycin, Eryc, EryDerm, Erythrocin, Erythromid ♣, Erythromycin Base, Ilotycin, Novorythro ♣, PCE, Robimycin, Ro-Mycin ♣, Staticin, T-Stat

E

ERYTHROMYCIN ESTOLATE

Ilosone, Nororythro ✦

ERYTHROMYCIN STEARATE

Apo-Erythro-S ✦, Eramycin, Erypar, Ethril, Erythrocin Stearate, SK-Erythromycin

Classifications: ANTIINFECTIVE; MACROLIDE ANTIBIOTIC

Pregnancy Category: B

AVAILABILITY Erythromycin 250 mg, 333 mg, 500 mg tablets, capsules; 1.5%, 2% topical solution; 2% gel; 2% ointment; 5% ophthalmic ointment; **Erythromycin Estolate** 250 mg capsules; 500 mg tablets; 125 mg/mL, 250 mg/mL suspension; **Erythromycin Stearate** 250 mg, 500 mg tablets

ACTIONS Macrolide antibiotic produced by a strain of *Streptomyces erythreus*. Bacteriostatic or bactericidal, depending on nature of organism and drug concentration used.

THERAPEUTIC EFFECTS More active against gram-positive than gram-negative bacteria. Effectiveness against *Chlamydia trachomatis* is basis for its topical use in prophylaxis of neonatal inclusion conjunctivitis.

USES Pneumococcal pneumonia, *Mycoplasma pneumoniae* (primary atypical pneumonia), acute pelvic inflammatory disease caused by *Neisseria gonorrhoeae* in females sensitive to penicillin, infections caused by susceptible strains of staphylococci, streptococci, and certain strains of *Haemophilus influenzae*. Also used in intestinal amebiasis, Legionnaires' disease, uncomplicated urethral, endocervical, and rectal infections caused by *Chlamydia trachomatis,* for prophylaxis of ophthalmia neonatorum caused by *N. gonorrhoeae, C. trachomatis,* and for chlamydial conjunctivitis in neonates. Considered an acceptable alternative to penicillin for treatment of streptococcal pharyngitis, for prophylaxis of rheumatic fever and bacterial endocarditis, for treatment of diphtheria as adjunct to antitoxin and for carrier state, and as alternate choice in treatment of primary syphilis in patients allergic to penicillins. **Topical applications:** Pyodermas, acne vulgaris, and external ocular infections, including neonatal chlamydial conjunctivitis and gonococcal ophthalmia.

CONTRAINDICATIONS Hypersensitivity to erythromycins. **Estolate:** History of erythromycin-associated hepatitis; liver dysfunction; treatment of skin disorders such as acne or furunculosis; prophylaxis of rheumatic fever.

CAUTIOUS USE Impaired liver function; pregnancy (category B), lactation.

ROUTE & DOSAGE

Moderate to Severe Infections

Adult: **PO** 250–500 mg q6h; 333 mg q8h
Child: **PO** 30–50 mg/kg/d divided q6h **Topical** Apply ointment to infected eye 1 or more times/d
Neonate: **PO** *≤7 d,* 10 mg/kg q12h; *>7 d,* 10 mg/kg q8–12h **Topical** 0.5–1 cm in conjunctival sac once

***Chlamydia trachomatis* Infections**

Adult: **PO** 500 mg q.i.d. or 666 mg q8h
Child: **Topical** Apply 0.5–1 cm ribbon in lower conjunctival sacs shortly after birth

ADMINISTRATION

Oral

- Give on an empty stomach 1 h before or 3 h after meals. Do not give with, or immediately before or after, fruit juices, and advise patient not to crush or chew tablets.
- Give enteric-coated tablets without regard to meals.
- Ensure that enteric-coated tablets are not chewed or crushed. They must be swallowed whole.
- Note: When switching from tablet to a PO liquid preparation, dosing may require adjustment.

Topical

- Prophylaxis for neonatal eye infection: Ribbon of ointment approximately 0.5–1 cm long is placed into lower conjunctival sac of neonate shortly after birth. Use a new tube of erythromycin for each neonate.
- Use only preparations labeled for ophthalmic use for treatment of eye infections.
- Store all forms at 15°–30° C (59°–86° F) in tightly capped containers unless otherwise directed by manufacturer.

ADVERSE EFFECTS (≥1%) **GI:** *Nausea, vomiting, abdominal cramping,* diarrhea, heartburn, anorexia. **Body as a Whole:** Fever, eosinophilia, urticaria, skin eruptions, fixed drug eruption, anaphylaxis. Superinfections by nonsusceptible bacteria, yeasts, or fungi. **Special Senses:** Ototoxicity: reversible bilateral hearing loss, tinnitus, vertigo. **Digestive:** (Estolate) Cholestatic hepatitis syndrome. **Skin:** (topical use) Erythema, desquamation, burning, tenderness, dryness or oiliness, pruritus.

DIAGNOSTIC TEST INTERFERENCE False elevations of ***urinary catecholamines, urinary steroids,*** and ***AST, ALT*** (by ***colorimetric methods***).

INTERACTIONS Drug: Serum levels and toxicities of **alfentanil, bexarotene, carbamazepine, cevimeline, cilostazol, clozapine, cyclosporine, disopyramide, estazolam, fentanyl, midazolam, methadone, modafinil, quinidine, sirolimus, digoxin, theophylline, triazolam, warfarin** are increased. **Ergotamine, dihydroergotamine** may increase peripheral vasospasm.

PHARMACOKINETICS Absorption: Erythromycin base is acid labile; most erythromycins are absorbed in small intestine. **Peak:** 1–4 h PO. **Distribution:** Widely distributed to most body tissues; low concentrations in CSF; concentrates in liver and bile; crosses placenta. **Metabolism:** Partially metabolized in liver. **Elimination:** Primarily excreted in bile; excreted in breast milk. **Half-Life:** 1.5–2 h.

NURSING IMPLICATIONS

Assessment & Drug Effects

- Report onset of GI symptoms after PO administration to physician. These are dose related; if symptoms persist after dosage reduction, physician may prescribe drug to be given with meals in spite of impaired absorption.
- Monitor for adverse GI effects. Pseudomembranous enterocolitis (see Appendix F), a potentially life-threatening condition, may occur during or after antibiotic therapy.
- Observe for S&S of superinfection by overgrowth of nonsusceptible bacteria or fungi. Emergence of resistant staphylococcal strains is highly predictable during prolonged therapy.

- Lab tests: Periodic liver function tests during prolonged therapy.
- Monitor for S&S of hepatotoxicity. Premonitory S&S include: Abdominal pain, nausea, vomiting, fever, leukocytosis, and eosinophilia; jaundice may or may not be present. Symptoms may appear a few days after initiation of drug but usually occur after 1–2 wk of continuous therapy. Symptoms are reversible with prompt discontinuation of erythromycin.
- Monitor for ototoxicity that appears to develop most frequently in patients receiving 4 g/d or more, older adults, female patients, and patients with kidney or liver dysfunction. It is reversible with prompt discontinuation of drug.

Patient & Family Education

- Notify physician for S&S of superinfection (see Appendix F).
- Notify physician immediately for S&S of pseudomembranous enterocolitis (see Appendix F), which may occur even after the drug is discontinued.
- Report any ototoxic effects including dizziness, vertigo, nausea, tinnitus, roaring noises, hearing impairment (see Appendix F).
- Do not breast feed while taking this drug without consulting physician.

ERYTHROMYCIN ETHYLSUCCINATE

(er-ith-roe-mye′sin)

Apo-Erythro-ES ✦, E.E.S., E.E.S.-200, E.E.S.-400, EryPed, Pediamycin

Classifications: ANTIINFECTIVE; MACROLIDE ANTIBIOTIC

Prototype: Erythromycin

Pregnancy Category: B

AVAILABILITY 200 mg chewable tablet, 400 mg tablets; 100 mg/2.5 mL, 200 mg/5 mL, 400 mg/5 mL suspension

ACTIONS Acid-stable ester salt of erythromycin.

THERAPEUTIC EFFECTS More active against gram-positive than gram-negative bacteria. Effectiveness against *Chlamydia trachomatis* is basis for its topical use in prophylaxis of neonatal inclusion conjunctivitis.

USES See erythromycin.

CONTRAINDICATIONS Hypersensitivity to erythromycins; history of erythromycin-associated hepatitis; preexisting liver disease.

CAUTIOUS USE Myasthenia gravis; pregnancy (category B), lactation.

ROUTE & DOSAGE

Infection

Adult: **PO** 400 mg q6h up to 4 g/d according to severity of infection
Child: **PO** 30–50 mg/kg/d in 4 divided doses (max: 100 mg/kg/d) for severe infections

ADMINISTRATION

Note: 400 mg erythromycin ethylsuccinate is approximately equal to 250 mg erythromycin base.

Oral

- Chewable tablets should be chewed and not swallowed whole.
- Suspensions are stable for 14 d at room temperature unless otherwise stated by manufacturer. Note expiration date.
- Store tablets in tight containers unless otherwise directed.

ADVERSE EFFECTS (≥1%) **GI:** Diarrhea, *nausea,* vomiting, stomatitis, *abdominal cramps,* anorexia, hepatotoxicity. **Skin:** Skin eruptions. **Special Senses:** Ototoxicity. **Body as a Whole:** Potential for superinfections.

INTERACTIONS Drug: Serum levels and toxicities of **alfentanil, bexarotene, carbamazepine, cevimeline, cilostazol, clozapine, cyclosporine, disopyramide, estazolam, fentanyl, midazolam, methadone, modafinil, quinidine, sirolimus, digoxin, theophylline, triazolam, warfarin** are increased. **Ergotamine** may increase peripheral vasospasm. May increase risk of arrhythmias with **terfenadine, astemizole.**

PHARMACOKINETICS Absorption: Readily absorbed from GI tract. **Peak:** 2 h. **Distribution:** Concentrates in liver; crosses placenta; distributed into breast milk. **Metabolism:** Metabolized in liver. **Elimination:** Excreted primarily in bile and feces. **Half-Life:** 2–5 h.

NURSING IMPLICATIONS

Assessment & Drug Effects

- Lab tests: Determine C&S prior to treatment. Periodic liver function tests and blood cell counts if therapy is prolonged 10 d.
- Cholestatic hepatitis syndrome is most likely to occur in adults who have received erythromycin estolate for >10 d or who have had repeated courses of therapy. The condition generally clears within 3–5 d after cessation of therapy.

Patient & Family Education

- Advise patient to report immediately the onset of adverse reactions and to be on the alert for signs and symptoms associated with jaundice (see Appendix F).
- Ototoxicity is most likely to occur in patients receiving high dosage or who have impaired kidney function. Report immediately the onset of tinnitus, vertigo, or hearing impairment.
- Do not breast feed while taking this drug without consulting physician.

ERYTHROMYCIN GLUCEPTATE

(er-ith-roe-mye′sin)

Ilotycin Gluceptate

ERYTHROMYCIN LACTOBIONATE

Erythrocin Lactobionate-I.V.

Classifications: ANTIINFECTIVE; MACROLIDE ANTIBIOTIC

Prototype: Erythromycin

Pregnancy Category: B

AVAILABILITY 500 mg, 1 g injection

ACTIONS Soluble salt of erythromycin. It binds to the 50s ribosome subunits of susceptible bacteria, resulting in the suppression of protein synthesis of bacteria.

THERAPEUTIC EFFECTS More active against gram-positive than gram-negative bacteria. Effectiveness against *Chlamydia trachomatis* is basis for its topical use in prophylaxis of neonatal inclusion conjunctivitis.

USES When oral administration is not possible or the severity of infection requires immediate high serum levels. See erythromycin.

CONTRAINDICATIONS Hypersensitivity to erythromycins; concurrent administration with terfenadine, astemizole, or cisapride.

CAUTIOUS USE Impaired liver function; pregnancy (category B), lactation.

E

ROUTE & DOSAGE

Infections

Adult: **IV** 250 mg–1 g q6h up to 4 g/d according to severity of infection
Child: **IV** 15–20 mg/kg/d in 4 divided doses up to 100 mg/kg/d for severe infections

ADMINISTRATION

Intravenous

PREPARE: **Intermittent/Continuous:** Initial solution is prepared by adding 10 mL sterile water for injection without preservatives to each 500 mg or fraction thereof. Shake vial until drug is completely dissolved. **Intermittent:** Further dilute each 1 gm dose in 100–250 mL of D5W or NS. **Continuous:** Further dilute each 1 gm in 1000 mL D5W or NS. Give within 4 h.

ADMINISTER: **Intermittent:** Give 1 gm or fraction thereof over 20–60 min. Slow rate if pain develops along course of vein. **Continuous:** Continuous infusion is administered slowly, usually over 6 h.

INCOMPATIBILITIES **Solution/additive: Dextrose**-containing solutions, **aminophylline, ampicillin,** TETRACYCLINES, **pentobarbital, secobarbital, streptomycin, heparin, cephalothin, colistimethate, floxacillin, furosemide, metaraminol, metoclopramide, vitamin B complex with C, ampicillin, amikacin. Y-site: Aminophylline, fluconazole, heparin,** TETRACYCLINES.

- Store: **Gluceptate**, reconstituted solution is stable up to 7 d if refrigerated at 2°–8° C (36°–46° F); use solution diluted for infusion within 4 h. **Lactobionate**, reconstituted solution is stable up to 14 d if refrigerated at 2°–8° C (36°–46° F); use solution diluted for infusion within 8 h.

ADVERSE EFFECTS (≥1%) **Body as a Whole:** *Pain and venous irritation after IV injection;* allergic reactions, anaphylaxis (rare); superinfections. **GI:** *Nausea,* vomiting, diarrhea, *abdominal cramps,* variations in liver function tests following prolonged or repeated therapy. [See also **erythromycin.**]

INTERACTIONS Drug: Serum levels and toxicities of **alfentanil, bexarotene, carbamazepine, cevimeline, cilostazol, clozapine, cyclosporine, disopyramide, estazolam, fentanyl, midazolam, methadone, modafinil, quinidine, sirolimus, digoxin, theophylline, triazolam, warfarin** are increased. **Ergotamine** may increase peripheral vasospasm. May increase risk of arrhythmias with **terfenadine, astemizole.**

PHARMACOKINETICS Peak: 1 h. **Distribution:** Concentrates in liver; crosses placenta; distributed into breast milk. **Metabolism:** Metabolized in liver. **Elimination:** Excreted primarily in bile and feces; 12%–15% excreted in urine. **Half-Life:** 3–5 h.

NURSING IMPLICATIONS

Assessment & Drug Effects

- Lab tests: Determine C&S prior to initiation of therapy. Periodic liver function tests with daily high doses or prolonged or repeated therapy.
- Monitor hearing impairment may occur with large doses of this drug. It may occur as early as the second day and as late as the third week of therapy.
- Monitor for S&S of thrombophlebitis (see Appendix F). IV infu-

sion of large doses is reported to increase risk.

Patient & Family Education

- Notify physician immediately of tinnitus, dizziness, or hearing impairment.
- Do not breast feed while taking this drug without consulting physician.

ESCITALOPRAM OXALATE

(es-ci-tal′o-pram)

Lexapro

Classifications: CENTRAL NERVOUS SYSTEM (CNS) AGENT; PSYCHOTHERAPEUTIC AGENT; SELECTIVE SEROTONIN-REUPTAKE INHIBITOR (SSRI)

Prototype: Fluoxetine

Pregnancy Category: C

AVAILABILITY 5 mg, 10 mg, 20 mg tablets; 5 mg/5 mL liquid

ACTIONS Selective serotonin reuptake inhibitor (SSRI) in the CNS. Antidepressant effect is presumed to be linked to its inhibition of CNS presynaptic neuronal uptake of serotonin which results in antidepressant activity. Does not produce any sympathomimetic response or anticholinergic activity.

THERAPEUTIC EFFECTS Does not inhibit MAOIS. Selective serotonin reuptake inhibition mechanism results in the antidepressant activity of escitalopram.

USES Depression, generalized anxiety disorder.

UNLABELED USES Treatment of panic disorders.

CONTRAINDICATIONS Hypersensitivity to citalopram; concurrent use of MAOIS or use within 14 d of discontinuing MAOIS; pregnancy (category C); volume depleted; lactation; children <18 y.

CAUTIOUS USE Hypersensitivity to other SSRIs; suicidal ideations, depression, mania, hyponatremia, ethanol intoxication, ECT, dehydration, renal or hepatic insufficiency; older adults; concurrent use of diuretics, cardiovascular disease (e.g., dysrhythmias, conduction defects, myocardial ischemia); history of seizure disorders or suicidal tendencies.

ROUTE & DOSAGE

Depression, Generalized Anxiety

Adult: **PO** 10 q.d., may increase to 20 mg q.d. if needed after 1 wk
Geriatric: **PO** 10 mg q.d.

Panic Disorder

Adult: **PO** 5 q.d., may increase to 20 mg q.d. if needed after 1 wk

Hepatic Impairment

Adult: **PO** 10 q.d.

ADMINISTRATION

Oral

- Do not begin this drug within 14 d of stopping an MAOI.
- Reduced doses are advised for the older adult and those with hepatic or renal impairment.
- Dose increments should be separated by at least 1 wk.
- Store at 15°–30° C (59°–86° F) in tightly closed container and protect from light.

ADVERSE EFFECTS (≥1%) **Body as a Whole:** Fatigue, fever, arthralgia, myalgia. **CV:** Palpitation, hypertension. **GI:** *Nausea,* diarrhea, dyspepsia, abdominal pain, dry mouth, vomiting, flatulence, reflux. **CNS:** Dizziness, *insomnia, somnolence,* paresthesia, migraine, tremor, vertigo. **Metabolic:** Increased or decreased weight. **Respiratory:** URI, rhinitis, sinusitis. **Skin:** Increased sweating. **Urogenital:** Dysmenorrhea, decreased libido, ejaculation disorder, impotence, menstrual cramps.

INTERACTIONS Drug: Combination with MAOI could result in hypertensive crisis, hyperthermia, rigidity, myoclonus, autonomic instability; **cimetidine** may increase escitalopram levels; **linezolid** may cause serotonin syndrome. **Herbal: St. John's wort** may cause serotonin syndrome.

PHARMACOKINETICS Absorption: Rapidly absorbed from GI tract. **Onset:** Approximately 1 week. **Peak:** 3 h. **Distribution:** 80% protein bound; crosses placenta; distributed into breast milk. **Metabolism:** Metabolized in liver by CYP3A4 2C19 and 2D6 enzymes. **Elimination:** 20% excreted in urine, 80% in bile. **Half-Life:** 25 h.

NURSING IMPLICATIONS

Assessment & Drug Effects

- Monitor for therapeutic effectiveness: Indicated by elevation of mood; 1–4 wk may be needed before improvement is noted.
- Closely observe for worsening of depression or emergence of suicidality.
- Lab tests: Monitor periodically hepatic functions, CBC, serum sodium, and lithium levels when the two drugs are given concurrently.
- Monitor periodically HR and BP, and carefully monitor complete cardiac status in person with known or suspected cardiac disease.
- Monitor closely older adult patients for adverse effects, especially with doses >20 mg/d.

Patient & Family Education

- Do not engage in hazardous activities until reaction to this drug is known.
- Avoid using alcohol while taking escitalopram.
- Inform physician of commonly used OTC drugs as there is potential for drug interactions.
- Report distressing adverse effects including any changes in sexual functioning or response.
- Periodic ophthalmology exams are advised with long-term treatment.
- Do not breast feed while taking this drug.

ESMOLOL HYDROCHLORIDE

(ess′moe-lol)

Brevibloc

Classifications: AUTONOMIC NERVOUS SYSTEM AGENT; BETA-ADRENERGIC ANTAGONIST (BLOCKING AGENT, SYMPATHOLYTIC)

Prototype: Propranolol

Pregnancy Category: C

AVAILABILITY 10 mg/mL, 250 mg/mL injection

ACTIONS Ultrashort-acting $beta_1$-adrenergic blocking agent with cardioselective properties but devoid of intrinsic sympathetic activity (ISA) or membrane-stabilizing (quinidine-like) activity. Hemodynamic effects are mild, with potency as a beta blocker about 1/100th that of propranolol. Inhibits the agonist effect of catecholamines by competitive binding at beta-adrenergic receptors.

THERAPEUTIC EFFECTS Blocks sympathetically mediated increases in cardiac rate and BP since it binds predominantly to $beta_1$-receptors in cardiac tissue.

USES Supraventricular tachyarrhythmias (SVT) in perioperative and postoperative periods or in other critical situations. Also short-term treatment of noncompensating sinus tachycardia and in the control of heart rate for patients with MI.

UNLABELED USES Moderate postoperative hypertension; treatment of intense transient adrenergic response to surgical stress in cardiac as well as noncardiac surgery.

CONTRAINDICATIONS Cardiac failure, heart block greater than first degree, sinus bradycardia, cardiogenic shock; pregnancy (category C), lactation. Safety in children is not established.

CAUTIOUS USE History of allergy or bronchial asthma, bronchospasm, emphysema; CHF; diabetes mellitus; kidney function impairment.

ROUTE & DOSAGE

Supraventricular Tachyarrhythmias
Adult: **IV** 500 mcg/kg loading dose followed by 50 mcg/kg/min, may increase dose q5–10min prn (max: 200 mcg/kg/min)

ADMINISTRATION

Note: Do not use the 2500 mg ampul for direct IV injection.

Intravenous

PREPARE: **Direct:** Use the 10 mg/mL vial undiluted for the loading dose. **IV Infusion:** Prepare maintenance infusion by adding 250 mL of diluent to each 2500 mg ampul to yield 10 mg/mL. Compatible diluents include D5W, D5/RL, D5/NS, D5/.45NS, RL.

ADMINISTER: **Direct:** Give loading dose over 1 min. **IV Infusion:** Give maintenance infusion over 4 min. If adequate response is noted, continue maintenance infusion with periodic adjustments as needed. If an adequate response has not occurred, repeat loading dose and follow with an increased maintenance infusion of 100 mcg/kg/min. May continue titration cycle with same loading dose while increasing maintenance infusion by 50 mcg/kg/min until desired end point is near. Then omit loading dose and titrate maintenance dose up or down by 25 to 50 mcg/kg/min until desired heart rate is reached.

INCOMPATIBILITIES **Solution/Additive: Procainamide. Y-site: Amphotericin B cholesteryl, furosemide, warfarin.**

- Diluted infusion solution is stable for at least 24 h at room temperature.

ADVERSE EFFECTS (≥1%) **CNS:** Headache, *dizziness,* somnolence, confusion, agitation. **CV:** *Hypotension* (dose related), cold hands and feet, bradyarrhythmias, flushing, myocardial depression. **GI:** Nausea, vomiting. **Respiratory:** Dyspnea, chest pain, rhonchi, <u>bronchospasm</u>. **Skin:** *Infusion site inflammation* (redness, swelling, induration).

INTERACTIONS Drug: May increase **digoxin** IV levels 10%–20%; **morphine** IV may increase esmolol levels by 45%; **succinylcholine** may prolong neuromuscular blockade.

PHARMACOKINETICS Onset: <5 min. **Peak:** 10–20 min. **Duration:** 10–30 min. **Metabolism:** Rapidly hydrolyzed by RBC esterases. **Elimination:** Eliminated in urine. **Half-Life:** 9 min.

NURSING IMPLICATIONS

Assessment & Drug Effects

- Monitor BP, pulse, ECG, during esmolol infusion. Hypotension may have its onset during the initial titration phase; thereafter the risk increases with increasing doses. Usually the hypotension experienced during esmolol infusion is resolved within 30 min after infusion is reduced or discontinued.

E

- Change injection site if local reaction occurs. IV site reactions (burning, erythema) or diaphoresis may develop during infusion. Both reactions are temporary. Blood chemistry abnormalities have not been reported.
- Overdose symptoms: Discontinue administration if the following symptoms occur: bradycardia, severe dizziness or drowsiness, dyspnea, bluish-colored fingernails or palms of hands, seizures.

ESOMEPRAZOLE MAGNESIUM

(e-so-me'pra-zole)

Nexium

Classifications: GASTROINTESTINAL AGENT; PROTON PUMP INHIBITOR

Prototype: Omeprazole

Pregnancy Category: B

AVAILABILITY 20 mg, 40 mg capsules

ACTIONS Isomer of omeprazole. A weak base that is converted to the active form in the highly acidic environment of the secretory surface of the gastric parietal cells. Inhibits the enzyme H^+K^+-ATPase (the acid pump).

THERAPEUTIC EFFECTS Due to inhibition of the H^+K^+-ATPase, esomeprazole substantially decreases both basal and stimulated acid secretion through inhibition of the acid pump in parietal cells.

USES Erosive esophagitis, gastrointestinal reflux disease (GERD), duodenal ulcer associated with *H. pylori* in combination with antibiotics.

CONTRAINDICATIONS Hypersensitivity to esomeprazole magnesium, omeprazole, or other proton pump inhibitors; gastric malignancy; lactation.

CAUTIOUS USE Severe renal insufficiency; sever hepatic impairment; treatment for more than a year; gastric ulcers; pregnancy (category C). Safety and efficacy in children are not established.

ROUTE & DOSAGE

Healing of Erosive Esophagitis

Adult: **PO** 20–40 mg q.d. at least 1 h before meals times 4–8 wks

GERD, Erosive Esophagitis Maintenance

Adult: **PO** 20 mg q.d.

Duodenal Ulcer

Adult: **PO** 40 mg q.d. times 10 d

ADMINISTRATION

Oral

- Give at least 1 h before eating.
- Do not crush or chew capsule. Must be swallowed whole.
- Open capsule and mix pellets with applesauce (cold or room temperature) if patient cannot swallow capsules. Do NOT crush pellets. Applesauce should be swallowed immediately after mixing without chewing.
- May take with antacids.
- Store in the original blister package 15°–30° C (59°–86° F)

ADVERSE EFFECTS (≥1%) **CNS:** Headache. **GI:** Nausea, vomiting, diarrhea, constipation, abdominal pain, flatulence, dry mouth.

INTERACTIONS Drug: May increase **diazepam, phenytoin, warfarin** levels. **Food:** Food decreases absorption by up to 35%.

PHARMACOKINETICS Absorption: Destroyed in acidic environment, therefore capsules are designed for delayed absorption in the small intestine. 70% reaches systemic circulation. **Metabolism:** Metabolized in liver by CYP2C19. **Elimination:** Inactive metabolites excreted in both urine and feces. **Half-Life:** 1.5 h.

NURSING IMPLICATIONS

Assessment & Drug Effects

- Monitor for S&S of adverse CNS effects (vertigo, agitation, depression) especially in severely ill patients.
- Monitor phenytoin levels with concurrent use.
- Monitor INR/PT with concurrent warfarin use.
- Lab tests: Periodic liver function tests, CBC, Hct & Hbg, urinalysis for hematuria and proteinuria.

Patient & Family Education

- Report any changes in urinary elimination such as pain or discomfort associated with urination to physician.
- Report severe diarrhea. Drug may need to be discontinued.
- Do not breast feed while taking this drug without consulting physician.

ESTAZOLAM

(es-ta-zo'lam)

Prosom

Classifications: CENTRAL NERVOUS SYSTEM (CNS) AGENT; ANXIOLYTIC; SEDATIVE-HYPNOTIC; BENZODIAZEPINE

Prototype: Lorazepam

Pregnancy Category: X

Controlled Substance: Schedule IV

AVAILABILITY 1 mg, 2 mg tablets

ACTIONS Benzodiazepine whose effects (anxiolytic, sedative, hypnotic, skeletal muscle relaxant) are mediated by the inhibitory neurotransmitter gamma-aminobutyric acid (GABA). GABA acts at the thalamic, hypothalamic, and limbic levels of CNS.

THERAPEUTIC EFFECTS Benzodiazepines generally decrease the number of awakenings from sleep. Stage 2 (unequivocal sleep) is increased with all benzodiazepines. Estazolam shortens stages 3 and 4 (slow-wave sleep), and REM sleep is shortened. The total sleep time, however, is increased with estazolam.

USES Short-term management of insomnia.

CONTRAINDICATIONS Known sensitivity to benzodiazepines; acute closed-angle glaucoma, primary depressive disorders or psychosis; abrupt discontinuation; children <18 y; coma, shock, acute alcohol intoxication; pregnancy (category X), lactation, obstetric delivery.

CAUTIOUS USE Renal and hepatic impairment, renal failure; organic brain syndrome, alcoholism, benzodiazepine dependence, suicidal ideations, CNS depression, seizure disorder, status epilepticus; substance abuse; shock, coma; dementia, mania, psychosis; myasthenia gravis, Parkinson's disease; sleep apnea; open-angle glaucoma, GI disorders, older adult and debilitated patients; limited pulmonary reserve, pulmonary disease.

ROUTE & DOSAGE

Insomnia

Adult: **PO** 1 mg h.s. may increase up to 2 mg if necessary (some debilitated older adult patients should start with 0.5 mg h.s.)

ADMINISTRATION

Oral

- For older adult patients in good health, a 1-mg dose is indicated;

reduce initial dose to 0.5 mg for debilitated or small older adult patients.
- Dosage reduction also may be needed in the presence of hepatic impairment.

ADVERSE EFFECTS (≥1%) **CNS:** Headache, dizziness, impaired coordination, hypokinesia, *somnolence,* hangover. **CV:** Palpitations, arrhythmias, syncope (all rare). **Hematologic:** Leukopenia, agranulocytosis. **GI:** Constipation, xerostomia, anorexia, flatulence, vomiting. **Musculoskeletal:** Arthritis, arthralgia, myalgia, muscle spasm.

INTERACTIONS Drug: Cimetidine may decrease metabolism of estazolam and increase its effects; alcohol and other CNS DEPRESSANTS may increase drowsiness; CYP3A4 inhibitors (**ketoconazole, itraconazole, nefazodone, diltiazem, fluvoxamine, cimetidine, isoniazid, erythromycin**) can increase concentrations and toxicity of estazolam; **carbamazepine, phenytoin, rifampin,** BARBITURATES may decrease estazolam concentrations. **Herbal: Kava-kava, valerian** may potentiate sedation.

PHARMACOKINETICS Absorption: Rapidly absorbed from GI tract. **Onset:** 20–30 min. **Peak:** 2 h. **Distribution:** Crosses rapidly into brain; crosses placenta; distributed into breast milk. **Metabolism:** Extensively metabolized in liver. **Elimination:** Excreted in urine. **Half-Life:** 10–24 h.

NURSING IMPLICATIONS

Assessment & Drug Effects
- Monitor for improvement in S&S of insomnia.
- Assess for excess CNS depression or daytime sedation.
- Assess for safety, especially with older adult or debilitated patients, as dizziness and impaired coordination are known adverse effects.

Patient & Family Education
- Learn adverse effects and report those experienced to the physician.
- Avoid using this drug in combination with other CNS depressant drugs or alcohol.
- Do not drive or engage in other potentially hazardous activities until response to drug is known.
- Do not breast feed while taking this drug.

ESTRADIOL (Pr)
(ess-tra-dye′ole)
Alora, Climara, Esclim, Estrace, Estraderm, Estrasorb, EstroGel, FemPatch, Menorest, Menostar, Vivelle, Vivelle DOT, Estring, Vagifem

ESTRADIOL ACETATE
Femring, Femtrace

ESTRADIOL CYPIONATE
Depo-Estradiol Cypionate, depGynogen, Depogen, Dura-Estrin, Estro-Cyp, Estroject-LA, and others

ESTRADIOL VALERATE
Delestrogen, Dioval, Duragen-10, Estraval, Femogex ♣, Gynogen LA, Valergen

Classifications: HORMONES & SYNTHETIC SUBSTITUTES; ESTROGENS
Pregnancy Category: X

AVAILABILITY Estradiol 0.025 mg, 0.0375 mg, 0.05 mg, 0.06 mg, 0.075 mg, 0.1 mg patch; 14 mcg/24 h transdermal patch; 0.5 mg, 1 mg, 2 mg tablets; 25 mcg vaginal tablets, 2 mg vaginal ring, 0.1 mg vaginal cream; 2.5 mg/g topical emulsion; 0.06% topical gel; **Cypionate** 5 mg/mL injection; **Valerate** 10 mg/mL, 20 mg/mL, 40 mg/mL injection; **Acetate** 0.45 mg, 0.9 mg, 1.8 mg tablets; 0.05 mg/d, 0.1 mg/d vaginal insert

ACTIONS Natural or synthetic steroid hormone secreted principally by the ovarian follicles, and also by the adrenals, corpus luteum, placenta, and testes. Estrogen binds to a specific intracellular receptor, forming a complex that stimulates synthesis of proteins responsible for estrogenic effects. Promotes endometrial lining development, but prolonged exposure leads to abnormal endometrial hyperplasia, a condition usually associated with an abnormal bleeding pattern. Conversely, estrogen-stimulated endometrium suddenly deprived of estrogen may bleed within 48–72 h.
THERAPEUTIC EFFECTS In general, estradiol (estrogens) effects simulate those produced by the endogenous hormone. May mask onset of climacteric.

USES Natural or surgical menopausal symptoms, kraurosis vulvae, atrophic vaginitis, primary ovarian failure, female hypogonadism, castration. Used adjunctively with diet, calcium, and physical therapy to prevent and treat postmenopausal osteoporosis; also for palliation in advanced prostatic carcinoma and inoperable metastatic breast cancer in women at least 5 y after menopause. Combined with progestins in many oral contraceptive formulations.

CONTRAINDICATIONS Known or suspected pregnancy (category X); estrogenic-dependent neoplasms, breast cancer (except in selected patients being treated for metastatic disease). History of thromboembolic disorders; active arterial thrombosis or thrombophlebitis; undiagnosed abnormal genital bleeding; history of cholestatic disease; thyroid dysfunction; blood dyscrasias.
CAUTIOUS USE Adolescents with incomplete bone growth; endometriosis; hypertension, cardiac insufficiency; diseases of calcium and phosphate metabolism (metabolic bone disease); cerebrovascular disease; mental depression; benign breast disease, family history of breast or genital tract neoplasm; diabetes mellitus; gall bladder disease; preexisting leiomyoma, abnormal mammogram, history of idiopathic jaundice of pregnancy; varicosities; asthma; epilepsy; migraine headaches; liver or kidney dysfunction; jaundice, acute intermittent porphyria, pyridoxine deficiency; lactation.

ROUTE & DOSAGE

Menopause, Atrophic Vaginitis, Kraurosis Vulvae, Female Hypogonadism, Female Castration, Primary Ovarian Failure

Adult: **PO** 0.45–2 mg/d in a cyclic regimen **Topical** 2–4 g vaginal cream intravaginally once/d for 1–2 wk, then 1–2 g/d for 1–2 wk, then 1 g 1–3 times/wk; Transdermal patch **Estraderm** twice weekly; **Climara, FemPatch, Menostar** qwk in a cyclic regimen; **Estrasorb** Apply 1 packet to the left thigh and calf and 1 packet to the right thigh and calf once daily in the morning; **EstroGel** Apply 1.25 g (one-half applicatorful) to one arm every day (usually in the morning). **IM Cypionate** 1–5 mg once q3–4wk; **Valerate** 10–25 mg once q4wk; **Acetate** Insert 1 vaginal ring into the upper third of the vaginal vault. Keep in place continuously for 3 mo, then remove.

Metastatic Breast Cancer

Adult: **PO** 10 mg t.i.d.

E

Prostatic Cancer

Adult: **PO** 1–2 mg t.i.d. **IM Valerate** 30 mg once q1–2wk

Postpartum Breast Engorgement

Adult: **IM Valerate** 10–25 mg at end of first stage of labor

ADMINISTRATION

Oral

- Give with or immediately after solid food to reduce nausea.
- Protect tablets from light and moisture in well-closed container. Protect from freezing, unless otherwise directed by manufacturer.

Intravaginal

- Insert calibrated dosage applicator approximately 5 cm (2 in.) into vagina, directing it slightly back toward sacrum. Instill medication by pushing plunger. Patient should remain in recumbent position about 30 min to prevent losing the medication. Observe perineal area before each administration: if mucosa is red, swollen, or excoriated or if there is a change in vaginal discharge, report to physician.

Topical

- Cleanse and dry selected skin area. Apply as directed under Route & Dosage.

Transdermal

- Cleanse and dry selected skin area on trunk of body, preferably the abdomen. Avoid application to the breasts, to an irritated, abraded, oily area, or to the waistline. If system falls off, it may be reapplied, or if necessary, a new one can be applied. Return to original treatment schedule. Rotate application site with an interval of at least 1 wk between applications to a particular site.

Intramuscular

- Give deep into a large muscle.
- Store at 15°–30° C (59°–86° F); protect from light and freezing.

ADVERSE EFFECTS (≥1%) **CNS:** Headache, migraine, dizziness, mental depression, chorea, convulsions. **CV:** Thromboembolic disorders, hypertension. **Special Senses:** Intolerance to contact lenses, worsening of myopia or astigmatism, scotomas. **GI:** *Nausea,* vomiting, anorexia, increased appetite, diarrhea, abdominal cramps or pain, constipation, bloating, colitis, acute pancreatitis, cholestatic jaundice, benign hepatoadenoma. **Urogenital:** Mastodynia, breast secretion, spotting, changes in menstrual flow, dysmenorrhea, amenorrhea, cervical erosion, altered cervical secretions, premenstrual-like syndrome, vaginal candidiasis, endometrial cystic hyperplasia, reactivation of endometriosis, increased size of preexisting fibromyomas, cystitis-like syndrome, hemolytic uremic syndrome, change in libido; in men: gynecomastia, testicular atrophy, feminization, impotence (reversible). **Metabolic:** Reduced carbohydrate tolerance, hyperglycemia, hypercalcemia, folic acid deficiency, fluid retention. **Skin:** Dermatitis, pruritus, seborrhea, oily skin, acne; photosensitivity, chloasma, loss of scalp hair, hirsutism. **Body as a Whole:** Pain and postinjection flare at injection site; sterile abscess; leg cramps, weight changes. **Hematologic:** Acute intermittent porphyria.

DIAGNOSTIC TEST INTERFERENCE Estradiol reduces response of ***metyrapone*** test and excretion of ***pregnanediol. Increases: BSP***

retention, norepinephrine-induced ***platelet aggregability, hydrocortisone, PBI, T_4, sodium, thyroxine-binding globulin (TBG), prothrombin and factors VII, VIII, IX,*** and ***X; serum triglyceride,*** and ***phospholipid*** concentrations, ***renin*** substrate. ***Decreases: antithrombin III, pyridoxine*** and ***serum folate*** concentrations, serum ***cholesterol,*** values for the ***T_3 resin uptake*** test, ***glucose tolerance.*** May cause false-positive test for ***LE cells*** or ***antinuclear antibodies (ANA).***

INTERACTIONS Drug: BARBITURATES, **phenytoin, rifampin** decrease estrogen effect by increasing its metabolism; ORAL ANTICOAGULANTS may decrease hypoprothrombinemic effects; interfere with effects of **bromocriptine**; may increase levels and toxicity of **cyclosporine,** TRICYCLIC ANTIDEPRESSANTS, **theophylline;** decrease effectiveness of **clofibrate.**

PHARMACOKINETICS Absorption: Rapid absorption from GI tract; readily absorbed through skin and mucous membranes; slow absorption from IM injections. **Distribution:** Distributed throughout body tissues, especially in adipose tissue; crosses placenta. **Metabolism:** Metabolized primarily in liver. **Elimination:** Excreted in urine; excreted in breast milk.

NURSING IMPLICATIONS

Assessment & Drug Effects

- Monitor adverse GI effects. Nausea, frequently at breakfast time, usually disappears after 1 or 2 wk of drug use.
- Check BP on a regular basis in patients with cardiac or kidney dysfunction or hypertension; monitored carefully.
- Note: Severe hypercalcemia (>15 mg/dL) may be caused by estradiol therapy in patients with breast cancer and bone metastasis.
- Interrupt estrogen treatment at least 4 wk before surgery associated with a prolonged period of immobilization or vascular complications.

Patient & Family Education

- Comply with established dosage schedule. Do not alter unless physician prescribes a change.
- Read patient package insert (PPI) carefully.
- Notify physician of intermittent breakthrough bleeding, spotting, bleeding, or unexplained and sudden pain.
- Determine weight under standard conditions 1 or 2 times/wk; report sudden weight gain or other signs of fluid retention.
- Notify physician of positive Homan's sign (calf pain upon flexing foot) and the following symptoms of thromboembolic disorders immediately: Tenderness, swelling, and redness in extremity; sudden, severe headache or chest pain; slurring of speech; change in vision; tenderness, pain, sudden shortness of breath.
- Monitor urine or blood glucose & HbA1c for glycemic control if diabetic.
- Decrease caffeine intake, since estrogen depresses caffeine metabolism.
- Learn self-examination of breasts and follow a monthly schedule.
- Reduce or terminate long-term or high-dosage therapy with estrogens gradually.
- Estrogen-induced feminization and impotence in male patients

E

are reversible with termination of therapy.

- Estrogen-primed or -stimulated endometrium may bleed 48–72 h after dose is discontinued. In cyclic therapy, estradiol is resumed on schedule before drug-induced vaginal bleeding stops.
- Withdrawal bleeding may occur even after oophorectomy and after menopause.
- Do not breast feed while taking this drug without consulting physician.

ESTRAMUSTINE PHOSPHATE SODIUM

(ess-tra-muss′teen)

Emcyt

Classifications: ANTINEOPLASTIC; ALKYLATING AGENT

Prototype: Cyclophosphamide

Pregnancy Category: X

AVAILABILITY 140 mg capsules

ACTIONS Conjugate of estradiol and the carbamate of nitrogen mustard. Extent of antitumor activity contributed by each, as well as precise mechanisms of action, unknown.

THERAPEUTIC EFFECTS Appears to act as a relatively weak alkylating agent and estrogen. Major effectiveness reported to be in patients who have been refractory to estrogen therapy alone.

USES Palliative treatment of metabolic or progressive carcinoma of prostate.

CONTRAINDICATIONS Hypersensitivity to either estradiol or nitrogen mustard; active thrombophlebitis or thromboembolic disorders; pregnancy (category X), lactation.

CAUTIOUS USE History of thrombophlebitis, thromboses, or thromboembolic disorders; cerebrovascular or coronary artery disease; gallstones or peptic ulcer; impaired liver function; metabolic bone diseases associated with hypercalcemia; diabetes mellitus; hypertension, conditions that might be aggravated by fluid retention (e.g., epilepsy, migraine, kidney dysfunction); older adult patients.

ROUTE & DOSAGE

Neoplasm

Adult: **PO** 14 mg/kg/d in 3–4 divided doses

ADMINISTRATION

Oral

- Give with meals to reduce incidence of GI adverse effects. Some patients require drug withdrawal because of intolerable GI effects.
- Store at 2°–8° C (38°–46° F) in tight, light-resistant containers, unless otherwise directed by manufacturer.

ADVERSE EFFECTS (≥1%) **CNS:** Lethargy, emotional lability, insomnia, headache, anxiety. **CV:** CVA, MI, *thrombophlebitis,* CHF, *peripheral edema.* **GI:** *Nausea,* diarrhea, anorexia, flatulence, vomiting, thirst, GI bleeding. **Hematologic:** Leukopenia, thrombocytopenia, *abnormalities in liver function tests,* hypercalcemia, bone marrow depression (rare). **Respiratory:** Hoarseness, burning sensation in throat, dyspnea, upper respiratory discharge, pulmonary emboli. **Skin:** Rash, pruritus, urticaria, dry skin, easy bruising, flushing, peeling skin and fingertips, thinning hair. **Special Senses:** Tearing of eyes. **Urogenital:** Gynecomastia, breast tenderness, impotence. **Endocrine:** Decrease in glucose tolerance. **Musculoskeletal:** Leg cramps.

INTERACTIONS Food: Milk, dairy products, calcium supplements may decrease estramustine absorption.

PHARMACOKINETICS Absorption: Readily absorbed from GI tract. **Peak:** 2–3 h. **Metabolism:** Dephosphorylated in intestines to estramustine, estradiol, estrone, and nitrogen mustard; further metabolized in liver. **Elimination:** Excreted in feces via bile. **Half-Life:** 20 h.

NURSING IMPLICATIONS

Assessment & Drug Effects

- Monitor weight and examine for peripheral edema. Be mindful that drug can cause CHF.
- Monitor I&O ratio and pattern to prevent dehydration and electrolyte imbalance, especially with vomiting or diarrhea.
- Observe diabetics closely because of possibility of estramustine-induced reduction in glucose tolerance. Monitor baseline and periodic glucose tolerance tests.
- Lab tests: Perform baseline and periodic liver enzymes and bilirubin tests; repeat after drug has been discontinued for 2 mo.

Patient & Family Education

- Eat small meals at frequent intervals to reduce drug-induced nausea, eat slowly, and try cold food if food odors are offensive.
- Drink liquids 1 h before or 1 h after rather than with meals; clear liquids may be more palatable.

ESTROGEN-PROGESTIN COMBINATIONS (CONTRACEPTIVES)

Oral

Monophasic: Apri, Alesse, Aviane, Demulen, Desogen, Lessina, Levlen, Levlite, Levora, Loestrin, Lo/Ovral, Low-Ogestrel, Microgestin, Modicon, Necon, Nordette, Norinyl, Nortrel, Ortho-Cept, Ortho-Cyclen, Ortho-Novum, Ogestrel, Ovcon, Ovral, Seasonale, Yasmin, Zovia

Biphasic: Jenest, Kariva, Mircette, Necon 10/11, Ortho-Novum 10/11

Triphasic: Estrostep, Ortho-Novum 7/7/7, Ortho Tri-Cyclen, Ortho Tri-Cyclen Lo, Tri-Levlen, Tri-Norinyl, Triphasil, Trivora

PostCoital Contraceptives: Plan B, Preven

Transdermal

Ortho Evra

Intravaginal

NuvaRing

Classifications: HORMONES AND SYNTHETIC SUBSTITUTES; ESTROGEN-PROGESTIN COMBINATIONS

Prototype: Estradiol, Progesterone

Pregnancy Category: X

AVAILABILITY Combination oral contraceptives contain one of the following estrogens and one of the following progestins. **Estrogen:** Ethinyl estradiol 10 mcg, 20 mcg, 25 mcg, 30 mcg, 35 mcg, 40 mcg, 50 mcg; mestranol 50 mcg; **Progestin:** Desogestrel 0.15 mg; drospirenone 3 mg; ethynodiol diacetate 1 mg; levonorgestrel 0.05 mg, 0.075 mg, 0.1 mg, 0.125 mg, 0.15 mg, 0.25 mg, 0.75 mg; norethindrone 0.4 mg, 0.5 mg, 0.75 mg, 1 mg; norethindrone acetate 1 mg, 1.5 mg; norgestimate 0.18 mg, 0.215 mg, 0.25 mg; norgestrel 0.3 mg, 0.5 mg; **Transdermal:** Norelgestromin 6 mg/0.75 mg ethinyl estradiol patch; **Vaginal:** Etonorgestrel 11.7 mg/2.7 mg ethinyl estradiol vaginal insert

ACTIONS Three types of estrogen-progestin combinations are available: (1) monophasic, fixed dosage of estrogen-progestin throughout the cycle; (2) biphasic, amount of estrogen remains the same throughout cycle, less progestin in first half of cycle and increased progestin in second half; (3) triphasic, estrogen amount is the same or varies throughout cycle, progestin amount varies.

THERAPEUTIC EFFECTS Fixed combination of estrogen and progestin produces contraception by preventing ovulation and rendering reproductive tract structures hostile to sperm penetration and zygote implantation.

USES To prevent conception and to treat hypermenorrhea and endometriosis; postcoital contraceptive or "morning after pill"; moderate acne in females ≥15 y (Tri-Cyclen).

CONTRAINDICATIONS Pregnancy (category X), lactation, missed abortion. Familial or personal history of or existence of breast or other estrogen-dependent neoplasm, recurrent chronic cystic mastitis, history of or existence of thrombophlebitis or thromboembolic disorders, cerebral vascular or coronary artery disease, MI, serious hepatic dysfunction, hepatic neoplasm, family history of hepatic porphyria, undiagnosed abnormal vaginal bleeding, women age 40 and over, adolescents with incomplete epiphyseal closure.

CAUTIOUS USE History of depression, preexisting hypertension, or cardiac or renal disease; impaired liver function, history of migraine, convulsive disorders, or asthma; multiparous women with grossly irregular menses, diabetes, or familial history of diabetes; gallbladder disease, lupus erythematosus, rheumatic disease, varicosities, smokers.

ROUTE & DOSAGE

Contraception

Adult: **PO** 1 active tablet daily for 21 d, then placebo tablet or no tablets for 7 d, repeat cycle **Continuous regimen** (Seasonale) 1 tablet daily × 84 consecutive days. Wait 7 d for withdrawal bleeding before starting next cycle **Topical** Apply one patch once weekly for 3 wk, then have 1 wk patch-free before repeating the cycle **Intravaginal** Insert 1 ring on or before day 5 of the cycle. Remove ring after 3 wk, followed by a 1/wk rest. Then insert new ring

Postcoital Contraception (Plan B, Preven, Ovral)

Adult: **PO** Ovral, 2 tablets within 72 h of intercourse, then 2 tablets 12 h later; 1 (Plan B) or 2 (Preven) tablets within 72 h of unprotected intercourse, take second dose of 1 (Plan B) or 2 (Preven) tablets 12 h later

ADMINISTRATION

- Give without regard to meals.
- Do not exceed 24-h intervals between the daily doses; taking with a meal or at bedtime is a helpful reminder.

ADVERSE EFFECTS (≥1%) **Body as a Whole:** Paresthesias. **CV:** Malignant hypertension, thrombotic and thromboembolic disorders, *mild to moderate increase in BP,* increase in size of varicosities, edema. **Endocrine:** Estrogen excess (*nausea,* bloating, menstrual tension, cervical mucorrhea, polyposis, *chloasma, hypertension,* migraine headache, breast fullness or tenderness, edema); estrogen deficiency (hypomenorrhea, *early or midcycle breakthrough bleeding,* increased spotting); progestin excess (hypomenorrhea, breast regression, *vaginal candidiasis,* depression, fatigue, weight gain, increased appetite, acne, oily scalp, hair loss); progestin deficiency (late-cycle breakthrough bleeding, amenorrhea). **GI:** *Nausea,* cholelithiasis, gallbladder disease, cholestatic jaundice, benign hepatic adenomas; diarrhea, constipation, abdominal cramps. **Metabolic:** *Decreased glucose tolerance,* pyridoxine deficiency (see also diagnostic test interferences), acute intermittent porphyria. **Skin:** Rash (allergic), photosensitivity (photoallergy or phototoxicity), irritation from patch. **Special Senses:** Unexplained loss of vision, optic neuritis, proptosis, diplopia, change in corneal curvature (steepening), intolerance to contact lenses, retinal thrombosis, papilledema. **Urogenital:** Ureteral dilation, increased incidence of urinary tract infection, hemolytic uremia syndrome, renal failure, increased risk of congenital anomalies, decreased quality and quantity of breast milk, dysmenorrhea, increased size of preexisting uterine fibroids, *menstrual disorders.* Foreign body sensation, coital problems, device expulsion, vaginal discomfort, vaginitis, leukorrhea from ring.

DIAGNOSTIC TEST INTERFERENCE Oral contraceptives (OCs) increase ***BSP*** retention, ***prothrombin*** and ***coagulation factors II, VII, VIII, IX, X; platelet agregability, thyroid-binding globulin, PBI,*** T_4: ***transcortin; corticosteroid, triglyceride*** and ***phospholipid*** levels; ***ceruloplasmin, aldosterone, amylase, transferrin; renin*** activity, ***vitamin A.*** OCs decrease ***antithrombin III,*** T_3 resin uptake, ***serum folate, glucose tolerance, albumin, vitamin*** B_{12} and reduce the ***metyrapone*** test response.

INTERACTIONS Drug: Aminocaproic acid may increase clotting factors, leading to hypercoagulable state; BARBITURATES, ANTICONVULSANTS, ANTIBIOTICS, **rifampin,** ANTIFUNGALS reduce efficacy of OCs and increase incidence of breakthrough bleeding and risk of pregnancy.

PHARMACOKINETICS Absorption: Oral: Readily absorbed from GI tract; readily absorbed from transdermal patch placed on abdomen, buttock, upper outer arm and upper torso (excluding breast). Vaginal insert: norgestrel 100% absorbed, ethinyl estradiol 56% absorbed. **Peak:** Patch: 48 h. **Duration:** Patch: 1 wk. **Distribution:** Widely distributed; crosses placenta; small amount distributed into breast milk. **Metabolism:** Metabolized in liver. **Elimination:** Excreted in urine and feces. **Half-Life:** 6–45 h oral. Following removal of the patch: norelgestromin 28 h, ethinyl estradiol 17 h; vaginal ring: norgestrel 29 h; ethinyl estradiol 45 h.

NURSING IMPLICATIONS

Assessment & Drug Effects

- Take complete medical and family history prior to initiation of OC therapy. Physical exam: Baseline and periodic BP, breasts, abdomen, pelvis, Pap smear, and other relevant tests.
- Rule out pregnancy before OC therapy is begun.
- Check BP periodically. In some women, changes in BP occur within each cycle; in others, slow

increase of pressure, particularly diastolic, over several months is significant. Drug-induced BP elevation is usually reversible with cessation of OC.

- Nausea with or without vomiting occurs in approximately 10% of patients during the first cycle and is reportedly one of the major reasons for voluntary discontinuation of therapy. Most adverse effects tend to disappear in third or fourth cycle of use. Instruct patient to report symptoms that persist after fourth cycle. Dose adjustment or a different product may be indicated.
- Hirsutism and loss of hair are reversible with discontinuation of OC or by change of selected combination.
- Acne may improve, worsen, or develop for first time. In women on OC for at least 1 y, postcontraceptive acne sometimes occurs 3–4 mo after stopping drug and may continue for 6–12 mo.
- Anovulation or amenorrhea following termination of OC regimen may persist more than 6 mo. The user with pretreatment oligomenorrhea or secondary amenorrhea is most apt to have oversuppression syndrome.

Patient & Family Education

- Use an additional method of birth control during the first week of the initial cycle.
- Missed dose: Take tablet as soon as remembered or take 2 tablets the next day. If 2 consecutive tablets are omitted, take 2 tablets daily for the next 2 d, then resume the regular schedule. If 3 consecutive tablets are missed, begin a new compact of tablets, starting 7 d after last tablet was taken.
- Use an additional form of birth control for 7 d after 2 missed doses; 14 d after 3 missed doses.
- Ovulation is unlikely with omission of 1 daily dose; however, the possibility of escaped ovulation, spotting, or breakthrough bleeding increases with each missed dose.
- Discontinue medication if intra-cycle bleeding resembling menstruation occurs. Begin taking tablets from a new compact on day 5. If bleeding persists, see physician.
- Transdermal patches: Apply only one patch at a time and never cut or otherwise alter a patch prior to application.
- See physician to rule out pregnancy if 2 consecutive periods are missed, before continuing on OC.
- Do not skip scheduled visits for physical checkups while on OC therapy. Learn breast self-examination and do every month.
- Record frequent weight checks to permit early recognition of fluid retention.
- Understand the increased risk of thromboembolic and cardiovascular problems and increased incidence of gallbladder disease with OC use. Be alert to manifestations of thrombotic or thromboembolic disorders: severe headache (especially if persistent and recurrent), dizziness, blurred vision, leg or chest pain, respiratory distress, unexplained cough. Discontinue drug if any of these symptoms appear and report them promptly to physician.
- Report sudden abdominal pain immediately to physician in order to rule out ectopic pregnancy.
- Be aware that ophthalmic sequelae can occur as soon as 24 h after initiation of OC. Stop drug and contact physician if unexplained partial or complete, sudden or gradual loss of vision, protrusion of eyeballs (proptosis), or diplopia occurs.

- Leukorrhea (increased clear discharge) is an expected physical reaction to the OC; however, if OC use is accompanied by vaginal itching and irritation, report to physician promptly to rule out candidiasis.
- Monitor urine and blood glucose closely if diabetic. Adjustment of antidiabetic medication may be necessary.
- Be aware that smokers using OC have a fivefold greater risk of fatal MI than nonsmoker OC users and a tenfold greater risk than non-OC users who are nonsmokers. The risk increases with age (marked in women >35 y) and with heavy smoking (15 or more cigarettes/d).
- Oral contraception can be started immediately after delivery in the nonlactating mother.
- Use alternate method of birth control when breast feeding until infant is weaned.
- Do not breast feed while taking this drug.

ESTROGENS, CONJUGATED

(ess'tro-jenz)

C.E.S. ♣, Cenestin, Enjuvia, Premarin, Progens

Classifications: HORMONES & SYNTHETIC SUBSTITUTES; ESTROGENS

Prototype: Estradiol

Pregnancy Category: X

AVAILABILITY 0.3 mg, 0.45 mg, 0.625 mg, 0.9 mg, 1.25 mg, 2.5 mg tablets; 25 mg injection; 0.625 mg vaginal cream

ACTIONS Short-acting estrogen mixture of conjugated estrogens including sodium estrone sulfate and sodium equilin sulfate.

THERAPEUTIC EFFECTS Binds to intracellular receptors that stimulate DNA and RNA to synthesize proteins responsible for effects of estrogen.

USES Atrophic vaginitis, kraurosis vulvae, and abnormal bleeding (hormonal imbalance); also female hypogonadism, primary ovarian failure, vasomotor symptoms associated with menopause; to retard progression of osteoporosis and as palliative therapy of breast and prostatic carcinomas.

UNLABELED USES Postcoital contraceptive.

CONTRAINDICATIONS Breast cancer; known or suspected pregnancy (category X), lactation.

CAUTIOUS USE Hypertension; gallbladder disease; diabetes mellitus; heart failure; liver or kidney dysfunction, history of thromboembolic disease.

ROUTE & DOSAGE

Menopause, Osteoporosis, Atrophic Vaginitis, Kraurosis Vulvae

Adult: **PO** 0.3–1.25 mg/d for 21 d each month, adjust to lowest level that gives symptom control (≤0.625 mg/d) **IV/IM** 25 mg, repeated in 6–12 h if needed **Topical** 2–4 g of cream/d

Female Hypogonadism

Adult: **PO** 2.5–7.5 mg/d in 1–3 divided doses for 20 d, followed by a 10 d rest period

Postcoital Contraception

Adult: **PO** 30 mg/d in divided doses for 5 consecutive days beginning within 72 h of coitus

Breast Cancer

Adult: **PO** 10 mg t.i.d. for at least 3 mo

Prostatic Cancer Palliation

Adult: **PO** 1.25–2.5 mg t.i.d.

E

ADMINISTRATION

Oral

- Give cyclically except when used for treatment of postpartum breast engorgement and for palliation of cancer. Cyclic regimen is to dose for 3 wk followed by 1 wk off.

Topical

- Use calibrated dosage applicator dispensed with the cream.

Intramuscular

- Reconstitute by first removing approximately 5 mL of air from the dry-powder vial, then slowly inject the supplied diluent to the vial by aiming it at the side of the vial. Gently agitate to dissolve but DO NOT SHAKE.
- Use within a few hours of reconstitution.

Intravenous

PREPARE: **Direct:** Reconstitute as for IM injection.

ADMINISTER: **Direct:** Give slowly at a rate of 5 mg/min. Estrogen solution is compatible with D5W and NS and may be added to IV tubing just distal to the needle if necessary.

- Store ampule and reconstituted solution at 2°–8° C (38°–46° F) and protected from light; stable for 60 d. Discard precipitated or discolored solution.

ADVERSE EFFECTS (≥1%) **CNS:** Headache, dizziness, depression, *libido changes*. **CV:** Thromboembolic disorders, hypertension. **GI:** *Nausea,* vomiting, diarrhea, bloating, cholestatic jaundice. **Urogenital:** Mastodynia, spotting, changes in menstrual flow, dysmenorrhea, amenorrhea. **Metabolic:** Reduced carbohydrate tolerance, fluid retention. **Other:** Leg cramps, intolerance to contact lenses.

INTERACTIONS Drug: BARBITURATES, **carbamazepine, phenytoin, rifampin** decrease estrogen effect by increasing its metabolism; ORAL ANTICOAGULANTS may decrease hypoprothrombinemic effects; interfere with effects of **bromocriptine;** may increase levels and toxicity of **cyclosporine,** TRICYCLIC ANTIDEPRESSANTS, **theophylline;** decrease effectiveness of **clofibrate.**

PHARMACOKINETICS Absorption: Rapid absorption from GI tract; readily absorbed through skin and mucous membranes (including vaginal mucosa); slow absorption from IM injections. **Distribution:** Distributed throughout body tissues, especially in adipose tissue; crosses placenta, excreted in breast milk. Conjugated estrogens are bound primarily to albumin. **Metabolism:** Metabolized primarily in liver to glucuronide and sulfate conjugates of estradiol, estrone, and estriol. **Elimination:** Excreted in urine. **Half-Life:** 4–18 h.

NURSING IMPLICATIONS

Assessment & Drug Effects

- See additional implications under estradiol.
- Monitor for and report breakthrough vaginal bleeding.
- Assess for relief of menopausal symptoms.
- Lab tests: Monitor serum phosphatase levels with prostate cancer.
- Monitor bone density annually when used for osteoporosis prophylaxis.

Patient & Family Education

- Be aware of importance of taking drug exactly as prescribed: Specifically, do not omit, increase, or decrease doses without advice of physician.

- Intravaginal administration: For self-administration, wash hands well before and after application, and avoid contact of denuded areas with the cream. Do not use tampons while on vaginal cream therapy.
- Notify physician promptly of adverse symptoms.
- Risk of blood clot formation is high with morning after pill. Know signs of thrombophlebitis (see Appendix F).
- Review package insert to ensure understanding of estrogen therapy.
- Do not breast feed while taking this drug.

ESTROGENS, ESTERIFIED

(ess'tro-jenz)

Estratab, Menest, Menrium, Neo-Estrone ♣

Classifications: HORMONES AND SYNTHETIC SUBSTITUTES; ESTROGEN

Prototype: Estradiol

Pregnancy Category: X

AVAILABILITY 0.3 mg, 0.625 mg, 1.25 mg, 2.5 mg tablets

ACTIONS Combination of same estrogens as found in conjugated estrogens, but in different proportions.

THERAPEUTIC EFFECTS Binds to intracellular receptors that stimulate DNA and RNA to synthesize proteins responsible for effects of estrogen.

USES Atrophic vaginitis, kraurosis vulvae and abnormal bleeding (hormonal imbalance), female hypogonadism, castration, primary ovarian failure, vasomotor symptoms associated with menopause, palliative therapy of breast and prostatic carcinomas; prevention of osteoporosis.

CONTRAINDICATIONS Breast cancer; known or suspected pregnancy (category X); lactation.

CAUTIOUS USE Hypertension; gallbladder disease; diabetes mellitus; heart failure; liver or kidney dysfunction; history of thromboembolic disease.

ROUTE & DOSAGE

Menopause

Adult: **PO** 0.3–1.25 mg/d for 21 d each month, adjust to lowest level that gives symptom control (≤0.625 mg/d)

Female Hypogonadism, Primary Ovarian Failure, Female Castration

Adult: **PO** 2.5–7.5 mg/d in 1–3 divided doses for 20 d followed by a 10-d rest period, during last 5 d of estrogen, give a PO progestin

Breast Cancer

Adult: **PO** 10 mg t.i.d. for 2–3 mo

Prostatic Cancer (palliation)

Adult: **PO** 1.25–2.5 mg t.i.d. for several weeks

Prevention of Osteoporosis

Adult: **PO** 0.3 mg q.d.

ADMINISTRATION

Oral

- Give with food or fluid of patient's choice.
- Give cyclically, except when used for palliation of cancer.
- Store tablets at 15°–30° C (59°–86° F) in a tightly closed container.

ADVERSE EFFECTS (≥1%) **CNS:** Headache, dizziness, depression, *libido changes*. **CV:** Thromboembolic disorders, hypertension. **GI:** *Nausea*, vomiting, diarrhea, bloating, cholestatic jaundice. **Urogeni-**

tal: Mastodynia, spotting, changes in menstrual flow, dysmenorrhea, amenorrhea. **Metabolic:** Reduced carbohydrate tolerance, fluid retention. **Other:** Leg cramps, intolerance to contact lenses.

E

INTERACTIONS Drug: BARBITURATES, **phenytoin, rifampin** decrease estrogen effect by increasing its metabolism; ORAL ANTICOAGULANTS may decrease hypoprothrombinemic effects; interfere with effects of **bromocriptine;** may increase levels and toxicity of **cyclosporine,** TCAS, **theophylline;** decrease effectiveness of **clofibrate.**

PHARMACOKINETICS Absorption: Well absorbed with first pass metabolism. **Metabolism:** Metabolized in GI mucosa and liver to estrone, further metabolized to inactive metabolites. **Elimination:** Excreted in urine and bile. **Half-Life:** 4–18.5 h.

NURSING IMPLICATIONS

Assessment & Drug Effects

- See nursing implications under estradiol.
- Monitor for and report breakthrough vaginal bleeding.
- Assess for relief of menopausal symptoms.
- Lab tests: Monitor serum phosphatase levels with prostate cancer.
- Monitor bone density annually when used for osteoporosis prophylaxis.

Patient & Family Education

- Be aware of importance of taking drug exactly as prescribed: Specifically, do not omit, increase, or decrease doses without advice of physician. Know what to do when a dose is missed.
- Review package insert to ensure understanding of estrogen therapy.
- Do not breast feed while taking this drug.

ESTRONE

(ess'trone)
Kestrone 5
Classifications: HORMONES AND SYNTHETIC SUBSTITUTES; ESTROGEN
Prototype: Estradiol
Pregnancy Category: X

AVAILABILITY 5 mg/mL injection

ACTIONS First sex hormone isolated in pure form; present in urine of pregnant mares along with other estrogens.
THERAPEUTIC EFFECTS Binds to intracellular receptors that stimulate DNA and RNA to synthesize proteins responsible for effects of estrogen.

USES Atrophic vaginitis, kraurosis vulvae, and abnormal bleeding (hormonal imbalance); also female hypogonadism, primary ovarian failure, vasomotor symptoms associated with menopause, and as palliative therapy of prostatic carcinoma.

CONTRAINDICATIONS Breast cancer; known or suspected pregnancy (category X), lactation.
CAUTIOUS USE Hypertension; gallbladder disease; diabetes mellitus; heart failure; liver or kidney dysfunction; history of thromboembolic disease.

ROUTE & DOSAGE

Menopause
Adult: **IM** 0.1–0.5 mg 2–3 times/wk

Female Hypogonadism, Primary Ovarian Failure
Adult: **IM** 0.1–1 mg/wk in single or divided doses

Inoperable Prostatic Cancer Palliation

Adult: **IM** 2–4 mg/d 2–3 times/wk

ADMINISTRATION

Intramuscular

- Shake vial and syringe well to suspend medication before withdrawing and injecting medication.
- Give deep into a large muscle.
- Store at 15°–30° C (59°–86° F); protect from light and do not freeze.

ADVERSE EFFECTS (≥1%) **CNS:** Headache, dizziness, depression, *libido changes.* **CV:** Thromboembolic disorders, hypertension. **GI:** *Nausea,* vomiting, diarrhea, bloating, cholestatic jaundice. **Urogenital:** Mastodynia, spotting, changes in menstrual flow, dysmenorrhea, amenorrhea. **Metabolic:** Reduced carbohydrate tolerance, fluid retention. **Other:** Leg cramps, intolerance to contact lenses.

INTERACTIONS Drug: Carbamazepine, phenytoin, rifampin decrease estrogen levels because they increase its metabolism; may enhance steroid effects of CORTICOSTEROIDS; may decrease anticoagulant effects of ORAL ANTICOAGULANTS.

PHARMACOKINETICS Absorption: Absorption occurs over several days. **Metabolism:** Converts to estradiol in GI mucosa. **Half-Life:** 4–18.5 h.

NURSING IMPLICATIONS

Assessment & Drug Effects

- See nursing implications under estradiol.
- Monitor for and report breakthrough vaginal bleeding.
- Assess for relief of menopausal symptoms.
- Lab tests: Monitor serum phosphatase levels with prostate cancer.
- Monitor patients with conditions that may be influenced by fluid retention carefully (e.g., migraine, cardiac or kidney dysfunction, asthma, epilepsy, hypertension). Check BP on a regular basis.
- Note: Spotting or breakthrough bleeding occurring when other drugs and estrone are taken concurrently indicates reduced availability of the estrogen.

Patient & Family Education

- Review package insert to assure understanding of estrogen therapy.
- Determine weight under standard conditions 1 or 2 times/wk and report sudden weight gain or other signs of fluid retention.
- Notify physician of positive Homan's sign (calf pain upon flexing foot) and the following symptoms of thromboembolic disorders immediately: Tenderness, swelling, and redness in extremity; sudden, severe headache or chest pain; slurring of speech; change in vision; sudden shortness of breath.
- Report symptoms of vaginal candidiasis (thick, white, curd-like secretions and inflamed, congested introitus) to permit appropriate treatment.
- Notify physician of severe abdominal pain and tenderness or abdominal mass.
- Do not breast feed while taking this drug.

ESTROPIPATE

(es-troe-pi′pate)

Ogen, Ortho-Est

Classifications: HORMONES AND SYNTHETIC SUBSTITUTES; ESTROGEN

Prototype: Estradiol

Pregnancy Category: X

E

AVAILABILITY 0.625 mg, 1.25 mg, 2.5 mg, 5 mg tablets; 1.5 mg/g cream

ACTIONS Water-soluble preparation of pure crystalline estrone (responsible for therapeutic actions).
THERAPEUTIC EFFECTS Binds to intracellular receptors that stimulate DNA and RNA to synthesize proteins responsible for effects of estrogen.

USES Atrophic vaginitis, kraurosis vulvae, and abnormal bleeding (hormonal imbalance); also female hypogonadism, primary ovarian failure, vasomotor symptoms associated with menopause, and as palliative therapy of prostatic carcinoma.

CONTRAINDICATIONS Estrogen hypersensitivity; breast cancer; known or suspected pregnancy (category X); lactation.
CAUTIOUS USE Hypertension; gallbladder disease; diabetes mellitus; heart failure; liver or kidney dysfunction; history of thromboembolic disease.

ROUTE & DOSAGE

Menopause, Atrophic Vaginitis, Kraurosis Vulvae

Adult: **PO** 0.75–6 mg/d for 21 d each month; adjust to lowest level that gives symptom control **Intravaginal** 2–4 g of cream once/d in a cyclic regimen

Female Hypogonadism, Primary Ovarian Failure, Female Castration

Adult: **PO** 1.5–9 mg/d in 1–3 divided doses for 21 d, followed by an 8–10-d drug-free period

ADMINISTRATION

Oral

- Give with food or fluid of patient's choice.

Intravaginal

- Apply vaginal cream using calibrated dosage applicator dispensed with drug. Squeeze tube of cream to force sufficient amount into applicator so that number on plunger indicating prescribed dose is level with top of barrel.
- Store at 15°–30° C (59°–86° F) in tightly closed containers unless otherwise directed.

ADVERSE EFFECTS (≥1%) **CNS:** Headache, dizziness, depression, *libido changes.* **CV:** Thromboembolic disorders, hypertension. **GI:** *Nausea,* vomiting, diarrhea, bloating, cholestatic jaundice. **Urogenital:** Mastodynia, spotting, changes in menstrual flow, dysmenorrhea, amenorrhea. **Metabolic:** Reduced carbohydrate tolerance, fluid retention. **Other:** Leg cramps, intolerance to contact lenses.

INTERACTIONS Drug: Carbamazepine, phenytoin, rifampin decrease estrogen levels because they increase its metabolism; may enhance steroid effects of CORTICOSTEROIDS; may decrease anticoagulant effects of ORAL ANTICOAGULANTS.

PHARMACOKINETICS Absorption: Absorbed with some metabolism occuring in GI tract. Some systemic absorption from vaginal administration. **Metabolism:** Metabolized in GI tract and liver. **Half-Life:** 4–18.5 h.

NURSING IMPLICATIONS

Assessment & Drug Effects

- See nursing implications under estradiol.
- Monitor for and report breakthrough vaginal bleeding.
- Assess for relief of menopausal symptoms.
- Lab tests: Monitor serum phosphatase levels with prostate cancer.

Patient & Family Education

- Do not use tampons while on vaginal cream therapy.
- Intravaginal administration: For self-administration, wash hands well before and after application, and avoid contact of denuded areas with the cream.
- Do not use tampons while on vaginal cream therapy. Pull plunger out of barrel and wash applicator in warm soapy water after use. Do not place plunger in hot or boiling water.
- Note: Sudden discontinuation of vaginal cream after high dosage or prolonged use may evoke withdrawal bleeding.
- Review patient package insert (PPI).
- Do not breast feed while taking this drug.

ESZOPICLONE

(es-zo'pi-clone)

Lunesta

Classifications: CENTRAL NERVOUS SYSTEM (CNS) AGENT; SEDATIVE-HYPNOTIC; NON-BENZODIAZEPINE

Prototype: Zolpidem

Pregnancy Category: C

Controlled Substance: Schedule Schedule IV

AVAILABILITY 1 mg, 2 mg, 3 mg tablets

ACTIONS Although the exact mechanism of action is unknown, its effects are thought to be modulated by an interaction with gamma aminobutyric acid (GABA) at the GABA-A-receptor complex in the brain.

THERAPEUTIC EFFECTS Among patients with chronic insomnia, a 6-mo course of eszopiclone provided improvements in relationship to sleep onset, and sleep maintenance.

USES Treatment of insomnia.

CONTRAINDICATIONS Hypersensitivity to zopiclone or eszopiclone; children <18 y.

CAUTIOUS USE Concomitant illness (i.e., condition that affects metabolism and/or hemodynamic responses); history of drug/alcohol abuse or psychiatric disorders (e.g., depression), new abnormal behavioral signs or symptoms; rapid dose reduction or abrupt withdrawal; pulmonary disease or disorders (e.g., sleep apnea syndrome), or patients with acute respiratory insufficiency; mild to moderate hepatic impairment; dosage adjustment with severe hepatic impairment, or coadministration of potent CYP3A4 inhibitors; older adults.

ROUTE & DOSAGE

Insomnia

Adult: **PO** 2 mg immediately before bedtime; may increase to 3 mg if needed.
Geriatric: **PO** If having difficulty falling asleep, 1 mg immediately before bedtime; if having difficulty staying asleep, 2 mg immediately before bedtime (max: 2 mg/d)

Adjustment for Hepatic Impairment

1 mg starting dose for severe hepatic impairment (also for patients concurrently on potent CYP3A4 inhibitors; see drug interactions)

ADMINISTRATION

Oral

- Do not exceed a 2 mg dose for geriatric patients.
- Store at 15°–30° C (59°–86° F).

ADVERSE EFFECTS (≥1%) **Body as a Whole:** Infection. **CNS:** *Headache,* anxiety, confusion, depression, dizziness, hallucinations, decreased libido, nervousness, somnolence, migraine. **CV:** Chest pain. **GI:** Dry mouth, dyspepsia, nausea, vomiting. **Endocrine:** Gynecomastia (women). **Metabolic:** Peripheral edema. **Skin:** Rash pruritus. **Special Senses:** *Unpleasant taste.* **Urogenital:** Dysmenorrhea.

INTERACTIONS Drug: Potent CYP-3A4 INHIBITORS (e.g., **clarithromycin, delavirdine, diltiazem, efavirenz, erythromycin, fluconazole, fluvoxamine, itraconazole, nefazodone, norfloxacin, omeprazole,** PROTEASE INHIBITORS, **quinine, verapamil, troleandomycin, voriconazole, zafirlukast**) may increase levels and toxicity of eszopiclone—max starting dose is 1 mg; additive CNS depressant effects with **alcohol; rifampin** may reduce effectiveness of eszopiclone. **Food:** Taking with or immediately after a high-fat meal may lead to a delay in onset.

PHARMACOKINETICS Absorption: Rapidly absorbed from GI tract. **Onset:** Onset may be delayed if taken with a high-fat meal. **Peak:** 1 h. **Metabolism:** Metabolized in liver by CYP3A4. **Elimination:** Primarily excreted in urine. **Half-Life:** 6 h.

NURSING IMPLICATIONS

Assessment & Drug Effects

- Monitor closely patients with sleep apnea or other pulmonary disorders.
- Monitor for CNS depression in patients with a history of drug/alcohol abuse or psychiatric disorders.
- Lab tests: LFTs pre/posttreatment in those with preexisting liver disease.

Patient & Family Education

- Drug effectiveness may be reduced when taken after a high-fat meal.
- Report promptly any of the following: confusion, lethargy, lack of balance or coordination, daytime sleepiness, or mood changes.
- Moderate alcohol consumption while taking this drug.
- Abruptly stopping the drug may result in restlessness and feelings of anxiety.
- Do not breast feed while taking this drug without consulting physician.

ETANERCEPT (Pr)

(e-tan'er-cept)

Enbrel

Classifications: BIOLOGIC RESPONSE MODIFIER; TUMOR NECROSIS FACTOR MODIFIER

Pregnancy Category: B

AVAILABILITY 25 mg, 50 mg injection; 50 mg/mL prefilled syringe

ACTIONS Produced by recombinant DNA technology. Binds specifically to tumor necrosis factor (TNF) and blocks it from attaching to cell surface TNF receptors.

THERAPEUTIC EFFECTS Indicated by improved RA symptomatology. This naturally occurring cytokine (e.g., IL-6) is part of the normal immune and inflammatory response. TNF mediates inflammation and modulates cellular immune responses. Elevated levels of TNF are found in the synovial fluids of rheumatoid arthritis (RA) patients.

USES Reduction of the signs and symptoms of RA and psoriatic RA in adults, and polyarticular juvenile RA (JRA) in children with inadequate response to other disease-modifying antirheumatic drugs. Treatment of ankylosing spondylitis.

CONTRAINDICATIONS Patients with sepsis or other active infection; agranulocytosis; hypersensitivity to etanercept; malignancy; benzyl alcohol hypersensitivity; bleeding, hematologic disease, fever, infection; intramuscular administration, intravenous administration; latex hypersensitivity; sepsis; varicella; lactation. **CAUTIOUS USE** Immunosuppression; autoimmune disease, bone marrow suppression; diabetes mellitus; hamster protein hypersensitivity; heart failure; multiple sclerosis, neoplastic disease, neurological disease, seizure disorder, seizures; pregnancy (category B). Safety and efficacy in children <4 y of age are not established.

ROUTE & DOSAGE

Rheumatoid Arthritis, Psoriatic Arthritis, Ankylosing Spondylitis

Adult: **SC** 25 mg twice weekly; or 0.08 mg/kg or 50 mg once weekly
Child: **SC** >4 y, 0.4 mg/kg (max: 25 mg/dose) twice weekly

ADMINISTRATION

Subcutaneous

- Do not administer to a patient who has known or suspected sepsis.
- Reconstitute by slowly injecting the supplied diluent into the vial. Swirl gently to dissolve and do not shake. Reconstituted solution should be clear and colorless. Use within 6 h.
- Inject into thigh, abdomen, upper arm; rotate injection sites and never inject into an old injection site or where skin is tender, bruised, red, or hard.
- Store reconstituted solution up to 6 h refrigerated at 2°–8° C (36°–46° F). Store unopened dose tray refrigerated at 2°–8° C (36°–46° F).

ADVERSE EFFECTS (≥1%) **Body as a Whole:** Asthenia, serious *infections,* sepsis, monitor for reactivation of tuberculosis. **CNS:** Headache, dizziness, cerebral ischemia, depression, demyelinating disorders (multiple sclerosis, myelitis, optic neuritis). **CV:** Heart failure, <u>MI</u>, myocardial ischemia, hypertension, hypotension. **GI:** Abdominal pain, dyspepsia, cholecystitis, pancreatitis, GI hemorrhage. **Respiratory:** Rhinitis, URI, pharyngitis, cough, respiratory disorder, sinusitis, dyspnea may reactivate latent tuberculosis (TB). **Skin:** Rash; injection site reactions (*erythema, itching, pain, swelling*). **Musculoskeletal:** Bursitis. **Hematologic:** <u>Pancytopenia</u>.

INTERACTIONS Drug: Concurrent or recent use with **azathioprine, cyclophosphamide, leflunomide, methotrexate** has been associated with pancytopenia.

PHARMACOKINETICS Onset: 1–2 wk. **Peak:** 72 h. **Half-Life:** 115 h.

NURSING IMPLICATIONS

Assessment & Drug Effects

- Monitor carefully for and immediately report S&S of infection.

Patient & Family Education

- A PPD test is recommended before starting therapy to check for TB.
- Discard all needles and syringes after use; do not reuse.
- Withhold etanercept and notify physician before resuming drug if you develop an infection or are exposed to varicella virus.
- Avoid vaccinations, in general, and live vaccines, in particular, while on etanercept.
- Note: Injection site reactions (e.g., redness, pain, swelling) are com-

mon in the first month of therapy but generally decrease over time.
- Do not breast feed while taking this drug.

E

ETHACRYNIC ACID
(eth-a-krin′ik)
Edecrin

ETHACRYNATE SODIUM
Sodium Edecrin
Classifications: ELECTROLYTIC AND WATER BALANCE AGENT; LOOP DIURETIC
Prototype: Furosemide
Pregnancy Category: B

AVAILABILITY 25 mg, 50 mg tablet; 50 mg injection

ACTIONS Inhibits sodium and chloride reabsorption in proximal tubule and most segments of Loop of Henle, promotes potassium and hydrogen ion excretion, and decreases urinary ammonium ion concentration and pH. Promotes calcium elimination in hypercalcemia and nephrogenic diabetes insipidus.
THERAPEUTIC EFFECTS Rapid and potent diuretic effect. Fluid and electrolyte loss may exceed that caused by thiazides. Hypotensive effect may be due to hypovolemia secondary to diuresis and in part to decreased vascular resistance.

USES Severe edema associated with CHF, hepatic cirrhosis, ascites of malignancy, kidney disease, nephrotic syndrome, lymphedema.
UNLABELED USES Treatment of nephrogenic diabetes insipidus, hypercalcemia, mild to moderate hypertension, and as adjunct in therapy of hypertensive crisis complicated by pulmonary edema.

CONTRAINDICATIONS History of hypersensitivity to ethacrynic acid; increasing azotemia, anuria; hepatic coma; severe diarrhea, dehydration, electrolyte imbalance, hypotension; lactation, infants, parenteral use in pediatric patients.
CAUTIOUS USE Hepatic cirrhosis; older adult cardiac patients; diabetes mellitus; history of gout; pulmonary edema associated with acute MI; hyperaldosteronism; nephrotic syndrome; history of pancreatitis; pregnancy (category B).

ROUTE & DOSAGE

Edema
Adult: **PO** 50–100 mg 1–2 times/d, may increase by 25–50 mg prn up to 400 mg/d **IV** 0.5–1 mg/kg or 50 mg up to 100 mg, may repeat if necessary
Child: **PO** 1 mg/kg q.d., may increase to 3 mg/kg/d

ADMINISTRATION

Oral
- Give after a meal or food to prevent gastric irritation.
- Schedule doses to avoid nocturia and thus sleep interference. Avoid administration within at least 4 h of bedtime, if possible. This recommendation may not apply to the patient who accumulates fluid and develops respiratory symptoms during sleep.

Intravenous

PREPARE: **Direct/Intermittent:** Reconstitute by adding 50 mL of D5W or NS to vial. Use solution within 24 h. Vials reconstituted with D5W may turn cloudy; if so, discard the vial.
ADMINISTER: **Direct:** Give at a rate of 10 mg/min. **Intermittent:** Give over 15–30 min. If a second IV dose is required, a new

site should be selected to prevent thrombophlebitis.

INCOMPATIBILITIES **Solution/additive: Hydralazine, procainamide, ranitidine, tolazoline, triflupromazine.**

▪ Store oral and parenteral form at 15°–30° C (59°–86° F) unless otherwise directed.

ADVERSE EFFECTS (≥1%) **CNS:** Headache, fatigue, apprehension, confusion. **CV:** *Postural hypotension* (dizziness, light-headedness). **Metabolic:** Hyponatremia, *hypokalemia,* hypochloremic alkalosis, hypomagnesemia, hypocalcemia, hypercalciuria, hyperuricemia, hypovolemia, hematuria, glycosuria, hyperglycemia, gynecomastia, elevated BUN, creatinine, and urate levels. **Special Senses:** Vertigo, tinnitus, sense of fullness in ears, temporary or permanent deafness. **GI:** Anorexia, diarrhea, nausea, vomiting, dysphagia, abdominal discomfort or pain, GI bleeding (IV use), abnormal liver function tests. **Hematologic:** Thrombocytopenia, agranulocytosis (rare), severe neutropenia (rare). **Skin:** Skin rash, pruritus. **Body as a Whole:** Fever, chills, acute gout; local irritation and thrombophlebitis with IV injection.

INTERACTIONS Drug: THIAZIDE DIURETICS increase potassium loss; increased risk of **digoxin** toxicity from hypokalemia; CORTICOSTEROIDS, **amphotericin B** increase risk of hypokalemia; decreased **lithium** clearance, so increased risk of lithium toxicity; SULFONYLUREA effect may be blunted, causing hyperglycemia; ANTIHYPERTENSIVE AGENTS increase risk of orthostatic hypotension; AMINOGLYCOSIDES may increase risk of ototoxicity; **warfarin** potentiates hypoprothrombinemia.

PHARMACOKINETICS Absorption: Rapidly absorbed from GI tract. **Onset:** 30 min PO; 5 min IV. **Peak:** 2 h PO; 15–30 min IV. **Duration:** 6–8 h PO; 2 h IV. **Distribution:** Does not cross CSF. **Metabolism:** Metabolized to cysteine conjugate. **Elimination:** 30%–65% excreted in urine; 35%–40% excreted in bile. **Half-Life:** 30–70 min.

NURSING IMPLICATIONS

Assessment & Drug Effects

- Observe closely when receiving the drug by IV infusion. Rapid, copious diuresis following IV administration can produce hypotension.
- Monitor IV site closely. Extravasation of IV drug causes local pain and tissue irritation from dehydration and blood volume depletion.
- Monitor BP during initial therapy. Because orthostatic hypotension can occur, supervise ambulation.
- Monitor BP and pulse throughout therapy in patients with impaired cardiac function. Diuretic-induced hypovolemia may reduce cardiac output, and electrolyte loss promotes cardiotoxicity in those receiving digitalis (cardiac) glycosides.
- Establish baseline weight prior to start of therapy; weigh patient under standard conditions. Keep physician informed of weight loss or gain in excess of 1 kg (2 lb)/d.
- Monitor I&O ratio. Drug should be discontinued if excessive diuresis, oliguria, hematuria, or sudden profuse diarrhea occurs. Report signs to physician.
- Lab tests: Determine baseline and periodic blood count, serum electrolytes, CO_2, BUN, creatinine, blood glucose, uric acid, and liver function.
- Observe for and report S&S of electrolyte imbalance: Anorexia,

nausea, vomiting, thirst, dry mouth, polyuria, oliguria, weakness, fatigue, dizziness, faintness, headache, muscle cramps , paresthesias, drowsiness, mental confusion. Instruct patient to report these symptoms promptly to physician.

- Report immediately possible signs of thromboembolic complications (see Appendix F).
- Impaired glucose tolerance with hyperglycemia and glycosuria has occurred in patients receiving doses in excess of 200 mg/d.

Patient & Family Education

- Learn S&S of hypokalemia and hyponatremia (see Appendix F), and report any of these promptly to physician.
- Make position changes slowly, particularly from lying to upright posture.
- Report GI adverse effects to physician; they occur most frequently after 1–3 mo of PO therapy or in patients on high dosage. The onset of loose stools or other GI symptoms at any time during therapy indicates possible need for dosage adjustment or discontinuation of drug.
- Notify physician immediately of any evidence of impaired hearing. Hearing loss may be preceded by vertigo, tinnitus, or fullness in ears; it may be transient, lasting 1–24 h, or it may be permanent.
- Do not breast feed while taking this drug.

ETHAMBUTOL HYDROCHLORIDE

(e-tham'byoo-tole)

Etibi ✤, Myambutol

Classifications: ANTIINFECTIVE; ANTITUBERCULOSIS AGENT

Prototype: Isoniazid

Pregnancy Category: B

AVAILABILITY 100 mg, 400 mg tablets

ACTIONS Mode of action not completely understood, but it appears to inhibit RNA synthesis and thus arrests multiplication of tubercle bacilli. The emergence of resistant strains is delayed by administering ethambutol in combination with other antituberculosis drugs.

THERAPEUTIC EFFECTS Synthetic antituberculosis agent with bacteriostatic effect.

USES In conjunction with at least one other antituberculosis agent in treatment of pulmonary tuberculosis.

UNLABELED USES Atypical mycobacterial infections.

CONTRAINDICATIONS Optic neuritis; hypersensitivity to ethambutol; optic neuritis, patients unable to report changes in vision (young children, or unconscious patients); children <6 y.

CAUTIOUS USE Renal impairment, hepatic disease; gout; ocular defects (e.g., cataract, recurrent ocular inflammatory conditions, diabetic retinopathy); pregnancy (category B), lactation.

ROUTE & DOSAGE

Tuberculosis

Adult: **PO** 15 mg/kg q24h; for retreatment start with 25 mg/kg/d for 60 d, then decrease to 15 mg/kg/d

Child: **PO** *6–12 y,* 10–15 mg/kg/d

ADMINISTRATION

Oral

- Give with food if GI irritation occurs.
- Protect ethambutol from light, moisture, and excessive heat.

Store at 15°–30° C (59°–86° F) in tightly closed container unless otherwise directed.

ADVERSE EFFECTS (≥1%) **CNS:** Headache, dizziness, confusion, hallucinations, paresthesias, joint pains. **Special Senses:** Ocular toxicity: *retrobulbar optic neuritis;* possibility of anterior optic neuritis with decrease in visual acuity, temporary loss of vision, constriction of visual fields, red–green color blindness, central and peripheral scotomas, eye pain, photophobia; retinal hemorrhage and edema. **GI:** Anorexia, nausea, vomiting, abdominal pain. **Body as a Whole:** Hypersensitivity (pruritus, dermatitis, anaphylaxis).

INTERACTIONS Drug: Aluminum-containing antacids can decrease absorption.

PHARMACOKINETICS Absorption: 70%–80% absorbed from GI tract. **Peak:** 2–4 h. **Distribution:** Distributes to most body tissues; highest concentrations in erythrocytes, kidney, lungs, saliva; crosses placenta; distributed into breast milk. **Metabolism:** Metabolized in liver. **Elimination:** 50% excreted in urine within 24 h; 20%–22% excreted in feces. **Half-Life:** 3–4 h.

NURSING IMPLICATIONS

Assessment & Drug Effects

- Perform C&S prior to and periodically throughout therapy.
- Perform ophthalmoscopic examination prior to and at monthly intervals during therapy. Test eyes separately as well as together.
- Note: Ocular toxicity generally appears within 1–7 mo after start of therapy. Symptoms usually disappear within several weeks to months after drug is discontinued, depending on degree of ocular damage.
- Monitor I&O ratio in patients with renal impairment. Report oliguria or any significant changes in ratio or in laboratory reports of kidney function. Systemic accumulation with toxicity can result from delayed drug excretion.
- Lab tests: Perform liver and kidney function tests, CBC, and serum uric acid levels at regular intervals throughout therapy.

Patient & Family Education

- Adhere to drug regimen exactly and keep follow-up appointments.
- Notify physician promptly of the onset of blurred vision, changes in color perception, constriction of visual fields, or any other visual symptoms. Have eyes checked periodically. Ethambutol can cause irreversible blindness due to optic neuritis.
- Do not breast feed while taking this drug.

ETHAVERINE HYDROCHLORIDE

(e′tha-ve-rine)

Ethaquin, Ethatab, Ethavex-100, Isovex

Classifications: CARDIOVASCULAR AGENT; NON-NITRATE VASODILATOR

Prototype: Hydralazine HCl

Pregnancy Category: C

AVAILABILITY 100 mg tablets

ACTIONS Alkaloid prepared synthetically from opium with no narcotic properties. Directly relaxes all smooth muscles, especially when they have been spasmodically contracted.

THERAPEUTIC EFFECTS Action is especially pronounced when spasm is present on coronary, cerebral, pulmonary, and peripheral arteries. Acts directly on myocardium like quinidine; depresses conduction and irritability, and prolongs refractory period.

USES Primarily for peripheral and cerebral vascular insufficiency associated with arterial spasm; also a smooth muscle spasmolytic in spastic conditions of the GI and GU tracts.

CONTRAINDICATIONS Complete atrioventricular dissociation (AV heart block) and severe liver disease; pregnancy (category C).
CAUTIOUS USE Patients with glaucoma; myocardial depression; lactation.

ROUTE & DOSAGE

Peripheral and Cerebral Vascular Insufficiency
Adult: **PO** 100 mg t.i.d., may increase up to 200 mg t.i.d.

ADMINISTRATION

Oral
- Monitor heart rate (apical pulse for 1 full minute) and BP; if significant changes occur (e.g., hypotension, arrhythmias), withhold drug and notify physician.
- Preserve in a tightly covered, light-resistant container.

ADVERSE EFFECTS (≥1%) **CNS:** Vertigo, *headache, drowsiness.* **CV:** *Hypotension,* arrhythmias. **GI:** Nausea, anorexia, abdominal distress, dry throat. **Other:** Malaise, *flushing,* sweating, lassitude, respiratory depression.

INTERACTIONS Drug: May decrease **levodopa** effectiveness; **morphine** may antagonize smooth muscle relaxation effect of ethaverine.

PHARMACOKINETICS Absorption: Readily absorbed from GI tract. **Peak:** 1–2 h. **Duration:** 6 h regular tablets. **Metabolism:** Metabolized in liver. **Elimination:** Excreted in urine chiefly as metabolites.

NURSING IMPLICATIONS

Assessment & Drug Effects
- Monitor apical pulse for changes in rate and rhythm routinely; drug may cause cardiac arrhythmias.
- Monitor BP for hypotension, and respiration rate for respiratory depression. Promptly report marked changes to physician.
- Lab tests: Periodic liver function and blood chemistry; hepatotoxicity (thought to be a hypersensitivity reaction) is reversible with prompt drug withdrawal.

Patient & Family Education
- Do not drive or engage in other potentially hazardous activities until response to drug is known.
- Avoid alcohol; it may increase drowsiness and dizziness.
- Notify physician if jaundice or skin rash appear. Liver function tests may be indicated.
- Be aware that drug may cause flushing, headache, and diaphoresis; notify physician if symptoms are pronounced.
- Notify physician if GI distress develops and persists.
- Do not breast feed while taking this drug without consulting physician.

ETHCHLORVYNOL

(eth-klor-vi'nole)
Placidyl
Classifications: CENTRAL NERVOUS SYSTEM AGENT; ANXIOLYTIC; SEDATIVE-HYPNOTIC; BARBITURATE
Prototype: Secobarbital
Pregnancy Category: C
Controlled Substance: Schedule IV

AVAILABILITY 200 mg, 500 mg, 750 mg capsules

ACTIONS CNS depressant effects similar to those of chloral hydrate and barbiturates. Mechanism of action not known. Also exhibits anticonvulsant and muscle relaxant activity. Has no analgesic properties. Effect on REM sleep not known. Not commonly used as a sedative because of its short duration of action.

THERAPEUTIC EFFECTS Hypnotic doses produce cerebral depression and quiet, deep sleep; sedative doses reduce anxiety and apprehension.

USES Short-term therapy of simple insomnia for periods up to 1 wk.

CONTRAINDICATIONS Porphyria; patients with uncontrolled pain; first and second trimesters of pregnancy (category C). Safety during lactation and in children is not established.

CAUTIOUS USE Third trimester of pregnancy; patients with mental depression or suicidal tendencies, addiction-prone individuals; impaired liver or kidney function; older adult or debilitated patients; patients who respond unpredictably to alcohol or barbiturates.

ROUTE & DOSAGE

Sedative

Adult: **PO** 200 mg b.i.d. or t.i.d.

Hypnotic

Adult: **PO** 500 mg–1 g h.s., may give an additional 200 mg if patient awakens early

ADMINISTRATION

Oral

- Minimize transient giddiness and ataxia by giving drug with milk or other food. Symptoms seen in patients who apparently absorb the drug rapidly.
- Store at 15°–30° C (59°–86° F) in tight, light-resistant containers (darkens on exposure to light; slight darkening does not affect potency).

ADVERSE EFFECTS (≥1%) **CNS:** Dizziness, facial numbness, headache, mild hangover, nightmares, coma, respiratory failure. **Special Senses:** Blurred vision. **GI:** Nausea, vomiting, aftertaste. **Body as a Whole:** Urticaria. **Musculoskeletal:** Muscle weakness, tremors.

DIAGNOSTIC TEST INTERFERENCE ***Phentolamine test:*** false-positive test results (ethchlorvynol should be withdrawn at least 24 h before the test).

INTERACTIONS Drug: Alcohol and other CNS DEPRESSANTS amplify CNS depression; decrease anticoagulation effect of ORAL ANTICOAGULANTS.

PHARMACOKINETICS Absorption: Readily absorbed from GI tract. **Onset:** 15–30 min. **Peak:** 1–2 h. **Duration:** 5 h. **Distribution:** Localizes in adipose tissue, liver, kidney, spleen, brain, CSF, bile; crosses placenta; distribution into breast milk unknown. **Metabolism:** Metabolized in liver with enterohepatic cycling and possibly in kidney. **Elimination:** 10% excreted in urine within 24 h. **Half-Life:** 20–100 h.

NURSING IMPLICATIONS

Assessment & Drug Effects

- Report mental confusion, hallucinations, or drowsiness in patients receiving daytime sedation; decrease in dosage or drug discontinuation is indicated.
- Observe intensity and duration of drug action, particularly in

older adults, who may not tolerate average adult doses.
- Do not discontinue abruptly; severe withdrawal symptoms may occur in patients taking regular doses.

Patient & Family Education
- Caution patient to avoid driving or engaging in other activities requiring mental alertness and physical coordination for at least 5 h after taking drug.
- Psychological and physical dependence is possible; therefore, prolonged administration is not recommended. Urge patient to adhere to established drug regimen.
- Do not breast feed while taking this drug without consulting physician.

ETHINYL ESTRADIOL

(eth′in-il ess-tra-dye′ole)
Estinyl, Feminone
Classifications: HORMONES AND SYNTHETIC SUBSTITUTES; ESTROGEN
Prototype: Estradiol
Pregnancy Category: X

AVAILABILITY 0.02 mg, 0.05 mg, 0.5 mg tablets

ACTIONS Oral estrogen with actions similar to those of estradiol. Given cyclically for short-term use.
THERAPEUTIC EFFECTS Binds to intracellular receptors that stimulate DNA and RNA to synthesize proteins responsible for effects of estrogen.

USES Moderate to severe vasomotor symptoms associated with menopause; also postmenopausal osteoporosis, female hypogonadism, and as palliation for inoperable, metastatic cancer of female breast (at least 5 y postmenopause) and of the prostate.

UNLABELED USES Postcoital contraceptive.

CONTRAINDICATIONS Breast cancer; known or suspected pregnancy (category X), lactation.
CAUTIOUS USE Hypertension; gallbladder disease; diabetes mellitus; heart failure; liver or kidney dysfunction, history of thromboembolic disease.

ROUTE & DOSAGE

Menopause, Postmenopausal Osteoporosis
Adult: **PO** 0.02–0.05 mg/d for 21 d each month, adjust to lowest level that gives symptom control

Female Hypogonadism
Adult: **PO** 0.05 mg 1–3 times/d for 2 wk, followed by 2 wk of progestin, continue this regimen for 3–6 mo

Breast Cancer
Adult: **PO** 1 mg t.i.d. for 2–3 mo

Prostatic Cancer Palliation
Adult: **PO** 0.15–2 mg/d

Postcoital Contraceptive
Adult: **PO** 5 mg/d for 5 consecutive days beginning within 72 h of coitus

ADMINISTRATION

Oral
- Morning-after pill: Start drug within 24 h and not later than 72 h after sexual exposure when used as an emergency postcoital contraceptive. Perform a pregnancy test prior to dosing.
- Store at 15°–30° C (59°–86° F) in tight, light-resistant container.

ADVERSE EFFECTS (≥1%) **CNS:** Headache, dizziness, depression, *li-*

bido changes. **CV:** Thromboembolic disorders, hypertension. **GI:** *Nausea,* vomiting, diarrhea, anorexia, weight changes, bloating, cholestatic jaundice. **Urogenital:** Mastodynia, breakthrough bleeding, changes in menstrual flow, dysmenorrhea, amenorrhea; in men: impotence, gynecomastia, testicular atrophy. **Metabolic:** Reduced carbohydrate tolerance, fluid retention. **Body as a Whole:** Leg cramps, edema, intolerance to contact lenses.

INTERACTIONS Drug: Carbamazepine, phenytoin, rifampin decrease estrogen levels because they increase its metabolism; may enhance steroid effects of CORTICOSTEROIDS; may decrease anticoagulant effects of ORAL ANTICOAGULANTS.

PHARMACOKINETICS Absorption: 83% absorbed. **Metabolism:** extensively metabolized in liver. **Elimination:** excreted in urine and feces. **Half-Life:** 3–27 h.

NURSING IMPLICATIONS

Assessment & Drug Effects

- Check BP on a regular basis in patients with conditions that may be influenced by fluid retention (migraine, cardiac or kidney dysfunction, asthma, epilepsy, hypertension).
- Supplement pyridoxine (vitamin B_6) in patients on long-term therapy, especially if undernourished; levels are lowered by estrogens.

Patient & Family Education

- Be aware that risk of blood clot formation is high. Notify physician immediately of positive Homan's sign (calf pain upon foot flexion) and the following symptoms of thromboembolic disorders: Tenderness, pain, swelling, and redness in extremity; sudden, severe headache or chest pain, slurring of speech; change in vision; sudden shortness of breath. If physician is not available, go to the nearest emergency room.
- Report severe abdominal pain and tenderness, or abdominal mass.
- Determine weight under standard conditions 1 or 2 times/wk and report sudden weight gain or other signs of fluid retention.
- Notify physician of yellow skin and sclera, pruritus, dark urine, and light-colored stools; history of jaundice in pregnancy increases the possibility of estrogen-induced jaundice. Estrogen therapy is usually interrupted pending clinical investigation.
- Abrupt withdrawal of vitamin C may lead to breakthrough bleeding; high vitamin C intake (e.g., 1 g/d) may increase ethinyl estradiol levels.
- Report symptoms of vaginal candidiasis (thick, white, curd-like secretions and inflamed congested introitus) to permit appropriate treatment.
- Note: Estrogen-induced feminization and impotence in male patients are reversible with termination of therapy.
- Decrease caffeine intake from sources such as tea, coffee, and cola; estrogenic depression of caffeine metabolism may cause caffeinism.
- Do not breast feed while taking this drug.

ETHIONAMIDE

(e-thye-on-am′ide)

Trecator-SC

Classifications: ANTIINFECTIVE; ANTITUBERCULOSIS AGENT; ANTILEPROSY (SULFONE) AGENT

Prototype: Isoniazid

Pregnancy Category: D

AVAILABILITY 250 mg tablets

ACTIONS Bacteriostatic or bactericidal depending on concentration used and susceptibility of organism. Emergence of resistant strains may be delayed or prevented when administered concurrently with other antituberculosis drugs.

THERAPEUTIC EFFECTS Effective against human and bovine strains of *Mycobacterium tuberculosis* and *M. kansasii* and some strains of *Mycobacterium avium-intracellulare complex*. Also active against *M. leprae*.

USES Any form of active tuberculosis when treatment with primary antituberculosis drugs (e.g., isoniazid, streptomycin, ethambutol, rifampin) has failed. Must be given with at least one other effective antituberculosis agent.

UNLABELED USES Atypical mycobacterial infections and tuberculous meningitis.

CONTRAINDICATIONS Hypersensitivity to ethionamide and chemically related drugs [e.g., isoniazid, niacin (nicotinamide)]; severe liver damage. Safety during pregnancy (category D), lactation, or in children and women of childbearing potential is not established.

CAUTIOUS USE Diabetes mellitus, liver dysfunction.

ROUTE & DOSAGE

Tuberculosis
Adult: **PO** 0.5–1 g/d divided q8–12h
Child: **PO** 15–20 mg/kg/d in 2–3 equally divided doses (max: 1 g/d)

ADMINISTRATION

Oral

- Give with or after meals to minimize GI adverse effects. Some patients tolerate ethionamide best when it is taken as a single dose after the evening meal or as a single dose at bedtime. GI symptoms appear to increase with divided doses, although serum concentrations may be higher.
- About 50% of patients cannot tolerate a single dose larger than 500 mg because of GI adverse effects. An antiemetic may be prescribed, but if symptoms persist, drug should be discontinued.
- Physician may prescribe pyridoxine (vitamin B_6) concurrently to prevent or relieve peripheral neuritis and other neurotoxic effects.
- Store in a cool, dry place at 8°–15° C (46°–59° F) in a tightly closed container unless otherwise directed.

ADVERSE EFFECTS (≥1%) **CNS:** Headache, restlessness, mental depression, drowsiness, dizziness, ataxia, hallucinations, paresthesias, convulsions. **GI:** Dose related and frequent; symptoms may be due to CNS stimulation rather than to GI irritation: anorexia, *epigastric distress, nausea, vomiting,* metallic taste, *diarrhea,* stomatitis, sialorrhea. **Metabolic:** Elevated ALT, AST; hepatitis (with jaundice), hypothyroidism. **Urogenital:** Menorrhagia, impotence. **Body as a Whole:** Postural hypotension.

INTERACTIONS Drug: Cycloserine, isoniazid may increase neurotoxic effects.

PHARMACOKINETICS Absorption: 80% absorbed from GI tract. **Peak:** 3 h. **Duration:** 9 h. **Distribution:** Widely distributed including CSF; crosses placenta; distribution into breast milk unknown. **Metabolism:** Metabolized in liver. **Elimination:** Excreted in urine. **Half-Life:** 3 h.

E

NURSING IMPLICATIONS

Assessment & Drug Effects

- Lab tests: Perform C&S prior to start of therapy. Baseline liver function tests (AST and ALT), CBC, and kidney function tests including urinalysis and every 2–4 wk during therapy.
- Report onset of skin rash. Progression to exfoliative dermatitis can occur if drug is not promptly discontinued.
- Monitor blood glucose & HbA1c closely in the diabetic until response to drug is established. These patients appear to be especially prone to hepatotoxicity (see Appendix F).

Patient & Family Education

- Avoid alcohol or use in moderation because ethionamide may increase potential for liver dysfunction.
- Notify physician of S&S of hepatotoxicity (see Appendix F); generally reversible if drug is promptly withdrawn.
- Make position changes slowly and in stages, particularly from lying to upright posture if experiencing hypotension.
- Do not breast feed while taking this drug without consulting physician.

ETHOSUXIMIDE Pr

(eth-oh-sux'i-mide)

Zarontin

Classifications: CENTRAL NERVOUS SYSTEM AGENT; SUCCINIMIDE ANTICONVULSANT

Pregnancy Category: C

AVAILABILITY 250 mg capsules; 250 mg/5 mL syrup

ACTIONS Succinimide anticonvulsant. Usually ineffective in management of psychomotor or major motor seizures.

THERAPEUTIC EFFECTS Reduces frequency of epileptiform attacks, apparently by depressing motor cortex and elevating CNS threshold to stimuli.

USES Management of absence (petit mal) seizures, myoclonic seizures, and akinetic epilepsy. May be administered with other anticonvulsants when other forms of epilepsy coexist with petit mal.

CONTRAINDICATIONS Hypersensitivity to succinimides; severe liver or kidney disease; use alone in mixed types of epilepsy (may increase frequency of grand mal seizures). Safety during pregnancy (category C), lactation, or in children <3 y is not established.

ROUTE & DOSAGE

Absence Seizures

Adult/Child: **PO** *6–12 y*, 250 mg b.i.d., may increase q4–7d prn (max: 1.5 g/d)
Child: **PO** *3–6 y*, 250 mg/d, may increase q4–7d prn (max: 1.5 g/d)

ADMINISTRATION

Oral

- Give with food if GI distress occurs.
- Store all forms at 15°–30° C (59°–86° F); capsules in tight containers, and syrup in light-resistant containers; avoid freezing.

ADVERSE EFFECTS (≥1%) **CNS:** Drowsiness, hiccups, ataxia, dizziness, headache, euphoria, restlessness, irritability, anxiety, hyperactivity, aggressiveness, inability to concentrate, lethargy, confusion, sleep disturbances, night terrors, hypochondriacal behavior, muscle

E

weakness, fatigue. **Special Senses:** Myopia. **GI:** Nausea, vomiting, *anorexia, epigastric distress,* abdominal pain, *weight loss,* diarrhea, constipation, gingival hyperplasia. **Urogenital:** Vaginal bleeding. **Hematologic:** Eosinophilia, leukopenia, thrombocytopenia, agranulocytosis, pancytopenia, aplastic anemia, positive direct Coombs' test. **Skin:** Hirsutism, pruritic erythematous skin eruptions, urticaria, alopecia, erythema multiforme, exfoliative dermatitis.

INTERACTIONS Drug: Carbamazepine decreases ethosuximide levels; **isoniazid** significantly increases ethosuximide levels; levels of both **phenobarbital** and ethosuximide may be altered with increased seizure frequency. **Herbal: Ginkgo** may decrease anticonvulsant effectiveness.

PHARMACOKINETICS Absorption: Readily absorbed from GI tract. **Peak:** 4 h; steady state: 4–7 d. **Metabolism:** Metabolized in liver. **Elimination:** Excreted slowly in urine; small amounts excreted in bile and feces. **Half-Life:** 30 h in children, 60 h in adults.

NURSING IMPLICATIONS

Assessment & Drug Effects

- Lab tests: Perform baseline and periodic hematologic studies, liver and kidney function.
- Monitor adverse drug effects. GI symptoms, drowsiness, ataxia, dizziness, and other neurologic adverse effects occur frequently and indicate the need for dosage adjustment.
- Observe closely during period of dosage adjustment and whenever other medications are added or eliminated from the drug regimen. Therapeutic serum levels: 40–80 mcg/mL.
- Observe patients with prior history of psychiatric disturbances for behavioral changes. Close supervision is indicated. Drug should be withdrawn slowly if these symptoms appear.

Patient & Family Education

- Discontinue drug only under physician supervision; abrupt withdrawal of ethosuximide (whether used alone or in combination therapy) may precipitate seizures or petit mal status.
- Do not drive or engage in other potentially hazardous activities until response to drug is known.
- Monitor weight on a weekly basis. Report anorexia and weight loss to physician; may indicate need to reduce dosage.
- Do not breast feed while taking this drug without consulting physician.

ETIDOCAINE HYDROCHLORIDE

(e-ti'doe-kane)

Duranest

Classifications: CENTRAL NERVOUS SYSTEM AGENT; LOCAL ANESTHETIC (AMIDE-TYPE)

Prototype: Procaine HCl

Pregnancy Category: B

AVAILABILITY 1% injection

ACTIONS Amide-type local anesthetic similar to bupivacaine in action and uses.

THERAPEUTIC EFFECTS Inhibits sodium fluxes into nerve cell required for initial depolarization, propagation, and conduction of nerve impulse.

USES Infiltration anesthesia, peripheral nerve blocks (intercostal, ulnar, inferior alveolar, brachial plexus) and central neural block (lumbar or caudal epidural blocks).

CONTRAINDICATIONS Known sensitivity to amide-type anesthetics, parabens, bisulfites; acidosis, heart block, severe hemorrhage, severe hypotension, hypertension; cerebrospinal deformities or disease; spinal block, epidural anesthesia in vaginal delivery; injection into inflamed or infected area. Safety during pregnancy (category B) (except during labor), lactation, or in children <14 y is not established.

CAUTIOUS USE Known drug sensitivities; impaired cardiac function; kidney or liver disease; severe shock; older adult, debilitated or severely ill patients.

ROUTE & DOSAGE

Percutaneous Infiltration

Adult: **IM** 0.5% solution (max: 300 mg, 400 mg if given with epinephrine)

Peripheral Nerve Block, Caudal

Adult: **IM** 0.5% or 1% solution (max: 300 mg, 400 mg if given with epinephrine)

Central Neural Block

Adult: **IM** 0.5% or 1.5% solution (max: 300 mg, 400 mg if given with epinephrine)

ADMINISTRATION

Intramuscular

- Aspirate prior to injection to avoid intravascular injection.
- Discard partially used vial of etidocaine, since it has no preservative.
- Store at 15°–30° C (59°–86° F); protect from freezing; protect solutions with epinephrine from direct light.

ADVERSE EFFECTS (≥1%) **Body as a Whole:** Anaphylaxis, anaphylactoid reactions. **CNS:** Nervousness, headache, anxiety, excitement, convulsions followed by drowsiness, unconsciousness, respiratory arrest. **CV:** Myocardial depression, arrhythmias, fetal cardiac arrest, bradycardia during delivery, maternal hypotension. **Special Senses:** Blurred vision, tinnitus, pupillary constriction. **GI:** Nausea, vomiting. **Skin:** Skin rash, injection site inflammation and pain. **Other:** Edema, backache.

INTERACTIONS **Drug:** MAOI, ANTIHYPERTENSIVES may increase risk of hypotension.

PHARMACOKINETICS **Absorption:** Readily absorbed from parenteral injection sites. **Onset:** 2–8 min. **Duration:** 4.5–13 h. **Distribution:** Crosses blood-brain barrier and placenta. **Metabolism:** Metabolized in liver. **Elimination:** Excreted in urine. **Half-Life:** 1–2 h.

NURSING IMPLICATIONS

Assessment & Drug Effects

- Note: When used for peridural analgesia, drug produces a profound degree of motor blockade and abdominal relaxation.
- Monitor patient's CV and respiratory status continuously during administration.
- Administer oxygen at first sign of CNS toxicity. Early warning S&S: Restlessness, anxiety, tinnitus, dizziness, blurred vision, tremors, and drowsiness.
- Note: Etidocaine may trigger familial malignant hyperthermia. Early unexplained signs of tachycardia, tachypnea, labile BP, metabolic acidosis, and skeletal muscle rigidity may precede temperature elevation.

E

Patient & Family Education

- Do not to chew solid foods or test the anesthetized region by biting or probing before anesthesia wears off to prevent traumatizing tongue, lip, and buccal mucosa.
- Note: Patient may experience temporary loss of sensation and motor activity, usually in the lower part of the body, after proper administration of epidural anesthesia.

ETIDRONATE DISODIUM Pr

(e-ti-droe'nate)

Didronel, Didronel IV, EHDP

Classifications: BISPHOSPHONATE; REGULATOR, BONE METABOLISM

Pregnancy Category: B (PO); C (parenteral)

AVAILABILITY 200 mg, 400 mg tablets; 300 mg ampule

ACTIONS Diphosphate preparation with primary action on bone. Reduces elevated cardiac output associated with Paget's disease by decreasing vascularity of bone. Induces reversible hyperphosphatemia without adverse effects.

THERAPEUTIC EFFECTS Slows rate of bone resorption and new bone formation in pagetic bone lesions and in normal remodeling process. Lowers serum alkaline phosphatase. Response of Paget's disease may be slow (1–3 mo) and may continue for months after treatment is discontinued.

USES Symptomatic Paget's disease and heterotopic ossification due to spinal cord injury or after total hip replacement.

UNLABELED USES To prevent parathyroid hormone-induced bone resorption, management of malignancy-associated hypercalcemia, treatment of osteoporosis.

CONTRAINDICATIONS Enterocolitis; children; pathologic fractures; pregnancy (category B, oral; category C, parenteral). Safety during lactation or in children is not established.

CAUTIOUS USE Renal impairment; patients on restricted calcium and vitamin D intake.

ROUTE & DOSAGE

Paget's Disease

Adult: **PO** 5–10 mg/kg/d for up to 6 mo or 11–20 mg/kg/d for up to 3 mo, may repeat after 3–6 mo off the drug if necessary

Heterotopic Ossification Due to Spinal Cord Injury

Adult: **PO** 20 mg/kg/d for 2 wk, then 10 mg/kg/d for an additional 10 wk

Heterotopic Ossification Due to Total Hip Arthroplasty

Adult: **PO** 20 mg/kg/d starting 1 mo before the procedure and continuing for 3 mo after

Malignancy-Associated Hypercalcemia

Adult: **IV** 7.5 mg/kg/d for 3–7 d diluted in at least 250 mL NS and infused over at least 2 h, may repeat after 7 d off the drug if necessary

ADMINISTRATION

Oral

- Give as single dose on empty stomach 2 h before meals with full glass of water or juice to reduce gastric irritation.
- Relieve GI adverse effects by dividing total oral daily dose.

Intravenous

PREPARE: **IV Infusion:** Dilute a single dose in at least 250 mL of NS.

ADMINISTER: **IV Infusion:** Give IV slowly over a period of at least 2 h.

- Store all forms at 15°–30° C (59°–86° F) in tightly closed container unless otherwise directed.

ADVERSE EFFECTS (≥1%) **GI:** Nausea, diarrhea, *loose bowel movements,* metallic or altered taste. **Musculoskeletal:** Increased or recurrent bone pain in pagetic sites, onset of bone pain in previously asymptomatic sites, increased risk of fractures in patient with Paget's disease. **Metabolic:** Hypocalcemia, hyperphosphatemia, elevated serum phosphatase, suppressed mineralization of uninvolved skeleton (focal osteomalacia). **Urogenital:** Renal insufficiency (high IV doses).

INTERACTIONS Drug: CALCIUM SUPPLEMENTS, ANTACIDS, IRON AND OTHER MINERAL SUPPLEMENTS may decrease absorption of etidronate (give etidronate 2 h before other drugs). **Food:** Food, especially milk and dairy products, will decrease absorption of etidronate (give 2 h before meals).

PHARMACOKINETICS Absorption: Variably absorbed from GI tract. **Distribution:** 50% of absorbed drug is distributed to bone. **Metabolism:** Not metabolized. **Elimination:** 50% of absorbed dose is excreted in urine. **Half-Life:** 6 h.

NURSING IMPLICATIONS

Assessment & Drug Effects

- Report persistent nausea or diarrhea; GI adverse effects may interfere with adequate nutritional status and need to be treated promptly.
- Monitor I&O ratio, serum creatinine, or BUN of patient with impaired kidney function.
- Lab tests: Periodic serum calcium and phosphate.
- Monitor for signs of hypocalcemia. Latent tetany (hypocalcemia) may be detected by Chvostek's and Trousseau's signs and a serum calcium value of 7–8 mg/dL.
- Note: Serum phosphate levels generally return to normal 2–4 wk after medication is discontinued.
- Note: Patients may experience a metallic taste during IV administration.

Patient & Family Education

- Avoid eating 2 h before or after taking PO etidronate. Drug absorption is decreased by food, especially milk, milk products, and other foods high in calcium, mineral supplements, and antacids.
- Notify physician promptly of sudden onset of unexplained pain. Risk of pathological fractures increases when daily dose of 20 mg/kg is taken longer than 3 mo.
- Report promptly if bone pain, restricted mobility, heat over involved bone site occur.
- Do not breast feed while taking this drug without consulting physician.

ETODOLAC

(e-to'do-lac)

Lodine, Lodine XL

Classifications: CENTRAL NERVOUS SYSTEM AGENT; ANALGESIC, NONSTEROIDAL ANTIINFLAMMATORY AGENT, NSAID; ANTIPYRETIC

Prototype: Ibuprofen

Pregnancy Category: C

AVAILABILITY 400 mg tablets; 200 mg, 300 mg capsules; 400 mg, 600 mg sustained release tablets

ACTIONS Exact mechanism of action is unknown but may inhibit cyclooxygenase activity and prostaglandin synthesis. NSAIDS may also suppress production of rheumatoid factor.

THERAPEUTIC EFFECTS Produces analgesic, antiinflammatory effects of a NSAID.

E

USES Osteoarthritis and acute pain, rheumatoid arthritis.

UNLABELED USES Temporal arteritis.

CONTRAINDICATIONS Hypersensitivity to NSAIDS and in GI ulceration or inflammation; lactation. Safety and efficacy in children <14 y are not established.

CAUTIOUS USE Renal impairment, liver function impairment, patients over 65 y, and pregnancy (category C).

ROUTE & DOSAGE

Acute Pain

Adult: **PO** 200–400 mg q6–8h prn

Osteoarthritis

Adult: **PO** 600–1200 mg/d in 2–4 divided doses, (max: 1200 mg/d or 20 mg/kg for patients ≤60 kg; Lodine XL 400–1000 mg once daily)

Rheumatoid Arthritis

Adult: **PO** 500 mg b.i.d.

ADMINISTRATION

Oral

- Give with food or antacid to reduce risk of GI ulceration.
- Ensure that sustained release form of drug is not chewed or crushed. It must be swallowed whole.
- Store at 15°–25° C (59°–77° F); tablets and capsules in bottles; sustained release capsules in unit-dose packages. Protect all forms from moisture.

ADVERSE EFFECTS (≥1%) **CV:** Fluid retention, edema. **CNS:** Dizziness, headache, drowsiness, insomnia. **GI:** *Dyspepsia, nausea, vomiting, diarrhea,* indigestion, heartburn, abdominal pain, constipation, flatulence, gastritis, melena, peptic ulcer, GI bleeding. **Hematologic:** Thrombocytopenia, increased bleeding time. **Skin:** Rash, pruritus. **Urogenital:** Urinary frequency. **Metabolic:** Hepatotoxicity. **Special Senses:** Blurred vision; tinnitus. **Respiratory:** Asthma.

DIAGNOSTIC TEST INTERFERENCE May cause a false-positive ***urinary bilirubin*** test and a false-positive ***ketone*** test done with the dipstick method. May cause a small decrease (1 to 2 mg/dL) in ***serum uric acid*** levels.

INTERACTIONS Drug: May reduce the effects of **diuretics** and the antihypertensive effects of **beta blockers** and other ANTIHYPERTENSIVE MEDICATIONS. May increase **digoxin** and **lithium** levels and nephrotoxicity due to **cyclosporine. Herbal: Feverfew, garlic, ginger, ginkgo** may increase bleeding.

PHARMACOKINETICS Absorption: Readily absorbed from GI tract. **Onset:** 30 min. **Peak:** 1–2 h. **Duration:** 4–12 h. **Distribution:** Widely distributed; 99% protein bound; not known if crosses placenta or if distributed into breast milk. **Metabolism:** Extensively metabolized in liver. **Elimination:** 72% excreted in urine, 16% in feces. **Half-Life:** 6–7 h.

NURSING IMPLICATIONS

Assessment & Drug Effects

- Assess for signs of GI ulceration and bleeding. Risk factors include high doses of etodolac, history of peptic ulcer disease, alcohol use, smoking, and concomitant use of aspirin.

- Assess carefully for fluid retention by monitoring weight and observing for edema in patients with a history of CHF.
- Monitor for decreased BP control in hypertensive patients.
- Lab tests: Periodic CBC and kidney and liver function.
- Monitor for drug toxicity when used concurrently with either digoxin or lithium.
- Monitor for rhinitis, urticaria, or other signs of allergic reactions. Discontinue drug and notify physician when present.
- Monitor carefully increases in etodolac dosage with older adult patients; adverse effects are more pronounced.
- Monitor for headaches, especially at high doses. Discontinuation of therapy may be indicated.

Patient & Family Education

- Learn S&S of GI ulceration. Stop medication in presence of bleeding and contact the physician immediately.
- Do not take aspirin, which may potentiate ulcerogenic effects.
- Do not breast feed while taking this drug.

ETOPOSIDE

(e-toe-po'side)

Etopophos, Toposar, VePesid, VP-16

Classifications: ANTINEOPLASTIC; MITOTIC INHIBITOR

Prototype: Vincristine

Pregnancy Category: D

AVAILABILITY 50 mg capsules; 20 mg/mL injection; 100 mg lyophilized powder for injection

ACTIONS Semisynthetic derivative of May apple plant. Produces cytotoxic action by unclear mechanism. Primary action is by arresting G_2 (resting or premitotic) phase of cell cycle; also acts on S phase of DNA synthesis. High doses cause lysis of cells entering mitotic phase, and lower doses inhibit cells from entering prophase.

THERAPEUTIC EFFECTS Antineoplastic effect is due to its ability to arrest mitosis (cell division).

USES Treatment of refractory testicular neoplasms, in patients who have already received appropriate surgical, chemotherapeutic, and radiation therapy; for treatment of choriocarcinoma in women and small cell carcinoma of the lung.

UNLABELED USES Hodgkin's and non-Hodgkin's lymphomas, acute myelogenous (nonlymphocytic) leukemia.

CONTRAINDICATIONS Severe bone marrow depression; severe hepatic or renal impairment; existing or recent viral infection, bacterial infection; intraperitoneal, intrapleural, or intrathecal administration. Safety during pregnancy (category D), lactation, or in children is not established.

CAUTIOUS USE Impaired kidney or liver function; gout.

ROUTE & DOSAGE

Testicular Carcinoma

Adult: **IV** 50–100 mg/m²/d for 5 consecutive days q3–4wk for 3–4 courses or 100 mg/m² on days 1, 3, and 5 q3–4wk for 3–4 courses **PO** Twice the IV dose rounded to the nearest 50 mg

Small Cell Lung Carcinoma

Adult: **IV** 35 mg/m²/d for 4 consecutive days to 50 mg/m²/d for 5 consecutive days q3–4wk **PO** Twice the IV dose rounded to the nearest 50 mg

E

ADMINISTRATION

Oral

- Oral dose is usually in the range of 70–100 mg/m^2 daily, rounded to nearest 50 mg.
- Refrigerate capsules at 2°–8° C (36°–46° F) unless otherwise directed. Do not freeze.

Intravenous

Note: Wear disposable surgical gloves when preparing or disposing of etoposide. Wash immediately with soap and water if skin comes in contact with drug.

PREPARE: **IV Infusion:** Each 100 mg must be diluted with 250–500 mL of D5W or NS to produce final concentrations of 0.2–0.4 mg/mL.

ADMINISTER: **IV Infusion:** Give by slow IV infusion over 30–60 min to reduce risk of hypotension and bronchospasm. Before administration, inspect solution for particulate matter and discoloration. Solution should be clear and yellow. If crystals are present, discard.

INCOMPATIBILITIES **Y-site: Amphotericin B, cefepime, chlorpromazine, filgrastim, idarubicin, imipenem-cilastatin, methylprednisolone, mitomycin, prochlorperazine.**

- Diluted solutions with concentration of 0.2 mg/mL are stable for 96 h, and the 0.4 mg/mL solutions are stable for 48 h under normal room fluorescent light in glass or plastic (PVC) containers.

ADVERSE EFFECTS (≥1%) **Body as a Whole:** Hypersensitivity (sweating, chills, fever, coryza, tachycardia; throat, back and general body pain; abdominal cramps, flushing, substernal chest pain, dyspnea, <u>bronchospasm</u>, pulmonary edema, <u>anaphylactoid reaction</u>). **CNS:** Peripheral neuropathy, paresthesias, weakness, somnolence, unusual tiredness, transient confusion. **CV:** Transient hypotension; thrombophlebitis with extravasation. **GI:** *Nausea, vomiting,* dyspepsia, anorexia, diarrhea, constipation, stomatitis. **Hematologic:** *Leukopenia (principally granulocytopenia), thrombocytopenia,* <u>severe myelosuppression</u>, *anemia, pancytopenia, neutropenia.* **Respiratory:** Pleural effusion, bronchospasm. **Skin:** *Reversible alopecia* (can progress to total baldness); radiation recall dermatitis; necrosis, *pain at IV site.*

INTERACTIONS Drug: ANTICOAGULANTS, ANTIPLATELET AGENTS, NSAIDS, **aspirin** may increase risk of bleeding.

PHARMACOKINETICS Absorption: Approximately 50% absorbed from GI tract. **Peak:** 1–1.5 h. **Distribution:** Variable penetration into CSF. **Metabolism:** Probably metabolized in liver. **Elimination:** 44%–60% excreted in urine, 2%–16% excreted in feces over 3 d. **Half-Life:** 5–10 h.

NURSING IMPLICATIONS

Assessment & Drug Effects

- Check IV site during and after infusion. Extravasation can cause thrombophlebitis and necrosis.
- Be prepared to treat an anaphylactoid reaction (see Appendix F). Stop infusion immediately if the reaction occurs.
- Monitor vital signs during and after infusion. Stop infusion immediately if hypotension occurs.
- Lab tests: Perform baseline all prior to and at regular intervals during therapy, and before each subsequent treatment course. Tests include: CBC with differential; liver and kidney function tests (AST, ALT, serum bilirubin, LDH, BUN, serum creatinine).
- Withhold therapy when an absolute neutrophil count is below

$500/mm^3$ or a platelet count below $50,000/mm^3$.

- Be alert to evidence of patient complaints that might suggest development of leukopenia (see Appendix F), infection (immunosuppression), and bleeding.
- Protect patient from any trauma that might precipitate bleeding during period of platelet nadir particularly. Withhold invasive procedures if possible.

Patient & Family Education

- Learn possible adverse effects of etoposide, such as blood dyscrasias, alopecia, carcinogenesis, before treatment begins.
- Make position changes slowly, particularly from lying to upright position because transient hypotension after therapy is possible.
- Inspect mouth daily for ulcerations and bleeding. Avoid obvious irritants such as hot or spicy foods, smoking, alcohol.
- Do not breast feed while taking this drug without consulting physician.

ETRETINATE

(e-tret′i-nate)

Tegison

Classifications: SKIN AND MUCOUS MEMBRANE AGENT; ANTIPSORIATIC; RETINOID

Prototype: Isotretinoin

Pregnancy Category: X

AVAILABILITY 10 mg, 25 mg capsules

ACTIONS Second-generation retinoid related to retinoic acid and retinol (vitamin A). Mechanism of action unknown.

THERAPEUTIC EFFECTS Reduces redness, scaling, and thickness of psoriasis lesions by normalizing epidermal differentiation; also decreases stratum corneum thickness and inflammation in epidermis and dermis.

USES Treatment of severe recalcitrant psoriasis in patients unresponsive to or intolerant of standard therapies.

CONTRAINDICATIONS Intolerance to isotretinoin, tretinoin, vitamin A derivatives, or to parabens (preservative in etretinate formulation); severe obesity; pregnancy (category X), lactation.

CAUTIOUS USE Cardiovascular disease or family history of; children (used only if all alternative therapies have been ineffective); hepatic impairment; diabetes mellitus, patients predisposed to hypertriglyceridemia.

ROUTE & DOSAGE

Psoriasis

Adult: **PO** 0.75–1 mg/kg/d in divided doses (max: 1.5 mg/kg/d), may be able to decrease to 0.5–0.75 mg/kg/d after 8–10 wk of therapy

ADMINISTRATION

Oral

- Give consistently with whole milk or other high-fat food increases drug absorption and allows smaller doses. This may allow easier titration to lowest effective dosage range. Discuss with physician.
- Store at 15°–30° C (59°–86° F); protect capsules from light and moisture.

ADVERSE EFFECTS (≥1%) **Body as a Whole:** Nearly all resemble those of hypervitaminosis A syndrome. **CNS:** *Fatigue, headache, fever,* dizziness, lethargy, amnesia, anxiety, depression, <u>pseudotumor cerebri</u>. **CV:** Edema; <u>cardiac thrombotic or</u>

E

obstructive events; postural hypotension, coagulation disorders, MI (rare). **Special Senses:** Dry nose, *nose bleeds,* change in hearing, earache, otitis externa; *Eye irritation,* decreased night vision, *eyelid abnormalities; double vision;* corneal erosion and abrasions; dry eyes, eye pain, blurred vision, excessive tearing, conjunctivitis, scotomas, photophobia. **GI:** Abdominal pain, *appetite change,* stomatitis, *sore tongue,* thirst, *nausea,* constipation, diarrhea, flatulence, weight loss, *gingival bleeding, dry mouth.* **Urogenital:** Abnormal menses, atrophic vaginitis, dysuria, polyuria. **Hematologic:** Anemia; increased or decreased serum potassium, calcium, sodium, *phosphorus, chloride, fasting blood sugars,* platelets, Hgb, Hct, *PTT, MCHC,* prothrombin time; increased BUN, creatinine. **Metabolic:** *Hypertriglyceridemia,* hepatitis (hepatotoxicity), *hypercholesterolemia,* lowered HDL, increased AST, ALT, bilirubin. **Musculoskeletal:** *Bone and joint pain,* muscle cramps, myalgia, gout, hyperkinesia, *hyperostosis.* **Respiratory:** Dyspnea, coughing. **Skin:** Nail disorders, *photosensitivity; skin fragility and peeling;* changes in perspiration, *hair loss,* dry skin, rash, itching, skin atrophy, fissures, ulcerations; hirsutism, herpes simplex. **Other:** *Chapped lips,* cheilitis; malignant neoplasms.

INTERACTIONS Drug: Alcohol may increase plasma triglyceride levels; **isotretinoin,** VITAMIN A PREPARATIONS compound toxic effects; **methotrexate** may increase risk of hepatotoxicity; TETRACYCLINES may increase risk of pseudotumor cerebri. **Food:** Milk will increase absorption of etretinate.

PHARMACOKINETICS Absorption: Readily absorbed from GI tract with significant first pass metabolism. **Peak:** 2.5–5 h. **Duration:** Detectable serum levels for years after discontinuation. **Distribution:** Accumulates in adipose tissue, liver, and subcutaneous fat; crosses placenta; distributed into breast milk. **Metabolism:** Metabolized in liver. **Elimination:** Excreted primarily in feces; some excretion in urine. **Half-Life:** 120 h.

NURSING IMPLICATIONS

Assessment & Drug Effects

- Monitor therapeutic effectiveness. Transient exacerbation of psoriasis may occur during the initial treatment.
- Lab tests: Perform baseline hepatic function tests prior to treatment, then at 1- to 2-wk intervals for 1–2 mo. Continue with periodic tests at intervals of 1–3 mo during treatment. Discontinue drug in presence of hepatitis. Determine blood lipid before treatment and repeat at 1- to 2-wk intervals until lipid response is established (usually 4–8 wk).

Patient & Family Education

- Use effective contraception at least 1 mo before starting treatment, throughout treatment, and for as long as 4 y after treatment ends.
- Note: Complete clearing of the disease has been observed after 4–9 mo of therapy in most patients.
- Notify physician immediately of pain and limitation of motion; drug will be discontinued. Common sites for drug-induced hyperostosis (abnormal growth of bone tissue) in adults are in the ankles, pelvis, and knees. Promptly report similar pain and limitation of motion when drug is prescribed for child.
- Notify physician immediately of S&S of hepatitis: jaundice (see Appendix F), flu-like symptoms.

- Discontinue drug if any visual difficulties develop and schedule an ophthalmic examination.
- Avoid high-fat foods in diet because this drug can cause hypertriglyceridemia and increased LDLs.
- Avoid vitamin A supplements because of the possibility of additive toxic effects.
- Report early symptoms of pseudotumor cerebri: Headache, vomiting, nausea, blurred vision.
- Avoid excessive sun exposure and sunlamp treatments because of potential drug-induced photosensitivity and photophobia.
- Notify physician of dry mouth; drug-induced effects on oral mucosa and gingiva need to be treated.
- Be completely aware of the teratogenic danger. Discuss the risk of becoming pregnant or continuing a pregnancy with your physician.
- Do not donate blood while taking etretinate or for several years after therapy.
- Do not breast feed while taking this drug.

EXEMESTANE

(ex-e-mes′tain)

Aromasin

Classifications: ANTINEOPLASTIC; HORMONES AND SYNTHETIC SUBSTITUTES; ANTIESTROGEN; STEROIDAL AROMATASE INHIBITOR

Prototype: Anastrozole

Pregnancy Category: D

AVAILABILITY 25 mg tablet

ACTIONS Steroidal aromatase inhibitor that suppresses plasma estrogens, estradiol and estrone without affecting cortisol or aldosterone synthesis in the adrenal glands. The enzyme, aromatase, converts estrone to estradiol.

THERAPEUTIC EFFECTS Breast tumor regression is possible in postmenopausal women. Effectiveness is indicated by evidence of tumor regression.

USES Treatment of advanced breast cancer in postmenopausal women whose disease has progressed following tamoxifen therapy.

CONTRAINDICATIONS Hypersensitivity to exemestane; pregnancy (category D), lactation.

CAUTIOUS USE Hepatic or renal insufficiency; GI disorders; cardiovascular disease; hyperlipidemia.

ROUTE & DOSAGE

Advanced Breast Cancer

Adult: **PO** 25 mg q.d. after a meal

ADMINISTRATION

Oral

- Give following a meal.
- Store at 15°–30° C (59°–86° F).

ADVERSE EFFECTS (≥1%) **Body as a Whole:** *Fatigue, hot flashes, pain,* flu-like symptoms; edema; fever; paresthesia. **CNS:** *Depression, insomnia, anxiety;* dizziness; headache. **CV:** Hypertension. **GI:** *Nausea,* vomiting, abdominal pain, anorexia, constipation, diarrhea, increased appetite. **Respiratory:** Dyspnea, cough, bronchitis, sinusitis. **Skin:** Increased sweating, rash, itching. **Other:** UTI; lymphedema.

PHARMACOKINETICS Absorption: Rapidly absorbed, approximately 42% reaches systemic circulation. **Distribution:** Extensive tissue distribution, 90% protein bound. **Metabolism:** Extensively metabolized in liver by CYP3A4. **Elimination:** Equally excreted in urine and feces. **Half-Life:** 24 h.

E

NURSING IMPLICATIONS

Assessment & Drug Effects

- Lab tests: Baseline liver function, BUN and creatinine; periodic WBC with differential, lipid profile, routine blood chemistry.

Patient & Family Education

- Review manufacturer's patient literature thoroughly to reinforce understanding of likely adverse effects.
- Report bothersome adverse effects to physician.
- Do not breast feed while taking this drug.

EZETIMIBE

(e-ze-ti'mibe)

Zetia, Ezetrol ✦

Classification: CARDIOVASCULAR AGENT; ANTILIPEMIC

Pregnancy Category: C

AVAILABILITY 10 mg tablets

ACTIONS Works at the lining of the small intestine inhibiting the absorption of cholesterol, but does not inhibit cholesterol synthesis in the liver or increases bile acid excretion. Thus it decreases the amount of intestinal cholesterol available to the liver.

THERAPEUTIC EFFECTS Lowers both total cholesterol and low-density lipid (LDL) cholesterol; its mechanism of action is complimentary to statins.

USES Treatment of primary hypercholesterolemia alone or with an HMG-CoA reductase inhibitor (statin); treatment of homozygous sitosterolemia as an adjunct to diet.

CONTRAINDICATIONS Hypersensitivity to ezetimibe; concurrent use with HMG-CoA reductase inhibitor in patients with active liver disease or elevated serum transaminases; hepatic insufficiency; concurrent administration with fibrates; lactation; pregnancy (category C); children <10 y.

CAUTIOUS USE Mild hepatic insufficiency.

ROUTE & DOSAGE

Hypercholesterolemia

Adult: **PO** 10 mg q.d.

ADMINISTRATION

Oral

- Give no sooner than 2 h before or 4 h after administration of a bile acid sequestrant such as cholestyramine.
- Store at 15°–30° C (59°–86° F). Protect from moisture.

ADVERSE EFFECTS (≥1%) **Body as a Whole:** Fatigue, arthralgia, back pain, myalgia, angioedema. **CNS:** Dizziness, headache. **GI:** Abdominal pain, diarrhea. **Respiratory:** Pharyngitis, sinusitis, cough. **Skin:** Rash.

INTERACTIONS Drug: BILE ACID SEQUESTRANTS (e.g., **cholestyramine**) may decrease absorption (give ezetimibe 2 h before or 4 h after these drugs); **cyclosporine** can significantly increase ezetimibe levels.

PHARMACOKINETICS Absorption: Well absorbed from the small intestine. **Peak:** 4–12 h. **Distribution:** Ezetimibe-glucuronide is 99% protein bound. **Metabolism:** Extensively conjugated to an active glucuronide compound (ezetimibe-glucuronide). Metabolized in small intestine and liver. **Elimination:** Primarily excreted in feces. **Half-Life:** 22 h.

NURSING IMPLICATIONS

Assessment & Drug Effects

- Lab tests: Monitor baseline and periodic lipid profile. Monitor

baseline LFTs and when used with a statin, monitor periodic LFTs in accordance with the monitoring schedule for that statin.
- Assess for and report unexplained muscle pain, especially when used in combination with a statin drug.
- Monitor closely patients who take both ezetimibe and cyclosporine.

Patient & Family Education
- Report unexplained muscle pain, tenderness, or weakness.
- Females should use effective methods of contraception to prevent pregnancy while taking this drug.
- Do not breast feed while taking this drug without consulting physician.

FAMCICLOVIR

(fam-ci'clo-vir)

Famvir

Classifications: ANTIINFECTIVE; ANTIVIRAL

Prototype: Acyclovir

Pregnancy Category: B

AVAILABILITY 125 mg, 250 mg, 500 mg tablets

ACTIONS Prodrug to the antiviral agent penciclovir; may have an advantage over acyclovir because of its greater stability intracellularly in infected cells. Prevents viral replication by inhibition of DNA synthesis in herpes virus-infected cells, and has longer-lasting antiviral activity than acyclovir.

THERAPEUTIC EFFECTS Indicated by decreasing pain and crusting of lesions followed by loss of vesicles, ulcers, and crusts. Interferes with DNA synthesis of herpes simplex virus type 1 and 2 (HSV-1 and HSV-2) infections, varicella-zoster virus and cytomegalovirus.

USES Management of acute herpes zoster, genital herpes, recurrent episodes of genital herpes in immunocompromised adults. Suppression of recurrent episodes of genital herpes in immunocompetent adults.

CONTRAINDICATIONS Hypersensitivity to famciclovir, lactation.

CAUTIOUS USE Renal or hepatic impairment, carcinoma, older adults, pregnancy (category B). Safety in children <18 y is not established.

ROUTE & DOSAGE

Herpes Zoster, Treatment

Adult: **PO** 500 mg q8h times 7 d, start within 48–72 h of onset of rash

Renal Impairment

Cl_{cr} 40–59 mL/min: 500 mg q12h; 20–39 mL/min: 500 mg q24h

Treatment of Recurrent Genital Herpes

Adult: **PO** 125 mg b.i.d. times 5 d

Suppression of Recurrent Genital Herpes

Adult: **PO** 250 mg b.i.d. for up to 1 y

ADMINISTRATION

Oral
- Reduce dosage in patients with reduced kidney function.
- Store at room temperature, 15°–30° C (59°–86° F).

ADVERSE EFFECTS (≥1%) **CNS:** *Headache,* somnolence, dizziness, paresthesias, fatigue, fever, rigors.

Hematologic: Purpura. **GI:** Nausea, diarrhea, vomiting, constipation, anorexia, abdominal pain. **Body as a Whole:** Pharyngitis, sinusitis, pruritus.

INTERACTIONS Drug: Probenecid may decrease elimination; famciclovir may increase **digoxin** levels.

F

PHARMACOKINETICS Absorption: Readily absorbed from GI tract and rapidly converted to penciclovir in intestinal and liver tissue. **Onset:** Median times to full crusting of lesions, loss of vesicles, loss of ulcers, and loss of crusts were 6, 5, 7, and 19 d, respectively; median time to loss of acute pain was 21 d. **Peak:** 1 h. **Distribution:** Distributes into breast milk of animals. **Metabolism:** Metabolized in liver and intestinal tissue to penciclovir, which is the active antiviral agent. **Elimination:** Approximately 60% recovered in urine as penciclovir. **Half-Life:** Penciclovir 2–3 h.

NURSING IMPLICATIONS

Assessment & Drug Effects

- Lab tests: Baseline CBC and routine blood chemistry studies prior to and after short courses of therapy; periodically during prolonged treatment.
- Monitor digoxin level and assess for S&S of digoxin toxicity when digoxin is used concurrently with famciclovir.

Patient & Family Education

- Learn potential adverse effects and report those that are bothersome to physician.
- Be aware that a full therapeutic response may take several weeks.
- Report S&S of hypersensitivity immediately to physician.
- Do not breast feed while taking this drug.

FAMOTIDINE

(fa-moe'ti-deen)
Pepcid, Pepcid AC
Classifications: GASTROINTESTINAL AGENT; ANTISECRETORY AGENT (H_2-RECEPTOR ANTAGONIST)
Prototype: Cimetidine
Pregnancy Category: B

AVAILABILITY 10 mg, 20 mg, 40 mg tablets; 40 mg/5 mL suspension; 10 mg/mL, 20 mg/50 mL injection

ACTIONS Thiazole derivative, structurally similar to histamine and pharmacologically similar to cimetidine. A potent competitive inhibitor of histamine at histamine (H_2) receptor sites in gastric parietal cells. Inhibits basal, nocturnal, meal-stimulated, and pentagastrin-stimulated gastric secretion; also inhibits pepsin secretion. Is 20–160 times more potent than cimetidine and 3–20 times more potent than ranitidine. Does not affect gastric emptying or exocrine pancreatic function.

THERAPEUTIC EFFECTS Reduces parietal cell output of hydrochloric acid; thus, detrimental effects of acid on gastric mucosa are diminished.

USES Short-term treatment of active duodenal ulcer. Maintenance therapy for duodenal ulcer patients on reduced dosage after healing of an active ulcer. Treatment of pathologic hypersecretory conditions (e.g., Zollinger-Ellison syndrome), benign gastric ulcer, gastroesophageal reflux disease (GERD), gastritis.

UNLABELED USES Stress ulcer prophylaxis.

CONTRAINDICATIONS Safe use during pregnancy (category B), by nursing mothers.
CAUTIOUS USE Renal insufficiency.

ROUTE & DOSAGE

Duodenal Ulcer

Adult: **PO** 40 mg h.s. or 20 mg b.i.d. **PO Maintenance Therapy** 20 mg h.s. **IV** 20 mg q12h
Child: **PO/IV** 0.5 mg/kg q8–12h (max: 40 mg/d)

Pathological Hypersecretory Conditions

Adult: **PO** 20–160 mg q6h

GERD, Gastritis

Adult: **PO** 10 mg b.i.d.
Child: **PO** 1 mg/kg/d in 2 divided doses (max: 40 mg b.i.d.)

Renal Impairment

Cl_{cr} <50 mL/min: 50% of usual dose or usual dose q36–48h for all indications

ADMINISTRATION

Oral

- Give with liquid or food of patient's choice; an antacid may also be given if patient is also on antacid therapy.
- Store at 15°–30° C (59°–86° F). Protect from moisture and strong light; do not freeze.

Intravenous

Note: Verify correct IV concentration and rate of infusion/injection with physician before administration to infants or children.

PREPARE: **Direct:** Dilute 20 mg (2 mL) famotidine IV solution (containing 10 mg/mL) with D5W, NS, or other compatible IV diluent (see manufacturer's directions) to a total volume of 5 or 10 mL. **IV Infusion:** Dilute 2 mL famotidine IV with 100 mL compatible IV solution.
ADMINISTER: **Direct:** Give over not less than 2 min. **IV Infusion:** Infuse over 15–30 min.
INCOMPATIBILITIES **Y-site: Amphotericin B cholesteryl complex**, **cefepime**

- Store IV solution at 2°–8° C (36°–46° F); reconstituted IV solution is stable for 48 h at room temperature 15°–30° C (59°–86° F).

ADVERSE EFFECTS (≥1%) **CNS:** Dizziness, headache, confusion, depression. **GI:** Constipation, diarrhea. **Skin:** Rash, acne, pruritus, dry skin, flushing. **Hematologic:** Thrombocytopenia. **Urogenital:** Increases in BUN and serum creatinine.

INTERACTIONS Drug: No clinically significant interactions established.

PHARMACOKINETICS Absorption: Incompletely absorbed from GI tract (40%–50% reaches systemic circulation). **Onset:** 1 h. **Peak:** 1–3 h PO; 0.5–3 h IV. **Duration:** 10–12 h. **Metabolism:** Metabolized in liver. **Elimination:** Excreted in urine. **Half-Life:** 2.5–4 h.

NURSING IMPLICATIONS

Assessment & Drug Effects

- Monitor for improvement in GI distress.
- Monitor for signs of GI bleeding.

Patient & Family Education

- Be aware that pain relief may not be experienced for several days after starting therapy.
- Do not breast feed while taking this drug without consulting physician.

FAT EMULSION, INTRAVENOUS

(fat e-mul'sion)

Intralipid, Liposyn, Nutralipid, Soyacal, Travamulsion

Classification: CALORIC AGENT

Pregnancy Category: B for Soyacal 10%; C for all others

AVAILABILITY 10%, 20% emulsion

ACTIONS Soybean oil in water emulsion containing egg yolk phospholipids and glycerin. Liposyn 10% is a safflower oil in water emulsion containing egg phosphatides and glycerin. Caloric value per milliliter of Intralipid 10% and Liposyn 10% is 1.1; Intralipid 20% is 2.

THERAPEUTIC EFFECTS Used as a nutritional supplement. Fat emulsions contain a mixture of neutral triglycerides, mostly unsaturated fatty acids.

USES Fatty acid deficiency. Also to supply fatty acids and calories in high-density form to patients receiving prolonged TPN therapy who cannot tolerate high dextrose concentrations or when fluid intake must be restricted as in renal failure, CHF, ascites.

CONTRAINDICATIONS Hyperlipemia; bone marrow dyscrasias; impaired fat metabolism as in pathological hyperlipemia, lipoid nephrosis, acute pancreatitis accompanied by hyperlipemia.

CAUTIOUS USE Severe hepatic or pulmonary disease; pregnancy (category C); coagulation disorders; anemia; newborns, premature neonates, infants with hyperbilirubinemia; when danger of fat embolism exists; diabetes mellitus; thrombocytopenia; history of gastric ulcer.

ROUTE & DOSAGE

Prevention of Essential Fatty Acid Deficiency

Adult: **IV** 500 mL of 10% or 250 mL of 20% solution infused over 8–12 h twice/wk (max: rate of 100 mL/h)
Child: **IV** 0.5–1 g/kg infused slowly over 8–12 h twice/wk (max: 3–4 g/kg/d; max: infusion 0.25 g/kg/h)

Calorie Source in Fluid-restricted Patients

Adult: **IV** up to 2.5 g/kg or 60% of nonprotein calories daily infused over at least 8–12 h (max: rate of 100 mL/h)
Child: **IV** up to 4 g/kg or 60% of nonprotein calories daily infused over at least 8–12 h (max: rate of 100 mL/h)
Premature neonate: **IV** 0.25–0.5 g/kg/d, increase by 0.25–0.5 g/kg/d (max: 3–4 g/kg/d; max: infusion 0.15 g/kg/h)

ADMINISTRATION

Intravenous

- Do not use if oil appears to be separating out of the emulsion.

PREPARE: **IV Infusion:** Allow preparations that have been refrigerated to stand at room temperature for about 30 min before using whenever possible. Check with a pharmacist before mixing fat emulsions with electrolytes, vitamins, drugs, or other nutrient solutions.

ADMINISTER: **IV Infusion:** Give fat emulsions via a separate peripheral site or by piggyback into same vein receiving amino acid injection and dextrose mixtures or give by piggyback through a Y-connector near infusion site so that the two solutions mix only in a short piece of tubing proximal to needle. ▪ Must hang fat emulsion higher than hyperalimentation solution bottle to prevent backup of fat emulsion into primary line. ▪ Do not use an in-line filter because size of fat particles is larger than pore size. Control flow rate of each solution by separate infusion pumps. Use a constant rate over 20–24 h to reduce risk of hyperlipemia in neonates and prematures because they tend to metabolize fat slowly.

INCOMPATIBILITIES **Solution/additive: Aminophylline, amphotericin B, ampicillin, calcium chloride, calcium gluconate, gentamicin, hetastarch, magnesium chloride methicillin, penicillin G, phenytoin, ranitidine, tetracycline, vitamin B complex. Y-site: Acyclovir, amphotericin B, cyclosporine, doxorubicin, doxycycline, droperidol, ganciclovir, haloperidol, heparin, hetastarch, hydromorphone, levorphanol, lorazepam, midazolam, minocycline, nalbuphine, ondansetron, pentobarbital, phenobarbital, phenytoin, potassium phosphate, sodium phosphate, tetracycline**.

▪ Discard contents of partly used containers. ▪ Store, unless otherwise directed by manufacturer, Intralipid 10% and Liposyn 10% at room temperature (25° C [77° F] or below); refrigerate Intralipid 20%. Do not freeze.

ADVERSE EFFECTS (≥1%) **Body as a Whole:** Hypersensitivity reactions (to egg protein), irritation at infusion site. **Hematologic:** Hypercoagulability, thrombocytopenia in neonates. **GI:** *Transient increases in liver function tests, hyperlipemia.* **[Long-Term Administration]** Sepsis, jaundice (cholestasis), hepatomegaly, kernicterus (infants with hyperbilirubinemia), shock (rare).

DIAGNOSTIC TEST INTERFERENCE Blood samples drawn during or shortly after fat emulsion infusion may produce abnormally high ***hemoglobin MCH and MCHC*** values. Fat emulsions may cause transient abnormalities in ***liver function tests*** and may interfere with estimations of ***serum bilirubin*** (especially in infants).

INTERACTIONS Drug: No clinically significant interactions established.

PHARMACOKINETICS Not studied.

NURSING IMPLICATIONS

Assessment & Drug Effects

- Observe patient closely. Acute reactions tend to occur within the first 2 1/2 h of therapy.
- Lab tests: Determine baseline values for hemoglobin, platelet count, blood coagulation, liver function, plasma lipid profile (especially serum triglycerides and cholesterol, free fatty acids in plasma). Repeat 1 or 2 times weekly during therapy in adults; more frequently in children. Report significant deviations promptly.
- Lab tests: Obtain daily platelet counts in neonates during first week of therapy, then every other day during second week, and 3 times a week thereafter because newborns are prone to develop thrombocytopenia.

- Note: Lipemia must clear after each daily infusion. Degree of lipemia is measured by serum triglycerides and cholesterol levels 4–6 h after infusion has ceased.

Patient & Family Education

- Report difficulty breathing, nausea, vomiting, or headache to physician.

F

FELBAMATE

(fel′ba-mate)

Felbatol

Classifications: CENTRAL NERVOUS SYSTEM AGENT; ANTICONVULSANT

Prototype: Phenytoin

Pregnancy Category: C

AVAILABILITY 400 mg, 600 mg tablets; 600 mg/5 mL suspension

ACTIONS Anticonvulsant mechanism has not been identified. Blocks repetitive firing of neurons and increases seizure threshold; prevents seizure spread. Less potent than phenytoin.

THERAPEUTIC EFFECTS Increases seizure threshold and prevents seizure spread.

USES Treatment of Lennox–Gastaut syndrome and partial seizures.

UNLABELED USES Monotherapy or in combination with other anticonvulsants for the treatment of generalized tonic/clonic seizures.

CONTRAINDICATIONS Hypersensitivity to felbamate or other carbamates, history of blood dyscrasia or hepatic dysfunction.

CAUTIOUS USE Pregnancy (category C), lactation, older adults. Safety and effectiveness in children other than those with Lennox–Gastaut syndrome are not established.

ROUTE & DOSAGE

Partial Seizures

Adult: **PO** Initiate with 1200 mg/d in 3–4 divided doses, may increase by 600 mg/d q2wk (max: 3600 mg/d); when converting to monotherapy, reduce dose of concomitant anticonvulsants by 1/3 when initiating felbamate, then continue to decrease other anticonvulsants by 1/3 with each increase in felbamate q2wk; when using as adjunctive therapy, decrease other anticonvulsants by 20% when initiating felbamate and note that further reductions in other anticonvulsants may be required to minimize side effects and drug interactions

Lennox–Gastaut Syndrome

Child: **PO** Start at 15 mg/kg/d in 3 or 4 divided doses, reduce concurrent antiepileptic drugs by 20%, further reductions may be required to minimize side effects due to drug interactions, may increase felbamate by 15 mg/kg/d at weekly intervals (max: 45 mg/kg/d)

ADMINISTRATION

Oral

- Do not give this drug to anyone with a history of blood dyscrasia or hepatic dysfunction.
- Titrate dose under close clinical supervision.
- Shake suspension well before giving a dose.
- Store in airtight container at room temperature, 15°–30° C (59°–86° F).

ADVERSE EFFECTS (≥1%) **CNS:** Mild tremors, headache, dizziness, ataxia, diplopia, blurred vision; agitation, aggression, hallucinations, fatigue, psychological disturbances. **Endocrine:** Slight elevation of serum cholesterol, hyponatremia, hypokalemia, weight gain and loss. **GI:** *Nausea and vomiting,* anorexia, constipation, hiccup, taste disturbance, indigestion, esophagitis, increased appetite, acute liver failure. **Hematologic:** *Aplastic anemia.*

INTERACTIONS Drug: Felbamate reduces serum **carbamazepine** levels by a mean of 25%, but increases levels of its active metabolite, increases serum **phenytoin** levels approximately 20%, and increases **valproic acid** levels. **Herbal: Gingko** may decrease anticonvulsant effectiveness.

PHARMACOKINETICS Absorption: 90% absorbed from GI tract. Absorption of tablet not affected by food. **Onset:** Therapeutic effect approximately 14 d. **Peak:** Peak plasma levels at 1–6 h. **Distribution:** 20%–25% protein bound, readily crosses the blood–brain barrier. **Metabolism:** Metabolized in the liver via the cytochrome P-450 system. **Elimination:** 40%–50% excreted unchanged in urine, rest excreted in urine as metabolites. **Half-Life:** 20–23 h.

NURSING IMPLICATIONS

Assessment & Drug Effects

- Lab tests: Obtain baseline values for liver function and complete hematologic studies before initiating therapy, repeat frequently during therapy, and for a lengthy period after discontinuation of felbamate. Monitor serum sodium and potassium levels periodically because hyponatremia and hypokalemia have been reported.
- Report immediately any hematologic abnormalities.
- Monitor results of hepatic function tests throughout therapy.
- Note: When used concomitantly with either phenytoin or carbamazepine, carefully monitor serum levels of these drugs when felbamate is added, when adjustments in felbamate dosing are made, or when felbamate is discontinued.
- Note: A reduction in phenytoin of 10%–40% is usually needed when felbamate is added to the regimen.
- Monitor weight, because both weight gain and loss have been reported.
- Monitor for S&S of drug toxicity including GI distress and CNS toxicity.

Patient & Family Education

- Note: It is highly recommended that patients and physicians review the indication for treatment, risks associated with the drug, and the importance of undergoing regular blood monitoring.
- Report unusual changes (e.g., blurred vision, dysplopia) to physician.
- Report S&S of hypersensitivity including pruritus, urticaria, and (rarely) photosensitivity allergic reaction to physician.
- Learn adverse effects and report these to physician immediately.
- Do not breast feed while taking this drug.

FELODIPINE

(fel-o′di-peen)
Plendil
Classifications: CARDIOVASCULAR AGENT; CALCIUM CHANNEL BLOCKER
Prototype: Nifedipine
Pregnancy Category: C

AVAILABILITY 2.5 mg, 5 mg, 10 mg sustained release tablets

F

ACTIONS Calcium antagonist with high vascular selectivity that reduces systolic, diastolic, and mean arterial pressure at rest and during exercise.

THERAPEUTIC EFFECTS BP reduction is due to a reduction in peripheral vascular resistance (afterload) against which the heart works. This reduces oxygen demand by the heart and consequently may account for its effectiveness in chronic stable angina.

USES Mild to moderate hypertension.

UNLABELED USES Severe hypertension, angina, CHF, pulmonary hypertension.

CONTRAINDICATIONS Hypersensitivity to felodipine and sick sinus rhythm or second- or third-degree heart block except with the use of a pacemaker. Safety and efficacy in children are not established.

CAUTIOUS USE Hypotension, CHF, hepatic impairment; pregnancy (category C), lactation.

ROUTE & DOSAGE

Hypertension

Adult: **PO** 5–10 mg once/d (max: 20 mg/d)

Hepatic Impairment Start older adults and patients with impaired liver function at 2.5 mg q.d.

ADMINISTRATION

Oral

- Give tablet whole. Do not crush or chew tablets.
- Store at or below 30° C (86° F) in a tightly closed, light-resistant container.

ADVERSE EFFECTS (≥1%) **Body as a Whole:** Most adverse effects appear to be dose dependent. **CV:** Tachycardia, *palpitations, flushing, peripheral edema*. **CNS:** *Dizziness, fatigue,* headache. **GI:** Nausea, flatulence, diarrhea, dyspepsia. **Hematologic:** Small but significant decreases in Hct, Hgb, and RBC count.

DIAGNOSTIC TEST INTERFERENCE Serum ***alkaline phosphatase*** may be slightly but significantly increased. Plasma total and ionized ***calcium*** levels rise significantly. Serum ***gamma-glutamyl transferase*** may increase.

INTERACTIONS Drug: Adenosine may cause prolonged bradycardia if it is used to treat patients with toxic concentrations of CALCIUM CHANNEL BLOCKERS. **Carbamazepine, phenobarbital, phenytoin** may decrease felodipine bioavailability and serum concentrations. **Cimetidine** may increase felodipine bioavailability (competes for hepatic metabolism). Concomitant felodipine and **digoxin** administration produces only transient increases in plasma **digoxin** concentrations (35%–40% increase), which are not sustained with continued administration. This interaction may be of clinical relevance in patients whose plasma **digoxin** concentration is in the upper portion of the therapeutic range or in patients with preexisting renal insufficiency.

PHARMACOKINETICS Absorption: Completely absorbed from GI tract; it undergoes extensive first-pass metabolism with only about 15% of dose reaching systemic circulation. **Onset:** <1 h. **Peak:** 2–4 h. **Duration:** 20–24 h (sustained release formulation). **Distribution:** >99% bound to plasma proteins. **Metabolism:** Metabolized via hepatic cytochrome P-450 mixed function oxidase system. **Elimination:** 60%–

70% of metabolites are excreted in urine within 72 h. **Half-Life:** 10 h.

NURSING IMPLICATIONS

Assessment & Drug Effects

- Monitor BP carefully, especially at initiation of drug therapy, in patients >64 y, and in those with impaired liver function.
- Anticipate BP reduction with possible reflex heart rate increase (5–10 bpm) 2–5 h after dosing.
- Report sustained hypotension promptly; more common with concurrent beta-blocker therapy.
- Assess for and report reflex tachycardia; may precipitate angina.
- Monitor patients for possible digoxin toxicity when taking concurrent digoxin.

Patient Education

- Report peripheral edema, headache, or flushing to physician. These may necessitate discontinuation of drug.
- Get up from lying down slowly and in stages; there is potential for dizziness and hypotension.
- Do not breast feed while taking this drug without consulting physician.

FENOFIBRATE

(fen-o-fi'brate)

Tricor, Luxacor, Lofibra

Classifications: CARDIOVASCULAR AGENT; ANTILIPEMIC

Prototype: Clofibrate

Pregnancy Category: C

AVAILABILITY 54 mg, 160 mg tablets; 67 mg, 134 mg, 200 mg capsules or 50 mg, 100 mg, 150 mg, 160 mg capsules

ACTIONS Fibric acid derivative with lipid-regulating properties. Lowers plasma triglycerides apparently by inhibiting triglyceride synthesis and, as a result, lowers VLDL production as well as stimulates the catabolism of triglyceride-rich lipoprotein (e.g., VLDL). Produces a moderate increase in HDL cholesterol levels in most patients.

THERAPEUTIC EFFECTS Indicated by reduction in the level of serum triglycerides; interferes with synthesis of serum triglycerides.

USES Adjunctive therapy to diet for patients with high triglycerides.

CONTRAINDICATIONS Hypersensitivity to fenofibrate or other fibric acid derivatives (e.g., clofibrate, benzofibrate); liver or severe kidney dysfunction; unexplained liver function abnormality; primary biliary cirrhosis; preexisting gallbladder disease; pregnancy (category C); lactation; thrombocytopenia. Safety and efficacy in children are not established.

CAUTIOUS USE Concomitant therapy with HMG-CoA reductase inhibitors (e.g., lovastatin, pravastatin, simvastatin), oral anticoagulant medications; renal impairment, older adults; history of bleeding disorders; myelosuppression.

ROUTE & DOSAGE

Hypertriglyceridemia

Adult: **PO** 54 mg q.d. (max: 160 mg/d)

ADMINISTRATION

Oral

- Give with meals.
- Limit dose to 54 mg/d in older adults or those with impaired kidney function.
- Give at least 1 h before or 4–6 h after cholestyramine.
- Store at 15°–30° C (59°–86° F) in a tightly closed container and protect from light.

F

ADVERSE EFFECTS (≥1%) **Body as a Whole:** Asthenia, fatigue, infections, flu-like syndrome, localized pain, arthralgia. **CNS:** Headache, paresthesia, dizziness, insomnia. **CV:** Arrhythmia. **GI:** Dyspepsia, eructation, flatulence, nausea, vomiting, abdominal pain, constipation, diarrhea, increased appetite. **Respiratory:** Cough, rhinitis, sinusitis. **Skin:** Pruritus, rash. **Special Senses:** Earache, eye floaters, blurred vision, conjunctivitis, eye irritation, **Urogenital:** Decreased libido, polyuria, vaginitis.

INTERACTIONS Drug: May potentiate anticoagulant effects of **warfarin;** combination with an HMG-COA REDUCTASE INHIBITOR (STATIN) may result in rhabdomyolysis or acute renal failure; **cholestyramine, colestipol** may decrease absorption (give fenofibrate 1 h before or 4–6 h after BILE ACID SEQUESTRANTS); may increase risk of nephrotoxicity of **cyclosporine.**

PHARMACOKINETICS Absorption: Well absorbed from the GI tract; absorption increased with food. **Peak:** 6–8 h. **Distribution:** 99% protein bound; excreted in breast milk. **Metabolism:** Rapidly hydrolyzed by esterases to active metabolite, fenofibric acid. **Elimination:** 60% excreted in urine, 25% in feces. **Half-Life:** 20 h.

NURSING IMPLICATIONS

Assessment & Drug Effects

- Lab tests: Periodically monitor lipid levels, liver functions, and CBC with differential.
- Discontinue therapy after 2 mo if adequate lipid reduction is not achieved with the maximum dose of 201 mg/d.
- Assess for muscle pain, tenderness, or weakness and, if present, monitor CPK level. Withdraw drug with marked elevations of CPK or if myopathy is suspected.
- Monitor patients on coumarin-type drugs closely for prolongation of PT/INR.

Patient & Family Education

- Contact physician immediately if any of the following develops: Unexplained muscle pain, tenderness, or weakness, especially with fever or malaise; yellowing of skin or eyes; nausea or loss of appetite; skin rash or hives.
- Inform physician regarding concurrent use of cholestyramine, oral anticoagulants, or cyclosporine.
- Do not breast feed while taking this drug.

FENOLDOPAM MESYLATE

(fen-ol′do-pam mes′y-late)

Corlopam

Classifications: CARDIOVASCULAR AGENT; ANTIHYPERTENSIVE; NON-NITRATE VASODILATOR; DOPAMINE AGONIST AGENT

Pregnancy Category: B

AVAILABILITY 10 mg/mL injection

ACTIONS Rapid-acting vasodilator that is a dopamine D_1-like receptor agonist. Exerts hypotensive effects by decreasing peripheral vascular resistance while increasing renal blood flow, diuresis, and natriuresis.

THERAPEUTIC EFFECTS Indicated by rapid reduction in BP. Decreases both systolic and diastolic pressures.

USES Short-term (up to 48 h) management of severe hypertension.

CONTRAINDICATIONS Hypersensitivity to fenoldopam. Avoid concomitant use with beta blockers.

F

CAUTIOUS USE Asthmatic patients; hepatic cirrhosis, portal hypertension, or variceal bleeding; arrhythmias, tachycardia, or angina, particularly unstable angina; elevated IOP; angular-closure glaucoma; hypotension; hypokalemia; acute cerebral infarct or hemorrhage; pregnancy (category B), lactation. Safety and efficacy in children are not established.

ROUTE & DOSAGE

Severe Hypertension

Adult: **IV** 0.025–0.3 mcg/kg/min by continuous infusion for up to 48 h, may increase by 0.05–0.1 mcg/kg/min q15min (dosage range: 0.01–1.6 mcg/kg/min)

ADMINISTRATION

Intravenous

PREPARE: **Continuous:** Dilute to a final concentration of 40 mcg/mL by adding 1 mL (10 mg), 2 mL (20 mg), or 3 mL (30 mg) of fenoldopam to 250, 500, or 1000 mL, respectively, of NS or D5W.
ADMINISTER: **Continuous:** Give only by continuous infusion; never give a direct or bolus dose. Titrate initial dose up or down no more frequently than q15min.
- Note: Diluted solution is stable under normal room temperature and light for 24 h. Discard any unused solution after 24 h.

- Store at 15°–30° C (59°–86° F) in a tightly closed container and protect from light.

ADVERSE EFFECTS (≥1%) **Body as a Whole:** Injection site reaction, pyrexia, nonspecific chest pain. **CNS:** Headache, nervousness, anxiety, insomnia, dizziness. **CV:** *Hypotension, tachycardia,* T-wave inversion, flushing, postural hypotension, extrasystoles, palpitations, bradycardia, heart failure, ischemic heart disease, MI, angina. **GI:** Nausea, vomiting, abdominal pain or fullness, constipation, diarrhea. **Metabolic:** Increased creatinine, BUN, glucose, transaminases, LDH; hypokalemia. **Respiratory:** Nasal congestion, dyspnea, upper respiratory disorder. **Skin:** Sweating. **Other:** UTI, leukocytosis, bleeding.

INTERACTIONS No clinically significant interactions established.

PHARMACOKINETICS Onset: 5 min. **Peak:** 15 min. **Duration:** 15–30 min. **Distribution:** Crosses placenta. **Metabolism:** Conjugated in liver. **Elimination:** 90% excreted in urine, 10% in feces. **Half-Life:** 5 min.

NURSING IMPLICATIONS

Assessment & Drug Effects

- Monitor BP and HR carefully at least q15min or more often as warranted; expect dose-related tachycardia.
- Lab tests: Carefully monitor serum electrolytes (especially serum potassium), BUN and creatinine, liver enzymes, and blood glucose & HbA_{1c}.

FENOPROFEN CALCIUM

(fen-oh-proe'fen)

Nalfon

Classifications: CENTRAL NERVOUS SYSTEM AGENT; ANALGESIC, ANTIPYRETIC; NSAID; COX-1

Prototype: Ibuprofen

Pregnancy Category: B (D in third trimester)

AVAILABILITY 200 mg, 300 mg capsules; 600 mg tablets

ACTIONS Exhibits antiinflammatory, analgesic, and antipyretic properties of an NSAID. Claimed to be comparable to aspirin in antiinflammatory activity and associated with lower incidence of adverse GI symptoms.

THERAPEUTIC EFFECTS Effectiveness evidenced within a few days with peak effect in 2–3 wk. Has nonsteroidal, antiinflammatory, antiarthritic properties which provides relief from mild to severe pain.

F

USES Antiinflammatory and analgesic effects in the symptomatic treatment of acute and chronic rheumatoid arthritis and osteoarthritis; relief of mild to moderate pain.

UNLABELED USES Juvenile rheumatoid arthritis, acute gouty arthritis, ankylosing spondylitis; fever associated with pulmonary tuberculosis, type A influenza, colds; neoplasms.

CONTRAINDICATIONS History of nephrotic syndrome associated with aspirin or other NSAIDS; patient in whom urticaria, severe rhinitis, bronchospasm, angioedema, nasal polyps are precipitated by aspirin or other NSAIDS; significant renal or hepatic dysfunction; pregnancy (category B, category D in third trimester). Safety in lactation or children is not established.

CAUTIOUS USE History of upper GI tract disorders; hemophilia or other bleeding tendencies; compromised cardiac function, hypertension; impaired hearing.

ROUTE & DOSAGE

Inflammatory Disease

Adult: **PO** 300–600 mg t.i.d. or q.i.d. (max: 3200 mg/d)
Child: **PO** 900 mg/m^2 in divided doses, may increase over 4 wk to 1.8 g/m^2

Mild to Moderate Pain

Adult: **PO** 200 mg q4–6h prn

ADMINISTRATION

Oral

- Give on an empty stomach 30–60 min before or 2 h after meals. Give with meals, milk, or antacid (prescribed) if patient experiences GI disturbances.
- May crush tablets or empty capsule and mix with fluid or mix with food.
- Store capsules and tablets in tightly closed containers at 15°–30° C (59°–86° F); avoid freezing.

ADVERSE EFFECTS (≥1%) **CNS:** *Headache, drowsiness,* dizziness, fatigue, lassitude, tremor, confusion, insomnia, nervousness, depression. **Special Senses:** Tinnitus, decreased hearing, deafness; blurred vision. **GI:** *Indigestion, nausea, vomiting,* anorexia, *constipation,* diarrhea, flatulence, abdominal pain, dry mouth; infrequent: gastritis, peptic ulcer, GI bleeding. **Urogenital:** Dysuria, cystitis, hematuria, oliguria, azotemia, anuria, allergic nephritis, papillary necrosis, nephrotoxicity (rare). **Hematologic:** (infrequent) Thrombocytopenia, hemolytic anemia, agranulocytosis, pancytopenia. **Skin:** (may or may not be hypersensitivity reaction) Pruritus, rash, purpura, increased sweating, urticaria. **Body as a Whole:** Dyspnea, malaise, anaphylaxis, edema.

INTERACTIONS Drug: Fenoprofen may prolong bleeding time; should not be given with ORAL ANTICOAGULANTS, **heparin;** action and side effects of **phenytoin,** SULFONYLUREAS, SULFONAMIDES, and fenoprofen may be potentiated. **Herbal: Feverfew, garlic, ginger, gingko** may increase bleeding potential.

PHARMACOKINETICS Absorption: 80% absorbed from GI tract. **Onset:** 2 h. **Peak:** 2 h. **Duration:** 4–6 h. **Distribution:** Small amounts distributed into breast milk. **Metabolism:** Metabolized in liver. **Elimination:** Excreted primarily in urine; some biliary excretion. **Half-Life:** 3 h.

NURSING IMPLICATIONS

Assessment & Drug Effects

- Lab tests: Baseline evaluations of Hct and Hgb, kidney and liver function.
- Baseline and periodic auditory and ophthalmic examinations are recommended in patients receiving prolonged or high dose therapy.
- Monitor for S&S of GI bleeding.
- Note: Dosage adjustment of fenoprofen may be required when phenobarbital is added to or withdrawn from patient's drug regimen.

Patient & Family Education

- Do not drive or engage in potentially hazardous activities until response to drug is known; fenoprofen may cause dizziness and drowsiness.
- Report immediately the onset of unexplained fever, rash, arthralgia, oliguria, edema, weight gain to physician. Possible symptoms of nephrotic syndrome are rapidly reversible if drug is promptly withdrawn.
- Understand that alcohol and aspirin may increase risk of GI ulceration and bleeding tendencies; avoid both unless otherwise advised by physician.
- Inform dentist or surgeon that you are taking fenoprofen because it may prolong bleeding time.
- Do not breast feed while taking this drug without consulting physician.

FENTANYL CITRATE

(fen'ta-nil)

Duragesic, Actiq Oralet, Sublimaze

Classifications: CENTRAL NERVOUS SYSTEM AGENT; ANALGESIC; NARCOTIC (OPIATE) AGONIST

Prototype: Morphine

Pregnancy Category: C

Controlled Substance: Schedule II

AVAILABILITY 0.05 mg/mL injection; 100 mcg, 200 mcg, 300 mcg, 400 mcg lozenges; 200 mcg, 400 mcg, 600 mcg, 800 mcg, 1200 mcg, 1600 mcg lozenges on a stick; 25 mcg/hr, 50 mcg/hr, 75 mcg/hr, 100 mcg/h transdermal patch

ACTIONS Synthetic, potent narcotic agonist analgesic with pharmacologic actions qualitatively similar to those of morphine and meperidine, but action is more prompt and less prolonged. Principal actions: analgesia and sedation. Drug-induced alterations in respiratory rate and alveolar ventilation may persist beyond the analgesic effect. Emetic effect is less than with either morphine or meperidine.

THERAPEUTIC EFFECTS Provides analgesia and sedation.

USES Short-acting analgesic during operative and perioperative periods, as a narcotic analgesic supplement in general and regional anesthesia, and with droperidol or with diazepam to produce neuroleptoanalgesia. Also given with oxygen and a skeletal muscle relaxant (neuroleptoanesthesia) to selected high-risk patients (e.g., those undergoing open heart surgery) when attenuation of the response to surgical stress without use of additional anesthesia agents is important.

CONTRAINDICATIONS Patients who have received MAO INHIBITORS within 14 d; myasthenia gravis; labor and delivery, lactation. Safety during pregnancy (category C) or in children <12 y is not established.

CAUTIOUS USE Head injuries, increased intracranial pressure; older adults, debilitated, poor-risk patients; COPD, other respiratory problems; liver and kidney dysfunction; bradyarrhythmias.

ROUTE & DOSAGE

Premedication

Adult: **IM** 50–100 mcg 30–60 min before surgery **PO** Suck on 400-mcg lozenge until sedated
Child: **PO** Suck on lozenge until sedated, *10–25 kg,* 200-mcg lozenge; *25–35 kg,* 300-mcg lozenge; *35–40 kg,* 400-mcg lozenge
Neonate: **IV** 1–4-mcg/kg slow IV push q2–4h or 1–2-mcg/kg bolus, then infuse at 0.5–1-mcg/kg/h
Child: **IV/IM** *1–12 y,* 1–2 mcg/kg q30–60 min or 1–2 mcg/kg followed by 1–3 mcg/kg/h infusion (max: 5 mcg/kg/h)

Adjunct for Regional Anesthesia

Adult: **IM** 50–100 mcg **IV** 2–20 mcg/kg over 1–2 min up to 50 mcg/kg

General Anesthesia

Adult: **IV** up to 150 mcg/kg as required

Postoperative Pain

Adult: **IM** 50–100 mcg q1–2h prn
Child: **IM** 1.7–3.3 mcg/kg q1–2h prn

Chronic Pain

Adult: **Transdermal** Individualize and regularly reassess doses of transdermal fentanyl; for patient not already receiving an opioid, the initial dose is 25 mcg/h patch q3d; for patients already on opioids, see package insert for conversions **Stick lozenge (Actiq)** Place in mouth between cheek and lower gum and suck on lozenge; should be consumed over 15-min period

ADMINISTRATION

Intravascular

PREPARE: **Direct:** Give parenteral doses undiluted or diluted in 5 mL sterile water or NS.
ADMINISTER: **Direct:** Infuse over 1–2 min.
INCOMPATIBILITIES **Solution/additive: Fluorouracil, pentobarbital, thiopental.**

- Store at 15°–30° C (59°–86° F) unless otherwise directed. Protect drug from light.

ADVERSE EFFECTS (≥1%) **CNS:** *Sedation,* euphoria, dizziness, diaphoresis, delirium, convulsions with high doses. **CV:** Hypotension, bradycardia, <u>circulatory depression, cardiac arrest</u>. **Special Senses:** Miosis, blurred vision. **GI:** *Nausea,* vomiting, constipation, ileus. **Respiratory:** Laryngospasm, bronchoconstriction, <u>respiratory depression or arrest</u>. **Body as a Whole:** Muscle rigidity, especially muscles of respiration after rapid IV infusion, urinary retention, **Skin:** Rash, contact dermatitis from patch.

INTERACTIONS Drug: Alcohol and other CNS DEPRESSANTS potentiate effects; MAO INHIBITORS may precipitate hypertensive crisis.

PHARMACOKINETICS Absorption: Absorbed through the skin, leveling off between 12–24 h. **Onset:** Immediate IV; 7–15 min IM; 12–24 h transdermal. **Peak:** 3–5 min IV; 24–72 h transdermal. **Duration:** 30–60 min IV; 1–2 h IM; 72 h transdermal. **Metabolism:** Metabolized in liver. **Elimination:** Excreted in urine. **Half-Life:** 17 h transdermal.

NURSING IMPLICATIONS

Assessment & Drug Effects

- Monitor vital signs and observe patient for signs of skeletal and thoracic muscle (depressed respirations) rigidity and weakness.
- Watch carefully for respiratory depression and for movements of various groups of skeletal muscle in extremities, external eye, and neck during postoperative period. These movements may present patient management problems; report promptly.
- Note: Duration of respiratory depressant effect may be considerably longer than narcotic analgesic effect. Have immediately available oxygen, resuscitative and intubation equipment, and an opioid antagonist such as naloxone.

FERROUS SULFATE Pr

(fer′rous sul′fate)

Feosol, Fer-In-Sol, Fer-Iron, Fero-Gradumet, Ferospace, Ferralyn, Ferra-TD, Fesofor, Hematinic, Mol-Iron, Novoferrosulfa ✦, Slow-Fe

FERROUS FUMARATE

(fer′rous foo′ma-rate)

Feco-T, Femiron, Feostat, Fersamal, Fumasorb, Fumerin, Hemocyte, Ircon-FA, Neo-Fer-50 ✦, Novofumar ✦, Palafer ✦, Palmiron

FERROUS GLUCONATE

(fer′rous gloo′koe-nate)

Fergon, Fertinic ✦, Novoferrogluc ✦, Simron

Classifications: BLOODS FORMERS, COAGULATORS, AND ANTICOAGULANTS; IRON PREPARATION

Pregnancy Category: A

AVAILABILITY Ferrous Sulfate 167 mg, 200 mg, 324 mg, 325 mg tablets; 160 mg sustained release tablets, capsules; 90 mg/5 mL syrup; 220 mg/5 ml elixir; 75 mg/0.6 mL drops **Ferrous Fumarate** 63 mg, 100 mg, 200 mg, 324 mg, 325 mg, 350 mg tablets; 100 mg/5 mL suspension; 45 mg/0.6 mL drops **Ferrous Gluconate** 240 mg, 325 mg tablets

ACTIONS ***Ferrous sulfate:*** Standard iron preparation against which other oral iron preparations are usually measured. Corrects erythropoietic abnormalities induced by iron deficiency but does not stimulate erythropoiesis. May reverse gastric, esophageal, and other tissue changes caused by lack of iron. ***Ferrous gluconate:*** Claimed to cause less gastric irritation and be better tolerated than ferrous sulfate.

THERAPEUTIC EFFECTS Experienced within 48 h as a sense of well-being, increased vigor, improved appetite, and decreased irritability (in children). Reticulocyte response begins in about 4 d; it usually peaks in 7–10 d (reticulocytosis) and returns to normal after 2 or 3 wk. Hemoglobin generally increases by 2 g/dL and hematocrit by 6% in 3 wk. Iron supplements correct erythropoietic abnormalities induced by iron deficiency but do not stimulate erythropoiesis.

USES To correct simple iron deficiency and to treat iron deficiency (microcytic, hypochromic) anemias. Also may be used prophylactically during periods of increased iron needs, as in infancy, childhood, and pregnancy.

CONTRAINDICATIONS Peptic ulcer, regional enteritis, ulcerative colitis; hemolytic anemias (in absence of iron deficiency), hemochromatosis, hemosiderosis, patients receiving repeated transfusions, pyridoxine-responsive anemia; cirrhosis of liver. **CAUTIOUS USE** Pregnancy (category A), lactation.

F

ROUTE & DOSAGE

Iron Deficiency

Adult: **PO Sulfate (30% elemental iron)** 750–1500 mg/d in 1–3 divided doses; **Fumarate (33% elemental iron)** 200 mg t.i.d. or q.i.d.; **Gluconate (12% elemental iron)** 325–600 mg q.i.d., may be gradually increased to 650 mg q.i.d. as needed and tolerated
Child: **PO Sulfate (30% elemental iron)** *<6 y,* 75–225 mg/d in divided doses; *6–12 y,* 600 mg/d in divided doses; **Fumarate (33% elemental iron)** 3 mg/kg t.i.d.; **Gluconate (12% elemental iron)** *<6 y,* 100–300 mg/d in divided doses; *6–12 y,* 100–300 mg t.i.d.

Iron Supplement

Adult: **PO Sulfate** *Pregnancy,* 300–600 mg/d in divided doses; **Fumarate** 200 mg once/d; **Gluconate** 325–600 mg once/d
Child: **PO Fumarate** 3 mg/kg once/d; **Gluconate** *<6 y,* 100–300 mg/d in divided doses; *6–12 y,* 100–300 mg once/d
Infant: **PO Fumarate** *Low birth weight,* 2 mg/kg/d up to 15 mg/d; *≤3 y,* 1 mg/kg/d (max: 15 mg/d)

ADMINISTRATION

Oral

- Give on an empty stomach if possible because oral iron preparations are best absorbed then (i.e., between meals). Minimize gastric distress if needed by giving with or immediately after meals with adequate liquid.
- Do not crush tablet or empty contents of capsule when administering.
- Do not give tablets or capsules within 1 h of bedtime.
- Consult physician about prescribing a liquid formulation or a less corrosive form, such as ferrous gluconate, if the patient experiences difficulty in swallowing tablet or capsule.
- Dilute liquid preparations well and give through a straw or placed on the back of tongue with a dropper to prevent staining of teeth and to mask taste. Instruct the patient to rinse mouth with clear water immediately after ingestion.
- Mix ferosol elixir with water; not compatible with milk or fruit juice. Fer-In-Sol (drops) may be given in water or in fruit or vegetable juice, according to manufacturer.
- Do not use discolored tablets.
- Store in tightly closed containers and protect from moisture. Store at 15°–30° C (59°–86° F).

ADVERSE EFFECTS (≥1%) **GI:** *Nausea, heartburn,* anorexia, *constipation,* diarrhea, epigastric pain, abdominal distress, *black stools.* **Special Senses:** Yellow-brown discoloration of eyes and teeth (liquid forms.) **Large Chronic Doses in Infants** Rickets (due to interference with phosphorus absorption). **Massive Overdosage** Lethargy, drowsiness, nausea, vomiting, abdominal pain, diarrhea, local corrosion of stomach and small intestines, pallor or cyanosis, metabolic acidosis, shock, cardiovascular collapse, convulsions, liver necrosis, coma, renal failure, death.

DIAGNOSTIC TEST INTERFERENCE By coloring feces black, large iron doses may cause false-positive tests for ***occult blood with orthotoluidine (Hematest, Occultist, Labstix); guaiac reagent benzidine test*** is reportedly not affected.

INTERACTIONS Drug: ANTACIDS decrease iron absorption; iron decreases absorption of TETRACYCLINES, **ciprofloxacin, ofloxacin; chloramphenicol** may delay iron's effects; iron may decrease absorption of **penicillamine. Food:** Food decreases absorption of iron; **ascorbic acid (vitamin C)** may increase iron absorption.

PHARMACOKINETICS Absorption: 5%–10% absorbed in healthy individuals; 10%–30% absorbed in iron-deficiency; food decreases amount absorbed. **Distribution:** Transported by transferrin to bone marrow, where it is incorporated into hemoglobin; crosses placenta. **Elimination:** Most of iron released from hemoglobin is reused in body; small amounts are lost in desquamation of skin, GI mucosa, nails, and hair; 12–30 mg/mo lost through menstruation.

NURSING IMPLICATIONS

Assessment & Drug Effects

- Lab tests: Monitor Hgb and reticulocyte values during therapy. Investigate the absence of satisfactory response after 3 wk of drug treatment.
- Continue iron therapy for 2–3 mo after the hemoglobin level has returned to normal (roughly twice the period required to normalize hemoglobin concentration).
- Monitor bowel movements as constipation is a common adverse effect.

Patient & Family Education

- Note: Ascorbic acid increases absorption of iron. Consuming citrus fruit or tomato juice with iron preparation (except the elixir) may increase its absorption.
- Be aware that milk, eggs, or caffeine beverages when taken with the iron preparation may inhibit absorption.
- Be aware that iron preparations cause dark green or black stools.
- Report constipation or diarrhea to physician; symptoms may be relieved by adjustments in dosage or diet or by change to another iron preparation.
- Do not breast feed while taking this drug without consulting physician.

FEXOFENADINE

(fex-o-fen′a-deen)

Allegra

Classifications: ANTIHISTAMINE; H_1-RECEPTOR ANTAGONIST; NON-SEDATING

Prototype: Lorataidine

Pregnancy Category: C

AVAILABILITY 60 mg capsules

ACTIONS Antihistamine competitively antagonizes histamine at the H_1-receptor site; does not bind with histamine to inactivate it. Not associated with anticholinergic or sedative properties.

THERAPEUTIC EFFECTS Inhibits antigen-induced bronchospasm and histamine release from mast cells. Efficacy is indicated by reduction of the following: nasal congestion and sneezing; watery or red eyes; itching nose, palate, or eyes.

USES Relief of symptoms associated with seasonal allergic rhinitis, and chronic urticaria.

CONTRAINDICATIONS Hypersensitivity to fexofenadine; pregnancy (category C).

CAUTIOUS USE Lactation; renal and hepatic insufficiency, hypertension, diabetes mellitus, ischemic heart disease, increased ocular pressure, hyperthyroidism, renal impairment, or prostatic hypertrophy. Safety and effectiveness in children <6 y are not established.

ROUTE & DOSAGE

Allergic Rhinitis
Adult/Child: >12 y, **PO** 60 mg b.i.d.
Child: **PO** 6–11, 30 mg b.i.d.

Chronic Urticaria
Adult: **PO** 60 mg b.i.d.
Child: **PO** >6 y, 30 mg b.i.d.

Renal Impairment
Cl_{cr} <80 mL/min
Adult: **PO** 60 mg q.d.
Child: **PO** 30 mg q.d.

ADMINISTRATION

Oral

- Reduce starting dose for those with decreased kidney function.
- Store at 20°–25° C (68°–77° F). Protect from excess moisture.

ADVERSE EFFECTS (≥1%) **CNS:** *Headache,* drowsiness, fatigue. **GI:** Nausea, dyspepsia, throat irritation.

INTERACTIONS Drug: No clinically significant interactions established.

PHARMACOKINETICS Absorption: Rapidly absorbed from GI tract, 33% reaches systemic circulation. **Onset:** 1 h. **Peak:** 2–3 h. **Duration:** At least 12 h. **Distribution:** 60%–70% bound to plasma proteins. **Metabolism:** Only 5% of dose metabolized in liver. **Elimination:** 80% excreted in urine, 11% in feces. **Half-Life:** 14.4 h.

NURSING IMPLICATIONS

Assessment & Drug Effects

- Monitor therapeutic effectiveness, which is indicated by decreased nasal congestion, sneezing, watery or red eyes, and itching nose, palate, or eyes.

Patient & Family Education

- Note: Drug is well tolerated and causes minimal adverse effects.
- Do not breast feed while taking this drug without consulting physician.

FILGRASTIM

(fil-gras'tim)
Neupogen
Classifications: BLOOD FORMERS, COAGULATORS, AND ANTICOAGULANTS; HEMATOPOIETIC GROWTH FACTOR
Prototype: Epoetin alfa
Pregnancy Category: C

AVAILABILITY 300 mcg/mL injection

ACTIONS Human granulocyte colony-stimulating factor (G-CSF) produced by recombinant DNA technology. Endogenous G-CSF regulates the production of neutrophils within the bone marrow; not species specific and primarily affects neutrophil proliferation, differentiation and selected end-cell functional activity (including enhanced phagocytic activity, antibody-dependent killing, and the increased expression of some functions associated with cell-surface antigens).

THERAPEUTIC EFFECTS Increases neutrophil proliferation and differentiation within the bone marrow.

USES To decrease the incidence of infection, as manifested by febrile neutropenia, in patients with nonmyeloid malignancies receiving myelosuppressive anticancer drugs associated with a significant incidence of severe neutropenia with fever; to decrease neutropenia associated with bone marrow transplant; to treat chronic neutropenia; to mobilize peripheral blood stem cells (PBSCs) for autologous transplantation.

CONTRAINDICATIONS Hypersensitivity to *Escherichia coli*–derived proteins, simultaneous administration with chemotherapy, and myeloid cancers.

CAUTIOUS USE Pregnancy (category C), lactation.

ROUTE & DOSAGE

Neutropenia

Adult/Child: **IV** 5 mcg/kg/d by 30 min infusion, may increase by 5 mcg/kg/d (max: 30 mcg/kg/d) **SC** 5 mcg/kg/d as single dose, may increase by 5 mcg/kg/d (max: 20 mcg/kg/d)

ADMINISTRATION

Subcutaneous & Intravenous

- Do not administer filgrastim 24 h before or after cytotoxic chemotherapy.
- Use only one dose per vial; do not reenter the vial.
- Prior to injection, filgrastim may be allowed to reach room temperature for a maximum of 6 h. Discard any vial left at room temperature for >6 h.

PREPARE: **Intermittent/Continuous:** May dilute with 10–50 mL D5W to yield 15 mcg/mL or greater. If more diluent is used to yield concentrations of 5–15 mcg/mL, 2 mL of 5% human albumin must be added for each 50 mL D5W (prior to adding filgrastim) to prevent adsorption to plastic IV infusion materials.

ADMINISTER: **Intermittent:** Give a single dose over 15–30 min. **Continuous:** Give a single dose over 4–24 h.

INCOMPATIBILITIES **Y-site: Amphotericin B, cefepime, cefoperazone, cefotaxime, cefoxitin, ceftizoxime, ceftriaxone, cefuroxime, clindamycin, dactinomycin, etoposide, fluorouracil, furosemide, gentamicin, heparin, imipenem, mannitol, methylprednisolone, metronidazole, mitomycin, piperacillin, prochlorperazine, thiotepa.**

- Store refrigerated at 2°–8° C (36°–46° F). Do not freeze. Avoid shaking.

ADVERSE EFFECTS (≥1%) **CV:** Abnormal ST segment depression. **Hematologic:** Anemia. **GI:** Nausea, anorexia. **Body as a Whole:** *Bone pain,* hyperuricemia, *fever.*

DIAGNOSTIC TEST INTERFERENCE Elevations in **leukocyte alkaline phosphatase, serum alkaline phosphatase, lactate dehydrogenase,** and **uric acid** have been reported. These elevations appear to be related to increased bone marrow activity.

INTERACTIONS Drug: Can interfere with activity of CYTOTOXIC AGENTS, do not use 24 h before or after CYTOTOXIC AGENTS

PHARMACOKINETICS Absorption: Readily absorbed from SC site. **Onset:** 4 h. **Peak:** 1 h. **Elimination:** Probably excreted in urine. **Half-Life:** 1.4–7.2 h.

F

NURSING IMPLICATIONS

Assessment & Drug Effects

- Lab tests: Obtain a baseline CBC with differential and platelet count prior to administering drug. Obtain CBC twice weekly during therapy to monitor neutrophil count and leukocytosis. Monitor Hct and platelet count regularly.
- Discontinue filgrastim if absolute neutrophil count exceeds 10,000/mm^3 after the chemotherapy-induced nadir. Neutrophil counts should then return to normal.
- Monitor patients with preexisting cardiac conditions closely. MI and arrhythmias have been associated with a small percent of patients receiving filgrastim.
- Monitor temperature q4h. Incidence of infection should be reduced after administration of filgrastim.
- Assess degree of bone pain if present. Consult physician if nonnarcotic analgesics do not provide relief.

Patient & Family Education

- Report bone pain and, if necessary, to request analgesics to control pain.
- Note: Proper drug administration and disposal is important. A puncture-resistant container for the disposal of used syringes and needles should be available to the patient.
- Do not breast feed while taking this drug without consulting physician.

FINASTERIDE Pr

(fin-as′te-ride)
Propecia, Proscar
Classifications: HORMONES & SYNTHETIC SUBSTITUTES; ANTIANDROGEN; 5-ALPHA REDUCTASE INHIBITOR
Pregnancy Category: X

AVAILABILITY 1 mg, 5 mg tablets

ACTIONS Specific inhibitor of the steroid 5-alpha-reductase, an enzyme necessary to convert testosterone into the potent androgen 5-alpha-dihydrotestosterone (DHT) in the prostate gland.
THERAPEUTIC EFFECTS Decreases the production of testosterone in the prostate gland.

USES Benign prostatic hypertrophy, male pattern hair loss (androgenetic alopecia).

CONTRAINDICATIONS Hypersensitivity to finasteride; pregnancy (category X), lactation, and children.
CAUTIOUS USE Hepatic impairment, obstructive uropathy.

ROUTE & DOSAGE

Benign Prostatic Hypertrophy
Adult: **PO** 5 mg/d
Male Pattern Hair Loss
Adult: **PO** 1 mg q.d.

ADMINISTRATION

Oral

- Crush tablets if necessary. Pregnant women should not handle the crushed drug; if absorbed through the skin it may be harmful to a male fetus.
- Store at 15°–30° C (59°–86° F) unless otherwise directed.

ADVERSE EFFECTS (≥1%) **Urogenital:** Impotence, decreased libido, decreased volume of ejaculate.

DIAGNOSTIC TEST INTERFERENCE Depresses levels of **DHT** and **prostate-specific antigen (PSA). Testosterone** levels usually are increased.

INTERACTIONS Drug: No clinically significant interactions established. **Herbal: Saw palmetto** may potentiate effects of finasteride.

PHARMACOKINETICS Absorption: Readily absorbed from GI tract. **Onset:** 3–6 mo **Duration:** 5–7 d. **Elimination:** 39% excreted in urine, 57% in feces. **Half-Life:** 5–7 h.

NURSING IMPLICATIONS

Assessment & Drug Effects

- Evaluate carefully any sustained increase in serum PSA levels while patient is taking finasteride. It may indicate the presence of prostate cancer or noncompliance with the therapy.
- Monitor patients with a large residual urinary volume or decreased urinary flow. These patients may not be candidates for this therapy.

Patient & Family Education

- Use a barrier contraceptive to prevent pregnancy in a sexual partner.
- Be aware that impotence and decreased libido may occur with treatment.
- Do not breast feed if exposed to this drug.

FLAVOXATE HYDROCHLORIDE

(fla-vox'ate)

Urispas

Classifications: AUTONOMIC NERVOUS SYSTEM AGENT; ANTICHOLINERGIC (PARASYMPATHOLYTIC); ANTISPASMODIC

Prototype: Atropine

Pregnancy Category: C

AVAILABILITY 100 mg tablets

ACTIONS Exerts spasmolytic (papaverine-like) action on smooth muscle. Reported to produce an increase in urinary bladder capacity in patients with spastic bladder, possibly by direct action on detrusor muscle. Also demonstrates local anesthetic and analgesic action.

THERAPEUTIC EFFECTS Has antispasmotic action on the urinary bladder.

USES Symptomatic relief of dysuria, frequency, urgency, nocturia, incontinence, and suprapubic pain associated with various urologic disorders.

CONTRAINDICATIONS Pyloric or duodenal obstruction, obstructive intestinal lesions, ileus, achalasia, GI hemorrhage; obstructive uropathies of lower urinary tract. Safety during pregnancy (category C) or in children <12 y is not established.

CAUTIOUS USE Suspected glaucoma.

ROUTE & DOSAGE

Dysuria, Nocturia, Incontinence

Adult: **PO** 100–200 mg t.i.d. or q.i.d.

ADMINISTRATION

Oral

- Give without regard to meals.
- Store at 15°–30° C (59°–86° F) unless otherwise directed.

ADVERSE EFFECTS (≥1%) **CNS:** Headache, vertigo, drowsiness, mental confusion (especially in older adults). **CV:** Palpitation, tachycardia. **Special Senses:** Blurred vision, increased intraocular tension, disturbances of eye accommodation. **GI:** Nausea, vomiting, dry mouth (and throat), constipation (with high doses). **Skin:** Dermatosis, urticaria. **Other:** Dysuria, hyperpyrexia, eosinophilia, leukopenia (rare).

INTERACTIONS Drug: May antagonize the GI motility effects of **cisapride, metoclopramide.**

PHARMACOKINETICS Elimination: 10%–30% excreted in urine within 6 h.

NURSING IMPLICATIONS

Assessment & Drug Effects

- Monitor heart rate. Take apical pulse for 1 full minute. Report tachycardia.
- Lab tests: Obtain periodic evaluation of blood counts during therapy.

Patient & Family Education

- Do not drive or engage in potentially hazardous activities until response to drug is known.
- Report adverse reactions to physician as well as clinical improvement or the lack of a favorable response.

FLECAINIDE

(fle-kay'nide)

Tambocor

Classifications: CARDIOVASCULAR AGENT; ANTIARRHYTHMIC, CLASS IC

Pregnancy Category: C

AVAILABILITY 50 mg, 100 mg, 150 mg tablets

ACTIONS Local (membrane) anesthetic and antiarrhythmic with electrophysiologic properties similar to other class IC antiarrhythmic drugs. Slows conduction velocity throughout myocardial conduction system, increases ventricular refractoriness; little effect on repolarization. Prolongs His-ventricular (HQ) and QRS intervals at therapeutic doses.

THERAPEUTIC EFFECTS Clinically, causes both hypotension and negative entropy (in higher dose ranges) and is an effective suppressant of PVCs and a variety of atrial and ventricular arrhythmias.

USES Life-threatening ventricular arrhythmias.

UNLABELED USES Atrial tachycardia and other arrhythmias unresponsive to standard agents (e.g., quinidine), Wolff-Parkinson-White syndrome, and recurrent ventricular tachycardias.

CONTRAINDICATIONS Hypersensitivity to flecainide; preexisting second- or third-degree AV block, right bundle branch block when associated with a left hemiblock unless a pacemaker is present; cardiogenic shock, significant hepatic impairment. Safety during pregnancy (category C), lactation, or in children <18 y is not established.

CAUTIOUS USE CHF, sick sinus syndrome, renal impairment.

ROUTE & DOSAGE

Life-threatening Ventricular Arrhythmias

Adult: **PO** 100 mg q12h, may increase by 50 mg b.i.d. q4d (max: 400 mg/d)

Child: **PO** 1–3 mg/kg/d in 3 divided doses (max: 8 mg/kg/d)

ADMINISTRATION

Oral

- Do not increase dosage more frequently than every 4 d.
- Store in tightly covered, light-resistant containers at 15°–30° C (59°–86° F) unless otherwise directed.

ADVERSE EFFECTS (≥1%) **CNS:** *Dizziness,* headache, light-headedness, unsteadiness, paresthesias, fatigue. **CV:** Arrhythmias, chest pain, worsening of CHF. **Special Senses:** *Blurred vision, difficulty in focusing,* spots before eyes. **GI:** *Nausea,* constipation, change in taste perception. **Body as a Whole:** Dyspnea, fever, edema.

INTERACTIONS Drug: Cimetidine may increase flecainide levels; may increase **digoxin** levels 15%–25%; BETA BLOCKERS may have additive negative inotropic effects.

PHARMACOKINETICS Absorption: Readily absorbed from GI tract. **Peak:** 2–3 h. **Distribution:** Crosses placenta; distributed into breast milk. **Metabolism:** Metabolized in liver. **Elimination:** Excreted mainly in urine. **Half-Life:** 7–22 h.

NURSING IMPLICATIONS

Assessment & Drug Effects

- Correct preexisting hypokalemia or hyperkalemia before treatment is initiated.
- Note: ECG monitoring, including Holter monitor for ambulating patients, is essential because of the possibility of drug-induced arrhythmias.
- Determine pacing threshold for patients with pacemakers before initiation of therapy, after 1 wk of therapy, and at regular intervals thereafter.
- Monitor plasma level recommended, especially in patients with severe CHF or renal failure because drug elimination may be delayed in these patients.
- Note: Effective trough plasma levels are between 0.7–1 mcg/mL. The probability of adverse reactions increases when trough levels exceed 1 mcg/mL.
- Attempt dosage reduction with caution after arrhythmia is controlled.

Patient & Family Education

- Note: It is VERY important to take this drug at the prescribed times.
- Report visual disturbances to physician.
- Do not breast feed while taking this drug without consulting physician.

FLOXURIDINE

(flox-yoor'i-deen)

FUDR

Classifications: ANTINEOPLASTIC; ANTIMETABOLITE

Prototype: Fluorouracil

Pregnancy Category: D

AVAILABILITY 500 mg powder for injection

ACTIONS Pyrimidine antagonist and cell-cycle specific. Catabolized to fluorouracil in the body; highly toxic by blocking an enzyme essential to normal DNA and RNA synthesis.

THERAPEUTIC EFFECTS Proliferative cells of neoplasms are affected more than healthy tissue cells.

USES Palliative agent in management of selected patients with GI metastasis to liver.

UNLABELED USES Carcinoma of breast, ovary, cervix, urinary bladder, and prostate not responsive to other antimetabolites.

CONTRAINDICATIONS Existing or recent viral infections. Pregnancy (category D); lactation.

CAUTIOUS USE Poor nutritional status, bone marrow depression, serious infections; high-risk patients: prior high-dose pelvic irradiation, use of alkylating agents; impaired kidney or liver function.

ROUTE & DOSAGE

Carcinoma

Adult: **Intraarterial** 0.1–0.6 mg/kg/d by continuous intraarterial infusion

ADMINISTRATION

Intraarterial Infusion

PREPARE: **Direct:** Reconstitute with 5 mL sterile distilled water for injection; further dilute with D5W or NS injection to a volume appropriate for the infusion apparatus to be used.

ADMINISTER: **Direct:** It is administered by pump to overcome pressure in large arteries and to ensure a uniform rate. Examine infusion site frequently for signs of extravasation. If this occurs, stop infusion and restart in another vessel.

INCOMPATIBILITIES **Y-site: Allopurinol**, **cefepime**

- Keep reconstituted solutions, which are stable at 2°–8° C (36°–46° F), for no more than 2 wk.
- Store at 15°–30° C (59°–86° F) unless otherwise directed.

ADVERSE EFFECTS (≥1%) **CNS:** Vertigo, convulsions, depression, hemiplegia. **CV:** Myocardial ischemia, angina. **GI:** *Nausea, vomiting, stomatitis,* diarrhea, cramps, anorexia, enteritis, gastritis, esophagopharyngitis. **Hematologic:** Leukopenia, *thrombocytopenia.* **Skin:** Dermatitis, alopecia (usually reversible), *erythema* or increased skin pigmentation (photosensitivity), dry skin, pruritic ulcerations, rash. **Body as a Whole:** Hiccups, fever, epistaxis, decreased resistance to disease. **Urogenital:** Renal insufficiency.

INTERACTIONS Drug: Metronidazole may increase general floxuridine toxicity; may increase or decrease serum levels of **phenytoin, fosphenytoin; hydroxyurea** can decrease conversion to active metabolite.

PHARMACOKINETICS Distribution: Distributed to tumor, intestinal mucosa, bone marrow, liver, and CSF; probably crosses placenta. **Metabolism:** Rapidly metabolized in liver to fluorouracil. **Elimination:** 15% excreted in urine, 60%–80% excreted through lungs as carbon dioxide. **Half-Life:** 16 min.

NURSING IMPLICATIONS

Assessment & Drug Effects

- Discontinue therapy promptly with onset of any of the following: Stomatitis, esophagopharyngitis, intractable vomiting, diarrhea, leukopenia (WBC <3500/mm^3), or rapidly falling WBC count, thrombocytopenia (platelets 100,000/mm^3), GI bleeding, hemorrhage from any site.
- Lab tests: Obtain baseline and periodic total and differential leukocyte counts, Hct, platelet count, serum uric acid creatinine, and liver function tests.

Patient & Family Education

- Be aware that floxuridine sometimes causes temporary thinning of hair.
- Do not breast feed while taking this drug.

FLUCONAZOLE (Pr)

(flu-con'a-zole)

Diflucan

Classifications: ANTIINFECTIVE; ANTIBIOTIC; ANTIFUNGAL

Pregnancy Category: C

AVAILABILITY 50 mg, 100 mg, 150 mg, 200 mg tablets; 10 mg/mL, 40 mg/mL suspension; 2 mg/mL injection

ACTIONS Fungistatic; may also be fungicidal depending on concentration. Interferes with formation of ergosterol, the principal sterol in the fungal cell membrane that, when depleted, interrupts membrane function.

THERAPEUTIC EFFECTS Antifungal properties are related to the drug effect on the fungal cell membrane functioning.

USES Cryptococcal meningitis and oropharyngeal and systemic candidiasis, both commonly found in AIDS and other immunocompromised patients; vaginal candidiasis.

CONTRAINDICATIONS Hypersensitivity to fluconazole or other azole antifungals; coadministration with cisapride; pregnancy (category C), lactation.

CAUTIOUS USE AIDS or malignancy; hepatic impairment.

ROUTE & DOSAGE

Oropharyngeal Candidiasis

Adult: **PO/IV** 200 mg day 1, then 100 mg q.d. × 2 wk
Child: **PO/IV** 3–6 mg/kg/d

Esophageal Candidiasis

Adult: **PO/IV** 200 mg day 1, then 100 mg q.d. × 3 wk
Child: **PO/IV** 3–6 mg/kg/d

Systemic Candidiasis

Adult: **PO/IV** 400 mg day 1, then 200 mg q.d. × 4 wk
Child: **PO/IV** 3–6 mg/kg/d

Vaginal Candidiasis

Adult: **PO** 150 mg × 1 dose

Cryptococcal Meningitis

Adult: **PO/IV** 400 mg day 1, then 200 mg q.d. × 10–12 wk
Child: **PO/IV** 3–6 mg/kg/d

ADMINISTRATION

Oral

- Take this medication for the full course of therapy, which may take weeks or months.
- Take next dose as soon as possible if you miss a dose; however, do not take a dose if it is almost time for next dose. Do not double dose.

Intravenous

PREPARE: **Continuous:** Packaged ready for use as a 2 mg/mL solution. Remove wrapper just prior to use.

ADMINISTER: **Continuous:** Give at a maximum rate of approximately 200 mg/h. Give after hemodialysis is completed.

- Do not use IV admixtures of fluconazole and other medications.

INCOMPATIBILITIES **Solution/additive: Trimethoprim-sulfamethoxazole. Y-site: Amphotericin B, amphotericin B cholesteryl, ampicillin, calcium gluconate, ceftazidime, ceftriaxone, cefuroxime, chloramphenicol, clindamycin, diazepam, digoxin, erythromycin, furosemide, haloperidol, hydroxyzine, imipenem-cilastatin, pentamidine, piperacillin, ticarcillin, trimethoprim-sulfamethoxazole.**

ADVERSE EFFECTS (≥1%) **CNS:** Headache. **GI:** Nausea, vomiting, abdominal pain, diarrhea, increase in AST in patients with cryptococcal meningitis and AIDS. **Skin:** Rash.

INTERACTIONS Drug: Increased PT in patients on **warfarin;** may increase **alosetron, bexarotene, phenytoin, cevimeline, cilostazol, cyclosporine, dofetilide, haloperidol, levobupivicaine, modafinil, zonisamide** levels and toxicity; hypoglycemic reactions with ORAL SULFONYLUREAS; decreased fluconazole levels with **rifampin, cimetidine;** may prolong the effects of **fentanyl, alfentanil, methadone;** increased ergotamine toxicity with **dihydroergotamine, ergotamine.**

F

PHARMACOKINETICS Absorption: 90% absorbed from GI tract. **Peak:** 1–2 h. **Distribution:** Widely distributed, including CSF. **Metabolism:** 11% of dose metabolized in liver. **Elimination:** Excreted in urine. **Half-Life:** 20–50 h.

NURSING IMPLICATIONS

Assessment & Drug Effects

- Monitor for allergic response. Patients allergic to other azole antifungals may be allergic to fluconazole.
- Lab tests: Monitor BUN, serum creatinine, and liver function.
- Note: Drug may cause elevations of the following laboratory serum values: ALT, AST, alkaline phosphatase, bilirubin.
- Monitor for S&S of hepatotoxicity.

Patient & Family Education

- Monitor carefully for loss of glycemic control if diabetic.
- Inform physician of all medications being taken.

FLUCYTOSINE

(floo-sye'toe-seen)

Ancobon, Ancotil ♣, 5-FC, 5-Fluorocytosine

Classifications: ANTIINFECTIVE; ANTIBIOTIC; ANTIFUNGAL

Prototype: Fluconazole

Pregnancy Category: C

AVAILABILITY 250 mg, 500 mg capsules

ACTIONS Ineffective for cancerous tumors possibly because it does not enter mammalian cells. Selectively penetrates fungal cell and is converted to fluorouracil, an antimetabolite believed to be responsible for antifungal activity.

THERAPEUTIC EFFECTS Has antifungal activity against *Cryptococcus* and *Candida* as well as *Chromomycosis.*

USES Alone or in combination with amphotericin B for serious systemic infections caused by susceptible strains of *Cryptococcus* and *Candida* species.

UNLABELED USES *Chromomycosis.*

CONTRAINDICATIONS Safety during pregnancy (category C) or lactation is not established.

CAUTIOUS USE Extreme caution in impaired kidney function; bone marrow depression, hematologic disorders, patients being treated with or having received radiation or bone marrow depressant drugs.

ROUTE & DOSAGE

Fungal Infection

Adult: **PO** 50–150 mg/kg/d divided q6h
Child: **PO** *<50 kg,* 1.5–4.5 g/m²/d divided q6h; *>50 kg,* 50–150 mg/kg/d divided q6h
Neonate: **PO** 50–100 mg/kg/d in 1–2 divided doses

ADMINISTRATION

Oral

- Give lower dosages with longer dosage intervals in patients with serum creatinine of 1.7 mg/dL or higher. Check with physician.

- Give capsules a few at a time over 15 min to decrease incidence and severity of nausea and vomiting.
- Store in light-resistant containers at 15°–30° C (59°–86° F).

ADVERSE EFFECTS (≥1%) **CNS:** Confusion, hallucinations, headache, sedation, vertigo. **GI:** Nausea, vomiting, diarrhea, abdominal bloating, enterocolitis. **Hematologic:** Hypoplasia of bone marrow: anemia, leukopenia, thrombocytopenia, agranulocytosis, eosinophilia. **Skin:** Rash. **Metabolic:** Elevated levels of serum alkaline phosphatase, AST, ALT, BUN, serum creatinine. **GI:** Hepatomegaly, hepatitis.

DIAGNOSTIC TEST INTERFERENCE False elevations of ***serum creatinine*** can occur with ***Ektachem analyzer.***

INTERACTIONS Drug: Amphotericin B produces additive or synergistic effects and can increase flucytosine toxicity by inhibiting its renal clearance.

PHARMACOKINETICS Absorption: Readily absorbed from GI tract. **Peak:** 2 h. **Distribution:** Widely distributed in body tissues including aqueous humor and CSF; crosses placenta. **Metabolism:** Minimally metabolized. **Elimination:** 75%–90% excreted in urine unchanged. **Half-Life:** 3–6 h.

NURSING IMPLICATIONS

Assessment & Drug Effects

- C&S tests should be performed before initiation of therapy and at weekly intervals during therapy. Organism resistance has been reported.
- Lab tests: Obtain baseline hematology, kidney and liver function on all patients before and at frequent intervals during therapy. Twice weekly leukocyte and differential counts with WBC with differential and platelet counts are recommended.
- Do frequent assays of blood drug level, especially in patients with impaired kidney function to determine adequacy of drug excretion (therapeutic range: 25–120 mg/mL).
- Monitor I&O. Report change in I&O ratio or pattern. Because most of drug is eliminated unchanged by kidneys, compromised function can lead to drug accumulation.

Patient & Family Education

- Report fever, sore mouth or throat, and unusual bleeding or bruising tendency to physician.
- Be aware that the general duration of therapy is 4–6 wk, but it may continue for several months.
- Do not breast feed while taking this drug without consulting physician.

FLUDROCORTISONE ACETATE

(floo-droe-kor′ti-sone)

Florinef Acetate

Classifications: HORMONE AND SYNTHETIC SUBSTITUTE; ADRENAL CORTICOSTEROID; MINERALOCORTICOID; ANTIINFLAMMATORY AGENT

Prototype: Hydrocortisone

Pregnancy Category: C

AVAILABILITY 0.1 mg tablets

ACTIONS Long-acting synthetic steroid with potent mineralocorticoid and moderate glucocorticoid activity. Small doses produce marked sodium retention, increased urinary potassium excretion, and elevated BP.

THERAPEUTIC EFFECTS Synthetic corticosteroid replacement product for adrenocortical insufficiency.

F

USES Partial replacement therapy for adrenocortical insufficiency and for treatment of salt-losing forms of congenital adrenogenital syndrome.
UNLABELED USES To increase systolic and diastolic blood pressure in patients with severe hypotension secondary to diabetes mellitus or to levodopa therapy.

CONTRAINDICATIONS Hypersensitivity to glucocorticoids, idiopathic thrombocytopenic purpura, psychoses, acute glomerulonephritis, viral or bacterial diseases of skin, infections not controlled by antibiotics, active or latent amebiasis, hypercorticism (Cushing's syndrome), smallpox vaccination or other immunologic procedures. Topical steroids are contraindicated in presence of varicella, vaccinia, on surfaces with compromised circulation, and in children <2 y.
CAUTIOUS USE Children; diabetes mellitus; chronic, active hepatitis positive for hepatitis B surface antigen; hyperlipidemia; cirrhosis; stromal herpes simplex; glaucoma, tuberculosis of eye; osteoporosis; convulsive disorders; hypothyroidism; diverticulitis; nonspecific ulcerative colitis; fresh intestinal anastomoses; active or latent peptic ulcer; gastritis; esophagitis; thromboembolic disorders; CHF; metastatic carcinoma; hypertension; renal insufficiency; history of allergies; active or arrested tuberculosis; systemic fungal infection; myasthenia gravis. Safety in pregnancy (category C) or lactation is not established.

ROUTE & DOSAGE

Adrenocortical Insufficiency
Adult: **PO** 0.1 mg/d, may range from 0.1 mg 3 times/wk to 0.2 mg/d
Child: **PO** 0.05–0.1 mg/d

Salt-losing Adrenogenital Syndrome
Adult: **PO** 0.1–0.2 mg/d
Child: **PO** 0.05–0.1 mg/d

ADMINISTRATION

Oral
- Note: Concomitant oral cortisone or hydrocortisone therapy may be advisable to provide substitute therapy approximating normal adrenal activity.
- Store in airtight containers at 15°–30° C (59°–86° F). Protect from light.

ADVERSE EFFECTS (≥1%) **CNS:** Vertigo, headache, nystagmus, increased intracranial pressure with papilledema (usually after discontinuation of medication), mental disturbances, aggravation of preexisting psychiatric conditions, insomnia, ataxia (rare). **CV:** CHF, hypertension, <u>thromboembolism</u> (rare), tachycardia. **Endocrine:** Suppressed linear growth in children, decreased glucose tolerance; hyperglycemia, manifestations of latent diabetes mellitus; hypocorticism; amenorrhea and other menstrual difficulties. **Special Senses:** Posterior subcapsular cataracts (especially in children), glaucoma, exophthalmos, increased intraocular pressure with optic nerve damage, perforation of the globe. **Metabolic:** Hypocalcemia; *sodium and fluid retention;* hypokalemia and hypokalemic alkalosis, negative nitrogen balance, decreased serum concentration of vitamins A and C. **GI:** *Nausea,* increased appetite, ulcerative esophagitis, pancreatitis, abdominal distension, peptic ulcer with perforation and hemorrhage, melena. **Hematologic:** Thrombocytopenia. **Musculoskeletal:** (long-term use) Osteoporosis, compression fractures, muscle wasting and weakness, tendon rupture, aseptic necrosis of femoral and humeral heads. **Skin:** Skin thinning and atrophy, *acne, impaired wound healing;* petechiae, ecchymosis, easy bruising; suppression of skin test reaction; hypopigmentation or hyperpigmentation, hirsutism, acneiform eruptions, subcutaneous fat atrophy; allergic dermatitis, urticaria, angioneurotic edema, increased sweating. **Body as a Whole:** Anaphylactoid reactions (rare), aggravation or masking of infections; malaise, weight gain, obesity. **Urogenital:** Increased or decreased motility and number of sperm.

INTERACTIONS Drug: The antidiabetic effects of **insulin** and SULFONYLUREAS may be diminished; **amphotericin B,** DIURETICS may increase **potassium** loss; **warfarin** may decrease prothrombin time; **indomethacin, ibuprofen** can potentiate the pressor effect of fludrocortisone; ANABOLIC STEROIDS increase risk of edema and acne; **rifampin** may increase the hepatic metabolism of fludrocortisone.

PHARMACOKINETICS Absorption: Readily absorbed from GI tract. **Peak:** 1.7 h. **Metabolism:** Metabolized in liver. **Half-Life:** 3.5 h.

NURSING IMPLICATIONS

Assessment & Drug Effects

- Monitor weight and I&O ratio to observe onset of fluid accumulation, especially if patient is on unrestricted salt intake and without potassium supplement. Report weight gain of 2 kg (5 lb)/wk.
- Monitor and record BP daily. If hypertension develops as a consequence of therapy, report to physician. Usually, the dose will be reduced to 0.05 mg/d.
- Check BP q4–6h and weight at least every other day during periods of dosage adjustment.
- Lab tests: Periodic serum electrolytes and ABGs during prolonged therapy.
- Monitor for S&S of hypokalemia and hyperkalemic metabolic alkalosis (see Appendix F).
- Monitor for signs of overdosage (hypercorticism): psychosis, excess weight gain, edema, congestive heart failure, ravenous appetite, severe insomnia, and increase in BP.
- Note: Signs of insufficient dosage (hypocorticism) are loss of weight and appetite, nausea, vomiting, diarrhea, muscular weakness, increased fatigue, and hypotension.

Patient & Family Education

- Report signs of hypokalemia (see Appendix F).
- Be aware of signs of potassium depletion associated with high sodium intake: Muscle weakness, paresthesias, circumoral numbness; fatigue, anorexia, nausea, mental depression, polyuria, delirium, diminished reflexes, arrhythmias, cardiac failure, ileus, ECG changes.
- Advise patient to eat foods with high potassium content.
- Signs of edema should be reported immediately. Sodium intake may or may not require regulation, depending on individual needs and clinical situation.
- Weigh daily under standard conditions and report steady weight gain.
- Report intercurrent infection, trauma, or unexpected stress of any kind promptly when taking maintenance therapy.
- Carry medical identification at all times. It needs to indicate medical diagnosis, medication(s),

physician's name, address, and telephone number.

- Do not breast feed while taking this drug without consulting physician.

FLUMAZENIL Pr

(flu-ma'ze-nil)

Mazicon ♣, Romazicon

Classifications: CENTRAL NERVOUS SYSTEM AGENT; BENZODIAZEPINE ANTAGONIST

Pregnancy Category: C

AVAILABILITY 0.1 mg/mL injection

ACTIONS Antagonizes the effects of benzodiazepine on the CNS, including sedation, impairment of recall, and psychomotor impairment. Does not reverse the effects of opioids.

THERAPEUTIC EFFECTS Reverses the action of a benzodiazepine.

USES Complete or partial reversal of sedation induced by benzodiazepine for anesthesia or diagnostic or therapeutic procedures and through overdose.

UNLABELED USES Seizure disorders, alcohol intoxication, hepatic encephalopathy, facilitation of weaning from mechanical ventilation.

CONTRAINDICATIONS Hypersensitivity to flumazenil or to benzodiazepines; patients given a benzodiazepine for control of a life-threatening condition; patients showing signs of cyclic antidepressant overdose; seizure-prone individuals during labor and delivery. Effects on children are not established.

CAUTIOUS USE Hepatic function impairment, older adults, pregnancy (category C), lactation, intensive care patients, head injury, drug- and alcohol-dependent patients, and physical dependence upon benzodiazepines.

ROUTE & DOSAGE

Reversal of Sedation

Adult: **IV** 0.2 mg over 15 s, may repeat 0.2 mg q60s for 4 additional doses or a cumulative dose of 1 mg

Benzodiazepine Overdose

Adult: **IV** 0.2 mg over 30 s, if no response after 30 s, then 0.3 mg over 30 s, may repeat with 0.5 mg q60s (max: cumulative dose of 3 mg)

ADMINISTRATION

Intravenous

PREPARE: **Direct:** May give undiluted or diluted. If diluted use D5W, Lactated Ringer's, NS.

ADMINISTER: **Direct:** ▪ Ensure patency of IV before administration of flumazenil, since extravasation will cause local irritation. ▪ Give through an IV that is freely flowing into a large vein. Give each 0.2 mg dose in small quantities over 15 s. Each 0.2 mg dose should be given in small quantities over 15 s. Repeat at 60 s intervals (see Route & Dosage). Do not give as a bolus dose. In high-risk patients, slow the rate to intervals of 6–10 min to provide the smallest effective dose. ▪ Give repeat doses at 20 min intervals if resedation occurs (max: 1 mg given at a rate of 0.2 mg/min, not to exceed 3 mg in any 1-h period). ▪ Use all diluted solutions within 24 h of dilution.

ADVERSE EFFECTS (≥1%) **CNS:** Emotional lability, headache, *dizziness,* agitation, *resedation,* seizures, blurred vision. **GI:** *Nausea, vomiting,* hiccups. **Other:** Shivering, pain at injection site, hypoventilation.

INTERACTIONS Drug: may antagonize effects of **zaleplon, zolpidem;** may cause convulsions or arrhythmias with TRICYCLIC ANTIDEPRESSANTS.

PHARMACOKINETICS Onset: 1–5 min. **Peak:** 6–10 min. **Duration:** 2–4 h. **Metabolism:** Metabolized in the liver to inactive metabolites. **Elimination:** 90%–95% excreted in urine, 5–10% in feces within 72 h. **Half-Life:** 54 min.

NURSING IMPLICATIONS

Assessment & Drug Effects

- Monitor respiratory status carefully until risk of resedation is unlikely (up to 120 min). Drug may not fully reverse benzodiazepine-induced ventilatory insufficiency.
- Monitor carefully for seizures and take appropriate precautions.

Patient & Family Education

- Do not drive or engage in potentially hazardous activities until at least 18–24 h after discharge following a procedure.
- Do not ingest alcohol or nonprescription drugs for 18–24 h after flumazenil is administered or if the effects of the benzodiazepine persist.
- Do not breast feed while taking this drug without consulting physician.

FLUNISOLIDE

(floo-niss′oh-lide)

AeroBid, Nasalide, Nasarel

Classifications: SKIN AND MUCOUS MEMBRANE AGENT; ANTIINFLAMMATORY; ADRENAL CORTICOSTEROID

Prototype: Hydrocortisone

Pregnancy Category: C

AVAILABILITY 250 mcg/spray aerosol; 0.025% (25 mcg/spray) nasal spray

See Appendix A-3.

FLUOCINOLONE ACETONIDE

(floo-oh-sin′oh-lone)

Fluoderm ♣, Fluolar, Fluonid, Flurosyn, Synalar, Synalar-HP, Synemol

Classifications: SKIN AND MUCOUS MEMBRANE AGENT; ANTIINFLAMMATORY; ADRENAL CORTICOSTEROID

Prototype: Hydrocortisone

Pregnancy Category: C

AVAILABILITY 0.025% ointment, cream; 0.2% cream; 0.01% cream, solution, shampoo, oil

See Appendix A-4.

FLUOCINONIDE

(floo-oh-sin′oh-nide)

Lidemol, Lidex, Lidex-E, Lyderm, Topsyn

Classifications: SKIN AND MUCOUS MEMBRANE AGENT; ANTIINFLAMMATORY; ADRENAL CORTICOSTEROID

Prototype: Hydrocortisone

Pregnancy Category: C

AVAILABILITY 0.05% cream, ointment, solution, gel

See Appendix A-4.

FLUORESCEIN SODIUM

(flure′e-seen)

Fluorescite, Fluor-I-Strip, Fluor-I-Ful-Glo, Funduscein

Classification: OPHTHALMIC DIAGNOSTIC AGENT

Pregnancy Category: C

AVAILABILITY 10%, 25% injection; 2% ocular solution; 0.6 mg, 1 mg, 9 mg strips

F

ACTIONS Mildly antiseptic fluorescent dye related chemically to phenolphthalein that demonstrates defects of the corneal epithelium.

THERAPEUTIC EFFECTS Any break in the epithelial tissue allows the dye to enter the tissue. Epithelial damage will appear as a bright green area.

USES An aid in fitting hard contact lenses, applanation tonometry, detecting corneal epithelial defects, and testing potency of lacrimal system. Used IV as a diagnostic aid in retinal angiography. Also used as an antidote for aniline dye.

CONTRAINDICATIONS Topical use with soft contact lenses not recommended.

CAUTIOUS USE History of hypersensitivity, allergies, bronchial asthma; pregnancy (category C), lactation.

ROUTE & DOSAGE

Diagnostic Aid

Adult: **Instillation** Instill 1–2 drops then have patient keep eyelid closed for 60 s or moisten strip with sterile water, touch conjunctiva or fornix with moistened tip, and have patient blink to distribute

Retinal Angiography

Adult: **IV** 5 mL of 10% solution or 3 mL of 25% solution injected rapidly in antecubital vein.
Child: **IV** 7.5 mg/kg injected rapidly in antecubital vein

ADMINISTRATION

Instillation

- Avoid touching eyelids or surrounding area with eyedropper when instilling medication.
- Fit hard contact lenses: Instill drug with contact lenses in place. Have patient blink several times to distribute dye. Under blue light, areas that lack fluorescein will appear black, indicating that contact lens is touching cornea at these points.
- Test for potency of lacrimal system: One drop of 2% solution is instilled into conjunctival sac. Have patient blink at least 4 times. After 6 min, nasal secretions are examined under blue light. Traces of dye in secretions indicate that nasolacrimal drainage system is open.
- Store below 27° C (80° F); keep tightly closed when not in use, and protect from light and freezing.

ADVERSE EFFECTS (≥1%) **Special Senses:** *Temporary stinging, burning sensation,* conjunctival redness. **CNS:** (IV administration) Headache, paresthesias, pyrexia, convulsions. **CV:** (IV administration) Hypotension, transient dyspnea, acute pulmonary edema, basilar artery ischemia, syncope, <u>severe shock, cardiac arrest</u>. **GI:** (IV administration) Nausea, vomiting, strong metallic taste following high dosage. **Body as a Whole:** (IV administration) Hypersensitivity (urticaria, pruritus, angioneurotic edema, <u>anaphylactic reaction</u>). **Skin:** (IV administration) Thrombophlebitis at injection site, temporary discoloration of skin and urine.

INTERACTIONS Drug: No clinically significant interactions established.

NURSING IMPLICATIONS

Assessment & Drug Effects

- Have facilities for treatment of anaphylactic reaction immediately available (e.g., epinephrine 1:1000 for IV or IM use, an antihistamine, and oxygen).
- Discontinue fluorescein immediately if S&S of sensitivity develop.

Patient & Family Education

- Note: IV administration may impart a yellowish orange discoloration to skin and to urine. Skin discoloration usually fades in 6–12 h; urine clears in 24–36 h.
- Do not breast feed while taking this drug without consulting physician.

FLUOROMETHOLONE

(flure-oh-meth'oh-lone)

Fluor-Op, FML Forte, FML Liquifilm Ophthalmic

Classifications: SKIN AND MUCOUS MEMBRANE AGENT; ANTIINFLAMMATORY; ADRENAL CORTICOSTEROID

Prototype: Hydrocortisone

Pregnancy Category: C

AVAILABILITY 0.1%, 0.25% suspension; 0.1% ointment

See Appendix A-1.

FLUOROURACIL [5-FLUOROURACIL (5-FU)] (Pr)

(flure-oh-yoor'a-sil)

Adrucil, Carac, Efudex, Fluoroplex

Classifications: ANTINEOPLASTIC AGENT; ANTIMETABOLITE

Pregnancy Category: D

AVAILABILITY 50 mg/mL injection; 1%, 2%, 5% topical solution; 0.5%, 1%, 5% topical cream

ACTIONS Pyrimidine antagonist and cell-cycle specific. Blocks action of enzymes essential to normal DNA and RNA synthesis and may become incorporated in RNA to form a fraudulent molecule; unbalanced growth and death of cell follow. Exhibits higher affinity for tumor tissue than healthy tissue.

THERAPEUTIC EFFECTS Highly toxic, especially to proliferative cells in neoplasms, bone marrow, and intestinal mucosa. Low therapeutic index with high potential for severe hematologic toxicity.

USES Systemically as single agent and in combination with other antineoplastics for palliative treatment of carefully selected patients with inoperable neoplasms of breast, colon or rectum, stomach, pancreas, urinary bladder, ovary, cervix, liver. Also topically for solar or actinic keratoses and superficial basal cell carcinoma.

UNLABELED USES To induce repigmentation in vitiligo; actinic cheilitis; malignant effusions; mucosal leukoplakia.

CONTRAINDICATIONS Poor nutritional status; myelosuppression. Safety during pregnancy (category D) or lactation is not established.

CAUTIOUS USE Major surgery during previous month; history of highdose pelvic irradiation, metastatic cell infiltration of bone marrow, previous use of alkylating agents; men and women in childbearing ages; hepatic or renal impairment.

ROUTE & DOSAGE

Carcinoma

Adult: **IV** 12 mg/kg/d for 4 consecutive days up to 800 mg or until toxicity develops or 12 d therapy, may repeat at 1 mo intervals; if toxicity occurs, 15 mg/kg once weekly can be given until toxicity subsides

Actinic and Solar Keratosis

Adult: **Topical** Apply cream or solution b.i.d. for 2–4 wk; apply Carac once daily

Superficial Basal Cell Carcinoma
Adult: **Topical** Apply 5% cream b.i.d. for 3–6 wk

ADMINISTRATION

Topical

- Use gloved fingers to apply topical drug.
- Do not use occlusive dressings with topical drug. Use a porous gauze dressing for cosmetic purposes; does not cause inflammation.
- Note: Second-degree burns resulting from contact between plastic eyeglass frames and treated skin have been reported. Reduce risk of burns or irritation by treating skin that contacts frames only at night when glasses are not worn, and using the lowest effective strength of topical preparation.
- Store at 15°–30° C (59°–86° F) unless otherwise directed. Protect from light and freezing.

Intravenous

Note: Parenteral dose is determined by actual weight unless patient is obese, in which case ideal weight is used.

- Safe Handling: Double-glove with latex gloves, and change the double set after every 30 min of exposure. If a drug spill occurs, change gloves immediately after it is cleaned up.

PREPARE: **Direct:** This drug may be given without dilution.

ADMINISTER: **Direct:** Give by direct IV injection over 1–2 min. Inspect injection site frequently; avoid extravasation. If it occurs, stop infusion and restart in another vein. Ice compresses may reduce danger of local tissue damage from infiltrated solution.

INCOMPATIBILITIES **Solution/additive: Carboplatin, cisplatin, cytarabine, diazepam, doxorubicin, droperidol, epirubicin, fentanyl, leucovorin calcium, metoclopramide, morphine. Y-site: Amphotericin B cholesteryl, droperidol, filgrastim, ondansetron,** TPN, **vinorelbine.**

- Fluorouracil solution is normally colorless to faint yellow. Slight discoloration during storage does not appear to affect potency or safety. Discard dark yellow solution. If a precipitate forms, redissolve drug by heating to 60° C (140° F) and shake vigorously. Allow to cool to body temperature before administration.

ADVERSE EFFECTS (≥1%) **CNS:** Euphoria, acute cerebellar syndrome (dysmetria, nystagmus, ataxia, severe mental deterioration); pustular contact hypersensitivity. **CV:** Cardiotoxicity (rare), angina. **GI:** Anorexia, *nausea, vomiting, stomatitis,* esophagopharyngitis, medicinal taste, *diarrhea,* proctitis. **Hematologic:** Anemia, <u>leukopenia</u>, thrombocytopenia, eosinophilia. **Body as a Whole:** Hypersensitivity: Pustular contact eruption, edema of face, eyes, tongue, legs. **Skin:** SLE-like dermatitis, *alopecia*, photosensitivity, erythema, increased pigmentation, skin dryness and fissuring, pruritic maculopapular rash. **[Topical]** Local pain, pruritus, hyperpigmentation, burning at site of application, dermatitis, suppuration, swelling, scarring, toxic granulation.

DIAGNOSTIC TEST INTERFERENCE Fluorouracil may increase excretion of ***5-hydroxyindoleacetic acid (5-HIAA)*** and decrease ***plasma albumin*** (because of drug-induced protein malabsorption).

INTERACTIONS Drug: Metronidazole may increase general floxuridine toxicity; may increase or decrease serum levels of **phenytoin, fosphenytoin; hydroxyurea** can decrease conversion to active metabolite.

PHARMACOKINETICS Distribution: Distributed to tumor, intestinal mucosa, bone marrow, liver, and CSF; probably crosses placenta. **Metabolism:** Rapidly metabolized in liver. **Elimination:** 15% excreted in urine, 60%–80% excreted through lungs as carbon dioxide. **Half-Life:** 16 min.

NURSING IMPLICATIONS

Assessment & Drug Effects

- Lab tests: Obtain total and differential leukocyte counts before each dose is administered. Discontinue drug if leukopenia occurs (WBC <3500/mm^3) or if patient develops thrombocytopenia (platelet count <100,000/mm^3). Baseline and periodic checks of Hct and liver and kidney function are also advised.
- Use protective isolation of patient during leukopenic period (WBC <3500/mm^3).
- Watch for and report signs of abnormal bleeding from any source during thrombocytopenic period (day 7–17); inspect skin for ecchymotic and petechial areas. Protect patient from trauma.
- Report disorientation or confusion; drug should be withdrawn immediately.
- Establish a reference data base for body weight, I&O ratio and pattern, food preferences and dietary habits, bowel habits, and condition of mouth.
- Report intractable vomiting to physician.
- Indications to discontinue drug: Severe stomatitis, leukopenia (WBC <3500/mm^3 or rapidly decreasing count), intractable vomiting, diarrhea, thrombocytopenia (platelets <100,000/mm^3), and hemorrhage from any site.
- Inspect patient's mouth daily. Promptly report cracked lips, xerostomia, white patches, and erythema of buccal membranes.
- Report development of maculopapular rash; it usually responds to symptomatic treatment and is reversible.
- Be aware of expected response of lesion to topical 5-FU: Erythema followed in sequence by vesiculation, erosion, ulceration, necrosis, epithelialization. Applications of drug are continued until ulcerative stage is reached (2–6 wk after initial applications) and then discontinued.
- Note: Systemic toxicity may follow use of topical drug on large ulcerated area. Report symptoms promptly.

Patient & Family Education

- Understand that it is very important to report the first signs of toxicity: Anorexia, vomiting, nausea, stomatitis, diarrhea, GI bleeding.
- Schedule and make sure to complete periodic checks on liver and kidney function.
- Do not change dosage regimen (i.e., do not increase or omit doses or change dosage intervals).
- Avoid exposure to sunlight or ultraviolet lamp treatments. Protect exposed skin. Photosensitivity usually subsides 2–3 mo after last dose.
- Report promptly to physician any difficulty in maintaining balance while ambulating.
- Be aware that your hair may fall out; new hair growth usually begins within 6–8 wk.

- Use contraception during 5-FU treatment. If you suspect you are pregnant, tell your physician.
- Do not breast feed while taking this drug without consulting physician.

F

FLUOXETINE HYDROCHLORIDE Pr

(flu'ox-e-tine)

Prozac, Prozac Weekly, Sarafem

Classifications: CENTRAL NERVOUS SYSTEM AGENT; PSYCHOTHERAPEUTIC AGENT; SELECTIVE SEROTONIN REUPTAKE INHIBITOR (SSRI)

Pregnancy Category: C

AVAILABILITY 10 mg tablets; 10 mg, 20 mg capsules; 20 mg/5 mL solution; 90 mg sustained-release capsules (Prozac Weekly)

ACTIONS Oral antidepressant chemically unrelated to tricyclic, tetracyclic, MAOI, or other available antidepressants. Antidepressant effect is presumed to be linked to its inhibition of CNS neuronal uptake of serotonin, a neurotransmitter. Known as a selective serotonin reuptake inhibitor (SSRI).

THERAPEUTIC EFFECTS Effectiveness may take from several days to 5 wk to develop fully. Drug has antidepressant, antiobsessive-compulsive, and antibulimic actions.

USES Depression, geriatric depression, obsessive-compulsive disorder (OCD), bulimia nervosa, premenstrual dysphoric disorder.

UNLABELED USES Obesity.

CONTRAINDICATIONS Hypersensitivity to fluoxetine or other SSRI drugs; concurrent administration with MAOIs, or thioridazine; pregnancy (category C), children <7 y for OCD, children <8 y for depression.

CAUTIOUS USE Hepatic and renal impairment, renal failure, abrupt discontinuation, anorexia nervosa, mania, bleeding, lactation; hyponatremia, cardiac disease, dehydration, diabetes mellitus, patients with history of suicidal ideations; seizure disorders, ECT, hepatic disease. Older adults may require dose adjustments.

ROUTE & DOSAGE

Depression, Obsessive-Compulsive Disorder

Adult: **PO** 20 mg/d in a.m., may increase by 20 mg/d at weekly intervals (max: 80 mg/d); 20 mg/d in a.m.; when stable may switch to 90 mg sustained-release capsule qwk (max: 90 mg/wk)
Child: **PO** > 7 y 10–20 mg/d in a.m. (max 60 mg/d for OCD)
Geriatric: **PO** Start with 10 mg/d

Premenstrual Dysphoric Disorder

Adult: **PO** 10–20 mg q.d. (max: 60 mg/d)

Bulimia Nervosa

Adult: **PO** 60 mg q.d.

ADMINISTRATION

Oral

- Give as a single dose in morning. Give in two divided doses; one in a.m. and one at noon to prevent insomnia, when more than 20 mg/d prescribed.
- Provide suicidal or potentially suicidal patient with small quantities of prescription medication.
- Monitor for worsening of depression or expression of suicidal ideations.
- Store at 15°–25° C (59°–77° F).

ADVERSE EFFECTS (≥1%) **CNS:** *Headache, nervousness, anxiety, insomnia,* drowsiness, fatigue, tremor, dizziness. **CV:** Palpitations, hot flushes, chest pain. **GI:** *Nausea, diarrhea,* anorexia, dyspepsia, increased appetite, dry mouth. **Skin:** Rash, pruritus, sweating, hypersensitivity reactions. **Special Senses:** Blurred vision. **Body as a Whole:** Myalgias, arthralgias, flu-like syndrome, hyponatremia. **Urogenital:** Sexual dysfunction, menstrual irregularities.

INTERACTIONS Drug: Concurrent use of **tryptophan** may cause agitation, restlessness, and GI distress; MAO INHIBITORS, **selegiline** may increase risk of severe hypertensive reaction and death; increases half-life of **diazepam;** may increase toxicity of TRICYCLIC ANTIDEPRESSANTS; AMPHETAMINES, **cilostazol, nefazodone, pentazocine, propafenone, sibutramine, tramadol, venlafaxine** may increase risk of serotonin syndrome; may inhibit metabolism of **carbamazepine, phenytoin, ritonavir;** increased ergotamine toxicity with **dihydroergotamine, ergotamine. Herbal: St. John's wort** may cause serotonin syndrome.

PHARMACOKINETICS Absorption: 60%–80% absorbed from GI tract. **Onset:** 1–3 wk. **Peak:** 4–8 h. **Distribution:** Widely distributed, including CNS. **Metabolism:** Metabolized in liver to active metabolite, norfluoxetine. **Elimination:** >80% excreted in urine; 12% in feces. **Half-Life:** Fluoxetine 2–3 d, norfluoxetine 7–9 d.

NURSING IMPLICATIONS

Assessment & Drug Effects

- Use with caution in the older adult patient or patient with impaired renal or hepatic function (may need lower dose).
- Use with caution in anorexic patient, since weight loss is a possible side effect.
- Monitor for S&S of anaphylactoid reaction (see Appendix F).
- Lab tests: Periodic serum electrolytes; monitor closely plasma glucose in diabetes.
- Monitor serum sodium level for development of hyponatremia, especially in patients who are taking diuretics or are otherwise hypovolemic.
- Monitor diabetics for loss of glycemic control; hypoglycemia has occurred during initiation of therapy, and hyperglycemia during drug withdrawal.
- Monitor for S&S of improved affect. Requires approximately 2–3 wk for therapeutic effects to be felt.
- Weigh weekly to monitor weight loss, particularly in the older adult or nutritionally compromised patient. Report significant weight loss to physician.
- Observe for and promptly report rash or urticaria and S&S of fever, leukocytosis, arthralgias, carpal tunnel syndrome, edema, respiratory distress, and proteinuria. Drug may have to be discontinued or adjunctive therapy instituted with steroids or antihistamines.
- Observe for dizziness and drowsiness and employ safety measures (up with assistance, side rails, etc.) as indicated.
- Monitor for and report increased anxiety, nervousness, or insomnia; may need modification of drug dose.
- Monitor for seizures in patients with a history of seizures. Use appropriate safety precautions.
- Supervise patients closely who are high suicide risks; especially during initial therapy.
- Monitor patients with hepatic or renal impairment carefully for S&S

of toxicity (e.g., agitation, restlessness, nausea, vomiting, seizures).

Patient & Family Education

- Notify physician of intent to become pregnant.
- Notify physician of any rash; possible sign of a serious group of adverse effects.
- Do not drive or engage in potentially hazardous activities until response to drug is known; especially if dizziness noted.
- Monitor blood glucose for loss of glycemic control if diabetic.
- Note: Drug may increase seizure activity in those with history of seizure.
- Do not breast feed while taking this drug without consulting physician.

F

FLUOXYMESTERONE

(floo-ox-ee-mess′te-rone)

Halotestin, Ora Testryl ♣

Classifications: HORMONES AND SYNTHETIC SUBSTITUTES; ANDROGEN/ANABOLIC STEROID

Prototype: Testosterone

Pregnancy Category: X

Controlled Substance: Schedule III

AVAILABILITY 2 mg, 5 mg, 10 mg tablets

ACTIONS Short-acting, orally effective derivative of testosterone with hypercholesterolemic effect. Retention of sodium is minimal; thus hypertension and edema rarely complicate therapy.

THERAPEUTIC EFFECTS Replacement therapy for endogenous testosterone. Promotes recalcification of osseous metastases and regression of soft tissue lesions.

USES In men as replacement therapy in conditions associated with testicular hormone deficiency; in women to antagonize effects of estrogen in androgen-responsive inoperable breast cancer. Also in combination with estrogens for management of severe postmenopausal vasomotor symptoms.

CONTRAINDICATIONS Breast cancer in men, prostatic cancer, benign obstructive prostatic hypertrophy; hypercalcemia; diabetes mellitus; severe cardiorenal disease or liver damage; nephrosis or nephrotic phase of nephritis; history of MI; athletes; infants; women with inoperable mammary cancer <1 y or >5 y after menopause; pregnancy (category X), lactation.

CAUTIOUS USE Children, older males, history of MI, or coronary disease, hepatic, renal or congestive heart failure, women.

ROUTE & DOSAGE

Male Hypogonadism

Adult: **PO** 2.5–20 mg/d

Metastatic Carcinoma of Female Breast

Adult: **PO** 10–40 mg/d in divided doses

Postpartum Breast Engorgement

Adult: **PO** 2.5 mg shortly after delivery, then 5–10 mg/d in divided doses for 4–5 d

ADMINISTRATION

Oral

- Give immediately before or with meals to diminish GI distress.

ADVERSE EFFECTS (≥1%) **Endocrine:** Virilization (women), gynecomastia (men). **Urogenital:** Priapism, impotence. **Metabolic:** Jaundice (reversible), hypoglycemia, hypercalcemia. **GI:** Hepatocellular carcinoma, peliosis hepatitis, nausea, vomiting, diarrhea, symptoms resembling peptic ulcer. **Body as a Whole:** Anaphylactic reactions (rare), *edema, acne.*

INTERACTIONS Drug: ORAL ANTICOAGULANTS increase risk of bleeding. Possibly increases risk of **cyclosporine** toxicity. **Insulin** and ORAL HYPOGLYCEMIC AGENTS may decrease **glucose** level; dose will need to be adjusted. **Herbal: echinacea** may increase hepatotoxicity.

PHARMACOKINETICS Absorption: Readily absorbed from GI tract. **Metabolism:** Metabolized in liver. **Half-Life:** 9.5 h.

NURSING IMPLICATIONS

Assessment & Drug Effects

- Lab test: Obtain baseline and periodic liver function and serum electrolytes, Hgb, Hct, and serum and urine calcium; also serial serum cholesterol in patients with history of MI or coronary artery disease.
- Monitor I&O ratio and pattern and weight, and check for edema; report significant changes.
- Monitor for S&S of hypercalcemia (see Appendix F); particularly likely in patients with metastatic breast carcinoma. Stop anabolic therapy if it develops.
- Be alert for voice change in female patient, an early sign of virilism. Virilism may be irreversible even after prompt discontinuation of therapy.
- Note: When used in pediatric patients, therapy is preceded by x-ray of wrist bones to establish level of bone maturation. During treatment, bone maturation may proceed more rapidly than linear growth; therefore, intermittent dosage schedule and periodic x-rays are usual.
- Observe children <7 y closely for precocious development of male sexual characteristics or masculinization because they are particularly sensitive to androgenic effects.
- Watch for symptoms of hypoglycemia (see Appendix F) and report to physician. Anabolic treatment may reduce blood glucose in diabetic patients.
- Observe patient on concomitant anticoagulant therapy for ecchymotic areas, petechiae, or abnormal bleeding from any site. Close monitoring of PT & INR is essential.
- Note: When used for palliation of mammary cancer, subjective effects of therapy may not be experienced for 1 mo; objective symptoms may be delayed for as long as 3 mo.
- Be aware that anabolic response may be evidenced by euphoria and gain in weight and appetite, especially in emaciated and debilitated patient.

Patient & Family Education

- Adhere to scheduled appointments for laboratory tests.
- Good personal hygiene, including meticulous skin care is very important (females and prepubertal males are especially likely to develop acne).
- Note and report symptoms of jaundice (see Appendix F) to physician. Dose adjustment may reverse the condition.
- Report menstrual irregularities.
- Keep child's appointments for bone maturation studies (usually every 3–6 mo) to prevent compromised adult height.
- Report priapism (prolonged erection) to physician promptly, it is a symptom of overdosage. A temporary interruption of regimen may be indicated. Also report persistent GI distress, diarrhea, or the onset of jaundice.

- Be aware that virilization usually occurs. Report to physician any voice change (hoarseness or deepening), increased libido (associated with clitoral enlargement), hirsutism immediately. Usually, stopping therapy will end further development of symptoms but will not reverse hirsutism or voice change.
- Do not breast feed while taking this drug.

FLUPHENAZINE DECANOATE

(floo-fen′a-zeen)

Prolixin Decanoate, Modecate Decanoate ✤

FLUPHENAZINE ENANTHATE

Moditen Enanthate ✤, Prolixin Enanthate

FLUPHENAZINE HYDROCHLORIDE

Moditen HCl ✤, Permitil, Prolixin

Classifications: CENTRAL NERVOUS SYSTEM AGENT; PSYCHOTHERAPEUTIC; ANTIPSYCHOTIC; PHENOTHIAZINE

Prototype: Chlorpromazine

Pregnancy Category: C

AVAILABILITY 1 mg, 2.5 mg, 5 mg, 10 mg tablets; 2.5 mg/5 mL elixir; 5 mg/mL oral concentrate; 2.5 mg/mL, 25 mg/mL injection

ACTIONS Potent phenothiazine, antipsychotic agent. Blocks postsynaptic dopamine receptors in the brain. Similar to other phenothiazines with the following exceptions: more potent per weight, higher incidence of extrapyramidal complications, and lower frequency of sedative, hypotensive, and antiemetic effects.

THERAPEUTIC EFFECTS Effective for treatment of antipsychotic symptoms including schizophrenia.

USES Management of manifestations of psychotic disorders.

UNLABELED USES As antineuralgia adjunct.

CONTRAINDICATIONS Known hypersensitivity to phenothiazines; subcortical brain damage, comatose or severely depressed states, blood dyscrasias, renal or hepatic disease. Safety during pregnancy (category C) or lactation is not established. Parenteral form not recommended for children <12 y.

CAUTIOUS USE With anticholinergic agents, other CNS depressants; older adults, previously diagnosed breast cancer; cardiovascular diseases; pheochromocytoma; history of convulsive disorders; patients exposed to extreme heat or phosphorous insecticides; peptic ulcer; respiratory impairment.

ROUTE & DOSAGE

Psychosis

Adult: **PO** 0.5–10 mg/d in 1–4 divided doses (max: of 20 mg/d) **IM/SC HCl** 2.5–10 mg/d divided q6–8h (max: 10 mg/d); **Decanoate** 12.5–25 mg q1–4wk; **Enanthate** 25 mg q2wk

Dementia Behavior

Geriatric: **PO** 1–2.5 mg/d, may increase every 4–7 d by 1–2.5 mg/d (max: 20 mg/d in 2–3 divided doses)

ADMINISTRATION

- Note: Fluphenazine hydrochloride (HCl) is given PO and IM. Fluphenazine enanthate and decanoate are given IM or SC.

Oral

- Give sustained release tablets whole (need to be swallowed whole; not recommended for children).

- Dilute oral concentrate in fruit juice, water, carbonated beverage, milk, soup. Avoid caffeine-containing beverages (cola, coffee) as a diluent, also tannic acid (tea) or pectinates (apple juice).
- Be careful not to contact skin or clothing with drug when preparing oral concentrate or liquid preparations for injection. Warn patient to avoid spilling drug. If drug contacts skin, rinse/flush skin promptly with warm water.
- Give oral preparations at least 1 h before or 2 h after the antacid. Antacids diminish absorption.
- Protect all preparations from light and freezing. Solutions may safely vary in color from almost colorless to light amber. Discard dark or otherwise discolored solutions.
- Store in tightly closed container at 15°–30° C (59°–86° F) unless otherwise specified by manufacturer. Protect all forms from light.

ADVERSE EFFECTS (≥1%) **CNS:** *Extrapyramidal symptoms* (resembling Parkinson's disease), tardive dyskinesia, sedation, drowsiness, dizziness, headache, mental depression, catatonic-like state, impaired thermoregulation, grand mal seizures. **CV:** Tachycardia, hypertension, hypotension. **GI:** Dry mouth, nausea, epigastric pain, constipation, fecal impaction, cholecystic jaundice. **Urogenital:** Urinary retention, polyuria, inhibition of ejaculation. **Hematologic:** Transient leukopenia, agranulocytosis. **Skin:** Contact dermatitis. **Body as a Whole:** Peripheral edema. **Special Senses:** Nasal congestion, blurred vision, increased intraocular pressure, *photosensitivity*. **Endocrine:** Hyperprolactinemia.

INTERACTIONS Drug: Alcohol and other CNS DEPRESSANTS may potentiate depressive effects; decreases seizure threshold, may need to adjust dosage of ANTICONVULSANTS. **Herbal: Kava-kava** may increase risk and severity of dystonic reactions.

PHARMACOKINETICS Absorption: HCl is readily absorbed PO and IM; decanoate, enanthate have delayed IM absorption. **Onset:** 1 h HCl; 24–72 h decanoate, enanthate. **Peak:** 0.5 h PO; 1.5–2 h IM HCl. **Duration:** 6–8 h HCl; 1–6 wk decanoate; 2–4 wk enanthate. **Distribution:** Crosses blood–brain barrier and placenta. **Metabolism:** Metabolized in liver. **Half-Life:** 15 h HCl; 3.6 d enanthate; 7–10 d decanoate.

NURSING IMPLICATIONS

Assessment & Drug Effects

- Report immediately onset of mental depression and extrapyramidal symptoms. Both occur frequently, particularly with long-acting forms (decanoate and enanthate).
- Be alert for appearance of acute dystonia (see Appendix F). Symptoms can be controlled by reducing dosage or by adding an antiparkinsonism drug such as benztropine.
- Be alert for red, dry, hot skin; full, bounding pulse, dilated pupils, dyspnea, mental confusion, elevated BP, temperature over 40.6° C (105° F). Inform physician and institute measures to reduce body temperature rapidly. Extended exposure to high environmental temperature, to sun's rays, or to a high fever places the patient taking this drug at risk for heat stroke.
- Lab tests: Monitor kidney function in patients on long-term treatment. Withhold drug and notify physician if BUN is elevated (normal BUN: 10–20 mg/dL). Also perform WBC with differential, liver function tests, periodically.

- Monitor BP during early therapy. If systolic drop is more than 20 mm Hg, inform physician.
- Monitor I&O ratio and bowel elimination pattern. Check for abdominal distension and pain. Monitor for xerostomia and constipation.
- Note: Patients on large doses who undergo surgery and those with cerebrovascular, cardiac, or renal insufficiency are especially prone to hypotensive effects.

Patient & Family Education

- Do not drive or engage in potentially hazardous activities until response to drug is known.
- Do not alter dosage regimen or stop taking drug abruptly. Do not give drug to any one else.
- Seek and obtain physician approval before taking any OTC drugs.
- Be alert for adverse effects, early detection is critical because both decanoate and enanthate have a long duration of action. Inform physician promptly if following symptoms appear: Light-colored stools, changes in vision, sore throat, fever, cellulitis, rash, any interference with your willful (volitional) movements.
- Make sure to eat and drink adequately in order to prevent constipation and dry mouth.
- Be aware that it may be difficult for you to adjust to extremes in temperature. Use caution because of this possible impaired thermoregulation.
- Avoid exposure to sun; wear protective clothing and cover exposed skin surfaces with sun screen lotion (SPF above 12).
- Avoid alcohol while on fluphenazine therapy.
- Note: Fluphenazine may discolor urine pink to red or reddish brown.
- Do not breast feed while taking this drug without consulting physician.
- Periodic ophthalmologic exams are recommended.

FLURANDRENOLIDE

(flure-an-dren′oh-lide)

Cordran, Cordran SP, Drenison ♣

Classifications: SKIN AND MUCOUS MEMBRANE AGENT; ANTIINFLAMMATORY; ADRENAL CORTICOSTEROID

Prototype: Hydrocortisone

Pregnancy Category: C

AVAILABILITY 0.025% ointment, cream; 0.05% ointment, cream, lotion

See Appendix A-4.

FLURAZEPAM HYDROCHLORIDE

(flure-az′e-pam)

Apo-Flurazepam ♣, Dalmane, Durapam, Novoflupam ♣

Classifications: CENTRAL NERVOUS SYSTEM AGENT; ANXIOLYTIC; SEDATIVE-HYPNOTIC; BENZODIAZEPINE

Prototype: Lorazepam

Pregnancy Category: X

Controlled Substance: Schedule IV

AVAILABILITY 15 mg, 30 mg capsules

ACTIONS Benzodiazepine derivative, with hypnotic activity equal to or greater than that produced by barbiturates or chloral hydrate. Mode and site of action not known; appears to act at limbic and subcortical levels of CNS to produce sedation, skeletal muscle relaxation, and anticonvulsant effects.

THERAPEUTIC EFFECTS Reduces sleep induction time; produces marked reduction of stage 4 sleep (deepest sleep stage) while at the same time increasing duration of total sleep time.

USES Hypnotic in management of all kinds of insomnia (e.g., difficulty in falling asleep, frequent nocturnal awakening or early morning awakening or both). Also for treatment of poor sleeping habits.

CONTRAINDICATIONS Prolonged administration; sleep apnea; intermittent porphyria; acute narrow-angle glaucoma; children <15 y; pregnancy (category X), lactation.
CAUTIOUS USE Impaired renal or hepatic function; mental depression, psychoses, history of suicidal tendencies, addiction-prone individuals; older adult or debilitated patients; COPD.

ROUTE & DOSAGE

Sedative, Hypnotic
Adult: **PO** ≥*15 y,* 15–30 mg h.s.
Geriatric: **PO** 15 mg h.s.

ADMINISTRATION

Oral
- Give once patient is in bed and ready to fall asleep.
- Store in light-resistant container with childproof cap at 15°–30° C (59°–86° F) unless otherwise specified.

ADVERSE EFFECTS (≥1%) **CNS:** *Residual sedation, drowsiness,* lightheadedness, dizziness, ataxia, headache, nervousness, apprehension, talkativeness, irritability, depression, hallucinations, nightmares, confusion, paradoxic reactions: excitement, euphoria, hyperactivity, disorientation, coma (overdosage). **Special Senses:** Blurred vision, burning eyes. **GI:** Heartburn, nausea, vomiting, diarrhea, abdominal pain. **Body as a Whole:** Immediate allergic reaction, hypotension, granulocytopenia (rare), jaundice (rare).

DIAGNOSTIC TEST INTERFERENCE Flurazepam may increase serum levels of ***total and direct bilirubin, alkaline phosphatase, AST,*** and ***ALT.*** False-negative ***urine glucose*** reactions may occur with ***Clinistix*** and ***Diastix;*** no effect with ***TesTape.***

INTERACTIONS Drug: Alcohol, CNS DEPRESSANTS, ANTICONVULSANTS potentiate CNS depression; **cimetidine, disulfiram** may increase flurazepam levels, thus increasing its toxicity. **Herbal: Kava-kava, valerian** may potentiate sedation.

PHARMACOKINETICS Absorption: Readily absorbed from GI tract. **Onset:** 15–45 min. **Duration:** 7–8 h. **Distribution:** Crosses blood–brain barrier and placenta; distributed into breast milk. **Metabolism:** Metabolized in liver to active metabolites. **Elimination:** Excreted primarily in urine. **Half-Life:** 47–100 h.

NURSING IMPLICATIONS

Assessment & Drug Effects
- Monitor effectiveness. Hypnotic effect is apparent on second or third night of consecutive use and continues 1–2 nights after drug is stopped (drug has a long half-life).
- Supervise ambulation. Residual sedation and drowsiness are relatively common. Excessive drowsiness, ataxia, vertigo, and falling occur more frequently in older adults or debilitated patients.
- Monitor drug ingestion if patient has a history of drug abuse. Prolonged use of large doses can result in psychic and physical dependence.

- Lab tests: Obtain blood counts and liver and kidney function with repeated use.
- Be aware that withdrawal symptoms have occurred 3 d after abrupt discontinuation after prolonged use and include worsening of insomnia, dizziness, blurred vision, anorexia, GI upset, nasal congestion, paresthesias.

Patient & Family Education

- Avoid potentially hazardous activities until response to drug is known.
- Avoid alcohol. Concurrent ingestion with flurazepam intensifies CNS depressant effects; symptoms may occur even when alcohol is ingested as long as 10 h after last flurazepam dose.
- Be aware of the possible additive depressant effects when drug is combined with barbiturates, tranquilizers, or other CNS depressants.
- Do not change dose intervals or dosage. Do not take for a self-diagnosed problem.
- Ask physician about the desirability of discontinuing the drug if you become or intend to become pregnant during therapy.
- Note: Prolonged use of this hypnotic is inadvisable because insomnia is usually transient.
- Do not breast feed while taking this drug.

FLURBIPROFEN SODIUM

(flure-bi′proe-fen)

Ansaid, Ocufen

Classifications: CENTRAL NERVOUS SYSTEM AGENT; ANALGESIC; NSAID; COX 1; ANTIPYRETIC

Prototype: Ibuprofen

Pregnancy Category: C

AVAILABILITY 50 mg, 100 mg tablets; 0.03% ophthalmic solution

ACTIONS Inhibits prostaglandin synthesis including in the conjunctiva and uvea; structurally and pharmacologically related to ibuprofen. When administered prophylactically, ocular flurbiprofen reduces miosis, permitting maintenance of drug-induced mydriasis during surgical procedures. Produces no significant effect on IOP.

THERAPEUTIC EFFECTS An antiinflammatory, nonsteroidal analgesic. Also inhibits migration of leukocytes into inflamed tissues, depresses monocyte function, and may inhibit platelet aggregation.

USES Inhibition of intraoperative miosis; arthritis and other inflammatory diseases; mild to moderate pain.

UNLABELED USES Management of postoperative ocular inflammation, prevention of postcystoid macular edema.

CONTRAINDICATIONS Epithelial herpes simplex keratitis. Safety during pregnancy (category C), lactation, or in children is not established. For contraindications to oral use, see ibuprofen.

CAUTIOUS USE Concomitant use with other NSAIDs; patient who may be adversely affected by prolonged bleeding time; patient in whom asthma, rhinitis, or urticaria is precipitated by aspirin or other NSAIDs.

ROUTE & DOSAGE

Inflammatory Disease

Adult: **PO** 200–300 mg/d in 2–4 divided doses (max: 300 mg/d)

Mild-to-Moderate Pain

Adult: **PO** 50–100 mg q6–8h

Inhibition of Intraoperative Miosis

Adult: **Topical** 1 drop in eye approximately q30min beginning 2 h before surgery for a total of 4 drops per affected eye

ADMINISTRATION

Topical

- Instill ophthalmic preparation with great care to avoid contamination of solution. Do not touch eye surface with dropper.

Oral

- Use the 300 mg dose for initiation of therapy or for acute exacerbations of disease.
- Store at 15°–30° C (59°–86° F) in tight, light-resistant container.

ADVERSE EFFECTS (≥1%) **Special Senses:** *Mild ocular stinging,* burning, itching, or foreign body sensation (transient). **Other:** Slowed corneal healing; increased bleeding time. **For adverse effects to oral preparations, see ibuprofen.**

INTERACTIONS Drug: ORAL ANTICOAGULANTS, **heparin** may prolong bleeding time; actions and side effects of both flurbiprofen and **phenytoin,** SULFONYLUREAS, or SULFONAMIDES may be potentiated. **Herbal: Feverfew, garlic, ginger, gingko** may increase bleeding potential.

PHARMACOKINETICS Absorption: 80% absorbed from GI tract. **Onset:** 2 h. **Peak:** 2 h. **Duration:** 6–8 h. **Distribution:** Small amounts distributed into breast milk. **Metabolism:** Metabolized in liver. **Elimination:** Excreted primarily in urine; some biliary excretion. **Half-Life:** 5 h.

NURSING IMPLICATIONS

Assessment & Drug Effects

- Observe patients with history of cardiac decompensation closely for evidence of fluid retention and edema.
- Lab tests: Baseline and periodic evaluations of Hgb, renal and hepatic function, and auditory and ophthalmologic examinations are recommended in patients receiving prolonged or high-dose therapy.
- Monitor for GI distress and S&S of GI bleeding.
- Note: Symptoms of acute toxicity in children include apnea, cyanosis, response only to painful stimuli, dizziness, and nystagmus.

Patient & Family Education

- Report ocular irritation that persists after flurbiprofen use during surgery (tearing, dry eye sensation, dull eye pain, photophobia) to physician.
- Be alert for bleeding tendency and report unexplained bleeding, prolongation of bleeding time, or bruises. Minor systemic absorption may temporarily increase bleeding time.
- Notify physician immediately of passage of dark tarry stools, "coffee ground" emesis, frankly bloody emesis, or other GI distress, as well as blood or protein in urine, and onset of skin rash, pruritus, jaundice.
- Do not drive or engage in potentially hazardous activities until response to the drug is known.
- Do not self-medicate with OTC drugs without consulting physician.
- Avoid alcohol and NSAIDS unless otherwise advised by physician. Concurrent use may increase risk of GI ulceration and bleeding tendencies.
- Do not breast feed while taking this drug without consulting physician.

FLUTAMIDE

(flu′ta-mide)

Eulexin

Classifications: ANTINEOPLASTIC; ANTIANDROGEN

Pregnancy Category: D

F

AVAILABILITY 125 mg capsules

ACTIONS Nonsteroidal, nonhormonal, antiandrogenic that inhibits androgen uptake or binding of androgen to target tissues (i.e., prostatic cancer cells).

THERAPEUTIC EFFECTS Interferes with the binding of both testosterone and dihydrotestosterone to target tissue (i.e., prostate cancer cells).

USES In combination with luteinizing hormone-releasing hormone agonists (i.e., leuprolide) or castration for early stage and metastatic prostate cancer.

CONTRAINDICATIONS Hypersensitivity to flutamide; severe liver impairment if ALT is equal to twice the normal value; pregnancy (category D), lactation.

ROUTE & DOSAGE

Prostate Cancer

Adult: **PO** 250 mg (2 caps) q8h

ADMINISTRATION

Oral

- Use with caution in patients with severe hepatic impairment.
- Store at 2°–30° C (36°–86° F) in a tightly closed, light-resistant container.

ADVERSE EFFECTS (≥1%) **CNS:** Drowsiness, confusion, depression, anxiety, nervousness. **GI:** Diarrhea, nausea, vomiting, anorexia, hepatitis, cholestatic jaundice, encephalopathy, hepatic necrosis, acute hepatic failure, may increase ALT, AST, bilirubin. **Urogenital:** *Hot flashes, loss of libido, impotence.* **Hematologic:** Anemia, leukopenia, thrombocytopenia. **Skin:** Rash. **Body as a Whole:** Edema. **Endocrine:** Gynecomastia, galactorrhea.

INTERACTIONS Drug: may increase INR in patients on **warfarin.**

PHARMACOKINETICS Absorption: Readily absorbed from GI tract. **Onset:** Antiandrogenic activity 2.2 h; symptomatic relief 2–4 wk. **Duration:** 3 mo–2.5 y, with an average of 10.5 mo. **Metabolism:** Metabolized in liver to at least 10 different metabolites; the major metabolite, 2-hydroxyflutamide (SCH-16423), is an alpha-hydroxylated derivative that is biologically active. **Elimination:** 98% excreted in urine. **Half-Life:** 5–6 h.

NURSING IMPLICATIONS

Assessment & Drug Effects

- Monitor therapeutic response with acid and alkaline phosphatase tests, bone and liver scans, chest x-ray, and physical exam.
- Monitor for symptomatic relief of bone pain.
- Assess for development of gynecomastia and galactorrhea; if these become bothersome, dosage reduction may be warranted.
- Lab tests: Monitor liver function and serum bilirubin periodically.
- Monitor for and report development of a lupus-like syndrome.

Patient & Family Education

- Be aware of potential adverse effects of therapy.
- Notify physician immediately of the following: Pain in upper abdomen, yellowing of skin and eyes, dark urine, respiratory problems, rashes on face, difficulty urinating, sore throat, fever, chills.
- Do not breast feed while taking this drug.

FLUTICASONE

(flu-ti-ca′sone)

Flonase, Flovent, Flovent HFA, Cutivate

Classifications: SKIN AND MUCOUS MEMBRANE AGENT; ANTIINFLAMMATORY; CORTICOSTEROID

Prototype: Hydrocortisone

Pregnancy Category: C

AVAILABILITY 44 mcg, 110 mcg, 220 mcg aerosol; 0.05%, 0.005% cream; 0.005% ointment

See Appendixes A-3, A-4.

FLUVASTATIN

(flu-vah-stat′in)

Lescol

Classifications: CARDIOVASCULAR AGENT; ANTILIPEMIC; HMG-COA REDUCTASE INHIBITOR (STATIN)

Prototype: Lovastatin

Pregnancy Category: X

AVAILABILITY 20 mg, 40 mg capsules

ACTIONS Inhibits therapeutic reductase 3-hydroxy-3-methylglutaryl coenzyme A (HMG-CoA), which is essential to hepatic production of cholesterol. Cholesterol-lowering effect triggers induction of LDL receptors, which promotes removal of LDL and VLDL remnants (precursors of LDL) from plasma.

THERAPEUTIC EFFECTS Results in an increase in plasma HDL concentration. HDLs collect excess cholesterol from body cells and transport it to the liver for excretion.

USES Adjunct to diet for the reduction of elevated total LDL cholesterol in patients with primary hypercholesterolemia (Types IIa and IIb).

UNLABELED USES Other types of hyperlipidemias.

CONTRAINDICATIONS Hypersensitivity to fluvastatin, lovastatin, pravastatin, or simvastatin; active liver disease or unexplained persistent elevated liver function tests; pregnancy (category X), lactation.

CAUTIOUS USE Patients who consume substantial quantities of alcohol; history of liver disease; renal impairment.

ROUTE & DOSAGE

Hypercholesterolemia
Adult: **PO** 20 mg h.s., may increase up to 80 mg/d in 1–2 doses

ADMINISTRATION

Oral

- Give at bedtime.
- Separate doses of this drug and bile-acid resin (e.g., cholestyramine) by at least 2 h when given concomitantly.
- Note: Dosage adjustments may be required in patients with significant renal or hepatic impairment.
- Store at room temperature, 15°–30° C (59°–86° F).

ADVERSE EFFECTS (≥1%) **CNS:** Headache. **GI:** Dyspepsia. **Skin:** Rash.

INTERACTIONS Drug: May increase risk of bleeding with **warfarin; cholestyramine** decreases fluvastatin absorption; **rifampin** increases metabolism of fluvastatin; may increase risk of myopathy and rhabdomyolysis with **gemfibrozil, fenofibrate, clofibrate.**

PHARMACOKINETICS Absorption: Readily absorbed from GI tract; about 24% reaches systemic circulation after first-pass metabolism **Onset:** 3–6 wk. **Peak:** Serum level 0.5–1 h. **Distribution:** 98% protein bound; distributed into breast milk. **Metabolism:** Metabolized in liver. **Elimination:** 95% excreted in bile; 5% excreted in urine. **Half-Life:** 0.5–1 h.

F

NURSING IMPLICATIONS

Assessment & Drug Effects

- Lab tests: Monitor lipoprotein levels; maximal lipid-lowering effect occurs in 4–6 wk. Monitor serum transaminase and CPK levels every 3–4 mo for the first year and periodically thereafter.
- Monitor PT & INR in patients on concurrent warfarin therapy; PT & INR may be prolonged.

Patient & Family Education

- Take fluvastatin at bedtime.
- Be alert & report signs of bleeding immediately when also taking warfarin.
- Notify physician immediately of the following: Fever; rash; muscle pain, weakness, tenderness, or cramping.
- Reduce or eliminate alcohol consumption while taking fluvastatin.
- Do not breast feed while taking this drug.

FLUVOXAMINE

(flu-vox'a-meen)

Luvox

Classifications: CENTRAL NERVOUS SYSTEM (CNS) AGENT; PSYCHOTHERAPEUTIC AGENT; SELECTIVE SEROTONIN REUPTAKE INHIBITOR (SSRI)

Prototype: Fluoxetine

Pregnancy Category: B

AVAILABILITY 25 mg, 50 mg, 100 mg tablets

ACTIONS Antidepressant with potent, selective, inhibitory activity on neuronal (5-HT) serotonin reuptake (SSRI); structurally unrelated to TCAs. Compared with TCAs, shows fewer anticholinergenic effects and no severe cardiovascular effects.

THERAPEUTIC EFFECTS Effective as an antidepressant and for control of obsessive-compulsive disorders.

USES Treatment of depression and obsessive-compulsive disorders.

UNLABELED USES Chronic tension-type headaches, panic attacks.

CONTRAINDICATIONS Hypersensitivity to fluvoxamine or fluoxetine; children <8 y.

CAUTIOUS USE Pregnancy (category B), lactation, liver disease, renal impairment, abrupt discontinuation; cardiac disease, dehydration, hyponatremia, older adults, ECT, seizure disorders, seizures, suicidal ideation, tobacco smoking.

ROUTE & DOSAGE

Depression, Obsessive-Compulsive Disorder

Adult: **PO** Start with 50 mg q.d., may increase slowly up to 300 mg/d given q.h.s. or divided b.i.d.
Child: **PO** *8–11 y,* Start with 25 mg q.h.s., may increase by 25 mg q4–7d (max: 200 mg/d in divided doses)

ADMINISTRATION

Oral

- Give starting doses at bedtime to improve tolerance to nausea and vomiting; both are common early in therapy.
- Store at room temperature, 15°–30° C (59°–86° F), away from moisture and light.

ADVERSE EFFECTS (≥1%) **CNS:** *Somnolence, headache, agitation, insomnia, dizziness,* seizures. **CV:** Orthostatic hypotension, slight bradycardia. **GI:** *Nausea, vomiting, dry mouth, constipation, anorexia.* **Urogenital:** Sexual dysfunction. **Skin:** Stevens-Johnson syndrome, toxic epidermal necrolysis (rare).

DIAGNOSTIC TEST INTERFERENCE ***Gamma-glutamyl transferase*** increased by more than 3-fold following 3 wk of therapy.

INTERACTIONS Drug: Fluvoxamine has been shown to significantly increase plasma levels of **amitriptyline, clomipramine,** and other TRICYCLIC ANTIDEPRESSANTS to mildly increase levels of their metabolites. May antagonize the blood pressure-lowering effects of **atenolol** and other BETA BLOCKERS. May increase levels and toxicity of **carbamazepine, mexiletine.** May increase **lithium** levels causing neurotoxicity, **serotonin** syndrome, somnolence, and mania. One report of increased **theophylline** levels with toxicity. Increases prothrombin time in patients on **warfarin;** increased ergotamine toxicity with **dihydroergotamine, ergotamine. Herbal: Melatonin** may increase and prolong drowsiness; **St. John's wort** may cause **serotonin** syndrome.

PHARMACOKINETICS Absorption: Almost completely absorbed from GI tract. **Onset:** 4–7 d. **Distribution:** Approximately 77% bound to plasma proteins; excreted in human breast milk but in an amount that poses little risk to the nursing infant. **Metabolism:** Metabolized in liver. **Elimination:** Completely excreted in urine. **Half-Life:** 16–24 h.

NURSING IMPLICATIONS

Assessment & Drug Effects

- Monitor for significant nausea and vomiting, especially during initial therapy.
- Monitor for worsening of depression or emergence of suicidal ideations.
- Assess safety; drowsiness and dizziness are common adverse effects.
- Monitor PT and INR carefully with concurrent warfarin therapy; adjust warfarin as needed.

Patient & Family Education

- Note: Nausea and vomiting are common in early therapy. Notify physician if these adverse effects last more than a few days.
- Exercise caution with hazardous activity until response to the drug is known.
- Do not breast feed while taking this drug without consulting physician.

FOLIC ACID (VITAMIN B_9, PTEROYLGLUTAMIC ACID)

(fol′ic)

Apo-Folic ♣, Folacin, Folvite, Novofolacid ♣

FOLATE SODIUM

Folvite Sodium

Classification: VITAMIN B_9

Pregnancy Category: A

AVAILABILITY 0.4 mg, 0.8 mg, 1 mg tablets; 5 mg/mL injection

ACTIONS Vitamin B complex essential for nucleoprotein synthesis and maintenance of normal erythropoiesis. Acts against folic acid deficiency that impairs thymidylate synthesis and results in production of defective DNA that leads to

F

megaloblast formation and arrest of bone marrow maturation.

THERAPEUTIC EFFECTS Stimulates production of RBCs, WBCs, and platelets in patients with megaloblastic anemias. Include improved symptoms of glossitis, diarrhea, constipation, weight loss, irritability, fatigue, restless legs, diffuse muscular pain, insomnia, forgetfulness, mental depression, pallor.

USES Folate deficiency, macrocytic anemia, and megaloblastic anemias associated with malabsorption syndromes, alcoholism, primary liver disease, inadequate dietary intake, pregnancy, infancy, and childhood.

CONTRAINDICATIONS Folic acid-alone for pernicious anemia or other vitamin B_{12} deficiency states; normocytic, refractory, aplastic, or undiagnosed anemia.

CAUTIOUS USE Pregnancy (category A), lactation.

ROUTE & DOSAGE

Therapeutic

Adult: **PO/IM/SC/IV** ≤1 mg/d
Child: **PO/IM/SC/IV** ≤1 mg/d

Maintenance

Adult: **PO/IM/SC/IV** ≤0.4 mg/d
Child: **PO/IM/SC/IV** *<4 y,* ≤0.3 mg/d; *>4 y,* ≤0.4 mg/d
Infant: **PO/IM/SC/IV** ≤0.1 mg/d

ADMINISTRATION

Intravenous

PREPARE: **Direct/Continuous:** Given undiluted.
ADMINISTER: **Direct/Continuous:** Give over 30–60 seconds. May also add to a continuous infusion.
INCOMPATIBILITIES **Solution/additive: Doxapram.**

- Store at 15°–30° C (59°–86° F) in tightly closed containers protected from light, unless otherwise directed.

ADVERSE EFFECTS (≥1%) [Reportedly nontoxic. Slight flushing and feeling of warmth following IV administration.]

DIAGNOSTIC TEST INTERFERENCE Falsely low serum ***folate levels*** may occur with ***Lactobacillus casei assay*** in patients receiving antibiotics such as TETRACYCLINES.

INTERACTIONS **Drug: Chloramphenicol** may antagonize effects of **folate** therapy; **phenytoin** metabolism may be increased, thus decreasing its levels in **folate**-deficient patients.

PHARMACOKINETICS **Absorption:** Readily absorbed from proximal small intestine. **Peak:** 30–60 min PO. **Distribution:** Distributed to all body tissues; high concentrations in CSF; crosses placenta; distributed into breast milk. **Metabolism:** Metabolized in liver to active metabolites. **Elimination:** Small amounts eliminated in urine in folate-deficient patients; large amounts excreted in urine with high doses.

NURSING IMPLICATIONS

Assessment & Drug Effects

- Obtain a careful history of dietary intake and drug and alcohol usage prior to start of therapy. Drugs reported to cause folate deficiency include oral contraceptives, alcohol, barbiturates, methotrexate, phenytoin, primidone, and trimethoprim. Folate deficiency may also result from renal dialysis.
- Keep physician informed of patient's response to therapy.

- Monitor patients on phenytoin for subtherapeutic plasma levels.

Patient & Family Education

- Remain under close medical supervision while taking folic acid therapy. Adjustment of maintenance dose should be made if there is threat of relapse.
- Do not breast feed while taking this drug without consulting physician.

FONDAPARINUX SODIUM

(fon-da-par'i-nux)

Arixtra

Classifications: BLOOD FORMERS, COAGULATORS & ANTICOAGULANTS; ANTICOAGULANT

Prototype: Enoxaparin

Pregnancy Category: B

AVAILABILITY 2.5 mg/0.5 mL syringe

ACTIONS Fondaparinux sodium causes antithrombin III (ATIII)-mediated selective inhibition of Factor Xa. Fondaparinux selectively binds to ATIII, potentiating the innate neutralization of Factor Xa by ATIII. Neutralization of Factor Xa by fondaparinux interrupts the blood coagulation cascade, inhibiting thrombin formation and, thus, thrombus development. Fondaparinux sodium does not inactivate thrombin (activated Factor II) and has no known effect on platelet function, therefore, it rarely causes thrombocytopenia.

THERAPEUTIC EFFECTS Fondaparinux is effective in the prevention and treatment of deep-vein thrombosis. The laboratory value utilized to determine the effectiveness of the drug is the amount of anti-Xa assay expressed in mg.

USES Prophylaxis for DVT or pulmonary embolism (PE) in patients undergoing hip or knee replacement surgery; treatment of acute DVT without PE with warfarin, treatment of PE with warfarin.

CONTRAINDICATIONS Hypersensitivity to fondaparinux; active bleeding; GI bleeding; severe renal impairment with a creatinine clearance of <30 mL/min; weight <50 kg; active major bleeding; bacterial endocarditis; intramuscular administration; thrombocytopenia associated with fondaparinux. Safety and effectiveness in children have not been established.

CAUTIOUS USE Renal impairment or disease; older adult; indwelling epidural catheter; dental disease, dental work; diabetic retinopathy; diverticulitis; endocarditis, epidural anesthesia; hemophilia, heparin-induced thrombocytopenia (HIT), hepatic disease, hypertension, idiopathic thrombocytopenia purpura (ITP); inflammatory bowel disease, lumbar puncture, spinal anesthesia; stroke, surgery; thrombocytopenia, thrombolytic therapy; vaginal bleeding, menstruation; peptic ulcer disease; pregnancy (category B); bleeding disorders including a history of GI ulceration, etc., history of heparin-induced thrombocytopenia; lactation.

ROUTE & DOSAGE

DVT, Pulmonary Embolism Prophylaxis

Adult: **SC** *>50 kg* 2.5 mg q.d. starting at least 6 h postsurgery times 5–9 days

Treatment of DVT, Pulmonary Embolism

Adult: **SC** *<50 kg,* 5 mg; *50–100 kg,* 7.5 mg; *>100 kg,* 10 mg once daily × 5–9 d

Renal Impairment

Cl_{cr} 30–50 mL/min, use with caution; <30 mL/min, use is contraindicated

F

ADMINISTRATION

Subcutaneous

- Consult physician about discontinuing other agents that may enhance the risk of hemorrhage prior to initiation of fondaparinux.
- Give no sooner than 6 h after surgery.
- Adjust doses in older adults based on renal function.
- Inspect visually for particulate matter and discoloration prior to administration.
- Do not expel the air bubble from the syringe before the injection.
- Use prefilled syringe to inject into fatty tissue, alternating injection sites (e.g., between L and R abdominal wall).
- Store at 25° C (77° F); excursions permitted to 15°–30° C (59°–86° F).

ADVERSE EFFECTS (≥1%) **Body as a Whole:** Fever, edema. **CNS:** Insomnia, dizziness, confusion, headache. **CV:** Hypotension. **GI:** Nausea, constipation, vomiting, diarrhea, dyspepsia, elevated LFTs. **Endocrine:** Hypokalemia. **Hematologic:** Hemorrhage, *anemia,* hematoma. **Skin:** Irritation at injection site, rash, purpura, bullous eruption. **Urogenital:** UTI, urinary retention.

INTERACTIONS Drug: ANTICOAGULANTS, NSAIDS, **aspirin** may increase risk of bleeding. **Herbal: Feverfew, ginkgo, ginger, valerian** may potentiate bleeding.

PHARMACOKINETICS Absorption: Rapidly and completely absorbed from SC injection site. **Peak:** 2–3 h. **Distribution:** Primarily in blood. **Metabolism:** Negligible metabolism. **Elimination:** Excreted in urine. **Half-Life:** 18 h.

NURSING IMPLICATIONS

Assessment & Drug Effects

- Monitor for S&S of bleeding or hemorrhage. If noted, withhold fondaparinux and notify physician immediately.
- Monitor closely patients with epidural catheters for signs of paralysis below catheter level.
- Withhold fondaparinux and notify physician if platelet count falls below 100,000/mm^3.
- Lab tests: Monitor baseline and periodic renal function rests; periodic CBC including platelet count, serum creatinine level, and stool occult blood tests. (Note: PT and aPTT are relatively insensitive measures of fondaparinux activity and unsuitable for monitoring.)

Patient & Family Education

- Report any of the following to a health care provider: signs of unexplained bleeding such as: pink, red, or dark brown urine; red or dark brown vomitus; bleeding gums or bloody sputum; dark, tarry stools.
- Learn proper injection technique if you are to self-administer this drug.
- Do not take any OTC drugs without first consulting physician.
- Do not breast feed while taking this drug without consulting physician.

FORMOTEROL FUMARATE

(for-mo-ter'ol)

Foradil Aerolizer

Classifications: AUTONOMIC NERVOUS SYSTEM AGENT; BETA-ADRENERGIC AGONIST (SYMPATHOMIMETIC); BRONCHODILATOR

Prototype: Albuterol

Pregnancy Category: C

AVAILABILITY 12 mcg inhalation capsules

ACTIONS Long-acting selective beta$_2$-adrenergic receptor agonist. Stimulates production of intracellular cyclic AMP, which causes relaxation of bronchial smooth muscle. Also inhibits release of mediators of immediate hypersensitivity (e.g., histamine and leukotrienes) from mast cells in the lung.
THERAPEUTIC EFFECTS Acts locally in lung as a bronchodilator; prevents bronchoconstriction that occurs during an asthma attack.

USES Treatment of asthma, prevention of exercise induced asthma, prevention of bronchospasm in COPD.
UNLABELED USES Bronchitis.

CONTRAINDICATIONS Hypersensitivity to formoterol; significantly worsening or acutely deteriorating asthma; severe asthmatic attacks; paradoxical bronchospasm; pregnancy (category C); lactation. Safety and efficiency in children <5 y are not established.
CAUTIOUS USE Cardiovascular disorders (especially coronary insufficiency, cardiac arrhythmias, and hypertension); convulsive disorders; thyrotoxicosis; heightened responsiveness to sympathomimetic amines; diabetes mellitus.

ROUTE & DOSAGE

Treatment of Asthma, COPD
Adult/Child: **Inhaled** ≥5 y, Inhale contents of 1 capsule q12h

Prevention of Exercise-Induced Asthma
Adult/Child: **Inhaled** ≥12 y, Inhale contents of 1 capsule at least 15 min before exercise, do not repeat for at least 12 h

ADMINISTRATION

Oral Inhalation
- Remove capsule from blister IMMEDIATELY before use.
- Avoid exposing capsules to moisture.
- Give capsules only by the oral inhalation route and only by using the Aerolizer Inhaler™. Review use of the Aerolizer Inhaler in *Patient Instructions for Use* provided by manufacturer. Do not use a spacer with the Aerolizer.
- Instruct patient not to swallow capsule and not to exhale into the Aerolizer.
- Patients who have been taking the inhaled form, short-acting beta$_2$-agonists regularly (e.g., 3–4 times a day) are usually instructed to use these drugs ONLY for symptomatic relief of acute asthma symptoms. Check with physician.
- Store capsules in the blister at 20°–25° C (86°–77° F).

ADVERSE EFFECTS (≥1%) **Body as a Whole:** *Viral infections,* chest infection, chest pain, fatigue. **CNS:** Headache, tremor, dizziness, insomnia. **GI:** Abdominal pain, dyspepsia, nausea. **Respiratory:** Pharyngitis, bronchitis, dyspnea, tonsillitis, dysphonia, fatal exacerbation of asthma. **Skin:** Rash.

INTERACTIONS Drug: Effects may be antagonized by NON-SELECTIVE BETA BLOCKERS; XANTHINES, STEROIDS; DIURETICS may potentiate hypokalemia.

PHARMACOKINETICS Absorption: Rapidly absorbed into plasma after oral inhalation. **Onset:** 1–3 min. **Peak:** 1–3 h. **Metabolism:** Metabolized by glucuronidation in the liver. **Elimination:** 60% excreted in urine, 33% in feces. **Half-Life:** 10 h.

F

NURSING IMPLICATIONS

Assessment & Drug Effects

- Monitor cardiovascular status with periodic ECG, BP, and HR determinations.
- Withhold drug and notify physician immediately of S&S of bronchospasm.
- Lab tests: Monitor serum potassium and blood glucose periodically.
- Monitor diabetics closely for loss of glycemic control.

Patient & Family Education

- Do not take this drug more frequently than every 12 h.
- Use a short-acting inhaler if symptoms develop between doses of formoterol.
- Seek medical care immediately if a previously effective dosage regimen fails to provide the usual response, or if swelling about the face and neck and difficulty breathing develop.
- Report any of the following immediately to the physician: Rash, hives, palpitations, chest pain, rapid heart rate, tremor or nervousness.
- Note to diabetics: Monitor blood glucose levels carefully since hyperglycemia is a possible adverse reaction.
- Do not breast feed while taking this drug.

FOSAMPRENAVIR CALCIUM

(fos-am-pre′na-vir)
Lexiva
Classifications: ANTI-INFECTIVE; ANTIRETROVIRAL AGENT; PROTEASE INHIBITOR
Prototype: Saquinavir
Pregnancy Category: C

AVAILABILITY 700 mg tablet

ACTIONS Fosamprenavir is a prodrug rapidly converted to amprenavir. Amprenavir is an HIV-1 protease inhibitor that binds to the active site of HIV-1 protease. Binding prevents processing of viral Gag and Gag-Pol polyprotein precursors, resulting in formation of immature noninfectious viral particles.
THERAPEUTIC EFFECTS Inhibits normal replication of the HIV virus rending the virus noninfectious.

USES Treatment of HIV infection in combination with other antiretroviral agents.

CONTRAINDICATIONS Hypersensitivity to any of the components of this product or to amprenavir; ergot derivatives, pimozide, midazolam, triazolam; coadministration of ritonavir, flecainide, and propafenone; severe hepatic impairment; pregnancy (category C), lactation. Safety and efficacy in pediatrics and patients >65 y have not been established.
CAUTIOUS USE Sulfa allergy; mild to moderate hepatic impairment; concurrent administration of amiodarone, astemizole, bepridil, cisapride, dihydroergotamine, ergotamine, flecainide, itraconazole, ketoconazole, lidocaine (systemic), midazolam, pimozide, propafenone, quinidine, triazolam, and tricyclic antidepressants; hepatic impairment; hemophilia.

ROUTE & DOSAGE

HIV Infection

Adult: **PO** 700 mg b.i.d. in combination with 100 mg ritonavir b.i.d. (preferred if previously on a protease inhibitor); or 1400 mg b.i.d.; or 1400 mg q.d. in combination with 200 mg ritonavir q.d.

Hepatic Impairment

Mild to Moderate Impairment
Reduce dose to 700 mg b.i.d. without ritonavir; not recommended in severe hepatic impairment

ADMINISTRATION

Oral

- Ensure that patient is not receiving drugs contraindicated with fosamprenavir.
- Store at 15°–30° C (59°–86° F) in a tightly closed container.

ADVERSE EFFECTS (≥1%) **Body as a Whole:** Fatigue. **CNS:** *Oral/perioral paresthesia,* peripheral paresthesia, depression, mood disorders. **GI:** *Nausea, vomiting, diarrhea,* abdominal pain, taste disorders, increased triglycerides, and hyperglycemia. **Skin:** *Rash,* pruritus, Stevens-Johnson Syndrome.

INTERACTIONS Note: Interaction profile can be significantly affected by coadministration with **ritonavir. Drug:** Administration with **amiodarone, astemizole, bepridil, cisapride, dihydroergotamine, ergotamine, flecainide, itraconazole, ketoconazole, lidocaine, midazolam, pimozide, propafenone, quinidine, triazolam,** and TRICYCLIC ANTIDEPRESSANTS may cause life-threatening reactions; **rifampin, rifabutin,** ORAL CONTRACEPTIVES, **phenobarbital, phenytoin, carbamazepine** decrease **amprenavir** concentrations; **amprenavir** may increase **dihydroergotamine, ergotamine, sildenafil** concentrations and toxicity; **amprenavir** may decrease **methadone** levels; monitor INR with **warfarin;** increased risk of myopathy and rhabdomyolysis with **lovastatin, simvastatin;** may decrease antiviral effectiveness of **delavirdine. Herbal: St. John's wort** may decrease antiretroviral activity.

PHARMACOKINETICS Absorption: Prodrug is rapidly hydrolyzed to amprenavir (active component) by gut enzymes during absorption. **Peak:** 2.5 h. **Metabolism:** Metabolized in liver by CYP3A4. **Elimination:** 14% excreted in urine, 75% excreted in feces. **Half-Life:** 7.7 h.

NURSING IMPLICATIONS

Assessment & Drug Effects

- Ensure that patient has provided a complete list of all prescription, nonprescription, or herbal drugs being used.
- Monitor closely diabetics for loss of glycemic control.
- Monitor males taking PDE5 inhibitors for erectile dysfunction for adverse events including hypotension, visual changes, and priapism. Report promptly.
- Lab test: Baseline and periodic LFTs; periodic lipid profile; periodic blood glucose.

Patient & Family Education

- If you miss a dose by >4 h, wait and take the next dose at the regular time.
- Do not take other prescription, nonprescription, or herbal drugs without consulting physician.
- Monitor blood glucose more often than usual if diabetic.
- To prevent pregnancy, use a barrier contraceptive in addition to hormonal contraception.
- Do not breast feed while taking this drug.

F

FOSCARNET

(fos′car-net)

Foscavir

Classifications: ANTIINFECTIVE; ANTIVIRAL

Prototype: Acyclovir

Pregnancy Category: C

AVAILABILITY 24 mg/mL injection

ACTIONS Inhibits the replication of all known herpes viruses in vitro.

THERAPEUTIC EFFECTS Acts against cytomegalovirus (CMV), herpes simplex virus types 1 and 2 (HSV-1, HSV-2), human herpesvirus 6 (HHV-6), Epstein-Barr virus (EBV), and varicella-zoster virus (VZV).

USES CMV retinitis, mucocutaneous HSV, acyclovir-resistant HSV in immunocompromised patients.

UNLABELED USES Other CMV infections, herpes zoster infections in AIDS patients.

CONTRAINDICATIONS Hypersensitivity to foscarnet.

CAUTIOUS USE Kidney function impairment, mineral and electrolyte imbalances, seizures, older adults; pregnancy (category C), lactation. Safety and efficacy in children are not established.

ROUTE & DOSAGE

CMV Retinitis

Adult: **IV Induction** 60 mg/kg infused over 1 h q8h for 2–3 wk; induction may be repeated if relapse occurs during maintenance therapy **Alternate Induction Therapies** 100 mg/kg q12h for 2–3 wk or 20–30 mg/kg infused over 30 min followed by a continuous infusion of 180–230 mg/kg/d for 2–3 wk **Maintenance Dose** 90–120 mg/kg/d infused over 2 h

Herpes Simplex Infections in AIDS

Adult: **IV** 40–60 mg/kg q8h for 2–3 wk, may be followed by 50 mg/kg/d for 5–7 d/wk for up to 15 wk

Acyclovir-Resistant HSV in Immunocompromised Patients

Adult: **IV** 40 mg/kg q8–12h for up to 3 wk or until lesions heal

Renal Impairment

See package insert

ADMINISTRATION

Note: Dose must be adjusted for renal insufficiency. See package insert for specific dosing adjustment.

Intravenous

PREPARE: **Direct:** Given undiluted (24 mg/mL) through a central line. For peripheral infusion, dilute to 12 mg/mL with D5W or NS. Do not give other IV solution or drug through the same catheter with foscarnet.

ADMINISTER: **Direct:** Give at a constant rate not to exceed 1 mg/kg/min over the specified period of infusion with an infusion pump. Do not increase the rate of infusion or shorten the specified interval between doses. ▪ Use prepared IV solutions within 24 h.

INCOMPATIBILITIES **Solution/additive:** **Ringer's lactate, acyclovir, amphotericin B, calcium, co-trimoxazole, diazepam, digoxin, diphenhydramine, dobutamine, droperidol, ganciclovir, haloperidol, leucovorin, lorazepam, midazolam, pentamidine, phenytoin, prochlorperazine, promethazine, trimetrexate, vancomycin.** **Y-site:** **Acyclovir, amphotericin B, calcium, co-trimoxazole, diazepam, digoxin, diphenhy-**

dramine, dobutamine, droperidol, ganciclovir, haloperidol, leucovorin, lorazepam, midazolam, pentamidine, phenytoin, prochlorperazine, promethazine, trimetrexate, vancomycin.

- Prehydrate and continue daily hydration with 2.5 L of NS to reduce nephrotoxicity.
- Store according to manufacturer's directions.

ADVERSE EFFECTS (≥1%) **CV:** Thrombophlebitis if infused through a peripheral vein. **CNS:** Tremor, muscle twitching, headache, weakness, fatigue, confusion, anxiety. **Endocrine:** *Hyperphosphatemia,* hypophosphatemia, hypocalcemia. **GI:** Nausea, vomiting, diarrhea. **Urogenital:** Penile ulceration. **Hematologic:** *Anemia,* leukopenia, thrombocytopenia. **Renal:** *Nephrotoxicity* (acute renal failure, tubular necrosis). **Skin:** Fixed drug eruption, rash.

DIAGNOSTIC TEST INTERFERENCE May cause increase or decrease in serum ***calcium, phosphorus,*** and ***magnesium.*** Decreases ***Hct*** and ***Hgb.*** Increased serum ***creatinine.***

INTERACTIONS Drug: AMINOGLYCOSIDES, **amphotericin B, vancomycin** may increase risk of nephrotoxicity. **Etidronate, pamidronate, pentamidine (IV)** may exacerbate hypocalcemia.

PHARMACOKINETICS Onset: 3–7 d. **Duration:** Relapse usually occurs 3–4 wk after end of therapy. **Distribution:** 3%–28% of dose may be deposited in bone; variable penetration into CSF; crosses placenta; distributed into breast milk. **Metabolism:** Does not appear to be metabolized. **Elimination:** 73%–94% excreted in urine. **Half-Life:** 3–4 h.

NURSING IMPLICATIONS

Assessment & Drug Effects

- Monitor for cardiac arrhythmias, especially in presence of known cardiac abnormalities.
- Lab tests: Periodic CBC, serum electrolytes, serum creatinine, and creatinine clearance throughout therapy.
- Monitor serum creatinine and creatinine clearance values. Drug dose will be decreased in response to decreased clearance.
- Monitor for electrolyte imbalances.
- Monitor for seizures and take appropriate precautions.
- Question patients regarding local irritation of the penile or vulvovaginal epithelium. If either occurs, increase hydration and better personal hygiene.

Patient & Family Education

- Report perioral tingling, numbness, and paresthesia to physician immediately.
- Understand that drug is not a cure for CMV retinitis; regular ophthalmologic exams are necessary.
- Note: Good hydration is important to maintain adequate output of urine.
- Do not breast feed while taking this drug without consulting physician.

FOSFOMYCIN TROMETHAMINE

(fos-fo-my'sin)

Monurol

Classifications: ANTIINFECTIVE; ANTIBIOTIC

Prototype: Nitrofurantoin

Pregnancy Category: B

AVAILABILITY 3 g packets

ACTIONS Synthetic, broad-spectrum, bactericidal antibiotic active

F

against gram-negative and gram-positive aerobic organisms that blocks the first steps in bacterial cell wall synthesis.

THERAPEUTIC EFFECTS Acts as a bactericidal against *Enterococcus faecalis, E. faecium,* and *Escherichia coli.* In addition, it is effective against *Klebsiella, Proteus,* and *Serratia.* Indicated by improvement in cystitis symptoms within 2–3 d.

F

USES Treatment of uncomplicated UTIs in women due to susceptible strains of *E. coli* and *E. faecalis.*

CONTRAINDICATIONS Hypersensitivity to fosfomycin; lactation.

CAUTIOUS USE Pregnancy (category B). Safety and efficiency in children <12 y are not established.

ROUTE & DOSAGE

UTI

Adult: **PO** 3 g sachet dissolved in 3–4 oz of water as a single dose given once

ADMINISTRATION

Oral

- Pour entire contents of a single dose into 3–4 oz water (not hot), stir to dissolve completely, and give immediately. Drug must not be taken in the dry form.
- Store at 15°–30° C (59°–86° F).

ADVERSE EFFECTS (≥1%) **Body as a Whole:** Pain. **CNS:** *Headache,* dizziness. **GI:** *Diarrhea,* nausea, abdominal pain, dyspepsia. **Respiratory:** Rhinitis, pharyngitis. **Urogenital:** Vaginitis, dysmenorrhea.

INTERACTIONS Drug: Metoclopramide may decrease urinary excretion of fosfomycin.

PHARMACOKINETICS Absorption: Rapidly absorbed from GI tract, 37% of dose reaches systemic circulation as free acid. **Peak Urine Concentration:** 2–4 h. **Distribution:** Not protein bound, distributed to kidneys, bladder wall, prostate, and seminal vesicles. **Elimination:** Primarily excreted in urine. **Half-Life:** 5.7 h.

NURSING IMPLICATIONS

Assessment & Drug Effects

- Lab tests: Obtain urine C&S before and after therapy.

Patient & Family Education

- Do not breast feed while taking this drug.

FOSINOPRIL

(fos-in′o-pril)

Monopril

Classifications: CARDIOVASCULAR AGENT; ANGIOTENSIN-CONVERTING ENZYME (ACE) INHIBITOR; ANTIHYPERTENSIVE AGENT

Prototype: Captopril

Pregnancy Category: C (first trimester); D (second and third trimesters)

AVAILABILITY 10 mg, 20 mg, 40 mg tablets

ACTIONS Lowers BP by interrupting conversion sequences initiated by renin that lead to formation of angiotensin II, a potent vasoconstrictor. Inhibition of ACE also leads to decreased circulating aldosterone, a secretory response to angiotensin II stimulation.

THERAPEUTIC EFFECTS Lowers blood pressure and reduces peripheral arterial resistance (afterload) and improves cardiac output as well as activity tolerance.

USES Mild to moderate hypertension, CHF.

CONTRAINDICATIONS Hypersensitivity to fosinopril or any other ACE inhibitor; pregnancy [category C (first trimester), category D (second or third trimesters)], lactation.
CAUTIOUS USE Impaired kidney function, hyperkalemia, or surgery and anesthesia. Safety in children is not established.

ROUTE & DOSAGE

Hypertension, CHF
Adult: **PO** 5–40 mg once/d (max: 80 mg/d)

ADMINISTRATION

Oral
- Discontinue diuretics 2–3 d before initiation of therapy if possible. If diuretics cannot be discontinued, start initial dose ≤10 mg.
- Store at 15°–30° C (59°–86° F) and protect from moisture.

ADVERSE EFFECTS (≥1%) **CV:** Hypotension. **CNS:** Headache, fatigue, dizziness. **Endocrine:** Hyperkalemia. **GI:** Nausea, vomiting, diarrhea. **Urogenital:** Proteinuria. **Respiratory:** Cough. **Skin:** Rash.

INTERACTIONS Drug: NSAIDS may decrease antihypertensive effects of fosinopril. POTASSIUM SUPPLEMENTS, POTASSIUM-SPARING DIURETICS increase risk of hyperkalemia. ACE inhibitors may increase **lithium** levels and toxicity.

PHARMACOKINETICS Absorption: Readily absorbed from GI tract; converted to its active form, fosinoprilat, in the liver. **Peak:** 3 h. **Duration:** 24 h. **Distribution:** Approximately 90% protein bound; crosses placenta. **Metabolism:** Hydrolyzed by intestinal and hepatic esterases to its active form, fosinoprilat. **Elimination:** 44% excreted in urine, 46% in feces. **Half-Life:** 3–4 h (fosinoprilat).

NURSING IMPLICATIONS

Assessment & Drug Effects
- Monitor BP at the time of peak effectiveness, 2–6 h after dosing and at the end of the dosing interval just before next dose.
- Report diminished antihypertensive effect toward the end of the dosing interval. An inadequate trough response may be an indication for dividing the daily dose.
- Monitor for first-dose hypotension, especially in salt- or volume-depleted patients.
- Lab tests: Obtain BUN and serum creatinine periodically. Increases may necessitate dose reduction or discontinuation of the drug. Monitor serum potassium.
- Observe for S&S of hyperkalemia (see Appendix F).

Patient & Family Education
- Discontinue fosinopril and report to physician any of the following: S&S of angioedema (e.g., swelling of face or extremities, difficulty breathing or swallowing); syncope; chronic, nonproductive cough.
- Maintain adequate fluid intake and avoid potassium supplements or salt substitutes unless specifically prescribed by the physician.
- Report vomiting or diarrhea to physician immediately.
- Do not breast feed while taking this drug.

FOSPHENYTOIN SODIUM

(fos-phen′i-toin)
Cerebyx
Classifications: CENTRAL NERVOUS SYSTEM AGENT; HYDANTOIN ANTICONVULSANT AGENT
Prototype: Phenytoin
Pregnancy Category: D

F

AVAILABILITY 150 mg, 750 mg vials

ACTIONS Prodrug of phenytoin that converts to the anticonvulsant, phenytoin, after parenteral administration. Thought to modulate the sodium channels of neurons, calcium flux across neuronal membranes, and enhance the sodium–potassium ATPase activity of neurons and glial cells.

THERAPEUTIC EFFECTS The cellular mechanism of phenytoin is thought to be responsible for the anticonvulsant activity of fosphenytoin.

USES Control of generalized convulsive status epilepticus and the prevention and treatment of seizures during neurosurgery, or as a parenteral short-term substitute for oral phenytoin.

UNLABELED USES Antiarrhythmic agent especially in treatment of digitalis-induced arrhythmia; treatment of trigeminal neuralgia (tic douloureux).

CONTRAINDICATIONS Hypersensitivity to hydantoin products, rash, seizures due to hypoglycemia, sinus bradycardia, complete or incomplete heart block; Adams–Stokes syndrome; pregnancy (category D), lactation.

CAUTIOUS USE Impaired liver or kidney function, alcoholism, hypotension, heart block, bradycardia, severe CAD, diabetes mellitus, hyperglycemia, respiratory depression, acute intermittent porphyria.

ROUTE & DOSAGE

Status Epilepticus

Adult: **IV Loading Dose** 15–20 mg PE/kg (PE = phenytoin sodium equivalents) administered at 100–150 mg PE/min **IV Maintenance Dose** is 4–6 mg PE/kg/d

Substitution for Oral Phenytoin Therapy

Adult: **IV/IM** Substitute fosphenytoin at the same total daily dose in mg PE as the oral dose at a rate of infusion not greater than 150 mg PE/min

ADMINISTRATION

Note: All dosing is expressed in phenytoin sodium equivalents (PE) to avoid the need to calculate molecular weight adjustments between fosphenytoin and phenytoin sodium doses. ALWAYS prescribe and fill Fosphenytoin in PE units.

Intramuscular

- Follow institutional policy regarding maximum volume to inject into one IM site.

Intravenous

PREPARE: **Direct:** Dilute in D5W or NS to a concentration of 1.5–25 mg PE/mL.

ADMINISTER: **Direct:** Do not administer at a rate >150 mg PE/min.

- Store at 2°–8° C (36°–46° F); may store at room temperature not to exceed 48 h.

ADVERSE EFFECTS (≥1%) **CNS:** Usually dose related. Paresthesia, tinnitus, *nystagmus, dizziness, somnolence, drowsiness,* ataxia, mental confusion, tremors, insomnia, headache, seizures, increased reflexes, dysarthria, intracranial hypertension. **CV:** Bradycardia, tachycardia, asystole, hypotension, hypertension, <u>cardiovascular collapse, cardiac arrest</u>, heart block, ventricular fibrillation, phlebitis. **Special Senses:** Photophobia, conjunctivitis, diplopia, blurred vision. **GI:** *Gingival hyperplasia,* nausea, vomiting, constipation, epigastric pain, dysphagia, loss of taste, weight loss, hepatitis, liver necrosis. **Hematologic:** Thrombocytopenia, leukopenia, leukocytosis, agranulocytosis, pancytopenia, eosinophilia; megaloblastic, hemolytic, or aplastic anemias. **Metabolic:** Fever, hyperglycemia, glycosuria, weight gain, edema, transient increase in serum thyrotropic (TSH) level, hyperkalemia, osteomalacia or rickets associated with hypocalcemia and elevated alkaline phosphatase activity. **Skin:** Alopecia, hirsutism (especially in young female); rash: scarlatiniform, maculopapular, urticarial, morbilliform (may be fatal); bullous, exfoliative, or purpuric dermatitis; Stevens–Johnson syndrome, toxic epidermal necrolysis, keratosis, neonatal hemorrhage, *pruritus*. **Urogenital:** Acute renal failure, Peyronie's disease. **Respiratory:** Acute pneumonitis, pulmonary fibrosis. **Musculoskeletal:** Periarteritis nodosum, acute systemic lupus erythematosus, craniofacial abnormalities (with enlargement of lips). **Other:** Lymphadenopathy, injection site pain, chills.

DIAGNOSTIC TEST INTERFERENCE Fosphenytoin may produce lower than normal values for ***dexamethasone*** or ***metyrapone*** tests; may increase serum levels of ***glucose, BSP,*** and ***alkaline phosphatase*** and may decrease ***PBI*** and ***urinary steroid*** levels.

INTERACTIONS Drug: Alcohol decreases fosphenytoin effects; OTHER ANTICONVULSANTS may increase or decrease fosphenytoin levels; fosphenytoin may decrease absorption and increase metabolism of ORAL ANTICOAGULANTS; fosphenytoin increases metabolism of CORTICOSTEROIDS and ORAL CONTRACEPTIVES, thus decreasing their effectiveness; **amiodarone, chloramphenicol, omeprazole** increase fosphenytoin levels; ANTITUBERCULOSIS AGENTS decrease fosphenytoin levels. **Food: folic acid, calcium, vitamin D** absorption may be decreased by fosphenytoin; fosphenytoin absorption may be decreased by enteral nutrition supplements. **Herbal: Ginkgo** may decrease anticonvulsant effectiveness.

PHARMACOKINETICS Absorption: Completely absorbed after IM administration. **Peak:** 30 min IM. **Distribution:** 95%–99% bound to plasma proteins, displaces phenytoin from protein binding sites; crosses placenta, small amount in breast milk. **Metabolism:** Converted to phenytoin by phosphatases; phenytoin is oxidized in liver to inactive metabolites. **Elimination:** Half-life 15 min to convert fosphenytoin to phenytoin, 22 h phenytoin; phenytoin metabolites excreted in urine.

NURSING IMPLICATIONS

Note: See **phenytoin** for additional nursing implications.

Assessment & Drug Effects

- Monitor ECG, BP, and respiratory function continuously during and for 10–20 min after infusion.
- Discontinue infusion and notify physician if rash appears. Be prepared to substite alternative therapy rapidly to prevent withdrawal-precipitated seizures.
- Lab tests: Monitor CBC with differential, platelet count, serum electrolytes, and blood glucose.
- Allow at least 2 h after IV infusion and 4 h after IM injection before monitoring total plasma phenytoin concentration.
- Monitor diabetics for loss of glycemic control.
- Monitor carefully for adverse effects, especially in patients with

renal or hepatic disease or hypoalbuminemia.

Patient & Family Education

- Be aware of potential adverse effects. Itching, burning, tingling, or paresthesia are common during and for some time following IV infusion.
- Do not breast feed while taking this drug.

F

FROVATRIPTAN

(fro-va-trip′tan)

Frova

Classifications: AUTONOMIC NERVOUS SYSTEM AGENT; ADRENERGIC AGONIST; SEROTONIN 5-HT_1-RECEPTOR AGONIST

Prototype: Sumatriptan

Pregnancy Category: C

AVAILABILITY 2.5 mg tablets

ACTIONS Selective agonist that binds with high affinity to 5-HT_{1D}, 5-HT_{1B}, 5-HT_{1F} serotonin receptors which are found on extracerebral and intracranial blood vessels, and on other structures in the central nervous system.

THERAPEUTIC EFFECTS Due primarily to agonist effects on 5-HT_{1D} and 5-HT_{1B} serotonin receptors on cranial blood vessels result in vasoconstriction and agonist effects on nerve terminals in the trigeminal system. Activation of these receptors results in constriction of cranial vessels which become dilated during a migraine attack, inhibition of neuropeptide release, and reduced signal transmission in the pain pathways.

USES Treatment of migraine headache with or without aura.

CONTRAINDICATIONS Hypersensitivity to frovatriptan; significant cardiovascular disease such as ischemic heart disease, coronary artery vasospasms, peripheral vascular disease, history of cerebrovascular events, or uncontrolled hypertension; within 24 h of receiving another 5-HT_1 agonist or an ergotamine-containing or ergot-type drug; basilar or hemiplegic migraine, pregnancy (category C).

CAUTIOUS USE Significant risk factors for coronary artery disease unless a cardiac evaluation has been done; hypertension; risk factors for cerebrovascular accident; impaired liver or kidney function; lactation. Safety and efficacy in children are not established.

ROUTE & DOSAGE

Migraine Headache

Adult: **PO** 2.5 mg. If headache returns, may repeat after at least 2 h (max: 7.5 mg/24 h)

ADMINISTRATION

Oral

- Do not give within 24 h of an ergot-containing drug.
- Administer any time after symptoms of migraine appear.
- Do not administer a second dose without consulting the physician for any attack during which the FIRST dose did NOT work.
- Give a second dose if headache was relieved by first dose but symptoms return; however, wait at least 2 h after the first dose before giving a second dose.
- Do not give more than two doses in 24 h.
- Store at 15°–30° C (59°–86° F).

ADVERSE EFFECTS (≥1%) **Body as a Whole:** Fatigue, hot or cold sensation, flushing. **CNS:** Dizziness, headache, paresthesia, somnolence, insomnia, anxiety. **CV:** Chest pain, palpitation. **GI:** Dyspepsia, nausea, vomiting, diarrhea, dry mouth. **Musculoskeletal:** Skeletal pain. **Special Senses:** Abnormal vision. **Skin:** Sweating.

INTERACTIONS Drug: Dihydroergotamine, methysergide, other 5-HT_1 AGONISTS may cause prolonged vasospastic reactions; SSRIS, **sibutramine** have rarely caused weakness, hyperreflexia, and incoordination; MAOIS should not be used with 5-HT_1 AGONISTS. **Herbal: Gingko, ginseng, echinacea, St. John's wort** may increase triptan toxicity.

PHARMACOKINETICS Absorption: 20–30% bioavailability. **Peak:** 2–4 h. **Distribution:** 15% protein bound. **Metabolism:** Metabolized in liver by CYP1A2. **Elimination:** 30% excreted renally, 60% excreted in feces. **Half-Life:** 26 h.

NURSING IMPLICATIONS

Assessment & Drug Effects

- Monitor cardiovascular status carefully following first dose in patients at relatively high risk for coronary artery disease (e.g., postmenopausal women, men over 40 years old, persons with known CAD risk factors), or who have coronary artery vasospasms.
- Report to physician immediately chest pain or tightness in chest or throat that is severe, or does not quickly resolve following a dose of frovatriptan.
- Pain relief usually begins within 10 min of ingestion, with complete relief in approximately 65% of all patients within 2 h.
- Monitor BP, especially in those being treated for hypertension.

Patient & Family Education

- Review patient information leaflet provided by the manufacturer carefully.
- Notify physician immediately if symptoms of severe angina (e.g., severe or persistent pain or tightness in chest, back, neck, or throat) or hypersensitivity (e.g., wheezing, facial swelling, skin rash, itching, or hives) occur.
- Do not take any other serotonin receptor agonist (e.g., Imitrex, Maxalt, Zomig, Amerge) within 24 h of taking frovatriptan.
- Advise physician of any drugs taken within 1 wk of beginning frovatriptan.
- Check with physician regarding drug interactions before taking any new OTC or prescription drugs.
- Report any other adverse effects (e.g., tingling, flushing, dizziness) at next physician visit.
- Do not breast feed while taking this drug without consulting physician.

FULVESTRANT

(ful-ves′trant)

Faslodex

Classifications: ANTINEOPLASTIC; HORMONE AND SYNTHETIC SUBSTITUTE; ANTIESTROGEN

Prototype: Tamoxifen Citrate

Pregnancy Category: D

AVAILABILITY 50 mg/mL in 2.5 mL, 5 mL syringes

ACTIONS Fulvestrant is an estrogen receptor antagonist that selectively binds to the estrogen receptors (ER) of breast cancer cells. It competes well with estradiol (estrogen) in binding to the estrogen receptor sites. Estrogen stimulates the tumor growth of estrogen-sensitive breast tissue cancer cells in postmenopausal women.

THERAPEUTIC EFFECTS In postmenopausal women, many breast cancers have estrogen receptors

(ERs), and the growth of these tumors is stimulated by estrogen. Therefore, fulvestrant decreases estrogen-sensitive breast tissue tumor growth.

USES Treatment of hormone receptor-positive metastatic breast cancer in postmenopausal women with disease progression following antiestrogen therapy.

CONTRAINDICATIONS Hypersensitivity to fulvestrant; pregnancy (category D); lactation.
CAUTIOUS USE Moderate to severe liver impairment; safety and effectiveness in children not established.

ROUTE & DOSAGE

Metastatic Breast Cancer
Adult: IM 250 mg once/mo

ADMINISTRATION

Intramuscular
- Do not administer unless the possibility of pregnancy has been ruled out.
- Break the seal of the white plastic cover on the syringe luer connector to remove the cover with the attached rubber tip cap. Twist to lock the needle to the luer connector. Remove excess gas from the syringe (a small gas bubble may remain).
- Administer slowly in the buttock.
- Immediately activate needle protection device upon withdrawal from patient by pushing lever arm completely forward until needle tip is fully covered.
- Store in a refrigerator, 2°–8° C (36°–46° F) in original container.

ADVERSE EFFECTS (≥1%) **Body as a Whole:** *Asthenia, pain, injection site pain,* flu-like syndrome, fever, peripheral edema. **CNS:** Dizziness, insomnia, paresthesia, depression, anxiety. **CV:** *Vasodilation.* **GI:** *Nausea, vomiting, constipation, diarrhea,* anorexia. **Hematologic:** Anemia. **Musculoskeletal:** *Bone pain,* arthritis. **Respiratory:** *Pharyngitis, dyspnea, cough.* **Skin:** Rash, sweating.

INTERACTIONS Drug: No clinically significant interactions reported.

PHARMACOKINETICS Peak: 7 d. **Duration:** 1 mo. **Distribution:** 99% protein bound. **Metabolism:** Metabolized via multiple pathways in liver. **Elimination:** Primarily excreted in bile. **Half-Life:** 40 d.

NURSING IMPLICATIONS

Assessment & Drug Effects
- Monitor for S&S of tumor progression.
- Lab tests: Monitor periodic CBC with differential.

Patient & Family Education
- Use two methods of contraception while taking this drug. Immediately notify physician if you think you are pregnant.
- Report vaginal bleeding to physician. Understand the possibility of drug-induced menstrual irregularities before starting treatment.
- Do not breast feed while taking this drug without consulting physician.

FURAZOLIDONE

(fur-a-zoe'li-done)
Furoxone
Classifications: ANTIINFECTIVE; NITROFURAN ANTIBIOTIC; MAO INHIBITOR
Pregnancy Category: C

AVAILABILITY 100 mg tablets; 50 mg/15 mL liquid

ACTIONS Synthetic nitrofuran with antibacterial and antiprotozoal prop-

erties. Acts by interfering with several bacterial enzyme systems including cell wall synthesis of the bacteria.
THERAPEUTIC EFFECTS A MAO INHIBITOR that is cumulative and dose related (occurring after 4 or 5 d of therapy). Bactericidal against majority of GI pathogens, including species of *Enterobacter aerogenes, Escherichia coli, Giardia lamblia, Proteus, Salmonella, Shigella, Staphylococcus,* and *Vibrio cholerae.*

USES Bacterial or protozoal diarrhea and enteritis caused by susceptible organisms.

CONTRAINDICATIONS Hypersensitivity to furazolidone, concurrent use with alcohol, other MAO INHIBITOR, tyramine-containing foods, indirect-acting sympathomimetic amines; infants <1 mo. Safety during pregnancy (category C) or lactation is not established.
CAUTIOUS USE If at all, patients with glucose-6-phosphate dehydrogenase (G6PD) deficiency.

ROUTE & DOSAGE

Diarrhea and Enteritis
Adult: **PO** 100 mg q.i.d.
Child: **PO** 1 mo–1 y, 8–17 mg q.i.d.; 1–4 y, 17–25 mg q.i.d.; ≥5 y, 25–50 mg q.i.d. (max: 8.8 mg/kg/d)

ADMINISTRATION

Oral
- Store in tight, light-resistant containers (drug darkens on exposure to light). Protect from excessive heat.

ADVERSE EFFECTS (≥1%) **GI:** *Nausea, vomiting,* abdominal pain, diarrhea. **Hypersensitivity:** Fever, arthralgia, hypotension, urticaria, angioedema, vesicular or morbilliform rash. **Body as a Whole:** Headache, malaise, dizziness, hypoglycemia. **Hematologic:** Intravascular hemolysis in patients with G6PD deficiency, agranulocytosis (rare). **Special Senses:** Partial deafness.

DIAGNOSTIC TEST INTERFERENCE Furazolidone metabolite reportedly may cause false-positive reactions for ***urine glucose*** with ***copper sulfate reduction methods,*** e.g., ***Benedict's reagent, Clinitest,*** and ***Fehling's solution.***

INTERACTIONS Drug: Alcohol may elicit disulfiram-type reaction up to 4 d after the drug is stopped; MAO INHIBITORS, NARCOTICS, SYMPATHOMIMETIC AMINES, **ephedrine**, **phenylpropanolamine** may cause a hypertensive reaction; TRICYCLIC ANTIDEPRESSANTS may cause toxic psychosis. **Food:** may interact with tyramine-containing foods, resulting in flushing, tachycardia, and hypertensive crisis. See **phenelzine** (MAO INHIBITOR prototype). **Herbal: Ginseng** may cause hypertension, manic symptoms, headaches, nervousness; **ma-huang, ephedra, St. John's wort** may lead to hypertensive crisis.

PHARMACOKINETICS Absorption: Poorly absorbed from GI tract. **Metabolism:** Metabolized in intestines. **Elimination:** Excreted in urine.

NURSING IMPLICATIONS

Assessment & Drug Effects
- Monitor for nausea and vomiting. Dosage reduction may be needed.
- Note: Bed rest, fluid and electrolyte replacement (as indicated) are important adjuncts to therapy. Consult physician regarding dietary allowances.
- Keep physician informed of S&S of dehydration (see Appendix F) and electrolyte imbalance.

- Monitor patients for lost glycemic control because drug may cause hypoglycemia (see Appendix F). Use glucose oxidase methods for urine testing (e.g., Clinistix, Diastix, TesTape).

Patient & Family Education

- Report the following to physician: Faintness, weakness, and light-headedness. These may be symptoms of hypersensitivity reaction or hypoglycemia.
- Be aware of and avoid foods high in tyramine (e.g., aged and fermented food and drinks) that may produce hypertensive reaction. Hypertensive crisis is most likely to occur when drug is continued beyond 5 d or when large doses are given.
- Do not drink alcohol during furazolidone therapy and for at least 4 d after drug is stopped. Ingestion of alcohol may cause disulfiram-type reaction (see Appendix F); symptoms may last up to 24 h.
- Note: Drug may impart a harmless brown color to urine.
- Monitor blood glucose for loss of glucemic control if diabetic.
- Do not breast feed while taking this drug without consulting physician.

FUROSEMIDE Pr

(fur-oh'se-mide)

Fumide ✦, Furomide ✦, Lasix, Luramide ✦

Classifications: ELECTROLYTIC AND WATER BALANCE AGENT; LOOP DIURETIC

Pregnancy Category: C

AVAILABILITY 20 mg, 40 mg, 80 mg tablets; 10 mg/mL, 40 mg/5 mL oral solution; 10 mg/mL injection

ACTIONS Rapid-acting potent sulfonamide "loop" diuretic and antihypertensive with pharmacologic effects and uses almost identical to those of ethacrynic acid. Exact mode of action not clearly defined; decreases renal vascular resistance and may increase renal blood flow.

THERAPEUTIC EFFECTS Inhibits reabsorption of sodium and chloride primarily in loop of Henle and also in proximal and distal renal tubules; an antihypertensive that decreases edema and intravascular volume. Reportedly less ototoxic than ethacrynic acid.

USES Treatment of edema associated with CHF, cirrhosis of liver, and kidney disease, including nephrotic syndrome. May be used for management of hypertension, alone or in combination with other antihypertensive agents, and for treatment of hypercalcemia. Has been used concomitantly with mannitol for treatment of severe cerebral edema, particularly in meningitis.

CONTRAINDICATIONS History of hypersensitivity to furosemide or sulfonamides; increasing oliguria, anuria, fluid and electrolyte depletion states; hepatic coma; pregnancy (category C), lactation.

CAUTIOUS USE Infants, older adults; hepatic cirrhosis, nephrotic syndrome; cardiogenic shock associated with acute MI; history of SLE, history of gout; patients receiving digitalis glycosides or potassium-depleting steroids.

ROUTE & DOSAGE

Edema

Adult: **PO** 20–80 mg in 1 or more divided doses up to 600 mg/d if needed **IV/IM** 20–40 mg in 1 or

more divided doses up to 600 mg/d
Child: **PO** 2 mg/kg, may be increased by 1–2 mg/kg q6–8h (max: 6 mg/kg/dose) **IV/IM** 1 mg/kg, may be increased by 1 mg/kg q2h if needed (max: mg/kg/dose)
Neonate: **PO** 1–4 mg/kg q12–24h **IV/IM** 1–2 mg/kg q12–24h

Hypertension

Adult: **PO** 10–40 mg b.i.d. (max: 480 mg/d)

ADMINISTRATION

Oral

- Give with food or milk to reduce possibility of gastric irritation.
- Schedule doses to avoid sleep disturbance (e.g., a single dose is generally given in the morning; twice-a-day doses at 8 a.m. and 2 p.m.).
- Note: Slight discoloration of tablets reportedly does not alter potency.
- Store tablets at controlled room temperature, preferably at 15°–30° C (59°–86° F) unless otherwise directed. Protect from light.
- Store oral solution in refrigerator, preferably at 2°–8° C (36°–46° F). Protect from light and freezing.

Intramuscular

- Protect syringes from light once they are removed from package.
- Discard yellow or otherwise discolored injection solutions.

Intravenous

Note: Verify correct IV concentration and rate of infusion/injection with physician before administration to infants or children.

PREPARE: **Direct:** Give undiluted.
ADMINISTER: **Direct:** Give undiluted at a rate of 20 mg or a fraction thereof over 1 min. With high doses a rate of 4 mg/min is recommended to decrease risk of ototoxicity.
INCOMPATIBILITIES **Solution/additive: Buprenorphine, chlorpromazine, ciprofloxacin, diazepam, diphenhydramine, dobutamine, doxapram, doxorubicin, droperidol, erythromycin, gentamicin, isoproterenol, labetalol, meperidine, metoclopramide, milrinone, netilmicin, pancuronium, prochlorperazine, promethazine, quinidine, thiamine vinblastine, vincristine. Y-site: Amrinone, amsacrine, ciprofloxacin, diazepam, diltiazem, dobutamine, diphenhydramine, dopamine, doxorubicin, droperidol, esmolol, filgrastim, fluconazole, gemcitabine, gentamicin, hydralazine, idarubicin, methocarbamol, metoclopramide, midazolam, milrinone, morphine, netilmicin, nicardipine, ondansetron, quinidine, thiopental, tobramycin, vecuronium, vinblastine, vincristine, vinorelbine,** TPN.

- Use infusion solutions within 24 h.
- Store parenteral solution at controlled room temperature, preferably at 15°–30° C (59°–86° F) unless otherwise directed. Protect from light.

ADVERSE EFFECTS (≥1%) **CV:** Postural hypotension, dizziness with excessive diuresis, acute hypotensive episodes, circulatory collapse. **Metabolic:** Hypovolemia, dehydration, hyponatremia *hypokalemia,* hypochloremia metabolic alkalosis, hypomagnesemia, hypocalcemia (tetany), hyperglycemia, glycosuria, elevated BUN, hyperuricemia. **GI:** Nausea, vomiting, oral and gastric burning, anorexia, diarrhea, constipation, abdominal

F

cramping, acute pancreatitis, jaundice. **Urogenital:** Allergic interstitial nephritis, irreversible renal failure, urinary frequency. **Hematologic:** Anemia, leukopenia, thrombocytopenic purpura; aplastic anemia, agranulocytosis (rare). **Special Senses:** Tinnitus, vertigo, feeling of fullness in ears, hearing loss (rarely permanent), blurred vision. **Skin:** Pruritus, urticaria, exfoliative dermatitis, purpura, photosensitivity, porphyria cutanea tarde, necrotizing angiitis (vasculitis). **Body as a Whole:** Increased perspiration; paresthesias; activation of SLE, muscle spasms, weakness; thrombophlebitis, pain at IM injection site.

DIAGNOSTIC TEST INTERFERENCE Furosemide may cause elevations in ***BUN, serum amylase, cholesterol, triglycerides, uric acid*** and ***blood glucose*** levels, and may decrease ***serum calcium, magnesium, potassium,*** and ***sodium*** levels.

INTERACTIONS Drug: OTHER DIURETICS enhance diuretic effects; with **digoxin** increased risk of toxicity because of hypokalemia; NONDEPOLARIZING NEUROMUSCULAR BLOCKING AGENTS (e.g., **tubocurarine**) prolong neuromuscular blockage; CORTICOSTEROIDS, **amphotericin B** potentiate hypokalemia; decreased **lithium** elimination and increased toxicity; SULFONYLUREAS, **insulin** blunt hypoglycemic effects; NSAIDS may attenuate diuretic effects.

PHARMACOKINETICS Absorption: 60 of oral dose absorbed from GI tract. **Peak:** 60–70 min PO; 20–60 min IV. **Onset:** 30–60 min PO; 5 min IV. **Duration:** 2 h. **Distribution:** Crosses placenta. **Metabolism:** Small amount metabolized in liver. **Elimination:** Rapidly excreted in urine; 50% of oral dose and 80% of IV dose excreted within 24 h; excreted in breast milk. **Half-Life:** 30 min.

NURSING IMPLICATIONS

Assessment & Drug Effects

- Observe patients receiving parenteral drug carefully; closely monitor BP and vital signs. Sudden death from cardiac arrest has been reported.
- Monitor BP during periods of diuresis and through period of dosage adjustment.
- Observe older adults closely during period of brisk diuresis. Sudden alteration in fluid and electrolyte balance may precipitate significant adverse reactions. Report symptoms to physician.
- Lab tests: Obtain frequent blood count, serum and urine electrolytes, CO_2, BUN, blood sugar, and uric acid values during first few months of therapy and periodically thereafter.
- Monitor for S&S of hypokalemia (see Appendix F).
- Monitor I&O ratio and pattern. Report decrease or unusual increase in output. Excessive diuresis can result in dehydration and hypovolemia, circulatory collapse, and hypotension. Weigh patient daily under standard conditions.
- Monitor urine and blood glucose & HbA_{1C} closely in diabetics and patients with decompensated hepatic cirrhosis. Drug may cause hyperglycemia.
- Note: Excessive dehydration is most likely to occur in older adults, those with chronic cardiac disease on prolonged salt restriction, or those receiving sympatholytic agents.

Patient & Family Education

- Consult physician regarding allowable salt and fluid intake.

- Ingest potassium-rich foods daily (e.g., bananas, oranges, peaches, dried dates) to reduce or prevent potassium depletion.
- Learn S&S of hypokalemia (see Appendix F). Report muscle cramps or weakness to physician.
- Make position changes slowly because high doses of antihypertensive drugs taken concurrently may produce episodes of dizziness or imbalance.
- Avoid replacing fluid losses with large amounts of water.
- Avoid prolonged exposure to direct sun.
- Do not breast feed while taking this drug.

GABAPENTIN

(gab-a-pen'tin)
Neurontin
Classifications: CENTRAL NERVOUS SYSTEM AGENT; ANTICONVULSANT
Prototype: Phenytoin
Pregnancy Category: C

AVAILABILITY 100 mg, 300 mg, 400 mg capsules; 600 mg, 800 mg tablets; 250 mg/5 mL solution.

ACTIONS Gabapentin is a GABA neurotransmitter analog; however, it does not interact with GABA receptors, and it does not inhibit GABA uptake or degradation. Mechanism of action is unknown. An effect of gabapentin on central serotonin metabolism has been postulated.

THERAPEUTIC EFFECTS Gabapentin is used in conjunction with other anticonvulsants to control certain types of seizures in patients with epilepsy.

USES Adjunctive therapy for partial seizures with or without secondary generalization in adults, postherpetic neuralgia.

UNLABELED USES Add-on therapy for generalized seizures.

CONTRAINDICATIONS Hypersensitivity to gabapentin; pregnancy (category C), lactation.

CAUTIOUS USE Status epilepticus, renal impairment, older adults. Safety and efficacy in children <3 y are not established.

ROUTE & DOSAGE

Adjunctive Therapy for Seizure Disorder

Adult/Child: **PO** *>12 y,* Initiate with 300 mg on day 1, 300 mg b.i.d. on day 2, 300 mg t.i.d. on day 3, and continue to increase over a week to an initial total dose of 400 mg t.i.d. (1200 mg/d); may increase to 1800–2400 mg/d depending on response (most patients receive 600–1800 mg/d in 3 divided doses) 400 mg t.i.d. (1200 mg/d); may increase to 1800–2400 mg/d depending on response (most patients receive 600–1800 mg/d in 3 divided doses) new content
Child: **PO** *3–12 y* Initiate with 10–15 mg/kg/d in 3 divided doses, titrate q3d to target dose of 40 mg/kg/d in pts 3–4 y or 25–35 mg/kg/d in pts ≥5 y in 3 divided doses

Post-Herpetic Neuralgia

Adult: **PO** Initiate with 300 mg day 1, 300 mg b.i.d. day 2, and 300 mg t.i.d. day 3; may increase up to 600 mg t.i.d. if needed

Renal Impairment

Cl_{cr} >60 mL/min: 400 mg t.i.d.; 30–60 mL/min: 300 mg b.i.d.; 15–30 mL/min: 300 mg q.d.; <15 mL/min: 300 mg q.o.d.; hemodialysis: 200–300 mg following dialysis

ADMINISTRATION

Oral

- Adjust dosage for patients with creatinine clearance of 60 mL/min or less. See manufacturer's recommendations.
- Separate doses of gabapentin and antacids by 2 h.
- Withdraw drug gradually over 1 wk; abrupt discontinuation may cause status epilepticus.
- Store at 15°–30° C (59°–86° F); protect from heat, moisture, and direct light.

ADVERSE EFFECTS (≥1%) **CNS:** *Drowsiness, fatigue,* dizziness, tremor, slurred speech, impaired concentration, headache, increased frequency of partial seizures. **Endocrine:** Weight gain. **GI:** Nausea, gastric upset, vomiting. **Special Senses:** Blurred vision, nystagmus, **Skin:** Rash, eczema.

INTERACTIONS Drug: Increase in **phenytoin** levels at higher doses (300–600 mg/d gabapentin). Does not appear to affect serum levels of other ANTICONVULSANTS. ANTACIDS reduce absorption of gabapentin about 20%.: **Herbal: Ginkgo** may decrease anticonvulsant effectiveness.

PHARMACOKINETICS Absorption: 50%–60% absorbed from GI tract. **Peak:** Peak level 1–3 h; peak effect 2–4 wk. **Distribution:** Crosses the blood–brain barrier comparable to other anticonvulsants; readily passes into cerebrospinal fluid; is not bound to plasma proteins; highest concentrations (in animal studies) found in pancreas and kidneys. **Metabolism:** Does not appear to be metabolized. **Elimination:** 76%–81% excreted unchanged in 96 h; 10%–23% recovered in feces. **Half-Life:** 5–6 h.

NURSING IMPLICATIONS

Assessment & Drug Effects

- Monitor for therapeutic effectiveness; may not occur until several weeks following initiation of therapy.
- Assess frequency of seizures: In rare cases, the drug has increased the frequency of partial seizures.
- Assess safety: Vision, concentration, and coordination may be impaired by gabapentin.

Patient & Family Education

- Learn potential adverse effects of drug.
- Notify physician immediately if any of the following occur: increased seizure frequency, visual changes, unusual bruising or bleeding.
- Do not drive or engage in other potentially hazardous activities until response to drug is known.
- Do not abruptly discontinue use of drug; do not take drug within 2 h of an antacid.
- Do not breast feed while taking this drug.

GALANTAMINE HYDROBROMIDE

(ga-lan'ta-meen)

Reminyl

Classifications: AUTONOMIC NERVOUS SYSTEM AGENT; CHOLINERGIC (PARASYMPATHOMIMETIC); CHOLINESTERASE INHIBITOR; CENTRAL ACTING

Prototype: Donezepril HCl

Pregnancy Category: B

AVAILABILITY 4 mg, 8 mg, 12 mg tablets

ACTIONS Competitive and reversible inhibitor of acetylcholinesterase which is the enzyme responsible for the hydrolysis (breakdown) of the neurotransmitter, acetylcholine.

THERAPEUTIC EFFECTS Believed to increase concentration of the neurotransmitter, acetylcholine, in the CNS. If this mechanism is correct, the effect of drug will lessen as disease progresses and since fewer neurons stimulated by acetylcholine remain functionally intact.

USES Treatment of mild to moderate dementia of Alzheimer's type.

CONTRAINDICATIONS Hypersensitivity to galantamine. Not recommended with severe renal or hepatic impairment; pregnancy (category B), lactation, or in children.

CAUTIOUS USE Bradycardia, heart block or other cardiac conduction disorders; asthma, COPD; potential bladder outflow obstruction; a history of seizures or GI bleeding; concurrent use of drugs which slow the heart rate, drugs which may cause syncope, NSAIDS, or neuromuscular blocking agents during anesthesia.

ROUTE & DOSAGE

Alzheimer's Disease

Adult: **PO** Initiate with 4 mg b.i.d. times at least 4 wks, if tolerated may increase by 4 mg b.i.d. q4wk to target dose of 12 mg b.i.d. (8–16 mg b.i.d.)

Hepatic Impairment

Not recommended with severe hepatic impairment

Renal Impairment

Cl_{cr} <9 mL/min: Not recommended

ADMINISTRATION

Oral

- Give with meals (breakfast and dinner) to reduce the risk of nausea.
- Make increases in dosage increments at four-week intervals.
- If drug is interrupted for several days or more, restart at the lowest dose and gradually increase to the current dose.
- Store at 15°–30° C (59°–86° F).

ADVERSE EFFECTS (≥1%) **Body as a Whole:** Weight loss, fatigue, rhinitis, syncope. **CNS:** Dizziness, headache, depression, insomnia, somnolence, tremor. **CV:** Bradycardia, chest pain. **GI:** *Nausea, vomiting,* diarrhea, anorexia, abdominal pain, dyspepsia, flatulence. **Hematologic:** Anemia. **Urogenital:** UTI, hematuria, incontinence.

INTERACTIONS Drug: Additive effects with other CHOLINESTERASE INHIBITORS (e.g., **succinylcholine, bethanecol**); **cimetidine, erythromycin, ketoconazole, paroxetine** may increase levels and toxicity.

PHARMACOKINETICS Absorption: Rapidly and completely absorbed. **Peak:** 1 h. **Distribution:** Mainly distributes to red blood cells. **Metabolism:** Metabolized in liver primarily by CYP2D6 and CYP3A4. **Elimination:** 95% excreted in urine. **Half-Life:** 7 h (4.4–10 h).

NURSING IMPLICATIONS

Assessment & Drug Effects

- Monitor cardiovascular status including baseline and periodic EKG and BP readings. Assess for postural hypotension.
- Monitor respiratory status; report worsening of preexisting asthma or COPD.
- Monitor I&O rates and pattern for urinary incontinence or urinary retention.
- Monitor appetite and food intake. Weigh weekly and report significant weight loss.
- Lab tests: Baseline ALT/AST, BUN and creatinine; periodic blood

glucose, alkaline phosphatase, urinalysis, stool for occult blood.

Patient & Family Education

- Report any of the following to a health care provider immediately: loss of weight, urinary retention, chest pain, palpitations, difficulty breathing, fainting, dark stools, blood in the urine.

GALLIUM NITRATE

(gal'li-um)

Ganite

Classification: BONE METABOLISM REGULATOR

Pregnancy Category: C

AVAILABILITY 25 mg/mL injection

ACTIONS The precise mechanism is not known.

THERAPEUTIC EFFECTS Induces hypocalcemia by inhibiting calcium resorption from bone.

USES Hypercalcemia of malignancy.

UNLABELED USES Paget's disease, painful bone metastases, adjuvant therapy for bladder cancer and lymphomas.

CONTRAINDICATIONS Severe renal impairment (serum creatinine >2.5 mg/dL), lactation.

CAUTIOUS USE Renal function impairment, pregnancy (category C). Safety and efficacy in children are not established.

ROUTE & DOSAGE

Hypercalcemia

Adult: **IV** 100–200 mg/m^2/d for 5–7 d, dilute in 1000 mL D5W or 0.9% NaCl and infuse continuously over 24 h

Bone Metastases

Adult: **IV** 200 mg/m^2/d for 7 d, dilute in 1000 mL D5W or 0.9% NaCl and infuse continuously over 24 h

ADMINISTRATION

Intravenous

Hydrate patient with oral or IV NS to produce a urine output of 2 L/d; maintain adequate hydration throughout treatment.

PREPARE: **Continuous:** Dilute each daily dose with 1000 mL NS (preferred if not contraindicated) or D5W.

ADMINISTER: **Continuous:** Infuse over 24 h taking care to avoid rapid infusion. Control rate with infusion pump or micro-drip device.

- Do not administer concurrently with potentially nephrotoxic drugs.
- Store IV solutions at 15°–30° C (59°–86° F) for 48 h or refrigerated at 2°–8° C (36°–46° F) for 7 d. Discard unused portions.

ADVERSE EFFECTS (≥1%) **CNS:** *Fatigue,* paresthesia, hyperthermia. **CV:** Hypotension. **GI:** *Nausea, vomiting, diarrhea,* anorexia, stomatitis, dysgeusia, mucositis, metallic taste. **Hematologic:** Anemia, granulocytopenia, thrombocytopenia. **Metabolic:** Hypocalcemia, hypophosphatemia, hypomagnesemia. **Urogenital:** <u>Nephrotoxicity</u>, acute renal failure. **Other:** Optic neuritis, maculopapular rash.

INTERACTIONS Drug: AMINOGLYCOSIDES, **amphotericin B, vancomycin** increase the risk of nephrotoxicity.

PHARMACOKINETICS Onset: 48 h. **Duration:** 4–14 d after discontinuation of therapy. **Distribution:** Concentrates in tumors; distributed to lung, skin, muscle, and heart with high concentrations in liver and kidney; not known if crosses placenta or is distributed into breast milk. **Metabolism:** Not metabolized. **Elimination:** 35%–71% is excreted through kidneys within first 24 h after administration. **Half-Life:** 25–111 h.

NURSING IMPLICATIONS

Assessment & Drug Effects

- Lab tests: Monitor BUN and serum creatinine throughout therapy. Notify physician if serum creatinine exceeds 2–5 mg/dL; discontinue drug if this occurs. Also, check baseline serum calcium and serum phosphorus; follow with assessments daily and twice weekly, respectively.
- Note: If hypocalcemia occurs, withhold gallium nitrate and notify physician.

Patient & Family Education

- Learn S&S of hypocalcemia (see Appendix F). Notify physician immediately if any occur.
- Do not breast feed while taking this drug.

GANCICLOVIR

(gan-ci'clo-vir)

Cytovene

Classifications: ANTIINFECTIVE; ANTIVIRAL AGENT

Prototype: Acyclovir

Pregnancy Category: C

AVAILABILITY 250 mg, 500 mg capsules; 500 mg powder for injection

ACTIONS Ganciclovir is an antiviral drug active against cytomegalovirus (CMV). It prevents the replication CMV DNA.

THERAPEUTIC EFFECTS Sensitive human viruses include CMV, herpes simplex virus-1 and -2 (HSV-1, HSV-2), Epstein-Barr virus, and varicella-zoster virus.

USES CMV retinitis, prophylaxis and treatment of systemic CMV infections in immunocompromised patients including HIV-positive and transplant patients.

CONTRAINDICATIONS Hypersensitivity to ganciclovir or acyclovir, lactation.

CAUTIOUS USE Renal impairment, older adults, pregnancy (category C). Safety and efficacy in children are not established.

G

ROUTE & DOSAGE

Induction Therapy

Adult/Child: **IV** >3 mo, 5 mg/kg over 1 h q12h for 14–21 d (doses may range from 2.5–5.0 mg/kg over 1 h q8–12h for 10–35 d)

Maintenance Therapy

Adult: **IV** 5 mg/kg over 1 h qd or 6 mg/kg over 1 h qd 5 d/wk
PO 1000 mg t.i.d. or 500 mg 6 times/d q3h while awake

Prevention of CMV Disease in Transplant Recipients

Adult/Child: **IV** 5 mg/kg q12h 7–14 d, then 5 mg/kg q.d. or 6 mg/kg/d 5 d/wk

CMV Infection after Bone Marrow Transplant

Child: **IV** 7.5–19.5 mg/kg/d divided q8h

Renal Impairment

See prescribing information for dosing in patients with renal impairment

ADMINISTRATION

- Note: Do not administer if neutrophil count falls below 500/

mm^3 or platelet count falls below 25,000/mm^3.

- Avoid direct contact of powder in capsules or solution with skin and mucous membranes. Wash thoroughly with soap and water if contact occurs.

Oral

- Give with food.

Intravenous

G

IV administration to infants and children: Verify correct IV concentration and rate of infusion with physician.

PREPARE: **Intermittent:** Reconstitute the 500-mg vial using only 10 mL of sterile water (supplied) for injection immediately before use to yield 50 mg/mL. ▪ Shake well to dissolve. ▪ Withdraw the ordered amount and add to 100 mL of NS, D5W, or RL (volume less than 100 mL may be used, but the final concentration should be <10 mg/mL).

ADMINISTER: **Intermittent:** Give at a constant rate over 1 h. Avoid rapid infusion or bolus injection.

INCOMPATIBILITIES **Solution/additive:** Amino acid solutions (TPN), bacteriostatic water for injection, **fludarabine, foscarnet, ondansetron. Y-site: Total parenteral nutrition.**

- Store reconstituted solutions refrigerated at 4° C; use within 12 h.
- Store infusion solution refrigerated up to 24 h of preparation.

ADVERSE EFFECTS (≥1%) **CNS:** *Fever,* headache, disorientation, mental status changes, ataxia, coma, confusion, dizziness, paresthesia, nervousness, somnolence, tremor. **CV:** Edema, phlebitis. **GI:** *Nausea, diarrhea,* anorexia, elevated liver enzymes. **Hematologic:** *Bone marrow suppression, thrombocytopenia, granulocytopenia, eosinophilia, leukopenia,* hyperbilirubinemia. **Metabolic:** Hyperthermia, hypoglycemia. **Urogenital:** Infertility. **Skin:** Rash.

INTERACTIONS Drug: ANTINEOPLASTIC AGENTS, **amphotericin B, didanosine, trimethoprim-sulfamethoxazole (TMP-SMZ), dapsone, pentamidine, probenecid, zidovudine** may increase bone marrow suppression and other toxic effects of ganciclovir; may increase risk of nephrotoxicity from **cyclosporine;** may increase risk of seizures due to **imipenem-cilastatin.**

PHARMACOKINETICS Onset: 3–8 d. **Duration:** Clinical relapse can occur 14 d to 3.5 mo after stopping therapy; positive blood and urine cultures recur 12–60 d after therapy. **Distribution:** Distributes throughout body including CSF, eye, lungs, liver, and kidneys; crosses placenta in animals; not known if distributed into breast milk. **Metabolism:** Not metabolized. **Elimination:** 94%–99% of dose is excreted unchanged in urine. **Half-Life:** 2.5–4.2 h.

NURSING IMPLICATIONS

Assessment & Drug Effects

- Lab tests: Neutrophil and platelet counts at least every other day during twice-daily dosing and weekly thereafter; more frequent monitoring may be indicated in certain patients. Monitor serum creatinine or creatinine clearance at least q2wk. Closely monitor renal function in the older adult.
- Inspect IV insertion site throughout infusion for signs and symptoms of phlebitis.

Patient & Family Education

- Note: Drug is not a cure for CMV retinitis; follow regular ophthalmologic examination schedule.
- Drink lots of fluids during therapy.

- Use barrier contraception throughout therapy and for at least 90 d afterwards.
- Maintain frequent hematologic monitoring.
- Do not breast feed while taking this drug.

GANIRELIX ACETATE

(gan-i-rel'ix)

Antagon

Classifications: HORMONES & SYNTHETIC SUBSTITUTES; GONADOTROPIN-RELEASING HORMONE ANTAGONIST

Prototype: Ganirelix

Pregnancy Category: X

AVAILABILITY 250 mcg/0.5 mL syringe

ACTIONS Ganirelix is a gonadotropin-releasing hormone (GnRH) antagonist which suppresses pituitary gonadotropins and sex hormones.

THERAPEUTIC EFFECTS It prevents LH surges in reproductive protocols, and causes shrinkage of uterine fibroids.

USES Infertility treatment.

CONTRAINDICATIONS Prior hypersensitivity to ganirelix, LHRH, or other LHRH analogs; pregnancy (category X), lactation.

CAUTIOUS USE History of current allergic disorders (e.g., asthma, hayfever, urticaria, eczema) or a history of allergic reactions to medications; renal/hepatic dysfunction; endocrine disorders.

ROUTE & DOSAGE

Infertility

Adult: **SC** After initiating follicle-stimulating hormone (FSH) therapy on day 2 or 3 of the cycle, give 250 mcg once daily during the early-to-mid-follicular phase

ADMINISTRATION

- Note: The packaging of the product, Antagon, contains natural rubber latex which may cause allergic reactions.

Subcutaneous

- Inject SC into the abdomen around the umbilicus or into the upper thigh.
- Rotate injection sites.
- Store at 5°–30° C (59°–86° F) and protect from light.

ADVERSE EFFECTS (≥1%) **CNS:** Headache. **GI:** Abdominal pain, nausea. **Endocrine:** Ovarian hyperstimulation syndrome. **Skin:** Injection site reaction. **Urogenital:** Vaginal bleeding.

INTERACTIONS Drug: No clinically significant interactions established.

PHARMACOKINETICS Absorption: 91% absorbed from SC site. **Peak:** 1 h. **Distribution:** 81% protein bound. **Elimination:** 75% excreted in feces; 22% in urine. **Half-Life:** 13–16 h.

NURSING IMPLICATIONS

Assessment & Drug Effects

- Exercise caution with patients with hypersensitivity to GnRH or with known allergic disorders (e.g., asthma, hay fever). These patients should be carefully monitored after the first injection for S&S of an anaphylactic reaction.
- Lab tests: Monitor baseline and periodic CBC with differential, and periodic total bilirubin.

Patient & Family Education

- Report menstrual disorders (e.g., spotting, frank vaginal bleeding) to physician.

- Notify physician immediately if you think you are pregnant.
- Do not breast feed while taking this drug.

GATIFLOXACIN

(gat-i-flox'a-sin)
Tequin
Classifications: ANTIINFECTIVE; ANTIBIOTIC; QUINOLONE
Prototype: Ciprofloxacin
Pregnancy Category: C

G

AVAILABILITY 200 mg, 400 mg tablets; 200 mg/20 mL, 400 mg/40 mL vials; 200 mg/100 mL, 400 mg/200 mL premixed bags

ACTIONS Synthetic quinolone that is a broad spectrum bactericidal agent. Inhibits DNA-gyrase, topoisomerase II, an enzyme necessary for bacterial replication, transcription, repair and recombination.
THERAPEUTIC EFFECTS Effectiveness indicated by normal C&S, WBC counts, and no systemic signs of infection. Effective against methicillin-resistant *Staphylococcus aureus* (MRSA) bacteria infections, penicillin resistant *Streptococcus pneumoniae,* and *Pseudomonas aeruginosa,* as well as cocci resistant to other quinolone antimicrobials.

USES Acute bacterial exacerbation of chronic bronchitis; acute sinusitis; community-acquired pneumonia; uncomplicated or complicated UTI; pyelonephritis; gonorrhea due to susceptible organisms.

CONTRAINDICATIONS Hypersensitivity to gatifloxacin or other quinolone antibiotics; pregnancy (category C).
CAUTIOUS USE Lactation; patients with central nervous system disorders including seizures or epilepsy; GI disorders, renal dysfunction; hypersensitivity to other medications; concurrent administration of aluminum-containing antacids. Safety and efficacy in children <18 y are unknown.

ROUTE & DOSAGE

Acute Bacterial Exacerbation of Chronic Bronchitis, Complicated
Adult: **PO/IV** 400 mg q.d. times 5 d

Complicated UTI, Acute Pyelonephritis
Adult: **PO/IV** 400 mg q.d. times 7–10 d

Acute Sinusitis
Adult: **PO/IV** 400 mg q.d. times 10 d

Community Acquired Pneumonia
Adult: **PO/IV** 400 mg q.d. times 7–14 d

Uncomplicated UTI
Adult: **PO/IV** 400 mg as a single dose or 200 mg q.d. times 3 d

Uncomplicated Gonorrhea
Adult: **PO/IV** 400 mg as a single dose

Renal Impairment
Cl_{cr} <40 mL/min or on dialysis: 400 mg times 1 d, then 200 mg q.d.

ADMINISTRATION

Oral
- Give at least 4 h before or after an aluminum- or magnesium-containing antacid, or iron-containing products.
- Store at 15°–30° C (59°–86° F).

Intravenous

PREPARE: **IV Infusion:** Dilute a 200 mg/20 mL or 400 mg/40 mL single-use vial by adding contents of the vial to either 80 mL or 160 mL, respectively, of D5W, NS, D5/NS, RL or other compatible IV solution. Resulting IV solution contains 2 mg/mL.

ADMINISTER: **IV Infusion:** Give a single dose over at least 60 min. Avoid rapid infusion.

INCOMPATIBILITIES **Y-site: Amphotericin B, amphotericin B cholesteryl sulfate, cefoperazone, cefonicid, cefoxitin, diazepam, furosemide, heparin, mezlocillin, phenytoin, piperacillin, piperacillin/tazobactam, potassium phosphate, vancomycin.**

ADVERSE EFFECTS (≥1%) **Body as a Whole:** Headache, allergic reactions, chills, fever; back pain, chest pain. **CNS:** Dizziness, abnormal dreams, insomnia, paresthesia, tremor, vasodilatation, vertigo. **CV:** Palpitation; peripheral edema. **GI:** Nausea, diarrhea, abdominal pain, constipation, dyspepsia, glossitis, oral moniliasis, stomatitis, vomiting. **Respiratory:** Dyspnea, pharyngitis. **Skin:** Rash, sweating. **Urogenital:** Vaginitis; dysuria; hematuria. **Special Senses:** Abnormal vision; taste perversion; tinnitus.

DIAGNOSTIC TEST INTERFERENCE May cause false positive on ***opiate screening tests.***

INTERACTIONS Drug: Probenecid decreases elimination of **gatifloxacin; ferrous sulfate,** ALUMINUM- or MAGNESIUM-CONTAINING ANTACIDS reduce absorption of **gatifloxacin; gatifloxacin** may cause slight increase in **digoxin** levels.

PHARMACOKINETICS Absorption: 96% absorbed from GI tract. **Peak:** 1–2 h PO. **Distribution:** 20% protein bound. **Metabolism:** Minimal metabolism (<1%). **Elimination:** Primarily excreted in urine. **Half-Life:** 7–14 h (up to 35–40 h in severe renal failure).

NURSING IMPLICATIONS

Assessment & Drug Effects

- Monitor for S&S of CNS disturbance especially with history of cerebrovascular disease or seizures.
- Lab tests: C&S prior to initiation of therapy; WBC with differential.
- Monitor for changes in digoxin blood levels with coadministered drugs.

Patient & Family Education

- Be aware that increased risk of seizures are associated with drug use in patient with history of seizures.
- Report unexplained dizziness or problems with balance, severe diarrhea, skin rash, mental status changes.
- Do not breast feed while taking this drug without consulting physician.

G

GEFITINIB Pr

(ge-fi′ti-nib)

Iressa

Classifications: ANTINEOPLASTIC AGENT; EPIDERMAL GROWTH FACTOR RECEPTOR (EGFR); TYROSINE KINASE INHIBITOR

Pregnancy Category: D

AVAILABILITY 250 mg tablets

ACTIONS Gefitinib is a selective epidermal growth factor receptor (EGFR) tyrosine kinase inhibitor (EGFR-TKI). EGFR is expressed or overexpressed in many cancers. EGFR expression is associated with poor prognosis, development of metastasis, and resistance to chemotherapy, hormonal therapy, and radiation therapy.

G

THERAPEUTIC EFFECTS Gefitinib inhibits up-regulation or overexpression of EGRF in cancer cells diminishing their capacity for cell proliferation, cell survival, and decreasing their invasive capacity and metastases.

USES Treatment of locally advanced or metastatic non-small cell lung cancer after failure of both platinum and docetaxel therapy.

UNLABELED USES Treatment of head and neck and other solid tumors.

CONTRAINDICATIONS Hypersensitivity to gefitinib; pregnancy (category D), lactation; children <18 y.

CAUTIOUS USE Severe renal impairment; hepatic impairment; bacterial/viral infection; dermatologic toxicities; GI disorders; hepatic insufficiency; interstitial lung disease (interstitial pneumonia, pneumonitis, and alveolitis), pulmonary fibrosis, respiratory insufficiency; myelosuppression; females of childbearing age; prior chemotherapy, radiation therapy; ocular toxicities (corneal ulcer, eye pain).

ROUTE & DOSAGE

Non-small Cell Lung Cancer

Adult: **PO** 250 mg q.d., may increase to 500 mg q.d. if on enzyme-inducing drugs

Head and Neck Cancers

Adult: **PO** 500 mg/day

ADMINISTRATION

Oral

- Give without regard to meals.
- Store tablets at 15°–30° C (59°–86° F).

ADVERSE EFFECTS (≥1%) **Body as a Whole:** Asthenia, peripheral edema. **GI:** *Diarrhea, nausea, vomiting,* anorexia, weight loss, stomatitis. **Respiratory:** Dyspnea, <u>interstitial lung disease.</u> **Skin:** *Acne/acneiform rash, dry skin,* pruritus, vesicular/bullous rash. **Special Senses:** Amblyopia, conjunctivitis, aberrant eyelash growth.

INTERACTIONS Drug: BARBITURATES, **bosentan, carbamazepine, dexamethasone, nevirapine, oxcarbazepine, phenytoin or fosphenytoin, rifampin, rifabutin, rifapentine** may increase metabolism and decrease levels of **gefitinib; amiodarone,** PROTEASE INHIBITORS, **cimetidine, clarithromycin, dalfopristin; quinupristin, delavirdine, efavirenz, erythromycin, fluconazole, fluvoxamine, fluoxetine, imatinib, itraconazole, ketoconazole, mifepristone, nefazodone and voriconazole** may increase levels and toxicity of gefitinib; may increase INR with **warfarin;** H_2-RECEPTOR ANTAGONISTS, PROTON PUMP INHIBITORS may decrease absorption of gefitinib. **Food: Grapefruit juice** may increase levels and toxicity of gefitinib. **Herbal: St. John's wort** may decrease levels of **gefitinib.**

PHARMACOKINETICS Absorption: Slowly absorbed, 60% reaches systemic circulation. **Peak:** 3–7 h. **Metabolism:** Metabolized in liver primarily by CYP3A4. **Elimination:** 86% eliminated in feces. **Half-Life:** 48 h.

NURSING IMPLICATIONS

Assessment & Drug Effects

- Monitor pulmonary status and report promptly dyspnea, cough, and fever.
- Withhold drug and notify physician for significant elevations of transaminases, bilirubin, or alkaline phosphatase.

- Monitor for adverse effects, especially with concurrent use of drugs that may inhibit CYP3A4 (e.g., amiodarone, cimetidine, erythromycin, fluconazole, grapefruit juice, etc.). See INTERACTIONS.
- Lab tests: Periodic LFTs; frequent PT/INR with concurrent warfarin.

Patient & Family Education

- Report promptly any of the following: eye pain or irritation; fever; breathing difficulty or shortness of breath; mouth sores.
- Inform physician of all prescription, nonprescription, or herbal drugs you are taking.
- Females should use reliable contraceptives while taking this drug.
- Minimize or avoid intake of grapefruit juice while taking this drug.
- Do not breast feed while taking this drug.

GEMCITABINE HYDROCHLORIDE

(gem-ci'ta-been)

Gemzar

Classifications: ANTINEOPLASTIC AGENT; ANTIMETABOLITE; IMMUNOSUPPRESSANT

Prototype: Fluorouracil

Pregnancy Category: D

AVAILABILITY 20 mg/mL injection

ACTIONS Pyrimidine analog with cell phase specificity by affecting rapidly dividing cells in S phase (DNA synthesis). It also blocks the progression of cells from G_1 phase to S phase of cell cycle. Gemcitabine interferes with DNA synthesis by inhibiting ribonucleotide reductase, which results in a reduction in the concentration of deoxynucleotides. In addition, if gemcitabine is incorporated into the DNA strand, it inhibits further growth of the DNA strand.

THERAPEUTIC EFFECTS Gemcitabine induces DNA fragmentation in cells resulting in the cell death of tumor cells.

USES Locally advanced or metastatic adenocarcinoma of the pancreas.

CONTRAINDICATIONS Hypersensitivity to gemcitabine, severe thrombocytopenia, acute infection, pregnancy (category D), lactation.

CAUTIOUS USE Myelosuppression, renal or hepatic dysfunction, history of bleeding disorders, infection, previous cytotoxic or radiation treatment. Safety and effectiveness in children are not established.

ROUTE & DOSAGE

Pancreatic Cancer

Adult: **IV** 1000 mg/m^2 once weekly for up to 7 wk, followed by 1 wk rest from treatment; may repeat once weekly for 3 of every 4 wk

ADMINISTRATION

Intravenous

PREPARE: **IV Infusion:** Dilute with NS without preservatives by adding 5 mL or 25 mL to the 200-mg or 1-g vial, respectively, to yield 40 mg/mL. ▪ Shake to dissolve. ▪ Dilute further if necessary with NS to concentrations as low as 0.1 mg/mL.

ADMINISTER: **IV Infusion:** Infuse over 30 min. Infusion time > 60 min is associated with increased toxicity.

- Store reconstituted solutions unrefrigerated at 20°–25° C (68°–77°

F). Use within 24 h of reconstitution.

ADVERSE EFFECTS (≥1%) **CNS:** *Fever, flu-like syndrome (anorexia, headache, cough, chills, myalgia),* paresthesias. **GI:** *Nausea, vomiting, diarrhea,* stomatitis, *transient elevations of liver transaminases.* **Hematologic:** *Myelosuppression (anemia, leukopenia, neutropenia, thrombocytopenia).* **Urogenital:** Mild proteinuria and hematuria. **Other:** *Dyspnea, edema, peripheral edema, infection.*

PHARMACOKINETICS Peak: Peak concentrations reached by 30 min after infusion; lower clearance in women and older adult results in higher concentrations at any given dose. **Distribution:** Crosses placenta, distributed into breast milk. **Metabolism:** Metabolized intracellularly by nucleoside kinases to active diphosphate (dFdCDP) and triphosphate (dFdCTP) nucleosides. **Elimination:** 92%–98% recovered in urine within 1 wk. **Half-Life:** 32–94 min.

NURSING IMPLICATIONS

Assessment & Drug Effects

- Lab tests: Monitor CBC with differential and platelet count prior to each dose. Monitor baseline and periodic renal and hepatic function.

Patient & Family Education

- Learn about common adverse effects and measures to control or minimize when possible. Notify physician immediately of any distressing adverse effects.
- Note: Fever with flu-like symptoms, rash, and GI distress are very common.
- Do not breast feed while taking this drug.

GEMFIBROZIL

(gem-fi'broe-zil)
Lopid
Classifications: CARDIOVASCULAR AGENT; ANTILIPEMIC; FIBRATE
Prototype: Clofibrate
Pregnancy Category: C

AVAILABILITY 600 mg tablets

ACTIONS Fibric acid derivative with lipid regulating properties. Blocks lipolysis of stored triglycerides in adipose tissue and inhibits hepatic uptake of fatty acids.
THERAPEUTIC EFFECTS Decreases VLDL and therefore triglyceride synthesis. Produces a moderate increase in HDL cholesterol levels and reduces levels of total and LDL cholesterol and triglycerides.

USES Patients with very high serum triglyceride levels (above 750 mg/dL) (type IV and V hyperlipidemia) who have not responded favorably to intensive diet restriction and who are at risk of pancreatitis and abdominal pain. Also severe familial hypercholesterolemia (type IIa or IIb) that developed in childhood and has failed to respond to dietary control or to other cholesterol-lowering drugs.

CONTRAINDICATIONS Gallbladder disease, biliary cirrhosis, hepatic or severe renal dysfunction; pregnancy (category C), lactation. Safety and efficacy in children <18 y are not established.
CAUTIOUS USE Diabetes mellitus, hypothyroidism; renal impairment, cholelithiasis.

ROUTE & DOSAGE

Hypertriglyceridemia
Adult: **PO** 600 mg b.i.d. 30 min before morning and evening

 Common adverse effects in *italic*, life-threatening effects underlined; generic names in **bold**; classifications in SMALL CAPS; ♣ Canadian drug name; ◉ Prototype drug

meal, may increase up to 1500 mg/d

ADMINISTRATION

Oral

- Give 30 min before breakfast and evening meal.
- Store at 15°–30° C (59°–86° F) unless otherwise directed.

ADVERSE EFFECTS (≥1%) **CNS:** Headache, dizziness, blurred vision. **GI:** *Abdominal* or *epigastric pain,* diarrhea, nausea, vomiting, flatulence. **Hematologic:** Eosinophilia, mild decreases in Hct, Hgb. **Musculoskeletal:** Painful extremities, back pain, muscle cramps, myalgia, arthralgia, swollen joints. **Skin:** Rash, dermatitis, pruritus, urticaria. **Endocrine:** Hypokalemia, moderate hyperglycemia.

INTERACTIONS Drug: May potentiate hypoprothrombinemic effects of ORAL ANTICOAGULANTS; **lovastatin** increases risk of myopathy and rhabdomyolysis; may increase **repaglinide** levels and duration of action.

PHARMACOKINETICS Absorption: Readily absorbed from GI tract. **Peak:** 1–2 h. **Metabolism:** Undergoes enterohepatic circulation. **Elimination:** Excreted primarily in urine; 6% excreted in feces. **Half-Life:** 1.3–1.5 h.

NURSING IMPLICATIONS

Assessment & Drug Effects

- Lab tests: Monitor baseline and at regular intervals during first year of therapy for serum LDL and VLDL, triglycerides, total cholesterol, CBC, blood glucose, liver function tests.
- Note: Mild decreases in WBC, Hgb, Hct may occur during early stage of treatment but generally stabilize with continued therapy.
- Notify physician if the lipid response is not adequate after 3 *mo* of therapy.
- Notify physician if patient presents S&S suggestive of cholelithiasis or cholecystitis; gallbladder studies may be indicated. Symptoms often occur during the night or early morning; jaundice may or may not be present.

Patient & Family Education

- Notify physician promptly if unexplained bleeding occurs (e.g., easy bruising, epistaxis, hematuria).
- Do not drive or engage in other potentially hazardous activities until response to drug is known.
- Note: Patients with high serum triglyceride levels are generally advised to lose excess weight and to restrict carbohydrate and alcohol intake (alcohol increases serum triglyceride levels).
- Do not breast feed while taking this drug without consulting physician.

GEMIFLOXACIN

(gem-i-flox'a-cin)
Factive
Classifications: ANTI-INFECTIVE; ANTIBIOTIC; QUINOLONE
Prototype: Ciprofloxacin HCl
Pregnancy Category: C

AVAILABILITY 320 mg tablet

ACTIONS Gemifloxacin inhibits bacterial DNA gyrases, enzymes essential in replication, transcription, and repair of bacterial DNA.
THERAPEUTIC EFFECTS Gemifloxacin is active against a wide range of gram-positive and gram-negative bacteria. Gemifloxacin has greater activity against gram-positive cocci and against penicillin-

and ciprofloxacin-resistant *Streptococcus pneumoniae* than other fluoroquinolones.

USES Treatment of acute exacerbations of chronic bronchitis, mild to moderate community-acquired pneumonia.

UNLABELED USES Acute sinusitis, UTI, acute pyelonephritis.

CONTRAINDICATIONS Hypersensitivity to gemifloxacin or other fluoroquinolone antibiotics; pregnancy (category C).

CAUTIOUS USE History of QT interval prolongation, hypokalemia, hypomagnesia, or concurrent use of Class IA or III antiarrhythmic agents; bradycardia, acute myocardial ischemia; concurrent use of other medications that may prolong the QT interval; central nervous system disorders such as epilepsy; glucose 6-phosphate dehydrogenase deficiency; tendonitis, elderly, concurrent use of corticosteroids; lactation; children.

ROUTE & DOSAGE

Acute Exacerbation of Chronic Bronchitis

Adult: **PO** 320 mg q.d. × 5 d

Community Acquired Pneumonia

Adult: **PO** 320 mg q.d. × 7 d

Sinusitus

Adult: **PO** 320 mg q.d. × 10 d

UTI

Adult: **PO** 320 mg q.d. × 3 d

Renal Impairment

Cl_{cr} ≤40 mL/min: 160 mg q.d.

ADMINISTRATION

Oral

- Give 2 h before/3 h after drugs containing aluminum, magnesium, iron, zinc, or buffered tablets of any type.
- Give at least 2 h before sucralfate.
- Store at 15°–30° C (59°–86° F) and protect from light.

ADVERSE EFFECTS (≥1%) **CNS:** Headache. **GI:** Nausea, vomiting, diarrhea, elevated liver enzymes. **Skin:** Rash.

INTERACTIONS Drug: ANTACIDS, **didanosine (tablets and powder), iron, sevelamer, sulcralfate** decrease absorption; may prolong the QT interval with **amiodarone, bretylium, disopyramide, dofetilide, ibutilide, quinidine, procainamide, sotalol** leading to arrhythmias; may augment photoxicity of RETINOIDS.

PHARMACOKINETICS Absorption: 71% absorbed. **Peak:** 0.5–2 h. **Metabolism:** Minimally metabolized in liver. **Elimination:** Primarily renal. **Half-Life:** 7 h.

NURSING IMPLICATIONS

Assessment & Drug Effects

- Monitor cardiac status, especially with concurrent use of drugs that may prolong the QT interval. Report immediately bradycardia or S&S of heart failure.
- Withhold drug and report to physician any of the following: tremors, restlessness, lightheadedness, confusion, hallucinations, paranoia, depression, nightmares, and insomnia.
- Lab tests: C&S prior to initiation of therapy; baseline and periodic serum electrolytes; frequent blood glucose levels in diabetics; CBC with differential and platelet count with prolonged treatment.

Patient & Family Education

- Use sunscreen and protective clothing outdoors. Avoid sun lamps.

- Stop gemifloxacin and notify physician for pain or swelling of a tendon or around a joint.
- Drink fluid liberally (unless contraindicated) while taking this drug.
- Do not drive or engage in other hazardous activities until reaction to drug is known.
- Do not breast feed without consulting physician.

GEMTUZUMAB OZOGAMICIN

(gem-tu'zu-mab)
Mylotarg
Classifications: IMMUNOSUPPRESSANT; MONOCLONAL ANTIBODY
Prototype: Basiliximab
Pregnancy Category: D

AVAILABILITY 5 mg vial

ACTIONS Chemotherapeutic agent composed of recombinant IgG antibodies which binds specifically to the CD33 antigens.
THERAPEUTIC EFFECTS Cytotoxic to the CD33 positive human leukemia cells in the bone marrow found on the surface of leukemic cells.

USES Treatment of CD33 positive acute myeloid leukemia (AML) in first relapse in patients ≥60 y.

CONTRAINDICATIONS Hypersensitivity to gemtuzumab or anti-CD33 antibody therapy, systemic infections; pregnancy (category D), lactation.
CAUTIOUS USE Hepatic impairment; renal dysfunction; moderate or severe thrombocytopenia or neutropenia. History of asthma or allergies; concurrent administration with antiplatelet agents or anticoagulants.

ROUTE & DOSAGE

Acute Myeloid Leukemia (AML)
Adult: **IV** 9 mg/m^2 infused over 2 h, repeat in 14 d

ADMINISTRATION

Intravenous

- Protect gemtuzumab from sunlight and unshielded fluorescent light during preparation and administration.
- Allow vials to come to room temperature before reconstitution.
- Acetaminophen 650 mg orally and diphenhydramine 25–50 mg IV are normally given prior to infusion to control adverse effects.

PREPARE: **Continuous:** Reconstitute each vial with 5 mL of sterile water for injection to yield 1 mg/mL. Gently swirl to dissolve. Dilute the reconstituted drug further just prior to administration by withdrawing the required amount of drug and adding it to 100 mL of NS. Cover the IV bag with a UV protectant cover.
ADMINISTER: **Continuous:** Infuse over 2 h through a separate IV line with a nonpyrogenic low-protein-binding 1.2 micron filter. Do not give push as a bolus dose.
INCOMPATIBILITIES **Solution/additive & Y-site:** Do not mix with other drugs.

- Store unopened vials refrigerated at 2°–8° C (36°–46° F). Store reconstituted drug refrigerated at 2°–8° C (36°–46° F) and protected for light for ≤8 h.

ADVERSE EFFECTS (≥1%) **Body as a Whole:** Severe hypersensitivity *anaphylaxis, chills, fever, asthenia, infection, sepsis.* **CV:** *Hypotension,*

G

hypertension, tachycardia. **GI:** *Nausea, vomiting, mucositis, abdominal pain, anorexia, constipation, diarrhea, stomatitis.* **Hematologic:** *Neutropenia, thrombocytopenia, anemia, bleeding,* epistaxis, cerebral hemorrhage, hematuria, ecchymosis. **Metabolic:** Hyperglycemia, *hyperbilirubinemia,* abnormal AST, ALT, hypokalemia, hypomagnesemia, increased lactic dehydrogenase. **Musculoskeletal:** Arthralgia. **CNS:** *Headache,* depression, dizziness, *insomnia.* **Respiratory:** Hypoxia, *dyspnea, cough,* pharyngitis, rhinitis, pneumonia, *fatal pulmonary events.* **Skin:** *Rash, herpes simplex, local reactions from infusion, peripheral edema, petechiae.*

INTERACTIONS No clinically significant interactions established.

PHARMACOKINETICS Metabolism: Hydrolyzed in liver to calicheamicin. **Half-Life:** 45–100 h.

NURSING IMPLICATIONS

Assessment & Drug Effects

- Monitor for S&S of postinfusion syndrome: fever, chills, and rigors which occur 2–4 h after initiation of infusion; hypotension and dyspnea which may occur during first 24 h after infusion.
- Monitor vital signs during and for at least 2 h after infusion.
- Lab tests: Monitor CBC with differential, platelet count, lymphoblast smears at least weekly. Periodically monitor liver functions and routine blood chemistry.

Patient & Family Education

- Report S&S of infection immediately to physician (e.g., chills, fever, sore throat, lower back or side pain).
- Report unusual bleeding or bruising, black tarry stools, or pinpoint red spots on skin to physician immediately.
- Avoid exposure to infections.
- Avoid immunizations unless approved by physician; avoid contact with anyone who has received oral polio virus vaccine.
- Avoid situations that could result in injury during periods of bone marrow suppression.

GENTAMICIN SULFATE (Pr)

(jen-ta-mye'sin)

Garamycin, Garamycin Ophthalmic, Genoptic

Classifications: ANTIINFECTIVE; AMINOGLYCOSIDE ANTIBIOTIC

Pregnancy Category: C

AVAILABILITY 10 mg/mL, 40 mg/mL; 0.1% ointment, cream; 3 mg/mL ophthalmic solution; 3 mg/g ophthalmic ointment

ACTIONS Broad-spectrum aminoglycoside antibiotic derived from *Micromonospora purpurea.* Action is usually bacteriocidal.

THERAPEUTIC EFFECTS Active against a wide variety of gram-negative bacteria, including *Citrobacter, Escherichia coli, Enterobacter, Klebsiella, Proteus* (including indole-positive and indole-negative strains), *Pseudomonas aeruginosa,* and *Serratia sp.* Also effective against certain gram-positive organisms, particularly penicillin-sensitive and some methicillin-resistant strains of *Staphylococcus aureus* (MRSA).

USES Parenteral use restricted to treatment of serious infections of GI, respiratory, and urinary tracts, CNS, bone, skin, and soft tissue (including burns) when other less toxic antimicrobial agents are ineffective or are contraindicated. Has been used in combination with other antibiotics. Also used topically for primary and secondary skin infections and for superficial infections of external eye and its adnexa.

UNLABELED USES Prophylaxis of bacterial endocarditis in patients undergoing operative procedures or instrumentation.

CONTRAINDICATIONS History of hypersensitivity to or toxic reaction with any aminoglycoside antibiotic. Safe use during pregnancy (category C) or lactation is not established.

CAUTIOUS USE Impaired renal function; history of eighth cranial (acoustic) nerve impairment; preexisting vertigo or dizziness or tinnitus; dehydration, fever; use in older adults, premature infants, neonates, and infants; obesity, neuromuscular disorders: myasthenia gravis, parkinsonian syndrome; hypocalcemia, heart failure, topical applications to widespread areas.

ROUTE & DOSAGE

Moderate to Severe Infection

Adult: **IV/IM** 1.5–2 mg/kg loading dose followed by 3–5 mg/kg/d in 2–3 divided doses **Intrathecal** 4–8 mg preservative free q.d. **Topical** 1–2 drops of solution in eye q4h up to 2 drops q1h or small amount of ointment b.i.d. or t.i.d.
Child: **IV/IM** 6–7.5 mg/kg/d in 3–4 divided doses **Intrathecal** *>3 mo,* 1–2 mg preservative free q.d.
Neonate: **IV/IM** 2.5 mg/kg q12–24h

Acute Pelvic Inflammatory Disease

Adult: **IV/IM** 2 mg/kg followed by 1.5 mg/kg q8h

Prophylaxis of Bacterial Endocarditis

Adult: **IV/IM** 1.5 mg/kg 30 min before procedure, may repeat in 8 h
Child: **IV/IM** *< 27 kg,* 2 mg/kg 30 min before procedure, may repeat in 8 h

ADMINISTRATION

Ophthalmic

- Apply pressure to inner canthus for 1 min immediately after instillation of drops.
- Have patient keep eyes closed for 1–2 min after administration of ophthalmic ointment to assure medication contact. Caution patient that vision will be blurred for a few minutes.

Topical

- Wash affected area with mild soap and water, rinse, and dry thoroughly. Gently apply small amount of medication to lesions; cover with sterile gauze.
- Do not apply topical preparations, particularly cream, to large denuded body surfaces because systemic absorption and toxicity are possible.

Intramuscular

- Give deep into a large muscle.
- Do not use solutions that are discolored or that contain particulate matter; drug for IV or IM is clear and colorless or slightly yellow.

Intrathecal

- Note: Intrathecal formulation is a clear and colorless solution.
- Use promptly after opening; contains no preservatives and any unused portion should be discarded.

Intravenous

PREPARE: **Intermittent:** Dilute a single dose with 50–200 mL of D5W or NS. For pediatric patients, amount of infusion fluid may be proportionately smaller depending on patient's needs but should be sufficient to be infused over the same time period as for adults.

ADMINISTER: **Intermittent:** Give over 30 min–2 h.

INCOMPATIBILITIES **Solution/additive:** Fat emulsion, TPN, **amphotericin B, ampicillin, carbenicillin,** CEPHALOSPORINS, **cytarabine, heparin. Y-site: Furosemide, iodipamide.**

- Store all gentamicin solutions between 2°–30° C (36°–86° F) unless otherwise directed by manufacturer.

G

ADVERSE EFFECTS (≥1%) **Special Senses:** Ototoxicity (vestibular disturbances, impaired hearing), optic neuritis. **CNS:** neuromuscular blockade: skeletal muscle weakness, apnea, respiratory paralysis (high doses); arachnoiditis (intrathecal use). **CV:** hypotension or hypertension. **GI:** Nausea, vomiting, transient increase in AST, ALT, and serum LDH and bilirubin; hepatomegaly, splenomegaly. **Hematologic:** Increased or decreased reticulocyte counts; granulocytopenia, thrombocytopenia (fever, bleeding tendency), thrombocytopenic purpura, anemia. **Body as a Whole:** Hypersensitivity (rash, pruritus, urticaria, exfoliative dermatitis, eosinophilia, burning sensation of skin, drug fever, joint pains, laryngeal edema, anaphylaxis). **Urogenital:** Nephrotoxicity: proteinuria, tubular necrosis, cells or casts in urine, hematuria, rising BUN, nonprotein nitrogen, serum creatinine; *decreased creatinine clearance.* **Other:** Local irritation and pain following IM use; thrombophlebitis, abscess, superinfections, syndrome of hypocalcemia (tetany, weakness, hypokalemia, hypomagnesemia). **Topical and Ophthalmic:** Photosensitivity, sensitization, erythema, pruritus; burning, stinging, and lacrimation (ophthalmic formulation).

INTERACTIONS Drug: Amphotericin B, capreomycin, cisplatin, methoxyflurane, polymyxin B, vancomycin, increase risk of nephrotoxicity. Ethacrynic acid and **furosemide** may increase risk of ototoxicity. GENERAL ANESTHETICS and NEUROMUSCULAR BLOCKING AGENTS (e.g., **succinylcholine**) potentiate neuromuscular blockade. **Indomethacin** may increase gentamicin levels in neonates.

PHARMACOKINETICS Absorption: Well absorbed from IM site. **Peak:** 30–90 min IM. **Distribution:** Widely distributed in body fluids, including ascitic, peritoneal, pleural, synovial, and abscess fluids; poor CNS penetration; concentrates in kidney and inner ear; crosses placenta. **Metabolism:** Not metabolized. **Elimination:** Excreted unchanged in urine; small amounts accumulate in kidney and are eliminated over 10–20 d; small amount excreted in breast milk. **Half-Life:** 2–4 h.

NURSING IMPLICATIONS

Assessment & Drug Effects

- Lab tests: Perform C&S and renal function prior to first dose and periodically during therapy; therapy may begin pending test results. Determine creatinine clearance and serum drug concentrations at frequent intervals, particularly for patients with impaired renal function, infants (renal immaturity), older adults, patients receiving high doses or therapy beyond 10 d, patients with fever or extensive burns, edema, obesity.
- Repeat C&S if improvement does not occur in 3–5 d; reevaluate therapy.

- Note: Dosages are generally adjusted to maintain peak serum gentamicin concentrations of 4–10 g/mL, and trough concentrations of 1–2 g/mL. Peak concentrations above 12 g/mL and trough concentrations above 2 g/mL are associated with toxicity.
- Draw blood specimens for peak serum gentamicin concentration 30 min–1h after IM administration, and 30 min after completion of a 30–60 min IV infusion. Draw blood specimens for trough levels just before the next IM or IV dose. Use nonheparinized tubes to collect blood.
- Check baseline weight and vital signs; determine vestibular and auditory function before therapy and at regular intervals. Check vestibular and auditory function again 3–4 wk after drug is discontinued (the time that deafness is most likely to occur).
- Monitor I&O. Keep patient well hydrated to prevent chemical irritation of renal tubules. Report oliguria, unusual appearance of urine, change in I&O ratio or pattern, and presence of edema (prolongs elimination time).
- Note: Ototoxic effect (see Appendix F) is greatest on the vestibular branch of eighth cranial (acoustic) nerve (symptoms: headache, dizziness or vertigo, nausea and vomiting with motion, ataxia, nystagmus). However, damage to the auditory branch (tinnitus, roaring noises, sensation of fullness in ears, hearing impairment) may also occur. Report promptly to prevent permanent damage.
- Watch for S&S of bacterial overgrowth (opportunistic infections) with resistant or nonsusceptible organisms (diarrhea, anogenital itching, vaginal discharge, stomatitis, glossitis).

Patient & Family Education

- Note: When using topical applications: Avoid excessive exposure to sunlight because of danger of photosensitivity; withhold medication and notify physician if condition fails to improve within 1 wk, worsens, or signs of irritation or sensitivity occur; and apply medication as directed and only for length of time prescribed (overuse can result in superinfections).
- Do not breast feed while taking this drug without consulting physician.

G

GLATIRAMER ACETATE

(gla-tir′a-mer)

Copaxone, Copolymer-1

Classification: IMMUNOMODULATOR

Pregnancy Category: B

AVAILABILITY 20 mg injection

ACTIONS Glatiramer (formerly Copolymer-1) is a random synthetic copolymer of L-alanine, L-glutamic acid, L-lysine, and L-tyrosine. Its mechanism of action is unknown.

THERAPEUTIC EFFECTS Its function is to reduce the relapse rate of multiple sclerosis (MS), a demyelinating disease of the CNS of unknown origin. During an autoimmune response, glatiramer is thought to divert immune cells away from their myelin target as occurs in multiple sclerosis.

USES Reduction of the frequency of relapses in patients with relapsing–remitting multiple sclerosis.

CONTRAINDICATIONS Hypersensitivity to glatiramer acetate or mannitol.

CAUTIOUS USE Pregnancy (category B), lactation, children <18 y of age, history of asthma or other respiratory disorders.

ROUTE & DOSAGE

Multiple Sclerosis
Adult: **SC** 20 mg q.d.

ADMINISTRATION

Subcutaneous
- Use recommended SC injection sites: Arms, abdomen, hips, and thighs.
- Reconstitute with supplied diluent, swirl gently, let stand at room temperature until completely dissolved, then use immediately.
- Do not store reconstituted drug. Before reconstitution, store vials at –20° to –10° C (–4° to –14° F).

ADVERSE EFFECTS (≥1%) **Body as a Whole:** *Asthenia, back pain,* chills, facial edema, fever, *flu-like syndrome, infection, pain, arthralgia.* **CNS:** Migraine, agitation, *anxiety, hypotonia.* **CV:** *Chest pain, palpitations,* syncope, tachycardia, *vasodilation.* **GI:** *Diarrhea, nausea,* anorexia, gastroenteritis, vomiting. **Respiratory:** *Dyspnea, rhinitis,* bronchitis. **Skin:** *Rash, pruritus, sweating.* **Other:** *Postinjection reaction (flushing, chest pain, palpitations, anxiety, dyspnea, constriction of throat, urticaria), injection site reactions (erythema, hemorrhage, pain, pruritus, urticaria, swelling),* ecchymoses, *lymphadenopathy,* ear pain, dysmenorrhea, urinary urgency.

PHARMACOKINETICS Not studied

NURSING IMPLICATIONS

Assessment & Drug Effects
- Monitor for therapeutic effectiveness: Indicated by longer remission periods and reduced frequency of attacks.
- Assess for systemic postinjection reactions (see PATIENT & FAMILY EDUCATION). Assure patient that reaction is self-limiting. Assess for local reactions at injection sites including erythema, itching, induration, and soreness.
- Monitor for S&S of compromised immune response (e.g., increasing frequency of infections).

Patient & Family Education
- Note: Systemic postinjection reaction with chest pain, palpitations, flushing, urticaria, anxiety, dyspnea, and laryngeal constriction may occur immediately after injection. These symptoms are transient (lasting from 30 s–30 min), require no treatment, and resolve spontaneously.
- Notify physician of a planned or suspected pregnancy.
- Report any distressing adverse drug effects.
- Do not breast feed while taking this drug without consulting physician.

GLIMEPIRIDE
(gli-me′pi-ride)
Amaryl
Classifications: HORMONES AND SYNTHETIC SUBSTITUTES; ANTIDIABETIC; SULFONYLUREA
Prototype: Glyburide
Pregnancy Category: C

AVAILABILITY 1 mg, 2 mg, 4 mg tablets

ACTIONS Second-generation sulfonylurea hypoglycemic agent used for once-a-day dosing.
THERAPEUTIC EFFECTS Directly stimulates functioning pancreatic beta cells to secrete insulin, leading to direct drop in blood glucose. Indirect action leads to in-

creased sensitivity of peripheral insulin receptors, resulting in increased insulin binding in peripheral tissues. Glimepiride improves postprandial glycemic control.

USES Adjunct to diet and exercise in patients with type 2 diabetes, may also be used in combination with insulin in type 2 diabetes.

CONTRAINDICATIONS Hypersensitivity to glimepiride, diabetic ketoacidosis, pregnancy (category C), lactation, nondiabetic patients with renal glycosuria.

CAUTIOUS USE Previous hypersensitivity to other sulfonylureas, sulfonamides, or thiazide diuretics; hypoglycemia or conditions predisposing to hypoglycemia (e.g., prolonged nausea and vomiting, alcohol ingestion, renal or hepatic function impairment, severe infections, surgery). Safe use in children is not established.

ROUTE & DOSAGE

Type 2 Diabetes mellitus

Adult: **PO** Start with 1–2 mg once daily with breakfast or first main meal, may increase to usual maintenance dose of 1–4 mg once daily (max: 8 mg/d)

ADMINISTRATION

Oral

- Give with breakfast or first main meal.
- Note: Maximum starting dose is ≤2 mg. With renal or hepatic insufficiency, initial recommended dose is 1 mg. Increase by ≤2 mg at 1- to 2-wk intervals maximum of 8 mg/d.
- Store in tightly closed container at 15°–30° C (59°–86° F).

ADVERSE EFFECTS (≥1%) **CNS:** Dizziness, asthenia, headache, blurred vision, changes in accommodation. **GI:** Nausea, vomiting, diarrhea, abdominal pain. **Hematologic:** Leukopenia, agranulocytosis (rare), thrombocytopenia. **Metabolic:** Hypoglycemia. **Skin:** Rash, pruritus, erythema, urticaria, maculopapular eruptions.

INTERACTIONS Drug: Hypoglycemic effects may be potentiated by other highly protein-bound drugs (e.g., ADRENERGIC ANTAGONISTS, **chloramphenicol,** MAO INHIBITORS, NSAIDS, **probenecid,** SALICYLATES, SULFONAMIDES, **warfarin**). CORTICOSTEROIDS, **phenytoin, isoniazid, nicotinic acid,** SYMPATHOMIMETIC AMINES, THIAZIDE DIURETICS may attenuate effects of glimepiride. **Herbal: Ginseng, garlic** may increase hypoglycemic effects.

PHARMACOKINETICS Absorption: Completely absorbed from GI tract. **Onset:** 1 h. **Peak:** 2–3 h. **Distribution:** >99.5% protein bound; probably secreted into breast milk. **Metabolism:** Metabolized in liver by cytochrome P4502C9 (CYP2C9). **Elimination:** 60% excreted in urine, 40% in feces. **Half-Life:** 5–9 h.

NURSING IMPLICATIONS

Assessment & Drug Effects

- Lab tests: monitor fasting and postprandial blood glucose and urinary glucose frequently. Monitor glycosylated hemoglobin every 3–6 mo. Monitor periodically during long-term therapy: Liver function tests, serum osmolarity, serum sodium, and CBC with differential.
- Monitor for hypoglycemia especially with concurrent drugs

G

which enhance hypoglycemic effects.

Patient & Family Education

- Take a missed dose as soon as possible unless it is almost time for next dose; NEVER take two doses at the same time.
- Avoid drinking alcohol or using OTC drugs without informing physician.
- Use sunscreen and avoid sunlamps.
- Learn about adverse reactions and drug interactions.
- Do not breast feed while taking this drug.

GLIPIZIDE

(glip′i-zide)

Glucotrol, Glucotrol XL

Classifications: HORMONES AND SYNTHETIC SUBSTITUTES; ANTIDIABETIC AGENT; SULFONYLUREA

Prototype: Glyburide

Pregnancy Category: C

AVAILABILITY 5 mg, 10 mg tablets; 5 mg, 10 mg sustained release tablets

ACTIONS Second generation sulfonylurea hypoglycemic agent. Potency is enhanced by as much as 200-fold over first generation agents.

THERAPEUTIC EFFECTS Directly stimulates functioning pancreatic beta cells to secrete insulin, leading to an acute drop in blood glucose. Indirect action leads to altered numbers and sensitivity of peripheral insulin receptors, resulting in increased insulin binding. It also causes inhibition of hepatic glucose production and reduction in serum glucagon levels.

USES Adjunct to diet for control of hyperglycemia in patient with type 2 diabetes mellitus after dietary control alone has failed; also used to treat transient loss of control in patient usually controlled well on diet.

CONTRAINDICATIONS Diabetic ketoacidosis. Safe use during pregnancy (category C), lactation, or in children is not established.

CAUTIOUS USE Impaired renal and hepatic function; older adults; debilitated, malnourished patients; patients with adrenal or pituitary insufficiency.

ROUTE & DOSAGE

Control of Hyperglycemia

Adult: **PO** 2.5–5 mg/d 30 min before breakfast, may increase by 2.5–5 mg q1–2wk; >15 mg/d in divided doses 30 min before morning and evening meal (max: 40 mg/d); 5–10 mg sustained release tablets once/d

ADMINISTRATION

Oral

- Give once-daily dosing 30 min before the first meal of the day.
- Ensure that sustained release form of drug is not chewed or crushed. It must be swallowed whole.
- Store in tightly closed, light-resistant container at 15°–30° C (59°–86° F).

ADVERSE EFFECTS (≥1%) **GI:** Nausea, diarrhea, constipation, gastralgia, cholestatic jaundice (rare). **Metabolic:** Hepatic porphyria, hypoglycemia. **Skin:** Erythema, morbilliform or maculopapular rash, pruritus, urticaria, eczema (transient). **Body as a Whole:** Hypersensitivity (fatigue, drowsiness, hunger, GI distress with heartburn, abdominal pain, anorexia). **CNS:** Transient drowsiness, headache, anxiety, ataxia, confusion; seizures, coma. **CV:** Tachycardia. **Special Senses:** Visual disturbances.

INTERACTIONS Drug: Alcohol produces **disulfiram**-like reaction in some patients; ORAL ANTICOAGULANTS, **chloramphenicol, clofibrate, phenylbutazone,** MAO INHIBITORS, SALICYLATES, **probenecid,** SULFONAMIDES may potentiate hypoglycemic actions; THIAZIDES may antagonize hypoglycemic effects; **cimetidine** may increase glipizide levels, causing hypoglycemia. **Herbal: Ginseng, garlic** may increase hypoglycemic effects.

PHARMACOKINETICS Absorption: Readily absorbed from GI tract. **Onset:** 15–30 min. **Peak:** 1–2 h. **Duration:** up to 24 h. **Metabolism:** Metabolized extensively in liver. **Elimination:** Excreted mainly in urine with some excretion via bile in feces. **Half-Life:** 3–5 h.

NURSING IMPLICATIONS

Assessment & Drug Effects

- Observe response to the initial dose and establish maintenance regimen cautiously in older adult or debilitated patients; early signs of hypoglycemia are easily overlooked.
- Lab tests: monitor periodically during long-term therapy: Liver function tests, serum electrolytes, and serum osmolarity.
- Note: Severe drug-induced skin rashes and pruritus may necessitate discontinuation of drug use. Symptoms usually subside rapidly when drug is withdrawn.
- Check urine for sugar and ketone bodies at least 3 times daily during insulin withdrawal and transfer to glipizide. Contact physician if tests are abnormal.
- Note: Patients transferred from a sulfonylurea with a long half-life (e.g., chlorpropamide, half-life: 30–40 h) must be observed for hypoglycemic responses (see Appendix F) for 1–2 wk because of potential overlapping of drug effect.
- Note: The first signs of hypoglycemia may be hard to detect in patients receiving concurrent beta blockers or older adults.

Patient & Family Education

- Overdose treatment: Treat mild hypoglycemia (reaction without loss of consciousness or neurologic symptoms) with PO glucose and adjustment of dosage and meal pattern; monitor closely for at least 5–7 d to assure reestablishment of safe control. Severe hypoglycemia requires emergency hospitalization to permit treatment to maintain a blood glucose level above 100 mg/dL.
- Note: Glipizide therapy accompanies (does NOT substitute for) continued control of diet and (if patient is obese) a weight-loss program.
- Test fasting and postprandial blood glucose frequently.
- Exercise is an important part of the total control program.
- When a drug that affects the hypoglycemic action of sulfonylureas (see DRUG INTERACTIONS) is withdrawn or added to the glipizide regimen, be alert to the added danger of loss of control. Urine and blood glucose tests and test for ketone bodies should be carefully monitored.
- Do not breast feed while taking this drug without consulting physician.

GLUCAGON

(gloo'ka-gon)

GlucaGen

Classification: HORMONES AND SYNTHETIC SUBSTITUTES

Pregnancy Category: B

G

AVAILABILITY 1 mg powder for injection

ACTIONS Polypeptide hormone produced by alpha cells of islets of Langerhans. Stimulates uptake of amino acids and their conversion to glucose precursors.

THERAPEUTIC EFFECTS Promotes lipolysis in liver and adipose tissue with release of free fatty acid and glycerol, which further stimulates ketogenesis and hepatic gluconeogenesis. Action in hypoglycemia relies on presence of adequate liver glycogen stores.

USES Emergency treatment of severe hypoglycemic reactions in diabetic patients who are unconscious or unable to swallow food or liquids and in psychiatric patients receiving insulin shock therapy. Also radiologic studies of GI tract to relax smooth muscle and thereby allow finer detail of mucosa; to diagnose insulinoma.

UNLABELED USES GI disturbances associated with spasm, cardiovascular emergencies, and to overcome cardiotoxic effects of beta blockers, quinidine, tricyclic antidepressants; as an aid in abdominal imaging.

CONTRAINDICATIONS Hypersensitivity to glucagon or protein compounds. Safe use during pregnancy (category B) or lactation is not established.

CAUTIOUS USE Insulinemia, pheochromocytoma.

ROUTE & DOSAGE

Hypoglycemia

Adult: **IM/IV/SC** 0.5–1 mg, may repeat q5–20 min if no response for 1–2 more doses
Child: **IM/IV/SC** 0.025 mg/kg (max: 1 mg/dose), may repeat q5–20 min if no response for 1–2 more doses
Neonate: **IM/IV/SC** 0.3 mg/kg (max: 1 mg)

Insulin Shock Therapy

Adult: **IM/IV/SC** 0.5–1 mg usually 1 h after coma develops, may repeat in 25 min if no response

Diagnostic Aid to Relax Stomach or Upper GI Tract

Adult: **IM/IV/SC** 0.25–2 mg 10 min before the procedure

Diagnostic Aid for Examination of Colon

Adult: **IM/IV/SC** 2 mg 10 min before the procedure

ADMINISTRATION

Note: 1 mg = 1 unit

Subcutaneous/Intramuscular

- Dilute 1 unit (1 mg) of glucagon with 1 mL of diluent supplied by manufacturer.
- Use immediately after reconstitution of dry powder. Discard any unused portion.
- Note: Glucagon is incompatible in syringe with any other drug.

Intravenous

PREPARE: **Direct:** Prepare as noted above. Do not use a concentration >1 unit/mL.

ADMINISTER: **Direct:** Give 1 unit or fraction thereof over 1 min. May be given through a Y-site D5W (not NS) infusing.

INCOMPATIBILITIES **Solution/additive:** Sodium chloride.

- Store unreconstituted vials and diluent at 20°–25° C (68°–77° F).

ADVERSE EFFECTS (≥1%) **GI:** Nausea and vomiting. **Body as a Whole:** Hypersensitivity reactions. **Skin:** Stevens-Johnson syndrome (erythema multiforme). **Metabolic:** hyperglycemia, hypokalemia.

PHARMACOKINETICS Onset: 5–20 min. **Peak:** 30 min. **Duration:** 1–1.5 h. **Metabolism:** Metabolized in liver, plasma, and kidneys. **Half-Life:** 3–10 min.

NURSING IMPLICATIONS

Assessment & Drug Effects

- Be prepared to give IV glucose if patient fails to respond to glucagon. Notify physician immediately.
- Note: Patient usually awakens from (diabetic) hypoglycemic coma 5–20 min after glucagon injection. Give PO carbohydrate as soon as possible after patient regains consciousness.
- Note: After recovery from hypoglycemic reaction, symptoms such as headache, nausea, and weakness may persist.

Patient & Family Education

- Note: Physician may request that a responsible family member be taught how to administer glucagon SC or IM for patients with frequent or severe hypoglycemic reactions. Notify physician promptly whenever a hypoglycemic reaction occurs so the reason for the reaction can be determined.
- Review package insert and directions (see ADMINISTRATION).
- Do not breast feed while taking this drug without consulting physician.

GLUTETHIMIDE

(gloo-teth'i-mide)
Doriglute
Classifications: CENTRAL NERVOUS SYSTEM AGENT; ANXIOLYTIC; SEDATIVE-HYPNOTIC
Prototype: Secobarbital
Pregnancy Category: C
Controlled Substance: Schedule III

AVAILABILITY 250 mg tablets

ACTIONS Pharmacologic actions similar to those of barbiturates. Can induce hypnosis without producing reliable analgesic, antitussive, or anticonvulsant action. Causes less respiratory depression but greater degree of hypotension than barbiturates. Addiction liability similar to that of barbiturates.
THERAPEUTIC EFFECTS Significantly suppresses REM sleep; but following drug withdrawal after chronic administration, REM rebound occurs, and patient may experience markedly increased dreaming, nightmares, insomnia.

USES Short-term treatment of insomnia and for sedative effect preoperatively and during first stage of labor. Not indicated for routine sedation or persistent insomnia.

CONTRAINDICATIONS Uncontrolled pain; intermittent porphyria; severe hepatic and renal impairment; prolonged administration; lactation; children <12 y. Safe use during pregnancy [(category C) except with caution during first stage of labor] is not established.
CAUTIOUS USE Older adult or debilitated patients; prostatic hypertrophy, bladder neck obstruction; pyloroduodenal obstruction, stenosing peptic ulcer; narrow-angle glau-

coma; hypotension, cardiac arrhythmias; mental depression (particularly in patients with suicidal tendencies), history of alcoholism or drug abuse.

ROUTE & DOSAGE

Insomnia

Adult: **PO** 250–500 mg h.s., may repeat prn but not <4 h before arising

Preoperative Sedation

Adult: **PO** 500 mg the night before surgery and 500 mg–1 g 1 h before anesthesia

ADMINISTRATION

Oral

- Give 4 h or more before the usual time of arising to avoid residual daytime effects when administered for insomnia.
- Withdraw drug gradually, using stepwise dose reduction over a period of several days or weeks. Abrupt withdrawal following regular use may produce nausea, vomiting, nervousness, tremors, abdominal cramps, nightmares, insomnia, tachycardia, chills, fever, numbness of extremities, dysphagia, delirium, hallucinations, or convulsions.

ADVERSE EFFECTS (≥1%) **Body as a Whole:** Acute hypersensitivity reactions. **CNS:** CNS depression in fetus; paradoxic excitement, headache, vertigo. **GI:** Gastric irritation, nausea, drug "hangover," dry mouth. **Hematologic:** Blood dyscrasias. **Skin:** Generalized skin rash (occasionally, purpuric or urticarial), exfoliative dermatitis (rare). **Other:** Hiccups, blurred vision. **Acute Overdosage:** CNS depression (coma; depressed reflexes, including corneal reflex; dilated, fixed pupils; hypotension; hypothermia followed by hyperpyrexia; tachycardia; respiratory depression, cyanosis, sudden apnea; decreased intestinal motility, adynamic ileus; facial twitching; intermittent spasticity; flaccid paralysis; pulmonary and cerebral edema; renal tubular necrosis; severe infections). **Chronic Ingestion:** Toxic psychosis (slurred speech, impaired memory, inability to concentrate, mydriasis, dry mouth, nystagmus, ataxia, hyporeflexia, tremors, peripheral neuropathy).

INTERACTIONS Drug: Alcohol, BARBITURATES, other CNS DEPRESSANTS compound depressant effects; TRICYCLIC ANTIDEPRESSANTS add to anticholinergic effects; decreases anticoagulant effects of ORAL ANTICOAGULANTS.

PHARMACOKINETICS Absorption: Erratic absorption from GI tract. **Onset:** 30 min. **Duration:** 4–8 h. **Distribution:** Widely distributed; localizes in adipose tissue, liver, kidney, brain, and bile; crosses placenta; distributed into breast milk in small quantities. **Metabolism:** Metabolized in liver. **Elimination:** Metabolites excreted in urine. **Half-Life:** 10–12 h.

NURSING IMPLICATIONS

Assessment & Drug Effects

- Inform physician of patient's response to drug. Smallest effective dosage should be used for the shortest period of time compatible with patient's needs.
- Note: Overdosage of glutethimide is difficult to treat. Patients tend to go in and out of toxicity, possibly because of delayed absorption of the drug.

Patient & Family Education

- Report onset of rash or any other unusual symptoms to physician.

Discontinuation of drug is indicated if a rash occurs.
- Do not drive or engage in other potentially hazardous activities requiring mental alertness for 7–8 h after drug ingestion.
- Note: Possible adverse reactions are increased when glutethimide is combined with alcohol or other CNS depressants.
- Understand that prolonged use of moderate to high doses of glutethimide can produce tolerance and psychologic and physical dependence.
- Do not breast feed while taking this drug.

GLYBURIDE (Pr)

(glye'byoor-ide)

DiaBeta, Euglucon ♣, Glynase, Micronase

Classifications: HORMONES AND SYNTHETIC SUBSTITUTES; ANTIDIABETIC AGENT; SULFONYLUREA

Pregnancy Category: C

AVAILABILITY 1.25 mg, 2.5 mg, 5 mg tablets; 1.5 mg, 3 mg, 4.5 mg, 6 mg micronized tablets

ACTIONS One of the most potent of the sulfonylurea hypoglycemic agents. Second-generation sulfonylurea closely related to tolbutamide. Potency is enhanced by as much as 200-fold over first-generation agents.

THERAPEUTIC EFFECTS Appears to lower blood sugar concentration in both diabetic and nondiabetic individuals by sensitizing functioning pancreatic beta cells to release insulin in the presence of elevated serum glucose levels. Blood glucose-lowering effect persists during long-term glyburide treatment, but there is a gradual decline in meal stimulated secretion of endogenous insulin toward pretreatment levels.

USES Adjunct to diet to lower blood glucose in patients with type 2 diabetes mellitus; after dietary control alone has failed.

CONTRAINDICATIONS Hypersensitivity to glyburide, diabetic ketoacidosis, as sole therapy for type 2 diabetes mellitus; pregnancy (category C); withhold 14 days before labor and delivery; lactation. Safe use in children is not established.

CAUTIOUS USE Limit use in patients with cardiovascular disease; renal or hepatic insufficiency; older adults, debilitated, or malnourished patients; adrenal or pituitary insufficiency.

ROUTE & DOSAGE

Control of Hyperglycemia

Adult: **PO** 1.25–5 mg/d with breakfast, may increase by 2.5–5 mg q1–2wk; >15 mg/d should be given in divided doses with morning and evening meal (max: 20 mg/d); Micronized 1.5–3 mg/d (max: 12 mg/d)

ADMINISTRATION

Oral
- Give once daily in the morning with breakfast or with first main meal.
- Store in tightly closed, light-resistant container at 15°–30° C (59°–86° F).

ADVERSE EFFECTS (≥1%) **Metabolic:** Hypoglycemia. **GI:** Epigastric fullness, heartburn, nausea, vomiting. **Skin:** Pruritus, erythema, urticarial or cholestatic jaundice (rare) morbilliform eruptions. **Special Senses:** Blurred vision.

INTERACTIONS Drug: Alcohol causes disulfiram-like reaction in some patients; ORAL ANTICOAGULANTS, **chloramphenicol, clofibrate, phenylbutazone,** MAO INHIBITORS, SALICYLATES, **probenecid,** SULFONAMIDES may potentiate hypoglycemic actions; THIAZIDES may antagonize hypoglycemic effects; **cimetidine** may increase glyburide levels, causing hypoglycemia. **Herbal: Ginseng, garlic** may increase hypoglycemic effects.

PHARMACOKINETICS Absorption: Readily absorbed from GI tract. **Onset:** 15–60 min. **Peak:** 1–2 h. **Duration:** Up to 24 h. **Distribution:** Distributed in highest concentrations in liver, kidneys, and intestines; crosses placenta. **Metabolism:** Metabolized extensively in liver. **Elimination:** Excreted equally in urine and feces. **Half-Life:** 10 h.

NURSING IMPLICATIONS

Assessment & Drug Effects

- Monitor blood glucose levels carefully during the dangerous early treatment period when dosage is being individualized. Older adults are especially vulnerable to glyburide-induced hypoglycemia (see Appendix F) because the antidiabetic agent is long-acting.
- Note: The first signs of hypoglycemia may be hard to detect when the patient is also receiving a beta blocker or is an older adult.
- Lab tests: Monitor at regular intervals: Blood and urine glucose, HbA1c, urine ketones, and liver function tests.

Patient & Family Education

- Eat or drink some form of sugar (e.g., corn syrup, orange juice with 2 or 3 tsp of table sugar) when symptoms of hypoglycemia occur. Report reaction to physician promptly.
- Remember that loss of control of diabetes may result from stress such as fever, surgery, trauma, or infection. Check blood glucose and urine for ketones more frequently during stress periods; transfer from the sulfonylurea to insulin may be necessary.
- Keep all follow-up medical appointments and adhere to dietary instructions, regular exercise program, and scheduled urine and blood testing.
- Report blurred vision to physician.
- Do not breast feed while taking this drug without consulting physician.

GLYCERIN

(gli'ser-in)

Fleet Babylax, Glycerol, Osmoglyn

GLYCERIN ANHYDROUS

Ophthalgan

Classifications: FLUID AND ELECTROLYTE AGENT; HYPEROSMOTIC LAXATIVE; ANTIGLAUCOMA

Pregnancy Category: C

AVAILABILITY 50% oral solution; suppositories; 4 mL/applicator, ophthalmic solution

ACTIONS When administered orally, glycerin raises plasma osmotic pressure by withdrawing fluid from extravascular spaces; lowers ocular tension by decreasing volume of intraocular fluid. Also may decrease CSF pressure and produce slight diuresis. Topical application to eye reduces edema by hydroscopic effect. Glycerin suppositories apparently work by causing dehydration of exposed tissue, which produces an irritant effect, and by absorbing water from tissues, thus creating more mass. Both actions stimulate peristalsis in the large bowel and thus increases peristalsis.

THERAPEUTIC EFFECTS Also reduces intraocular pressure by lowering intraocular fluid. Relieves constipation by absorption of water and stimulation of peristalsis.

USES Orally to reduce elevated intraocular pressure (IOP) before or after surgery in patients with acute narrow-angle glaucoma, retinal detachment, or cataract and to reduce elevated CSF pressure. Sterile glycerin (anhydrous) is used topically to reduce superficial corneal edema resulting from trauma, surgery, or disease and to facilitate ophthalmoscopic examination. Used rectally (suppository or enema) to relieve constipation.

UNLABELED USES To reduce mortality due to strokes in older adults.

CONTRAINDICATIONS Safe use during pregnancy (category C) or lactation is not established.

CAUTIOUS USE Cardiac, renal, or hepatic disease; diabetes mellitus; dehydrated or older adult patients.

ROUTE & DOSAGE

Decrease IOP

Adult/Child: **PO** 1–1.8 g/kg 1–1.5 h before ocular surgery, may repeat q5h

Constipation

Adult/Child: **PR** ≥6 y, Insert 1 suppository or 5–15 mL of enema high into rectum and retain for 15 min
Child: **PR** <6 y, Insert 1 infant suppository or 2–5 mL of enema high into rectum and retain for 15 min
Neonate: **PR** 0.5 mL of rectal solution (enema)

Reduction of Corneal Edema

Adult: **Topical** 1–2 drops instilled into eye q3–4h

ADMINISTRATION

Oral

- Pour commercially available flavored solution over crushed ice, then sip through a straw. Lemon or lime juice and NS (if allowed) may be added to unflavored solution for palatability.
- Prevent or relieve headache (from cerebral dehydration) by having patient lie down during and after administration of drug.

Rectal

- Ensure that suppository is inserted beyond rectal sphincter.

ADVERSE EFFECTS (≥1%) **CNS:** Headache, dizziness, disorientation. **CV:** Irregular heartbeat. **GI:** Nausea, vomiting, thirst, diarrhea, abdominal cramps, rectal discomfort, hyperemia of rectal mucosa. **Metabolic:** Hyperglycemia, glycosuria, dehydration, hyperosmolar nonketotic coma.

PHARMACOKINETICS Absorption: Readily absorbed from GI tract after oral administration; rectal preparations are poorly absorbed. **Onset:** 10 min PO. **Peak:** 30 min–2 h. **Duration:** 4–8 h. **Metabolism:** 80% metabolized in liver; 10%–20% metabolized in kidneys to CO_2 and water or utilized in glucose or glycogen synthesis. **Elimination:** 7%–14% excreted unchanged in urine. **Half-Life:** 30–40 min.

NURSING IMPLICATIONS

Assessment & Drug Effects

- Consult physician regarding fluid intake in patients receiving drug

for elevated IOP. Although hypotonic fluids will relieve thirst and headache caused by the dehydrating action of glycerin, these fluids may nullify its osmotic effect.
- Monitor glycemic control in diabetics. Drug may cause hyperglycemia (see Appendix F).

Patient & Family Education
- Evacuation usually comes 15–30 min after administration of glycerin rectal suppository or enema.
- Note: Slight hyperglycemia and glycosuria may occur with PO use; adjustment in antidiabetic medication dosage may be required.
- Do not breast feed while taking this drug without consulting physician.

G

GLYCOPYRROLATE

(glye-koe-pye'roe-late)
Robinul, Robinul Forte
Classifications: AUTONOMIC NERVOUS SYSTEM AGENT; ANTICHOLINERGIC (PARASYMPATHOLYTIC); ANTIMUSCARINIC; ANTISPASMODIC
Prototype: Atropine
Pregnancy Category: B

AVAILABILITY 1 mg, 2 mg tablets; 0.2 mg/mL injection

ACTIONS Synthetic anticholinergic (antimuscarinic) compound with pharmacologic effects similar to those of atropine. Inhibits muscarinic action of acetylcholine or autonomic neuroeffector sites innervated by postganglionic cholinergic nerves.
THERAPEUTIC EFFECTS Inhibits motility of GI tract and genitourinary tract and decreases volume of gastric and pancreatic secretions, saliva, and perspiration.

USES Adjunctive management of peptic ulcer and other GI disorders associated with hyperacidity, hypermotility, and spasm. Also used parenterally as preanesthetic and intraoperative medication and to reverse neuromuscular blockade.

CONTRAINDICATIONS Glaucoma; asthma; prostatic hypertrophy, obstructive uropathy; obstructive lesions or atony of GI tract; severe ulcerative colitis; myasthenia gravis; tachycardia; during cyclopropane anesthesia; children <12 y (except parenteral use in conjunction with anesthesia). Safe use during pregnancy (category B) or lactation is not established.
CAUTIOUS USE Autonomic neuropathy, hepatic or renal disease.

ROUTE & DOSAGE

Peptic Ulcer
Adult: **PO** 1 mg t.i.d or 2 mg b.i.d. or t.i.d. in equally divided intervals (max: 8 mg/d), then decrease to 1 mg b.i.d. **IM/IV** 0.1–0.2 mg as single dose t.i.d. or q.i.d.

Reversal of Neuromuscular Blockade
Adult/Child: **IV** 0.2 mg glycopyrrolate administered with 1 mg of neostigmine or 5 mg pyridostigmine

Control of Secretions
Child: **PO** 40–100 mcg/kg t.i.d.–q.i.d. **IM/IV** 4–10 mcg/kg t.i.d.–q.i.d.
Adult: **PO** 1–2 mg/dose b.i.d. or t.i.d. **IM/IV** 0.1–0.2 mg/dose given q4–8h

ADMINISTRATION

Oral
- Give without regard to meals.

Intramuscular
- Give undiluted, deep into a large muscle.

Intravenous

PREPARE: **Direct:** Give undiluted.

- Inspect for cloudiness and discoloration. Discard if present.

ADMINISTER: **Direct:** Give 0.2 mg or fraction thereof over 1–2 min.

INCOMPATIBILITIES **Solution/additive: Methylprednisolone, chloramphenicol, dexamethasone, diazepam, dimenhydrinate, methohexital, pentazocine, phenobarbital, secobarbital, sodium bicarbonate, thiopental. Y-site: Diazepam, dimenhydrinate, methohexital, pentazocine, phenobarbital, secobarbital, thiopental.**

- Store at 20°–25° C (68°–77° F).

ADVERSE EFFECTS (≥1%) **Body as a Whole:** *Decreased sweating,* weakness. **CNS:** Dizziness, drowsiness, overdosage (neuromuscular blockade with curare-like action leading to muscle weakness and paralysis is possible). **CV:** Palpitation, tachycardia. **GI:** *Xerostomia,* constipation. **GU:** *Urinary hesitancy or retention.* **Special Senses:** Blurred vision, mydriasis.

INTERACTIONS Drug: Amantadine, ANTIHISTAMINES, TRICYCLIC ANTIDEPRESSANTS, **quinidine, disopyramide, procainamide** compound anticholinergic effects; decreases **levodopa** effects; **methotrimeptrazine** may precipitate extrapyramidal effects; decreases antipsychotic effects (decreased absorption) of PHENOTHIAZINES.

PHARMACOKINETICS Absorption: Poorly and incompletely absorbed from GI tract. **Onset:** 1 min IV; 15–30 min IM/SC; 1 h PO. **Peak:** 30–45 min IM/SC; 1 h PO. **Duration:** 2–7 h IM/SC; 8–12 h PO. **Distribution:** Crosses placenta. **Metabolism:** Minimally metabolized in liver. **Elimination:** 85% excreted in urine.

NURSING IMPLICATIONS

Assessment & Drug Effects

- Incidence and severity of adverse effects are generally dose related.
- Monitor I&O ratio and pattern particularly in older adults. Watch for urinary hesitancy and retention.
- Monitor vital signs, especially when drug is given parenterally. Report any changes in heart rate or rhythm.

Patient & Family Education

- Avoid high environmental temperatures (heat prostration can occur because of decreased sweating).
- Do not drive or engage in other potentially hazardous activities requiring mental alertness until response to drug is known.
- Use good oral hygiene, rinse mouth with water frequently and use a saliva substitute to lessen effects of dry mouth.
- Do not breast feed while taking this drug without consulting physician.

GOLD SODIUM THIOMALATE

(thye-oh-mah'late)

Myochrysine

Classification: GOLD COMPOUND
Prototype: Aurothioglucose
Pregnancy Category: C

AVAILABILITY 50 mg/mL injection

ACTIONS Water-soluble gold compound similar to aurothioglucose in actions and uses. Has immunomodulatory and antiinflammatory effects. Action mechanism unclear. Drug appears to act by suppression of phagocytosis, altered immune responses, and possibly by inhibition of prostaglandin synthesis.

THERAPEUTIC EFFECTS Has immunomodulatory and antiinflammatory effects.

USES Selected patients (adults and juveniles) with acute rheumatoid arthritis.

UNLABELED USES Psoriatic arthritis, Felty's syndrome.

CONTRAINDICATIONS History of severe toxicity from previous exposure to gold or other heavy metals; severe debilitation; SLE, Sjögren's syndrome in rheumatoid arthritis; renal disease; hepatic dysfunction, history of infectious hepatitis or hematologic disorders; uncontrolled diabetes or CHF. Safe use during pregnancy (category C) and lactation is not established.

CAUTIOUS USE History of drug allergies or hypersensitivity, hypertension.

ROUTE & DOSAGE

Rheumatoid Arthritis

Adult: **IM** 10 mg wk 1, 25 mg wk 2, then 25–50 mg/wk to a cumulative dose of 1 g (if improvement occurs, continue at 25–50 mg q2 wk for 2–20 wk, then q3–4 wk indefinitely or until adverse effects occur)
Child: **IM** 10 mg test dose, then 1 mg/kg/wk or 2.5–5 mg for wk 1 and 2, followed by 1 mg/kg q1–4 wk (max: single dose 50 mg)

ADMINISTRATION

Intramuscular

- Agitate vial before withdrawing dose to ensure uniform suspension.
- Give deep into upper outer quadrant of gluteus maximus with patient lying down. Patient should remain recumbent for at least 30 min after injection because of the danger of "nitritoid reaction" (transient giddiness, vertigo, facial flushing, fainting).
- Observe for allergic reactions.
- Store in tight, light-resistant containers at 15°–30° C (59°–86° F). Do not use if any darker than pale yellow.

ADVERSE EFFECTS (≥1%) **CNS:** Dizziness, syncope, sweating, flushing. **CV:** Bradycardia. **GI:** Hepatitis, metallic taste, *stomatitis,* nausea, vomiting. **Hematologic:** <u>Agranulocytosis, aplastic anemia</u>, eosinophilia (all rare). **Urogenital:** Nephrotic syndrome, glomerulitis with hematuria, *proteinuria.* **Skin:** Transient pruritus, *erythema, dermatitis,* fixed drug eruption, alopecia, shedding of nails, gray to blue pigmentation of skin (chrysiasis). **Special Senses:** Gold deposits in ocular tissues, *photosensitivity.* **Body as a Whole:** Peripheral neuritis, angioneurotic edema, interstitial pneumonitis, <u>anaphylaxis</u> (rare). **Respiratory:** Pulmonary fibrosis.

INTERACTIONS Drug: ANTIMALARIALS, IMMUNOSUPPRESSANTS, **penicillamine, phenylbutazone** increase risk of blood dyscrasias.

PHARMACOKINETICS Absorption: Slowly and irregularly absorbed from IM site. **Peak:** 3–6 h. **Distribution:** Widely distributed, especially to synovial fluid, kidney, liver, and spleen; does not cross blood–brain barrier; crosses placenta. **Metabolism:** Not studied. **Elimination:** 60%–90% of dose ultimately excreted in urine; also eliminated in feces; traces may be found in urine for 6 mo. **Half-Life:** 3–168 d.

NURSING IMPLICATIONS

Assessment & Drug Effects

- Lab tests: Prior to each injection, urinalysis for protein, blood, and sediment. Withhold drug and notify physician promptly if proteinuria or hematuria develops. Also do baseline Hgb and RBC, WBC count, differential count, platelet count before initiation of therapy and at regular intervals.

- Note: Rapid reduction in hemoglobin level, WBC count below $4000/mm^3$, eosinophil count above 5%, and platelet count below $100,000/mm^3$ signify possible toxicity.
- Interview and examine patient before each injection to detect occurrence of transient pruritus or dermatitis (both are common early indications of toxicity), stomatitis (sore tongue, palate, or throat), metallic taste, indigestion, or other signs and symptoms of possible toxicity. Interrupt treatment immediately and notify physician if any of these reactions occurs.
- Observe for allergic reaction, which may occur almost immediately after injection, 10 min after injection, or at any time during therapy. Withhold drug and notify physician if observed. Keep antidote dimercaprol (BAL) on hand during time of injection.

Patient & Family Education

- Therapeutic effects may not appear until after 2 mo of therapy.
- Notify physician of rapid improvement in joint swelling; this is indicative that you are closely approaching drug tolerance level.
- Use protective measures in sunlight. Exposure to sunlight may aggravate gold dermatitis.
- Notify physician at the appearance of purpura or ecchymoses; this is always an indication for doing a platelet count.
- Know possible adverse reactions and report any symptom suggestive of toxicity immediately to physician.
- Do not breast feed while taking this drug without consulting physician.

GONADORELIN HYDROCHLORIDE

(goe-nad-oh-rell'in)

Factrel

Classifications: HORMONES AND SYNTHETIC SUBSTITUTES; DIAGNOSTIC AGENT

Pregnancy Category: B

AVAILABILITY 100 mcg/vial

ACTIONS Synthetic luteinizing hormone–releasing hormone (LHRH) with structure identical to the natural hormone; also referred to as gonadotropin-releasing hormone (GnRH).

THERAPEUTIC EFFECTS Stimulates anterior pituitary to release the gonadotropin LH.

USES To evaluate functional capacity and response of the gonadotropes of anterior pituitary and in suspected gonadotropic deficiency. Also used to evaluate residual gonadotropic function of the pituitary following surgical or radiologic removal of a pituitary tumor.

UNLABELED USES Treatment of delayed puberty, amenorrhea, and infertility in males.

CONTRAINDICATIONS Lactation; concurrent use of other drugs having effect on pituitary gonadotropic function; children <18 y; disorders of reproductive organs; anterior pituitary and the CNS. Safe use during pregnancy (category B) is not established.

ROUTE & DOSAGE

Evaluation of Functional Capacity of Anterior Pituitary

Adult: **SC/IV** 100 mcg administered in women during early phase of menstrual cycle (days 1–7) if it can be determined

G

ADMINISTRATION

Subcutaneous

- Reconstitute 100-g vial with 1 mL sterile diluent (supplied by manufacturer), and the 500-g vial with 2 mL. Use immediately after preparation for best results.

Intravenous

PREPARE: **Direct:** Reconstitute as for SC injection.

ADMINISTER: **Direct:** Give a single dose by direct IV over 15–30 s.

- Store ampule and reconstituted drug at room temperature. Use reconstituted drug within 24 h. Discard unused diluted solution and diluent.

ADVERSE EFFECTS (≥1%) **CNS:** Headache, light-headedness. **GI:** Nausea, abdominal discomfort. **Other:** Flushing, local inflammation at injection site if given SC, hypersensitivity reaction (rare).

DIAGNOSTIC TEST INTERFERENCE ***Baseline LH levels*** are elevated in menopausal and postmenopausal women. Patients clinically diagnosed or with suspected pituitary or hypothalamus dysfunction often demonstrate subnormal or absent LH response after test dose.

INTERACTIONS Drug: ANDROGENS, ESTROGENS, PROGESTINS, GLUCOCORTICOIDS may cause false test results; **digoxin** may suppress gonadotropin levels; DOPAMINE ANTAGONISTS, PHENOTHIAZINES increase **prolactin** and blunt response to gonadorelin; **spironolactone, levodopa** increase gonadotropin levels.

PHARMACOKINETICS Duration: 3–5 h. **Distribution:** Distributed into breast milk. **Metabolism:** Hydrolyzed in plasma. **Elimination:** Metabolites excreted in urine. **Half-Life:** 10–40 min.

NURSING IMPLICATIONS

Assessment & Drug Effects

- Subnormal or absent LH response indicates pituitary or hypothalamus dysfunction.

Patient & Family Education

- Do not breast feed while taking this drug.

GOSERELIN ACETATE

(gos-er′e-lin)

Zoladex

Classifications: HORMONE AND SYNTHETIC SUBSTITUTE; GONADOTROPIN-RELEASING HORMONE ANALOG

Prototype: Leuprolide

Pregnancy Category: X

AVAILABILITY 3.6 mg, 10.8 mg SC implant

ACTIONS A synthetic form of luteinizing hormone-releasing hormone (LHRH or GnRH) that inhibits pituitary gonadotropin secretion. **THERAPEUTIC EFFECTS** With chronic administration, serum testosterone levels fall into the range normally seen with surgically castrated men.

USES Prostate cancer, breast cancer. Endometrial thinning agent prior to endometrial ablation for dysfunctional uterine bleeding. **UNLABELED USES** Endometriosis, uterine leiomyomas.

CONTRAINDICATIONS Pregnancy (category X); lactation; known hypersensitivity to a LHRH; endometriosis or endometrial thinning; hypercalcemia.
CAUTIOUS USE Urinary tract obstruction and children; family history of osteoporosis; concurrent use with anticonvulsants or corticosteroids. Safety and efficacy in children <18 y are not established.

ROUTE & DOSAGE

Prostate Cancer, Breast Cancer, Endometriosis, Uterine Leiomyomas
Adult: **SC** 3.6 mg once q28d. 10.8 mg depot q12 wk
Endometrial Thinning Prior to Endometrial Ablation
Adult: **SC** 3.6 mg once q28d

ADMINISTRATION

Subcutaneous
- Follow manufacturer's directions exactly for implanting the drug SC in the upper abdominal wall.
- Store at room temperature not to exceed 25° C (77° F).

ADVERSE EFFECTS (≥1%) **CNS:** Headache, tumor flare. **Endocrine:** Gynecomastia, breast swelling and tenderness, *postmenopausal symptoms* (*hot flashes*, vaginal dryness). **GI:** Nausea. **Urogenital:** Vaginal spotting, breakthrough bleeding, decreased libido, *impotence*. **Musculoskeletal:** Bone pain, bone loss.

DIAGNOSTIC TEST INTERFERENCE Increased levels of ***alkaline phosphatase*** and ***estradiol*** in the first 1–8 d; initial increase then decrease in ***FSH, LH,*** and ***testosterone.***

INTERACTIONS Drug: No clinically significant interactions established.

PHARMACOKINETICS Absorption: Rapidly absorbed following SC administration. **Duration:** 29 d. **Elimination:** Excreted by kidneys. **Half-Life:** 4.9 h.

NURSING IMPLICATIONS

Assessment & Drug Effects
- Monitor carefully during the first month of therapy for S&S of spinal cord compression or ureteral obstruction in patients with prostate cancer. Report immediately to physician.
- Anticipate a transient worsening of symptoms (e.g., bone pain) during the first weeks of therapy in patients with prostate cancer.

Patient & Family Education
- Note: Sexual dysfunction in men and hot flashes may accompany drug use.
- Notify physician immediately of symptoms of spinal cord compression or urinary obstruction.
- Do not breast feed while taking this drug.

GRANISETRON

(gran'i-se-tron)
Kytril
Classifications: GASTROINTESTINAL AGENT; ANTIEMETIC; 5-HT_3 ANTAGONIST
Prototype: Ondansetron
Pregnancy Category: B

AVAILABILITY 1 mg tablets; 1 mg/mL injection

ACTIONS Granisetron is a selective serotonin (5-HT_3) receptor antagonist. Serotonin receptors of the 5-HT_3 type are located centrally in the chemoreceptor trigger zone, and peripherally on the vagal nerve terminals. Serotonin is released from the wall of the small intestine, stimulates the vagal afferent neurons through the serotonin (5-HT_3) receptors, and initiates the vomiting reflex.

THERAPEUTIC EFFECTS This selective serotonin (5-HT_3) receptor antagonist is used for the prevention of nausea and vomiting associated with cancer chemotherapy.

USES Prevention of nausea and vomiting associated with initial and repeat courses of emetogenic cancer therapy, including high-dose cisplatin.

CONTRAINDICATIONS Hypersensitivity to granisetron.

CAUTIOUS USE Liver disease, pregnancy (category B), lactation, children <2 y.

ROUTE & DOSAGE

Nausea and Vomiting

Adult/Child: **IV** >2 y, 10 mcg/kg infused over 30 s–5 min, beginning at least 30 min before initiation of chemotherapy (up to 40 mcg/kg per dose has been used) **PO** 1 mg b.i.d., start 1 mg up to 1 h prior to chemotherapy, then second tab 12 h later or 2 mg q.d.

ADMINISTRATION

Oral

- Give only on the day of chemotherapy.

Intravenous

PREPARE: **Direct:** Give undiluted. **IV Infusion:** Dilute in NS or D5W to a total volume of 20–50 mL. Prepare infusion at time of administration; do not mix in solution with other drugs.

ADMINISTER: **Direct:** Give a single dose over 30 sec. **IV Infusion:** Infuse diluted drug over 5 min or longer; complete infusion 20–30 min prior to initiation of chemotherapy.

- Store at 15°–30° C (59°–86° F) for 24 h after dilution under normal lighting conditions.

ADVERSE EFFECTS (≥1%) **CNS:** *Headache,* dizziness, somnolence, insomnia, labile mood, anxiety, fatigue. **GI:** Constipation, diarrhea, elevated liver function tests.

PHARMACOKINETICS **Onset:** Several minutes. **Duration:** Approximately 24 h. **Distribution:** Widely distributed in body tissues. **Metabolism:** Appears to be metabolized in liver. **Elimination:** Excreted in urine as metabolites. **Half-Life:** 10–11 h in cancer patients, 4–5 h in healthy volunteers.

NURSING IMPLICATIONS

Assessment & Drug Effects

- Monitor the frequency and severity of nausea and vomiting.
- Lab tests: Monitor liver function; elevated AST and ALT values usually normalize within 2 wk of last dose.
- Assess for headache, which usually responds to nonnarcotic analgesics.

Patient & Family Education

- Note: Headache requiring an analgesic for relief is a common adverse effect.
- Learn ways to manage constipation.
- Do not breast feed while taking this drug without consulting physician.

GRISEOFULVIN MICRO-SIZE

(gri-see-oh-ful'vin)

Fulvicin-U/F, Grifulvin V, Grisactin, Grisovin-FP ♣

GRISEOFULVIN ULTRAMICROSIZE

Fulvicin P/G, Grisactin Ultra, Gris-PEG

Classifications: ANTIINFECTIVE; ANTIBIOTIC; ANTIFUNGAL

Prototype: Fluconazole

Pregnancy Category: C

AVAILABILITY **Griseofulvin Micro-Size** 250 mg, 500 mg tablets, 250 mg capsules; 125 mg/5 ml Suspension **Griseofulvin Ultramicrosize** 125 mg, 165 mg, 250 mg, 330 mg tablets.

ACTIONS Fungistatic antibiotic derived from species of *Penicillium.* Arrests metaphase of cell division by disrupting mitotic spindle structure in fungal cells. Deposits in keratin precursor cells and has special affinity for diseased tissue. It is tightly bound to new keratin of skin, hair, and nails, which becomes highly resistant to fungal invasion. Theoretically cross sensitivity with penicillin is a possibility.

THERAPEUTIC EFFECTS Effective against various species of *Epidermophyton, Microsporum,* and *Trichophyton* (has no effect on other fungi, including *Candida,* bacteria, and yeasts).

USES Mycotic disease of skin, hair, and nails not amenable to conventional topical measures. Concomitant use of appropriate topical agent may be required, particularly for tinea pedis.

UNLABELED USES Raynaud's disease, angina pectoris, and gout.

CONTRAINDICATIONS Porphyria; hepatic disease; SLE. Safe use during pregnancy (category C), lactation, children ≤2 y, or for prophylaxis against fungal infections is not established.

CAUTIOUS USE Penicillin-sensitive patients (possibility of cross-sensitivity with penicillin exists; however, reportedly penicillin-sensitive patients have been treated without difficulty).

ROUTE & DOSAGE

Tinea Corporis, Tinea Cruris, Tinea Capitis

Adult: **PO** 500 mg micro-size or 330–375 mg ultramicrosize daily in single or divided doses
Child: **PO** 10–20 mg/kg/d micro-size or 5–10 mg/kg/d ultramicrosize in single or divided doses

Tinea Pedis, Tinea Unguium

Adult: **PO** 0.75–1 g micro-size or 660–750 mg ultramicrosize daily in single or divided doses (decrease micro-size dose to 500 mg/d after response is noted)
Child: **PO** 10–20 mg/kg/d micro-size or 5–10 mg/kg/d ultramicrosize in single or divided doses

ADMINISTRATION

Oral

- Give with or after meals to allay GI disturbances.
- Give the micro-size formulations with a high fat content meal (increases drug absorption rate) to enhance serum levels. Consult physician.
- Store at 15°–30° C (59°–86° F) in tightly covered containers unless otherwise directed.

ADVERSE EFFECTS (≥1%) **Body as a Whole:** Hypersensitivity (urticaria, photosensitivity, skin rashes, pruritus, fixed drug eruption, serum sickness syndromes, severe angioedema). **CNS:** *Severe headache,* insomnia, fatigue, mental confusion, impaired performance of routine functions, psychotic symptoms, vertigo. **GI:** Heartburn, nausea, vomiting, diarrhea, flatulence, dry mouth, thirst, decreased taste acuity, anorexia, unpleasant taste, furred tongue, oral thrush. **Hematologic:** Leukopenia, neutropenia, granulocytopenia, punctate basophilia, monocytosis. **Urogenital:** Nephrotoxicity (proteinuria); hepatotoxicity; estrogen-like effects (in children); aggravation of SLE. **Other:** Overgrowth of nonsusceptible organisms; candidal intertrigo.

INTERACTIONS Drug: Alcohol may cause flushing and tachycardia; BARBITURATES may decrease activity of griseofulvin; may decrease hypoprothrombinemic effects of ORAL ANTICOAGULANTS; may increase **estrogen** metabolism, resulting in break through bleeding, and decrease contraceptive efficacy of ORAL CONTRACEPTIVES.

PHARMACOKINETICS Absorption: Absorbed primarily from duodenum; micro-size is variably and unpredictably absorbed; ultramicrosize is almost completely absorbed. **Peak:** 4–8 h. **Distribution:** Concentrates in skin, hair, nails, fat, and skeletal muscle; crosses placenta. **Metabolism:** Metabolized in liver. **Elimination:** Excreted mainly in urine; some excretion in perspiration. **Half-Life:** 9–24 h.

NURSING IMPLICATIONS

Assessment & Drug Effects

- Inquire about history of sensitivity to griseofulvin, penicillins, or other allergies prior to initiating treatment.
- Monitor food intake. Drug may alter taste sensations, and this may cause appetite suppression and inadequate nutrient intake.
- Lab tests: WBC with differential at least once weekly during first month of therapy or longer; periodic renal and hepatic function tests are also advised.
- Continue treatment until there is clinical improvement or until 2 or 3 consecutive weekly cultures are negative.

Patient & Family Education

- Continuing treatment as prescribed to prevent relapse, even if you experience symptomatic relief after 48–96 h of therapy.
- Note: Duration of treatment depends on time required to replace infected skin, hair, or nails, and thus varies with infection site. Average duration of treatment for tinea capitis (scalp ringworm), 4–6 wk; tinea corporis (body ringworm), 2–4 wk; tinea pedis (athlete's foot), 4–8 wk; tinea unguium (nail fungus), at least 4 mo for fingernails, depending on rate of growth, and 6 mo or more for toenails.
- Avoid exposure to intense natural or artificial sunlight, because photosensitivity-type reactions may occur.
- Note: Headaches often occur during early therapy but frequently disappear with continued drug administration.
- Disulfiram-type reaction (see Appendix F) are possible with ingestion of alcohol during therapy.
- Pharmacologic effects of oral contraceptives may be reduced. Breakthrough bleeding and pregnancy may occur. Alternative forms of birth control should be used during therapy.
- Do not breast feed while taking this drug without consulting physician.

GUAIFENESIN (Pr)

(gwye-fen′e-sin)

Amonidrin, Anti-Tuss, Breonesin, Gee-Gee, GG-Cen, Glyceryl Guaiacolate, Glycotuss, Glytuss, Guaituss, Hytuss, Malotuss, Mytussin, Mucinex, Nortussin, Resyl ♣, Robitussin

Classifications: ANTITUSSIVE; EXPECTORANT

Pregnancy Category: C

AVAILABILITY 100 mg/5 mL syrup; 100 mg/5 mL, 200 mg/5 mL liquid; 200 mg capsules; 300 mg sustained release capsules; 100 mg, 200 mg, 1200 mg tablets; 600 mg sustained release tablets

ACTIONS Enhances reflex outflow of respiratory tract fluids by irritation of gastric mucosa.

THERAPEUTIC EFFECTS Aids in expectoration by reducing adhesiveness and surface tension of secretions.

USES To combat dry, nonproductive cough associated with colds and bronchitis. A common ingredient in cough mixtures.

CONTRAINDICATIONS Hypersensitivity to guaifenesin; pregnancy (category C), lactation.

ROUTE & DOSAGE

Cough

Adult: **PO** 200–400 mg q4h up to 2.4 g/d

Child: **PO** *<2 y:* 12 mg/kg/d in 6 divided doses; *2–5 y:* 50–100 mg q4h up to 600 mg/d; *6–11 y,* 100–200 mg q4h up to 1.2 g/d

ADMINISTRATION

Oral

- Ensure that sustained release form of drug is not chewed or crushed. It must be swallowed whole.
- Follow dose with a full glass of water if not contraindicated.
- Carefully observe maximum daily doses for adults and children.

ADVERSE EFFECTS (≥1%) **GI:** Low incidence of nausea. **CNS:** Drowsiness.

DIAGNOSTIC TEST INTERFERENCE Guaifenesin may produce color interference with certain laboratory determinations of ***urinary 5-hydroxyindoleacetic acid (5-HIAA)*** and ***vanillylmandelic acid (VMA).***

INTERACTIONS Drug: By inhibiting platelet function, guaifenesin may increase risk of hemorrhage in patients receiving **heparin** therapy.

PHARMACOKINETICS Not studied.

NURSING IMPLICATIONS

Assessment & Drug Effects

- Monitor for therapeutic effectiveness. Persistent cough may indicate a serious condition requiring further diagnostic work.
- Notify physician if high fever, rash, or headaches develop.

Patient & Family Education

- Increase fluid intake to help loosen mucus; drink at least 8 glasses of fluid daily.
- Contact physician if cough persists beyond 1 wk.
- Contact physician if high fever, rash, or headache develops.
- Do not breast feed while taking this drug.

GUANABENZ ACETATE

(gwan'a-benz)

Wytensin

Classifications: CARDIOVASCULAR AGENT; CENTRAL-ACTING ANTIHYPERTENSIVE

Prototype: Methyldopa

Pregnancy Category: C

G

AVAILABILITY 4 mg, 8 mg tablets

ACTIONS Centrally acting alpha$_2$-adrenergic agonist. Pharmacologic actions closely resemble those of clonidine. Lowers BP, primarily, by stimulating central alpha-adrenergic receptors which leads to inhibition of sympathetic outflow from brain. Has no effect on exercise tolerance or on potassium levels. It does not cause sodium retention or excretion; however, it appears to enhance urinary dilution and free water diuresis.

THERAPEUTIC EFFECTS Given the fact that central adrenergic hyperactivity causes symptoms of narcotic withdrawal, guanabenz appears to help control abstinence symptoms by reducing norepinephrine output. Reduces both supine and standing BP, usually without producing postural hypotension, and slightly lowers pulse rate.

USES Used alone in treatment of hypertension or in combination with a thiazide diuretic.

UNLABELED USES Opiate detoxification, analgesic for chronic pain.

CONTRAINDICATIONS Safe use during pregnancy (category C), lactation, or in children is not established.

CAUTIOUS USE Severe coronary insufficiency, recent MI, cerebrovascular disease, severe hepatic or renal failure.

ROUTE & DOSAGE

Hypertension

Adult: **PO** 4 mg b.i.d., may increase by 4–8 mg/d q 1–2 wk up to 32 mg b.i.d.
Geriatric: **PO** 4 mg once daily, may increase every 1–2 wk

Opiate Withdrawal

Adult: **PO** 4 mg b.i.d. to q.i.d.

ADMINISTRATION

Oral

- Give one dose at bedtime to ensure overnight control and reduce possibility of daytime drowsiness or sedation.
- Store at 15°–30° C (59°–86° F) in tightly closed containers unless otherwise directed.

ADVERSE EFFECTS (≥1%) **CNS:** *Drowsiness* or *sedation,* dizziness, weakness, headache, anxiety, ataxia, depression, sleep disturbances, somnolence. **CV:** Chest pain, edema, arrhythmias, palpitation, hypotension, bradycardia, nervousness. **GI:** *Dry mouth,* nausea, epigastric pain, diarrhea, vomiting, constipation, abdominal discomfort, taste disorders. **Urogenital:** Increased urination, urinary frequency, sexual dysfunction. **Special Senses:** Blurred vision, miosis, nasal congestion. **Body as a Whole:** Dyspnea, muscle aches, aches in extremities, lethargy, irritability, unusual fatigue or weakness. **Skin:** Rash, pruritus.

INTERACTIONS Drug: Alcohol and other CNS DEPRESSANTS compound CNS depression; TRICYCLIC ANTIDEPRESSANTS may reduce antihypertensive effects of guanabenz.

PHARMACOKINETICS Absorption: 75% absorbed from GI tract. **Onset:** 60 min. **Peak:** 2–5 h. **Dura-**

Common adverse effects in *italic*, life-threatening effects underlined: generic names in **bold**; classifications in SMALL CAPS; ♣ Canadian drug name; ● Prototype drug

tion: 6–12 h. **Distribution:** Widely distributed; crosses blood–brain barrier; not known if crosses placenta or distributed into breast milk. **Metabolism:** Extensively metabolized. **Elimination:** 80% excreted in urine; 20% in feces. **Half-Life:** 4–14 h.

NURSING IMPLICATIONS

Assessment & Drug Effects

- Monitor BP and HR. Report palpitations or hypotension to physician.
- Evaluate mental status and alertness.
- Lab tests: Baseline and periodic blood chemistry (serum potassium, CBC, creatinine, uric acid, cholesterol, glucose), urinalysis for protein and sugar, and ECG.
- Give early attention and specific treatment to dry mouth. It can interfere with patient's food and fluid intake; deprivation of normal salivary flow is a potential dental hazard since it favors demineralization of teeth; and it can be a factor in noncompliance.

Patient & Family Education

- Make all position changes slowly and in stages in the event that you experience orthostatic hypotension. This is important in older adults, who tend to be more sensitive to normal adult doses of antihypertensive drugs because of deficient baroreceptor reflexes.
- Do not omit a dose or stop drug therapy without consulting physician. Do not discontinue therapy abruptly; can cause sympathetic overactivity (anxiety, nervousness, palpitation, chest pain, fast or irregular heartbeat, trembling, flushing, headache, increased sweating and salivation, elevation of BP, usually above basal level).
- Do not drive or engage in potentially hazardous activities until response to drug is known. Also, guanabenz may reduce tolerance to alcohol and other CNS depressants.
- Do not breast feed while taking this drug without consulting physician.

GUANADREL SULFATE

(gwahn'a-drel)

Hylorel

Classifications: CARDIOVASCULAR AGENT; CENTRALLY ACTING ANTIHYPERTENSIVE

Prototype: Methyldopa

Pregnancy Category: B

AVAILABILITY 10 mg, 25 mg tablets

ACTIONS Adrenergic ganglionic blocking agent structurally and pharmacologically related to guanethidine. It blocks the release of norepinephrine from adrenal medulla and adrenergic nerve endings that normally follows sympathetic nerve stimulation.

THERAPEUTIC EFFECTS Blocking the release of norepinephrine leads to catecholamine depletion with resulting relaxation of vascular smooth muscle, reduction of peripheral vascular resistance, lowering of systolic and diastolic BP, and a relative increase in parasympathetic tone. Decreases standing more than supine BP and is more effective in lowering systolic than diastolic BP.

USES Stepped-care approach: Step 2 treatment of hypertension, usually with a diuretic.

CONTRAINDICATIONS Pheochromocytoma, CHF, patients taking MAO INHIBITORS. Safe use during pregnancy (category B), lactation, or in children is not established.

CAUTIOUS USE Cerebrovascular, coronary artery, or peripheral vas-

G

cular disease, bronchial asthma, history of peptic ulcer, diarrhea, older adult patients.

ROUTE & DOSAGE

Hypertension
Adult: **PO** 5 mg b.i.d., may increase up to 20–75 mg/d in 2–4 divided doses
Geriatric: **PO** Start with 5 mg once daily

G

ADMINISTRATION

Oral

- Because serum half-life of guanadrel averages about 10 h, dosage adjustments are generally made weekly or monthly.
- Store at 15°–30° C (59°–86° F) unless otherwise directed.

ADVERSE EFFECTS (≥1%) **Body as a Whole:** Musculoskeletal aches, pains, or inflammation; excessive weight gain or loss, peripheral edema. **CNS:** *Fatigue, headache, drowsiness,* paresthesias, tremors, confusion, depression or other psychologic problems, sleep disorders. **CV:** *Morning orthostatic hypotension* (light-headedness, weakness), *orthostatic hypotension during the day,* palpitation, chest pain. **GI:** *Diarrhea,* or increased number of stools, indigestion, constipation, dry mouth and thirst, anorexia, glossitis, nausea, vomiting, abdominal distress or pain. **Urogenital:** Nocturia, urine retention, urinary urgency or frequency, hematuria, *impaired ejaculation,* impotence. **Special Senses:** Visual disturbances, nasal stuffiness. **Respiratory:** Cough, *shortness of breath at rest or with exercise.*

INTERACTIONS Drug: Alcohol intensifies orthostatic hypotension and sedation; ALPHA- OR BETA-ADRENERGIC BLOCKERS, **reserpine** may intensify orthostatic hypotension and bradycardia; may enhance the action of **epinephrine, norepinephrine, methoxamine;** MAO INHIBITORS, PHENOTHIAZINES, TRICYCLIC ANTIDEPRESSANTS, **ephedrine, phenylpropanolamine** may antagonize hypotensive effects of guanadrel.

PHARMACOKINETICS Absorption: Readily absorbed from GI tract. **Onset:** 0.5–2 h. **Peak:** 4–6 h. **Duration:** 4–14 h. **Distribution:** Widely distributed. **Elimination:** 85% excreted in urine within 24 h. **Half-Life:** 10–12 h.

NURSING IMPLICATIONS

Assessment & Drug Effects

- Monitor and record BP in supine position and after standing 2–20 min. Record baseline measurements for future comparison purposes.
- Evaluate the full effect of guanadrel on standing (orthostatic) BP carefully before discharging the hospitalized patient. For ambulatory patients, take BP measurements following exercise for complete assessment.
- Monitor patients closely with cerebrovascular, coronary artery, or peripheral vascular disease because they are particularly prone to orthostatic hypotension.
- Monitor weight gain and assess for edema formation. Guanadrel tends to enhance sodium and water retention, but these effects are generally controlled by concurrent diuretic therapy.

Patient & Family Education

- Be aware of the possibility of orthostatic hypotension; do not get out of bed without assistance during initial dosage adjustment

period. Make position changes slowly and in stages, especially from recumbent to upright posture throughout drug therapy.
- Lie down immediately at first hint of faintness, dizziness, weakness, or light-headedness. All are possible manifestations of orthostatic hypotension.
- Monitor weight, check legs and ankles for edema, and note if rings or shoes suddenly seem too tight. Notify physician of peripheral edema or unexpected weight gain of ≥1 kg (2 lb)/day.
- Take drug at the same time(s) each day, in relation to a daily routine activity.
- Note: Most adverse effects disappear or at least diminish in intensity after about 8 wk of therapy.
- Do not use OTC drugs for treatment of colds, allergy, asthma, or appetite suppressants without consulting the physician or pharmacist. Many of these products contain adrenergic (sympathomimetic) amines, which may interfere with hypotensive action of guanadrel.
- Do not breast feed while taking this drug without consulting physician.

GUANETHIDINE SULFATE

(gwahn-eth'i-deen)
Ismelin, Apo-Guanethidine ♣
Classifications: CARDIOVASCULAR AGENT; CENTRALLY ACTING ANTIHYPERTENSIVE
Prototype: Methyldopa
Pregnancy Category: C

AVAILABILITY 10 mg, 25 mg tablets

ACTIONS Potent, long-acting, adrenergic blocking agent. Competes with norepinephrine for reuptake into adrenergic neurons; displaces stored norepinephrine, thus exposing it to degradation by MAO. Produces a gradual prolonged fall in BP, usually associated with bradycardia and decreased pulse pressure. Drug-induced sodium retention and expansion of plasma volume, with resulting tolerance to antihypertensive effect, may occur unless concomitant diuretic therapy is administered.
THERAPEUTIC EFFECTS It is more effective in lowering orthostatic than supine BP. Antihypertensive effect results from venous dilatation with peripheral pooling, decreased venous return, and decreased cardiac output.

USES Stepped care approach to treatment of moderate to severe hypertension either alone or in conjunction with a thiazide diuretic or hydralazine.
UNLABELED USES Chronic open-angle glaucoma, endocrine ophthalmopathy. **Orphan Drug:** Reflex sympathetic dystrophy syndrome; causalgia.

CONTRAINDICATIONS Pheochromocytoma, frank CHF (not due to hypertension). Safe use during pregnancy (category C) is not established.
CAUTIOUS USE Diabetes mellitus, impaired renal or hepatic function, sinus bradycardia, limited cardiac reserve, coronary disease with insufficiency, recent MI, cerebrovascular insufficiency, febrile illnesses, older adults; lactation; history of peptic ulcer, colitis, or bronchial asthma.

ROUTE & DOSAGE

Hypertension
Adult: **PO** 10 mg once/d, may be increased by 10 mg q5–7d up to 300 mg/d (start with 25–50 mg/d in hospitalized patients, increase by 25–50 mg q1–3d)

Geriatric: **PO** Start with 5 mg once daily
Child: **PO** 0.2 mg/kg/d, may increase by 0.2 mg/kg q1–3wk if needed (max: 1–1.6 mg/kg/d)

G

ADMINISTRATION

Oral

- Crush tablet before administration if needed to enable swallowing and give with fluid of patient's choice.
- Increase dosage slowly (at intervals of no less than 5–7 d for adults and 1–3 wk in children) and only if there has been no reduction in standing BP from previous levels. BP should be monitored during dosage adjustment period.

ADVERSE EFFECTS (≥1%) **CV:** *Marked orthostatic and exertional hypotension* with dizziness, lightheadedness; bradycardia, symptomatic sick sinus syndrome (weakness, dizziness, blurred vision); angina, *edema with weight gain,* CHF, complete heart block. **Special Senses:** Blurred vision, ptosis of eyelids, parotid tenderness, nasal congestion. **GI:** *Severe diarrhea,* nausea, vomiting, constipation, dry mouth. **Urogenital:** Nocturia, urinary retention, incontinence, inhibition of ejaculation, impotence. **Skin:** Skin eruptions, loss of scalp hair. **Other:** Dyspnea, psychic depression, weakness, fatigue, myalgia, tremor, chest paresthesias, asthma, rise in BUN, polyarteritis nodosa.

INTERACTIONS Drug: Alcohol, levodopa, DIURETICS and other HYPOTENSIVE AGENTS increase hypotensive effects; MAO INHIBITORS may antagonize hypotensive effects; **norepinephrine, pseudoephedrine,** OTHER DECONGESTANTS, TRICYCLIC ANTIDEPRESSANTS, PHENOTHIAZINES block hypotensive effects. **Herbal: Ma-huang, ephedra** may cause enhanced sympathomimetic effects.

PHARMACOKINETICS Absorption: Completely absorbed, but undergoes significant first pass metabolism by liver; 3%–50% of dose reaches systemic circulation. **Peak:** 1–3 wk. **Distribution:** Rapidly distributed to adrenergic neuron storage sites; does not cross blood–brain barrier. **Metabolism:** Metabolized in liver to inactive metabolites. **Elimination:** Excreted in urine. **Half-Life:** 5 d.

NURSING IMPLICATIONS

Assessment & Drug Effects

- Take BP first in supine position and then again after patient has been standing for 10 min. Ideal dosage reduces standing BP to within normal range without faintness, dizziness, weakness, or fatigue.
- Monitor I&O, especially in older adults and patients with limited cardiac reserve or impaired renal function. Report changes in I&O ratio.
- Observe for evidence of edema and weight gain. Sudden weight gain of 1 kg (2 lb) in 24 h or more should be reported to physician. Patients with limited cardiac reserve are particularly susceptible to guanethidine-induced sodium and water retention, with resulting edema, CHF, and drug resistance.
- Observe patients on antidiabetic therapy closely for signs of hypoglycemia.

Patient & Family Education

- Do not stop drug without consulting physician.
- Ask for assistance with walking; older adults are prone to develop orthostatic hypotension.

- Understand that orthostatic hypotension is most prominent shortly after arising from sleep and when too rapid changes are made to sitting or upright positions. Move gradually to sitting position and make all position changes slowly and in stages. Flex arms and legs slowly before standing to augment venous return. Orthostatic hypotension is intensified by prolonged standing, hot baths or showers, hot weather, alcohol ingestion, and strenuous physical exercise (particularly if followed by immobility).
- Lie down or sit down (in head-low position) immediately at the onset of dizziness, weakness, or faintness.
- Consult physician regarding allowable salt intake.
- Reduced dosage in presence of febrile illnesses. Report fever to physician.
- Consult physician or pharmacist before taking any OTC drug; guanethidine may sensitize the patient to some sympathomimetic agents found in OTC cold remedies and cause hypertensive crisis.
- Do not breast feed while taking this drug.

GUANFACINE HYDROCHLORIDE

(gwahn'fa-seen)

Tenex

Classifications: CARDIOVASCULAR AGENT; CENTRAL-ACTING ANTIHYPERTENSIVE

Prototype: Methyldopa

Pregnancy Category: B

AVAILABILITY 1 mg, 2 mg tablets

ACTIONS Central-acting antihypertensive with alpha$_2$-adrenergic agonist properties. In cerebral cortex, stimulation of alpha$_2$-adrenoceptors triggers inhibitory neurons to reduce central sympathetic outflow (i.e., impulses from vasomotor center to heart and blood vessels).

THERAPEUTIC EFFECTS Results in decreased peripheral vascular resistance and a slightly reduced (5 bpm) heart rate. Cardiac output is not altered by this agent.

USES Management of mild to moderate hypertension.

UNLABELED USES Adjunct in heroin withdrawal.

CONTRAINDICATIONS Treatment of acute hypertension associated with toxemia of pregnancy; pregnancy (category B); children <12 y.

CAUTIOUS USE Severe coronary insufficiency, recent MI, cerebrovascular disease; chronic renal or hepatic failure; lactation.

ROUTE & DOSAGE

Hypertension

Adult: **PO** 1 mg/d h.s., may be gradually increased to 3 mg/d if needed

ADMINISTRATION

Oral

- Take single dose at bedtime to reduce effect of somnolence.
- Discontinue treatment gradually with planned tapering of schedule.
- Store tablets at 15°–30° C (59°–86° F) in tightly closed container; protect from light.

ADVERSE EFFECTS (≥1%) **CNS:** Confusion, amnesia, mental depression, drowsiness, *dizziness, sedation,* headache, asthenia, *fatigue,* insomnia. **CV:** Bradycardia, palpitation, substernal pain. **Special Senses:** Rhinitis, tinnitus, taste change; vision disturbances, conjunctivitis, iritis. **GI:** *Dry mouth, constipation,* abdominal pain, diarrhea, dysphagia, nausea. **Urogenital:** *Impotence,* testicular disorder, urinary incontinence. **Musculoskeletal:** Leg cramps, hypokinesia. **Skin:** Dermatitis, pruritus, purpura, sweating. **Other:** Dyspnea.

INTERACTIONS Drug: Alcohol and other CNS DEPRESSANTS compound sedation and CNS depression.

PHARMACOKINETICS Absorption: Readily absorbed from GI tract. **Onset:** 2 h. **Peak:** 6 h. **Duration:** Up to 24 h. **Distribution:** Crosses placenta. **Metabolism:** Metabolized in liver. **Elimination:** 80% excreted in the urine in 24 h. **Half-Life:** 17 h.

NURSING IMPLICATIONS

Assessment & Drug Effects

- Do not discontinue abruptly; may cause plasma and urinary catecholamine increases leading symptoms of tachycardia, insomnia, anxiety, nervousness. Rebound hypertension (i.e., increases in BP to levels significantly greater than those before therapy) may occur 2–7 d after abrupt drug withdrawal, but serious effects rarely develop.
- Monitor BP until it is stabilized. Report a rise in pressure that occurs toward end of dose interval; a divided dose schedule may be ordered.
- Assess mental status and alertness. Adverse effects tend to be dose-dependent, increasing significantly with doses above 3 mg/d.

Patient & Family Education

- Continue drug even after you feel well. This is a maintenance dosage regimen (dose and dose intervals). If 2 or more doses are missed, consult physician about how to reestablish dosage regimen.
- Employ measures to keep mouth moist; saliva substitutes (e.g., Moi-Stir, Xero-Lube) are available OTC. If dry mouth persists >2 wk, patient should check with dentist.
- Do not drive or engage in other potentially hazardous tasks requiring alertness until response to drug is known.
- Avoid alcohol and do not self-medicate with OTC drugs such as sleeping medications, or cough medications without consulting physician.
- Do not breast feed while taking this drug without consulting physician.

HAEMOPHILUS b CONJUGATE VACCINE (HIB)

(hee-mof′il-us)

HibTITER, PedvaxHIB, ProHIBiT

Classifications: ANTIINFECTIVE; VACCINE

Prototype: Hepatitis B vaccine

Pregnancy Category: C

AVAILABILITY 7.5 mcg, 10 mcg, 15 mcg, 25 mcg injection

ACTIONS A highly purified capsular polysaccharide extracted from *Haemophilus influenzae* type b (Hib). Hib capsular polysaccharide, principal antigen in the vaccine, promotes production of Hib anticapsular antibodies. It mediates complement-dependent bacteriolyses of *H. influenzae* type b organism. Serum antibody response is age dependent; i.e., response is poor in infants, increasing significantly between 12–24 mo.

THERAPEUTIC EFFECTS The vaccine produces antibodies effective against *H. influenza* type b.

USES To provide active immunity to *H. influenzae* type b (Hib) infection in children 2 mo–5 y.

UNLABELED USES Adults at risk of Hib infection who have Hodgkin's disease, before immunosuppressive chemotherapy.

CONTRAINDICATIONS Hypersensitivity to any component of vaccine (e.g., thiomersal); febrile illness (other than upper respiratory tract infection); active infection. Safe use during pregnancy (category C) or lactation is not established.

ROUTE & DOSAGE

Immunoprophylaxis for *H. influenzae* type b Infection

Child: **IM** *2–6 mo,* HibTITER 0.5 mL, 3 doses 2 mo apart with booster at 15 mo; PedvaxHIB 0.5 mL, 2 doses 2 mo apart with booster at 12 mo *7–11 mo,* HibTITER 0.5 mL, 2 doses 2 mo apart with booster at 15 mo; PedvaxHIB 0.5 mL, 2 doses 2 mo apart with booster at 15 mo *12–14 mo,* HibTITER 0.5 mL, 1 dose with booster at 15 mo; PedvaxHIB 0.5 mL, 1 dose with booster at 15 mo *15 mo–5 y,* all vaccines 0.5 mL as 1 dose

ADMINISTRATION

Intramuscular

- Reconstitute lyophilized powder with supplied diluent to yield 25 mcg/0.5 mL.
- Note: Use different sites when giving Hib polysaccharide vaccine and DPT (diphtheria, pertussis, tetanus) at the same time.
- Store at 2°–8° C (36°–46° F); may be frozen without loss of potency. Do not freeze the diluent.

ADVERSE EFFECTS (≥1%) **Skin:** Irritation at injection site (4%–9%). **Other:** Acute febrile reactions (13%), irritability, anorexia, anaphylactoid reaction (rare).

DIAGNOSTIC TEST INTERFERENCE Hib polysaccharide vaccine may interfere with interpretation of ***antigen detection tests*** (e.g., latex agglutination) used in diagnosis of systemic Hib disease.

INTERACTIONS Drug: IMMUNOSUPPRESSANT DRUGS, STEROIDS may decrease antibody response.

PHARMACOKINETICS Onset: Antibody levels detected within 2 wk. **Peak:** 3 wk. **Duration:** 1.5–3.5 y. **Distribution:** Crosses placenta; distributed into breast milk.

H

NURSING IMPLICATIONS

Assessment & Drug Effects

- Be prepared for anaphylactoid reaction (see Appendix F) by having epinephrine 1:1000 available.

Patient & Family Education

- Note: Local reactions to the vaccine at the injection site (erythema, tenderness, induration, swelling, pain) may appear within 6 h after administration; usually symptoms are mild and disappear in 24 h.
- Monitor temperature after injection. An acute febrile reaction with temperature above 38.3° C (101° F) may follow vaccination (less than 1% of recipients). Notify physician.
- Do not breast feed while taking this drug without consulting physician.

HALAZEPAM

(hal-az'e-pam)

Paxipam

Classifications: CENTRAL NERVOUS SYSTEM AGENT; ANXIOLYTIC; SEDATIVE-HYPNOTIC; BENZODIAZEPINE

Prototype: Lorazepam

Pregnancy Category: D

Controlled Substance: Schedule IV

AVAILABILITY 20 mg, 40 mg tablets

ACTIONS Psychotropic drug that shares antianxiety action of other short-term benzodiazepine derivatives. Effects (anxiolytic, sedative, hypnotic, and skeletal muscle relaxant) are mediated by the inhibitory neurotransmitter GABA.

THERAPEUTIC EFFECTS Clinically it produces a dose-related CNS depressant effect ranging from mild improvement of psychomotor activity, decreased anxiety to sedative hypnotic effects.

USES To manage anxiety disorders or for short-term relief of anxiety symptoms.

CONTRAINDICATIONS Hypersensitivity to halazepam or other benzodiazepines; psychosis, anxiety-free psychiatric disorders; acute narrow-angle glaucoma.

CAUTIOUS USE Abnormal kidney or liver function. Safe use during pregnancy (category D), lactation, or in children <8 y is not established.

ROUTE & DOSAGE

Anxiety
Adult: **PO** 20–40 mg t.i.d. or q.i.d.
Geriatric: **PO** 20 mg 1–2 times daily

ADMINISTRATION

Oral

- Note: Patients with renal or hepatic impairment may require lower doses. Consult physician.
- Store at 2°–30° C (36°–86° F) unless directed otherwise.

ADVERSE EFFECTS (≥1%) **CNS:** *Drowsiness, sedation,* headache, confusion, ataxia, paresthesia, motion sickness. **CV:** Hypotension, tachycardia, bradycardia. **GI:** Dry mouth, increased salivation, nausea, vomiting, constipation, abnormal liver values. **Special Senses:** Visual disturbances. **Urogenital:** GU distress. **Respiratory:** Respiratory disturbances.

INTERACTIONS Drug: Cimetidine, disulfiram, ORAL CONTRACEPTIVES may increase effects of halazepam; **alcohol,** other CNS DEPRESSANTS compound CNS depression. **Herbal: Kava-kava, valerian** may potentiate sedation.

PHARMACOKINETICS Absorption: Readily absorbed from GI tract. **Peak:** 1–3 h. **Distribution:** Crosses placenta; distributed into breast milk. **Metabolism:** Metabolized in liver to active form. **Elimination:** Excreted in urine. **Half-Life:** 30–200 h (active metabolite).

NURSING IMPLICATIONS

Assessment & Drug Effects

- Monitor for adverse effects. Ataxia, confusion, or oversedation may be symptoms of overdosage and can occur at relatively low dosage in older adult or debilitated patient.
- Reassess response to halazepam periodically.

Patient & Family Education

- Discuss with physician desirability of discontinuing drug because of its potential hazard to the fetus if you become or plan to become pregnant.
- Do not stop taking drug suddenly. Barbiturate-like withdrawal symptoms may occur (dysphoria, insomnia, abdominal and muscle cramps, vomiting, sweating, tremors, convulsions).
- Note: Smoking decreases sedative effects of halazepam.
- Do not drive or engage in other potentially hazardous activities until response to drug is known.

- Be aware that alcohol or other CNS depressants can produce additive effects.
- Do not breast feed while taking this drug without consulting physician.

HALCINONIDE

(hal-sin'oh-nide)
Halog
Classifications: SKIN AND MUCOUS MEMBRANE AGENT; ANTIINFLAMMATORY STEROID
Prototype: Hydrocortisone
Pregnancy Category: C

AVAILABILITY 0.1% ointment, cream, solution; 0.025% cream

ACTIONS Fluorinated steroid with substituted 17-hydroxyl group, chemically similar to flurandrenolide (Cordran).
THERAPEUTIC EFFECTS Crosses cell membranes, complexes with nuclear DNA and stimulates synthesis of enzymes thought to be responsible for antiinflammatory effects.

USES Relief of pruritic and inflammatory manifestations of corticosteroid-responsive dermatoses.

CONTRAINDICATIONS Use on large body surface area; long term use.
CAUTIOUS USE Children, lactation, pregnancy (category C).

ROUTE & DOSAGE

Inflammation
Adult: **Topical** Apply thin layer b.i.d. or t.i.d.
Child: **Topical** Apply thin layer once/d

ADMINISTRATION

Topical
- Wash skin gently and dry thoroughly before each application.
- Note: Ointment is preferred for dry scaly lesions. Moist lesions are best treated with solution.
- Do not apply in or around the eyes.
- Do not apply occlusive dressings over areas covered with halcinonide unless specifically prescribed.
- Store at 15°–30° C (59°–86° F).

ADVERSE EFFECTS (≥1%) **Endocrine:** Reversible HPA axis suppression, hyperglycemia, glycosuria. **Skin:** Burning, itching, irritation, erythema, dryness, folliculitis, hypertrichosis, pruritus, acneiform eruptions, hypopigmentation, perioral dermatitis, allergic contact dermatitis, stinging cracking/tightness of skin, secondary infection, skin atrophy, striae, miliaria, telangiectasia.

PHARMACOKINETICS Absorption: Minimum absorption through intact skin; increased absorption from axilla, eyelid, face, scalp, scrotum, or with occlusive dressing.

NURSING IMPLICATIONS

Assessment & Drug Effects
- Discontinue if signs of infection or irritation occur.
- Monitor for systemic corticosteroid effects that may occur with occlusive dressings or topical applications over large areas of skin.

Patient & Family Education
- Do not breast feed while using this drug without consulting physician.

H

HALOPERIDOL

(ha-loe-per′i-dole)
Haldol, Peridol ♣

HALOPERIDOL DECANOATE

Haldol LA
Classifications: CENTRAL NERVOUS SYSTEM AGENT; PSYCHOTHERAPEUTIC; ANTIPSYCHOTIC; BUTYROPHENONE
Pregnancy Category: C

H

AVAILABILITY 0.5 mg, 1 mg, 2 mg, 5 mg, 10 mg, 20 mg tablets; 2 mg/mL oral solution; 5 mg/mL, 50 mg/mL, 100 mg/mL injection

ACTIONS Potent, long-acting butyrophenone derivative with pharmacologic actions similar to those of piperazine phenothiazines but with higher incidence of extrapyramidal effects and less hypotensive and relatively low sedative activity.
THERAPEUTIC EFFECTS Decreases psychotic manifestations and exerts strong antiemetic effect.

USES Management of manifestations of psychotic disorders and for control of tics and vocal utterances of Gilles de la Tourette's syndrome; for treatment of agitated states in acute and chronic psychoses. Used for short-term treatment of hyperactive children and for severe behavior problems in children of combative, explosive hyperexcitability.
UNLABELED USES Cancer chemotherapy as an antiemetic in doses smaller than those required for antipsychotic effects; treatment of autism; alcohol dependence; chorea.

CONTRAINDICATIONS Parkinson's disease, parkinsonism, seizure disorders, coma; alcoholism; severe mental depression, CNS depression; thyrotoxicosis. Safe use during pregnancy (category C), lactation, or in children <3 y is not established.
CAUTIOUS USE Older adult or debilitated patients, urinary retention, glaucoma, severe cardiovascular disorders; patients receiving anticonvulsant, anticoagulant, or lithium therapy.

ROUTE & DOSAGE

Psychosis
Adult: **PO** 0.2–5 mg b.i.d. or t.i.d. **IM** 2–5 mg repeated q4h prn; Decanoate 50–100 mg q4wk
Child: **PO** 0.5 mg/d in 2–3 divided doses, may be increased by 0.5 mg q5–7d to 0.05–0.15 mg/kg/d

Severe Psychosis
Adult: **PO** 3–5 mg b.i.d. or t.i.d., may need up to 100 mg/d **IM** 2–5 mg, may repeat q.h. prn; Decanoate: 50–100 mg q4wk
Child: **PO** 0.05–0.15 mg/kg/d in 2–3 divided doses

Dementia
Geriatric: **PO** 0.25–0.5 mg 1–2 times daily, may increase every 4–7 d (max: 4 mg/d in 2–3 divided doses)

Tourette's Disorder
Adult: **PO** 0.2–5 mg b.i.d. or t.i.d.
Child: **PO** 0.05–0.075 mg/kg/d in 2–3 divided doses

ADMINISTRATION

Oral
- Give with a full glass (240 mL) of water or with food or milk.
- Taper dosing regimen when discontinuing therapy. Abrupt termination can initiate extrapyramidal symptoms.

Intramuscular

- Give by deep injection into a large muscle. Do not exceed 3 mL per injection site.
- Have patient recumbent at time of parenteral administration and for about 1 h after injection. Assess for orthostatic hypotension.
- Store in light-resistant container at 15°–30° C (59°–86° F), unless otherwise specified by manufacturer. Discard darkened solutions.

ADVERSE EFFECTS (≥1%) **CNS:** *Extrapyramidal reactions:* Parkinsonian symptoms, dystonia, akathisia, tardive dyskinesia (after long-term use); insomnia, restlessness, anxiety, euphoria, agitation, drowsiness, mental depression, lethargy, fatigue, weakness, tremor, ataxia, headache, confusion, vertigo; neuroleptic malignant syndrome, hyperthermia, grand mal seizures, exacerbation of psychotic symptoms. **CV:** Tachycardia, ECG changes, hypotension, hypertension (with overdosage). **Endocrine:** Menstrual irregularities, galactorrhea, lactation, gynecomastia, impotence, increased libido, hyponatremia, hyperglycemia, hypoglycemia. **Special Senses:** Blurred vision. **Hematologic:** Mild transient leukopenia, agranulocytosis (rare). **GI:** Dry mouth, anorexia, nausea, vomiting, constipation, diarrhea, hypersalivation. **Urogenital:** Urinary retention, priapism. **Respiratory:** Laryngospasm, bronchospasm, increased depth of respiration, bronchopneumonia, respiratory depression. **Skin:** Diaphoresis, maculopapular and acneiform rash, photosensitivity. **Other:** Cholestatic jaundice, variations in liver function tests, decreased serum cholesterol.

INTERACTIONS Drug: CNS DEPRESSANTS, OPIATES, **alcohol** increase CNS depression; may antagonize activity of ORAL ANTICOAGULANTS; ANTICHOLINERGICS may increase intraocular pressure; **methyldopa** may precipitate dementia.

PHARMACOKINETICS Absorption: Well absorbed from GI tract; 60% reaches systemic circulation. **Onset:** 30–45 min IM. **Peak:** 2–6 h PO; 10–20 min IM; 6–7 d decanoate. **Distribution:** distributes mainly to liver with lower concentration in brain, lung, kidney, spleen, heart. **Metabolism:** Metabolized in liver. **Elimination:** 40% excreted in urine within 5 d; 15% eliminated in feces; excreted in breast milk. **Half-Life:** 13–35 h.

NURSING IMPLICATIONS

Assessment & Drug Effects

- Monitor for therapeutic effectiveness. Because of long half-life, therapeutic effects are slow to develop in early therapy or when established dosing regimen is changed. "Therapeutic window" effect (point at which increased dose or concentration actually decreases therapeutic response) may occur after long period of high doses. Close observation is imperative when doses are changed.
- Target symptoms expected to decrease with successful haloperidol treatment include hallucinations, insomnia, hostility, agitation, and delusions.
- Monitor patient's mental status daily.
- Monitor for neuroleptic malignant syndrome (NMS) (see Appendix F), especially in those with hypertension or taking lithium. Symptoms of NMS can appear suddenly after initiation of therapy or after months or years of taking neuroleptic (antipsychotic) medication. Immediately discontinue drug if NMS suspected.

- Monitor for parkinsonism and tardive dyskinesia (see Appendix F). Risk of tardive dyskinesia appears to be greater in women receiving high doses and in older adults. It can occur after long-term therapy and even after therapy is discontinued.
- Monitor for extrapyramidal (neuromuscular) reactions that occur frequently during first few days of treatment. Symptoms are usually dose related and are controlled by dosage reduction or concomitant administration of antiparkinson drugs.
- Be alert for behavioral changes in patients who are concurrently receiving antiparkinson drugs.
- Monitor for exacerbation of seizure activity.
- Observe patients closely for rapid mood shift to depression when haloperidol is used to control mania or cyclic disorders. Depression may represent a drug adverse effect or reversion from a manic state.
- Lab tests: Monitor WBC count with differential and liver function in patients on prolonged therapy.

Patient & Family Education

- Avoid use of alcohol during therapy.
- Do not drive or engage in other potentially hazardous activities until response to drug is known.
- Discuss oral hygiene with health care provider; dry mouth may promote dental problems. Drink adequate fluids.
- Avoid overexposure to sun or sunlamp and use a sunscreen; drug can cause a photosensitivity reaction.
- Do not breast feed while taking this drug without consulting physician.

HALOPROGIN

(ha-loe-proe'jin)

Halotex

Classifications: ANTIINFECTIVE; ANTIBIOTIC; ANTIFUNGAL

Prototype: Fluconazole

Pregnancy Category: B

AVAILABILITY 1% cream, solution

ACTIONS Synthetic iodinated phenolic ether which is fungicidal or fungistatic against certain species.

THERAPEUTIC EFFECTS Fungicidal or fungistatic against various species of *Trichophyton, Epidermophyton, Microsporum, Malassezia,* and *Candida*. Also active in vitro against *Staphylococcus aureus* and *Streptococcus pyogenes.*

USES Superficial fungal infections such as tinea pedis, tinea cruris, tinea corporis, and tinea manus. Also tinea versicolor caused by *Malassezia furfur*. May be used in combination antiinfective therapy for mixed infections.

CONTRAINDICATIONS Lactation; children <5 y.

CAUTIOUS USE Older adults; severe cardiovascular disease; history of seizures of abnormal EEG; thyrotoxicosis; bipolar disorder. Safe use during pregnancy (category B) is not established.

ROUTE & DOSAGE

Superficial Fungal Infections

Adult: **Topical** Apply liberally to affected area b.i.d. for 2–3 wk

ADMINISTRATION

Topical

- Wash skin gently and dry thoroughly before each application.

- Avoid contact of medication with eyes.

ADVERSE EFFECTS (≥1%) **Body as a Whole:** Low incidence of systemic toxicity. **Skin:** Local irritation, burning sensation, vesiculation, increased maceration, exacerbation of preexisting lesions, sensitization, pruritus.

INTERACTIONS Drug: No clinically significant interactions established.

PHARMACOKINETICS Absorption: Minimum absorption through intact skin.

NURSING IMPLICATIONS

Assessment & Drug Effects

- Discontinue medication if signs of infection or irritation occur.
- Reevaluate therapy if no improvement is noted after 2–3 wk.

Patient & Family Education

- Discontinue medication if condition worsens or if burning, irritation, or signs of sensitization occur, and consult physician.
- Do not wear occlusive foot-wear with tinea pedis (athlete's foot) because it promotes drug absorption and enhances fungal growth.
- Do not breast feed while using this drug.

HEMIN

(hee'min)

Panhematin

Classifications: BLOOD FORMERS AND COAGULANTS; ENZYME INHIBITOR; BLOOD DERIVATIVE

Pregnancy Category: C

AVAILABILITY 7 mg/mL injection

ACTIONS Sterile, nonpyrogenic ferric iron complex of protoporphyrin IX; derived from processed red blood cells.

THERAPEUTIC EFFECTS Represses synthesis of porphyrin in liver or bone marrow by blocking production of delta-aminolevulinic acid (ALA) synthetase, an essential enzyme in the porphyrin-heme biosynthetic pathway.

USES Recurrent attacks of acute intermittent porphyria (AIP) only after an appropriate period of alternate therapy has been tried (i.e., glucose 400 g/d for 1–2 d).

CONTRAINDICATIONS History of hypersensitivity to hemin; porphyria cutanea tarda.

CAUTIOUS USE Safe use during pregnancy (category C), lactation, or in children is not established.

ROUTE & DOSAGE

Acute Intermittent Porphyria

Adult: **IV** 1–4 mg/kg/d administered over 10–15 min for 3–14 d, do not repeat dose earlier than q12h (max: 6 mg/kg in 24 h)

ADMINISTRATION

Intravenous

- Administer via a large arm vein or central venous catheter to reduce risk of phlebitis. Terminal filtration through a sterile 0.45 micron or smaller filter is recommended.

PREPARE: **IV Infusion:** Reconstitute immediately before use by aseptically adding 43 mL sterile water for injection to vial to yield 7 mg/mL. ▪ Shake well for 2–3 min to dissolve all particles. ▪ Discard unused portions.

ADMINISTER: **IV Infusion:** Give a single dose over 10–15 min.

- Freeze and store lyophilized powder until time of use.

H

ADVERSE EFFECTS (≥1%) **Body as a Whole:** *Phlebitis* (when administered into small veins). **Hematologic:** Decreased Hct, anticoagulant effect (prolonged PT, thromboplastin time, thrombocytopenia, hypofibrinogenemia). **Urogenital:** Reversible renal shutdown (with excessive doses).

INTERACTIONS Drug: Potentiates anticoagulant effects of ANTICOAGULANTS; BARBITURATES, ESTROGENS, SULFONAMIDES may antagonize hemin effect.

PHARMACOKINETICS Duration: Can be detected in plasma up to 5 d. **Elimination:** Excess amounts eliminated in bile and urine.

NURSING IMPLICATIONS

Assessment & Drug Effects

- Monitor IV site for signs and symptoms of thrombophlebitis (see Appendix F).
- Monitor throughout therapy (decrease in these values indicates favorable clinical response): ALA, UPG (uroporphyrinogen), PBG (porphobilinogen or coproporphyrin).
- Monitor clinical effect of drug therapy by checking patient's symptoms and complaints associated with acute porphyria, which may include depression, insomnia, anxiety, disorientation, hallucinations, psychoses; dark urine, nausea, vomiting, abdominal pain, low back and leg pain, pareses (neuropathy), seizures.
- Monitor I&O and promptly report the onset of oliguria or anuria.

Patient & Family Education

- Notify physician of bruising, hematuria, tarry black stools, and nosebleeds.
- Do not breast feed while taking this drug without consulting physician.

HEPARIN SODIUM (Pr)

Hepalean ♣, Heparin Sodium Lock Flush Solution, Hep-Lock, Lipo-Hepin, Liquaemin Sodium

Classification: BLOOD FORMERS, COAGULATORS, AND ANTICOAGULANTS

Pregnancy Category: C

AVAILABILITY 10 units/mL, 100 units/mL, 1000 units/mL 2000 units/mL, 5000 units/mL, 10,000 units/mL, 20,000 units/mL, 40,000 units/mL injection

ACTIONS Strongly acidic, high molecular weight mucopolysaccharide with rapid anticoagulant effect. Prepared from bovine lung tissue or porcine intestinal mucosa.

THERAPEUTIC EFFECTS Exerts direct effect on blood coagulation (clotting) by enhancing the inhibitory actions of antithrombin III (heparin cofactor) on several factors essential to normal blood clotting, thereby blocking the conversion of prothrombin to thrombin and fibrinogen to fibrin. Does not lyse already existing thrombi but may prevent their extension and propagation. Inhibits formation on new clots.

USES Prophylaxis and treatment of venous thrombosis and pulmonary embolism and to prevent thromboembolic complications arising from cardiac and vascular surgery, frostbite, and during acute stage of MI. Also used in treatment of disseminated intravascular coagulation (DIC), atrial fibrillation with embolization, and as anticoagulant in blood transfusions, extracorporeal circulation, and dialysis procedures.

UNLABELED USES Prophylaxis in hip and knee surgery. Heparin Sodium Lock Flush Solution is used to maintain potency of indwelling IV catheters in intermittent IV therapy or blood sampling. It is not intended for anticoagulant therapy.

CONTRAINDICATIONS History of hypersensitivity to heparin (white clot syndrome); active bleeding, bleeding tendencies (hemophilia, purpura, thrombocytopenia); jaundice; ascorbic acid deficiency; inaccessible ulcerative lesions; visceral carcinoma; open wounds, extensive denudation of skin, suppurative thrombophlebitis; advanced kidney, liver, or biliary disease; active tuberculosis; bacterial endocarditis; continuous tube drainage of stomach or small intestines; threatened abortion; suspected intracranial hemorrhage, severe hypertension; recent surgery of eye, brain, or spinal cord; spinal tap; shock.

CAUTIOUS USE Alcoholism; history of allergy (asthma, hives, hay fever, eczema); during menstruation; pregnancy (category C) especially the last trimester, and immediate postpartum period; patients with indwelling catheters; older adults; use of acid-citrate-dextrose (ACD)-converted blood (may contain heparin); patients in hazardous occupations; cerebral embolism.

ROUTE & DOSAGE

Treatment of Thromboembolism

Adult: **IV** 5000-U bolus dose, then 20,000–40,000 U infused over 24 h, dose adjusted to maintain desired APTT or 5000–10,000 U IV piggyback q4–6h **SC** 10,000–20,000 U followed by 8000–20,000 U q8–12h

Child: **IV** 50 U/kg bolus, then 20,000 U/m^2/24 h or 50–100 U/kg q4h or 15–25 U/kg/h

Open Heart Surgery

Adult: **IV** 150–300 U/kg

Prophylaxis of Embolism

Adult: **SC** 5000 U q8–12h

ADMINISTRATION

- Note: Before administration, check coagulation test values; if results are not within therapeutic range, notify physician for dosage adjustment. Do not use solutions of heparin or heparin lock-flush that contain benzyl alcohol preservative in neonates.

Subcutaneous

- Use more concentrated heparin solutions for SC injection.
- Make injections into the fatty layer of the abdomen or just above the iliac crest. Avoid injecting within 5 cm (2 in) of umbilicus or in a bruised area. Insert needle into tissue roll perpendicular to skin surface. Do not withdraw plunger to check entry into blood vessel. Systematically rotate injection sites and keep record.
- Exercise caution to avoid IM injection.

Intravenous

PREPARE: **Direct:** Give undiluted. **Intermittent/Continuous:** May add to any amount of NS, D5W, or Ringer's for injection. ▪ Invert IV solution container at least 6 times to ensure adequate mixing.
ADMINISTER: **Direct:** Give a single dose over 60 sec. **Intermittent/Continuous:** Use infusion pump and give over 4–24 h.
INCOMPATIBILITIES **Solution/additive: Amikacin, codeine, chlorpromazine, cytarabine, diazepam, dobutamine, dox-**

H

orubicin, droperidol, erythromycin, gentamicin, haloperidol, hyaluronidase, hydrocortisone, kanamycin, levorphanol, mepbreak eridine, methadone, methicillin, methotrimeprazine, morphine, netilmicin, nitroglycerin, pentazocine, polymyxin B, promethazine, streptomycin, tetracycline, tobramycin, triflupromazine, vancomycin. Y-site: Amikacin, dacarbazine, diazepam, diphenhydramine, doxycycline, doxorubicin, droperidol, ergotamine, erythromycin, gentamicin, haloperidol, kanamycin, methotrimeprazine, netilmicin, nitroglycerin, phenytoin, polymyxin B, streptomycin, tobramycin, triflupromazine, vancomycin.

- Store at 15°–30° C (59°–86° F). Protect from freezing.

ADVERSE EFFECTS (≥1%) **Hematologic:** Spontaneous bleeding, *transient thrombocytopenia,* hypofibrinogenemia, "white clot syndrome." **Body as a Whole:** Fever, chills, urticaria, pruritus, skin rashes, itching and burning sensations of feet, numbness and tingling of hands and feet, elevated BP, headache, nasal congestion, lacrimation, conjunctivitis, chest pains, arthralgia, bronchospasm, anaphylactoid reactions. **Endocrine:** Osteoporosis, hypoaldosteronism, suppressed renal function, hyperkalemia; rebound hyperlipidemia (following termination of heparin therapy). **GI:** increased AST, ALT. **Urogenital:** Priapism (rare). **Skin:** Injection site reactions: pain, itching, ecchymoses, tissue irritation and sloughing; cyanosis and pains in arms or legs (vasospasm), reversible transient alopecia (usually around temporal area).

DIAGNOSTIC TEST INTERFERENCE Notify laboratory that patient is receiving heparin, when a test is to be performed. Possibility of false-positive rise in ***BSP*** test and in ***serum thyroxine;*** and increases in ***resin T_3*** **uptake;** false-negative ***^{125}I fibrinogen uptake.*** Heparin prolongs ***PT.*** Valid readings may be obtained by drawing blood samples at least 4–6 h after an IV dose (but at any time during heparin infusion) and 12–24 h after an SC heparin dose.

INTERACTIONS Drug: May prolong PT, which is used to monitor therapy with ORAL ANTICOAGULANTS; **aspirin,** NSAIDS increase risk of bleeding; **nitroglycerin** IV may decrease anticoagulant activity; **protamine** antagonizes effects of heparin. **Herbal: Feverfew, ginkgo, ginger, valerian** may potentiate bleeding.

PHARMACOKINETICS Onset: 20–60 min SC. **Peak:** Within minutes. **Duration:** 2–6 h IV; 8–12 h SC. **Distribution:** Does not cross placenta; not distributed into breast milk. **Metabolism:** Metabolized in liver and by reticuloendothelial system. **Elimination:** Excreted slowly in urine. **Half-Life:** 90 min.

NURSING IMPLICATIONS

Assessment & Drug Effects

- Lab tests: Baseline blood coagulation tests, Hct, Hgb, RBC, and platelet counts prior to initiation of therapy and at regular intervals throughout therapy.
- Monitor APTT levels closely.
- Note: In general, dosage is adjusted to keep APTT between 1.5–2.5 times normal control level.
- Draw blood for coagulation test 30 min before each scheduled SC or intermittent IV dose and approximately q4h for patients re-

ceiving continuous IV heparin during dosage adjustment period. After dosage is established, tests may be done once daily.
- Patients vary widely in their reaction to heparin; risk of hemorrhage appears greatest in women, all patients >60 y, and patients with liver disease or renal insufficiency.
- Monitor vital signs. Report fever, drop in BP, rapid pulse, and other S&S of hemorrhage.
- Observe all needle sites daily for hematoma and signs of inflammation (swelling, heat, redness, pain).
- Antidote: Have on hand protamine sulfate (1% solution), specific heparin antagonist.

Patient & Family Education
- Protect from injury and notify physician of pink, red, dark brown, or cloudy urine; red or dark brown vomitus; red or black stools; bleeding gums or oral mucosa; ecchymoses, hematoma, epistaxis, bloody sputum; chest pain; abdominal or lumbar pain or swelling; unusual increase in menstrual flow; pelvic pain; severe or continuous headache, faintness, or dizziness.
- Note: Menstruation may be somewhat increased and prolonged; usually, this is not a contraindication to continued therapy if bleeding is not excessive.
- Learn correct technique for SC administration if discharged from hospital on heparin.
- Engage in normal activities such as shaving with a safety razor in the absence of a low platelet (thrombocyte) count. Usually, heparin does not affect bleeding time.
- Caution: Smoking and alcohol consumption may alter response to heparin and are not advised.
- Do not take aspirin or any other OTC medication without physician's approval.

HEPATITIS A VACCINE

(hep'a-ti-tis)
Havrix, Vaqta
Classifications: ANTIINFECTIVE; VACCINE
Prototype: Hepatitis B vaccine
Pregnancy Category: C

AVAILABILITY 720 EIU/0.5 mL, 1440 EIU/1 mL (Havrix); 25 U/0.5 mL, 50 U/1 mL (Vaqta)

ACTIONS Anti-hepatitis A virus antibody titers following administration of hepatitis A vaccine (inactivated) are comparable to those observed after natural hepatitis A virus infection.
THERAPEUTIC EFFECTS Antibody levels are 50- to 300-fold higher with inactivated hepatitis A vaccine than with passive immunity with human immune globulin.

USES Active immunization against hepatitis A.

CONTRAINDICATIONS Hypersensitivity to any component in vaccine, pregnancy (category C), children <2 y.
CAUTIOUS USE Lactation.

ROUTE & DOSAGE

Hepatitis A Immunization
Adult: **IM** 1 mL in deltoid muscle; booster dose (1 mL) at 6–12 mo after primary dose
Child: **IM** *2–18 y,* 2 doses of 0.5 mL in deltoid muscle given 1 mo apart; booster dose (0.5 mL) at 6–12 mo after primary doses

ADMINISTRATION

Intramuscular
- Give only in deltoid for adults and children older than 2 y. DO

NOT give IV, SC, or intradermally.
- Use vaccine as packaged without dilution.
- Shake vial and syringe well before withdrawal and injection, respectively. Vaccine should be an opaque white suspension; discard if it looks otherwise.
- Store at 2°–8° C (36°–47° F). Discard vaccine if it has been frozen.

ADVERSE EFFECTS (≥1%) **CNS:** *Headache,* fatigue, fever, malaise, somnolence vertigo, insomnia, photophobia, convulsions, neuropathy, paresthesia. **GI:** Anorexia, nausea, abdominal pain, diarrhea, dysgeusia, vomiting. **Skin:** Pruritus, rash, urticaria, erythema multiforme, hyperhidrosis, angioedema (rare). **Other:** *Soreness at injection site, pain, swelling, redness at injection site,* pharyngitis, lymphadenopathy.

INTERACTIONS Drug: No clinically significant interactions established.

PHARMACOKINETICS Onset: 3 wk. **Duration:** 1–3 y with single dose, 5–10 y with booster.

NURSING IMPLICATIONS

Assessment & Drug Effects

- Do not administer during a febrile illness.
- Assess for S&S of anaphylaxis and have epinephrine available.

Patient & Family Education

- Note: Injection site soreness is common; most adverse reactions are mild and usually last less than 24 h.
- Get booster injection within 6–12 mo if risk of exposure is still present.
- Do not breast feed while taking this drug without consulting physician.

HEPATITIS B IMMUNE GLOBULIN

(hep'a-ti-tis)

H-BIG, Hep-B-Gammagee, HyperHep

Classifications: ANTIINFECTIVE; VACCINE

Prototype: Hepatitis B vaccine

Pregnancy Category: C

AVAILABILITY 1 mL, 4 mL, 5 mL vials

ACTIONS Sterile solution of immunoglobulins [immunoglobulin G (IgG)] prepared by a special process using pooled human plasma. Serum has also been tested for and found free of antibody to HIV. The possibility of transmission of hepatitis infection or AIDS from H-BIG is remote.

THERAPEUTIC EFFECTS Preparation contains a high antibody titer specific to hepatitis B surface antigen (anti-HBs); plasma does not show serologic evidence of hepatitis B surface antigen (HBsAg).

USES Prophylactically to provide passive immunity to hepatitis B infection in individuals exposed to HBV or HBsAg-positive materials (blood plasma, serum). Also as postexposure prophylaxis after bite or percutaneous exposure, ingestion, direct mucous membrane contact, sexual or intimate contact, and in neonates born to HBsAg-positive women.

CONTRAINDICATIONS Pregnancy (category C).

CAUTIOUS USE History of systemic allergic reactions to immune globulin, concurrent administration of immunosuppression drugs; thrombocytopenia or bleeding disorders, HBsAg-positive individuals, patients with specific immunoglobulin A (IgA) deficiency; lactation.

ROUTE & DOSAGE

Hepatitis B Prophylaxis

Adult/Child: **IM** 0.06 mL/kg as soon as possible after exposure, preferably within 24 h, but no later than 7 d, repeat 28–30 d after exposure

Newborn Exposure

Child: **IM** 0.5 mL as soon as possible after birth, but no later than 24 h, repeat dose 3 and 6 mo later

ADMINISTRATION

Intramuscular

- Give Hepatitis B immune globulin at the same time or up to 1 mo preceding hepatitis B vaccination (hepatitis B vaccine) does not impair the active immune response from the vaccination.
- Give preferably into deltoid muscle or anterolateral aspect of thigh.
- Note: For neonates and small children the preferred injection site is the anterolateral aspect of the thigh.
- Do NOT administer by IV; inadvertent IV or intravascular administration can cause a precipitous fall in BP and an anaphylactic reaction.
- Store at 2°–8° C (36°–46° F) unless otherwise directed. Avoid freezing.

ADVERSE EFFECTS (≥1%) **Body as a Whole:** Muscle stiffness; pain, tenderness, swelling, erythema of injection site, nausea, faintness, fever, dizziness, malaise, lassitude, body and joint pain, leg cramps. **Skin:** Urticaria, rash, angioedema, pruritus, erythema, sensitization (following large or repeated doses), anaphylaxis (rare).

INTERACTIONS Drug: May interfere with immune response to LIVE-VIRUS VACCINES (measles/mumps/rubella/poliovirus).

PHARMACOKINETICS Absorption: Slowly absorbed from IM site. **Onset:** 1–6 d. **Peak:** 3–11 d. **Duration:** 2–6 mo. **Elimination:** Half-life 21 d.

NURSING IMPLICATIONS

Assessment & Drug Effects

- Have epinephrine 1:1000 readily available; hypersensitivity reactions are most likely to occur in patients receiving large doses or repeated injections.

Patient & Family Education

- Learn potential adverse reactions.
- Do not breast feed after taking this drug without consulting physician.

HEPATITIS B VACCINE (RECOMBINANT) Pr

(hep'a-ti-tis)

Engerix-B, Recombivax HB

Classifications: ANTIINFECTIVE; VACCINE

Pregnancy Category: C

AVAILABILITY 10 mcg/mL, 5 mcg/0.5 mL, 40 mcg/mL (Recombivax); 20 mcg/mL, 10 mcg/0.5 mL (Engerix-B)

ACTIONS Suspension of inactivated and purified hepatitis B surface antigen (HBsAg) derived from human plasma of screened asymptomatic HBsAg-positive carriers of hepatitis B virus. Hepatitis B vaccine recombinant is the first vaccine produced by gene splicing. No human plasma is used in its production.

THERAPEUTIC EFFECTS The recommended 3-dose regimen produces active immunity against hepatitis B infection by inducing protective antibody (anti-HBs) formation.

USES To promote active immunity in individuals at high risk of potential exposure to hepatitis B virus or HBsAg-positive materials. Has been used simultaneously (into different sites) with hepatitis B immune globulin (H-BIG) for post-exposure prophylaxis in selected patients and in infants born to HBsAg-positive mothers.

H

CONTRAINDICATIONS History of allergic reaction to hepatitis B vaccine or to any ingredient in the formulation; HBsAg carriers. Safe use during pregnancy (category C) and lactation is not established.
CAUTIOUS USE Compromised cardiopulmonary status, serious active infection or fever; thrombocytopenia or other bleeding disorders.

ROUTE & DOSAGE

Hepatitis B Prophylaxis

Adult: **IM** Recombivax 1 mL (10 mcg) at 0, 1, and 6 mo; Engerix-B 1 mL (20 mcg) at 0, 1, and 6 mo or 0, 1, 2, and 12 mo
Child: **IM** Recombivax 0.5 mL (5 mcg) at 0, 1, and 6 mo; Engerix-B 0.5 mL (10 mcg) at 0, 1, and 6 mo or 0, 1, 2, and 12 mo

Dialysis and Immunodeficient Patients

Adult: **IM** Recombivax 2 mL (20 mcg) at 0, 1, and 6 mo Engerix-B 2 mL (40 mcg) at 0, 1, and 6 mo or 0, 1, 2, and 12 mo

ADMINISTRATION

Intramuscular

- Give preferably into the deltoid and in neonates into the anterolateral thigh, avoiding blood vessels and nerves. Carefully aspirate to prevent inadvertent intravascular injection.
- Have epinephrine immediately available to treat anaphylaxis.
- Shake vial well before withdrawing dose to assure uniform suspension.
- Store unopened and opened vials at 2°–8° C (36°–46° F) unless otherwise directed. Avoid freezing (freezing destroys potency).

ADVERSE EFFECTS (≥1%) **Body as a Whole:** *Mild local tenderness at injection site, local inflammatory reaction* (swelling, heat, redness, induration, pain); *fever, malaise, fatigue,* headache, dizziness, faintness, leg cramps, myalgia, arthralgia. **GI:** Nausea, vomiting, diarrhea. **Skin:** Rash, urticaria, pruritus.

INTERACTIONS Drug: No clinically significant interactions established.

PHARMACOKINETICS Absorption: Slowly absorbed from IM site. **Onset:** 2 wk. **Peak:** 6 mo. **Duration:** At least 3 y.

NURSING IMPLICATIONS

Assessment & Drug Effects

- Note: The ACIP recommends serologic confirmation of postvaccination immunity in patients undergoing dialysis and in immunodeficient patients.
- Monitor temperature. Some patients develop a temperature elevation of 38.3° C (101° F) following vaccination that may last 1 or 2 d.

Patient & Family Education

- Learn potential adverse reaction.
- Do not breast feed while taking this drug without consulting physician.

HETASTARCH

(het'a-starch)

HES, Hespan, Hydroxyethyl Starch, Hextend

Classification: PLASMA VOLUME EXPANDER

Prototype: Albumin

Pregnancy Category: C

AVAILABILITY 6 g/100 mL injection

ACTIONS Synthetic starch closely resembling human glycogen. Acts much like albumin and dextran but is claimed to be less likely to produce anaphylaxis or to interfere with cross matching or blood typing procedures. Causes no significant alterations in fibrinogen or clotting time but may prolong the PTT and PT. Not a substitute for blood or plasma.

THERAPEUTIC EFFECTS Colloidal osmotic properties are approximately equal to those of human serum albumin. In hypovolemic patients, it increases arterial and venous pressures, heart rate, cardiac output, urine output, and colloidal osmotic pressure.

USES Early fluid replacement and plasma volume expansion when whole blood is not available or when there is no time for necessary cross matching. Used to expand plasma volume during cardiopulmonary bypass and in adjunctive treatment of shock caused by hemorrhage, burns, surgery, sepsis, or other trauma. Also used as sedimenting agent in preparation of granulocytes by leukopheresis.

UNLABELED USES As a priming fluid in pump oxygenators for perfusion during extracorporeal circulation and as a cryoprotective agent for long-term storage of whole blood.

CONTRAINDICATIONS Severe bleeding disorders, CHF, renal failure with oliguria and anuria, treatment of shock not accompanied by hypovolemia, pregnancy (category C). Safe use in children is not established.

CAUTIOUS USE Hepatic or renal insufficiency, pulmonary edema in the very young or older adults, patients on sodium restriction.

ROUTE & DOSAGE

Plasma Volume Expansion

Adult: **IV** 500–1000 mL at a maximum rate of 20 mL/kg/h (max: 1500 mL/d)

Child: **IV** 10 mL/kg/dose (max: 20 mL/kg/24 h)

Leukapheresis

Adult: **IV** 250–750 mL infused at a constant fixed ratio of 8:1 to venous whole blood

ADMINISTRATION

Intravenous

PREPARE: **IV Infusion:** Use undiluted as prepared by manufacturer.

ADMINISTER: **IV Infusion:** Specific flow rate is prescribed by physician. Rate may be as high as 20 mL/kg/h in acute hemorrhagic shock. Rate is usually reduced in patients with burns or septic shock.

- Store at room temperature; avoid extremes of heat or cold.
- Discard partially used bags.

ADVERSE EFFECTS (≥1%) **CV:** Peripheral edema, circulatory overload, heart failure. **Hematologic:** With large volumes, prolongation of PT, PTT, clotting time, and bleeding time; decreased Hct, Hgb, platelets, calcium, and fibrinogen; dilution of plasma proteins, hyperbilirubinemia, increased sedimentation rate. **Body as a Whole:** Pruritus, anaphylactoid reactions (periorbital edema, urticaria, wheezing), vomiting, mild fever, chills, influenza-like symptoms, headache, muscle pains, submaxillary and parotid glandular swelling.

INTERACTIONS Drug: No clinically significant interactions established.

H

PHARMACOKINETICS Duration: 24–36 h. **Distribution:** Remains in intravascular space. **Metabolism:** Metabolized in reticuloendothelial system. **Elimination:** Excreted in urine with some biliary excretion.

NURSING IMPLICATIONS

Assessment & Drug Effects

- Monitor for S&S of hypersensitivity reaction (see Appendix F).
- Measure and record I&O. Report oliguria or significant changes in I&O ratio.
- Monitor BP and vital signs and observe patient for unusual bruising or bleeding.
- Lab tests: Monitor WBC count with differential, platelet count, and PT & PTT during leukapheresis.
- Observe for signs of circulatory overload (see Appendix F).
- Check laboratory reports of Hct values. Notify physician if there is an appreciable drop in Hct or if value approaches 30% by volume. Hct should not be allowed to drop below 30%.

Patient & Family Education

- Notify physician for any of the following: Difficulty breathing, nausea, chills, headache, itching.

HOMATROPINE HYDROBROMIDE (Pr)

(hoe-ma′troe-peen)

AK-Homatropine, Homatropine, Isopto Homatropine

Classifications: EYE PREPARATION; MYDRIATIC; AUTONOMIC NERVOUS SYSTEM AGENT; ANTICHOLINERGIC (PARASYMPATHOLYTIC)

Pregnancy Category: C

AVAILABILITY 2%, 5% solution

See Appendix A-1.

HYDRALAZINE HYDROCHLORIDE (Pr)

(hye-dral′a-zeen)

Alazine, Apresoline

Classifications: CARDIOVASCULAR AGENT; NONNITRATE VASODILATOR; ANTIHYPERTENSIVE

Pregnancy Category: C

AVAILABILITY 10 mg, 25 mg, 50 mg, 100 mg tablets; 20 mg/mL vial

ACTIONS Reduces BP mainly by direct effect on vascular smooth muscles of arterial-resistance vessels, resulting in vasodilation. Has little effect on venous-capacitance vessels. Hypotensive effect may be limited by sympathetic reflexes, which increase heart rate, stroke volume, and cardiac output.

THERAPEUTIC EFFECTS Diastolic response is often greater than systolic response. Vasodilation reduces peripheral resistance and substantially improves cardiac output, and renal and cerebral blood flow. Postural hypotensive effect is reportedly less than that produced by ganglionic blocking agents.

USES Most commonly in stepped-care approach to treat moderate to severe hypertension. Also in early malignant hypertension and resistant hypertension that persists after sympathectomy.

UNLABELED USES Conjunctively with cardiac glycosides and other vasodilators in short-term treatment of acute CHF; unexplained pulmonary hypertension.

CONTRAINDICATIONS Coronary artery disease, mitral valvular rheumatic heart disease, MI, tachycardia, SLE. Safe use during pregnancy (category C) or lactation is established.

CAUTIOUS USE Cerebrovascular accident, advanced renal impairment, use with MAO INHIBITORS.

ROUTE & DOSAGE

Hypertension

Adult: **PO** 10–50 mg q.i.d. **IM** 10–50 mg q4–6h **IV** 10–20 mg q4–6h

Geriatric: **PO** start with 10 mg 2–3 times/d

Child: **PO** 3–7.5 mg/kg/d in 4 divided doses **IV/IM** 1.7–3.5 mg/kg/d in 4 divided doses

ADMINISTRATION

Oral

- Give with food; bioavailability is increased by taking it with food.
- Discontinue gradually to avoid sudden rise in BP and acute heart failure.
- Inform patients of the dangers of abrupt withdrawal.

Intramuscular

- Give deep into a large muscle.

Intravenous

PREPARE: **Direct:** Give undiluted. Use immediately after being drawn into syringe. Do not add to IV solutions.

ADMINISTER: **Direct:** Give each 10 mg or fraction thereof over 1 min.

INCOMPATIBILITIES **Solution/additive: Aminophylline, ampicillin, chlorothiazide, edetate calcium disodium, hydrocortisone, mephentermine, methohexital, nitroglycerin, phenobarbital, verapamil.**

- Store at 15°–30° C (59°–86° F) in tight, light-resistant containers unless otherwise directed. Avoid freezing.

ADVERSE EFFECTS (≥1%) **Body as a Whole:** Hypersensitivity (rash, urticaria, pruritus, fever, chills, arthralgia, eosinophilia, cholangitis, hepatitis, obstructive jaundice). **CNS:** *Headache,* dizziness, tremors. **CV:** *Palpitation,* angina, *tachycardia,* flushing, paradoxical pressor response. Overdose: arrhythmia, shock. **Special Senses:** Lacrimation, conjunctivitis. **GI:** Anorexia, nausea, vomiting, diarrhea, constipation, abdominal pain, paralytic ileus. **Urogenital:** Difficulty in urination, glomerulonephritis. **Hematologic:** Decreased hematocrit and hemoglobin, anemia, agranulocytosis (rare). **Other:** Nasal congestion, muscle cramps, SLE-like syndrome, fixed drug eruption, edema.

DIAGNOSTIC TEST INTERFERENCE Positive ***direct Coombs' tests*** in patients with hydralazine-induced SLE. Hydralazine interferes with urinary ***17-OHCS*** determinations ***(modified Glenn-Nelson technique).***

INTERACTIONS Drug: BETA BLOCKERS and other ANTIHYPERTENSIVE AGENTS compound hypotensive effects.

PHARMACOKINETICS Absorption: Readily absorbed from GI tract. **Onset:** 20–30 min. **Peak:** 2 h. **Dura-**

H

tion: 2–6 h. **Distribution:** Crosses placenta; distributed into breast milk. **Metabolism:** Metabolized in intestinal wall and liver. **Elimination:** 90% rapidly excreted in urine; 10% excreted in feces. **Half-Life:** 2–8 h.

NURSING IMPLICATIONS

Assessment & Drug Effects

- Lab tests: Determine antinuclear antibody titer before initiation of therapy and periodically during prolonged therapy.
- Make baseline and periodic determinations of BUN, creatinine clearance, uric acid, serum potassium, blood glucose, and ECG.
- Monitor for S&S of SLE, especially with prolonged therapy.
- Monitor BP and HR closely. Check every 5 min until it is stabilized at desired level, then every 15 min thereafter throughout hypertensive crisis.
- Monitor I&O when drug is given parenterally and in those with renal dysfunction.

Patient & Family Education

- Monitor weight, check for edema, and report weight gain to physician.
- Note: Some patients experience headache and palpitations within 2–4 h after first PO dose; symptoms usually subside spontaneously.
- Make position changes slowly and avoid standing still, hot baths/showers, strenuous exercise, and excessive alcohol intake.
- Do not drive or engage in other potentially hazardous activities until response to drug is known.
- Do not breast feed while taking this drug without consulting physician.

HYDROCHLOROTHIAZIDE (Pr)

(hye-droe-klor-oh-thye′a-zide)

Apo-Hydro ♣, Diaqua, Esidrix, Hydro-Chlor, HydroDIURIL, Hydromal, Hydro-T, Oretic, SK-Hydrochlorothiazide, HCTZ, Urozide ♣

Classifications: ELECTROLYTIC AND WATER BALANCE AGENT; DIURETIC; THIAZIDE

Pregnancy Category: B

AVAILABILITY 12.5 mg capsules; 25 mg, 50 mg, 100 mg tablets; 50 mg/5 mL oral solution

ACTIONS Similar to chlorothiazide. Diuretic action is associated with drug interference with absorption of sodium ions across the distal renal tubular segment of the nephron. This enhances excretion of sodium, chloride, potassium, bicarbonates, and water.

THERAPEUTIC EFFECTS It has hypotensive action, elevates plasma renin activity, and precipitates diabetes in the prediabetic patient.

USES Adjunct in treatment of edema associated with CHF, hepatic cirrhosis, renal failure, and in the stepped-care management of hypertension (step 1 and 2 agent).

UNLABELED USES Nephrogenic diabetes insipidus, hypercalciuria, and treatment of electrolyte disturbances associated with renal tubular acidosis.

CONTRAINDICATIONS Hypersensitivity to thiazides or other sulfonamides; anuria, pregnancy (category B), lactation.

CAUTIOUS USE Bronchial asthma, allergy; hepatic cirrhosis; renal dysfunction; history of gout, SLE; diabetes mellitus; older adults.

ROUTE & DOSAGE

Edema
Adult: **PO** 25–200 mg/d in 1–3 divided doses

Hypertension
Adult: **PO** 12.5–100 mg/d in 1–2 divided doses
Child: **PO** 2.2 mg/kg/d in 2 divided doses
Neonate: **PO** *<6 mo,* 2–4 mg/kg/d in 2 divided doses

ADMINISTRATION

Oral

- Give with food or milk to reduce GI upset.
- Schedule doses to avoid nocturia and interrupted sleep. If given in 2 doses, schedule second dose no later than 3 p.m.
- Store tablets in tightly closed container at 15°–30° C (59°–86° F) unless otherwise directed.

ADVERSE EFFECTS (≥1%) **CNS:** Mood changes, unusual tiredness or weakness, dizziness, light-headedness, paresthesias. **CV:** Irregular heartbeat, weak pulse, orthostatic hypotension. **GI:** Dry mouth, increased thirst, nausea, vomiting, anorexia, diarrhea, pancreatitis, jaundice. **Hematologic:** Agranulocytosis, thrombocytopenia, aplastic anemia, leukopenia. **Metabolic:** *Hyperglycemia,* glycosuria, *hyperuricemia, hypokalemia.* **Other:** Hypersensitivity reactions, photosensitivity, blurred vision, yellow vision (xanthopsia), muscle spasm.

DIAGNOSTIC TEST INTERFERENCE Falsely decreased value in ***total-urinary estrogen*** by ***spectrophotometric assay.*** See ***chlorothiazide.***

INTERACTIONS Drug: Amphotericin B, CORTICOSTEROIDS increase hypokalemic effects; SULFONYLUREAS, **insulin** may antagonize hypoglycemic effects; **cholestyramine, colestipol** decrease THIAZIDE absorption; **diazoxide** intensifies hypoglycemic and hypotensive effects; increased **potassium** and **magnesium** loss may cause **digoxin** toxicity; decreases **lithium** excretion and increases toxicity; increases risk of NSAID-induced renal failure and may attenuate diuresis.

PHARMACOKINETICS Absorption: Incompletely absorbed. **Onset:** 2 h. **Peak:** 4 h. **Duration:** 6–12 h. **Distribution:** Distributed throughout extracellular tissue; concentrates in kidney; crosses placenta; distributed in breast milk. **Metabolism:** Does not appear to be metabolized. **Elimination:** Excreted in urine. **Half-Life:** 45–120 min.

NURSING IMPLICATIONS

Assessment & Drug Effects

- Monitor for therapeutic effectiveness. Antihypertensive effects may be noted in 3–4 d; maximal effects may require 3–4 wk.
- Lab tests: Baseline and periodic determinations of serum electrolytes, blood counts, BUN, blood glucose, uric acid, CO_2, are recommended.
- Check BP before initiation of therapy and at regular intervals.
- Monitor closely for hypokalemia; it increases the risk of digoxin toxicity.
- Monitor I&O and check for edema.
- Note: Drug may cause hyperglycemia and loss of glycemic control in diabetics.
- Note: Drug may cause orthostatic hypotension, dizziness.

Patient & Family Education

- Consult physician before using OTC drugs. Many contain large

H

amounts of sodium as well as potassium.

- Monitor weight daily.
- Note: Diabetic patients need to monitor blood glucose closely. This drug causes impaired glucose tolerance.
- Report signs of hypokalemia (see Appendix F) to physician.
- Change positions slowly; avoid hot baths or showers, extended exposure to sunlight, and sitting or standing still for long periods.
- Note: Photosensitivity reaction may occur 10–14 d after initial sun exposure.
- Do not breast feed while taking this drug.

H

HYDROCODONE BITARTRATE

(hye-droe-koe'done)

Dihydrocodeinone Bitartrate, Hycodan, Robidone A, Vicodin (with acetaminophen)

Classifications: CENTRAL NERVOUS SYSTEM AGENT; NARCOTIC (OPIATE) AGONIST ANALGESIC; ANTITUSSIVE

Prototype: Morphine

Pregnancy Category: C

Controlled Substance: Schedule III

AVAILABILITY 5 mg hydrocodone usually with 500 mg or more acetaminophen

ACTIONS Morphine derivative similar to codeine but more addicting and with slightly greater antitussive activity, and analgesic effect. CNS depressant with moderate to severe relief of pain. Available in the United States only in combination with other drugs.

THERAPEUTIC EFFECTS Suppresses cough reflex by direct action on cough center in medulla. CNS depressant with moderate to severe relief of pain.

USES Symptomatic relief of hyperactive or nonproductive cough and for relief of moderate to moderately severe pain. A common ingredient in a variety of proprietary mixtures.

CONTRAINDICATIONS Hypersensitivity to hydrocodone; lactation.

CAUTIOUS USE Respiratory depression, asthma, emphysema; history of drug abuse or dependence; postoperative patients; debilitated patients; children <1 y; pregnancy (category C); patients with preexisting increased intracranial pressure.

ROUTE & DOSAGE

Mild to Moderate Pain, Cough

Adult: **PO** 5–10 mg q4–6h prn (max: 15 mg/dose)

Child: **PO** *2–12 y,* 1.25–5 mg q4–6h (max: 10 mg/dose)

ADMINISTRATION

Oral

- Give with food or milk to prevent GI irritation.
- Preserve in tight, light-resistant containers.

ADVERSE EFFECTS (≥1%) **GI:** Dry mouth, *constipation, nausea,* vomiting. **CNS:** light-headedness, sedation, dizziness, *drowsiness,* euphoria, dysphoria. **Respiratory:** <u>*Respiratory depression*</u>. **Skin:** Urticaria, rash, pruritus.

INTERACTIONS Drug: Alcohol and other CNS DEPRESSANTS compound sedation and CNS depression. **Herbal: St. John's wort** increases sedation.

PHARMACOKINETICS Onset: 10–20 min. **Duration:** 3–6 h. **Distribution:** Crosses placenta; distributed into breast milk. **Metabolism:** Metabolized in liver. **Elimination:** Excreted in urine. **Half-Life:** 3.8 h.

NURSING IMPLICATIONS

Assessment & Drug Effects

- Monitor for effectiveness of drug for pain relief.
- Monitor for nausea and vomiting, especially in ambulatory patients.
- Monitor respiratory status and bowel elimination.

Patient & Family Education

- Avoid hazardous activities until response to drug is determined.
- Do not use alcohol or other CNS depressants; may cause additive CNS depression.
- Drink plenty of liquids for adequate hydration.
- Do not take larger doses than prescribed since abuse potential is high.
- Do not breast feed while taking this drug.

HYDROCORTISONE (Pr)

(hye-droe-kor'ti-sone)

Aeroseb-HC, Alphaderm, Cetacort, Cortaid, Cort-Dome, Cortenema, Cortril, Dermacort, Dermolate, Hydrocortone, Hytone, Proctocort, Rectocort ✦, Synacort

HYDROCORTISONE ACETATE

Anusol HC, CaldeCort, Carmol HC, Colifoam, Cortaid, Cortamed, Cort-Dome, Cortef Acetate, Corticaine, Cortifoam, Cortiment ✦, Epifoam, Hydrocortone Acetate

HYDROCORTISONE CYPIONATE

Cortef Fluid

HYDROCORTISONE SODIUM PHOSPHATE

Hydrocortone Phosphate

HYDROCORTISONE SODIUM SUCCINATE

A-Hydrocort, Solu-Cortef

HYDROCORTISONE VALERATE

Westcort

Classifications: SKIN AND MUCOUS MEMBRANE AGENT; ANTIINFLAMMATORY; SYNTHETIC HORMONE; ADRENAL CORTICOSTEROIDS; GLUCOCORTICOID; MINERALOCORTICOID

Pregnancy Category: C

AVAILABILITY **Hydrocortisone** 5 mg, 10 mg, 20 mg tablets; 0.5%, 1%, 2.5% cream, lotion, ointment, spray **Hydrocortisone Acetate** 25 mg/mL, 50 mg/mL suspension; 0.5%, 1% cream, ointment **Hydrocortisone Cypionate** 10 mg/5 mL oral suspension **Hydrocortisone Sodium Phosphate** 50 mg/mL injection **Hydrocortisone Sodium Succinate** 100 mg/2 mL, 250 mg/2 mL, 500 mg/4 mL, 1000 mg/8 mL vials **Hydrocortisone Valerate** 0.2% cream, ointment

ACTIONS Short-acting synthetic steroid with both glucocorticoid and mineralocorticoid properties that affect nearly all systems of the body. **Antiinflammatory (glucocorticoid) action:** Stabilizes leukocyte lysosomal membranes; inhibits phagocytosis and release of allergic substances; suppresses fibroblast formation and collagen deposition; reduces capillary dilation and permeability; and increases responsiveness of cardiovascular system to circulating catecholamines. **Immunosuppressive action:** Modifies immune response to various stimuli; reduces antibody titers; and suppresses cell-mediated hypersensitivity reactions. **Mineralocorticoid action:** Promotes sodium retention, but under certain circumstances (e.g., sodium loading), enhances sodium excretion; promotes potassium excretion; and increases glomerular filtration rate (GFR). **Metabolic action:** Promotes he-

H

patic gluconeogenesis, protein catabolism, redistribution of body fat, and lipolysis.

THERAPEUTIC EFFECTS Hydrocortisone has antiinflammatory, immunosuppressive, and metabolic functions in the body.

USES Replacement therapy in adrenocortical insufficiency; to reduce serum calcium in hypercalcemia, to suppress undesirable inflammatory or immune responses, to produce temporary remission in nonadrenal disease, and to block ACTH production in diagnostic tests. Use as antiinflammatory or immunosuppressive agent largely replaced by synthetic glucocorticoids that have minimal mineralocorticoid activity.

CONTRAINDICATIONS Hypersensitivity to glucocorticoids, idiopathic thrombocytopenic purpura, psychoses, acute glomerulonephritis, viral or bacterial diseases of skin, infections not controlled by antibiotics, active or latent amebiasis, hypercorticism (Cushing's syndrome), smallpox vaccination or other immunologic procedures. Topical steroids contraindicated in presence of varicella, vaccinia, on surfaces with compromised circulation, and in children <2 y. Safe use during pregnancy (category C) or lactation is not established.

CAUTIOUS USE Children; diabetes mellitus; chronic, active hepatitis positive for hepatitis B surface antigen; hyperlipidemia; cirrhosis; stromal herpes simplex; glaucoma, tuberculosis of eye; osteoporosis; convulsive disorders; hypothyroidism; diverticulitis; nonspecific ulcerative colitis; fresh intestinal anastomoses; active or latent peptic ulcer; gastritis; esophagitis; thromboembolic disorders; CHF; metastatic carcinoma; hypertension; renal insufficiency; history of allergies; active or arrested tuberculosis; systemic fungal infection; myasthenia gravis.

ROUTE & DOSAGE

Adrenal Insufficiency, Antiinflammatory

Adult: **PO** 10–320 mg/d in 3–4 divided doses **IV/IM** 15–800 mg/d in 3–4 divided doses (max: 2 g/d) **SC** Sodium phosphate only, 15–240 mg/d
Child: **PO** 2.5–10 mg/kg/d in 3–4 divided doses **IV/IM** 1–5 mg/kg/d divided q12–24 h

Intraarticular, Intralesional (Acetate Salt)

Adult: **IM** 5–50 mg q3–5d for bursae; 5–50 mg once q1–4 wk for joints

Antiinflammatory Agent

Adult: **Topical** apply a small amount to the affected area 1–4 times/d **PR** insert 1% cream, 10% foam, 10–25 mg suppository, or 100 mg enema nightly

ADMINISTRATION

Note: Hydrocortisone phosphate may be given SC, IM, or IV. Hydrocortisone succinate may be given IM or IV.

Oral

- Give oral drug with food.

Rectal

- Administer retention enema preferably after a bowel movement; retain at least 1 h or all night if possible.

Topical

- Apply medication sparingly, rub until it disappears, and then reapply, leaving a thin coat over lesion. Completely cover area with transparent plastic or other occlusive device or vehicle when so ordered.

- Avoid covering a weeping or exudative lesion.
- Note: Occlusive dressings usually are not applied to face, scalp, scrotum, axilla, and groin.
- Inspect skin carefully between applications for ecchymotic, petechial, and purpuric signs, maceration, secondary infection, skin atrophy, striae or miliaria; if present, stop medication and notify physician.
- Store medication at 15°–30° C (59°–86° F) unless otherwise directed by manufacturer; protect from light and freezing.

Intramuscular

- Inject deep into gluteal muscle.

Intravenous

- IV administration to infants, children: Verify correct IV concentration and rate of infusion/injection with physician.

PREPARE: **Direct:** Give undiluted (preferred). **Intermittent:** Dilute in 50–100 mL of D5W, NS, or D5/NS.

ADMINISTER: **Direct:** Give each dose at a rate of 25 mg or fraction thereof (phosphate) or 500 mg or fraction thereof (succinate) over 1 min. **Intermittent:** Give over 10 min.

INCOMPATIBILITIES **Solution/additive: Amobarbital, ampicillin, bleomycin, colistimethate, dimenhydrinate, doxapram, doxorubicin, ephedrine, heparin, hydralazine, metaraminol, methicillin, nafcillin, pentobarbital, phenobarbital, prochlorperazine, promethazine, secobarbital, tetracyclines. Y-site: Ergotamine, phenytoin.**

- Administer solutions that have been diluted for IV infusion within 24 h.

ADVERSE EFFECTS (≥1%) **Body as a Whole:** Hypersensitivity or anaphylactoid reactions; aggravation or masking of infections; malaise, weight gain, obesity; urogenital urinary frequency and urgency, enuresis increased or decreased motility and number of sperm. **CNS:** Vertigo, headache, nystagmus, ataxia (rare), increased intracranial pressure with papilledema (usually after discontinuation of medication), mental disturbances, aggravation of preexisting psychiatric conditions, insomnia, anxiety, mental confusion, depression. **CV:** Syncopal episodes, thrombophlebitis, thromboembolism or fat embolism, palpitation, tachycardia, necrotizing angiitis, CHF, hypertension edema. **Endocrine:** Suppressed linear growth in children, decreased glucose tolerance; hyperglycemia, manifestations of latent diabetes mellitus; hypocorticism; amenorrhea and other menstrual difficulties moonfacies. **GI:** Cramping, bleeding. **Special Senses:** Posterior subcapsular cataracts (especially in children), glaucoma, exophthalmos, increased intraocular pressure with optic nerve damage, perforation of the globe, fungal infection of the cornea, decreased or blurred vision. **Metabolic:** Hypocalcemia; *sodium* and *fluid retention;* hypokalemia and hypokalemic alkalosis decreased serum concentration of vitamins A and C; hyperglycemia, hypernatremia. **GI:** *Nausea,* increased appetite, ulcerative esophagitis, pancreatitis, abdominal distention, peptic ulcer with perforation and hemorrhage, melena. **Hematologic:** Thrombocytopenia, polycythemia, ecchymoses. **Musculoskeletal:** Osteoporosis, compression fractures, muscle wasting and weakness, tendon rupture, aseptic necrosis of femoral and humeral heads. **Skin:** Skin thinning and atrophy, *acne, impaired wound healing;* petechiae, ecchymosis, easy bruising; suppression of skin test reaction; hypopigmentation or hyperpigmentation, hirsutism, acneiform eruptions, subcutaneous fat atrophy; allergic dermatitis, urticaria, angioneurotic edema, increased sweating. With parenteral therapy at IV site–pain, irritation, necrosis, atrophy, sterile abscess; Charcot-like arthropathy following intraarticular use; burning and tingling in perineal area (after IV injection).

DIAGNOSTIC TEST INTERFERENCE Hydrocortisone (corticosteroids) may increase serum ***cholesterol, blood glucose,*** serum ***sodium, uric acid*** (in acute leukemia) and ***calcium*** (in bone metastasis). It may decrease serum ***calcium, potassium, PBI, thyroxin (T_4), triiodothyronine (T_3) and reduce thyroid I 131*** uptake. It increases ***urine glucose*** level and ***calcium*** excretion; decreases ***urine 17-OHCS*** and ***17-KS*** levels. May produce false-negative results with **nitroblue tetrazolium test** for systemic bacterial infection and may suppress reactions to skin tests.

INTERACTIONS Drug: BARBITURATES, **phenytoin, rifampin** may increase hepatic metabolism, thus decreasing cortisone levels; ESTROGENS potentiate the effects of hydrocortisone; NSAIDS compound ulcerogenic effects; **cholestyramine, colestipol** decrease hydrocortisone absorption; DIURETICS, **amphotericin b** exacerbate hypokalemia; ANTICHOLINESTERASE AGENTS (e.g., **neostigmine**) may produce severe weakness; immune response to VACCINES and TOXOIDS may be decreased.

PHARMACOKINETICS Absorption: Readily absorbed from GI tract and IM injection site. **Onset:** 1–2 h PO; immediately IV; 3–5 d PR. **Peak:** 1 h PO; 4–8 h IM. **Duration:** 1–1.5 d PO/IM; 0.5–4 wk intraarticular. **Distribution:** Distributed primarily to muscles, liver, skin, intestines, kidneys; crosses placenta. **Metabolism:** Hepatically metabolized. **Elimination:** HPA suppression 8–12 h; metabolites excreted in urine; excreted in breast milk. **Half-Life:** 1.5–2 h.

NURSING IMPLICATIONS

Assessment & Drug Effects

- Establish baseline and continuing data on BP, weight, fluid and electrolyte balance, and blood glucose.
- Lab tests: Periodic serum electrolytes blood glucose, Hct and Hgb, platelet count, and WBC with differential.
- Monitor for adverse effects. Older adults and patients with low serum albumin are especially susceptible to adverse effects.
- Be alert to signs of hypocalcemia (see Appendix F).
- Ophthalmoscopic examinations are recommended every 2–3 mo, especially if patient is receiving ophthalmic steroid therapy.
- Monitor for persistent backache or chest pain; compression and spontaneous fractures of long bones and vertebrae present hazards.
- Monitor for and report changes in mood and behavior, emotional instability, or psychomotor activity, especially with long-term therapy.
- Be alert to possibility of masked infection and delayed healing (antiinflammatory and immunosuppressive actions).
- Note: Dose adjustment may be required if patient is subjected to severe stress (serious infection, surgery, or injury).

- Note: Single doses of corticosteroids or use for a short period (<1 wk) do not produce withdrawal symptoms when discontinued, even with moderately large doses.

Patient & Family Education

- Expect a slight weight gain with improved appetite. After dosage is stabilized, notify physician of a sudden slow but steady weight increase [2 kg (5 lb)/wk].
- Avoid alcohol and caffeine; may contribute to steroid-ulcer development in long-term therapy.
- Do not ignore dyspepsia with hyperacidity. Report symptoms to physician and do NOT self-medicate to find relief.
- Do NOT use aspirin or other OTC drugs unless prescribed specifically by the physician.
- Note: A high protein, calcium, and vitamin D diet is advisable to reduce risk of corticosteroid-induced osteoporosis.
- Notify physician of slow healing, any vague feeling of being sick, or return to pretreatment symptoms.
- Do not abruptly discontinue drug; doses are gradually reduced to prevent withdrawal symptoms.
- Report exacerbation of disease during drug withdrawal.
- Carry medical identification at all times. It needs to indicate medical diagnosis, drug therapy, and name of physician.
- Apply topical preparations sparingly in small children. The hazard of systemic toxicity is higher because of the greater ratio of skin surface area to body weight.
- Check shelf-life date on topical corticosterone during long-term use.
- Do not breast feed while taking/using this drug without consulting physician.

HYDROFLUMETHIAZIDE

(hye-droe-floo-meth-eye'a-zide)

Diucardin, Saluron

Classifications: ELECTROLYTIC AND WATER BALANCE AGENT; DIURETIC; THIAZIDE

Prototype: Hydrochlorothiazide

Pregnancy Category: B

AVAILABILITY 50 mg tablets

ACTIONS Thiazide diuretic chemically related to sulfonamides. Diuretic action results in excretion of sodium, chloride, potassium bicarbonate, and water.

THERAPEUTIC EFFECTS Results in antihypertensive activity, and decreased edema.

USES Mild hypertension, management of edema associated with CHF.

CONTRAINDICATIONS Hypersensitivity to other thiazides or sulfonamide derivatives; anuria; lactation; hypokalemia.

CAUTIOUS USE Pregnancy (category B).

ROUTE & DOSAGE

Edema

Adult: **PO** 25 mg–200 mg/d in 1–2 divided doses

Hypertension

Adult: **PO** 50–100 mg/d in 1–2 divided doses

Child: **PO** 1 mg/kg/d once/d

ADMINISTRATION

Oral

- Give diuretic dose early in the morning to prevent interrupted sleep. If two doses are taken each day, schedule second dose no later than 3 p.m.

- Store tablets in tightly closed container at 15°–30° C (59°–86° F) unless otherwise directed.

ADVERSE EFFECTS (≥1%) **CV:** Postural hypotension. **Skin:** Photosensitivity. **Metabolic:** *Hypokalemia, hyperglycemia,* hyponatremia, *asymptomatic hyperuricemia*. (See also hydrochlorothiazide.)

INTERACTIONS Drug: Amphotericin B, CORTICOSTEROIDS increase hypokalemic effects; may antagonize hypoglycemic effects of ORAL HYPOGLYCEMIC AGENTS, **insulin; cholestyramine, colestipol** decrease thiazide absorption; **diazoxide** intensifies hypoglycemic and hypotensive effects; increased potassium and magnesium loss may cause **digoxin** toxicity; decreases **lithium** excretion, thus increasing **lithium** toxicity; increases risk of NSAID-induced renal failure (NSAIDS may attenuate diuresis).

PHARMACOKINETICS Absorption: Incompletely absorbed. **Onset:** 1–2 h. **Peak:** 3–4 h. **Duration:** 18–24 h. **Distribution:** Distributed throughout extracellular tissue; concentrates in kidney; crosses placenta; distributed in breast milk. **Metabolism:** Does not appear to be metabolized. **Elimination:** Excreted in urine. **Half-Life:** 17 h.

NURSING IMPLICATIONS

Assessment & Drug Effects

- Monitor for therapeutic effectiveness. Antihypertensive effects may be noted in 3–4 d, maximal effects may require 3–4 wk.
- Lab tests: Make baseline and periodic determinations for serum electrolytes, blood counts, BUN, blood glucose, uric acid, and CO_2.
- Monitor patient for hypokalemia and hyponatremia (see Appendix F).
- Note: Older adults are especially susceptible to the hypotensive effects that accompany excessive diuresis.
- Report onset of joint pain and limitation of motion to physician; asymptomatic hyperuricemia can result from interference with uric acid excretion.
- Monitor for S&S of diabetes. Watch diabetic patients for loss of glycemic control.

Patient & Family Education

- Note: Thiazide-related photosensitivity is considered a photoallergy. It occurs 1 1/2–2 wk after initial sun exposure. Inform physician.
- Do not breast feed while taking this drug.

HYDROMORPHONE HYDROCHLORIDE

(hye-droe-mor'fone)

Dilaudid, Dilaudid-HP, Palladone

Classifications: CENTRAL NERVOUS SYSTEM (CNS) AGENT; ANALGESIC; NARCOTIC (OPIATE) AGONIST

Prototype: Morphine

Pregnancy Category: C

Controlled Substance: Schedule II

AVAILABILITY 1 mg, 2 mg, 3 mg, 4 mg, 8 mg tablets; 12 mg, 16 mg, 24 mg, 32 mg extended-release capsules; 5 mg/5 mL oral liquid; 1 mg/mL, 2 mg/mL, 4 mg/mL, 10 mg/mL injection; 3 mg suppositories

ACTIONS Semisynthetic derivative structurally similar to morphine but with 8–10 times more potent analgesic effect. Has more rapid onset and shorter duration of action than morphine and is reported to have less hypnotic action and less tendency to produce nausea and vomiting.

THERAPEUTIC EFFECTS Is a narcotic analgesic which controls mild to moderate pain. Has antitussive properties.

USES Relief of moderate to severe pain and control of persistent nonproductive cough.

CONTRAINDICATIONS Intolerance to opiate agonists; pregnancy (category C), acute bronchial asthma, COPD, upper airway obstruction, decreased respiratory reserve, severe respiratory depression, opiate-naïve patients.

CAUTIOUS USE Abrupt discontinuation, alcoholism; angina; biliary tract disease; older adults; epidural administration; GI disease, GI obstruction; head trauma; heart failure; hepatic disease; hypotension, hypovolemia, oliguria, prostatic hypertrophy; pulmonary disease; renal disease, renal impairment; paralytic ileus; increased intracranial pressure; inflammatory bowel disease; labor; latex hypersensitivity; obstetric delivery; bladder obstruction; cardiac arrhythmias, cardiac disease; respiratory depression; seizure disorder, seizures; substance abuse; surgery; ulcerative colitis; urethral stricture, urinary retention; lactation, neonates, and infants <6 mo.

ROUTE & DOSAGE

Moderate to Severe Pain

Adult: **PO/SC/IM/IV** 1–4 mg q4–6h prn. **Extended release** 12–32 mg q24h (see prescribing information for conversion from other opioid analgesics) **Rectal** 3 mg q4–6h
Child: **PO** 0.03–0.08 mg/kg q4–6h (max: 5 mg/dose) **IV** 0.015 mg/kg q4–6h

Antitussive

Adult: **PO** 1 mg q3–4h prn
Child: **PO** *6–12 y,* 0.5 mg q3–4h prn

ADMINISTRATION

Note: A fixed schedule when narcotic therapy is initiated provides more effective management than a prn schedule.

Intravenous

IV administration to infants, children: Verify correct IV concentration and rate of infusion with physician.

PREPARE: **Direct:** Dilute each dose in at least 5 mL of sterile water or NS. **IV Infusion:** Using Dilaudid-HP, reconstitute 250 mg dry powder vial immediately prior to use with 25 mL sterile water for injection to yield 10 mg/mL. Final dilution of Dilaudid-HP 250 and HP 500 (supplied 500 mg/50 mL) must be ordered by physician.

ADMINISTER: **Direct:** Give 2 mg or fraction thereof over 3–5 min. **IV Infusion:** Both final volume and rate of infusion must be ordered by physician.

INCOMPATIBILITIES **Solution/additive: Prochlorperazine, sodium bicarbonate, thiopental. Y-site: Minocycline, prochlorperazine, tetracycline.**

- A slight discoloration in ampules or multidose vials causes no loss of potency.
- Store in tight, light-resistant containers at 15°–30° C (59°–86° F).

ADVERSE EFFECTS (≥1%) **GI:** Nausea, vomiting, constipation. **CNS:** Euphoria, dizziness, sedation, *drowsiness.* **CV:** Hypotension, bradycardia or tachycardia. **Respiratory:** <u>Respiratory depression</u>. **Special Senses:** Blurred vision.

INTERACTIONS Drug: Alcohol and other CNS DEPRESSANTS compound sedation and CNS depression. **Herbal: St. John's wort** may increase sedation.

PHARMACOKINETICS Absorption: 60% absorbed from GI tract. **Onset:** 15 min IV, 30 min PO/rectal. **Peak:** 30–90 min. **Duration:** 3–4 h. **Distribution:** Crosses placenta; distributed into breast milk. **Metabolism:** Metabolized in liver. **Elimination:** Excreted in urine. **Half-life:** 2–3 h; 18 h extended release.

NURSING IMPLICATIONS

Assessment & Drug Effects

- Note baseline respiratory rate, rhythm, and depth and size of pupils before administration. Respirations of 12/min or less and mitosis are signs of toxicity. Withhold drug and promptly notify physician.
- Monitor vital signs at regular intervals. Drug-induced respiratory depression may occur even with small doses and increases progressively with higher doses.
- Assess effectiveness of pain relief 30 min after medication administration.
- Monitor drug effects carefully in older adult or debilitated patients and those with impaired renal and hepatic function.
- Assess effectiveness of cough. Drug depresses cough and sigh reflexes and may induce atelectasis, especially in postoperative patients and those with pulmonary disease.
- Note: Nausea and orthostatic hypotension most often occur in ambulatory patients or when a supine patient assumes the head-up position.
- Monitor I&O ratio and pattern. Assess lower abdomen for bladder distension. Report oliguria or urinary retention.
- Monitor bowel pattern; drug-induced constipation may require treatment.

Patient & Family Education

- Request medication at the onset of pain and do not wait until pain is severe.
- Use caution with activities requiring alertness; drug may cause drowsiness, dizziness, and blurred vision.
- Avoid alcohol and other CNS depressants while taking this drug.
- Do not breast feed while taking this drug.

HYDROQUINONE

(hye′droe-kwin-one)

Eldopaque, Eldoquin, Esoterica Regular, Melanex, Porcelana, Solaquin

Classifications: SKIN AND MUCOUS MEMBRANE AGENT; DEPIGMENTOR

Pregnancy Category: C

AVAILABILITY 1.5%, 2%, 3%, 4% cream, gel, solution

ACTIONS Topical agent that causes reversible bleaching of hyperpigmented skin due to increased melanin. Interferes with formation of new melanin but does not destroy existing pigment. Depresses melanin synthesis and melanocytic growth, possibly by increasing excretion of melanin from melanocytes.

THERAPEUTIC EFFECTS Interferes with formation of new melanin but does not destroy existing pigment.

USES Gradual bleaching of hyperpigmented skin conditions such as chloasma or melasma, severe freckling, senile lentigines (age spots or liver spots). Also as an antioxidant in topical preparations. Some formulations include a sunscreening agent (e.g., Porcelana with Sunscreen, Mercolized Cocrema, Pabaquinone, and Solaquin).

CONTRAINDICATIONS Prickly heat, sunburn, irritated skin, depilatory usage; lactation.
CAUTIOUS USE Safe use during pregnancy (category C) or in children ≤12 y is not established.

ROUTE & DOSAGE

Bleaching of Hyperpigmented Skin
Adult: **Topical** Apply thin layer and rub into hyperpigmented skin b.i.d., a.m. and p.m.

ADMINISTRATION

Topical
- Test skin for sensitivity before treatment is initiated. Apply small amount of drug (about 25 mm in diameter) to an unbroken patch of skin and check in 24 h. Do not use drug if vesicle formation, itching, or excessive inflammation occur. Minor redness is not a contraindication.
- Limit applications to an area no larger than that of face and neck.

ADVERSE EFFECTS (≥1%) **Skin:** Dryness and fissuring of paranasal and infraorbital areas, inflammatory reaction, erythema; stinging, tingling, burning sensations; irritation, sensitization, and contact dermatitis.

INTERACTIONS Drug: No clinically significant interactions established.

NURSING IMPLICATIONS

Assessment & Drug Effects
- Monitor for therapeutic effectiveness: In general, complete depigmentation occurs in 1–4 mo and lasts 2–6 mo after hydroquinone is discontinued. Once desired results are obtained, reduce amount and frequency of applications to the least that will maintain depigmentation.
- Discontinue if bleaching or skin lightening does not occur after 2 or 3 mo of therapy.

Patient & Family Education
- Use a sunscreen agent or a hydroquinone formulation containing a sunscreen for daytime applications.
- Wash drug off if rash or irritation develops and consult physician.
- Avoid contact with the eyes and not to use on open lesions, sunburned, irritated, or otherwise damaged skin.
- Continue use of protective clothing and sunscreening agent after treatment is terminated to reduce possibility of repigmentation.
- Do not breast feed while taking/using this drug.

HYDROXOCOBALAMIN (VITAMIN $B_{12\,alpha}$)

(hye-drox-oh-koe-bal'a-min)
Hydrobexan, Hydroxo-12, LA-12
Classifications: HORMONES AND SYNTHETIC SUBSTITUTES; VITAMIN B_{12}
Prototype: Cyanocobalamin
Pregnancy Category: A (C if >RDA)

AVAILABILITY 1000 mcg/mL injection

ACTIONS Cobalamin derivative similar to cyanocobalamin (vitamin B_{12}). More slowly absorbed from injection site than cyanocobalamin and may be taken up by liver in larger quantities. Essential for normal cell growth, cell reproduction maturation of RBCs, myelin synthesis, and believed to be involved in protein synthesis.
THERAPEUTIC EFFECTS Vitamin B_{12} deficiency results in megaloblastic anemia.

USES Treatment of Vitamin B_{12} deficiency.

UNLABELED USES Cyanide poisoning and tobacco amblyopia.

CONTRAINDICATIONS History of sensitivity to vitamin B_{12}, other cobalamins, or cobalt; indiscriminate use in folic acid deficiency.

CAUTIOUS USE Safe use during pregnancy [category A, category C (parenteral)], lactation, or in children is not established.

H

ROUTE & DOSAGE

Vitamin B_{12} Deficiency

Adult: **IM** 30 mcg/d for 5–10 d and then 100–200 mcg/mo or 1000 mcg qod until remission and then 1000 mcg/mo

Child: **IM** 100 mcg doses to a total of 1–5 mg over 2 wk and then 30–50 mcg/mo

ADMINISTRATION

Intramuscular

- Give deep into a large muscle.

INTERACTIONS Drug: Chloramphenicol may interfere with therapeutic response to hydroxocobalamin.

PHARMACOKINETICS Distribution: Widely distributed; principally stored in liver, kidneys, and adrenals; crosses placenta. **Metabolism:** Converted in tissues to active coenzymes; enterohepatically cycled. **Elimination:** 50%–95% of doses ≥100 mcg are excreted in urine in 48 h; excreted in breast milk.

NURSING IMPLICATIONS

Assessment & Drug Effects

- Monitor for therapeutic effectiveness: Response to drug therapy is usually dramatic, occurring within 48 h. Effectiveness is measured by laboratory values and improvement in manifestations of vitamin B_{12} deficiency. Characteristically, reticulocyte concentration rises in 3–4 d, peaks in 5–8 d, and then gradually declines as erythrocyte count and hemoglobin rise to normal levels (in 4–6 wk).
- Lab tests: Prior to therapy determine reticulocyte and erythrocyte counts, Hgb, Hct, vitamin B_{12}, and serum folate levels; repeated 5–7 d after start of therapy and at regular intervals during therapy.
- Obtain a careful history of sensitivities. Sensitization can take as long as 8 y to develop.
- Monitor potassium levels during the first 48 h, particularly in patients with Addisonian pernicious anemia or megaloblastic anemia. Conversion to normal erythropoiesis increases erythrocyte potassium requirement and can result in severe hypokalemia and sudden death.
- Monitor vital signs in patients with cardiac disease and in those receiving parenteral cyanocobalamin, and be alert to symptoms of pulmonary edema; generally occur early in therapy.
- Note: Some patients experience mild pain at injection site after administration.
- Monitor bowel function. Bowel regularity is essential for consistent absorption of oral preparations.
- Note: Smokers appear to have increased requirements for vitamin B_{12}.

Patient & Family Education

- Notify physician of any intercurrent disease or infection. Increased dosage may be required.
- Note: It is imperative to understand that drug therapy must be continued throughout life for pernicious anemia to prevent irreversible neurologic damage.

- Neurologic damage is considered irreversible if there is no improvement after 1–1 1/2 y of adequate therapy.
- Dietary deficiency of vitamin B_{12} has been observed in strict vegetarians (vegans) and their breast-fed infants and in the elderly.
- Do not breast feed while taking this drug without consulting physician.

HYDROXYAMPHETAMINE HBr

(hy-drox′ee-am-phe′-ta-meen)
Paredrine
Classifications: EYE PREPARATION; MYDRIATIC
Prototype: Homatropine HBr
Pregnancy Category: C

AVAILABILITY 1% ophthalmic solution; 1% hydroxyamphetamine/ 0.25% tropicamide solution

See Appendix A-1.

HYDROXYCHLOROQUINE SULFATE

(hye-drox-ee-klor′oh-kwin)
Plaquenil Sulfate
Classifications: ANTIINFECTIVE; ANTIMALARIAL
Prototype: Chloroquine
Pregnancy Category: C

AVAILABILITY 200 mg tablets

ACTIONS Derivative closely related to chloroquine. Antimalarial activity is believed to be based on ability to form complexes with DNA of parasite, thereby inhibiting replication and transcription to RNA and DNA synthesis of the parasite.
THERAPEUTIC EFFECTS of the parasite. Effective against *Plasmodium vivax* and *Plasmodium malariae*.

USES Suppressive prophylaxis and treatment of acute malarial attacks due to all forms of susceptible malaria. Used adjunctively with primaquine for eradication of *Plasmodium vivax* and *Plasmodium malariae*. More commonly prescribed than chloroquine for treatment of rheumatoid arthritis and lupus erythematosus (usually in conjunction with salicylate or corticosteroid therapy).
UNLABELED USES Porphyria cutanea tarda.

CONTRAINDICATIONS Known hypersensitivity to, or retinal or visual field changes associated with quinoline compounds; psoriasis, porphyria, long-term therapy in children; pregnancy (category C). Safe use in juvenile arthritis or lactation is not established.
CAUTIOUS USE Hepatic disease; alcoholism, use with hepatotoxic drugs; impaired renal function; metabolic acidosis; patients with tendency to dermatitis.

ROUTE & DOSAGE

Note: Doses are expressed in terms of hydroxychloroquine base: 400-mg tablet = 310-mg base; 800-mg tablet = 620-mg base

Acute Malaria

Adult: **PO** 620-mg base followed by 310-mg base at 6, 18, and 24 h
Child: **PO** 10-mg base/kg, then 5-mg base/kg at 6, 18, and 24 h

Malaria Suppression

Adult: **PO** 310-mg base the same day each week starting 2 wk before exposure and continuing for 4–6 wk after leaving the area of exposure
Child: **PO** 5-mg base/kg the same day each week starting 2

wk before exposure and continuing for 4–6 wk after leaving the area of exposure

Lupus Erythematosus

Adult: **PO** 310-mg base 1–2 times/d

Child: **PO** 3–5 mg/kg/d in 1–2 divided doses (max: 400 mg/d or 7 mg/kg/d)

Rheumatoid Arthritis

Adult: **PO** 400–600 mg/d until response, then decrease to lowest maintenance levels possible

Child: **PO** 3–5 mg/kg/d in 1–2 divided doses (max: 400 mg/d or 7 mg/kg/d)

H

ADMINISTRATION

Oral

- Give drug with meals or milk to reduce incidence of GI distress.
- Give antacids and laxatives at least 4 h before or after hydroxychloroquine.
- Store at 15°–30° C (59°–86° F) unless otherwise directed.

ADVERSE EFFECTS (≥1%) **CNS:** Fatigue, vertigo, headache, mood or mental changes, anxiety, *retinopathy,* blurred vision, difficulty focusing. **GI:** Anorexia, nausea, vomiting, diarrhea, abdominal cramps, weight loss. **Hematologic:** Hemolysis in patients with G6PD deficiency, <u>agranulocytosis</u> (rare), <u>aplastic anemia</u> (rare), thrombocytopenia. **Skin:** Bleaching or loss of hair, unusual pigmentation (blue-black) of skin or inside mouth, skin rash, itching.

INTERACTIONS Drug: Aluminum- and **magnesium**-containing ANTACIDS and LAXATIVES decrease hydroxychloroquine absorption; separate administrations by at least 4 h; hydroxychloroquine may interfere with response to **rabies vaccine.**

PHARMACOKINETICS Absorption: Rapidly and almost completely absorbed. **Peak:** 1–2 h. **Distribution:** Widely distributed; concentrates in lungs, liver, erythrocytes, eyes, skin, and kidneys; crosses placenta. **Metabolism:** Partially metabolized in liver to active metabolite. **Elimination:** Eliminated in urine; excreted in breast milk. **Half-Life:** 70–120 h.

NURSING IMPLICATIONS

Assessment & Drug Effects

- Monitor for therapeutic effectiveness; may not appear for several weeks, and maximal benefit may not occur for 6 mo.
- Do baseline and periodic ophthalmoscopic examinations and blood cell counts on all patients on long-term therapy.
- Discontinue drug if weakness, visual symptoms, hearing loss, unusual bleeding, bruising, or skin eruptions occur.

Patient & Family Education

- Learn about adverse effects and their symptoms when taking prolonged therapy.
- Follow drug regimen exactly as prescribed by the physician.
- Make sure to keep this drug out of reach of children.
- Do not breast feed while taking this drug without consulting physician.

HYDROXYPROGESTERONE CAPROATE

(hye-drox-ee-proe-jess'te-rone)

Duralutin, Gesterol L. A., Hylutin, Hyprogest 250, Pro-Depo

Classifications: HORMONES AND SYNTHETIC SUBSTITUTES; PROGESTIN

Prototype: Progesterone

Pregnancy Category: X

AVAILABILITY 125 mg/mL; 250 mg/mL injection

ACTIONS Long-acting synthetic progestational hormone. Has slower onset and longer action than progesterone. Has minimal estrogenic and androgenic activity.

THERAPEUTIC EFFECTS Induces and maintains endometrium, preventing uterine bleeding. Inhibits production of pituitary gonadotropin, preventing ovulation. Also produces thick cervical mucus resistant to passage of sperm.

USES Amenorrhea, abnormal uterine bleeding, advanced uterine cancer, and as "medical D & C" (conversion of proliferative endometrium to secretory endometrium and desquamation). Also as a test for endogenous estrogen production.

CONTRAINDICATIONS Severe hepatic disease, carcinoma of breast or genital region; thromboembolic disorders, pregnancy (category X), lactation, missed abortion, abnormal vaginal bleeding.

CAUTIOUS USE Diabetes mellitus; asthma; epilepsy; migraine; cardiac or renal dysfunction; mental depression.

ROUTE & DOSAGE

Amenorrhea

Adult: **IM** 375 mg started anytime during cycle, after 4 d of desquamation or if no bleeding (21 d after injection, start cyclic therapy, repeat cyclic therapy q4wk and stop after 4 cycles)

Advanced Uterine Adenocarcinoma

Adult: **IM** ≥1 g at once, and repeat 1 or more times/wk, stop at time of relapse or if no desirable results obtained after a total of 12 wk of therapy

Test for Endogenous Estrogen Production

Adult: **IM** 250 mg at any time during cycle, repeat for confirmation 4 wk after first injection, stop after second injection

ADMINISTRATION

Intramuscular

- Inject deep into a large muscle. Drug may cause local irritation at injection site.
- Store preparation away from light at 15°–30° C (59°–86° F).

ADVERSE EFFECTS (≥1%) **CNS:** Cerebral thrombosis or hemorrhage, migraine, depression. **CV:** Hypertension, thromboembolic disorders, e.g., <u>pulmonary embolism</u>. **GI:** Nausea, vomiting, cholestatic jaundice, abdominal cramps. **Urogenital:** Breakthrough bleeding; changes in cervical erosion and secretions, changes in menstrual flow, dysmenorrhea; breast tenderness, enlargement, or secretion; vaginal candidiasis; female fetus masculinization. **Respiratory:** Coughing, dyspnea, chest constriction. **Skin:** Photosensitivity, acne, melasma, hirsutism, some loss of scalp hair, rash. **Body as a Whole:** Edema, weight changes; allergy-like reactions (especially at high doses). **Metabolic:** Decreased glucose tolerance.

INTERACTIONS Drug: Rifampin may decrease pharmacologic effects of progestins.

PHARMACOKINETICS Duration: 9–17 d. **Distribution:** Crosses placenta; distributed into breast milk. **Metabolism:** Metabolized in liver. **Elimination:** Eliminated in urine.

NURSING IMPLICATIONS

Assessment & Drug Effects

- Record onset and duration of menstrual flow when drug is used to treat amenorrhea.

Patient & Family Education

- Notify physician immediately of suspected pregnancy, onset of vaginal bleeding, or thromboembolic implications (pain or numbness of legs, sudden onset of chest pain or shortness of breath, sudden severe headache or dizziness, visual problems).
- Learn and perform breast self-examination.
- Monitor blood glucose closely with diabetes.
- Use sunscreen and protective clothing to reduce risk of photosensitivity.
- Note: The onset of normal menstrual cycles may not occur for 2 or 3 mo after cessation of drug.
- Do not breast feed while taking this drug.

HYDROXYUREA

(hye-drox'ee-yoo-ree-ah)

Hydrea, Droxia

Classifications: ANTINEOPLASTIC; ANTIMETABOLITE

Prototype: Fluorouracil

Pregnancy Category: D

AVAILABILITY 500 mg capsules

ACTIONS Synthetic analog of urea with antimetabolite activity. Blocks incorporation of thymidine into DNA and may damage already formed DNA molecules; does not affect synthesis of RNA or protein. May reduce iron use by erythrocytes; has no effect on erythrocyte survival time.

THERAPEUTIC EFFECTS Cytotoxic effect limited to tissues with high rates of cell proliferation. No cross resistance with other antineoplastics has been demonstrated.

USES Palliative treatment of metastatic melanoma, chronic myelocytic leukemia; recurrent metastatic, or inoperable ovarian cancer. Also used as adjunct to x-ray therapy for treatment of advanced primary squamous cell (epidermoid) carcinoma of head (excluding lip), neck, lungs.

UNLABELED USES Psoriasis; combination therapy with radiation of lung carcinoma; sickle cell anemia.

CONTRAINDICATIONS Pregnancy (category D), lactation, children, myelosuppression.

CAUTIOUS USE Recent use of other cytotoxic drugs or irradiation; renal dysfunction; older adults; history of gout.

ROUTE & DOSAGE

Palliative Therapy

Adult: **PO** 80 mg/kg q3d or 20–30 mg/kg/d

Sickle Cell Anemia

Adult: **PO** 15 mg/kg/d, may increase by 5 mg/kg/d (max: of 35 mg/kg/d or until toxicity develops)

ADMINISTRATION

Oral

- Open, mix with water, and give immediately when patient has difficulty swallowing capsule.
- Store in tightly covered container at 15°–30° C (59°–86° F) unless otherwise directed.

ADVERSE EFFECTS (≥1%) **CNS:** Rare: Headache, dizziness, hallucinations, convulsions. **GI:** Stomatitis, anorexia, nausea, vomiting, diarrhea, constipation. **Hematologic:** Bone marrow suppression (*leukopenia,* anemia, thrombocytopenia), megaloblastic erythropoiesis. **Skin:** Maculopapular rash, facial erythema, postirradiation erythema. **Urogenital:** Renal tubular dysfunction, elevated BUN, serum, creatinine levels, hyperuricemia. **Body as a Whole:** Fever, chills, malaise.

INTERACTIONS Drug: No clinically significant interactions established.

PHARMACOKINETICS Absorption: Readily absorbed from GI tract. **Peak:** 2 h. **Distribution:** Crosses blood–brain barrier. **Metabolism:** Metabolized in liver. **Elimination:** Eliminated as respiratory CO_2 and as urea in urine.

NURSING IMPLICATIONS

Assessment & Drug Effects

- Lab tests: Determine status of kidney, liver, and bone marrow function before and periodically during therapy; monitor hemoglobin, WBC, platelet counts at least once weekly.
- Interrupt therapy if WBC drops to 2500/mm^3 or platelets to 100,000/mm^3.
- Monitor I&O. Advise patients with high serum uric acid levels to drink at least 10–12 240 mL (8 oz) glasses of fluid daily to prevent uric acid nephropathy.
- Note: Patients with marked renal dysfunction may rapidly develop visual and auditory hallucinations and hematologic toxicity.

Patient & Family Education

- Note: Incidence of toxicity is as high as 66% with doses of 40 mg/kg body weight.
- Notify physician of fever, chills, sore throat, nausea, vomiting, diarrhea, loss of appetite, and unusual bruising or bleeding.
- Use barrier contraceptive during therapy. Drug is teratogenic.
- Do not breast feed while taking this drug.

H

HYDROXYZINE HYDROCHLORIDE (Pr)

(hye-drox′i-zeen)

Atarax, Hyzine-50, Quiess, Vistaril Intramuscular, Vistacon, Vistaject-25 & -50

HYDROXYZINE PAMOATE

Hy-Pam, Vamate, Vistaril Oral

Classifications: ANTIHISTAMINE; ANTIPRURITIC

Pregnancy Category: C

AVAILABILITY Hydroxyzine HCl 10 mg, 25 mg, 50 mg, 100 mg tablets; 10 mg/5 mL syrup; 25 mg/5 mL oral suspension; 25 mg/mL, 50 mg/mL injection **Hydroxyzine Pamoate** 25 mg, 50 mg, 100 mg capsules

ACTIONS Piperazine derivative structurally and pharmacologically related to other cyclizines (e.g., buclizine, chlorcyclizine). In common with such agents, it causes CNS depression.

THERAPEUTIC EFFECTS Its tranquilizing (ataractic) effect is produced primarily by depression of hypothalamus and brain-stem reticular formation, rather than cortical areas. In addition it is an effective agent for pruritus.

USES Emotional or psychoneurotic states characterized by anxiety, tension, or psychomotor agitation; to relieve anxiety, control nausea and emesis, and reduce narcotic requirements before or after surgery or delivery. Also used in management of pruritus due to allergic conditions, e.g., chronic urticaria, atopic and contact dermatoses, and in treatment of acute and chronic alcoholism with withdrawal symptoms or delirium tremens.

CONTRAINDICATIONS Known hypersensitivity to hydroxyzine; use as sole treatment in psychoses or depression. Safe use during early pregnancy (category C) or lactation is not established.

CAUTIOUS USE History of allergies; older adults.

ROUTE & DOSAGE

Anxiety

Adult: **PO** 25–100 mg t.i.d. or q.i.d. **IM** 25–100 mg q4–6h
Child: **PO** <6 y, 50 mg/d in divided doses; >6 y, 50 mg/d in divided doses **IM** 1.1 mg/kg q4–6h

Pruritus

Adult: **PO** 25 mg t.i.d. or q.i.d. **IM** 25 mg q4–6h
Geriatric: **PO** 10 mg 3–4 times daily
Child: **PO** >6 y, 50–100 mg/d in divided doses; <6 y, 50 mg/d in divided doses **IM** 1.1 mg/kg q4–6h

Nausea

Adult: **IM** 25–100 mg q4–6h
Child: **IM** 1.1 mg/kg q4–6h

ADMINISTRATION

Oral

- Note: Tablets may be crushed and taken with fluid of patient's choice. Capsule may be emptied and contents swallowed with water or mixed with food. Liquid formulations are available.

Intramuscular

- Give deep into body of a relatively large muscle. The Z-track technique of injection is recommended to prevent SC infiltration.
- Recommended site: In adult, the gluteus maximus or vastus lateralis; in children, the vastus lateralis.
- Protect all forms from light. Store at 15°–30° C (59°–86° F) unless otherwise specified.

INCOMPATIBILITIES **Solution/additive: Aminophylline, amobarbital, chloramphenicol, dimenhydrinate, penicillin G, pentobarbital, phenobarbital.**

ADVERSE EFFECTS (≥1%) **CNS:** *Drowsiness* (usually transitory), sedation, dizziness, headache. **CV:** Hypotension. **GI:** *Dry mouth*. **Body as a Whole:** Urticaria, dyspnea, chest tightness, wheezing, involuntary motor activity (rare). **Hematologic:** Phlebitis, hemolysis, thrombosis. **Skin:** Erythematous macular eruptions, erythema multiforme, digital gangrene from inadvertent IV or intraarterial injection, injection site reactions.

DIAGNOSTIC TEST INTERFERENCE Possibility of false-positive ***urinary 17-hydroxycorticosteroid*** determinations (modified ***Glenn-Nelson technique***).

INTERACTIONS Drug: Alcohol and CNS DEPRESSANTS add to CNS depression; TRICYCLIC ANTIDEPRESSANTS and other ANTICHOLINERGICS have additive anticholinergic effects; may inhibit pressor effects of **epinephrine.**

PHARMACOKINETICS Absorption: Readily absorbed from GI tract. **Onset:** 15–30 min PO. **Duration:** 4–6 h. **Distribution:** Not known if it crosses placenta or is distributed into breast milk. **Metabolism:** Metabolized in liver. **Elimination:** Probably excreted in bile.

NURSING IMPLICATIONS

Assessment & Drug Effects

- Evaluate alertness. Drowsiness may occur and usually disappears with continued therapy or following reduction of dosage.
- Monitor condition of oral membranes daily when patient is on high dosage of hydroxyzine.
- Reevaluate usefulness of drug periodically.
- Reduce dosage of the depressant up to 50% when CNS depressants are prescribed concomitantly.

Patient & Family Education

- Do not drive or engage in other potentially hazardous activities until response to drug is known.
- Do NOT take alcohol and hydroxyzine at the same time.
- Notify physician immediately if you become pregnant.
- Relieve dry mouth by frequent warm water rinses, increasing fluid intake, and use of a salivary substitute (e.g., Moi-Stir, Xero-Lube).
- Give teeth scrupulous care. Avoid irritation or abrasion of gums and other oral tissues.
- Consult physician before self-dosing with OTC medications.
- Do not breast feed while taking this drug without consulting physician.

HYOSCYAMINE SULFATE

(hye-oh-sye′a-meen)

Anaspaz, Cystospaz, Levsin, Levsinex, Neoquess, NuLev

Classifications: ANTICHOLINERGIC (PARASYMPATHOLYTIC); ANTIMUSCARINIC; ANTISPASMODIC

Prototype: Atropine

Pregnancy Category: C

AVAILABILITY 0.125 mg, 0.150 mg tablets; 0.125 mg sublingual tablets; 0.375 sustained release capsules; 0.125 mg orally disintegrating tablet 0.125 mg/mL oral solution; 0.125 mg/5 mL elixir; 0.5 mg/mL injection

ACTIONS Extremely potent belladonna alkaloid with anticholinergic and antispasmodic activity. Anticholinergic effect chiefly related to the levo isomer.

THERAPEUTIC EFFECTS Anticholinergic and antispasmodic action is produced by competitive inhibition of acetylcholine at the parasympathetic neuroeffector junctions.

USES GI tract disorders caused by spasm and hypermotility, as conjunct therapy with diet and antacids for peptic ulcer management, and as an aid in the control of gastric hypersecretion and intestinal hypermotility. Also symptomatic relief of biliary and renal colic, as a "drying agent" to relieve symptoms of acute rhinitis, to control preanesthesia salivation and respiratory tract secretions, to treat symptoms of parkinsonism, and to reduce pain and hypersecretion in pancreatitis.

CONTRAINDICATIONS Hypersensitivity to belladonna alkaloids, narrow-angle glaucoma, prostatic

H

hypertrophy, obstructive diseases of GI or GU tract, paralytic ileus or intestinal atony, myasthenia gravis; children <2 y.

CAUTIOUS USE Diabetes mellitus, cardiac disease; pregnancy (category C).

ROUTE & DOSAGE

GI Spasms

Adult: **IV/IM/SC** 0.25–0.5 mg q6h **PO/SL** 0.125–0.25 mg t.i.d. or q.i.d. prn

Child: **PO** *2–12 y,* 0.0625–0.125 mg q4h prn (max: 0.75 mg/d)

ADMINISTRATION

Note: Dose for older adults may need to be less than the standard adult dose. Observe patient carefully for signs of paradoxic reactions.

Oral

- Give preparations about 1 h before meals and at bedtime (at least 2 h after last meal).
- Ensure that sustained release form of drug is not chewed or crushed. It must be swallowed whole.

Intravenous

PREPARE: **Direct:** Give undiluted.
ADMINISTER: **Direct:** Give a single dose over 60 sec.

- Store 15°–30° C (59°–86° F).

ADVERSE EFFECTS (≥1%) **CNS:** Headache, unusual tiredness or weakness, confusion, *drowsiness,* excitement in older adult patients. **CV:** Palpitations, tachycardia. **Special Senses:** *Blurred vision,* increased intraocular tension, cycloplegia, mydriasis. **GI:** *Dry mouth, constipation,* paralytic ileus. **Other:** *Urinary retention,* anhidrosis, suppression of lactation.

INTERACTIONS Drug: Amantadine, ANTIHISTAMINES, TRICYCLIC ANTI-DEPRESSANTS, **quinidine, disopyramide, procainamide** add anticholinergic effects; decreases **levodopa** effects; **methotrimeprazine** may precipitate extrapyramidal effects; decreases antipsychotic effects of PHENOTHIAZINES (decreased absorption).

PHARMACOKINETICS Absorption: Well absorbed from all administration sites. **Onset:** 2–3 min IV; 20–30 min PO. **Peak:** 15–30 min IV; 30–60 min PO. **Duration:** 4–6 h (up to 12 h with sustained release form). **Distribution:** Distributed in most body tissues; crosses blood–brain barrier and placenta; distributed in breast milk. **Metabolism:** Metabolized in liver. **Elimination:** Excreted in urine. **Half-Life:** 3.5–13 h.

NURSING IMPLICATIONS

Assessment & Drug Effects

- Monitor bowel elimination; may cause constipation.
- Monitor urinary output.
- Lessen risk of urinary retention by having patient void prior to each dose.
- Assess for dry mouth and recommend good practices of oral hygiene.

Patient & Family Education

- Avoid excessive exposure to high temperatures; drug-induced heatstroke can develop.
- Do not drive or engage in other potentially hazardous activities until response to drug is known.
- Use dark glasses if experiencing blurred vision, but if this adverse effect persists, notify physician for dose adjustment or possible drug change.

IBUPROFEN (Pr)

(eye-byoo'proe-fen)

Advil, Amersol ♣, Children's Motrin, Haltran, Ibuprin, Junior Strength Motrin Caplets, Medipren, Motrin, Nuprin, Pediaprofen, Pamprin-IB, Rufen, Trendar

Classifications: CENTRAL NERVOUS SYSTEM AGENT; NSAID (COX-1); ANALGESIC; ANTIPYRETIC

Pregnancy Category: B

AVAILABILITY 100 mg, 200 mg, 400 mg, 600 mg, 800 mg tablets; 50 mg, 100 mg chewable tablets; 100 mg/5 mL, 100 mg/2.5 mL suspension; 40 mg/mL drops

ACTIONS Prototype of the propionic acid NSAIDS (COX-1) inhibitor with nonsteroidal antiinflammatory activity and significant antipyretic and analgesic properties. Blocks prostaglandin synthesis. Ibuprofen activity also includes modulation of T-cell function, inhibition of inflammatory cell chemotaxis, decreased release of superoxide radicals, or increased scavenging of these compounds at inflammatory sites.

THERAPEUTIC EFFECTS Has nonsteroidal antiinflammatory, analgesic, and antipyretic effects. Inhibits platelet aggregation and prolongs bleeding time but does not affect prothrombin or whole blood clotting times. Cross-sensitivity with aspirin and other nonsteroidal antiinflammatory drugs has been reported.

USES Chronic, symptomatic rheumatoid arthritis and osteoarthritis; relief of mild to moderate pain; primary dysmenorrhea; reduction of fever.

UNLABELED USES Gout, juvenile rheumatoid arthritis, psoriatic arthritis, ankylosing spondylitis, vascular headache.

CONTRAINDICATIONS Patient in whom urticaria, severe rhinitis, bronchospasm, angioedema, nasal polyps are precipitated by aspirin or other NSAIDS; active peptic ulcer, bleeding abnormalities. Safe use during pregnancy (category B), lactation, or children <6 mo is not established.

CAUTIOUS USE Hypertension, history of GI ulceration, impaired hepatic or renal function, chronic renal failure, cardiac decompensation, patients with SLE.

ROUTE & DOSAGE

Inflammatory Disease

Adult: **PO** 400–800 mg t.i.d. or q.i.d. (max: 3200 mg/d)
Child: **PO** *<20 kg,* up to 400 mg/d in divided doses; *20–30 kg,* up to 600 mg/d in divided doses; *30–40 kg,* up to 800 mg/d in divided doses

Mild to Moderate Pain, Dysmenorrhea

Adult: **PO** 400 mg q4–6h up to 1200 mg/d

Fever

Adult: **PO** 200–400 mg t.i.d. or q.i.d. (max: 1200 mg/d)
Child: **PO** *6 mo–12 y,* 5–10 mg/kg q4–6h up to 40 mg/kg/d

ADMINISTRATION

Oral

- Give on an empty stomach, 1 h before or 2 h after meals. May be taken with meals or milk if GI intolerance occurs.
- Ensure that chewable tablets are chewed or crushed before being swallowed.

- Note: Tablet may be crushed if patient is unable to swallow it whole and mixed with food or liquid before swallowing.
- Store in tightly closed, light-resistant container unless otherwise directed by manufacturer.

ADVERSE EFFECTS (≥1%) **CNS:** Headache, dizziness, light-headedness, anxiety, emotional lability, fatigue, malaise, drowsiness, anxiety, confusion, depression, aseptic meningitis. **CV:** Hypertension, palpitation, congestive heart failure (patient with marginal cardiac function); peripheral edema. **Special Senses:** Amblyopia (blurred vision, decreased visual acuity, scotomas, changes in color vision); nystagmus, visual-field defects; tinnitus, impaired hearing. **GI:** Dry mouth, gingival ulcerations, dyspepsia, *heartburn, nausea,* vomiting, anorexia, diarrhea, constipation, bloating, flatulence, epigastric or abdominal discomfort or pain, GI ulceration, *occult blood loss*. **Hematologic:** Thrombocytopenia, neutropenia, hemolytic or aplastic anemia, leukopenia; decreased Hgb, Hct; transitory rise in AST, ALT, serum alkaline phosphatase; rise in (Ivy) bleeding time. **GU:** Acute renal failure, polyuria, azotemia, cystitis, hematuria, nephrotoxicity, decreased creatinine clearance. **Skin:** Maculopapular and vesicobullous skin eruptions, erythema multiforme, pruritus, rectal itching, acne. **Body as a Whole:** Fluid retention with edema, Stevens-Johnson syndrome, toxic hepatitis, hypersensitivity reactions, anaphylaxis, bronchospasm, serum sickness, SLE, angioedema.

INTERACTIONS Drug: ORAL ANTICOAGULANTS, **heparin** may prolong bleeding time; may increase **lithium** and **methotrexate** toxicity. **Herbal: Feverfew, garlic, ginger, ginkgo** may increase bleeding potential.

PHARMACOKINETICS Absorption: 80% absorbed from GI tract. **Onset:** 1 h antipyretic effect. **Peak:** 1–2 h. **Duration:** 6–8 h. **Metabolism:** Metabolized in liver. **Elimination:** Excreted primarily in urine; some biliary excretion. **Half-Life:** 2–4 h.

NURSING IMPLICATIONS

Assessment & Drug Effects

- Monitor for therapeutic effectiveness. Optimum response generally occurs within 2 wk (e.g., relief of pain, stiffness, or swelling; or improved joint flexion and strength).
- Observe patients with history of cardiac decompensation closely for evidence of fluid retention and edema.
- Lab tests: Baseline and periodic evaluations of Hgb, renal and hepatic function, and auditory and ophthalmologic examinations are recommended in patients receiving prolonged or high-dose therapy.
- Monitor for GI distress and S&S of GI bleeding.
- Note: Symptoms of acute toxicity in children include apnea, cyanosis, response only to painful stimuli, dizziness, and nystagmus.

Patient & Family Education

- Notify physician immediately of passage of dark tarry stools, "coffee ground" emesis, frankly bloody emesis, or other GI distress, as well as blood or protein in urine, and onset of skin rash, pruritus, jaundice.
- Do not drive or engage in other potentially hazardous activities until response to the drug is known.
- Do not self-medicate with ibuprofen if taking prescribed drugs or being treated for a serious condition without consulting physician.

- Do not take aspirin concurrently with ibuprofen.
- Avoid alcohol and NSAIDS unless otherwise advised by physician. Concurrent use may increase risk of GI ulceration and bleeding tendencies.
- Do not breast feed while taking this drug without consulting physician.

IBUTILIDE FUMARATE

(i-bu'ti-lide)

Corvert

Classifications: CARDIOVASCULAR AGENT; ANTIARRHYTHMIC AGENT, CLASS III

Prototype: Amiodarone HCl

Pregnancy Category: C

AVAILABILITY 0.1 mg/mL injection

ACTIONS Ibutilide is a Class III antiarrhythmic agent. It prolongs the cardiac action potential and increases both atrial and ventricular refractoriness without effecting conduction (i.e., Class III antiarrhythmic electrophysiologic effects).

THERAPEUTIC EFFECTS It is used to treat recently occurring atrial arrhythmias. Like other Class III antiarrhythmic drugs it may produce proarrhythmic effects that can be life threatening.

USES Rapid conversion of atrial fibrillation or atrial flutter of recent onset.

CONTRAINDICATIONS Hypersensitivity to ibutilide, pregnancy (category C), hypokalemia, hypomagnesia.

CAUTIOUS USE History of CHF, ejection fraction of 35% or less, recent MI, prolonged QT intervals, liver disease, cardiovascular disorder other than atrial arrhythmias, other drugs that prolong QT interval, lactation. Safety and effectiveness in children <18 y is not established.

ROUTE & DOSAGE

Atrial Fibrillation or Flutter

Adult: **IV** *<60 kg,* 0.01 mg/kg (0.1 mL/kg), may repeat in 10 min if inadequate response; *≥60 kg,* 1 mg (10 mL), may repeat in 10 min if inadequate response

ADMINISTRATION

- Hypokalemia and hypomagnesemia should be corrected prior to treatment with ibutilide.
- Class Ia and other class III antiarrhythmic drugs should not be given concurrently or within 4 h of ibutilide.

Intravenous

PREPARE: **Direct:** Give undiluted. **IV Infusion:** Contents of 1 mg vial may be diluted in 50 mL of D5W or NS to yield 0.017 mg/mL.

ADMINISTER: **Direct/IV Infusion:** Give a single dose by direct injection or infusion over 10 min. ■ Stop injection/infusion as soon as presenting arrhythmia is terminated or with appearance of ventricular tachycardia or marked prolongation of QT or QT_C.

- Store diluted solution up to 24 h at 15°–30° C (59°–86° F) or 48 h refrigerated at 2°–8° C (36°–46° F).

ADVERSE EFFECTS (≥1%) **CNS:** Headache. **CV:** Proarrhythmic effects (sustained and nonsustained polymorphic ventricular tachycardia), AV block, bundle branch block, ventricular extrasystoles, hypotension, postural hypotension, bradycardia, tachycardia, palpitations, prolonged QT segment. **GI:** Nausea.

INTERACTIONS Drug: Increased potential for proarrhythmic effects when administered with **astemizole,** PHENOTHIAZINES, TRICYCLIC ANTIDEPRESSANTS, **terfenadine, amiodarone, disopyramide, quinidine, procainamide, sotalol** may cause prolonged refractoriness if given within 4 h of ibutilide.

PHARMACOKINETICS Onset: 30 min. **Metabolism:** Metabolized in liver. **Elimination:** 82% excreted in urine, 19% in feces. **Half-Life:** 6 h (range 2–21 h).

I

NURSING IMPLICATIONS

Assessment & Drug Effects

- Monitor for therapeutic effectiveness. Conversion to normal sinus rhythm normally occurs within 30 min of initiation of infusion.
- Observe with continuous ECG, BP, and HR monitoring during and for at least 4 h after infusion or until QT_C has returned to baseline. Monitor for longer periods with liver dysfunction or if proarrhythmic activity is observed.

Patient & Family Education

- Consult physician and understand the potential risks of ibutilide therapy.
- Do not breast feed while taking this drug without consulting physician.

IDARUBICIN

(i-da-a-roo'bi-cin)

Idamycin, Idamycin PFS

Classification: ANTINEOPLASTIC, ANTIBIOTIC

Prototype: Doxorubicin

Pregnancy Category: D

AVAILABILITY 5 mg, 10 mg, 20 mg vials; 1 mg/mL injection

ACTIONS Cytotoxic anthracycline antibiotic and derivative of daunorubicin. Potency of idarubicin is greater than that of daunorubicin or doxorubicin. It may be less cardiotoxic than other anthracyclines. Idarubicin exhibits inhibitory effects on DNA and RNA polymerase and, therefore, on nucleic acid synthesis. Intensive maintenance with idarubicin is not recommended due to its considerable toxicity, including deaths while patient was in remission of acute myelogenous leukemia (AML).

THERAPEUTIC EFFECTS Idarubicin exhibits inhibitory effects on DNA and RNA polymerase and, therefore, on nucleic acid synthesis.

USES In combination with other antineoplastic drugs for treatment of AML.

UNLABELED USES Breast cancer, other solid tumors.

CONTRAINDICATIONS Myelosuppression, hypersensitivity to idarubicin or doxorubicin, pregnancy (category D), lactation.

CAUTIOUS USE Impaired renal or hepatic function; patients who have received irradiation or radiotherapy to areas surrounding heart. Safety and efficacy in children not established.

ROUTE & DOSAGE

Acute Myelogenous Leukemia (AML)

Adult: **IV** 8–12 mg/m^2 daily for 3 d injected slowly over 10–15 min

Acute Nonlymphocytic Leukemia, Acute Lymphocytic Leukemia

Child: **IV** 10–12 mg/m^2/d for 3 d

ADMINISTRATION

Intravenous

IV administration to infants, children: Verify correct IV concentration and rate of infusion with physician.

PREPARE: **IV Infusion:** Reconstitute 5- and 10-mg vials with 5 and 10 mL, respectively, of nonbacteriostatic NS to yield 1 mg/mL. ▪ Vials are under negative pressure, therefore, carefully insert needle into vial to reconstitute. ▪ Wash skin accidentally exposed with soap and water.

ADMINISTER: **IV Infusion:** Give slowly over 10–15 min into tubing of free flowing IV of NS or D5W. ▪ If extravasation is suspected, immediately stop infusion, elevate the arm, and apply ice pack for 1/2 h then q.i.d. for 1/2 h × 3 d.

INCOMPATIBILITIES **Solution/additive: Acyclovir,** ALKALINE SOLUTIONS (i.e., **sodium bicarbonate**), **ampicillin/sulbactam, cefazolin, ceftazidime, clindamycin, dexamethasone, etoposide, furosemide, gentamicin, heparin, hydrocortisone, imipenem/cilastatin, meperidine, methotrexate, mezlocillin, sargramostim, sodium bicarbonate, vancomycin, vincristine. Y-site:** Same as above.

▪ Store reconstituted solutions up to 7 d refrigerated at 2°–8° C (36°–46° F) and 72 h at room temperature 15°–30° C (59°–86° F).

ADVERSE EFFECTS (≥1%) **CV:** CHF, atrial fibrillation, chest pain, MI. **GI:** *Nausea, vomiting, diarrhea, abdominal pain,* mucositis. **Hematologic:** *Anemia, leukopenia,* thrombocytopenia. **Other:** Nephrotoxicity, hepatotoxicity, *alopecia,* rash.

INTERACTIONS Drug: IMMUNOSUPPRESSANTS cause additive bone marrow suppression; ANTICOAGULANTS, NSAIDS, SALICYLATES, **aspirin,** THROMBOLYTIC AGENTS increase risk of bleeding; idarubicin may blunt the effects of **filgrastim, sargramostim.**

PHARMACOKINETICS Onset: Median time to remission 28 d. **Peak:** Serum level 4 h. **Duration:** Serum levels 120 h. **Distribution:** Concentrates in nucleated blood and bone marrow cells. **Metabolism:** Metabolized in liver to idarubicinol, which may be as active as idarubicin. **Elimination:** 16% excreted in urine; 17% excreted in bile. **Half-Life:** Idarubicin 15–45 h, idarubicinol 45 h.

NURSING IMPLICATIONS

Assessment & Drug Effects

- Monitor infusion site closely, as extravasation can cause severe local tissue necrosis. Notify physician if pain, erythema, or edema develops at insertion site.
- Lab tests: Monitor hepatic and renal function, CBC with differential and coagulation studies periodically.
- Monitor cardiac status closely, especially in older adult patients or those with preexisting cardiac disease.
- Monitor hematologic status carefully; during the period of myelosuppression, patients are at high risk for bleeding and infection.
- Monitor for development of hyperuricemia secondary to lysis of leukemic cells.

Patient & Family Education

- Learn all potential adverse reactions to idarubicin.
- Anticipate possible hair loss.
- Discuss interventions to minimize nausea, vomiting, diarrhea, and stomatitis with health care providers.

- Do not breast feed while taking this drug.

IDOXURIDINE (IDU)

(eye-dox-yoor′i-deen)
Herplex Liquifilm, IDU, Stoxil
Classifications: ANTIINFECTIVE; ANTIVIRAL
Prototype: Acyclovir
Pregnancy Category: C

AVAILABILITY 0.1% ophthalmic solution

ACTIONS Topical antiviral agent. Pyrimidine nucleoside structurally related to thymidine, a nucleic acid essential for synthesis of viral DNA. Antiviral activity is primarily due to inhibition of viral replication.
THERAPEUTIC EFFECTS Inhibits growth of *Herpes simplex types I* and *II, varicella-zoster, vaccinia, cytomegalovirus,* and small animal viruses containing DNA. Not effective against RNA viruses. Epithelial viral infections characterized by a dendritic figure respond well to the antiviral activity especially during initial attacks. Chronic or recurrent viral infections that involve deep stromal structures (e.g., herpetic iritis) respond less well and do not heal. Some resistant strains of *Herpes simplex* have been reported.

USES *Herpes simplex* keratitis as single agent or conjunctively with a corticosteroid.
UNLABELED USES Cutaneous *Herpes simplex.*

CONTRAINDICATIONS Hypersensitivity to idoxuridine, iodine or iodine-containing preparations, or any components in the formulation, lactation.
CAUTIOUS USE Pregnancy (category C), corticosteroid therapy.

ROUTE & DOSAGE

Herpes Simplex Keratitis
Adult/Child: **Topical** 1 drop instilled in conjunctival sac q1h during the day and q2h at night until improvement occurs, then decrease to q2h during the day and q4h at night; use ointment q4h during the day with the last dose at bedtime (5 applications/d)

ADMINISTRATION

Topical
- Prevent the possibility of systemic absorption by applying light finger pressure to head of lacrimal duct for 1 min when eyedrop is instilled.
- Follow manufacturer's directions regarding storage. Decomposed idoxuridine not only has reduced antiviral activity but also may be toxic.
- Store ophthalmic solution refrigerated at 2°–8° C (36°–46° F) in a tight, light-resistant container unless otherwise directed. The ointment should be stored at 2°–15° C (36°–59° F).

ADVERSE EFFECTS (≥1%) **Body as a Whole:** [Sensitization. Systemic absorption (stomatitis, anorexia, nausea, vomiting, alopecia, leukopenia, thrombocytopenia, iodism, hepatotoxicity).] **Special Senses:** [Local irritation, pain, burning, lacrimation, pruritus, inflammation, or edema of eyes, lids, and surrounding face; follicular] conjunctivitis, photophobia; corneal ulceration and swelling; delayed healing, small defects in corneal epithelium (local overdosage).

INTERACTIONS Drug: Boric acid-containing solutions may cause precipitation.

PHARMACOKINETICS Absorption: Poorly absorbed from eye tissues. **Distribution:** Crosses placenta. **Metabolism:** Metabolized in liver.

NURSING IMPLICATIONS

Assessment & Drug Effects

- Monitor for therapeutic effectiveness. Epithelial infections usually improve within 7–8 d. If patient continues to improve, therapy is generally continued ≤21 d.
- Supervise patients closely by ophthalmologist.

Patient & Family Education

- Learn proper technique for eye drop instillation.
- Do not exceed the recommended frequency and duration of therapy.
- Wear sunglasses if photosensitivity is troublesome.
- Do not breast feed while taking this drug.

IFOSFAMIDE

(i-fos′-fa-mide)

Ifex

Classifications: ANTINEOPLASTIC; ALKYLATING AGENT

Prototype: Cyclophosphamide

Pregnancy Category: D

AVAILABILITY 1 g, 3 g vials

ACTIONS Ifosfamide is a chemotherapeutic agent chemically related to nitrogen mustards. The alkylated metabolites of ifosfamide interact with DNA.

THERAPEUTIC EFFECTS Antineoplastic or cytotoxic action is primarily due to cross-linking of strands of DNA and RNA as well as inhibition of protein synthesis.

USES In combination with other agents in various regimens for germ cell testicular cancer, soft tissue sarcomas, Ewing's sarcoma, and non-Hodgkin's lymphoma. Also for lung and pancreatic sarcoma.

CONTRAINDICATIONS Patients with severe bone marrow depression or who have demonstrated previous hypersensitivity to ifosfamide; pregnancy (category D) and lactation.

CAUTIOUS USE Impaired renal function, prior radiation or prior therapy with other cytotoxic agents.

ROUTE & DOSAGE

Antineoplastic

Adult: **IV** 1.2 $g/m^2/d$ for 5 consecutive d; administer over at least 30 min, repeat q3 wk or after recovery from hematologic toxicity (platelets ≥100,000/mm^3; WBC ≥4,000/mm^3)

ADMINISTRATION

Intravenous

PREPARE: **IV Infusion:** Dilute each 1 g in 20 mL of sterile water or bacteriostatic water to yield 50 mg/mL. ▪ Shake well to dissolve. ▪ May be further diluted with D5W, NS, or RL to achieve concentrations of 0.6–20 mg/mL. ▪ Use solution prepared with sterile water within 6 h.

ADMINISTER: **IV Infusion:** Give slowly over 30 min.

- Store reconstituted solution prepared with bacteriostatic solution up to a week at 30° C (86° F) or 6 wk at 5° C (41° F).

ADVERSE EFFECTS (≥1%) **CNS:** *Somnolence, confusion, hallucinations,* coma, dizziness, seizures, cranial nerve dysfunction. **GI:** *Nausea, vomiting,* anorexia, diarrhea, metabolic acidosis, hepatic dysfunction. **Hematologic:** Neutropenia, thrombocytopenia. **Urogenital:** Hemorrhagic cystitis, nephrotoxicity. **Skin:** *Alopecia,* skin necrosis with extravasation.

INTERACTIONS Drug: HEPATIC ENZYME INDUCERS (BARBITURATES, **phenytoin, chloral hydrate**) may increase hepatic conversion of ifosfamide to active metabolite; CORTICOSTEROIDS may inhibit conversion to active metabolites.

PHARMACOKINETICS Distribution: Distributed into breast milk. **Metabolism:** Metabolized in liver to active form. **Elimination:** 70%–86% excreted in urine. **Half-Life:** 7–15 h.

I

NURSING IMPLICATIONS

Assessment & Drug Effects

- Lab tests: Monitor CBC with differential prior to each dose and at regular intervals; urinalysis prior to each dose for microscopic hematuria.
- Hold drug and notify physician if WBC count is below $2000/mm^3$ or platelet count is below $50{,}000/mm^3$.
- Reduce risk of hemorrhagic cystitis by hydrating with 3000 mL of fluid daily prior to therapy and for at least 72 h following treatment to ensure ample urine output.
- Discontinue therapy if any of the following CNS symptoms occur: Somnolence, confusion, depressive psychosis, and hallucinations.

Patient & Family Education

- Void frequently to lessen contact of irritating chemical with bladder mucosa.
- Note: Susceptibility to infection may increase. Avoid people with infection. Notify physician of any infection, fever or chills, cough or hoarseness, lower back or side pain, painful or difficult urination.
- Check with physician immediately if there is any unusual bleeding or bruising, black tarry stools, or blood in urine or if pinpoint red spots develop on skin.
- Discuss possible adverse effects (e.g., alopecia, nausea, and vomiting) and measures that can minimize them with health care provider.
- Do not breast feed while taking this drug.

IMATINIB MESYLATE

(i-ma′ti-nib)

Gleevec

Classifications: IMMUNOSUPPRESSANT; MONOCLONAL ANTIBODY

Prototype: Basiliximab

Pregnancy Category: D

AVAILABILITY 100 mg capsule

ACTIONS Tyrosine kinase inhibitor; inhibits the Bcr-Abl tyrosine kinase, an abnormal tyrosine kinase created by the Philadelphia chromosome abnormality in chronic myeloid leukemia (CLM). Tyrosine kinase is required for activation of a wide variety of intracellular activities vital to cell functioning; thus drug interferes with vital intracellular metabolic pathways.

THERAPEUTIC EFFECTS Inhibits WBC cell proliferation and induces cell death in Bcr-Abl positive cells as well as in newly formed leukemic cells. Thus, it interferes with progression of chronic myeloid leukemia (CML).

USES Treatment of CML in blast crisis, or in chronic phase after failure of interferon-alpha therapy; unresectable and/or metastatic malignant gastrointestinal stromal tumors (GISTs).

UNLABELED USES Acute lymphocytic leukemia (ALL), soft tissue sarcoma.

CONTRAINDICATIONS Hypersensitivity to imatinib or any of its components; viral infections, including herpes and chickenpox; intramuscular injections with concurrent thrombocytopenia; pregnancy (category D), lactation; children <3 y.
CAUTIOUS USE History of hypersensitivity to other monoclonal antibodies; hepatic or renal impairment; bleeding, bone marrow suppression; cardiac disease; dental disease, dental work; older adults, females of childbearing age; fungal infections; GI bleeding; heart failure; hepatic disease; herpes infection, immunosuppression, infection; jaundice; neutropenia; peripheral edema, renal disease; thrombocytopenia, vaccination, varicella, viral infection; concurrent administration of drugs which are CYP3A4 inhibitors (i.e., ketoconazole, itraconazole, erythromycin, clarithromycin).

ROUTE & DOSAGE

CML Chronic Phase

Adult: **PO** 400–800 mg q.d. with a meal and large glass of water
Child: **PO** *>3 y,* 260 mg/m^2/d in 1 or 2 divided dose(s) (max: 340 mg/m^2/d)

CML Accelerated Phase or Blast Crisis

Adult: **PO** 600 mg q.d. with a meal and large glass of water

GISTs

Adult: **PO** 400–600 mg q.d. times up to 24 mo

Hepatic Impairment

Reduce dose to 300 mg q.d. (chronic) or 400 mg q.d. (accelerated, blast crisis)

ADMINISTRATION

Oral

- Give with meal and large glass of water (at least 8 oz).
- Store at 15°–30° C (59°–86° F).

ADVERSE EFFECTS (≥1%) **Body as a Whole:** *Fluid retention, edema, fatigue,* weight gain, *fever,* night sweats, weakness. **CNS:** CNS hemorrhage, *headache.* **GI:** *Nausea, vomiting, diarrhea,* GI hemorrhage, dyspepsia, *abdominal pain, constipation, anorexia,* increased AST, ALT, and bilirubin. **Hematologic:** Hemorrhage, *neutropenia, thrombocytopenia,* petechiae, epistaxis, pancytopenia (rare), thrombocytopenia (rare). **Metabolic:** Hypokalemia. **Musculoskeletal:** *Muscle cramps, pain, arthralgia,* myalgia. **Respiratory:** *Cough, dyspnea,* pharyngitis, pneumonia. **Skin:** *Rash,* pruritus.

INTERACTIONS Drug: Clarithromycin, erythromycin, ketoconazole, itraconazole may increase imatinib levels and toxicity; **carbamazepine, dexamethasone, phenobarbital, phenytoin, rifampin** may decrease imatinib levels; may increase levels of BENZODIAZEPINES, DIHYDROPYIDINE, CALCIUM CHANNEL BLOCKERS (e.g., **nifedipine**), **warfarin. Herbal: St. John's wort** may decrease imatinib levels.

PHARMACOKINETICS Absorption: Well absorbed, 98% reaches systemic circulation. **Peak:** 2–4 h. **Metabolism:** Metabolized primarily by CYP3A4 in liver. **Elimination:** Primarily excreted in feces. **Half-Life:** 18 h imatinib, 40 h active metabolite.

NURSING IMPLICATIONS

Assessment & Drug Effects

- Monitor for S&S of fluid retention. Weigh daily and report rapid weight gain immediately.

- Lab tests: CBC with platelet count and differential weekly times 1 mo, biweekly for the 2nd mo, periodically thereafter as clinically indicated; baseline and monthly AST, ALT, alkaline phosphatase, bilirubin; periodic serum creatinine and electrolytes.
- Withhold drug and notify physician for any of the following: bilirubin >3 times ULN, AST/ALT >5 times ULN; treatment may be reinstituted when bilirubin <1.5 times ULN and AST/ALT <2.5 times ULN.
- Review concurrent medications. Consult physician about switching patients taking warfarin to low-molecular weight or standard heparin. Patients taking ketoconazole and other CYP3A4 inhibitors may experience increased adverse drug reactions.

Patient & Family Education

- Do not take any OTC drugs (e.g., acetaminophen, St. John's wort) without consulting physician.
- Report any S&S of bleeding immediately to physician (e.g., black tarry stool, bright red or coke colored urine, bleeding from gums).
- Report immediately to physician any unexplained change in mental status.
- Use effective means of contraception while taking this drug. Women of childbearing age should avoid becoming pregnant.
- Do not breast feed while taking this drug.

IMIPENEM-CILASTATIN SODIUM (Pr)

(i-mi-pen'em sye-la-stat'in)

Primaxin

Classifications: ANTIINFECTIVE; BETA-LACTAM ANTIBIOTIC

Pregnancy Category: C

AVAILABILITY 250 mg, 500 mg, 750 mg vials

ACTIONS Fixed combination of imipenem, a beta-lactam antibiotic, and cilastatin. Action of imipenem: inhibition of mucopeptide synthesis in bacterial cell walls leading to cell death. Cilastatin increases the serum half life of imipenem.

THERAPEUTIC EFFECTS Has the greatest microbiologic spectrum of any beta-lactam antibiotic, surpassing that of all the third-generation cephalosporins. Acts synergistically with aminoglycoside antibiotics against some isolates of *Pseudomonas aeruginosa*. Infections resistant to cephalosporins, penicillins, and aminoglycosides have responded to treatment with this combination.

USES Treatment of serious infections caused by susceptible organisms in the urinary tract, lower respiratory tract, bones and joints, skin and skin structures; also intra-abdominal, gynecologic, and mixed infections; bacterial septicemia and endocarditis.

CONTRAINDICATIONS Hypersensitivity to any component of product, multiple allergens. Safe use in pregnancy (category C) is not established.

CAUTIOUS USE Lactation; patients with CNS disorders (e.g., seizures, brain lesions, history of recent head injury); renal impairment; patients with history of penicillin allergies.

ROUTE & DOSAGE

Serious Infections

Adult: **IV** 250–500 mg infused over 20–30 min q6–8h, up to 1 g infused over 40–60 min q6h
IM 500 or 750 mg q12h
Child: **IV** 10–15 mg/kg q6h
IM 15–25 mg/kg q12h

Neonate: **IV** 20–40 mg/kg/d divided q12–24h

Renal Impairment

Cl_{cr} 20–30 mL/min, dose q8–12h; <20 mL/min, dose q12h

ADMINISTRATION

Caution: IM and IV solutions are NOT interchangeable; do NOT give IM solution by IV, and do NOT give IV solution as IM.

Intramuscular

- Reconstitute powder for IM injection as follows: Add 2 mL or 3 mL of 1% lidocaine HCl solution without epinephrine, respectively, to the 500 mg vial or the 750 mg vial. Agitate to form a suspension then withdraw and inject entire contents of the vial IM.
- Give IM suspension by deep injection into the gluteal muscle or lateral thigh.
- Use reconstituted IM injection within 1 h after preparation.

Intravenous

PREPARE: **Intermittent:** Dilute each dose with 10 mL of D5W, NS, or other compatible infusion solution. ▪ Agitate the solution until clear. Color should range from colorless to yellow. ▪ Further dilute with 100 mL of same solution used for initial dilution.

ADMINISTER: **Intermittent:** Give each 500 mg or fraction thereof over 20–30 min. DO NOT give as a bolus dose. Nausea appears to be related to infusion rate, and if it presents during infusion, slow the rate (occurs most frequently with 1-g doses).

INCOMPATIBILITIES **Solution/additive: Ringer's lactate,** stable in **dextrose**-containing solutions for only 4 h.

- Store according to manufacturer's recommendations; stability of IV solutions depends on diluent used for reconstitution. ▪ Most IV solutions retain potency for 4 h at 15°–30° C (59°–86° F) or for 24 h if refrigerated at 4° C (39° F). Avoid freezing.

ADVERSE EFFECTS (≥1%) **Body as a Whole:** Hypersensitivity (rash, fever, chills, dyspnea, pruritus), weakness, oliguria/anuria, polyuria, polyarthralgia; *phlebitis and pain at injection site,* superinfections. **CNS:** Seizures, dizziness, confusion, somnolence, encephalopathy, myoclonus, tremors, paresthesia, headache. **GI:** *Nausea, vomiting,* diarrhea, pseudomembranous colitis, hemorrhagic colitis, gastroenteritis, abdominal pain, glossitis, heartburn. **Respiratory:** Chest discomfort, hyperventilation, dyspnea. **Skin:** Rash, pruritus, urticaria, candidiasis, flushing, increased sweating, skin texture change, facial edema. **Metabolic:** Hyponatremia, hyperkalemia. **Special Senses:** Transient hearing loss; increased WBC, AST, ALT, alkaline phosphatase, BUN, LDH, creatinine; decreased Hgb, Hct, eosinophilia.

INTERACTIONS Drug: Aztreonam, cephalosporins, penicillins may antagonize the antibacterial effects.

PHARMACOKINETICS Distribution: Widely distributed; limited concentrations in CSF; crosses placenta; in breast milk. **Elimination:** 70% of dose excreted in urine within 10 h. **Half-Life:** 1 h.

NURSING IMPLICATIONS

Assessment & Drug Effects

- Determine previous hypersensitivity reaction to beta-lactam antibiotics (penicillins and cephalosporins) or to other allergens.
- Monitor for S&S of hypersensitivity (see Appendix F). Discon-

tinue drug and notify physician if S&S occur.

- Monitor closely patients vulnerable to CNS adverse effects.
- Notify physician if focal tremors, myoclonus, or seizures occur; dosage adjustment may be needed.
- Monitor for S&S of superinfection (see Appendix F).
- Notify physician promptly to rule out pseudomembranous enterocolitis if severe diarrhea accompanied by abdominal pain and fever occurs (see Appendix F).
- Note: Sodium content derived from drug is high; consider in patient on restricted sodium intake.
- Monitor renal, hematologic, and liver function periodically.

Patient & Family Education

- Notify physician immediately to report pruritus or symptoms of respiratory distress.
- Report pain or discomfort at IV infusion site.
- Report loose stools or diarrhea promptly.
- Do not breast feed while taking this drug without consulting physician.

IMIPRAMINE HYDROCHLORIDE (Pr)

(im-ip′ra-meen)

Impril ✦, Janimine, Novopramine ✦, Tofranil

IMIPRAMINE PAMOATE

Tofranil-PM

Classifications: CENTRAL NERVOUS SYSTEM AGENT; PSYCHOTHERAPEUTIC; TRICYCLIC ANTIDEPRESSANT

Pregnancy Category: C

AVAILABILITY 10 mg, 25 mg, 50 mg tablets; 75 mg, 100 mg, 125 mg, 150 mg capsules

ACTIONS Tricyclic antidepressant (TCA) and tertiary amine, structurally related to the phenothiazines. In contrast with phenothiazines, which act on dopamine receptors, TCAs potentiate both norepinephrine and serotonin in the CNS by blocking their reuptake by presynaptic neurons. Decreases number of awakenings from sleep, markedly reduces time in REM sleep, and increases stage 4 sleep.

THERAPEUTIC EFFECTS As a TCA antidepressant, imipramine potentiates the effects of both norepinephrine and serotonin in the CNS by blocking their reuptake by the neurons. Relief of nocturnal enuresis is perhaps due to anticholinergic activity and to nervous system stimulation, resulting in earlier arousal to sensation of full bladder.

USES Endogenous depression and occasionally for reactive depression. Imipramine is the only TCA used as temporary adjuvant treatment of enuresis in children >6 y.

UNLABELED USES Certain syndromes that mimic or overlap diagnostically with depression: alcoholism, cocaine withdrawal; attention deficit disorder with or without hyperactivity (children >6 y and adolescents); with amphetamines or methylphenidate for narcolepsy; phobic anxiety syndromes such as panic disorders and agoraphobia; obsessive-compulsive neurosis; chronic intractable pain.

CONTRAINDICATIONS Hypersensitivity to tricyclic drugs; acute recovery period after MI, defects in bundle-branch conduction; severe renal or hepatic impairment; use of imipramine HCl in children <12 y except to treat enuresis; use of pamoate in children of any age. Safe use during pregnancy (category D) or lactation is not established.

CAUTIOUS USE Children, adolescents, older adults; respiratory difficulties; cardiovascular, hepatic, or GI diseases; blood disorders; increased intraocular pressure, narrow-angle glaucoma; schizophrenia, hypomania or manic episodes, patient with suicidal tendency, seizure disorders; prostatic hypertrophy, urinary retention; alcoholism, hyperthyroidism; electroshock therapy.

ROUTE & DOSAGE

Depression

Adult: **PO** 75–100 mg/d (max: 300 mg/d) in 1 or more divided doses **IM** 50–100 mg/d in divided doses
Child: **PO** 1.5 mg/kg/d, may increase by 1 mg/kg/d q3–4d (max: 5 mg/kg/d)

Enuresis in Childhood

Child: **PO** 25 mg 1 h before bedtime; *<12 y*, may increase to 50 mg nightly (max: 2.5 mg/kg); *>12 y*, may increase to 75 mg nightly (max: 2.5 mg/kg)

ADMINISTRATION

Oral

- Do NOT make dosage adjustments more frequently than q4d.
- Give with or immediately after food.
- Note: Single doses can be given h.s. or qa.m., respectively, if drowsiness or insomnia results.

Intramuscular

- Use IM form only for those unable/unwilling to take oral form.
- Dissolve crystals by immersing intact ampule in warm water for about 1 min.

ADVERSE EFFECTS (≥1%) **Body as a Whole:** Hypersensitivity (skin rash, erythema, petechiae, urticaria, pruritus, photosensitivity, angioedema of face, tongue, or generalized; drug fever). **CNS:** *Sedation, drowsiness,* dizziness, headache, fatigue, numbness, tingling (paresthesias) of extremities; incoordination, ataxia, tremors, peripheral neuropathy, extrapyramidal symptoms (including parkinsonism effects and tardive dyskinesia); lowered seizure threshold, altered EEG patterns, delirium, disturbed concentration, confusion, hallucinations, anxiety, nervousness, insomnia, vivid dreams, restlessness, agitation, shift to hypomania, mania; exacerbation of psychoses; hyperpyrexia. **CV:** *Orthostatic hypotension,* mild sinus tachycardia; *arrhythmias,* hypertension or hypotension, palpitation, MI, CHF, *heart block,* ECG changes, stroke, flushing, cold cyanotic hands and feet (peripheral vasospasm). **Endocrine:** Testicular swelling, gynecomastia (men), galactorrhea and breast enlargement (women), increased or decreased libido, ejaculatory and erectile disturbances, delayed or absent orgasm (male and female); elevation or depression of blood glucose levels. **Special Senses:** Nasal congestion, tinnitus; *blurred vision,* disturbances of accommodation, *slight mydriasis,* nystagmus. **GI:** *Dry mouth,* constipation, heartburn, excessive appetite, weight gain, nausea, vomiting, diarrhea, slowed gastric emptying time, flatulence, abdominal cramps, esophageal reflux, anorexia, stomatitis, increased salivation, black tongue, peculiar taste, paralytic ileus. **Urogenital:** *Urinary retention,* delayed micturition, nocturia, paradoxic urinary frequency. **Hematologic:** Bone marrow depression; agranulocytosis, eosinophilia, thrombocytopenia. **Other:** Excessive perspiration, cholestatic jaundice, precipitation of acute intermittent porphyria; dyspnea, changes in heat and cold tolerance, hair loss, syndrome of inappropriate antidiuretic hormone secretion (SIADH).

DIAGNOSTIC TEST INTERFERENCE Imipramine elevates ***serum bilirubin, alkaline phosphatase*** and may increase or decrease ***blood glucose.*** It decreases ***urinary 5-HIAA*** and ***VMA*** excretion and may falsely increase excretion of ***urinary catecholamines.***

I

INTERACTIONS Drug: MAO INHIBITORS may precipitate hyperpyrexic crisis, tachycardia, or seizures; ANTIHYPERTENSIVE AGENTS potentiate orthostatic hypotension; CNS DEPRESSANTS, **alcohol** add to CNS depression; **norepinephrine** and other SYMPATHOMIMETICS may increase cardiac toxicity; **cimetidine** decreases hepatic metabolism, thus increasing imipramine levels; **methylphenidate** inhibits metabolism of imipramine and thus may increase its toxicity. **Herbal: Ginkgo** may decrease seizure threshold; **St. John's wort** may cause **serotonin** syndrome.

PHARMACOKINETICS Absorption: Completely absorbed from GI tract. **Peak:** 1–2 h PO; 30 min IM. **Metabolism:** Metabolized to the active metabolite desipramine in liver. **Elimination:** Primarily excreted in urine, small amount in feces; crosses placenta; may be secreted in breast milk. **Half-Life:** 8–16 h.

NURSING IMPLICATIONS

Assessment & Drug Effects

- Monitor for therapeutic effectiveness: May not occur for 2 wk or more.
- Prevent serious adverse effects by accurate early reporting to physician about patient's response to drug.
- Note: Dose sensitivity and adverse effects are most likely to occur in adolescents and older adults; use a lower initial dose in these patients.
- Lab tests: Monitor hepatic and renal function, CBC with differential, and fluid and electrolyte balance periodically.
- Monitor HR and BP frequently. Orthostatic hypotension may be marked in pretreatment hypertensive or cardiac patients.
- Monitor for potential signs of toxicity: QRS prolongation (to 100 millisecond or greater), arrhythmias, hypotension, respiratory depression, altered level of consciousness, seizures. Overdose onset may be sudden.
- Note: During the first 2 wk of therapy, older adults may develop confusion, restlessness, disturbed sleep, forgetfulness. Symptoms last 3–20 d. Report to physician.
- Weigh patient under standard conditions biweekly: report a gain of 0.5–1.0 kg (1 1/2–2 lb) within 2–3 d and frank edema.
- Monitor urinary and bowel elimination, at least until maintenance dosage is stabilized, to detect urinary retention or frequency, constipation, or paralytic ileus.
- Report promptly early signs of agranulocytosis (see Appendix F).
- Report signs of cholestatic jaundice: flu-like symptoms, yellow skin or sclerae, dark urine, light-colored stools, pruritus.
- Notify physician of extrapyramidal symptoms (tremors, twitching, ataxia, incoordination, hyperreflexia, drooling) in patients receiving large doses and especially in older adults.
- Monitor diabetic patients for loss of glycemic control. Hyperglycemia or hypoglycemia (see Appendix F) occur in some patients.

- Inspect oral mucosa frequently, especially gingival surfaces under dentures.

Patient & Family Education

- Change position slowly and in stages, especially from lying down to upright posture and dangle legs over bed for a few minutes before walking.
- Note: Effectiveness can decrease with continued drug administration in some patients. Inform physician if this occurs.
- Do NOT use OTC drugs while on a TCA without physician approval.
- Do not drive or engage in other potentially hazardous activities until response to drug is known.
- Avoid exposure to strong sunlight because of potential photosensitivity. Use sunscreen with at least SPF of 12–15 if allowed.
- Do not breast feed while taking this drug without consulting physician.

IMIQUIMOD

(i-mi'qui-mod)

Aldara

Classifications: SKIN & MUCOUS MEMBRANE AGENT; KERATOLYTIC AGENT

Pregnancy Category: C

AVAILABILITY 5% cream in 250 mg single use packets

ACTIONS An "immune response modifier"; exact mechanism of action is unknown. Induces cytokine production, including interferon-alfa, which may interfere with viral replication.

THERAPEUTIC EFFECTS Does not totally eradicate HPV. Despite destruction of HPV warts, latent or subclinical HPV infection can persist, and recurrence of visible warts is common.

USES Treatment of external genital and perianal warts *(Condylomata acuminate),* actinic keratosis on the face and scalp of immunocompetent adults, and superficial basal cell carcinoma.

CONTRAINDICATIONS Occlusive dressing; ocular exposure; excessive sun exposure or sunburn; UV exposure; surgery or drug treatment on affected area; pregnancy (category C); children <12 y.

CAUTIOUS USE Hypersensitivity to benzyl alcohol or paraben; HIV infection; lactation

ROUTE & DOSAGE

Genital and Perianal Warts

Adult/Adolescent: **Topical** >*12 y* Apply a thin layer to the affected areas once daily 3 times per week just before bedtime. Wash off cream after 6–10 h (max: 16 wk therapy).

Actinic Keratosis

Adult: **Topical** Apply a thin layer to the affected areas once daily 2 times per week just before sleep for 16 wks. Wash off cream after 8 h.

Superficial Basal Cell Carcinoma

Adult: **Topical** Apply a thin layer to the affected areas once daily 5 times per week just before sleep for 6 wk. Wash off cream after 8 h.

ADMINISTRATION

Topical

- Hand washing before and after application is recommended.
- Wash treatment area with soap and water and allow to dry thoroughly (at least 10 min).
- Single-use packets contain sufficient cream to cover an area of up to 20 cm^2 (approx. 8 in. by 8 in.).

- Instruct patient to apply a thin layer of cream (avoid using excessive cream), and work into area until no longer visible. Do not occlude the application site.
- After each treatment period, remove the cream by washing the treated area with soap and water.
- Store below 25° C (77° F).

ADVERSE EFFECTS (≥1%) **Body as a Whole:** Fungal infections, flu-like symptoms, myalgia. **CNS:** Headache. **Skin:** *Application site reactions, pruritus,* burning, bleeding, stinging, redness, tender- ness, irritation, *erythema,* edema, weeping/exudates, dry skin, scabbing/crusting, hyperkeratosis.

INTERACTIONS Drug: None reported.

PHARMACOKINETICS Absorption: Minimal absorption through intact skin.

NURSING IMPLICATIONS

Patient & Family Education

- Uncircumcised males with warts under the foreskin: Pull back the foreskin and clean the area daily to help avoid penile skin reactions.
- Females should not apply cream directly into the vagina. Application to the labia may cause pain or swelling and may cause difficulty in passing urine.
- Avoid or minimize UV light exposure (artificial and sunlight) during treatment of actinic keratosis. Wear protective clothing. If sunburn develops, avoid using imiquimod cream until fully recovered.
- Do not breast feed without consulting physician.

IMMUNE GLOBULIN INTRAMUSCULAR [IGIM, GAMMA GLOBULIN, IMMUNE SERUM GLOBULIN (ISG)] Pr

(im′mune glob′u-lin)

BayGam

IMMUNE GLOBULIN INTRAVENOUS (IGIV)

Gamimune N, Gammagard, Gammar-P IV, Gamunex, IGIV, Iveegam, Octagam, Sandoglobulin, Venoglobulin-S

Classifications: BIOLOGIC RESPONSE MODIFIER; IMMUNOGLOBULIN

Pregnancy Category: C

AVAILABILITY IGIM 2 mL, 10 mL vials **IGIV** 5%, 10% solution; 50 mg/mL powder for injection

ACTIONS Sterile concentrated solution containing globulin (primarily IgG) prepared from large pools of normal human plasma of either venous or placental origin and processed by a special fractionating technique.

THERAPEUTIC EFFECTS Like hepatitis B immune globulin (H-BIG), contains antibodies specific to hepatitis B surface antigen but in lower concentrations. Therefore, not considered treatment of first choice for postexposure prophylaxis against hepatitis B but usually an acceptable alternative when H-BIG is not available. Also much less expensive than H-BIG. Nonreactive when tested for hepatitis B.

USES IGIM: In susceptible persons to provide passive immunity or to modify severity of certain infectious diseases, e.g., rubeola (measles), rubella (German measles), varicella-zoster (chickenpox), type

A (infectious) hepatitis, and as replacement therapy in congenital agammaglobulinemia or IgG deficiency diseases. May be used as an alternative to H-BIG to provide passive immunity in hepatitis B infection. Also for postexposure prophylaxis of hepatitis non-A, non-B, and nonspecific hepatitis. **IGIV:** Principally as maintenance therapy in patients unable to manufacture sufficient quantities of IgG antibodies, in patients requiring an immediate increase in immunoglobulin levels, and when IM injections are contraindicated as in patients with bleeding disorders or who have small muscle mass. Also in chronic autoimmune thrombocytopenia and idiopathic thrombocytopenic purpura (ITP).

UNLABELED USES Kawasaki syndrome, chronic lymphocytic leukemia, AIDS, premature and low-birth-weight neonates, autoimmune neutropenia, or hemolytic anemia.

CONTRAINDICATIONS History of anaphylaxis or severe reaction to human immune serum globulin (IG) or to any ingredient in the formulation such as thimerosal (mercury derivative) preservative in IM formulations and maltose (stabilizing agent) in IV formulations; persons with clinical hepatitis A; IGIV for patients with class-specific anti-IgA deficiencies; IGIM in severe thrombocytopenia or other bleeding disorders; intramuscular injection, pregnancy (category C), lactation.

CAUTIOUS USE Dehydration, diabetes mellitus, children, older adults, hypovolemia, IgA deficiency, infection; renal disease, renal failure, renal impairment; sepsis; sucrose hypersensitivity; vaccination, viral infection.

ROUTE & DOSAGE

Hepatitis A Exposure

Adult/Child: **IM** 0.02 mL/kg as soon as possible after exposure; if period of exposure will be ≥3 mo, give 0.05–0.06 mL/kg once q4–6mo

Hepatitis B Exposure

Adult/Child: **IM** 0.02–0.06 mL/kg as soon as possible after exposure if H-BIG is unavailable

Rubella Exposure

Adult: **IM** 20 mL as single dose in susceptible pregnant women

Rubeola Exposure

Adult/Child: **IM** 0.25 mL/kg within 6 d of exposure

Varicella-zoster Exposure

Adult/Child: **IM** 0.6–1.2 mL/kg promptly

Immunoglobulin Deficiency

Adult/Child: **IV** Gammagard, Gamimune, 100 mg/kg/mo; Sandoglobulin, Venoglobulin-S 200 mg/kg/mo **IM** 1.2 mL/kg followed by 0.6 mL/kg q2–4wk

Idiopathic Thrombocytopenia Purpura

Adult/Child: **IV** 400 mg/kg/d for 5 consecutive d or 1 g/kg q.o.d. for up to 3 doses

ADMINISTRATION

Note: In hepatitis A (infectious hepatitis), immune globulin is most effective when given before or as soon as possible after exposure but not more than 2wk after (incubation period for hepatitis A is 15–50 d). Do not give immune globulin to those presenting clinical manifestations of hepatitis A. For hepatitis B (serum hepatitis), give immune globulin within 24 h and not more than 7 d after exposure. IGIM and IGIV formulations are NOT interchangeable.

Intramuscular

- Give adults and older children injections into deltoid or anterolateral aspect of thigh; neonates and small children, into anterolateral aspect of thigh.
- Avoid gluteal injections; however, when large volumes of immune globulin are prescribed or when large doses must be divided into several injections, the upper outer quadrant of the gluteus has been used in adults.

Intravenous

PREPARE: **IV Infusion:** Refer to manufacturer's directions for information on reconstitution, dilution, and flow IV rates. ▪ Venoglobulin-S and Gammagard are packaged with the diluent and transfer device. ▪ Gamimune N may be given undiluted or diluted to a 5% solution. ▪ Sandoglobulin is provided with enough diluent to make a 3% solution.

ADMINISTER: **IV Infusion:** Flow rates vary with product being infused. ▪ Gamimune N is generally started at 0.01–0.02 mL/kg/min for 30 min; if tolerated, rate is increased to 0.02–0.04 mL/kg/min. ▪ The initial flow rate for Sandoglobulin is 0.5–1 mL/min; if tolerated after 15–30 min, rate is increased to 1.5–2.5 mL/min.

▪ Store Gamimune N at 2°–8° C (36°–46° F); store Sandoglobulin below 20° C (68° F) unless otherwise directed. ▪ Avoid freezing. Do not use if turbidity has occurred or if product has been frozen. ▪ Do not mix with other drugs. ▪ Discard partially used vial.

ADVERSE EFFECTS (≥1%) **Body as a Whole:** *Pain, tenderness, muscle stiffness at IM site;* local inflammatory reaction, erythema, urticaria, angioedema, headache, malaise, fever, arthralgia, nephrotic syndrome, hypersensitivity (fever, chills, anaphylactic shock), infusion reactions (*nausea, flushing, chills,* headache, chest tightness, wheezing, skeletal pain, back pain, abdominal cramps, anaphylaxis).

INTERACTIONS Drug: May interfere with antibody response to LIVE VIRUS VACCINES (measles/mumps/rubella); give VACCINES 14 d before or 3 mo after IMMUNE GLOBULINS.

PHARMACOKINETICS Peak: 2 d. **Distribution:** Rapidly and evenly distributed to intravascular and extravascular fluid compartments. **Half-Life:** 21–23 d.

NURSING IMPLICATIONS

Assessment & Drug Effects

- Make sure emergency drugs and appropriate emergency facilities are immediately available for treatment of anaphylaxis or sensitization.
- Note: Hypersensitivity reactions (see Appendix F) are most likely in patients receiving large IM doses, repeated injections, or rapid IV infusion.
- Monitor vital signs and infusion rate closely when patient is receiving IGIV.
- Note: IGIV has a mild diuretic effect in some patients due to presence of maltose.

Patient & Family Education

- Report immediately S&S of hypersensitivity (see Appendix F).
- Report immediately infusion symptoms of nausea, chills, headache, and chest tightness; these are indications to slow rate of infusion.
- Note: Passive immunity to measles (rubeola) lasts about 3–4 wk

after immune globulin. In general, children ≤15 mo need active immunization with measles virus vaccine 3 mo after IGIM.

- Do not breast feed while taking this drug without consulting physician.

INAMRINONE LACTATE Pr

(in-am'ri-none)

Inocor

Classifications: CARDIOVASCULAR AGENT; INOTROPIC AGENT; VASODILATOR

Pregnancy Category: C

AVAILABILITY 5 mg/mL injection

ACTIONS A new chemical class of cardiac inotropic agents with vasodilator activity. Mode of action appears to differ from that of the digitalis glycosides and beta-adrenergic stimulants. In patients with depressed myocardial function, it enhances myocardial contractility, increases cardiac output and stroke volume, and reduces right and left ventricular filling pressure, pulmonary capillary wedge pressure (PCWP), and systemic vascular resistance.

THERAPEUTIC EFFECTS It reduces afterload and preload by its direct relaxant effect on vascular smooth muscle. Inamrinone produces hemodynamic improvements and symptomatic relief in patients in CHF due to ischemic heart disease.

USES Short-term management of CHF in patients not adequately controlled by traditional therapy, such as digitalis, diuretics, and vasodilators, and may be used in conjunction with these agents.

CONTRAINDICATIONS Hypersensitivity to inamrinone or to bisulfites; severe aortic or pulmonic valvular disease in lieu of appropriate surgery, acute MI; uncorrected hypokalemia or dehydration. Safe use during pregnancy (category C), lactation, or children is not established.

CAUTIOUS USE Compromised renal or hepatic function, arrhythmias, hypertrophic subaortic stenosis; decreased platelets. Concomitant cardiac glycoside therapy recommended in patients with atrial flutter or fibrillation.

ROUTE & DOSAGE

Congestive Heart Failure

Adult: **IV** 0.75 mg/kg bolus given slowly over 2–3 min, then start infusion at 5–10 mcg/kg/min, may repeat bolus in 30 min (max: 10 mg/kg/d)

ADMINISTRATION

Intravenous

PREPARE: **Direct:** Give loading dose undiluted or diluted by adding 1 mL of NS or 0.45% NS to each 5 mg (1 mL). **IV Infusion:** Dilute 300 mg (60 mL) in 60 mL of NS or 0.45% NS to yield 2.5 mg/mL. ▪ Natural color is clear yellow. Discard discolored solutions and those with precipitate.

ADMINISTER: **Direct:** Give loading dose over 2–3 min. May inject into a running D5W infusion through Y-connector or directly. **IV Infusion:** Give diluted solution at a rate of 5–10 mg/kg/min. ▪ Use infusion pump to regulate rate.

INCOMPATIBILITIES **Solution/additive: Sodium bicarbonate, dextrose**-containing solutions. **Y-site: Furosemide.**

▪ Use all diluted solutions within 24 h. ▪ Protect ampules from light.

ADVERSE EFFECTS (≥1%) **Body as a Whole:** Hypersensitivity (pericarditis, pleuritis; myositis with interstitial shadows on chest x-ray and elevated sedimentation rate; vasculitis with nodular pulmonary densities, hypoxemia, ascites, jaundice). **CV:** Hypotension, arrhythmias. **Endocrine:** Nephrogenic diabetes insipidus. **GI:** Nausea, vomiting, anorexia, abdominal cramps, hepatotoxicity. **Hematologic:** Asymptomatic thrombocytopenia.

I

INTERACTIONS Drug: Possibility of excessive hypotension with disopyramide.

PHARMACOKINETICS Onset: 2–5 min. **Peak:** 10 min. **Duration:** About 2 h. **Distribution:** Unknown if it crosses placenta or into breast milk. **Metabolism:** Metabolized in liver. **Elimination:** Excreted primarily in urine. **Half-Life:** 3.6–7.5 h.

NURSING IMPLICATIONS

Assessment & Drug Effects

- Monitor for therapeutic effectiveness: Increased cardiac output, decreased PCWP, relief of symptoms of CHF. Central venous pressure may be used to assess hypotension and blood volume.
- Monitor BP, heart rate, and respirations and keep physician informed. Rate of administration and duration of therapy are prescribed according to clinical response and adverse effects.
- Consult physician for guidelines. In general, rate of infusion should be slowed or stopped with excessive drop in BP or arrhythmias.
- Monitor infusion site to prevent extravasation.
- Monitor I&O ratio and pattern and daily weights. Improvement in cardiac output enhances diuresis with consequent danger of hypokalemia and arrhythmias, particularly in digitalized patients.
- Lab tests: Monitor closely platelet counts, liver enzymes, fluid and electrolyte balances, renal function.
- Correct hypokalemia before and during therapy.
- Note: If platelet count falls below 150,000/mm^3, report immediately to physician; may indicate thrombocytopenia.
- Allergy alert: IV preparation contains sodium metabisulfite, a reducing agent to which certain susceptible individuals are allergic. Discontinue immediately if patient shows hypersensitivity reactions.
- Observe patient closely when drug is withdrawn after prolonged therapy; clinical deterioration may occur within hours.

Patient & Family Education

- Do not breast feed without consulting physician.

INDAPAMIDE

(in-dap'a-mide)

Lozide ✦, Lozol

Classifications: ELECTROLYTIC AND WATER BALANCE AGENT; THIAZIDE-LIKE DIURETIC

Prototype: Hydrochlorothiazide

Pregnancy Category: B

AVAILABILITY 1.25, 2.5 mg tablets

ACTIONS Sulfonamide derivative which has both diuretic and direct vascular effects. Action mechanism is similar to that of the thiazide diuretics. Principal site of action is on the proximal portion of the distal renal tubules. Enhances excretion of sodium, potassium, and water by interfering with sodium transfer across renal epithelium of the tubules.

THERAPEUTIC EFFECTS Hypotensive activity in the hypertensive patient appears to result from a decrease in plasma and extracellular fluid volume, decreased peripheral vascular resistance, direct arteriolar dilation, and calcium channel blockade. Augments the action of other hypotensive agents.

USES Alone or with other antihypertensives as step 1 agent in the management of hypertension in patients who have failed to respond to diet, exercise, or weight reduction.

UNLABELED USES Edema associated with CHF.

CONTRAINDICATIONS Hypersensitivity to indapamide or other sulfonamide derivatives, anuria.

CAUTIOUS USE Electrolyte imbalance, hypokalemia, severe renal disease; impaired hepatic function or progressive liver disease; prediabetic and type II diabetic patient, hyperparathyroidism, thyroid disorders; SLE; sympathectomized patient; history of gout. Safe use during pregnancy (category B), lactation, or children is not established.

ROUTE & DOSAGE

Hypertension, Edema

Adult: **PO** 2.5 mg once/d, may increase to 5 mg/d if needed

ADMINISTRATION

Oral

- Give with food or milk to reduce GI irritation.
- Administer in a.m. to prevent nocturia. Urge patient to take at least 240 mL (8 oz) of fluid (if allowed) with the medication.
- Store in tight, light-resistant container unless otherwise directed.

ADVERSE EFFECTS (≥1%) **CNS:** Headache, dizziness, fatigue, weakness, muscle cramps or spasm, paresthesia, tension, anxiety, nervousness, agitation, vertigo, insomnia, mental depression, blurred vision, drowsiness. **CV:** Orthostatic hypotension, PVCs, dysrhythmias, flushing, palpitation. **GI:** Dry mouth, anorexia, nausea, vomiting, diarrhea, constipation, abdominal cramps or pain. **Urogenital:** Urinary frequency, nocturia, polyuria, glycosuria, impotence or reduced libido. **Skin:** Rash, hives, pruritus, vasculitis, photosensitivity. **Metabolic:** Dilutional hyponatremia, *hyperuricemia,* exacerbation of gout; *hypokalemia,* hyperglycemia, hypochloremia, hypercalcemia, increased BUN or creatinine, weight loss, exacerbation of SLE; increased cholesterol.

DIAGNOSTIC TEST INTERFERENCE Since indapamide may cause hypercalcemia (and hypophosphatemia), it is generally withheld before tests for ***parathyroid function*** are performed.

INTERACTIONS Drug: Effects of **diazoxide** and indapamide intensified; increased risk of **digoxin** toxicity with hypokalemia; decreased renal **lithium** clearance may increase risk of lithium toxicity.

PHARMACOKINETICS Absorption: Readily absorbed from GI tract. **Peak:** 2–2.5 h. **Duration:** Up to 36 h. **Metabolism:** Metabolized in liver. **Elimination:** 60% excreted in urine; 16%–23% excreted in feces. **Half-Life:** 14–18 h.

NURSING IMPLICATIONS

Assessment & Drug Effects

- Monitor BP periodically throughout therapy.
- Lab tests: Obtain baseline and periodic BUN, serum creatinine, uric acid, blood glucose, serum electrolytes, and fluid balance.

- Monitor for digitalis toxicity with concurrent therapy.
- Note: Electrolyte imbalances may be clinically serious with protracted vomiting and diarrhea, excessive sweating, GI drainage, and paracentesis.
- Report promptly signs of hyponatremia or hypokalemia (see Appendix F).
- Monitor diabetics for loss of glycemic control.

Patient & Family Education

- Notify physician of decreased urine output, dizziness, weakness or muscle cramps, nausea, jaundice, or blurred vision.
- Take precautions from sun exposure because of risk of photosensitivity.
- Record weight at least every other day; inspect ankles and legs for edema. Report unexplained, progressive weight gain (e.g., 1–1.5 kg [2–3 lb] in 2–3 d).
- Do not breast feed while taking this drug without consulting physician.

INDINAVIR SULFATE

(in-din'a-vir)

Crixivan

Classifications: ANTIINFECTIVE; ANTIVIRAL AGENT; PROTEASE INHIBITOR

Prototype: Saquinavir

Pregnancy Category: C

AVAILABILITY 100 mg, 200 mg, 333 mg, 400 mg capsules

ACTIONS Indinavir is an HIV protease inhibitor. HIV protease is an enzyme required to produce the polyprotein precursors of the functional proteins in infectious HIV.

THERAPEUTIC EFFECTS Protease inhibitors prevent cleavage of the HIV viral polyproteins, resulting in formation of immature noninfectious virus particles. Indinavir binds to the protease active site and thus inhibits activity of the enzyme.

USES Treatment of HIV infection, usually in combination with other antiretroviral agents or protease inhibitors.

CONTRAINDICATIONS Hypersensitivity to indinavir; pregnancy (category C), lactation.

CAUTIOUS USE Hepatic dysfunction, renal impairment, history of nephrolithiasis, history of adverse responses to other protease inhibitors. Safety and efficacy in children are not established.

ROUTE & DOSAGE

HIV

Adult: **PO** 800 mg (2 × 400 mg) q8h 1 h before or 2 h after meal

ADMINISTRATION

Oral

- Give with water on an empty stomach 1 h before or 2 h after meal; if needed, may be given with a very light meal or beverage.
- Note: When didanosine and indinavir are ordered concurrently, give each on empty stomach at least 1 h apart.
- Do not administer concurrently with astemizole, cisapride, midazolam, terfenadine, or triazolam.
- Store tightly closed with desiccant in original bottle.

ADVERSE EFFECTS (≥1%) **CNS:** Fatigue, headache, insomnia, dizziness, somnolence, nervousness, agitation, anxiety, paresthesia, peripheral neuropathy, tremor, vertigo. **CV:** Palpitations. **Hematologic:** Anemia, splenomegaly, lymphadenopathy. **GI:** *Nausea,* diarrhea, abdominal discomfort, dyspepsia, stomatitis, anorexia, dry mouth, cholecystitis, cholestasis, constipation, flatulence. **Skin:** Body odor, rash, pruritus, seborrhea, skin ulceration, dry skin, sweating, urticaria. **Other:** Myalgia, allergic reaction, bronchitis, cough, rhinitis, taste alterations, visual disturbances, hyperglycemia, diabetes, kidney stones.

INTERACTIONS Drug: Rifabutin, rifampin significantly decrease indinavir levels. **Ketoconazole** significantly increases indinavir levels. Indinavir could inhibit the metabolism and increase the toxicity of **astemizole, cisapride, midazolam, sildenafil, tadalafil, terfenadine, trazodone, triazolam, vardenafil.** Indinavir and **didanosine** should be administered at least 1 h apart on empty stomach to permit full absorption of each; increased ergotamine toxicity with indinavir. **Herbal: St. John's wort** decreases antiretroviral activity of indinavir.

PHARMACOKINETICS Absorption: Rapidly absorbed from GI tract; a meal high in calories, fat, and protein significantly reduces absorption. **Distribution:** 60% protein bound. **Metabolism:** Metabolized in liver by cytochrome P4503A4 (CYP3A4). **Elimination:** Excreted primarily in feces (>80%), 20% excreted in urine.

NURSING IMPLICATIONS

Assessment & Drug Effects

- Lab tests: Monitor CBC with differential and platelet count, liver function tests, CPK, urinalysis, and serum amylase periodically.
- Assess for S&S of renal dysfunction, respiratory dysfunction, GI distress, and other common adverse effects.

Patient & Family Education

- Learn drug interactions and potential adverse reactions. Drink plenty of liquid to minimize risk of renal stones.
- Notify physician of flank pain, hematuria, S&S of jaundice, or other distressing adverse effects.
- Do not breast feed while taking this drug.

INDOMETHACIN

(in-doe-meth'a-sin)

Indameth, Indocid ♣, Indocin, Indocin SR

Classifications: CENTRAL NERVOUS SYSTEM AGENT; ANALGESIC, ANTIPYRETIC; NSAID

Prototype: Ibuprofen

Pregnancy Category: B (D in third trimester)

AVAILABILITY 25 mg, 50 mg capsules; 75 mg sustained release capsules; 25 mg/5 mL oral suspension; 50 mg suppositories; 1 mg injection

ACTIONS Potent nonsteroidal compound with antiinflammatory, analgesic, and antipyretic effects similar to those of aspirin. Appears to reduce motility of polymorphonuclear leukocytes, development of cellular exudates, and vascular permeability in injured tissue resulting in its antiinflammatory effects.

THERAPEUTIC EFFECTS Antipyretic and antiinflammatory actions may be related to its ability to inhibit prostaglandin biosynthesis. It is a potent analgesic.

USES Palliative treatment in active stages of moderate to severe rheumatoid arthritis, ankylosing rheumatoid spondylitis, acute gouty arthritis, and osteoarthritis of hip in patients intolerant to or unresponsive to adequate trials with salicyl-

I

ates and other therapy. Also used IV to close patent ductus arteriosus in the premature infant.
UNLABELED USES To relieve biliary pain and dysmenorrhea, Paget's disease, athletic injuries, juvenile arthritis, idiopathic pericarditis.

CONTRAINDICATIONS Allergy to indomethacin, aspirin, or other NSAID; nasal polyps associated with angioedema, history of GI lesions; pregnancy (category B; D in third trimester), lactation, children (≤14 y).
CAUTIOUS USE History of psychiatric illness, epilepsy, parkinsonism; impaired renal or hepatic function; uncontrolled infections; coagulation defects, CHF; older adults, persons in hazardous occupations.

I

ROUTE & DOSAGE

Rheumatoid Arthritis

Adult: **PO** 25–50 mg b.i.d or t.i.d. (max: 200 mg/d) or 75 mg sustained release 1–2 times/d

Pediatric Arthritis

Child: **PO** 1–2 mg/kg/d in 2–4 divided doses (max: 4 mg/kg/d) or 150–200 mg/d

Acute Gouty Arthritis

Adult: **PO/PR** 50 mg t.i.d. until pain is tolerable, then rapidly taper

Bursitis

Adult: **PO** 25–50 mg t.i.d. or q.i.d. (max: 200 mg/d) or 75 mg sustained release 1–2 times/d

Close Patent Ductus Arteriosus

Premature neonate: **IV** *<48 h,* 0.2 mg/kg followed by 2 doses of 0.1 mg/kg q12–24h; *2–7 d,* 0.2 mg/kg followed by 2 doses of 0.2 mg/kg q12–24h; *<7 d,* 0.2 mg/kg followed by 2 doses of 0.25 mg/kg q12–24h

ADMINISTRATION

Oral

- Give immediately after meals, or with food, milk, or antacid (if prescribed) to minimize GI side effects.

Rectal

- Indomethacin rectal suppository use is contraindicated with history of proctitis or recent bleeding.

Intravenous

PREPARE: **Direct:** Dilute 1 mg with 1 mL of NS or sterile water for injection without preservatives. Resulting concentration (1 mg/mL) may be further diluted with an additional 1 mL for each 1 mg to yield 0.5 mg/mL.

ADMINISTER: **Direct:** Give by direct IV with a single dose given over 5–10 s. ▪ Avoid extravasation or leakage; drug can be irritating to tissue. ▪ Discard any unused drug, since it contains no preservative.

- Store oral and rectal forms in tight, light-resistant containers unless otherwise directed. Do not freeze.

ADVERSE EFFECTS (≥1%) **Body as a Whole:** Hypersensitivity (rash, purpura, pruritus, urticaria, angioedema, angiitis, rapid fall in blood pressure, dyspnea, asthma syndrome in aspirin-sensitive patients), edema, weight gain, flushing, sweating. **CNS:** Headache, *dizziness,* vertigo, light-headedness, syncope, fatigue, muscle weakness, ataxia, insomnia, nightmares, drowsiness, confusion, coma, convulsions, peripheral neuropathy, psychic disturbances (hallucinations, depersonalization, depression), aggravation of epilepsy, parkinsonism. **CV:** Elevated BP, palpitation, chest pains, tachycardia, bradycardia, CHF. **Special Senses:** Blurred vision, lacrimation, eye pain, visual field changes, corneal deposits, retinal disturbances including macula, *tinnitus,* hearing disturbances, epistaxis. **GI:** *Nausea, vomiting,* diarrhea, anorexia, bloating, abdominal distention, ulcerative stomatitis, proctitis, rectal bleeding, GI ulceration, hemorrhage, perforation, toxic hepatitis. **Hematologic:** Hemolytic anemia, aplastic anemia (sometimes fatal), agranulocytosis, leukopenia, thrombocytopenic purpura, inhibited platelet aggregation. **Urogenital:** Renal function impairment, hematuria, urinary frequency; vaginal bleeding, breast changes. **Skin:** Hair loss, exfoliative dermatitis, erythema nodosum, tissue irritation with extravasation. **Metabolic:** Hyponatremia, hypokalemia, hyperkalemia, hypoglycemia or hyperglycemia, glycosuria (rare).

DIAGNOSTIC TEST INTERFERENCE Increased ***AST, ALT, bilirubin, BUN;*** positive direct ***Coombs' test.***

INTERACTIONS Drug: ORAL ANTICOAGULANTS, **heparin, alcohol** may prolong bleeding time; may increase **lithium** toxicity; effects of ORAL ANTICOAGULANTS, **phenytoin,** SALICYLATES, SULFONAMIDES, SULFONYLUREAS increased because of protein-binding displacement; increased toxicity including GI bleeding with SALICYLATES, NSAIDS; may blunt effects of ANTIHYPERTENSIVES and DIURETICS. **Herbal: Feverfew, garlic, ginger, ginkgo** may increase bleeding potential.

PHARMACOKINETICS Absorption: Completely absorbed from GI tract. **Onset:** 1–2 h. **Peak:** 3 h. **Duration:** 4–6 h. **Metabolism:** Metabolized in liver. **Elimination:** Excreted primarily in urine. **Half-Life:** 2.5–124 h.

NURSING IMPLICATIONS

Assessment & Drug Effects

- Monitor for therapeutic effectiveness: In acute gouty attack, relief of joint tenderness and pain is usually apparent in 24–36 h; swelling generally disappears in 3–5 d. In rheumatoid arthritis: Reduced fever, increased strength, reduced stiffness, and relief of pain, swelling, and tenderness.
- Question patient carefully regarding aspirin sensitivity before initiation of therapy.
- Observe patients carefully; instruct to report adverse reactions promptly to prevent serious and sometimes irreversible or fatal effects.
- Lab tests: Monitor renal function, hepatic function, CBC with differential, BP and HR, visual and hearing acuity periodically.
- Monitor weight and observe dependent areas for signs of edema in patients with underlying cardiovascular disease.
- Monitor I&O closely and keep physician informed during IV administration for patent ductus arteriosus. Significant impairment of renal function is possible; urine output may decrease by 50% or more. Also monitor BUN, serum creatinine, glomerular filtration rate, creatinine clearance, and serum electrolytes.

Patient & Family Education

- Notify physician of S&S of GI bleeding, visual disturbance, tinnitus, weight gain, or edema.
- Do not take aspirin or other NSAIDS; they increase possibility of ulcers.
- Note: Frontal headache is the most frequent CNS adverse effect; if it persists, dosage reduction or drug withdrawal may be indicated. Take drug at bedtime

I

with milk to reduce the incidence of morning headache.
- Do not drive or engage in other potentially hazardous activities until response to drug is known.
- Do not breast feed while taking this drug.

INFLIXIMAB

(in-flix'i-mab)
Remicade
Classifications: BIOLOGIC RESPONSE MODIFIER; TUMOR NECROSIS FACTOR MODIFIER
Prototype: Etanercept
Pregnancy Category: B

I

AVAILABILITY 100 mg powder for injection

ACTIONS IgG_1-K monoclonal antibody that binds specifically to tumor necrosis factor-alpha (TNF-alpha), a cytokine. Thus, it prevents TNF-alpha from binding to its receptors. TNF-alpha induces proinflammatory cytokines such as interleukin-1 (IL-1) and IL-6.
THERAPEUTIC EFFECTS Treatment with infliximab reduces infiltration of inflammatory cells and TNF-alpha production in inflamed areas of the intestine. Elevated concentrations of TNF-alpha have been found in the stools of Crohn's disease patients and correlated with disease activity.

USES Moderately to severely active Crohn's disease, including fistulizing Crohn's disease, rheumatoid arthritis.

CONTRAINDICATIONS Hypersensitivity to infliximab; CHF; infection, sepsis; murine protein hypersensitivity; lactation.
CAUTIOUS USE History of allergic phenomena or untoward responses to monoclonal antibody preparation; renal or hepatic impairment; multiple sclerosis (potential exacerbation); fungal infection; heart failure, human antichimeric antibody (HACA); leukopenia, thrombocytopenia; immunosuppressed patients; neoplastic disease; tuberculosis; vaccination; vasculitis; neurological disease; neutropenia; seizure disorder, seizures; older adults; pregnancy (category B). Safety and effectiveness in pediatric patients are not established.

ROUTE & DOSAGE

Crohn's Disease
Adult: **IV** 5 mg/kg infused over at least 2 h, may repeat at 2 and 6 wk for fistulizing disease
Rheumatoid Arthritis
Adult: **IV** 3 mg/kg infused over at least 2 h, followed by 2 mg/kg on weeks 2 and 6, then 2 mg/kg q8wk

ADMINISTRATION

Note: Do not administer to a patient who has known or suspected sepsis.

Intravenous

PREPARE: **IV Infusion:** Reconstitute each vial with 10 mL of sterile water for injection using a 21-gauge or smaller syringe. Inject sterile water against wall of vial, then gently swirl to dissolve but do not shake. ▪ Let stand for 5 min. ▪ Solution should be colorless to light yellow with a few translucent particles. Discard if particles are opaque. ▪ Further dilute by first removing from a 250-mL IV bag of NS a volume of NS equal to the volume of reconstituted infliximab to be added to the IV bag. Slowly add the total volume of reconstituted infliximab solution to the 250-mL infusion bag and gently mix. ▪ Infusion concentration should be 0.4 to 4 mg/mL. ▪ Begin infusion within 3 h of preparation.

ADMINISTER: **IV Infusion:** Give over at least 2 h using a polyethylene-lined infusion set with an in-line, low-protein-binding filter (pore size 1.2 micron or less). ▪ Infliximab is INCOMPATIBLE with PVC equipment or devices. ▪ Discard unused infusion solution.

INCOMPATIBILITIES **Solution/additive:** Incompatible with PVC bags and tubing. **Y-site:** Do not infuse with any other drugs.

▪ Store unopened vials at 2°–8° C (36°–46° F).

ADVERSE EFFECTS (≥1%) **Body as a Whole:** Fatigue, fever, pain, myalgia, back pain, chills, hot flashes, arthralgia; infusion-related reactions (fever, chills, pruritus, urticaria, chest pain, hypotension, hypertension, dyspnea). Increased risk of opportunistic infections, including tuberculosis. **CNS:** Headache, dizziness, involuntary muscle contractions, paresthesias, vertigo, anxiety, depression, insomnia. **CV:** Chest pain, peripheral edema, hypotension, hypertension, tachycardia, anemia, CHF, pericardial effusion, systemic and cutaneous vasculitis. **GI:** Nausea, diarrhea, abdominal pain, vomiting, constipation, dyspepsia, flatulence, intestinal obstruction, ulcerative stomatitis, increased hepatic enzymes. **Hematologic:** Leukopenia, neutropenia, thrombocytopenia, pancytopenia. **Respiratory:** URI, pharyngitis, bronchitis, rhinitis, coughing, sinusitis, dyspnea. **Skin:** Rash, pruritus, acne, alopecia, fungal dermatitis, eczema, dry skin, increased sweating, urticaria. **Other:** Infections, development of autoantibodies, lupus-like syndrome, conjunctivitis, dysuria, urinary frequency.

INTERACTIONS Drug: May blunt effectiveness of VACCINES given concurrently.

PHARMACOKINETICS Distribution: Distributed primarily to the vascular compartment. **Half-Life:** 9.5 d.

NURSING IMPLICATIONS

Assessment & Drug Effects

- Discontinue IV infusion and notify physician for fever, chills, pruritus, urticaria, chest pain, dyspnea, hypo/hypertension.
- Monitor for and immediately report S&S of local IV site or more generalized infection.

Patient & Family Education

- Report any infection to your physician promptly.
- Do not breast feed while taking this drug.

INSULIN ASPART

(in′su-lyn)

NovoLog

Classifications: HORMONE AND SYNTHETIC SUBSTITUTE; ANTIDIABETIC AGENT; INSULIN

Prototype: Insulin Injection

Pregnancy Category: C

AVAILABILITY 100 U/mL injection

ACTIONS A recombinant insulin analog that is more rapidly absorbed than human insulin, with a more rapid onset and shorter duration than regular human insulin.

THERAPEUTIC EFFECTS Provides better blood glucose control than regular human insulin when given before a meal.

USES Treatment of diabetes mellitus.

CONTRAINDICATIONS Systemic allergic reactions; history of allergic reactions to insulin; hypoglycemia; pregnancy (category C).

CAUTIOUS USE Fever, hyperthyroidism, surgery or trauma; decreased insulin requirements due to diarrhea, nausea, or vomiting, malabsorption; renal or hepatic impairment, hypokalemia; lactation.

ROUTE & DOSAGE

Diabetes

Adult: **SC** 0.25–0.7 units/kg/d injected 5–10 min before each meal

ADMINISTRATION

Subcutaneous

- Note: Must give 5–10 min before a meal.
- Draw up insulin aspart first when mixing with NPH insulin. Give injection immediately after it is mixed. Do not give NPH mixture by IV.
- Store refrigerated at 2°–8° C (36°–46° F); may be stored at room temperature, 15°–30° C (59°–86° F) for up to 28 d. Do not expose to excessive heat or sunlight, and do not freeze.

ADVERSE EFFECTS (≥1%) **Body as a Whole:** Allergic reactions. **Endocrine:** Hypoglycemia, hypokalemia. **Skin:** Injection site reaction, lipodystrophy, pruritus, rash.

INTERACTIONS Drug: ORAL ANTIDIABETIC AGENTS, ACE INHIBITORS, **disopyramide, fluoxetine,** MAO INHIBITORS, **propoxyphene,** SALICYLATES, SULFONAMIDE ANTIBIOTICS, **octreotide** may enhance hypoglycemia; CORTICOSTEROIDS, **niacin, danazol,** DIURETICS, SYMPATHOMIMETIC AGENTS, PHENOTHIAZINES, THYROID HORMONES, ESTROGENS, PROGESTOGENS, **isoniazid, somatropin** my decrease hypoglycemic effects; BETA-BLOCKERS, **clonidine, lithium, alcohol** may either potentiate or weaken effects of insulin; **pentamidine** may cause hypoglycemia followed by hyperglycemia. **Herbal: Garlic, ginseng** may potentiate hypoglycemic effects.

PHARMACOKINETICS Absorption: Rapidly absorbed from SC injection site. **Onset:** 15 min. **Peak:** 40–50 min. **Duration:** 3–5 h. **Distribution:** Low protein binding. **Metabolism:** Metabolized primarily in liver with some metabolism in the kidneys. **Half-Life:** 81 min.

NURSING IMPLICATIONS

Assessment & Drug Effects

- Monitor for S&S of hypoglycemia (see Appendix F). Initial hypoglycemic response begins within 15 min and peaks 45–90 min after injection.
- Lab tests: Periodically monitor fasting blood glucose and HbA_{1C}.
- Withhold drug and notify physician if patient is hypokalemic.

Patient & Family Education

- Do not inject into areas with redness, swelling, itching, or dimpling.
- Ingest some form of sugar (e.g., orange juice, dissolved table sugar, honey) if symptoms of hypoglycemia develop, and seek medical assistance.
- Check blood sugar as prescribed, especially postprandial values; notify physician of fasting blood glucose <80 and >120 mg/dL.
- Notify the physician of any of the following: Fever, infection, trauma, diarrhea, nausea or vomiting. Dosage adjustment may be needed.
- Do not take any other medication unless approved by the physician.

- Do not breast feed while taking this drug without consulting physician.

INSULIN GLARGINE

(in'su-lin glar'geen)

Lantus

Classifications: HORMONES & SYNTHETIC SUBSTITUTES; ANTIDIABETIC AGENT; INSULIN

Prototype: Insulin Injection

Pregnancy Category: C

AVAILABILITY 100 U/mL injection; 3 mL cartridge

ACTIONS A recombinant human insulin analog with a long duration of action. Enhances transmembrane passage of glucose across cell membranes.

THERAPEUTIC EFFECTS Lowers blood glucose levels over an extended period of time by stimulating peripheral glucose uptake especially in muscle and fat tissue. In addition, insulin inhibits hepatic glucose production.

USES Bedtime dosing of adults and children with type 1 diabetes, or adults with type 2 diabetes.

CONTRAINDICATIONS Prior hypersensitivity to insulin glargine; hypoglycemia.

CAUTIOUS USE Renal and hepatic impairment; pregnancy (category C), lactation; safety and efficacy in children <6 y of age are not established.

ROUTE & DOSAGE

Type 1 Diabetes

Adult/Child: **SC** If not taking insulin, give 10 U at same time each day (usually at bedtime) once daily; if taking NPH or ultralente insulin once daily, give same dose at same time each day (usually at bedtime); if taking NPH insulin twice daily, give 80% of total daily dose at same time each day (usually at bedtime)

Type 2 Diabetes

Adult: **SC** If already taking oral hypoglycemic drugs, start with 10 U at same time each day (usually at bedtime) once daily and adjust according to patient's needs

ADMINISTRATION

Subcutaneous

- Do not give this product IV.
- Give at same time each day (usually at bedtime) and do not mix with any other insulin product.
- Store in refrigerator at 2°–8° C (36°–46° F), may store at room temperature, 15°–30° C (59°–86° F). Discard opened refrigerated vials after 28 d and unrefrigerated vials after 14 d. Do not expose to excessive heat or sunlight, and do not freeze.

ADVERSE EFFECTS (≥1%) **Body as a Whole:** Allergic reactions. **Endocrine:** Hypoglycemia, hypokalemia. **Skin:** Injection site reaction, lipodystrophy, pruritus, rash.

INTERACTIONS Drug: ORAL ANTIDIABETIC AGENTS, ACE INHIBITORS, **disopyramide, fluoxetine,** MAO INHIBITORS, **propoxyphene,** SALICYLATES, SULFONAMIDE ANTIBIOTICS, **octreotide** may enhance hypoglycemia; CORTICOSTEROIDS, **niacin, danazol,** DIURETICS, SYMPATHOMIMETIC AGENTS, PHENOTHIAZINES, THYROID HORMONES, ESTROGENS, PROGESTOGENS, **isoniazid, somatropin** may decrease hypoglycemic effects; BETA-BLOCKERS, **clonidine, lithium, alcohol** may either potentiate or weaken effects of insulin; **pentamidine** may cause hypoglycemia followed by hyperglycemia. **Herbal: Garlic, ginseng** may potentiate hypoglycemic effects.

PHARMACOKINETICS Absorption: Slowly absorbed from SC injection site. **Duration:** 10.4–24 h. **Metabolism:** Metabolized primarily in liver to active metabolites.

NURSING IMPLICATIONS

Assessment & Drug Effects

- Monitor for S&S of hypoglycemia (see Appendix F), especially after changes in insulin dose or type.
- Lab tests: Monitor fasting blood glucose and HbA_{1C} periodically.
- Withhold drug and notify physician if patient is hypokalemic.

Patient & Family Education

- Do not inject into areas with redness, swelling, itching, or dimpling.
- Absorption patterns for this drug are not dependent on the injection site.
- Ingest some form of sugar (e.g., orange juice, dissolved table sugar, honey) if symptoms of hypoglycemia develop; and seek medical assistance.
- Check blood sugar as prescribed; notify physician of fasting blood glucose <80 and >120 mg/dL.
- Notify the physician of any of the following: fever, infection, trauma, diarrhea, nausea, or vomiting. Dosage adjustment may be needed.
- Do not take any other medication unless approved by physician.
- Do not breast feed while taking this drug without consulting physician.

INSULIN GLULISINE

(in′su-lin glu-li′seen)

Apidra

Classifications: HORMONES & SYNTHETIC SUBSTITUTES; ANTIDIABETIC AGENT; INSULIN

Prototype: Insulin Injection (Regular)

Pregnancy Category: C

AVAILABILITY 100 units/mL multidose (10 mL) vials

ACTIONS Insulin glulisine, formed by recombinant DNA, is a rapid-acting insulin. Insulin lowers blood glucose by stimulating peripheral glucose uptake by skeletal muscle and fat and by inhibiting hepatic glucose production. Insulin causes lipolysis in the adipocyte, inhibits proteolysis, and enhances protein synthesis.

THERAPEUTIC EFFECTS Insulin glulisine has a more rapid onset of action and a shorter duration of action than regular human insulin; thus, it provides good postprandial blood glucose control.

USES Treatment of diabetes mellitus.

CONTRAINDICATIONS Hypoglycemia; systemic allergy to insulin; pregnancy (category C). Safety and effectiveness in children <18 y have not been established.

CAUTIOUS USE Renal impairment, hepatic dysfunction; lactation.

ROUTE & DOSAGE

Diabetes

Adult: **SC** 5–10 units within 15 min before starting a meal or within 20 min after starting a meal. Dose should be individualized.

ADMINISTRATION

Subcutaneous

- Give within 15 min before or up to 20 min after a meal.
- Store refrigerated at 36° F to 46° F (2° C to 8° C). Discard vial if frozen. Protect from light.

ADVERSE EFFECTS (≥1%) [see INSULIN (REGULAR)] **Body as a Whole:** Allergic reactions. **Metabolic:** Hypoglycemia. **Skin:** Injection site reactions, lipodystrophy, pruritus, rash.

DIAGNOSTIC TEST INTERFERENCE See Insulin Injection (Regular)

PHARMACOKINETICS Absorption: 70% bioavailable from injection sites. **Peak:** 55 min. **Duration:** 140–150 min. **Metabolism:** Metabolized primarily in liver with some metabolism in the kidney. **Half-Life:** 42 min SC.

NURSING IMPLICATIONS

Assessment & Drug Effects

- Monitor for S&S of hypoglycemia (see Appendix F). Initial hypoglycemic response begins within 15 min and peaks, on average, 40–60 min after injection.
- Lab tests: Periodically monitor fasting and postprandial blood glucose and HbA_{1C}.

Patient & Family Education

- Do not inject into areas with redness, swelling, itching, or dimpling.
- If mixing with NPH human insulin, draw up insulin glulisine first. Inject immediately after mixing.
- Ingest some form of sugar (e.g., orange juice, dissolved table sugar, honey) if symptoms of hypoglycemia develop, and seek medical assistance.
- Check blood sugar as prescribed, especially postprandial values; notify physician of fasting blood glucose <80 and >140 mg/dL.
- Notify the physician of any of the following: fever, infection, trauma, diarrhea, nausea, or vomiting. Dosage adjustment may be needed.
- Do not take any other medication unless approved by the physician.
- Do not breast feed while taking this drug without consulting physician.

INSULIN (REGULAR) Ⓟ

(in′su-lin)

Humulin R, Novolin R, Regular Insulin, Pork Regular Iletin II, Regular Purified Pork Insulin, Velosulin, Velosulin BR, Velosulin Human

Classifications: HORMONE AND SYNTHETIC SUBSTITUTE; ANTIDIABETIC AGENT; INSULIN

Pregnancy Category: B

AVAILABILITY 100 units/mL

ACTIONS Short-acting, clear, colorless solution of exogenous unmodified insulin extracted from beta cells in pork pancreas or synthesized by recombinant DNA technology (human). Enhances transmembrane passage of glucose across cell membranes of most body cells and by unknown mechanism may itself enter the cell to activate selected intermediary metabolic processes. Promotes conversion of glucose to glycogen.

THERAPEUTIC EFFECTS It lowers blood glucose levels by increasing peripheral glucose uptake, especially by skeletal muscle and fat tissue, and by inhibiting the liver from changing glycogen to glucose.

USES Emergency treatment of diabetic ketoacidosis or coma, to initiate therapy in patient with insulin-dependent diabetes mellitus, and in

I

combination with intermediate-acting or long-acting insulin to provide better control of blood glucose concentrations in the diabetic patient. Used IV to stimulate growth hormone secretion (glucose counter regulatory hormone) to evaluate pituitary growth hormone reserve in patient with known or suspected growth hormone deficiency. Other uses include promotion of intracellular shift of potassium in treatment of hyperkalemia (IV) and induction of hypoglycemic shock as therapy in psychiatry.

CONTRAINDICATIONS Hypersensitivity to insulin animal protein.

CAUTIOUS USE Pregnancy (category B), lactation, renal impairment, hepatic impairment, and older adults. Safety and efficacy in children <2 y are not established.

ROUTE & DOSAGE

Diabetes Mellitus

Adult: **SC** 5–10 U 15–30 min a.c. and h.s. (dose adjustments based on blood glucose determinations)
Child: **SC** 2–4 U 15–30 min a.c. and h.s. (dose adjustments based on blood glucose determinations)

Ketoacidosis

Adult: **IV** 2.4–7.2 U loading dose, followed by 2.4–7.2 U/h continuous infusion
Child: **IV** 0.1 U/kg loading dose, followed by 0.1 U/h continuous infusion

ADMINISTRATION

Note: Insulins should not be mixed unless prescribed by physician. In general, regular insulin is drawn up into syringe first. Any change in the strength (e.g., U-40, U-100), brand (manufacturer), purity, type (regular, etc.), species (pork, human), or sequence of mixing two kids of insulin is made by the physician only, since a simultaneous change in dosage may be necessary.

Subcutaneous

- Use an insulin syringe.
- Give regular insulin 30 min before a meal.
- Avoid injection of cold insulin; it can lead to lipodystrophy, reduced rate of absorption, and local reactions.
- Common injection sites: Upper arms, thighs, abdomen (avoid area over urinary bladder and 2 in. [5 cm] around navel), buttocks, and upper back (if fat is loose enough to pick up). Rotate sites.

Intravenous

PREPARE: **Direct:** Give undiluted. **Continuous:** Typically diluted in NS or 0.45% NaCl. 100 U added to 1000 mL yields 0.1 U/mL.

ADMINISTER: **Direct:** Give 50 U or a fraction thereof over 1 min. **Continuous:** Rate must be ordered by physician.

INCOMPATIBILITIES **Solution/additive: Aminophylline, amobarbital, chlorothiazide, cytarabine, dobutamine, pentobarbital, phenobarbital, phenytoin, secobarbital, sodium bicarbonate, thiopental. Y-site: Dobutamine.**

- Regular insulin may be adsorbed into the container or tubing when added to an IV infusion solution. Amount lost is variable and depends on concentration of insulin, infusion system, contact duration, and flow rate. ■ Monitor patient response closely.

- Insulin is stable at room temperature up to 1 mo. Avoid exposure to direct sunlight or to temperature extremes (safe range is wide:

5°–38° C [40°–100° F]). Refrigerate but do not freeze stock supply. Insulin tolerates temperatures above 38° C with less harm than freezing.

ADVERSE EFFECTS (≥1%) **Body as a Whole:** Most adverse effects are related to hypoglycemia; anaphylaxis (rare), hyperinsulinemia [*Profuse sweating,* hunger, headache, *nausea, tremulousness,* tremors, *palpitation,* tachycardia, weakness, fatigue, nystagmus, circumoral pallor; numb mouth, tongue, and other paresthesias; visual disturbances (diplopia, blurred vision, mydriasis), staring expression, confusion, personality changes, ataxia, incoherent speech, apprehension, irritability, inability to concentrate, personality changes, uncontrolled yawning, loss of consciousness, delirium, hypothermia, convulsions, Babinski reflex, coma. (Urine glucose tests will be negatives). **CNS:** With overdose, psychic disturbances (i.e., aphasia, personality changes, maniacal behavior). **Metabolic:** Posthypoglycemia or rebound hyperglycemia (Somogyi effect), lipoatrophy and lipohypertrophy of injection sites; insulin resistance. **Skin:** Localized allergic reactions at injection site; generalized urticaria or bullae, lymphadenopathy.

DIAGNOSTIC TEST INTERFERENCE Large doses of insulin may increase urinary excretion of ***VMA.*** Insulin can cause alterations in ***thyroid function tests*** and ***liver function test*** and may decrease ***serum potassium*** and ***serum calcium.***

INTERACTIONS Drug: Alcohol, ANABOLIC STEROIDS, MAO INHIBITORS, **guanethidine,** SALICYLATES may potentiate hypoglycemic effects; **dextrothyroxine,** CORTICOSTEROIDS, **epinephrine** may antagonize hypoglycemic effects; **furosemide,** THIAZIDE DIURETICS increase **serum glucose** levels; **propranolol** and other BETA BLOCKERS may mask symptoms of hypoglycemic reaction. **Herbal: Garlic, ginseng** may potentiate hypoglycemic effects.

PHARMACOKINETICS Absorption: Rapidly absorbed from IM and SC injections. **Onset:** 0.5–1 h. **Peak:** 2–3 h. **Duration:** 5–7 h. **Distribution:** Throughout extracellular fluids. **Metabolism:** Metabolized primarily in liver with some metabolism in kidneys. **Elimination:** <2% excreted in urine. **Half-Life:** Biological, up to 13 h.

NURSING IMPLICATIONS

Assessment & Drug Effects

- Note: Frequency of blood glucose monitoring is determined by the type of insulin regimen and health status of the patient.
- Lab tests: Periodic postprandial blood glucose, and HbA_{1C}. Test urine for ketones in new, unstable, and type 1 diabetes; if patient has lost weight, exercises vigorously, or has an illness; whenever blood glucose is substantially elevated.
- Notify physician promptly for presence of acetone with sugar in the urine; may indicate onset of ketoacidosis. Acetone without sugar in the urine usually signifies insufficient carbohydrate intake.
- Monitor for hypoglycemia (see Appendix F) at time of peak action of insulin. Onset of hypoglycemia (blood sugar: 50–40 mg/dL) may be rapid and sudden.
- Check BP, I&O ratio, and blood glucose and ketones every hour during treatment for ketoacidosis with IV insulin.
- Give patients with severe hypoglycemia glucagon, epinephrine, or IV glucose 10%–50%. As soon as patient is fully conscious, give oral

carbohydrate (e.g., dilute corn syrup or orange juice with sugar, Gatorade, or Pedialyte) to prevent secondary hypoglycemia.

Patient & Family Education

- Learn correct injection technique.
- Inject insulin into the abdomen rather than a near muscle that will be heavily taxed, if engaged in active sports.
- Notify physician of local reactions at injection site; may develop 1–3 wk after therapy starts and last several hours to days, usually disappear with continued use.
- Do not change prescription lenses during early period of dosage regulation; vision stabilizes, usually 3–6 wk.
- Note: Hypoglycemia can result from excess insulin, insufficient food intake, vomiting, diarrhea, unaccustomed exercise, infection, illness, nervous or emotional tension, or overindulgence in alcohol.
- Respond promptly to beginning symptoms of hypoglycemia. Severe hypoglycemia is an emergency situation. Take 4 oz (120 mL) of any fruit juice or regular carbonated beverage [1.5–3 oz (45–90 mL) for child] followed by a meal of longer-acting carbohydrate or protein food. Failure to show signs of recovery within 30 min indicates need for emergency treatment.
- Carry some form of fast-acting carbohydrate (e.g., lump sugar, Life-Savers or other candy) at all times to treat hypoglycemia.
- Check blood glucose regularly during menstrual period; loss of diabetes control (hyperglycemia or hypoglycemia) is common; adjust insulin dosage accordingly, as prescribed by physician.
- Notify physician of S&S of diabetic ketoacidosis.
- Continue taking insulin during an illness, go to bed, and drink noncaloric liquids liberally (every hour if possible). Consult physician for insulin regulation if unable to eat prescribed diet.
- Avoid OTC medications unless approved by physician.
- Do not breast feed while taking this drug without consulting physician.

INSULIN INJECTION CONCENTRATED

(in'su-lin)

Iletin II Regular (Concentrated), U-500

Classifications: HORMONE AND SYNTHETIC SUBSTITUTE; ANTIDIABETIC AGENT

Prototype: Insulin

Pregnancy Category: B

AVAILABILITY 500 units/mL

ACTIONS Concentrated insulin from purified pork pancreas unmodified by any agent that might prolong its action. Because of its high concentration, duration of action is similar to that of an intermediate-acting insulin.

THERAPEUTIC EFFECTS It lowers blood glucose levels by increasing peripheral glucose uptake, especially by skeletal muscle and fat tissue, and by inhibiting the liver from changing glycogen to glucose.

USES Only for the occasional patient who develops insulin resistance and requires daily doses greater than 200 U (even as high as several thousand units).

CONTRAINDICATIONS During episodes of hypoglycemia or in patients sensitive to any ingredient in the formulation.

CAUTIOUS USE In insulin resistant patients, hyperthyroidism or hypothyroidism; lactation, older adults, pregnancy (category B), renal or hepatic impairment. Safety and efficacy in children <12 y are not established.

ROUTE & DOSAGE

Diabetes Mellitus
Adult: **SC** Individualized doses (see INSULIN, REGULAR)

ADMINISTRATION

Subcutaneous
- Do NOT give this preparation by IV because of a high risk of allergic or anaphylactoid reaction.
- Use a tuberculin syringe for accuracy in measurement. Even a slight variation can cause a large overdose or underdose.
- Store in a cold place, preferably a refrigerator, unless otherwise directed. Avoid freezing.

INCOMPATIBILITIES **Solution/additive: Regular insulin with aminophylline, amobarbital, chlorothiazide, dobutamine, pentobarbital, phenobarbital, phenytoin, secobarbital, sodium bicarbonate, thiopental.**

ADVERSE EFFECTS (≥1%) (see INSULIN INJECTION, REGULAR).

INTERACTIONS (see INSULIN INJECTION, REGULAR).

PHARMACOKINETICS Onset: 0.5–1 h regular. **Peak:** 2–3 h regular. **Duration:** 5–7 h regular. **Metabolism:** Metabolized in liver and kidney. **Elimination:** <2% excreted unchanged in urine. **Half-Life:** Up to 13 h.

NURSING IMPLICATIONS

(see INSULIN INJECTION, REGULAR)

Assessment & Drug Effects
- Keep patients receiving concentrated insulin under close surveillance until dosage is established. Close monitoring for symptoms of hypoglycemia, hyperglycemia, allergic or anaphylactoid reactions, and of water and electrolyte imbalance is essential.
- Have on hand glucagon, IV dextrose, epinephrine. Severe secondary hypoglycemia reactions may develop 18–24 h after administration of drug.

Patient & Family Education
- Be alert for and immediately report S&S of severe hypoglycemia, which may develop up to 24 h after administration of drug.
- Note: Responsiveness to insulin effect is frequently regained after a short period of therapy with concentrated insulin.
- Do not breast feed while taking this drug without consulting physician.

INSULIN, ISOPHANE (NPH)

(in'su-lin)

Humulin N, Iletin II (pork), Insulatard NPH, Mixtard, Novolin 70/30, Novolin

Classifications: HORMONE AND SYNTHETIC SUBSTITUTE; ANTIDIABETIC AGENT

Prototype: Insulin

Pregnancy Category: B

AVAILABILITY 100 units/mL

ACTIONS Intermediate-acting, cloudy suspension of zinc insulin crystals modified by protamine in a neutral buffer. NPH Iletin II (pork), and Insulatard NPH are "purified" or "single component" insulins that have been purified and are less likely to cause allergic reactions than nonpurified preparations.

THERAPEUTIC EFFECTS Lowers blood glucose levels by increasing peripheral glucose uptake, especially by skeletal muscle and fat tissue, and by inhibiting the liver from changing glycogen to glucose. Therapeutic effect controls postprandial hyperglycemia, usually without supplemental doses of insulin injection.

USES Used to control hyperglycemia in the diabetic patient. Mixtard and Novolin 70/30 are fixed combinations of purified regular insulin 30% and NPH 70%.

CONTRAINDICATIONS During episodes of hypoglycemia or in patients sensitive to any ingredient in the formulation.

CAUTIOUS USE In insulin resistant patients, hyperthyroidism or hypothyroidism; lactation, older adults, pregnancy (category B), renal or hepatic impairment. Safety and efficacy in children <3 y are not established.

ROUTE & DOSAGE

Diabetes Mellitus

Adult: **SC** Individualized doses (see INSULIN, REGULAR)

ADMINISTRATION

Subcutaneous

- Give isophane insulin 30 min before first meal of the day. If necessary, a second smaller dose may be prescribed 30 min before supper or at bedtime.
- Ensure complete dispersion by mixing thoroughly by gently rotating vial between palms and inverting it end to end several times. Do not shake.
- Do NOT mix insulins unless prescribed by physician. In general, when insulin injection (regular insulin) is to be combined, it is drawn first.
- Note: Isophane insulin may be mixed with insulin injection without altering either solution. Do NOT mix with Lente forms.
- Store unopened vial at 2°–8° C (36°–46° F). Avoid freezing and exposure to extremes in temperature or to direct sunlight.

ADVERSE EFFECTS (≥1%) (see INSULIN, REGULAR).

INTERACTIONS (see INSULIN, REGULAR).

PHARMACOKINETICS **Onset:** 1–2 h. **Peak:** 4–12 h NPH. **Duration:** 18–24 h NPH. **Metabolism:** Metabolized in liver and kidney. **Elimination:** <2% excreted unchanged in urine. **Half-Life:** up to 13 h.

NURSING IMPLICATIONS

(see INSULIN, REGULAR)

Assessment & Drug Effects

- Suspect hypoglycemia if fatigue, weakness, sweating, tremor, or nervousness occur.

Patient & Family Education

- If insulin was given before breakfast, a hypoglycemic episode is most likely to occur between mid-afternoon and dinnertime, when insulin effect is peaking. Advise to eat a snack in mid-afternoon and to carry sugar or candy to treat a reaction. A snack at bedtime will prevent insulin reaction during the night.
- Learn the S&S of hypoglycemia and hyperglycemia (see Appendix F).
- Do not breast feed while taking this drug without consulting physician.

INSULIN LISPRO

(in'su-lin lis'pro)

Humalog

Classifications: HORMONE AND SYNTHETIC SUBSTITUTE; ANTIDIABETIC AGENT

Prototype: Insulin Injection

Pregnancy Category: B

AVAILABILITY 100 units/mL

ACTIONS Insulin lispro of recombinant DNA origin is a human insulin that is a rapid-acting, glucose-lowering agent.

THERAPEUTIC EFFECTS It lowers blood glucose levels by increasing peripheral glucose uptake, especially by skeletal muscle and fat tissue, and by inhibiting the liver from changing glycogen to glucose. One unit of insulin lispro has the same glucose-lowering ability as human regular insulin, but the effect is more rapid and of shorter duration.

USES Treatment of diabetes mellitus.

CONTRAINDICATIONS During episodes of hypoglycemia or in patients sensitive to any ingredient in the formulation.

CAUTIOUS USE In insulin resistant patients, hyperthyroidism or hypothyroidism; lactation, older adults, pregnancy (category B), renal or hepatic impairment. Safety and efficacy in children <3 y are not established.

ROUTE & DOSAGE

Diabetes Mellitus (type 1)

Adult: **SC** 5–10 U 0–15 min a.c. (dose adjustments based on blood glucose determinations)

ADMINISTRATION

Subcutaneous

- Give 0–15 min before meals.
- Note: May be given in same syringe with longer-acting insulins but absorption may be delayed.

ADVERSE EFFECTS (≥1%) (see INSULIN INJECTIONS, REGULAR).

INTERACTIONS (see INSULIN INJECTION, REGULAR).

PHARMACOKINETICS Absorption: Rapidly absorbed from IM and SC injection sites. **Onset:** <15 min. **Peak:** 0.5–1 h. **Duration:** 3–4 h. **Distribution:** Throughout extracellular fluids. **Metabolism:** Metabolized in liver with some metabolism in kidneys. **Elimination:** <2% excreted in urine. **Half-Life:** Biological, up to 13 h.

NURSING IMPLICATIONS

(see INSULIN INJECTION, REGULAR)

Assessment & Drug Effects

- Assess for hypoglycemia from 1 to 3 h after injection.
- Assess highly insulin-dependent patients for need for increases in intermediate/long-acting insulins.

Patient & Family Education

- Note: Risk of hypoglycemia is greatest 1–3 h after injection.
- Do not breast feed while taking this drug without consulting physician.

INSULIN, PROTAMINE ZINC (PZI)

(in'su-lin)

Iletin II

Classifications: HORMONE AND SYNTHETIC SUBSTITUTE; ANTIDIABETIC AGENT

Prototype: Insulin Injection

Pregnancy Category: B

AVAILABILITY 100 units/mL

ACTIONS Long-acting, cloudy suspension of insulin modified by addition of zinc chloride and protamine sulfate, which has poor solubility and thus delays absorption. It is derived from pork pancreas.

THERAPEUTIC EFFECTS Iletin II lowers blood glucose levels by increasing peripheral glucose uptake, especially by skeletal muscle and fat tissue, and by inhibiting the liver from changing glycogen to glucose. May be used in combination with a shorter acting form.

USES Diabetes mellitus in patients who are not adequately controlled by unmodified insulin.

CONTRAINDICATIONS During episodes of hypoglycemia or in patients sensitive to any ingredient in the formulation.

CAUTIOUS USE In insulin resistant patients, hyperthyroidism or hypothyroidism; lactation, older adults, pregnancy (category B), renal or hepatic impairment. Safety and efficacy in children <2 y are not established.

ROUTE & DOSAGE

Diabetes Mellitus

Adult: **IM/SC** Individualized doses (see INSULIN INJECTION, REGULAR)

ADMINISTRATION

Subcutaneous/Intramuscular

- Give PZI 30 min before breakfast.
- Ensure complete dispersion by mixing thoroughly, then gently rotating vial between palms and inverting it end to end several times. Do not shake.
- Note: PZI is compatible with regular insulin. Do NOT mix insulins unless prescribed by physician.
- Prepare solution immediately before administration when mixing regular insulin with PZI. Withdraw insulin injection into syringe before PZI.
- Store unopened vial at 2°–8° C (36°–46° F); store vial in use at 15°–30° C (59°–86° F). Avoid freezing and exposure to extremes in temperature or to direct sunlight.

ADVERSE EFFECTS (≥1%) (see INSULIN INJECTION).

INTERACTIONS (see INSULIN INJECTION).

PHARMACOKINETICS Onset: 4–8 h. **Peak:** 14–24 h. **Duration:** 36 h. **Metabolism:** Metabolized in liver and kidney. **Elimination:** <2% excreted unchanged in urine. **Half-Life:** Up to 13 h.

NURSING IMPLICATIONS

(see INSULIN INJECTION, REGULAR)

Assessment & Drug Effects

- Monitor therapeutic effectiveness: May be delayed several days following institution of treatment.

Patient & Family Education

- Distribute carbohydrates carefully in a balanced diet to prolong insulin effect.
- Note: Between-meal snacks may be necessary; bedtime snacks are essential.
- Note: If injection is given in the morning, hypoglycemia is most likely to occur during the night or early morning.
- Learn to be alert to the significance of sweating or fatigue unwarranted by activity, as well as other vague symptoms such as lassitude, drowsiness, tremulousness. Blood glucose levels fall slowly after injection of PZI; marked hypoglycemia may develop without an apparent cluster of symptoms.

- Learn to treat PZI-induced hypoglycemia, first with fast acting and complex carbohydrate (e.g., corn syrup or honey with bread), followed in 1–2 h by additional "slow" carbohydrates, such as milk and crackers.
- Do not breast feed while taking this drug without consulting physician.

INSULIN ZINC SUSPENSION (LENTE)

(in′su-lin)

Humulin L, Lente Iletin II (pork), Lente Purified Pork Insulin, Novolin

Classifications: HORMONE AND SYNTHETIC SUBSTITUTE; ANTIDIABETIC AGENT

Prototype: Insulin Injection

Pregnancy Category: B

AVAILABILITY 100 units/mL

ACTIONS Intermediate-acting, cloudy insulin suspension, equivalent to a mixture of 30% prompt insulin zinc (Semilente) and 70% extended zinc insulin (Ultralente) suspensions. Obtained from pork pancreas. Allergic reactions are rare. Time action is intermediate between those of prompt and extended insulins and is so close to that of isophane (NPH) insulin that the two forms may be used interchangeably.

THERAPEUTIC EFFECTS It lowers blood glucose levels by increasing peripheral glucose uptake, especially by skeletal muscle and fat tissue, and by inhibiting the liver from changing glycogen to glucose.

USES Hyperglycemia in diabetic patients allergic to other preparations of insulin. Also for patients with evidence of thrombotic phenomena in which protamine may be a factor.

CONTRAINDICATIONS During episodes of hypoglycemia or in patients sensitive to any ingredient in the formulation.

CAUTIOUS USE In insulin resistant patients, hyperthyroidism or hypothyroidism; lactation, older adults, pregnancy (category B), renal or hepatic impairment. Safety and efficacy in children <12 y have not been established.

ROUTE & DOSAGE

Diabetes Mellitus

Adult: **IM/SC** Individualized doses (see INSULIN INJECTION, REGULAR)

ADMINISTRATION

Subcutaneous/Intramuscular

- Give insulin zinc suspensions 30 min before breakfast. Some patients require another injection 30 min before supper time or at bedtime.
- Note: Zinc insulin preparations (Ultralente, Lente, Semilente) can be mixed with one another if prescribed by physician, but they must NOT be mixed with other modified insulins. Compatible with regular insulin.
- Ensure complete dispersion by mixing thoroughly by gently rotating the vial between the palms and by inverting it end-to-end several times. Do not shake.
- Note: Time of action of insulin zinc suspension (Lente) approximates that of isophane insulin suspension (NPH) allowing patients usually to be transferred directly to the latter on a unit-for-unit basis.
- Store unopened vial at 2°–8° C (36°–46° F). Avoid freezing and exposure to extremes in temperature or to direct sunlight.

ADVERSE EFFECTS (≥1%) (see INSULIN INJECTION, REGULAR).

INTERACTIONS (see INSULIN INJECTION).

PHARMACOKINETICS **Onset:** 1–2 h. **Peak:** 8–12 h. **Duration:** 18–24 h. **Metabolism:** Metabolized in liver and kidney. **Elimination:** <2% excreted unchanged in urine. **Half-Life:** Up to 13 h.

NURSING IMPLICATIONS

(see INSULIN INJECTION, REGULAR)

I

Patient & Family Education

- Be alert for S&S of hypoglycemia (see Appendix F); most apt to occur between mid-afternoon and dinner time (an early symptom may be a sense of extreme fatigue). Immediately take soluble carbohydrate (e.g., orange juice, honey). If the time between the midday and evening meal is prolonged, an afternoon snack may be needed.
- Do not overlook possibility of nocturnal hypoglycemia, especially during dose adjustment. Signs include restlessness or profuse sweating during sleep.
- Do not breast feed while taking this drug without consulting physician.

INSULIN ZINC SUSPENSION, EXTENDED (ULTRALENTE)

(in′su-lin)

Humulin U, Ultralente, Ultralente Insulin

Classifications: HORMONE AND SYNTHETIC SUBSTITUTE; ANTIDIABETIC AGENT

Prototype: Insulin Injection

Pregnancy Category: B

AVAILABILITY 100 units/mL

ACTIONS Long-acting cloudy suspension of insulin modified by addition of zinc chloride. Large particle size and high zinc content delay absorption and prolong action. Obtained from pork pancreas. Incidence of allergic reactions is low. Similar to protamine zinc insulin suspension (PZI) in actions and indications.

THERAPEUTIC EFFECTS It lowers blood glucose levels by increasing peripheral glucose uptake, especially by skeletal muscle and fat tissue, and by inhibiting the liver from changing glycogen to glucose. Usually administered in combination with a shorter acting insulin preparation.

USES Diabetes mellitus type 1.

CONTRAINDICATIONS During episodes of hypoglycemia or in patients sensitive to any ingredient in the formulation.

CAUTIOUS USE In insulin resistant patients, hyperthyroidism or hypothyroidism; lactation, older adults, pregnancy (category B), renal or hepatic impairment. Safety and efficacy in children <3 y are not established.

ROUTE & DOSAGE

Diabetes Mellitus

Adult: **IM/SC** Individualized doses (see INSULIN INJECTION, REGULAR)

ADMINISTRATION

Subcutaneous/Intramuscular

- Give 30 min before breakfast by deep SC injection.
- Ensure complete dispersion by mixing thoroughly by gently rotating vial between palms and by inverting it end-to-end several times. Do not shake.
- Note: Ultralente may be mixed with Semilente but not with

other modified insulin preparations. Compatible with regular insulin. Do NOT mix insulins unless prescribed by physician.
- Store unopened vial at 2°–8° C (36°–46° F). Avoid freezing and exposure to extremes in temperature or to direct sunlight.

ADVERSE EFFECTS (≥1%) (see INSULIN INJECTION, REGULAR).

INTERACTIONS (see INSULIN INJECTION).

PHARMACOKINETICS Onset: 4–8 h. **Peak:** 16–18 h. **Duration:** 36 h. **Metabolism:** Metabolized in liver and kidney. **Elimination:** <2% excreted unchanged in urine. **Half-Life:** Up to 13 h.

NURSING IMPLICATIONS

(see INSULIN INJECTION, REGULAR)

Patient & Family Education
- Be aware that restlessness or profuse sweating during sleep are S&S of hypoglycemia. Notify physician. Treat by eating soluble carbohydrate (orange juice, sugar, honey) plus a slowly digestible carbohydrate (bread, crackers). Supplemental feedings may be prescribed.
- Do not breast feed while taking this drug without consulting physician.

INSULIN ZINC SUSPENSION, PROMPT (SEMILENTE)

(in'su-lin)

Semilente Insulin, Semilente Purified Pork Insulin

Classifications: HORMONE AND SYNTHETIC SUBSTITUTE; ANTIDIABETIC AGENT

Prototype: Insulin Injection

Pregnancy Category: B

AVAILABILITY 100 units/mL

ACTIONS Rapid-acting cloudy suspension of insulin modified by addition of zinc chloride so that suspension is amorphous and therefore more quickly absorbed. Obtained from pork pancreas. Incidence of allergic reactions is low.

THERAPEUTIC EFFECTS It lowers blood glucose levels by increasing peripheral glucose uptake, especially by skeletal muscle and fat tissue, and by inhibiting the liver from changing glycogen to glucose.

USES Most commonly to supplement intermediate and long-acting insulins. Also for routine management of diabetes, especially for patients allergic to other types of insulin, and for patients with evidence of thrombotic phenomena in which protamine may be a factor.

CONTRAINDICATIONS During episodes of hypoglycemia or in patients sensitive to any ingredient in the formulation.

CAUTIOUS USE In insulin resistant patients, hyperthyroidism or hypothyroidism; lactation, older adults, pregnancy (category B), renal or hepatic impairment. Safety and efficacy in children <12 y are not established.

ROUTE & DOSAGE

Diabetes Mellitus

Adult: **IM/SC** Individualized doses (see INSULIN INJECTION, REGULAR)

ADMINISTRATION

Subcutaneous/Intramuscular
- Give Semilente once daily, 30 min before breakfast. Additional doses may be required for some patients 30 min before a meal or at bedtime.

- Ensure complete dispersion by mixing thoroughly by gently rotating vial between palms and by inverting it end-to-end several times. Do not shake.
- Note: Zinc insulin preparations (Ultralente, Lente, Semilente) can be mixed with one another but they must NOT be mixed with other modified insulins. Do NOT mix insulins unless prescribed by physician.
- Store unopened vial at 2°–8° C (36°–46° F). Avoid freezing and exposure to extremes in temperature or to direct sunlight.

I

ADVERSE EFFECTS (≥1%) (see INSULIN INJECTION, REGULAR).

INTERACTIONS (see INSULIN INJECTION).

PHARMACOKINETICS Onset: 0.5–1 h. **Peak:** 4–7 h. **Duration:** 12–16 h. **Metabolism:** Metabolized in liver and kidney. **Elimination:** <2% excreted unchanged in urine. **Half-Life:** Up to 13 h.

NURSING IMPLICATIONS

(see INSULIN INJECTION, REGULAR)

Patient & Family Education

- Be alert for symptoms of hypoglycemia that are most apt to appear before lunch; glycosuria is most apt to appear during the night.
- Do not breast feed while taking this drug without consulting physician.

INTERFERON ALFA-2a Pr

(in-ter-feer′on)

Roferon-A Injection

Classifications: IMMUNOMODULATOR; INTERFERON

Pregnancy Category: C

AVAILABILITY 3 million IU/mL, 6 million IU/mL, 9 million IU/mL, 36 million IU/mL, 6 million IU/0.5 mL, 9 million IU/0.5 mL injection.

ACTIONS Interferon (IFN) alfa-2a, one of 4 types of alpha interferon, is a highly purified protein and natural product of human leukocytes within 4–6 h after viral stimulation. Also produced by recombinant DNA technology (rIFN-A). ***Antiviral action:*** Reprograms virus-infected cells to inhibit various stages of virus replication. ***Antitumor action:*** Suppresses cell proliferation. ***Immunomodulating action:*** Enhances phagocytic activity of macrophages and augments specific cytotoxicity of lymphocytes for target cells. IFN is species specific but not virus specific; it partially inhibits viral replication and is immediately produced at site of viral entry by any cell; thus, the immune system and the interferon system of defense are complementary.

THERAPEUTIC EFFECTS Has a broad spectrum of antiviral, cytotoxic, and immunomodulating activity (i.e., favorably adjusts immune system to better combat foreign invasion of antigens and viruses).

USES To induce hairy cell leukemia remission in splenectomized and nonsplenectomized patients; treatment of hepatitis C, adjunct to surgery for malignant melanoma.

UNLABELED USES Chronic hepatitis B virus infection, solid tumors, human papillomavirus (HPV)-associated diseases, AIDS associated Kaposi's sarcoma.

CONTRAINDICATIONS Hypersensitivity to alpha interferons or any component of product and to mouse immunoglobulin. Safe use during pregnancy (category C), lactation, or by children <18 y is not established.

CAUTIOUS USE Cardiac disease or history of cardiac illness, severe cardiac, renal, or hepatic disease; seizure disorders, compromised CNS function; myelosuppression; chickenpox (existing or recent, including recent exposure), herpes zoster.

ROUTE & DOSAGE

Hairy Cell Leukemia

Adult: **SC/IM** 3 million U/d for 16–24 wk, may be reduced to 3 times/wk for maintenance therapy

AIDS-related Kaposi's Sarcoma

Adult: **SC/IM** 36 million U/d for 10–12 wk, may then be reduced to 3 times/wk

Genital and Anal Warts

Adult: **Intralesional** 1 million U injected in each lesion 3 times/wk on alternate days for 3 wk

Chronic Viral Hepatitis

Adult: **SC/IM** 1–3 million U/d for 1 wk, then 3 times/wk for 48–52 wk

ADMINISTRATION

Note: IFN should be administered under the guidance of a qualified physician.

Subcutaneous/Intramuscular

- Reconstitute by adding supplied diluent to the sterile powder vial.
- Use reconstituted solutions within 30 d. Inspect solution for particulate matter and discoloration before administration.
- Note: SC administration is recommended especially for patient who is at risk for bleeding (platelet count less than 50,000).
- Store sterile powder and its accompanying diluent, reconstituted solution, and injectable solution in refrigerator at 2°–8° C (36°–46° F). Do not freeze or shake solution.

ADVERSE EFFECTS (≥1%) **Body as a Whole:** *Flu-like syndrome (fever, chills, myalgia, headache).* **CNS:** *Fatigue, dizziness,* confusion, paresthesias, lethargy, psychosis, depression, nervousness, forgetfulness. **CV:** Dyspnea, edema, hypertension, palpitations. **GI:** *Nausea,* vomiting, *diarrhea, anorexia,* abdominal pain, change in taste, mild to moderate hepatotoxicity. **Hematologic:** Leukopenia, neutropenia, thrombocytopenia, myelosuppression. **Skin:** *Rash,* dry skin, pruritus, partial alopecia (eyelash growth increases), urticaria, reactivation of herpes labialis. **Respiratory:** Dryness or inflammation of oropharynx, *coughing.* **Other:** Transient impotence, arthralgia.

I

DIAGNOSTIC TEST INTERFERENCE Decreased Hgb, Hct; elevated fasting blood sugar, serum phosphorus, serum creatinine, AST, ALT, alkaline phosphatase, LDH; hypocalcemia.

INTERACTIONS Drug: May increase **theophylline** levels; additive myelosuppression with ANTINEOPLASTICS, **zidovudine** may increase hematologic toxicity, increase **doxorubicin** toxicity, increase neurotoxicity with **vinblastine. Aldesleukin (IL-2)** may potentiate the risk of renal failure.

PHARMACOKINETICS Absorption: Well absorbed after IM or SC injection. **Peak:** 15–60 min IV; 1–8 h IM. **Distribution:** Widely distributed, concentrating in spleen, kidney, liver, and lung. **Metabolism:** Metabolized principally in kidney. **Half-Life:** 5.1 h.

NURSING IMPLICATIONS

Assessment & Drug Effects

- Lab tests: Establish baseline data for CBC and platelet count, peripheral and bone marrow hairy

cells, liver and renal function. Monitor monthly during treatment.
- Monitor I&O ratio and pattern. Patient should be well hydrated during early stages of treatment. Encourage increased intake to at least 2500 mL if tolerated.
- Be aware of potential side effects. If detected early, most are reversible.
- Note: Flu-like syndrome (fever, chills) occurs in most patients 2–6 h after a dose of IFN. Anorexia may persist after such an episode. Symptoms tend to lessen with continued therapy.
- Monitor for ecchymoses, petechiae, unexplained bleeding.
- Monitor BP, vital signs, and cardiac function. Older adults are particularly susceptible to cardiotoxicity.
- Monitor for gait difficulty, dizziness, and hypotension. Advise against hazardous activity until response to drug is known.
- Monitor for oral superinfection with *Candida albicans*. Alert physician if stomatitis (sore mouth with ulceration), gingivitis, or white patches on oropharyngeal membrane surfaces are evidenced.

Patient & Family Education
- Understand the risks of severe and even fatal adverse reactions as well as the benefits from IFN therapy.
- Learn to self-administer after therapy is well established. Read and keep handy patient information sheet about IFN.
- Avoid exposure to infection during nadir period.
- Follow up with careful periodic neuropsychiatric monitoring.
- Notify physician promptly if symptoms of infection develop (sore throat, fever, vomiting, diarrhea).
- Note: Fertile, nonpregnant women need to use effective contraception.
- Do not change brands of interferon alfa without first consulting the physician (because of risk of dosage change).
- Do not breast feed while taking this drug without consulting physician.

INTERFERON ALFA-2b

(in-ter-feer′on)
Intron A
Classifications: IMMUNOMODULATOR; INTERFERON
Prototype: Interferon alfa-2a
Pregnancy Category: C

AVAILABILITY 5 million IU, 10 million IU, 18 million IU, 25 million IU, 50 million IU vials

ACTIONS Alpha (leukocyte) interferon is a natural product induced virally in peripheral WBC or lymphoblastoid cells. The drug interferon alfa-2b is obtained by recombinant DNA technology from a strain of *Escherichia coli* bearing an interferon alfa-2b gene from human leukocytes.
THERAPEUTIC EFFECTS Has the same actions (antiviral, immunomodulating, antiproliferative) as interferon alfa-2a.

USES Hairy cell leukemia in splenectomized and nonsplenectomized patients ≥18 y, chronic hepatitis B or C.
UNLABELED USES Multiple sclerosis, condylomata acuminata, AIDS-related Kaposi's sarcoma.

CONTRAINDICATIONS Hypersensitivity to interferon alfa-2b or to any components of the product. Safe use during pregnancy (category C), lactation, or children <18 y is not established.
CAUTIOUS USE Severe, preexisting cardiac, renal, or hepatic disease;

pulmonary disease (e.g., COPD); diabetes mellitus patients prone to ketoacidosis; coagulation disorders; severe myelosuppression; recent MI; previous dysrhythmias.

ROUTE & DOSAGE

Hairy Cell Leukemia
Adult: **IM/SC** 2 million U/m^2 3 times/wk

Kaposi's Sarcoma
Adult: **IM/SC** 30 million U/m^2 3 times/wk

Condylomata Acuminata
Adult: **IM/SC** 1 million U/m^2 3 times/wk

Chronic Hepatitis B or C
Adult: **SC** 3 million U 3 times/wk x 18–24 mo

ADMINISTRATION

Note: Interferon alfa-2b should be administered under the guidance of a qualified physician.

Subcutaneous/Intramuscular

- Reconstitution: The final concentration with the amount of required diluent is determined by the condition being treated (see manufacturer's directions). Inject diluent (bacteriostatic water for injection) into interferon alfa-2b vial; gently agitate solution before withdrawing dose with a sterile syringe.
- Make sure reconstituted solution is clear and colorless to light yellow and free of particulate material; discard if there are particles or solution is discolored.
- Store vials and reconstituted solutions at 2°–8° C (36°–46° F); remains stable for 1 mo.

ADVERSE EFFECTS (≥1%) **Body as a Whole:** *Flu-like syndrome (fever, chills) associated with myalgia and arthralgia,* leg cramps. **CNS:** Depression, nervousness, anxiety, confusion, *dizziness, fatigue,* somnolence, insomnia, altered mental states, ataxia, tremor, paresthesias, *headache.* **CV:** Hypertension, dyspnea, *hot flushes.* **Special Senses:** Epistaxis, pharyngitis, sneezing; abnormal vision. **GI:** Taste alteration, *anorexia,* weight loss, *nausea,* vomiting, stomatitis, *diarrhea,* flatulence. **Hematologic:** Mild thrombocytopenia, transient granulocytopenia, <u>leukemia</u>. **Skin:** Mild pruritus, mild alopecia, rash, dry skin, herpetic eruptions, nonherpetic cold sores, urticaria.

INTERACTIONS Drug: May increase **theophylline** levels; additive myelosuppression with ANTINEOPLASTICS, **zidovudine** may increase hematologic toxicity, increase **doxorubicin** toxicity, increase neurotoxicity with **vinblastine.**

PHARMACOKINETICS Peak: 6–8 h. **Metabolism:** Metabolized in kidneys. **Half-Life:** 6–7 h.

NURSING IMPLICATIONS

(see INTERFERON ALFA-2A)

Assessment & Drug Effects

- Lab tests: Monitor CBC with differential and platelet counts closely.
- Monitor for ecchymoses, petechiae, and bruising.
- Assess hydration status; patient should be well hydrated especially during initial stage of treatment and if vomiting or diarrhea occurs.
- Assess for flu-like symptoms, which may be relieved by acetaminophen (if prescribed).
- Monitor level of GI distress and ability to consume fluids and food.
- Monitor mental status and alertness; implement safety precautions if needed.

I

Patient & Family Education

- Learn techniques for reconstitution and administration of drug.
- Do NOT change brands of interferon without first consulting the physician.
- Note: If flu-like symptoms develop, take acetaminophen as advised by physician and take interferon at bedtime.
- Note: Fertile, nonpregnant women need to use effective contraception.
- Use caution with hazardous activities until response to drug is known.
- Learn about adverse effects and notify physician about those that cause significant discomfort.
- Do not breast feed while taking this drug without consulting physician.

I

INTERFERON ALFA-n1 LYMPHOBLASTOID

(in-ter-fer′on)

Wellferon

Classifications: IMMUNOMODULATOR; ANTIVIRAL

Prototype: Interferon alfa-2a

Pregnancy Category: C

AVAILABILITY 3 MU/mL vial

ACTIONS Interferon alfa-n1 is a blend of human alpha interferons following induction of a virus into leukocytes. **Antiviral Action:** Wellferon reprograms virus-infected cells to inhibit various stages of viral replication.

THERAPEUTIC EFFECTS Effectiveness indicated by reduction in serum ALT and HCV viral load. **Antitumor Action:** Suppresses cell proliferation. **Immunomodulating Action:** Enhances phagocytic activity of macrophages and augments cytotoxicity of lymphocyte natural killer (NK) cells.

USES Treatment of chronic hepatitis C.

CONTRAINDICATIONS Hypersensitivity to alpha interferons; history of anaphylaxis to bovine immunoglobulins, egg protein, polymycin B, or neomycin B; pregnancy (category C); lactation.

CAUTIOUS USE Hepatitis from causes other than hepatitis C; psychiatric disorder; hypertension, supraventricular arrhythmias, MI, hypotension; seizures; hypothyroidism; hepatic dysfunction; older adults; autoimmune disease; leukopenia; pulmonary dysfunction; concurrent use of immunosuppressive agents. Safety and efficacy in children <18 y are unknown.

ROUTE & DOSAGE

Chronic Hepatitis C
Adult: **SC/IM** 3 MU 3 times/wk times 48 wk

ADMINISTRATION

Subcutaneous/Intramuscular

- Administer undiluted IM or SC as ordered. Do not shake vial.
- Do not initiate therapy unless acceptable baseline lab values have been attained. Platelet count ≥75 × 10^9/L, Hgb ≥100 g/L, ANC ≥1500 × 10^6/L, serum creatinine <2.0 mg/dL, serum albumin ≥25 g/L, bilirubin WNL, TSH, and T_4 WNL.
- Refrigerate between 2°–8° C (36°–46° F) and protect from light.

ADVERSE EFFECTS (≥1%) **Body as a Whole:** *Asthenia, headache, fever, chills, injection site reaction (pain, edema, hemorrhage, inflammation), pain, myalgia, arthralgia.* **CNS:** *Anxiety, nervousness, insomnia, somnolence, depression,* dizziness, confusion, abnormal thinking, amnesia, paresthesia. **GI:** *Nausea, diarrhea, abdominal pain,* anorexia, vomiting, weight loss, hepatotoxicity, **Hematologic:** Thrombocytopenia, leukopenia, anemia. **Respiratory:** Cough, bronchitis, dyspnea, pneumonia, rhinitis, pharyngitis. **Skin:** *Alopecia,* rash, dry skin, pruritus, urticaria, sweat.

INTERACTIONS No clinically significant interactions established.

PHARMACOKINETICS Absorption: 40%–100% absorbed from SC or IM site. **Peak:** 6–9 h. **Metabolism:** Renal and cellular catabolism. **Half-Life:** 7–10 h.

NURSING IMPLICATIONS

Assessment & Drug Effects

- Monitor for S&S of depression, suicidal ideation, other CNS effects.
- Monitor cardiovascular status carefully especially with preexisting CV disease. Do baseline and periodic EKG throughout therapy.
- Lab tests: Monitor baseline and q3mo TSH and T_4; monitor baseline and periodic Hgb and Hct, CBC with differential, platelet count, liver functions.
- Assess hydration status; good hydration especially important during initial stage of treatment.

Patient & Family Education

- Learn appropriate self-injection techniques. Do not reuse syringes.
- Relieve flu-like symptoms with acetaminophen or anti-inflammatory analgesic.
- Drink plenty of fluids especially in the initial weeks of treatment.
- Do not accept interferon brand changes without first consulting physician.
- Use reliable contraception.
- Do not breast feed while taking this drug.

INTERFERON ALFACON-1

(in-ter-fer'on al'fa-con)

Infergen

Classifications: IMMUNOMODULATOR; ANTIVIRAL

Prototype: Interferon alfa-2a

Pregnancy Category: C

AVAILABILITY 9 mcg, 15 mcg injection

ACTIONS DNA recombinant Type 1 interferon. Its antiviral, antiproliferative, and natural killer (NK) cell activity is five times greater than interferon alpha-2a or interferon alpha-2b.

THERAPEUTIC EFFECTS Normalization of ALT level and serum HCV RNA <100 copies/mL. Type 1 interferons bind to the cell surface receptors inducing biologic responses including antiviral, antiproliferative, and immunomodulatory activities.

USES Treatment of chronic hepatitis C.

CONTRAINDICATIONS Hypersensitivity to alpha interferons or *E.coli* products; patients with decompensated liver disease such as jaundice, ascites, etc.; pregnancy (category C), lactation, children <18 y.

CAUTIOUS USE History of severe psychiatric disorder, depression, or suicidal ideation; pre-existing cardiac disease, myelosuppression, previous hypersensitivity to interferon therapy; history of endocrine disorders; ophthalmic disorders or autoimmune disorders.

ROUTE & DOSAGE

Chronic Hepatitis C

Adult: **SC** 9 mcg 3 times/wk times 24 wk

ADMINISTRATION

Subcutaneous

- Allow at least 24 h to elapse between doses of interferon alfacon-1.
- Give only one dose per vial or per prefilled syringe. Enter each vial only once. Discard unused portion of a vial or prefilled syringe immediately.
- Initiate treatment only if acceptable baseline lab values are obtained: Platelet count ≥75 × 10^9/L, Hgb ≥100 g/L, ANC ≥1500 × 10^6/L, serum creatinine <2.0 mg/dL, serum albumin ≥25 g/L, bilirubin WNL, TSH, and T_4 WNL.
- Store vials and syringes at 2°–8° C (36°–46° F). Avoid direct sunlight and vigorous shaking.

ADVERSE EFFECTS (≥1%) **Body as a Whole:** *Asthenia, headache, fatigue, fever, chills, injection site reaction (pain, edema, hemorrhage, inflammation), pain, myalgia, arthralgia,* increased sweating. **CNS:** *Insomnia, depression, dizziness, paresthesia nervousness, depression, anxiety,* agitation. **CV:** Hypertension, palpitation. **GI:** *Nausea, diarrhea, abdominal pain, anorexia, vomiting, dyspepsia,* constipation, flatulence, toothache, hemorrhoids, weight loss, hepatotoxicity. **Hematologic:** *Granulocytopenia, thrombocytopenia, leukopenia,* ecchymosis, lymphadenopathy, lymphocytosis. **Respiratory:** *Cough, bronchitis, dyspnea, pneumonia, rhinitis,* pharyngitis. **Skin:** *Alopecia, rash,* dry skin, *pruritus,* erythema. **Urogenital:** Dysmenorrhea, vaginitis, menstrual disorder.

INTERACTIONS No clinically significant interactions established.

PHARMACOKINETICS Peak: 24–36 h.

NURSING IMPLICATIONS

Assessment & Drug Effects

- Monitor for and report any of the following S&S immediately: Depression, suicidal ideation, suicide attempt, or other indications of psychiatric disturbance.
- Withhold drug and notify physician if symptoms of hepatic decompensation such as jaundice or ascites develop. Withhold drug and notify physician if any other severe adverse reaction occurs.
- Lab tests: Baseline, 2 wk after initiation of therapy, and periodically thereafter: platelet count, Hgb and Hct, WBC and ANC, serum creatinine, serum albumin, bilirubin, thyroid function, and triglyceride; periodic ALT to determine liver functions.

Patient & Family Education

- Report immediately any signs of psychiatric disturbance including depression, thoughts of suicide, nervousness, anxiety, agitation, apathy, or significant mood swings to physician.
- Do not breast feed while taking this drug.

INTERFERON BETA-1a

(in-ter-fer'on)

Avonex, Rebif

Classifications: IMMUNOMODULATOR; INTERFERON

Prototype: Interferon alfa-2a

Pregnancy Category: C

AVAILABILITY Avonex 33 mcg vial; 30 mcg/5 mL prefilled syringe; **Rebif** 22 mcg, 44 mcg vial

ACTIONS Interferon beta-1a is produced by recombinant DNA technology. Interferon beta exerts its biological effects by binding to specific receptors on the surface of human cells.

THERAPEUTIC EFFECTS The mechanisms by which interferon beta-1a exerts its effect on multiple sclerosis is not fully defined; however, time of onset of progression in disability was significantly longer in patients treated with interferon beta-1a.

USES Relapsing-remitting multiple sclerosis.

CONTRAINDICATIONS Previous hypersensitivity to interferon beta or human albumin, pregnancy (category C) but may cause a spontaneous abortion, lactation.

CAUTIOUS USE Suicidal tendencies, depression, preexisting psychiatric disorders; hepatic impairment. Safety and efficacy in children <18 y are not established.

ROUTE & DOSAGE

Multiple Sclerosis

Adult: **IM Avonex** 30 mcg qwk
SC Rebif 44 mcg 3 times/wk

ADMINISTRATION

Intramuscular

- Avonex: Reconstitute single use Avonex vial (33 mcg of lyophilized powder) with 1.1 mL of supplied diluent and swirl gently to dissolve. Withdraw 1.0 mL for administration. Discard any residual drug as the product contains no preservatives.
- Use within 6 h of reconstitution.

Subcutaneous

- Rebif: Give at the same time each day (preferably in the late afternoon or evening) on the same three days of the week at least 48 h apart each week. Dose is usually titrated up from 8.8 mcg to 44 mcg three times a week over a four-week period.
- Inject SC using either a 22 or 44 mcg prefilled syringe. Discard any residual drug as the product contains no preservatives.
- Store unreconstituted vials or prefilled syringes at 2°–8° C (36°–46° F). May store for ≤30 d at room temperature up to 25° C (77° F). Do not use beyond expiration date.

ADVERSE EFFECTS (≥1%) **Body as a Whole:** Alopecia, myalgias, *flu-like syndrome,* anaphylaxis. **CNS:** Headache, *fever,* fatigue, lethargy, depression, somnolence, weakness, agitation, malaise, confusion or reduced ability to concentrate, anxiety, dementia, emotional lability, depersonalization, suicide attempts, worsening of psychiatric disorders. **CV:** Tachycardia, CHF (rare). **GI:** Nausea, vomiting, *diarrhea, hepatic injury.* **Hematologic:** *Leukopenia, thrombocytopenia,* anemia, pancytopenia (rare), thrombocytopenia (rare). **Metabolic:** Hypocalcemia, elevated serum creatinine, elevated liver transaminases. **Skin:** Local skin necrosis at injection site, *pain at injection site.*

PHARMACOKINETICS Peak: Avonex 7.8–9.8 h; **Rebif** 16 h. **Metabolism:** Rapidly inactivated in body fluids and tissue. **Half-Life: Avonex** 8.6–10 h; **Rebif** 69 h.

NURSING IMPLICATIONS

Assessment & Drug Effects

- Withhold drug and notify physician if depression or suicidal ideation develops or if there is a worsening of psychiatric symptoms.
- Monitor patients with cardiac disease carefully for worsening cardiac function.
- Lab tests: Monitor periodically liver function tests, renal function tests, routine blood chemistry,

I

and CBC with differential, and platelet count. Monitor thyroid function tests q6mo with preexisting thyroid dysfunction or when clinically indicated.

Patient & Family Education

- Take a missed dose as soon as possible but not within 48 h of next scheduled dose.
- Learn about common adverse effects, especially flu-like syndrome (headache, fatigue, fever, rigors, chest pain, back pain, myalgia).
- Withhold drug and notify physician of depression or suicidal ideation or exacerbation of a preexisting seizure disorder.
- Note: Women who wish to become pregnant must discontinue therapy.
- Do not breast feed while taking this drug.

INTERFERON BETA-1b

(in-ter-fer'on)

Betaseron

Classifications: IMMUNOMODULATOR; INTERFERON

Prototype: Interferon alfa-2a

Pregnancy Category: C

AVAILABILITY 0.3 mg vial

ACTIONS Interferon beta-1b is a glycoprotein produced by recombinant DNA techniques using a strain of *E. coli*. Naturally occurring interferon beta-1b is produced principally by fibroblasts and macrophages.

THERAPEUTIC EFFECTS Both natural and recombinant DNA interferon beta-1b possess antiviral, antiproliferative, antitumor, and immunomodulatory activity. The use of interferon beta-1b for multiple sclerosis (MS) is based on the assumption that MS is an immunologically mediated illness.

USES Relapsing and relapsing-remitting multiple sclerosis.

UNLABELED USES AIDS, AIDS-related Kaposi's sarcoma, metastatic renal cell carcinoma, malignant melanoma, cutaneous T-cell lymphoma, acute hepatitis C.

CONTRAINDICATIONS Previous hypersensitivity to interferon beta-1b or human albumin, pregnancy (category C) but may cause a spontaneous abortion, lactation.

CAUTIOUS USE Suicidal/mental disorders especially chronic depression; seizures; cardiac disease. Safety and efficacy in children <18 y are not established. Safety and efficacy in chronic progressive MS not evaluated.

ROUTE & DOSAGE

Multiple Sclerosis

Adult: **SC** 0.25 mg (8 million IU) q.o.d.

ADMINISTRATION

Subcutaneous

- Reconstitute by adding 1.2 mL of the supplied diluent (0.54% NaCl) to vial and gently swirl. Do NOT shake. The resultant solution contains 0.25 mg (8 million units)/mL.
- Discard reconstituted solution if it contains particulate matter or is discolored. Also discard unused solution.
- Rotate injection sites; use 27-gauge needle to administer drug.
- Store vials under refrigeration, 2°–8° C (36°–46° F) or at room temperature.

ADVERSE EFFECTS (≥1%) **CNS:** Headache, *fever,* fatigue, lethargy, depression, somnolence, weakness, agitation, malaise, confusion or reduced ability to concentrate, anxiety, dementia, emotional lability, depersonalization, suicide attempts. **CV:** Tachycardia, CHF (rare). **GI:** Nausea, vomiting, *diarrhea.* **Hematologic:** *Leukopenia, thrombocytopenia,* anemia. **Metabolic:** Hypocalcemia, elevated serum creatinine, elevated liver transaminases. **Skin:** Local skin necrosis at injection site, *pain at injection site.* **Body as a Whole:** Alopecia, myalgias, *flu-like syndrome.*

INTERACTIONS Drug: Zidovudine (AZT) levels are increased, resulting in toxicity.

PHARMACOKINETICS Absorption: About 50% absorbed from SC sites. **Distribution:** Penetrates intact blood–brain barrier poorly; crosses placenta; distributed into breast milk. **Metabolism:** Rapidly inactivated in body fluids and tissue.

NURSING IMPLICATIONS

Assessment & Drug Effects

- Monitor vital signs, neurologic status, and neuropsychiatric status frequently during therapy.
- Lab tests: Monitor liver function, renal function, complete blood counts, and serum electrolytes periodically.
- Assess for and promptly treat flu-like symptom complex (fever, chills, myalgia, etc.).
- Assess injection sites; pain and redness are common reactions. Report tissue ulceration promptly.

Patient & Family Education

- Learn and understand potential adverse drug reactions.
- Learn proper technique for solution preparation and injection.
- Self-medicate with acetaminophen (if not contraindicated) if flu-like symptom complex develops.
- Avoid prolonged exposure to sunlight.
- Use caution when performing hazardous activities until response to drug is known.
- Do not breast feed while taking this drug.

INTERFERON GAMMA-1b

(in-ter-feer′on)
Actimmune
Classifications: IMMUNOMODULATOR; INTERFERON
Prototype: Interferon alfa-2a
Pregnancy Category: C

AVAILABILITY 100 mcg (2 million IU)/0.5 mL vial

ACTIONS Has potent phagocyte-activating effects that include stimulating macrophages and generation of toxic oxygen metabolites (i.e., free radicals) capable of destroying virally infected cells. It also exerts antitumor effects by increasing expression of tumor suppressor genes and activating macrophages to lyse tumor cells.
THERAPEUTIC EFFECTS Is a naturally occurring cytokine with antiviral, immunomodulatory, and antiproliferative activity. It enhances phagocyte function in chronic granulomatous disease and improves killing of viruses; also enhances osteoclast function in malignant osteopetrosis.

USES Chronic granulomatous disease, severe malignant osteopetrosis
UNLABELED USES Idiopathic pulmonary fibrosis, refractory mycobacterium infection, ovarian cancer.

CONTRAINDICATIONS Hypersensitivity to interferon gamma or products derived from *E. coli;* pregnancy (category C); lactation.
CAUTIOUS USE Preexisting cardiac disease; seizure disorders and

I

compromised CNS function; myelosuppression. Safety and efficacy in children are unknown.

ROUTE & DOSAGE

Chronic Granulomatous Disease, Osteopetrosis
Adult/Child: **SC** *BSA ≥0.5 m² 50 mcg/m²* 3 times weekly
Adult/Child: **SC** *BSA ≤0.5 m² 1.5 mcg/kg* 3 times weekly

Idiopathic Pulmonary Fibrosis
Adult: **SC** 180–200 mcg 3 times weekly

ADMINISTRATION

- Note: Pretreatment (4 h before) with acetaminophen is recommended to reduce headache, myalgia, and fever. Treatment should be continued 24 h postinjection.

Subcutaneous

- Do not shake vial. Inject SC undiluted into right or left deltoid area or anterior thigh area
- Avoid intradermal or IV injection. Rotate injection sites.
- Store 2°–8° C (36°–46° F); do not freeze. Discard any unused portions or any vial left at room temperature for >12 h.

ADVERSE EFFECTS (≥1%) **Body as a Whole:** *Fever, fatigue, chills,* myalgia, arthralgia, night sweats. **CNS:** *Headache,* altered mental status, ataxia, confusion, dizziness, Parkinsonian symptoms, disorientation, seizures, hallucinations. **CV:** Heart block, heart failure, DVT, hypotension, MI, syncope, tachyarrhythmia. **GI:** *Nausea, vomiting, diarrhea.* **Hematologic:** *Leukopenia, thrombocytopenia.* **Respiratory:** Bronchospasm, interstitial pneumonitis, pulmonary embolism, tachypnea. **Skin:** Local skin necrosis at injection site, *pain at injection site, rash.* **Urogenital:** Reversible renal insufficiency.

INTERACTIONS Drug: Use cautiously with **amiophylline, fosphenytoin, phenytoin, theophylline, warfarin.**

PHARMACOKINETICS Absorption: 90% absorbed from SC site. **Peak:** 7 h **Half-Life:** 5.9 h.

NURSING IMPLICATIONS

Assessment & Drug Effects

- Monitor CV status frequently. Report promptly severe hypotension and/or syncope.
- Monitor for and report S&S of infection.
- Lab tests: Baseline and at 3 mo CBC with differential and platelet counts; complete blood chemistry (including renal and liver function tests), and urinalysis.

Patient & Family Education

- Report promptly: skin rash, itching, unusual weakness or tiredness, chest pain or palpitations, or signs of an infection.
- Do not accept vaccination with a live vaccine during or for 3 mo following the end of therapy.
- Do not breast feed while taking this drug.

IODOQUINOL

(eye-oh-do-kwin'ole)
Diiodohydroxyquin, Dioquinol, Sebaquin, Yodoxin
Classifications: ANTIINFECTIVE; AMEBICIDE; ANTIPROTOZOAL
Prototype: Emetine
Pregnancy Category: C

AVAILABILITY 210 mg, 650 mg tablets

ACTIONS Direct-acting (contact) amebicide.

THERAPEUTIC EFFECTS Effective against both trophozoites and cyst forms of *Entamoeba histolytica* in intestinal lumen. Not useful for extraintestinal amebiasis. Range of antiprotozoal action includes *Trichomonas vaginalis* and *Balantidium coli;* also has some antibacterial and antifungal properties.

USES Intestinal amebiasis and for asymptomatic passers of cysts. Commonly used either concurrently or in alternating courses with another intestinal amebicide.

UNLABELED USES *Balantidiasis* and *Acrodermatitis enteropathica;* traveler's diarrhea; shampoo preparation (Sebaquin) used for control of seborrheic dermatitis of scalp.

CONTRAINDICATIONS Hypersensitivity to any 8-hydroxyquinoline or to iodine-containing preparations or foods; hepatic or renal damage; preexisting optic neuropathy. Safe use during pregnancy (category C) or lactation is not established.

CAUTIOUS USE Severe thyroid disease; minor self-limiting problems; prolonged high-dosage therapy.

ROUTE & DOSAGE

Intestinal Amebiasis

Adult: **PO** 630–650 mg t.i.d. for 20 d (max: 2 g/d); may repeat after a 2–3 wk drug-free interval
Child: **PO** 30–40 mg/kg/d in 2–3 divided doses for 20 d (max: 1.95 g/d); may repeat after a 2–3 wk drug-free interval

ADMINISTRATION

Oral

- Give drug after meals. If patient has difficulty swallowing tablet, crush and mix with applesauce.

ADVERSE EFFECTS (≥1%) **Body as a Whole:** Hypersensitivity (urticaria, pruritus). **CNS:** Headache, agitation, retrograde amnesia, vertigo, ataxia, peripheral neuropathy (especially in children); muscle pain, weakness usually below T_{12} vertebrae, dysesthesias especially of lower limbs, paresthesias, increased sense of warmth. **Special Senses:** Blurred vision, optic atrophy, optic neuritis, permanent loss of vision. **GI:** Nausea, vomiting, anorexia, abdominal cramps, diarrhea, constipation, rectal irritation and itching. **Skin:** Discoloration of hair and nails, acne, hair loss, urticaria, various forms of skin eruptions. **Hematologic:** Agranulocytosis (rare). **Endocrine:** Thyroid hypertrophy, iodism [generalized furunculosis (iodine toxiderma), skin eruptions, fever, chills, weakness].

DIAGNOSTIC TEST INTERFERENCE Iodoquinol can cause elevations of ***PBI*** and decrease of ***I-131 uptake*** (effects may last for several weeks to 6 mo even after discontinuation of therapy). ***Ferric chloride test for PKU*** (phenylketonuria) may yield false-positive results if iodoquinol is present in urine.

INTERACTIONS No clinically significant interactions established.

PHARMACOKINETICS Absorption: Small amount absorbed from GI tract. **Elimination:** Excreted in feces.

NURSING IMPLICATIONS

Assessment & Drug Effects

- Monitor I&O ratio. Record characteristics of stools: color, consistency, frequency, presence of blood, mucus, or other material.
- Note: ophthalmologic examinations are recommended at regu-

I

lar intervals during prolonged therapy.

- Monitor and report immediately the onset of blurred or decreased vision or eye pain. Also report symptoms of peripheral neuropathy: pain, numbness, tingling, or weakness of extremities.

Patient & Family Education

- Report skin rash and symptoms of agranulocytosis (see Appendix F).
- Complete full course of treatment. Stool needs be examined again 1, 3, and 6 mo after termination of treatment.
- Note: Intestinal amebiasis is spread mainly by contaminated water, raw fruits or vegetables, flies, roaches, and hand-to-mouth transfer of infected feces. It is very important to wash hands after defecation and before eating.
- Do not breast feed while taking this drug without consulting physician.

I

IPECAC SYRUP

(ip'e-kak)

Ipecac Syrup

Classifications: GASTROINTESTINAL AGENT; EMETIC

Pregnancy Category: C

AVAILABILITY 15 mL, 30 mL doses

ACTIONS Derived from dried rhizomes and roots of *Cephaelis ipecacuanha*. Contains cephaeline (produces emesis) and emetine, a toxic alkaloid that is excreted slowly from the body. Emetine can cause potentially fatal cumulative toxicity with repeated use. It appears to inhibit protein synthesis and energy production in muscle tissue with resultant skeletal and cardiac muscle toxicity.

THERAPEUTIC EFFECTS Acts locally on gastric mucosa and centrally on chemoreceptor trigger zone (CTZ) in the medulla to induce vomiting.

USES Emergency emetic to remove unabsorbed ingested poisons.

CONTRAINDICATIONS Comatose, semicomatose, inebriated, deeply sedated patients; patients in shock; patients with depressed gag reflex; seizures, active or impending; impaired cardiac function; arteriosclerosis; treatment of ingested strong alkali, acids, or other corrosives, strychnine, petroleum distillates, volatile oils, or rapid-acting CNS depressants.

CAUTIOUS USE Safe use in pregnancy (category C), lactation, or infants <6 mo is not established.

ROUTE & DOSAGE

Emergency Emesis

Adult: **PO** 30 mL followed by 1–2 240 mL (8 oz) glasses of water, may repeat once in 20 min if necessary

Child: **PO** *>1 y,* 15 mL followed by 1–2 240 mL (8 oz) glasses of water, may repeat once in 20 min if necessary; *<1 y,* 5–10 mL followed by 120–240 mL (4–8 oz) of water, may repeat once in 20 min if necessary

ADMINISTRATION

Oral

- Do not confuse with ipecac fluid extract, which is 14 times stronger and has caused deaths when mistakenly given at the same dosage as ipecac syrup.
- Do not induce vomiting if victim is unconscious, semiconscious, or convulsing.

- Store in tight containers at temperature not exceeding 25° C (77° F).

ADVERSE EFFECTS (≥1%) **Body as a Whole:** Achy, stiff muscles, severe myopathy, convulsions, coma. **CV:** Cardiomyopathy, cardiotoxicity, cardiac arrhythmias, atrial fibrillation, tachycardia, chest pain, dyspnea, hypotension, fatal myocarditis. **GI:** Diarrhea, mild GI upset. If drug is not vomited but absorbed or if ipecac overdosage: *persistent vomiting,* gastroenteritis, bloody diarrhea, sensory disturbances, stomach cramps, tremor.

PHARMACOKINETICS Onset: 15–30 min. **Duration:** 25 min. **Elimination:** Metabolite can be detected in urine up to 60 d after excessive doses.

NURSING IMPLICATIONS

Assessment & Drug Effects

- Note: Emetic effect occurs in 15–30 min and continues for 20–25 min. If vomiting does not occur in 20–30 min, repeat dose once.
- Contact physician immediately if vomiting does not occur within 15–20 min after a second dose. Dosage should be recovered by gastric lavage and activated charcoal if necessary.
- Note: Ipecac syrup can be cardiotoxic if not vomited and allowed to be absorbed.
- Report immediately to physician if vomiting persists longer than 2–3 h after ipecac syrup is given.

Patient & Family Education

- Call an emergency room, poison control center, or physician before using ipecac syrup.
- Do not breast feed after using this drug without consulting physician.

IPRATROPIUM BROMIDE

(i-pra-troe′pee-um)

Atrovent

Classifications: AUTONOMIC NERVOUS SYSTEM AGENT; ANTICHOLINERGIC (PARASYMPATHOLYTIC); BRONCHODILATOR

Prototype: Atropine

Pregnancy Category: B

AVAILABILITY 0.02% solution for inhalation; 18 mcg inhaler; 0.03%, 0.06% nasal spray

I

ACTIONS Quaternary compound, chemically related to atropine, with low solubility; does not cross blood–brain barrier. Produces local, site-specific effects on the larger central airways including bronchodilation and prevention of bronchospasms.

THERAPEUTIC EFFECTS Bronchodilation inhibits acetylcholine at its receptor sites, thereby blocking cholinergic bronchomotor tone (bronchoconstriction); also abolishes vagally mediated reflex bronchospasm triggered by such nonspecific agents as cigarette smoke, inert dusts, cold air, and a range of inflammatory mediators (e.g., histamine).

USES Maintenance therapy in COPD including chronic bronchitis and emphysema; nasal spray for perennial rhinitis and symptomatic relief of rhinorrhea associated with the common cold.

UNLABELED USES Perennial nonallergic rhinitis.

CONTRAINDICATIONS Use as primary treatment for acute episodes; hypersensitivity to atropine or derivatives. Safe use in children <12 y is not established.

CAUTIOUS USE Pregnancy (category B), lactation; narrow-angle glaucoma; prostatic hypertrophy, bladder neck obstruction.

ROUTE & DOSAGE

COPD

Adult: **Inhalation** 2 inhalations of MDI q.i.d. at no less than 4 h intervals (max: 12 inhalations in 24 h) **Nebulizer** 500 mcg (1 unit dose vial) q6–8h
Child: **Inhalation** *3–12 y,* 1–2 inhalations t.i.d. (max: 6/d) **Nebulizer** 125–250 mcg t.i.d.

Rhinitis

Adult: **Intranasal** ≥*5 y,* 2 sprays of 0.03% each nostril b.i.d. or t.i.d.

Common Cold

Adult: **Intranasal** 2 sprays of 0.06% each nostril t.i.d. or q.i.d. up to 4 d

I

ADMINISTRATION

Intranasal/Inhalation/Nebulizer
- Demonstrate aerosol use and check return demonstration.
- Wait 3 min between inhalations if more than one inhalation per dose is ordered.
- Avoid contact with eyes.

ADVERSE EFFECTS (≥1%) **Special Senses:** Blurred vision (especially if sprayed into eye), difficulty in accommodation, acute eye pain, worsening of narrow-angle glaucoma. **GI:** Bitter taste, dry oropharyngeal membranes. With higher doses: nausea, constipation. **Respiratory:** *Cough,* hoarseness, exacerbation of symptoms, drying of bronchial secretions, mucosal ulcers, epistaxis, nasal dryness. **Skin:** Rash, hives. **Urogenital:** Urinary retention. **CNS:** Headache.

PHARMACOKINETICS Absorption: 10% of inhaled dose reaches lower airway; approximately 0.5% of dose is systemically absorbed. **Peak:** 1.5–2 h. **Duration:** 4–6 h. **Elimination:** 48% of dose excreted in feces; <5% excreted in urine. **Half-Life:** 1.5–2 h.

NURSING IMPLICATIONS

Assessment & Drug Effects
- Monitor respiratory status; auscultate lungs before and after inhalation.
- Report treatment failure (exacerbation of respiratory symptoms) to physician.

Patient & Family Education
- Note: This medication is not an emergency agent because of its delayed onset and the time required to reach peak bronchodilation.
- Review patient information sheet on proper use of nasal spray.
- Allow 30–60 s between puffs for optimum results. Do not let medication contact your eyes.
- Wait 5 min between this and other inhaled medications. Check with physician about sequence of administration.
- Take medication only as directed, noting some leniency in number of puffs within 24 h. Supervise child's administration until certain all of dose is being administered.
- Rinse mouth after medication puffs to reduce bitter taste.
- Discuss changes in normal urinary pattern with the physician (more common in older adults).
- Call physician if you note changes in sputum color or amount, ankle edema, or significant weight gain.
- Do not breast feed while taking this drug without consulting physician.

IRBESARTAN

(ir-be-sar′tan)

Avapro

Classifications: CARDIOVASCULAR AGENT; ANGIOTENSIN II RECEPTOR ANTAGONIST

Prototype: Losartan

Pregnancy Category: C (first trimester); D (second and third trimesters)

AVAILABILITY 75 mg, 150 mg, 300 mg tablets

ACTIONS Irbesartan is an angiotensin II receptor (type AT_1) antagonist. Angiotensin II is a hormone of the renin–angiotensin–aldosterone system. Irbesartan selectively blocks the binding of angiotensin II to the AT_1 receptors found in many tissues (e.g., vascular smooth muscle, adrenal glands).

THERAPEUTIC EFFECTS Binding to the receptors results in blocking the vasoconstricting and aldosterone-secreting effects of angiotensin II, thus resulting in an antihypertensive effect.

USES Hypertension, treatment of diabetic nephropathy in patients with hypertension and type 2 diabetes.

UNLABELED USES CHF.

CONTRAINDICATIONS Hypersensitivity to irbesartan, losartan, or valsartan; pregnancy [(category C first trimester), category D (second and third trimesters)], lactation.

CAUTIOUS USE Patients on diuretics, arterial stenosis of the renal artery, severe CHF.

ROUTE & DOSAGE

Hypertension

Adult: **PO** Start with 150 mg once daily, may increase to 300 mg/d

ADMINISTRATION

Oral

- Correct volume depletion prior to initiation of therapy to prevent hypotension. Titrate daily dose up to 300 mg; larger doses, however, are not likely to provide additional benefit.

ADVERSE EFFECTS (≥1%) **Body as a Whole:** Edema, fatigue, pain. **CNS:** Dizziness, headache, anxiety, nervousness. **CV:** Tachycardia, chest pain. **GI:** Diarrhea, dyspepsia, nausea, vomiting, abdominal pain. **Respiratory:** Upper respiratory infection, cough, sinus disorder, pharyngitis, rhinitis. **Skin:** Rash. **Other:** UTI.

PHARMACOKINETICS Absorption: Rapidly absorbed from GI tract, 60%–80% bioavailability. **Distribution:** 90% protein bound. **Metabolism:** Metabolized in the liver primarily by CYP2C9. **Elimination:** Primarily excreted in feces (80%). **Half-Life:** 11–15 h.

NURSING IMPLICATIONS

Assessment & Drug Effects

- Monitor for therapeutic effectiveness: Maximum pressure lowering effect may not be evident for 6–12 wk; indicated by decreases in systolic and diastolic BP.
- Monitor BP periodically; trough readings, just prior to the next scheduled dose, should be made when possible.
- Lab tests: Monitor periodically BUN and creatinine, serum potassium, and CBC with differential.

Patient & Family Education

- Inform physician immediately if you become pregnant.
- Notify physician of episodes of dizziness, especially when making position changes.
- Do not breast feed while taking this drug.

IRINOTECAN HYDROCHLORIDE

(eye-ri-no'te-can)

Camptosar

Classifications: ANTINEOPLASTIC; CAMPTOTHECIN

Prototype: Topotecan

Pregnancy Category: D

AVAILABILITY 20 mg/mL injection

ACTIONS Irinotecan is a camptothecin analog that displays antitumor activity by inhibiting the intranuclear enzyme topoisomerase I. Thus, it is a strong inhibitor of DNA and RNA synthesis. Topoisomerase I is an essential intranuclear enzyme that relaxes the supercoiled DNA, thus enabling replication and transcription to take place.

THERAPEUTIC EFFECTS By inhibiting topoisomerase I, irinotecan and its active metabolite SN-38 cause double-stranded DNA damage during the synthesis (S) phase of DNA. This inhibits both DNA and RNA synthesis.

USES Metastatic carcinoma of colon or rectum.

CONTRAINDICATIONS Previous hypersensitivity to irinotecan, topotecan, or other camptothecin analogs; acute infection, diarrhea, pregnancy (category D), lactation.

CAUTIOUS USE Gastrointestinal disorders, myelosuppression, renal or hepatic function impairment, history of bleeding disorders, previous cyotoxic or radiation therapy. Safety and effectiveness in children are not established.

ROUTE & DOSAGE

Metastatic Carcinoma

Adult: **IV** 125 mg/m^2 once weekly for 4 wk, then a 2-wk rest period (future courses may be adjusted to range from 50 to 150 mg/m^2 depending on tolerance; see complete prescribing information for specific dosage adjustment recommendations based on toxic effects)

ADMINISTRATION

Intravenous

Administer only after premedication (at least 30 min prior) with an antiemetic. ▪ Wash immediately with soap and water if skin contacts drug during preparation.

PREPARE: **IV Infusion:** Dilute the ordered dose in enough D5W (preferred) or NS to yield a concentration of 0.12–1.1 mg/mL. Typical amount of diluent used is 500 mL.

ADMINISTER: **IV Infusion:** Infuse over 90 min. Closely monitor IV site; if extravasation occurs, immediately flush with sterile water and apply ice.

▪ Store undiluted at 15°–30° C (59°–86° F) and protect from light. Use reconstituted solutions within 24 h.

ADVERSE EFFECTS (≥1%) **Body as a Whole:** *Asthenia, fever, pain,* chills, edema, abdominal enlargement, back pain. **CNS:** Headache, *insomnia, dizziness.* **CV:** Vasodilation/flushing. **GI:** *Diarrhea (early and late onset), dehydration, nausea, vomiting, anorexia, weight loss, constipation, abdominal cramping and pain,* flatulence, stomatitis, dyspepsia, increased alkaline phosphatase and AST. **Hematologic:** *Leukopenia, neutropenia, anemia.* **Respiratory:** *Dyspnea,* cough, rhinitis. **Skin:** *Alopecia,* sweating, rash.

INTERACTIONS Drug: ANTICOAGULANTS, ANTIPLATELET AGENTS, NSAIDS may increase risk of bleeding; **carbamazepine, phenytoin, phenobarbital** may decrease irinotecan levels. **Herbal: St. John's wort** may decrease irinotecan levels.

PHARMACOKINETICS Peak: 1 h. **Distribution:** Irinotecan is 30% bound to plasma proteins; active metabolite SN-38 is 95% protein bound. **Metabolism:** Metabolized in liver by carboxylesterase enzyme to active metabolite SN-38. **Elimination:** 10 h for SN-38; approximately 20% excreted in urine. **Half-Life:** 6 h.

NURSING IMPLICATIONS

Assessment & Drug Effects

- Lab tests: Monitor WBC with differential, Hgb, and platelet count before each dose; monitor closely coagulation parameters especially with concurrent use of other drugs which affect these parameters.
- Lab tests: Monitor fluid and electrolyte balance closely during and after periods of diarrhea. Monitor liver and renal function tests and blood glucose periodically.
- Monitor for acute GI distress, especially early diarrhea (within 24 h of infusion), which may be preceded by diaphoresis and cramping, and late diarrhea (>24 h after infusion).

Patient & Family Education

- Learn about common adverse effects and measures to control or minimize when possible.
- Notify physician immediately when you experience diarrhea, vomiting, and S&S of infection. Diarrhea requires prompt treatment to prevent serious fluid and electrolyte imbalances.
- Do not breast feed while taking this drug.

IRON DEXTRAN

(i'ern dek'stran)

Dexferrum, Imfed, Imferon

Classifications: BLOOD FORMERS, COAGULATORS, AND ANTICOAGULANTS; IRON PREPARATION

Prototype: Ferrous sulfate

Pregnancy Category: C

AVAILABILITY 50 mg/mL

ACTIONS A dark brown, slightly viscous liquid complex of ferric hydroxide with dextran in 0.9% NaCl solution for injection.

THERAPEUTIC EFFECTS Reticuloendothelial cells of liver, spleen, and bone marrow dissociate iron from iron dextran complex. The released ferric ion combines with transferrin and is transported to bone marrow, where it is incorporated into hemoglobin.

USES Only in patients with clearly established iron deficiency anemia when oral administration of iron is unsatisfactory or impossible. Each milliliter of iron dextran contains 50 mg elemental iron.

CONTRAINDICATIONS Hypersensitivity to the product; all anemias except iron-deficiency anemia. Safe use during pregnancy (category C) is not established.

CAUTIOUS USE Lactation; rheumatoid arthritis, ankylosing spondylitis; impaired hepatic function; history of allergies or asthma.

ROUTE & DOSAGE

Iron Deficiency

Adult: **IM/IV** dose is individualized and determined from a table

of correlations between patient's weight and hemoglobin (see package insert); do not administer more than 100 mg (2 mL) of iron dextran within 24 h
Child: **IM/IV** *<5 kg,* no more than 0.5 mL (25 mg)/d; *5–10 kg,* no more than 1 mL (50 mg)/d; *>10 kg,* no more than 2 mL (100 mg)/d

ADMINISTRATION

Note: The multiple-dose vial is used ONLY for IM injections. It is not suitable for IV use because it contains a preservative (phenol).

Test Dose

- Give a test dose of 0.5 mL over a 5 min period before the first IM or IV therapeutic dose to observe patient's response to the drug. Have epinephrine (0.5 mL of a 1:1000 solution) immediately available for hypersensitivity emergency.
- Note: Although anaphylactic reactions (see Appendix F) usually occur within a few minutes after injection, it is recommended that 1 h or more elapse before remainder of initial dose is given following test dose.

Intramuscular

- Use the multiple-dose vial ONLY for IM injections. It is not suitable for IV use because it contains a preservative (phenol).
- Give injection only into the muscle mass in upper outer quadrant of buttock (never in the upper arm). In small child, use the lateral thigh. Use a 2- or 3-inch, 19- or 20-gauge needle. The Z-track technique is recommended. Use one needle to withdraw drug from container and another needle for injection.
- Note: If patient is receiving IM in standing position, patient should be bearing weight on the leg opposite the injection site; if in bed, patient should be in the lateral position with injection site uppermost.

Intravenous

Ensure that ONLY the vial for IV use is selected.

PREPARE: **Direct:** If the IV injection does not exceed 100 mg, it is administered undiluted. **IV Infusion:** Dilute in 250–1000 mL of NS.

ADMINISTER: **Direct:** Give 50 mg (1 mL) or fraction thereof over 60 sec. **IV Infusion:** Give test dose of 25 mg (0.5 mL) over 5 min. If no adverse reactions occur, infuse remainder over 1–8 h.

- After infusion is completed, flush vein with 10 mL of NS.
- Have patient remain in bed for at least 30 min after IV administration to prevent orthostatic hypotension. ▪ Monitor BP and pulse.

- Store below 30° C (86° F) unless otherwise directed.

ADVERSE EFFECTS (≥1%) **Body as a Whole:** Hypersensitivity (urticaria, skin rash, allergic purpura, pruritus, fever, chills, dyspnea, arthralgia, myalgia; anaphylaxis). **CNS:** Headache, shivering, transient paresthesias, syncope, dizziness, coma, seizures. **CV:** *Peripheral vascular flushing (rapid IV), hypotension,* precordial pain or pressure sensation, tachycardia, fatal cardiac arrhythmias, circulatory collapse. **GI:** Nausea, vomiting, transient loss of taste perception, metallic taste, diarrhea, melena, abdominal pain, hemorrhagic gastritis, intestinal necrosis, hepatic damage. **Skin:** Sterile abscess and brown skin discoloration (IM site), local phlebitis (IV site), lymphadenopathy, *pain at IM injection site.* **Metabolic:** Hemosiderosis, metabolic acidosis, hyperglycemia, reactivation of quiescent rheumatoid arthritis, exogenous hemosiderosis. **Hematologic:** Bleeding disorder with severe toxicity.

DIAGNOSTIC TEST INTERFERENCE Falsely elevated ***serum bilirubin*** and falsely decreased ***serum calcium*** values may occur. Large doses of iron dextran may impart a brown color to serum drawn 4 h after iron administration. ***Bone scans*** involving Tc-99m diphosphonate have shown dense areas of activity along contour of iliac crest 1–6 d after IM injections of iron dextran.

INTERACTIONS May decrease absorption of oral **iron, chloramphenicol** may decrease effectiveness of iron, a toxic complex may form with **dimercaprol.**

PHARMACOKINETICS Absorption: 60% absorbed from IM site by 3 d; 90% absorbed by 1–3 wk. **Distribution:** Crosses placenta; distributed into breast milk. **Metabolism:** Metabolized in reticuloendothelial system. **Half-Life:** 6 h.

NURSING IMPLICATIONS

Assessment & Drug Effects

- Monitor for therapeutic effectiveness: Anticipated response to parenteral iron therapy is an average weekly hemoglobin rise of about 1 g/d. Peak levels are generally reached in about 4–8 wk.
- Note: Systemic reactions may occur over 24 h after parenteral iron has been administered. Large IV doses are associated with increased frequency of adverse effects.
- Lab tests: Periodic determinations of Hgb and Hct, and reticulocyte count should be made.

Patient & Family Education

- Do not take oral iron preparations when receiving iron injections.
- Eat foods high in iron and vitamin C.
- Notify physician of any of the following: backache or muscle ache, chills, dizziness, fever, headache, nausea or vomiting, paresthesias, pain or redness at injection site, skin rash or hives, or difficulty breathing.
- Do not breast feed while taking this drug without consulting physician.

IRON SUCROSE INJECTION

(i'ron su'crose)
Venofer
Classifications: BLOOD FORMERS, COAGULATORS, AND ANTICOAGULANTS; IRON PREPARATION
Prototype: Ferrous Sulfate
Pregnancy Category: B

AVAILABILITY 100 mg elemental iron/5 mL vial

ACTIONS A complex of polynuclear iron (III) hydroxide in sucrose. It is dissociated by the reticuloendothelial system (RES) into iron and sucrose.

THERAPEUTIC EFFECTS Hemodialysis patients on erythropoietin therapy showed significant increases in serum iron and serum ferritin after 4 weeks of treatment with Venofer.

USES Treatment of iron deficiency anemia in patients on chronic hemodialysis.

CONTRAINDICATIONS Patients with iron overload, hypersensitivity to Venofer, or for anemia not caused by iron deficiency; concomitant use with an oral iron preparation.

CAUTIOUS USE Patients with a history of hypotension; pregnancy (category B), lactation; older adults, decreased renal, hepatic, or cardiac function. Safety and effectiveness in children are not established.

ROUTE & DOSAGE

Iron Deficiency Anemia

Adult: **IV** 1 mL (20 mg) injected in dialysis line at rate of 1 mL/min up to 5 mL (100 mg) or infuse 100 mg in NS over 15 min 1–3 times/wk

ADMINISTRATION

Intravenous

PREPARE: **Direct:** Give undiluted. **IV Infusion:** Dilute one vial (100 mg) in a maximum of 100 mL NS immediately prior to infusion.

ADMINISTER: **Direct:** Give undiluted by IV push at a rate of 1 mL (20 mg) per min during dialysis. Do not exceed one vial (100 mg) per injection. Avoid rapid injection. **IV Infusion:** Infusion diluted solution into dialysis line at a rate of 100 mg over at least 15 min. Avoid rapid infusion.

INCOMPATIBILITIES **Solution/additive:** Do not mix with other medications or parenteral nutrition solutions.

- Store unopened vials preferably at 25° C (77° F), but room temperature permitted. Discard unused portion in opened vial.

ADVERSE EFFECTS (≥1%) **Body as a Whole:** Fever, pain, asthenia, malaise, anaphylactoid reactions. **Cardiovascular:** *Hypotension,* chest pain, hypertension, hypervolemia. **Digestive:** Nausea, vomiting, diarrhea, abdominal pain, elevated liver function tests. **Musculoskeletal:** *Leg cramps,* muscle pain. **CNS:** Headache, dizziness. **Respiratory:** Dyspnea, pneumonia, cough. **Skin:** Pruritus, injection site reaction.

INTERACTIONS Drug: May reduce absorption of ORAL IRON PREPARATIONS.

PHARMACOKINETICS Peak: 4 wk. **Distribution:** Primarily to blood with some distribution to liver, spleen, bone marrow. **Metabolism:** Dissociated to iron and sucrose in reticuloendothelial system. **Elimination:** Sucrose is eliminated in urine, 5% of iron excreted in urine. **Half-Life:** 6 h.

NURSING IMPLICATIONS

Assessment & Drug Effects

- Withhold drug and notify physician when serum ferritin level equals or exceeds established guidelines.
- Stop infusion and notify physician for S&S overdosage or infusing too rapidly: hypotension, edema; headache, dizziness, nausea, vomiting, abdominal pain, joint or muscle pain, and paresthesia.
- Lab tests: Periodic serum ferritin, transferrin saturation, Hct, and Hgb.
- Monitor patient carefully during the first 30 min after initiation of IV therapy for signs of hypersensitivity and anaphylactoid reaction (see Appendix F).

Patient & Family Education

- Report any of the following promptly: Itching, rash, chest pain, headache, dizziness, nausea, vomiting, abdominal pain, joint or muscle pain, and numbness and tingling.
- Do not breast feed while taking this drug without consulting physician.

ISOCARBOXAZID

(eye-soe-kar-box'a-zid)

Marplan

Classifications: CENTRAL NERVOUS SYSTEM AGENT; PSYCHOTHERAPEUTIC; ANTIDEPRESSANT; MONOAMINE OXIDASE (MAO) INHIBITOR

Prototype: Phenelzine

Pregnancy Category: C

Common adverse effects in *italic*, life-threatening effects underlined: generic names in **bold**; classifications in SMALL CAPS; ♣ Canadian drug name; ● Prototype drug

AVAILABILITY 10 mg tablets

ACTIONS MAO INHIBITOR of the hydrazine group. Inhibits monoamine oxidase, the enzyme involved in the catabolism of catecholamine neurotransmitters and serotonin.
THERAPEUTIC EFFECTS Marplan increases concentration of catecholamine neurotransmitters as well as serotonin and dopamine within presynaptic neurons and at receptor sites, the proposed basis for the antidepressant effect of MAOIS.

USES Symptomatic treatment of depressed patients refractory to or intolerant of TCAs or electroconvulsive therapy.

CONTRAINDICATIONS Hypersensitivity to MAO INHIBITORS; pheochromocytoma; CHF; children (<16 y); older adults (>60 y) or debilitated patients; severe renal or hepatic impairment. Safe use during pregnancy (category C) or lactation is not established.
CAUTIOUS USE Hypertension, hyperthyroidism, parkinsonism, cardiac arrhythmias, epilepsy, suicidal risks.

ROUTE & DOSAGE

Refractory Depression
Adult: **PO** 10–30 mg/d in 1–3 divided doses (max: 30 mg/d)

ADMINISTRATION

Oral
- Note: Dosage is individualized on the basis of patient response. Lowest effective dosage should be used.
- Store in a tight, light-resistant container.

ADVERSE EFFECTS (≥1%) **CNS:** Dizziness, light-headedness, tiredness, weakness, *drowsiness,* vertigo, headache, *overactivity,* hyperreflexia, muscle twitching, tremors, mania hypomania, *insomnia,* confusion, memory impairment. **CV:** *Orthostatic hypotension,* paradoxical hypertension, palpitation, tachycardia, other arrhythmias. **Special Senses:** *Blurred vision,* nystagmus, glaucoma. **GI:** Increased appetite, weight gain, *nausea,* diarrhea, *constipation, anorexia,* black tongue, *dry mouth,* abdominal pain. **Urogenital:** Dysuria, *urinary retention,* incontinence, sexual disturbances. **Body as a Whole:** Peripheral edema, excessive sweating, chills, skin rash, hepatitis, jaundice.

INTERACTIONS Drug: TRICYCLIC ANTIDEPRESSANTS, **fluoxetine,** AMPHETAMINES, **ephedrine, phenylpropanolamine, reserpine, guanethidine, buspirone, methyldopa, dopamine, levodopa, tryptophan** may precipitate hypertensive crisis, headache, or hyperexcitability; **alcohol** and other CNS DEPRESSANTS compound CNS depressant effects; **meperidine** can cause fatal cardiovascular collapse; ANESTHETICS exaggerate hypotensive and CNS depressant effects; **metrizamide** increases risk of seizures; compounds hypotensive effects of DIURETICS and other ANTIHYPERTENSIVE AGENTS. **Food:** All **tyramine**-containing foods (aged cheeses, processed cheeses, sour cream, wine, champagne, beer, pickled herring, anchovies, caviar, shrimp, liver, dry sausage, figs, raisins, overripe bananas or avocados, chocolate, soy sauce, bean curd, yeast extracts, yogurt, papaya products, meat tenderizers, broad beans) may precipitate hypertensive crisis. **Herbal: Ginseng, Ephedra, ma huang, St. John's wort** may precipitate hypertensive crisis.

PHARMACOKINETICS Duration: Up to 2 wk. **Metabolism:** Metabolized in liver.

NURSING IMPLICATIONS

Assessment & Drug Effects

- Monitor for therapeutic effectiveness: May be apparent within 1 wk or less, but in some patients there may be a time lag of 3–4 wk before improvement occurs.
- Monitor BP. Monitor for orthostatic hypotension by evaluating BP with patient recumbent and standing.
- Check for peripheral edema daily and monitor weight several times weekly.
- Note: Toxic symptoms from overdosage or from ingestion of contraindicated substances (e.g., foods high in tyramine) may occur within hours.
- Monitor I&O and bowel elimination patterns.

Patient & Family Education

- Make position changes slowly and in stages; lie down or sit down if faintness occurs.
- Use caution when performing potentially hazardous activities.
- Consult physician before self-medicating with OTC agents (e.g., cough, cold, hay fever, or diet medications).
- Avoid alcohol and excessive caffeine-containing beverages and tryptophan and tyramine-containing foods including cheeses, yeast, meat extracts, smoked or pickled meat, poultry, or fish, fermented sausages, and overripe fruit.
- Do not breast feed while taking this drug without consulting physician.

ISOETHARINE HYDROCHLORIDE

(eye-soe-eth'a-reen)

Arm-a-Med Isoetharine, Beta-2, Bronkosol, Dey-Lute, Dispos-a-Med Isoetharine

Classifications: AUTONOMIC NERVOUS SYSTEM AGENT; BETA-ADRENERGIC AGONIST (SYMPATHOMIMETIC); BRONCHODILATOR

Prototype: Albuterol

Pregnancy Category: C

AVAILABILITY 1% solution

ACTIONS Synthetic sympathomimetic stimulant with relatively rapid onset and long duration of action. Has selective affinity for $beta_2$ adreno-receptors on bronchial and selected arteriolar musculature.

THERAPEUTIC EFFECTS Relieves reversible bronchospasm and by bronchodilation facilitates expectoration of pulmonary secretions. Increases vital capacity and decreases airway resistance.

USES Bronchial asthma and reversible bronchospasm occurring with bronchitis and emphysema.

CONTRAINDICATIONS Known hypersensitivity to sympathomimetic amines and to bisulfites; concomitant use with epinephrine or other sympathomimetic amines; patients with preexisting cardiac arrhythmias associated with tachycardia. Use during pregnancy (category C) or lactation requires judgment of risk/benefit ratio.

CAUTIOUS USE Older adults; hypertension; acute coronary artery disease; CHF; cardiac asthma; hyperthyroidism, diabetes mellitus; tuberculosis; history of seizures.

ROUTE & DOSAGE

Bronchospasm

Adult: **Inhalation** 0.5–1 mL 0.5% or 0.5 mL 1% solution diluted 1:3 with normal saline or 2–4 mL 0.125% solution undiluted or 2–5 mL 0.2% solution undiluted or 2 mL 0.25% solution undiluted per nebulizer q4h (max: 5 times/d); 1–2 inhalations from an MDI q4h up to 5 times/d
Child: **Inhalation** 0.01 mL/kg of 1% solution (max: 0.5 mL) diluted in 2–3 mL normal saline

ADMINISTRATION

Inhalation

- Give on arising in morning and before meals to reduce fatigue from activity by improving lung ventilation.
- Wait 1 full min after initial 1 or 2 inhalations (Bronkometer) to be sure of necessity for another dose. Action should begin immediately and peak within 5–15 min.
- Alternate therapy with concurrent epinephrine administration but do not administer simultaneously because of danger of excessively rapid heartbeat.
- Do not use discolored or precipitated solutions.
- Protect solutions from light, freezing, and heat.

ADVERSE EFFECTS (≥1%) **CV:** *Tachycardia, palpitations,* changes in BP, cardiac arrest. **GI:** Nausea, vomiting. **CNS:** Headache, *anxiety,* tension, restlessness, insomnia, *tremor,* weakness, dizziness, excitement. **Respiratory:** Cough, bronchial irritation and edema; tachyphylaxis.

INTERACTIONS Drug: Epinephrine, other SYMPATHOMIMETIC BRONCHODILATORS possibly have additive effects; MAO INHIBITORS, TRICYCLIC ANTIDEPRESSANTS potentiate action on vascular system; effects of both BETA-ADRENERGIC BLOCKERS and isoetharine antagonized when given together.

PHARMACOKINETICS Onset: Immediate. **Peak:** 5–15 min. **Duration:** 1–4 h. **Metabolism:** Metabolized in lungs, liver, GI tract, and other tissues. **Elimination:** Excreted by kidneys.

NURSING IMPLICATIONS

Assessment & Drug Effects

- Do not use this product if patient has a history of allergy to sulfite agents. The preservative sodium bisulfite is in the hydrochloride formulation.
- Monitor cardiac status and report tachycardia and palpitations. Older adults may be especially sensitive to adrenergic drug effects.

Patient & Family Education

- Close eyes when actuating the nebulizer.
- Use inhalation therapy according to prescribed regimen. Overuse may decrease desired effect and cause symptoms including tachycardia, palpitations, headache, nausea, dizziness.
- Read information and instructions furnished with the aerosol form of isoetharine.
- Increase daily fluid intake to aid in liquefaction of bronchial secretions.
- Discontinue drug and notify physician if a sudden increase in dyspnea occurs.
- Do not discard drug applicator. Refill units are available.
- Do not breast feed while taking this drug without consulting physician.

ISOMETHEPTENE/ DICHLORALPHENAZONE/ ACETAMINOPHEN

(i-so-meth'ep-tene/di-chlor-al-phen'a-zone/a-cet'a-min-o-phen)

Isopap, Duradrin, Midrin, Migratine

Classifications: CENTRAL NERVOUS SYSTEM AGENT; ANALGESIC, NONNARCOTIC

Prototype: Isometheptene/dichloralphenazone/acetaminophen

Pregnancy Category: C

AVAILABILITY 65 mg **isometheptene mucate,** 100 mg **dichloralphenazone,** 325 mg **APAP** capsules

ACTIONS Isometheptene is a sympathomimetic amine that acts by constricting cranial and cerebral arterioles.

THERAPEUTIC EFFECTS Isometheptene relieves vascular headaches. Dichloralphenazone is a mild sedative that helps reduce headache pain. Acetaminophen is a mild analgesic.

USES Relief for tension, vascular, and migraine headaches.

CONTRAINDICATIONS Patients with glaucoma; severe renal disease, organic heart disease; hepatic disease; concurrent MAO inhibitors.

CAUTIOUS USE Hypertension; peripheral vascular disease, and recent cardiovascular attacks.

ROUTE & DOSAGE

Tension Headache

Adult: **PO** 1–2 capsules q4h up to 8 capsules/24 h

Migraine Headache

Adult: **PO** 2 capsules at onset, then 1 capsule qh until relief (max: 5 capsules/12 h)

ADMINISTRATION

Oral

- Do not give this drug to anyone who is concurrently using a MAOI. Allow 14 days to elapse between discontinuation of the MAOI and administration of this drug.
- Do not give more than 8 capsules in a 24 h period.
- Store at 15°–30° C (59°–86° F) in a dry place.

ADVERSE EFFECTS (≥1%) **CNS:** Transient dizziness. **GI:** Acetaminophen hepatotoxicity. **Skin:** Rash.

INTERACTIONS Drug: MAOIS may cause hypertensive crisis; other **acetaminophen**-containing drugs (including OTC) may increase risk of hepatotoxicity.

PHARMACOKINETICS Absorption: Rapidly absorbed. **Metabolism:** Dichloralphenazone is metabolized to chloral hydrate and antipyrine. See ACETAMINOPHEN and CHLORAL HYDRATE for more detail. **Elimination:** Renal and hepatic. **Half-Life:** 12 h.

NURSING IMPLICATIONS

Assessment & Drug Effects

- Monitor BP closely with preexisting hypertension.
- Monitor lower extremity perfusion with a history of PVD.

Patient & Family Education

- Avoid, or moderate, alcohol use while taking this drug.
- Do not drive or engage in other potentially hazardous activities until response to drug is known.

- Report any decrease in tolerance to walking if you have a history of PVD.

ISONIAZID (ISONICOTINIC ACID HYDRAZIDE) Pr

(eye-soe-nye'a-zid)

INH, Isotamine ♣, Laniazid, Nydrazid, PMS Isoniazid ♣, Teebaconin

Classifications: ANTIINFECTIVE; ANTITUBERCULOSIS AGENT

Pregnancy Category: C

AVAILABILITY 50 mg, 100 mg, 300 mg tablets; 50 mg/5 mL syrup; 100 mg/mL injection

ACTIONS Hydrazide of isonicotinic acid with highly specific action against *Mycobacterium tuberculosis*. Postulated to act by interfering with biosynthesis of bacterial proteins, nucleic acid, and lipids.

THERAPEUTIC EFFECTS Exerts bacteriostatic action against actively growing tubercle bacilli; may be bactericidal in higher concentrations.

USES Treatment of all forms of active tuberculosis caused by susceptible organisms and as preventive in high-risk persons (e.g., household members, persons with positive tuberculin skin test reactions). May be used alone or with other tuberculostatic agents.

UNLABELED USES Treatment of atypical mycobacterial infections; tuberculous meningitis; action tremor in multiple sclerosis.

CONTRAINDICATIONS History of isoniazid-associated hypersensitivity reactions, including hepatic injury; acute liver damage of any etiology; pregnancy (category C) unless risk is warranted.

CAUTIOUS USE Chronic liver disease; renal dysfunction; history of convulsive disorders; chronic alcoholism; persons over 35 y; lactation.

ROUTE & DOSAGE

Treatment of Active Tuberculosis

Adult: **PO/IM** 5 mg/kg (max: 300 mg/d)
Child: **PO/IM** 10–20 mg/kg (max: 300–500 mg/d)

Preventive Therapy

Adult: **PO** 300 mg/d
Child: **PO** 10 mg/kg up to 300 mg/d or 15 mg/kg 3 times/wk

ADMINISTRATION

Oral

- Give on an empty stomach at least 1 h before or 2 h after meals. If GI irritation occurs, drug may be taken with meals.

Intramuscular

- Note: Isoniazid solution for IM injection tends to crystallize at low temperatures; if this occurs, solution should be allowed to warm to room temperature to redissolve crystals before use.
- Give deep into a large muscle and rotate injection sites; local transient pain may follow IM injections.
- Store in tightly closed, light-resistant containers.

ADVERSE EFFECTS (≥1%) **Body as a Whole:** Drug-related fever, rheumatic and lupus erythematosus-like syndromes, irritation at injection site; hypersensitivity (fever, chills, skin eruption, vasculitis). **CNS:** *Paresthesias, peripheral neuropathy,* headache, unusual tiredness or weakness, tinnitus, dizziness, hallucinations. **Special Senses:** Blurred vision, visual disturbances, optic neuritis, atrophy. **GI:** Nausea, vomiting, epigastric distress, dry mouth, constipation; hepatotoxicity (*elevated AST, ALT;* bilirubinemia, jaundice, hepatitis). **Hematologic:** Agranulocytosis, hemolytic or aplastic anemia, thrombocytopenia, eosinophilia, methemoglobinemia. **Metabolic:** Decreased vitamin B_{12} absorption, pyridoxine (vitamin B_6) deficiency, pellagra, gynecomastia, hyperglycemia, glycosuria, hyperkalemia, hypophosphatemia, hypocalcemia, acetonuria, metabolic acidosis, proteinuria. **Other:** Dyspnea, urinary retention (males).

I

DIAGNOSTIC TEST INTERFERENCE Isoniazid may produce false-positive results using ***copper sulfate tests*** (e.g., ***Benedict's solution, Clinitest***) but not with **glucose oxidase methods** (e.g., **Clinistix, Dextrostix, TesTape**).

INTERACTIONS Drug: Cycloserine, ethionamide enhance CNS toxicity; may increase **phenytoin** levels, resulting in toxicity; ALUMINUM-CONTAINING ANTACIDS decrease GI absorption; **disulfiram** may cause coordination difficulties or psychotic reactions; **alcohol** increases risk of hepatotoxicity. **Food:** Food decreases rate and extent of isoniazid absorption; should be taken 1 h before meals.

PHARMACOKINETICS Absorption: Readily absorbed from GI tract; food may reduce rate and extent of absorption. **Peak:** 1–2 h. **Distribution:** Distributed to all body tissues and fluids including the CNS; crosses placenta. **Metabolism:** Inactivated by acetylation in liver. **Elimination:** 75%–96% excreted in urine in 24 h; excreted in breast milk. **Half-Life:** 1–4 h.

NURSING IMPLICATIONS

Assessment & Drug Effects

- Monitor for therapeutic effectiveness: Evident within the first 2–3 wk of therapy. Over 90% of patients receiving optimal therapy have negative sputum by the sixth month.
- Perform appropriate susceptibility tests before initiation of therapy and periodically thereafter to detect possible bacterial resistance.
- Lab tests: Monitor hepatic function periodically. Isoniazid hepatitis (sometimes fatal) usually develops during the first 3–6 mo of treatment, but may occur at any time during therapy; much more frequent in patients 35 y or older, especially in those who ingest alcohol daily.
- Monitor for visual disturbance. An eye examination may be warranted.
- Note: Inactivation of the drug is genetically determined. Slow inactivation leads to high plasma drug levels and increased risk of toxicity.
- Isoniazid-induced pyridoxine (vitamin B_6) depletion causes neurotoxic effects. B_6 supplementation (10–50 mg) usually accompanies isoniazid use.
- Peripheral neuritis, the most common toxic effect, is usually preceded by paresthesias of feet and hands (numbness, tingling, burning). Patients particularly susceptible include alcoholics and patients with liver disease, malnourished patients, diabetics, slow inactivators, pregnant women, and older adults.
- Monitor BP during period of dosage adjustment. Some experience orthostatic hypotension; therefore, caution against rapid positional changes.

- Monitor diabetics for loss of glycemic control.
- Check weight at least twice weekly under standard conditions.

Patient & Family Education

- Note: Eating tyramine-containing foods (e.g., aged cheeses, smoked fish) may cause palpitation, flushing, and blood pressure elevation. Histamine-containing foods (e.g., skipjack, tuna, sauerkraut juice, yeast extracts) may cause exaggerated drug response (headache, hypotension, palpitation, sweating, itching, flushing, diarrhea).
- Withhold medication and notify physician if S&S of hepatotoxicity develop (e.g., dark urine, jaundice, clay-colored stools).
- Avoid or at least reduce alcohol intake while on isoniazid therapy because of increased risk of hepatotoxicity.
- Withhold all drugs and notify physician of hypersensitivity reaction immediately; generally occurs within 3–7 wk after initiation of therapy.
- Do not breast feed while taking this drug without consulting physician.

ISOPROTERENOL HYDROCHLORIDE

(eye-soe-proe-ter′e-nole)

Dispos-a-Med, Isoproterenol, Isuprel

ISOPROTERENOL SULFATE

Medihaler-Iso

Classifications: AUTONOMIC NERVOUS SYSTEM AGENT; BETA-ADRENERGIC AGONIST (SYMPATHOMIMETIC); BRONCHODILATOR

Prototype: Albuterol

Pregnancy Category: C

AVAILABILITY **Isoproterenol HCl** 0.5%, 1% solution for inhalation; 103 mcg aerosol; 0.2 mg/mL, 0.02 mg/mL injection; **Isoproterenol Sulfate** 80 mcg aerosol

ACTIONS Synthetic sympathomimetic amine. Acts directly on beta$_1$-adrenergic receptors with little or no effect on alpha-adrenoceptors. Drug induced stimulation of beta$_1$-adrenergic receptors results in increased cardiac output and cardiac work by increasing strength of contraction and, to a slight degree, rate of contraction of the heart. Produces slight increase in systolic BP and decrease in diastolic pressure.

THERAPEUTIC EFFECTS Reduces total peripheral resistance and increases venous return to the heart by mobilizing blood from vascular reservoirs and increases cardiac contractions. Stimulation of beta$_2$-adrenoceptors relaxes bronchospasm and, by increasing ciliary motion, facilitates expectoration of pulmonary secretions. May dilate trachea and main bronchi past the resting diameter.

USES Bronchodilator in treatment of bronchial asthma and reversible bronchospasm induced by anesthesia. Also used as cardiac stimulant in cardiac arrest, carotid sinus hypersensitivity, cardiogenic and bacteremic shock, Adams-Stokes syndrome, or ventricular arrhythmias. Used in treatment of shock that persists after replacement of blood volume.

UNLABELED USES Treatment of status asthmaticus in children.

CONTRAINDICATIONS Preexisting cardiac arrhythmias associated with tachycardia; tachycardia caused by digitalis intoxication, central hyperexcitability, cardiogenic shock secondary to coronary artery occlusion and MI; simultaneous administration

I

with epinephrine. Safe use during pregnancy (category C) or lactation is not established.

CAUTIOUS USE Sensitivity to sympathomimetic amines; older adult and debilitated patients, hypertension, coronary insufficiency and other cardiovascular disorders, renal dysfunction, hyperthyroidism, diabetes, prostatic hypertrophy, glaucoma, tuberculosis, during anesthesia by cyclopropane.

ROUTE & DOSAGE

Bronchospasms

Adult/Child: **MDI** 1–2 inhalations 4–6 times/d (max: 6 inhalations in any hour during a 24 h period). **Compressed Air or IPPB** 0.5 mL of 0.5% solution diluted to 2–2.5 mL with water or saline over 10–20 min up to 5 times/d
Adult: **IV** 0.01–0.02 mg prn

Cardiac Arrhythmias/Cardiac Resuscitation

Adult: **IV** 0.02–0.06 mg bolus, followed by 5 mcg/min infusion **SC** 0.15–0.2 mg prn
Child: **IV** 2.5 mcg/min *or* 0.1 mcg/kg/min by continuous infusion

ADMINISTRATION

MDI

- Shake MDI thoroughly to activate.
- Breathe out through nose expelling as much air from lungs as possible.
- Close lips and teeth around open end of mouthpiece placed well into mouth aimed at back of throat.
- Inhale deeply while pressing down on canister to activate spray mechanism.
- Try to hold breath for 10 s; then slowly exhale through nose or pursed lips.
- Wait 2 full min before starting a second inhalation, if it is necessary.

IPPB

- Follow IPPB manufacturer's instructions.
- Have patient sit erect in chair or, if not able, lie in semi-Fowler's position.
- Instruct patient to ALLOW MACHINE TO DO THE WORK (deliver medication into air passages and breathe for the patient).
- Leave dentures in place.
- Rinse mouth immediately after inhalation therapy to prevent dryness and throat irritation.
- Store all formulations in tight, light-resistant containers.

Intravenous

PREPARE: **Direct:** Dilute 1 mL of 1:5000 solution with 9 mL NS or D5W to produce a 1:50,000 (0.02 mg/mL) solution. **IV Infusion:** Dilute 10 mL of 1:5000 solution in 500 mL D5W to produce a 1:250,000 (4 mcg/mL) solution.

ADMINISTER: **Direct:** Give each 1 ml of 1:50,000 solution over 1 min. Flush with 15–20 mL NS. **IV Infusion:** Infusion rate is generally decreased or infusion may be temporarily discontinued if heart rate exceeds 110 bpm, because of the danger of precipitating arrhythmias. Microdrip or constant-infusion pump is recommended to prevent sudden influx of large amounts of drug. IV administration is regulated by continuous ECG monitoring. Patient must be observed and response to therapy must be monitored continuously.

INCOMPATIBILITIES **Solution/additive:** Sodium bicarbonate, **aminophylline.**

- Isoproterenol solutions lose potency with standing. Discard if precipitate or discoloration is present.

ADVERSE EFFECTS (≥1%) **CNS:** Headache, mild tremors, nervousness, anxiety, insomnia, excitement, fatigue. **CV:** Flushing, palpitations, tachycardia, unstable BP, anginal pain, ventricular arrhythmias. **GI:** Swelling of parotids (prolonged use), bad taste, buccal ulcerations (sublingual administration), nausea. **Other:** Severe prolonged asthma attack, sweating, bronchial irritation and edema. **Acute Poisoning:** Overdosage, especially after excessive use of aerosols (*tachycardia,* palpitations, nervousness, nausea, vomiting).

INTERACTIONS Drug: Epinephrine and other SYMPATHOMIMETIC AMINES increase effects and cause cardiac toxicity. HALOGENATED GENERAL ANESTHETICS exacerbate arrhythmias; while BETA BLOCKERS antagonize effects.

PHARMACOKINETICS Absorption: Rapidly absorbed from oral inhalation or parenteral administration. **Onset:** Immediate. **Duration:** 1 h oral inhalation; 2 h SC. **Metabolism:** Action terminated by tissue uptake and metabolized by COMT in liver, lungs, and other tissues. **Elimination:** 40%–50% excreted in urine unchanged.

NURSING IMPLICATIONS

Assessment & Drug Effects

- Check pulse before and during IV administration. Rate >110 usually indicates need to slow infusion rate or discontinue infusion. Consult physician for guidelines. Incidence of arrhythmias is high, particularly when drug is administered IV to patients with cardiogenic shock or ischemic heart disease, digitalized patients, or to those with electrolyte imbalance.
- Note: Tolerance to bronchodilating effect and cardiac stimulant effect may develop with prolonged use.
- Discontinue drug if parotid swelling occurs; has been reported after prolonged use.
- Note: Once tolerance has developed, continued use can result in serious adverse effects including rebound bronchospasm.

Patient & Family Education

- Take medication as prescribed; (i.e., do not increase, decrease, or omit doses or change intervals between doses). Notify physician if treatment fails to give satisfactory relief.
- Learn with responsible family members about adverse effects and report onset of such reactions to physician.
- Be aware that saliva and sputum may appear pink after inhalation treatment.
- Do not breast feed while taking this drug without consulting physician.

ISOSORBIDE

(eye-soe-sor′bide)

Ismotic

Classifications: OSMOTIC DIURETIC; ANTIGLAUCOMA

Prototype: Mannitol

Pregnancy Category: B

AVAILABILITY 45% solution

ACTIONS Actions similar to those of other osmotic agents, e.g., mannitol, but produces greater diuresis and does not cause hyperglycemia. **THERAPEUTIC EFFECTS** Reduces intraocular pressure (IOP) by increasing plasma osmotic pressure.

USES Short-term emergency treatment of acute angle-closure glaucoma and for reducing IOP before and after surgery for glaucoma and cataract.

CONTRAINDICATIONS Hypersensitivity to isosorbide; severe renal disease, anuria; severe dehydration; frank or impending pulmonary edema; hemorrhagic glaucoma. Safe use during pregnancy (category B) is not established.
CAUTIOUS USE Diseases associated with sodium retention, lactation.

ROUTE & DOSAGE

Acute Angle-closure Glaucoma
Adult: **PO** 1–3 g/kg b.i.d. to q.i.d.

ADMINISTRATION

Oral
- Pour over ice and have patient sip in order to make more palatable.

ADVERSE EFFECTS (≥1%) **CNS:** Headache, lethargy, vertigo, dizziness, light-headedness, syncope, *confusion, disorientation,* irritability. **GI:** *Nausea, vomiting,* diarrhea, anorexia, gastric discomfort, thirst. **Respiratory:** Hiccups. **Skin:** Rash. **Metabolic:** Hypernatremia, hyperosmolality.

INTERACTIONS No clinically significant interactions established.

PHARMACOKINETICS Absorption: Readily absorbed from GI tract. **Onset:** 30 min. **Peak:** 1–1.5 h. **Duration:** Up to 5–6 h. **Elimination:** Eliminated unchanged in urine.

NURSING IMPLICATIONS

Assessment & Drug Effects
- Monitor fluid and electrolyte balance carefully.
- Monitor IOP frequently.

Patient & Family Education
- Keep follow-up appointments.
- Do not breast feed while taking this drug without consulting physician.

ISOSORBIDE DINITRATE

(eye-soe-sor′bide)
Coronex ♣, Dilatrate-SR, Iso-Bid, Isordil, Isotrate, Novosorbide ♣, Sorbitrate, Sorbitrate SA
Classifications: CARDIOVASCULAR AGENT; NITRATE VASODILATOR
Prototype: Nitroglycerin
Pregnancy Category: C

AVAILABILITY 2.5 mg, 5 mg, 10 mg sublingual tablets; 5 mg, 10 mg chewable tablets; 5 mg, 10 mg, 20 mg, 30 mg, 40 mg tablets; 40 mg sustained release tablets, capsules

ACTIONS Organic nitrate with pharmacologic actions similar to those of nitroglycerin. Relaxes vascular smooth muscle with resulting vasodilation. Dilation of peripheral blood vessels tends to cause peripheral pooling of blood, decreased venous return to heart, and decreased left ventricular end-diastolic pressure, with consequent reduction in myocardial oxygen consumption.
THERAPEUTIC EFFECTS Has an antianginal effect by causing vasodilation of the coronary arteries.

USES Relief of acute anginal attacks and for management of long-term angina pectoris.
UNLABELED USES Alone or in combination with a cardiac glycoside or with other vasodilators (e.g., hydralazine, prazosin, for refractory CHF; diffuse esophageal spasm without gastroesophageal reflux and heart failure).

CONTRAINDICATIONS Hypersensitivity to nitrates or nitrites; severe anemia; head trauma; increased intracranial pressure. Safe use during pregnancy (category C) or lactation is not established.

CAUTIOUS USE Glaucoma, hypotension, hyperthyroidism.

ROUTE & DOSAGE

Angina Prophylaxis

Adult: **PO** Regular tablets 2.5–30 mg q.i.d. a.c. and h.s.; Sublingual tablet 2.5–10 mg q4–6h; Chewable tablet 5–30 mg chewed q2–3h; Sustained release tablets 40 mg q6–12h

Acute Anginal Attack

Adult: **PO** Sublingual tablet 2.5–10 mg q2–3h prn; Chewable tablet 5–30 mg chewed prn for relief

ADMINISTRATION

Oral

- Do not confuse with isosorbide, an oral osmotic diuretic.
- Give regular oral forms on an empty stomach (1 h a.c. or 2 h p.c.). If patient complains of vascular headache, however, it may be taken with meals.
- Advise patient not to eat, drink, talk, or smoke while sublingual tablet is under tongue.
- Instruct patient to place sublingual tablet under tongue at first sign of an anginal attack. If pain is not relieved, repeat dose at 5–10 min intervals to a maximum of 3 doses. If pain continues, notify physician or go to nearest hospital emergency room.
- Chewable tablet must be thoroughly chewed before swallowing.
- Do not crush sustained release form. It must be swallowed whole.
- Have patient sit when taking rapid-acting forms of isosorbide dinitrate (sublingual and chewable tablets) because of the possibility of faintness.
- Store in tightly closed container in a cool, dry place. Do not expose to extremes of temperature.

ADVERSE EFFECTS (≥1%) **Body as a Whole:** Hypersensitivity reaction, paradoxical increase in anginal pain, methemoglobinemia (overdose). **CNS:** Headache, dizziness, weakness, *lightheadedness,* restlessness. **CV:** Palpitation, postural hypotension, tachycardia. **GI:** Nausea, vomiting. **Skin:** *Flushing,* pallor, perspiration, rash, exfoliative dermatitis.

INTERACTIONS Drug: Alcohol may enhance hypotensive effects and lead to cardiovascular collapse; ANTIHYPERTENSIVE AGENTS, PHENOTHIAZINES add to hypotensive effects.

PHARMACOKINETICS Absorption: Significant first pass metabolism with PO absorption, with 10%–90% reaching systemic circulation. **Onset:** 2–5 min SL; within 1 h regular tabs; within 3 min chewable tabs; 30 min sustained release tabs. **Duration:** 1–2 h SL; 4–6 h regular tabs; 0.5–2 h chewable tabs; 6–8 h sustained release tabs. **Metabolism:** Metabolized in liver. **Elimination:** 80%–100% excreted in urine within 24 h.

NURSING IMPLICATIONS

Assessment & Drug Effects

- Monitor effectiveness of drug in relieving angina.
- Note: Headaches tend to decrease in intensity and frequency with continued therapy but may require administration of analgesic and reduction in dosage.
- Note: Chronic administration of large doses may produce tolerance and thus decrease effectiveness of nitrate preparations.

Patient & Family Education

- Make position changes slowly, particularly from recumbent to upright posture, and dangle feet and ankles before walking.
- Lie down at the first indication of light-headedness or faintness.
- Keep a record of anginal attacks and the number of sublingual tablets required to provide relief.
- Do not drink alcohol because it may increase possibility of light-headedness and faintness.
- Do not breast feed while taking this drug without consulting physician.

ISOSORBIDE MONONITRATE

(eye-soe-sor'bide)

Ismo, Imdur, Monoket

Classifications: CARDIOVASCULAR AGENT; NITRATE VASODILATOR

Prototype: Nitroglycerin

Pregnancy Category: C (category B for sustained release form)

AVAILABILITY 10 mg, 20 mg tablets; 30 mg, 60 mg, 120 mg sustained release tablets

ACTIONS Isosorbide mononitrate is a long-acting metabolite of the coronary vasodilator isosorbide dinitrate. It decreases preload as measured by pulmonary capillary wedge pressure (PCWP), and left ventricular end volume and diastolic pressure (LVEDV), with a consequent reduction in myocardial oxygen consumption.

THERAPEUTIC EFFECTS It is equally or more effective than isosorbide dinitrate in the treatment of chronic, stable angina. It is a potent vasodilator with antianginal and antiischemic effects.

USES Prevention of angina. Not indicated for acute attacks.

CONTRAINDICATIONS Hypersensitivity to nitrates; severe anemia; closed-angle glaucoma, postural hypotension, head trauma, cerebral hemorrhage (increases intracranial pressure). Safe use during pregnancy [(category C) and (category B) for sustained form] or lactation is not established.

CAUTIOUS USE Older adults, hypotension.

ROUTE & DOSAGE

Prevention of Angina

Adult: **PO** Regular release (ISMO, Monoket) 20 mg b.i.d. 7 h apart; Sustained release (Imdur) 30–60 mg every morning, may increase up to 120 mg once daily after several days if needed (max: dose 240 mg)

ADMINISTRATION

Oral

- Give first dose in morning on arising and second dose 7 h later with twice daily dosing regimen. Give in morning on arising with once daily dosing.
- Store sustained release tablets in a tight container.

ADVERSE EFFECTS (≥1%) **CNS:** Headache, agitation, anxiety, confusion, loss of coordination, hypoesthesia, hypokinesia, insomnia or somnolence, nervousness, migraine headache, paresthesia, vertigo, ptosis, tremor. **CV:** Aggravation of angina, abnormal heart sounds, murmurs, MI, transient hypotension, palpitations. **Hematologic:** Hypochromic anemia, purpura, thrombocytopenia, methemoglobinemia (high doses). **GI:** Nausea, vomiting, dry mouth, abdominal pain, constipation, diarrhea, dyspepsia, flatulence, tenesmus, gastric ulcer, hemorrhoids, gastritis, glossitis. **Metabolic:** Hyperuricemia, hypokalemia. **GU:** Renal calculus, UTI, atrophic vaginitis, dysuria, polyuria, urinary frequency, decreased libido, impotence. **Respiratory:** Bronchitis, pneumonia, upper respiratory tract infection, nasal congestion, bronchospasm, coughing, dyspnea, rales, rhinitis. **Skin:** Rash, pruritus, hot flashes, acne, abnormal texture. **Special Senses:** Diplopia, blurred vision, photophobia, conjunctivitis.

INTERACTIONS Drug: Alcohol may cause severe hypotension and cardiovascular collapse. **Aspirin** may increase nitrate serum levels. CALCIUM CHANNEL BLOCKERS may cause orthostatic hypotension.

PHARMACOKINETICS Absorption: Completely and rapidly absorbed from GI tract; 93% reaches systemic circulation. **Onset:** 1 h. **Peak:** Regular release 30–60 min; sustained release 3–4 h. **Duration:** Regular release 5–12 h; sustained release 12 h. **Metabolism:** Metabolized in liver by denitration and conjugation to inactive metabolites. **Elimination:** Excreted primarily by kidneys. **Half-Life:** 4–5 h.

NURSING IMPLICATIONS

Assessment & Drug Effects

- Monitor cardiac status, frequency and severity of angina, and BP.
- Assess for and report possible S&S of toxicity, including orthostatic hypotension, syncope, dizziness, palpitations, light-headedness, severe headache, blurred vision, and difficulty breathing.
- Lab tests: Monitor serum electrolytes periodically.

Patient & Family Education

- Do not crush or chew sustained release tablets. May break tablets in two and take with adequate fluid (4–8 oz).
- Do not withdraw drug abruptly; doing so may precipitate acute angina.
- Maintain correct dosing interval with twice daily dosing.
- Note: Geriatric patients are more susceptible to the possibility of developing postural hypotension.
- Avoid alcohol ingestion and aspirin unless specifically permitted by physician.
- Do not breast feed while taking this drug without consulting physician.

ISOTRETINOIN (13-*cis*-RETINOIC ACID) Pr

(eye-soe-tret′i-noyn)

Accutane, Claravis

Classifications: SKIN AND MUCOUS MEMBRANE AGENT; ANTIACNE (RETINOID)

Pregnancy Category: X

AVAILABILITY 10 mg, 20 mg, 40 mg capsules

ACTIONS Highly toxic metabolite of retinol (vitamin A). Principal actions: regulation of cell (e.g., epithelial) differentiation and proliferation and of altered lipid composition on skin surface.

THERAPEUTIC EFFECTS Decreases sebum secretion by reducing sebaceous gland size; inhibits gland cell differentiation; blocks follicular keratinization. Has antiacne properties and may be used as a chemotherapeutic agent for epithelial carcinomas.

USES Treatment of severe recalcitrant cystic or conglobate acne in patient unresponsive to conventional treatment, including systemic antibiotics.

UNLABELED USES Lamellar ichthyosis, oral leukoplakia, hyperkeratosis, acne rosacea, scarring gram-negative folliculitis; adjuvant therapy of basal cell carcinoma of lung and cutaneous T-cell lymphoma (mycosis fungoides); psoriasis; chemoprevention for prostate cancer.

CONTRAINDICATIONS Tinnitus; hypersensitivity to parabens (preservatives in the formulation), retinoid hypersensitivity, leukopenia, neutropenia; UV exposure; pregnancy (category X), females of childbearing age, lactation.

CAUTIOUS USE Coronary artery disease; major depression, psychosis, history of suicides, alcoholism; hepatitis, hepatic disease; visual disturbance; rheumatologic disorders, osteoporosis; history of pancreatitis, inflammatory bowel disease; diabetes mellitus; obesity; retinal disease; elevated triglycerides, hyperlipidemia.

ROUTE & DOSAGE

Cystic Acne

Adult: **PO** 0.5–1 mg/kg/d in 2 divided doses (max: recommended dose 2 mg/kg/d)

Disorders of Keratinization

Adult: **PO** up to 4 mg/kg/d in divided doses

ADMINISTRATION

Oral

- Give with or shortly after meals.
- Reassess regimen after 2 wk of treatment and dose adjusted as warranted.
- Note: A single course of therapy provides adequate control in many patients. If a second course is necessary, it is delayed at least 8 wk because improvement may continue without the drug.
- Store in tight, light-resistant container. Capsules remain stable for 2 y.

ADVERSE EFFECTS (≥1%) **Body as a Whole:** Most are dose-related (i.e., occurring at doses >1 mg/kg/d), reversible with termination of therapy. **CNS:** Lethargy, headache, fatigue, visual disturbances, pseudotumor cerebri, paresthesias, dizziness, depression, psychosis, suicide (rare). **Special Senses:** Reduced night vision, dry eyes, papilledema, eye irritation, *conjunctivitis,* corneal opacities. **GI:** *Dry mouth,* anorexia, nausea, vomiting, abdominal pain, nonspecific GI symptoms, acute hepatotoxic reactions (rare), inflammation and bleeding of gums, increased AST, ALT, acute pancreatitis. **Hematologic:** Decreased Hct, Hgb, elevated sedimentation rate. **Musculoskeletal:** Arthralgia; bone, joint, and muscle pain and stiffness; chest pain, skeletal hyperostosis (especially in athletic people and with prolonged therapy), mild bruising. **Skin:** *Cheilitis,* skin fragility, dry skin, pruritus, peeling of face, palms, and soles; photosensitivity (photoallergic and phototoxic), erythema, skin infections, petechiae, rash, urticaria, exaggerated healing response (painful exuberant granulation tissue with crusting), brittle nails, thinning hair. **Respiratory:** Epistaxis, *dry nose.* **Metabolic:** Hyperuricemia, *increased serum concentrations of triglycerides by 50% – 70%,* serum cholesterol by 15%–20%, VLDL cholesterol by 50–60%, LDL cholesterol by 15%–20%.

INTERACTIONS Drug: VITAMIN A SUPPLEMENTS increase toxicity; decreases effectiveness of ESTROGEN hormonal contraceptives in oral form as well as topical/injectable/implantable/insertable ESTROGEN hormonal birth control.

PHARMACOKINETICS Absorption: Rapid absorption after slow dissolution in GI tract; 25% of administered drug reaches systemic circulation. **Peak:** 3.2 h. **Distribution:** Not fully understood; appears in liver, ureters, adrenals, ovaries and lacrimal glands. **Metabolism:** Metabolized in liver; enterohepatically cycled. **Elimination:** Excreted in urine and feces in equal amounts. **Half-Life:** 10–20 h.

NURSING IMPLICATIONS

Assessment & Drug Effects

- Lab tests: Determine baseline blood lipids at outset of treatment, then at 2 wk, 1 mo, and every month thereafter throughout course of therapy; liver function tests at 2- or 3-wk intervals for 6 mo and once a month thereafter during treatment.
- Report signs of liver dysfunction (jaundice, pruritus, dark urine) promptly.
- Monitor closely for loss of glycemic control in diabetic and diabetic-prone patients.
- Note: Persistence of hypertriglyceridemia (levels above 500–800 mg/dL) despite a reduced dose indicates necessity to stop drug to prevent onset of acute pancreatitis.

Patient & Family Education

- Maintain drug regimen even if during the first few weeks transient exacerbations of acne occur. Recurring symptoms may signify response of deep unseen lesions.
- Discontinue medication at once and notify physician to rule out benign intracranial hypertension if visual disturbances occur along with nausea, vomiting, and headache.
- Note: Visual disturbances may also signify development of corneal opacities, which should be ruled out by ophthalmic examination. Discontinue drug if corneal opacities are present. Return for a follow-up examination.
- Rule out pregnancy within 2 wk of starting treatment. Use a reliable contraceptive 1 mo before, throughout, and 1 mo after therapy is discontinued.
- Reduce weight and restrict alcohol and dietary fat intake as prophylactic measures against development of hypertriglyceridemia.
- Do not self-medicate with multivitamins, which usually contain vitamin A. Toxicity of isotretinoin is enhanced by vitamin A supplements.
- Avoid or minimize exposure of the treated skin to sun or sunlamps. Photosensitivity (photoallergic and phototoxic) potential is high; risk of skin cancer may be increased by this drug.
- Notify physician of abdominal pain, rectal bleeding, or severe diarrhea, which are possible symptoms of drug-induced inflammatory bowel disease. Drug treatment will be discontinued.
- Keep lips moist and softened (use thin layer of lubricant such as petroleum jelly); dry mouth and cheilitis (inflamed, chapped lips), frequent adverse effects of isotretinoin, are distressing and are potential preconditions to infections.
- Notify physician of joint pain, such as pain in the great toe (symptom of gout and hyperuricemia).
- Do not share drug with friend(s) because it is associated with adverse effects that necessitate medical supervision.
- Do not breast feed while taking this drug.

ISOXSUPRINE HYDROCHLORIDE

(eye-sox'syoo-preen)

Vasodilan, Vasoprine

Classifications: AUTONOMIC NERVOUS SYSTEM AGENT; BETA-ADRENERGIC AGONIST; VASODILATOR

Prototype: Albuterol

Pregnancy Category: C

AVAILABILITY 10 mg, 20 mg tablets

ACTIONS Sympathomimetic with beta-adrenergic stimulant activity and with slight effect on alpha receptors. Vasodilating action on arteries within skeletal muscles is greater than on cutaneous vessels. Also causes cardiac stimulation and may produce bronchodilation, mild inhibition of GI motility, and uterine relaxation.

THERAPEUTIC EFFECTS Has both cerebral and peripheral vasodilatory properties.

USES Adjunctive therapy in treatment of cerebral vascular insufficiency and peripheral vascular disease, such as arteriosclerosis obliterans, thromboangitis obliterans (Buerger's disease), and Raynaud's disease.

UNLABELED USES Dysmenorrhea and threatened abortion and premature labor, but efficacy has not been established.

CONTRAINDICATIONS Immediately postpartum; presence of arterial bleeding; parenteral use in presence of hypotension, tachycardia. Safe use in pregnancy (category C) or lactation is not established.

CAUTIOUS USE Bleeding disorders; severe cerebrovascular disease, severe obliterative coronary artery disease, recent MI.

ROUTE & DOSAGE

Cerebral Vascular Insufficiency, Peripheral Vascular Disease

Adult: **PO** 10–20 mg t.i.d. or q.i.d.

ADMINISTRATION

Oral

- When used with premature labor: Do not give immediately after delivery because it causes uterine relaxation, or in the presence of arterial bleeding.

ADVERSE EFFECTS (≥1%) **CV:** Flushing, orthostatic hypotension with light-headedness, faintness; palpitation, tachycardia. **CNS:** Dizziness, nervousness, trembling, weakness. **GI:** Nausea, vomiting, abdominal distress, abdominal distention.

INTERACTIONS Drug: No clinically significant interactions established.

PHARMACOKINETICS Absorption: Readily absorbed from GI tract. **Peak:** 1 h. **Duration:** 3 h. **Distribution:** Crosses placenta. **Metabolism:** Metabolized in blood. **Elimination:** Excreted in urine. **Half-Life:** 1.25 h.

NURSING IMPLICATIONS

Assessment & Drug Effects

- Monitor for therapeutic effectiveness: Response to treatment of peripheral vascular disorders may take several weeks. Evaluate clinical manifestations of arterial insufficiency.
- Monitor BP and pulse; may cause hypotension and tachycardia. Supervise ambulation.
- Observe both mother and baby for hypotension and irregular and rapid heartbeat if isoxsuprine is used to delay premature labor. Hypocalcemia, hypoglycemia, and ileus have been ob-

served in babies born of mothers taking isoxsuprine.

Patient & Family Education

- Notify physician of adverse reactions (skin rash, palpitation, flushing) promptly; symptoms are usually effectively controlled by dosage reduction or discontinuation of drug.
- Prevent orthostatic hypotension by making position changes slowly and in stages, particularly from lying down to sitting upright and avoid standing still.
- Note: For treatment of menstrual cramps, isoxsuprine is usually started 1–3 d before onset of menstruation and continued until pain is relieved or menstrual flow stops.
- Do not breast feed while taking this drug without consulting physician.

ISRADIPINE

(is-ra′di-peen)

DynaCirc, DynaCirc CR

Classifications: CARDIOVASCULAR AGENT; CALCIUM CHANNEL BLOCKER

Prototype: Nifedipine

Pregnancy Category: C

AVAILABILITY 2.5 mg, 5 mg capsules; 5 mg, 10 mg sustained release tablets

ACTIONS Inhibits calcium ion influx into cardiac muscle and smooth muscle without changing calcium concentrations, thus affecting contractility.

THERAPEUTIC EFFECTS Isradipine relaxes coronary vascular smooth muscle with little or no negative inotropic effect. It significantly decreases systemic vascular resistance and reduces BP at rest and during isometric and dynamic exercise.

USES Mild to moderate hypertension.

UNLABELED USES Angina, CHF.

CONTRAINDICATIONS Hypersensitivity to isradipine.

CAUTIOUS USE Patients with CHF, pregnancy (category C), and lactation. Safety and effectiveness in children are not established.

ROUTE & DOSAGE

Hypertension

Adult: **PO** 1.25–10 mg b.i.d. (max: 20 mg/d); DynaCirc CR dosed q.d.

Angina

Adult: **PO** 2.5–7.5 mg t.i.d. (max: 15 mg/d)

ADMINISTRATION

Oral

- Do not crush sustained release form. It must be swallowed whole.
- Note: After the first 2–4 wk of therapy, dose may be increased for improved BP control in increments of 5 mg/d at 2–4 wk intervals up to a maximum dose of 20 mg/d.
- Store in tight, light-resistant container.

ADVERSE EFFECTS (≥1%) **CNS:** Headache, dizziness, fainting, fatigue, sleep disturbances, vertigo. **CV:** Flushing, ankle edema, palpitations, tachycardia, hypotension, chest pain, CHF. **GI:** Nausea, vomiting, abdominal discomfort, constipation, increased liver enzymes. **Respiratory:** Dyspnea. **Skin:** Rash, decreased skin sensation.

INTERACTIONS Drug: Adenosine may prolong bradycardia. May increase **cyclosporine** levels and toxicity.

PHARMACOKINETICS Absorption: Rapidly and completely absorbed from GI tract, but only 15%–24% reaches systemic circulation be-

I

cause of first-pass metabolism. **Onset:** 1 h. **Peak:** 2–3 h. **Duration:** 12 h. **Distribution:** Not known if crosses placenta or is distributed into breast milk. **Metabolism:** Extensive first-pass metabolism in liver. **Elimination:** 70% excreted in urine as inactive metabolites; 30% excreted in feces. **Half-Life:** 5–11 h.

NURSING IMPLICATIONS

Assessment & Drug Effects

- Monitor BP throughout course of therapy.
- Monitor patients with a history of CHF carefully, especially with concurrent beta blocker use. Promptly report S&S of worsening heart failure.
- Monitor ambulation, especially with older adult patients, until response to drug is known.

Patient & Family Education

- Notify physician promptly of shortness of breath, palpitations, or other signs of adverse cardiovascular effects.
- Do not drive or engage in other potentially hazardous activities until response to drug is known.
- Do not breast feed while taking this drug without consulting physician.

ITRACONAZOLE

(i-tra-con′a-zole)

Sporanox

Classifications: ANTIINFECTIVE; ANTIBIOTIC; ANTIFUNGAL

Prototype: Fluconazole

Pregnancy Category: C

AVAILABILITY 100 mg capsules; 10 mg/mL oral solution; 10 mg/mL injection

ACTIONS Synthetic antifungal agent active against many fungi, including yeast and dermatophytes.

THERAPEUTIC EFFECTS Antifungal spectrum of activity is similar to fluconazole.

USES Treatment of systemic fungal infections caused by blastomycosis, histoplasmosis, aspergillosis, onychomycosis due to dermatophytes of the toenail with or without fingernail involvement; oropharyngeal and esophageal candidiasis; orally to treat superficial mycoses (*Candida,* pityriasis versicolor). IV for treatment of blastomycosis, histoplasmosis, and aspergillosis.

UNLABELED USES Systemic and vaginal candidiasis.

CONTRAINDICATIONS Coadministration of terfenadine; hypersensitivity to itraconazole; renal failure; pregnancy (category C), lactation.

CAUTIOUS USE Hypersensitivity to other azole antifungal agents, achlorhydria, angina, cardiac disease; COPD, cystic fibrosis; dialysis; older adults, females of childbearing age; hepatic disease, hepatitis, HIV infection; hypochlorhydria; pulmonary disease; renal disease, renal impairment; valvular heart disease, ventricular dysfunction, children.

ROUTE & DOSAGE

Pulmonary and Extrapulmonary Blastomycosis, Nonmeningeal Histoplasmosis

Adult: **PO** 200 mg once daily (increase to max: 200 mg b.i.d. if no apparent improvement). Continue for at least 3 mo; for life-threatening infections, start with 200 mg t.i.d. for 3 d, then 200–400 mg/d
IV 200 mg b.i.d. infused over 1 h for 4 doses, then 200 mg q.d.
Child: **PO** 3–5 mg/kg/d for 3–6 mo

Oropharyngeal Candidiasis
Adult: **PO** 200 mg daily for 1–2 wk
Esophageal Candidiasis
Adult: **PO** 100 mg daily for at least 3 wk (max: 200 mg/d)
Vaginal Candidiasis
Adult: **PO** 200 mg q.d. for 3 d
Onychomycosis
Adult: **PO** 200 mg q.d. for 3 mo

ADMINISTRATION

Oral

- Give capsules with a full meal.
- Give oral solution without food. Liquid should be vigorously swished for several seconds and swallowed.
- Do not interchange oral solution and capsules.
- Divide dosages greater than 200 mg/d into two doses.
- Store liquid at or below 25° C (77° F).

Intravenous

PREPARE: **Intermittent:** Withdraw 25 mL from the ampule and add to infusion bag provided (contains 50 mL of NS). Mix gently to disperse evenly. IV solution contains 3.33 mg/mL.

ADMINISTER: **Intermittent:** Use a flow control device and the infusion set provided to infuse 60 mL (200 mg) of the diluted solution over 60 min. Stop the infusion and flush set with 15–20 mL NS over 1–15 min via the 2-way stopcock. Then discard the entire infusion set.

INCOMPATIBILITIES **Solution/additive or Y-site:** Do not mix with any other drugs or infuse other drugs concomitantly through the same line.

ADVERSE EFFECTS (≥1%) **CV:** Hypertension with higher doses. **CNS:** Headache, dizziness, fatigue, somnolence (euphoria, drowsiness <1%). **Endocrine:** Gynecomastia, hypokalemia (especially with higher doses), hypertriglyceridemia. **GI:** *Nausea, vomiting, dyspepsia, abdominal pain, diarrhea, anorexia, flatulence, gastritis;* elevations of serum transaminases, alkaline phosphatase, and bilirubin. **Urogenital:** Decreased libido, impotence. **Skin:** Rash, pruritus. **Acute Poisoning:** Severe toxicity (doses exceeding 400 mg daily have been associated with higher risk of hypokalemia, hypertension, adrenal insufficiency).

INTERACTIONS Drug: Itraconazole may increase levels and toxicity of **ergotamine, dihydroergotamine,** ORAL HYPOGLYCEMIC AGENTS **warfarin, ritonavir, indinavir, vinca alkaloids, busulfan, ergonovine, methylergonovine, midazolam, triazolam, diazepam, nifedipine, nicardipine, amlodipine, felodipine, lovastatin, simvastatin, cyclosporine, tacrolimus, methylprednisolone, digoxin.** Combination with **cisapride, dofetilide, levomethadyl, oral midazolam, pimozide, quinidine, triazolam** may cause severe cardiac events including cardiac arrest or sudden death. Itraconazole levels are decreased by **carbamazepine, phenytoin, phenobarbital, isoniazid, rifabutin, rifampin.**

PHARMACOKINETICS Absorption: Well absorbed from GI tract when taken with food. **Onset:** 2 wk–3 mo. **Peak:** Peak levels at 1.5–5 h. Steady-state concentrations reached in 10–14 d. **Distribution:** Highly protein bound, minimal concentrations in CSF. Higher concentrations in tissues than in plasma. **Metabolism:** Extensively metabolized in liver by CYP3A4, may undergo enterohepatic recirculation. **Elimination:** 35%

in urine, 55% excreted in feces. **Half-Life:** 34–42 h.

NURSING IMPLICATIONS

Assessment & Drug Effects

- Lab tests: C&S tests should be done before initiation of therapy. Drug may be started pending results. Monitor hepatic functions especially in those with preexisting hepatic abnormalities.
- Monitor for digoxin toxicity when given concurrently with digoxin.
- Monitor PT and INR carefully when given concurrently with warfarin.
- Monitor for S&S of hypersensitivity (see Appendix F); discontinue drug and notify physician if noted.

Patient & Family Education

- Take capsules, but NOT oral solution, with food.
- Notify physician promptly for S&S of liver dysfunction, including anorexia, nausea, and vomiting; weakness and fatigue; dark urine and clay-colored stool.
- Note: Risk of hypoglycemia may increase in diabetics on oral hypoglycemic agents.
- Do not breast feed while taking this drug.

IVERMECTIN

(i-ver-mec'tin)

Stromectol

Classifications: ANTIINFECTIVE; ANTHELMINTIC

Prototype: Mebendazole

Pregnancy Category: C

AVAILABILITY 6 mg tablets

ACTIONS A semisynthetic anthelmintic agent which is a broad-spectrum antiparasitic agent with a unique mode of action. It leads to an increase in the permeability to chloride ions of the cell membrane of the parasites, resulting in hyperpolarization of the nerve or muscle cell.

THERAPEUTIC EFFECTS Hyperpolarization of nerve and muscle cells of the parasites results in its paralysis and death.

USES Treatment of strongyloidiasis of the intestinal tract, onchocerciasis.

CONTRAINDICATIONS Hypersensitivity to ivermectin; pregnancy (category C).

CAUTIOUS USE Lactation. Safety and efficacy in children ≤15 kg are not established.

ROUTE & DOSAGE

Strongyloides

Adult/Child: **PO** *≥15 kg,* 200 mcg/kg times 1 dose (supplied as 6-mg tablets)

Onchocerciasis

Adult/Child: **PO** *≥15 kg,* 150 mcg/kg times 1 dose, may repeat q3–12 mo prn

ADMINISTRATION

Oral

- Give tablets with water rather than any other type of liquid.
- Store below 30° C (86° F).

ADVERSE EFFECTS (≥1%) **Body as a Whole:** *Fever,* peripheral edema. **CNS:** Dizziness. **CV:** Tachycardia. **GI:** Diarrhea, nausea. **Skin:** *Pruritus, rash.* **Other:** Arthralgia/synovitis, lymphadenopathy.

INTERACTIONS No clinically significant interactions established.

PHARMACOKINETICS Peak: 4 h. **Distribution:** Distributed into breast milk. **Metabolism:** Metabolized in the liver. **Elimination:** Excreted in feces over 12 d. **Half-Life:** 16 h.

NURSING IMPLICATIONS

Assessment & Drug Effects

- Monitor for therapeutic effectiveness: Indicated by negative stool samples.
- Monitor for cardiovascular effects such as orthostatic hypotension and tachycardia.
- Monitor for and report inflammatory conditions of the eyes.

Patient & Family Education

- Get a follow-up stool examination to determine effectiveness of treatment. Treatment for worms does not kill adult parasites; repeated follow-up and retreatment are usually needed.
- Notify physician if eye discomfort develops.
- Do not breast feed while taking this drug without consulting physician.

KANAMYCIN

(kan-a-mye'sin)

Kantrex

Classifications: ANTIINFECTIVE; ANTIBIOTIC; AMINOGLYCOSIDE

Prototype: Gentamicin

Pregnancy Category: D

AVAILABILITY 75 mg, 500 mg; 1 g vials

ACTIONS Broad-spectrum, aminoglycoside antibiotic derived from *Streptomyces kanamyceticus*. Usually bacteriocidal in action.

THERAPEUTIC EFFECTS Active against many gram-negative microorganisms, especially *Acinetobacter, Escherichia coli, Enterobacter aerogenes, Klebsiella pneumoniae, Proteus sp,* and *Serratia marcescens*. Also effective against many strains of *Staphylococcus aureus,* but it is not the drug of choice. Inhibits growth of *Mycobacterium tuberculosis* in vitro.

USES Orally to reduce ammonia-producing bacteria in intestinal tract, as adjunctive treatment of hepatic coma, and for preoperative bowel antisepsis; parenterally for short-term treatment of serious infections; intraperitoneally after fecal spill during surgery; as irrigation solution; and as aerosol treatment. In conjunction with other drugs to treat tuberculosis in patients resistant to conventional therapy.

CONTRAINDICATIONS History of hypersensitivity to kanamycin or other aminoglycosides; history of drug-induced ototoxicity, preexisting hearing loss, vertigo, or tinnitus; long-term therapy; PO use in intestinal obstruction or ulcerative bowel lesions; intraperitoneally to patients under effects of inhalation anesthetics or skeletal muscle relaxants. Safety during pregnancy (category D) or lactation is not established.

CAUTIOUS USE Impaired renal function; older adults, neonates, and infants (immature renal systems); myasthenia gravis; parkinsonian syndrome.

ROUTE & DOSAGE

Preoperative Intestinal Antisepsis

Adult: **PO** 1 g q1h for 4 doses then q6h for 36–72 h

Hepatic Coma

Adult: **PO** 8–12 g/d in divided doses

Serious Infection

Adult/Child: **IV/IM** 15 mg/kg/d in equally divided doses q8–12h
Adult: **Intraperitoneal** 500 mg diluted in 20 mL sterile water instilled through wound catheter
Inhalation 250 mg diluted in 3 mL

NS administered per nebulizer q6–12h **Irrigation** 0.25% solution prn

ADMINISTRATION

Oral

- Give on a full or empty stomach.
- Store capsules at 15°–30° C (59°–86° F) unless otherwise directed.

Intramuscular

- Administer IM injection deep into upper outer quadrant of gluteal muscle (often painful).
- Observe sites daily for signs of irritation; rotate injection sites.

Intravenous

PREPARE: **Intermittent:** Dilute each 500 mg with at least 100 mL NS, D5W, D5/NS.

ADMINISTER: **Intermittent:** Over 30–60 min.

INCOMPATIBILITIES **Solution/additive: Cephalothin, cephapirin, chlorpheniramine, colistimethate, heparin, hydrocortisone, methohexital, ampicillin, carbenicillin, methicillin, penicillin, mezlocillin, piperacillin. Y-site: Heparin, methohexital.**

- Store vials at 15°–30° C (59°–86° F) unless otherwise directed. Some vials may darken with time, but this does not affect potency. Discard partially used vials within 48 h.

ADVERSE EFFECTS (≥1%) **All:** Dose related. **Body as a Whole:** Eosinophilia, maculopapular rash, pruritus, urticaria, drug fever, anaphylaxis. **CNS:** Dizziness, circumoral and other paresthesias, optic neuritis, peripheral neuritis, headache, restlessness, tremors, lethargy, convulsions; neuromuscular paralysis, respiratory depression (rarely). **Special Senses:** Deafness (can be irreversible), *tinnitus, vertigo* or *dizziness,* ataxia, nystagmus. **GI:** Nausea, vomiting, diarrhea, appetite changes, abdominal discomfort, stomatitis, proctitis, malabsorption syndrome (with prolonged oral administration). **Hematologic:** Anemia, increased or decreased reticulocytes, granulocytopenia, agranulocytosis, thrombocytopenia, purpura. **Urogenital:** Nephrotoxicity; hematuria, urine casts and cells, proteinuria; elevated serum creatinine and BUN. **Other:** Superinfections; local pain; nodular formation at injection site.

INTERACTIONS Drug: Amphotericin B, cisplatin, methoxyflurane, vancomycin add to nephrotoxicity; GENERAL ANESTHETICS, SKELETAL MUSCLE RELAXANTS add to neuromuscular blocking effects; **capreomycin** compounds ototoxicity and nephrotoxicity; LOOP AND THIAZIDE DIURETICS may increase risk of ototoxicity.

PHARMACOKINETICS Absorption: Poorly absorbed from GI tract; readily absorbed from peritoneal cavity, bronchial tree, and wounds. **Peak:** 1–2 h. **Distribution:** Crosses placenta; distributed into breast milk. **Elimination:** 80%–90% excreted in urine within 24 h. **Half-Life:** 2–4 h.

NURSING IMPLICATIONS

Assessment & Drug Effects

- Lab tests: Monitor baseline C&S, urinalysis, and kidney function prior to initiation of therapy and periodically thereafter. Monitor serum sodium, potassium, calcium, and magnesium.
- Notify physician immediately of signs of renal irritation: albuminuria, casts, red and white cells in urine, increasing BUN, and serum creatinine, decreasing creatinine clearance, oliguria, and edema.
- Monitor peak and trough serum kanamycin concentrations: Assess peak specimen 30–60 min af-

ter IM administration; 30 min after completion of a 30–60 min IV infusion. Assess trough levels just before the next IM or IV dose.

- Keep patient well hydrated to prevent chemical irritation of renal tubules.
- Monitor I&O. Report decrease in urine output or change in I&O ratio.
- Determine baseline weight and vital signs and monitor at regular intervals during therapy.
- Report signs of superinfection (see Appendix F).
- Monitor for hearing and balance problems; stop drug if ototoxicity occurs. Tinnitus is not a reliable index of ototoxicity in the very elderly. Risk of ototoxicity is high in patients with impaired renal function, older adults, poorly hydrated patients, and with therapy ≥5 d.
- Note: Deafness has occurred 2–7 d or more after termination of therapy in patients with impaired renal function.

Patient & Family Education

- Report ototoxic symptoms such as dizziness, hearing loss, weakness, or loss of balance; drug may need to be discontinued.
- Do not breast feed while taking this drug without consulting physician.

KAOLIN AND PECTIN

(kay'oh-lin and pek'tin)

Kao-Span, Kaolin w/Pectin, K-C

Classifications: GASTROINTESTINAL AGENT; ANTIDIARRHEAL

Prototype: Diphenoxylate with atropine

Pregnancy Category: C

AVAILABILITY 5.2 g Kaolin/260 mg pectin/30 mL, 90 g Kaolin/2 g pectin/30 mL

ACTIONS Kaolin is hydrated aluminum silicate. Efficacy of kaolin or pectin in diarrhea is not clearly established.

THERAPEUTIC EFFECTS Kaolin is reported to have adsorbent, protectant, and demulcent properties. Mechanism of action of pectin may help consolidate stool.

USES Adjunct in symptomatic treatment of mild to moderately severe acute diarrhea. Commonly used in antidiarrheal combination products.

CONTRAINDICATIONS Suspected obstructive bowel lesion, pseudomembranous colitis, diarrhea associated with bacterial toxins; presence of fever; use for more than 48 h without medical direction. Safety during pregnancy (category C) or lactation is not established.

CAUTIOUS USE Infants or children ≤3 y, older adults.

ROUTE & DOSAGE

Diarrhea

Adult: **PO** 60–120 mL of regular suspension or 45–90 mL of concentrated suspension after each loose bowel movement

Child: **PO** *3–5 y,* 15–30 mL regular suspension or 15 mL concentrated suspension after each loose bowel movement; *6–11 y,* 30–60 mL regular suspension or 30 mL concentrated suspension after each loose bowel movement; *≥12 y,* 60 mL regular suspension or 45 mL concentrated suspension after each loose bowel movement

ADMINISTRATION

Oral

- Administer at least 2–4 h before other oral medications.

- Shake suspension well before pouring.
- Store in tightly closed container at 15°–30° C (59°–86° F) unless otherwise directed. Protect from freezing.

ADVERSE EFFECTS (≥1%) **GI:** Constipation usually mild and transient.

INTERACTIONS Drug: Chloroquine, digoxin, penicillamine, tetracycline, ciprofloxacin, and most other drugs.

PHARMACOKINETICS Absorption: Not absorbed from GI tract.

NURSING IMPLICATIONS

Assessment & Drug Effects

- Assess for abdominal distension and number of stools per day.
- Note: Fecal impaction may result from taking kaolin and pectin, especially in older adults.
- Note: Drug may decrease absorption of any orally administered medication.

Patient & Family Education

- Do not to exceed prescribed dosage.
- Notify physician if diarrhea is not controlled within 48 h or if fever develops.
- Do not breast feed infants while taking this drug without consulting physician.

KETOCONAZOLE

(ke-to-con'a-zol)

Nizoral, Nizoral A–D

Classifications: ANTIINFECTIVE; ANTIBIOTIC; AZOLE ANTIFUNGAL

Prototype: Fluconazole

Pregnancy Category: C

AVAILABILITY 200 mg tablets; 2% cream; 2% shampoo

ACTIONS Synthetic imidazole derivative and broad-spectrum antifungal agent closely related to miconazole. Studies suggest mode of action interferes with synthesis of ergosterol which results in an increase in cell membrane permeability and ultimately inhibition of fungal growth.

THERAPEUTIC EFFECTS Usually fungistatic, but may be fungicidal in high concentrations.

USES Oral—Severe systemic fungal infections including candidiasis (e.g., oral thrush, candiduria), chronic mucocutaneous candidiasis, pulmonary and disseminated coccidioidomycosis, histoplasmosis, paracoccidioidomycosis, blastomycosis, and chromomycosis. **Topical**—Tinea corporis and tinea cruris (caused by *Epidermophyton floccosum, Trichophyton mentagrophytes,* and *Trichophyton rubrum*) and in treatment of tinea versicolor (pityriasis) caused by *Malassezia furfur (Pityrosporum obiculare),* seborrheic dermatitis.

UNLABELED USES Oral—Onychomycosis, vaginal candidiasis, Cushing's syndrome associated with adrenal or pituitary adenoma; precocious puberty, dysfunctional hirsutism, and as swish and swallow preparation for prophylaxis against fungal infections in patients with neutropenia induced by cancer chemotherapy and in patients with AIDS.

CONTRAINDICATIONS Hypersensitivity to ketoconazole or any component in the formulation; chronic alcoholism, fungal meningitis; onychomycosis; ocular exposure, ophthalmic administration. Safety during pregnancy (category C), lactation, or in children <2 y is not established.

CAUTIOUS USE Achlorhydria, hypochlorhydria; history of hepatic disease, HIV infection; alcoholism; azole antifungal hypersensitivity.

ROUTE & DOSAGE

Fungal Infections

Adult: **PO** 200–400 mg once/d **Topical** Apply 1–2 times/d to affected area and surrounding skin
Child: **PO** >2 y, 3.3–6.6 mg/kg/d as single dose

Dandruff

Adult/Child: **Topical** Shampoo twice a week for 4 wk with at least 3 d between shampoos

ADMINISTRATION

Oral

- Give with water, fruit juice, coffee, or tea; drug requires an acid medium for dissolution and absorption.
- Relieve nausea and vomiting during early therapy by taking drug with food and dividing into 2 daily doses.
- Do not give with antacids.
- Store in tightly covered container at 15°–30° C (59°–86° F) unless otherwise directed.

Topical

- Apply sufficient shampoo to produce lather to wash scalp and hair and gently massage over entire scalp area for 1 min, rinse hair thoroughly and repeat, leaving shampoo on scalp for 3 min. Rinse thoroughly.

ADVERSE EFFECTS (≥1%) **Oral—Body as a Whole:** Skin rash, erythema, urticaria, pruritus, angioedema, anaphylaxis. **GI:** *Nausea, vomiting,* anorexia, epigastric or abdominal pain, constipation, diarrhea, transient elevation in serum liver enzymes, fatal hepatic necrosis (rare). **Hematologic:** With high doses, lowers serum testosterone and ACTH-induced corticosteroid serum levels, transient decreases in serum cholesterol and triglycerides; hyponatremia (rare). **Urogenital:** Gynecomastia (males), breast pain; uterine bleeding, loss of libido, impotence, oligospermia, hair loss. **Other:** Acute hypoadrenalism (reduction of adrenal stress syndrome), renal hypofunction. **Topical—Skin:** Mild transient erythema, severe irritation, pruritus, stinging.

INTERACTIONS Drug: Alcohol may cause sunburnlike reaction; ANTACIDS, ANTICHOLINERGICS, H_2-RECEPTOR ANTAGONISTS decrease ketoconazole absorption; **isoniazid, rifampin** increase ketoconazole metabolism, thus decreasing its activity; levels of **phenytoin** and ketoconazole decreased; may increase **cyclosporine** levels and toxicity; **warfarin** may potentiate hypoprothrombinemia; may increase levels of **carbamazepine, cisapride,** resulting in arrhythmias; may increase ergotamine toxicity of **dihydroergotamine, ergotamine;** may increase concentration and toxicity of **trazodone. Herbal: Echinacea** may increase risk of hepatotoxicity.

PHARMACOKINETICS Absorption: Erratically absorbed from GI tract (needs an acid pH); minimal absorption topically. **Peak:** 1–2 h. **Distribution:** Distributed to saliva, urine, sebum, and cerumen; CSF levels unpredictable; distributed into breast milk. **Metabolism:** Metabolized in liver. **Elimination:** Primarily excreted in feces, 13% in urine. **Half-Life:** 8 h.

NURSING IMPLICATIONS

Assessment & Drug Effects

- Lab tests: Monitor baseline liver function tests (AST, ALT, alkaline phosphatase, and bilirubin) and repeat at least monthly throughout therapy.

- Monitor for S&S of hepatotoxicity (see Appendix F). Discontinue drug immediately to prevent irreversible liver damage and report to physician.

Patient & Family Education

- Report S&S of hepatotoxicity promptly to physician (see Appendix F).
- Note: Drowsiness and dizziness are early and time-limited adverse effects.
- Do not drive or engage in potentially hazardous activities until response to drug is known.
- Avoid OTC drugs for gastric distress, such as Rolaids, Tums, Alka-Seltzer and check with physician before taking any other nonprescribed medicines.
- Do not alter dose or dose interval and do not stop taking ketoconazole before consulting the physician.
- Notify physician if skin condition fails to respond to topical therapy or worsens or if signs of irritation or sensitivity occur.
- Do not breast feed infants while taking this drug without consulting physician.

KETOPROFEN

(kee-toe-proe'fen)

Actron, Orudis, Orudis KT, Oruvail, Rhodis A

Classifications: CENTRAL NERVOUS SYSTEM AGENT; ANALGESIC; ANTIPYRETIC; NSAID

Prototype: Ibuprofen

Pregnancy Category: B

AVAILABILITY 12.5 mg, 25 mg, 50 mg, 75 mg capsules; 100 mg, 150 mg, 200 mg sustained release capsules

ACTIONS Nonsteroidal antiinflammatory drug (NSAID) structurally related to ibuprofen. Analgesic potency matches that of indomethacin and is stronger than that of aspirin. Inhibits platelet aggregation and prolongs bleeding time. Has fewer adverse GI effects than aspirin.

THERAPEUTIC EFFECTS Has analgesic, antiinflammatory, and antiplatelet properties.

USES Acute or long-term treatment of rheumatoid arthritis and osteoarthritis; primary dysmenorrhea; headache; symptomatic relief of postoperative, dental, and postpartum pain; visceral pain associated with cancer.

UNLABELED USES Reiter's syndrome, juvenile arthritis, acute gouty arthritis, biliary pain, renal colic.

CONTRAINDICATIONS Patient in whom aspirin or another NSAID induces asthma, urticaria, bronchospasm, severe rhinitis, shock. Safety during pregnancy (category B), lactation, or in children <12 y is not established.

CAUTIOUS USE History of GI disease, GI bleeding, active ulcer; renal or hepatic impairment, patient who may be adversely affected by prolongation of bleeding time; heart failure, hypertension; patient receiving diuretics; geriatric patient; myasthenia gravis.

ROUTE & DOSAGE

Inflammatory Disease

Adult: **PO** 75 mg t.i.d. or 50 mg q.i.d. (max: 300 mg/d) or 200 mg sustained release q.d.

Geriatric: **PO** Start with 25 mg q.i.d., may also start with 50 mg t.i.d.

Mild to Moderate Pain, Dysmenorrhea

Adult: **PO** 12.5–50 mg q6–8h

ADMINISTRATION

Oral

- Do not crush.
- Give with food, milk, or prescribed antacid to reduce GI irritation.
- Store drug at 15°–30° C (59°–86° F) in tightly closed, light-resistant container unless otherwise directed.

ADVERSE EFFECTS (≥1%) **CNS:** Trouble in sleeping, nervousness, *headache,* dizziness; depression, drowsiness, confusion, migraine, vertigo. **CV:** Peripheral edema, palpitations, hypertension, tachycardia. **Special Senses:** Visual disturbances, conjunctivitis, eye pain, retinal hemorrhage, pigmentation changes; Dry nose or throat, tinnitus, hearing impairment. **GI:** *Dyspepsia,* drug-induced peptic ulcer, GI bleeding, nausea, vomiting, diarrhea, constipation, flatulence, stomach pain, anorexia, dry mouth, gingivitis, rectal burning and hemorrhage, melena, jaundice, elevated ALT, AST. **Hematologic:** Prolonged bleeding time, anemia, purpura, agranulocytosis, thrombocytosis. **Urogenital:** Gynecomastia, changes in libido, urinary tract irritation (dysuria, frequency/urgency), renal impairment. **Respiratory:** Laryngospasm, bronchospasm, laryngeal edema, pharyngitis. **Skin:** Rash, pruritus, urticaria, erythema, photosensitivity. **Endocrine:** Aggravation of diabetes mellitus.

INTERACTIONS Drug: ORAL ANTICOAGULANTS, **heparin** may prolong bleeding time; may increase **lithium** toxicity; may increase **methotrexate** toxicity. **Herbal: Feverfew, garlic, ginger, ginkgo** increases bleeding potential.

PHARMACOKINETICS Absorption: Readily absorbed from GI tract. **Onset:** 1–2 h. **Peak:** 1–2 h. **Duration:** 4–6 h. **Metabolism:** Metabolized in liver. **Elimination:** Excreted primarily in urine, with some biliary excretion. **Half-Life:** 1.1–4 h.

NURSING IMPLICATIONS

Assessment & Drug Effects

- Lab tests: Monitor baseline and periodic evaluations of hemoglobin, renal and hepatic function.
- Monitor for and report tinnitus, hearing impairment, and visual disturbance, especially during prolonged or high-dose therapy.
- Monitor for S&S of GI ulceration (e.g., stool for occult blood, persistent indigestion).

Patient & Family Education

- Report promptly signs of jaundice (see Appendix F) as well as the following: blurred vision, tinnitus, urinary urgency or frequency, unexplained bleeding, weight gain with edema.
- Note: Possible CNS adverse effects (e.g., light-headedness, dizziness, drowsiness).
- Do not drive or engage in potentially hazardous activities until response to drug is known.
- Note: Alcohol, aspirin, or other NSAIDS may increase risk of GI ulceration and bleeding tendencies and therefore should be avoided.
- Tell dentist or surgeon that you are taking ketoprofen.
- Do not breast feed infants while taking this drug without consulting physician.

KETOROLAC TROMETHAMINE

(ke-tor′o-lac)

Toradol, Acular, Acular LS

Classifications: CENTRAL NERVOUS SYSTEM AGENT; NSAID, ANALGESIC; ANTIPYRETIC

Prototype: Ibuprofen

Pregnancy Category: B

AVAILABILITY 10 mg tablets; 15 mg/mL, 30 mg/mL injection; 0.4%, 0.5% ophthalmic solution

ACTIONS It inhibits synthesis of prostaglandins and is a peripherally acting analgesic. Ketorolac does not have any known effects on opiate receptors.

THERAPEUTIC EFFECTS Ketorolac exhibits analgesic, antiinflammatory, and antipyretic activity.

USES *Short-term* management of pain; ocular itching due to seasonal allergic conjunctivitis, reduction of post-operative pain and photophobia after refractive surgery.

CONTRAINDICATIONS Hypersensitivity to ketorolac; individuals with complete or partial syndrome of nasal polyps, angioedema, and bronchospastic reaction to aspirin or other NSAIDS; during labor and delivery; patients with severe renal impairment or at risk for renal failure due to volume depletion; patients with risk of bleeding; active peptic ulcer disease; pre- or intraoperatively; intrathecal or epidural administration; in combination with other NSAIDS; lactation.

CAUTIOUS USE History of peptic ulcers; impaired renal or hepatic function; older adults; debilitated patients; pregnancy (category B). Safety and effectiveness in children is not established.

ROUTE & DOSAGE

Pain

Adult: **IV Loading Dose** 30 mg (15 mg <50 kg) **IM** 30–60 mg loading dose, then 15–30 mg q6h (max: 150 mg/d on first day, then 120 mg subsequent days [30 mg load, then 15 mg q6h if <50 kg]) **PO** 10 mg q6h prn (max: 40 mg/d) max duration all routes 5 d

Geriatric: **IV Loading Dose** 15 mg **IM** 30 mg loading dose, then 15 mg q6h **PO** 5–10 mg q6h prn (max: 40 mg/d) max duration all routes 5 d

Pain after Refractive Surgery

Adult: **Ophthalmic** *Acular LS only* 1 drop in operative eye q.i.d. up to 4 d

Allergic Conjunctivitis

Adult: **Ophthalmic** 1 drop 0.5% solution q.i.d.

ADMINISTRATION

WARNING: Do not administer IV, IM, or PO ketorolac longer than 5 d.

Oral

- Give with food to reduce GI effects.

Instillation

- Do not touch container to the eye when applying ophthalmic drops.

Intramuscular

- Inject IM drug slowly and deeply into a large muscle.
- Rotate injection sites to avoid injection site pain in patients receiving multiple doses.

Intravenous

PREPARE: **Direct:** Give undiluted.
ADMINISTER: **Direct:** Give IV bolus dose over at least 15 s. Pre-

ferred method is to give through a Y-tube in a free-flowing IV.

- Store all forms at 15°–30° C (59°–86° F).

ADVERSE EFFECTS (≥1%) **CNS:** *Drowsiness,* dizziness, headache. **GI:** *Nausea,* dyspepsia, GI pain, hemorrhage. **Other:** Edema, sweating, pain at injection site.

INTERACTIONS Drug: May increase **methotrexate** levels and toxicity; may increase **lithium** levels and toxicity. **Herbal: Feverfew, garlic, ginger, ginkgo** increased bleeding potential.

PHARMACOKINETICS Peak: 45–60 min. **Distribution:** Distributed into breast milk. **Metabolism:** Metabolized in liver. **Elimination:** Excreted in urine. **Half-Life:** 4–6 h.

NURSING IMPLICATIONS

Assessment & Drug Effects

- Correct hypovolemia prior to administration of ketorolac.
- Lab tests: Periodic serum electrolytes and liver functions; urinalysis (for hematuria and proteinuria) with long-term use.
- Monitor urine output in older adults and patients with a history of cardiac decompensation, renal impairment, heart failure, or liver dysfunction as well as those taking diuretics. Discontinuation of drug will return urine output to pretreatment level.
- Monitor for S&S of GI distress or bleeding including nausea, GI pain, diarrhea, melena, or hematemesis. GI ulceration with perforation can occur anytime during treatment. Drug decreases platelet aggregation and thus may prolong bleeding time.
- Monitor for fluid retention and edema in patients with a history of CHF.

Patient & Family Education

- Watch for S&S of GI ulceration and bleeding (e.g., bloody emesis, black tarry stools) during long-term therapy.
- Note: Possible CNS adverse effects (e.g., light-headedness, dizziness, drowsiness).
- Do not drive or engage in potentially hazardous activities until response to drug is known.
- Do not use other NSAIDS while taking this drug.
- Do not breast feed while taking this drug.

KETOTIFEN FUMARATE

(kee-toe-tye′fen)

Zaditor

Classifications: EYE PREPARATION; OCULAR ANTIHISTAMINE

Prototype: Levocabastine HCl

Pregnancy Category: C

AVAILABILITY 0.025% solution

See Appendix A-1.

LABETALOL HYDROCHLORIDE

(la-bet′a-lole)

Normodyne, Trandate

Classifications: AUTONOMIC NERVOUS SYSTEM AGENT; ALPHA- AND BETA-ADRENERGIC ANTAGONIST (SYMPATHOLYTIC); ANTIHYPERTENSIVE AGENT

Prototype: Propranolol

Pregnancy Category: C

AVAILABILITY 100 mg, 200 mg, 300 mg tablet; 5 mg/mL injection

ACTIONS The alpha blockade results in vasodilation, decreased peripheral resistance, and orthostatic hypotension and only slightly affects cardiac output and coronary artery blood flow. It has beta-blocking effects on the sinus node, AV node, and ventricular muscle, which lead to bradycardia, delay in AV conduction, and depression of cardiac contractility.

THERAPEUTIC EFFECTS Acts as an adrenergic receptor blocking agent that combines selective alpha activity and nonselective beta-adrenergic blocking actions. Both actions contribute to blood pressure reduction.

USES Mild, moderate, and severe hypertension. May be used alone or in combination with other antihypertensive agents, especially thiazide diuretics.

CONTRAINDICATIONS Bronchial asthma; uncontrolled cardiac failure, heart block (greater than first degree), cardiogenic shock, severe bradycardia. Safe use during pregnancy (category C), lactation, or in children is not established.

CAUTIOUS USE Nonallergic bronchospastic disease (COPD), well-compensated patients with history of heart failure; pheochromocytoma; impaired liver function, jaundice; diabetes mellitus; peripheral vascular disease.

ROUTE & DOSAGE

Hypertension

Adult: **PO** 100 mg b.i.d., may gradually increase to 200–400 mg b.i.d. (max: 1200–2400 mg/d). **IV** 20 mg slowly over 2 min, with 40–80 mg q10min if needed up to 300 mg total or 2 mg/min continuous infusion (max: 300 mg total dose)
Geriatric: **PO** Start with 100 mg daily **IV** 20 mg slowly over 2 min, with 40–80 mg q10min if needed up to 300 mg total or 2 mg/min continuous infusion (max: 300 mg total dose)

ADMINISTRATION

Oral

- Give with or immediately after food consistently. Food increases drug bioavailability.

Intravenous

Note: Amount of IV solution may be changed depending on patient status.

PREPARE: **Direct:** Give undiluted. **Continuous:** Dilute 300 mg in 240 of D5W, NS, D5/NS, RL, or other compatible IV solution to yield 1 mg/mL.

ADMINISTER: **Direct:** Give a 20-mg dose slowly over 2 min. Maximum hypotensive effect occurs 5–15 min after each administration. **Continuous:** Normal rate is 2 mg/min. Keep patient supine when receiving labetalol IV. Take BP immediately before administration. Rate is adjusted according to BP response. Discontinue drug once the desired BP is attained.

INCOMPATIBILITIES **Solution/additive: Sodium bicarbonate. Y-site: Furosemide, heparin, nafcillin, thiopental, warfarin.**

- Controlled infusion pump device is recommended for maintaining accurate flow rate during IV infusion. Usually administered at rate of 2 mg/min.

- Store at 2°–30° C (36°–86° F) unless otherwise advised. Do not freeze. Protect tablets from moisture.

ADVERSE EFFECTS (≥1%) **CNS:** Dizziness, fatigue/malaise, headache, tremors, transient paresthesias (especially scalp tingling), hypoesthesia (numbness) following IV, mental depression, drowsiness, sleep disturbances, nightmares. **CV:** *Postural hypotension,* angina pectoris, palpitation, bradycardia, syncope, pedal or peripheral edema, pulmonary edema, CHF, flushing, cold extremities, arrhythmias (following IV), paradoxical hypertension (patients with pheochromocytoma). **Special Senses:** Dry eyes, vision disturbances, nasal stuffiness, rhinorrhea. **GI:** Nausea, vomiting, dyspepsia, constipation, diarrhea, taste disturbances, cholestasis with or without jaundice, increases in serum transaminases, dry mouth. **Urogenital:** Acute urinary retention, difficult micturition, impotence, ejaculation failure, loss of libido, Peyronie's disease. **Respiratory:** Dyspnea, bronchospasm. **Skin:** Rashes of various types, increased sweating, pruritus. **Body as a Whole:** Myalgia, muscle cramps, toxic myopathy, antimitochondrial antibodies, positive antinuclear antibodies (ANA), SLE syndrome, pain at IV injection site.

DIAGNOSTIC TEST INTERFERENCE False increases in ***urinary catecholamines*** when measured by ***nonspecific trihydroxyindole (THI) reaction*** (due to labetalol metabolites) but not with specific ***radioenzymatic*** or ***high-performance liquid chromatography assay techniques.***

INTERACTIONS Drug: Cimetidine may increase effects of labetalol; **glutethimide** decreases effects of labetalol; **halothane** adds to hypotensive effects; may mask symptoms of hypoglycemia caused by ORAL SULFONYLUREAS, **insulin;** BETA AGONISTS antagonize effects of labetalol.

PHARMACOKINETICS Absorption: Readily absorbed from GI tract, but only 25% reaches systemic circulation because of first pass metabolism. **Onset:** 20 min–2 h PO; 2–5 min IV. **Peak:** 1–4 h PO; 5–15 min IV. **Duration:** 8–24 h PO; 2–4 h IV. **Distribution:** Crosses placenta; distributed into breast milk. **Metabolism:** Metabolized in liver. **Elimination:** 60% excreted in urine, 40% in bile. **Half-Life:** 3–8 h.

NURSING IMPLICATIONS

Assessment & Drug Effects

- Monitor BP and pulse during dosage adjustment period. Use standing BP as indicator for making dosage adjustments for oral drugs and assessing patient's tolerance of dosage increases. Take after patient stands for 10 min. Clarify with physician.
- Monitor BP at 5 min intervals for 30 min after IV administration; then at 30 min intervals for 2 h; then hourly for about 6 h; and as indicated thereafter.
- Monitor diabetic patients closely; drug may mask usual cardiovascular response to acute hypoglycemia (e.g., tachycardia).
- Convert from IV to PO therapy only when supine diastolic pressure rises about 10 mm Hg.
- Maintain patient in supine position for at least 3 h after IV administration. Then determine patient's ability to tolerate elevated and upright positions before allowing ambulation. Manage this slowly.

Patient & Family Education

- Note: Postural hypotension is most likely to occur during peak plasma levels (i.e., 2–4 h after drug administration).
- Make all position changes slowly and in stages, particularly from lying to upright position. Older adult patients are especially sensitive to hypotensive effects.
- Do not drive or engage in other potentially hazardous activities until response to drug is known.
- Note: Most adverse effects (e.g., scalp tingling) are mild, transient,

and dose related and occur early in therapy.

- Be sure to keep follow-up appointments. Get liver and kidney function tests periodically during therapy.
- Discontinue drug gradually over 1–2 wk period after chronic administration. Close monitoring during this time is very important.
- Do not breast feed while taking this drug without consulting physician.

LACTULOSE

(lak'tyoo-lose)

Cephulac, Chronulac

Classifications: GASTROINTESTINAL AGENT; HYPEROSMOTIC LAXATIVE

Pregnancy Category: C

AVAILABILITY 10 g/15 mL solution, syrup

ACTIONS Reduces blood ammonia; appears to involve metabolism of lactose to organic acids by resident intestinal bacteria.

THERAPEUTIC EFFECTS Acidifies colon contents, which retards diffusion of nonionic ammonia (NH_3) from colon to blood while promoting its migration from blood to colon. In the acidic colon, NH_3 is converted to nonabsorbable ammonium ions (NH_4) and is then expelled in feces by laxative action. Decreased blood ammonia in a patient with hepatic encephalopathy is marked by improved EEG patterns and mental state (clearing of confusion, apathy, and irritation). Osmotic effect of organic acids causes laxative action, which moves water from plasma to intestines, softens stools, and stimulates peristalsis by pressure from water content of stool.

USES Prevention and treatment of portal-systemic encephalopathy (PSE), including stages of hepatic precoma and coma, and by prescription for relief of chronic constipation.

UNLABELED USES to restore regular bowel habit posthemorrhoidectomy; to evacuate bowel in older adult patients with severe constipation after barium studies; and for treatment of chronic constipation in children.

CONTRAINDICATIONS Low galactose diet; pregnancy (category C). Safe use in lactation or children is not established.

CAUTIOUS USE Diabetes mellitus; concomitant use with electrocautery procedures (proctoscopy, colonoscopy); older adult and debilitated patients; pediatric use.

ROUTE & DOSAGE

Prevention and Treatment of Portal-Systemic Encephalopathy

Adult: **PO** 30–45 mL t.i.d. or q.i.d. adjusted to produce 2–3 soft stools/d

Adolescent/Child: **PO** 40–90 mL/d in divided doses adjusted to produce 2–3 soft stools/d

Infant: **PO** 2.5–10 mL/d in 3–4 divided doses adjusted to produce 2–3 soft stools/d

Management of Acute Portal-Systemic Encephalopathy

Adult: **PO** 30–45 mL q1–2 h until laxation is achieved, then adjusted to produce 2–3 soft stools/d. **Rectal** 300 mL diluted with 700 mL water given via rectal balloon catheter, and retained for 30–60 min, may repeat in 4–6 h if necessary or until patient can take PO

Chronic Constipation
Adult: **PO** 30–60 mL/d prn
Child: **PO** 7.5 mL/d after breakfast

ADMINISTRATION

Oral

- Give with fruit juice, water, or milk (if not contraindicated) to increase palatability. Laxative effect is enhanced by taking with ample liquids. Avoid meal times.

Rectal

- Administer as a retention enema via a rectal balloon catheter. If solution is evacuated too soon, instillation may be promptly repeated.
- Do not freeze. Avoid prolonged exposure to temperatures above 30° C (86° F) or to direct light. Normal darkening does not affect action, but discard solution that is very dark or cloudy.

ADVERSE EFFECTS (≥1%) **GI:** Flatulence, borborygmi, belching, abdominal cramps, pain, and distention (initial dose); *diarrhea* (excessive dose); nausea, vomiting, colon accumulation of hydrogen gas; hypernatremia.

INTERACTIONS Drug: LAXATIVES may incorrectly suggest therapeutic action of lactulose.

PHARMACOKINETICS Absorption: Poorly absorbed from GI tract. **Metabolism:** Metabolized in gut by intestinal bacteria.

NURSING IMPLICATIONS

Assessment & Drug Effects

- In children if the initial dose causes diarrhea, dosage is reduced immediately. Discontinue if diarrhea persists.
- Promote fluid intake (≥1500–2000 mL/d) during drug therapy for constipation; older adults often self-limit liquids. Lactulose-induced osmotic changes in the bowel support intestinal water loss and potential hypernatremia. Discuss strategy with physician.

Patient & Family Education

- Laxative action is not instituted until drug reaches the colon; therefore, about 24–48 h is needed.
- Do not self-medicate with another laxative due to slow onset of drug action.
- Notify physician if diarrhea (i.e., more than 2 or 3 soft stools/d) persists more than 24–48 h. Diarrhea is a sign of overdosage. Dose adjustment may be indicated.
- Do not breast feed while taking this drug without consulting physician.

LAMIVUDINE

(lam-i-vu'deen)

Epivir, Epivir-HBV, Heptovir ♣

Classifications: ANTIINFECTIVE; ANTIRETROVIRAL AGENT

Prototype: Zidovudine (AZT)

Pregnancy Category: C

AVAILABILITY 100 mg, 150 tablets; 5 mg/mL, 10 mg/mL oral solution

ACTIONS Lamivudine (formerly 3TC) is a synthetic nucleoside analog.

THERAPEUTIC EFFECTS Its phosphorylated metabolite (L-TP) inhibits the transcription of the HIV viral DNA chain.

USES HIV infection in combination with zidovudine; treatment of chronic hepatitis B.

CONTRAINDICATIONS Hypersensitivity to lamivudine, lactation.
CAUTIOUS USE Renal impairment, pregnancy (category C), children.

ROUTE & DOSAGE

HIV Infection

Adult: Epivir **PO** 150 mg b.i.d.
Child: Epivir **PO** *3 mo–16 y*, 4 mg/kg b.i.d. (max: of 150 mg b.i.d.)

Renal Impairment

Cl_{cr} 30–49 mL/min: 150 mg q.d.; 15–29 mL/min: 150 mg first dose, then 100 mg q.d.; 5–14 mL/min: 150 mg first dose, then 50 mg q.d.; <5 mL/min: 50 mg first dose, then 25 mg q.d.

L

Chronic Hepatitis B

Adult: Epivir-HBV: **PO** 100 mg q.d.

Renal Impairment

Cl_{cr} 30–49 mL/min: 100 mg first dose, then 50 mg q.d.; 15–29 mL/min: 100 mg first dose, then 25 mg q.d.; 5–14 mL/min: 35 mg first dose, then 15 mg q.d.; <5 mL/min: 35 mg first dose, then 10 mg q.d.

ADMINISTRATION

Oral

- Give Epivir b.i.d. in combination with AZT. The recommended dose for adults who weigh <50 kg (110 lb) is 2 mg/kg. Give Epivir-HBV qd; do NOT give in combination with AZT.
- Store solution at 2°–25° C (36°–77° F) tightly closed.

ADVERSE EFFECTS (≥1%) **CNS:** *Neuropathy, insomnia,* sleep disorders, *dizziness,* depression, *headache,* fatigue, *fever, chills.* **GI:** *Nausea, diarrhea,* vomiting, anorexia, abdominal pain, cramps, dyspepsia, increased LFTs (ALT, amylase), hepatomegaly with steatosis. **Hematologic:** Neutropenia, anemia, thrombocytopenia. **Musculoskeletal:** Myalgia, arthralgia, malaise, pain. **Skin:** Rash. **Respiratory:** Nasal symptoms, cough. **Metabolic:** Lactic acidosis.

INTERACTIONS Drug: Increases the C_{max} of **zidovudine. Trimethoprim-sulfamethoxazole** increases serum levels of lamivudine. Increased risk of lactic acidosis in combination with other REVERSE TRANSCRIPTASE INHIBITORS and ANTIRETROVIRAL AGENTS.

PHARMACOKINETICS Absorption: Rapidly absorbed from GI tract (86% reaches systemic circulation). **Distribution:** Low binding to plasma proteins. **Metabolism:** Minimal metabolism. **Elimination:** Excreted primarily unchanged in urine. **Half-Life:** 2–4 h.

NURSING IMPLICATIONS

Assessment & Drug Effects

- Monitor children closely for S&S of pancreatitis; if they occur, immediately stop drug and notify physician.
- Lab tests: Monitor CBC with differential, kidney & liver function, and serum amylase throughout therapy.
- Monitor for and report all significant adverse reactions.

Patient & Family Education

- Report any of the following immediately: nausea, vomiting, anorexia, abdominal pain, jaundice.
- Note: The long-term effects of lamivudine are unknown.
- Do not breast feed while taking this drug.

LAMOTRIGINE

(la-mo′tri-geen)
Lamictal
Classifications: CENTRAL NERVOUS SYSTEM AGENT; ANTICONVULSANT
Prototype: Phenytoin
Pregnancy Category: C

AVAILABILITY 25 mg, 100 mg, 150 mg, 200 mg tablets; 5 mg, 25 mg chewable tablets

ACTIONS Anticonvulsant. The exact mechanism of action is not known; thought to act by inhibiting the release of glutamate, an excitatory neurotransmitter, at voltage-sensitive sodium channels.

THERAPEUTIC EFFECTS Stabilizes neuronal membranes and inhibits neurotransmitter release (i.e., glutamate) in brain tissue.

USES Adjunctive therapy for partial seizures in adults and children (>2 y). Generalized tonic–clonic, absence, or myoclonic seizures in adults, treatment of bipolar disorder.

CONTRAINDICATIONS Hypersensitivity to lamotrigine, lactation. Safety and efficacy in children ≤2 y are not established.

CAUTIOUS USE Renal insufficiency, concomitant administration of other anticonvulsants, pregnancy (category C), cardiac or liver function impairment. Note: Fatal rash has been reported in children <16 y.

ROUTE & DOSAGE

Partial Seizures, Patients Receiving Anticonvulsants Other Than Valproic Acid

Adult: **PO** Start with 50 mg q.d. for 2 wk, then 50 mg b.i.d. for 2 wk, may titrate up to 300–500 mg/d in 2 divided doses (max: 700 mg/d)
Child: **PO** *2–16 y,* 1 mg/kg b.i.d. times 2 wk, then 2.5 mg/kg b.i.d. times 2 wk, then 5 mg/kg b.i.d. (max: 15 mg/kg/d or 400 mg/d)

Partial Seizures, Patients Receiving Valproic Acid

Adult: **PO** Start with 25 mg q.o.d. for 2 wk, then 25 mg q.d. for 2 wk, may titrate up to 150 mg/d in 2 divided doses (max: 200 mg/d)
Child: **PO** *2–16 y,* 0.2 mg/kg/d × 2 wk, then 0.5 mg/kg/d × 2 wk, then 1 mg/kg/d (max: 5 mg/kg/d or 250 mg/d)

Bipolar Disorder, Patients Not Receiving Valproate or Carbamazepine

Adult: **PO** Start with 25 mg q.d. for 2 wk, then 50 mg q.d. for 2 wk, then 100 mg/d for 1 wk, then 200 mg q.d.

Bipolar Disorder, Patients Receiving Valproic Acid

Adult: **PO** Start with 25 mg q.o.d. for 2 wk, then 25 mg q.d. for 2 wk, then 50 mg q.d. for 1 wk, then 100 mg q.d.

Bipolar Disorder, Patients Receiving Carbamazepine

Adult: **PO** Start with 50 mg q.d. for 2 wk, then 50 mg b.i.d. for 2 wk, then 100 b.i.d for 1 wk, then 150 mg b.i.d. for 1 wk, then 200 mg b.i.d.

ADMINISTRATION

Oral

- Note: Reduced dose may be warranted with renal and hepatic impairment.
- Ensure that chewable tablets are chewed or crushed before being swallowed with a liquid.
- When discontinued, drug should be tapered off gradually over a 2-wk period, unless patient safety is at risk.

ADVERSE EFFECTS (≥1%) **CNS:** *Dizziness, ataxia, somnolence, headache,* aphasia, vertigo, confusion, slurred speech, irritability, depression, incoordination, hostility. **GI:** *Nausea,* vomiting, anorexia, abdominal pain, diarrhea, dyspepsia, constipation. **Urogenital:** Hematuria, dysmenorrhea, vaginitis. **Special Senses:** *Diplopia, blurred vision.* **Musculoskeletal:** Peripheral neuropathy, chills, tremor, arthralgia. **Skin:** Rash (including Stevens-Johnson syndrome, toxic epidermal necrolysis), urticaria, pruritus, alopecia, acne. **Respiratory:** *Rhinitis,* pharyngitis, cough.

INTERACTIONS Drug: Carbamazepine, phenobarbital, primidone, phenytoin, fosphenytoin, ORAL CONTRACEPTIVES may decrease lamotrigine levels. **Valproic acid** may increase lamotrigine levels. Lamotrigine may decrease serum levels of **valproic acid. Herbal: Ginkgo** may decrease anticonvulsant effectiveness.

PHARMACOKINETICS Absorption: Readily absorbed from GI tract; 98% reaches systemic circulation. **Onset:** 12 wk. **Peak:** 1–4 h. **Distribution:** 55% protein bound; crosses placenta; distributed into breast milk. **Metabolism:** Metabolized in liver to inactive metabolite. **Elimination:** Can induce own metabolism; excreted in urine. **Half-Life:** 25–30 h.

NURSING IMPLICATIONS

Assessment & Drug Effects

- Withhold drug if rash develops and immediately report to physician.
- Monitor the plasma levels of lamotrigine and other anticonvulsants when given concomitantly.
- Monitor for adverse reactions when lamotrigine is used with other anticonvulsants, especially valproic acid.
- Be aware of drug interactions and closely monitor when interacting drugs are added or discontinued.

Patient & Family Education

- Notify physician for any of the following: Worsening seizure control, skin rash, ataxia, blurred vision or diplopia, fever or flu-like symptoms.
- Do not drive or engage in other potentially hazardous activities until response to the drug is known.
- Use protection from sunlight or ultraviolet light until tolerance is known; drug increases photosensitivity.
- Schedule periodic ophthalmologic exams with long-term use.
- Do not discontinue lamotrigine abruptly.
- Do not breast feed while taking this drug.

LANSOPRAZOLE

(lan′so-pra-zole)

Prevacid, Prevacid IV, Prevacid SoluTab

Classifications: GASTROINTESTINAL AGENT; ANTISECRETORY; PROTON PUMP INHIBITOR

Prototype: Omeprazole

Pregnancy Category: B

AVAILABILITY 15 mg, 30 mg sustained release capsules; 15 mg, 30 mg orally disintegrating tablets; 15 mg, 30 mg packets for suspension; 30 mg powder for injection

ACTIONS Belongs to a class of antisecretory compounds that are gastric acid pump inhibitors. Specifically, it suppresses gastric acid secretion by inhibiting the H^+, K^+-ATPase enzyme (the acid [proton H^+] pump) in the

parietal cells. Lansoprazole does not exhibit anticholinergic or H_2-histamine antagonist properties.
THERAPEUTIC EFFECTS Suppresses gastric acid formation in the stomach.

USES Short-term treatment of duodenal ulcer (up to 4 wk) and erosive esophagitis (up to 8 wk), pathologic hypersecretory disorders, gastric ulcers; in combination with clarithromycin and amoxicillin for *Helicobacter pylori.* Gastroesophageal reflux disease.

CONTRAINDICATIONS Hypersensitivity to lansoprazole, severe hepatic impairment, proton pump inhibitors (PPIs) hypersensitivity, lactation, infants.
CAUTIOUS USE Hepatic disease, pregnancy (category B).

ROUTE & DOSAGE

Duodenal Ulcer

Adult: **PO** 15 mg once daily times 4 wk

Erosive Esophagitis

Adult: **PO** 30 mg once daily times 8 wk, then decrease to 15 mg once daily. **IV** 30 mg once daily for up to 7 days

GERD

Adult: **PO** 15 mg once daily for up to 8 wk
Child: **PO** *1–11 y* 1.5 mg/kg/d (max 30 mg/d)

Hypersecretory Disorder

Adult: **PO** 60 mg once daily (max: 120 mg/d in divided doses), may need to be adjusted for hepatic impairment

H. pylori

Adult: **PO** 30 mg b.i.d. times 2 wk, in combination with 2 antibiotics

ADMINISTRATION

Oral

- *All forms:* Administer dosage 30 min a.c. Give once daily dose before breakfast.
- Give at least 30 min prior to any concurrent sucralfate therapy.
- Do not crush or chew capsules. Capsules can be opened and granules sprinkled on food or mixed with 40 mL of apple juice and administered through an NG tube. Do not crush or chew granules.
- Note: Disintegrating tablets contain phenylalanine and should not be used for patients with PKU. Capsule and syrup formulations do not contain phenylalanine.

Intravenous

PREPARE: **IV Infusion:** Add 5 mL of sterile water for injection to each 30 mg vial to yield 6 mg/mL. Swirl gently to mix. Further dilute in 50 mL of NS, RL, or D5W. If reconstituted with NS or LR, administer within 24 h. If reconstituted with D5W, administer within 12 h.
ADMINISTER: **IV Infusion:** Infuse over 30 min through the in-line filter provided. Use a dedicated line or a Y-site; flush Y-site with NS before and after administration. Do NOT give IV push. Immediately stop infusion if precipitation or discoloration occurs.

INCOMPATIBILITIES **Solution/additive, Y-site:** Do not administer with other drugs or diluents.

- Reconstituted solution can be held for 1 h at 25° C (77° F) before further dilution.

ADVERSE EFFECTS (≥1%) **CNS:** Fatigue, dizziness, headache. **GI:** Nausea, *diarrhea,* constipation, anorexia, increased appetite, thirst elevated serum transaminases (AST, ALT). **Skin:** Rash.

INTERACTIONS Drug: May decrease **theophylline** levels. **Sucralfate** decreases lansoprazole bioavailability. May interfere with absorption of **ketoconazole, digoxin, ampicillin,** or IRON SALTS. **Food:** Food reduces peak lansoprazole levels by 50%.

PHARMACOKINETICS Absorption: Rapidly absorbed from GI tract after leaving stomach; unstable in acidic media. **Onset:** Acid reduction within 2 h; ulcer relief within 1 wk. **Peak:** 1.5–3 h. **Duration:** 24 h. **Distribution:** 97% bound to plasma proteins. **Metabolism:** Metabolized in liver by cytochrome P450 system. **Elimination:** 14%–25% excreted in urine as metabolites; part of dose eliminated in bile and feces. **Half-Life:** 1.5 h.

L

NURSING IMPLICATIONS

Assessment & Drug Effects

- Lab tests: Monitor CBC, kidney & liver function tests, and serum gastric levels periodically.
- Monitor for therapeutic effectiveness of concurrently used drugs that require an acid medium for absorption (e.g., digoxin, ampicillin, ketoconazole).

Patient & Family Education

- Inform physician of significant diarrhea.
- Do not breast feed while taking this drug.

LANTHANUM CARBONATE

(lan-tha′num)

Fosrenol

Classifications: ELECTROLYTE AND WATER BALANCE AGENT; PHOSPHATE BINDER

Prototype: Sevelamer Hydrochloride

Pregnancy Category: C

AVAILABILITY 250 mg, 500 mg chewable tablets

ACTIONS Lanthanum is used for the management of hyperphosphatemia in patients with end-stage renal disease; it is a calcium-/aluminum-free phosphate binding agent. It has a higher affinity for binding to phosphate than calcium or aluminum. Low systemic absorption minimizes the risk of aluminum intoxication and hypercalcemia.

THERAPEUTIC EFFECTS Lanthanum decreases phosphate absorption from the diet. Dietary phosphate bound to lanthanum carbonate is excreted in the feces and results in lowering of serum phosphate and urinary excretion of phosphate.

USES Reduce serum phosphate levels in patients with end-stage renal disease.

CONTRAINDICATIONS Prior hypersensitivity to lanthanum carbonate; pregnancy (category C); children <18 y.

CAUTIOUS USE Bowel obstruction, Crohn's disease, acute peptic ulcer, ulcerative colitis; lactation.

ROUTE & DOSAGE

Hyperphosphatemia

Adult: **PO** 250–500 mg t.i.d. with or immediately after meals; may titrate up every 2–3 wk in increments of 750 mg/d to achieve acceptable serum phosphate levels (max: 3750 mg/d)

ADMINISTRATION

Oral

- Give with or immediately after a meal.
- Tablets must be chewed completely before swallowing. Whole tablets should not be swallowed.

- Store at 15°–30° C (59°–86° F).

ADVERSE EFFECTS (≥1%) **CNS:** Headache. **CV:** Hypotension. **GI:** *Nausea, vomiting, diarrhea,* abdominal pain, constipation. **Respiratory:** Bronchitis, rhinitis. **Other:** Dialysis graft occlusion.

PHARMACOKINETICS Absorption: Minimal absorption from GI tract. **Metabolism:** Not metabolized. **Elimination:** Excreted in feces. **Half-Life:** 53 h.

NURSING IMPLICATIONS

Assessment & Drug Effects

- Monitor for dialysis graft occlusion, as lanthanum therapy may increase occlusion risk.
- Lab tests: serum phosphate levels during dosage titration and regularly throughout treatment; periodic serum calcium, bicarbonate, and chloride.

Patient & Family Education

- Chew chewable tablets completely, then swallow.
- Report promptly any of the following: headache, drowsiness, dizziness, fainting, confusion, irritability, nausea, vomiting, or loss of appetite.
- Do not breast feed while taking this drug without consulting physician.

LARONIDASE

(la-ron'i-dase)

Aldurazyme

Classifications: ENZYME; ENZYME REPLACEMENT THERAPY

Prototype: Pancrelipase

Pregnancy Category: B

AVAILABILITY 2.9 mg/5 mL injection

ACTIONS Laronidase is a recombinant form of human alpha-L-iduronidase used for enzyme replacement therapy in individuals with mucopolysaccharidosis I (MPSI). This is an inherited lysosomal storage disease caused by deficiency of the enzyme alpha-L-iduronidase.

THERAPEUTIC EFFECTS Laronidase has been shown to improve pulmonary function and walking capacity.

USES Treatment of Hurler and Hurler-Scheie forms of mucopolysaccharidosis I (MPS I); treatment of moderate to severe Scheie form of MPS I.

CONTRAINDICATIONS Hypersensitivity to laronidase; lactation; children <5 y.

CAUTIOUS USE Renal or hepatic dysfunction; history of allergies, asthma; hypersensitivity to drugs, especially recombinant forms; pregnancy (category B).

ROUTE & DOSAGE

Mucopolysaccharidosis

Adult/Child: **IV** > *5 y,* 0.58 mg/kg infused over 3–4 h once/wk

ADMINISTRATION

Intravenous

- Pretreatment with antipyretics and/or antihistamines 60 min prior to infusion is recommended.

PREPARE: **IV Infusion:** Determine volume of infusion based on the patient's body weight (100 mL if ≤20 kg or 250 mL if >20 kg). Prepare IV infusion of 0.1% albumin (human) in NS injection as follows: 1) remove and discard a volume of NS injection equal to the volume of albumin (human) to be added to the IV bag (for 100 mL infusion use 2 mL of 5% albumin

L

of 0.4 mL or 25% albumin, for 250 mL infusion use 5 mL of 5% albumin or 1 mL of 25% albumin); 2) add the appropriate volume of albumin to the IV bag and gently rotate; 3) add the albumin to IV bag and gently rotate to mix; 4) withdraw and discard a volume of the 0.1% albumin in NS injection from the IV bag equal to the volume of laronidase concentrate to be added; 5) slowly withdraw the required amount of laronidase from vials (avoid excessive agitation), then slowly add laronidase to the IV solution. Use immediately.

ADMINISTER: **IV Infusion:** Infuse initially at 10 mcg/kg/hr; may increase q15min during first h, as tolerated, to a max rate of 200 mcg/kg/hr. Maintain max for remainder of the infusion (2–3 h).

- Store at 2°–8° C (36°–46° F). Do not freeze or shake. Discard any unused drug.

INCOMPATIBILITIES **Solution/additive:** No compatibility data available. Do not recommend mixing or infusing with other drugs.

ADVERSE EFFECTS (≥1%) **Body as a Whole:** Infusion reactions (flushing, fever, headache, rash), injection site pain, hypersensitivity reactions. **CNS:** Hyperreflexia, paresthesias. **CV:** Chest pain, hypotension, edema. **Hematologic:** Thrombocytopenia. **Respiratory:** Upper respiratory tract infection. **Skin:** Rash.

PHARMACOKINETICS Half-Life: 1.5–3.6 h.

NURSING IMPLICATIONS

Assessment & Drug Effects

- Monitor for infusion-related reactions. Slow or stop infusion and notify physician for any of the following: cough, bronchospasm, dyspnea, urticaria, angioedema, pruritus, or other signs of hypersensitivity.
- Lab tests: Periodic platelet count.

Patient & Family Education

- Report promptly difficulty breathing, rash, or itching.
- Do not breast feed while taking this drug without consulting physician.

LATANOPROST Pr

(la-tan′o-prost)

Xalatan

Classifications: EYE PREPARATION; PROSTAGLANDIN

Pregnancy Category: C

AVAILABILITY 0.005% solution

ACTIONS Prostaglandin analog that is thought to reduce intraocular pressure (IOP) by increasing the outflow of aqueous humor.

THERAPEUTIC EFFECTS Reduces elevated intraocular pressure in patients with open-angle glaucoma.

USES Treatment of open-angle glaucoma, ocular hypertension and elevated intraocular pressure (IOP).

CONTRAINDICATIONS Hypersensitivity to latanoprost or another component in the solution; pregnancy (category C); intraocular infection; conjunctivitis.

CAUTIOUS USE Lactation; active intraocular inflammation such as: iritis or uveitis; patients at risk for macular edema; hepatic or renal impairment. Safety and effectiveness in children are not established.

ROUTE & DOSAGE

Glaucoma

Adult: **Ophthalmic** 1 drop in affected eye(s) q.d. in evening

Common adverse effects in *italic*, life-threatening effects underlined: generic names in **bold**; classifications in SMALL CAPS; ♣ Canadian drug name; Pr Prototype drug

ADMINISTRATION

Installation

- Ensure that contact lenses are removed prior to installation and not reinserted for 15 min after installation.
- Apply only to affected eye(s). Ensure that only one drop is instilled.
- Do not allow tip of dropper to touch eye.
- Wait at least 5 min before/after instillation of other eye drops.
- Refrigerate at 2°–8° C (36°–46° F). Protect from light.

ADVERSE EFFECTS (≥1%) **Body as a Whole:** Headaches, asthenia, flu-like symptoms. **GI:** Abnormal liver function tests. **Skin:** Rash. **Special Senses:** *Conjunctival hyperemia, growth of eyelashes, ocular pruritus,* ocular dryness, visual disturbance, ocular burning, foreign body sensation, eye pain, pigmentation of the periocular skin, blepharitis, cataract, superficial punctate keratitis, eyelid erythema, ocular irritation, and eyelash darkening, eye discharge, tearing, photophobia, allergic conjunctivitis, increases in iris pigmentation (brown pigment), conjunctival edema.

INTERACTIONS Drug: Precipitation may occur if mixed with eye drops containing **thimerosal;** space other EYE PREPARATIONS at least 5 min apart.

PHARMACOKINETICS Absorption: Absorbed through the cornea. **Onset:** 3–4 h. **Peak IOP reduction:** 8–12 h. **Distribution:** Minimal systemic distribution. **Metabolism:** Hydrolyzed in aqueous humor to active form. **Elimination:** Renally excreted. **Half-Life:** 17 min.

NURSING IMPLICATIONS

Assessment & Drug Effects

- Withhold eye drops and notify physician if acute intraocular inflammation (iritis or uveitis) or external eye inflammation are noted.
- Note that increased pigmentation of the iris and eyelid, and additional growth of eyelashes on the treated eye are adverse effects that may develop gradually over months to years.

Patient & Family Education

- Contact physician immediately if any ocular reaction occurs, especially conjunctivitis and lid reactions.
- Note: Increased pigmentation of the iris and eyelid, and additional growth of eyelashes on the treated eye, are possible adverse effects of this drug. Persons with light colored eyes receiving treatment to one eye may develop a darker eye.
- Do not breast feed while using this drug.

L

LEFLUNOMIDE

(le-flu'no-mide)

Arava

Classifications: BIOLOGIC RESPONSE MODIFIER; TUMOR NECROSIS FACTOR MODIFIER

Prototype: Etanercept

Pregnancy Category: X

AVAILABILITY 10 mg, 20 mg, 100 mg tablets

ACTIONS An immunomodulator that demonstrates antiinflammatory effects.

THERAPEUTIC EFFECTS Reduces the S&S of rheumatoid arthritis (RA).

USES Active RA.

CONTRAINDICATIONS Hepatic disease; jaundice; lactase deficiency; hypersensitivity to leflunomide; pregnancy (category X); lactation; patients with positive hepatitis B

or C serology; malignancy, particularly lymphoproliferative disorders; severe immunosuppression; vaccination, infants. Use in patients <18 y has not been fully studied.
CAUTIOUS USE Renal insufficiency; renal failure; alcoholism; immunosuppression; infection.

ROUTE & DOSAGE

Rheumatoid Arthritis
Adult: **PO** Initiate with a loading dose of 100 mg/d times 3 d, then maintenance dose of 20 mg q.d., may decrease to 10 mg/d if higher dose is not tolerated

ADMINISTRATION

Oral
- Initiate with a 3-d loading dose followed by a lower maintenance dose.

ADVERSE EFFECTS (≥1%) **Body as a Whole:** Allergic reaction, asthenia, flu-like syndrome, infection, pain, back pain, arthralgia, leg cramps, synovitis, tenosynovitis. **CNS:** Dizziness, headache, paresthesias, peripheral neuropathy. **CV:** Hypertension, chest pain. **GI:** *Diarrhea,* increased LFTs (ALT and AST), abdominal pain, anorexia, dyspepsia, gastroenteritis, nausea, mouth ulcer, vomiting, weight loss, hepatotoxicity. **Metabolic:** Hypokalemia. **Respiratory:** Bronchitis, cough, respiratory infection, pharyngitis, pneumonia, rhinitis, sinusitis. **Skin:** Rash, alopecia, eczema, pruritus, dry skin, Stevens-Johnson syndrome, toxic epidermal necrolysis (rare). **Urogenital:** UTI.

INTERACTIONS Drug: Rifampin may significantly increase leflunomide levels; **cholestyramine, charcoal** decrease absorption; caution should be used with other hepatotoxic drugs.

PHARMACOKINETICS Absorption: Approximately 80% reaches systemic circulation. **Peak:** 6–12 h for active metabolite. **Distribution:** >99% protein bound. **Metabolism:** Metabolized primarily to M1 (active metabolite). **Elimination:** 43% excreted in urine, 48% in feces. **Half-Life:** 19 d for active metabolite.

NURSING IMPLICATIONS

Assessment & Drug Effects
- Lab tests: Baseline screening to rule out hepatitis B or C; baseline and monthly liver enzymes × 12 mo, then every 6 mo thereafter.
- Monitor carefully for and report immediately S&S of infection; withhold leflunomide if infection is suspected.
- Monitor BP and weight periodically. Doses greater than 25 mg/d are associated with a greater incidence of side effects such as alopecia, weight loss, and elevated liver enzymes.

Patient & Family Education
- Use reliable contraception while taking leflunomide.
- Note: Both women and men need to discontinue leflunomide and undergo a drug elimination procedure prescribed by the physician BEFORE conception.
- Withhold drug if you develop an infection and notify the physician before resuming the drug.
- Notify physician about any of the following: hair loss, weight loss, GI distress, rash, or itching.
- Do not breast feed while taking this drug.

LEPIRUDIN (Pr)

(le-pir'u-din)

Refludan

Classifications: BLOOD FORMERS, COAGULATORS, AND ANTICOAGULANTS; DIRECT THROMBIN INHIBITOR

Pregnancy Category: B

AVAILABILITY 50 mg powder for injection

ACTIONS Highly specific direct inhibitor of thrombin. One molecule of lepirudin binds to one molecule of thrombin and thereby blocks the thrombogenic activity of thrombin.

THERAPEUTIC EFFECTS Increases PT/INR and aPTT values in relation to the dose given. Effectiveness is indicated by aPTT ratio in target range of 1.5 to 2.5.

USES Anticoagulation in patients with heparin-induced thrombocytopenia (HIT).

CONTRAINDICATIONS Hypersensitivity to lepirudin; lactation; pregnancy (category B); intracranial bleeding; patients with increased risk of bleeding (e.g., recent surgery, CVA, advanced kidney impairment). Safety and efficacy in children not established.

CAUTIOUS USE Serious liver injury (e.g., cirrhosis); concomitant administration with streptokinase; renal impairment.

ROUTE & DOSAGE

Anticoagulation

Adult: **IV** 0.4 mg/kg initial bolus (max: 44 mg) followed by 0.15 mg/kg/h (max: 16.5 mg/h) for 2–10 d, adjust rate to maintain aPTT of 1.5–2.5

ADMINISTRATION

Intravenous

PREPARE: **Direct:** Reconstitute by adding 1 mL of sterile water for injection or NS to the 50-mg vial. To prepare bolus dose, withdraw reconstituted solution into a 10-cc syringe and dilute to 10 mL with sterile water for injection, NS or D5W to yield 5 mg/mL. **Continuous:** Transfer the contents of two reconstituted vials into 250 or 500 mL of D5W or NS to yield of 0.4 or 0.2 mg/mL, respectively.

ADMINISTER: **Direct:** Give over 15–20 s. **Continuous:** Give at a rate determined by body weight.

- Diluted solution is stable for 24 h during infusion. Store unopened vials at 2°–25° C (36°–77° F).

L

ADVERSE EFFECTS (≥1%) **CNS:** Intracranial bleeding. **CV:** Heart failure, ventricular fibrillation, pericardial effusion, MI. **GI:** Abnormal LFTs. **Hematologic:** Bleeding from injection site, anemia, hematoma, bleeding, hematuria, GI and rectal bleeding, epistaxis, hemothorax, vaginal bleeding. **Respiratory:** Pneumonia, cough, bronchospasm, stridor, dyspnea. **Skin:** Allergic skin reactions. **Body as a Whole:** Sepsis, abnormal kidney function, multiorgan failure.

INTERACTIONS Drug: Warfarin, NSAIDS, SALICYLATES, ANTIPLATELET AGENTS increases risk of bleeding. **Herbal: Feverfew, ginkgo, ginger, valerian** may potentiate bleeding.

PHARMACOKINETICS Distribution: Distributed primarily to extracellular compartment. **Metabolism:** Metabolized by catabolic hydrolysis in serum. **Elimination:** 48% excreted in urine. **Half-Life:** 1.3 h.

NURSING IMPLICATIONS

Assessment & Drug Effects

- Lab tests: Baseline PT/INR and aPTT prior to initiation of therapy (withhold therapy and notify physician if baseline aPTT ratio ≥2.5); aPTT 4 h after start of therapy and at least once daily (more often with renal or hepatic impairment) thereafter.
- Give with extreme caution to those at increased risk for bleeding.
- Monitor carefully for bleeding events (e.g., from puncture wounds, hematoma, hematuria); and report immediately.
- Do not give oral anticoagulants until lepirudin dose has been reduced and aPTT ratio lowered to just above 1.5.

Patient & Family Education

- Do not breast feed while taking this drug.

LETROZOLE

(le'tro-zole)

Femara

Classifications: ANTINEOPLASTIC; HORMONE AND SYNTHETIC SUBSTITUTE; AROMATASE INHIBITOR

Prototype: Anastrozole

Pregnancy Category: D

AVAILABILITY 2.5 mg tablets

ACTIONS Nonsteroid competitive inhibitor of the enzyme system that converts androgens to estrogens.

THERAPEUTIC EFFECTS Results in the regression of estrogen-dependent tumors.

USES Advanced breast cancer in postmenopausal women following antiestrogen therapy.

CONTRAINDICATIONS Hypersensitivity to letrozole; pregnancy (category D).

CAUTIOUS USE Moderate to severe hepatic impairment; lactation. Safety and efficacy in children are not established.

ROUTE & DOSAGE

Breast Cancer

Adult: **PO** 2.5 mg q.d.

ADMINISTRATION

Oral

- Give without regard to food.

ADVERSE EFFECTS (≥1%) **Body as a Whole:** Fatigue, peripheral edema, asthenia, weight increase, *musculoskeletal pain,* arthralgia. **CNS:** Headache, somnolence, dizziness. **CV:** Chest pain, hypertension, hypercholesterolemia. **GI:** Nausea, vomiting, constipation, diarrhea, abdominal pain, anorexia, dyspepsia. **Respiratory:** Dyspnea, cough. **Skin:** Hot flushes, rash, pruritus.

INTERACTIONS Drug: ESTROGENS, ORAL CONTRACEPTIVES could interfere with the pharmacologic action of letrozole.

PHARMACOKINETICS Absorption: Rapidly absorbed from GI tract. **Metabolism:** Metabolized in liver by cytochromes P450 3A4 and 2A6. **Elimination:** 90% excreted in urine. **Half-Life:** 2 d.

NURSING IMPLICATIONS

Assessment & Drug Effects

- Lab tests: Periodically monitor serum calcium and CBC with differential.
- Monitor carefully for S&S of thrombophlebitis or thromboembolism; report immediately.

Patient & Family Education

- Notify physician immediately if S&S of thrombophlebitis develop (see Appendix F).

- Do not breast feed while taking this drug without consulting physician.

LEUCOVORIN CALCIUM

(loo-koe-vor'in)

Calcium Folinate, Citrovorum Factor, Folinic Acid, Wellcovorin

Classifications: BLOOD FORMERS, COAGULATORS, AND ANTICOAGULANTS; ANTIANEMIC AGENT; ANTIDOTE

Pregnancy Category: C

AVAILABILITY 5 mg, 15 mg, 25 mg tablets; 3 mg/mL ampule; 50 mg, 100 mg, 350 mg vials

ACTIONS A reduced form of folic acid; unlike folic acid, it does not require enzymatic reduction and therefore is readily available to participate in reactions.

THERAPEUTIC EFFECTS Functions as an essential cell growth factor. When given during antineoplastic therapy, it prevents serious toxicity by protecting cells from the action of folic acid antagonists such as methotrexate.

USES Folate-deficient megaloblastic anemias due to sprue, pregnancy, and nutritional deficiency when oral therapy is not feasible. Also to prevent or diminish toxicity of antineoplastic folic acid antagonists, particularly methotrexate; and as adjunct with antifols (e.g., pyrimethamine) in pneumocystosis or toxoplasmosis to prevent significant bone marrow toxicity.

CONTRAINDICATIONS Undiagnosed anemia, pernicious anemia, or other megaloblastic anemias secondary to vitamin B_{12} deficiency. Safe use during pregnancy (category C) or lactation is not established.

CAUTIOUS USE Renal dysfunction.

ROUTE & DOSAGE

Megaloblastic Anemia

Adult/Child: **IV/IM** No more than 1 mg/d

Leucovorin Rescue for Methotrexate Toxicity

Adult/Child: **PO/IM/IV** 10 mg/m^2 followed by 10 mg/m^2 q6h for 72 h, further doses based on serum methotrexate concentrations

Leucovorin Rescue for Other Folate Antagonist Toxicity

Adult/Child: **PO/IM/IV** 5–15 mg/d

Adjunct for Treatment of Pneumocystosis or Toxoplasmosis

Adult/Child: **PO/IM/IV** 3–6 mg t.i.d.

ADMINISTRATION

Note: Oral route is NOT recommended for doses higher than 25 mg or if patient is likely to vomit.

Intramuscular

- Use 3 mg ampules for IM injection.
- Give deep into a large muscle.

Intravenous

PREPARE: **Direct:** Give 1 mL (3 mg) ampules, which contain benzyl alcohol, undiluted. **IV Infusion:** For doses <10 mg/m^2, reconstitute each 50 mg in 5 mL (10 mg per 1 mL in 10 mL) of bacteriostatic water for injection with benzyl alcohol. For doses >10 mg/m^2 reconstitute, as above, but with sterile water for injection without a preservative. Final concentration is 10 mg/mL. Further dilute in 100–500 mL of IV solutions (e.g., D5W, NS, RL) to yield a concentration of 10–20 mg/mL of IV solution.

ADMINISTER: **Direct:** Give 160 mg or fraction thereof over 1 min. **IV Infusion:** Do not exceed direct IV rate. Give more slowly if the volume of IV solution to be infused is large; over 15–60 min, depending on the volume of solution.
INCOMPATIBILITIES **Solution/additive: Droperidol, fluorouracil. Y-site: Amphotericin B cholesteryl complex, droperidol, foscarnet, sodium bicarbonate.**

- Use solution reconstituted with bacteriostatic water within 7 d. Use solution reconstituted with sterile water for injection immediately.
- Protect from light.

ADVERSE EFFECTS (≥1%) **Body as a Whole:** Allergic sensitization (urticaria, pruritus, rash, wheezing). **Hematologic:** Thrombocytosis.

INTERACTIONS Drug: May enhance adverse effects of **fluorouracil;** may reverse therapeutic effects of **methotrexate, trimethoprim-sulfamethoxazole.**

PHARMACOKINETICS Onset: Within 30 min. **Duration:** 3–6 h. **Distribution:** Crosses placenta; distributed into breast milk. **Metabolism:** Metabolized in liver and intestinal mucosa to tetrahydrofolic acid derivatives. **Elimination:** 80%–90% excreted in urine, 5%–8% in feces.

NURSING IMPLICATIONS

Assessment & Drug Effects

- Monitor neurologic status. Use of leucovorin alone in treatment of pernicious anemia or other megaloblastic anemias associated with vitamin B_{12} deficiency can result in an apparent hematological remission while allowing already present neurologic damage to progress.
- Lab tests: Do Cl_{cr} determinations prior to initiation of leucovorin, urine pH prior to and about every 6 h throughout therapy; daily serum creatinine levels are recommended to detect onset of kidney function impairment.

Patient & Family Education

- Notify physician of S&S of a hypersensitivity reaction immediately (see Appendix F).
- Do not breast feed while taking this drug without consulting physician.

LEUPROLIDE ACETATE (Pr)

(loo-proe′lide)
Eligard, Lupron, Lupron Depot, Lupron Depot-Ped, Viadur
Classifications: HORMONE AND SYNTHETIC SUBSTITUTE; GONADOTROPIN-RELEASING HORMONE ANALOG
Pregnancy Category: X

AVAILABILITY 5 mg/mL injection; 3.75 mg, 7.5 mg, 11.25 mg, 15 mg, 22.5 mg, 30 mg microspheres for injection (depot formulations); 65 mg implant

ACTIONS Occupies and desensitizes pituitary GnRH receptors, resulting initially in release of gonadotropins LH and FSH and stimulation of ovarian and testicular steroidogenesis.
THERAPEUTIC EFFECTS Long-term administration suppresses both gonadotropin secretion and steroidogenesis and leads to prostatic and testicular atrophy. **Antitumor effect:** May inhibit growth of hormone-dependent tumors as indicated by reduction in concentrations of PSA and serum testosterone to levels equal to or less than pretreatment levels. **Contraceptive effect:** By inhibiting gonadotropin release,

ovulation or spermatogenesis is suppressed.

USES Palliative treatment of advanced prostatic carcinoma as alternative to orchiectomy or estrogen administration; endometriosis; anemia caused by leiomyomata.
UNLABELED USES Breast cancer; male contraceptive; delayed puberty.

CONTRAINDICATIONS Following orchiectomy or estrogen therapy; metastatic cerebral lesions; pregnancy (category X), lactation.
CAUTIOUS USE Life-threatening carcinoma in which rapid symptomatic relief is necessary; known hypersensitivity to benzyl alcohol.

ROUTE & DOSAGE

Palliative Treatment for Prostate Cancer

Adult: **SC** 1 mg/d **IM** 7.5 mg/mo or 22.5 mg q3mo or 30 mg q4mo (depot preparation)
Implant one implant q12mo

Endometriosis, Anemia

Adult: **IM** 3.75 mg qmo or 11.25 mg q3mo

Precocious Puberty

Child: **IM** Depot-Ped, 0.15–0.3 mg/kg q28d (min: 7.5 mg), titrate by 3.75-mg increments q4wk

ADMINISTRATION

Subcutaneous

- Do not use Depot-Ped form for SC injection.
- Rotate injection sites.

Intramuscular

- Prepare solution for Depot-Ped injection using a 22-gauge needle (or syringe provided by manufacturer), withdraw 1.5 mL of diluent from the supplied ampul and inject it into the vial. Shake well to form a uniform suspension. Withdraw entire contents and administer immediately.
- Do not administer parenteral drug formulation if particulate matter or discoloration is present.
- Refrigerate unopened vials. Store vial in use at room temperature for several months with minimal loss of potency. Protect from light and freezing.

ADVERSE EFFECTS (≥1%) **Body as a Whole:** *Disease flare (worsening of S&S of carcinoma),* injection site irritation, asthenia, fatigue, fever, facial swelling. **CNS:** Dizziness, pain, headache, paresthesia. **CV:** *Peripheral edema,* cardiac arrhythmias, MI. **Endocrine:** *Hot flushes, impotence, decreased libido,* gynecomastia, breast tenderness, amenorrhea, vaginal bleeding, thyroid enlargement, hypoglycemia. **GI:** Nausea, vomiting, constipation, anorexia, sour taste, GI bleeding, diarrhea. **Musculoskeletal:** Increased bone pain, myalgia. **Renal:** Increased hematuria, dysuria, flank pain. **Respiratory:** Pleural rub, pulmonary fibrosis flare. **Hematologic:** Decreased Hct, Hgb. **Skin:** Pruritus, rash, hair loss.

INTERACTIONS Drug: ANDROGENS, ESTROGENS would counteract therapeutic effects.

PHARMACOKINETICS Absorption: Readily absorbed from SC or IM sites. **Metabolism:** Metabolized by enzymes in hypothalamus and anterior pituitary. **Half-Life:** 3 h.

NURSING IMPLICATIONS

Assessment & Drug Effects

- Monitor PSA and testosterone levels in males with prostate cancer. A gradual rise in values after their decrease may signify treatment failure.

L

- Inspect injection site. If local hypersensitivity reactions occur (erythema, induration), suspect sensitivity to benzyl alcohol. Report to physician.
- Monitor I&O ratio and pattern. Report hematuria and decreased output. Carefully monitor voiding problems.

Patient & Family Education

- When used for prostate cancer, bone pain and voiding problems (i.e., symptoms of tumor obstruction) usually increase during first several weeks of continuous treatment but are transient. Hot flushes also may be experienced.
- Notify physician of neurologic S&S (paresthesia and weakness in lower limbs). Exercise caution when walking without assistance.
- When used for endometriosis. Continuous treatment may cause amenorrhea and other menstrual irregularities.
- Do not breast feed while taking this drug.

L

LEVALBUTEROL HYDROCHLORIDE

(lev-al-bu'ter-ole)

Xopenex, Xopenex HFA

Classifications: AUTONOMIC NERVOUS SYSTEM AGENT; BETA-ADRENERGIC AGONIST (SYMPATHOMIMETIC); BRONCHODILATOR (RESPIRATORY SMOOTH MUSCLE RELAXANT)

Prototype: Albuterol

Pregnancy Category: C

AVAILABILITY 0.63 mg/3 mL, 1.25 mg/3 mL inhalation solution

ACTIONS An isomer of albuterol with $beta_2$-adrenergic agonist properties, drug acts on the $beta_2$ receptors of the smooth muscles of the bronchial tree, thus resulting in bronchodilation.

THERAPEUTIC EFFECTS Decreases airway resistance, facilitates mucous drainage, and increases vital capacity.

USES Treatment or prevention of bronchospasm in patients with reversible obstructive airway disease.

CONTRAINDICATIONS Hypersensitivity to levalbuterol or albuterol; angioedema; pregnancy (category C); children <6 y; lactation.

CAUTIOUS USE Cardiovascular disorders especially coronary insufficiency, cardiac arrhythmias, hypertension, QT elongation, convulsive disorders; diabetes mellitus, diabetic ketoacidosis; older adults; seizures, status asthmaticus, tachycardia; hypersensitivity to sympathetic amines; hyperthyroidism, thyrotoxicosis.

ROUTE & DOSAGE

Bronchospasm

Adult: **Inhalation** 0.63 mg by nebulization t.i.d. every 6–8 h, may increase to 1.25 mg t.i.d. if needed

Child: **Inhalation** *6–11 y* 0.31 mg by nebulization t.i.d. every 6–8 h (max 0.63 mg t.i.d.)

ADMINISTRATION

Inhalation

- Use vials within 2 wk of opening pouch. Protect vial from light and use within one wk after removal from pouch. Use only if solution in vial is colorless.

INCOMPATIBILITIES **Solution/additive:** Compatibility when mixed with other drugs in a nebulizer has not been established.

- Store at 15°–25° C (59°–77° F) in protective foil pouch.

ADVERSE EFFECTS (≥1%) **Body as a Whole:** Allergic reactions, flu syndrome, pain. **CNS:** Migraine, dizziness, nervousness, tremor, anxiety. **CV:** Tachycardia. **GI:** Dyspepsia. **Respiratory:** Increased cough, viral infection, rhinitis, sinusitis, turbinate edema, paradoxical bronchospasm. **Endocrine:** Increase in serum glucose.

INTERACTIONS Drug: BETA-ADRENERGIC BLOCKERS may antagonize **levalbuterol** effects; MAOI, TRICYCLIC ANTIDEPRESSANTS may potentiate **levalbuterol** effects on vascular system; ECG changes or hypokalemia may be exacerbated by LOOP or THIAZIDE DIURETICS.

PHARMACOKINETICS Onset: 5–15 min. **Duration:** 3–6 h. **Half-Life:** 3.3 h.

NURSING IMPLICATIONS

Assessment & Drug Effects

- Monitor for S&S of CNS or cardiovascular stimulation (e.g., BP, HR, respiratory status).
- Lab tests: Periodic serum potassium levels especially with coadministered loop or thiazide diuretics.
- Monitor diabetics for loss of glycemic control.

Patient & Family Education

- Seek medical advice immediately if a previously effective dose becomes ineffective.
- Report immediately to physician: chest pains or palpitations, swelling of the eyelids, tongue, lips or face; increased wheezing or difficulty breathing.
- Do not use drug more frequently than prescribed.
- Exercise caution with hazardous activities; dizziness and vertigo are possible side effects.
- Check with physician before taking OTC cold medication.
- Do not breast feed while taking this drug.

LEVETIRACETAM

(lev-e-tir′a-ce-tam)

Keppra

Classifications: CENTRAL NERVOUS SYSTEM AGENT; ANTICONVULSANT

Pregnancy Category: C

AVAILABILITY 250 mg, 500 mg, 750 mg tablets; 100 mg/mL oral solution

ACTIONS The precise mechanism of antiepileptic effects is unknown. It is a broad spectrum antiepileptic agent, which does not involve GABA inhibition.

THERAPEUTIC EFFECTS Inhibits complex partial seizures and prevents epileptic and seizure activity.

USES Adjunctive therapy for partial onset seizures in adults.

CONTRAINDICATIONS Hypersensitivity to levetiracetam; labor and delivery.

CAUTIOUS USE Renal impairment; older adults; pregnancy (category C), lactation; suicidal tendencies. Safety & efficacy in children <16 y are not established.

ROUTE & DOSAGE

Partial Onset Seizures

Adult: **PO** 500 mg b.i.d., may increase by 500 mg b.i.d. q2wks (max: 3000 mg/d)

Renal Impairment

Cl_{cr} 50–80 mL/min: 500–1000 mg q12h; 30–50 mL/min: 250–750 mg q12h; <30 mL/min: 250–500 mg q12h; hemodialysis: 500–1000 mg q24h

ADMINISTRATION

Oral

- Reduced doses are indicated when creatinine clearance is <80 mL/min.
- Make dosage increment changes at 2-wk intervals.
- Taper dose if discontinued.
- Give supplemental doses to dialysis patients after dialysis.
- Store at 15°–30° C (59°–86° F).

ADVERSE EFFECTS (≥1%) **Body as a Whole:** *Asthenia, headache, infection,* pain. **CNS:** *Somnolence,* amnesia, anxiety, ataxia, depression, dizziness, emotional lability, hostility, nervousness, vertigo, paradoxical increase in seizures (as add-on therapy). **GI:** Anorexia. **Respiratory:** Cough, pharyngitis, rhinitis, sinusitis. **Special Senses:** Diplopia.

INTERACTIONS **Drug:** Levetiracetam does not decrease **estrogen** levels.

PHARMACOKINETICS **Absorption:** Rapidly and almost completely absorbed. **Peak:** 1 h; steady-state 2 d. **Distribution:** <10% protein bound. **Metabolism:** Minimal hepatic metabolism. **Elimination:** Renally eliminated. **Half-Life:** 7.1 h (9.6 h in older adults).

NURSING IMPLICATIONS

Assessment & Drug Effects

- Monitor & notify physician of difficulty with gait or coordination.
- Lab tests: Periodic CBC with differential, Hct & Hgb, LFTs.
- Monitor for changes in phenytoin blood levels with coadministered drugs.

Patient & Family Education

- Do not drive or engage in potentially hazardous activities until response to drug is known.
- Do not abruptly discontinue drug. MUST use gradual dose reduction/taper.
- Notify physician of intention to become pregnant.
- Do not breast feed while taking this drug without consulting physician.

LEVOBETAXOLOL HYDROCHLORIDE

(le-vo-be-tax′oh-lol)

Betaxon

Classifications: EYE PREPARATION; MIOTIC (ANTIGLAUCOMAL AGENT); AUTONOMIC NERVOUS SYSTEM AGENT; BETA-ADRENERGIC BLOCKER

Prototype: Propranolol

Pregnancy Category: C

AVAILABILITY 0.5% ophthalmic suspension

See Appendix A-1.

LEVOBUNOLOL

(lee-voe-byoo′noe-lole)

Betagan

Classifications: EYE PREPARATION; AUTONOMIC NERVOUS SYSTEM AGENT; BETA-ADRENERGIC ANTAGONIST (SYMPATHOLYTIC)

Prototype: Propranolol

Pregnancy Category: C

AVAILABILITY 0.25%, 0.5% ophthalmic solution

See Appendix A-1.

LEVOBUPIVACAINE

(lev-o-bu-piv′a-cane)

Chirocaine

Classifications: CENTRAL NERVOUS SYSTEM AGENT; LOCAL ANESTHETIC (ESTER TYPE)

Prototype: Procaine HCl

Pregnancy Category: B

AVAILABILITY 2.5 mg/mL, 5 mg/mL, 7.5 mg/mL injection

ACTIONS Decreases sodium flux into nerve cell, inhibiting initial depolarization, and prevents propagation and conduction of nerve impulse.

THERAPEUTIC EFFECTS Progression of anesthesia is manifested clinically as sequential loss of nerve function: pain, temperature, touch, proprioception and skeletal muscle tone.

USES Local or regional anesthesia for surgery and obstetrics, and for postoperative pain management.

CONTRAINDICATIONS Hypersensitivity to levobupivacaine or any other local anesthetic of the amide type (e.g., procaine, bupivacaine); acidosis; cardiac heart block; severe hemorrhaging; cerebral spinal disease; septicemia. Safe use during pregnancy (category B) other than labor and delivery, or in children is not established.

ROUTE & DOSAGE

Surgical Anesthesia

Adult: **Epidural** 25–50 mg **Nerve Block** 1–2 mg/kg **Infiltration** 150 mg

Pain Management

Adult: **Epidural** 5–25 mg/h

ADMINISTRATION

Epidural

- Aspirate for blood and cerebrospinal fluid prior to original dose and all subsequent doses to avoid injection into intravascular and intrathecal spaces.
- Use lowest effective dose to achieve desired outcome.
- Use either the 0.125% or 0.25% solution for postoperative pain management; give 5–25 mg/h (4–10 mL/hr).

INCOMPATIBILITIES **Solution/additive:** ALKALINE SOLUTIONS (e.g., **aminophylline, phenobarbital, sodium bicarbonate**). **Y-site:** ALKALINE SOLUTIONS (e.g., **aminophylline, phenobarbital, sodium bicarbonate**).

- Store at 20°–25° C (86°–77° F); brief excursions beyond this range are tolerated.

ADVERSE EFFECTS (≥1%) **Body as a Whole:** Fever, pain, back pain, paresthesia. **CV:** *Hypotension,* abnormal ECG, bradycardia, tachycardia. **GI:** *Nausea, vomiting,* constipation, enlarged abdomen, dyspepsia. **Hematologic:** *Anemia.* **Metabolic:** Hypothermia. **CNS:** Headache, dizziness. **Skin:** Pruritus. **Urogenital:** Albuminuria, hematuria, fetal distress, delivery delayed.

INTERACTIONS **Drug:** CALCIUM CHANNEL BLOCKERS, **clarithromycin, erythromycin, ketoconazole, ritonavir** may potentiate effect. **Omeprazole, phenobarbital, phenytoin, rifampin** may decrease effect. Additive adverse effects and toxicity with other LOCAL ANESTHETICS.

PHARMACOKINETICS **Peak:** 30 min. **Distribution:** >97% protein bound. **Metabolism:** Metabolized in liver by CYP3A4 and CYP1A2. **Elimination:** 71% excreted in urine, 24% excreted in feces. **Half-Life:** 3.3 h.

NURSING IMPLICATIONS

Assessment & Drug Effects

- Monitor for and immediately report: Hypotension, bradycardia, heart block (seen with inadvertent intravascular injection).
- Monitor continuously cardiovascular status, respiratory function,

L

level of consciousness, and sensory/motor function.

- Supervise ambulation as dizziness is a common side effect.

Patient & Family Education

- Report any of the following to physician: Tremors, lightheadedness, numbness and tingling around the mouth.

LEVOCABASTINE HYDROCHLORIDE Pr

(lev-o-ca-bas'teen)

Livostin

Classifications: EYE PREPARATION; OCULAR ANTIHISTAMINE; H_1-RECEPTOR ANTAGONIST

Pregnancy Category: C

L

AVAILABILITY 0.05% ophthalmic suspension

ACTIONS Potent antihistamine that competes for H_1-receptor sites on effector cells, thus blocking histamine release.

THERAPEUTIC EFFECTS Blocks histamine release as an antihistamine H_1 receptor antagonist.

USES Temporary relief of seasonal allergic conjunctivitis.

CONTRAINDICATIONS Hypersensitivity to levocabastine, soft contact lenses.

CAUTIOUS USE Hypersensitivity to other antihistamines, kidney disease, pregnancy (category C), or lactation. Safety and efficacy in children <12 y are not established.

ROUTE & DOSAGE

Allergic Conjunctivitis

Adult: **Ophthalmic** 1 drop in affected eye q.i.d.

ADMINISTRATION

Instillation

- Shake well before using. Apply drops in the center of the lower conjunctional sac. Do not touch eyelids with dropper.
- Store in a tightly closed bottle. Do not use if discolored.

ADVERSE EFFECTS (≥1%) **CNS:** Drowsiness, fatigue, headache. **GI:** Dry mouth. **Special Senses:** *Ocular irritation, mild transient stinging and burning,* conjunctival congestion, eyelid edema, eye pain, photophobia, abnormal lacrimation.

INTERACTIONS Drug: No clinically significant interactions established.

PHARMACOKINETICS Absorption: Significant systemic absorption; 30%–60% reaches systemic circulation. **Onset:** 15 min. **Duration:** 4 h. **Distribution:** Slight distribution into breast milk. **Metabolism:** Minimal metabolism in liver. **Elimination:** 65%–73% excreted in urine unchanged; up to 20% excreted in bile. **Half-Life:** 33–40 h.

NURSING IMPLICATIONS

Assessment & Drug Effects

- Monitor for S&S of hypersensitivity to the drug (see Appendix F).
- Evaluate safety of engaging in hazardous activities since drowsiness is a potential adverse effect.

Patient & Family Education

- Learn potential adverse responses to drug.
- Eye drops contain benzalkonium chloride, which may damage soft contact lenses.
- Do not breast feed while using this drug without consulting physician.

LEVODOPA (L-DOPA) Pr

(lee-voe-doe'pa)

Dopar, Larodopa

Classifications: AUTONOMIC NERVOUS SYSTEM AGENT; ANTICHOLINERGIC (PARASYMPATHOLYTIC); ANTIPARKINSONISM AGENT

Pregnancy Category: C

AVAILABILITY 100 mg, 250 mg, 500 mg tablets and capsules

ACTIONS Drug is a metabolic precursor of dopamine, a catecholamine neurotransmitter. Unlike dopamine, levodopa readily crosses the blood–brain barrier. Precise mechanism of action unknown.

THERAPEUTIC EFFECTS Levodopa restores dopamine levels in extrapyramidal centers (believed to be depleted in parkinsonism).

USES Idiopathic Parkinson's disease, postencephalitic and arteriosclerotic parkinsonism, and parkinsonism symptoms associated with manganese and carbon monoxide poisoning.

UNLABELED USES To relieve pain of herpes zoster (shingles), liver coma (caused by cirrhosis or fulminating hepatitis), bone pain in metastatic breast carcinoma, adjunctive therapy in CHF.

CONTRAINDICATIONS Known hypersensitivity to levodopa; narrow-angle glaucoma patients with suspicious pigmented lesion or history of melanoma; acute psychoses, severe psychoneurosis, within 2 wk of use of MAO INHIBITORS. Safe use during pregnancy (category C), lactation, or in children <2 y is not established.

CAUTIOUS USE Cardiovascular, kidney, liver, or endocrine disease, history of MI with residual arrhythmias; peptic ulcer; convulsions: psychiatric disorders; chronic wide-angle glaucoma; diabetes; pulmonary diseases, bronchial asthma; patients receiving antihypertensive drugs.

ROUTE & DOSAGE

Parkinson's Disease

Adult: **PO** 500 mg to 1 g daily in 2 or more equally divided doses, may be increased by 100–750 mg q3–7d (max: 8 g/d); used in combination with carbidopa, decrease levodopa dose by 75%–80%

ADMINISTRATION

Oral

- Give with food to reduce nausea. Absorption is decreased with high-protein meals.
- Crush tablets or empty capsule content into fruit juice as needed.
- Store in tight, light-resistant containers.

ADVERSE EFFECTS (≥1%) **CNS:** *Choreiform and involuntary movements,* increased hand tremor, bradykinetic episodes (on–off phenomena), trismus, grinding of teeth (bruxism), ataxia, muscle twitching, numbness, weakness, fatigue, headache, opisthotonos, confusion, agitation, anxiety, euphoria, insomnia, nightmares; psychotic episodes with paranoid delusions or hallucinations, severe depression, including suicidal tendencies, hypomania. **CV:** *Orthostatic hypotension;* palpitations, tachycardia, hypertension. **Special Senses:** *Blepharospasm,* diplopia, blurred vision, dilated pupils. **GI:** *Anorexia, nausea, vomiting,* abdominal distress, flatulence, dry mouth, dysphagia, sialorrhea; burning sensation of tongue, bitter taste, diarrhea or constipation; GI bleeding, hepatotoxicity. **Body as a Whole:** Flushing, increased sweating, weight

L

gain or loss, edema, dark sweat or urine. **Urogenital:** Urinary retention or incontinence, increased sexual drive, priapism, postmenopausal bleeding. **Skin:** Skin rashes, loss of hair. **Respiratory:** Rhinorrhea, bizarre breathing patterns.

DIAGNOSTIC TEST INTERFERENCE Altered laboratory values: Elevated ***BUN, AST, ALT, alkaline phosphatase, LDH, bilirubin, protein-bound iodine,*** serum level of ***growth hormone;*** decreased ***glucose tolerance; hypokalemia,*** *decreased* ***WBC, Hgb, Hct.*** **Urine glucose:** False-negative tests may result with use of ***glucose oxidase methods*** (e.g., ***Clinistix, TesTape***) and false-positive results with the ***copper reduction method*** (e.g., ***Clinitest***), especially in patients receiving large doses. It is reported that ***Clinistix*** and ***TesTape*** may be used if reading is taken at margin of wet and dry tape. **Urinary ketones:** There is possibility of false-positive tests by dipsticks, e.g., ***Acetest*** (equivocal), ***Ketostix, Labstix;*** **Serum and urinary uric acid:** False elevations by ***colorimetric methods,*** but not with ***uricase;*** **Urinary protein:** False increases by ***Lowry method;*** **Urinary VMA:** False decreases by ***Pisano method;*** **Urinary catecholamine:** False increases by ***Hingerty method.*** **PKU urine test:** Interference.

INTERACTIONS Drug: MAO INHIBITORS may precipitate hypertensive crisis; TRICYCLIC ANTIDEPRESSANTS augment postural hypotension; PHENOTHIAZINES, **haloperidol** may antagonize the therapeutic effects of levodopa; **pyridoxine** can reverse effects of levodopa; ANTICHOLINERGICS may exacerbate abnormal involuntary movements; **methyldopa** may increase toxic CNS effects; HALOGENATED GENERAL ANESTHETICS increase risk of arrhythmias. **Food:** food decreases the rate and extent of levodopa absorption. **Herbal: Kava-kava** may worsen parkinsonian symptoms.

PHARMACOKINETICS Absorption: Rapidly and well absorbed from GI tract; lower absorption if taken with food. **Peak:** 1–3 h. **Distribution:** Widely distributed in body. **Metabolism:** Most of drug is decarboxylated to dopamine in lumen of GI tract, liver, and serum. **Elimination:** 80%–85% of dose excreted in urine in 24 h. **Half-Life:** 1 h.

NURSING IMPLICATIONS

Assessment & Drug Effects

- Monitor vital signs, particularly during period of dosage adjustment. Report alterations in BP, pulse, and respiratory rate and rhythm.
- Supervise ambulation as indicated. Orthostatic hypotension is usually asymptomatic, but some patients experience dizziness and syncope. Tolerance to this effect usually develops within a few months of therapy.
- Make accurate observations and report adverse reactions and therapeutic effects promptly. Rate of dosage increase is determined primarily by patient's tolerance and response to drug.
- Monitor all patients closely for behavior changes.
- Monitor patients with chronic wide-angle glaucoma for changes in intraocular pressure.
- Monitor diabetics for loss of glycemic control.
- Lab tests: Monitor blood glucose & HbA_{1c}, CBC, Hgb and Hct, serum potassium, and liver & kidney function periodically.

- Report promptly muscle twitching and spasmodic winking (blepharospasm); these are early signs of overdosage. Patients on full therapeutic doses for >1 y may develop such abnormal involuntary movements as well as jerky arm and leg movements. Symptoms tend to increase if dosage is not reduced.
- Report to physician any S&S of the on–off phenomenon sometimes associated with chronic management: Rapid unpredictable swings in intensity of motor symptoms of parkinsonism evidenced by increase in bradykinesia (attacks of "leg freezing" or slow body movement).
- Monitor mental status for S&S of drug-induced neuropsychiatric adverse reactions.

Patient & Family Education

- Do not take with high-protein foods. Also avoid high consumption of food sources of pyridoxine, including wheat germ, green vegetables, banana, whole-grain cereals, muscular and glandular meats (especially liver), legumes. Learn good dietary practices.
- Do not take OTC preparations or fortified cereals unless approved by physician. Multivitamins, antinauseants, and fortified cereals usually contain vitamin B_6.
- Make positional changes slowly, particularly from lying to upright position, and dangle legs a few minutes before standing.
- Resume activities gradually, observing safety precautions to avoid injury. Elevation of mood and sense of well-being may precede objective improvement. Significant improvement usually occurs during second or third week of therapy, but may not occur for 6 mo or more in some patients.
- Follow prescribed drug regimen. Sudden withdrawal of medication can lead to parkinsonism crisis (with return of marked rigidity, akinesia, tremor, hyperpyrexia) or neuroleptic malignant syndrome (NMS).
- A metabolite of levodopa may cause urine to darken and sweat to be dark-colored.
- Do not breast feed while taking this drug without consulting physician.

LEVOFLOXACIN

(lev-o-flox′a-sin)

Levaquin, Iquix, Quixin

Classifications: ANTIINFECTIVE; ANTIBIOTIC; QUINOLONE

Prototype: Ciprofloxacin

Pregnancy Category: C

AVAILABILITY 250 mg, 500 mg tablets; 250 mg, 500 mg injection; 0.5% ophthalmic solution

ACTIONS A broad-spectrum fluoroquinolone antibiotic that inhibits DNA bacterial topoisomerase II, an enzyme required for DNA replication, transcription, repair, and recombination.

THERAPEUTIC EFFECTS Prevents replication of certain bacteria resistant to beta-lactam antibiotics.

USES Treatment of maxillary sinusitis, acute exacerbations of bacterial bronchitis, community-acquired pneumonia, uncomplicated skin/skin structure infections, UTI, acute pyelonephritis caused by susceptible bacteria; chronic bacterial prostatitis; bacterial conjunctivitis.

CONTRAINDICATIONS Hypersensitivity to levofloxacin and quinolone antibiotics; hypokalemia,

L

tendon pain, pregnancy (category C); syphilis; viral infections; phototoxicity; lactation.

CAUTIOUS USE Known or suspected CNS disorders predisposed to seizure activity (e.g., severe cerebral atherosclerosis), risk factors associated with potential seizures (e.g., some drug therapy, renal insufficiency), dehydration, colitis; QT prolongation, cardiac arrhythmias; renal impairment; diabetes; patients receiving theophylline or caffeine; older adults. Safety and efficacy in children <18 y are not established.

ROUTE & DOSAGE

Infections

Adult: **PO** 500 mg q24h × 10 d
IV 500 mg infused over 60 min q24h × 7–14 d

Community-Acquired Pneumonia

Adult: **PO/IV** 750 mg q24h × 5 d

Uncomplicated UTI

Adult: **PO** 250 mg q24h × 14 d

Complicated UTI, Pyelonephritis

Adult: **PO** 250 mg q24h × 10 d
IV 250 mg infused over 60 min q24h × 10 d

Chronic Bacterial Prostatitis

Adult: **PO** 500 mg q24h × 28 d

Renal Impairment

Give an initial dose of 500 mg with adjusted maintenance doses as follows; Cl_{cr} 20–50 mg/min: 250 mg q24h; <20 mL/min: 250 mg q48h

Skin & Skin Structure Infections

Adult: **PO** 750 mg q24h × 14 d

Renal Impairment

Give an initial dose of 250 mg with adjusted maintenance doses as follows; Cl_{cr} <20 mL/min: 250 mg q48h

Bacterial Conjunctivitis

Adult: **Ophthalmic** days 1–2, 1–2 drops in affected eye(s) q2h while awake (max: 8 times/d), days 3–7, 1–2 drops in affected eye(s) q4h while awake (max: 4 times/d)

ADMINISTRATION

Oral

- Do not give oral drug within 2 h of drugs containing aluminum or magnesium (antacids), iron, zinc, or sucralfate.

Intravenous

PREPARE: **Intermittent:** Withdraw the desired dose from 500 mg (25 mg/mL) single-use vial. Add to enough D5W, NS, D5/NS, D5/RL, or other compatible solutions to produce a concentration of 5 mg/mL [e.g., 500 mg (or 20 mL) added to 80 mL]. Discard any unused drug remaining in the vial.

ADMINISTER: **Intermittent:** Give over ≥60 min. Do NOT give a bolus dose or infuse too rapidly.

INCOMPATIBILITIES **Y-site:** Do not add any drugs to levofloxacin solution or infuse simultaneously through the same line (manufacturer recommendation).

- Store tablets in a tightly closed container. IV solution is stable for 72 h at 25° C (77° F).

ADVERSE EFFECTS (≥1%) **CNS:** Headache, insomnia, dizziness. **GI:** Nausea, diarrhea, constipation, vomiting, abdominal pain, dyspepsia. **Skin:** Rash, pruritus. **Special Senses:** Decreased vision, foreign body sensation, transient ocular burning, ocular pain, photophobia. **Urogenital:** Vaginitis. **Body as a Whole:** Injection site pain or inflammation, chest or back pain, fever, pharyngitis.

DIAGNOSTIC TEST INTERFERENCE May cause false positive on ***opiate screening tests.***

INTERACTIONS Drug: Magnesium or **aluminum**-containing antacids, **sucralfate, iron, zinc** may decrease levofloxacin absorption; NSAIDS may increase risk of CNS reactions, including seizures; may cause hyper- or hypoglycemia in patients on ORAL HYPOGLYCEMIC AGENTS.

PHARMACOKINETICS Absorption: Rapidly absorbed from GI tract. **Peak:** PO 1–2 h. **Distribution:** Penetrates lung tissue, 24%–38% protein bound. **Metabolism:** Minimally metabolized in the liver. **Elimination:** Primarily excreted unchanged in urine. **Half-Life:** 6–8 h.

NURSING IMPLICATIONS

Assessment & Drug Effects

- Lab tests: Do C&S test prior to beginning therapy and periodically.
- Withhold therapy and report to physician immediately any of the following: Skin rash or other signs of a hypersensitivity reaction (see Appendix F); CNS symptoms such as seizures, restlessness, confusion, hallucinations, depression; skin eruption following sun exposure; symptoms of colitis such as persistent diarrhea; joint pain, inflammation, or rupture of a tendon; hypoglycemic reaction in diabetic on an oral hypoglycemic agent.

Patient & Family Education

- Learn important indications for discontinuing drug and immediately notifying physician.
- Consume fluids liberally while taking levofloxacin.
- Allow a minimum of 2 h between drug dosage and taking any of the following: Aluminum or magnesium antacids, iron supplements, multivitamins with zinc, or sucralfate.
- Avoid exposure to excess sunlight or artificial UV light.
- Avoid NSAIDS while taking levofloxacin, if possible.
- Do not breast feed while taking this drug.

LEVOMETHADYL ACETATE HYDROCHLORIDE

(lev-o-meth′a-dil)

Orlaam

Classifications: CENTRAL NERVOUS SYSTEM AGENT; NARCOTIC AGONIST ANALGESIC; OPIOID DETOXIFICATION AGENT

Prototype: Morphine

Pregnancy Category: C

AVAILABILITY 10 mg/mL oral solution

ACTIONS Used as a cross-substitute for morphine-like agents, including heroin, because its actions/pharmacologic effects are similar to those opioid analgesics. Tolerance to the analgesic and sedative effects of levomethadyl occurs with prolonged usage.

THERAPEUTIC EFFECTS Provides a long duration of action as a synthetic opioid analgesic (methadone derivative).

USES Management of opiate dependence.

CONTRAINDICATIONS Hypersensitivity to levomethadyl, lactation, pregnancy (category C).

CAUTIOUS USE Concurrent use of other CNS depressants, renal or hepatic insufficiency, older adults, cardiac disease or hypertension, head injury or increased intracranial pressure, respiratory disorders (asthma, cor pulmonale, COPD), hypothyroidism, Addison's disease, pros-

L

tatic hypertrophy, acute abdomen, anesthesia, previous hypersensitivity to methadone or other opioids. Safety and effectiveness in children <18 y are not established.

ROUTE & DOSAGE

Opiate Detoxification

Adult: **PO** 20–40 mg diluted in liquid q48–72h, may be adjusted by 5–10 mg in 1- to 2-wk intervals (doses have ranged from 10 to 140 mg 3 times/wk)

ADMINISTRATION

Oral

- Do not give daily doses; recommended doses are intended for q.o.d./q3d dosing only; daily use will lead to serious and potentially fatal overdose.
- Treatment of overdose: Cautiously give naloxone beginning with small doses of 0.1–0.2 mg; increase if needed at 2- to 3-min intervals (max: of 10 mg). Keep under prolonged observation following initial reversal; levomethadyl has longer duration of action than naloxone.
- See manufacturer's guidelines for reinduction following a lapse of one or more doses.
- Protect from direct light.

ADVERSE EFFECTS (≥1%) **Body as a Whole:** Withdrawal reactions (nasal congestion, abdominal symptoms, diarrhea, muscle aches, anxiety); asthenia, arthralgia, back pain, chills, edema, hot flashes (especially males), flu syndrome, *malaise*, cough, rhinitis, yawning, rash, *sweating*. **CV:** Prolonged QTc interval leading to severe arrhythmias. **CNS:** Abnormal dreams, anxiety, decreased libido, depression, euphoria, headache, *insomnia, nervousness*, somnolence. **GI:** *Abdominal pain, constipation*. diarrhea, dry mouth, nausea, vomiting. **Special Senses:** Blurred vision. **Urogenital:** *Difficult ejaculation, impotence*.

INTERACTIONS Drug: NARCOTIC ANTAGONISTS **(naloxone, naltrexone)** or PARTIAL ANTAGONISTS **(buprenorphine, butorphanol, nalbuphine, pentazocine)** can induce withdrawal symptoms. **Carbamazepine, phenobarbital, phenytoin, rifabutin, rifampin** may increase peak activity or shorten the duration of action of levomethadyl. **Cimetidine, erythromycin, ketoconazole** may slow onset, lower activity, or increase duration of action of levomethadyl.

PHARMACOKINETICS Absorption: Rapidly absorbed from GI tract. **Onset:** 15–30 min. **Peak:** 1.5–2 h. **Duration:** 48–72 h. **Distribution:** Approximately 80% protein bound, crosses placenta. **Metabolism:** Extensive first-pass metabolism to active metabolite, norlaam. **Elimination:** 72% eliminated in urine. **Half-Life:** 2.6 d.

NURSING IMPLICATIONS

Assessment & Drug Effects

- Monitor carefully throughout induction period for overdose and respiratory depression.
- Dosage adjustment is complex due to delayed onset of action; monitor for excessive opioid effect (i.e., sedation, incoordination, orthostatic hypotension).
- Monitor for and report S&S of withdrawal during interdose periods; changes in dosing may be needed.

Patient & Family Education

- Full effect of drug requires 7–10 d. Avoid abuse of psychoactive drugs and alcohol, especially during initial induction period; may potentiate drug effect.

- Learn common adverse effects and possible drug interactions.
- Do not drive or engage in other potentially hazardous activities until response to drug is known.
- Do not breast feed while taking this drug.

LEVONORGESTREL-RELEASING INTRAUTERINE SYSTEM

(lev-o-nor-ges′te-rel)
Mirena
Classifications: HORMONE AND SYNTHETIC SUBSTITUTE; PROGESTIN
Prototype: Progesterone
Pregnancy Category: X

AVAILABILITY 52 mg unit

ACTIONS A progestogen that induces morphological changes in the endometrium including glandular atrophy, a leukocytic infiltration, and decrease in glandular and stromal mitoses. Mechanisms of action not fully understood.
THERAPEUTIC EFFECTS Contraceptive. May act by preventing follicular maturation and ovulation, thickening of the cervical mucus of the uterus, thus preventing passage of sperm into the uterus, or decreasing ability of sperm to survive in an environment of altered endometrium.

USES Hormonal contraception.

CONTRAINDICATIONS Hypersensitivity to any component of the product; previously inserted IUD which has not been removed; pregnancy (category X), suspicion of pregnancy, within 6 weeks of giving birth or prior to complete involution of the uterus; history of ectopic pregnancy or any condition which predisposes to ectopic pregnancy; history of uterine anomalies which distort the uterine cavity; acute PID or history of PID unless there has been a subsequent intrauterine pregnancy; cervicitis or vaginitis or other lower genital tract infection; genital actinomycosis; woman or partner has multiple sex partners; vaginal bleeding of unknown etiology; postpartum endometriosis or septic abortion in past 3 mo; abnormal Pap or suspected/known cervical neoplasm; known or suspected carcinoma of the breast; acute liver disease or liver tumor; immune deficiency states; lactation.
CAUTIOUS USE Women at risk for venereal disease; anemia; diabetes mellitus; history of psychic depression; persons susceptible to acute intermittent porphyria; fluid retention; history of migraines; impaired liver function; presence or history of salpingitis; venereal disease; genital bleeding of unknown etiology; previous pelvic surgery.

ROUTE & DOSAGE

Contraception
Adult: **Intrauterine** Insert device on 7th day of menstrual cycle, may leave in place up to 5 years

ADMINISTRATION

Intrauterine
- Inserted only by physician or other person qualified by special training in the intrauterine system.

ADVERSE EFFECTS (≥1%) **CV:** Hypertension. **GI:** Abdominal pain, nausea. **Endocrine:** Breast tenderness/pain. **Hematologic:** Anemia. **Metabolic:** Weight gain. **CNS:** Depression, emotional lability, headache (including migraine), nervousness. **Skin:** Acne, alopecia, eczema. **Urogenital:** Amenorrhea, dysmenorrhea, leukorrhea, decreased libido, vaginal moniliasis, vulvovaginal disorders, cervicitis, dyspareunia.

INTERACTIONS Drug: No clinically significant interactions established.

PHARMACOKINETICS Peak: Few weeks. **Duration:** 5 years. **Distribution:** 86% protein bound. **Metabolism:** Metabolized in liver. **Elimination:** Excreted in both urine and feces. **Half-Life:** 37 h.

NURSING IMPLICATIONS

Assessment & Drug Effects

- Monitor for decreased pulse, perspiration, or pallor during insertion. Keep patient supine until these signs have disappeared.
- Monitor BP especially with preexisting hypertension.
- Monitor diabetics for loss of glycemic control.

L

Patient & Family Education

- Report S&S of PID immediately: (e.g., prolonged or heavy bleeding, unusual vaginal discharge, abdominal or pelvic pain or tenderness, painful sexual intercourse, chills, fever, and flu-like symptoms).
- Report any of the following to physician immediately: Migraine (if not experienced before) or exceptionally severe headache, or jaundice.
- Note: Diabetics should monitor closely blood glucose for indications of loss of control.
- Do not breast feed while taking this drug.

LEVORPHANOL TARTRATE

(lee-vor′fa-nole)

Levo-Dromoran

Classifications: CENTRAL NERVOUS SYSTEM AGENT; ANALGESIC; NARCOTIC (OPIATE) AGONIST

Prototype: Morphine Sulfate

Pregnancy Category: B

Controlled Substance: Schedule II

AVAILABILITY 2 mg tablets; 2 mg/mL injection

ACTIONS A potent synthetic morphine derivative with agonist activity only. Reported to cause less nausea, vomiting, and constipation than equivalent doses of morphine but may produce more sedation, smooth-muscle stimulation, and respiratory depression.

THERAPEUTIC EFFECTS More potent as an analgesic and has somewhat longer duration of action than morphine.

USES To relieve moderate to severe pain. Also preoperatively to allay apprehension.

CONTRAINDICATIONS Hypersensitivity to levorphanol; labor and delivery, lactation. Safety and effectiveness in children <18 are not established.

CAUTIOUS USE Patients with impaired respiratory reserve, or depressed respirations from another cause (e.g., severe infection, obstructive respiratory conditions, chronic bronchial asthma). Patients with head injury or increased intracranial pressure; acute MI, cardiac dysfunction; liver disease, biliary surgery, alcohol or delirium tremens; liver or kidney dysfunction, hypothyroidism, Addison's Disease, toxic psychosis, prostatic hypertrophy, or urethral stricture. Concurrent use with CNS depressant drugs; pregnancy (category C); older adults, other vulnerable populations.

ROUTE & DOSAGE

Moderate to Severe Pain

Adult: **PO** 2–3 mg q6–8h prn **SC/IM** 1–2 mg q6–8h prn **IV** up to 1 mg q3–6h prn

ADMINISTRATION

Oral/Subcutaneous/ Intramuscular

- Give in the smallest effective dose to minimize the possibility of tolerance and physical dependence.
- Rotate injection sites.
- Store tablets and injection at 15°–30° C (59°–86° F) unless otherwise directed. Store tablets in tightly covered, light-resistant containers.

Intravenous

***PREPARE:* Direct:** Dilute in 3–5 mL sterile water or NS.

***ADMINISTER:* Direct:** Give slowly over 4–5 min.

***INCOMPATIBILITIES* Solution/additive: Aminophylline, ammonium chloride,** BARBITURATES, **chlorothiazide, heparin, methicillin, phenytoin, sodium bicarbonate.**

ADVERSE EFFECTS (≥1%) **CNS:** Euphoria, *sedation, drowsiness,* nervousness, confusion. **CV:** Hypotension, fast, slow, or pounding heartbeat. **GI:** *Nausea,* vomiting, dry mouth, cramps, *constipation.* **Urogenital:** Urinary frequency, urinary retention, sedation. **Special Senses:** Blurred vision. **Respiratory:** Respiratory depression. **Body as a Whole:** Physical dependence.

INTERACTIONS Drug: Alcohol and other CNS DEPRESSANTS compound sedation and CNS depression. **Herbal: St. John's wort** may increase sedation.

PHARMACOKINETICS Peak: 60–90 min. **Duration:** 6–8 h. **Distribution:** Crosses placenta; distributed into breast milk. **Metabolism:** Metabolized in liver. **Elimination:** Excreted in urine. **Half-Life:** 1.2 h.

NURSING IMPLICATIONS

Assessment & Drug Effects

- Assess degree of pain relief. Drug is most effective when peaks and valleys of pain relief are avoided.
- Monitor bowel function.
- Monitor ambulation, especially in older adult patients.

Patient & Family Education

- Do not drive or engage in other potentially hazardous activities.
- Avoid alcohol and other CNS depressants unless approved by physician.
- Note: Ambulation may increase frequency of nausea and vomiting.
- Increase fluid and fiber intake to offset constipating effects of the drug.
- Do not breast feed while taking this drug.

L

LEVOTHYROXINE SODIUM (T_4) Pr

(lee-voe-thye-rox'een)

Eltroxin ♣, Levothroid, Levoxyl, Levo-T, Synthroid

Classifications: HORMONES AND SYNTHETIC SUBSTITUTES; THYROID AGENT

Pregnancy Category: A

AVAILABILITY 25 mcg, 50 mcg, 75 mcg, 88 mcg, 100 mcg, 112 mcg, 125 mcg, 137 mcg, 150 mcg 175 mcg, 200 mcg, 300 mcg tablets; 200 mcg, 500 mcg vials

ACTIONS Synthetically prepared monosodium salt and levo-isomer of thyroxine, with similar actions and uses (thyroxine, principal component of thyroid gland secretions, determines normal thyroid function).

THERAPEUTIC EFFECTS Principal effects includes diuresis, loss of weight and puffiness, increased sense of well-being and activity tolerance, and rise of T_3 and T_4 serum levels toward normal.

USES Specific replacement therapy for diminished or absent thyroid function resulting from primary or secondary atrophy of gland, surgery, excessive radiation or antithyroid drugs, congenital defect. Administered orally for hypothyroid state; administered IV for myxedematous coma or other thyroid dysfunctions demanding rapid replacement, as well as in failure to respond to oral therapy.

CONTRAINDICATIONS Hypersensitivity to levothyroxine; thyrotoxicosis, severe cardiovascular conditions, adrenal insufficiency.

CAUTIOUS USE Angina pectoris, hypertension, impaired kidney function, pregnancy (category A), lactation.

ROUTE & DOSAGE

Thyroid Replacement

Adult: **PO** 25–50 mcg/d, gradually increased by 50–100 mcg q1–4wk to usual dose of 100–400 mcg/d **IV** 1/2 of usual PO dose

Child: **PO** *0–6 mo,* 8–10 mcg/kg/d or 25–50 mcg/d; *6–12 mo,* 6–8 mcg/kg/d or 50–75 mcg/d; *1–5 y,* 5–6 mcg/kg/d or 75–100 mcg/d; *6–12 y,* 4–5 mcg/kd/d or 100–150 mcg/d; *>12 y,* 2–3 mcg/kg/d or >150 mcg/d **IV** 1/2 of usual PO dose

Myxedema Coma

Adult: **IV** 250–500 mcg IV stat, then 100–300 mcg after 24 h if needed, then 50–200 mcg/d until patient is stable and can take drug PO

ADMINISTRATION

Oral

- Give as a single dose, preferably 1 h before or 2 h after breakfast, to prevent insomnia. Give consistently with respect to meals.
- Maintenance dosage for older adults may be 25% lower than for heavier and younger adults.

Intravenous

PREPARE: **Direct:** Reconstitute by adding 5 mL NS for injection immediately before administration. Shake vial until solution is clear. Do NOT mix with IV solutions. Discard unused portion.

ADMINISTER: **Direct:** Give at a rate of 0.1 mg or a fraction thereof over 1 min into a Y-site closest to needle insertion. Give IMMEDIATELY after reconstitution.

- Store in tight, light-resistant container.

ADVERSE EFFECTS (≥1%) **CNS:** Irritability, nervousness, *insomnia,* headache (pseudotumor cerebri in children), tremors, craniosynostosis (excessive doses in children). **CV:** Palpitations, tachycardia, arrhythmias, angina pectoris, hypertension. **GI:** Nausea, diarrhea, change in appetite. **Urogenital:** Menstrual irregularities. **Body as a Whole:** Weight loss, heat intolerance, sweating, fever, leg cramps, temporary hair loss (children).

INTERACTIONS Drug: Cholestyramine, colestipol decrease absorption of levothyroxine; **epinephrine, norepinephrine** increase risk of cardiac insufficiency; ORAL ANTICOAGULANTS may potentiate hypoprothrombinemia.

PHARMACOKINETICS Absorption: Variable and incompletely absorbed from GI tract (50%–80%). **Peak:** 3–4 wk. **Duration:** 1–3 wk. **Distribution:** Gradually released into tissue cells. **Half-Life:** 6–7 d.

NURSING IMPLICATIONS

Assessment & Drug Effects

- Monitor pulse before each dose during dose adjustment. If rate is >100, consult physician.
- Monitor for adverse effects during early adjustment. If metabolism increases too rapidly, especially in older adults and heart disease patients, symptoms of angina or cardiac failure may appear.
- Note: Levothyroxine may aggravate severity of previously obscured symptoms of diabetes mellitus, Addison's disease, or diabetes insipidus. Therapy for these disorders may require adjustment.
- Lab tests: Baseline and periodic tests of thyroid function. Closely monitor PT/INR and assess for evidence of bleeding if patient is receiving concurrent anticoagulant therapy. A decrease in anticoagulant dosage may be needed 1–4 wk after concurrent levothyroxine is started.
- Monitor bone age, growth, and psychomotor function in children.
- Some children have partial hair loss after a few months; it returns even with continued therapy.
- Synthroid 0.1 and 0.3 mg tablets contain tartrazine, which may cause an allergic-type reaction in certain patients; particularly those who are hypersensitive to aspirin.

Patient & Family Education

- Thyroid replacement therapy is usually lifelong.
- Learn how to self-monitor pulse rate. Notify physician if rate begins to increase above 100 or if rhythm changes are noted.
- Notify physician immediately of signs of toxicity (e.g., chest pain, palpitations, nervousness).
- Avoid OTC medications unless approved by physician.
- Do not breast feed while taking this drug without consulting physician.

LIDOCAINE HYDROCHLORIDE (Pr)

(lye'doe-kane)

Anestacon, Dilocaine, L-Caine, Lidoderm, Lida-Mantle, Lido-ject-1, LidoPen Auto Injector, Nervocaine, Octocaine, Xylocaine, Xylocard ♣

Classifications: CARDIOVASCULAR AGENT; ANTIARRHYTHMIC, CLASS IB; CENTRAL NERVOUS SYSTEM AGENT; LOCAL ANESTHETIC (AMIDE TYPE)

Pregnancy Category: B

AVAILABILITY Antidysrhythmic 300 mg/3 mL auto-injector; 0.2%, 0.4%, 0.8%, 1%, 2%, 4%, 10%, 20% injections **Local Anesthetic** 0.5%, 1%, 1.5%, 2%, 4% **Topical** 2%, 2.5%, 4%, 5% solution; 2.5%, 5% ointment; 0.5%, 4% cream; 0.5%, 2.5% gel; 0.5%, 10% spray; 2% jelly; 0.5% patch

ACTIONS Similar to those of procainamide and quinidine, but has little effect on myocardial contractility, AV and intraventricular conduction, cardiac output, and systolic arterial pressure in equivalent doses. Exerts antiarrhythmic action (Class IB) by suppressing automaticity in His-Purkinje system and by elevating electrical stimulation threshold of ventricle during diastole. Action as local anesthetic is more prompt, more intense, and longer lasting than that of procaine.

THERAPEUTIC EFFECTS Suppresses automaticity in His-Purkinje system and elevates electrical stimulation threshold of ventricle during diastole. Prompt, intense, and long-lasting local anesthetic.

USES Rapid control of ventricular arrhythmias occurring during acute MI, cardiac surgery, and cardiac catheterization and those caused by digitalis intoxication. Also as surface and infiltration anesthesia and for nerve block, including caudal and spinal block anesthesia and to relieve local discomfort of skin and mucous membranes. Patch for relief of pain associated with post-herpetic neuralgia.
UNLABELED USES Refractory status epilepticus.

CONTRAINDICATIONS History of hypersensitivity to amide-type local anesthetics; application or injection of lidocaine anesthetic in presence of severe trauma or sepsis, blood dyscrasias, supraventricular arrhythmias, Stokes-Adams syndrome, untreated sinus bradycardia, severe degrees of sinoatrial, atrioventricular, and intraventricular heart block. Safe use during pregnancy (category B), lactation, or in children is not established.
CAUTIOUS USE Liver or kidney disease, CHF, marked hypoxia, respiratory depression, hypovolemia, shock; myasthenia gravis; debilitated patients, older adults; family history of malignant hyperthermia (fulminant hypermetabolism). Topical use in eyes, over large body areas, over prolonged periods, in severe or extensive trauma or skin disorders.

ROUTE & DOSAGE

Ventricular Arrhythmias

Adult: **IV** 50–100 mg bolus at a rate of 20–50 mg/min, may repeat in 5 min, then start infusion of 20–50 mcg/kg/min (1–4 mg/min) immediately after first bolus **IM/SC** 200–300 mg IM, may repeat once after 60–90 min
Child: **IV** 0.5–1 mg/kg bolus dose, then 10–50 mcg/kg/min infusion

Anesthetic Uses

Adult: **Infiltration** 0.5%–1% solution **Nerve Block** 1%–2% solution **Epidural** 1%–2% solution **Caudal** 1%–1.5% solution **Spinal** 5% with glucose **Saddle Block** 1.5% with dextrose **Topical** 2.5%–5% jelly, ointment, cream, or solution

Post-Herpetic Neuralgia

Adult: **Topical** Apply up to 3 patches over intact skin in most painful areas once for up to 12 h per 24 h period

ADMINISTRATION

Intramuscular
- Give in deltoid muscle as preferred site.

Topical
- Do not apply topical lidocaine to large areas of skin or to broken or abraded surfaces. Consult physician about covering area with a dressing.
- Avoid topical preparation contact with eyes.

Intravenous

Note: Do not use lidocaine solutions containing preservatives for spinal or epidural (including caudal) block. Use ONLY lidocaine HCl injection without preservatives or epinephrine that is specifically labeled for IV injection or infusion.

PREPARE: **Direct:** Give undiluted. **IV Infusion:** Use D5W for infusion. For adults, add 1 g to 250 or 500 mL to yield 2 or 4 mg/mL, respectively; for children, add 120 mg to 100 m to yield 1.2 mg/mL.

- Do not use solutions with particulate matter or discoloration.

ADMINISTER: **Direct:** Give at a rate of 50 mg or fraction thereof over 1 min. **IV Infusion:** Use microdrip and infusion pump. Rate of flow is usually ≤4 mg/min.

INCOMPATIBILITIES **Solution/additive: Phenytoin, ampicillin, cefazolin. Y-site: Amphotericin B cholesteryl complex, phenytoin, thiopental.**

- Discard partially used solutions of lidocaine without preservatives.

ADVERSE EFFECTS (≥1%) **CNS:** Drowsiness, dizziness, light-headedness, restlessness, confusion, disorientation, irritability, apprehension, euphoria, wild excitement, numbness of lips or tongue and other paresthesias including sensations of heat and cold, chest heaviness, difficulty in speaking, difficulty in breathing or swallowing, muscular twitching, tremors, psychosis. With high doses: convulsions, respiratory depression and arrest. **CV:** With high doses, hypotension, bradycardia, conduction disorders including heart block, cardiovascular collapse, cardiac arrest. **Special Senses:** Tinnitus, decreased hearing; blurred or double vision, impaired color perception. **Skin:** Site of topical application may develop erythema, edema. **GI:** Anorexia, nausea, vomiting. **Body as a Whole:** Excessive perspiration, soreness at IM site, local thrombophlebitis (with prolonged IV infusion), hypersensitivity reactions (urticaria, rash, edema, anaphylactoid reactions).

DIAGNOSTIC TEST INTERFERENCE Increases in ***creatine phosphokinase (CPK)*** level may occur for 48 h after IM dose and may interfere with test for presence of MI.

INTERACTIONS Drug: Lidocaine patch may increase toxic effects of **tocainide, mexiletine;** BARBITURATES decrease lidocaine activity; **cimetidine,** BETA BLOCKERS, **quinidine** increase pharmacologic effects of lidocaine; **phenytoin** increases cardiac depressant effects; **procainamide** compounds neurologic and cardiac effects.

PHARMACOKINETICS Absorption: Topical application is 3% absorbed through intact skin. **Onset:** 45–90 s IV; 5–15 min IM; 2–5 min topical. **Duration:** 10–20 min IV; 60–90 min IM; 30–60 min topical; >100 min injected for anesthesia. **Distribution:** Crosses blood–brain barrier and placenta; distributed into breast milk. **Metabolism:** Metabolized in liver. **Elimination:** Excreted in urine. **Half-Life:** 1.5–2 h.

L

NURSING IMPLICATIONS

Assessment & Drug Effects

- Stop infusion immediately if ECG indicates excessive cardiac depression (e.g., prolongation of PR interval or QRS complex and the appearance or aggravation of arrhythmias).
- Monitor BP and ECG constantly; assess respiratory and neurologic status frequently to avoid potential overdosage and toxicity.
- Auscultate lungs for basilar rales, especially in patients who tend to metabolize the drug slowly (e.g., CHF, cardiogenic shock, hepatic dysfunction).
- Watch for neurotoxic effects (e.g., drowsiness, dizziness, confusion, paresthesias, visual disturbances, excitement, behavioral changes) in patients receiving IV infusions or with high lidocaine blood levels.
- Note: Lidocaine blood levels of 1.5–6 mcg/mL are reported to provide "usually effective" antiar-

rhythmic activity. Blood levels greater than 7 mcg/mL are potentially toxic.

Patient & Family Education

- Swish and spit out when using lidocaine solution for relief of mouth discomfort; gargle for use in pharynx, may be swallowed (as prescribed).
- Oral topical anesthetics (e.g., Xylocaine Viscous) may interfere with swallowing reflex. Do NOT ingest food within 60 min after drug application; especially pediatric, geriatric, or debilitated patients. Do not chew gum while buccal and throat membranes are anesthetized to prevent biting trauma.
- Do not breast feed while taking this drug without consulting physician.

L

LINCOMYCIN HYDROCHLORIDE

(lin-koe-mye'sin)

Lincocin

Classifications: ANTIINFECTIVE; CLINDAMYCIN ANTIBIOTIC

Prototype: Clindamycin

Pregnancy Category: B

AVAILABILITY 500 mg capsules; 300 mg injection

ACTIONS Derived from *Streptomyces lincolnensis*. Similar to clindamycin in antibacterial activity and demonstrates some cross-resistance with it. Bacteriostatic or bactericidal depending on concentration used and sensitivity of organism.

THERAPEUTIC EFFECTS Effective against most of the common gram-positive pathogens, particularly streptococci, pneumococci, and staphylococci. Also effective against Bacteroides and other anaerobes; however, it has little activity against most gram-negative organisms and ineffective against viruses, yeasts, or fungi. Resistance by *Staphylococcus* is acquired in stepwise manner.

USES Reserved for treatment of serious infections caused by susceptible bacteria in penicillin-allergic patients or patients for whom penicillin is inappropriate.

CONTRAINDICATIONS Previous hypersensitivity to lincomycin and clindamycin; impaired liver function, known monilial infections (unless treated concurrently); use in newborns. Safe use in pregnancy (category B) or lactation is not established.

CAUTIOUS USE Impaired kidney function; history of GI disease, particularly colitis; history of liver, endocrine, or metabolic diseases; history of asthma, hay fever, eczema, drug or other allergies; older adult patients.

ROUTE & DOSAGE

Infections

Adult: **PO** 500 mg q6–8h (max: 8 g/d) **IM** 600 mg q12–24 h **IV** 600 mg–1 g q8–12h
Child: **PO** *>1 mo,* 30–60 mg/kg in 3–4 divided doses **IM** 10 mg/kg q12–24h **IV** 10–20 mg/kg/d in 2–3 divided doses

ADMINISTRATION

Oral/Intramuscular

- Give with a full glass (240 mL [8 oz]) of water at least 1 h before or 2 h after meals; absorption is reduced and delayed by presence of food in stomach.
- Give injection deep into large muscle mass; inject slowly to minimize pain. Rotate injection sites.

Intravenous

PREPARE: **Intermittent:** Dilute 1 g of lincomycin in at least 100 mL of D5W, NS, or other compatible solution.

ADMINISTER: **Intermittent:** Give at a rate ≤1 g/h.

INCOMPATIBILITIES **Solution/additive: Penicillin G, phenytoin, ampicillin, carbenicillin, methicillin.**

- Follow manufacturer's directions for further information on reconstitution, storage time, compatible IV fluids, and IV administration rates.

ADVERSE EFFECTS (≥1%) **Body as a Whole:** Hypersensitivity (pruritus, urticaria, skin rashes, exfoliative and vesiculobullous dermatitis, erythema multiforme [rare], angioedema, photosensitivity, <u>anaphylactoid reaction</u>, serum sickness); superinfections (proctitis, pruritus ani, vaginitis); vertigo, dizziness, headache, generalized myalgia, thrombophlebitis following IV use; pain at IM injection site. **CV:** Hypotension, syncope, <u>cardiopulmonary arrest</u> (particularly after rapid IV). **GI:** Glossitis, stomatitis, *nausea, vomiting,* anorexia, decreased taste acuity, unpleasant or altered taste, abdominal cramps, *diarrhea,* acute enterocolitis, <u>pseudomembranous colitis (potentially fatal)</u>. **Hematologic:** Neutropenia, leukopenia, <u>agranulocytosis</u>, thrombocytopenic purpura, <u>aplastic anemia</u>. **Special Senses:** Tinnitus.

INTERACTIONS Drug: Kaolin and pectin decreases lincomycin absorption; **tubocurarine, pancuronium** may enhance neuromuscular blockade.

PHARMACOKINETICS Absorption: Partially absorbed from GI tract (20%–30%). **Peak:** 2–4 h PO; 30 min IM. **Duration:** 6–8 h PO; 12–14 h IM; 14 h IV. **Distribution:** High concentrations in bone, aqueous humor, bile, and peritoneal, pleural, and synovial fluids; crosses placenta; distributed into breast milk. **Metabolism:** Partially metabolized in liver. **Elimination:** Excreted in urine and feces. **Half-Life:** 5 h.

NURSING IMPLICATIONS

Assessment & Drug Effects

- Lab tests: Perform C&S initially and during therapy to determine continued microbial susceptibility. Periodic liver & kidney function tests and CBC are indicated during prolonged drug therapy.
- Take a careful history of previous sensitivities to drugs or other allergens.
- Monitor BP and pulse. Have patient remain recumbent following drug administration until BP stabilizes.
- Monitor closely and report changes in bowel frequency. Discontinue drug if significant diarrhea occurs.
- Diarrhea, acute colitis, or pseudomembranous colitis (see Appendix F) may occur up to several weeks after cessation of therapy.
- Examine IM/IV injection sites daily for signs of inflammation.
- Monitor serum drug levels closely in patients with severe impairment of kidney function (levels tend to be higher).
- Superinfections by nonsusceptible organisms are most likely to occur when duration of therapy exceeds 10 d (see Appendix F).

Patient & Family Education

- Notify physician immediately of symptoms of hypersensitivity (see Appendix F). Drug should be discontinued.
- Notify physician promptly of the onset of perianal irritation, diarrhea, or blood and mucus in stools.

Do not self-medicate for diarrhea—anti-diarrheal agents may prolong and worsen diarrhea by delaying removal of toxins from colon.
- Take drug as prescribed for full course of therapy.
- Do not breast feed while taking this drug without consulting physician.

LINDANE (Pr)

(lin'dane)

Gamma Benzene, Kwell, Scabene

Classifications: SKIN AND MUCOUS MEMBRANE AGENT; SCABICIDE; PEDICULICIDE

Pregnancy Category: C

AVAILABILITY 1% lotion, shampoo

ACTIONS Related to its direct absorption by parasites and ova (nits). Drug absorption through the exoskeleton stimulates the nervous system of the parasites, resulting in seizures and death.

THERAPEUTIC EFFECTS Has ectoparasitic and ovicidal activity against the two variants of *Pediculus humanus, Pediculus capitis* (head louse) and *Pediculus pubis* (crab louse), and the arthropod *Sarcoptes scabiei* (scabies). Lindane is not prophylactic for pediculosis.

USES To treat head and crab lice and scabies infestations and to eradicate their ova.

CONTRAINDICATIONS Premature neonates, patient with known seizure disorders; application to eyes, face, mucous membranes, urethral meatus, open cuts or raw, weeping surfaces; prolonged or excessive applications or simultaneous application of creams, ointments, oils. Use during pregnancy (category B) or lactation is not recommended by CDC.

CAUTIOUS USE Children <10 y.

ROUTE & DOSAGE

Lice and Scabies Infestation

Adult/Child: **Topical** Apply to all body areas except the face, leave lotion on 8–12 h, then rinse off; leave shampoo on 5 min, then rinse thoroughly; do NOT repeat in <1 wk

ADMINISTRATION

Note: Caregiver needs to wear plastic disposable or rubber gloves when applying lindane, especially if pregnant or applying medication to more than one patient, to avoid prolonged skin contact.

Topical
- Remove all skin lotions, creams, and oil-based hair dressings completely and allow skin to dry and cool before applying lindane; this will reduce percutaneous absorption.
- Shake cream or lotion container well. *Scabies:* Apply thin film from neck down over entire body surface including soles of feet. Avoid face and urethral meatus. Pay particular attention to intertriginous areas (finger webs and other body creases and folds), wrists, elbows, and belt line. Rub drug in; allow skin to dry and cool after application. After 8–12 h, remove medication by bath or shower. *Crab lice:* Apply thin film of drug to hair and skin of pubic area and, if infected, to thighs, trunk, axillary areas. Leave in place 8–12 h and follow with bath or shower. Observation of living lice after 7 d indicates the need for reapplication.
- Shampoo *(head lice):* Apply sufficient quantity to wet hair and skin. Work drug thoroughly onto hair shafts and scalp and allow to remain in place 4 min. Add small

amounts of water sufficient to make a thick lather; then rinse well with water. Pay particular attention to areas above and behind ears and occipital region. Use fine-tooth comb or tweezers to remove remaining nit shells. If necessary, treatment may be repeated after 7 d but not more than twice in 1 wk. *Crab lice:* See above. Repeat treatment after 7 d only if live lice can be demonstrated.
- Store in tight container away from direct light and heat. Protect from freezing.

ADVERSE EFFECTS (≥1%) **CNS:** CNS stimulation (usually after accidental ingestion or misuse of product): restlessness, dizziness, tremors, convulsions. **Body as a Whole:** Inhalation (headache, nausea, vomiting, irritation of ENT). **Skin:** Eczematous eruptions.

INTERACTIONS Drug: No clinically significant interactions established.

PHARMACOKINETICS Absorption: Slowly and incompletely absorbed through intact skin; maximum absorption from face, scalp, axillae. **Distribution:** Stored in body fat. **Metabolism:** Metabolized in liver. **Elimination:** Excreted in urine and feces.

NURSING IMPLICATIONS

Assessment & Drug Effects
- Suspect scabies if a person complains of nocturnal itching (classic symptom). Infestation sources: Sex partner, other family members, people and animals in close contact.
- Identify and treat the sex partner simultaneously because both scabies and *P. pubis* infestation are sexually transmitted diseases.
- Burrows made by scabies mites (may or may not be visible) appear as grayish black straight or S-shaped lines with a papule containing the mite at one end and surrounded by a mild erythematous area.

Patient & Family Education
- Lindane is highly toxic drug if topical applications are excessive or if swallowed or inhaled. Keep out of reach of children.
- Note: Lindane shampoo is an effective disinfectant for personal items such as combs, brushes.
- Skin penetration with scabies mites causes an intolerable itching that may persist 2–3 wk after they have been killed.
- Discontinue medication and notify physician if skin eruptions appear.
- Do not apply medication to face, mouth, open skin lesions, or to eyelashes; avoid contact with eyes. If accidental eye contact occurs, flush with water.
- Recurring limited infestations of scabies may indicate a domestic animal source (e.g., cat, dog, cattle, poultry).
- Do not breast feed while taking this drug.

LINEZOLID Pr

(lin-e-zo'lid)

Zyvox, Zyvoxam ♣

Classifications: ANTIINFECTIVE; ANTIBIOTIC; OXAZOLIDINONE

Pregnancy Category: C

AVAILABILITY 400 mg, 600 mg tablets; 100 mg/5 mL suspension; 200 mg, 400 mg, 600 mg injection

ACTIONS Synthetic antibiotic of a new class, the oxazolidinone group, that is bacteriocidal against gram-positive, gram-negative, and anaerobic bacteria. It binds to a site on the bacterial 23S ribosomal

RNA of the bacteria which prevents the bacterial RNA translation process.

THERAPEUTIC EFFECTS Bacteriostatic against *enterococci* and *staphylococci,* and bacteriocidal against *streptococci*. These include *Enterococcus faecium* [vancomycin-resistant strains (VREF) only, *Staphylococcus aureus* including methicillin-resistant (MRSA)] strains.

USES Treatment of vancomycin-resistant (VREF) *Enterococcus faecium,* nosocomial pneumonia, complicated and uncomplicated skin and skin structure infections, community-acquired pneumonia due to susceptible gram-positive organisms.

CONTRAINDICATIONS Hypersensitivity to linezolid, pregnancy (category C), lactation, neonates. Safety and effectiveness in children <2 y not established.

CAUTIOUS USE Lactation, history of thrombocytopenia, thrombocytopenia; patients on MAOI, or serotonin reuptake inhibitors, or adrenergic agents, active alcoholism, anemia, bleeding, bone marrow suppression, cardiac arrhythmias, cardiac disease, cerebrovascular disease, chemotherapy, coagulopathy, colitis, diarrhea, hypertension, hyperthyroidism, leukopenia, MI, PKU disorder, radiographic contrast administration, spinal anesthesia, surgery, hypertension; phenylketonuria; carcinoid syndrome.

ROUTE & DOSAGE

Vancomycin-Resistant *Enterococcus faecium*

Adult/Adolescent: **PO/IV** *>12 y,* 600 mg q12h × 14–28 d
Child: **PO/IV** *2–11 y, 10* mg/kg q8 h × 14–28 d

Nosocomial or Community-Acquired Pneumonia, Complicated Skin Infections

Adult/Adolescent: **PO/IV** *>12 y,* 600 mg q12h × 10–14 d
Child: **PO/IV** *5–11 y,* 10 mg/kg q8h × 10–14 d

Uncomplicated Skin Infections

Adult/Adolescent: **PO** *>12 y,* 600 mg q12h × 10–14 d
Child: **PO** *< 5 y,* 10 mg/kg q8h × 10–14 d *5–11 y,* 10 mg/kg q12h × 10–14 d

ADMINISTRATION

Note: No dosage adjustment is necessary when switching from IV to oral administration.

Oral

- Reconstitute suspension by adding 123 mL distilled water in two portions; after adding first half, shake to wet all of the powder, then add second half of water and shake vigorously to produce a uniform suspension with a concentration of 100 mg/5 mL.
- Before each use, mix suspension by inverting bottle 3–5 times, but DO NOT SHAKE. Discard unused suspension after 21 d.

Intravenous

PREPARE: **Intermittent:** IV solution is supplied in a single-use, ready-to-use infusion bag. Remove from protective wrap immediately prior to use. Check for minute leaks by firmly squeezing bag. Discard if leaks are detected.

ADMINISTER: **Intermittent:** Do not use infusion bag in a series connection. Give over 30–120 min. If IV line is used to infuse other drugs, flush before and after with D5W, NS, or LR.

INCOMPATIBILITIES **Solution/additive: Ceftriaxone, erythromycin, trimethoprim-sulfamethoxazole. Y-site: Amphotericin B, ceftriaxone, chlorpromazine, diazepam, pentamidine, erythromycin, phenytoin, trimethoprim-sulfamethoxazole.**

- Store at 25° C (77° F) preferred; 15°–30° C (59°–86° F) permitted. Protect from light and keep bottles tightly closed.

ADVERSE EFFECTS (≥1%) **Body as a Whole:** Fever. **GI:** Diarrhea, nausea, vomiting, constipation, taste alteration, abnormal LFTs, tongue discoloration. **Hematologic:** Thrombocytopenia, leukopenia. **CNS:** Headache, insomnia, dizziness. **Skin:** Rash. **Urogenital:** Vaginal moniliasis.

INTERACTIONS Drug: MAO INHIBITORS may cause hypertensive crisis; **pseudoephedrine** may cause elevated BP; may cause **serotonin** syndrome with **citalopram, escitalopram. Food:** TYRAMINE CONTAINING FOOD may cause elevated BP. **Herbal: Ginseng, ephedra, ma huang** may lead to elevated BP, headache, nervousness.

PHARMACOKINETICS Absorption: Rapidly or extensively absorbed, 100% bioavailable. **Peak:** 1–2 h PO. **Distribution:** 31% protein bound. **Metabolism:** Metabolized by oxidation. **Elimination:** Primarily excreted in urine. **Half-Life:** 6–7 h.

NURSING IMPLICATIONS

Assessment & Drug Effects

- Monitor for S&S of: Bleeding; hypertension; or pseudomembranous colitis that begins with diarrhea.
- Lab tests: C&S before initiating therapy and during therapy as indicated; drug may be started pending results. Monitor complete blood count, including platelet count and Hgb & Hct, in those at risk for bleeding or with >2 wk of linezolid therapy.

Patient & Family Education

- Report any of the following to physician promptly: Onset of diarrhea; easy bruising or bleeding of any type; or S&S of superinfection (see Appendix F).
- Avoid foods and beverages high in tyramine (e.g., aged, fermented, pickled, or smoked foods, and beverages). Limit tyramine intake to >100 mg per meal (see *Information for Patients* provided by the manufacturer).
- Do not take OTC cold remedies or decongestants without consulting physician.
- Note for phenylketonurics: Each 5 mL oral suspension contains 20 mg phenylalanine.
- Do not breast feed while taking this drug without consulting physician.

L

LIOTHYRONINE SODIUM (T_3)

(lye-oh-thye'roe-neen)

Cytomel, Triostat

Classifications: HORMONES AND SYNTHETIC SUBSTITUTES; THYROID AGENT

Prototype: Levothyroxine Sodium

Pregnancy Category: A

AVAILABILITY 5 mcg, 25 mcg, 50 mcg tablets; 10 mcg/mL injection

ACTIONS Synthetic form of natural thyroid hormone. Shares actions and uses of thyroid but has more rapid action and more rapid disappearance of effect, permitting quick dosage adjustment if necessary.

THERAPEUTIC EFFECTS Used in T_3 suppression test to differentiate suspected hyperthyroidism from euthyroidism. Principal effect: increase in the metabolic rate of all body tissues.

USES Replacement or supplemental therapy for cretinism, myxedema, goiter, secondary (pituitary) or tertiary (hypothalamic) hypothyroidism, and T_3 suppression test.

CONTRAINDICATIONS Hypersensitivity to liothyronine; thyrotoxicosis, severe cardiovascular conditions, adrenal insufficiency.
CAUTIOUS USE Angina pectoris, hypertension, impaired kidney function; pregnancy (category A), lactation.

ROUTE & DOSAGE

Thyroid Replacement
Adult: **PO** 25–75 mcg/d
Geriatric: **PO** 5 mcg/d, increase by 5 mcg/d every 1–2 wk
Child: **PO** 5 mcg/d gradually increased by 5 mcg/d q3–4d until desired response

Myxedema
Adult: **PO** 5–100 mcg/d **IV** 25–50 mcg, may repeat >4 h and <12 h after previous dose. Target dose >65 mcg/d (max: 100 mcg/d)
Geriatric: **PO** Start at 5 mcg/d

Goiter
Adult: **PO** 5–75 mcg/d
Geriatric: **PO** Start at 5 mcg/d
Child: **PO** 5 mcg/d, increase by 5 mcg q1–2 wk (usual maintenance dose 15–20 mcg/d)

T_3 Suppression Test
Adult: **PO** 75–100 mcg/d times 7 d

ADMINISTRATION

Oral
- Give daily before breakfast.
- Discontinue other thyroid drug when changing to liothyronine; initiate liothyronine at low dosage with gradual increases according to patient's response.

Intravenous

PREPARE: **Direct:** Give undiluted.
ADMINISTER: **Direct:** Give each 10 mcg or fraction thereof over 1 min.

- Store tablets in heat-, light-, and moisture-proof container.

ADVERSE EFFECTS (≥1%) **Endocrine:** Result from overdosage evidenced as S&S of hyperthyroidism (see Appendix F). **Musculoskeletal:** Accelerated rate of bone maturation in children.

INTERACTIONS Drug: Cholestyramine, colestipol decrease absorption; **epinephrine, norepinephrine** increase risk of cardiac insufficiency; ORAL ANTICOAGULANTS may potentiate hypoprothrombinemia.

PHARMACOKINETICS Absorption: Completely absorbed from GI tract. **Peak:** 24–72 h. **Duration:** Up to 72 h. **Distribution:** Gradually released into tissue cells. **Half-Life:** 6–7 d.

NURSING IMPLICATIONS

Assessment & Drug Effects
- Watch for possible additive effects during the early period of liothyronine substitution for another preparation, particularly in older adults, children, and patients with cardiovascular disease. Residual actions of other thyroid preparations may persist for weeks.
- Metabolic effects of liothyronine persist a few days after drug withdrawal.
- Withhold drug for 1–2 d at onset of overdosage symptoms (hyper-

thyroidism, see Appendix F); usually therapy can be resumed with lower dosage.

Patient & Family Education

- Take medication exactly as ordered.
- Learn S&S of hyperthyroidism (see Appendix F); notify physician promptly if they appear.
- Do not breast feed while taking this drug without consulting physician.

LIOTRIX (T_3-T_4)

(lye'oh-trix)

Euthroid, Thyrolar

Classifications: HORMONES & SYNTHETIC SUBSTITUTES; THYROID AGENT

Prototype: Levothyroxine Sodium

Pregnancy Category: A

AVAILABILITY 0.0125 mcg, 3.1 mcg, 6.25 mcg, 12.5 mcg, 25 mcg, 37.5 mcg

ACTIONS Synthetic levothyroxine (T_4) and liothyronine (T_3) combined in a constant 4:1 ratio by weight. Products by different manufacturers differ in total amounts of each drug included in the formulation.

THERAPEUTIC EFFECTS Increases metabolic rate of all body tissues.

USES Replacement or supplemental therapy for cretinism, myxedema, goiter, and secondary (pituitary) or tertiary (hypothalamic) hypothyroidism. Also with antithyroid agents in thyrotoxicosis and to prevent goitrogenesis and hypothyroidism.

CONTRAINDICATIONS Untreated thyrotoxicosis, acute MI, morphologic hypogonadism, nephrosis, adrenal deficiency due to hypopituitarism; tartrazine dye hypersensitivity, obesity treatment.

CAUTIOUS USE Concomitant anticoagulant therapy; myxedema; hypertension, angina, cardiac arrhythmias, cardiac disease, coronary artery disease; older adults; hypertension; neonates, infants, children; arteriosclerosis; kidney dysfunction, pregnancy (category A), lactation.

ROUTE & DOSAGE

Thyroid Replacement

Adult/Child: **PO** 12.5–30 mcg/d, gradually increase to desired response

ADMINISTRATION

Oral

- Give as a single daily dose, preferably before breakfast.
- Make dose increases at 1- to 2-wk intervals.
- Store in heat-, light-, and moisture-proof container. Shelf-life: 2 y.

ADVERSE EFFECTS (≥1%) **CNS:** Nervousness, headache, tremors, insomnia. **CV:** Palpitation, tachycardia, angina pectoris, cardiac arrhythmias, hypertension, CHF. **GI:** Nausea, abdominal cramps, diarrhea. **Body as a Whole:** Weight loss, heat intolerance, fever, sweating, menstrual irregularities. **Musculoskeletal:** Accelerated rate of bone maturation in infants and children.

INTERACTIONS Drug: Cholestyramine, colestipol decrease absorption; **epinephrine, norepinephrine** increase risk of cardiac insufficiency; ORAL ANTICOAGULANTS may potentiate hypoprothrombinemia.

PHARMACOKINETICS Not studied

NURSING IMPLICATIONS

Assessment & Drug Effects

- Watch for possible additive effects during the early period of liothyronine substitution for an-

L

other preparation, particularly in older adults, children, and patients with cardiovascular disease. Residual actions of other thyroid preparations may persist for weeks.

- Note: Metabolic effects of liotrix persist a few days after drug withdrawal.
- Withhold drug for 1–2 d at onset of overdosage symptoms (hyperthyroidism, see Appendix F); usually therapy can be resumed with lower dosage.
- Monitor diabetics for glycemic control; an increase in insulin or oral hypoglycemic may be required.

Patient & Family Education

- Follow directions for taking this drug (see ADMINISTRATION).
- Notify physician of headache (euthyroid patients); may indicate need for dosage adjustment or change to another thyroid preparation.
- Take medication exactly as ordered.
- Learn S&S of hyperthyroidism (see Appendix F); notify physician if they appear.
- Do not breast feed while taking this drug without consulting physician.

L

LISINOPRIL

(ly-sin′o-pril)

Prinivil, Zestril

Classifications: CARDIOVASCULAR AGENT; ANGIOTENSIN-CONVERTING ENZYME (ACE) INHIBITOR; ANTIHYPERTENSIVE AGENT

Prototype: Captopril

Pregnancy Category: D

AVAILABILITY 2.5 mg, 5 mg, 10 mg, 20 mg, 40 mg tablets

ACTIONS Lowers BP by specific inhibition of the angiotensin-converting enzyme (ACE). This interrupts conversion sequences initiated by renin that form angiotensin II, a potent vasoconstrictor. ACE inhibition alters hemodynamics without compensatory reflex tachycardia or changes in cardiac output (except in patients with CHF).

THERAPEUTIC EFFECTS Improved cardiac output and exercise tolerance due to inhibition of ACE also decreases circulating aldosterone, which is normally released in response to angiotensin II stimulation. Reduced aldosterone is associated with a potassium-sparing effect. Also decreases peripheral resistance (afterload) and pulmonary vascular resistance.

USES Hypertension, alone or concomitantly with other classes of antihypertensive agents; CHF; to improve MI survival.

CONTRAINDICATIONS Patients with a history of angioedema related to treatment with an ACE inhibitor, ACE inhibitor hypersensitivity; pregnancy (category D), children <6 y; lactation.

CAUTIOUS USE Impaired kidney function, hyperkalemia, patients on diuretic therapy; aortic stenosis, cardiomyopathy; cerebrovascular disease; collagen vascular disease; coronary artery disease, dialysis; older adults; heart failure, hyperkalemia, hypotension, hypovolemia; African Americans; renal artery stenosis, renal disease, renal failure, renal impairment; autoimmune diseases, especially systemic lupus erythematosus (SLE).

ROUTE & DOSAGE

Hypertension
Adult: **PO** 10 mg once/d, may increase up to 20–40 mg 1–2 times/d (max: 80 mg/d)
Child: **PO** *6–16 y,* Start at 0.07 mg/kg (max 5 mg) once/d (max: 40 mg/d)
Geriatric: **PO** Initial 2.5–5 mg/d, may increase by 2.5–5 mg/d every 1–2 wk (max: 40 mg/d).

ADMINISTRATION

Oral

- Give an initial dose of 5 mg for diuretic-treated patients. Monitor drug effect for 2 h or until the BP is stabilized for at least 1 additional hour. Concurrent administration with a diuretic may compound hypotensive effect.
- Give before dialysis; lisinopril is removed from blood by hemodialysis.
- Store away from both moisture and heat.

ADVERSE EFFECTS (≥1%) **CNS:** Headache, dizziness, fatigue. **CV:** Hypotension, chest pain. **GI:** Nausea, vomiting, diarrhea, anorexia, constipation, intestinal angioedema. **Hematologic:** Neutropenia. **Respiratory:** Dyspnea, cough. **Skin:** Rash. **Metabolic:** Azotemia, hyperkalemia, increased BUN, and creatinine levels.

INTERACTIONS Drug: Indomethacin and other NSAIDS may decrease antihypertensive activity; POTASSIUM SUPPLEMENTS, POTASSIUM-SPARING DIURETICS may cause hyperkalemia; may increase **lithium** levels and toxicity.

PHARMACOKINETICS Absorption: 25% absorbed from GI tract. **Onset:** 1 h. **Peak:** 6–8 h. **Duration:** 24 h. **Distribution:** Limited amount crosses blood–brain barrier; crosses placenta; small amount distributed in breast milk. **Metabolism:** Is not metabolized. **Elimination:** Excreted primarily in urine. **Half-Life:** 12 h.

NURSING IMPLICATIONS

Assessment & Drug Effects

- Place patient in supine position and notify physician if sudden and severe hypotension occurs within the first 1–5 h after initial drug dose; possible particularly in patients who are sodium- or volume-depleted because of diuretic therapy.
- Measure BP just prior to dosing to determine whether satisfactory control is being maintained for 24 h. If the antihypertensive effect is diminished in less than 24 h, an increase in dosage may be necessary.
- Monitor closely for angioedema of extremities, face, lips, tongue, glottis, and larynx. Discontinue drug promptly and notify physician if such symptoms appear; carefully monitor for airway obstruction until swelling is relieved.
- Monitor serum sodium and serum potassium levels for hyponatremia and hyperkalemia.
- Lab tests: Determine WBC count prior to initiation of treatment, every month for the first 3–6 mo of therapy, and at periodic intervals for 1 y. Withhold therapy and notify physician if neutropenia (neutrophil count <1000/mm^3) develops; kidney function tests at periodic intervals, especially in patients with severe volume or sodium replacement or those with severe CHF.

Patient & Family Education

- Discontinue drug and contact physician immediately for severe hypersensitivity reaction (e.g., hoarseness, swelling of the face, mouth, hands, or feet, or sudden trouble breathing).

- Be aware of importance of proper diet, including sodium and potassium restrictions. Do NOT use salt substitute containing potassium.
- Continued compliance with high BP medication is very important. If a dose is missed, take it as soon as possible but not too close to next dose.
- Do not drive or engage in other potentially hazardous activities until response to the drug is known.
- With concomitant therapy, lisinopril increases the risk of lithium toxicity.
- Notify physician promptly of any indication of infection (e.g., sore throat, fever).
- Do not store drug in a moist area. Heat and moisture may cause the medicine to break down.
- Do not breast feed while taking this drug.

LITHIUM CARBONATE (Pr)

(li'thee-um)

Eskalith, Eskalith CR, Lithane, Lithobid, Lithonate, Lithotabs

LITHIUM CITRATE

Cibalith-S

Classifications: CENTRAL NERVOUS SYSTEM (CNS) AGENT; PSYCHOTHERAPEUTIC AGENT; MOOD STABILIZER

Pregnancy Category: D

AVAILABILITY **Lithium Carbonate** 150 mg, 300 mg, 600 mg capsules; 300 mg tablets; 300 mg, 450 mg sustained release tablets **Lithium Citrate** 300 mg/5 mL syrup

ACTIONS The lithium ion behaves in the body much like the sodium ion; but its exact mechanism of action is unclear. Competes with various physiologically important cations: Na^+, K^+, Ca^{++}, Mg^{++}; therefore, it affects cell membranes, body water, and neurotransmitters. At the synapse, it accelerates catecholamine destruction, inhibits the release of neurotransmitters and decreases sensitivity of postsynaptic receptors.

THERAPEUTIC EFFECTS Inhibits neurotransmitters; decreases overactivity of receptors involved in stimulating manic states. Response evidenced by changed facial affect, improved posture, assumption of self-care, improved ability to concentrate, improved sleep pattern.

USES Control and prophylaxis of acute mania and the acute manic phase of mixed bipolar disorder.

UNLABELED USES Acute and recurrent depression (unipolar affective disorder), schizophrenic disorders, disorders of impulse control, alcohol dependence, antineoplastic drug-induced neutropenia, aplastic anemia, SIADH, cyclic neutropenia.

CONTRAINDICATIONS Significant cardiovascular or kidney disease, brain damage, severe debilitation, dehydration or sodium depletion; patients on low-salt diet or receiving diuretics; pregnancy, especially first trimester (category D), lactation, children <12 y.

CAUTIOUS USE Older adults; thyroid disease; epilepsy; concomitant use with haloperidol and other antipsychotics; cardiac disease, cardiac arrhythmias, dehydration, diarrhea; older adults; fever, hyponatremia, hypothyroidism, concurrent infection; leukemia; mental status changes, organic brain syndrome, parkinsonism; psoriasis; renal disease, renal impairment; seizure disorder, sick sinus syndrome, sodium restriction, suicidal ideation, thyroid disease, urinary retention; diabetes mellitus; severe infections; urinary retention.

ROUTE & DOSAGE

Mania

Adult: **PO Loading Dose** 600 mg t.i.d. or 900 mg sustained-release b.i.d. or 30 mL (48 mEq) of solution t.i.d. **PO Maintenance Dose** 300 mg t.i.d. or q.i.d. or 15–20 mL (24–32 mEq) solution in 2–4 divided doses (max: 2.4 g/d)
Child: **PO** 15–60 mg/kg/d in divided doses

ADMINISTRATION

Oral

- Give with meals.
- Ensure that sustained release tablets are not chewed or crushed; must be swallowed whole.
- Protect from light and moisture.

ADVERSE EFFECTS (≥1%) **CNS:** Dizziness, *headache, lethargy,* drowsiness, *fatigue,* slurred speech, psychomotor retardation, giddiness, incontinence, restlessness, seizures, confusion, blackout spells, disorientation, *recent memory loss,* stupor, coma, EEG changes. **CV:** Arrhythmias, hypotension, vasculitis, <u>peripheral circulatory collapse</u>, ECG changes. **Special Senses:** Impaired vision, transient scotomas, tinnitus. **Endocrine:** Diffuse thyroid enlargement, hypothyroidism, *nephrogenic diabetes insipidus,* transient hyperglycemia, glycosuria, hyponatremia. **GI:** *Nausea, vomiting, anorexia, abdominal pain, diarrhea, dry mouth,* metallic taste. **Musculoskeletal:** *Fine hand tremors,* coarse tremors, choreoathetotic movements; fasciculations, clonic movements, incoordination including ataxia, *muscle weakness,* hyperreflexia, encephalopathic syndrome (weakness, lethargy, fever, tremors, confusion, extrapyramidal symptoms). **Skin:** Thought to be toxicity rather than allergy: Pruritus, maculopapular rash, hyperkeratosis, chronic folliculitis, transient acneiform papules (face, neck, intertriginous areas), anesthesia of skin, cutaneous ulcers, drying and thinning of hair, allergic vasculitis. **Hematologic:** *Reversible leukocytosis* (14,000 to 18,000/mm^3). **Urogenital:** Albuminuria, oliguria, urinary incontinence, polyuria, polydipsia, increased uric acid excretion. **Body as a Whole:** Edema, weight gain (common) or loss, exacerbation of psoriasis; flu-like symptoms.

INTERACTIONS Drug: Carbamazepine, haloperidol, PHENOTHIAZINES increase risk of neurotoxicity, extrapyramidal effects, and tardive dyskinesias; DIURETICS, NSAIDS, **methyldopa, probenecid,** TETRACYCLINES decrease renal clearance of lithium, increasing pharmacologic and toxic effects; THEOPHYLLINES, **urea, sodium bicarbonate, sodium or potassium citrate** increase renal clearance of lithium, decreasing its pharmacologic effects.

PHARMACOKINETICS Absorption: Readily absorbed from GI tract. **Peak:** 0.5–3 h carbonate; 15–60 min citrate. **Distribution:** Crosses blood–brain barrier and placenta; distributed into breast milk. **Metabolism:** Not metabolized. **Elimination:** 95% excreted in urine, 1% in feces, 4%–5% in sweat. **Half-Life:** 20–27 h.

NURSING IMPLICATIONS

Assessment & Drug Effects

- Monitor response to drug. Usual lag of 1–2 wk precedes response to lithium therapy. Keep physician informed of progress.
- Monitor lithium level: Generally dosage regimen is designed to maintain serum lithium levels of 1.0–1.5 mEq/L in acute mania and 0.6–1.6 mEq/L during maintenance treatment; blood sample

L

to determine serum lithium level is drawn prior to next dose (8–12 h after last dose) when lithium level is fairly stable.

- Monitor for S&S of lithium toxicity, often when lithium levels are 1.5–2.0 mEq/L (e.g., vomiting, diarrhea, lack of coordination, drowsiness, muscular weakness, slurred speech). Withhold one dose and call physician. Drug should not be stopped abruptly.
- When lithium levels are above 2.0 mEq/L, symptoms may include ataxia, blurred vision, giddiness, tinnitus, muscle twitching or coarse tremors, and a large output of dilute urine.
- Weigh patient daily; check ankles, tibiae, and wrists for edema. Report changes in I&O ratio, sudden weight gain, or edema.
- Polydipsia and polyuria, apparently not dose-related, are common early adverse effects, particularly in older adults. Symptoms may lessen but reappear after several months or even years of maintenance.
- Report early signs of extrapyramidal reactions promptly to physician. The encephalopathic syndrome may be induced when lithium is given concomitantly with haloperidol or with other antipsychotic medication, particularly in older adults.
- Keep physician informed of all presenting S&S. The fine tremor of hand or jaw, polyuria, mild thirst, transient mild nausea, and general discomfort that may occur in early treatment of mania sometimes persist throughout therapy. Usually, however, symptoms subside with temporary reduction of dose. If symptoms persist, drug is withdrawn.
- Monitor thyroid function periodically. Be alert to and report symptoms of hypothyroidism (see Appendix F).
- Neonates born of mothers who took lithium during pregnancy may have high serum lithium level manifested by flaccidity, poor reflexes, cardiac dysrhythmia, and chronic twitching.
- Lithane contains tartrazine, which may cause an allergic-type reaction in susceptible patients.
- Monitor older adults carefully to prevent toxicity, which may occur at serum levels ordinarily tolerated by other patients.

Patient & Family Education

- Be alert to increased output of dilute urine and persistent thirst. Dose reduction may be indicated.
- Contact physician if diarrhea or fever develops. Avoid practices that may encourage dehydration: hot environment, excessive caffeine beverages (diuresis).
- Drink plenty of liquids (2–3 L/d) during stabilization period and at least 1–1/2 L/d during ongoing of therapy.
- Avoid self-prescribed low-salt regimen, self-dosing with Rolaids, Soda-mints, or other sodium antacids, high-sodium foods (e.g., prepared meats and diet soda). Avoid also crash diets or diet pills that reduce appetite and food, salt, and fluid intake.
- Reduced intake of fluid and sodium can accelerate lithium retention with subsequent toxicity. Conversely, marked increase in sodium intake can increase lithium excretion and reduce drug effect.
- Do not drive or engage in other potentially hazardous activities until response to drug is known. Lithium may impair both physical and mental ability.
- Use effective contraceptive measures during lithium therapy. If therapy is continued during preg-

nancy, serum lithium levels must be closely monitored to prevent toxicity. Kidney clearance of lithium increases during pregnancy but reverts to lower rate immediately after delivery; dosage is reduced to prevent toxicity.
- Follow a regular clinical evaluation schedule on serum lithium levels to ensure safe and effective treatment. It is important to you and your family to keep all clinic appointments.
- Do not breast feed while taking this drug.

LODOXAMIDE
(lo-dox'a-mide)
Alomide
Classifications: MAST CELL STABILIZER; ANTIALLERGIC AGENT
Prototype: Cromolyn Sodium
Pregnancy Category: B

AVAILABILITY 0.1% solution
See Appendix A-1.

LOMEFLOXACIN
(lo-me-flox'a-cin)
Maxaquin
Classifications: ANTIINFECTIVE; QUINOLONE ANTIBIOTIC
Prototype: Ciprofloxacin
Pregnancy Category: C

AVAILABILITY 400 mg tablets

ACTIONS An oral fluoroquinolone broad spectrum bactericidal agent that inhibits DNA gyrase, an enzyme necessary for bacterial DNA replication and some aspects of its transcription, repair, recombination, and transposition.
THERAPEUTIC EFFECTS Inhibits replication of susceptible gram-negative and gram-positive bacteria. Antibiotic spectrum of activity is similar to that of other fluoroquinolones.

USES Urinary tract infections, transurethral surgery prophylaxis.
UNLABELED USES Lower respiratory tract infections.

CONTRAINDICATIONS Known hypersensitivity to lomefloxacin or any other quinolone, lactation.
CAUTIOUS USE Kidney disease; patients with a history of epilepsy, psychosis, or increased intracranial pressure; pregnancy (category C); children and adolescents.

ROUTE & DOSAGE

Urinary Tract & Lower Respiratory Tract Infections
Adult: **PO** 400 mg q.d. times 10 d
Transurethral Surgery Prophylaxis
Adult: **PO** 400 mg 2–6 h before surgery

ADMINISTRATION

Oral
- Avoid giving mineral supplements or vitamins with iron or zinc within 2 h of lomefloxacin.
- Do not give antacids with magnesium, aluminum, or sucralfate within 4 h before or 2 h after drug.
- Give hemodialysis patients an initial 400 mg loading dose followed by a 200 mg/d maintenance dose.

ADVERSE EFFECTS (≥1%) **CNS:** *Headache*. **GI:** Nausea, abdominal discomfort. **Skin:** Photosensitivity.

DIAGNOSTIC TEST INTERFERENCE May cause false positive on ***opiate screening tests.***

INTERACTIONS Drug: ALUMINUM and MAGNESIUM-CONTAINING ANTACIDS decrease systemic bioavailability of lomefloxacin.

L

PHARMACOKINETICS Absorption: Readily absorbed from GI tract. **Peak:** 1–2 h. **Distribution:** Crosses placenta; distributed into breast milk. **Elimination:** 76% excreted in urine within 48 h. **Half-Life:** 6.35–7.77 h.

NURSING IMPLICATIONS

Assessment & Drug Effects

- Lab tests: Draw C&S prior to first dose; drug may be started pending results of C&S.
- Take thorough history of hypersensitivity reactions to quinolones or other drugs prior to therapy.
- Discontinue lomefloxacin and notify physician at the first sign of a skin rash or other allergic reaction.
- Monitor for seizures, especially in patients with known or suspected CNS disorders. Discontinue lomefloxacin and notify physician immediately if a seizure occurs.
- Assess for S&S of superinfection (see Appendix F).

Patient & Family Education

- Notify physician of loose stools or diarrhea promptly.
- Drink fluids liberally, if not contraindicated.
- Take appropriate cautions, dizziness or light-headedness may occur.
- Be aware of the possibility of phototoxicity; avoid excessive sunlight or artificial ultraviolet light.
- Do not breast feed while taking this drug.

LOMUSTINE

(loe-mus'teen)

CeeNU, CCNU

Classifications: ANTINEOPLASTIC; ALKYLATING AGENT

Prototype: Cyclophosphamide

Pregnancy Category: D

AVAILABILITY 10 mg, 40 mg, 100 mg capsules

ACTIONS Lipid-soluble alkylating nitrosourea with actions like those of carmustine (e.g., cell-cycle-nonspecific activity against rapidly proliferating cell populations).

THERAPEUTIC EFFECTS Inhibits synthesis of both DNA and RNA; has antineoplastic and myelosuppressive effect.

USES Palliative therapy in addition to other modalities or with other chemotherapeutic agents in primary and metastatic brain tumors and as secondary therapy in Hodgkin's disease.

UNLABELED USES GI, lung, and renal carcinomas, non-Hodgkin's lymphomas, malignant melanoma, and multiple myelomas.

CONTRAINDICATIONS Immunization with live virus vaccines, viral infections. Safe use during pregnancy (category D) or lactation is not established. Reported to be carcinogenic in laboratory animals.

CAUTIOUS USE Patients with decreased circulating platelets, leukocytes, or erythrocytes; kidney or liver function impairment; infection; previous cytotoxic or radiation therapy.

ROUTE & DOSAGE

Palliative Therapy

Adult: **PO** 130 mg/m^2 as single dose, repeated in 6 wk; subsequent doses based on hematologic response (WBC >4000/mm^3, platelets >100,000/mm^3)
Child: **PO** 75–150 mg/m^2 q6wk

ADMINISTRATION

Oral

- Give on an empty stomach to reduce possibility of nausea, may

also give an antiemetic before drug to prevent nausea.
- Store capsules away from excessive heat (over 40° C).

ADVERSE EFFECTS (≥1%) **CNS:** Lethargy, ataxia, disorientation. **GI:** Anorexia, *nausea, vomiting,* stomatitis, transient elevations of LFTs. **Hematologic:** Delayed (cumulative) myelosuppression: (thrombocytopenia, leukopenia); anemia. **Skin:** Alopecia, skin rash, itching. **Urogenital:** Nephrotoxicity. **Respiratory:** Pulmonary toxicity (rare).

INTERACTIONS Drug: Cimetidine can increase bone marrow toxicity; ANTICOAGULANTS, NSAIDS, SALICYLATES increase risk of bleeding.

PHARMACOKINETICS Absorption: Readily absorbed from GI tract. **Peak:** 1–6 h. **Distribution:** Readily crosses blood–brain barrier; crosses placenta; distributed into breast milk. **Metabolism:** Metabolized in liver to several active metabolites. **Elimination:** Excreted in urine. **Half-Life:** 16–48 h.

NURSING IMPLICATIONS

Assessment & Drug Effects

- Lab tests: Monitor blood counts weekly for at least 6 wk after last dose. Liver and kidney function tests should be performed periodically.
- A repeat course is not given until platelets have returned to above 100,000/mm^3 and leukocytes to above 4000/mm^3.
- Avoid invasive procedures during nadir of platelets.
- Thrombocytopenia occurs about 4 wk and leukopenia about 6 wk after a dose, persisting 1–2 wk.
- Inspect oral cavity daily for S&S of superinfections (see Appendix F) and stomatitis or xerostomia.

Patient & Family Education

- Nausea and vomiting may occur 3–5 h after drug administration, usually lasting less than 24 h.
- Anorexia may persist for 2 or 3 d after a dose.
- Notify physician of signs of sore throat, cough, fever. Also report unexplained bleeding or easy bruising.
- Use reliable contraceptive measures during therapy.
- Be aware of the possibility of hair loss while taking this drug.
- A given dose may include capsules of different colors; the pharmacist prepares prescribed dose by combining various capsule strengths.
- Do not breast feed while taking this drug without consulting physician.

L

LOPERAMIDE

(loe-per′a-mide)

Imodium, Imodium AD, Kaopectate III, Maalox Anti-diarrheal, Pepto Diarrhea Control

Classifications: GASTROINTESTINAL AGENT; ANTIDIARRHEAL

Prototype: Diphenoxylate HCl with atropine sulfate

Pregnancy Category: B

AVAILABILITY 2 mg tablets, capsules; 1 mg/mL, 1 mg/5 mL liquid

ACTIONS Effective antidiarrheal; synthetic piperidine derivative chemically related to diphenoxylate and to meperidine. Reportedly has longer duration of action.

THERAPEUTIC EFFECTS Inhibits GI peristaltic activity by direct action on circular and longitudinal intestinal muscles. Prolongs transit time of intestinal contents, increases consistency of stools, and reduces fluid and electrolyte loss.

USES Acute nonspecific diarrhea, chronic diarrhea associated with inflammatory bowel disease, and to reduce fecal volume from ileostomies.

CONTRAINDICATIONS Conditions in which constipation should be avoided, severe colitis, acute diarrhea caused by broad-spectrum antibiotics (pseudomembranous colitis) or associated with microorganisms that penetrate intestinal mucosa (e.g., toxigenic *Escherichia coli, Salmonella,* or *Shigella*). Safe use during pregnancy (category B), lactation, or in children <2 y is not established.

CAUTIOUS USE Dehydration; diarrhea caused by invasive bacteria; impaired liver function; prostatic hypertrophy; history of narcotic dependence.

L

ROUTE & DOSAGE

Acute Diarrhea

Adult: **PO** 4 mg followed by 2 mg after each unformed stool (max: 16 mg/d)
Child: **PO** *2–6 y,* 1 mg t.i.d.; *6–8 y,* 2 mg b.i.d.; *8–12 y,* 2 mg t.i.d.

Chronic Diarrhea

Adult: **PO** 4 mg followed by 2 mg after each unformed stool until diarrhea is controlled (max: 16 mg/d)
Child: **PO** 0.1 mg/kg after each unformed stool (usually 1 mg)

ADMINISTRATION

Oral

- Do not give prn doses to a child with acute diarrhea.

ADVERSE EFFECTS (≥1%) **Body as a Whole:** Hypersensitivity (skin rash); fever. **CNS:** Drowsiness, fatigue, dizziness, CNS depression (overdosage). **GI:** Abdominal discomfort or pain, abdominal distention, bloating, constipation, nausea, vomiting, anorexia, dry mouth; <u>toxic megacolon</u> (patients with ulcerative colitis).

INTERACTIONS Drug: No clinically significant interactions established.

PHARMACOKINETICS Absorption: Poorly absorbed from GI tract. **Onset:** 30–60 min. **Peak:** 2.5 h solution; 4–5 h capsules. **Duration:** 4–5 h. **Metabolism:** Metabolized in liver. **Elimination:** Primarily excreted in feces, <2% excreted in urine. **Half-Life:** 11 h.

NURSING IMPLICATIONS

Assessment & Drug Effects

- Monitor therapeutic effectiveness. Chronic diarrhea usually responds within 10 d. If improvement does not occur within this time, it is unlikely that symptoms will be controlled by further administration.
- Discontinue if there is no improvement after 48 h of therapy for acute diarrhea.
- Monitor fluid and electrolyte balance.
- Notify physician promptly if the patient with ulcerative colitis develops abdominal distention or other GI symptoms (possible signs of potentially fatal toxic megacolon).

Patient & Family Education

- Notify physician if diarrhea does not stop in a few days or if abdominal pain, distension, or fever develops.
- Record number and consistency of stools.
- Do not drive or engage in other potentially hazardous activities until response to drug is known.
- Do not take alcohol and other CNS depressants concomitantly unless otherwise advised by physician; may enhance drowsiness.

- Learn measures to relieve dry mouth; rinse mouth frequently with water, suck hard candy.
- Do not breast feed while taking this drug without consulting physician.

LOPINAVIR/RITONAVIR

(lop-i-na′ver/rit-o-na′ver)
Kaletra
Classifications: ANTIINFECTIVE; ANTIRETROVIRAL AGENT; PROTEASE INHIBITOR
Prototype: Saquinavir Mesylate
Pregnancy Category: C

AVAILABILITY 133.3 mg lopinavir/ 33.3 mg ritonavir capsules; 400 mg lopinavir/100 mg ritonavir/5 mL suspension

ACTIONS Lopinavir, an HIV protease inhibitor that inhibits the activity of HIV protease and prevents the cleavage of viral polyproteins essential for the maturation of HIV. Ritonavir in the formulation inhibits the CYP3A metabolism of lopinavir, thereby, increasing the blood level of lopinavir.
THERAPEUTIC EFFECTS Decreases plasma HIV RNA level; elevates CD_4 cell counts as a result of the combined therapy of the two drugs in HIV infected patients.

USES Treatment of HIV infection in combination with other antiretroviral agents.

CONTRAINDICATIONS Hypersensitivity to lopinavir or ritonavir; concurrent administration with drugs that utilize CYP3A or CYP2D6 for metabolism (e.g., ergotamine, pimozide); lactation.
CAUTIOUS USE Hepatic impairment, patients with hepatitis B or C, older adults; pregnancy (category C). Safety and efficacy in children <6 mo are not established.

ROUTE & DOSAGE

HIV Infection

Adult: **PO** 400/100 mg (3 capsules or 5 mL suspension) b.i.d., increase dose to 533/133 mg (4 capsules or 6.5 mL) b.i.d., with concurrent efavirenz or nevirapine
Child: **PO** *6 mo–12 y,* 7–15 kg, 12/3 mg/kg; 15–40 kg, 10/2.5 mg/kg; >40 kg, 400/100 mg b.i.d., increase dose 7–15 kg, 13/3.25 mg/kg; 15–40 kg, 11/2.75 mg/kg; >40 kg, 533/ 133 mg b.i.d., with concurrent efavirenz or nevirapine

ADMINISTRATION

Note: Take with food.

Oral
- Give with a meal or light snack.
- Note: If didanosine is concurrently ordered, give didanosine 1 h before or 2 h after lopinavir/ritonavir.
- Store refrigerated at 2°–8° C (36°–46° F). If stored at room temperature ≤25° C (77° F), discard after 2 mo.

ADVERSE EFFECTS (≥1%) **Body as a Whole:** Asthenia, pain. **GI:** Abdominal pain, abnormal stools, *diarrhea, nausea,* vomiting. **CNS:** Headache, insomnia. **Skin:** Rash.

INTERACTIONS Drug: flecainide, propafenone, pimozide may lead to life-threatening arrhythmias; **rifampin** may decrease antiretroviral response; **dihydroergotamine, ergonovine, ergotamine, methylergonovine** may lead to acute ergot toxicity; HMG-COA REDUCTASE INHIBITORS may increase risk of myopathy and rhabdomyolysis; BENZODIAZEPINES may have prolonged sedation or respiratory depression; **efavirenz, nevirapine,** ANTICONVULSANTS, STER-

OIDS may decrease lopinavir levels; **delavirdine, ritonavir** may increase lopinavir levels; may increase levels of **amprenavir, indinavir, saquinavir, ketoconazole, itraconazole, midazolam, triazolam, rifabutin, sildenafil, atorvastatin, cerivastatin,** IMMUNOSUPPRESSANTS; may decrease levels of **atovaquone, methadone, ethinyl estradiol.** Also see Interactions in **ritonavir** monograph. **Herbal: St. John's wort** may decrease antiretroviral activity.

PHARMACOKINETICS Absorption: Increased absorption when taken with food. **Peak:** 4 h. **Distribution:** 98%–99% protein bound. **Metabolism:** Extensively metabolized by CYP3A. **Elimination:** Excreted primarily in feces. **Half-Life:** 5–6 h lopinavir.

L

NURSING IMPLICATIONS

Assessment & Drug Effects

- Monitor for S&S of: Pancreatitis, especially with marked triglyceride elevations; new onset diabetes or loss of glycemic control; hypothyroidism or Cushing's syndrome.
- Lab test: Periodically monitor fasting blood glucose, AST & ALT, total cholesterol & triglycerides, serum amylase, inorganic phosphorus, CBC with differential, and thyroid functions.

Patient & Family

- Report all prescription and nonprescription drugs being taken. Do not use herbal products, especially St. John's wort, without first consulting the physician.
- Become familiar with the potential adverse effects of this drug; report those that are bothersome to physician.
- Concurrent use of sildenafil (Viagra) increases risk for adverse effects such as hypotension, changes in vision, and sustained erection; promptly report any of these to the physician.
- Use additional or alternative contraceptive measures if estrogen-based hormonal contraceptives are being used.
- Do not breast feed while taking this drug.

LORACARBEF

(lor-a-car'bef)

Lorabid

Classifications: ANTIINFECTIVE; ANTIBIOTIC; BETA-LACTAM

Prototype: Imipenem

Pregnancy Category: B

AVAILABILITY 200 mg, 400 mg capsules; 100 mg/5 mL, 200 mg/5 mL suspension

ACTIONS Second-generation cephalosporin antibiotic with drug structure characterized by a beta-lactam ring (like the penicillin structure). Generally resistant to hydrolysis by beta-lactamases.

THERAPEUTIC EFFECTS Effective against gram-positive and gram-negative bacteria including *staphylococci, beta-hemolytic streptococci, Streptococcus pneumoniae, Haemophilus influenzae, Moraxella catarrhalis.*

USES Upper and lower respiratory tract infections, skin and skin structure infections, urinary tract infections.

CONTRAINDICATIONS Hypersensitivity to cephalosporins and related antibiotics.

CAUTIOUS USE Renal impairment, seizures, pregnancy (category B), lactation.

ROUTE & DOSAGE

Upper & Lower Respiratory Tract Infections

Adult: **PO** 200–400 mg q12h taken 1 h a.c. or 2 h p.c.
Child: **PO** 15–30 mg/kg/d divided q12h taken 1 h a.c. or 2 h p.c.

Skin & Skin Structure Infections

Adult: **PO** 200 mg q12h taken 1 h a.c. or 2 h p.c.
Child: **PO** 15 mg/kg/d divided q12h taken 1 h a.c. or 2 h p.c.

Urinary Tract Infections

Adult: **PO** 200 mg q24h or 400 mg q12h taken 1 h a.c. or 2 h p.c.

Otitis Media

Child: **PO** 30 mg/kg/d divided q12h taken 1 h a.c. or 2 h p.c.

Renal Impairment

Cl_{cr} 10–49 mL/min: reduce recommended dose by 50% or give standard dose q24h; <10 mL/min: extend dosing interval to every 3–5 d

ADMINISTRATION

Oral

- Reconstitute suspension by adding 30 or 60 mL of water to the 50- or 100-mL bottles, respectively, of dry mixture. Add the water in 2 portions and shake bottle after each portion.
- Give at least 1 h before or 2 h after meals.
- Give half of the normal dose if Cl_{cr} lies between 10 and 49 mL/min.
- Store suspension in a tightly closed container. Discard after 14 d.

ADVERSE EFFECTS (≥1%) **CNS:** Headache. **GI:** Nausea, vomiting, diarrhea, diaper rash, abdominal pain. **Other:** Rash, candidiasis.

INTERACTIONS Drug: May have prolonged bleeding time with **warfarin.**

PHARMACOKINETICS Absorption: Readily absorbed from GI tract. **Peak:** 45–60 min. **Distribution:** Distributes into middle ear fluid. **Elimination:** Excreted in urine. **Half-Life:** 0.78–0.85 h.

NURSING IMPLICATIONS

Assessment & Drug Effects

- Take a careful history to determine previous hypersensitivity reaction to beta-lactam antibiotics (penicillins and cephalosporins) or to other allergens.
- Discontinue drug and notify the physician immediately if allergic reaction occurs (e.g., hives, wheezing, rash, pruritus).
- Inspect patient's mouth on a regular basis to detect superinfection (see Appendix F).
- Rule out pseudomembranous enterocolitis (see Appendix F) if severe diarrhea accompanied by abdominal pain and fever occurs. Notify physician immediately.
- Monitor kidney function throughout therapy with concurrent diuretic use.

Patient & Family Education

- Notify physician immediately of rash or any other allergic reaction.
- Report loose stools or diarrhea promptly.
- Do not breast feed while taking this drug without consulting physician.

LORATADINE (Pr)

(lor'a-ta-deen)

Alavert, Claritin, Claritin Reditabs

Classifications: ANTIHISTAMINE; H_1-RECEPTOR ANTAGONIST; NONSEDATING

Pregnancy Category: B

AVAILABILITY 10 mg tablets; 1 mg/mL syrup

ACTIONS Long-acting antihistamine with selective peripheral H_1-receptor sites, thus blocking histamine release.

THERAPEUTIC EFFECTS Long-acting H_1-receptor antagonist of histamine that disrupts capillary permeability and edema formation and constriction of respiratory, GI, and vascular smooth muscle.

USES Relief of symptoms of seasonal allergic rhinitis; idiopathic chronic urticaria.

CONTRAINDICATIONS Hypersensitivity to loratadine.

CAUTIOUS USE Hepatic and renal impairment, pregnancy (category B), lactation. Safety and effectiveness in children <2 y are not established.

L

ROUTE & DOSAGE

Allergic Rhinitis

Adult: **PO** 10 mg once/d on an empty stomach; Start patients with liver disease with 10 mg every other day

Child: **PO** *<30 kg,* 5 mg q.d.; *>30 kg,* 10 mg q.d.

ADMINISTRATION

Oral

- Give on an empty stomach, 1 h before or 2 h after a meal.
- Store in a tightly closed container.

ADVERSE EFFECTS (≥1%) **CNS:** Dizziness, dry mouth, fatigue, headache, somnolence, altered salivation and lacrimation, thirst, flushing, anxiety, depression, impaired concentration. **CV:** Hypotension, hypertension, palpitations, syncope, tachycardia. **GI:** Nausea, vomiting, flatulence, abdominal distress, constipation, diarrhea, weight gain, dyspepsia. **Body as a Whole:** Arthralgia, myalgia. **Special Senses:** Blurred vision, earache, eye pain, tinnitus. **Skin:** Rash, pruritus, photosensitivity.

INTERACTIONS Drug: No clinically significant interactions established.

PHARMACOKINETICS Absorption: Readily absorbed from GI tract. **Onset:** 1–3 h. **Peak:** 8–12 h; reaches steady state levels in 3–5 d. **Duration:** 24 h. **Distribution:** Distributed into breast milk. **Metabolism:** Metabolized to active metabolite, descarboethoxyloratidine, in the liver. **Elimination:** Excreted in urine and feces. **Half-Life:** 12–15 h.

NURSING IMPLICATIONS

Assessment & Drug Effects

- Assess carefully for and report distressing or dangerous S&S that occur after initiation of the drug. A variety of adverse effects, although not common, are possible. Some are an indication to discontinue the drug.
- Monitor cardiovascular status and report significant changes in BP and palpitations or tachycardia.

Patient & Family Education

- Drug may cause significant drowsiness in older adult patients and those with liver or kidney impairment.
- Note: Concurrent use of alcohol and other CNS depressants may have an additive effect.
- Do not breast feed while taking this drug without consulting physician.

LORAZEPAM

(lor-a'ze-pam)
Ativan
Classifications: CENTRAL NERVOUS SYSTEM AGENT; ANXIOLYTIC; SEDATIVE-HYPNOTIC; BENZODIAZEPINE
Pregnancy Category: D
Controlled Substance: Schedule IV

AVAILABILITY 0.5 mg, 1 mg, 2 mg tablets; 2 mg/mL oral solution; 2 mg/mL, 4 mg/mL injection

ACTIONS Most potent of the available benzodiazepines. Effects (anxiolytic, sedative, hypnotic, and skeletal muscle relaxant) are mediated by the inhibitory neurotransmitter GABA. Action sites: thalamic, hypothalamic, and limbic levels of CNS.
THERAPEUTIC EFFECTS Antianxiety agent that also causes mild suppression of REM sleep, while increasing total sleep time.

USES Management of anxiety disorders and for short-term relief of symptoms of anxiety. Also used for preanesthetic medication to produce sedation and to reduce anxiety and recall of events related to day of surgery; for management of status epilepticus.
UNLABELED USES Chemotherapy-induced nausea and vomiting.

CONTRAINDICATIONS Known sensitivity to benzodiazepines; acute narrow-angle glaucoma; primary depressive disorders or psychosis; children <12 y (PO preparation); coma, shock, acute alcohol intoxication; pregnancy (category D), and lactation.
CAUTIOUS USE Renal or hepatic impairment; organic brain syndrome; myasthenia gravis; narrow-angle glaucoma; suicidal tendency; GI disorders; older adult and debilitated patients; limited pulmonary reserve.

ROUTE & DOSAGE

Antianxiety
Adult: **PO** 2–6 mg/d in divided doses (max: 10 mg/d)
Geriatric: **PO** 0.5–1 mg/d (max: 2 mg/d)
Child: **PO/IV** 0.05 mg/kg q4–8h (max: 2 mg/dose)

Insomnia
Adult: **PO** 2–4 mg at bedtime
Geriatric: **PO** 0.5–1 mg h.s.

Premedication
Adult: **IM** 2–4 mg (0.05 mg/kg) at least 2 h before surgery **IV** 0.044 mg/kg up to 2 mg 15–20 min before surgery
Child: **PO/IV/IM** 0.05 mg/kg (range: 0.02–0.09 mg/kg)

Status Epilepticus
Adult: **IV** 4 mg injected slowly at 2 mg/min, may repeat dose once if inadequate response after 10 min
Child: **IV** 0.1 mg/kg slow IV over 2–5 min (max: 4 mg/dose), may repeat with 0.05 mg in 10–15 min if needed
Neonate: **IV** 0.05 mg/kg over 2–5 min, may repeat in 10–15 min

ADMINISTRATION

Oral
- Increase the evening dose when higher oral dosage is required, before increasing daytime doses.

Intramuscular
- Injected undiluted, deep into a large muscle mass.

Intravenous
- IV administration to neonates, infants, children: Verify cor-

L

rect IV concentration and rate of infusion with physician.
- Patients >50 y may have more profound and prolonged sedation with IV lorazepam (usual max: initial dose of 2 mg).

PREPARE: **Direct:** Prepare lorazepam immediately before use. Dilute with an equal volume of sterile water, D5W, or NS.

ADMINISTER: **Direct:** Inject directly into vein or into IV infusion tubing at rate not to exceed 2 mg/min and with repeated aspiration to confirm IV entry. Take extreme precautions to PREVENT intraarterial injection and perivascular extravasation.

INCOMPATIBILITIES **Y-site: Idarubicin, omeprazole, ondansetron, sargramostim, sufentanil, TPN with albumin.**

L

- Keep parenteral preparation in refrigerator; do not freeze. ▪ Do not use a discolored solution or one with a precipitate.

ADVERSE EFFECTS (≥1%) **Body as a Whole:** Usually disappear with continued medication or with reduced dosage. **CNS:** Anterograde amnesia, *drowsiness, sedation,* dizziness, weakness, unsteadiness, disorientation, depression, sleep disturbance, restlessness, confusion, hallucinations. **CV:** Hypertension or hypotension. **Special Senses:** Blurred vision, diplopia; depressed hearing. **GI:** Nausea, vomiting, abdominal discomfort, anorexia.

INTERACTIONS Drug: Alcohol, CNS DEPRESSANTS, ANTICONVULSANTS potentiate CNS depression; **cimetidine** increases lorazepam plasma levels, increases toxicity; lorazepam may decrease antiparkinsonism effects of **levodopa;** may increase **phenytoin** levels; smoking decreases sedative and antianxiety effects. **Herbal: Kava-kava, valerian** may potentiate sedation.

PHARMACOKINETICS Absorption: Readily absorbed from GI tract. **Onset:** 1–5 min IV; 15–30 min IM. **Peak:** 60–90 min IM; 2 h PO. **Duration:** 12–24 h. **Distribution:** Crosses placenta; distributed into breast milk. **Metabolism:** Not metabolized in liver. **Elimination:** Excreted in urine. **Half-Life:** 10–20 h.

NURSING IMPLICATIONS

Assessment & Drug Effects

- Have equipment for maintaining patent airway immediately available before starting IV administration.
- IM or IV lorazepam injection of 2–4 mg is usually followed by a depth of drowsiness or sleepiness that permits patient to respond to simple instructions whether patient appears to be asleep or awake.
- Supervise ambulation of older adult patients for at least 8 h after lorazepam injection to prevent falling and injury.
- Lab tests: Assess CBC and liver function tests periodically for patients on long-term therapy.
- Supervise patient who exhibits depression with anxiety closely; the possibility of suicide exists, particularly when there is apparent improvement in mood.

Patient & Family Education

- Do not drive or engage in other hazardous activities for a least 24–48 h after receiving IM injection of lorazepam.
- Do not drink large volumes of coffee. Anxiolytic effects of lorazepam can significantly be altered by caffeine.
- Do not consume alcoholic beverages for at least 24–48 h after an

injection and avoid when taking an oral regimen.
- Notify physician if daytime psychomotor function is impaired; a change in regimen or drug may be needed.
- Terminate regimen gradually over a period of several days. Do not stop long-term therapy abruptly; withdrawal may be induced with feelings of panic, tonic–clonic seizures, tremors, abdominal and muscle cramps, sweating, vomiting.
- Do not self-medicate with OTC drugs; seek physician guidance.
- Discuss discontinuation of drug with physician if you wish to become pregnant.
- Do not breast feed while taking this drug.

LOSARTAN POTASSIUM Pr

(lo-sar'tan)

Cozaar

Classifications: CARDIOVASCULAR AGENT; ANGIOTENSIN II RECEPTOR ANTAGONIST; ANTIHYPERTENSIVE

Pregnancy Category: C (first trimester); D (second and third trimesters)

AVAILABILITY 25 mg, 50 mg tablet

ACTIONS Angiotensin II receptor (type AT_1) antagonist acts as a potent vasoconstrictor and primary vasoactive hormone of the renin–angiotensin–aldosterone system.

THERAPEUTIC EFFECTS Selectively blocks the binding of angiotensin II to the AT_1 receptors found in many tissues (e.g., vascular smooth muscle, adrenal glands). Antihypertensive effect results from blocking the vasoconstricting and aldosterone-secreting effects of angiotensin II.

USES Hypertension.

CONTRAINDICATIONS Hypersensitivity to losartan, pregnancy [category C (first trimester), category D (second and third trimesters)], lactation.

CAUTIOUS USE Patients on diuretics, renal or hepatic impairment.

ROUTE & DOSAGE

Hypertension

Adult: **PO** 25–50 mg in 1–2 divided doses (max: 100 mg/d); start with 25 mg/d if volume depleted (i.e., on diuretics)

ADMINISTRATION

Oral
- Note: Starting dose is reduced 50% in patients with possible volume depletion or a history of liver disease.

ADVERSE EFFECTS (≥1%) **CNS:** Dizziness, insomnia, headache. **GI:** Diarrhea, dyspepsia. **Musculoskeletal:** Muscle cramps, myalgia, back or leg pain. **Respiratory:** Nasal congestion, cough, upper respiratory infection, sinusitis.

INTERACTIONS Drug: Phenobarbital decreases serum levels of losartan and its metabolite.

PHARMACOKINETICS Absorption: Rapidly absorbed from GI tract; approximately 25%–33% reaches systemic circulation. **Peak:** 6 h. **Duration:** 24 h. **Distribution:** Highly bound to plasma proteins; does not appear to cross blood–brain barrier. **Metabolism:** Extensively metabolized in liver by cytochrome P450 enzymes to an active metabolite. **Elimination:** 35% excreted in urine, 60% in feces. **Half-Life:** Losartan 1.5–2 h; metabolite 6–9 h.

NURSING IMPLICATIONS

Assessment & Drug Effects

- Monitor BP at drug trough (prior to a scheduled dose).
- Monitor drug effectiveness, especially in African-Americans when losartan is used as monotherapy.
- Inadequate response may be improved by splitting the daily dose into twice-daily dose.
- Lab tests: Monitor CBC, electrolytes, liver & kidney function with long-term therapy.

Patient & Family Education

- Notify physician of symptoms of hypotension (e.g., dizziness, fainting).
- Notify physician immediately of pregnancy.
- Do not breast feed while taking this drug.

L

LOTEPREDNOL ETABONATE

(lo-te'pred-nol e-ta-bo'nate)

Alrex, Lotemax

Classifications: EYE PREPARATION; HORMONE AND SYNTHETIC SUBSTITUTE; ANTIINFLAMMATORY; ADRENAL CORTICOSTEROID

Prototype: Hydrocortisone

Pregnancy Category: C

AVAILABILITY 0.2%, 0.5% suspension

See Appendix A-1.

LOVASTATIN (Pr)

(loe-vah-stat'in)

Altoprev, Mevacor, Mevinolin

Classifications: CARDIOVASCULAR AGENT; ANTILIPEMIC; LIPID-LOWERING AGENT; HMG-CoA REDUCTASE INHIBITOR (STATIN)

Pregnancy Category: X

AVAILABILITY 10 mg, 20 mg, 40 mg tablets; 10 mg, 20 mg, 40 mg, 60 mg extended-release tablets

ACTIONS Reduces plasma cholesterol levels by interfering with body's ability to produce its own cholesterol. This cholesterol-lowering effect triggers induction of LDL receptors, which promote removal of LDL and VLDL remnants (precursors of LDL) from plasma. Also results in an increase in plasma HDL concentrations (HDL collects excess cholesterol from body cells and transports it to liver for excretion).

THERAPEUTIC EFFECTS Reduces plasma cholesterol levels by interfering with body's ability to produce its own cholesterol, and it also lowers LDL and VLDL cholesterol.

USES Adjunct to diet for treatment of primary moderate hypercholesterolemia (types IIa and IIb) when diet and other nonpharmacologic measures have failed to reduce elevated total LDL cholesterol levels. Lovastatin is less effective in treatment of homozygous familial hypercholesterolemia than primary hypercholesterolemia, possibly because in these persons LDL receptors are not functional.

CONTRAINDICATIONS Active liver disease, unexplained elevations of serum transaminases; cholestasis, hepatic encephalopathy, hepatic disease, hepatitis, jaundice; rhabdomyolysis; surgery, trauma; hypotension, renal failure; pregnancy (category X), lactation, children <10 y.

CAUTIOUS USE Patient who consumes substantial quantities of alcohol; history of liver disease; electrolyte imbalance, endocrine disease, females of childbearing age, infection, myopathy, renal disease, renal impairment, seizure disorder. Patient with risk factor predisposing to development of kidney failure secondary to rhabdomyolysis.

ROUTE & DOSAGE

Hypercholesterolemia
Adult: **PO** 20–40 mg 1–2 times/d

ADMINISTRATION

Oral

- Give with the evening meal if q.d. Give the first of 2 daily doses with breakfast.
- Store tablets at 5°–30° C (41°–86° F) in light-resistant, tightly closed container.
- Ensure that extended-release tablets are not crushed or chewed. They must be swallowed whole.

ADVERSE EFFECTS (≥1%) **Body as a Whole:** Generally well tolerated. **CNS:** Dizziness, mild transient headache, insomnia, fatigue. **Special Senses:** Blurred vision. **GI:** Dyspepsia, dysgeusia, heartburn, nausea, constipation, diarrhea, flatus, abdominal pain, and cramps. **Metabolic:** Increases in serum transaminases, elevated creatine phosphokinase (CPK). **Skin:** Rash, pruritus.

INTERACTIONS Drug: Clarithromycin, clofibrate, cyclosporine, danazol, erythromycin, fenofibrate, fluconazole, gemfibrozil, itraconazole, ketoconazole, miconazole, niacin, and PROTEASE INHIBITORS increase risk of myopathy and rhabdomyolysis; potentiate hypoprothrombinemia with **warfarin. Food: Grapefruit juice** (>1 qt/d) may increase risk of myopathy and rhabdomyolysis.

PHARMACOKINETICS Absorption: Approximately 30% absorbed from GI tract; extensive first-pass metabolism. **Onset:** 2 wk. **Peak:** 4–6 wk. **Distribution:** Crosses blood–brain barrier and placenta; distributed into breast milk. **Metabolism:** Metabolized in liver to active metabolites. **Elimination:** 83% excreted in feces; 10% excreted in urine. **Half-Life:** 1.1–1.7 h.

NURSING IMPLICATIONS

Assessment & Drug Effects

- Lab tests: Perform liver function tests q4–6wk during first 15 mo of therapy. Monitor blood cholesterol levels and lipid profile periodically.
- Drug-induced increases in serum transaminases, usually not associated with jaundice or other clinical S&S, return to normal when drug is discontinued. If these values rise and remain at 3 times upper level of normal, drug will be discontinued and liver biopsy considered.

Patient & Family Education

- Do not interrupt, increase, decrease, or omit dosage without advice of physician.
- Notify physician promptly of muscle tenderness or pain, especially if accompanied by fever or malaise. If CPK is elevated or if myositis is diagnosed, drug will be discontinued.
- Avoid or at least reduce alcohol consumption.
- Understand that lovastatin is not a substitute for, but an addition to, diet therapy.
- Do not breast feed while taking this drug without consulting physician.

LOXAPINE HYDROCHLORIDE

(lox'a-peen)
Loxitane C, Loxitane IM

LOXAPINE SUCCINATE

Loxitane, Loxapac ♣
Classifications: CENTRAL NERVOUS SYSTEM AGENT; PSYCHOTHERAPEUTIC; ANTIPSYCHOTIC
Prototype: Chlorpromazine
Pregnancy Category: C

AVAILABILITY 5 mg, 10 mg, 25 mg, 50 mg capsules; 25 mg/mL oral solution; 50 mg/mL injection

ACTIONS This dibenzoxazepine antipsychotic is chemically distinct from other antipsychotics. Its exact mode of action is not established. Sedative action is less than that produced by chlorpromazine, but anticholinergic effects are comparable and extrapyramidal effects may be more intense. Also has antiemetic activity; lowers seizure threshold in patients with history of convulsive disorders.

THERAPEUTIC EFFECTS Stabilizes emotional component of schizophrenia by acting on subcortical level of CNS.

L

USES Manifestations of psychotic disorders.

UNLABELED USES Anxiety associated with mental depression.

CONTRAINDICATIONS Severe drug-induced CNS depression; comatose states, children <16 y. Safe use during pregnancy (category C) or lactation is not established.

CAUTIOUS USE Glaucoma, prostatic hypertrophy, urinary retention, history of convulsive disorders, cardiovascular disease.

ROUTE & DOSAGE

Psychosis

Adult: **PO** Start with 10 mg b.i.d. and rapidly increase to maintenance levels of 60–100 mg/d in 2–4 divided doses (max: 250 mg/d) **IM** 12.5–50 mg q4–6h

Dementia Behavior

Geriatric: **PO** 5–10 mg 1–2 times/d, may increase q4–7d (max: 125 mg/d)

ADMINISTRATION

Oral

- Give with food, milk, or water to reduce possibility of stomach irritation.
- Dilute oral concentrate in about 2–3 oz (60–90 mL) water or orange or grapefruit juice shortly before administration. Measure concentrate with calibrated dropper dispensed with drug. Do not store diluted solution.

Intramuscular

- Use only with acute psychosis or when oral route not feasible.
- Reduce dosage gradually over period of several days when therapy is to be terminated.
- Protect from light and freezing. Intensification of straw color to light amber is acceptable. Discard if solution is noticeably discolored.

ADVERSE EFFECTS (≥1%) **CNS:** *Drowsiness,* sedation, dizziness, syncope, EEG changes, paresthesias, staggering gait, muscle weakness, *extrapyramidal effects,* akathisia, tardive dyskinesia, neuroleptic malignant syndrome. **CV:** *Orthostatic hypotension,* hypertension, tachycardia. **Special Senses:** Nasal congestion, tinnitus; blurred vision, ptosis. **GI:** Constipation, dry mouth. **Skin:** Dermatitis, facial edema, pruritus, photosensitivity. **Urogenital:** Urinary retention, menstrual irregularities. **Body as a Whole:** Polydipsia, weight gain or loss, hyperpyrexia, transient leukopenia.

INTERACTIONS Drug: Alcohol and other CNS DEPRESSANTS potentiate CNS depression; will inhibit vasopressor effects of **epinephrine.**

PHARMACOKINETICS Absorption: Readily absorbed from GI tract. **Onset:** 20–30 min. **Peak:** 1.5–3 h. **Duration:** 12 h. **Distribution:** Widely distributed; crosses placenta; distributed into breast milk. **Metabolism:** Metabolized in liver. **Elimination:** 50% excreted in urine, 50% excreted in feces. **Half-Life:** 19 h.

NURSING IMPLICATIONS

Assessment & Drug Effects

- Monitor baseline BP pattern prior and during therapy; both hypotension and hypertension have been reported as adverse reactions.
- Observe carefully for extrapyramidal effects such as acute dystonia (see Appendix F) during early therapy. Most symptoms disappear with dose adjustment or with antiparkinsonism drug therapy.
- Discontinue therapy and report promptly to physician the first signs of impending tardive dyskinesia (fine vermicular movements of the tongue) when patient is on long-term treatment.
- Monitor I&O and bowel elimination patterns and check for bladder distention. Depressed patients often fails to report urinary retention or constipation.
- Risk of seizures is increased in those with history of convulsive disorders.

Patient & Family Education

- Do NOT change dosage regimen in any way without physician approval.
- Avoid self-dosing with OTC drugs unless approved by the physician.
- Drowsiness usually decreases with continued therapy. If it persists and interferes with daily activities, consult physician. A change in time of administration or dose may help.
- Avoid potentially hazardous activity until response to drug is known.
- Learn measures to relieve dry mouth; rinse mouth frequently with water, suck hard candy. Avoid commercial products that may contain alcohol and enhances drying and irritation.
- Notify physician of blurred or colored vision.
- Do not take drug dose and notify physician of following: Light-colored stools, bruising, unexplained bleeding, prolonged constipation, tremor, restlessness and excitement, sore throat and fever, rash.
- Stay out of bright sun; cover exposed skin with sunscreen.
- Do not breast feed while taking this drug without consulting physician.

LYMPHOCYTE IMMUNE GLOBULIN

(lymph'o-site)

Antithymocyte Globulin, ATG, Atgam

Classifications: BIOLOGIC RESPONSE MODIFIER; IMMUNOGLOBULIN

Prototype: Immune globulin

Pregnancy Category: C

L

AVAILABILITY 50 mg/mL injection

ACTIONS An immunoglobulin (IgG) and lymphocyte-selective immunosuppressant derived from serum of healthy horses that have been immunized with human thymus lymphocytes. Action mechanism is not clear. Produces little effect on B-lymphocyte cells and is not associated with severe lymphopenia. Increases susceptibility of patient to viral infections; it may reactivate or support infection with cytomegalovirus, herpes simplex virus (especially labial infections), or with Epstein-Barr virus (EBV). As with other immunosuppressant agents, carcinogenicity of this drug may be expressed.

THERAPEUTIC EFFECTS Alters the formation of T lymphocytes (killer cells) and reduces their number.

USES Primarily to prevent or delay onset or to reverse acute renal allograft rejection.

UNLABELED USES Moderate and severe aplastic anemia in patients unsuitable for bone marrow transplantation, T-cell malignancy, acute and chronic graft-vs-host disease, and to prevent rejection of skin allografts.

CONTRAINDICATIONS Hypersensitivity to thimerosal (preservative) or to other equine gamma globulin preparations; history of previous systemic reaction to ATG, hemorrhagic diatheses; leporine protein hypersensitivity; use in kidney transplant patient not receiving a concomitant immunosuppressant; fungal or viral infections; pregnancy (category C), lactation.

L

CAUTIOUS USE Children (experience limited); hypotension, infection, leukopenia, lymphoma, neoplastic disease, thrombocytopenia, vaccination, varicella.

ROUTE & DOSAGE

Renal Allotransplantation

Adult: **IV** 10–30 mg/kg/d by slow **IV** infusion
Child: **IV** 5–25 mg/kg/d by slow **IV** infusion

Prevention of Allograft Rejection

Adult: **IV** 15 mg/kg/d for 14 d followed by 15 mg/kg q.o.d. for 14 d

Treatment of Allograft Rejection

Adult: **IV** 10–15 mg/kg/d for 14 d followed by 15 mg/kg q.o.d. for 14 d if needed

Aplastic Anemia

Adult: **IV** 15 mg/kg/d for 14 d followed by 15 mg/kg q.o.d. for 14 d or 15 mg/kg/d for 10 d
Child: **IV** 10–20 mg/kg/d for 8–14 d, then 10–30 mg/kg q.o.d. for 7 more doses

ADMINISTRATION

Intravenous

▪ Administer lymphocyte immune globulin (ATG) ONLY if experienced with immunosuppressant therapy and management of kidney transplant patients.
▪ Do an intradermal skin test to rule out allergy to the drug before first dose. Inject 0.1 mL of a 1:1000 dilution (5 mcg equine IgG in normal saline) and a saline control. If local reaction occurs (wheal or erythema more than 10 mm) or if there is pseudopod formation, itching, or local swelling, use caution during infusion. Discontinue infusion if systemic reaction develops (generalized rash, tachycardia, dyspnea, hypotension, anaphylaxis).

PREPARE: **IV Infusion:** Withdraw required dose of ATG concentrate and inject into IV solution container of 0.45% NaCl or NS. Invert IV container during injection of ATG to prevent its contact with air inside container. Use enough IV solution to create a concentration ≤4 mg/mL. ▪ Inspect concentrate and diluted solution for particulate matter (may develop during storage) and discoloration; discard if present.

ADMINISTER: **IV Infusion:** Give through an in-line 0.2–1.0 mcg filter into a high-flow vein to decrease potential for phlebitis and thrombosis. Give over ≥4 h (usually 4–8 h). Must finish infusion within 12 h of preparation.

▪ Total storage time for diluted solutions: NO MORE than 12 h (including storage time and actual infusion time). Refrigerate ampules and diluted solutions (if prepared before time of infusion) at 2°–8° C (35°–46° F). Do not freeze.

ADVERSE EFFECTS (≥1%) **CNS:** Headache, paresthesia, seizures. **CV:** Peripheral thrombophlebitis, hypotension, hypertension. **GI:** Nausea, vomiting, diarrhea, stomatitis, hiccups, epigastric pain, abdominal distension. **Hematologic:** *Leukopenia, thrombocytopenia.* **Musculoskeletal:** Arthralgia, myalgias, chest or back pain. **Respiratory:** Dyspnea, laryngospasm, pulmonary edema. **Skin:** *Rash, pruritus,* urticaria, wheal and flare. **Body as a Whole:** *Chills, fever,* night sweats, pain at infusion site, hyperglycemia, systemic infection, wound dehiscence; anaphylaxis, *serum sickness,* herpes simplex virus reactivation.

INTERACTIONS Drug: Azathioprine, CORTICOSTEROIDS, other IMMUNOSUPPRESSANTS increase degree of immunosuppression.

PHARMACOKINETICS Distribution: Poorly distributed into lymphoid tissues (spleen, lymph nodes); probably crosses placenta and into breast milk. **Elimination:** About 1% of dose is excreted in urine. **Half-Life:** Approximately 6 d.

NURSING IMPLICATIONS

Assessment & Drug Effects

- Discontinue infusion and initiate appropriate therapy promptly with onset of anaphylactic response (respiratory distress; pain in chest, flank, back; hypotension, anxiety).
- Monitor BP, vital signs, and patient's complaints during entire administration period carefully. Prompt treatment is indicated for observed and reported symptoms of anaphylaxis (incidence: 1%), serum sickness, or allergic response. Always have equipment for assisted respiration, epinephrine, antihistamines, corticosteroid, and vasopressor available at bedside.
- Predictive value of skin test is not proven. Observe patient carefully; allergic reaction can occur even when test is negative.
- Watch closely for S&S of serum sickness: fever, malaise, arthralgia, nausea, vomiting, lymphadenopathy and morbilliform eruptions on trunk and extremities. Rash begins as asymptomatic pale pink macules in periumbilical region, axilla, and groin, then rapidly becomes generalized, erythematous, and confluent. Bands of progressive erythema along the sides of hands, fingers, feet, toes, and at margins of palm or plantar skin are characteristic. In ATG-induced serum sickness, when platelet count is low, petechiae and purpura rapidly replace rash distribution over the body. Petechial areas are especially noticeable on legs but also on palms and soles. Serum sickness usually occurs 6–18 d after initiation of therapy; may occur during drug administration or when treatment is stopped.
- Monitor carefully for S&S of thrombocytopenia, concurrent infection, and leukopenia; patient usually receives concomitant corticosteroids and antimetabolites.
- Monitor patient's temperature and attend to complaints of sore throat or rhinorrhea. Report to physician; ATG treatment may be stopped.

Patient & Family Education

- Notify physician immediately of pain in chest, flank, or back; chills; pruritus; night sweats; sore throat.
- Do not breast feed while taking this drug without consulting physician.

L

MAFENIDE ACETATE

(ma'fe-nide)
Sulfamylon
Classifications: ANTIINFECTIVE; ANTIBIOTIC; SULFONAMIDE DERIVATIVE
Prototype: Sulfisoxazole
Pregnancy Category: C

AVAILABILITY 5% solution; cream

ACTIONS Topical sulfonamide derivative effective against both gram-positive and gram-negative drugs. Topical applications produce marked reduction of bacterial growth in vascular tissue. Active in presence of pus and serum and not affected by changes in pH of tissue environment. Cross-sensitivity with other sulfonamides not established.

THERAPEUTIC EFFECTS Bacteriostatic against many gram-positive and gram-negative organisms, including *Pseudomonas aeruginosa,* and certain strains of anaerobes.

USES Adjunctive therapy in second- and third-degree burns to prevent sepsis.

CONTRAINDICATIONS History of hypersensitivity to mafenide or any ingredients in the formulation (e.g., metabisulfite); respiratory (inhalation) injury, pulmonary infection; pregnancy (category C), lactation, children <3 mo.

CAUTIOUS USE Impaired kidney or pulmonary function, burn patients with acute kidney failure.

ROUTE & DOSAGE

Burns

Adult: **Topical** Apply aseptically to burn areas to a thickness of approximately 15 mm (1/16 in) once or twice daily

ADMINISTRATION

Topical

- Apply cream or solution aseptically to cleansed, debrided burn areas with sterile gloved hand.
- Cover burn areas with cream at all times. Make reapplications to areas from which cream has been removed as necessary.
- Store in tight, light-resistant containers. Avoid extremes of temperature.

ADVERSE EFFECTS (≥1%) **Hypersensitivity:** Pruritus, rash, urticaria, blisters, facial edema, eosinophilia. **Skin:** *Intense pain, burning, or stinging at application sites,* bleeding of skin, excessive body water loss, delayed eschar separation, excoriation of new skin, superinfections. **Hematologic:** <u>Hemolytic anemia, bone marrow suppression</u> (rare). **Other:** Metabolic acidosis.

INTERACTIONS Drug: No clinically significant interactions established.

PHARMACOKINETICS Absorption: Rapidly absorbed from burn surface. **Peak:** 2–4 h. **Metabolism:** Rapidly inactivated in blood to a weak carbonic anhydrase inhibitor. **Elimination:** Eliminated through kidneys.

NURSING IMPLICATIONS

Assessment & Drug Effects

- Monitor vital signs. Report immediately changes in BP, pulse, and respiratory rate and volume.
- Monitor I&O. Report oliguria or changes in I&O ratio and pattern.
- Lab tests: Monitor fluid and electrolyte status throughout therapy; acid–base balance should be monitored in patients with extensive burns and in those with pulmonary or kidney dysfunction.

M

- Be alert to S&S of metabolic acidosis (see Appendix F).
- Be alert to evidence of superinfections (see Appendix F), particularly in and below burn eschar.
- Observe carefully; accuracy is critical. It is frequently difficult to distinguish between adverse reactions to mafenide and the effects of severe burns.
- Note: Allergic reactions have reportedly occurred 10–14 d after initiation of mafenide therapy. Temporary discontinuation of drug may be necessary.
- Report intense local pain to physician; pain caused by drug may require administration of analgesic.

Patient & Family Education

- Apply only a thin dressing over burns unless otherwise directed.
- Therapy is usually continued until healing is progressing well (usually 60 d) or site is ready for grafting (after about 35–40 d). It is not withdrawn while there is a possibility of infection unless adverse reactions intervene.
- Report any of the following to the physician immediately: Foul smelling drainage from wounds, bleeding at wound site, unexplained fever.
- Do not breast feed while using this drug.

MAGALDRATE

(mag′al-drate)

Hydromagnesium Aluminate, Lowsium, Riopan

Classifications: GASTROINTESTINAL AGENT; ANTACID

Prototype: Aluminum Hydroxide

Pregnancy Category: C

AVAILABILITY 540 mg/5 mL suspension

ACTIONS By reducing gastric acidity, stomach pH increases and proteolytic activity of pepsin is inhibited. Reportedly does not produce alkalosis or acid rebound and is not as likely to produce alterations of bowel function that occur with either aluminum or magnesium hydroxide alone.

THERAPEUTIC EFFECTS Nonsystemic antacid with true buffering action and high acid-neutralizing capacity.

USES Symptomatic relief of hyperacidity associated with peptic ulcer, gastritis, peptic esophagitis, and hiatal hernia, particularly in patients who need to restrict sodium.

CONTRAINDICATIONS Sensitivity to components; hypermagnesia; pregnancy (category C).

CAUTIOUS USE Impaired kidney function, dialysis patients; lactation.

ROUTE & DOSAGE

Antacid

Adult: **PO** 480–1080 mg (5–10 mL suspension or 1–2 tablets) q.i.d. (max: 20 tablets or 100 mL/d)

ADMINISTRATION

Oral

- Shake suspension vigorously before pouring. Preferably give between meals and at bedtime.
- Give suspension with sufficient water to ensure passage of drug into stomach.
- Make sure chewable tablets are chewed thoroughly before being swallowed. Give tablet to be swallowed whole with enough water to ensure prompt swallowing without chewing.

ADVERSE EFFECTS (≥1%) **GI:** Infrequent constipation or diarrhea (with prolonged use). **Urogenital:** Hyper-

M

magnesemia (in patients with impaired kidney function).

INTERACTIONS Drug: Will decrease absorption of TETRACYCLINES.

PHARMACOKINETICS Absorption: Minimally absorbed from GI tract. **Duration:** Buffering action may persist for 60 min.

NURSING IMPLICATIONS

Assessment & Drug Effects

- Question patient about effectiveness of medication in relieving GI distress.
- Lab tests: Check patients on prolonged therapy periodically for electrolyte imbalance (i.e., hypermagnesemia).

Patient & Family Education

- Be aware that, in common with other antacids, magaldrate may cause premature dissolution and absorption of enteric-coated tablets and interfere with the absorption of oral tetracyclines and other oral medications.
- Do not take other oral drugs, generally, within 1–2 h of an antacid.
- Do not breast feed while taking this drug without consulting physician.

M

MAGNESIUM CITRATE

(mag-nes'i-um)

Citrate of Magnesia, Citroma, Citro-Nesia

Classifications: GASTROINTESTINAL AGENT; SALINE CATHARTIC

Prototype: Magnesium Hydroxide

Pregnancy Category: B

AVAILABILITY 1.75 g/30 mL solution

ACTIONS Promotes bowel evacuation by causing osmotic retention of fluid, which distends colon and stimulates peristaltic activity.

THERAPEUTIC EFFECTS Evacuates bowels.

USES To evacuate bowel prior to certain surgical and diagnostic procedures and to help eliminate parasites and toxic materials after treatment with a vermifuge.

CONTRAINDICATIONS Kidney disease; nausea, vomiting, diarrhea, abdominal pain, acute surgical abdomen; intestinal impaction, obstruction or perforation; rectal bleeding; use of solutions containing sodium bicarbonate in patients on sodium-restricted diets; lactation. **CAUTIOUS USE** Pregnancy (category B).

ROUTE & DOSAGE

Bowel Evacuation
Adult: **PO** 240 mL once
Child: **PO** *2–6 y,* 4–12 mL; *6–12 y,* 50–100 mL

ADMINISTRATION

Oral

- Give on an empty stomach with a full (240 mL) glass of water. Time dosing so that it does not interfere with sleep. Drug produces a watery or semifluid evacuation in 2–6 h.
- Chill solution by pouring it over ice or refrigerate it until ready to use to increase palatability.
- Be aware that once container is opened, effervescence will decrease. This does not effect the quality of preparation.
- Store at 2°–30° C (36°–86° F) in tightly covered containers.

ADVERSE EFFECTS (≥1%) **GI:** Abdominal cramps, nausea, fluid and electrolyte imbalance, hypermagnesemia (prolonged use).

INTERACTIONS Drug: May decrease effectiveness of **digoxin,** ORAL ANTI-

COAGULANTS, PHENOTHIAZINES; will decrease absorption of **ciprofloxacin,** TETRACYCLINES; **sodium polystyrene sulfonate** will bind magnesium, decreasing its effectiveness.

PHARMACOKINETICS Onset: 0.5–2 h.

NURSING IMPLICATIONS

Assessment & Drug Effects

- Monitor for dehydration, hypokalemia, and hyponatremia (see Appendix F) since drug may cause intense bowel evacuation.

Patient & Family Education

- Do not use for routine treatment of constipation (especially older adult).
- Expect some degree of abdominal cramping.
- Do not breast feed while using this drug.

MAGNESIUM HYDROXIDE (Pr)

(mag-nes'i-um)

Magnesia, Magnesia Magma, Milk of Magnesia, M.O.M.

Classifications: GASTROINTESTINAL AGENT; SALINE CATHARTIC; ANTACID

Pregnancy Category: B

AVAILABILITY 311 mg tablets; 400 mg/5 mL, 800 mg/5 mL suspension

ACTIONS Aqueous suspension of magnesium hydroxide with rapid and long-acting neutralizing action. May cause slight acid rebound.

THERAPEUTIC EFFECTS Acts as antacid in low doses and as mild saline laxative at higher doses. Causes osmotic retention of fluid which distends colon, resulting in mechanical stimulation of peristaltic activity.

USES Short-term treatment of occasional constipation, for relief of GI symptoms associated with hyperacidity, and as adjunct in treatment of peptic ulcer. Also has been used in treatment of poisoning by mineral acids and arsenic, and as mouthwash to neutralize acidity.

CONTRAINDICATIONS Abdominal pain, nausea, vomiting, diarrhea, severe kidney dysfunction, fecal impaction, intestinal obstruction or perforation, rectal bleeding, colostomy, ileostomy, lactation. Safety during pregnancy (category B) and in children <2 y is not established.

ROUTE & DOSAGE

Laxative

Adult: **PO** 2.4–4.8 g (30–60 mL)/d in 1 or more divided doses
Child: **PO** *2–5 y,* 0.4–1.2 g (5–15 mL)/d in 1 or more divided doses; *6–11 y,* 1.2–2.4 g (15–30 mL)/d in 1 or more divided doses

ADMINISTRATION

Oral

- Shake bottle well before pouring to assure mixing of suspension.
- Follow drug with at least a full glass of water to enhance drug action for laxative effect. Administer in the morning or at bedtime. Most effective when taken on an empty stomach.
- Store at 15°–30° C (59°–86° F) in tightly covered container. Slowly absorbs carbon dioxide on exposure to air. Avoid freezing.

ADVERSE EFFECTS (≥1%) **GI:** Nausea, vomiting, abdominal cramps, *diarrhea*. **Urogenital:** Alkalinization of urine. **Body as a Whole:** Weakness, lethargy, mental depression, hyporeflexia, dehydration, coma. **Metabolic:** Electrolyte imbalance with prolonged use. **CV:** Hypotension, bradycardia, complete heart block and other ECG abnormalities. **Respiratory:** Respiratory depression.

INTERACTIONS Drug: Milk of Magnesia decreases absorption of **chlordiazepoxide, dicumarol, digoxin, isoniazid,** QUINOLONES, TETRACYCLINES.

PHARMACOKINETICS Absorption: 15%–30% of magnesium is absorbed. **Onset:** 3–6 h. **Distribution:** Small amounts of magnesium distributed in saliva and breast milk. **Elimination:** Excreted in feces; some renal excretion.

NURSING IMPLICATIONS

Assessment & Drug Effects

- Evaluate the patient's continued need for drug. Prolonged and frequent use of laxative doses may lead to dependence. Additionally, even therapeutic doses can raise urinary pH and thereby predispose susceptible patients to urinary infection and urolithiasis.
- Lab tests: Monitor serum magnesium with signs of hypermagnesemia such as bradycardia (see Appendix F), especially with frequent use or any degree of renal impairment.

Patient & Family Education

- Investigate the cause of persistent or recurrent constipation or gastric distress with physician.
- Do not breast feed while using this drug.

MAGNESIUM OXIDE

(mag-nes'i-um)

Mag-Ox, Maox, Par-Mag, Uro-Mag

Classifications: GASTROINTESTINAL AGENT; ANTACID; SALINE CATHARTIC

Prototype: Magnesium Hydroxide

Pregnancy Category: B

AVAILABILITY 400 mg, 420 mg, 500 mg tablets; 140 mg capsules

ACTIONS Nonsystemic antacid with high neutralizing capacity and relatively long duration of action.

THERAPEUTIC EFFECTS Antacid in low doses and a mild saline laxative at higher doses. Causes osmotic retention of fluid, which distends colon, resulting in mechanical stimulation of peristaltic activity.

USES Essentially the same as magnesium hydroxide. May also be used as magnesium supplement.

CONTRAINDICATIONS Abdominal pain, nausea, vomiting, diarrhea, severe kidney dysfunction, fecal impaction, intestinal obstruction or perforation, rectal bleeding, colostomy, ileostomy; lactation. Safety during pregnancy (category B) or in children <2 y is not established.

ROUTE & DOSAGE

Antacid

Adult: **PO** 280–1500 mg with water or milk q.i.d., p.c. and h.s.

Laxative

Adult: **PO** 2–4 g with water or milk h.s.

Magnesium Supplement

Adult: **PO** 400–1200 mg/d in divided doses

ADMINISTRATION

Oral

- Separate administration of this drug from other oral drugs by 1–2 h.
- Store at 15°–30° C (59°–86° F) in airtight containers. On exposure to air, magnesium oxide rapidly absorbs moisture and carbon dioxide.

ADVERSE EFFECTS (≥1%) **GI:** *Diarrhea,* abdominal cramps, nausea; hypermagnesemia, kidney stones (chronic use).

INTERACTIONS Drug: See magnesium hydroxide.

PHARMACOKINETICS Absorption: 30%–50% absorbed from GI tract. **Elimination:** Eliminated in urine.

NURSING IMPLICATIONS

Assessment & Drug Effects

- Monitor for dehydration, hypokalemia, and hyponatremia (see Appendix F) since drug may cause intense bowel evacuation.
- Lab tests: Check patients on prolonged therapy periodically for electrolyte imbalance (i.e., hypermagnesemia).

Patient & Family Education

- Liquid preparation is reportedly more effective than the tablet form, as with other antacids.
- Do not breast feed while using this drug.

MAGNESIUM SALICYLATE

(mag-nes′i-um)

Doan's Pills, Magan, Mobidin

Classifications: CENTRAL NERVOUS SYSTEM AGENT; ANALGESIC; SALICYLATE; NSAID; ANTIPYRETIC

Prototype: Aspirin

Pregnancy Category: C

AVAILABILITY 467 mg, 500 mg, 580 mg caplets; 545 mg, 600 mg tablets

ACTIONS Sodium-free salicylate derivative with low incidence of GI irritation. Unlike aspirin, not associated with asthmatic reactions and does not inhibit platelet aggregation or increase bleeding time.

THERAPEUTIC EFFECTS In equal doses, less potent than aspirin as an analgesic and antipyretic.

USES Relief of pain and inflammation in rheumatoid arthritis, osteoarthritis, bursitis, and other musculoskeletal disorders.

CONTRAINDICATIONS Hypersensitivity to salicylates; erosive gastritis, peptic ulcer; advanced renal insufficiency, liver damage; bleeding disorders; before surgery.

CAUTIOUS USE Safety during pregnancy (category C), lactation, or in children <12 y is not established.

ROUTE & DOSAGE

Analgesic/Antipyretic

Adult: **PO** 650 mg t.i.d. or q.i.d.

Arthritic Conditions

Adult: **PO** Up to 9.6 g/d in divided doses

ADMINISTRATION

Oral

- Give with a full glass of water, food, or milk to minimize gastric irritation.

ADVERSE EFFECTS (≥1%) **Body as a Whole:** Salicylism [dizziness, drowsiness, tinnitus, hearing loss, nausea, vomiting, hypermagnesemia (with high doses in patients with renal insufficiency)].

INTERACTIONS Drug: Aminosalicylic acid increases risk of SALICYLATE toxicity; **ammonium chloride** and other ACIDIFYING AGENTS decrease renal elimination and increase risk of SALICYLATE toxicity; anticoagulants—added risk of bleeding with ANTICOAGULANTS; CARBONIC ANHYDRASE INHIBITORS enhance SALICYLATE toxicity; CORTICOSTEROIDS compound ulcerogenic effects; increases **metho-**

M

trexate toxicity; low doses of SALICYLATES may antagonize uricosuric effects of **probenecid, sulfinpyrazone.**

PHARMACOKINETICS Absorption: Well absorbed from the GI tract. **Peak:** 20 min. **Distribution:** Widely distributed with high levels of salicylic acid in liver and kidney, crosses placenta, excreted in breast milk. **Metabolism:** Salicylic acid is metabolized in liver. **Elimination:** Excreted in kidneys. **Half-Life:** 2–3 h with single dose, 15–30 h with chronic dosing.

NURSING IMPLICATIONS

Assessment & Drug Effects

- Lab tests: Monitor serum magnesium levels hypermagnesemia if used in high dosages or patients with any degree of renal impairment.
- Do not use salicylates in children or teenagers with influenza or chickenpox because of association with development of Reye's syndrome.

Patient & Family Education

- Report to physician promptly tinnitus, hearing loss, or dizziness.
- Do not to take aspirin-containing drugs without consent of physician.
- Check ingredients. Doan's pills may contain acetaminophen plus salicylamide.
- Do not breast feed while taking this drug without consulting physician.

MAGNESIUM SULFATE

(mag-nes′i-um)

Epsom Salt

Classifications: GASTROINTESTINAL AGENT; SALINE CATHARTIC; REPLACEMENT AGENT; ANTICONVULSANT

Prototype: Magnesium Hydroxide

Pregnancy Category: A

AVAILABILITY 0.8 mEq/mL, 1 mEq/mL, 4 mEq/mL injection

ACTIONS *Orally:* Acts as a laxative by osmotic retention of fluid, which distends colon, increases water content of feces, and causes mechanical stimulation of bowel activity. *Parenterally:* Acts as a CNS depressant and also as a depressant of smooth, skeletal, and cardiac muscle function. Anticonvulsant properties thought to be produced by CNS depression, principally by decreasing the amount of acetylcholine liberated from motor nerve terminals, thus producing peripheral neuromuscular blockade.

THERAPEUTIC EFFECTS Effective parenterally as a CNS depressant, smooth muscle relaxant and anticonvulsant in labor and delivery, and cardiac disorders. It is a laxative when taken orally.

USES Orally to relieve acute constipation and to evacuate bowel in preparation for x-ray of intestines. Parenterally to control seizures in toxemia of pregnancy, epilepsy, and acute nephritis and for prophylaxis and treatment of hypomagnesemia. Topically to reduce edema, inflammation, and itching.

UNLABELED USES To inhibit premature labor (tocolytic action) and as adjunct in hyperalimentation.

CONTRAINDICATIONS Myocardial damage; heart block; cardiac arrest except for certain arrhythmias; IV administration during the 2 h preceding delivery; PO use in patients with abdominal pain, nausea, vomiting, fecal impaction, or intestinal irritation, obstruction, or perforation.

CAUTIOUS USE Impaired kidney function; digitalized patients; concomitant use of other CNS depressants; neuromuscular blocking agents, or cardiac glycosides;

pregnancy (category A), lactation, children.

ROUTE & DOSAGE

Laxative
Adult: **PO** 10–15 g once/d
Preeclampsia, Eclampsia
Adult: **IM/IV** 4 g in 250 mL D5W infused slowly, followed by 4–5 g IM in alternate buttocks q4h
Hypomagnesemia Seizures
Adult: **IM/IV** *Mild,* 1 g q6h for 4 doses; *Severe,* 250 mg/kg infused over 4 h
Child: **IV** 20–100 mg/kg q4–6h prn
Total Parenteral Nutrition
Adult: **IV** 0.5–3 g/d

ADMINISTRATION

Oral

- Give in the morning or mid-afternoon in a glass of water for laxative action. Disguise bitter, salty taste by chilling or flavoring with lemon or orange juice.

Intramuscular

- Give deep using the 50% concentration for adults and the 20% concentration for children.

Intravenous

Note: Verify correct IV concentration and rate of infusion for administration to infants, children with physician.

PREPARE: **Direct/IV Infusion:** Give solutions with concentrations of ≤20% undiluted.

ADMINISTER: **Direct:** Give at a rate of 150 mg over at least 1 min. Note: 20% solution contains 200 mg/mL, 10% solution contains 100 mg/mL. **IV Infusion:** Give required dose over 4 h. Do not exceed the direct rate.

INCOMPATIBILITIES **Solution/additive: 10% fat emulsion; amphotericin B, calcium gluceptate, clindamycin, cyclosporine, dobutamine, polymyxin B sulfate, procaine, sodium bicarbonate. Y-site: Amphotericin B cholesteryl, cefepime.**

ADVERSE EFFECTS (≥1%) **Body as a Whole:** Flushing, sweating, extreme thirst, sedation, confusion, depressed reflexes or no reflexes, muscle weakness, flaccid paralysis, hypothermia. **CV:** Hypotension, depressed cardiac function, <u>complete heart block, circulatory collapse</u>. **Respiratory:** <u>Respiratory paralysis</u>. **Metabolic:** Hypermagnesemia, hypocalcemia, dehydration, electrolyte imbalance including hypocalcemia with repeated laxative use.

INTERACTIONS Drug: NEUROMUSCULAR BLOCKING AGENTS add to respiratory depression and apnea.

PHARMACOKINETICS Onset: 1–2 h PO; 1 h IM. **Duration:** 30 min IV; 3–4 h PO. **Distribution:** Crosses placenta; distributed into breast milk. **Elimination:** Eliminated in kidneys.

NURSING IMPLICATIONS

Assessment & Drug Effects

- Observe constantly when given IV. Check BP and pulse q10–15 min or more often if indicated.
- Lab tests: Monitor plasma magnesium levels in patients receiving drug parenterally (normal: 1.8–3.0 mEq/L). Plasma levels in excess of 4 mEq/L are reflected in depressed deep tendon reflexes and other symptoms of magnesium intoxication (see ADVERSE EFFECTS). Cardiac arrest occurs at levels in excess of 25 mEq/L. Monitor calcium and phosphorus levels also.
- Early indicators of magnesium toxicity (hypermagnesemia) include

M

cathartic effect, profound thirst, feeling of warmth, sedation, confusion, depressed deep tendon reflexes, and muscle weakness.

- Monitor respiratory rate closely. Report immediately if rate falls below 12.
- Test patellar reflex before each repeated parenteral dose. Depression or absence of reflexes is a useful index of early magnesium intoxication.
- Check urinary output, especially in patients with impaired kidney function. Therapy is generally not continued if urinary output is less than 100 mL during the 4 h preceding each dose.
- Observe newborns of mothers who received parenteral magnesium sulfate within a few hours of delivery for signs of toxicity, including respiratory and neuromuscular depression.
- Observe patients receiving drug for hypomagnesemia for improvement in these signs of deficiency: Irritability, choreiform movements, tremors, tetany, twitching, muscle cramps, tachycardia, hypertension, psychotic behavior.
- Have calcium gluconate readily available in case of magnesium sulfate toxicity.

Patient & Family Education

- Drink sufficient water during the day when drug is administered orally to prevent net loss of body water.
- Recommended daily allowances of magnesium are obtained in a normal diet. Rich sources are whole-grain cereals, legumes, nuts, meats, seafood, milk, most green leafy vegetables, and bananas.
- Do not breast feed while taking this drug without consulting physician.

M

MANNITOL (Pr)

(man'i-tole)

Osmitrol

Classifications: ELECTROLYTIC AND WATER BALANCE AGENT; OSMOTIC DIURETIC

Pregnancy Category: C

AVAILABILITY 5%, 10%, 15%, 20%, 25% injection

ACTIONS In large doses, increases rate of electrolyte excretion by the kidney, particularly sodium, chloride, and potassium.

THERAPEUTIC EFFECTS Induces diuresis by raising osmotic pressure of glomerular filtrate, thereby inhibiting tubular reabsorption of water and solutes. Reduces elevated intraocular and cerebrospinal pressures by increasing plasma osmolality, thus inducing diffusion of water from these fluids back into plasma and extravascular space.

USES To promote diuresis in prevention and treatment of oliguric phase of acute kidney failure following cardiovascular surgery, severe traumatic injury, surgery in presence of severe jaundice, hemolytic transfusion reaction. Also used to reduce elevated intraocular (IOP) and intracranial pressure (ICP), to measure glomerular filtration rate (GFR), to promote excretion of toxic substances, to relieve symptoms of pulmonary edema, and as irrigating solution in transurethral prostatic reaction to minimize hemolytic effects of water. Commercially available in combination with sorbitol for urogenital irrigation.

CONTRAINDICATIONS Anuria; marked pulmonary congestion or edema; severe CHF; metabolic edema; organic CNS disease, intracranial bleeding; shock, severe dehydration, history of allergy; pregnancy (category C), lactation; concomitantly with blood.

ROUTE & DOSAGE

Acute Kidney Failure

Adult: **IV Test Dose** 0.2 g/kg or 12.5 g as a 15%–20% solution over 3–5 min **Positive Response** 30–50 mL of urine over next 2–3 h, may repeat test dose 1 time. If still negative, do not use. **Treatment** 50–100 g as 15%–20% solution over 90 min to several hours
Child: **IV Test Dose** 200 mg/kg (max: 12.5 g) over 3–5 min **Positive Response** Urine flow of 1 mL/kg/h for 1–2 h **Maintenance** 0.25–0.5 g/kg q4–6 h

Edema, Ascites

Adult: **IV** 100 g as a 10%–20% solution over 2–6 h

Elevated IOP or ICP

Adult: **IV** 1.5–2 mg/kg as a 15%–25% solution over 30–60 min

Acute Chemical Toxicity

Adult: **IV** 100–200 g depending on urine output

Measurement of GFR

Adult: **IV** 100 mL of 20% solution diluted with 180 mL NaCl injection infused at a rate of 20 mL/min

ADMINISTRATION

Intravenous

Note: Verify correct IV concentration and rate of infusion for administration to infants, children with physician.

PREPARE: **IV Infusion:** Give undiluted.

ADMINISTER: **IV Infusion:** Give a single dose over 30–90 min. Oliguria: A test dose is given to patients with marked oliguria to check adequacy of kidney function. Response is considered satisfactory if urine flow of at least 30–50 mL/h is produced over 2–3 h after drug administration; then rate is adjusted to maintain urine flow at 30–50 mL/h with a single dose usually being infused over ≥90 min. Concentrations higher than 15% have a greater tendency to crystallize. Use an administration set with an in-line IV filter when infusing concentrations of 15% or above.

INCOMPATIBILITIES **Solution/additive: Imipenem-cilastatin. Y-site: Cefepime, doxorubicin liposome, filgrastim.**

- Store at 15°–30° C (59°–86° F) unless otherwise directed. Avoid freezing.

M

ADVERSE EFFECTS (≥1%) **CNS:** Headache, tremor, convulsions, dizziness, transient muscle rigidity. **CV:** Edema, CHF, angina-like pain, hypotension, hypertension, thrombophlebitis. **Eye:** Blurred vision. **GI:** Dry mouth, nausea, vomiting. **Urogenital:** Marked diuresis, urinary retention, nephrosis, uricosuria. **Metabolic:** *Fluid and electrolyte imbalance,* especially hyponatremia; dehydration, acidosis. **Other:** With extravasation (local edema, skin necrosis; chills, fever, allergic reactions).

INTERACTIONS Drug: Increases urinary excretion of **lithium,** SALICYLATES, BARBITURATES, **imipramine, potassium.**

PHARMACOKINETICS Onset: 1–3 h diuresis; 30–60 min IOP; 15 min ICP. **Duration:** 4–6 h IOP; 3–8 h ICP. **Distribution:** Confined to extracellular space; does not cross blood–brain barrier except with very high plasma levels in the presence of acidosis. **Metabolism:** Small quantity metabolized to glycogen in liver. **Elimination:** Rapidly excreted by kidneys. **Half-Life:** 100 min.

NURSING IMPLICATIONS

Assessment & Drug Effects

- Take care to avoid extravasation. Observe injection site for signs of inflammation or edema.
- Lab tests: Monitor closely serum and urine electrolytes and kidney function during therapy.
- Measure I&O accurately and record to achieve proper fluid balance.
- Monitor vital signs closely. Report significant changes in BP and signs of CHF.
- Monitor for possible indications of fluid and electrolyte imbalance (e.g., thirst, muscle cramps or weakness, paresthesias, and signs of CHF).
- Be alert to the possibility that a rebound increase in ICP sometimes occurs about 12 h after drug administration. Patient may complain of headache or confusion.
- Take accurate daily weight.

Patient & Family Education

- Report any of the following: Thirst, muscle cramps or weakness, paresthesia, dyspnea, or headache.
- Family members should immediately report any evidence of confusion.
- Do not breast feed while using this drug.

MAPROTILINE HYDROCHLORIDE

(ma-proe'ti-leen)

Maprotiline HCl

Classifications: CENTRAL NERVOUS SYSTEM AGENT; PSYCHOTHERAPEUTIC; TETRACYCLIC ANTIDEPRESSANT

Prototype: Mirtazapine

Pregnancy Category: B

AVAILABILITY 25 mg, 50 mg, 75 mg tablets

ACTIONS Tetracyclic antidepressant pharmacologically and therapeutically similar to the tricyclic antidepressants. Has significant sedative effect and less prominent anticholinergic action; may lower seizure threshold. Precise mechanism is unknown, however, it blocks the reuptake of norepinephrine at the neural membranes.

THERAPEUTIC EFFECTS Useful in depression associated with anxiety and sleep disturbances.

USES Treatment of depressive neurosis (dysthymic disorder) and manic-depressive illness, depressed type (major depressive disorder).

CONTRAINDICATIONS Patients <18 y; history of seizure disorder; pregnancy (category B), lactation.

CAUTIOUS USE History of seizure activity. Also see precautions under imipramine HCl.

ROUTE & DOSAGE

Mild to Moderate Depression

Adult: **PO** Start at 75 mg/d and gradually increase q2wk up to 150 mg/d in single or divided doses

Geriatric: **PO** Start with 25 mg h.s. and gradually increase to 50–75 mg/d

Severe Depression

Adult: **PO** Start at 100–150 mg/d and gradually increase up to 300 mg/d in single or divided doses if needed

ADMINISTRATION

Oral

- Give as single dose or in divided doses. Initiate therapy with low dosages to reduce risk of seizures.

- Store at 15°–30° C (59°–86° F) unless otherwise specified.

ADVERSE EFFECTS (≥1%) **CNS:** Seizures, exacerbation of psychosis, hallucinations, tremors, excitement, confusion, dizziness, *drowsiness*. **CV:** *Orthostatic hypotension,* hypertension, tachycardia. **Special Senses:** Accommodation disturbances, blurred vision, mydriasis. **GI:** Nausea, vomiting, epigastric distress, *constipation, dry mouth*. **Urogenital:** *Urinary retention,* frequency. **Skin:** Hypersensitivity reactions (skin rash, urticaria, photosensitivity).

INTERACTIONS Drug: May decrease some response to ANTIHYPERTENSIVES; CNS DEPRESSANTS, **alcohol,** HYPNOTICS, BARBITURATES, SEDATIVES potentiate CNS depression; may increase hypoprothrombinemic effect of ORAL ANTICOAGULANTS; transient delirium with **ethchlorvynol;** with **levodopa,** SYMPATHOMIMETICS (e.g., **epinephrine**, **norepinephrine**) there is possibility of sympathetic hyperactivity with hypertension and hyperpyrexia; with MAO INHIBITORS there is possibility of severe reactions, toxic psychosis, cardiovascular instability; **methylphenidate** increases plasma TCA levels; THYROID DRUGS increase possibility of arrhythmias; **cimetidine** may increase plasma TCA levels.

PHARMACOKINETICS Absorption: Slowly absorbed from GI tract. **Peak:** 12 h. **Distribution:** Distributed chiefly to brain, lungs, liver, and kidneys. **Metabolism:** Metabolized in liver. **Elimination:** 70% excreted in urine, 30% in feces. **Half-Life:** 51 h.

NURSING IMPLICATIONS

Assessment & Drug Effects

- Monitor for therapeutic effectiveness; 2–3 wk are usually necessary for full effect.
- Assess level of sedative effect. If recovering patient becomes too lethargic to care for personal hygiene or to maintain food intake and interactions with others, report to physician.
- Monitor bowel elimination pattern and I&O ratio. Severe constipation and urinary retention are potential problems, especially in the older adult. Advise increased fluid intake (at least 1500 mL/d).
- Observe seizure precautions; risk of seizures appears to be high in heavy drinkers.
- Bear in mind that if patient uses excessive amounts of alcohol, potentiated effects of maprotiline may increase the danger of overdosage or suicide attempt.

Patient & Family Education

- Report symptoms of stomatitis and dry mouth when taking high doses. Sore or dry mouth can lead to lack of compliance.
- Use caution with tasks that require alertness and skill; ability may be impaired during early therapy.
- Do not change dose or dose schedule without consulting physician.
- Do not use OTC drugs unless approved by physician.
- Avoid alcohol; the effects of maprotiline are potentiated when both are used together and for 2 wk after maprotiline is discontinued.
- Do not breast feed while using this drug.

MASOPROCOL CREAM

(mas-o-pro′col)

Actinex

Classification: SKIN AND MUCOUS MEMBRANE AGENT

Pregnancy Category: B

AVAILABILITY 10% Cream

ACTIONS Mechanism of action of masoprocol in the treatment of actinic keratoses is unknown. Dispensed as 10% cream.
THERAPEUTIC EFFECTS Antiproliferative activity against keratinocytes.

USES Treatment of actinic keratosis.
UNLABELED USES Malignant melanoma.

CONTRAINDICATIONS Hypersensitivity to masoprocol.
CAUTIOUS USE Pregnancy (category B) and lactation. Safety and efficacy in children are not established.

ROUTE & DOSAGE

Actinic Keratosis
Adult: **Topical** Apply to lesions b.i.d. for 14–28 d

ADMINISTRATION

Topical
- Use externally only. Do not apply on mucous membranes. In case of eye contact, wash eye with water immediately.
- Wash and dry affected areas before application. Gently massage into area until it is evenly distributed.
- Wash hand immediately if cream is applied without a glove.
- Do not apply occlusive dressings over cream.
- Store at 15°–30° C (59°–86° F) unless otherwise directed.

ADVERSE EFFECTS (≥1%) **Skin:** *Inflammation, erythema, dryness, flaking,* itching, burning, tightness, bleeding, edema.

INTERACTIONS Drug: No clinically significant interactions established.

PHARMACOKINETICS Absorption: <2% absorbed through intact skin. **Onset:** 2–4 wk.

NURSING IMPLICATIONS

Assessment & Drug Effects
- Assess for allergic contact dermatitis, which is an indication to discontinue.
- Report severe skin reactions of any kind to physician.

Patient & Family Education
- Learn proper technique for application of the cream.
- Be prepared for a transient local burning sensation immediately following application.
- Local skin reactions are common but usually disappear within 2 wk of discontinuing cream application.
- Be aware that this product contains sulfites.
- Masoprocol may stain clothing.
- Do not breast feed while taking this drug without consulting physician.

MAZINDOL
(may'zin-dole)
Mazanor, Sanorex
Classifications: CENTRAL NERVOUS SYSTEM AGENT; CEREBRAL STIMULANT; ANOREXIANT
Prototype: Amphetamine Sulfate
Pregnancy Category: C
Controlled Substance: Schedule IV

AVAILABILITY 1 mg, 2 mg tablets

ACTIONS Pharmacologic properties are similar to those of amphetamines. Produces CNS and cardiac stimulation in addition to amphetamine-like effects. Appears to exert primary effects on limbic system and to alter norepinephrine metabolism by inhibiting normal neuronal uptake mechanism.
THERAPEUTIC EFFECTS CNS and cardiac stimulant; also results in increased motor activity, dimin-

ished sense of fatigue, alertness, wakefulness, and mood elevation.

USES Short-term management of exogenous obesity.

CONTRAINDICATIONS Glaucoma; severe hypertension; symptomatic cardiovascular disease, including arrhythmias; agitated states; history of drug abuse; during or within 14 d after administration of MAO inhibitors; children <12 y. Safety during pregnancy (category C) or lactation is not established.
CAUTIOUS USE Hyperexcitability states.

ROUTE & DOSAGE

Obesity
Adult: **PO** 1 mg t.i.d. a.c. or 2 mg q.d. 1 h before lunch

ADMINISTRATION

Oral
- Given 1 h before meals if t.i.d. or 1 h before lunch if q.d. dose.
- Give with meals if GI discomfort occurs.

ADVERSE EFFECTS (≥1%) **CNS:** *Restlessness,* dizziness, insomnia, dysphoria, depression, tremor, headache, drowsiness, weakness. **CV:** Palpitation, tachycardia. **Endocrine:** Impotence. **GI:** *Dry mouth,* unpleasant taste, diarrhea, constipation, nausea, vomiting. **Skin:** Rash, excessive sweating, clamminess.

INTERACTIONS Drug: Acetazolamide, sodium bicarbonate decrease mazindol elimination; **ammonium chloride, ascorbic acid** increase mazindol elimination; the effects of mazindol and BARBITURATES may be antagonized; **furazolidone** may increase BP effects of mazindol, and interaction may persist for several weeks after discontinuing **furazolidone;** antihypertensive effects of **guanethidine, guanadrel** antagonized; MAO INHIBITORS, **selegiline** can cause hypertensive crisis—do not administer mazindol during or within 14 d of administration of these drugs; PHENOTHIAZINES may inhibit mood elevating effects of mazindol; BETA-ADRENERGIC AGONISTS increase adverse cardiovascular effects of mazindol.

PHARMACOKINETICS Absorption: Readily absorbed from GI tract. **Onset:** 30–60 min. **Duration:** 8–15 h. **Metabolism:** Metabolized in liver. **Elimination:** 95% excreted in feces, 2%–5% in urine. **Half-Life:** 2.5–9 h.

NURSING IMPLICATIONS

Assessment & Drug Effects
- Monitor weight periodically.
- Give drug early in the day if patient experiences excessive restlessness or insomnia.

Patient & Family Education
- Rate of weight loss is greatest during first few weeks of therapy and tends to decrease thereafter.
- Be aware that insulin requirements (for diabetics) may be decreased in association with mazindol.
- Do not drive or engage in potentially hazardous activities until response to drug is known.
- Do not take more medication than prescribed.
- Report excessively dry mouth or constipation.
- Do not breast feed while taking this drug without consulting physician.

M

MEBENDAZOLE (Pr)

(me-ben′da-zole)
Vermox
Classifications: ANTIINFECTIVE; ANTHELMINTIC
Pregnancy Category: C

AVAILABILITY 100 mg tablets

ACTIONS Carbamate with unusually broad spectrum of anthelmintic activity. Mechanism of action not known.
THERAPEUTIC EFFECTS Inhibits formation of worm's microtubules and inhibits glucose and other nutrient uptake by susceptible helminths.

USES Treatment of *Trichuris trichiura* (whipworm), *Enterobius vermicularis* (pinworm), *Ascaris lumbricoides* (roundworm), *Ancylostoma duodenale* (common hookworm), *Necator americanus* (American hookworm) in single or mixed infections.
UNLABELED USES Beef, dwarf, and pork tapeworm and threadworm infections.

CONTRAINDICATIONS Safety during pregnancy (category C), lactation, or in children <2 y is not established.

ROUTE & DOSAGE

Enterobiasis
Adult: **PO** 100 mg as single dose
Child: **PO** 100 mg as single dose

Other Infestations
Adult: **PO** 100 mg b.i.d. times 3 d
Child: **PO** 100 mg b.i.d. times 3 d

ADMINISTRATION

Oral
- Allow tablets to be chewed and swallowed, or crushed and mixed with food if needed.

ADVERSE EFFECTS (≥1%) **GI:** Transient abdominal pain, diarrhea. **Body as a Whole:** Dizziness, fever (possibly due to tissue necrosis in cysts).

INTERACTIONS Drug: Carbamazepine, phenytoin can increase metabolism of mebendazole.

PHARMACOKINETICS Absorption: Minimal absorption from GI tract (2%–10% of oral dose). **Metabolism:** Metabolized to inactive metabolite. **Elimination:** Primarily eliminated in feces. **Half-Life:** 3–9 h.

NURSING IMPLICATIONS

Assessment & Drug Effects
- Initiate second course of treatment if cure does not occur within 3 wk.
- Examine and treat all family members simultaneously because pinworms are readily transmitted from person to person.

Patient & Family Education
- Practice thorough hand washing after touching any potentially contaminated item.
- Change underclothing, bedclothes, towels, and facecloths daily; bathe frequently, preferably by showering. Infected person should sleep alone.
- Do not breast feed while taking this drug without consulting physician.

MECAMYLAMINE HYDROCHLORIDE

(mek-a-mill′a-meen)
Inversine
Classifications: CARDIOVASCULAR AGENT; CENTRAL ACTING ANTIHYPERTENSIVE
Prototype: Methyldopa
Pregnancy Category: C

AVAILABILITY 2.5 mg tablets

ACTIONS Potent, long-acting secondary amine nondepolarizing ganglionic blocking agent. Blocks neurotransmission at both sympathetic and parasympathetic ganglia by competing with acetylcholine (Ach) for cholinergic receptor sites on postsynaptic membranes.

THERAPEUTIC EFFECTS Reduces BP in both normotensive and hypertensive individuals, generally with greater decrease in standing or sitting BP than in supine BPs.

USES Moderately severe to severe hypertension and uncomplicated malignant hypertension.

CONTRAINDICATIONS Coronary insufficiency, pyloric stenosis; glaucoma; uremia, chronic pyelonephritis; recent MI; mild labile hypertension; unreliable uncooperative patients; pregnancy (category C), lactation.

CAUTIOUS USE Rising or elevated BUN; renal, cerebral, or coronary vascular pathology; recent CVA; prostatic hypertrophy, bladder neck obstruction, urethral stricture.

ROUTE & DOSAGE

Moderately Severe to Severe Hypertension

Adult: **PO** 2.5 mg b.i.d. p.c. for 2 d, increased by increments of 2.5 mg at intervals of ≥2 d until desired BP response is attained (2.5–25 mg/d in 2–4 divided doses)

ADMINISTRATION

Oral

- Give after meals for more gradual absorption and smoother control of BP. Schedule consistently relative to meals.
- Note: Because of diurnal variations in BP, physician may prescribe a relatively small dose in the morning or omission of morning dose (morning BP usually lower) and larger doses for afternoon or evening.
- Do not suddenly discontinue drug; may result in severe hypertensive rebound with CVA and acute CHF. Usually, other antihypertensive therapy must be substituted gradually, and patient must be supervised daily during period of dosage adjustment.
- Store at 15°–30° C (59°–86° F) unless otherwise directed.

ADVERSE EFFECTS (≥1%) **CNS:** Weakness, fatigue, sedation, headache, paresthesias. confusion, depression, choreiform movements, tremor. **CV:** *Orthostatic hypotension,* changes in heart rate, dizziness, syncope, precipitation of angina. **Special Senses:** Mydriasis, *blurred vision,* cycloplegia, nasal congestion, *dry mouth* with dysphagia, glossitis. **GI:** *Anorexia, nausea, vomiting, constipation, diarrhea,* <u>adynamic ileus</u>. **Urogenital:** Decreased libido, impotence, *urinary retention.*

INTERACTIONS Drug: Alcohol, other ANTIHYPERTENSIVE AGENTS, **bethanechol,** THIAZIDE DIURETICS potentiate hypotensive effects; **acetazolamide, sodium bicarbonate** increase mecamylamine toxicity because they decrease its elimination.

PHARMACOKINETICS Absorption: Almost completely absorbed from GI tract. **Onset:** 30 min–2 h. **Peak:** 3–5 h. **Duration:** 6–12 h. **Distribution:** Crosses blood-brain barrier and placenta; distributed into breast milk. **Metabolism:** Metabolized in

M

liver. **Elimination:** Primarily excreted in urine.

NURSING IMPLICATIONS

Assessment & Drug Effects

- Monitor therapeutic effectiveness by taking BP readings in standing position at time of maximal drug effect. Assess for symptoms of orthostatic hypotension (faintness, dizziness, light-headedness). Also note any changes in pulse rate.
- Monitor BP closely. Partial tolerance may develop in some patients, necessitating dosage adjustment.
- Report promptly constipation, frequent loose stools with abdominal distension, or decreased bowel sounds; may be the first signs of paralytic ileus (relatively frequent). Paralytic ileus is sometimes preceded by small, frequent stools.

Patient & Family Education

- Make position changes slowly and in stages, particularly from recumbent to upright posture; sit on edge of bed and move ankles and feet before walking.
- Lie down immediately if feeling light-headed or dizzy. Report adverse reactions immediately because drug effects may last hours to days after drug is discontinued.
- Seasonal variations may alter the hypotensive effect (e.g., usually smaller doses are required in summer than in winter).
- Do not drive or engage in potentially hazardous activities until response to drug is known.
- Learn measures to relieve dry mouth; rinse mouth frequently with water, suck hard candy.
- Do not breast feed while using this drug.

MECHLORETHAMINE HYDROCHLORIDE (Pr)

(me-klor-eth′a-meen)

Mustargen

Classifications: ANTINEOPLASTIC; ALKYLATING AGENT; NITROGEN MUSTARD

Pregnancy Category: D

AVAILABILITY 10 mg powder for injection

ACTIONS Analog of mustard gas and standard of reference for nitrogen mustards. Forms highly reactive carbonium ion, which causes cross-linking and abnormal base-pairing in DNA, thereby interfering with DNA replication and RNA and protein synthesis.

THERAPEUTIC EFFECTS Cell-cycle nonspecific inhibitor of DNA and RNA synthesis. Simulates actions of x-ray therapy, but nitrogen mustards produce more acute tissue damage and more rapid recovery.

USES Generally confined to nonterminal stages of neoplastic disease. Employed as single agent or in combination with other agents in palliative treatment of Hodgkin's disease (stages III and IV), lymphosarcoma, mycosis fungoides, polycythemia vera, bronchogenic carcinoma, chronic myelocytic or chronic lymphocytic leukemia. Also for intrapleural, intrapericardial and intraperitoneal palliative treatment of metastatic carcinoma resulting in effusion.

CONTRAINDICATIONS Myelosuppression; infectious granuloma; known infectious diseases, acute herpes zoster; intracavitary use with other systemic bone marrow suppressants; pregnancy (category D), lactation.

M

CAUTIOUS USE Bone marrow infiltration with malignant cells, chronic lymphocytic leukemia; men or women in childbearing age; use with x-ray treatment or other chemotherapy in alternating courses.

ROUTE & DOSAGE

Advanced Hodgkin's Disease
Adult: **IV** 6 mg/m^2 on day 1 and 8 of a 28 d cycle
Other Neoplasms
Adult: **IV** 0.4 mg/kg given as a single dose or in divided doses of 0.1–0.2 mg/kg/d, may repeat course in 3–6 wk

ADMINISTRATION

Intravenous

- Wear surgical gloves during preparation and administration of solution. ▪ Avoid inhalation of vapors and dust and contact of drug with eyes and skin. ▪ Flush contaminated area immediately if drug contacts the skin. Use copious amounts of water for at least 15 min, followed by 2% sodium thiosulfate solution. Irritation may appear after a latent period. ▪ Irrigate immediately if eye contact occurs. Use copious amounts of NS followed by ophthalmologic examination as soon as possible.

PREPARE: **IV Infusion:** Reconstitute immediately before use by adding 10 mL sterile water for injection or NS injection to vial to yield 1 mg/mL. With needle still in stopper, shake vial several times to dissolve. Discard colored solution or contents of any vial which has drops of moisture.
ADMINISTER: **IV Infusion:** To reduce risk of severe infections from extravasation or high concentration of the drug, inject into tubing or sidearm of freely flowing IV infusion. Flush vein with running IV solution for 2–5 min to clear tubing of any remaining drug.
INCOMPATIBILITIES **Solution/additive: Methohexital. Y-site: Allopurinol, cefepime.**

- Be alert for extravasation. Treat promptly with subcutaneous or intradermal injection with isotonic sodium thiosulfate solution (1/6 molar) and application of ice compresses intermittently for a 6–12 h period to reduce local tissue damage and discomfort. Tissue induration and tenderness may persist 4–6 wk, and tissue may slough.

ADVERSE EFFECTS (≥1%) **CNS:** Neurotoxicity: vertigo, tinnitus, headache, drowsiness, peripheral neuropathy, light-headedness, paresthesias, cerebral deterioration, coma. **GI:** Stomatitis, xerostomia, anorexia, *nausea, vomiting,* diarrhea. **Hematologic:** Leukopenia, *thrombocytopenia,* lymphocytopenia, agranulocytosis, *anemia,* hyperheparinemia. **Skin:** Pruritus, hyperpigmentation, herpes zoster, alopecia. **Urogenital:** Amenorrhea, azoospermia, chromosomal abnormalities, hyperuricemia. **Body as a Whole:** Weakness, hypersensitivity reactions. *With extravasation: painful inflammatory reaction, tissue sloughing, thrombosis, thrombophlebitis.*

INTERACTIONS Drug: Mechlorethamine (NITROGEN MUSTARDS) may reduce effectiveness of ANTIGOUT AGENTS by raising serum **uric acid** levels; dosage adjustments may be necessary; may prolong neuromuscular blocking effects of **succinylcholine;** may potentiate bleeding effects of ANTICOAGULANTS, SALICYLATES, NSAIDS, PLATELET INHIBITORS.

PHARMACOKINETICS Metabolism: Rapid transformation to metabolites. **Elimination:** Not detectable in blood within a few minutes; <0.01% excreted in urine.

NURSING IMPLICATIONS

Assessment & Drug Effects

- Establish baseline data for body weight, I&O ratio and pattern, and blood labs as reference for design of drug and care regimens.
- Lab tests: Monitor CBC with differential and platelet count.
- Determine dosage on basis of ideal dry body weight (i.e., not augmented by edema or ascites). Record daily weight. Alert physician to sudden or slow, steady weight gain.
- Monitor cardiac function during and after treatment until cardiac status is stable. Pain is rare with intrapleural injection, but transient cardiac irregularities may occur.
- Schedule treatments, other drugs, and meals to avoid peak times of nausea. Nausea and vomiting may occur 1–3 h after drug injection; vomiting usually subsides within 8 h, but nausea may persist.
- Monitor and record patient's fluid losses carefully. Prolonged vomiting and diarrhea can produce volume depletion.
- Report immediately petechiae, ecchymoses, or abnormal bleeding from intestinal and buccal membranes. Keep injections and other invasive procedures to a minimum during period of thrombocytopenia.
- Report symptoms of unexplained fever, chills, sore throat, tachycardia, and mucosal ulceration; may signal onset of agranulocytosis (see Appendix F).
- Prevent exposure of patient to people with infection, especially upper respiratory tract infections, and plan nursing interventions to keep patient's expenditure of energy at a minimum.
- Herpes zoster may be precipitated by mechlorethamine treatment and usually necessitates withdrawal of the drug. It occurs commonly in patients with lymphoma.
- Be aware that rapid neoplastic cell and leukocyte destruction leads to elevated serum uric acid (hyperuricemia, see Appendix F) and potential renal urate calculi.
- Use preventive measures against incidence of hyperuricemia: Increased fluid intake, alkalinizing of urine, and administration of allopurinol.
- Note and record state of hydration of oral mucosa, condition of gingiva, teeth, tongue, mucosa, and lips. If prosthetic devices do not fit properly, record.

Patient & Family Education

- Keep appointments for clinical evaluation. Laboratory studies of peripheral blood are essential guides for determining when to give another course of therapy.
- Report any signs of bleeding immediately because of the significance of thrombocytopenia with the development of bleeding tendencies.
- Use caution to prevent falls or other traumatic injuries, especially during periods of thrombocytopenia.
- Increase fluid intake up to 3000 mL/d if allowed to minimize risk of kidney stones. Report promptly all symptoms including flank or joint pain, swelling of lower legs and feet, changes in voiding pattern.
- Report symptoms tinnitus and deafness promptly when taking high doses and regional infusion of drug.
- Do not breast feed while using this drug.

MECLIZINE HYDROCHLORIDE Pr

(mek'li-zeen)

Antivert, Antrizine, Bonamine ✦, Bonine, Dizmiss, RuVert-M

Classifications: ANTIHISTAMINE; H_1-RECEPTOR ANTAGONIST; ANTI-VERTIGO AGENT

Pregnancy Category: B

AVAILABILITY 12.5 mg, 25 mg, 50 mg tablets; 25 mg, 30 mg capsules

ACTIONS Long-acting piperazine antihistamine, structurally and pharmacologically related to cyclizine compounds. Marked effect in blocking histamine-induced vasopressive response but only slight anticholinergic action. Marked depressant action on labyrinthine excitability and on conduction in vestibular-cerebellar pathways.

THERAPEUTIC EFFECTS Exhibits CNS depression, antispasmodic, antiemetic, and local anesthetic activity.

USES Management of nausea, vomiting, and dizziness associated with motion sickness and in vertigo associated with diseases affecting vestibular system.

CONTRAINDICATIONS Hypersensitivity to meclizine; pregnancy (category B).

CAUTIOUS USE Angle-closure glaucoma, prostatic hypertrophy. Safety in lactation or children <12 y is not established.

ROUTE & DOSAGE

Motion Sickness

Adult: **PO** 25–50 mg 1 h before travel, may repeat q24h if necessary for duration of journey

Vertigo

Adult: **PO** 25–100 mg/d in divided doses

ADMINISTRATION

Oral

- Give without regard to meals.
- Ensure that chewable tablets are chewed or crushed before being swallowed with a liquid.

ADVERSE EFFECTS (≥1%) **CNS:** *Drowsiness.* **GI:** Dry mouth. **Special Senses:** Blurred vision. **Body as a Whole:** Fatigue.

INTERACTIONS Drug: alcohol, CNS DEPRESSANTS may potentiate sedative effects of meclizine.

PHARMACOKINETICS Absorption: Readily absorbed from GI tract. **Onset:** 1 h. **Duration:** 8–24 h. **Distribution:** Crosses placenta. **Elimination:** Excreted primarily in feces. **Half-Life:** 6 h.

NURSING IMPLICATIONS

Assessment & Drug Effects

- Supervision of ambulation, particularly with the older adult, since drug may cause drowsiness.
- Assess effectiveness of drug and inform physician when prescribed for vertigo; dosage adjustment may be required.

Patient & Family Education

- Do not drive or engage in potentially hazardous activities until response to drug is known.
- Be aware that sedative action may add to that of alcohol, barbiturates, narcotic analgesics, or other CNS depressants.
- Take 1 h before departure when prescribed for motion sickness.
- Do not breast feed while taking this drug without consulting physician.

M

MECLOCYCLINE SULFOSALICYLATE

(me-kloe-sye'kleen)
Meclan
Classifications: ANTIINFECTIVE; ANTIBIOTIC; TETRACYCLINE
Prototype: Tetracycline
Pregnancy Category: B

AVAILABILITY 1% cream

ACTIONS Synthetic derivative of oxytetracycline. Antibacterial action appears to be related to ability to suppress growth of susceptible organisms.

THERAPEUTIC EFFECTS Suppresses growth of *Propionibacterium acnes,* an anaerobic organism in sebaceous glands and follicles. Inactive against viruses and fungi.

M

USES Inflammatory acne vulgaris.

CONTRAINDICATIONS Hypersensitivity to tetracyclines or any ingredients in the formulation (e.g., formaldehyde). Safety during pregnancy (category B), lactation, or in children <11 y is not established.

ROUTE & DOSAGE

Inflammatory Acne Vulgaris
Adult: **Topical** Apply to affected areas b.i.d., a.m. and p.m.

ADMINISTRATION

Topical
- Apply cream generously morning and evening over affected skin areas.
- Use less frequent applications depending on patient's response.

ADVERSE EFFECTS (≥1%) **Skin:** Skin irritation; stinging, burning sensation; temporary yellow staining of skin around hair follicles (with excessive applications), superinfections.

INTERACTIONS Drug: No clinically significant interactions established.

PHARMACOKINETICS Absorption: Not absorbed systemically in measurable amounts.

NURSING IMPLICATIONS

Assessment & Drug Effects
- Monitor patients with kidney or liver dysfunction carefully since significant percutaneous absorption may result with prolonged use.
- Monitor for S&S of superinfection (see Appendix F).

Patient & Family Education
- Keep follow-up appointments. Overuse of tetracycline preparations can result in overgrowth of nonsusceptible organisms.
- Be aware that excessive applications may cause temporary staining around hair roots and also can stain fabrics.
- Avoid use near or in eyes, ears, nose, mouth, or other mucous membranes.
- Notify physician if noticeable improvement has not occurred by 6–8 wk. Maximum benefit may not be apparent for ≥12 wk.
- Treated skin areas will be fluorescent under ultraviolet light.
- Take care using abrasive or medicated soaps and cleaners, other topical acne preparations, alcohol-containing preparations (e.g., after-shave astringents, lotions), "cover-up" medications, peeling agents (e.g., benzoyl peroxide, resorcinol, sulfur, salicylic acid, tretinoin). Possible cumulative drying or irritant effects can occur. Use such preparations with caution and only under medical guidance.
- Do not breast feed while taking this drug without consulting physician.

MECLOFENAMATE SODIUM

(me-kloe-fen-am′ate)
Meclofen, Meclomen
Classifications: CENTRAL NERVOUS SYSTEM AGENT; ANALGESIC; NSAID; ANTIPYRETIC
Prototype: Ibuprofen
Pregnancy Category: B (D in third trimester)

AVAILABILITY 50 mg, 100 mg capsules

ACTIONS Action mechanism unclear, but thought to inhibit prostaglandin synthesis and competition for binding at prostaglandin receptor sites. Does not appear to alter course of arthritis.
THERAPEUTIC EFFECTS Palliative antiinflammatory, analgesic, and antipyretic activity.

USES Symptomatic treatment of acute or chronic rheumatoid arthritis and osteoarthritis. Also in combination with gold salts or corticosteroids in treatment of rheumatoid arthritis.
UNLABELED USES Management of psoriatic arthritis, mild to moderate postoperative pain, dysmenorrhea.

CONTRAINDICATIONS Patient in whom bronchospasm, urticaria, and allergic rhinitis are induced by aspirin or other NSAIDS; pregnancy [first trimester (category B) and third trimester (category D)], lactation, children <14 y, patient designated as functional class IV rheumatoid arthritis (incapacitated, bedridden, or confined to wheelchair, little or no self-care); active peptic ulcer.
CAUTIOUS USE History of upper GI tract disease; compromised cardiac and kidney function, or other conditions predisposing to fluid retention.

ROUTE & DOSAGE

Inflammatory Disease
Adult: **PO** 200–400 mg/d in 3–4 divided doses (max: 400 mg/d)

ADMINISTRATION

Oral
- Give with food or milk if patient complains of GI distress. An aluminum and magnesium hydroxide antacid (Maalox) also may be prescribed. Consult physician if symptoms persist.
- Withhold dose and report to physician if significant diarrhea occurs.
- Store at 15°–30° C (59°–86° F) in airtight, light-resistant container.

ADVERSE EFFECTS (≥1%) **CNS:** *Dizziness,* vertigo, lack of concentration, confusion, *headache,* tinnitus. **CV:** Edema. **GI:** *Severe diarrhea (dose-related),* peptic ulceration, <u>GI bleeding</u>, dyspepsia, abdominal pain, *nausea,* vomiting (may be severe), flatulence, eructation, pyrosis, anorexia, constipation. **GI:** *Abnormal liver function tests,* cholestatic jaundice. **Special Senses:** Blurred vision. **Urogenital:** Elevated BUN and creatinine, kidney failure. **Skin:** Rash, pruritus, urticaria.

INTERACTIONS Drug: ORAL ANTICOAGULANTS, **heparin** may prolong bleeding time; may increase **lithium** toxicity; increases pharmacologic and toxic activity of **phenytoin,** SULFONYLUREAS, SULFONAMIDES, **warfarin** through protein-binding displacement. **Herbal: Feverfew, garlic, ginger, ginkgo** increase bleeding potential.

PHARMACOKINETICS Absorption: Rapidly and completely absorbed from GI tract. **Peak:** 1–2 h. **Duration:** 2–4 h. **Distribution:** Crosses placenta.

M

Metabolism: Metabolized in liver. **Elimination:** 60% excreted in urine, 30% in feces. **Half-Life:** 2–3.3 h.

NURSING IMPLICATIONS

Assessment & Drug Effects

- Expect clinical improvement in the rheumatoid patient within 2–3 wk with reduction in number of tender joints, severity of tenderness, and duration of morning stiffness.
- Observe improvement in the osteoarthritic patient as reflected by reduced night pain, pain on walking, starting pain, and pain with passive motion and improved joint function.
- Report diarrhea promptly. It is the most frequent adverse effect and usually dose related.
- Lab tests: Monitor kidney function where incidence of adverse reactions is potentially high because drug is excreted primarily by the kidneys. Monitor PT, PTT, and INR frequently with concurrent anticoagulant therapy.
- Monitor I&O ratio. Encourage fluid intake of at least 8 glasses of liquid a day.
- Consider sodium content of meclofenamate tablets if patient is on restricted sodium intake.

Patient & Family Education

- Stop taking drug and promptly notify the physician if nausea, vomiting, severe diarrhea, and abdominal pain occur. Generally dose reduction or temporary withdrawal will control symptoms.
- Report to physician without delay: Blurred vision, tinnitus, or taste disturbances.
- Schedule ophthalmic examinations before and periodically during treatment and whenever you experience visual disturbances.
- Notify physician if you become pregnant.
- Weigh under standard conditions (similar clothing, same time of day) twice weekly. Report weight gain of more than 2.5 to 3.5 kg (3–4 lb)/wk as well as signs of edema: Swollen ankles, tibiae, hands, feet.
- Do not use OTC drugs without approval of physician.
- Dizziness, a troublesome early side effect, frequently disappears in time. Avoid driving a car or potentially hazardous activities until response to drug is known.
- Report immediately to physician any sign of bleeding (e.g., melena, epistaxis, ecchymosis) when taking concomitant oral anticoagulant.
- Do not breast feed while using this drug.

MEDROXYPROGESTERONE ACETATE

(me-drox'ee-proe-jess'te-rone)

Amen, Cycrin, Depo-Provera, Provera

Classifications: HORMONES AND SYNTHETIC SUBSTITUTES; PROGESTIN

Prototype: Progesterone

Pregnancy Category: X

AVAILABILITY 2.5 mg, 5 mg, 10 mg tablets; 400 mg/mL injection

ACTIONS Synthetic derivative of progesterone with prolonged, variable duration of action and androgenic and antiestrogenic activity. No deleterious effects on lipid metabolism.

THERAPEUTIC EFFECTS Induces and maintains endometrium, preventing uterine bleeding; inhibits production of pituitary gonadotropin, preventing ovulation; and produces thick cervical mucus resistant to passage of sperm.

USES Dysfunctional uterine bleeding; secondary amenorrhea; paren-

teral form (Depo-Provera) used in adjunctive, palliative treatment of inoperable, recurrent, and metastatic endometrial or renal carcinoma; contraception.
UNLABELED USES Obstructive sleep apnea.

CONTRAINDICATIONS History of thromboembolic disorders; pregnancy (category X), lactation.
CAUTIOUS USE Asthma, seizure disorders, migraine, cardiac or kidney dysfunction, liver disease.

ROUTE & DOSAGE

Secondary Amenorrhea

Adult: **PO** 5–10 mg/d for 5–10 d beginning any time if endometrium is adequately estrogen primed (withdrawal bleeding occurs in 3–7 d after discontinuing therapy)

Abnormal Bleeding due to Hormonal Imbalance

Adult: **PO** 5–10 mg/d for 5–10 d beginning on the assumed or calculated 16th or 21st day of menstrual cycle; if bleeding is controlled, administer 2 subsequent cycles

Carcinoma

Adult: **IM** 400–1000 mg/wk; continue at 400 mg/mo if improvement occurs and disease stabilizes

Contraceptive

Adult: **IM** 100 mg q3mo

Sleep Apnea

Adult: **PO** 20 mg t.i.d.

ADMINISTRATION

Oral

- Oral drug may be given with food to minimize GI distress.

Intramuscular

- Administer IM deep into a large muscle.
- Store both formulations at 15°–30° C (59°–86° F); protect from freezing.

ADVERSE EFFECTS (≥1%) **CNS:** <u>Cerebral thrombosis or hemorrhage</u>, depression. **CV:** Hypertension, pulmonary embolism, edema. **GI:** Vomiting, nausea, cholestatic jaundice, abdominal cramps. **Urogenital:** *Breakthrough bleeding,* changes in menstrual flow, dysmenorrhea, vaginal candidiasis. **Skin:** Angioneurotic edema. **Body as a Whole:** Weight changes; *breast tenderness,* enlargement or secretion.

INTERACTIONS Drug: aminoglutethimide decreases serum concentrations of medroxyprogesterone; BARBITURATES, **carbamazepine, oxcarbazepine, phenytoin, primidone, rifampin, modafinil, rifabutin, topiramate** can increase metabolism and decrease serum levels of medroxyprogesterone. **Herbal:** intermenstrual bleeding and loss of contraceptive efficacy may occur with **St. John's wort.**

PHARMACOKINETICS Peak: 2–4 h PO, 3 wk IM. **Distribution:** >90% protein bound. **Metabolism:** Metabolized in liver. **Elimination:** Excreted primarily in feces. **Half-Life:** 30 d PO, 50 d IM.

NURSING IMPLICATIONS

Assessment & Drug Effects

- See progesterone for numerous additional nursing implications.
- Be aware that IM injection may be painful. Monitor sites for evidence of sterile abscess. A residual lump and discoloration of tissue may develop.
- Monitor for S&S of thrombophlebitis (see Appendix F).

M

- Note: Planned menstrual cycling with medroxyprogesterone may benefit the patient with a history of recurrent episodes of abnormal uterine bleeding.

Patient & Family Education

- Be aware that after repeated IM injections, infertility and amenorrhea may persist as long as 18 mo.
- Learn breast self-examination.
- Review package insert to ensure complete understanding of progestin therapy.
- Do not breast feed while using this drug.

MEDROXYPROGESTERONE ACETATE/ESTRADIOL CYPIONATE

(med-rox′y-pro-ges′te-rone/ es-tra-di′ol)

Lunelle

Classifications: HORMONE AND SYNTHETIC SUBSTITUTE; ESTROGEN; PROGESTIN

Prototype: Estradiol/Progesterone

Pregnancy Category: X

AVAILABILITY 25 mg medroxyprogesterone/5 mg estradiol cypionate per 0.5 mL

ACTIONS Progesterone prevents follicular maturation and ovulation. In addition, it induces morphological changes in the endometrium including thinning of its lining, which may result in decreased likelihood of implantation. Mechanism of action is not fully understood.

THERAPEUTIC EFFECTS Contraceptive that may act by preventing follicular maturation and ovulation, thickening of the cervical mucus, which prevents passage of sperm into the uterus, and decreases ability of sperm to survive in an environment of altered endometrium.

USES Hormonal contraception.

CONTRAINDICATIONS Hypersensitivity of any component of the product; pregnancy (category X), suspicion of pregnancy; genital bleeding of unknown etiology; thrombophlebitis or history of thrombophlebitic disorders: CVA or coronary artery disease (CAD); liver dysfunction, jaundice associated with pregnancy or contraceptive use; carcinoma of the endometrium, breast or other known estrogen dependent neoplasia; severe hypertension; diabetes with vascular involvement; headaches with focal neurological symptoms; valvular heart disease with complications; history of hypertension or hypertensive related diseases (i.e., renal disease or renal failure); liver dysfunction; lactation.

CAUTIOUS USE Diabetes mellitus; history of depression; disorders involving fluid retention; history of hyperlipidemia.

ROUTE & DOSAGE

Contraception

Adult/Adolescent: **IM** 0.5 mL q month or 28 d

ADMINISTRATION

Intramuscular

- Shake vial or prefilled syringe vigorously before use to ensure a uniform suspension.
- Give into the deltoid, gluteus maximus, or anterior thigh.
- Store at 20°–25° C (68°–77° F).

ADVERSE EFFECTS (≥1%) **Body as a Whole:** Asthenia, dizziness. **CV:** Hypertension, MI, thrombophlebitis. **GI:** Abdominal pain, nausea, gallbladder disease, hepatic adenomas or benign liver tumors, enlarged abdomen. **Endocrine:** Breast tenderness/pain. **Hematologic:** Arterial thromboembolism. **Metabolic:** Weight gain. **CNS:** Cerebral hemorrhage, cerebral thrombosis, depression, emotional lability, headache, nervousness. **Respiratory:** Pulmonary embolism. **Skin:** Acne, alopecia. **Urogenital:** Amenorrhea, dysmenorrhea, menorrhagia, metrorrhagia, decreased libido, vaginal moniliasis, vulvovaginal disorders. (Also see ORAL CONTRACEPTIVES.)

DIAGNOSTIC TEST INTERFERENCE Increase ***BSP*** retention, ***prothrombin, platelet aggregability, thyroid-binding globulin, PBI, T4, transcortin, corticosteroid, triglyceride, phospholipid*** levels; may increase ***ceruloplasmin, aldosterone, amylase transferrin, renin*** activity; May decrease ***antithrombin III, T3 resin uptake, serum folate, glucose tolerance, albumin, vitamin B_{12};*** may reduce ***metapyrone*** test response.

INTERACTIONS Drug: Aminoglutethimide, ANTIBIOTICS, BARBITURATES, **carbamazepine, fosphenytoin, griseofulvin, modafinil, oxcarbazepine, phenytoin, pioglitazone, primidone,** PROTEASE INHIBITORS, **rifampin, rifabutin, rifapentine, topiramate, troglitazone** may decrease contraceptive effectiveness; may decrease effectiveness of ORAL HYPOGLYCEMIC AGENTS, **clofibrate;** may increase toxicity of **cyclosporine;** may increase hypercoagulability with **aminocaproic acid;** may interfere with activity of AROMATASE INHIBITORS. **Herbal: St. John's wort** may decrease contraceptive effectiveness.

PHARMACOKINETICS Absorption: Slowly absorbed from IM site. **Peak:** 1–10 d. **Duration:** 1 month. **Distribution:** 86% protein bound. **Metabolism:** Extensively metabolized by hydrolysis in liver. **Elimination:** Primarily excreted in urine. **Half-Life:** 14–15 d.

NURSING IMPLICATIONS

Assessment & Drug Effects

- Monitor for and report immediately S&S of thrombophlebitis or thromboembolism (e.g., pulmonary embolism, CVA, TIA, retinal embolism).
- Monitor BP especially with preexisting hypertension.
- Monitor weight and degree of fluid retention.
- Monitor for S&S of bronchospasm in asthma patients; notify physician immediately.
- Lab tests: HgA_{1C} q3mo, and frequent fasting blood glucose and postprandial blood glucose in diabetics; periodic lipid profile and liver function tests.

Patient & Family Education

- Follow the schedule for receiving this drug. Drug must be administered every 28–30 days to remain effective.
- Use alternative forms of barrier contraception while taking antibiotics.
- Avoid smoking while using this form of contraception. Smoking greatly increases the risk of serious cardiovascular adverse effects.
- Diabetics should closely monitor blood glucose for loss of glycemic control.
- Do not use OTC drugs, including St. John's wort, vitamin C, or acetaminophen without consulting the physician.
- Report episodes of calf pain or tenderness, shortness of breath, chest pain, visual disturbances, drooping eyelid, double vision, or any other unusual symptom to the physician.
- Do not breast feed while taking this drug.

MEFENAMIC ACID

(me-fe-nam′ik)

Ponstan, Ponstel

Classifications: CENTRAL NERVOUS SYSTEM AGENT; ANALGESIC; NSAID; ANTIPYRETIC

Prototype: Ibuprofen

Pregnancy Category: C

AVAILABILITY 250 mg tablets

ACTIONS Anthranilic acid derivative. Like ibuprofen inhibits prostaglandin synthesis and affects platelet function. No evidence that it is superior to aspirin.

THERAPEUTIC EFFECTS Analgesic, antiinflammatory, and antipyretic actions similar to those of ibuprofen.

M

USES Short-term relief of mild to moderate pain including primary dysmenorrhea.

CONTRAINDICATIONS Hypersensitivity to drug; GI inflammation, or ulceration. Safety in children <14 y, during pregnancy (category C), or lactation is not established.

CAUTIOUS USE History of kidney or liver disease; blood dyscrasias; asthma; diabetes mellitus; hypersensitivity to aspirin. Long term use increases risk of serious adverse events (see DRUG INTERACTIONS).

ROUTE & DOSAGE

Mild to Moderate Pain

Adult: **PO Loading Dose** 500 mg **PO Maintenance Dose** 250 mg q6h prn

ADMINISTRATION

Oral

- Give with meals, food, or milk to minimize GI adverse effects.
- Do not use drug for a period exceeding 1 wk (manufacturer's warning).

ADVERSE EFFECTS (≥1%) **CNS:** Drowsiness, insomnia, dizziness, nervousness, confusion, headache. **GI:** *Severe diarrhea,* ulceration, and bleeding; *nausea, vomiting,* abdominal cramps, flatus, constipation, hepatic toxicity. **Hematologic:** Prolonged prothrombin time, severe autoimmune hemolytic anemia (long-term use), leukopenia, eosinophilia, agranulocytosis, thrombocytopenic purpura, megaloblastic anemia, pancytopenia, bone marrow hypoplasia. **Urogenital:** Nephrotoxicity, dysuria, albuminuria, hematuria, elevation of BUN. **Skin:** Urticaria, rash, facial edema. **Special Senses:** Eye irritation, loss of color vision (reversible), blurred vision, ear pain. **Body as a Whole:** Perspiration. **CV:** Palpitation. **Respiratory:** Dyspnea; acute exacerbation of asthma; bronchoconstriction (in patients sensitive to aspirin).

DIAGNOSTIC TEST INTERFERENCE False-positive reactions for ***urinary bilirubin*** (using ***diazo tablet test***).

INTERACTIONS Drug: Mefenamic acid may prolong bleeding time with ORAL ANTICOAGULANTS, **heparin;** may increase **lithium** toxicity; increases pharmacologic and toxic activity of **phenytoin,** SULFONYLUREAS, SULFONAMIDES, **warfarin** because of protein binding displacement. **Herbal: Feverfew, garlic, ginger, ginkgo** increase bleeding potential.

PHARMACOKINETICS Absorption: Rapidly and completely absorbed from GI tract. **Peak:** 2–4 h. **Duration:** 6 h. **Distribution:** Distributed in breast milk. **Metabolism:** Partially metabolized in liver. **Elimination:** 50% excreted in urine, 50% in feces. **Half-Life:** 2 h.

NURSING IMPLICATIONS

Assessment & Drug Effects

- Assess patients who develop severe diarrhea and vomiting for dehydration and electrolyte imbalance.
- Lab tests: With long-term therapy (not recommended) obtain periodic complete blood counts, Hct and Hgb, and kidney function tests.

Patient & Family Education

- Discontinue drug promptly if diarrhea, dark stools, hematemesis, ecchymoses, epistaxis, or rash occur and do not use again. Contact physician.
- Notify physician if persistent GI discomfort, sore throat, fever, or malaise occur.
- Do not drive or engage in potentially hazardous activities until response to drug is known. It may cause dizziness and drowsiness.
- Monitor blood glucose for loss of glycemic control if diabetic.
- Do not breast feed while taking this drug without consulting physician.

MEFLOQUINE HYDROCHLORIDE

(me-flo′quine)
Lariam
Classifications: ANTIINFECTIVE; ANTIMALARIAL
Prototype: Chloroquine
Pregnancy Category: C

AVAILABILITY 250 mg tablets

ACTIONS Antimalarial agent, structurally related to quinine.
THERAPEUTIC EFFECTS Effective against all types of malaria, including chloroquine resistant malaria.

USES Treatment of mild to moderate acute malarial infections, prevention of chloroquine-resistant malaria caused by *Plasmodium falciparum* and *P. vivax*.

CONTRAINDICATIONS Hypersensitivity to mefloquine or a related compound; with a calcium channel blocking agent, severe heart arrhythmias, history of QTc prolongation; aggressive behavior; active depression, or history of depression, suicidal ideation; generalized anxiety disorder, psychosis, schizophrenia, or other major psychiatric disorders; seizure disorders; pregnancy (category C); infancy.
CAUTIOUS USE Lactation; persons piloting aircraft or operating heavy machinery. Safety and efficacy in children are not established.

ROUTE & DOSAGE

Note: FDA has NOT approved use of mefloquine in children, and the U.S. Public Health Service does NOT recommend its use in children <15 kg or in pregnant women

Treatment of Malaria

Adult: **PO** 1250 mg (5 tablets) as single oral dose taken with at least 8 oz of water
Child: **PO** 20–30 mg/kg as single dose

Prophylaxis for Malaria

Adult: **PO** 250 mg once/wk × 4 wk (beginning 1 wk before travel), then 250 mg every other wk for duration of exposure and for 2 doses after leaving endemic area
Child: **PO** *15–19 kg*, 1/4 tablet; *20–30 kg*, 1/2 tablet; *31–45 kg*, 3/4 tablet

ADMINISTRATION

Oral

- Give with food and at least 8 oz water.

- Do not give concurrently with quinine or quinidine; wait at least 12 h beyond last dose of either drug before administering mefloquine.
- Store at 15°–30° C (59°–86° F).

ADVERSE EFFECTS (≥1%) **Body as a Whole:** Arthralgia, chills, fatigue, fever. **CNS:** Dizziness, nightmares, visual disturbances, headache, syncope, confusion, psychosis, aggression, suicide ideation (rare). **CV:** Bradycardia, ECG changes (including QTc prolongation), first-degree AV block. **GI:** Nausea, vomiting, abdominal pain, anorexia, diarrhea. **Skin:** Rash, itching.

DIAGNOSTIC TEST INTERFERENCE Transient increase in liver transaminases.

INTERACTIONS Drug: Mefloquine can prolong cardiac conduction in patients taking BETA BLOCKERS, CALCIUM CHANNEL BLOCKERS, and possibly **digoxin. Quinine** may decrease plasma mefloquine concentrations. Mefloquine may decrease **valproic acid** serum concentrations by increasing its hepatic metabolism. Administration with **chloroquine** may increase risk of seizures. Increased risk of cardiac arrest and seizures with **quinidine.**

PHARMACOKINETICS Absorption: 85% absorbed, concentrates in red blood cells. **Onset:** 59 and 28 h for parasite and fever clearance times in patients with *P. vivax* infections, respectively; 166 and 93 h in patients with *P. malariae* infections. **Distribution:** Concentrated in red blood cells due to high-affinity binding to red blood cell membranes; 98% protein bound; distributed minimally into breast milk. **Metabolism:** Metabolized in liver. **Elimination:** Eliminated primarily in bile and feces. **Half-Life:** 10–21 d (shorter in patients with acute malaria).

NURSING IMPLICATIONS

Assessment & Drug Effects

- Monitor carefully during prophylactic use for development of unexplained anxiety, depression, restlessness, or confusion; such manifestations may indicate a need to discontinue the drug.
- Evaluate cardiac and liver functions periodically with prolonged use.
- Lab tests: Monitor periodically CBC with differential during prolonged use.
- Monitor blood levels of anticonvulsants with concomitant therapy closely.

Patient & Family Education

- Take drug on the same day each week when used for malaria prophylaxis.
- Do not perform potentially hazardous activities until response to drug is known.
- Report any of the following immediately: Fever, sore throat, muscle aches, visual problems, anxiety, confusion, mental depression, hallucinations.
- Do not breast feed while taking this drug without consulting physician.

MEGESTROL ACETATE

(me-jess'trole)

Megace

Classifications: ANTINEOPLASTIC; HORMONE AND SYNTHETIC SUBSTITUTE; PROGESTIN

Prototype: Progesterone

Pregnancy Category: X

AVAILABILITY 40 mg/mL suspension; 20 mg, 40 mg tablets

ACTIONS Progestational hormone with antineoplastic properties. Mechanism of action unclear; however, an antiluteinizing effect mediated via the pituitary has been postulated.

THERAPEUTIC EFFECTS Moderate disease effects. Local effect when instilled directly into the endometrial cavity.

USES Palliative agent for treatment of advanced carcinoma of breast or endometrium.

UNLABELED USES Appetite stimulant in patients with AIDS.

CONTRAINDICATIONS Diagnostic test for pregnancy; use in neoplastic diseases other than cancer of endometrium and breast; first 4 mo of pregnancy (category X).

ROUTE & DOSAGE

Palliative Treatment for Advanced Breast Cancer
Adult: **PO** 40 mg q.i.d.

Palliative Treatment for Advanced Endometrial Cancer
Adult: **PO** 40–320 mg/d in divided doses

Appetite Stimulation
Adult: **PO** 200 mg q6h

ADMINISTRATION

Oral

- Give with meals or food if GI distress occurs.
- Shake oral suspension well before use.
- Store at 15°–30° C (59°–86° F) in tightly closed container.

ADVERSE EFFECTS (≥1%) **Urogenital:** Vaginal bleeding. **Body as a Whole:** Breast tenderness, headache, increased appetite, weight gain, allergic-type reactions (including bronchial asthma). **GI:** Abdominal pain, nausea, vomiting. **Hematologic:** DVT.

INTERACTIONS Drug: May increase levels of **warfarin;** may decrease renal clearance of **dofetilide.**

PHARMACOKINETICS Absorption: Appears to be well absorbed from GI tract. **Onset:** Onset of objective response in breast cancer in 6–8 wk. **Peak:** 1–3 h. **Duration:** 3–12 mo. **Metabolism:** Completely metabolized in liver. **Elimination:** 57%–78% of dose excreted in urine within 10 d.

NURSING IMPLICATIONS

Assessment & Drug Effects

- Monitor weight periodically.
- Notify physician if abdominal pain, headache, nausea, vomiting, or breast tenderness become pronounced.
- Monitor for allergic reactions, including breathing distress characteristic of asthma, rash, urticaria, anaphylaxis, tachypnea, anxiety. Stop medication if they appear and notify physician.

Patient & Family Education

- Use contraception measures during therapy for carcinoma.
- Learn breast self-examination.
- Learn S&S of thrombophlebitis (see Appendix F).
- Review package insert to ensure understanding of megestrol therapy.

MELOXICAM

(mel-ox′-i-cam)

Mobic

Classifications: CENTRAL NERVOUS SYSTEM AGENT (CNS); ANALGESIC; NONSTEROIDAL ANTI-INFLAMMATORY DRUG (NSAID)

Prototype: Ibuprofen

Pregnancy Category: C (first and second trimesters) D (third trimester)

AVAILABILITY 7.5 mg tablets

ACTIONS Is a nonsteroidal anti-inflammatory drug (NSAID) that exhibits anti-inflammatory, analgesic, and antipyretic activities. The mechanism of action, like other NSAIDs, may be related to prostaglandin synthetase (cyclooxygenase) inhibition.

THERAPEUTIC EFFECTS Exhibits antiinflammatory, analgesic, and antipyretic actions.

USES Relief of the signs and symptoms of osteoarthritis, rheumatoid arthritis.

CONTRAINDICATIONS Hypersensitivity to meloxicam; rhinitis, urticaria/angioedema, asthma; allergic reactions to aspirin or other antiinflammatory agents; NSAID hypersensitivity, severe renal or hepatic disease; salicylate hypersensitivity, pregnancy [(category C) first and second trimester, (category D) third trimester)], lactation; bleeding.

CAUTIOUS USE *Helicobacter pylori* infections; history of coagulation defects, liver dysfunction, gastrointestinal disease or ulceration, anemia, anticoagulant therapy; asthma; bone marrow suppression; corticosteroid therapy, dehydration, edema, older adults; females of childbearing age; GI bleeding, GI diseases, GI perforation; heart failure; hepatic disease, hypertension, hypovolemia, immunosuppression; jaundice, lactase deficiency, advanced renal dysfunction; hypertension or cardiac conditions aggravated by fluid retention and edema.

M

ROUTE & DOSAGE

Osteoarthritis
Adult: **PO** 7.5–15 mg once daily

Rheumatoid Arthritis
Adult: **PO** 15 mg once daily

ADMINISTRATION

Oral

- Do not exceed the maximum recommended daily dose of 15 mg.
- Use the lowest effective dose for the shortest duration to minimize risk of serious adverse effects.
- Store at 15°–30° C (59°–86° F).

ADVERSE EFFECTS (≥1%) **Body as a Whole:** Edema, fall, flu-like syndrome, pain. **GI:** Abdominal pain, diarrhea, dyspepsia, flatulence, nausea, constipation, ulceration, GI bleed. **Hematologic:** Anemia. **Musculoskeletal:** Arthralgia. **CNS:** Dizziness, headache, insomnia. **Respiratory:** Pharyngitis, upper respiratory tract infection, cough. **Skin:** Rash, pruritus. **Urogenital:** Micturition frequency, urinary tract infection.

INTERACTIONS Drug: May decrease effectiveness of ACE INHIBITORS, DIURETICS; **aspirin** may increase risk of GI bleed; may increase **lithium** levels and toxicity; **warfarin** may increase risk of bleeding. **Herbal: Feverfew, garlic, ginger, ginkgo** may increase bleeding potential.

PHARMACOKINETICS Absorption: 89% bioavailable. **Peak:** 4–5 h. **Distribution:** >99% protein bound, distributes into synovial fluid. **Metabolism:** Metabolized in liver by CYP2C9. **Elimination:** Equally eliminated in urine and feces. **Half-Life:** 15–20 h.

NURSING IMPLICATIONS

Assessment & Drug Effects

- Monitor for and immediately report S&S of GI ulceration or bleeding, including black, tarry stool, abdominal or stomach pain; hepatotoxicity, including fatigue, lethargy, pruritus, jaundice, flu-like symptoms; skin rash; weight gain and edema.
- Withhold drug and notify physician if hepatotoxicity or GI bleeding is suspected.

- Monitor carefully patients with a history of CHF, HTN, or edema for fluid retention.
- Monitor diabetics using sulfonylureas for hypoglycemia.
- Lab tests: Hgb & Hct, CBC with differential, liver function tests, serum electrolytes, BUN, and creatinine within 3 mo of initiating therapy and every 6–12 mo thereafter; with high-risk patients (e.g., >60 yr, history of peptic ulcer disease, prolonged or high-dose NSAID therapy, concurrent use of corticosteroids or anticoagulants) monitor within first 3–4 wk and every 3–6 mo thereafter.
- Coadministered drugs: With warfarin, closely monitor INR when meloxicam is initiated or dose changed; monitor for lithium toxicity, especially during addition, withdrawal, or change in dose of meloxicam.

Patient & Family Education

- Report any of the following to the physician immediately: nausea, black tarry stool, abdominal or stomach pain, unexplained fatigue or lethargy, itching, jaundice, flu-like symptoms, skin rash, weight gain, or edema.
- Minimize alcohol intake and use of tobacco. Discontinue drug if hepatotoxicity or GI bleeding is suspected. Note that GI bleeding may occur without forewarning and is more likely in older adults, in those with a history of ulcers or GI bleeding, and with alcohol consumption and cigarette smoking.
- Do not take aspirin or other NSAIDs while on this medication.
- Do not breast feed while taking this drug.

MELPHALAN

(mel'fa-lan)

Alkeran, L-Pam, Phenylalanine Mustard, Alkeran IV

Classifications: ANTINEOPLASTIC; ALKYLATING AGENT

Prototype: Mechlorethamine

Pregnancy Category: D

AVAILABILITY 2 mg tablets; 50 mg powder for injection

ACTIONS Nitrogen mustard chemically and pharmacologically related to mechlorethamine. Forms a highly reactive carbonium ion which causes cross-linking and abnormal base-pairing in DNA thereby interfering with DNA replication as well as RNA and protein synthesis.

THERAPEUTIC EFFECTS Strong immunosuppressive and myelosuppressive effects but, unlike mechlorethamine, lacks vesicant properties. Carcinogenic potential suspected.

USES Chiefly for palliative treatment of multiple myeloma. Also many other neoplasms, including Hodgkin's disease and carcinomas of breast and ovary.

UNLABELED USES Polycythemia vera.

CONTRAINDICATIONS Lactation. Safety during pregnancy (category D) or in men and women of childbearing age is not established.

CAUTIOUS USE Recent treatment with other chemotherapeutic agents; concurrent administration with radiation therapy; severe anemia, neutropenia, or thrombocytopenia, Impaired kidney function.

ROUTE & DOSAGE

Multiple Myeloma

Adult: **PO** 6 mg/d for 2–3 wk, drug then withdrawn for 4–5 wk,

M

restart at 2 mg/d when WBC and platelet counts start to rise **IV** 16 mg/m^2 over 15 min q2wk for 4 doses

Epithelial Ovarian Cancer

Adult: **PO** 0.2 mg/kg/d in divided doses for 5 d as single course, may repeat course q4–5 wk, depending on hematologic tolerance

ADMINISTRATION

Oral

- Give with meals to reduce nausea and vomiting. An antiemetic may be ordered.

Intravenous

PREPARE: **IV Infusion:** Reconstitute melphalan powder by RAPIDLY injecting 10 mL of the provided diluent into the vial to yield 5 mg/mL. Shake vigorously until clear. Immediately dilute further with NS to a concentration of 0.45 mg/mL or less. Note: 45 mg in 100 mL yields 0.45 mg/mL. Do not refrigerate reconstituted solution prior to infusion.

ADMINISTER: **IV Infusion:** Give over ≥15 min. Administration MUST be completed within 60 min of reconstitution of drug because both reconstituted and diluted solutions are unstable.

INCOMPATIBILITIES **Y-site: Amphotericin B, chlorpromazine.**

- Store at 15°–30° C (59°–86° F) in light-resistant, airtight containers.

ADVERSE EFFECTS (≥1%) **Hematologic:** Leukopenia, agranulocytosis, thrombocytopenia, anemia, acute nonlymphatic leukemia. **Body as a Whole:** Uremia, angioneurotic peripheral edema. **GI:** Nausea, vomiting, stomatitis. **Skin:** Temporary alopecia. **Respiratory:** Pulmonary fibrosis.

INTERACTIONS Drug: Increases risk of nephrotoxicity with **cyclosporine.**

PHARMACOKINETICS Absorption: Incompletely and variably absorbed from GI tract. **Peak:** 2 h. **Distribution:** Widely distributed to all tissues. **Metabolism:** Metabolized by spontaneous hydrolysis in plasma. **Elimination:** 25%–50% excreted in feces. **Half-Life:** 1.5 h; 25%–30% excreted in urine.

NURSING IMPLICATIONS

Assessment & Drug Effects

- Lab tests: Monitor WBC and platelet counts 2–3 times/wk during dosage adjustment period; determine WBC each week for 6–8 wk during maintenance therapy. Monitor serum uric acid levels.
- Monitor laboratory reports to anticipate leukopenic and thrombocytopenic periods.
- A degree of myelosuppression is maintained during therapy so as to keep leukocyte count in range of 3000–3500/mm^3.
- Assess for flank and joint pains that may signal onset of hyperuricemia.

Patient & Family Education

- Be alert to onset of fever, profound weakness, chills, tachycardia, cough, sore throat, changes in kidney function, or prolonged infections and report to physician.
- Understand that reversible hair loss is an expected adverse effect.
- Do not breast feed while using this drug.

MEMANTINE

(me-man'teen)

Namenda

Classifications: CENTRAL NERVOUS SYSTEM AGENT; N-METHYL-D-ASPARTATE (NMDA) RECEPTOR ANTAGONIST

Pregnancy Category: B

AVAILABILITY 5 mg, 10 mg tablets

ACTIONS Glutamate activation at the (*N*-methyl-*D*-aspartate) NMDA receptor is needed for memory and learning processes in the brain. Excess glutamate may play a role in Alzheimer's disease by over-stimulating NMDA receptors, thus causing increased Ca^{2+} movement into neurons leading to neuronal damage. Memantine is a low-affinity, uncompetitive antagonist at NMDA receptors in the brain. Blockade of NMDA receptors by memantine may slow intracellular calcium accumulation, and help to prevent further nerve damage without interfering with the physiological actions of glutamate that are required for memory and learning.

THERAPEUTIC EFFECTS Improves cognitive functioning in moderate-to-severe Alzheimer's disease (AD) and in mild-to-moderate vascular dementia.

USES Treatment of symptoms of moderate to severe Alzheimer's disease

UNLABELED USES Treatment of moderate to severe vascular dementia

CONTRAINDICATIONS Safety and efficacy in children are unknown.

CAUTIOUS USE Moderate to severe renal impairment; concurrent use with carbonic anhydrase inhibitors, or sodium bicarbonate, pregnancy (category B), lactation.

ROUTE & DOSAGE

Alzheimer's Disease

Adult: **PO** Initiate with 5 mg once daily, increase dose by 5 mg/wk over a 3-wk period to target dose of 10 mg b.i.d.

ADMINISTRATION

Oral

- Note: The recommended interval between dose increases is 1 wk.
- Dose reductions should be considered with moderate renal impairment.
- Store between 15°–30° C (59°–86° F).

ADVERSE EFFECTS (≥1%) **Body as a Whole:** Fatigue, pain, flu-like symptoms, peripheral edema. **CNS:** Dizziness, headache, confusion, somnolence, hallucinations, agitation, insomnia, abnormal gait, depression, anxiety, syncope, TIA, vertigo, ataxia, hypokinesia, aggressive reaction. **CV:** Hypertension, cardiac failure. **GI:** Constipation, vomiting, diarrhea, nausea, anorexia. **Hematologic:** Anemia. **Metabolic:** Weight loss, increased alkaline phosphatase. **Musculoskeletal:** Back pain, arthralgia. **Respiratory:** Coughing, dyspnea, bronchitis, upper respiratory infections, pneumonia. **Skin:** Rash. **Special Senses:** Conjunctivitis. **Urogenital:** Urinary incontinence, UTI, frequent micturition.

INTERACTIONS Drug: Drugs that increase the pH of the urine (CARBONIC ANHYDRASE INIBITORS, **sodium bicarbonate**) may increase levels of memantine; may enhance the effects of **amantadine, dextromethorphan, ketamine, bromocriptine, pergolide, pramipexole,** and **ropinirole;** may enhance the adverse effects of **levodopa**-containing drugs.

M

PHARMACOKINETICS Absorption: 100% absorbed from GI tract. **Duration:** 4–6 h. **Distribution:** Easily crosses the blood-brain barrier. **Metabolism:** Minimal metabolism. **Elmination:** Primarily excreted unchanged in urine. Increases in urinary pH can decrease elimination of drug. **Half-Life:** 60–80 h.

NURSING IMPLICATIONS

Assessment & Drug Effects

- Monitor respiratory and CV status, especially with preexisting heart disease.
- Assess for and report S&S of focal neurologic deficits (e.g., TIA, ataxia, vertigo).
- Lab tests: Periodic Hct & Hgb, serum sodium, alkaline phosphatase, and blood glucose.
- Monitor diabetics for loss of glycemic control.

Patient & Family Education

- Report any of the following to the physician: problems with vision, skin rash, shortness of breath, swelling in throat or tongue, agitation or restlessness, confusion, dizziness, or incontinence.
- Do not drive or engage in other hazardous activities until reaction to drug is known.
- Do not breast feed while taking this drug.

MEPERIDINE HYDROCHLORIDE

(me-per'i-deen)

Demerol, Pethadol ✦, Pethidine Hydrochloride ✦

Classifications: CENTRAL NERVOUS SYSTEM AGENT; NARCOTIC (OPIATE) AGONIST ANALGESIC

Prototype: Morphine

Pregnancy Category: B (D at term)

Controlled Substance: Schedule II

AVAILABILITY 50 mg, 100 mg tablets; 50 mg/5 mL syrup; 10 mg/mL, 25 mg/mL, 50 mg/mL, 75 mg/mL, 100 mg/mL injection

ACTIONS Synthetic morphine-like compound. Chemically dissimilar to morphine, but in equianalgesic doses it is qualitatively comparable. Usual doses produce either no pupillary change or slight miosis, but overdosage results in marked miosis or mydriasis. Also, unlike morphine, has little or no antidiarrheic or antitussive action. Produces CNS stimulation in toxic doses.

THERAPEUTIC EFFECTS Control of moderate to severe pain.

USES Relief of moderate to severe pain, for preoperative medication, for support of anesthesia, and for obstetric analgesia.

CONTRAINDICATIONS Hypersensitivity to meperidine; convulsive disorders; acute abdominal conditions prior to diagnosis; pregnancy prior to labor [(category B), at term (category D)], lactation.

CAUTIOUS USE Head injuries, increased intracranial pressure; asthma and other respiratory conditions; supraventricular tachycardias; prostatic hypertrophy; urethral stricture; glaucoma; older adult or debilitated patients; impaired kidney or liver function, hypothyroidism, Addison's disease.

ROUTE & DOSAGE

Moderate to Severe Pain

Adult: **PO/SC/IM/IV** 50–150 mg q3–4h prn

Child: **PO/SC/IM/IV** 1–1.5 mg/kg q3–4h (max: ≤100 mg q4h) prn

Preoperative

Adult: **IM/SC** 50–150 mg 30–90 min before surgery
Child: **IM/SC** 1–2.2 mg/kg 30–90 min before surgery

Obstetric Analgesia

Adult: **IM/SC** 50–100 mg when pains become regular, may be repeated q1–3h

ADMINISTRATION

Oral

- Give syrup formulation in half a glass of water. Undiluted syrup may cause topical anesthesia of mucous membranes.

Subcutaneous and Intramuscular Injections

- Be aware that SC route is painful and can cause local irritation. IM route is generally preferred when repeated doses are required.
- Aspirate carefully before giving IM injection to avoid inadvertent IV administration. IV injection of undiluted drug can cause a marked increase in heart rate and syncope.

Intravenous

Note: Verify correct IV concentration and rate of infusion/injection for administration to infants or children with physician.

PREPARE: **Direct:** Dilute 50 mg in at least 5 mL of NS or sterile water to yield 10 mg/mL. **IV Infusion:** Dilute to a concentration of 1–10 mg/mL in NS, D5W, or other compatible solution.

ADMINISTER: **Direct:** Give at a rate not to exceed 25 mg/min. Slower injection preferred. **IV Infusion:** Usually given through a controlled infusion device at a rate not to exceed 25 mg/min.

INCOMPATIBILITIES **Solution/additive:** **Aminophylline,** BARBITURATES, **floxacillin, furosemide, heparin, methicillin, morphine, phenytoin, sodium bicarbonate.** **Y-site:** **Allopurinol, amphotericin B cholesteryl complex, cefepime, cefoperazone, doxorubicin liposome, furosemide, heparin, idarubicin, imipenem-cilastatin, mezlocillin, minocycline, tetracycline.**

- Store at 15°–30° C (59°–86° F) in tightly closed, light-resistant containers unless otherwise directed by manufacturer.

ADVERSE EFFECTS

(≥1%) **Body as a Whole:** Allergic (*Pruritus,* urticaria, skin rashes, wheal and flare over IV site), profuse perspiration. **CNS:** *Dizziness,* weakness, euphoria, dysphoria, *sedation,* headache, uncoordinated muscle movements, disorientation, decreased cough reflex, miosis, corneal anesthesia, <u>respiratory depression</u>. Toxic doses: muscle twitching, tremors, hyperactive reflexes, excitement, hypersensitivity to external stimuli, agitation, confusion, hallucinations, dilated pupils, <u>convulsions</u>. **CV:** Facial flushing, light-headedness, hypotension, syncope, palpitation, bradycardia, tachycardia, <u>cardiovascular collapse, cardiac arrest (toxic doses)</u>. **GI:** Dry mouth, *nausea,* vomiting, *constipation,* biliary tract spasm. **Urogenital:** Oliguria, urinary retention. **Respiratory:** <u>Respiratory depression in newborn, bronchoconstriction</u> (large doses). **Skin:** Phlebitis (following IV use), pain, tissue irritation and induration, particularly following subcutaneous injection. **Metabolic:** Increased levels of serum amylase, BSP retention, bilirubin, AST, ALT.

DIAGNOSTIC TEST INTERFERENCE

High doses of meperidine may interfere with ***gastric emptying***

studies by causing delay in gastric emptying.

INTERACTIONS Drug: Alcohol and other CNS DEPRESSANTS, **cimetidine** cause additive sedation and CNS depression; AMPHETAMINES may potentiate CNS stimulation; MAO INHIBITORS, **selegiline, furazolidone** may cause excessive and prolonged CNS depression, convulsions, cardiovascular collapse; **phenytoin** may increase toxic meperidine metabolites. **Herbal: St. John's Wort** may increase sedation.

PHARMACOKINETICS Absorption: 50%–60% absorbed from GI tract. **Onset:** 15 min PO; 10 min IM, SC; 5 min IV. **Peak:** 1 h PO, IM, SC. **Duration:** 2–4 h PO, IM, SC; 2 h IV. **Distribution:** Crosses placenta; distributed into breast milk. **Metabolism:** Metabolized in liver. **Elimination:** excreted in urine. **Half-Life:** 3–5 h.

NURSING IMPLICATIONS

Assessment & Drug Effects

- Give narcotic analgesics in the smallest effective dose and for the least period of time compatible with patient's needs.
- Assess patient's need for prn medication. Record time of onset, duration, and quality of pain.
- Note respiratory rate, depth, and rhythm and size of pupils in patients receiving repeated doses. If respirations are 12/min or below and pupils are constricted or dilated (see ACTIONS AND USES) or breathing is shallow, or if signs of CNS hyperactivity are present, consult physician before administering drug.
- Monitor vital signs closely. Heart rate may increase markedly, and hypotension may occur. Meperidine may cause severe hypotension in postoperative patients and those with depleted blood volume.
- Schedule deep breathing, coughing (unless contraindicated), and changes in position at intervals to help to overcome respiratory depressant effects.
- Chart patient's response to drug and evaluate continued need.
- Repeated use can lead to tolerance as well as psychic and physical dependence of the morphine type.
- Be aware that abrupt discontinuation following repeated use results in morphine-like withdrawal symptoms. Symptoms develop more rapidly (within 3 h, peaking in 8–12 h) and are of shorter duration than with morphine. Nausea, vomiting, diarrhea, and pupillary dilatation are less prominent, but muscle twitching, restlessness, and nervousness are greater than produced by morphine.

Patient & Family Education

- Do not smoke and walk without assistance after receiving the drug. Bed side rails may be advisable.
- Be aware nausea, vomiting, dizziness, and faintness associated with fall in BP are more pronounced when walking than when lying down (these symptoms may also occur in patients without pain who are given meperidine). Symptoms are aggravated by the head-up position.
- Do not drive or engage in potentially hazardous activities until any drowsiness and dizziness have passed.
- Do not take other CNS depressants or drink alcohol because of their additive effects.
- Do not breast feed while using this drug.

MEPHENTERMINE SULFATE

(me-fen′ter-meen)
Wyamine
Classifications: AUTONOMIC NERVOUS SYSTEM AGENT; BETA-ADRENERGIC AGONIST (SYMPATHOMIMETIC)
Prototype: Isoproterenol
Pregnancy Category: D

AVAILABILITY 15 mg/mL 30 mg/mL injection

ACTIONS Synthetic sympathomimetic with alpha- and predominant beta-adrenergic activity. Acts by releasing norepinephrine from tissue storage sites. Produces a positive inotropic action and increases cardiac output. Elevation of BP results primarily from increased cardiac output, and to a lesser extent from increased peripheral vasoconstriction. Antiarrhythmic action results from decrease in AV conduction time, atrial refractory period, and conduction time in ventricular muscle.
THERAPEUTIC EFFECTS Heart rate may be reflectively slowed; BP elevated. Antiarrhythmic.

USES Mainly as pressor agent in treatment of hypotension secondary to ganglionic blockade or spinal anesthesia. Also has been used as an emergency measure in therapy of shock secondary to hemorrhage until whole blood replacement is available; as adjunct in treatment of cardiogenic shock, and to abolish certain cardiac arrhythmias.

CONTRAINDICATIONS Shock secondary to hemorrhage (except in emergency). Safety during pregnancy (category D) or lactation is not established.
CAUTIOUS USE Arteriosclerosis; cardiovascular disease; hypovolemia; hypertension; hyperthyroidism; patients with known hypersensitivities; chronically ill patients.

ROUTE & DOSAGE

Hypotension
Adult: **IM/IV** 10–80 mg
Child: **IM/IV** 0.4 mg/kg

Hypotensive Emergency
Adult: **IV** 20–60 mg as an IV infusion (1.2 mg/mL in D5W)

ADMINISTRATION

Intravenous

PREPARE: **Direct:** May give undiluted. **IV Infusion:** Further dilute by adding 600 mg to 50 mL of D5W.
ADMINISTER: **Direct:** Give at a rate of 30 mg/min. **IV Infusion:** Give at a rate of 1–5 mg/min (rate is usually prescribed by physician).
INCOMPATIBILITIES **Solution/additive: Epinephrine, hydralazine.**

- Store at 15°–30° C (59°–86° F) in tightly closed, light-resistant containers unless otherwise directed by manufacturer.

ADVERSE EFFECTS (≥1%) **CNS:** Euphoria, anorexia, weeping, nervousness, anxiety, tremor, seizures, incoherence, drowsiness. **CV:** Tachycardia. With large doses: cardiac arrhythmias, marked elevation of BP.

INTERACTIONS Drug: Mephentermine may be ineffective in patients receiving **reserpine, guanethidine,** PHENOTHIAZINES; MAO INHIBITORS, SYMPATHOMIMETIC AMINES, **furazolidone, isoniazid** may potentiate pressor response; **methyldopa,** TRICYCLIC ANTIDEPRESSANTS may potentiate or inhibit pressor response; **cyclopropane, halothane** may cause serious arrhyth-

M

mia; may increase risk of **digoxin**-induced arrhythmias.

PHARMACOKINETICS Onset: 5–15 min IM; immediate IV. **Duration:** 1–4 h IM; 15–30 min IV. **Metabolism:** Rapidly metabolized in liver. **Elimination:** Excreted in urine.

NURSING IMPLICATIONS

Assessment & Drug Effects

- Observe and monitor BP, HR, ECG, and CVP carefully.
- IV administration: Check BP and pulse q2min until stabilized at prescribed level, then q5min during therapy. Continue monitoring vital signs for at least 45–60 min and longer if indicated after therapy.

MEPHENYTOIN

(me-fen'i-toyn)

Mesantoin

Classifications: CENTRAL NERVOUS SYSTEM AGENT; ANTICONVULSANT; HYDANTOIN

Prototype: Phenytoin

Pregnancy Category: D

AVAILABILITY 100 mg tablets

ACTIONS Precise mechanism of anticonvulsant action unknown, but drug use is accompanied by reduced voltage, frequency and spread of electrical discharges within the motor cortex, resulting in seizure activity inhibition. Reported to have more sedative and hypnotic action than phenytoin. Causes serious toxic reactions more frequently than phenytoin, including fatal blood dyscrasias.

THERAPEUTIC EFFECTS Controls seizure activity of the cortex of the brain. Relatively ineffective for petit mal seizures.

USES Control of grand mal, focal, Jacksonian, and psychomotor seizures in patients refractory to less toxic anticonvulsants. Usually used concomitantly with other antiepilepsy agents.

CONTRAINDICATIONS Use in conjunction with oxazolidinedione anticonvulsant agents [e.g., paramethadione, trimethadione (toxic synergism)] lactation. Safety during pregnancy (category D) is not established.

CAUTIOUS USE History of drug hypersensitivities.

ROUTE & DOSAGE

Seizures

Adult: **PO** 50–100 mg/d during first week, increase weekly to 200–600 mg/d in 3 divided doses
Child: **PO** 3–15 mg/kg/d in 3 divided doses, increase weekly to 100–400 mg/d in 3 divided doses

ADMINISTRATION

Oral

- Given with food to reduce GI distress.
- Do not increase dose until it is taken for at least 1 wk.
- Change from another anticonvulsant agent gradually by increasing dose at weekly intervals and reducing dose of drug to be discontinued over 3–6 wk.

ADVERSE EFFECTS (≥1%) **CNS:** Drowsiness, dizziness. **Skin:** Skin and mucous membrane manifestations (<u>exfoliative dermatitis</u>, erythema multiforme, toxic epidermal necrolysis, other skin rashes). **Hematologic:** <u>Blood dyscrasias (leukopenia, eutropenia, agranulocytosis, thrombocytopenia, aplastic anemia)</u>. **GI:** Hepatic damage. **Body as a Whole:** Periarteritis nodosa, systemic lupus erythematosus syndrome.

DIAGNOSTIC TEST INTERFERENCE Phenytoin (hydantoins) may produce lower than normal values for ***dexamethasone*** or ***metyrapone*** tests; may increase serum levels of ***glucose, BSP,*** and ***alkaline phosphatase*** and may decrease ***PBI*** and ***urinary steroid*** levels.

INTERACTIONS Drug: Alcohol decreases mephenytoin effects; OTHER ANTICONVULSANTS may increase or decrease mephenytoin levels; may decrease absorption and increase metabolism of ORAL ANTICOAGULANTS; increases metabolism of CORTICOSTEROIDS, ORAL CONTRACEPTIVES, and **nisoldipine,** thus decreasing their effectiveness; **amiodarone, chloramphenicol, omeprazole,** and **ticlopidine** increase mephenytoin levels; ANTITUBERCULOSIS AGENTS decrease mephenytoin levels. **Food:** Folic acid, calcium, and vitamin D absorption may be decreased mephenytoin absorption may be decreased by enteral nutrition supplements. **Herbal: Ginkgo** may decrease anticonvulsant effectiveness.

PHARMACOKINETICS Absorption: Readily absorbed from GI tract. **Onset:** 30 min. **Duration:** 24–48 h. **Metabolism:** Metabolized in liver. **Elimination:** Excreted in urine. **Half-Life:** 144 h.

NURSING IMPLICATIONS

Assessment & Drug Effects

- Keep patients under close supervision at all times; drug is associated with severe adverse effects. Serious blood dyscrasias have occurred 2 wk–30 mo after initiation of therapy.
- Lab tests: Baseline liver function, total white cell count, and differential count prior to initiation of therapy. Perform blood studies q2 wk and continue until patient is on maintenance dosage for 2 wk; then repeat monthly for 1 y, and thereafter every 3 mo (unless neutrophil count drops to 2500/mm^3 or 1600/mm^3, then performed every 2 wk).
- Discontinue if neutrophil count falls to 1600/mm^3.

Patient & Family Education

- Avoid potentially hazardous activities until response to drug is known. Be aware that supervision of ambulation may be indicated for some patients during early therapy.
- Report immediately to physician: Onset of drowsiness, ataxia, skin rash, sore throat, fever, mucous membrane bleeding, or glandular swelling. All are indications of developing toxic reaction.
- Discontinue drug gradually to minimize the risk of precipitating seizures or status epilepticus.
- Do not breast feed while using this drug.

M

MEPHOBARBITAL

(me-foe-bar'bi-tal)

Mebaral, Methylphenobarbital

Classifications: CENTRAL NERVOUS SYSTEM AGENT; ANTICONVULSANT; BARBITURATE; SEDATIVE-HYPNOTIC

Prototype: Phenobarbital

Pregnancy Category: D

Controlled Substance: Schedule IV

AVAILABILITY 32 mg, 50 mg, 100 mg tablets

ACTIONS Long-acting barbiturate with pharmacologic properties similar to those of phenobarbital; however, larger doses are required to produce comparable anticonvulsant effects

THERAPEUTIC EFFECTS Limits the spread of seizure activity by increasing the threshold for motor cortex stimuli. Exerts strong sedative effect, but relatively mild hypnotic effect.

USES To control grand mal and petit mal epilepsy, alone or in combination with other anticonvulsant agents, and for sedative effect in management of delirium tremens and other acute agitation and anxiety states.

CONTRAINDICATIONS Hypersensitivity to barbiturates; lactation. Safety during pregnancy (category D) is not established.
CAUTIOUS USE Fever, hyperthyroidism, alcoholism; liver, kidney, or cardiac dysfunction.

ROUTE & DOSAGE

Anticonvulsant
Adult: **PO** 400–600 mg/d in divided doses
Child: **PO** ≤*5 y,* 16–32 mg t.i.d. or q.i.d.; ≥*5 y,* 32–64 mg t.i.d. or q.i.d.

Sedative
Adult: **PO** 32–100 mg t.i.d. or q.i.d.
Child: **PO** ≤*5 y,* 16–32 mg t.i.d. or q.i.d.; ≥*5 y,* 32–64 mg t.i.d. or q.i.d.

Delirium Tremens
Adult: **PO** 200 mg t.i.d. or q.i.d.

ADMINISTRATION

Oral
- Change from other anticonvulsant by gradually tapering off the former as mephobarbital doses are increased to maintain seizure control.
- When prescribed concurrently with phenobarbital, dose should be about one-half the amount of each used alone. When prescribed concurrently with phenytoin, the dose of phenytoin is usually reduced.
- Reduce discontinued drug dosage gradually over 4 or 5 days to avoid precipitating seizures of status epilepticus.

ADVERSE EFFECTS (≥1%) **CNS:** *Drowsiness,* dizziness, unsteadiness, hangover, paradoxical excitement. **GI:** Nausea, vomiting, constipation. **Body as a Whole:** Hypersensitivity reactions, respiratory depression.

INTERACTIONS Drug: Alcohol, CNS DEPRESSANTS compound CNS depression; may decrease absorption and increase metabolism of ORAL ANTICOAGULANTS; increases metabolism of CORTICOSTEROIDS, ORAL CONTRACEPTIVES, ANTICONVULSANTS, **digitoxin,** possibly decreasing their effects; ANTIDEPRESSANTS potentiate adverse effects; **griseofulvin** decreases absorption of mephobarbitol. **Herbal: Kava-kava, valerian** may potentiate sedation.

PHARMACOKINETICS Absorption: 50% absorbed from GI tract. **Onset:** 60 min. **Duration:** 10–12 h. **Metabolism:** Metabolized in liver to phenobarbital. **Elimination:** Excreted in urine. Alkalinization of urine or increase of urinary flow significantly increases the rate of phenobarbital excretion. **Half-Life:** 34 h.

NURSING IMPLICATIONS

Assessment & Drug Effects
- Monitor respiratory status, especially with concurrent CNS therapy with other drugs.
- Be prepared for paradoxical response to barbiturate therapy (i.e., irritability, marked excitement, aggression in children, depression, confusion) in older adults, debilitated patients, or children.

Patient & Family Education

- Be aware that abrupt cessation after prolonged therapy may result in withdrawal symptoms (tremulousness, weakness, insomnia, delirium, convulsions).
- Avoid driving and potentially hazardous activities until response to drug has stabilized.
- Do not take alcohol in any amount with a barbiturate.
- Do not breast feed while using this drug.

MEPROBAMATE Pr

(me-proe-ba'mate)

Equanil, Meprospan, Miltown

Classifications: CENTRAL NERVOUS SYSTEM AGENT; PSYCHOTHERAPEUTIC; CARBAMATE; ANXIOLYTIC; SEDATIVE-HYPNOTIC

Pregnancy Category: D

Controlled Substance: Schedule IV

AVAILABILITY 200 mg, 400 mg 600 mg tablets

ACTIONS Propanediol carbamate derivative structurally and pharmacologically related to carisoprodol. CNS depressant actions similar to those of barbiturates. Acts on multiple sites in CNS and appears to block corticothalamic impulses. No effect on medulla, reticular activating system, or autonomic nervous system.

THERAPEUTIC EFFECTS Antianxiety agent. Hypnotic doses suppress REM sleep.

USES To relieve anxiety and tension of psychoneurotic states and as adjunct in disease states associated with anxiety and tension. Also used to promote sleep in anxious, tense patients.

CONTRAINDICATIONS History of hypersensitivity to meprobamate or related carbamates such as carisoprodol and tybamate; history of acute intermittent porphyria; pregnancy (category D), lactation, children <6 y.

CAUTIOUS USE Impaired kidney or liver function; convulsive disorders; history of alcoholism or drug abuse; patients with suicidal tendencies.

ROUTE & DOSAGE

Sedative

Adult: **PO** 1.2–1.6 g/d in 3–4 divided doses (max: 2.4 g/d)
Child: **PO** 100–200 mg b.i.d. or t.i.d.

Hypnotic

Adult: **PO** 400–800 mg
Geriatric: **PO** 200 mg 2–3 times/d
Child: **PO** 200 mg

ADMINISTRATION

Oral

- Give with food to minimize gastric distress.
- Treatment physical dependence by gradual drug withdrawal over 1–2 wk to prevent onset of withdrawal symptoms.
- Store at 15°–30° C (59°–86° F) unless otherwise specified by manufacturer.

ADVERSE EFFECTS (≥1%) **Body as a Whole:** Allergy or idiosyncratic reactions (itchy, urticarial, or erythematous maculopapular rash; exfoliative dermatitis, petechiae, purpura, ecchymoses, eosinophilia, peripheral edema, angioneurotic edema, adenopathy, fever, chills, proctitis, bronchospasm, oliguria, anuria, Stevens-Johnson syndrome); anaphylaxis. **CNS:** *Drowsiness* and *ataxia,* dizziness, vertigo, slurred speech, headache, weakness, paresthesias, impaired visual accommodation, paradoxic euphoria and rage reactions, seizures in epileptics, panic re-

M

action, rapid EEG activity. **CV:** Hypotensive crisis, syncope, palpitation, tachycardia, arrhythmias, transient ECG changes, circulatory collapse (toxic doses). **GI:** Anorexia, nausea, vomiting, diarrhea. **Hematologic:** Aplastic anemia (rare): leukopenia, agranulocytosis, thrombocytopenia, exacerbation of acute intermittent porphyria. **Respiratory:** Respiratory depression.

DIAGNOSTIC TEST INTERFERENCE Meprobamate may cause falsely high ***urinary steroid*** determinations. ***Phentolamine*** tests may be falsely positive; meprobamate should be withdrawn at least 24 h and preferably 48–72 h before the test.

INTERACTIONS Drug: Alcohol entacapone, TRICYCLIC ANTIDEPRESSANTS, ANTIPSYCHOTICS, OPIATES, SEDATING ANTIHISTAMINES, **pentazocine, tramadol,** MAOIS, SEDATIVE-HYPNOTICS, ANIXIOLYTICS may potentiate CNS depression. **Herbal: Kava-kava, valerian** may potentiate sedation.

PHARMACOKINETICS Absorption: Well absorbed from GI tract. **Peak:** 1–3 h. **Onset:** 1 h. **Distribution:** Uniformly distributed throughout body; crosses placenta. **Metabolism:** Rapidly metabolized in liver. **Elimination:** Renally excreted; excreted in breast milk. **Half-Life:** 10–11 h.

NURSING IMPLICATIONS

Assessment & Drug Effects

- Supervise ambulation, if necessary. Older adults and debilitated patients are prone to oversedation and to the hypotensive effects, especially during early therapy.
- Utilize safety precautions for hospitalized patients. Hypnotic doses may cause increased motor activity during sleep.
- Consult physician if daytime psychomotor function is impaired. A change in regimen or drug may be indicated.
- Withdraw gradually in physically dependent patients to prevent preexisting symptoms or withdrawal reactions within 12–48 h: Vomiting, ataxia, muscle twitching, mental confusion, hallucinations, convulsions, trembling, sleep disturbances, increased dreaming, nightmares, insomnia. Symptoms usually subside within 12–48 h.

Patient & Family Education

- Take drug as prescribed. Psychic or physical dependence may occur with long-term use of high doses.
- Be aware that tolerance to alcohol will be lowered.
- Make position changes slowly, especially from lying down to upright; dangle legs for a few minutes before standing.
- Avoid driving or engaging in hazardous activities until response to drug is known.
- Report immediately onset of skin rash, sore throat, fever, bruising, unexplained bleeding.
- Do not breast feed while using this drug.

MEQUINOL/TRETINOIN

(me-qui′nol/tre-ti′noyn)
Solagé
Classifications: SKIN AND MUCOUS MEMBRANE AGENT; RETINOID
Prototype: Isotretinoin
Pregnancy Category: X

AVAILABILITY Mequinol 2%/tretinoin 0.01% 30 mL solution

ACTIONS Mequinol is a depigmenting agent and tretinoin is a retinoid used to improve dermatologic changes (e.g., fine wrinkling, mottled hyperpigmentation, roughness) associated with photo-damage and aging. Sun avoidance, as well as a comprehensive skin care plan (e.g., emollient creams, sunscreen, protective clothing), is very important in controlling age spots.

THERAPEUTIC EFFECTS Mequinol's mechanism of depigmentation is probably due to oxidation by tyrosine to cytotoxic products in metanocytes, and/or inhibition of melanin formation. Tretinoin, a retinoid, is used to improve photodamage to the skin by acting via retinoic acid receptors (RARs).

USES Treatment of solar lentigines.

CONTRAINDICATIONS Pregnancy (category X), lactation, hypersensitivity to mequinol, tretinoin.

CAUTIOUS USE History of hypersensitivity to acitretin, isotretinoin, etretinate, or other vitamin A derivatives, or hydroquinone; patients with eczema, moderate to severe skin pigmentation, vitiligo; concurrent use of photosensitive medications (e.g., thiazide diuretics, fluoroquinolones, phenothiazines, sulfonamides), concurrent use of astringents; cold weather.

ROUTE & DOSAGE

Solar Lentigines

Adult: **Topical** Apply to solar lentigines b.i.d. at least 8 h apart

ADMINISTRATION

Topical

- Apply doses at least 8 h apart; avoid application to unaffected areas.
- Avoid contact with eyes, lips, mucus membranes, or paranasal creases.
- Protect from light.

ADVERSE EFFECTS (≥1%) **Skin:** *Erythema, burning, stinging, tingling, desquamation, pruritus,* skin irritation, temporary hypopigmentation, rash, dry skin, crusting, application site reaction.

INTERACTIONS Drug: THIAZIDE DIURETICS, TETRACYCLINES, FLUOROQUINOLONES, PHENOTHIAZINES, SULFONAMIDES may augment phototoxicity.

PHARMACOKINETICS Absorption: 4.4% absorbed through skin. **Peak:** 1–2 h.

NURSING IMPLICATIONS

Assessment & Drug Effects

- Monitor for and report peeling, erythema, or hypopigmentation.
- Monitor for signs of tretinoin toxicity: headache, fever, weakness, and fatigue.

Patient & Family Education

- Do not apply larger than recommended amounts.
- Do not wash affected area for at least 6 h after drug application; do not apply cosmetics to affected area for at least 30 min after drug application.
- Minimize exposure to sunlight or sunlamps. Use extra caution if also taking concurrently other drugs that are photosensitizing (e.g., thiazide diuretics, phenothiazines).
- Notify physician if vitiligo (hypopigmentation of skin) or S&S of tretinoin toxicity develop (see ASSESSMENT & DRUG EFFECTS).
- Do not breast feed while taking this drug.

M

MERCAPTOPURINE (6-MP, 6-MERCAPTOPURINE)

(mer-kap-toe-pyoor′een)

Purinethol

Classifications: ANTINEOPLASTIC; ANTIMETABOLITE; IMMUNOSUPPRESSANT

Prototype: Fluorouracil

Pregnancy Category: D

AVAILABILITY 50 mg tablets

ACTIONS Antimetabolite and purine antagonist. Inhibits purine metabolism by unclear mechanism. Blocks conversion of inosinic acid to adenine and xanthine ribotides within sensitive tumor cells. Also inhibits adenine-containing coenzymes, suggesting an influence over multiple cellular reactions.

THERAPEUTIC EFFECTS Delayed immunosuppressive properties and carcinogenic potential.

USES Primarily for acute lymphocytic and myelogenous leukemia. Response in adults is less than in children, but mercaptopurine is initial drug of choice. In chronic granulocytic leukemia, produces temporary remission.

UNLABELED USES Prevention of transplant graft rejection; SLE; rheumatoid arthritis; Crohn's disease.

CONTRAINDICATIONS Prior resistance to mercaptopurine; first trimester of pregnancy (category D); lactation; infections.

CAUTIOUS USE Impaired kidney or liver function; concomitant use with allopurinol.

ROUTE & DOSAGE

Leukemias

Adult/Child: **PO Loading Dose** 2.5 mg/kg/d, may increase up to 5 mg/kg/d after 4 wk if needed **PO Maintenance Dose** 1.25–2.5 mg/kg/d

ADMINISTRATION

Oral

- Give total daily dose at one time.
- Reduce dose of mercaptopurine usually by 1/3–1/4 when given concurrently with allopurinol.
- Store tablets in light- and air-resistant container.

ADVERSE EFFECTS (≥1%) **GI:** Stomatitis, esophagitis, anorexia, nausea, vomiting, diarrhea, intestinal ulcerations, impaired liver function, hepatic necrosis. **Hematologic:** Leukopenia, anemia, eosinophilia, pancytopenia, thrombocytopenia, abnormal bleeding, bone marrow hypoplasia. **Urogenital:** Hyperuricemia, oliguria, renal impairment. **Skin:** Rash. **Body as a Whole:** Drug fever.

INTERACTIONS Drug: Allopurinol may inhibit metabolism and thus increase toxicity of mercaptopurine; may potentiate or antagonize anticoagulant effects of **warfarin.**

PHARMACOKINETICS Absorption: Approximately 50% absorbed from GI tract. **Peak:** 2 h. **Distribution:** Distributes into total body water. **Metabolism:** Rapidly metabolized by xanthine oxidase in liver. **Elimination:** 11% excreted in urine within 6 h. **Half-Life:** 20–50 min.

NURSING IMPLICATIONS

Assessment & Drug Effects

- Lab tests: Monitor CBC with differential, platelet count, Hgb, Hct, and liver functions closely.
- Monitor for S&S of liver damage. Hepatic toxicity occurs most often when dose exceeds 2.5 mg/kg/d. Jaundice signals onset of hepatic toxicity and may necessitate terminating use.
- Withhold drug and notify physician at the first sign of an abnormally large or rapid fall in platelet and leukocyte counts.
- Record baseline data related to I&O ratio and pattern and body weight.
- Check vital signs daily. Report febrile states promptly.
- Protect patient from exposure to trauma, infections, or other

stresses (restrict visitors and personnel who have colds) during periods of leukopenia.
- Report nausea, vomiting, or diarrhea. These may signal excessive dosage, especially in adults.
- Watch for signs of abnormal bleeding (ecchymoses, petechiae, melena, bleeding gums) if thrombocytopenia develops; report immediately.

Patient & Family Education
- Report any signs of bleeding (e.g., hematuria, bruising, bleeding gums).
- Report signs of hepatic toxicity (see Appendix F).
- Increase hydration (10–12 glasses of fluid daily) to reduce risk of hyperuricemia. Consult physician about desirable volume.
- Notify physician of onset of chills, nausea, vomiting, flank or joint pain, swelling of legs or feet, or symptoms of anemia.
- Do not breast feed while using this drug.

MEROPENEM

(mer-o′pe-nem)
Merrem
Classifications: ANTIINFECTIVE; CARBAPENEM ANTIBIOTIC
Prototype: Imipenem
Pregnancy Category: B

AVAILABILITY 500 mg, 1 g injection

ACTIONS Broad-spectrum carbapenem antibiotic that inhibits the cell wall synthesis of gram-positive and gram-negative bacteria by its strong affinity for penicillin-binding proteins of bacterial cell wall.
THERAPEUTIC EFFECTS Effective against both gram-positive and gram-negative bacteria. High resistance to most bacterial beta-lactamases. Do not use to treat methicillin-resistant *Staphylococci* (MRSA).

USES Complicated appendicitis and peritonitis, bacterial meningitis caused by susceptible bacteria.
UNLABELED USES Other intraabdominal infections, skin/soft tissue infections, febrile neutropenia.

CONTRAINDICATIONS Hypersensitivity to meropenem, other carbapenem antibiotics including imipenem, penicillins, cephalosporins, or other beta-lactams; lactation.
CAUTIOUS USE History of asthma or allergies, renal impairment, epileptics, history of neurologic disorders, older adult, pregnancy (category B). Safety and effectiveness in infants <3 mo not established.

ROUTE & DOSAGE

Intraabdominal Infections
Adult: **IV** 1 g q8h
Child: **IV** *≥3 mo,* 20 mg/kg q8h (max: 1 g q8h)
Bacterial Meningitis
Adult: **IV** 2 g q8h
Child: **IV** *≥3 mo,* 40 mg/kg q8h (max: 2 g q8h)
Renal Impairment
Cl_{cr} 26–50 mL/min: 1 g q12h; 10–25 mL/min: 500 mg q12h; <10 mL/min: 500 mg q24h

ADMINISTRATION

Intravenous

Note: Dosage reduction is recommended for older adults.

PREPARE: **Direct:** Reconstitute the 500-mg or 1-g vial, respectively, by adding 10 or 20 mL sterile water for injection to yield approximately 50 mg/mL. Shake to dissolve and let stand until clear.

M

IV Infusion: Further dilute in 50–100 mL of D5W, NS, or D5/NS.
ADMINISTER: **Direct:** Give over 3–5 min. **IV Infusion:** Give over 15–30 min.
INCOMPATIBILITIES **Solution/additive: Ringers lactate, mannitol, amphotericin B, metronidazole, multivitamins. Y-site: Amphotericin B, diazepam, metronidazole.**

- Store undiluted at 15°–30° C (59°–86° F), diluted IV solutions should generally be used within 1 h of preparation.

ADVERSE EFFECTS (≥1%) **GI:** Diarrhea, nausea, vomiting, constipation. **Other:** Inflammation at injection site, phlebitis, thrombophlebitis. **CNS:** Headache. **Skin:** Rash, pruritus, diaper rash. **Body as a Whole:** Apnea, oral moniliasis, sepsis, shock. **Hematologic:** Anemia.

M

INTERACTIONS Drug: Probenecid will delay meropenem excretion; may decrease **valproic acid** serum levels.

PHARMACOKINETICS Distribution: Attains high concentrations in bile, bronchial secretions, cerebrospinal fluid. **Metabolism:** Undergoes renal and extrarenal metabolism via dipeptidases or nonspecific degradation. **Elimination:** Excreted primarily in urine. **Half-Life:** 0.8–1 h.

NURSING IMPLICATIONS

Assessment & Drug Effects

- Lab tests: Perform C&S tests prior to therapy. Monitor periodically liver and kidney function.
- Determine history of hypersensitivity reactions to other beta-lactams, cephalosporins, penicillins, or other drugs.
- Discontinue drug and immediately report S&S of hypersensitivity (see Appendix F).
- Report S&S of superinfection or pseudomembranous colitis (see Appendix F).
- Monitor for seizures especially in older adults and those with renal insufficiency.

Patient & Family Education

- Learn S&S of hypersensitivity, superinfection, and pseudomembranous colitis; report any of these to physician promptly.
- Do not breast feed while using this drug.

MESALAMINE Pr

(me-sal′a-meen)

Asacol, Canasa, Rowasa, Salofalk ✤, Pentasa

Classifications: SKIN AND MUCOUS MEMBRANE AGENT; ANTIINFLAMMATORY; PROSTAGLANDIN INHIBITOR

Pregnancy Category: B

AVAILABILITY 250 mg controlled release capsule (Pentasa); 400 mg delayed release tablet (Asacol); 500 mg suppository, 4 g/60 mL rectal suspension (Rowasa); 500 mg suppositories (Canasa)

ACTIONS Thought to diminish inflammation by blocking cyclooxygenase and inhibiting prostaglandin synthesis in the colon.
THERAPEUTIC EFFECTS Provides topical antiinflammatory action in the colon of patients with ulcerative colitis.

USES Indicated in active mild to moderate distal ulcerative colitis, proctosigmoiditis, or proctitis; maintenance of remission of ulcerative colitis.
UNLABELED USES Crohn's disease.

CONTRAINDICATIONS Hypersensitivity to mesalamine, aminosalicylates, or salicylates.

CAUTIOUS USE Renal impairment, renal disease, renal failure, pregnancy (category B), lactation; older adults; sulfite hypersensitivity; sensitivity to sulfasalazine.

ROUTE & DOSAGE

Ulcerative Colitis
Adult: **Rectal** (Rowasa) 4 g once/d h.s., enema should be retained for about 8 h if possible or 1 suppository (500 mg) b.i.d.; (Canasa) 500 mg b.i.d., may increase up to 500 mg t.i.d. **PO** (Asacol) 800 mg t.i.d. times 6 wk; (Pentasa) 500 mg t.i.d. times 6 wk. **Maintenance Dose** (Asacol) 800 mg b.i.d. or 400 mg q.i.d.
Child: **PO** 50 mg/kg/d divided q6–12h

ADMINISTRATION

Oral
- Ensure that controlled-release and enteric forms of the drug are not crushed or chewed.
- Shake the bottle well to make sure the suspension is mixed.

Rectal
- Use rectal suspension at bedtime with the objective of retaining it all night.
- Store at 15°–30° C (59°–86° F) away from heat and light.

ADVERSE EFFECTS (≥1%) **CNS:** *Headache,* fatigue, asthenia, malaise, weakness, dizziness. **GI:** *Abdominal pain, cramps,* or *discomfort,* flatulence, nausea, diarrhea, constipation, hemorrhoids, rectal pain, hepatitis (rare). **Skin:** Sensitivity reactions, rash, pruritus, alopecia. **Body as a Whole:** Fever. **Hematologic:** Thrombocytopenia (rare), eosinophilia. **Urogenital:** Interstitial nephritis.

PHARMACOKINETICS Absorption: PR 5%–35% absorbed from colon depending on retention time of enema or suppository. PO Asacol, approximately 28% absorbed; 80% of drug is released in colon 12 h after ingestion. PO Pentasa, 50% of drug is released in colon at a pH <6. **Peak:** 3–6 h. **Distribution:** Rectal administration may reach as high as the ascending colon. Asacol is released in the ileum and colon; Pentasa is released in the jejunum, ileum, and colon. Low concentrations of mesalamine and higher concentrations of its metabolites are excreted in breast milk. **Metabolism:** Rapidly acetylated in the liver and colon wall. **Elimination:** Excreted primarily in feces; absorbed drug excreted in urine. **Half-Life:** 2–15 h (depending on formulation).

NURSING IMPLICATIONS

Assessment & Drug Effects
- Lab tests: Monitor carefully urinalysis, BUN, and creatinine, especially in patients with preexisting kidney disease. The kidney is the major target organ for toxicity.
- Assess for S&S of allergic-type reactions (e.g., hives, itching, wheezing, anaphylaxis). Suspension contains a sulfite that may cause reactions in asthmatics and some nonasthmatic persons.
- Expect response to therapy within 3–21 d; however, the usual course of therapy is from 3–6 wk depending on symptoms and sigmoidoscopic examinations.

Patient & Family Education
- Report to physician promptly: Cramping, abdominal pain, or bloody diarrhea, which are indications for immediate drug withdrawal.
- Check with doctor if rectal irritation (e.g., bleeding, blistering, pain, burning, itching) occurs while using this drug.

- Check with physician before using any new medicine (prescription or OTC).
- Continue medication for full time of treatment even if you are feeling better.
- Do not breast feed while taking this drug without consulting physician.

MESNA

(mes'na)

Mesnex

Classifications: ANTIDOTE; DETOXIFYING AGENT

Pregnancy Category: B

AVAILABILITY 100 mg/mL injection

ACTIONS Detoxifying agent used to inhibit the hemorrhagic cystitis induced by ifosfamide. Analogous to the physiological cysteine-cystine system.

THERAPEUTIC EFFECTS In the kidney, thiol compound reacts chemically with urotoxic ifosfamide metabolites, resulting in their detoxification, and thus significantly decreases the incidence of hematuria.

USES Prophylaxis for ifosfamide-induced hemorrhagic cystitis. Not effective in preventing hematuria due to other pathologic conditions such as thrombocytopenia.

UNLABELED USES Reduces the incidence of cyclophosphamide-induced hemorrhagic cystitis.

CONTRAINDICATIONS Hypersensitivity to mesna or other thiol compounds; lactation.

CAUTIOUS USE Pregnancy (category B); only if the benefits clearly outweigh any possible risk to fetus.

ROUTE & DOSAGE

Use with Ifosfamide

Adult: **IV** Dose = 20% of ifosfamide dose and is given at time of ifosfamide administration and 4 and 8 h after ifosfamide administration

Child: Not established

ADMINISTRATION

Note: To be effective, mesna must be administered with each dose of ifosfamide.

Intravenous

PREPARE: **Direct:** Add 4 mL of D5W, NS, or RL for each 100 mg of mesna to yield 20 mg/mL.

ADMINISTER: **Direct:** Give a single dose by direct IV over 60 s.

INCOMPATIBILITIES **Solution/additive: Carboplatin, cisplatin, ifosfamide with epirubicin. Y-site: Amphotericin B cholesteryl complex.**

- Inspect parenteral drug products visually for particulate matter and discoloration prior to administration. ■Discard any unused portion of the ampul because drug oxidizes on contact with air.

- Refrigerate diluted solutions or use within 6 h of mixing even though diluted solutions are chemically and physically stable for 24 h at 25° C (77° F). ■Store unopened ampul at 15°–30° C (59°–86° F) unless otherwise specified.

ADVERSE EFFECTS (≥1%) **GI:** *Bad taste in mouth, soft stools,* nausea, vomiting.

DIAGNOSTIC TEST INTERFERENCE May produce a false-positive result in test for ***urinary ketones.***

INTERACTIONS No clinically significant interactions established.

PHARMACOKINETICS Metabolism: Rapidly oxidized in liver to active metabolite dimesna; dimesna is further metabolized in kidney. **Elimination:** 65% excreted in urine within 24 h. **Half-Life:** Mesna 0.36 h, dimesna 1.17 h.

NURSING IMPLICATIONS

Assessment & Drug Effects

- Monitor urine for hematuria.
- Be aware that a false-positive test for urinary ketones may arise in patients treated with mesna. In this test, a red-violet color develops that, with the addition of glacial acetic acid, will turn to violet.
- About 6% of patients treated with mesna along with ifosfamide still develop hematuria.

Patient & Family Education

- Mesna prevents ifosfamide-induced hemorrhagic cystitis; it will not prevent or alleviate other adverse reactions or toxicities associated with ifosfamide therapy.
- Report any unusual or allergic reactions to physician.
- Check with physician before using any new prescription or OTC medicine.
- Do not breast feed while using this drug.

MESORIDAZINE BESYLATE

(mez-oh-rid'a-zeen)

Serentil

Classifications: CENTRAL NERVOUS SYSTEM AGENT; PSYCHOTHERAPEUTIC; PHENOTHIAZINE; ANTIPSYCHOTIC

Prototype: Chlorpromazine

Pregnancy Category: C

AVAILABILITY 10 mg, 25 mg, 50 mg, 100 mg tablets; 25 mg/mL oral solution; 25 mg/mL injection

ACTIONS Piperidine derivative of phenothiazine. Tranquilizer with stronger sedative action than produced by chlorpromazine, but has more antiemetic action and lower incidence of extrapyramidal adverse effects.

THERAPEUTIC EFFECTS Antipsychotic effect due to psychomotor slowing and reduction of emotional stress.

USES Second-line therapy for schizophrenia, behavioral problems in mental deficiency and chronic brain syndrome, acute and chronic alcoholism. Also to reduce symptoms of anxiety and tension associated with many neurotic disorders.

CONTRAINDICATIONS Known sensitivity to other phenothiazines; severely depressed (drug-induced) patient; comatose state; children <12 y. Safety during pregnancy (category C) or lactation is not established.

CAUTIOUS USE Previously detected cancer of breast; glaucoma; prostatic hypertrophy, urinary retention; history of cardiovascular disease (can prolong QTc interval).

ROUTE & DOSAGE

Psychotic Disorders

Adult: **PO** 10–50 mg b.i.d. or t.i.d., may increase as needed up to 400 mg/d **IM** 25 mg, may repeat in 30–60 min if necessary

Dementia Behavior

Geriatric: **PO** 10 mg 1–2 times/d, may gradually increase q4–7d (max: 250 mg/d)

Management of Hyperactivity

Adult: **PO** 25 mg t.i.d. up to 75–300 mg/d

Alcohol Dependence

Adult: **PO** 25 mg b.i.d. up to 50–200 mg/d

Anxiety & Tension
Adult: **PO** 10 mg b.i.d. up to 150 mg/d

ADMINISTRATION

Oral

- Measure drug with calibrated dispenser included in original package. Dilute oral concentrate in about 1/2 glass (120 mL) of fluid just before administration. Use fruit juices, water, soup, carbonated beverage.

Intramuscular

- Inject IM solution slowly and deeply into upper outer quadrant of buttock. Advise patient to lie still for 20–30 min after the injection to minimize possible dizziness.
- Slight yellowing of the solution will not change potency; however, darkened solution should be discarded.
- Store at 15°–30° C (59°–86° F); refrigeration is not necessary. Protect solution from light and freezing.

M

ADVERSE EFFECTS (≥1%) **CNS:** Dizziness, *sedation,* fainting, extrapyramidal effects, dystonic reactions, akathisia, tardive dyskinesia, neuroleptic malignant syndrome. **Special Senses:** Blurred vision, xerostomia, nasal congestion. **Urogenital:** Urinary retention or incontinence, ejaculation dysfunction, impotence, priapism. **GI:** Constipation. **Body as a Whole:** Decreased sweating. **Skin:** Rash, exfoliative dermatitis photosensitivity. **CV:** Tachycardia, *orthostatic hypotension,* arrhythmias (prolong QTc interval) heart block.

INTERACTIONS Drug: amiodarone, amoxapine, astemizole, bepridil, cisapride, clarithromycin, daunorubicin, diltiazem, disopyramide, dofetilide, dolasetron, doxorubicin, encainide, erythromycin, flecainide, gatifloxacin, grepafloxacin, haloperidol, ibutilide, indapamide, LOCAL ANESTHETICS, **maprotiline, moxifloxacin, octreotide, pentamidine, pimozide, procainamide, probucol, quinidine, risperidone, sotalol, sparfloxacin, tocainide,** TRICYCLIC ANTIDEPRESSANTS, **verapamil,** and **ziprasidone** prolong the QTc interval and can cause arrhythmias; **amantadine, clozapine, cyclobenzaprine, diphenoxylate, olanzapine, orphenadrine,** SEDATING H_1-BLOCKERS may have additive anticholinergic effects; **entacapone, tolcapone, pramipexole, ropinirole** ANTICONVULSANTS may cause additive drowsiness and CNS depressant effects. **Herbal: Kava-kava** may increase risk and severity of dystonic reactions.

PHARMACOKINETICS Absorption: Readily absorbed from GI tract. **Peak:** 2 h PO; 30 min IM. **Duration:** 4–6 h PO; 6–8 h IM. **Metabolism:** Metabolized in liver. **Elimination:** Excreted in urine and bile. **Half-Life:** 24–48 h.

NURSING IMPLICATIONS

Assessment & Drug Effects

- Monitor I&O and bowel elimination patterns and check bladder for distension. Depressed patients often fail to report urinary discomfort or constipation.
- Report to physician if patient complains of blurred vision. Periodic ophthalmic examinations are advisable with long-term therapy.
- Monitor BP with patient supine and standing.

Patient & Family Education

- Avoid spilling drug on skin since it may cause contact dermatitis. Thoroughly rinse off with water if spilling occurs.
- Do not drive or engage in potentially hazardous activities until re-

sponse to drug is known. Dizziness and drowsiness are possible during early period of therapy.

- Expect drowsiness to decrease with continued therapy. If it persists consult physician. A change in time of administration or dose may help to prevent interference with normal physical activities.
- Dangle legs at bedside when rising because of possible orthostatic hypotension.
- Avoid alcohol during therapy.
- Relieve dry mouth by rinsing frequently with water, sucking hard candy.
- Do not breast feed while taking this drug without consulting physician.

METAPROTERENOL SULFATE

(met-a-proe-ter′e-nole)

Alupent, Metaprel

Classifications: AUTONOMIC NERVOUS SYSTEM AGENT; BETA-ADRENERGIC AGONIST; BRONCHODILATOR

Prototype: Albuterol

Pregnancy Category: C

AVAILABILITY 10 mg, 20 mg tablet; 10 mg/5 mL syrup; 75 mg, 150 mg metered dose inhaler; 0.4%, 0.6%, 5% solution for inhalation

ACTIONS Potent synthetic sympathomimetic amine similar to isoproterenol in chemical structure and pharmacologic actions. Acts selectively on beta$_2$-adrenergic receptors to relax smooth muscle of bronchi, uterus, and blood vessels supplying skeletal muscles.

THERAPEUTIC EFFECTS Bronchodilator; controls bronchospasm in asthmatics.

USES Bronchodilator in symptomatic relief of asthma and reversible bronchospasm associated with bronchitis and emphysema.

UNLABELED USES Treatment and prophylaxis of heart block and to avert progress of premature labor (tocolytic action).

CONTRAINDICATIONS Sensitivity to other sympathomimetic agents; cardiac arrhythmias associated with tachycardia; hyperthyroidism; pregnancy (category C), lactation. Safety in children <12 y (for aerosol use) is not established.

CAUTIOUS USE Older adults; hypertension, cardiovascular disorders including coronary artery disease; hyperthyroidism; diabetes.

ROUTE & DOSAGE

Bronchospasm

Adult: **PO** 20 mg q6–8h **Metered Dose Inhaler** 2–3 inhalations q3–4h (max: 12 inhalations/d) **Nebulizer** 5–10 inhalations of undiluted 5% solution **IPPB** 2.5 mL of 0.4–0.6% solution q4–6h
Geriatric: **PO** 10 mg 3–4 times/d, may increase to 20 mg 3–4 times/d
Child: **PO** *<2 y,* 0.4 mg/kg t.i.d.–q.i.d.; *2–6 y,* 1.2–2.6 mg/kg/d in 3–4 divided doses; *6–9 y,* 10 mg q6–8h; *>9 y,* 20 mg q6–8h

ADMINISTRATION

- Note: Patient may use tablets and aerosol concomitantly.

Oral

- Give with food to reduce GI distress.

Inhalation

- Instruct patient to shake metered dose aerosol container, exhale through nose as completely as possible, administer aerosol while inhaling deeply through mouth, and to hold breath about 10 seconds

before exhaling slowly. Administer second inhalation 10 min after first.
- Store all forms at 15°–30° C (59°–86° F); protect from light and heat.

ADVERSE EFFECTS (≥1%) **CNS:** Nervousness, weakness, drowsiness, *tremor (particularly after PO administration),* headache, fatigue. **CV:** *Tachycardia,* hypertension, cardiac arrest, palpitation. **GI:** Nausea, vomiting, bad taste. **Urogenital:** Occasional difficulty in micturition and muscle cramps. **Respiratory:** Throat irritation, cough, exacerbation of asthma.

INTERACTIONS Drug: Epinephrine other SYMPATHOMIMETIC BRONCHODILATORS may compound effects of metaproterenol; MAO INHIBITORS, TRICYCLIC ANTIDEPRESSANTS potentiate action of metaproterenol on vascular system; the effects of both metaproterenol and BETA-ADRENERGIC BLOCKERS are antagonized.

PHARMACOKINETICS Absorption: 40% of PO doses reach systemic circulation. **Onset:** Inhaled: 1 min; PO 15 min. **Peak:** 1 h all routes. **Duration:** Inhaled: 1–5 h; PO 4 h. **Metabolism:** Metabolized in liver. **Elimination:** Excreted in urine.

NURSING IMPLICATIONS

Assessment & Drug Effects
- Monitor respiratory status. Auscultate lungs before and after inhalation to determine efficacy of drug in decreasing airway resistance.
- Monitor cardiac status. Report tachycardia and hypotension.

Patient & Family Education
- Report failure to respond to usual dose. Drug may have shorter duration of action after long-term use.
- Do not increase dose or frequency unless ordered by physician; there is the possibility of serious adverse effects.
- Anticipate tremor as a possible adverse effect.
- Do not breast feed while taking this drug without consulting physician.

METFORMIN (Pr)
(met-for'min)
Fortamet, Glucophage, Glucophage XR, Riomet
Classifications: HORMONES & SYNTHETIC SUBSTITUTES; ANTIDIABETIC AGENT; BIGUANIDES
Pregnancy Category: B

AVAILABILITY 500 mg, 850 mg tablets; 500 mg, 750 mg, 1000 mg sustained-release tablets; 100 mg/mL oral solution

ACTIONS Biguanide oral hypoglycemic agent. Unlike sulfonylureas, biguanides do not stimulate the release of insulin from the beta cells of the pancreas. Mechanism of action is thought to be due to both increasing the binding of insulin to its receptor and potentiating insulin action.
THERAPEUTIC EFFECTS Improves tissue sensitivity to insulin, increases glucose transport into skeletal muscles and fat, and suppresses gluconeogenesis and hepatic production of glucose, thus lowering blood glucose levels.

USES Treatment of type 2 diabetes mellitus in patients not controlled with diet alone. May be used with an oral sulfonylurea.

CONTRAINDICATIONS Hypersensitivity to metformin; hepatic or cardiopulmonary insufficiency; alcoholism; concurrent infection; acute MI, cardiogenic shock; diabetic ketoacidosis; hypoxemia, lactic acidosis; radiographic contrast administration; renal disease, renal failure, renal impairment; sepsis; surgery; children <10 y, lactation.

CAUTIOUS USE Previous hypersensitivity to phenformin or buformin; anemia; coma; dehydration, diarrhea; older adults; ethanol intoxication; fever; gastroparesis, GI obstruction; heart failure; hyperthyroidism, pituitary insufficiency; polycystic ovary syndrome; trauma, emesis; pregnancy (category B).

ROUTE & DOSAGE

Type 2 Diabetes Mellitus

Adult: **PO** Start with 500 mg q.d. to t.i.d. or 850 mg q.d. to b.i.d. with meals, may increase by 500–850 mg/d every 1–3 wk (max: 2550 mg/d); or start with 500 mg sustained-release with p.m. meal, may increase by 500 mg/d at p.m. meal qwk (max: 2000 mg/d)

ADMINISTRATION

Oral

- Ensure that extend-release tablets are not crushed or chewed. They must be swallowed whole.
- Use a calibrated oral syringe or container to measure the oral solution for accurate dosing.
- Give with or shortly after main meals.
- Withhold metformin 48 h before and 48 h after receiving IV contrast dye.
- Make dose increment, if needed, at 2- to 3-wk intervals.
- Store at 15°–30° C (59°–86° F).

ADVERSE EFFECTS (≥1%) **CNS:** Headache, dizziness, agitation, fatigue. **Metabolic:** Lactic acidosis. **GI:** *Nausea, vomiting, abdominal pain, bitter or metallic taste, diarrhea, bloatedness, anorexia;* malabsorption of amino acids, vitamin B_{12}, and folic acid possible.

INTERACTIONS Drug: Captopril, furosemide, nifedipine may increase risk of hypoglycemia. **Cimetidine** reduces clearance of metformin. Concomitant therapy with AZOLE ANTIFUNGAL AGENTS **(fluconazole, ketoconazole, itraconazole)** and ORAL HYPOGLYCEMIC DRUGS has been reported in severe hypoglycemia. IODINATED RADIOCONTRAST DYES can cause lactic acidosis and acute kidney failure. **Amiloride, cimetidine digoxin, dofetilide, midodrine, morphine, procainamide, quinidine, quinine, ranitidine, triamterene, trimethoprim, or vancomycin** may decrease metformin elimination by competing for common renal tubular transport systems. **Acarbose** may decrease metformin levels. **Iodinated contrast dyes** may cause lactic acidosis or acute kidney failure. **Herbal: Garlic, ginseng** may increase hypoglycemic effects.

PHARMACOKINETICS Absorption: 50%–60% of dose reaches systemic circulation. **Peak:** 1–3 h. **Distribution:** Not bound to plasma proteins. **Metabolism:** Not metabolized. **Elimination:** Excreted in urine. **Half-Life:** 6.2–17.6 h.

NURSING IMPLICATIONS

Assessment & Drug Effects

- Lab tests: Obtain baseline and periodic kidney and liver function tests; drug contraindicated in the presence of renal or hepatic insufficiency. Monitor blood glucose and HbA_{1C}, and lipid profile periodically.
- Monitor known or suspected alcoholics carefully for decreased liver function.
- Monitor cardiopulmonary status throughout course of therapy;

M

cardiopulmonary insufficiency may predispose to lactic acidosis.

Patient & Family Education

- Be aware that hypoglycemia is not a risk when drug is taken in recommended therapeutic doses unless combined with other drugs which lower blood glucose.
- Report to physician immediately S&S of infection, which increase the risk of lactic acidosis (e.g., abdominal pains, nausea, and vomiting, anorexia).
- Do not breast feed while taking this drug without consulting physician.

METHADONE HYDROCHLORIDE

(meth'a-done)

Dolophine, Methadone

Classifications: CENTRAL NERVOUS SYSTEM AGENT; NARCOTIC (OPIATE) AGONIST; ANALGESIC

Prototype: Morphine

Pregnancy Category: B (D for use of high doses at term)

Controlled Substance: Schedule II

AVAILABILITY 5 mg, 10 mg, 40 mg tablets; 5 mg/5 mL, 10 mg/5 mL, 10 mg/mL oral solution; 10 mg/mL injection

ACTIONS Synthetic derivative similar to morphine but is orally effective and has longer duration of action. A single oral dose produces less sedation and euphoria than does morphine, but repeated doses produce marked sedation. Causes less constipation than morphine, but respiratory depressant effect and antitussive actions are comparable. Highly addictive, with abuse potential that matches that of morphine; abstinence syndrome develops more slowly; withdrawal symptoms are less intense but more prolonged.

THERAPEUTIC EFFECTS Relieves severe pain and manages withdrawal therapy from narcotics.

USES To relieve severe pain; for detoxification and temporary maintenance treatment in hospital and in federally controlled maintenance programs for ambulatory patients with narcotic abstinence syndrome.

CONTRAINDICATIONS Obstetric analgesia. Safety during pregnancy (category B, category D for use of high doses at term), lactation, or for treatment of narcotic addiction in patients <18 y is not established.
CAUTIOUS USE Liver, kidney, or cardiac dysfunction.

ROUTE & DOSAGE

Moderate to Severe Acute Pain

Adult: **PO/SC/IM** 2.5–10 mg q3–4h prn
Child: **PO/IV** 0.1 mg/kg q4h times 2–3 doses, then q6–12h prn (max: 10 mg/dose)

Chronic Pain

Adult: **PO/SC/IM** 5–20 mg q6–8h

Detoxification Treatment

Adult: **PO/SC/IM** 15–40 mg once/d, usually maintained at 20–120 mg/d
Neonate: **PO/IV** 0.05–0.2 mg/kg q12–24h or 0.5 mg/kg/d divided q8h; taper dose by 10%–20%/wk over 1–11/2 mo

ADMINISTRATION

Oral

- Give for analgesic effect in the smallest effective dose to minimize the possible tolerance and physical and psychic dependence.
- Dilute dispersible tablets in 120 mL of water or fruit juice and allow at least 1 min for dispersion.

Subcutaneous/Intramuscular

- Note: IM route is preferred over SC when repeated parenteral administration is required (SC injections may cause local irritation and induration). Rotate injection sites.

Intravenous

Verify correct IV concentration and rate of infusion for administration to neonates, infants, children with physician.

- IV route is used rarely. Get specific orders from physician.

INCOMPATIBILITIES **Solution/additive: Aminophylline, ammonium chloride,** BARBITURATES, **chlorothiazide, heparin, methicillin, phenytoin, sodium bicarbonate.**

- Store at 15°–30° C (59°–86° F) in tight, light-resistant containers.

ADVERSE EFFECTS (≥1%) **CNS:** *Drowsiness,* light-headedness, dizziness, hallucinations. **GI:** Nausea, vomiting, dry mouth, *constipation.* **Body as a Whole:** Transient fall in BP, bone and muscle pain. **Urogenital:** Impotence. **Respiratory:** <u>Respiratory depression</u>.

INTERACTIONS Drug: Alcohol and other CNS DEPRESSANTS, **cimetidine** add to sedation and CNS depression; AMPHETAMINES may potentiate CNS stimulation; with MAO INHIBITORS, **selegiline, furazolidone** causes excessive and prolonged CNS depression, convulsions, cardiovascular collapse.

PHARMACOKINETICS Absorption: Well absorbed from GI tract. **Onset:** 30–60 min PO; 10–20 min IM/SC. **Peak:** 1–2 h. **Duration:** 6–8 h PO, IM, SC; may last 22–48 h with chronic dosing. **Distribution:** Crosses placenta; distributed into breast milk. **Metabolism:** Metabolized in liver. **Elimination:** Excreted in urine. **Half-Life:** 15–25 h.

NURSING IMPLICATIONS

Assessment & Drug Effects

- Evaluate patient's continued need for methadone for pain. Adjustment of dosage and lengthening of between-dose intervals may be possible.
- Monitor respiratory status. Principal danger of overdosage, as with morphine, is extreme respiratory depression.
- Be aware that because of the cumulative effects of methadone, abstinence symptoms may not appear for 36–72 h after last dose and may last 10–14 d. Symptoms are usually of mild intensity (e.g., anorexia, insomnia, anxiety, abdominal discomfort, weakness, headache, sweating, hot and cold flashes).
- Observe closely for recurrence of respiratory depression during use of narcotic antagonists such as naloxone, naltrexone, and levallorphan to terminate methadone intoxication. Since antagonist action is shorter (1–3 h) than that of methadone (36–48 h or more), repeated doses for 8–24 h may be required.

Patient & Family Education

- Be aware that orthostatic hypotension, sweating, constipation, drowsiness, GI symptoms, and other transient adverse effects of therapeutic doses appear to be more prominent in ambulatory patients. Most adverse effects disappear over a period of several weeks.
- Make position changes slowly, particularly from lying down to upright position; sit or lie down if you feel dizzy or faint.
- Do not drive or engage in potentially hazardous activities until response to drug is known.
- Do not breast feed while taking this drug without consulting physician.

METHAMPHETAMINE HYDROCHLORIDE

(meth-am-fet'a-meen)

Desoxyephedrine, Desoxyn

Classifications: CENTRAL NERVOUS SYSTEM AGENT; CEREBRAL STIMULANT; ANOREXIANT; AMPHETAMINE

Prototype: Amphetamine Sulfate

Pregnancy Category: C

Controlled Substance: Schedule II

AVAILABILITY 5 mg tablets; 5 mg, 10 mg, 15 mg long-acting tablets

ACTIONS Sympathomimetic amine chemically related to amphetamine. CNS stimulant actions approximately equal to those of amphetamine, but accompanied by less peripheral activity. However, larger doses produce increased cardiac output, possibly reflex slowing of heart rate, and sustained increase in BP, chiefly by cardiac stimulation.

THERAPEUTIC EFFECTS CNS stimulant actions approximately equal to those of amphetamine, but accompanied by less peripheral activity.

USES Short-term adjunct in management of exogenous obesity, as adjunctive therapy in attention deficit disorder (ADD), narcolepsy, epilepsy, and postencephalitic parkinsonism, and in treatment of certain depressive reactions, especially when characterized by apathy and psychomotor retardation.

CONTRAINDICATIONS During pregnancy, especially first trimester (category C), lactation; as anorexiant in children <12 y; patients receiving MAO INIBITORS; arteriosclerotic parkinsonism.

CAUTIOUS USE Mild hypertension; psychopathic personalities; hyperexcitability states; history of suicide attempts; older adult or debilitated patients.

ROUTE & DOSAGE

Attention Deficit Disorder

Child: **PO** ≥6 y, 2.5–5 mg 1–2 times/d, may increase by 5 mg at weekly intervals up to 20–25 mg/d

Obesity

Adult: **PO** 2.5–5 mg 1–3 times/d 30 min before meals or 5–15 mg of long-acting form once/d

ADMINISTRATION

Oral

- Give early in the day to avoid insomnia, if possible.
- Ensure that long-acting tablets are not chewed or crushed; these need to be swallowed whole.
- Give 30 min before each meal when used for treatment of obesity. If insomnia results, advise patient to inform physician.
- Preserve in tight, light-resistant containers.

ADVERSE EFFECTS (≥1%) **CNS:** Restlessness, tremor, hyperreflexia, insomnia, headache, nervousness, anxiety, dizziness, euphoria or dysphoria. **CV:** Palpitation, arrhythmias, hypertension, hypotension, <u>circulatory collapse</u>. **GI:** Dry mouth, unpleasant taste, nausea, vomiting, diarrhea, constipation. **Special Senses:** Increased intraocular pressure.

INTERACTIONS Drug: Acetazolamide, sodium bicarbonate decreases methamphetamine elimination; **ammonium chloride, ascorbic acid** increases methamphetamine elimination; effects of both methamphetamine and BARBITURATES may be antagonized; **furazolidone** may increase BP effects of AMPHETAMINES—interaction may persist for several weeks after discontinuing **furazolidone;** antagonizes antihypertensive effects of **guanethidine, guanadrel;** MAO INHIBITORS, **selegiline** can cause hypertensive crisis (fatalities reported)—do not administer AMPHETAMINES during or within 14 d of administration of these drugs; PHENOTHIAZINES may inhibit mood elevating effects of AMPHETAMINES; TRICYCLIC ANTIDEPRESSANTS enhance methamphetamine effects because they increase norepinephrine release; BETA-ADRENERGIC AGONISTS increase adverse cardiovascular effects of AMPHETAMINES.

PHARMACOKINETICS Absorption: Readily absorbed from the GI tract. **Duration:** 6–12 h. **Distribution:** All tissues especially the CNS; excreted in breast milk. **Metabolism:** Metabolized in liver. **Elimination:** Renal elimination.

NURSING IMPLICATIONS

Assessment & Drug Effects

- Monitor weight throughout period of therapy.
- Be alert for paradoxic increase in depression or agitation in depressed patients. Report immediately; drug should be withdrawn.
- Do not exceed duration of a few weeks for treatment of obesity.

Patient & Family Education

- Be alert for development of tolerance; happens readily, and prolonged use may lead to drug dependence. Abuse potential is high. Methamphetamine is commonly known as "speed" or "crystal" among drug abusers.
- Withdrawal after prolonged use is frequently followed by lethargy that may persist for several weeks.
- Weigh every other day under standard conditions and maintain a record of weight loss.
- Do not breast feed while using this drug.

METHAZOLAMIDE

(meth-a-zoe'la-mide)

Neptazane

Classifications: EYE PREPARATION; CARBONIC ANHYDRASE INHIBITOR; SULFONAMIDE DERIVATIVE; ANTI-GLAUCOMA

Prototype: Acetazolamide

Pregnancy Category: C

AVAILABILITY 25 mg, 50 mg tablets

ACTIONS Nonbactericidal sulfonamide derivative similar to acetazolamide but with slower onset and longer duration of action. Appears to cause more drowsiness and fatigue than acetazolamide does, and has less diuretic activity.

THERAPEUTIC EFFECTS Inhibits carbonic anhydrase activity in eye by reduces rate of aqueous humor formation with consequent lowering of intraocular pressure.

USES Adjunctive treatment in chronic simple (open-angle) glaucoma and secondary glaucoma and preoperatively in acute angle-closure glaucoma when delay of surgery is desired in order to lower intraocular pressure. May be used concomitantly with miotic and osmotic agents.

CONTRAINDICATIONS Glaucoma due to severe peripheral anterior synechiae, severe or absolute glaucoma, hemorrhagic glaucoma; hypokalemia, hyponatremia.

CAUTIOUS USE Pregnancy (category C), lactation.

ROUTE & DOSAGE

Glaucoma

Adult: **PO** 50–100 mg b.i.d. or t.i.d.

ADMINISTRATION

Oral

- Give with meals to minimize GI distress.

ADVERSE EFFECTS (≥1%) **Body as a Whole:** Malaise, drowsiness, fatigue, lethargy. **GI:** Mild GI disturbance, anorexia. **CNS:** Headache, vertigo, paresthesias, mental confusion, depression.

INTERACTIONS Drug: Renal excretion of AMPHETAMINES, **ephedrine, flecainide, quinidine, procainamide,** TRICYCLIC ANTIDEPRESSANTS may be decreased, thereby enhancing or prolonging their effects; increases renal excretion of **lithium;** excretion of **phenobarbital** may be increased; **amphotericin B,** CORTICOSTEROIDS may add to potassium loss; hypokalemia caused by methazolamide may predispose patients on DIGITALIS GLYCOSIDES to **digitalis** toxicity; patients on high doses of SALICYLATES are at higher risk for SALICYLATE toxicity.

PHARMACOKINETICS Absorption: Slowly absorbed from GI tract. **Onset:** 2–4 h. **Peak:** 6–8 h. **Duration:** 10–18 h. **Distribution:** Distributed throughout body, concentrating in RBCs, plasma, and kidneys; crosses placenta. **Metabolism:** Partially metabolized in liver. **Elimination:** Excreted primarily in urine.

NURSING IMPLICATIONS

Assessment & Drug Effects

- Supervise ambulation in older adult, since drug may cause vertigo.
- Assess patient's ability to perform ADL since drug may cause fatigue and lethargy.
- Lab tests: Obtain periodic serum electrolytes, especially in older adults. Monitor lithium levels with concurrent administration of lithium and methazolamide.

Patient & Family Education

- Be aware that drug may cause drowsiness. Advise caution with hazardous activities until response to drug is known.
- Do not breast feed while taking this drug without consulting physician.

METHENAMINE HIPPURATE

(meth-en'a-meen hip'yoo-rate)

Hiprex, Urex

METHENAMINE MANDELATE

Mandelamine, Mandameth

Classification: URINARY TRACT ANTIINFECTIVE

Prototype: Trimethoprim

Pregnancy Category: C

AVAILABILITY Methenamine Hippurate 1 g tablets **Methenamine Mandelate** 0.5 g, 1 g tablets; 0.5 g/5 mL suspension

ACTIONS Tertiary amine liberates formaldehyde in an acid medium. Nonspecific antibiotic agent with bactericidal activity.

THERAPEUTIC EFFECTS Most bacteria and fungi are susceptible to formaldehyde; however, bacteria that are urease-positive (e.g., *Proteus sp*) convert urea to ammonium hydroxide, which prevents the generation of formaldehyde from methenamine.

USES Prophylactic treatment of recurrent urinary tract infections (UTIs). Also long-term prophylaxis when residual urine is present (e.g., neurogenic bladder).

CONTRAINDICATIONS Renal insufficiency; liver disease; gout; severe dehydration; combined therapy with sulfonamides. Safety during

pregnancy (category C) or lactation is not established.
CAUTIOUS USE Oral suspension for patients susceptible to lipoid pneumonia (e.g., older adults, debilitated patients).

ROUTE & DOSAGE

UTI Prophylaxis
Adult: **PO** (Hippurate) 1 g b.i.d.; (Mandelate) 1 g q.i.d.
Child: **PO** *≤6 y,* (Mandelate) 18.4 mg/kg q.i.d.; *6–12 y,* (Hippurate) 0.5–1 g b.i.d.; (Mandelate) 500 mg q.i.d. or 50 mg/kg/d in 3 divided doses

ADMINISTRATION

Oral
- Give after meals and at bedtime to minimize gastric distress.
- Give oral suspension with caution to older adult or debilitated patients because of the possibility of lipid (aspiration) pneumonia; it contains a vegetable oil base.
- Store at 15°–30° C (59°–86° F) in tightly closed container; protect from excessive heat.

ADVERSE EFFECTS (≥1%) **GI:** Nausea, vomiting, diarrhea, abdominal cramps, anorexia. **Renal:** Bladder irritation, dysuria, frequency, albuminuria, hematuria, crystalluria.

DIAGNOSTIC TEST INTERFERENCE Methenamine (formaldehyde) may produce falsely elevated values for ***urinary catecholamines*** and ***urinary steroids (17-hydroxycorticosteroids)*** (by ***Reddy method***). Possibility of false ***urine glucose determinations*** with ***Benedict's*** test. Methenamine interferes with ***urobilinogen*** and possibly ***urinary VMA*** determinations.

INTERACTIONS Drug: Sulfamethoxazole forms insoluble precipitate in acid urine; **acetazolamide, sodium bicarbonate** may prevent hydrolysis to formaldehyde.

PHARMACOKINETICS Absorption: Readily absorbed from GI tract, although 10%–30% of dose is hydrolyzed to formaldehyde in stomach. **Peak:** 2 h. **Duration:** Up to 6 h or until patient voids. **Distribution:** Crosses placenta; distributed into breast milk. **Metabolism:** Hydrolyzed in acid pH to formaldehyde. **Elimination:** Excreted in urine. **Half-Life:** 4 h.

NURSING IMPLICATIONS

Assessment & Drug Effects
- Monitor urine pH; value of 5.5 or less is required for optimum drug action.
- Monitor I&O ratio and pattern; drug most effective when fluid intake is maintained at 1500 or 2000 mL/d.
- Do not force fluids with this drug; copious amounts may increase diuresis, elevate urine pH, and dilute formaldehyde concentration to subinhibitory levels.
- Consult physician about changing to enteric-coated tablet if patient complains of gastric distress.
- Supplemental acidification to maintain pH of 5.5 or below required for drug action may be necessary. Accomplish by drugs (ascorbic acid, ammonium chloride) or by foods.

Patient & Family Education
- Do not self-medicate with OTC antacids containing sodium bicarbonate or sodium carbonate (to prevent raising urine pH).
- Achieve supplementary acidification by limiting intake of foods that can increase urine pH [e.g., vegetables, fruits, and fruit juice (except

cranberry, plum, prune)] and increasing intake of foods that can decrease urine pH (e.g., proteins, cranberry juice, plums, prunes).
- Do not breast feed while taking this drug without consulting physician.

METHIMAZOLE

(meth-im′a-zole)
Tapazole
Classifications: HORMONES AND SYNTHETIC SUBSTITUTES; ANTITHYROID AGENT
Prototype: Propylthiouracil
Pregnancy Category: D

AVAILABILITY 5 mg, 10 mg tablets

ACTIONS Thioamide with actions and uses similar to those of propylthiouracil but 10 times as potent. Actions are less consistent, but effects appear more promptly than with propylthiouracil. Inhibits synthesis of thyroid hormones as the drug accumulates in the thyroid gland. Does not affect existing T_3 or T_4 levels.
THERAPEUTIC EFFECTS Corrects hyperthyroidism by inhibiting synthesis of the thyroid hormone.

USES Hyperthyroidism and prior to surgery or radiotherapy of the thyroid; may be used cautiously to treat hyperthyroidism in pregnancy.

CONTRAINDICATIONS Pregnancy (category D), lactation.
CAUTIOUS USE Other drugs known to cause agranulocytosis.

ROUTE & DOSAGE

Hyperthyroidism
Adult: **PO** 5–15 mg q8h
Child: **PO** 0.2–0.4 mg/kg/d divided q8h

ADMINISTRATION

Oral
- Give at same time each day relative to meals.
- Store at 15°–30° C (59°–86° F) in light-resistant container.

ADVERSE EFFECTS (≥1%) **GI:** hepatotoxicity (rare). **Endocrine:** Hypothyroidism. **Hematologic:** *Leukopenia,* agranulocytosis, granulocytopenia, thrombocytopenia, pancytopenia, and aplastic anemia. **Musculoskeletal:** Arthralgia. **CNS:** Peripheral neuropathy, drowsiness, neuritis, paresthesias, vertigo. **Skin:** Rash, alopecia, skin hyperpigmentation, urticaria, and pruritus. **Urogenital:** Nephrotic syndrome.

INTERACTIONS Drug: can reduce anticoagulant effects of **warfarin;** may increase serum levels of **digoxin;** may alter **theophylline** levels; may need to decrease dose of BETA-BLOCKERS.

PHARMACOKINETICS Absorption: Readily absorbed from GI tract. **Onset:** 30–40 min. **Peak:** 1 h. **Duration:** 2–4 h. **Distribution:** Crosses placenta; distributed into breast milk. **Elimination:** 12% excreted in urine within 24 h. **Half-Life:** 5–13 h.

NURSING IMPLICATIONS

Assessment & Drug Effects
- Lab tests: Periodic blood work, since agranulocytosis is a rare, but possible adverse effect.
- Closely monitor PT and INR in patients on oral anticoagulants. Anticoagulant activity may be potentiated.

Patient & Family Education
- Adhere to established dosage regimen (i.e., not to double, decrease, or omit doses and not to alter the interval between doses).

- Be aware that skin rash or swelling of cervical lymph nodes may indicate need to discontinue drug and change to another antithyroid agent. Consult physician.
- Notify physician promptly if the following symptoms appear: Bruising, unexplained bleeding, sore throat, fever, jaundice.
- Drug-induced jaundice may persist up to 10 wk after withdrawal of drug.
- Methimazole does not induce hypothyroiditis.
- Do not breast feed while using this drug.

METHOCARBAMOL

(meth-oh-kar'ba-mole)
Marbaxin, Robaxin
Classification: SOMATIC NERVOUS SYSTEM AGENT; SKELETAL MUSCLE RELAXANT; CENTRAL-ACTING
Prototype: Cyclobenzaprine
Pregnancy Category: C

AVAILABILITY 500 mg, 750 mg tablet; 100 mg/mL injection

ACTIONS Similar to cyclobenzaprine, but it produces higher plasma levels more rapidly and for longer periods. Exerts skeletal muscle relaxant action by depressing multisynaptic pathways in the spinal cord and possibly by sedative effect.

THERAPEUTIC EFFECTS No direct action on skeletal muscles; just on multisynaptic pathways in spinal cord that control muscular spasm.

USES Adjunct to physical therapy and other measures in management of discomfort associated with acute musculoskeletal disorders. Also used intravenously as adjunct in management of neuromuscular manifestations of tetanus.

CONTRAINDICATIONS Comatose states; CNS depression; acidosis, kidney dysfunction (injectable methocarbamol contains polyethylene glycol 300 in vehicle, which may cause urea retention and acidotic problems); pregnancy (category C).

CAUTIOUS USE Epilepsy; older adults; females of childbearing age; renal disease, renal failure, renal impairment, seizure disorder; lactation, children <16 y.

ROUTE & DOSAGE

Acute Musculoskeletal Disorders

Adult: **PO** 1.5 g q.i.d. for 2–3 d, then 4–4.5 g/d in 3–6 divided doses **IM** 0.5–1 g q8h **IV** 1–3 g/d in divided doses (max: rate of 300 mg/min)

Tetanus

Adult: **PO** Up to 24 g/d in divided doses crushed and suspended in saline, flushed down a nasogastric tube **IV** 1–2 g/d directly into IV tubing (max: rate of 300 mg/min), may be repeated q6h until nasogastric tube is possible
Child: **PO** 15 mg/kg repeated q6h as needed up to 1.8 g/m^2/d for 3 consecutive d if necessary

ADMINISTRATION

Intramuscular

- Do not exceed IM dose of 5 mL (0.5 g) into each gluteal region. Insert needle deep and carefully aspirate. Inject drug slowly. Rotate injection sites and observe daily for evidence of irritation.

Intravenous

PREPARE: **Direct:** May be given undiluted or diluted in up to 250 mL of NS or D5W.

ADMINISTER: **Direct:** Give at a rate of 300 mg or fraction thereof over 1 min or longer.
▪ Keep patient recumbent during and for at least 15 min after IV injection in order to reduce possibility of orthostatic hypotension and other adverse reactions. ▪ Monitor vital signs and IV flow rate. ▪ Take care to avoid extravasation of IV solution, which may result in thrombophlebitis and sloughing.
▪ Store at 15°–30° C (59°–86° F).

ADVERSE EFFECTS (≥1%) **Body as a Whole:** Fever, anaphylactic reaction, flushing, syncope, convulsions. **Skin:** Urticaria, pruritus, rash, thrombophlebitis, pain, sloughing (with extravasation). **Special Senses:** Conjunctivitis, blurred vision, nasal congestion. **CNS:** *Drowsiness, dizziness, light-headedness,* headache. **CV:** Hypotension, bradycardia. **GI:** Nausea, metallic taste. **Hematologic:** Slight reduction of white cell count with prolonged therapy. **Renal:** Polyethylene glycol in the injection may increase preexisting acidosis and urea retention in patients with renal impairment.

DIAGNOSTIC TEST INTERFERENCE Methocarbamol may cause false increases in ***urinary 5-HIAA*** (with ***nitrosonaphthol reagent***) and ***VMA (Gitlow method).***

INTERACTIONS Drug: Alcohol and other CNS DEPRESSANTS enhance CNS depression.

PHARMACOKINETICS Absorption: Readily absorbed from GI tract. **Onset:** 30 min. **Peak:** 1–2 h. **Metabolism:** Metabolized in liver. **Elimination:** Excreted in urine. **Half-Life:** 1–2 h.

NURSING IMPLICATIONS

Assessment & Drug Effects

- Lab tests: Obtain periodic WBC counts during prolonged therapy.
- Monitor vital signs closely during IV infusion.
- Supervise ambulation following parenteral administration.

Patient & Family Education

- Make position changes slowly, particularly from lying down to upright position; dangle legs before standing.
- Be aware that adverse reactions after oral administration are usually mild and transient and subside with dosage reduction. Use caution regarding drowsiness and dizziness. Avoid activities requiring mental alertness and physical coordination until response to drug is known.
- Urine may darken to brown, black, or green on standing.
- Do not breast feed while taking this drug without consulting physician.

METHOHEXITAL SODIUM

(meth-oh-hex′i-tal)

Brevital Sodium

Classifications: CENTRAL NERVOUS SYSTEM (CNS) AGENT; GENERAL ANESTHETIC; BARBITURATE
Prototype: Thiopental
Pregnancy Category: B
Controlled Substance: Schedule IV

AVAILABILITY 500 mg, 2.5 g, 5 g powder for injection

ACTIONS Rapid, ultra-short-acting barbiturate anesthetic agent. More potent than thiopental but has less cumulative effect and shorter duration of action, and recovery is more rapid.

THERAPEUTIC EFFECTS Induces brief general anesthesia without analgesia by depression of the CNS.

USES Induction of anesthesia, as supplement for other anesthetics, and as general anesthetic for brief operative procedures.

CONTRAINDICATIONS Hypersensitivity to methohexital sodium; agranulocytosis; barbiturate hypersensitivity; hepatic encephalopathy; intraarterial administration; shock, heart failure, PVD, severe hypo- and hypertension, respiratory depression, infants <1 mo; neonates.

CAUTIOUS USE Pregnancy (category B), labor, lactation; adrenal insufficiency, anemia, carbamazepine hypersensitivity; cardiac disease, COPD; uncontrolled asthma, status asthmaticus, sleep apnea, respiratory insufficiency, CNS depression; depression, ethanol intoxication; exfoliative dermatitis; hepatic disease; hydantoin hypersensitivity, older adult; neuromuscular disease; obesity; porphyria; pulmonary disease, renal disease, uremia, renal impairment; seizure disorders, status epilepticus, seizures; shock.

ROUTE & DOSAGE

Induction of Anesthesia

Adult: **IV** 5–12 mL of 1% solution (50–120 mg) at a rate of 1 mL (5 mg) q5min, then 2–4 mL (20–40 mg) q4–7min prn
Child: **IV** 1–2 mg/kg **PR** 20–35 mg/kg as 10% solution (max: 500 mg/dose)

ADMINISTRATION

Intravenous

- Give to recumbent patient. Fall in BP may occur in susceptible patients receiving drug in upright position.

PREPARE: **Direct:** Prepare a 1% solution (10 mg/mL) by diluting with sterile water for injection, D5W, or NS. Use only clear, colorless solutions. Do not allow contact with rubber stoppers or parts of syringes treated with silicone because solution is incompatible with acid solutions (see IMCOMPATIBILITIES).

ADMINISTER: **Direct:** Give 5 mg over 5–10 sec.

INCOMPATIBILITIES **Solution/additive: Atropine, chlorpromazine, clindamycin, fentanyl, glycopyrrolate, hydralazine, kanamycin, lidocaine, methicillin, mechlorethamine, methyldopa, pentazocine, prochlorperazine, promazine, promethazine, streptomycin,** TETRACYCLINES.

- Store drug in sterile water for injection at room temperature for at least 6 wk. Solutions prepared with isotonic NaCl injection or 5% dextrose injection are stable for ONLY about 24 h.

ADVERSE EFFECTS (≥1%) **CV:** Hypotension, cardiac arrhythmias, cardiac arrest. **Musculoskeletal:** Muscle spasm. **CNS:** Postoperative psychomotor impairment that persists for 24 hours, anxiety, drowsiness, emergence delirium, restlessness, and seizures. **Respiratory:** Bronchospasm, cough, hiccups, respiratory depression, apnea, dyspnea, respiratory arrest. **Skin:** Phlebitis and nerve injury adjacent to the injection site, local irritation, edema, ulceration, necrosis.

INTERACTIONS Drug: Alcohol and other CNS DEPRESSANTS enhance CNS depression.

PHARMACOKINETICS Absorption: 17% absorbed PR. **Distribution:** Crosses CNS, placenta and excreted

M

in breast milk. **Metabolism:** Oxidized in liver. **Elimination:** Primarily excreted in urine.

NURSING IMPLICATIONS

Assessment & Drug Effects

- Hiccups are common, particularly with rapid injection; they sometimes persist after anesthesia.
- Keep facilities for assisting respiration and administration of oxygen readily available in the event of respiratory distress.

METHOTREXATE

(meth-oh-trex′ate)

Amethopterin, Mexate, MTX, Rheumatrex

METHOTREXATE SODIUM

Folex, Mexate

Classifications: ANTINEOPLASTIC AGENT; ANTIMETABOLITE; IMMUNOSUPPRESSANT

Prototype: Fluorouracil

Pregnancy Category: D

AVAILABILITY 2.5 mg tablets; 20 mg, 1 g powder for injection; 2.5 mg/mL, 25 mg/mL injection

ACTIONS Antimetabolite and folic acid antagonist. Blocks folic acid participation in nucleic acid synthesis, thereby interfering with mitotic process.

THERAPEUTIC EFFECTS Rapidly proliferating tissues (malignant cells, bone marrow) are sensitive to interference of the mitotic process by this drug. In psoriasis, reproductive rate of epithelial cells is higher than in normal cells. Induces remission slowly; use often preceded by other antineoplastic therapies.

USES Principally in combination regimens to maintain induced remissions in neoplastic diseases. Effective in treatment of gestational choriocarcinoma and hydatidiform mole and as immunosuppressant in kidney transplantation, for acute and subacute leukemias and leukemic meningitis, especially in children. Used in lymphosarcoma, in certain inoperable tumors of head, neck, and pelvis, and in mycosis fungoides. Also used to treat severe psoriasis nonresponsive to other forms of therapy, rheumatoid arthritis.

UNLABELED USES Psoriatic arthritis, SLE, polymyositis.

CONTRAINDICATIONS Pregnancy (category D), men and women in childbearing age; lactation; hepatic and renal insufficiency; concomitant administration of hepatotoxic drugs and hematopoietic depressants; alcohol; ultraviolet exposure to psoriatic lesions; pre-existing blood dyscrasias.

CAUTIOUS USE Infections; peptic ulcer, ulcerative colitis; very young or old patients; cancer patients with preexisting bone marrow impairment; poor nutritional status.

ROUTE & DOSAGE

Trophoblastic Neoplasm

Adult: **PO** 15–30 mg/d for 5 d, repeat q12wk for 3–5 courses **IM/IV** 15–30 mg/d for 5 d, repeat q12wk for 3–5 courses

Leukemia

Adult: **IM/IV Loading Dose** 3.3 $mg/m^2/d$ **PO/IM/IV Maintenance Dose** 20–30 mg/m^2 2 times/wk

Child: **PO/IM** 7.5–30 mg/m^2 q1–2 wk

Lymphoma

Adult: **PO** 12–25 mg/d for 4–8 d with 7–10 d rest intervals

Psoriasis

Adult: **PO** 2.5–5 mg q12h for 3 doses each wk up to 25–30 mg/wk **IM/IV** 10–25 mg/wk

Rheumatoid Arthritis

Adult: **PO** 2.5–5 mg q12h for 3 doses each wk or 7.5 mg once/wk

Child: **PO/IM** 5–15 mg/m²/wk as single dose or in 3 divided doses 12 h apart

ADMINISTRATION

Oral

- Give 1 h before or 2 h after meals.
- Use a test dose (5–10 mg parenterally) 1 wk before therapy for treatment of psoriasis.
- Avoid skin exposure and inhalation of drug particles.

Intravenous

Note: Verify correct IV concentration and rate of infusion for administration to children with physician.

PREPARE: **Direct:** Reconstitute powder vial by adding 2 mL of NS or D5W without preservatives to each 5 mg to yield 2.5 mg/mL. Reconstitute 1 g high-dose vial with 19.4 mL D5W or NS to yield 50 mg/mL. **IV Infusion:** Further dilute contents of high-dose vial in D5W or NS.

ADMINISTER: **Direct:** Give at rate of 10 mg or fraction thereof over 60 s. **IV Infusion:** Give over 1–4 h or as prescribed.

INCOMPATIBILITIES **Solution/additive: Bleomycin, prednisolone, droperidol, heparin, metoclopramide, ranitidine. Y-site: Chlorpromazine, droperidol, gemcitabine, idarubicin, ifosfamide, midazolam, nalbuphine, promethazine, propofol.**

- Preserve drug in tight, light-resistant container.

ADVERSE EFFECTS

(≥1%) **CNS:** *Headache,* drowsiness, blurred vision, dizziness, aphasia, hemiparesis; arachnoiditis, convulsions (after intrathecal administration); mental confusion, tremors, ataxia, coma. **GI:** Hepatotoxicity, GI ulcerations and hemorrhage, *ulcerative stomatitis, glossitis, gingivitis,* pharyngitis, nausea, vomiting, diarrhea, hepatic cirrhosis. **Urogenital:** Defective oogenesis or spermatogenesis, nephropathy, hematuria, menstrual dysfunction, infertility, abortion, fetal defects. **Hematologic:** *Leukopenia, thrombocytopenia,* anemia, marked myelosuppression, aplastic bone marrow, telangiectasis, thrombophlebitis at intraarterial catheter site, hypogammaglobulinemia, and hyperuricemia. **Skin:** Erythematous rashes, pruritus, urticaria, folliculitis, vasculitis, photosensitivity, depigmentation, hyperpigmentation, alopecia. **Body as a Whole:** Malaise, undue fatigue, systemic toxicity (after intrathecal and intraarterial administration), chills, fever, decreased resistance to infection, septicemia, osteoporosis, metabolic changes precipitating diabetes and sudden death, pneumonitis, pulmonary fibrosis.

DIAGNOSTIC TEST INTERFERENCE

Severe reactions may occur when ***live vaccines*** are administered because of immunosuppressive activity of methotrexate.

INTERACTIONS

Drug: Alcohol, azathioprine, sulfasalazine increase risk of hepatotoxicity; **chloramphenicol, etretinate,** SALICYLATES, NSAIDS, SULFONAMIDES, SULFONYLUREAS, **phenylbutazone, phenytoin,** TETRACYCLINES, **PABA, penicillin, probenecid** may increase methotrexate levels with increased toxicity; **folic acid** may alter response to methotrexate. May increase **theophylline** levels; **cholestyramine** enhances methotrexate clearance. **Herbal: Echinacea** may increase risk of hepatotoxicity. **Food: Caffeine** >180 mg/d (3–4 cups) may decrease effectiveness for rheumatoid arthritis.

PHARMACOKINETICS Absorption: Readily absorbed from GI tract. **Peak:** 0.5–2 h IM/IV; 1–4 h PO. **Distribution:** Widely distributed with highest concentrations in kidneys, gallbladder, spleen, liver, and skin; minimal passage across blood–brain barrier; crosses placenta; distributed into breast milk. **Metabolism:** Metabolized in liver. **Elimination:** Excreted primarily in urine. **Half-Life:** 2–4 h.

NURSING IMPLICATIONS

Assessment & Drug Effects

- Lab tests: Obtain baseline liver and kidney function, CBC with differential, platelet count, and chest x-rays. Repeat weekly during therapy.
- Prolonged treatment with small frequent doses may lead to hepatotoxicity, which is best diagnosed by liver biopsy.
- Monitor for and report ulcerative stomatitis with glossitis and gingivitis, often the first signs of toxicity. Inspect mouth daily; report patchy necrotic areas, bleeding and discomfort, or overgrowth (black, furry tongue).
- Keep patient well hydrated (about 2000 mL/24 h).
- Monitor I&O ratio and pattern. Severe nephrotoxicity (hematuria, dysuria, azotemia, oliguria) fosters drug accumulation and kidney damage and requires dosage adjustment or discontinuation.
- Prevent exposure to infections or colds during leukopenia periods. Be alert to onset of agranulocytosis (cough, extreme fatigue, sore throat, chills, fever) and report symptoms promptly. Therapy will be interrupted and appropriate antibiotic drugs prescribed.
- Be alert for and report symptoms of thrombocytopenia (e.g., ecchymoses, petechiae, epistaxis, melena, hematuria, vaginal bleeding, slow and protracted oozing following trauma).
- Report bloody diarrhea to physician; necessitates interruption of therapy to prevent perforation or hemorrhagic enteritis.
- Monitor blood glucose and HbA1c periodically in diabetics.

Patient & Family Education

- Be aware of dangers of drug and report promptly any abnormal symptoms to physician.
- Alcohol ingestion increases the incidence and severity of methotrexate hepatotoxicity.
- Practice fastidious mouth care to prevent infection, provide comfort, and maintain adequate nutritional status.
- Report joint pains to physician; drug may precipitate gouty arthritis.
- Do not self-medicate with vitamins. Some OTC compounds may include folic acid (or its derivatives), which alters methotrexate response.
- Use contraceptive measures during and for at least 8 wk following therapy.
- Avoid exposure to sunlight and ultraviolet light. Wear sunglasses and sunscreen.
- Do not breast feed while using this drug.

METHOTRIMEPRAZINE

(meth-oh-trye-mep'ra-zeen)

Levoprome, Nozinan ♣

Classifications: CENTRAL NERVOUS SYSTEM AGENT; NONNARCOTIC ANALGESIC; PHENOTHIAZINE; ANXIOLYTIC; SEDATIVE-HYPNOTIC

Prototype: Chlorpromazine

Pregnancy Category: C

AVAILABILITY 20 mg/mL injection

ACTIONS Tranquilizes and produces sedative effects; also has prominent analgesic properties. Extrapyramidal symptoms and dry mouth reportedly uncommon, but orthostatic hypotension and sedation effects are more prominent.

THERAPEUTIC EFFECTS Raises pain threshold, produces amnesia, as well as sedative effects.

USES To relieve moderate to severe pain in nonambulatory patients and for analgesia and sedation when respiratory depression is to be avoided, as in obstetrics and pre- and postoperatively.

CONTRAINDICATIONS Hypersensitivity to phenothiazines and ingredients in the formulation (e.g., bisulfite); severe cardiac, kidney, or liver disease; history of convulsive disorders; significant hypotension; comatose states; premature labor; children <12 y; concomitant use with antihypertensive agents, including MAO inhibitors.

CAUTIOUS USE Older adult and debilitated patients with heart disease; early pregnancy (category C), lactation.

ROUTE & DOSAGE

Analgesia, Sedation

Adult: **IM** 10–20 mg q4–6h

Preoperative Medication

Adult: **IM** 2–20 mg 45 min–3 h before surgery

Postoperative Analgesia

Adult: **IM** 2.5–7.5 mg q4–6h as needed

ADMINISTRATION

Intramuscular

- Give IM injection deep into large muscle mass.
- Pain at injection site and local inflammatory reaction commonly occur. Rotate injection sites and observe daily.
- Mix in same syringe with either atropine or scopolamine, but not with any other drug. Reduce dosage of atropine or scopolamine.
- Protect drug from light.

INCOMPATIBILITIES **Solution/additive: Ranitidine. Y-site: Heparin.**

M

ADVERSE EFFECTS (≥1%) **CNS:** *Excessive sedation, drowsiness, amnesia,* disorientation, euphoria, delirium, extrapyramidal symptoms, headache. **CV:** *Orthostatic hypotension with faintness,* weakness, dizziness; tachycardia, bradycardia, palpitation. **Special Senses:** Blurred vision, nasal congestion. **GI:** Nausea, vomiting, abdominal discomfort, dry mouth, jaundice. **Urogenital:** Dysuria, hematuria. **Body as a Whole:** Slurred speech, fever, chills, injection site reactions, increased weight. **Respiratory:** Respiratory depression. **Hematologic:** Blood dyscrasias including agranulocytosis and pancytopenia.

INTERACTIONS Drug: Alcohol and other CNS DEPRESSANTS enhance CNS depression; with ANTICHOLINERGIC AGENTS, aggravation of extrapyramidal symptoms, CNS stimulation, delirium, tachycardia, and hypotension; ANTIHYPERTENSIVE AGENTS, MAO

INHIBITORS add to hypotensive effects; **epinephrine** may antagonize pressor effects; SKELETAL MUSCLE RELAXANTS may prolong duration of muscle relaxation.

PHARMACOKINETICS Onset: 20–40 min. **Peak:** 1–2 h. **Duration:** 4 h. **Distribution:** Crosses CSF and placenta; distributed into breast milk. **Metabolism:** Metabolized in liver. **Elimination:** Slowly excreted in urine; elimination may continue for 1 wk after a single dose.

NURSING IMPLICATIONS

Assessment & Drug Effects

- Carefully supervise ambulation for at least 6 h, but preferably 12 h. Orthostatic hypotension with faintness, weakness, and dizziness may occur within 10–20 min after drug administration and may last 4–6 h and occasionally as long as 12 h. Tolerance to effects usually develops with successive doses.
- Excessive sedation and amnesia also occur commonly during early drug therapy.
- Assess BP and pulse frequently until dosage requirements and response are stabilized. Monitor older adult and debilitated patients closely.
- Methotrimeprazine injection contains a bisulfite, an allergen for some patients.
- Do not treat severe hypotension with epinephrine; it is specifically contraindicated.

M

METHOXAMINE HYDROCHLORIDE (Pr)

(meth-ox'a meen)

Vasoxyl

Classifications: AUTONOMIC NERVOUS SYSTEM AGENT; ALPHA-ADRENERGIC AGONIST (SYMPATHOMIMETIC)

Pregnancy Category: C

AVAILABILITY 20 mg/mL ampules

ACTIONS Direct-acting sympathomimetic amine pharmacologically related to phenylephrine. Acts almost exclusively on alpha-adrenergic receptors. Pressor action is due primarily to direct peripheral vasoconstriction, which in turn causes rise in arterial BP. Has no direct effect on heart. Markedly reduces renal blood flow. Tends to slow ventricular rate by vagal stimulation in response to elevated BP.

THERAPEUTIC EFFECTS Terminates episodes of paroxysmal supraventricular tachycardia. Large doses may produce bradycardia. CNS-stimulating action. True tachyphylaxis not reported.

USES To support, restore, or maintain BP during anesthesia and to terminate some episodes of paroxysmal supraventricular tachycardia.

CONTRAINDICATIONS Severe coronary or cardiovascular disease; hypovolemia, in combination with local anesthetics for tissue infiltration; within 2 wk of MAO inhibitors; pregnancy (category C).

CAUTIOUS USE History of hypertension or hyperthyroidism; following use of ergot alkaloids; lactation. Safety and effectiveness in children are not established.

ROUTE & DOSAGE

Hypotension During Anesthesia

Adult: **IM** 5–20 mg **IV** 3–5 mg
Child: **IM** 0.25 mg/kg **IV** 0.08 mg/kg

Paroxysmal Supraventricular Tachycardia

Adult: **IM** 10–20 mg **IV** 5–15 mg over 3–5 min

ADMINISTRATION

Intramuscular

- Give supplemental IM, as needed, after emergency IV infusion.

Intravenous

PREPARE: **Direct:** Give undiluted. **IV Infusion:** May be diluted in 250 mL D5W.

ADMINISTER: **Direct:** Give at a rate of 5 mg/min if systolic BP is less than 60 mm Hg. **IV Infusion:** Give at rate needed to maintain BP.

- Be alert for extravasation. Antidote: Infiltrate area as soon as possible with 10–15 mL NS saline solution containing 5–10 mg phentolamine.
- Protect drug from light.

ADVERSE EFFECTS (≥1%) **Body as a Whole:** Paresthesias, feeling of coldness (particularly with high dosage), restlessness, nervousness. **CV:** High BP, bradycardia. **GI:** Projectile vomiting. **CNS:** Severe headache, pilomotor erection (gooseflesh). **Urogenital:** Urinary urgency.

INTERACTIONS Drug: Phentolamine and PHENOTHIAZINES block vasopressor response. BETA BLOCKERS may increase amount of methoxamine available to receptor sites. **Atropine** blocks reflex bradycardia and enhances vasopressor effects. MAO INHIBITORS, **vasopressin,** and ERGOT ALKALOIDS may cause hypertensive crisis.

PHARMACOKINETICS Onset: Immediately after IV. **Peak:** 0.5–2 min IV; 15–20 min IM. **Duration:** 5–15 min IV; 60–90 min IM. **Metabolism:** Unknown. **Elimination:** Unknown.

NURSING IMPLICATIONS

Assessment & Drug Effects

- Supervise patients closely.
- Monitor vital signs continuously. Report any increase in BP above level prescribed by physician; report slowing of HR.
- Be alert for sudden changes in BP and pulse after drug has been discontinued.
- Monitor I&O. Urinary frequency with retention is a possibility. Report oliguria or change in I&O ratio.
- Methoxamine injection contains a bisulfite, an allergen for some patients.

Patient & Family Education

- Report headache to physician; it may be severe. This adverse effect may require analgesia for relief.
- Report nausea to physician; it may be accompanied by projectile vomiting.

METHOXSALEN (Pr)

(meth-ox'a-len)

8-MOP, Oxsoralen, UltraMOP, Uvadex

Classifications: SKIN AND MUCOUS MEMBRANE AGENT; PSORALEN

Pregnancy Category: C

AVAILABILITY 10 mg capsules, 20 mcg/mL solution; 1% lotion

ACTIONS Psoralen derivative with strong photosensitizing effects: used with ultraviolet-A light (UVA) in therapeutic regimens called PUVA (P-psoralen). After photoactivation by long wavelength, UVA, methoxsalen combines with epidermal cell DNA causing photodamage (cytotoxic action).

THERAPEUTIC EFFECTS Photodamage inhibits rapid and uncontrolled epidermal cell turnover characteristic of psoriasis. Results in an inflammatory reaction with erythema. Strongly melanogenic.

USES With controlled exposure to UVA to repigment vitiliginous skin

and for symptomatic treatment of severe disabling psoriasis that is refractory to other forms of therapy.
UNLABELED USES (PUVA therapy) mycosis fungoides.

CONTRAINDICATIONS Sunburn, sensitivity (or its history) to psoralens, diseases associated with photosensitivity (e.g., LE, albinism, melanoma or its history); invasive squamous cell cancer; cataract; aphakia; previous exposure to arsenic or ionizing radiation; pregnancy (category C). Safety (oral) in children is not established.
CAUTIOUS USE Hepatic insufficiency; GI disease; chronic infection; treatment with known photosensitizing agents; immunosuppressed patient; cardiovascular disease; lactation. Safety (lotion) in children <12 y is not established.

M

ROUTE & DOSAGE

Idiopathic Vitiligo
Adult: **Topical** Apply lotion 1–2 h before exposure to UV light once/wk
Psoriasis
Adult: **PO** Give 1.5–2 h before exposure to UV light 2–3 times/wk: *<30 kg,* 10 mg; *30–50 kg,* 20 mg; *51–65 kg,* 30 mg; *66–80 kg,* 40 mg; *81–90 kg,* 50 mg; *91–115 kg,* 60 mg; *>115 kg,* 70 mg

ADMINISTRATION

Note: Methoxsalen therapy with UV light (PUVA therapy) should be done under the complete control of a physician with special competence and experience in photochemotherapy.

Oral
- Give with milk or food to prevent GI distress.
- Maintain consistent time relationship between food–drug ingestion. Food digestion and absorption appear to affect drug serum levels.

Topical
- Only small (less than 10 cm^2), well-defined areas are treated with lotion. Systemic treatment is used for large areas.
- Apply lotion with cotton swabs, allow to dry 1–2 min, then reapply. Protect borders of the lesion with petrolatum and sunscreen lotion to prevent hyperpigmentation.
- Use finger cots or gloves to apply lotion and prevent photosensitization and burned skin.
- Apply sunscreen lotion to the skin for about one third of the initial exposure time during PUVA therapy until there is sufficient tanning. Do not apply to psoriatic areas before treatment.
- Store lotion and capsules at 15°–30° C (59°–86° F) in light-resistant containers unless otherwise directed by manufacturer.

ADVERSE EFFECTS (≥1%) **CNS:** Nervousness, dizziness, headache, mental depression or excitation, vertigo, insomnia. **Special Senses:** Cataract formation, ocular damage. **GI:** Cheilitis, *nausea* and other GI disturbances, toxic hepatitis. **Skin:** Phototoxic effects: severe edema and erythema, *pruritus,* painful blisters; burning, peeling, thinning, freckling, and accelerated aging of skin; hyper- or hypopigmentation; severe skin pain (lasting 1–2 mo), photoallergic contact dermatitis (with topical use), exacerbation of latent photosensitive dermatoses, malignant melanoma (rare). **Body as a Whole:** Transient loss of muscular coordination, edema, leg cramps, systemic immune effects, drug fever.

INTERACTIONS Drug: Anthralin, coal tar, griseofulvin, PHENOTHIAZINES, **naladixic acid,** SULFONAMIDES, BACTERIOSTATIC SOAPS, TETRACYCLINES, THIAZIDES compound photosensitizing effects. **Food:** Food will increase peak and extent of absorption.

PHARMACOKINETICS Absorption: Variably absorbed from GI tract. **Peak:** 2 h. **Duration:** 8–10 h. **Distribution:** Preferentially taken up by epidermal cells; distributes into lens of eye. **Elimination:** 80%–90% excreted in urine within 8 h. **Half-Life:** 0.75–2.4 h.

NURSING IMPLICATIONS

Assessment & Drug Effects

- Schedule a pretreatment ophthalmologic exam to rule out cataracts; repeat periodically during treatment and at yearly intervals thereafter.
- Lab tests: Monitor CBC, kidney and liver function, and antinuclear antibody tests during oral therapy.
- Fair-skinned patients appear to be at greatest risk for phototoxicity from PUVA therapy (see ADVERSE EFFECTS).
- Be aware that repigmentation is more rapid on fleshy areas (i.e., face, abdomen, buttocks) than on hands or feet.

Patient & Family Education

- Expect that effective repigmentation may require 6–9 mo of treatment; periodic treatment usually is necessary to retain pigmentation. If, after 3 mo of treatment, there is no apparent response, drug is discontinued.
- Avoid additional exposure to UV light (direct or indirect) for at least 8 h after oral drug ingestion and UVA exposure.
- Understand intended treatment schedule: After topical application, the initial sunlight exposure is limited to 1 min, with subsequent gradual and incremental exposures by prescription.
- Avoid additional UV light for 24–48 h after topical application and UVA exposure.
- Wear sunscreen lotion (with SPF 15 or higher) and protective clothing (hat, gloves) to cover all exposed areas including lips, to prevent burning or blistering if sunlight cannot be avoided after the treatment.
- Do not sunbathe for at least 48 h after PUVA treatment. Sunburn and photochemotherapy are additive in the production of burning and erythema.
- Wear wraparound sunglasses with UVA-absorbing properties both indoors and outdoors during daylight hours for 24 h. Do not substitute prescription sunglasses or photosensitive darkening glasses; they may actually increase danger of cataract formation.
- Alert physician to appearance of new psoriatic areas, flares, or regressed cleared skin areas during treatment and maintenance periods.
- Do not breast feed while taking this drug without consulting physician.

METHSCOPOLAMINE BROMIDE

(meth-skoe-pol'a-meen)

Pamine

Classifications: AUTONOMIC NERVOUS SYSTEM AGENT; ANTICHOLINERGIC (PARASYMPATHOLYTIC); ANTIMUSCARINIC; ANTISPASMODIC

Prototype: Atropine

Pregnancy Category: C

AVAILABILITY 2.5 mg tablets

ACTIONS Quaternary ammonium derivative of scopolamine that lacks the

M

CNS actions of scopolamine. Its spasmolytic and antisecretory actions are quantitatively similar to those of atropine but they last longer.

THERAPEUTIC EFFECTS Greater selectivity in blocking vagal impulses from GI tract than either scopolamine or atropine.

USES Adjunct in treatment of peptic ulcer, irritable bowel syndrome, and a variety of other GI conditions. Also may be used to control excessive sweating and salivation, migraine headaches, and premenstrual cramps.

CONTRAINDICATIONS Hypersensitivity to any of the drug's constituents; prostatic hypertrophy; pyloric obstruction; intestinal atony; tachycardia, cardiac disease; pregnancy (category C), lactation.

CAUTIOUS USE Older adult and debilitated patients.

M

ROUTE & DOSAGE

Irritable Bowel Syndrome

Adult: **PO** 2.5–5 mg 30 min a.c. and h.s.

ADMINISTRATION

Oral

- Give 30 min before meals and at bedtime.
- Preserve in tight, light-resistant containers.

ADVERSE EFFECTS (≥1%) **GI:** Dry mouth, constipation. **Special Senses:** Blurred vision. **CNS:** Dizziness, drowsiness, flushing of skin. **Urogenital:** Urinary hesitancy or retention.

INTERACTIONS Drug: Amantadine, TRICYCLIC ANTIDEPRESSANTS increase anticholinergic effects; may increase effects of **atenolol, digoxin;** may decrease effectiveness of PHENOTHIAZINES.

PHARMACOKINETICS Absorption: Erratic after PO administration. **Onset:** Approximately 1 h. **Duration:** 4–6 h. **Elimination:** Excreted primarily in urine and bile; some unchanged drug excreted in feces.

NURSING IMPLICATIONS

Assessment & Drug Effects

- Incidence and severity of adverse effects are generally dose-related. Dosage is usually maintained at a level that produces slight dryness of mouth.
- Report urinary retention promptly; may indicate discontinuation.

Patient & Family Education

- Do not drive or engage in potentially hazardous activities until response to drug is known.
- Make position changes slowly and in stages.
- Learn measures to relieve dry mouth; rinse mouth frequently with water, suck hard candy.
- Do not breast feed while taking this drug.

METHYCLOTHIAZIDE

(meth-i-kloe-thye′a-zide)

Aquatensen, Duretic ♣, Enduron, Ethon

Classifications: ELECTROLYTIC AND WATER BALANCE AGENT; THIAZIDE DIURETIC; ANTIHYPERTENSIVE AGENT

Prototype: Hydrochlorothiazide

Pregnancy Category: C

AVAILABILITY 2.5 mg, 5 mg tablets

ACTIONS Thiazide diuretic which is similar to hydrochlorothiazide. Diuretic effect results from a drug-induced inhibition of the renal tubular reabsorption of electrolytes. The excretion of sodium and chloride is enhanced. There is also a loss of potassium ions via the kidney.

THERAPEUTIC EFFECTS BP is lowered, probably by the loss of sodium and water, and consequently blood volume. Edema is also decreased in CHF patients by the same mechanism.

USES Antihypertensive treatment and adjunctively in the management of edema associated with CHF, renal pathology, and hepatic cirrhosis.

CONTRAINDICATIONS Hypersensitivity to thiazides, and sulfonamide derivatives; anuria, hypokalemia, pregnancy (category C), lactation.

CAUTIOUS USE Impaired kidney or liver function; gout; SLE; hypercalcemia; diabetes mellitus.

ROUTE & DOSAGE

Edema

Adult: **PO** 2.5–10 mg once/d or 3–5 times/wk

Hypertension

Adult: **PO** 2.5–10 mg/d
Child: **PO** 0.05–0.2 mg/kg/d

ADMINISTRATION

Oral

- Give early in a.m. after eating (reduces gastric irritation) to prevent sleep interruption because of diuresis. If 2 doses are ordered, administer second dose no later than 3 p.m.
- Store at 15°–30° C (59°–86° F) unless otherwise instructed.

ADVERSE EFFECTS (≥1%) **Body as a Whole:** Postural hypotension, sialadenitis, unusual fatigue, dizziness, paresthesias. **Skin:** Photosensitivity. **Special Senses:** Yellow vision. **Metabolic:** *Hypokalemia*. **Hematologic:** Agranulocytosis.

INTERACTIONS Drug: Amphotericin B, CORTICOSTEROIDS increase hypokalemic effects; may antagonize hypoglycemic effects of **insulin,** SULFONYLUREAS; **cholestyramine, colestipol** decrease thiazide absorption; intensifies hypoglycemic and hypotensive effects of **diazoxide;** increased potassium and magnesium loss may cause **digoxin** toxicity; decreases **lithium** excretion, increasing its toxicity; NSAIDS may attenuate diuresis, and risk of NSAID-induced kidney failure increased.

PHARMACOKINETICS Absorption: Incompletely absorbed. **Onset:** 2 h. **Peak:** 6 h. **Duration:** >24 h. **Distribution:** Distributed throughout extracellular tissue; concentrates in kidney; crosses placenta; distributed in breast milk. **Metabolism:** Does not appear to be metabolized. **Elimination:** Excreted in urine.

NURSING IMPLICATIONS

Assessment & Drug Effects

- Expect antihypertensive effects in 3–4 d; maximal effects may require 3–4 wk.
- Monitor BP and I&O ratio during first phase of antihypertensive therapy. Report a sudden fall in BP, which may initiate severe postural hypotension and potentially dangerous perfusion problems, especially in the extremities.
- Lab tests: Periodic serum electrolytes and CBC with differential.
- Monitor patient for S&S of hypokalemia (see Appendix F). Report promptly. Physician may change dose and institute replacement therapy.

Patient & Family Education

- Eat a balanced diet to protect against hypokalemia; generally

M

not severe even with long-term therapy. Prevent onset by eating potassium-rich foods including a banana (about 370 mg potassium) and at least 180 mL (6 oz) orange juice (about 330 mg potassium) every day.

- Watch carefully for loss of glycemic control (diabetics) and early signs of hyperglycemia (see Appendix F). Symptoms are slow to develop.
- Avoid OTC drugs unless the physician approves them. Many preparations contain both potassium and sodium, and may induce electrolyte imbalance adverse effects.
- Older adults are more responsive to excessive diuresis; orthostatic hypotension may be a problem.
- Change positions slowly and in stages from lying down to upright positions; avoid hot baths or showers, extended exposure to sunlight, and standing still. Accept assistance as necessary to prevent falling.
- Do not drive or engage in potentially hazardous activities until adjustment to the hypotensive effects of drug has been made.
- Do not breast feed while taking this drug.

M

METHYLDOPA Pr

(meth-ill-doe'pa)

Aldomet, Apo-Methyldopa ♣, Dopamet ♣, Novomedopa ♣

METHYLDOPATE HYDROCHLORIDE

(meth-ill-doe'pate)

Aldomet

Classifications: CARDIOVASCULAR AGENT; CENTRAL-ACTING ANTIHYPERTENSIVE; AUTONOMIC NERVOUS SYSTEM AGENT; ALPHA-ADRENERGIC AGONIST (SYMPATHOMIMETIC)

Pregnancy Category: C

AVAILABILITY 125 mg, 250 mg, 500 mg tablets; 50 mg/mL oral suspension; 50 mg/mL injection

ACTIONS Structurally related to catecholamines and their precursors. Has weak neurotransmitter properties; inhibits decarboxylation of dopa, thereby reducing concentration of dopamine, a precursor of norepinephrine. It also inhibits the precursor of serotonin.

THERAPEUTIC EFFECTS Lowers standing and supine BP, and unlike adrenergic blockers, is not so prone to produce orthostatic hypotension, diurnal BP variations, or exercise hypertension. Reduces renal vascular resistance; maintains cardiac output without acceleration, but may slow heart rate; tends to support sodium and water retention.

USES Treatment of sustained moderate to severe hypertension, particularly in patients with kidney dysfunction. Also used in selected patients with carcinoid disease. Parenteral form has been used for treatment of hypertensive crises but is not preferred because of its slow onset of action.

CONTRAINDICATIONS Active liver disease (hepatitis, cirrhosis); pheochromocytoma; blood dyscrasias. Safety during pregnancy (category C) is not established.

CAUTIOUS USE History of impaired liver or kidney function or disease; angina pectoris; history of mental depression; lactation; young or older adult patients.

ROUTE & DOSAGE

Hypertension

Adult: **PO** 250 mg b.i.d. or t.i.d., may be increased up to 3 g/d in divided doses **IV** 250–500 mg q6h, may be increased up to 1 g q6h

Geriatric: **PO** 125 mg b.i.d. or t.i.d., may increase gradually (max: 3 g/d)
Child: **PO** 10–65 mg/kg/d in 2–4 divided doses (max: 3 g/d) **IV** 20–65 mg/kg/d in 4 divided doses

ADMINISTRATION

Oral

- Make dosage increases in evening to minimize daytime sedation. Some patients maintain adequate BP control with a single evening dose.

Intravenous

PREPARE: **Intermittent:** Dilute in 100–200 mL of D5W, as needed, to yield 10 mg/mL.

ADMINISTER: **Intermittent:** Give over 30–60 min.

INCOMPATIBILITIES **Solution/additive: Amphotericin B**, **methohexital**, **verapamil. Y-site: Fat emulsion**.

ADVERSE EFFECTS (≥1%) **Body as a Whole:** Hypersensitivity (*Fever,* skin eruptions, ulcerations of soles of feet, flu-like symptoms, lymphadenopathy, eosinophilia). **CNS:** *Sedation, drowsiness,* sluggishness, headache, weakness, fatigue, dizziness, vertigo, *decrease in mental acuity,* inability to concentrate, amnesia-like syndrome, parkinsonism, mild psychoses, depression, nightmares. **CV:** Orthostatic hypotension, syncope, bradycardia, myocarditis, edema, weight gain *(sodium and water retention),* paradoxic hypertensive reaction (especially with IV administration). **GI:** Diarrhea, constipation, abdominal distension, malabsorption syndrome, nausea, vomiting, dry mouth, sore or black tongue, sialadenitis, abnormal liver function tests, jaundice, hepatitis, hepatic necrosis (rare). **Hematologic:** *Positive direct Coombs' test* (common especially in African-Americans), granulocytopenia. **Special Senses:** *Nasal stuffiness.* **Endocrine:** Gynecomastia, lactation, *decreased libido, impotence,* hypothermia (large doses), positive tests for lupus and rheumatoid factors. **Skin:** Granulomatous skin lesions.

DIAGNOSTIC TEST INTERFERENCE Methyldopa may interfere with ***serum creatinine*** measurements using ***alkaline picrate method, AST*** by ***colorimetric methods,*** and ***uric acid*** measurements by ***phosphotungstate method*** (with high methyldopa blood levels); it may produce false elevations of ***urinary catecholamines*** and increase in ***serum amylase*** in methyldopa-induced sialadenitis.

INTERACTIONS Drug: AMPHETAMINES, TRICYCLIC ANTIDEPRESSANTS, PHENOTHIAZINES may attenuate antihypertensive response; methyldopa may inhibit effectiveness of **ephedrine; haloperidol** may exacerbate psychiatric symptoms; with **levodopa** additive hypotension, increased CNS toxicity, especially psychosis; increases risk of **lithium** toxicity; **methotrimeprazine** causes excessive hypotension; MAO INHIBITORS may cause hallucinations; **phenoxybenzamine** may cause urinary incontinence.

PHARMACOKINETICS Absorption: About 50% absorbed from GI tract. **Peak:** 4–6 h. **Duration:** 24 h PO; 10–16 h IV. **Distribution:** Crosses placenta, distributed into breast milk. **Metabolism:** Metabolized in liver and GI tract. **Elimination:** Excreted primarily in urine. **Half-Life:** 1.7 h.

NURSING IMPLICATIONS

Assessment & Drug Effects

- Check BP and pulse at least q30min until stabilized during IV

M

infusion and observe for adequacy of urinary output.

- Take BP taken at regular intervals in lying, sitting, and standing positions during period of dosage adjustment if physician requests.
- Be aware that transient sedation, drowsiness, mental depression, weakness, and headache commonly occur during first 24–72 h of therapy or whenever dosage is increased. Symptoms tend to disappear with continuation of therapy or dosage reduction.
- Supervision of ambulation in older adults and patients with impaired kidney function; both are particularly likely to manifest orthostatic hypotension with dizziness and light-headedness during period of dosage adjustment.
- Monitor fluid and electrolyte balance and I&O. Report oliguria and changes in I&O ratio. Weigh patient daily, and check for edema because methyldopa favors sodium and water retention.
- Lab tests: Schedule baseline and periodic blood counts and liver function tests especially during first 6–12 wk of therapy or if patient develops unexplained fever; periodic serum electrolytes.
- Be alert to and report symptoms of mental depression (e.g., anorexia, insomnia, inattention to personal hygiene, withdrawal). Drug-induced depression may persist after drug is withdrawn.
- Be alert that rising BP indicating tolerance to drug effect may occur during week 2 or 3 of therapy.

Patient & Family Education

- Exercise caution with hot baths and showers, prolonged standing in one position, and strenuous exercise that may enhance orthostatic hypotension. Make position changes slowly, particularly from lying down to upright posture; dangle legs a few minutes before standing.
- Avoid potentially hazardous tasks such as driving until response to drug is known; drug may affect ability to perform activities requiring concentrated mental effort, especially during first few days of therapy or whenever dosage is increased.
- Do not to take OTC medications unless approved by physician.
- Do not breast feed while taking this drug without consulting physician.

METHYLERGONOVINE MALEATE

(meth-ill-er-goe-noe'veen)

Methergine

Classifications: AUTONOMIC NERVOUS SYSTEM AGENT; ADRENERGIC ANTAGONIST (SYMPATHOLYTIC); ERGOT ALKALOID; OXYTOCIC

Prototype: Ergotamine

AVAILABILITY 0.2 mg tablet; 0.2 mg/mL injections

ACTIONS Ergot alkaloid that induces rapid, sustained tetanic uterine contraction that shortens third stage of labor and reduces blood loss.

THERAPEUTIC EFFECTS Administered after delivery of the placenta. It minimizes the risk of postpartal hemorrhage.

USES Routine management after delivery of placenta and for postpartum atony, subinvolution, and hemorrhage. With full obstetric supervision, may be used during second stage of labor.

CONTRAINDICATIONS Hypersensitivity to ergot preparations; to induce labor; use prior to delivery of placenta; threatened spontaneous abortion; prolonged use; uterine sepsis; hypertension; toxemia; lactation.

ROUTE & DOSAGE

Postpartum Hemorrhage

Adult: **PO** 0.2–0.4 mg q6–12h until danger of atony passes (2–7 d) **IM/IV** 0.2 mg q2–4h (max: 5 doses)

ADMINISTRATION

- Use parenteral routes only in emergencies.

Oral

- Note: Dosing should not exceed 1 wk.

Intravenous

PREPARE: **Direct:** Give undiluted or diluted in 5 mL of NS.

ADMINISTER: **Direct:** Give 0.2 mg or fraction thereof over 60 sec.

- Do not use ampuls containing discolored solution or visible particles.
- Store at 15°–30° C (59°–86° F) unless otherwise directed. Protect from light.

ADVERSE EFFECTS (≥1%) **GI:** *Nausea, vomiting* (especially with IV doses). **CV:** Severe hypertensive episodes, bradycardia. **Body as a Whole:** Allergic phenomena including <u>shock</u>, ergotism.

INTERACTIONS Drug: PARENTERAL SYMPATHOMIMETICS, other ERGOT ALKALOIDS, TRIPTANS add to pressor effects and carry risk of hypertension; **amprenavir, delavirdine, efavirenz, indinavir, nelfinavir, ritonavir,** and **saquinavir** may decrease metabolism of **ergot** derivatives.

PHARMACOKINETICS Absorption: Readily absorbed from GI tract. **Onset:** 5–15 min PO; 2–5 min IM; immediate IV. **Duration:** 3 or more h PO; 3 h IM; 45 min IV. **Distribution:** Distributed into breast milk. **Metabolism:** Slowly metabolized in liver. **Elimination:** Excreted mainly in feces, small amount in urine. **Half-Life:** 0.5–2 h.

NURSING IMPLICATIONS

Assessment & Drug Effects

- Monitor vital signs (particularly BP) and uterine response during and after parenteral administration of methylergonovine until partum period is stabilized (about 1–2 h).
- Notify physician if BP suddenly increases or if there are frequent periods of uterine relaxation.

Patient & Family Education

- Report severe cramping for increased bleeding.
- Report any of the following: Cold or numb fingers or toes, nausea or vomiting, chest or muscle pain.
- Do not breast feed while taking this drug.

M

METHYLPHENIDATE HYDROCHLORIDE

(meth-ill-fen'i-date)

Concerta, Metadate CD, Metadate ER, Methylin, Ritalin, Ritalin LA, Ritalin SR

Classifications: CENTRAL NERVOUS SYSTEM (CNS) AGENT; CEREBRAL STIMULANT

Prototype: Amphetamine

Pregnancy Category: C

Controlled Substance: Schedule II

AVAILABILITY 5 mg, 10 mg, 20 mg tablets; 2.5 mg, 5 mg, 10 mg chewable tablets; 5 mg/5 mL, 10 mg/5 mL oral solution; 20 mg, 30 mg, 40 mg sustained release capsules; 18 mg, 27 mg, 36 mg, 54 mg sustained release tablet

ACTIONS Piperidine derivative with actions and abuse potential qualitatively similar to those of amphetamine. Acts mainly on cerebral cortex exerting a stimulant effect.

THERAPEUTIC EFFECTS Results in mild CNS and respiratory stimulation with potency intermediate between amphetamine and caffeine. More prominent on mental than on motor activities. Also believed to have an anorexiant effect.

USES Adjunctive therapy in hyperkinetic syndromes characterized by attention deficit disorder, narcolepsy, mild depression, and apathetic or withdrawn senile behavior.

CONTRAINDICATIONS Hypersensitivity to drug; history of marked anxiety, agitation; motor tics or Tourette's disease; substance abuse; severe anxiety, psychosis, major depression, suicidal ideation; glaucoma; pregnancy (category C), lactation, children <6 y of age.

CAUTIOUS USE Alcoholic; emotionally unstable patient; abrupt discontinuation; recent MI, anxiety, cardiac arrhythmias, cardiac disease, dysphagia, older adults; esophageal stricture, GI obstruction, heart failure, hepatic disease, hyperthyroidism, history of paralytic ileus, cystic fibrosis, mania, radiographic contrast administration, seizure disorder, hypertension; history of seizures.

ROUTE & DOSAGE

Narcolepsy

Adult: **PO** 10 mg b.i.d. or t.i.d. 30–45 min p.c. (range: 20–40 mg/d)

Attention Deficit Disorder

Child: **PO** 5–10 mg before breakfast and lunch, with a gradual increase of 5–10 mg/wk as needed (max: 60 mg/d) or 20–40 mg sustained release q.d. before breakfast

Depression

Geriatric: **PO** 2.5 mg in morning before 9 a.m., may increase by 2.5–5 mg q2–3d (max: 20 mg/d) divided 7 a.m. and noon

ADMINISTRATION

Oral

- Give 30–45 min before meals. To avoid insomnia, give last dose before 6 p.m.
- Ensure that sustained-release form is not chewed or crushed. It must be swallowed whole.
- Can open Metadate CD capsules and sprinkle on food
- Store at 15°–30° C (59°–86° F).

ADVERSE EFFECTS (≥1%) **CNS:** Dizziness, drowsiness, *nervousness, insomnia.* **CV:** Palpitations, changes in BP and pulse rate, angina, cardiac arrhythmias. **Special Senses:** Difficulty with accommodation, blurred vision. **GI:** Dry throat, anorexia, nausea; HEPATOTOXICITY; abdominal pain. **Body as a Whole:** Hypersensitivity reactions (rash, fever, arthralgia, urticaria, exfoliative dermatitis, erythema multiforme); growth suppression.

INTERACTIONS Drug: MAO INHIBITORS may cause hypertensive crisis; antagonizes hypotensive effects of **guanethidine, bretylium;** potentiates action of CNS STIMULANTS (e.g. **amphetamine, caffeine**); may inhibit metabolism and increase serum levels of **fosphenytoin, phenytoin, phenobarbital, and primidone, warfarin,** TRICYCLIC ANTIDEPRESSANTS.

PHARMACOKINETICS Absorption: Readily absorbed from GI tract. **Peak:** 1.9 h; 4–7 h sustained release. **Duration:** 3–6 h; 8 h sustained release. **Elimination:** Excreted in urine.

NURSING IMPLICATIONS

Assessment & Drug Effects

- Monitor BP and pulse at appropriate intervals.
- Lab tests: Obtain periodic CBC with differential and platelet counts during prolonged therapy.
- Chronic abusive use can lead to tolerance, psychic dependence, and psychoses.
- Assess patient's condition with periodic drug-free periods during prolonged therapy.
- Supervise drug withdrawal carefully following prolonged use. Abrupt withdrawal may result in severe depression and psychotic behavior.

Patient & Family Education

- Report adverse effects to physician, particularly nervousness and insomnia. These effects may diminish with time or require reduction of dosage or omission of afternoon or evening dose.
- Check weight at least 2 or 3 times weekly and report weight loss. Check height and weight in children; failure to gain in either should be reported to physician.
- Do not breast feed while taking this drug without consulting physician.

METHYLPREDNISOLONE

(meth-ill-pred-niss'oh-lone)
Medrol

METHYLPREDNISOLONE ACETATE

Depoject, Depo-Medrol, Depopred, Duralone, M-Prednisol, Rep-Pred

METHYLPREDNISOLONE SODIUM SUCCINATE

A-Methapred, Solu-Medrol
Classifications: HORMONES AND SYNTHETIC SUBSTITUTES; ADRENAL CORTICOSTEROID; GLUCOCORTICOID; ANTIINFLAMMATORY
Prototype: Prednisone
Pregnancy Category: C

AVAILABILITY **Methylprednisolone** 2 mg, 4 mg, 8 mg, 16 mg, 24 mg, 32 mg tablets **Methylprednisolone Acetate** 20 mg/mL, 40 mg/mL, 80 mg/mL injection **Methylprednisolone Sodium Succinate** 40 mg, 125 mg, 500 mg, 1 g, 2 g powder for injection

ACTIONS Intermediate-acting synthetic adrenal corticosteroid with similar glucocorticoid activity; has considerably fewer sodium and water retention effects than hydrocortisone. Acetate has longer duration of action and more rapid onset of activity than parent compound. Sodium succinate form is characterized by rapid onset of action and is used for emergency therapy of short duration. It inhibits phagocytosis, and release of allergic substances. Also modifies the immune response of the body to various stimuli.

THERAPEUTIC EFFECTS Antiinflammatory and immunosuppressive properties.

USES An antiinflammatory agent in the management of acute and chronic inflammatory diseases, for palliative management of neoplastic diseases, and for control of severe acute and chronic allergic processes. High-dose, short-term therapy: management of acute bronchial asthma, prevention of fat embolism in patient with long-bone fracture.

UNLABELED USES Acetate form used as a long-acting contracep-

M

tive and for spinal cord injury, lupus nephritis, multiple sclerosis.

CONTRAINDICATIONS Systemic fungal infections. Safety during pregnancy (category C) or lactation is not established.

CAUTIOUS USE Cushing's syndrome; GI ulceration; hypertension; varicella, vaccinia; diabetes mellitus; emotional instability or psychotic tendencies.

ROUTE & DOSAGE

Inflammation

Adult: **PO** 2–60 mg/d in 1 or more divided doses **IM** (Acetate) 4–80 mg/wk for 1–4 wk; (Succinate) 10–250 mg q6h **IV** 10–250 mg q6h
Child: **PO/IM/IV** 0.5–1.7 mg/kg/d divided q6–12h

Acute Spinal Cord Injury

Adult/Child: **IV** 30 mg/kg over 15 min, followed in 45 min by 5.4 mg/kg/h times 23 h

ADMINISTRATION

Oral

- Crush tablet before and give with fluid of patient's choice.
- Note: Preparation less irritating if given with food.
- Use alternate day therapy when given over long period.

Intramuscular

- Give injection deep into large muscle (not deltoid).

Intravenous

Note: Do NOT use methylprednisolone acetate for IV.

PREPARE: **Direct/Intermittent:** Available in ACT-O-Vial from which the desired dose may be withdrawn after initial dilution with supplied diluent. May be further diluted according to physician's orders.

ADMINISTER: **Direct/Intermittent:** Give each 500 mg or fraction thereof over 2–3 min.

INCOMPATIBILITIES **Solution/additive: Dextrose 5%/sodium chloride 0.45%, calcium gluconate, glycopyrrolate, metaraminol, nafcillin, penicillin G sodium, doxapram. Y-site: Allopurinol, amsacrine, ciprofloxacin, cisatracurium** (≥2 mg/mL concentration), **diltiazem, etoposide, filgrastim, gemcitabine, ondansetron, paclitaxel, potassium chloride, propofol, sargramostim, vinorelbine.**

- Store at 15°–30° C (59°–86° F). Do not freeze.

ADVERSE EFFECTS (≥1%) **CNS:** Euphoria, headache, insomnia, confusion, psychosis. **CV:** CHF, edema. **GI:** Nausea, vomiting, peptic ulcer. **Musculoskeletal:** Muscle weakness, delayed wound healing, muscle wasting, osteoporosis, aseptic necrosis of bone, spontaneous fractures. **Endocrine:** Cushingoid features, growth suppression in children, carbohydrate intolerance, hyperglycemia. **Special Senses:** Cataracts. **Hematologic:** Leukocytosis. **Metabolic:** Hypokalemia.

INTERACTIONS Drug: Amphotericin B, furosemide, THIAZIDE DIURETICS increase potassium loss; with ATTENUATED VIRUS VACCINES, may enhance virus replication or increase vaccine adverse effects; **isoniazid, phenytoin, phenobarbital, rifampin** decrease effectiveness of methylprednisolone because they increase metabolism of STEROIDS.

PHARMACOKINETICS Absorption: Readily absorbed from GI tract. **Peak:** 1–2 h PO; 4–8 d IM. **Duration:** 1.25–1.5 d PO; 1–5 wk IM. **Metabolism:** Metabolized in liver.

Half-Life: >3.5 h; HPA suppression: 18–36 h.

NURSING IMPLICATIONS

Assessment & Drug Effects

- Lab tests: Monitor periodically kidney and liver function, thyroid function, CBC, serum electrolytes, weight, and total cholesterol.
- Monitor diabetics for loss of glycemic control.
- Monitor serum potassium and report S&S of hypokalemia (see Appendix F).
- Monitor for and report S&S of Cushing's syndrome (see Appendix F).

Patient & Family Education

- Consult physician for any of the following: slow wound healing, significant insomnia or confusion, or unexplained bone pain.
- Do not alter established dosage regimen (i.e., not to increase, decrease, or omit doses or change dose intervals). Withdrawal symptoms (rebound inflammation, fever) can be induced with sudden discontinuation of therapy.
- Report onset of signs of hypocorticism adrenal insufficiency immediately: Fatigue, nausea, anorexia, joint pain, muscular weakness, dizziness, fever.
- Do not breast feed while taking this drug without consulting physician.

METHYLTESTOSTERONE

(meth-ill-tess-toss'te-rone)

Android, Metandren ♣, Testred, Virilon

Classifications: HORMONES AND SYNTHETIC SUBSTITUTES; ANDROGEN/ANABOLIC STEROID

Prototype: Testosterone

Pregnancy Category: X

Controlled Substance: Schedule III

AVAILABILITY 10 mg, 25 mg tablets; 10 mg buccal tablet

ACTIONS Short-acting steroid with androgen/anabolic activity ratio (1:1) similar to that of testosterone but less effective than its esters. Fails to produce full sexual maturation when administered to preadolescent male with complete testicular failure unless preceded by testosterone therapy.

THERAPEUTIC EFFECTS Androgen activity is similar to testosterone; used in replacement therapy, and palliative treatment of postmenopausal female breast cancer.

USES Androgen replacement therapy, delayed puberty (male), palliation of female mammary cancer (1–5 y postmenopausal), postpartum breast engorgement.

CONTRAINDICATIONS Liver dysfunction; prostate cancer; pregnancy (category X), lactation.

CAUTIOUS USE Liver, kidney, or cardiac dysfunction.

ROUTE & DOSAGE

Replacement

Adult: **PO** 10–50 mg/d in divided doses

Breast Cancer

Adult: **PO** 50–200 mg/d in divided doses for duration of therapeutic response or no longer than 3 mo if no remission

Postpartum Breast Engorgement

Adult: **PO** 80 mg/d for 3–5 d

ADMINISTRATION

Oral

- Place buccal tablets between cheek and gum. Ensure that tablet is absorbed, not chewed or swallowed; and eating or drink-

M

ing avoided until absorption is complete.

- Store at 15°–30° C (59°–86° F). Avoid freezing.

ADVERSE EFFECTS (≥1%) **GI:** Cholestatic hepatitis with jaundice, irritation of oral mucosa with buccal administration. **Urogenital:** Renal calculi (especially in immobilized patient), priapism. **Endocrine:** *Acne, gynecomastia, edema,* oligospermia, menstrual irregularities.

INTERACTIONS Drug: Increases risk of bleeding associated with ORAL ANTICOAGULANTS; possibly increases risk of **cyclosporine** toxicity; may decrease glucose level, making adjustment of doses of **insulin,** SULFONYLUREAS necessary. **Herbal: Echinacea** may increase risk of hepatotoxicity.

M

PHARMACOKINETICS Absorption: Readily absorbed from GI tract. **Metabolism:** Metabolized in liver. **Elimination:** Excreted in urine.

NURSING IMPLICATIONS

Assessment & Drug Effects

- Lab tests: Monitor liver function periodically; report signs of hepatic toxicity (see Appendix F).
- Monitor for flank pain, abdominal pain radiating to groin, or other symptoms of renal calculi.

Patient & Family Education

- Be prepared for distressing and undesirable adverse effects of virilization (women) since dosage sufficient to produce remission in breast cancer is quantitatively similar to that used for androgen replacement in the male.
- Report signs of virilism promptly. Voice change and hirsutism may be irreversible, even after drug is withdrawn.
- Report priapism (men) or other signs of excess sexual stimulation. The physician will terminate therapy.
- Report symptoms of jaundice with or without pruritus to physician; appears to be dose related. If liver function tests are altered at the same time, this drug will be withdrawn.
- Do not breast feed while taking this drug.

METIPRANOLOL HYDROCHLORIDE

(me-ti-pran′ol-ol)

OptiPranolol

Classifications: AUTONOMIC NERVOUS SYSTEM AGENT; BETA-ADRENERGIC ANTAGONIST (SYMPATHOLYTIC); EYE PREPARATION; MITOTIC (ANTIGLAUCOMA AGENT)

Prototype: Propranolol

Pregnancy Category: C

AVAILABILITY 0.3% ophthalmic solution

See Appendix A-1.

METOCLOPRAMIDE HYDROCHLORIDE (Pr)

(met-oh-kloe-pra′mide)

Clopra, Emex ♣, Maxeran ♣, Maxolon, Reglan

Classifications: GASTROINTESTINAL AGENT; PROKINETIC AGENT (GI STIMULANT)

Pregnancy Category: B

AVAILABILITY 5 mg, 10 mg tablets; 5 mg/5 mL solution; 5 mg/mL injection

ACTIONS Potent central dopamine receptor antagonist. Structurally related to procainamide but has little antiarrhythmic or anesthetic activity. Exact mechanism of action not clear but appears to sensitize GI smooth muscle to effects of acetylcholine by direct action.

THERAPEUTIC EFFECTS Increases resting tone of esophageal sphincter, and tone and amplitude of upper GI contractions. As a result, gastric emptying and intestinal transit are accelerated with little effect, if any, on gastric, biliary, or pancreatic secretions. Antiemetic action results from drug-induced elevation of CTZ threshold and enhanced gastric emptying. In diabetic gastroparesis, indicated by relief of anorexia, nausea, vomiting, persistent fullness after meals.

USES Management of diabetic gastric stasis (gastroparesis); to prevent nausea and vomiting associated with emetogenic cancer chemotherapy (e.g., cisplatin, dacarbazine); to facilitate intubation of small bowel; symptomatic treatment of gastroesophageal reflux.

CONTRAINDICATIONS Sensitivity or intolerance to metoclopramide; allergy to sulfiting agents; history of seizure disorders; concurrent use of drugs that can cause extrapyramidal symptoms; pheochromocytoma; mechanical GI obstruction or perforation; ileus; history of breast cancer; pregnancy (category B), lactation, children <6 y, infants, and neonates.

CAUTIOUS USE CHF, cardiac disease; sulfite hypersensitivity, asthma, hypokalemia, hypertension; depression; hepatic disease, infertility, methemoglobin reductase deficiency, Parkinson's disease, kidney dysfunction; GI hemorrhage; G6PD deficiency, procainamide hypersensitivity, seizure disorder, seizures, tardive dyskinesia; children; history of intermittent porphyria.

ROUTE & DOSAGE

Gastroesophageal Reflux

Adult: **PO** 10–15 mg q.i.d. a.c. and h.s.
Child: **PO/IV/IM** 0.4–0.8 mg/kg/d in 4 divided doses

Diabetic Gastroparesis

Adult: **PO** 10 mg q.i.d. a.c. and h.s. for 2–8 wk
Geriatric: **PO** 5 mg a.c and h.s.

Small-bowel Intubation, Radiologic Examination

Adult: **IM/IV** 10 mg administered over 1–2 min
Child: **IM/IV** *<6 y,* 0.1 mg/kg over 1–2 min; *6–14 y,* 2.5–5 mg over 1–2 min

Chemotherapy-induced Emesis

Adult/Child: **PO** 2 mg/kg 1 h before antineoplastic administration, may repeat q2h for 3 more doses if needed **IM/IV** 2 mg/kg 30 min before antineoplastic administration, may repeat q2h for 2 doses, then q3h for 3 doses if needed

ADMINISTRATION

Oral

- Give 30 min before meals and at bedtime.

Intravenous

Note: Verify correct IV concentration and rate of infusion for administration to infants or children with physician.

PREPARE: **Direct:** Doses of 10 mg or less may be given undiluted. **IV Infusion:** Doses >10 mg IV should be diluted in at least 50 mL of D5W, NS, D5/.45% NaCl, RL or other compatible solution.

ADMINISTER: **Direct:** Give over 1–2 min. **IV Infusion:** Give over 15 min. Note: Bags of metoclopramide should be protected from light during IV infusion (use of aluminum foil or a thick cotton cover).

INCOMPATIBILITIES **Solution/additive: Ampicillin, calcium gluconate, cephalothin, chloramphenicol, cisplatin, erythromycin, floxacillin, fluorouracil, furosemide, methotrexate, penicillin G potassium, sodium bicarbonate,** TETRACYCLINES. **Y-site: Allopurinol, amphotericin B cholesteryl complex, amsacrine, cefepime, doxorubicin liposome, furosemide, propofol.**

- Discard open ampules; do not store for future use.
- Store at 15°–30° C (59°–86° F) in light-resistant bottle. Tablets are stable for 3 y; solutions and injections, for 5 y.

M

ADVERSE EFFECTS (≥1%) **CNS:** *Mild sedation, fatigue, restlessness,* agitation, headache, insomnia, disorientation, *extrapyramidal symptoms* (acute dystonic type), neurologic malignant syndrome with injection. **GI:** Nausea, constipation, *diarrhea,* dry mouth, altered drug absorption. **Skin:** Urticarial or maculopapular rash. **Body as a Whole:** Glossal or periorbital edema. **Hematologic:** Methemoglobinemia. **Endocrine:** Galactorrhea, gynecomastia, amenorrhea, impotence. **CV:** Hypertensive crisis (rare).

DIAGNOSTIC TEST INTERFERENCE Metoclopramide may interfere with gonadorelin test by increasing ***serum prolactin*** levels.

INTERACTIONS Drug: Alcohol and other CNS DEPRESSANTS add to sedation; ANTICHOLINERGICS, OPIATE ANALGESICS may antagonize effect on GI motility; PHENOTHIAZINES may potentiate extrapyramidal symptoms; may decrease absorption of **acetaminophen, aspirin, atovaquone, diazepam, digoxin, lithium, tetracycline;** may antagonize the effects of **amantadine, bromocriptine, levodopa, pergolide, ropinirole, pramipexole;** may cause increase in extrapyramidal and dystonic reactions with PHENOTHIAZINES, THIOXANTHENES, **droperidol, haloperidol, loxapine, metyrosine;** may prolong neuromuscular blocking effects of **succinylcholine.**

PHARMACOKINETICS Absorption: Readily absorbed from GI tract. **Onset:** 30–60 min PO; 10–15 min IM; 1–3 min IV. **Peak:** 1–2 h. **Duration:** 1–3 h. **Distribution:** Distributed to most body tissues including CNS; crosses placenta; distributed into breast milk. **Metabolism:** Minimally metabolized in liver. **Elimination:** 95% Excreted in urine, 5% in feces. **Half-Life:** 2.5–6 h.

NURSING IMPLICATIONS

Assessment & Drug Effects

- Report immediately the onset of restlessness, involuntary movements, facial grimacing, rigidity, or tremors. Extrapyramidal symptoms are most likely to occur in children, young adults, and the older adult and with high-dose treatment of vomiting associated with cancer chemotherapy. Symptoms can take months to regress.
- Be aware that during early treatment period, serum aldosterone may be elevated; after prolonged administration periods, it returns to pretreatment level.
- Lab tests: Periodic serum electrolyte.
- Monitor for possible hypernatremia and hypokalemia (see Ap-

pendix F), especially if patient has CHF or cirrhosis.
- Adverse reactions associated with increased serum prolactin concentration (galactorrhea, menstrual disorders, gynecomastia) usually disappear within a few weeks or months after drug treatment is stopped.

Patient & Family Education
- Avoid driving and other potentially hazardous activities for a few hours after drug administration.
- Avoid alcohol and other CNS depressants.
- Report S&S of acute dystonia, such as trembling hands and facial grimacing (see Appendix F), immediately.
- Do not breast feed while taking this drug without consulting physician.

METOCURINE IODIDE

(met-oh-kyoo'reen)
Metubine Iodide
Classifications: AUTONOMIC NERVOUS SYSTEM AGENT; SKELETAL MUSCLE RELAXANT; NONDEPOLARIZING
Prototype: Tubocurarine
Pregnancy Category: C

AVAILABILITY 2 mg/mL injection

ACTIONS Semisynthetic nondepolarizing neuromuscular blocking agent. Pharmacologic effects almost identical to those of tubocurarine but is reportedly 2–3 times more potent. Has a slightly shorter duration of action, less histamine-releasing effect, and produces less ganglionic blockade.
THERAPEUTIC EFFECTS Produces skeletal muscle relaxation or paralysis by competing with acetylcholine at cholinergic receptor sites on skeletal muscle endplates, and thus blocks nerve impulse transmission.

USES Adjunct to anesthesia to induce skeletal muscle relaxation. Has been used to reduce intensity of skeletal muscle contractions in drug- or electrically induced convulsions and to facilitate endotracheal intubation.

CONTRAINDICATIONS Hypersensitivity to metocurine or to iodides; allergies, asthma; lactation.
CAUTIOUS USE Myasthenia gravis; renal, hepatic, or pulmonary impairment; respiratory depression; electrolyte disturbances; pregnancy (category C).

ROUTE & DOSAGE

Adjunct to General Anesthesia
Adult: **IV** 0.1–0.3 mg/kg over 30–60 s with 0.5–1 mg q30–90 min prn
Adjunct for Intubation
Adult: **IV** 0.2–0.4 mg/kg over 30–60 s
Electroshock Therapy
Adult: **IV** 1.75–5.5 mg/kg

ADMINISTRATION

Intravenous

PREPARE: **Direct:** Give undiluted.
ADMINISTER: **Direct:** Give over 30–60 s.
INCOMPATIBILITIES **Solution/additive:** ALKALINE SOLUTIONS. **Y-site:** BARBITURATES, **meperidine, morphine.**

- Protect solution from prolonged exposure to heat and direct sunlight. ▪ Store at 15°–30° C (59°–86° F).

ADVERSE EFFECTS (≥1%) **Body as a Whole:** Slight dizziness, feeling of warmth, malignant hyperthermia, hypersensitivity reactions. **CV:** *Hy-*

potension, circulatory collapse. **GI:** Decreased GI motility. **Musculoskeletal:** Profound and prolonged muscle weakness and flaccidity. **Respiratory:** Respiratory depression, hypoxia, apnea, increased bronchial and salivary secretions, bronchospasm.

INTERACTIONS Drug: Carbamazepine, phenytoin can lengthen time to neuromuscular blockade; may potentiate the effects of **botulinum toxin.**

PHARMACOKINETICS Onset: 1–4 min. **Peak:** 3–5 min. **Duration:** 35–90 min. **Distribution:** Crosses placenta. **Elimination:** Primarily excreted in urine, small amount in feces. **Half-Life:** 3.6 h.

NURSING IMPLICATIONS

Assessment & Drug Effects

- Note: Complete recovery from IV dose may require several hours.
- Use a peripheral nerve stimulator to monitor response.

METOLAZONE

(me-tole'a-zone)

Diulo, Mykrox, Zaroxolyn

Classifications: ELECTROLYTIC AND WATER BALANCE AGENT; THIAZIDE-LIKE DIURETIC; ANTIHYPERTENSIVE

Prototype: Hydrochlorothiazide

Pregnancy Category: D

AVAILABILITY 0.5 mg, 2.5 mg, 5 mg, 10 mg tablets

ACTIONS Diuretic structurally and pharmacologically similar to hydrochlorothiazide. Diuretic action is associated with drug interference with transport of sodium ions across renal tubular epithelium. This enhances excretion of sodium, chloride, potassium, bicarbonate, and water.

THERAPEUTIC EFFECTS Produces a decrease in the systolic and diastolic BPs, and reduces edema in CHF and kidney failure patients. Appears to be more effective as a diuretic than thiazides in patients with severe kidney failure.

USES Management of hypertension as sole agent or to enhance effectiveness of other antihypertensives in severe form of hypertension; also edema associated with CHF and kidney disease.

CONTRAINDICATIONS Anuria, hypokalemia; hepatic coma or precoma; hypersensitivity to metolazone and sulfonamides; pregnancy (category D), lactation.

CAUTIOUS USE History of gout; allergies; concomitant use of digitalis glycosides; kidney and liver dysfunction.

ROUTE & DOSAGE

Edema

Adult: **PO** 5–20 mg/d
Child: **PO** 0.2–0.4 mg/kg/d divided q12–24h

Hypertension

Adult: **PO** 2.5–5 mg/d; (Mykrox) 0.5–1 mg/d

ADMINISTRATION

Oral

- Do not interchange slow availability tablets and rapid availability tablets. They are not equivalent.
- Schedule doses to avoid nocturia and interrupted sleep. Give early in a.m. after eating to prevent gastric irritation (if given in 2 doses, schedule second dose no later than 3 p.m.).

- Store at 15°–30° C (59°–86° F) in tightly closed container.

ADVERSE EFFECTS (≥1%) **GI:** Cholestatic jaundice. **Body as a Whole:** Vertigo, orthostatic hypotension. **Hematologic:** Venous thrombosis, leukopenia. **Metabolic:** Dehydration, *hypokalemia, hyperuricemia, hyperglycemia.*

INTERACTIONS Drug: Amphotericin B, CORTICOSTEROIDS increase hypokalemic effects; may antagonize hypoglycemic effects of SULFONYLUREAS, **insulin; cholestyramine, colestipol** decrease thiazide absorption; intensifies hypoglycemic and hypotensive effects of **diazoxide;** because of increased potassium and magnesium loss, may cause **digoxin** toxicity; decreases **lithium** excretion, increasing its toxicity; NSAIDS may attenuate diuresis—increased risk of NSAID-induced kidney failure.

PHARMACOKINETICS Absorption: Incompletely absorbed; Mykrox has greater absorption. **Onset:** 1 h. **Peak:** 2–8 h. **Duration:** 12–24 h. **Distribution:** Distributed throughout extracellular tissue; concentrates in kidney; crosses placenta; distributed in breast milk. **Metabolism:** Does not appear to be metabolized. **Elimination:** Excreted in urine. **Half-Life:** 14 h.

NURSING IMPLICATIONS

Assessment & Drug Effects

- Anticipate overdosage and adverse reactions in geriatric patients; may be more sensitive to effects of usual adult dose.
- Terminate therapy when adverse reactions are moderate to severe.
- Expect possible antihypertensive effects in 3 or 4 d, but 3–4 wk are required for maximum effect.
- Lab tests: Determine serum potassium at regular intervals. Prolonged treatment and inadequate potassium intake increase potential for hypokalemia (see Appendix F). Periodic plasma glucose and urinalysis determinations.

Patient & Family Education

- Do not drink alcohol; it potentiates orthostatic hypotension.
- Antihypertensive therapy may require as adjunct a high-potassium, low-sodium, and low-calorie diet.
- Include potassium-rich foods in the diet.
- Be aware that if hypokalemia develops, dietary potassium supplement of 1000–2000 mg (25–50 mEq) is usually adequate treatment.
- Do not breast feed while taking this drug.

M

METOPROLOL TARTRATE

(me-toe′proe-lole)

Apo-Metoprolol ♣, Betaloc ♣, Lopressor, Norometoprol ♣, Toprol XL

Classifications: AUTONOMIC NERVOUS SYSTEM AGENT; BETA-ADRENERGIC ANTAGONIST (SYMPATHOLYTIC); ANTIHYPERTENSIVE

Prototype: Propranolol

Pregnancy Category: C

AVAILABILITY 50 mg, 100 mg tablets; 50 mg, 100 mg, 200 mg sustained release tablets; 1 mg/mL injection

ACTIONS Beta-adrenergic blocking agent with preferential effect on $beta_1$ adrenoreceptors located primarily on cardiac muscle. At higher doses, metoprolol also inhibits $beta_2$ receptors located chiefly on bronchial and vascular musculature. Antihypertensive action may be due to competitive antagonism of catecholamines at cardiac adrenergic neuron sites, drug-induced reduction of sympathetic outflow to the periphery, and to suppression of renin activity.

THERAPEUTIC EFFECTS Reduces heart rate and cardiac output at rest and during exercise; lowers both supine and standing BP, slows sinus rate and decreases myocardial automaticity. Antianginal effect is like that of propranolol.

USES Management of mild to severe hypertension (monotherapy or in combination with a thiazide or vasodilator or both); long-term treatment of angina pectoris and prophylactic management of stable angina pectoris reduce the risk of mortality after an MI.

UNLABELED USES CHF

CONTRAINDICATIONS Cardiogenic shock, sinus bradycardia, heart block greater than first degree, overt cardiac failure, right ventricular failure secondary to pulmonary hypertension. Safety during pregnancy (category C), lactation, or in children is not established.

CAUTIOUS USE Impaired liver or kidney function; cardiomegaly, CHF controlled by digitalis and diuretics; AV conduction defects; bronchial asthma and other bronchospastic diseases; history of allergy; thyrotoxicosis; diabetes mellitus; peripheral vascular disease.

ROUTE & DOSAGE

Hypertension

Adult: **PO** 50–100 mg/d in 1–2 divided doses, may increase weekly up to 100–450 mg/d
Geriatric: **PO** 25 mg/d (range: 25–300 mg/d)

Angina Pectoris

Adult: **PO** 100 mg/d in 2 divided doses, may increase weekly up to 100–400 mg/d

Myocardial Infarction

Adult: **IV** 5 mg q2min for 3 doses, followed by PO therapy **PO** 50 mg q6h for 48 h, then 100 mg b.i.d.

ADMINISTRATION

Oral

- Ensure that sustained-release form is not chewed or crushed. It must be swallowed whole.
- Give with food to slightly enhance absorption; however, administration with food not essential. It is important to give with or without food consistently to minimize possible variations in bioavailability.

Intravenous

PREPARE: **Direct:** Give undiluted.
ADMINISTER: **Direct:** Give at a rate of 5 mg over 60 seconds. Note conditions which are contraindications to drug administration.
INCOMPATIBILITIES **Y-site:** **Amphotericin B cholesteryl complex**

- Store at 15°–30° C (59°–86° F). Protect from heat, light, and moisture.

ADVERSE EFFECTS (≥1%) **Body as a Whole:** Hypersensitivity (erythematous rash, fever, headache, muscle aches, sore throat, laryngospasm, respiratory distress). **CNS:** *Dizziness, fatigue, insomnia,* increased dreaming, mental depression. **CV:** *Bradycardia,* palpitation, cold extremities, Raynaud's phenomenon, intermittent claudication, angina pectoris, CHF, intensification of AV block, AV dissociation, complete heart block, cardiac arrest. **GI:** Nausea, *heartburn,* gastric pain, diarrhea or constipation, flatulence. **Hematologic:** Eosinophilia, thrombocytopenic and nonthrombocytopenic purpura, agranulocytosis (rare). **Skin:** Dry skin, pruritus, skin eruptions. **Special Senses:** Dry mouth and mucous membranes. **Metabolic:** Hypoglycemia. **Respiratory:** Bronchospasm (with high doses), *shortness of breath*.

DIAGNOSTIC TEST INTERFERENCE In common with other beta blockers, metoprolol may cause elevated ***BUN*** and ***serum creatinine levels*** (patients with severe heart disease), elevated ***serum transaminase, alkaline phosphatase, lactate dehydrogenase,*** and ***serum uric acid.***

INTERACTIONS Drug: BARBITURATES, **rifampin** may decrease effects of metoprolol; **cimetidine, methimazole, propylthiouracil,** ORAL CONTRACEPTIVES may increase effects of metoprolol; additive bradycardia with **digoxin;** effects of both metoprolol and **hydralazine** may be increased; **indomethacin** may attenuate hypotensive response; BETA AGONISTS and metoprolol mutually antagonistic; **verapamil** may increase risk of heart block and bradycardia.

PHARMACOKINETICS Absorption: Readily absorbed from GI tract; 50% of dose reaches systemic circulation. **Onset:** 15 min. **Peak:** 1.5 h. **Duration:** 13–19 h. **Distribution:** Crosses blood–brain barrier and placenta; distributed into breast milk. **Metabolism:** Extensively metabolized in liver. **Elimination:** Excreted in urine. **Half-Life:** 3–4 h.

NURSING IMPLICATIONS

Assessment & Drug Effects

- Take apical pulse and BP before administering drug. Report to physician significant changes in rate, rhythm, or quality of pulse or variations in BP prior to administration.
- Monitor BP, HR, and ECG carefully during IV administration.
- Expect maximal effect on BP after 1 wk of therapy.
- Take several BP readings close to the end of a 12 h dosing interval to evaluate adequacy of dosage for patients with hypertension, particularly in patients on twice daily doses. Some patients require doses 3 times a day to maintain satisfactory control.
- Observe hypertensive patients with CHF closely for impending heart failure: Dyspnea on exertion, orthopnea, night cough, edema, distended neck veins.
- Lab tests: Obtain baseline and periodic evaluations of blood cell counts, blood glucose, liver and kidney function.
- Monitor I&O, daily weight; auscultate daily for pulmonary rales.
- Withdraw drug if patient presents symptoms of mental depression because it can progress to catatonia. Possible symptoms of depression: disinterest in people, surroundings, food, personal hygiene; withdrawal, apathy, sadness, difficulty in concentrating, insomnia.
- Monitor patients with thyrotoxicosis closely since drug masks signs of hyperthyroidism (see Appendix F). Abrupt withdrawal may precipitate thyroid storm.

Patient & Family Education

- Learn how to take radial pulse before each dose. Report to physician if pulse is slower than base rate (e.g., 60 bpm) or becomes irregular. Consult physician for parameters.

M

- Reduce insomnia or increased dreaming by avoiding late evening doses.
- Monitor blood glucose (diabetics) for loss of glycemic control. Drug may mask some symptoms of hypoglycemia (e.g., BP and HR changes) and prolong hypoglycemia. Be alert to other possible signs of hypoglycemia not affected by metoprolol and report to physician if present: Sweating, fatigue, hunger, inability to concentrate.
- Protect extremities from cold and do not smoke. Report cold, painful, or tender feet or hands or other symptoms of Raynaud's disease (intermittent pallor, cyanosis or redness, paresthesias). Physician may prescribe a vasodilator.
- Report immediately to physician the onset of problems with vision.
- Learn measures to relieve dry mouth; rinse mouth frequently with water, increase noncalorie liquid intake if inadequate, suck sugarless gum or hard candy.
- Relieve eye dryness by using sterile artificial tears available OTC.
- Do not drive or engage in potentially hazardous activities until response to drug is known.
- Do not alter established dosage regimen; compliance is very important.
- Reduce dosage reduced gradually over a period of 1–2 wk when drug is discontinued. Sudden withdrawal can result in increase in anginal attacks and MI in patients with angina pectoris and thyroid storm in patients with hyperthyroidism.
- Do not breast feed while taking this drug without consulting physician.

METRONIDAZOLE (Pr)

(me-troe-ni'da-zole)

Flagyl, Flagyl ER, Flagyl IV RTU, Flagyl 375, Metizol, Metric 21, Metro I.V., MetroGel, MetroGel Vaginal, MetroLotion, Noritate, Protostat

Classifications: ANTIINFECTIVE; ANTITRICHOMONAL; AMEBICIDE; ANTIBIOTIC

Pregnancy Category: B

AVAILABILITY 250 mg, 500 mg tablets; 375 mg capsules; 750 mg sustained release tablets; 500 mg vials; 0.75% lotion; 1% cream; 0.75% gel

ACTIONS Synthetic compound with direct trichomonacidal and amebicidal activity as well as antibacterial activity against anaerobic bacteria and some gram-negative bacteria.

THERAPEUTIC EFFECTS Effective against *Trichomonas vaginalis, Entamoeba histolytica,* and *Giardia lamblia*. Exhibits antibacterial activity against obligate anaerobic bacteria, gram-negative anaerobic bacilli, and *Clostridia*. Microaerophilic *Streptococci* and most aerobic bacteria are resistant.

USES Asymptomatic and symptomatic trichomoniasis in females and males; acute intestinal amebiasis and amebic liver abscess; preoperative prophylaxis in colorectal surgery, elective hysterectomy or vaginal repair, and emergency appendectomy. IV metronidazole is used for the treatment of serious infections caused by susceptible anaerobic bacteria in intraabdominal infections, skin infections, gynecologic infections, septicemia, and for both pre- and postoperative prophylaxis, bacterial vaginosis. ***Topical:*** Rosacea.

UNLABELED USES Treatment of pseudomembranous colitis, Crohn's disease, *H. pylori* eradication.

CONTRAINDICATIONS Blood dyscrasias; active CNS disease; first trimester of pregnancy (category B), lactation.

CAUTIOUS USE Coexistent candidiasis; second and third trimesters of pregnancy (category B); alcoholism; liver disease.

ROUTE & DOSAGE

Trichomoniasis, Giardiasis, *Gardnerella*

Adult: **PO** 2 g once or 250 mg t.i.d.; 375 mg b.i.d. or 500 mg b.i.d. for 7 d **Vaginal** Apply once or twice daily times 5 d
Child: **PO** 15 mg/kg/d in 3 divided doses for 7–10 d
Infant: **PO** 10–30 mg/kg/d for 5–8 d

Amebiasis

Adult: **PO** 500–750 mg t.i.d.
Child: **PO** 35–50 mg/kg/d in 3 divided doses

Anaerobic Infections

Adult: **PO** 7.5 mg/kg q6h (max: 4 g/d) **IV Loading Dose** 15 mg/kg **IV Maintenance Dose** 7.5 mg/kg q6h (max: 4 g/d)
Child: **PO/IV** 30 mg/kg/d divided q6h (max: 4 g/d)
Neonate: **PO/IV** 7.5–15 mg/kg/d divided q12–48h

Pseudomembranous Colitis

Adult: **PO** 250–500 mg t.i.d. **IV** 250–500 mg t.i.d. or q.i.d.
Child: **PO** 30 mg/kg/d divided q6h times 7 d

Bacterial Vaginosis

Adult: **PO** (Flagyl ER) 750 mg q.d. times 7 d

Rosacea

Adult: **Topical** apply thin film to affected area b.i.d.

ADMINISTRATION

Oral

- Crush tablets before ingestion if patient cannot swallow whole.
- Ensure that Flagyl ER (extend-release form) is not chewed or crushed. It must be swallowed whole. Give on an empty stomach, 1 h before or 2 h after meals.
- Give immediately before, with, or immediately after meals or with food or milk to reduce GI distress.
- Give lower than normal doses in presence of liver disease.

Intravenous

Note: Verify correct IV concentration and rate of infusion for administration to neonates, infants, or children with physician.

PREPARE: **Intermittent:** Sequence for preparing solution (important) consists of (1) reconstitution with 4.4 mL sterile water or NS, (2) dilution in IV solution to yield 8 mg/mL in NS, D5W, or RL, (3) pH neutralization with approximately 5 mEq sodium bicarbonate injection for each 500 mg of Flagyl I.V. used. Avoid use of aluminum-containing equipment when manipulating IV product (including syringes equipped with aluminum needles or hubs). Note: Flagyl IV RTU does not require mixing, diluting, or neutralizing. Each container contains 14 mEq of sodium.

ADMINISTER: **Intermittent:** Give IV solution slowly at a rate of one dose per hour.

INCOMPATIBILITIES **Solution/additive:** TPN, **amoxicillin/clavulanate, aztreonam, dopamine, meropenem. Y-site: Amphotericin B cholesteryl complex, aztreonam, filgrastim, meropenem, warfarin.**

M

▪ Note: Precipitation occurs if neutralized solution is refrigerated. Use diluted and neutralized solution within 24 h of preparation.

▪ Store at 15°–30° C (59°–86° F); protect from light. Reconstituted Flagyl I.V. is chemically stable for 96 h when stored below 30° C (86° F) in room light. Diluted and neutralized IV solutions containing Flagyl I.V. should be used within 24 h of mixing.

ADVERSE EFFECTS (≥1%) **Body as a Whole:** hypersensitivity (rash, urticaria, pruritus, flushing), fever, fleeting joint pains, overgrowth of *Candida*. **CNS:** Vertigo, headache, ataxia, confusion, irritability, depression, restlessness, weakness, fatigue, drowsiness, insomnia, paresthesias, sensory neuropathy (rare). **GI:** *Nausea,* vomiting, anorexia, epigastric distress, abdominal cramps, diarrhea, constipation, dry mouth, metallic or bitter taste, proctitis. **Urogenital:** Polyuria, dysuria, pyuria, incontinence, cystitis, decreased libido, dyspareunia, dryness of vagina and vulva, sense of pelvic pressure. **Special Senses:** Nasal congestion. **CV:** ECG changes (flattening of T wave).

DIAGNOSTIC TEST INTERFERENCE **Metronidazole** may interfere with certain chemical analyses for ***AST,*** resulting in decreased values.

INTERACTIONS Drug: ORAL ANTICOAGULANTS potentiate hypoprothrombinemia; **alcohol** may elicit disulfiram reaction; oral solutions of **citalopram, ritonavir; lopinavir/ritonavir,** and IV formulations of **sulfamethoxazole; trimethoprim, SMX-TMP, nitroglycerin** may elicit disulfiram reaction due to the alcohol content of the dosage form; **disulfiram** causes acute psychosis; **phenobarbital** increases metronidazole metabolism; may increase **lithium** levels; **fluorouracil, azathioprine** may cause transient neutropenia.

PHARMACOKINETICS Absorption: 80% of dose absorbed from GI tract. **Peak:** 1–3 h. **Distribution:** Widely distributed to most body tissues, including CSF, bone, cerebral and hepatic abscesses; crosses placenta; distributed in breast milk. **Metabolism:** 30%–60% metabolized in liver. **Elimination:** 77% excreted in urine; 14% excreted in feces within 24 h. **Half-Life:** 6–8 h.

NURSING IMPLICATIONS

Assessment & Drug Effects

- Discontinue therapy immediately if symptoms of CNS toxicity (see Appendix F) develop. Monitor especially for seizures and peripheral neuropathy (e.g., numbness and paresthesia of extremities).
- Lab tests: Obtain total and differential WBC counts before, during, and after therapy, especially if a second course is necessary.
- Monitor for S&S of sodium retention, especially in patients on corticosteroid therapy or with a history of CHF.
- Monitor patients on lithium for elevated lithium levels.
- Report appearance of candidiasis or its becoming more prominent with therapy to physician promptly.
- Repeat feces examinations, usually up to 3 mo, to ensure that amebae have been eliminated.

Patient & Family Education

- Adhere closely to the established regimen without schedule interruption or changing the dose.
- Refrain from intercourse during therapy for trichomoniasis unless

male partner wears a condom to prevent reinfection.
- Have sexual partners receive concurrent treatment. Asymptomatic trichomoniasis in the male is a frequent source of reinfection of the female.
- Do not drink alcohol during therapy; may induce a disulfiram-type reaction (see Appendix F). Avoid alcohol or alcohol-containing medications for at least 48 h after treatment is completed.
- Urine may appear dark or reddish brown (especially with higher than recommended doses). This appears to have no clinical significance.
- Report symptoms of candidal overgrowth: Furry tongue, color changes of tongue, glossitis, stomatitis; vaginitis, curd-like, milky vaginal discharge; proctitis. Treatment with a candidacidal agent may be indicated.
- Do not breast feed while taking this drug.

METYROSINE

(me-tye'roe-seen)
Demser
Classifications: HORMONES AND SYNTHETIC SUBSTITUTES; ENZYME INHIBITOR
Pregnancy Category: C

AVAILABILITY 250 mg capsules

ACTIONS Blocks the enzyme tyrosine hydroxylase to inhibit the conversion of tyrosine to DOPA, which is the initial and rate-setting step in synthesis of catecholamines (dopamine, epinephrine, norepinephrine).
THERAPEUTIC EFFECTS In patients with pheochromocytoma, reduces catecholamine synthesis as much as 80%, ameliorating hypertensive attacks and associated symptoms.

USES Short-term management of pheochromocytoma until surgery is performed, in long-term control when surgery is contraindicated, and in patients with malignant pheochromocytoma.
UNLABELED USES Has been used in selected patients with schizophrenia to potentiate antipsychotic effects of phenothiazines.

CONTRAINDICATIONS Control of essential hypertension. Safety during pregnancy (category C), lactation, or in children <12 y is not established.
CAUTIOUS USE Impaired liver or kidney function.

ROUTE & DOSAGE

Pheochromocytoma
Adult: **PO** 250 mg q.i.d., may increase to 2–3 g/d in divided doses (max: 4 g/d)

ADMINISTRATION

Oral
- Give each dose with a full glass of water and be consistent about time medication is to be taken.
- Store at 15°–30° C (59°–86° F).

ADVERSE EFFECTS (≥1%) **CNS:** *Sedation,* fatigue; *extrapyramidal signs: drooling, difficulty in speaking (dysarthria), tremors,* jaw stiffness (trismus); frank parkinsonism, psychic disturbances (anxiety, depression, hallucinations, disorientation, confusion), headache, muscle spasms. **GI:** *Diarrhea,* nausea, vomiting, abdominal pain, dry mouth. **Skin:** Rash, urticaria. **Urogenital:** Transient dysuria, crystalluria, hematuria, impotence, failure of ejaculation. **Endocrine:** Breast swelling, galactorrhea. **Body as a Whole:** Peripheral edema, nasal stuffiness, shortness of breath. **Hematologic:** Eosinophilia.

DIAGNOSTIC TEST INTERFERENCE False increases in ***urinary catecholamines*** may occur because of catechol metabolites of metyrosine.

INTERACTIONS Drug: Alcohol and other CNS DEPRESSANTS add to sedation and CNS depression; **droperidol, haloperidol,** PHENOTHIAZINES potentiate extrapyramidal effects.

PHARMACOKINETICS Absorption: Readily absorbed from GI tract. **Peak:** 2–3 d. **Duration:** 3–4 d. **Distribution:** Crosses blood–brain barrier. **Elimination:** Excreted in urine. **Half-Life:** 3.4–7.2 h.

NURSING IMPLICATIONS

Assessment & Drug Effects

- Monitor therapeutic effectiveness with frequent assessment of vital signs.
- Monitor I&O ratio and pattern. Fluid intake must be enough (e.g., 10–12 glasses or more) to maintain urinary output of 2000 mL or more to minimize risk of crystalluria.
- Perform routine urinalysis; if crystals occur, increase fluid intake further. If crystalluria persists, decrease drug dosage or discontinued.
- Lab tests: Obtain baseline and periodic measurements of urinary catecholamines and their metabolites (metanephrines and VMA). Metabolite excretion should decrease in patients with pheochromocytoma. Other baseline and regular determinations include kidney and liver function tests (in patients with dysfunction), and blood and urine glucose tests.
- Supervise ambulation. Sedative effects occur commonly within the first 24 h after drug is started. Maximal sedative effects in 2 or 3 d.

Patient & Family Education

- Notify physician if following adverse effects occur: Diarrhea, particularly if it is severe or persists, painful urination, jaw stiffness, drooling, difficult speech, tremors, disorientation. Dosage reduction or discontinuation of drug may be indicated.
- Avoid driving and potentially hazardous activities until response to drug is known.
- Be aware that abrupt withdrawal of metyrosine may result in psychic stimulation, feeling of increased energy, temporary changes in sleep pattern (usually insomnia). Symptoms may last for 2 or 3 d.
- Carry medical identification at all times if on prolonged therapy and notify all physicians and dentists involved in care about drug regimen.
- Do not breast feed while taking this drug without consulting physician.

MEXILETINE

(mex-il′e-teen)

Mexitil

Classifications: CARDIOVASCULAR AGENT; ANTIARRHYTHMIC, CLASS IB

Prototype: Lidocaine

Pregnancy Category: C

AVAILABILITY 150 mg, 200 mg, 250 mg capsules

ACTIONS Analog of lidocaine with class IB electrophysiologic properties similar to those of procainamide. Shortens action potential refractory period duration and improves resting potential.

THERAPEUTIC EFFECTS Has little or no effect on atrial tissue and produces modest suppression of sinus node automatically and AV nodal conduction. Prolongs the

His-to-ventricular interval (HQ) only if patient has preexisting conduction disturbance.

USES Acute and chronic ventricular arrhythmias; prevention of recurrent cardiac arrests; suppression of PVCs due to ventricular tachyarrhythmias.
UNLABELED USES Wolff-Parkinson-White syndrome and supraventricular arrhythmias.

CONTRAINDICATIONS Severe left ventricular failure, cardiogenic shock, severe bradyarrhythmias. Preexisting second- or third-degree heart block; pregnancy (category C), lactation; concurrent administration of drugs which alter urinary pH.
CAUTIOUS USE Patients with sinus node conduction irregularities, intraventricular conduction abnormalities; hypotension; severe congestive heart failure; liver dysfunction.

ROUTE & DOSAGE

Ventricular Arrhythmias
Adult: **PO** 200–300 mg q8h (max: 1200 mg/d)
Child: **PO** 1.4–5 mg/kg q8h

ADMINISTRATION

Oral
- Give with food or milk to reduce gastric distress.

ADVERSE EFFECTS (≥1%) **CNS:** *Dizziness, tremor, nervousness, incoordination,* headache, blurred vision, paresthesias, numbness. **CV:** Exacerbated arrhythmias, palpitations, chest pain, syncope, hypotension. **GI:** *Nausea, vomiting, heartburn,* diarrhea, constipation, dry mouth, abdominal pain. **Skin:** Rash. **Body as a Whole:** Dyspnea, edema, arthralgia, fever, malaise, hiccups. **Urogenital:** Impotence, urinary retention.

INTERACTIONS Drug: Phenytoin, phenobarbital, rifampin may decrease mexiletine levels; **cimetidine, fluvoxamine** may increase mexiletine levels; may increase **theophylline** levels; may increase proarrhythmic effects of **dofetilide** (separate administration by at least one week).

PHARMACOKINETICS Absorption: Readily absorbed from GI tract. **Peak:** 2–3 h. **Distribution:** Distributed into breast milk. **Metabolism:** Metabolized in liver. **Elimination:** Excreted in urine; renal elimination increases with urinary acidification. **Half-Life:** 10–12 h.

NURSING IMPLICATIONS

Assessment & Drug Effects
- Check pulse and BP before administration; make sure both are stabilized.
- Effective serum concentration range is 0.5–2 mcg/mL.
- Lab tests: Baseline and periodic liver function tests.
- Supervise ambulation in the weak, debilitated patient or the older adult during drug stabilization period. CNS adverse reactions predominate (e.g., intention tremors, nystagmus, blurred vision, dizziness, ataxia, confusion, nausea).
- Encourage drug compliance; affected particularly by the distressing adverse effects of tremor, ataxia, and eye symptoms.
- Check frequently with patient about adherence to drug regimen. If adverse effects are increasing, consult physician. Dose adjustment or discontinuation may be needed.

Patient & Family Education
- Learn about pulse parameters to be reported: Changes in rhythm and rate (bradycardia = pulse below 60); symptomatic bradycardia

M

(light-headedness, syncope, dizziness), and postural hypotension.
- Do not breast feed while taking this drug.

MEZLOCILLIN SODIUM

(mez-loe-sill'in)
Mezlin
Classifications: ANTIINFECTIVE; ANTIBIOTIC; ANTIPSEUDOMONAL PENICILLIN
Pregnancy Category: B

AVAILABILITY 1 g, 2 g, 3 g, 4 g, 20 g injection

ACTIONS Semisynthetic penicillin with extended spectrum. Structurally resembles ampicillin and has similar but wider antibacterial spectrum than either ampicillin, carbenicillin, or ticarcillin. In common with other penicillins, mezlocillin is bactericidal and acts by interfering with bacterial cell wall synthesis. Active against a wide variety of gram-negative and gram-positive bacteria including aerobic and anaerobic strains.

THERAPEUTIC EFFECTS Broadened spectrum of activity includes strains of pathogenic aerobic gram-negative bacteria (e.g., *Bacteroides, Enterobacter, Escherichia, Haemophilus, Klebsiella, Pseudomonas, Proteus*, and *Serratia*) and gram-positive organisms [e.g., *Streptococcus faecalis* (enterococcus)]. Inactive against penicillinase-producing strains of *Staphylococcus aureus*.

USES Primarily for serious infections caused by *Pseudomonas aeruginosa* alone or in combination with an aminoglycoside or a cephalosporin. Also used to treat other infections caused by susceptible strains.

CONTRAINDICATIONS History of hypersensitivity to penicillins or cephalosporins. Safety during pregnancy (category B) or lactation is not established.

CAUTIOUS USE Patients with known or suspected allergies to drugs or other substances; renal impairment, uremia; hypokalemia; bleeding tendencies.

ROUTE & DOSAGE

Uncomplicated UTI
Adult: **IM/IV** 1.5–2 g q6h (100–125 mg/kg/d)

Moderate to Severe Infections
Adult: **IM/IV** 4 g q6h (150–200 mg/kg/d)

Life-threatening Infection, *Pseudomonas* Infections
Adult: **IM/IV** 3 g q4h (max: 24 g/d)
Child: **IM/IV** *<1 mo,* 75 mg/kg q8–12h; *1 mo–12 y,* 50–75 mg/kg q4h

ADMINISTRATION

Intramuscular
- Give IM injection into a relatively large muscle such as the gluteus maximus (upper outer quadrant). Do not exceed 2 g per IM injection site.
- Lessen discomfort associated with IM administration lessened by giving injection slowly (over 12–15 seconds) and by reconstituting solution with lidocaine 0.5%–1% (lessens pain).

Intravenous

PREPARE: **Direct:** Dilute each 1 g with 10 mL of sterile water, D5W, or NS. Shake to dissolve. **Intermittent:** Further dilute with selected IV fluid to a volume of 50–100 mL.

ADMINISTER: **Direct:** Give over 3–5 min. **Intermittent:** Give over 30 min.

INCOMPATIBILITIES **Solution/additive: Ciprofloxacin,** AMINOGLYCOSIDES. **Y-site: Ciprofloxacin, meperidine, verapamil,** AMINOGLYCOSIDES.

- Store unopened vials and infusion bottles at or below 30° C (86° F) unless otherwise directed. Powder and reconstituted solutions may darken slightly, but this does not indicate loss of potency. Solutions should be clear. If a precipitate should form under refrigeration, warm solution to 37° C (98.6° F) in a water bath and shake well.

ADVERSE EFFECTS (≥1%) **CNS:** Convulsive seizures, neuromuscular hyperirritability. **GI:** Abnormal taste sensations, nausea, vomiting, *diarrhea*. **Hematologic:** Neutropenia, leukopenia, eosinophilia, thrombocytopenia (infrequent); increases in AST, ALT, alkaline phosphatase, serum bilirubin, creatinine, BUN; decreased Hct and Hgb. **Body as a Whole:** Hypersensitivity (*Rash,* pruritus, urticaria, drug fever, anaphylactic reactions). Local, pain (following IM), thrombophlebitis (IV injection); superinfections.

INTERACTIONS Drug: Mezlocillin increases risk of bleeding associated with ANTICOAGULANTS; **probenecid** decreases elimination of mezlocillin.

PHARMACOKINETICS Peak: 45 min IM; 5 min IV. **Distribution:** Widely distributed with highest concentrations in urine and bile; adequate CSF penetration with inflamed meninges; crosses placenta; distributed into breast milk. **Metabolism:** Slightly metabolized in liver. **Elimination:** 75% excreted in urine, up to 25% excreted in bile. **Half-Life:** 50–55 min.

NURSING IMPLICATIONS

Assessment & Drug Effects

- Obtain a detailed history before initiation of therapy to determine previous hypersensitivity, especially to penicillins and cephalosporins but also to other substances.
- Lab tests: Perform C&S tests prior to and periodically during therapy. Perform baseline and regularly scheduled studies of blood, kidney and liver function during long-term therapy.
- Observe IV sites for evidence of thrombophlebitis (see Appendix F).
- Monitor carefully during first 30 min after initiation of IV therapy for S&S of hypersensitivity and anaphylactoid reaction (see Appendix F).
- Observe and report ecchymoses, petechiae, bleeding gums, nosebleeds, or any other evidence of bleeding. Bleeding abnormalities (thrombocytopenia), although rare, are particularly likely to occur in patients with impaired kidney function.
- Be alert to signs of superinfections (see Appendix F).

Patient & Family Education

- Understand that therapy generally continues for at least 2 d after S&S of infection have subsided. Usual duration of therapy for serious infections is 7–10 d, but it may be longer in complicated infections.
- Report (women) onset of symptoms of *Candida* vaginitis. *Candida* vaginitis symptoms are moderate amount of white, cheesy, nonodorous vaginal discharge, vaginal inflammation, and itching.
- Report skin rash or pruritus to physician, who will assess for other signs of hypersensitivity (see Appendix F). Drug may need to be discontinued.

M

- Do not breast feed while taking this drug without consulting physician.

MICONAZOLE NITRATE

(mi-kon'a-zole)

Monistat-Derm, Monistat 3, Monistat 7, Femizol-M, M-Zole, Micatin, Tetterine, Fungoid, Lotrimin AF, Desenex

Classifications: ANTIINFECTIVE; ANTIBIOTIC; ANTIFUNGAL

Prototype: Fluconazole

Pregnancy Category: B

AVAILABILITY 100 mg, 200 mg vaginal suppositories; 2% cream; 2% ointment; 2% powder; 2% spray; 2% solution

M

ACTIONS Broad-spectrum agent with fungicidal activity. Mode of action is unclear but appears to inhibit uptake of components essential for cell reproduction and growth as well as cell wall structure, thus promoting cell death of fungi.

THERAPEUTIC EFFECTS Effective against *Candida albicans* and other species of this genus. Inhibits growth of common dermatophytes *Trichophyton rubrum, Trichophyton mentagrophytes, Epidermophyton floccosum,* and the organism responsible for tinea versicolor *(Malassezia furfur).*

USES Vulvovaginal candidiasis, tinea pedis (athlete's foot), tinea cruris, tinea corporis, and tinea versicolor caused by dermatophytes.

CONTRAINDICATIONS Hypersensitivity to miconazole.

CAUTIOUS USE Pregnancy (category B), lactation.

ROUTE & DOSAGE

Fungal Infection

Adult: **Topical** Apply cream sparingly to affected areas twice a day, and once daily for tinea versicolor, for 2 wk (improvement expected in 2–3 d, tinea pedis is treated for 1 mo to prevent recurrence) **Intravaginal** Insert suppository or vaginal cream q h.s. times 7 d (100 mg) or 3 d (200 mg)

ADMINISTRATION

Topical

- Apply cream sparingly to intertriginous areas (between skin folds) to avoid maceration of skin.
- Massage affected area gently until cream disappears.
- Store at 15°–30° C (59°–86° F) unless otherwise directed.

ADVERSE EFFECTS (≥1%) **Urogenital:** Vulvovaginal burning, itching, or irritation; maceration, allergic contact dermatitis.

INTERACTIONS Drug: may increase INR with **warfarin;** may inactivate **nonoxynol-9** spermicides.

PHARMACOKINETICS Absorption: Small amount absorbed from vagina. **Metabolism:** Rapidly metabolized in liver. **Elimination:** Excreted in urine and feces. **Half-Life:** 2.1–24 h.

NURSING IMPLICATIONS

Assessment & Drug Effects

- Expect clinical improvement from topical application in 1 or 2 wk. If no improvement in 4 wk, diagnosis is reevaluated. Treat tinea pedis infection for 1 mo to assure permanent recovery.

Patient & Family Education

- Complete full course of treatment to ensure recovery.
- Do not interrupt vaginal application during menstrual period.
- Avoid contact of drug with eyes.
- Do not breast feed while taking this drug without consulting physician.

MIDAZOLAM HYDROCHLORIDE

(mid'az-zoe-lam)

Versed

Classifications: CENTRAL NERVOUS SYSTEM AGENT; BENZODIAZEPINE ANXIOLYTIC; SEDATIVE-HYPNOTIC

Prototype: Lorazepam

Pregnancy Category: D

Controlled Substance: Schedule IV

AVAILABILITY 2 mg/mL syrup; 1 mg/mL, 5 mg/mL injection

ACTIONS Short-acting parenteral benzodiazepine. Mechanism of action unclear. Intensifies activity of gamma-aminobenzoic acid (GABA), a major inhibitory neurotransmitter of the brain, by interfering with its reuptake and promoting its accumulation at neuronal synapses. This calms the patient, relaxes skeletal muscles, and in high doses produces sleep.

THERAPEUTIC EFFECTS CNS depressant with muscle relaxant, sedative-hypnotic, anticonvulsant, and amnestic properties.

USES Sedation before general anesthesia, induction of general anesthesia; to impair memory of perioperative events (anterograde amnesia); for conscious sedation prior to short diagnostic and endoscopic procedures; and as the hypnotic supplement to nitrous oxide and oxygen (balanced anesthesia) for short surgical procedures.

CONTRAINDICATIONS Intolerance to benzodiazepines; acute narrow-angle glaucoma; shock, coma; acute alcohol intoxication; intraarterial injection. Safety in pregnancy (category D), labor and delivery, or lactation is not established.

CAUTIOUS USE Patient with COPD; chronic kidney failure; CHF; the older adult.

ROUTE & DOSAGE

Conscious Sedation

Adult: **IM** 0.07–0.08 mg/kg 30–60 min before procedure **IV** 1–1.5 mg, may repeat in 2 min prn; *Intubated Patients,* 0.05–0.2 mg/kg/h by continuous infusion

Child: **IM** 0.08 mg/kg times 1 dose **PR** 0.3 mg/kg times 1 dose; *Intubated Patients,* 2 mcg/kg/min by continuous infusion, may increase by 1 mcg/kg/min q30 min until light sleep is induced

Neonate: **IV** 0.5–1 mcg/kg/min

IV Induction for General Anesthesia

Adult: **IV** *Premedicated,* 0.15–0.25 mg/kg over 20–30 s, allow 2 min for effect **IV** *Nonpremedicated,* 0.3–0.35 mg/kg over 20–30 s, allow 2 min for effect

Child: **IV** 0.15 mg/kg followed by 0.05 mg/kg q2 min times 1–3 doses

Status Epilepticus

Child: **IV Loading Dose** *>2 mo,* 0.15 mg/kg **IV Maintenance Dose** 1 mcg/kg/min infusion, may titrate upward as needed q5min

Preoperative Sedation

Child: **PO** *<5 y,* 0.5 mg/kg; *>5 y,* 0.4–0.5 mg/kg

ADMINISTRATION

Intramuscular

- Inject IM drug deep into a large muscle mass.

Intravenous

PREPARE: **Direct:** Dilute in D5W or NS to a concentration of 0.25 mg/mL (e.g., 1 mg in 4 mL or 5 mg in 20 mL) **IV Infusion:** Add 5 mL of the 5 mg/mL concentration to 45 mL of D5W or NS to yield 0.5 mg/mL.

ADMINISTER: **Direct:** *Sedation,* Give over ≥2 min; *Induction of Anesthesia,* Give over 20–30 sec. **IV Infusion:** Give at a rate based on weight.

INCOMPATIBILITIES **Solution/additive: Lactated ringers, dimenhydrinate, pentobarbital, perphenazine, prochlorperazine, ranitidine. Y-site: Albumin, amoxicillin, amoxicillin/clavulanate, amphotericin B cholesteryl complex, ampicillin, bumetanide, butorphanol, ceftazidime, cefuroxime, clonidine, dexamethasone, dimenhydrinate, floxacillin, foscarnet, fosphenytoin, furosemide, hydrocortisone, imipenem/cilastatin, methotrexate, nafcillin, omeprazole, pentobarbital, perphenazine, prochlorperazine, sodium bicarbonate, thiopental, TPN.**

- Store at 15°–30° C (59°–86° F), therapeutic activity is retained for 2 y from date of manufacture.

ADVERSE EFFECTS (≥1%) **CNS:** *Retrograde amnesia,* headache, euphoria, drowsiness, excessive sedation, confusion. **CV:** Hypotension. **Special Senses:** Blurred vision, diplopia, nystagmus, pinpoint pupils. **GI:** Nausea, vomiting. **Respiratory:** Coughing, laryngospasm (rare), respiratory arrest. **Skin:** Hives, swelling, burning, pain, induration at injection site, tachypnea. **Body as a Whole:** Hiccups, chills, weakness.

INTERACTIONS Drug: Alcohol, CNS DEPRESSANTS, ANTICONVULSANTS potentiate CNS depression; **cimetidine** increases midazolam plasma levels, increasing its toxicity; may decrease antiparkinsonism effects of **levodopa;** may increase **phenytoin** levels; **smoking** decreases sedative and antianxiety effects. **Herbal: Kava-kava, valerian** may potentiate sedation.

PHARMACOKINETICS Onset: 1–5 min IV; 5–15 min IM, 20–30 min PO. **Peak:** 20–60 min. **Duration:** <2 h IV; 1–6 h IM. **Distribution:** Crosses blood–brain barrier and placenta. **Metabolism:** Metabolized in liver. **Elimination:** Excreted in urine. **Half-Life:** 1–4 h.

NURSING IMPLICATIONS

Assessment & Drug Effects

- Inspect insertion site for redness, pain, swelling, and other signs of extravasation during IV infusion.
- Monitor for hypotension, especially if the patient is premedicated with a narcotic agonist analgesic.
- Monitor vital signs for entire recovery period. In obese patient, half-life is prolonged during IV infusion; therefore, duration of effects is prolonged (i.e., amnesia, postoperative recovery).
- Be aware that overdose symptoms include somnolence, confusion, sedation, diminished reflexes, coma, and untoward effects on vital signs.

Patient & Family Education

- Do not drive or engage in potentially hazardous activities until response to drug is known. You may

feel drowsy, weak, or tired for 1–2 d after drug has been given.
- Be prepared for amnesia to prevent an upsetting postoperative period.
- Review written instructions to assure future understanding and compliance. Patient teaching during amnestic period may not be remembered. Even if dose is small and depth of amnesia is unclear, relearn information.

MIDODRINE HYDROCHLORIDE

(mid′o-dreen)

ProAmatine

Classifications: AUTONOMIC NERVOUS SYSTEM AGENT; ALPHA$_1$ AGONIST

Prototype: Methoxamine

Pregnancy Category: C

AVAILABILITY 2.5 mg, 5 mg tablets

ACTIONS Vasopressor and alpha$_1$ agonist. Activates the alpha-adrenergic receptors of the arteries and veins, resulting in increased vascular tone and elevation in blood pressure.

THERAPEUTIC EFFECTS Affects standing, sitting, and supine systolic and diastolic blood pressures. Indicated by an increase in 1-min standing systolic BP and subjective feelings of clinical improvement.

USES Treatment of symptomatic orthostatic hypotension.

CONTRAINDICATIONS Severe organic heart disease; acute kidney disease; urinary retention; pheochromocytoma; thyrotoxicosis; persistent and excessive supine hypertension.

CAUTIOUS USE Renal impairment, hepatic impairment; history of visual problems; diabetes with hypotension or visual disorders; pregnancy (category C), lactation. Safety and efficacy in children are not established.

ROUTE & DOSAGE

Orthostatic Hypotension

Adult: **PO** 10 mg t.i.d. during the daytime hours, dosed not less that 3 h apart with last dose at least 4 h before bedtime (max: 20 mg/dose)

ADMINISTRATION

Oral
- Do not give at bedtime or before napping (within 4 h of lying supine for any length of time)
- Give with caution in persons with pretreatment, supine systolic BP ≥170 mm Hg.
- Store at 15°–30° C (59°–86° F).

ADVERSE EFFECTS (≥1%) **Body as a Whole:** *Paresthesia,* chills, pain, facial flushing. **CNS:** Confusion, nervousness, anxiety. **CV:** *Hypertension.* **GI:** Dry mouth. **Skin:** *Pruritus, piloerection,* rash. **Urogenital:** *Dysuria, urinary retention, urinary frequency.*

INTERACTIONS Drug: may antagonize effects of **doxazosin, prazosin, terazosin;** may potentiate vasoconstrictive effects of **ephedrine, phenylephrine, phenylpropanolamine, pseudoephedrine;** may cause hypertensive crisis with MAOIS.

PHARMACOKINETICS Absorption: Rapidly absorbed from GI tract. **Peak:** Midodrine 0.5 h; desglymidodrine 1–2 h. **Metabolism:** Rapidly metabolized to desglymidodrine, the active metabolite. **Elimination:** Excreted in urine. **Half-Life:** Midodrine 25 min, desglymidodrine 3–4 h.

NURSING IMPLICATIONS

Assessment & Drug Effects
- Lab tests: Evaluate kidney and liver function prior to initiating therapy.

M

- Monitor regularly supine and standing BP. Stop drug if supine BP increases excessively; determine acceptable parameters.
- Monitor carefully effect of the drug in diabetics with orthostatic hypotension and those taking fludrocortisone acetate, which may increase intraocular pressure.

Patient & Family Education

- Take last daily dose 4 h before bedtime.
- Report immediately to physician sensations associated with supine hypertension (e.g., pounding in ears, headache, blurred vision, awareness of heart beating).
- Discontinue drug and report to physician if S&S of bradycardia develop (e.g., dizziness, pulse slowing, fainting).
- Do not take allergy drugs, cold preparations, or diet pills without consulting physician.
- Do not breast feed while taking this drug without consulting physician.

MIGLITOL

(mig'li-tol)

Glyset

Classifications: HORMONES AND SYNTHETIC SUBSTITUTES; ANTIDIABETIC AGENT; ALPHA-GLUCOSIDASE INHIBITOR

Prototype: Acarbose

Pregnancy Category: B

AVAILABILITY 25 mg, 50 mg, 100 mg tablets

ACTIONS Enzyme inhibition of intestinal glucosidases that delays the formation of glucose from saccharides in the small intestine. Miglitol does not enhance insulin secretion.

THERAPEUTIC EFFECTS It delays the digestion of carbohydrates, lowers the postprandial hyperglycemia, and reduces the levels of glysylated hemoglobin (HbA_{1C}) in type 2 diabetics.

USES Adjunct to diet for control of type 2 diabetes; may be used alone or with a sulfonylurea.

CONTRAINDICATIONS Diabetic ketoacidosis; digestive or absorptive disorders; history of or partial intestinal obstruction, inflammatory bowel disease; hypersensitivity to miglitol; lactation.

CAUTIOUS USE Hypersensitivity to acarbose; creatinine clearance above 2 mg/dL; concomitant use with sulfonylurea; high stress conditions (i.e., surgery, trauma, etc.); pregnancy (category B). Safety and efficacy in children <18 y unknown.

ROUTE & DOSAGE

Type 2 Diabetes Mellitis

Adult: **PO** 25 mg t.i.d. at the start of each meal, may increase after 4–8 wk to 50 mg t.i.d. (max: 100 mg t.i.d.)

ADMINISTRATION

Oral

- Give drug with first bite of each of the three main meals.
- Store at 15°–30° C (59°–86° F).

ADVERSE EFFECTS (≥1%) **GI:** *Abdominal pain, diarrhea, flatulence.* **Skin:** Rash. **Metabolic:** Hypoglycemia.

INTERACTIONS Drug: Miglitol may reduce bioavailability of **propranolol, ranitidine; charcoal, pancreatin, amylase, pancrelipase** may decrease effectiveness of **miglitol. Herbal: Garlic, ginseng** may potentiate hypoglycemic effects.

PHARMACOKINETICS Absorption: 25 mg dose is completely absorbed, amount absorbed decreases with increasing dose to where 100 mg dose is 50–70% absorbed. **Peak:** 2–3 h. **Distribution:** Minimal protein binding (<4%). **Metabolism:** Not metabolized. **Elimination:** Half-life 2 h; 95% excreted unchanged in urine, lower doses should be used in patients with renal impairment.

NURSING IMPLICATIONS

Assessment & Drug Effects

- Monitor for therapeutic effectiveness: Indicated by improved blood glucose levels and decreased HbA_{1C}.
- Monitor for S&S of hypoglycemia when used in combination with sulfonylureas, insulin, other hypoglycemia agents.
- Lab tests: Monitor HbA_{1C} q3mo.
- Treat hypolgycemia with oral glucose (dextrose); miglitol interferes with the breakdown of sucrose (table sugar).

Patient & Family Education

- Keep a source of oral glucose available to treat low blood sugar; miglitol prevents digestive breakdown of table sugar.
- Abdominal discomfort, flatulence, and diarrhea tend to diminish with continued therapy.
- Do not breast feed while taking this drug.

MILRINONE LACTATE

(mil′ri-none)

Primacor

Classifications: CARDIOVASCULAR AGENT; INOTROPIC AGENT; VASODILATOR

Prototype: Inamrinone

Pregnancy Category: C

AVAILABILITY 1 mg/mL, 200 mcg/mL injection

ACTIONS Member of a class of inotropic/vasodilator agents. Positive inotropic action and vasodilator, with little chronotropic activity; mode of action and structure are different from digitalis and catecholamines as well as beta-adrenergic agonists. Inhibitory action against cyclic-AMP phosphodiesterase in cardiac and smooth vascular muscle. Increases cardiac contractility.

THERAPEUTIC EFFECTS In therapeutic dose, increases myocardial contractility. Therefore, increases cardiac output and decreases pulmonary wedge pressure and vascular resistance, without increasing myocardial oxygen demand or significantly increasing heart rate.

USES Short-term management of CHF.

UNLABELED USES Short-term use to increase the cardiac index in patients with low cardiac output after surgery. To increase cardiac function prior to heart transplantation.

CONTRAINDICATIONS Hypersensitivity to milrinone.

CAUTIOUS USE Older adult; pregnancy (category C), lactation. Safety and efficacy in children are not established.

ROUTE & DOSAGE

Heart Failure

Adult: **IV Loading Dose** 50 mcg/kg IV over 10 min **IV Maintenance Dose** 0.375–0.75 mcg/kg/min

ADMINISTRATION

Intravenous

Note: Correct preexisting hypokalemia before administering

milrinone. See manufacturer's information for dosage reduction in the presence of renal impairment.

PREPARE: **Loading Dose:** Give undiluted or dilute each 1 mg in 1 mL NS or 0.45% NaCl. **IV Infusion:** Dilute 20 mg of milrinone in D5W, NS, or 0.45% NaCl to yield: 100 mcg/mL with 180 mL diluent; 150 mcg/mL with 113 mL diluent; 200 mcg/mL with 80 mL diluent.

ADMINISTER: **Loading Dose:** Give 50 mcg/kg over 10 min. **IV Infusion:** Give at a rate based on weight. Use a microdrip set and infusion pump.

INCOMPATIBILITIES **Solution/additive: Furosemide, procainamide. Y-site: Furosemide, procainamide.**

- Store according to manufacturer's directions.

ADVERSE EFFECTS (≥1%) **CV:** Increased ectopic activity, PVCs, ventricular tachycardia, ventricular fibrillation, supraventricular arrhythmias; possible increase in angina symptoms, hypotension.

INTERACTIONS Drug: Disopyramide may cause excessive hypotension.

PHARMACOKINETICS Peak: 2 min. **Duration:** 2 h. **Distribution:** 70% protein bound. **Elimination:** 80%–85% excreted unchanged in urine within 24 h. Active renal tubular secretion is primary elimination pathway. **Half-Life:** 1.7–2.7 h.

NURSING IMPLICATIONS

Assessment & Drug Effects

- Monitor cardiac status closely during and for several hours following infusion. Supraventricular and ventricular arrhythmias have occurred.
- Monitor BP and promptly slow or stop infusion in presence of significant hypotension. Closely monitor those with recent aggressive diuretic therapy for decreasing blood pressure.
- Monitor fluid and electrolyte status. Hypokalemia should be corrected whenever it occurs during administration.

Patient & Family Education

- Report immediately angina that occurs during infusion to physician.
- Be aware that drug may cause a headache, which can be treated with analgesics.

MINERAL OIL

Agoral Plain, Heavy Mineral Oil, Kondremul Plain, Milkinol, Neo-Cultol, Zymenol

Classifications: GASTROINTESTINAL AGENT; STOOL SOFTENER

Prototype: Docusate

Pregnancy Category: C

AVAILABILITY Liquid and emulsion

ACTIONS Mixture of hydrocarbons obtained from petroleum. Aids passage of stool by lubricating it and by slowing the rate of water absorption from the feces while it is in the large intestine.

THERAPEUTIC EFFECTS Lubricates and softens feces, retards water absorption from fecal content, eases passage of stool.

USES Temporary relief of constipation, when straining at stool is contraindicated (e.g., hypertension, certain cardiac disorders, following anorectal surgery), and to relieve fecal impaction. Also used as pharmaceutical solvent and vehicle.

CONTRAINDICATIONS Nausea, vomiting, abdominal pain, intestinal obstruction; oral administration to dysphagic patients; use with emollients. **CAUTIOUS USE** Oral use in older adult or debilitated patients; pregnancy (category C), lactation.

ROUTE & DOSAGE

Constipation
Adult: **PO** 15–30 mL prn **PR** 90–120 mL
Child: **PO** ≥6 *y*, 5–15 mL once/d

ADMINISTRATION

Oral
- Give preferably in the evening. Digestion and passage of food from stomach may be delayed if taken within 2 h of mealtime.
- Give with patient in upright position and avoid giving just before patient retires. Potential of lipid pneumonia from aspiration is especially high in older adult and debilitated patients.
- Use as retention enema is generally followed by a cleansing enema in 30–60 min. Consult physician.

ADVERSE EFFECTS (≥1%) **Body as a Whole:** Pruritus ani; interference with postoperative anorectal wound healing. **Respiratory:** With aspiration: pulmonary granuloma, lipid pneumonitis. **GI:** Anorexia, nausea, vomiting. **Metabolic:** Nutritional deficiencies (with prolonged use). **Hematologic:** Hypoprothrombinemia (with prolonged use).

INTERACTIONS Drug: May potentiate effects of ORAL ANTICOAGULANTS by decreasing the absorption of Vitamin K; large doses may decrease the absorption of **warfarin;** STOOL SOFTENERS may form a concretion in the GI tract.

PHARMACOKINETICS Absorption: Limited absorption from GI tract. **Distribution:** Distributes to mesenteric lymph nodes, intestinal mucosa, liver, and spleen. **Elimination:** Eliminated in stool in 6–10 h.

NURSING IMPLICATIONS

Assessment & Drug Effects
- Monitor bowel movements.

Patient & Family Education
- Be aware that prolonged use (>2 wk) can reduce absorption of fat-soluble vitamins A, D, E, and K, carotene, calcium, and phosphates.
- Frequent or prolonged use of mineral oil may result in dependence.
- Do not breast feed while taking this drug without consulting physician.

MINOCYCLINE HYDROCHLORIDE

(mi-noe-sye'kleen)
Minocin, Dynacin, Vectrin
Classifications: ANTIINFECTIVE; TETRACYCLINE ANTIBIOTIC
Prototype: Tetracycline
Pregnancy Category: D

AVAILABILITY 50 mg, 100 mg capsules; 50 mg/5 mL suspension; 100 mg injection

ACTIONS Semisynthetic tetracycline derivative which appears to be active against strains of *Staphylococci* resistant to other tetracyclines; photosensitivity occurs only rarely. Reported to be more completely absorbed than other TETRACYCLINES because it is more lipid-soluble.
THERAPEUTIC EFFECTS Effective against *Mycobacterium marinum* infections, *U. urealyticum, N. gonorrhoeae.*

USES Treatment of mucopurulent cervicitis, granuloma inguinale, lymphogranuloma venereum, proctitis, bronchitis, lower respiratory tract in-

M

fections caused by *Mycoplasma pneumoniae,* Rickettsial infections, chlamydial infections, non-gonococcal urethritis, chlamydial conjunctivitis, plague, brucellosis, bartonellosis, tularemia, UTI, and prostatitis; *acne vulgaris,* gonorrhea, cholera, meningococcal carrier state,

CONTRAINDICATIONS Hypersensitivity to tetracyclines; oral administration in meningococcal infections; pregnancy (category D), lactation, children <8 y.
CAUTIOUS USE Renal and hepatic impairment.

ROUTE & DOSAGE

Antiinfective

Adult: **PO/IV** 200 mg followed by 100 mg q12h
Child: **PO/IV** >8 y, 4.4 mg/kg followed by 2 mg/kg q12h

Acne

Adult: **PO** 50 mg 1–3 times/d

Meningococcal carrier state

Adult: **PO** 100 mg q12h times 5 d
Child: **PO** >8 y, 4 mg/kg followed by 2 mg/kg q12h times 5 d (max: 100 mg/dose)

ADMINISTRATION

Oral

- Shake suspension well before administration.
- Oral therapy is the preferred route; institute as soon as possible.
- Check expiration date. Outdated tetracycline can cause severe adverse effects.

Intravenous

PREPARE: **Intermittent:** Reconstitute 100 mg with 5 mL of sterile water for injection; further dilute with 500–1000 mL of D5W, NS, D5/NS, or RL.

ADMINISTER: **Intermittent:** Start infusion immediately after preparation. Avoid rapid infusion. Give at a rate determined by the total volume of solution.

INCOMPATIBILITIES **Solution/additive: Doxapram, rifampin. Y-site: Allopurinol, amifostine, hydromorphone, meperidine, morphine, piperacillin/tazobactam, propofol, thiotepa, TPN.**

- Reconstituted solution is stable at room temperature for 24 h; further diluted solution should be used immediately.

ADVERSE EFFECTS (≥1%) **CNS:** *Weakness, light-headedness, ataxia, dizziness, or vertigo.* **GI:** Nausea, cramps, diarrhea, flatulence.

INTERACTIONS Drug: ANTACIDS, **iron, calcium, magnesium, zinc, kaolin and pectin, sodium bicarbonate, bismuth subsalicylate** can significantly decrease minocycline absorption; effects of both **desmopressin** and minocycline antagonized; increases **digoxin** absorption, increasing risk of **digoxin** toxicity; **methoxyflurane** increases risk of kidney failure. **Food:** Dairy products significantly decrease minocycline absorption; food may also decrease its absorption.

PHARMACOKINETICS Absorption: 90%–100% absorbed from GI tract. **Peak:** 2–3 h. **Distribution:** Tends to accumulate in adipose tissue; crosses placenta; distributed into breast milk. **Metabolism:** Partially metabolized. **Elimination:** 20%–30% excreted in feces; about 12% excreted in urine. **Half-Life:** 11–26 h.

NURSING IMPLICATIONS

Assessment & Drug Effects

- Obtain history of hypersensitivity reactions prior to administration;

drug is contraindicated with known tetracycline hypersensitivity.

- Lab: C&S should be drawn prior to initiation of therapy.
- Monitor IV infusion site carefully, since thrombophlebitis occurs relatively often (see Appendix F).
- Monitor carefully for signs of hypersensitivity response (see Appendix F), particularly in patients with history of allergies, especially to drugs.
- Monitor at-risk patients for S&S of superinfection (see Appendix F).
- Assess risk of toxic effects carefully; increases with renal and hepatic impairment.
- Determine serum drug level in patients receiving prolonged therapy.
- Supervise ambulation, since lightheadedness, dizziness, and vertigo occur frequently.

Patient & Family Education

- Avoid hazardous activities or those requiring alertness while taking minocycline.
- Use sunscreen when outdoors and otherwise protect yourself from direct sunlight since photosensitivity reaction may occur.
- Report vestibular adverse effects (e.g., dizziness), which usually occur during first week of therapy. Effects are reversible if drug is withdrawn.
- Report loose stools or diarrhea or other signs of superinfection promptly to physician.
- Use or add barrier contraceptive while they are taking drug if using hormonal contraceptive.
- Do not breast feed while taking this drug.

MINOXIDIL

(mi-nox'i-dill)

Loniten, Rogaine

Classifications: CARDIOVASCULAR AGENT; NONNITRATE VASODILATOR; ANTIHYPERTENSIVE

Prototype: Hydralazine

Pregnancy Category: C

AVAILABILITY 2.5 mg, 10 mg tablets; 2% solution

ACTIONS Direct-acting vasodilator similar to other drugs of this class, but hypotensive effect is more pronounced. Appears to act by blocking calcium uptake through cell membrane. Reduces elevated systolic and diastolic blood pressures in supine and standing positions, by decreasing peripheral vascular resistance.

THERAPEUTIC EFFECTS Hypotensive action accompanied by reflex activation of sympathetic, vagal inhibitory, and renal homeostatic mechanisms; increased sympathetic stimulation also activates the renin-angiotensin-aldosterone system. Net result is increased heart rate and cardiac output, sodium retention, and edema, which usually necessitates concomitant supportive drug therapy. Drug-induced hair growth with systemic minoxidil usually develops after 1 y of therapy: it is nonvirilizing, involving face and limbs of the female and generalized increase in body hair in men. Topical minoxidil reverses balding to some degree.

USES Treat severe hypertension that is symptomatic or associated with damage to target organs and is not manageable with maximum therapeutic doses of a diuretic plus two other antihypertensive drugs. Used with a diuretic to prevent fluid retention and a beta adrenergic blocking agent (e.g.,

M

propranolol) or an alpha-adrenergic agonist (e.g., clonidine or methyldopa) to prevent tachycardia. *(Topical)* to treat alopecia areata and male pattern alopecia.

CONTRAINDICATIONS Pheochromocytoma; acute MI, dissecting aortic aneurysm, valvular dysfunction, heart failure. Safety during pregnancy (category C) or lactation is not established.

CAUTIOUS USE Severe renal impairment; recent MI (within preceding month); coronary artery disease, chronic CHF.

ROUTE & DOSAGE

Hypertension

Adult: **PO** 5 mg/d, increased q3–5d up to 40 mg/d in single or divided doses as needed (max: 100 mg/d)
Child: **PO** 0.2 mg/kg/d (max: 5 mg/d) initially, gradually increased to 0.25–1 mg/kg/d in divided doses (max: 50 mg/d)

Alopecia

Adult: **Topical** Apply 1 mL of 2% solution to affected area b.i.d.

ADMINISTRATION

Oral

- Dose increments at usually made at 3–5 day intervals. If more rapid adjustment is necessary, adjustments can be made q6h with careful monitoring.

Topical

- Do not apply topical product to an irritated scalp (e.g., sunburn, psoriasis).
- Store at 15°–30° C (59°–86° F) in tightly covered container unless otherwise directed.

ADVERSE EFFECTS (≥1%) **CV:** *Tachycardia,* angina pectoris, *ECG changes,* pericardial effusion and tamponade, rebound hypertension (following drug withdrawal); *edema,* including pulmonary edema; *CHF (salt and water retention).* **Skin:** *Hypertrichosis,* transient pruritus, darkening of skin, hypersensitivity rash, Stevens-Johnson syndrome. With topical use: itching, flushing, scaling, dermatitis, folliculitis. **Body as a Whole:** Fatigue.

DIAGNOSTIC TEST INTERFERENCE ***Hct, Hgb,*** and ***erythrocyte count*** usually decrease (about 7%) during early therapy; ***serum alkaline phosphatase, BUN,*** and ***creatinine*** may increase during early therapy.

INTERACTIONS Drug: Epinephrine, norepinephrine cause excessive cardiac stimulation; **guanethidine** causes profound orthostatic hypotension.

PHARMACOKINETICS Absorption: Readily absorbed from GI tract. **Onset:** 30 min PO; at least 4 mo topical. **Peak:** 2–8 h PO. **Duration:** 2–5 d PO; new hair growth will remain 3–4 mo after withdrawal of topical. **Distribution:** Widely distributed including into breast milk. **Metabolism:** Metabolized in liver. **Elimination:** 97% excreted in urine and feces. **Half-Life:** 4.2 h.

NURSING IMPLICATIONS

Assessment & Drug Effects

- Take BP and apical pulse before administering medication and report significant changes. Consult physician for parameters.
- Lab tests: Periodic serum electrolytes.
- Do not stop drug abruptly. Abrupt reduction in BP can result in CVA and MI. Keep physician informed.
- Monitor fluid and electrolyte balance closely throughout ther-

apy. Sodium and water retention commonly occur. Consult physician regarding sodium restriction. Monitor potassium intake and serum potassium levels in patient on diuretic therapy.
- Monitor I&O and daily weight. Report unusual changes in I&O ratio or daily weight gain, greater than 1 kg (2 lb).
- Observe patient daily for edema and auscultate lungs for rales. Be alert to signs and symptoms of CHF (see Appendix F).
- Observe for symptoms of pericardial effusion or tamponade. Symptoms are similar to those of CHF, but additionally patient may have paradoxical pulse (normal inspiratory reduction in systolic BP may fall as much as 10–20 mm Hg).

Patient & Family Education
- Learn about usual pulse rate and count radial pulse for one full minute before taking drug. Report an increase of 20 or more bpm.
- Notify physician promptly if the following S&S appear: Increase of 20 or more bpm in resting pulse; breathing difficulty; dizziness; light-headedness; fainting; edema (tight shoes or rings, puffiness, pitting); weight gain, chest pain, arm or shoulder pain; easy bruising or bleeding.
- Be aware of possibility of hypertrichosis: Elongation, thickening, and increased pigmentation of fine body hair, especially of face, arms, and back. Develops 3–9 wk after start of therapy and occurs in approximately 80% of patients; reversible within 1–6 mo after drug withdrawal.
- Report any dermatologic adverse effects or any other adverse effect promptly to physician.
- Schedule follow-up examinations for q4–6 mo.
- Comply strictly with regular regimen; maximizes chance of at least some hair regrowth.
- Do not breast feed while taking this drug without consulting physician.

MIRTAZAPINE (Pr)

(mir-taz'a-peen)

Remeron, Remeron SolTab

Classifications: CENTRAL NERVOUS SYSTEM (CNS) AGENT; PSYCHOTHERAPEUTIC AGENT; ANTIDEPRESSANT, TETRACYCLIC

Pregnancy Category: C

AVAILABILITY 15 mg, 30 mg, 45 mg tablets and orally disintegrating tablets

ACTIONS Tetracyclic antidepressant pharmacologically and therapeutically similar to the tricyclic antidepressants. Tetracyclics enhance central nonadrenergic and serotonergic activity; thought to be due to normalizing of neurotransmission efficacy. Mirtazapine is a potent antagonist of 5-HT_2 and 5-HT_3 serotonin receptors.

THERAPEUTIC EFFECTS Acts as antidepressant. Effectiveness is indicated by mood elevation.

USES Treatment of depression.

CONTRAINDICATIONS Hypersensitivity to mirtazapine or mianserin; hypersensitivity to other antidepressants (e.g., tricyclic antidepressants and MAOI depressants), acute MI; fever, infection; agranulocytosis, neutropenia, hematologic disease; suicidal ideation; jaundice, ethanol intoxication; pregnancy (category C), lactation.

CAUTIOUS USE History of cardiovascular or GI disorders; BPH, urinary retention; narrow-angle glaucoma, increased intraocular pressure; hepatic or renal impair-

M

ment, renal failure; hypercholesterolemia, hypertriglyceridemia, thrombocytopenia; older adults; angina, cardiac arrhythmias, anticholinergic medications; bipolar disorder, mania, bone marrow suppression, PKU, history of MI; cerebrovascular disease, seizure disorder, seizures, stroke; depression; hypovolemia, surgery; closed-angle glaucoma; ileus, GI obstruction, dehydration; diabetes mellitus, diabetic ketoacidosis. Safety and effectiveness in children are not established.

ROUTE & DOSAGE

Depression
Adult: **PO** 15 mg/d in single dose h.s., may increase q1–2wk (max: 45 mg/d)
Geriatric: **PO** use lower doses
Renal or Hepatic Impairment
Use lower doses

ADMINISTRATION

Oral

- Give preferably prior to sleep to minimize injury potential.
- Begin drug no sooner than 14 d after discontinuation of an MAO inhibitor.
- Reduce dosage as warranted with severe renal or hepatic impairment and in older adults.
- Store at 20°–25° C (68°–77° F) in tight, light-resistant container.

ADVERSE EFFECTS (≥1%) **Body as a Whole:** Asthenia, flu syndrome, back pain, general and peripheral edema, malaise. **CNS:** *Somnolence,* dizziness, abnormal dreams, abnormal thinking, tremor, confusion, depression, agitation, vertigo, twitching. **CV:** Hypertension, vasodilation. **GI:** Nausea, vomiting, abdominal pain, *increased appetite*/weight gain, *dry mouth, constipation,* anorexia, cholecystitis, stomatitis, colitis, abnormal liver function tests. **Respiratory:** Dyspnea, cough, sinusitis. **Skin:** Pruritus, rash. **Urogenital:** Urinary frequency.

INTERACTIONS Drug: Additive cognitive and motor impairment with **alcohol** or BENZODIAZEPINES; increase risk of hypertensive crisis with MAOIS. **Herbal: Kava-kava, valerian** may potentiate sedative effects.

PHARMACOKINETICS Absorption: Rapidly absorbed from GI tract, 50% reaches systemic circulation. **Peak:** 2 h. **Distribution:** 85% protein bound. **Metabolism:** Metabolized in liver by cytochrome P450 system (CYP2D6, CYP1A2, CYP3A). **Elimination:** 75% excreted in urine, 15% in feces. **Half-Life:** 20–40 h.

NURSING IMPLICATIONS

Assessment & Drug Effects

- Lab tests: Monitor WBC count with differential, lipid profile, and ALT/AST periodically.
- Patients should be monitored for worsening of depression or emergence of suicidality.
- Assess for weight gain and excessive somnolence or dizziness.
- Monitor for orthostatic hypotension with a history of cardiovascular or cerebrovascular disease. Periodically monitor ECG especially in those with known cardiovascular disease.
- Monitor those with a history of increased intraocular pressure or urinary retention carefully for worsening or recurrence.
- Monitor those with history of seizures for lowering of the seizure threshold.

Patient & Family Education

- Do not drive or engage in potentially hazardous activities until response to drug is known.

- Do not use alcohol while taking drug.
- Report immediately unexplained fever or S&S of infection, especially flu-like symptoms, to physician.
- Do not take other prescription or OTC drugs without consulting physician.
- Make position changes slowly especially from lying or sitting to standing. Report dizziness, palpitations, and fainting.
- Notify (women) physician immediately if you become pregnant.
- Monitor weight periodically and report significant weight gains.
- Do not breast feed while taking this drug without consulting physician.

MISOPROSTOL

(my-so-prost'ole)

Cytotec

Classification: PROSTAGLANDIN
Prototype: Dinoprostone
Pregnancy Category: X

AVAILABILITY 100 mcg, 200 mcg tablets

ACTIONS Synthetic prostaglandin E_1 analog, with both antisecretory (inhibiting gastric acid secretion) and mucosal protective properties. Increases bicarbonate and mucosal protective properties. Also increases bicarbonate and mucous production.

THERAPEUTIC EFFECTS Inhibits basal and nocturnal gastric acid secretion and acid secretion in response to a variety of stimuli, including meals, histamine, pentagastrin, and coffee. Produces uterine contractions that may endanger pregnancy and cause a miscarriage.

USES Prevention of NSAID (including aspirin-induced) gastric ulcers in patients at high risk of complications from a gastric ulcer (e.g., the older adult and patients with a concomitant debilitating disease or a history of ulcers). Drug is taken for the duration of NSAID therapy and does not interfere with the efficacy of the NSAID.

UNLABELED USES Short-term treatment of duodenal ulcers; cervical ripening and induction of labor.

CONTRAINDICATIONS History of allergies to prostaglandins; pregnancy (category X), lactation.

CAUTIOUS USE Renal impairment. Safety in children <18 y is not established.

ROUTE & DOSAGE

Prevention of NSAID-induced Ulcers

Adult: **PO** 100–200 mcg q.i.d. p.c. and h.s. or 200 mcg b.i.d. or t.i.d.

ADMINISTRATION

Oral

- Give with food to minimize GI adverse effects (manufacturer recommendation).
- Store away from heat, light, and moisture.

ADVERSE EFFECTS (≥1%) **CNS:** Headache. **GI:** *Diarrhea, abdominal pain,* nausea, flatulence, dyspepsia, vomiting, constipation. **Urogenital:** Spotting, cramps, dysmenorrhea, uterine contractions.

INTERACTIONS Drug: MAGNESIUM-CONTAINING ANTACIDS may increase diarrhea.

PHARMACOKINETICS Absorption: Readily absorbed from GI tract; extensive first pass metabolism. **Onset:** 30 min. **Peak:** 60–90 min. **Duration:** At least 3 h. **Metabolism:** Metabolized in liver. **Elimination:** Pri-

M

marily excreted in urine; small amount excreted in feces. **Half-Life:** 20–40 min.

NURSING IMPLICATIONS

Assessment & Drug Effects

- Monitor for diarrhea; may be minimized by giving drug after meals and at bedtime. Diarrhea is a common adverse effect that is dose related and usually self-limiting (often resolving in 8 d).

Patient & Family Education

- Avoid using concurrent magnesium-containing antacids because of increased incidence of diarrhea.
- Report postmenopausal bleeding to physician; it may be drug related.
- Avoid pregnancy during misoprostol therapy; use an effective contraception method while taking drug.
- Drug has abortifacient property. Contact physician and immediately discontinue drug if you becomes pregnant.
- Do not breast feed while taking this drug.

MITOMYCIN

(mye-toe-mye′sin)
Mutamycin
Classifications: ANTINEOPLASTIC; ANTIBIOTIC
Prototype: Doxorubicin
Pregnancy Category: D

AVAILABILITY 5 mg, 20 mg, 40 mg injection

ACTIONS Potent antibiotic antineoplastic compound. Effective in certain tumors unresponsive to surgery, radiation, or other chemotherapeutic agents. Action mechanism unclear but reportedly combines with DNA, thereby interfering with cellular and enzymatic RNA and protein synthesis.

THERAPEUTIC EFFECTS Highly destructive to rapidly proliferating cells and slowly developing carcinomas.

USES In combination with other chemotherapeutic agents in palliative, adjunctive treatment of disseminated adenocarcinoma of breast, pancreas, or stomach, squamous cell carcinoma of head, neck, lung, and cervix. Not recommended to replace surgery or radiotherapy or as a single primary therapeutic agent.

CONTRAINDICATIONS Hypersensitivity or idiosyncrasy reaction; thrombocytopenia; coagulation disorders or bleeding tendencies; pregnancy (category D), lactation.

CAUTIOUS USE Renal impairment; myelosuppression.

ROUTE & DOSAGE

Cancer

Adult/Child: **IV** 20 mg/m²/d as a single dose q6–8wk, additional doses based on hematologic response

ADMINISTRATION

Intravenous

Note: Verify correct IV concentration and rate of infusion/injection for administration to children with physician.

PREPARE: **IV Infusion:** Dilute each 5 mg with 10 mL sterile water for injection. Shake to dissolve. If product does not clear immediately, allow to stand at room temperature until solution is obtained. Reconstituted solution is purple.

ADMINISTER: **IV Infusion:** Give reconstituted solution over 5–10 min or longer as determined by total volume of solution. Monitor

IV site closely. Avoid extravasation to prevent extreme tissue reaction (cellulitis) to the toxic drug.

INCOMPATIBILITIES **Solution/additive:** DEXTROSE-CONTAINING SOLUTIONS, **bleomycin. Y-site: Aztreonam, cefepime, etoposide, filgrastim, gemcitabine, sargramostim, vinorelbine.**

- Store drug reconstituted with sterile water for injection (0.5 mg/mL) for 14 d refrigerated or 7 d at room temperature. Drug diluted in D5W (20–40 mcg/mL) is stable at room temperature for 3 h.

ADVERSE EFFECTS (≥1%) **CNS:** Paresthesias. **GI:** Stomatitis, *nausea, vomiting,* anorexia, hematemesis, diarrhea. **Hematologic:** Bone marrow toxicity (*thrombocytopenia, leukopenia* occurring 4–8 wk after treatment onset), thrombophlebitis, anemia. **Respiratory:** Acute bronchospasm, hemoptysis, dyspnea, nonproductive cough, pneumonia, interstitial pneumonitis. **Skin:** Desquamation; induration, pain, necrosis, cellulitis at injection site; reversible alopecia, purple discoloration of nail beds. **Body as a Whole:** Pain, headache, fatigue, edema. **Urogenital:** Hemolytic uremic syndrome, renal toxicity.

PHARMACOKINETICS Metabolism: Metabolized rapidly in liver. **Elimination:** Excreted in urine. **Half-Life:** 17 min.

NURSING IMPLICATIONS

Assessment & Drug Effects

- Lab tests: Perform WBC with differential, platelet count, PT, INR, aPTT, Hgb, Hct, and serum creatinine frequently during and for at least 7 wk after treatment.
- Do not administer if serum creatinine is >1.7 mg/dL or if platelet count falls below 150,000/mm^3 and WBC is down to 4000/mm^3 or if prothrombin or bleeding times are prolonged.
- Monitor I&O ratio and pattern. Report any sign of impaired kidney function: Change in ratio, dysuria, hematuria, oliguria, frequency, urgency. Keep patient well hydrated (at least 2000–2500 mL orally daily if tolerated). Drug is nephrotoxic.
- Observe closely for signs of infection. Monitor body temperature frequently.
- Inspect oral cavity daily for signs of stomatitis or superinfection (see Appendix F).

Patient & Family Education

- Report respiratory distress to physician immediately.
- Report signs of common cold to physician immediately.
- Understand that hair loss is reversible after cessation of treatment.
- Do not breast feed while taking this drug.

M

MITOTANE

(mye'toe-tane)

Lysodren

Classifications: ANTINEOPLASTIC; ADRENOCORTICAL CYTOTOXIC

Pregnancy Category: C

AVAILABILITY 500 mg tablets

ACTIONS Cytotoxic agent with suppressant action on the adrenal cortex. Modifies peripheral metabolism of steroids and reduces production of adrenal steroids. Extra-adrenal metabolism of cortisol is altered, leading to reduction in 17-hydroxycorticosteroids (17-OHCS); however, plasma levels of corticosteroids do not fall.

THERAPEUTIC EFFECTS Cytotoxic agent with suppressant action on the adrenal cortex.

USES Inoperable adrenal cortical carcinoma (functional and nonfunctional).

UNLABELED USES Cushing's syndrome secondary to pituitary disorders.

CONTRAINDICATIONS Pregnancy (category C) or lactation (only after risk-benefit ratio to mother and fetus has been assessed).

CAUTIOUS USE Liver disease.

ROUTE & DOSAGE

Adrenocortical Carcinoma

Adult: **PO** 9–10 g/d in divided doses t.i.d. or q.i.d. (tolerated doses range: 2–16 g/d)

ADMINISTRATION

Oral

- Withhold temporarily and consult physician if emergency occurs, since adrenal suppression is its prime action. Exogenous steroids may be required until the already depressed adrenal starts secreting steroids.
- Store at 15°–30° C (59°–86° F) in tight, light-resistant containers.

ADVERSE EFFECTS (≥1%) **CNS:** Vertigo, dizziness, drowsiness, tiredness, depression, *lethargy, sedation,* headache, confusion, tremors. **CV:** Hypertension, hypotension, flushing. **GI:** *Anorexia, nausea, vomiting, diarrhea.* **Urogenital:** Hematuria, hemorrhagic cystitis, albuminuria. **Endocrine:** Adrenocortical insufficiency. **Special Senses:** Blurred vision, diplopia, lens opacity, toxic retinopathy. **Body as a Whole:** Generalized aching, fever, muscle twitching, hypersensitivity reactions, hyperpyrexia. **Skin:** *Rash,* cutaneous eruptions and pigmentation. **Metabolic:** *Hypouricemia, hypercholesterolemia.*

DIAGNOSTIC TEST INTERFERENCE Mitotane decreases ***protein-bound iodine (PBI)*** and ***urinary 17-OHCS levels***.

INTERACTIONS Drug: Potentiates sedative effects of **alcohol** and other CNS DEPRESSANTS; may increase the metabolism of **phenytoin, phenobarbital, warfarin,** decreasing their effectiveness.

PHARMACOKINETICS Absorption: Approximately 40% absorbed from GI tract. **Onset:** 2–4 wk. **Peak:** 3–5 h. **Distribution:** Deposits in most body tissues, especially adipose tissue. **Metabolism:** Metabolized in liver. **Elimination:** Small amount excreted in bile. **Half-Life:** 18–159 d.

NURSING IMPLICATIONS

Assessment & Drug Effects

- Monitor pulse and BP for early signs of shock (adrenal insufficiency).
- Observe for symptoms of hepatotoxicity (see Appendix F). Report them promptly, since reduced hepatic capacity can increase toxicity of mitotane and because dose may have to be decreased.
- Notify physician if following persist and become more severe: Aching muscles, fever, flushing, and muscle twitching.
- Monitor obese patient for symptoms of adrenal hypofunction. Because a large portion of the drug deposits in fatty tissue, the obese are particularly susceptible to prolonged adverse effects.
- Make neurologic and behavioral assessments at regular intervals throughout therapy.

Patient & Family Education

- Be aware that mitotane does not cure but does reduce tumor mass, pain, weakness, anorexia, and steroid symptoms.

- Report symptoms of adrenal insufficiency (weakness, fatigue, orthostatic hypotension, pigmentation, weight loss, dehydration, anorexia, nausea, vomiting, and diarrhea) to physician.
- Exercise caution when driving or performing potentially hazardous tasks requiring alertness because of drug-induced drowsiness, tiredness, dizziness. Symptoms tend to recede with continuation in therapy.
- Use contraceptive measures during therapy because of teratogenic properties of drug. Notify physician if you suspect you are pregnant.
- Do not breast feed while taking this drug.

MITOXANTRONE HYDROCHLORIDE

(mi-tox′an-trone)

Novantrone

Classifications: ANTINEOPLASTIC; ANTIBIOTIC; IMMUNOSUPPRESSANT

Prototype: Doxorubicin

Pregnancy Category: D

AVAILABILITY 2 mg/mL injection

ACTIONS Noncell-cycle specific antitumor agent with less cardiotoxicity than doxorubicin. Interferes with DNA synthesis by intercalating with the DNA double helix, blocking effective DNA and RNA transcription.

THERAPEUTIC EFFECTS Highly destructive to rapidly proliferating cells in all stages of cell division.

USES In combination with other drugs for the treatment of acute nonlymphocytic leukemia (ANLL) in adults, bone pain in advanced prostate cancer. Reducing neurologic disability and/or the frequency of clinical relapses in patients with secondary progressive, progressive relapsing, or worsening relapsing-remitting multiple sclerosis.

UNLABELED USES Breast cancer, refractory lymphomas.

CONTRAINDICATIONS Hypersensitivity to mitoxantrone; myelosuppression; pregnancy (category D), lactation.

CAUTIOUS USE Impaired cardiac function; impaired liver and kidney function; systemic infections.

ROUTE & DOSAGE

Combination Therapy for ANLL

Adult: **IV Induction Therapy:** 12 mg/m²/d on days 1–3, may need to repeat induction course. **IV Consolidation therapy:** 12 mg/m² on days 1 and 2 (max: lifetime dose 80–120 mg/m²)

Child: **IV** 8–33 mg/m² q3–4wk

Solid Tumors

Child: **IV** 5–8 mg/m² once a week or 18–20 mg/m² q3–4wk

Multiple Sclerosis

Adult: **IV** 12 mg/m² over 5–15 min q3mo (max: lifetime dose 140 mg/m²)

ADMINISTRATION

Intravenous

- If mitoxantrone touches skin, wash immediately with copious amounts of warm water.

PREPARE: **IV Infusion:** Withdraw contents of vial and add to at least 50 mL of D5W or NS. Use of goggles, gloves, and protective gown during drug preparation and administration.

ADMINISTER: **IV Infusion:** Give into the tubing as a freely running IV of D5W or NS and infused over at least 3 min or

longer (i.e., 30–60 min) depending on the total volume of IV solution. If extravasation occurs, stop infusion and immediately restart in another vein.
INCOMPATIBILITIES **Solution/additive: Heparin, hydrocortisone, paclitaxel. Y-site: amphotericin B cholesteryl complex, aztreonam, doxorubicin liposome, paclitaxel, piperacillin/tazobactam, propofol, TPN.**

- Discard unused portions of diluted solution. ■ Once opened, multiple use vials may be stored refrigerated at 2°–8° C (35°–46° F) for 14 d.

ADVERSE EFFECTS (≥1%) **CV:** Arrhythmias, decreased left ventricular function, *CHF,* tachycardia, ECG changes, MI (occurs with cumulative doses of >80–100 mg/m²), edema. **GI:** *Nausea, vomiting,* diarrhea, hepatotoxicity. **Hematologic:** *Leukopenia, thrombocytopenia*. **Other:** Discolors urine and sclera a blue-green color. **Skin:** Mild phlebitis, blue skin discoloration, alopecia.

INTERACTIONS Drug: May impair immune response to VACCINES such as influenza and pneumococcal infections. May have increased risk of infection with **yellow fever vaccine.**

PHARMACOKINETICS Distribution: Rapidly taken up by tissues and slowly released into plasma, resulting in low renal, hepatic, and metabolic clearance rates; 95% protein bound. **Metabolism:** Metabolized in liver. **Elimination:** Excreted primarily in bile. **Half-Life:** 37 h.

NURSING IMPLICATIONS

Assessment & Drug Effects

- Monitor IV insertion site. Transient blue skin discoloration may occur at site if extravasation has occurred.
- Monitor cardiac functioning throughout course of therapy; report signs and symptoms of CHF or cardiac arrhythmias.
- Lab tests: Perform liver function tests prior to and during course of treatment. Monitor serum uric acid levels and initiate hypouricemic therapy before antileukemic therapy. Monitor carefully CBC with differential prior to and during therapy.

Patient & Family Education

- Understand potential adverse effects of mitoxantrone therapy.
- Expect urine to turn blue-green for 24 h after drug administration; sclera may also take on a bluish color.
- Be aware that stomatitis/mucositis may occur within 1 wk of therapy.
- Do not to risk exposure to those with known infections during the periods of myelosuppression.
- Do not breast feed while taking this drug.

MIVACURIUM CHLORIDE

(miv-a-cur'i-um)

Mivacron

Classifications: AUTONOMIC NERVOUS SYSTEM AGENT; MUSCLE RELAXANT; NONDEPOLARIZING

Prototype: Tubocurarine

Pregnancy Category: C

AVAILABILITY 0.5 mg/mL, 2 mg/mL injection

ACTIONS Short-acting, skeletal muscle relaxant that combines competitively to cholinergic receptors on the motor neuron end-plate. Antagonizes action of acetylcholine, and blocks neuromuscular transmission. Neuromuscular blocking action is readily reversible with an anticholinesterase agent.

THERAPEUTIC EFFECTS Blocks nerve impulse transmission, which results in skeletal muscle relaxation and paralysis.

USES Adjunct to general anesthesia, to facilitate tracheal intubation, and to provide skeletal muscle relaxation during surgery or mechanical ventilation.

CONTRAINDICATIONS Allergic reactions to mivacurium or its ingredients.

CAUTIOUS USE Kidney function impairment, liver function impairment; older adult patients; pregnancy (category C), lactation.

ROUTE & DOSAGE

Tracheal Intubation and Mechanical Ventilation

Adult: **IV Loading Dose** 0.15 mg/kg given over 5–15 s (over 60 s in patients with cardiovascular disease) **IV Maintenance Dose:** 0.1 mg/kg generally q15min **IV Continuous Infusion:** Initial infusion of 9–10 mcg/kg/min, reduce infusion to 4 mcg/kg/min if started with initial bolus
Child: **IV Loading Dose** *2–12 y,* 0.2 mg/kg given over 5–15 s (range: 0.09–0.2 mg/kg) **IV Maintenance Dose** Same as adult **IV Continuous Infusion** 10–15 mcg/kg/min

Renal Impairment

Cl_{cr} Decrease infusion rates by 50%

ADMINISTRATION

Intravenous

PREPARE: **Direct:** Add 3 mL of D5W, NS, D5/NS, RL, or D5/RL to each 1 mL mivacurium to yield 0.5 mg/mL. **IV Infusion:** Available premixed (50 mL of 0.5 mg/mL).

ADMINISTER: **Direct:** Give over 15–60 sec. **IV Infusion:** Refer to manufacturer's infusion rate tables. The use of a peripheral nerve stimulator permits optimal dosing and minimizes risks of overdose or underdose.

INCOMPATIBILITIES **Solution/additive:** ALKALINE SOLUTIONS pH >8.5 (BARBITURATES).

- Store diluted solution at 5°–25° C (41°–77° F) for up to 24 h.

ADVERSE EFFECTS (≥1%) **CV:** Transient decrease in arterial BP, hypotension, increases and decreases in heart rate. **Skin:** *Transient flushing about the face, neck, and/or chest* (especially with rapid administration).

INTERACTIONS Drug: GENERAL ANESTHETICS **(enflurane, halothane, isoflurane)** may enhance the degree of neuromuscular blockade produced by mivacurium. AMINOGLYCOSIDES, TETRACYCLINES, **bacitracin,** POLYMYXINS, **lincomycin, clindamycin, colistin, magnesium salts, lithium,** LOCAL ANESTHETICS, **procainamide,** and **quinidine** may enhance the neuromuscular blockade.

PHARMACOKINETICS Peak: 2–6 min. **Duration:** 25–30 min in adults, 8–16 min in children. **Distribution:** Limited tissue distribution. **Metabolism:** Rapidly hydrolyzed by plasma cholinesterase.

NURSING IMPLICATIONS

Assessment & Drug Effects

- Assess patients with neuromuscular disease carefully and adjust drug dosage using a peripheral nerve stimulator when they experience prolonged neuromuscular blocks.
- Monitor hemodynamic status carefully in patients with significant cardiovascular disease or those

M

with potentially greater sensitivity to release of histamine-type mediators (e.g., asthma).
- Monitor for significant drop in BP because overdose may increase the risk of hemodynamic adverse effects.

MODAFINIL Pr

(mod-a′fi-nil)

Provigil, Alertec ♣

Classifications: CENTRAL NERVOUS SYSTEM (CNS) AGENT; CEREBRAL STIMULANT

Pregnancy Category: C

Controlled Substance: Schedule IV

AVAILABILITY 100 mg, 200 mg capsules

ACTIONS CNS stimulant; the precise mechanism of action is unknown. Modafinil causes an increase in extracellular dopamine.

THERAPEUTIC EFFECTS Modafinil causes wakefulness, increased locomotor activity, and psychoactive and euphoric effects.

USES Improve wakefulness in patients with narcolepsy or excessive sleepiness associated with shift work sleep disorder, obstructive sleep apnea/hypnea syndrome.

UNLABELED USES Fatigue related to organic brain syndrome or multiple sclerosis.

CONTRAINDICATIONS Hypersensitivity to modafinil; acute MI, valvular heart disease; pregnancy (category C); lactation. Safety and efficacy in children <16 y are unknown.

CAUTIOUS USE Cardiovascular disease including left ventricular hypertrophy; cardiac disease, ischemic ECG changes, chest pain, arrhythmias, mitral valve prolapse, recent MI, unstable angina; older adults; history of drug or alcohol abuse; psychosis or emotional instability; leukopenia, MI, neurological disease, hypertension, severe hepatic disease, severe renal impairment, renal failure, seizure disorder, sleep apnea.

ROUTE & DOSAGE

Narcolepsy, Fatigue

Adult: **PO** 200 mg/d as single dose in the morning

Hepatic Impairment

Reduce dose by 50%

ADMINISTRATION

Oral
- Give in the morning shortly after awakening.
- Store at 15°–30° C (59°–86° F).

ADVERSE EFFECTS (≥1%) **Body as a Whole:** Chest pain, neck pain, chills, eosinophilia. **CNS:** *Headache,* nervousness, dizziness, depression, anxiety, cataplexy, insomnia, paresthesia, dyskinesia, hypertonia. **CV:** Hypotension, hypertension, vasodilation, arrhythmia, syncope. **GI:** *Nausea,* diarrhea, dry mouth, anorexia, abnormal LFTs, vomiting, mouth ulcer, gingivitis, thirst. **Respiratory:** Rhinitis, pharyngitis, lung disorder, dyspnea. **Skin:** Dry skin. **Special Senses:** Amblyopia, abnormal vision.

INTERACTIONS Drug: Methylphenidate may delay absorption of **modafinil; modafinil** may decrease levels of **cyclosporine,** ORAL CONTRACEPTIVES; **modafinil** may increase levels of **clomipramine, phenytoin, warfarin,** TRICYCLIC ANTIDEPRESSANTS.

PHARMACOKINETICS Absorption: Rapidly absorbed. **Peak:** 2–4 h. **Distribution:** Approximately 60%

protein bound. **Metabolism:** Metabolized in liver to inactive metabolites. **Elimination:** Excreted in urine. **Half-Life:** 15 h.

NURSING IMPLICATIONS

Assessment & Drug Effects

- Therapeutic effectiveness: Indicated by improved daytime wakefulness.
- Monitor BP and cardiovascular status, especially with preexisting hypertension and mitral valve prolapse or other CV condition.
- Monitor for S&S of psychosis, especially when history of psychotic episodes exists.
- Lab tests: Periodic liver function tests.
- Coadministered drugs: Monitor INR with warfarin for first several months and when dosage is changed; monitor for toxicity with phenytoin.

Patient & Family Education

- Use barrier contraceptive instead of/in addition to hormonal contraceptive.
- Inform physician of all prescription or OTC drugs in/added to your regimen.
- Notify physician if any S&S of an allergic reaction appear.
- Do not breast feed while taking this drug without consulting physician.

MOEXIPRIL HYDROCHLORIDE

(mo-ex′i-pril)

Univasc

Classifications: CARDIOVASCULAR AGENT; ANGIOTENSIN-CONVERTING ENZYME INHIBITOR; ANTIHYPERTENSIVE

Prototype: Captopril

Pregnancy Category: C (first trimester); D (second and third trimesters)

AVAILABILITY 7.5 mg, 15 mg tablets

ACTIONS ACE inhibitor that results in decreased conversion of angiotensin I to angiotensin II. Results in decreased vasopressor activity and aldosterone secretion.

THERAPEUTIC EFFECTS ACE inhibition and decreased aldosterone secretion. Antihypertensive effect.

USES Hypertension.

UNLABELED USES CHF.

CONTRAINDICATIONS Hypersensitivity to moexipril; history of angioedema related to an ACE inhibitor; pregnancy [(category C) first trimester; (category D) second and third trimesters].

CAUTIOUS USE Hypersensitivity to any other ACE inhibitor; renal impairment, renal artery stenosis, volume-depleted patients; hypertensive patient with CHF; history of autoimmune disease; severe liver dysfunction; immunosuppressed patients; hyperkalemia; patients undergoing surgery/anesthesia; preexisting neutropenia; concurrent lithium therapy; lactation. Safety and efficacy in children are not established.

ROUTE & DOSAGE

Hypertension

Adult: **PO** 7.5 mg once/d, may increase up to 30 mg/d in divided doses

Renal Impairment

Cl_{cr} ≤40 mL/min: Start with 3.75 mg q.d. (also if patient is volume depleted or on diuretics)

ADMINISTRATION

Oral

- Give 1 h before or 2 h after meals. Food greatly reduces absorption of moexipril.

- May need to reduce starting dose 50% in patients with possible volume depletion or a history of renal insufficiency.
- Store at 15°–30° C (59°–86° F).

ADVERSE EFFECTS (≥1%) **CNS:** Headache, *dizziness,* drowsiness, sleep disturbances, nervousness, anxiety, mood changes. **CV:** Hypotension, chest pain, angina, peripheral edema, MI, palpitations, arrhythmias. **Endocrine:** Hyperkalemia. **GI:** Diarrhea, nausea, dyspepsia, abdominal pain, taste disturbances, constipation, vomiting, dry mouth, pancreatitis. **Urogenital:** Urinary frequency, increased BUN and serum creatinine. **Hematologic:** Neutropenia, hemolytic anemia. **Respiratory:** Cough, pharyngitis, rhinitis, flu-like symptoms. **Skin:** Angioedema (rare), rash, flushing.

INTERACTIONS Drug: Capsaicin may exacerbate cough. NSAIDS may reduce antihypertensive effects. May increase **lithium** levels and toxicity. POTASSIUM SUPPLEMENTS and POTASSIUM-SPARING DIURETICS may increase risk of hyperkalemia. **Food:** Food greatly reduces absorption of moexipril.

PHARMACOKINETICS Absorption: Readily absorbed from GI tract; approximately 13% of active metabolite reaches systemic circulation; absorption greatly reduced by food. **Onset:** 1 h. **Duration:** 24 h. **Distribution:** Approximately 50% protein bound. **Metabolism:** Metabolized in liver to moexiprilat (active metabolite). **Elimination:** 13% excreted in urine, 53% excreted in feces. **Half-Life:** 2–9 h.

NURSING IMPLICATIONS

Assessment & Drug Effects

- Monitor closely for systematic hypotension that may occur within 1–3 h of first dose, especially in those with high blood pressure, on a diuretic or restricted salt intake, or otherwise volume depleted.
- Monitor BP and HR frequently during initiation of therapy, whenever a diuretic is added, and periodically throughout therapy.
- Determine trough BP (just before next dose) before dose adjustments are made.
- Lab tests: Monitor serum electrolytes, WBC with differential, Hct and Hgb, UA, and kidney and liver function tests periodically throughout therapy.
- Supervise therapeutic response closely in patients with CHF.

Patient & Family Education

- Report to physician immediately swelling around face or neck or in extremities.
- Report S&S of hypotension (e.g., dizziness, weakness, syncope); nonproductive cough; skin rash; flu-like symptoms; jaundice; irregular heartbeat or chest pains; and dehydration from vomiting, diarrhea, or diaphoresis.
- Consult physician before using potassium-containing salt substitutes.
- Do not breast feed while taking this drug without consulting physician.

MOLINDONE HYDROCHLORIDE

(moe-lin′done)

Moban

Classifications: CENTRAL NERVOUS SYSTEM AGENT; PSYCHOTHERAPEUTIC; ANTIPSYCHOTIC PHENOTHIAZINE

Prototype: Chlorpromazine

Pregnancy Category: C

AVAILABILITY 5 mg, 10 mg, 25 mg, 50 mg, 100 mg tablets; 20 mg/mL liquid

ACTIONS Tranquilizer structurally unrelated but pharmacologically similar to the piperazine phenothiazines; thought to block postsynaptic dopamine receptors in the brain. Has less sedative but comparable anticholinergic activity and greater incidence of extrapyramidal adverse effects than chlorpromazine. EEG studies suggest ascending reticular system is chief site of action.

THERAPEUTIC EFFECTS Reportedly lowers convulsive threshold and produces tranquilization without compromising alertness. Antipsychotic effect includes reduction in bizarre behavior, and control of aggressiveness.

USES Management of manifestations of psychotic disorders.

CONTRAINDICATIONS Known hypersensitivity to molindone or to phenothiazines; severe CNS depression; comatose states; children <12 y. Safety during pregnancy (category C) or lactation is not established.

CAUTIOUS USE Those harmed by increase in physical activity; prostatic hypertrophy; cardiovascular disease; previously detected cancer of breast.

ROUTE & DOSAGE

Psychotic Disorders

Adult: **PO** 50–75 mg/d in 3–4 divided doses, may be increased to 100 mg/d in 3–4 d or may be able to decrease to 15–60 mg/d in divided doses (max: 225 mg/d)

ADMINISTRATION

Oral

- Be certain patient swallows the medication.
- Store medication in tightly capped, light-resistant bottles. Protect from heat and moisture.

ADVERSE EFFECTS (≥1%) **CNS:** *Transient drowsiness,* insomnia, *extrapyramidal symptoms* (dose related), euphoria, neuroleptic malignant syndrome. **GI:** Dry mouth, constipation, hepatotoxicity. **Special Senses:** Tinnitus, blurred vision, nasal congestion. **Urogenital:** Urinary retention. **Skin:** Mild photosensitivity. **CV:** Tachycardia. **Body as a Whole:** Change in weight. **Endocrine:** SLE-like syndrome, heavy menses, amenorrhea, galactorrhea, gynecomastia, increased libido, premature ejaculation.

INTERACTIONS Drug: May potentiate CNS depression with CNS DEPRESSANTS, **alcohol. Herbal: Kava-kava** may increase risk and severity of dystonic reactions.

PHARMACOKINETICS Absorption: Readily absorbed from GI tract. **Peak:** 1 h. **Duration:** 24–36 h. **Distribution:** Distributed into breast milk. **Metabolism:** Metabolized in liver. **Elimination:** Excreted in urine and feces. **Half-Life:** 1.5 h.

NURSING IMPLICATIONS

Assessment & Drug Effects

- Withhold dose and consult with physician if the following symptoms occur: Tremor, involuntary twitching, exaggerated restlessness, changes in vision, light-colored stools, sore throat, fever, rash.
- Monitor bowel pattern and urinary output. The depressed pa-

M

tient may not report constipation or urinary retention, both adverse effects of this medicine.

- Supervise ambulation and other ADL in the older adult or debilitated or patient with impaired vision to prevent injury or falling because drug increases motor activity.
- Be alert early during treatment to onset of parkinsonism (extrapyramidal) symptoms: Rigidity, immobility, reduction of voluntary movements, tremors, fine vermicular tongue movements. Withhold dose and report promptly to physician.

Patient & Family Education

- Take drug as prescribed: do not alter dose regimen or stop medication without consulting physician.
- Dizziness during early therapy usually disappears as treatment continues.
- Do not drive or engage in potentially hazardous activities requiring mental or physical coordination until response to drug is known.
- Avoid alcohol and self-medication with other depressants during therapy. Get physician approval before using any OTC drug.
- Relieve dry mouth by rinsing frequently with warm water, increasing noncaloric fluid intake, sucking hard candy.
- Avoid overexertion (patient with angina) and report increase in frequency of precordial pain.
- Schedule periodic ophthalmic examinations when treatment is long-term.
- Do not breast feed while taking this drug without consulting physician.

MOMETASONE FUROATE

(mo-met'a-sone)

Elocon, Nasonex

Classifications: SKIN AND MUCOUS MEMBRANE AGENT; ANTIINFLAMMATORY; HORMONES AND SYNTHETIC SUBSTITUTES; STEROID

Prototype: Hydrocortisone

Pregnancy Category: C

AVAILABILITY 50 mcg spray; 0.1% ointment; cream; lotion

See Appendix A-3.

MONOCTANOIN

(mon-oh-ock'ta-noyn)

Moctanin

Classifications: GASTROINTESTINAL AGENT; CHOLELITHOLYTIC

Pregnancy Category: C

AVAILABILITY 120 mL infusion

ACTIONS Cholesterol solubilizing agent that shrinks, softens, and dissolves cholesterol gallstones, depending on size and number. An effective alternative to gallstones removal in some patients, superior to other solvent-type medications (e.g., chenodiol).

THERAPEUTIC EFFECTS Clinical efficacy related mainly to amount of cholesterol in the stones. Complete dissolution is more likely when there is only one stone than when multiple stones are present.

USES To dissolve cholesterol (radiolucent) gallstones retained in the biliary tract after cholecystectomy when other means are not viable or are unsuccessful.

CONTRAINDICATIONS Noncholesterol gallstones; impaired liver function; obstructive jaundice; pancreatitis; history of intolerance of vegetable oils; recent duodenal ulcer, or jejunitis, infection. Safety during pregnancy (category C) or in children ≤2 y is not established. **CAUTIOUS USE** Bile duct obstruction; lactation.

ROUTE & DOSAGE

Radiolucent Gallstones
Adult: **Biliary Instillation** 3–5 mL/h at pressure of 10 cm H_2O for 2–10 d (avg: 5 d)

ADMINISTRATION

Instillation

- Give by continuous perfusion through a percutaneous transhepatic catheter directly inserted into the common bile duct.
- Administer (usually) with a positive pressure or peristaltic perfusion pump equipped with an overflow manometer. Monitor pressure to prevent exceeding 15 cm H_2O.
- Monitor flow rate carefully and adjust if necessary. If rate is too fast, incidence of GI adverse effects are apt to increase. Be alert to persistent nausea and diarrhea.
- Note: Perfusion temperature is brought to room temperature (21°–27° C [70°–80° F]) before the perfusion is started.
- Interrupt perfusion for 1–2 h at mealtimes to reduce GI adverse effects.
- Store at 15°–30° C (59°–86° F).

ADVERSE EFFECTS (≥1%) **CNS:** Drowsiness, depression. **GI:** *Abdominal pain,* epigastric burning, anorexia, *nausea, vomiting, diarrhea,* reversible irritability of duodenal mucosa, pancreatitis (rare). **Hematologic:** Bleeding from duodenal ulcer, hypokalemia, increase in serum amylase. **Body as a Whole:** Shortness of breath, pruritus, fatigue, diaphoresis, fever, facial flushing.

INTERACTIONS Drug: No clinically significant interactions established.

PHARMACOKINETICS Metabolism: Metabolized by pancreatic lipase and other digestive enzymes to fatty acids and glycerol, which are readily absorbed by the portal vein.

NURSING IMPLICATIONS

Assessment & Drug Effects

- Relieve discomfort from adverse effects by temporary interruption of the treatment. Abdominal pain does not appear to be dose- or perfusion-rate dependent. If adverse effects persist, drug may be discontinued.
- Monitor vital signs. An elevated temperature with chills combined with severe right upper quadrant abdominal pain and jaundice suggest onset of ascending cholangitis. Report to physician.
- Correlate lab studies of WBC with patient's complaint of sore throat accompanied by fever and chills; rule out leukopenia.

MONTELUKAST

(mon-te-lu'cast)
Singulair
Classifications: BRONCHODILATOR (RESPIRATORY SMOOTH MUSCLE RELAXANT); LEUKOTRIENE RECEPTOR ANTAGONIST
Prototype: Zafirlukast
Pregnancy Category: B

AVAILABILITY 5 mg, 10 mg tablets; 4 mg chewable tablets; 4 mg oral granules

ACTIONS Selective receptor antagonist of leukotriene D_4, thus inhibiting bronchoconstriction. Leukotrienes are considered more important than prostaglandins as inflammatory agents; they induce bronchoconstriction and mucus production. Elevated sputum and blood levels of leukotrienes have been documented during acute asthma attacks.

THERAPEUTIC EFFECTS Controls asthmatic attacks by inhibiting leukotriene release as well as inflammatory action associated with the attack. Indicated by improved pulmonary functions and better controlled asthmatic symptoms.

USES Prophylaxis and chronic treatment of asthma or allergic rhinitis.

CONTRAINDICATIONS Hypersensitivity to montelukast; severe asthma attacks; bronchoconstriction due to asthma or NSAIDs; status asthmaticus; lactation.

CAUTIOUS USE Hypersensitivity to other leukotriene receptor antagonists (e.g., zafirlukast, zileuton); severe liver disease; severe asthma; pregnancy (category B); children <12 mo.

M

ROUTE & DOSAGE

Asthma

Adult: **PO** 10 mg q.d. in evening
Child: **PO** *12 mo–5 y,* 4 mg q.d. in evening; *6–14 y,* 5 mg chewable tablet q.d. in evening

ADMINISTRATION

Oral

- Give in the evening for maximum effectiveness.
- Ensure chewable tablets for children are not swallowed whole.
- Store at 15°–30° C (59°–86° F) in a tightly closed container and protect from light.

ADVERSE EFFECTS (≥1%) **Body as a Whole:** Asthenia, fever, trauma. **CNS:** Dizziness, *headache.* **GI:** Abdominal pain, dyspepsia, gastroenteritis, dental pain, abnormal liver function tests (ALT, AST), diarrhea, nausea. **Respiratory:** Nasal congestion, cough, influenza, laryngitis, pharyngitis, sinusitis. **Skin:** Rash. **Urogenital:** Pyuria.

PHARMACOKINETICS Absorption: Rapidly absorbed from GI tract, bioavailability 64%. **Peak:** 3–4 h for oral tablet, 2–2.5 h for chewable tablet. **Distribution:** >99% protein bound. **Metabolism:** Extensively metabolized by cytochromes P450 3A4 and 2C9. **Elimination:** Excreted in feces. **Half-Life:** 2.7–5.5 h.

NURSING IMPLICATIONS

Assessment & Drug Effects

- Monitor effectiveness carefully when used in combination with phenobarbital or other potent cytochrome P450 enzyme inducers.
- Lab test: Periodic liver function tests.

Patient & Family Education

- Do not use for reversal of an acute asthmatic attack.
- Inform physician if short-acting inhaled bronchodilators are needed more often than usual with montelukast.
- Use chewable tablets (contain phenylalanine) with caution with PKU.
- Do not breast feed while taking this drug.

MORICIZINE

(mor-i′ci-zeen)
Ethmozine
Classifications: CARDIOVASCULAR AGENT; ANTIARRHYTHMIC AGENT, CLASS IC
Prototype: Flecainide
Pregnancy Category: B

AVAILABILITY 200 mg, 250 mg, 300 mg tablets

ACTIONS Class IC antiarrhythmic agent with potent local anesthetic effect and myocardial membrane stabilizing effects. Shortens phase II and phase III repolarization, resulting in a decreased action potential duration and effective refractory period of the cardiac muscle. Decrease in the maximum rate of phase 0 depolarization (V_{max}) occurs. Sinus node and atrial tissue are not affected.

THERAPEUTIC EFFECTS Prolongs atrioventricular conduction in patients with ventricular tachycardia. In patients with impaired left ventricular functioning, has minimal effects on cardiac index, pulmonary wedge pressure, and ejection fraction, either at rest or during exercise.

USES Treatment of ventricular tachycardia and ventricular premature depolarizations.

UNLABELED USES Supraventricular arrhythmias.

CONTRAINDICATIONS Preexisting second- and third-degree AV block, right bundle branch block unless a pacemaker is used; cardiogenic shock; hypersensitivity to moricizine; lactation.

CAUTIOUS USE Non-life-threatening arrhythmia; hypokalemia, hyperkalemia, hypomagnesia; sick sinus syndrome; hepatic impairment, renal impairment; pregnancy (category B). Safety and efficacy in children <18 y are not established.

ROUTE & DOSAGE

Ventricular and Supraventricular Arrhythmias

Adult: **PO** 200–300 mg q8h

Renal Hepatic or Impairment

Start with 600 mg/d or less

ADMINISTRATION

Oral

- Withdraw previous drug for 1–2 half-lives before transferring to moricizine.
- Dose increments are usually limited to 150 mg/d at 3-d intervals.
- Store at 15°–30° C (59°–86° F) unless otherwise directed by manufacturer.

ADVERSE EFFECTS (≥1%) **CV:** <u>Arrhythmias, including PVCs and ventricular tachycardia</u>. **CNS:** *Dizziness, light-headedness, anxiety, headache, euphoria, perioral numbness.* **GI:** Nausea, diarrhea, dry mouth, abdominal discomfort. **Body as a Whole:** Hyperthermia (rare).

INTERACTIONS Drug: May decrease **theophylline** concentrations. May increase the hypoprothrombinemic effects of **warfarin.**

PHARMACOKINETICS Absorption: Readily absorbed from GI tract. 30%–40% reaches systemic circulation due to extensive first-pass metabolism. **Onset:** 2 h. **Peak:** 10–14 h. **Duration:** 10 h. **Distribution:** 92%–95% bound to plasma proteins. Distributed into breast milk. **Metabolism:** Extensively metabolized in the liver. **Elimination:** 39% excreted in urine over 2 d, 56% excreted in feces over 4–5 d. **Half-Life:** elimination 10 h.

NURSING IMPLICATIONS

Assessment & Drug Effects

- Lab tests: Baseline serum electrolytes, liver and kidney function tests.
- Correct electrolyte imbalances, especially hypo/hyperkalemia and hypomagnesemia prior to beginning drug.
- Monitor cardiac status at beginning and throughout therapy

closely because drug may cause serious new arrhythmias or worsening of preexisting arrhythmias.
- Monitor patients with liver or kidney dysfunction closely for adverse effects.
- Monitor patients with sick sinus syndrome or conduction abnormalities carefully. Drug may interfere with sinus activity or cause AV block, both of which may necessitate prompt withdrawal of drug.
- Use precautions for dizziness; it occurs ≥15% of those taking drug.

Patient & Family Education
- Understand seriousness of taking moricizine exactly as prescribed.
- Take drug consistently with respect to meals.
- Keep regular follow-up appointments while taking this drug.
- Report immediately palpitations, irregular heartbeat, chest pains, or fever to physician.
- Do not breast feed while taking this drug.

MORPHINE SULFATE (Pr)

(mor'feen)

Astramorph PF, Avinza, DepoDur, Duramorph, Epimorph ♣, Kadian, MSIR, MS Contin, Oramorph SR, Roxanol, RMS, Statex ♣

Classifications: CENTRAL NERVOUS SYSTEM (CNS) AGENT; ANALGESIC; NARCOTIC (OPIATE) AGONIST

Pregnancy Category: B (D in long-term use or high dose)

Controlled Substance: Schedule II

AVAILABILITY 10 mg, 15 mg, 30 mg tablets/capsules; 15 mg, 20 mg, 30 mg, 60 mg, 100 mg, 120 mg, 200 mg controlled release tablets/capsules; 10 mg/2.5 mL, 10 mg/5 ml, 20 mg/mL, 20 mg/5 mL, 30 mg/1.5 mL, 100 mg/5 mL oral solution; 0.5 mg/mL, 1 mg/mL, 2 mg/mL, 4 mg/mL, 5 mg/mL, 8 mg/mL, 10 mg/mL, 15 mg/mL, 25 mg/mL, 50 mg/mL injection; 10 mg/mL, 15 mg/1.5 mL, 20 mg/2 mL extended-release lysosomal injection; 5 mg, 10 mg, 20 mg, 30 mg suppositories

ACTIONS Natural opium alkaloid with agonist activity by binding with the same receptors as endogenous opioid peptides. Narcotic agonist effects are identified with 3 types of receptors: Analgesia at supraspinal level, euphoria, respiratory depression and physical dependence; analgesia at spinal level, sedation and miosis; and dysphoric, hallucinogenic and cardiac stimulant effects.

THERAPEUTIC EFFECTS Controls severe pain; also used as an adjunct to anesthesia.

USES Symptomatic relief of severe acute and chronic pain after nonnarcotic analgesics have failed and as preanesthetic medication; also used to relieve dyspnea of acute left ventricular failure and pulmonary edema and pain of MI.

CONTRAINDICATIONS Hypersensitivity to opiates; increased intracranial pressure; convulsive disorders; acute alcoholism; acute bronchial asthma, chronic pulmonary diseases, severe respiratory depression; chemical-irritant induced pulmonary edema; prostatic hypertrophy; diarrhea caused by poisoning until the toxic material has been eliminated; undiagnosed acute abdominal conditions; following biliary tract surgery and surgical anastomosis; pancreatitis; acute ulcerative colitis; severe liver or renal insufficiency; Addison's disease; hypothyroidism; during labor for delivery of a premature infant, in premature infants; pregnancy (category B; D in long-term use or when high dose is used); lactation.

CAUTIOUS USE Toxic psychosis; cardiac arrhythmias, cardiovascular disease; emphysema; kyphoscoliosis; cor pulmonale; severe obesity; reduced blood volume; very old, very young, or debilitated patients; labor.

ROUTE & DOSAGE

Pain Relief

Adult: **PO** 10–30 mg q4h prn or 15–30 mg sustained release q8–12h; (Kadian) dose q12–24h, increase dose prn for pain relief **IV** 2.5–15 mg q4h or 0.8–10 mg/h by continuous infusion, may increase prn to control pain or 5–10 mg given epidurally q24h **Epidural** (DepoDur only) 10–15 mg as single dose 30 min before surgery (max: 20 mg) **IM/SC** 5–20 mg q4h **PR** 10–20 mg q4h prn
Child: **IV** 0.05–0.1 mg/kg q4h or 0.025–2.6 mg/kg/h by continuous infusion **IM/SC** 0.1–0.2 mg/kg q4h (max: 15 mg/dose) **PO** 0.2–0.5 mg/kg q4–6h; 0.3–0.6 mg/kg sustained release q12h
Neonate: **IV/IM/SC** 0.05 mg/kg q4–8h (max: 0.1 mg/kg) or 0.01–0.02 mg/kg/h

ADMINISTRATION

Oral

- Use a fixed, individualized schedule when narcotic analgesic therapy is started to provide effective management; blood levels can be maintained and peaks of pain can be prevented (usually a 4-h interval is adequate).
- Use lower dosage for older adult or debilitated patients than for adults.
- Do not break in half, crush, or allow sustained release tablet to be chewed.
- Do not give patient sustained release tablet within 24 h of surgery.
- Dilute oral solution in approximately 30 mL or more of fluid or semisolid food. A calibrated dropper comes with the bottle. Read labels carefully when using liquid preparation; available solutions: 20 mg/mL; 100 mg/mL.

Intravenous

Note: Verify correct IV concentration and rate of infusion/injection for administration to neonates, infants, or children with physician.

PREPARE: **Direct:** Dilute 2–10 mg in at least 5 mL of sterile water for injection.

ADMINISTER: **Direct:** Give a single dose over 4–5 min. Avoid rapid administration.

INCOMPATIBILITIES **Solution/additive: Aminophylline, amobarbital, chlorothiazide, floxacillin, fluorouracil, haloperidol, heparin, meperidine, pentobarbital, phenobarbital, phenytoin, sodium bicarbonate, thiopental. Y-site: Amphotericin B cholesteryl complex, cefepime, doxorubicin liposome, minocycline, sargramostim, tetracycline.**

- Store at 15°–30° C (59°–86° F). Avoid freezing. Refrigerate suppositories. Protect all formulations from light.

ADVERSE EFFECTS (≥1%) **Body as a Whole:** Hypersensitivity [*Pruritus,* rash, urticaria, edema, hemorrhagic urticaria (rare), anaphylactoid reaction (rare)], sweating, skeletal muscle flaccidity; cold, clammy skin, hypothermia. **CNS:** Euphoria, insomnia, disorientation, visual

M

disturbances, dysphoria, paradoxic CNS stimulation (restlessness, tremor, delirium, insomnia), convulsions (infants and children); decreased cough reflex, drowsiness, dizziness, deep sleep, coma, continuous intrathecal infusion may cause granulomas leading to paralysis. **Special Senses:** Miosis. **CV:** Bradycardia, palpitations, syncope; flushing of face, neck, and upper thorax; orthostatic hypotension, cardiac arrest. **GI:** *Constipation,* anorexia, dry mouth, biliary colic, *nausea,* vomiting, elevated transaminase levels. **Urogenital:** Urinary retention or urgency, dysuria, oliguria, reduced libido or potency (prolonged use). **Other:** Prolonged labor and respiratory depression of newborn. **Hematologic:** Precipitation of porphyria. **Respiratory:** Severe respiratory depression (as low as 2–4/min) or arrest; pulmonary edema.

DIAGNOSTIC TEST INTERFERENCE False-positive ***urine glucose*** determinations may occur using ***Benedict's solution. Plasma amylase*** and ***lipase*** determinations may be falsely positive for 24 h after use of morphine; ***transaminase levels*** may be elevated.

INTERACTIONS Drug: CNS DEPRESSANTS, SEDATIVES, BARBITURATES, **alcohol,** BENZODIAZEPINES, and TRICYCLIC ANTIDEPRESSANTS potentiate CNS depressant effects. Use MAO INHIBITORS cautiously; they may precipitate hypertensive crisis. PHENOTHIAZINES may antagonize analgesia. **Herbal: Kava-kava, valerian, St. John's wort** may increase sedation.

PHARMACOKINETICS Absorption: Variably absorbed from GI tract. **Peak:** 60 min PO; 20–60 min PR; 50–90 min SC; 30–60 min IM; 20 min IV. **Duration:** Up to 7 h. **Distribution:** Crosses blood–brain barrier and placenta; distributed in breast milk. **Metabolism:** Metabolized primarily in liver. **Elimination:** 90% of drug and metabolites excreted in urine in 24 h; 7%–10% excreted in bile.

NURSING IMPLICATIONS

Assessment & Drug Effects

- Obtain baseline respiratory rate, depth, and rhythm and size of pupils before administering the drug. Respirations of 12/min or below and miosis are signs of toxicity. Withhold drug and report to physician.
- Observe patient closely to be certain pain relief is achieved. Record relief of pain and duration of analgesia.
- Be alert to elevated pulse or respiratory rate, restlessness, anorexia, or drawn facial expression that may indicate need for analgesia.
- Differentiate among restlessness as a sign of pain and the need for medication, restlessness associated with hypoxia, and restlessness caused by morphine-induced CNS stimulation (a paradoxic reaction that is particularly common in women and older adult patients).
- Monitor for respiratory depression; it can be severe for as long as 24 h after epidural or intrathecal administration.
- Monitor carefully those at risk for severe respiratory depression after epidural or intrathecal injection: Older adult or debilitated patients or those with decreased respiratory reserve (e.g., emphysema, severe obesity, kyphoscoliosis).
- Continue monitoring for respiratory depression for at least 24 h

after each epidural or intrathecal dose.

- Assess vital signs at regular intervals. Morphine-induced respiratory depression may occur even with small doses, and it increases progressively with higher doses (generally max: 90 min after SC, 30 min after IM, and 7 min after IV).
- Encourage changes in position, deep breathing, and coughing (unless contraindicated) at regularly scheduled intervals. Narcotic analgesics also depress cough and sigh reflexes and thus may induce atelectasis, especially in postoperative patients.
- Be alert for nausea and orthostatic hypotension (with light-headedness and dizziness) in ambulatory patients or when a supine patient assumes the head-up position or in patients not experiencing severe pain.
- Monitor I&O ratio and pattern. Report oliguria or urinary retention. Morphine may dull perception of bladder stimuli; therefore, encourage the patient to void at least q4h. Palpate lower abdomen to detect bladder distention.

Patient & Family Education

- Avoid alcohol and other CNS depressants while receiving morphine.
- Do not use of any OTC drug unless approved by physician.
- Do not smoke or ambulate without assistance after receiving drug. Bedside rails are advised.
- Use caution or avoid tasks requiring alertness (e.g., driving a car) until response to drug is known since morphine may cause drowsiness, dizziness, or blurred vision.
- Do not breast feed while taking this drug.

MOXIFLOXACIN HYDROCHLORIDE

(mox-i-flox′a-sin)
Avelox, Vigamox
Classifications: ANTIINFECTIVE; ANTIBIOTIC; QUINOLONE
Prototype: Ciprofloxacin
Pregnancy Category: C

AVAILABILITY 400 mg tablets/injection; 0.5% ophthalmic solution

ACTIONS Moxifloxacin is a synthetic broad-spectrum antibiotic belonging to the fluoroquinolone class of drugs. It is bactericidal against gram-positive and gram-negative organisms. It inhibits topoisomerase II and IV (DNA gyrase) required for DNA replication, transcription, repair, and recombination of bacterial DNA.

THERAPEUTIC EFFECTS It is effective against *Staphylococcus aureus, Streptococcus pneumonia, Haemophilus influenzae, Klebsiella pneumoniae, Moraxella catarrhalis, Chlamydia pneumoniae,* and *Mycoplasma pneumoniae,* as well as other microbes.

USES Treatment of acute bacterial sinusitis, acute bacterial exacerbation of chronic bronchitis, community-acquired pneumonia, skin and skin structure infections, bacterial conjunctivitis.

CONTRAINDICATIONS Hypersensitivity to moxifloxacin or other quinolones; moderate to severe hepatic insufficiency; syphilis; pregnancy (category C); lactation; patients with history of prolonged QT_C interval on ECG, history of ventricular arrhythmias, atrial fibrillation, hypokalemia, bradycardia, acute myocardial ischemia, acute MI, patients receiving Class IA or Class III antiarrhythmic drugs; tendon pain; viral

M

infection; torsade de pointes; ocular preparation use in children <1 y.
CAUTIOUS USE CNS disorders; cerebrovascular disease, colitis, diarrhea, GI disease; diabetes mellitus; mild or moderate heart insufficiency; myasthenia gravis; seizure disorder; sunlight (UV) exposure. Safety and efficacy in children <18 y are unknown.

ROUTE & DOSAGE

Acute Bacterial Sinusitis, Acute Bacterial Exacerbation of Chronic Bronchitis, Community-Acquired Pneumonia, Skin Infections

Adult: **PO/IV** 400 mg q.d. × 5–10 d

Bacterial Conjunctivitis

Adult/Child: **Ophthalmic** >1 y, 1 drop in affected eye(s) t.i.d. × 7 d

M

ADMINISTRATION

Note: Do not administer to persons with QT_C prolongation, hypokalemia, or those receiving Class IA or Class III antiarrhythmic drugs.

Intravenous

PREPARE: **IV Infusion:** Avelox (400 mg) is supplied in ready-to-use 250 mL IV bags. No further dilution is necessary.
ADMINISTER: **IV Infusion:** Give over 60 min. AVOID RAPID OR BOLUS DOSE.

Oral

- Administer at least 4 h before or 8 h after multivitamins containing iron or zinc, or antacids containing magnesium, calcium, aluminum, or sucralfate.
- Store at 15°–30° C (59°–86° F); protect from high humidity.

ADVERSE EFFECTS (≥1%) **CNS:** Dizziness, headache, peripheral neuropathy. **GI:** Nausea, diarrhea, abdominal pain, vomiting, taste perversion, abnormal liver function tests, dyspepsia. **Musculoskeletal:** Tendon rupture.

DIAGNOSTIC TEST INTERFERENCE May cause false positive on ***opiate screening tests.***

INTERACTIONS Drug: Iron, zinc, ANTACIDS, **aluminum, magnesium, calcium, sucralfate** decrease absorption; **atenolol, cisapride, erythromycin,** ANTIPSYCHOTICS, TRICYCLIC ANTIDEPRESSANTS, **quinidine, procainamide, amiodarone, sotalol** may cause prolonged QT_C interval.

PHARMACOKINETICS Absorption: Well absorbed, 90% bioavailable. **Steady State:** 3 d. **Distribution:** 50% protein bound. **Metabolism:** Metabolized in liver. **Elimination:** Unchanged drug: 20% in urine, 25% in feces; metabolites: 38% in feces, 14% in urine. **Half-Life:** 12 h.

NURSING IMPLICATIONS

Assessment & Drug Effects

- Monitor therapeutic effectiveness indicated by clinical improvement of infection.
- Monitor for and notify physician immediately of adverse CNS effects.
- Notify physician immediately for S&S of hypersensitivity (see Appendix F).
- Lab tests: C&S before initiation of therapy and baseline serum potassium with history of hypokalemia.

Patient & Family Education

- Exercise care in timing of consumption of vitamins and antacids (see ADMINISTRATION).
- Drink fluids liberally, unless directed otherwise.
- Increased seizure potential is possible, especially when history of seizure exists.
- Stop taking drug and notify physician if experiencing palpita-

tions, fainting, skin rash, severe diarrhea, ankle/foot pain, agitation, insomnia.
- Avoid engaging in hazardous activities until reaction to drug is known.
- Do not breast feed while taking this drug.

MUPIROCIN

(mu-pi-ro'sin)

Bactroban, Bactroban Nasal

Classifications: ANTIINFECTIVE; PSEUDOMONIC ACID ANTIBIOTIC

Pregnancy Category: B

AVAILABILITY 2% ointment; cream

ACTIONS Topical antibacterial produced by fermentation of *Pseudomonas fluorescens*.

THERAPEUTIC EFFECTS Inhibits bacterial protein synthesis by binding with the bacterial transfer-RNA. Susceptible bacteria are *Staphylococcus aureus* [including methicillin-resistant (MRSA) and beta-lactamase-producing strains], *Staphylococcus epidermidis, Staphylococcus saprophyticus,* and *Streptococcus pyogenes*.

USES Impetigo due to *Staphylococcus aureus, beta-hemolytic Streptococci*, and *Streptococcus pyogenes;* nasal carriage of *S. aureus*.

UNLABELED USES Superficial skin infections.

CONTRAINDICATIONS Hypersensitivity to any of its components and for ophthalmic use.

CAUTIOUS USE Burn patients; pregnancy (category B) or lactation.

ROUTE & DOSAGE

Impetigo

Adult/Child: **Topical** Apply to affected area t.i.d., if no response in 3–5 d, reevaluate (usually continue for 1–2 wk)

Elimination of Staphylococcal Nasal Carriage

Child: **Intranasal** Apply intranasally b.i.d. to q.i.d. for 5–14 d

ADMINISTRATION

Topical
- Apply thin layer of medication to affected area.
- Cover area being treated with a gauze dressing if desired.

ADVERSE EFFECTS (≥1%) **Skin:** Burning, stinging, pain, pruritus, rash, erythema, dry skin, tenderness, swelling. **Special Senses:** Intranasal, local stinging, soreness, dry skin, pruritus.

INTERACTIONS Drug: Incompatible with **salicylic acid 2%**; do not mix in HYDROPHILIC VEHICLES (e.g., **Aquaphor**) or COAL TAR SOLUTIONS; **chloramphenicol** may interfere with bactericidal action of mupirocin.

PHARMACOKINETICS Absorption: Not systemically absorbed.

NURSING IMPLICATIONS

Assessment & Drug Effects
- Watch for signs and symptoms of superinfection (see Appendix F). Prolonged or repeated therapy may result in superinfection by nonsusceptible organisms.
- Reevaluate drug use if patient does not show clinical response within 3–5 d.
- Discontinue the drug and notify physician if signs of contact dermatitis develop or if exudate production increases.

Patient & Family Education
- Discontinue drug and contact physician if a sensitivity reaction or chemical irritation occurs (e.g., increased redness, itching, burning).
- Do not breast feed while taking this drug without consulting physician.

MUROMONAB-CD3

(myoo-roe-moe′nab)
Orthoclone OKT3
Classifications: IMMUNOSUPPRESSANT; MONOCLONAL ANTIBODY
Prototype: Cyclosporine
Pregnancy Category: C

AVAILABILITY 5 mg/mL injection

ACTIONS Murine monoclonal antibody (purified IgG_2). Specifically targets the T_3 (CD_3) molecule in the antigenic recognition site of the human T-cell membrane. Following this antigenic challenge, CD_3-positive T-cells are rapidly removed from circulation, and T-lymphocyte action leading to renal inflammation and destruction is blocked, thus reversing graft rejection. Lymphomas may follow immunosuppression therapy with muromonab-CD_3; incidence is related to intensity and duration of drug-induced immunosuppression.

THERAPEUTIC EFFECTS CD_3-positive T-lymphocytes immunosuppression results in reversing graft rejection of a transplanted kidney.

USES Acute allograft rejection in kidney transplant patients.

UNLABELED USES Acute allograft rejection in heart and liver transplant patients.

CONTRAINDICATIONS Intolerance to any product of murine origin; patient with fluid overload; weight gain of more than 3% within week prior to treatment; infection: chickenpox (existing, recent, including recent exposure), herpes zoster. Safety during pregnancy (category C) or lactation is not established.

CAUTIOUS USE Repeated courses.

ROUTE & DOSAGE

Transplant Rejection
Adult: **IV** 5 mg/d administered in <1 min for 10–14 d
Child: **IV** *<12 y,* 0.1 mg/kg q.d. times 10–14 d or *≤30 kg,* 2.5 mg q.d.; *>30 kg,* 5 mg q.d.

ADMINISTRATION

Note: Only persons experienced with immunosuppressive therapy and management of kidney transplant patients should administer Muromonab-CD_3 and only in an area equipped with staff and facilities to deal with cardiac resuscitation.

Intravenous

Note: Verify correct rate of IV injection for administration to infants or children with physician. ▪ Administer IV methylprednisolone sodium succinate before and IV hydrocortisone sodium succinate 30 min after muromonab-CD_3 to decrease incidence of first dose reaction. ▪ Be aware that concomitant maintenance immunosuppressive therapy is reduced or discontinued during drug therapy with muromonab-CD_3 and resumed about 3 d prior to end of therapy.

PREPARE: **Direct:** Give undiluted. Do not shake ampule. Draw sterile solution into syringe through a low protein-binding 0.2- or 0.22-micron filter. Discard filter; attach syringe to an appropriate needle for IV bolus injection.

ADMINISTER: **Direct:** Give by rapid (bolus) injection. Do not give by IV infusion or in conjunction with other drug solutions.

▪ Store at 2°–8° C (36°–46° F) unless otherwise stipulated. Avoid freezing.

ADVERSE EFFECTS (≥1%) **All:** Especially during first 2 d of therapy.

GI: *Nausea, vomiting, diarrhea.* **Respiratory:** Severe pulmonary edema, *dyspnea, chest pain, wheezing.* **Body as a Whole:** *Fever, chills,* malaise, *tremor, increased susceptibility to cytomegalovirus, herpes simplex, Pneumocystis carinii, Legionella, Cryptococcus, Serratia* organisms, and gram negative bacteria. **CV:** Tachycardia.

PHARMACOKINETICS Onset: The number of circulating CD_3-positive T-cells decreases within minutes. **Peak:** 2–7 d. **Duration:** 7 d.

NURSING IMPLICATIONS

Assessment & Drug Effects

- Assess and monitor vital signs. If temperature rises above 37.8° C (100° F), suspect infection (commonly observed in first 45 d of therapy). Take temperature before treatment and several hours after drug administration to detect first signs of infection.
- Consult physician if patient has a fever exceeding 37.8° C (100° F) before treatment. Make immediate attempts to lower temperature to at least 37.8° C (100° F) with antipyretics before muromonab-CD_3 is administered.
- Be alert to susceptibility of patient with pretreatment fluid over-load to acute pulmonary edema (may be fatal). Be prepared for prompt intubation, oxygenation, and corticosteroid drug administration should it occur.
- Monitor patient's response closely for 48 h for first dose reaction (occurs within 45–60 min after first dose and lasts several hours). It may occur (less severe) after second dose; then usually does not occur with subsequent doses. Symptoms: Chills, dyspnea, malaise, high fever.

Patient & Family Education

- Report any of the following to physician: Chest pain, difficulty breathing, wheezing, nausea and vomiting, significant weight gain, an infection, or fever.
- Use an effective method of birth control for 12 weeks following the end of therapy.

MYCOPHENOLATE MOFETIL

(my-co-phen′o-late mo′fe-till)

CellCept

MYCOPHENOLATE SODIUM

Myfortic

Classifications: BIOLOGIC RESPONSE MODIFIER; IMMUNOSUPPRESSANT

Prototype: Cyclosporine

Pregnancy Category: C

AVAILABILITY 250 mg capsules; 500 mg tablets; 180 mg, 360 mg delayed-release tablets; 500 mg injection

ACTIONS Prodrug with immunosuppressant properties; inhibits T- and B-lymphocyte proliferation responses inhibits antibody formation, and blocks the generation of cytotoxic T-cells.

THERAPEUTIC EFFECTS Antirejection effects attributed to decreased number of activated lymphocytes in the graft site. Synergistic with cyclosporine.

USES Prophylaxis of organ rejection in patients receiving allogenic kidney transplants or heart transplants.

UNLABELED USES Rejection prophylaxis for liver transplants, treatment of rheumatoid arthritis and psoriasis.

CONTRAINDICATIONS Hypersensitivity to mycophenolate mofetil; vaccination, varicella; pregnancy (category C), lactation; children <5 y.

CAUTIOUS USE Viral or bacterial infections; presence or history of carcinoma; bone marrow suppression;

M

active peptic ulcer disease; cholestasis; gallbladder disease; GI disease, severe diarrhea; malabsorption syndromes; hepatic encephalopathy, hepatic or renal impairment; renal failure, uremia; herpes infection, infection; hypoalbuminemia; PKU; lactase deficiency.

ROUTE & DOSAGE

Note: CellCept and Myfortic are not interchangeable.

Prophylaxis for Kidney Transplant Rejection

Adult: **PO/IV** Start within 24 h of transplant, 1 g (mofetil) or 720 mg (sodium) b.i.d. in combination with corticosteroids and cyclosporine
Child: **PO** 600 mg/m^2 (mofetil) or 400 mg/m^2 (sodium) b.i.d. (max: 2 g/d mofetil, 720 mg/d sodium)

Prophylaxis for Heart Transplant Rejection

Adult: **PO/IV** 1.5 g b.i.d. started within 24 h of transplant

ADMINISTRATION

Oral

- Give oral drug on an empty stomach.
- Adjust dosage with severe chronic kidney failure.
- Do not open or crush capsules; avoid contact with powder in capsules, and wash thoroughly with soap and water if contact occurs.

Intravenous

PREPARE: **IV Infusion:** Reconstitute each vial with 14 mL D5W. Further dilute vial used in an additional 70 mL with D5W to yield 6 mg/mL.

ADMINISTER: **IV Infusion:** Slowly infuse over ≥2 h. Avoid rapid injection.

INCOMPATIBILITIES **Solution/additive & Y-site:** Do not mix or infuse with other medications.

- Begin IV mycophenolate mofetil within 24 h of transplant and continued for up to 14 d.
- Switch patient to oral drug as soon as possible.
- Store at 15°–30° C (59°–86° F).

ADVERSE EFFECTS (≥1%) **CNS:** *Headache, tremor,* insomnia, dizziness, weakness. **CV:** *Hypertension.* **Endocrine:** Hyperglycemia, hypercholesterolemia, hypophosphatemia, hypokalemia, hyperkalemia, *peripheral edema.* **GI:** *Diarrhea, constipation, nausea,* anorexia, vomiting, *abdominal pain, dyspepsia.* **Urogenital:** *UTI, hematuria,* renal tubular necrosis, burning, frequency, vaginal burning or itching, vaginal bleeding, kidney stones. **Hematologic:** *Leukopenia, anemia, thrombocytopenia,* hypochromic anemia, leukocytosis. **Respiratory:** *Respiratory infection, dyspnea,* increased cough, pharyngitis. **Skin:** Rash. **Body as a Whole:** Leg or hand cramps, bone pain, myalgias, *sepsis (bacterial, fungal, viral).*

INTERACTIONS Drug: Acyclovir, ganciclovir may increase mycophenolate serum levels. ANTACIDS, **cholestyramine** decreases mycophenolate absorption. **Mycophenolate** may decrease protein binding of **phenytoin** or **theophylline,** causing increased serum levels.

PHARMACOKINETICS Absorption: Rapidly absorbed from GI tract; 94% reaches systemic circulation; absorption decreased by food. **Onset:** 4 wk. **Metabolism:** Metabolized in liver to active form, mycophenolic acid. **Elimination:** 87% excreted in urine. **Half-Life:** 11 h.

NURSING IMPLICATIONS

Assessment & Drug Effects

- Lab tests: Monitor CBC weekly for first month, biweekly for second and third months, then once per month for first year. If neutropenia develops (ANC <1.3 × 10^3/mcL), withhold dose and notify physician. Periodically monitor and report abnormalities for any of the following: Kidney and liver function, serum electrolytes, lipase, and amylase; blood glucose; routine urinalysis.
- Monitor for and report any S&S of sepsis or infection.

Patient & Family Education

- Comply exactly with dosing regimen and scheduled laboratory tests.
- Report to physician immediately S&S of infection, such as UTI or respiratory infection.
- Report all troubling adverse reactions (e.g., blood in urine and swelling in arms and legs) to physician as soon as possible.
- Avoid taking OTC antacids simultaneously with mycophenolate mofetil. Separate the two drugs by 2 h.
- Do not breast feed while taking this drug.

NABUMETONE

(na-bu-me'tone)
Relafen
Classifications: CENTRAL NERVOUS SYSTEM AGENT; ANALGESIC, NSAID; ANTIPYRETIC
Prototype: Ibuprofen
Pregnancy Category: C

AVAILABILITY 500 mg, 750 mg tablets

ACTIONS Blocks prostaglandin synthesis by inhibiting cyclooxygenase, an enzyme that converts arachidonic acid to precursors of prostaglandins.

THERAPEUTIC EFFECTS Antiinflammatory, analgesic, and antipyretic effects. Inhibits platelet aggregation and prolongs bleeding time but does not affect prothrombin or whole blood clotting times. Cross-sensitivity with aspirin and other nonsteroidal antiinflammatory drugs has been reported.

USES Rheumatoid arthritis and osteoarthritis.

CONTRAINDICATIONS Patients in whom urticaria, severe rhinitis, bronchospasm, angioedema, or nasal polyps are precipitated by aspirin or other NSAIDS; active peptic ulcer; bleeding abnormalities. Safety during pregnancy (category C), lactation, or in children <6 mo is not established.

CAUTIOUS USE Hypertension, history of GI ulceration, impaired liver or kidney function, chronic kidney failure, cardiac decompensation, patients with SLE.

ROUTE & DOSAGE

Rheumatoid & Osteoarthritis
Adult: **PO** 1000 mg/d as a single dose, may increase (max: of 2000 mg/d in 1–2 divided doses)

ADMINISTRATION

Oral

- Give with food, milk, or antacid (if prescribed) to reduce the possibility of GI upset.
- Store at 15°–30° C (59°–86° F).

ADVERSE EFFECTS (≥1%) **GI:** Diarrhea, abdominal pain, nausea, dyspepsia, flatulence, melena, ulcers, constipation, dry mouth, gastritis. **CNS:** Tinnitus, dizziness, headache, insomnia, vertigo, fa-

N

tigue, diaphoresis, nervousness, somnolence. **Skin:** Rash, pruritus.

INTERACTIONS Drug: May attenuate the antihypertensive response to DIURETICS. NSAIDS increase the risk of **methotrexate** toxicity. **Food:** Food may increase the peak but not the overall absorption of nabumetone. **Herbal: Feverfew, garlic, ginger, ginkgo** may increase bleeding potential.

PHARMACOKINETICS Absorption: Readily absorbed from GI tract; approximately 35% is converted to its active metabolite on first pass through the liver. **Onset:** 1–3 wk for antirheumatic action. **Peak:** 3–6 h. **Distribution:** 99% protein bound; distributes into synovial fluid. **Metabolism:** Metabolized in liver to its active metabolite, 6-methoxy-2-naphthylacetic acid (6MNA). **Elimination:** 80% of dose is excreted in urine as 6MNA; 10% excreted in feces. **Half-Life:** 24 h (6MNA).

N

NURSING IMPLICATIONS

Assessment & Drug Effects

- Lab tests: Obtain baseline and periodic evaluation of Hgb and Hct levels with prolonged or high-dose therapy.
- Monitor for signs and symptoms of GI bleeding.

Patient & Family Education

- Use caution with hazardous activities since nabumetone may cause dizziness, drowsiness, and blurred vision.
- Report abdominal pain, nausea, dyspepsia, or black tarry stools.
- Be aware that alcohol and aspirin will increase the risk of GI ulceration and bleeding.
- Notify your physician if any of the following occur: persistent headache, skin rash or itching, visual disturbances, weight gain, or edema.
- Do not breast feed while taking this drug without consulting physician.

NADOLOL

(nay-doe'lole)

Corgard

Classifications: AUTONOMIC NERVOUS SYSTEM AGENT; BETA-ADRENERGIC ANTAGONIST (SYMPATHOLYTIC, ADRENERGIC BLOCKING AGENT); ANTIHYPERTENSIVE

Prototype: Propranolol

Pregnancy Category: C

AVAILABILITY 20 mg, 40 mg, 80 mg, 120 mg, 160 mg tablets

ACTIONS Nonselective beta-adrenergic blocking agent pharmacologically and chemically similar to propranolol. Inhibits response to adrenergic stimuli by competitively blocking beta-adrenergic receptors within heart.

THERAPEUTIC EFFECTS Reduces heart rate and cardiac output at rest and during exercise, and also decreases conduction velocity through AV node and myocardial automaticity. Decreases both systolic and diastolic BP at rest and during exercise. Suppression of $beta_2$-adrenergic receptors in bronchial and vascular smooth muscle can cause bronchospasm and a Raynaud's-like phenomenon.

USES Hypertension, either alone or in combination with a diuretic. Also long-term prophylactic management of angina pectoris.

CONTRAINDICATIONS Bronchial asthma, severe COPD, inadequate myocardial function, sinus bradycardia, greater than first-degree conduction block, overt cardiac failure, cardiogenic shock. Safety during pregnancy (category C), lactation, and in children <18 y is not established.

CAUTIOUS USE CHF; diabetes mellitus; hyperthyroidism; renal impairment.

ROUTE & DOSAGE

Hypertension, Angina
Adult: **PO** 40 mg once/d, may increase up to 240–320 mg/d in 1–2 divided doses

ADMINISTRATION

Note: Dose is usually titrated up in 40–80 mg increments until optimum dose is achieved.

Oral

- Do not discontinue abruptly; reduce dosage over a 1–2-wk period. Abrupt withdrawal can precipitate MI or thyroid storm in susceptible patients.
- Store at 15°–30° C (59°–86° F); protect drug from light.

ADVERSE EFFECTS (≥1%) **Body as a Whole:** Hypersensitivity (rash, pruritus, laryngospasm, respiratory disturbances). **CV:** *Bradycardia, peripheral vascular insufficiency (Raynaud's type),* palpitation, postural hypotension, conduction or rhythm disturbances, CHF. **GI:** Dry mouth. **CNS:** *Dizziness, fatigue,* sedation, headache, paresthesias, behavioral changes. **Special Senses:** Blurred vision, dry eyes. **Skin:** Dry skin. **Urogenital:** Impotence.

INTERACTIONS Drug: NSAIDS may decrease hypotensive effects; may mask symptoms of a hypoglycemic reaction to **insulin,** SULFONYLUREAS; **prazosin, terazosin** may increase severe hypotensive response to first dose.

PHARMACOKINETICS Absorption: 30%–40% of PO dose absorbed. **Peak:** 2–4 h. **Duration:** 17–24 h. **Distribution:** Widely distributed; crosses placenta; distributed in breast milk. **Metabolism:** No hepatic metabolism. **Elimination:** 70% excreted in urine; also excreted in feces. **Half-Life:** 10–24 h.

NURSING IMPLICATIONS

Assessment & Drug Effects

- Assess heart rate and BP before administration of each dose. Withhold drug and notify physician if apical pulse drops below 60 bpm or systolic BP below 90 mm Hg.
- Monitor weight. Advise patient to report weight gain of 1–1.5 kg (2–3 lb) in a day and any other possible signs of CHF (e.g., cough, fatigue, dyspnea, rapid pulse, edema).
- Evaluate effectiveness for patients with angina by reduction in frequency of anginal attacks and improved exercise tolerance. Improvement should coincide with steady state serum concentration reached within 6–9 d. Keep physician informed of drug effect.
- Monitor patients with diabetes mellitus closely. Beta-adrenergic blockade produced by nadolol may prevent important clinical manifestations of hypoglycemia (e.g., tachycardia, BP changes).
- Monitor I&O ratio and creatinine clearance in patients with impaired kidney function or with cardiac problems. Dosage intervals will be lengthened with decreases in creatinine clearance.

Patient & Family Education

- Check pulse before taking each dose. Do not take your medication if pulse rate drops below 60 (or other parameter set by physician) or becomes irregular. Consult your physician right away.

N

- Do not stop taking your medication or alter dosage without consulting your physician.
- Do not drive or engage in potentially hazardous activities until response to drug is known.
- Do not breast feed while taking this drug without consulting physician.

NAFARELIN ACETATE

(na-fa're-lin)

Synarel

Classifications: HORMONE AND SYNTHETIC SUBSTITUTE; GONADOTROPIN-RELEASING HORMONE ANALOG

Prototype: Leuprolide

Pregnancy Category: X

AVAILABILITY 2 mg/mL nasal solution

ACTIONS Potent agonist analog of gonadotropin-releasing hormone (GnRH). Inhibits pituitary gonadotropin secretion of LH and FSH.

THERAPEUTIC EFFECTS Decrease in serum estradiol or testosterone concentrations results in the quiescence of tissues and functions that depend on LH and FSH.

USES Endometriosis and precocious puberty.

UNLABELED USES Uterine leiomyomas, benign prostatic hypertrophy.

CONTRAINDICATIONS Hypersensitivity to GnRH or GnRH agonist analog; undiagnosed abnormal vaginal bleeding; pregnancy (category X), lactation.

CAUTIOUS USE Polycystic ovarian disease.

ROUTE & DOSAGE

Endometriosis

Adult: **Inhalation** 2 inhalations/d (200 mcg/inhalation), one in each nostril, begin between days 2 and 4 of menstrual cycle; in patients with persistent regular menstruation after 2 mo of therapy, may increase to 800 mcg/d as 2 inhalations (one in each nostril) b.i.d.; continue therapy for 6 mo, retreatment is not advised because of lack of safety data

Precocious Puberty

Child: **Inhalation** 800–1200 mcg/d divided q8h

ADMINISTRATION

Inhalation

- Withhold any topical nasal decongestant, if being used, until at least 30 min after nafarelin administration.
- Store at 15°–30° C (59°–86° F); protect from light.

ADVERSE EFFECTS (≥1%) **GI:** *Bloating, abdominal cramps,* weight gain, nausea. **Endocrine:** *Hot flashes, anovulation, amenorrhea, vaginal dryness,* galactorrhea. **Metabolic:** Decreased bone mineral content (reversible). **CNS:** Transient headache, inertia, mild depression, moodiness, fatigue. **Respiratory:** Nasal irritation. **Urogenital:** *Impotence, decreased libido,* dyspareunia.

DIAGNOSTIC TEST INTERFERENCE Increased ***alkaline phosphatase;*** marked increase in ***estradiol*** in first 2 wk, then decrease to below baseline; decreased ***FSH*** and ***LH*** levels; decreased ***testosterone*** levels.

INTERACTIONS Drug: No clinically significant interactions established.

PHARMACOKINETICS Absorption: 21% absorbed from nasal mucosa. **Onset:** 4 wk. **Peak:** 12 wk. **Duration:** 30–50 d after discontinuing drug. **Distribution:** 78%–84% bound to plasma proteins; crosses placenta. **Metabolism:** Hydrolyzed in kidney. **Elimination:** 44%–55% excreted in urine over 7 d, 19%–44% in feces. **Half-Life:** 2.7 h.

NURSING IMPLICATIONS

Assessment & Drug Effects

- Make appropriate inquiries about breakthrough bleeding, which may indicate that patient has missed successive drug doses.

Patient & Family Education

- Read the information pamphlet provided with nafarelin.
- Inform physician if breakthrough bleeding occurs or menstruation persists.
- Use or add barrier contraceptive during treatment.
- Do not breast feed while taking this drug.

NAFCILLIN SODIUM

(naf-sill′in)

Nafcil, Nallpen, Unipen

Classifications: ANTIINFECTIVE; BETA-LACTAM ANTIBIOTIC; PENICILLIN; ANTISTAPHYLOCOCCAL PENICILLIN

Prototype: Penicillin G potassium

Pregnancy Category: B

AVAILABILITY 250 mg capsules; 500 mg, 1 g, 2 g injection

ACTIONS Semisynthetic, acid-stable, penicillinase-resistant penicillin. Mechanism of bactericidal action is by interfering with synthesis of mucopeptides essential to formation and integrity of bacterial cell wall.

THERAPEUTIC EFFECTS Effective against both penicillin-sensitive and penicillin-resistant strains of *Staphylococcus aureus*. Also active against pneumococci and group A beta-hemolytic *Streptococci*. Highly active against penicillinase-producing *Staphylococci* but less potent than penicillin G against penicillin-sensitive microorganisms and generally ineffective against Methicillin-Resistant *Staphylococcus aureus* (MRSA).

USES Primarily, infections caused by penicillinase-producing *Staphylococci*. May also be used to initiate treatment in suspected staphylococcal infections pending culture and sensitivity test results. As with other penicillins, serum concentrations are considerably enhanced by concurrent use of probenecid.

CONTRAINDICATIONS Hypersensitivity to penicillins, cephalosporins, and other allergens; use of oral drug in severe infections, gastric dilatation, cardiospasm, or intestinal hypermotility; lactation. Safety during pregnancy (category B) is not established.

CAUTIOUS USE History of or suspected atopy or allergy (eczema, hives, hay fever, asthma).

N

ROUTE & DOSAGE

Staphylococcal Infections

Adult: **IM/IV** 500 mg–2 g q4–6h up to 12 g/d **PO** 250–1000 mg q4–6h
Child: **IM/IV** 100–300 mg/kg/d divided q4–6h **PO** 50–100 mg/kg/d in 4 divided doses
Neonate: **IM/IV** 50–100 mg/kg/d divided q6–12h

ADMINISTRATION

Oral

- Give on empty stomach (at least 1 h before or 2 h after meals).

Intramuscular

- Reconstitute each 500 mg with 1.7 mL of sterile water for injection or NaCal injection to yield 250 mg/mL. Shake vigorously to dissolve.

- In adults: Make certain solution is clear. Select site carefully. Inject deeply into gluteal muscle. Rotate injection sites.
- In children: The preferred IM site in children <3 y is the midlateral or anterolateral thigh. Check agency policy.
- Label and date vials of reconstituted solution. Remains stable for 7 d under refrigeration and for 3 d at 15°–30° C (59°–86° F).

Intravenous

Note: Verify correct IV concentration and rate of infusion in neonates, infants, children with physician.

PREPARE: **Direct:** Reconstitute as for IM injection. Further dilute with 15–30 mL of D5W, NS, or 0.45% NaCl. **Intermittent:** Dilute reconstituted solution in 100–150 mL of compatible IV solution. **Continuous:** Add desired dose to a volume of IV solution that maintains concentration of drug between 2–40 mg/mL.

ADMINISTER: **Direct:** Give over at least 10 min. **Intermittent:** Give over 30–90 min. **Continuous:** Give at ordered rate.

INCOMPATIBILITIES **Solution/additive:** **Aminophylline, ascorbic acid, aztreonam, bleomycin, cytarabine, hydrocortisone, methylprednisolone, promazine.** **Y-site:** **Droperidol, Innovar, labetalol, nalbuphine, pentazocine, verapamil.**

- Note: Usually, limit IV therapy to 24–48 h because of the possibility of thrombophlebitis (see Appendix F), particularly in older adults.
- Discard unused portions 24 h after reconstitution.

ADVERSE EFFECTS (≥1%) **Body as a Whole:** Drug fever, anaphylaxis (particularly following parenteral therapy). **GI:** Nausea, vomiting, *diarrhea,* increase in serum transaminase activity (following IM). **Hematologic:** Eosinophilia, thrombophlebitis following IV; neutropenia (long-term therapy). **Metabolic:** Hypokalemia (with high IV doses). **Skin:** Urticaria, pruritus, rash, pain and tissue irritation. **Urogenital:** Allergic interstitial nephritis.

DIAGNOSTIC TEST INTERFERENCE Nafcillin in large doses can cause false-positive ***urine protein*** tests using ***sulfosalicylic acid method.***

INTERACTIONS Drug: May antagonize hypoprothrombinemic effects of **warfarin**.

PHARMACOKINETICS Absorption: Incompletely and erratically absorbed orally. **Peak:** 30–120 min IM; 15 min IV. **Duration:** 4 h PO; 4–6 h IM. **Distribution:** Distributes into CNS with inflamed meninges; crosses placenta; distributed into breast milk. **Metabolism:** Enters enterohepatic circulation. **Elimination:** Primarily excreted in bile; 10%–30% excreted in urine. **Half-Life:** 1 h.

NURSING IMPLICATIONS

Assessment & Drug Effects

- Lab tests: Perform C&S prior to initiation of therapy and periodically thereafter. Obtain twice weekly differential WBC counts in patients receiving IV nafcillin therapy for longer than 2 wk.
- Obtain a careful history before therapy to determine any prior allergic reactions to penicillins, cephalosporins, and other allergens.
- Inspect IV site for inflammatory reaction. Also check IV site for leakage; in the older adult patient especially, loss of tissue elasticity with aging may promote extravasation around the needle.

- Note: Allergic reactions, principally rash, occur most commonly. Nausea, vomiting, and diarrhea may occur with oral therapy.
- Monitor neutrophil count. Nafcillin-induced neutropenia (agranulocytosis) occurs commonly during third week of therapy. It may be associated with malaise, fever, sore mouth, or throat. Perform periodic assessments of liver and kidney functions during prolonged therapy.
- Be alert for signs of bacterial or fungal superinfections (see Appendix F) in patients on prolonged therapy.
- Determine IV sodium intake for patients with sodium restriction. Nafcillin sodium contains approximately 3 mEq of sodium per gram.

Patient & Family Education

- Report promptly S&S of neutropenia (see Assessment & Drug Effects), superinfection, or hypokalemia (see Appendix F).
- Do not breast feed while taking this drug.

NAFTIFINE

(naf′ti-feen)

Naftin

Classifications: ANTIINFECTIVE; ANTIBIOTIC; ANTIFUNGAL

Prototype: Fluconazole

Pregnancy Category: B

AVAILABILITY 1% cream, gel

ACTIONS Synthetic broad-spectrum antifungal agent that may be fungicidal depending on the organism. Interferes in the synthesis of ergosterol, the principal sterol in the fungus cell membrane. Ergosterol becomes depleted and membrane function is affected.

THERAPEUTIC EFFECTS Effective against topical infections caused by *Candida albicans, Epidermophyton floccosum, Microsporum canis, M. audouinii, M. gypseum, Trichophyton rubrum, T. mentagrophytes,* and *T. tonsurans.*

USES *Tinea pedis, tinea cruris,* and *tinea corporis.*

CONTRAINDICATIONS Hypersensitivity to naftifine.

CAUTIOUS USE Pregnancy (category B), lactation. Safety and efficacy in children are not established.

ROUTE & DOSAGE

Tinea Infections

Adult: **Topical** Apply cream once daily, or apply gel twice daily, may use up to 4 wk

ADMINISTRATION

Topical

- Gently massage into affected area and surrounding skin. Wash hands before and after application.
- Do not apply occlusive dressing unless specifically directed to do so.
- Store at 15°–30° C (59°–86° F).

ADVERSE EFFECTS (≥1%) **Skin:** Burning or stinging, dryness, erythema, itching, local irritation.

INTERACTIONS No clinically significant interactions established.

PHARMACOKINETICS Absorption: 2.5%–6% absorbed through intact skin. **Onset:** 7 d. **Metabolism:** Metabolized in liver. **Elimination:** Excreted in urine and feces. **Half-Life:** 2–3 d.

NURSING IMPLICATIONS

Assessment & Drug Effects

- Assess for irritation or sensitivity to cream; these are indications to discontinue use.

- Reevaluate use of drug if no improvement is noted after 4 wk.

Patient & Family Education

- Learn correct application technique.
- Avoid contact with eyes or mucous membranes.
- Do not breast feed while taking this drug without consulting physician.

NALBUPHINE HYDROCHLORIDE

(nal'byoo-feen)

Nubain

Classifications: CENTRAL NERVOUS SYSTEM AGENT; ANALGESIC; NARCOTIC (OPIATE) AGONIST-ANTAGONIST

Prototype: Pentazocine

Pregnancy Category: C

AVAILABILITY 10 mg/mL, 20 mg/mL injection

ACTIONS Synthetic narcotic analgesic with agonist and weak antagonist properties. Analgesic potency is about 3 or 4 times greater than that of pentazocine and approximately equal to that produced by equivalent doses of morphine. On a weight basis, produces respiratory depression about equal to that of morphine; however, in contrast to morphine, doses >30 mg produce no further respiratory depression. Antagonistic potency is approximately one fourth that of naloxone and about 10 times greater than that of pentazocine.

THERAPEUTIC EFFECTS Analgesic action that relieves moderate to severe pain with apparently low potential for dependence.

USES Symptomatic relief of moderate to severe pain. Also preoperative sedation analgesia and as a supplement to surgical anesthesia.

CONTRAINDICATIONS History of hypersensitivity to drug. Safety during pregnancy (category C) or lactation is not established. Prolonged use during pregnancy could result in neonatal withdrawal.

CAUTIOUS USE History of emotional instability or drug abuse; head injury, increased intracranial pressure; impaired respirations; impaired kidney or liver function; MI; biliary tract surgery.

ROUTE & DOSAGE

Moderate to Severe Pain

Adult: **IV/IM/SC** 10–20 mg q3–6h prn (max 160 mg/d)
Child: **IV/IM/SC** 0.1–0.15 mg/kg q3–6h prn

ADMINISTRATION

Intramuscular/Subcutaneous

- Inject undiluted.

Intravenous

Note: Verify correct rate of IV injection in infants, children with physician.

PREPARE: **Direct:** Give undiluted.

ADMINISTER: **Direct:** Give at a rate of 10 mg or fraction thereof over 3–5 min.

INCOMPATIBILITIES **Solution/additive: Diazepam, pentobarbital, promethazine, thiethylperazine. Y-site: Nafcillin.**

- Store at 15°–30°C (59°–86°F), avoid freezing.

ADVERSE EFFECTS (≥1%) **CV:** Hypertension, hypotension, bradycardia, tachycardia, flushing. **GI:** Abdominal cramps, bitter taste, *nausea, vomiting,* dry mouth. **CNS:** *Sedation, dizziness,* nervousness, depression, restlessness, crying, euphoria, dysphoria, distortion of body image, unusual dreams, confusion, hallucinations; numbness and tingling sensations, headache, vertigo. **Respiratory:** Dyspnea, asthma, respiratory depression. **Skin:** Pruritus, urticaria, burning sensation, *sweaty, clammy skin*. **Special Senses:** Miosis, blurred vision, speech difficulty. **Urogenital:** Urinary urgency.

INTERACTIONS Drug: Alcohol and other CNS DEPRESSANTS add to CNS depression.

PHARMACOKINETICS Onset: 2–3 min IV; 15 min IM. **Peak:** 30 min IV. **Duration:** 3–6 h. **Distribution:** Crosses placenta. **Metabolism:** Metabolized in liver. **Elimination:** Eliminated in urine. **Half-Life:** 5 h.

NURSING IMPLICATIONS

Assessment & Drug Effects

- Assess respiratory rate before drug administration. Withhold drug and notify physician if respiratory rate falls below 12.
- Watch for allergic response in persons with sulfite sensitivity.
- Administer with caution to patients with hepatic or renal impairment.
- Monitor ambulatory patients; nalbuphine may produce drowsiness.
- Watch for respiratory depression of newborn if drug is used during labor and delivery.
- Avoid abrupt termination of nalbuphine following prolonged use, which may result in symptoms similar to narcotic withdrawal: nausea, vomiting, abdominal cramps, lacrimation, nasal congestion, piloerection, fever, restlessness, anxiety.

Patient & Family Education

- Do not drive or engage in potentially hazardous activities until response to drug is known.
- Avoid alcohol and other CNS depressants.
- Do not breast feed while taking this drug without consulting physician.

NALIDIXIC ACID

(nal-i-dix'ik)

NegGram

Classifications: URINARY TRACT ANTIINFECTIVE; ANTIBIOTIC; QUINOLONE

Prototype: Ciprofloxacin

Pregnancy Category: B (second and third trimester)

AVAILABILITY 250 mg, 500 mg, 1 g tablets; 250 mg/5 mL suspension

ACTIONS Synthetic quinolone. Intracellular action (by unknown mechanism) inhibits microbial DNA replication and RNA synthesis.

THERAPEUTIC EFFECTS Marked bactericidal activity against most gram-negative urinary tract pathogens with the exception of strains of *Pseudomonas*. Also effective against some strains of *Shigella* and *Salmonella*. Gram-positive bacteria are relatively resistant to drug action.

USES Urinary tract infections caused by susceptible gram-negative organisms including most *Proteus* strains, *Klebsiella, Enterobacter,* and *Escherichia coli*.

UNLABELED USES GI tract infections caused by susceptible strains of *Shigella sonnei;* prophylaxis of bacteriuria and in bladder irrigation for low-grade cystitis.

CONTRAINDICATIONS History of convulsive disorders; first trimester of pregnancy; infants <3 mo.

CAUTIOUS USE Prepubertal child; second and third trimesters of pregnancy (category B); kidney or liver disease; epilepsy; cerebral arteriosclerosis; respiratory insufficiency; patients and breast-feeding infants with G6PD deficiency.

ROUTE & DOSAGE

Urinary Tract Infections
Adult: **PO** Acute therapy: 1 g q.i.d. Chronic therapy: 500 mg q.i.d.
Child: **PO** *>3 mo,* Acute therapy: 55 mg/kg/d in 4 divided doses; Chronic therapy: 33 mg/kg/d in 4 divided doses

ADMINISTRATION

Oral

- Give with food or milk if drug causes GI distress. Otherwise, give on an empty stomach 1 h before or 2 h after meals.
- Store at 15°–30° C (59°–86° F) in tight container and avoid freezing.

ADVERSE EFFECTS (≥1%) **Body as a Whole:** Angioedema, fever, chills, arthralgia, hypersensitivity pneumonitis, anaphylaxis (rare). **CNS:** Drowsiness, headache, malaise, dizziness, vertigo, syncope, weakness, myalgia, peripheral neuritis, confusion, excitement, mental depression, seizures, insomnia. **GI:** Abdominal pain, *nausea, vomiting,* diarrhea, cholestasis, transient increase in AST. **Hematologic:** Eosinophilia, hemolytic anemia (especially in G6PD deficiency). **Skin:** Photosensitivity, pruritus, urticaria, rash.

DIAGNOSTIC TEST INTERFERENCE False-positive urine tests for ***glucose*** with ***cupric sulfate reagent*** (e.g., ***Benedict's*** or ***Clinitest***) but not with ***glucose oxidase methods*** (e.g., ***Clinistix, TesTape***). May cause elevation of ***urinary 17-ketosteroids (Zimmerman method)*** and ***urine vanillylmandelic acid (VMA).***

INTERACTIONS Drug: ANTACIDS, **sucralfate, calcium, magnesium, didanosine,** MULTIVITAMINS (containing **iron** or **zinc**) may decrease absorption of nalidixic acid; may increase hypoprothrombinemic effects of **warfarin.**

PHARMACOKINETICS Absorption: Readily absorbed from GI tract. **Peak:** Urine: 3–4 h. **Distribution:** Crosses placenta; distributed into breast milk. **Metabolism:** Partially metabolized in liver; some metabolism in kidneys. **Elimination:** Excreted in urine. **Half-Life:** 1.1–2.5 h.

NURSING IMPLICATIONS

Assessment & Drug Effects

- Lab tests: Perform C&S tests prior to initiation of treatment and periodically thereafter. Obtain blood counts and kidney or liver function tests if therapy is continued longer than 2 wk.
- Watch for CNS reactions, which tend to occur 30 min after initiation of treatment or after second or third dose. Infants, children, and older adults are especially susceptible. Report immediately the onset of marked irritability, vomiting, bulging of anterior fontanelle, headache, excitement or drowsiness, papilledema, vertigo.

Patient & Family Education

- Use drug exactly as prescribed and do not change dosage. Omitted doses, especially in early days of therapy, may promote development of bacterial resistance. Take full amount of medication.
- Contact physician immediately for unexplained behavior changes or severe headaches.
- Maintain adequate hydration (2000–3000 mL/d if tolerated) during treatment period. Consult physician if you notice a change in your urination pattern.

- Avoid exposure to direct sunlight or ultraviolet light while receiving drug. Contact physician if photosensitivity occurs. You may be photosensitive up to 3 mo after termination of drug.
- Contact your physician if you notice visual disturbances during first few days of therapy. Symptoms usually disappear promptly with reduction of dosage or discontinuation of therapy.
- Do not breast feed while taking this drug without consulting physician.

NALMEFENE HYDROCHLORIDE

(nal'me-feen)

Revex

Classifications: CENTRAL NERVOUS SYSTEM AGENT; NARCOTIC (OPIATE) ANTAGONIST

Prototype: Naloxone

Pregnancy Category: B

AVAILABILITY 100 mcg/mL, 1 mg/mL injection

ACTIONS Opiate antagonist that has no opioid agonist activity; also has no pharmacologic activity when given in the absence of an opioid agonist.

THERAPEUTIC EFFECTS Prevents or reverses the effects of opiates, including respiratory depression, sedation, and hypotension; these effects are dose related.

USES Complete or partial reversal of opioid drug effects, management of opioid overdose.

CONTRAINDICATIONS Hypersensitivity to nalmefene.

CAUTIOUS USE Patients at high cardiovascular risk or who have received potential cardiotoxic drugs; patients with known physical dependence on opioids; renal or hepatic impairment; pregnancy (category B), lactation. Safety and efficacy in children are not established.

ROUTE & DOSAGE

Reversal of Postoperative Opioid Depression

Adult: **IV/IM/SC** Use 100 mcg/mL concentration, 0.25 mcg/kg followed by 0.25 mcg/kg incremental doses q2–5min until desired degree of reversal or 1 mcg/kg cumulative dose is reached

Known/Suspected Opioid Overdose

Adult: **IV/IM/SC** Use 1 mg/mL concentration, then for nonopioid-dependent patients: 0.5 mg/70 kg, may repeat with 1 mg/70 kg 2–5 min later; for opioid-dependent patients: 0.1 mg/70 kg, if no evidence of withdrawal in 2 min, continue with 0.5 mg/70 kg, may repeat with 1 mg/70 kg 2–5 min later (doses >1.5 mg/70 kg not likely to be more effective)

ADMINISTRATION

Note: When using the 100 mcg/mL concentration, calculate the volume of a dose equal to 0.25 mcg/kg by multiplying the weight in kilograms by 0.0025. When using the 1 mg/mL concentration, calculate the volume of a dose equal to 0.1, 0.5, or 1 mg/70 kg by dividing the weight in kilograms by 70, then multiplying that result by the number of milligrams ordered per 70 kg.

Intramuscular/Subcutaneous

- Note: If IV access is lost, a single 1-mg dose may be given IM or SC. Allow 5–15 min for effect to occur.

Intravenous

PREPARE: **Direct:** Give undiluted.
ADMINISTER: **Direct:** Give over 15–30 sec. In patients with kidney failure give over 60 sec.

ADVERSE EFFECTS (≥1%) **Body as a Whole:** Fever, chills. **CV:** Tachycardia, hypotension, hypertension, pulmonary edema, ventricular arrhythmias (especially in patients with preexisting cardiovascular disease). **GI:** *Nausea, vomiting,* diarrhea, dry mouth, dyspepsia, elevation of liver function tests. **CNS:** Dizziness, headache, irritability, tremor, paresthesias, confusion, paranoia, drowsiness, fatigue, vertigo, agitation, nervousness. **Special Senses:** Blurred vision.

INTERACTIONS Drug: Potential risk of seizures when combined with **flumazenil.**

N

PHARMACOKINETICS Absorption: Well absorbed from IM and SC sites. **Onset:** 2–5 min IV; 15 min IM/SC. **Peak:** 5 min IV; 2 h IM/SC. **Duration:** 4–8 h. **Distribution:** Approximately 45% protein bound; blocks >80% of brain opioid receptors within 5 min; distributed into breast milk of rats. **Metabolism:** Metabolized in liver by glucuronidation. **Elimination:** Metabolites excreted primarily in urine, 17% excreted in feces. **Half-Life:** 8.5–10.8 h.

NURSING IMPLICATIONS

Assessment & Drug Effects

- Monitor carefully for reversal of opioid depression within 2–5 min of an IV dose or 5–15 min of an IM/SC dose.
- Note: If recurrent respiratory depression following the reversal, titrate the dose again to avoid over-reversal.
- Monitor cardiovascular status closely, assessing for changes in blood pressure and heart rate and development of arrhythmias.

Patient & Family Education

- Do not breast feed while taking this drug without consulting physician.

NALOXONE HYDROCHLORIDE Pr

(nal-ox'one)

Narcan

Classifications: CENTRAL NERVOUS SYSTEM AGENT; NARCOTIC (OPIATE) ANTAGONIST

Pregnancy Category: B

AVAILABILITY 0.02 mg/mL, 0.4 mg/mL, 1 mg/mL injection

ACTIONS Analog of oxymorphone. A "pure" narcotic antagonist, essentially free of agonistic (morphine-like) properties. Thus, it produces no significant analgesia, respiratory depression, psychotomimetic effects, or miosis when administered in the absence of narcotics and possesses more potent narcotic antagonist action.

THERAPEUTIC EFFECTS Reverses the effects of opiates, including respiratory depression, sedation, and hypotension.

USES Narcotic overdosage; complete or partial reversal of narcotic depression including respiratory depression induced by natural and synthetic narcotics and by pentazocine and propoxyphene. Drug of choice when nature of depressant drug is not known and for diagnosis of suspected acute opioid overdosage.

UNLABELED USES Shock and to reverse alcohol-induced or clonidine-induced coma or respiratory depression.

CONTRAINDICATIONS Respiratory depression due to nonopioid drugs. Safety during pregnancy (other than labor) (category B) or lactation is not established.

CAUTIOUS USE Neonates and children; known or suspected narcotic dependence; cardiac irritability.

ROUTE & DOSAGE

Opiate Overdose

Adult: **IV** 0.4–2 mg, may be repeated q2–3min up to 10 mg if necessary
Child: **IV** 0.01 mg/kg, may be repeated q2–3min up to 10 mg if necessary

Postoperative Opiate Depression

Adult: **IV** 0.1–0.2 mg, may be repeated q2–3min for up to 3 doses if necessary
Child: **IV** 0.005–0.01 mg/kg, may be repeated q2–3min up to 3 doses if necessary

Asphyxia Neonatorum

Child: **IV** 0.01 mg/kg into umbilical vein, may be repeated q2–3min up to 3 doses if necessary

ADMINISTRATION

Intravenous

PREPARE: **Direct:** May be given undiluted. **IV Infusion:** Dilute 2 mg in 500 mL of D5W or NS to yield 4 mcg/mL (0.004 mg/mL).

ADMINISTER: **Direct:** Give 0.4 mg or fraction thereof over 10–15 sec. **IV Infusion:** Adjust rate according to patient response.

INCOMPATIBILITIES **Y-site: Amphotericin B cholesteryl complex.**

- Use IV solutions within 24 h.
- Store at 15°–30° C (59°–86° F), protect from excessive light.

ADVERSE EFFECTS (≥1%) **Body as a Whole:** Reversal of analgesia, tremors, hyperventilation, slight drowsiness, sweating. **CV:** Increased BP, tachycardia. **GI:** Nausea, vomiting. **Hematologic:** Elevated partial thromboplastin time.

INTERACTIONS Drug: Reverses analgesic effects of NARCOTIC (OPIATE) AGONISTS and NARCOTIC (OPIATE) AGONIST-ANTAGONISTS.

PHARMACOKINETICS Onset: 2 min. **Duration:** 45 min. **Distribution:** Crosses placenta. **Metabolism:** Metabolized in liver. **Elimination:** Excreted in urine. **Half-Life:** 60–90 min.

NURSING IMPLICATIONS

Assessment & Drug Effects

- Observe patient closely; duration of action of some narcotics may exceed that of naloxone. Keep physician informed; repeat naloxone dose may be necessary.
- Note: Narcotic abstinence symptoms induced by naloxone generally start to diminish 20–40 min after administration and usually disappear within 90 min.
- Monitor respirations and other vital signs.
- Monitor surgical and obstetric patients closely for bleeding. Naloxone has been associated with abnormal coagulation test results. Also observe for reversal of analgesia, which may be manifested by nausea, vomiting, sweating, tachycardia.

Patient & Family Education

- Report postoperative pain that emerges after administration of this drug to physician.

NALTREXONE HYDROCHLORIDE

(nal-trex'one)

Trexan, ReVia, Depade

Classifications: CENTRAL NERVOUS SYSTEM AGENT; NARCOTIC (OPIATE) ANTAGONIST

Prototype: Naloxone HCl

Pregnancy Category: C

AVAILABILITY 50 mg tablets

ACTIONS Pure opioid antagonist with prolonged pharmacologic effect, structurally and pharmacologically similar to naloxone. Mechanism of action not clearly delineated, but it appears that its competitive binding at opioid receptor sites reduces euphoria and drug craving without supporting the addiction.

THERAPEUTIC EFFECTS Weakens or completely and reversibly blocks the subjective effects (the "high") of IV opioids and analgesics possessing both agonist and antagonist activity.

USES Adjunct to the maintenance of an opioid-free state in detoxified addicts who are and desire to remain narcotic free. Management of alcohol dependence as an adjunct to social and psychotherapeutic methods.

UNLABELED USES Obesity.

CONTRAINDICATIONS Patients receiving opioid analgesics or in acute opioid withdrawal; opioid-dependent patient; acute hepatitis, liver failure. Also contraindicated in any individual who (1) fails naloxone challenge, (2) has a positive urine screen for opioids, or (3) has a history of sensitivity to naltrexone. Safety during pregnancy (category C), lactation, or in children <18 y is not established.

ROUTE & DOSAGE

Treatment of Opiate Cessation

Adult: **PO** 25 mg followed by another 25 mg in 1 h if no withdrawal response; maintenance regimen is individualized (max: 800 mg/d)

Alcohol Dependence

Adult: **PO** 50 mg once/d

ADMINISTRATION

Challenge Test

Give the naloxone challenge test (administered IV of SC) before starting the abstinence program with naltrexone.

- SC dose: The SC dose is followed by an observation period of 45 min for symptoms of withdrawal (see below).
- IV dose: A portion of the IV dose is injected and, with the needle left in place, the patient is observed for 30 sec for withdrawal symptoms. If none are observed, remainder of dose is injected and patient is observed for the next 20 min.
- Withdrawal symptoms: Stuffiness or runny nose; tearing; yawning; sweating; tremors; vomiting; gooseflesh; feeling of temperature change; bone, joint, and muscle pains; abdominal cramps.
- Interpretation: Evidence of withdrawal symptoms indicates that the patient is a potential risk and should not enter a naltrexone program.
- Do not give naltrexone until patient is opiate free for at least 7–10 days.

Oral

- Give without regard to food.

ADVERSE EFFECTS (≥1%) **GI:** Dry mouth, anorexia, *nausea, vomiting,* constipation, *abdominal cramps/*

pain, hepatotoxicity. **Musculoskeletal:** *Muscle and joint pains.* **CNS:** *Difficulty sleeping, anxiety, headache, nervousness,* reduced or increased energy, irritability, dizziness, depression. **Skin:** Skin rash. **Body as a Whole:** Chills.

INTERACTIONS Drug: Increased somnolence and lethargy with PHENOTHIAZINES; reverses analgesic effects of NARCOTIC (OPIATE) AGONISTS and NARCOTIC (OPIATE) AGONIST-ANTAGONISTS.

PHARMACOKINETICS Absorption: Rapidly absorbed from GI tract; 20% reaches systemic circulation (first pass effect). **Onset:** 15–30 min. **Peak:** 1 h. **Duration:** 24–72 h. **Metabolism:** Metabolized in liver to active metabolite. **Elimination:** Excreted in urine. **Half-Life:** 10–13 h.

NURSING IMPLICATIONS

Assessment & Drug Effects

- Lab tests: Check liver function before the treatment is started, at monthly intervals for 6 mo, and then periodically as indicated.

Patient & Family Education

- Note: Naltrexone therapy may put you in danger of overdosing if you use opiates. Small doses even at frequent intervals will give no desired effects; however, a dose large enough to produce a high is dangerous and may be fatal.
- It may be possible to transfer from methadone to naltrexone. This can be done after gradual withdrawal and final discontinuation of methadone.
- Report promptly onset of signs of hepatic toxicity (see Appendix F) to physician. The drug will be discontinued.
- Do not self-dose with OTC drugs for treatment of cough, colds, diarrhea, or analgesia. Many available preparations contain small doses of an opioid. Consult physician for safe drugs if they are needed.
- Tell a doctor or dentist before treatment that you are using naltrexone.
- Wear identification jewelry indicating naltrexone use.
- Do not breast feed while taking this drug without consulting physician.

NANDROLONE DECANOATE

(nan′droe-lone)

Androlone-D, Deca-Durabolin, Hybolin Decaneate

NANDROLONE PHENPROPIONATE

Durabolin, Hybolin Improved, Nandrobolic

Classifications: HORMONE AND SYNTHETIC SUBSTITUTE; ANABOLIC/ANDROGEN STEROID
Prototype: Testosterone
Pregnancy Category: X
Controlled Substance: Schedule III

AVAILABILITY 100 mg/mL, 200 mg/mL injection

ACTIONS Synthetic steroid with high ratio of anabolic activity to androgenic activity. Both esters have same actions and uses but differ in duration of action. Decanoate actions last 3–4 wk; phenpropionate ester continues to exert anabolic effect for 1–3 wk.

THERAPEUTIC EFFECTS Increase hemoglobin and red cell mass and increase lean body mass in patients with cachexia (muscle wasting).

USES Control of metastatic breast cancer, management of anemia of renal insufficiency.

CONTRAINDICATIONS Males with prostate or breast cancer; liver dysfunction, nephrotic syndrome,

hypercalcemia; pregnancy (category X), lactation.
CAUTIOUS USE Benign prostatic hypertrophy, history of MI.

ROUTE & DOSAGE

Anemia (Decanoate)
Adult: **IM** 50–200 mg/wk
Child: **IM** *2–13 y,* 25–50 mg q3–4wk

Metastatic Breast Cancer (Phenpropionate)
Adult: **IM** 50–100 mg/wk

ADMINISTRATION

Intramuscular

- Inject drug deep IM, preferably into gluteal muscle in adult. Follow agency policy regarding IM site in small child.
- Intermittent therapy is usually recommended (4-mo course of treatment followed by 6–8-wk rest period).

ADVERSE EFFECTS (≥1%) **Body as a Whole:** Muscle cramps. **GI:** *Nausea, vomiting,* diarrhea, anorexia, abdominal fullness, cholestatic jaundice, <u>hepatic necrosis, hepatocellular neoplasms</u>. **Hematologic:** Leukopenia. **Metabolic:** Sodium, chloride, water, potassium, phosphate, and calcium retention, ankle edema, glucose intolerance, increased cholesterol. **CNS:** Excitation, insomnia, chills, toxic confusion. **Endocrine:** *Acne, virilization.*

INTERACTIONS Drug: May increase hypoprothrombinemic effects of **warfarin;** may decrease **insulin** and SULFONYLUREA requirements; CORTICOSTEROIDS may increase edema. **Herbal: Echinacea** may increase risk of hepatotoxicity.

PHARMACOKINETICS Absorption: Slowly absorbed from IM injection site over 4 days. **Peak:** 3–6 d. **Metabolism:** Metabolized in liver to active metabolite. **Half-Life:** 6–8 d.

NURSING IMPLICATIONS

Assessment & Drug Effects

- Lab tests: Obtain baseline and periodic liver function evaluations and electrolyte levels.
- Monitor for S&S of hepatic toxicity (see Appendix F) and electrolyte imbalance, especially hyperkalemia and hypercalcemia (see Appendix F).
- Monitor diabetics for loss of glycemic control.

Patient & Family Education

- Note: In women, the drug may cause virilization (e.g., increased facial and body hair, deepening of voice).
- Do not breast feed while taking this drug.

NAPHAZOLINE HYDROCHLORIDE (Pr)

(naf-az′oh-leen)

Ak-Con, Albalon, Allerest, Clear Eyes, Comfort, Degest-2, Muro's Opcon, Nafazair, Naphcon, Privine, VasoClear, Vasocon

Classifications: EYE, EAR, NOSE AND THROAT (EENT) PREPARATION; VASOCONSTRICTOR; DECONGESTANT; AUTONOMIC NERVOUS SYSTEM AGENT; ALPHA-ADRENERGIC AGONIST (SYMPATHOMIMETIC)

Pregnancy Category: C

AVAILABILITY 0.012%, 0.02%, 0.03%, 0.1% ophthalmic solution; 0.05% nasal solution

ACTIONS Direct-acting imidazoline derivative with marked alpha-adrenergic activity. Differs from other sympathomimetic amines in that systemic absorption may cause CNS depression rather than stimulation.

THERAPEUTIC EFFECTS Produces rapid and prolonged vasoconstriction of arterioles, thereby decreasing fluid exudation and mucosal engorgement.

USES Nasal decongestant and ocular vasoconstrictor.

CONTRAINDICATIONS Narrow-angle glaucoma; concomitant use with MAO inhibitors or tricyclic antidepressants. Safety during pregnancy (category C), lactation, or in infants is not established.

CAUTIOUS USE Hypertension, cardiac irregularities, advanced arteriosclerosis; diabetes; hyperthyroidism; older adult patients.

ROUTE & DOSAGE

Congestion

Adult: **Intranasal** 2 drops or sprays of 0.05% solution in each nostril q3–6h for no more than 3–5 d. **Ophthalmic** See Appendix A
Child: **Intranasal** 1–2 drops or sprays of 0.025% solution q3–6h for no more than 3–5 d

ADMINISTRATION

Instillation

- Instill nasal spray with patient in upright position. If administered in reclining position, a stream rather than a spray may be ejected, with possibility of systemic reaction.
- Minimize amount of drug swallowed by taking care not to direct the flow toward nasopharynx and by positioning patient properly with the head tilted slightly downward.
- Store at 15°–30° C (59°–86° F), protect from freezing.

ADVERSE EFFECTS (≥1%) **Body as a Whole:** Hypersensitivity reactions, headache, nausea, weakness, sweating, drowsiness, hypothermia, coma. **CV:** Hypertension, bradycardia, shock-like hypotension. **Special Senses:** Transient nasal stinging or burning, dryness of nasal mucosa, pupillary dilation, increased intraocular pressure, rebound redness of the eye.

INTERACTIONS Drug: TRICYCLIC ANTIDEPRESSANTS, **maprotiline** may potentiate pressor effects.

PHARMACOKINETICS Onset: Within 10 min. **Duration:** 2–6 h.

NURSING IMPLICATIONS

Assessment & Drug Effects

- Watch for rebound congestion and chemical rhinitis with frequent and continued use.
- Monitor BP periodically for development or worsening of hypertension, especially with ophthalmic route.
- Overdose: Bradycardia and hypotension can result. Report promptly.

Patient & Family Education

- Do not exceed prescribed regimen. Systemic effects can result from swallowing excessive medication.
- Discontinue medication and contact physician if nasal congestion is not relieved after 5 d.
- Prevent contamination of eye solution by taking care not to touch eyelid or surrounding area with dropper tip.
- Do not breast feed while taking this drug without consulting physician.

NAPROXEN

(na-prox'en)

Apo-Naproxen ♣, EC-Naprosyn, Naprelan, Naprosyn, Naxen ♣, Novonaprox ♣

NAPROXEN SODIUM

Aleve, Anaprox, Anaprox DS

Classifications: CENTRAL NERVOUS SYSTEM AGENT; ANALGESIC; NSAID; ANTIPYRETIC

Prototype: Ibuprofen

Pregnancy Category: B

AVAILABILITY 200 mg, 250 mg, 375 mg, 500 mg tablets; 375 mg, 500 mg sustained release tablets

ACTIONS Propionic acid derivative. NSAID with properties similar to those of other propionic acid derivatives, e.g., ibuprofen, fenoprofen, ketoprofen. Mechanism of action thought to be related to inhibition of prostaglandin synthesis.

THERAPEUTIC EFFECTS Analgesic, antiinflammatory and antipyretic effects; also inhibits platelet aggregation and prolongs bleeding time but does not alter whole blood clotting, prothrombin time or platelet count. Cross-sensitivity with other NSAIDs has been reported.

USES Antiinflammatory and analgesic effects in symptomatic treatment of acute and chronic rheumatoid arthritis, juvenile arthritis (naproxen only), and for treatment of primary dysmenorrhea. Also management of ankylosing spondylitis, osteoarthritis, and gout.

UNLABELED USES Paget's disease of bone, Bartter's syndrome.

CONTRAINDICATIONS Active peptic ulcer; patients in whom asthma, rhinitis, urticaria, bronchospasm, or shock is precipitated by aspirin or other NSAIDs. Safety during pregnancy (category B), lactation, or in children <2 y is not established.

CAUTIOUS USE History of upper GI tract disorders; impaired kidney, liver, or cardiac function; patients on sodium restriction (naproxen sodium); low pretreatment Hgb concentration; fluid retention, hypertension, heart failure; older adults.

ROUTE & DOSAGE

Note: 275 mg naproxen sodium = 250 mg naproxen

Inflammatory Disease

Adult: **PO** 250–500 mg b.i.d. (max: 1000 mg/d naproxen, 1100 mg/d naproxen sodium); Naprelan is dosed q.d.

Child: **PO** >2 *y,* 10–15 mg/kg/d in 2 divided doses (max: 1000 mg/d)

Mild to Moderate Pain, Dysmenorrhea

Adult: **PO** 500 mg followed by 200–250 mg q6–8h prn up to 1250 mg/d

Child: **PO** >2 *y,* 5–7 mg/kg q8–12h

ADMINISTRATION

Oral

- Ensure that extended release or enteric-coated form is not chewed or crushed. It must be swallowed whole.
- Give with food or an antacid (if prescribed) to reduce incidence of GI upset.
- Store at 15°–30° C (59°–86° F) in tightly closed container; protect from freezing.

ADVERSE EFFECTS (≥1%) **CNS:** *Headache, drowsiness, dizziness,* lightheadedness, depression. **CV:** Palpitation, dyspnea, peripheral edema, CHF, tachycardia. **Special Senses:** Blurred vision, tinnitus, hearing loss. **GI:** *Anorexia, heartburn,* indigestion, *nausea,* vomiting, thirst, GI bleeding, elevated serum ALT, AST. **Hematologic:** Thrombocytopenia, leukopenia, eosinophilia, inhibited platelet aggregation, agranulocytosis (rare). **Skin:** Pruritus, rash, ecchymosis. **Urogenital:** Nephrotoxicity. **Respiratory:** Pulmonary edema.

DIAGNOSTIC TEST INTERFERENCE Transient elevations in ***BUN*** and serum ***alkaline phosphatase*** may occur. Naproxen may interfere with some urinary assays of ***5-HIAA*** and may cause falsely high ***urinary 17-KGS*** levels (using ***m-dinitrobenzene reagent***). Naproxen should be withdrawn 72 h before adrenal function tests.

INTERACTIONS Drug: Bleeding time effects of ORAL ANTICOAGULANTS, **heparin** may be prolonged; may increase **lithium** toxicity. **Herbal: Feverfew, garlic, ginger, ginkgo** may increase bleeding potential.

PHARMACOKINETICS Absorption: Almost completely absorbed from GI tract when taken on empty stomach. **Peak:** 2 h naproxen; 1 h naproxen sodium. **Duration:** 7 h. **Metabolism:** Metabolized in liver. **Elimination:** Excreted primarily in urine; some biliary excretion (<1%). **Half-Life:** 12–15 h.

NURSING IMPLICATIONS

Assessment & Drug Effects

- Take detailed drug history prior to initiation of therapy. Observe for signs of allergic response in those with aspirin or other NSAID sensitivity.
- Lab tests: Obtain baseline and periodic evaluations of Hgb and kidney and liver function in patients receiving prolonged or high dose therapy.
- Schedule baseline and periodic auditory and ophthalmic examinations in patients receiving prolonged or high dose therapy.
- Monitor therapeutic effectiveness. Patients with arthritis may experience symptomatic relief (reduction in joint pain, swelling, stiffness) within 24–48 h with naproxen sodium therapy and in 2–4 wk with naproxen.

Patient & Family Education

- Be aware that the therapeutic effect of naproxen may not be experienced for 3–4 wk.
- Do not drive or engage in potentially hazardous activities until response to drug is known.
- Avoid alcohol and aspirin (as well as other NSAIDS) unless otherwise advised by a physician. Potential to increase risk of GI ulceration and bleeding.
- Tell your dentist or surgeon if you are taking naproxen before any treatment; it may prolong bleeding time.
- Do not breast feed while taking this drug without consulting physician.

NARATRIPTAN

(nar-a-trip'tan)

Amerge

Classifications: AUTONOMIC NERVOUS SYSTEM AGENT; ADRENERGIC ANTAGONIST (SYMPATHOLYTIC); 5-HT_1 SEROTONIN AGONIST

Prototype: Sumatriptan

Pregnancy Category: C

AVAILABILITY 1 mg, 2.5 mg tablets

ACTIONS Binds to the serotonin receptors ($5HT_{1D}$ and $5HT_{1B}$) on intracranial blood vessels, resulting in se-

N

lective vasoconstriction of dilated vessels in the carotid circulation.
THERAPEUTIC EFFECTS Inhibits vasoconstriction of dilated vessels selectively and also the release of proinflammatory neuropeptides. This results in the relief of acute migraine headache attacks.

USES Acute migraine headaches with or without aura.

CONTRAINDICATIONS Severe renal impairment (creatinine clearance <15 mL/min); severe hepatic impairment; history of ischemic heart disease (i.e., angina pectoris, MI); cerebrovascular syndromes (i.e., strokes or TIA); uncontrolled hypertension; patients with hemiplegic or basilar migraine; hypersensitivity to naratriptan; older adults.
CAUTIOUS USE Cardiovascular disease; renal or hepatic insufficiency; pregnancy (category C), lactation. Safety and efficacy in children <18 y are not established.

N

ROUTE & DOSAGE

Acute Migraine
Adult: **PO** 1–2.5 mg; may repeat in 4 h if necessary (max: 5 mg/24 h); patients with mild or moderate renal or hepatic impairment should not exceed 2.5 mg/24 h

ADMINISTRATION

Oral
- Give any time after symptoms of migraine appear. If the first tablet was effective but symptoms return, a second tablet may be given, but no sooner than 4 h after the first. Do not exceed 5 mg in 24 h.
- If there is no response to the first tablet, contact physician before administering a second tablet.
- Do not give within 24 h of an ergot-containing drug or other 5-HT_1 agonist.
- Store at 2°–25° C (36°–77° F); protect from light.

ADVERSE EFFECTS (≥1%) **Body as a Whole:** Asthenia, fatigue, malaise, pain, pressure sensation, paresthesias, throat pressure, warm/cold sensations, hot flushes. **CNS:** Somnolence, dizziness, drowsiness, headache, hypesthesia, decreased mental acuity, euphoria, tremor. **CV:** Coronary artery vasospasm, transient myocardial ischemia, MI, ventricular tachycardia, ventricular fibrillation, chest pain/tightness/heaviness, palpitations. **GI:** Dry mouth, nausea, vomiting, diarrhea. **Respiratory:** Dyspnea. **Skin:** Flushing.

INTERACTIONS Drug: Dihydroergotamine, methysergide, and other 5-HT_1 AGONISTS may cause prolonged vasospastic reactions; SSRIS have rarely caused weakness, hyperreflexia, and incoordination; MAOIS should not be used with 5-HT_1 agonists. **Herbal: Gingko, ginseng, echinacea, St. John's wort** may increase triptan toxicity.

PHARMACOKINETICS Absorption: Rapidly absorbed, 70% bioavailability. **Peak:** 2–4 h. **Distribution:** 28%–31% protein bound. **Metabolism:** Metabolized in liver. **Elimination:** Excreted primarily in urine. **Half-Life:** 6 h.

NURSING IMPLICATIONS

Assessment & Drug Effects
- Monitor carefully cardiovascular status following first dose in patients at risk for CAD (e.g., postmenopausal women, men over 40 y, persons with known CAD risk factors) or coronary artery vasospasms.

- Be aware that ECG is recommended following first administration of naratriptan to someone with known CAD risk factors and periodically with long-term use.
- Report immediately to the physician: chest pain, nausea, or tightness in chest or throat that is severe or does not quickly resolve.
- Obtain periodic cardiovascular evaluation with continued use.

Patient & Family Education

- Carefully review patient information leaflet and guidelines for administration.
- Contact physician immediately for any of the following: symptoms of angina (e.g., severe and/or persistent pain or tightness in chest or throat, severe nausea); hypersensitivity (e.g., wheezing, facial swelling, skin rash, or hives); or abdominal pain.
- Report any other adverse effects (e.g., tingling, flushing, dizziness) at next physician visit.
- Do not breast feed while taking this drug without consulting physician.

NATALIZUMAB

(na-tal′-i-zu-mab)

Tysabri

Classifications: BIOLOGIC RESPONSE MODIFIER; MONOCLONAL ANTIBODY

Prototype: Basiliximab

Pregnancy Category: C

AVAILABILITY 300 mg/15 mL injection

ACTIONS Natalizumab is a recombinant immunoglobulin-G4 (IgG4) monoclonal antibody thought to interfere with the migration of lymphocytes and monocytes into the CNS endothelium of patients with multiple sclerosis, thereby reducing inflammation and demyelination of CNS white matter.

THERAPEUTIC EFFECTS Inhibition of T-cell infiltration into the brain is thought to impede the demyelinating process of multiple sclerosis. Natalizumab is also thought to attenuate T-lymphocyte–mediated intestinal inflammation in Crohn's disease and possibly ulcerative colitis.

USES Treatment of relapsing forms of multiple sclerosis.

UNLABELED USES Treatment of Crohn's disease.

CONTRAINDICATIONS Safety and efficacy of the drug have not been established for chronic progressive multiple sclerosis. Prior hypersensitivity to natalizumab; murine protein hypersensitivity; active infection; lactation; females of childbearing age; pregnancy (category C); children <18 y.

CAUTIOUS USE Coadministration with other immunosuppressive medication; diabetes mellitus, immunocompromised patients; exposure to infection or tuberculosis.

ROUTE & DOSAGE

Multiple Sclerosis

Adult: **IV** 300 mg infused over 1 h every 4 wk

ADMINISTRATION

Intravenous

PREPARE: **IV Infusion:** Before and after dilution, solution should be colorless and clear to slightly opaque. Do not use if the solution has visible particles, flakes, color, or is cloudy. Withdraw 15 mL from the vial and add to an IV bag with 100 mL of NS. Do not use with any other diluent.

Gently invert the bag to mix; do not shake. The IV solution must be used within 8 h.
ADMINISTER: **IV Infusion:** Flush IV line before/after with NS. Infuse over 1 h. Do not give a bolus dose. Stop infusion immediately if S&S of hypersensitivity appear.
INCOMPATIBILITIES **Solution/additive/Y-site:** Do not mix or infuse with other drugs.

- Store IV solution for up to 8 h at 2°–8° C (36°–46° F). Allow solution to warm to room temperature before administration

ADVERSE EFFECTS (≥1%) **Body as a Whole:** Anaphylaxis (rare, usually within 2 h of infusion), infections, fatigue, rigors. **CNS:** Depression, headache, syncope, tremor. **CV:** Chest discomfort. **GI:** Abdominal discomfort, abnormal liver function tests. **Hematologic:** Local bleeding from infusion site. **Musculoskeletal:** Arthralgia. **Respiratory:** Pneumonia. **Skin:** Acute urticaria. **Urogenital:** Urinary frequency, irregular menstruation, amenorrhea, dysmenorrhea. **Other:** Infusion-related reactions (headache, dizziness, fatigue, hypersensitivity reactions, urticaria, pruritus, and rigors).

INTERACTIONS Drug: May reduce the effectiveness of VACCINES and TOXOIDS; may increase risk of infection with IMMUNOSUPPRESSANTS.

PHARMACOKINETICS Half-Life: 11 d.

NURSING IMPLICATIONS

Assessment & Drug Effects

- During IV infusion and for 1–2 h after, monitor closely for S&S of hypersensitivity (e.g., urticaria, dizziness, fever, rash, chills, pruritus, nausea, flushing, hypotension, dyspnea, and chest pain).

Patient & Family Education

- Report immediately any of the following during/after IV infusion: difficulty breathing, wheezing or shortness of breath, swelling or tightness about the neck and throat, chest pain, skin rash or hives.
- Report promptly S&S of infection (e.g., cough, fever, chills, or sore throat).
- Do not breast feed while taking this drug.

NATAMYCIN

(na-ta-mye′sin)
Natacyn
Classifications: ANTIINFECTIVE; ANTIFUNGAL AGENT
Prototype: Fluconazole
Pregnancy Category: C

AVAILABILITY 5% suspension

ACTIONS Derived from *Streptomyces natalensis.* Action mechanism simulates that of amphotericin B and nystatin by binding to sterols in the fungal cell membrane.
THERAPEUTIC EFFECTS Effective against many yeasts and filamentous fungi including *Candida, Aspergillus, Cephalosporium, Fusarium,* and *Penicillium.* Limited activity in vivo against *Trichomonas vaginalis;* not active against gram-positive or gram-negative bacteria or viruses.

USES Blepharitis, conjunctivitis, and keratitis caused by susceptible fungi. Drug of choice for *Fusarium solani* keratitis.
UNLABELED USES Oral, cutaneous, and vaginal candidiasis; intranasal treatment of pulmonary aspergillosis.

CONTRAINDICATIONS Concomitant administration of a corticosteroid.
CAUTIOUS USE Pregnancy (category C) or lactation. Safety and ef-

ficacy in children are not established.

ROUTE & DOSAGE

Fungal Keratitis
Adult: **Ophthalmic** 1 drop in conjunctival sac of infected eye q1–2h for 3–4 d, then decrease to 1 drop q6–8h, then gradually decrease to 1 drop q4–7d

ADMINISTRATION

Instillation
- Wash hands thoroughly before and after treatment. Infection is easily transferred from infected to noninfected eye and to other individuals.
- Shake well before using.
- Store at 2°–24° C (36°–75° F).

ADVERSE EFFECTS (≥1%) **Special Senses:** Blurred vision, photophobia, eye pain. Uneven adherence of suspension to epithelial ulcerations or in fornices.

INTERACTIONS Drug: No clinically significant interactions established.

PHARMACOKINETICS Absorption: Drug adheres to ulcerated surface of the cornea and is retained in conjunctival fornices. Does not appear to be systemically absorbed.

NURSING IMPLICATIONS

Assessment & Drug Effects
- Inspect eye for response and tolerance at least twice weekly.
- Note: Lack of improvement in keratitis within 7–10 d suggests that causative organisms may not be susceptible to natamycin. Reevaluation is indicated and possibly a change in therapy.

Patient & Family Education
- Learn appropriate technique for application of eye drops.
- Expect temporary light sensitivity. Be prepared to wear sunglasses outdoors after drug administration and perhaps for a few hours indoors.
- Return to ophthalmologist for reevaluation of eye problem if you experience symptoms of conjunctivitis: pain, discharge, itching, scratching "foreign body sensation," changes in vision.
- Do not share facecloths and hand towels; this will help prevent transmission of the fungal infection.
- Do not breast feed while taking this drug without consulting physician.

NATEGLINIDE

(nat-e′gli-nide)
Starlix
Classifications: HORMONE AND SYNTHETIC SUBSTITUTE; ANTIDIABETIC; MEGLITINIDE
Prototype: Repaglinide
Pregnancy Category: D

AVAILABILITY 60 mg, 120 mg tablets

ACTIONS Lowers blood glucose levels by stimulating the release of insulin from the pancreatic cells of a type 2 diabetic.
THERAPEUTIC EFFECTS Significantly reduces postprandial blood glucose in type 2 diabetics and improves glycemic control when given before meals. There is minimal risk of hypoglycemia. Indicated by preprandial blood glucose between 80–120 mg/dL and HbA_{1c} <7%.

USES Alone or in combination with metformin for the treatment of non-insulin dependent diabetes mellitus.

CONTRAINDICATIONS Prior hypersensitivity to nateglinide. Type 1 (insulin-dependent) diabetes mel-

N

litus, diabetic ketoacidosis; pregnancy (category B), lactation.

CAUTIOUS USE Renal impairment; liver dysfunction; adrenal or pituitary insufficiency; malnutrition; infection, trauma, surgery or unusual stress; concurrent therapy of drugs which inhibit cytochrome P450-3A4 (e.g. erythromycin, ketoconazole); concurrent therapy with drugs which are inducers of cytochrome P450-3A4 (e.g. rifampin); other medications, especially beta-adrenergic blocking agents.

ROUTE & DOSAGE

Diabetes Mellitus
Adult: **PO** 60–120 mg t.i.d. 1–30 min prior to meals

ADMINISTRATION

Oral

- Give, preferably, 10 min before meals. Omit the dose if the meal is skipped. Add a dose if an extra meal is eaten. Never double the dose.
- Store at 15°–30° C (59°–86° F).

N

ADVERSE EFFECTS (≥1%) **Body as a Whole:** Back pain, flu-like symptoms. **CV:** Dizziness. **GI:** Diarrhea. **Metabolic:** Hypoglycemia. **Musculoskeletal:** Arthropathy. **Respiratory:** Upper respiratory infection, bronchitis, cough.

INTERACTIONS Drug: NSAIDS, SALICYLATES, MAO INHIBITORS, BETA-ADRENERGIC BLOCKERS, may potentiate hypoglycemic effects; THIAZIDE DIURETICS, CORTICOSTEROIDS, THYROID PREPARATIONS, SYMPATHOMIMETIC AGENTS may attenuate hypoglycemic effects. **Herbal: Garlic, ginseng** may potentiate hypoglycemic effects.

PHARMACOKINETICS Absorption: Rapidly absorbed, 73% bioavailability. **Peak:** 1 h. **Distribution:** 98% protein bound. **Metabolism:** Metabolized in liver by CYP2C9 (70%) and CYP3A4 (30%). **Elimination:** Primarily excreted in urine. **Half-Life:** 1.5 h.

NURSING IMPLICATIONS

Assessment & Drug Effects

- Lab tests: Frequent FBS monitoring and HbA_{1C} q3mo to determine effective dose.
- Monitor carefully for S&S of hypoglycemia especially during the one-week period following transfer from a longer acting sulfonylurea such as chlorpropamide.

Patient & Family Education

- Take only before a meal to lessen the chance of hypoglycemia.
- When transferred to nateglinide from another oral hypoglycemia drug, start nateglinide the morning after the other agent is stopped, unless directed otherwise by physician.
- Watch for S&S of hyperglycemia or hypoglycemia (see Appendix F); report poor blood glucose control to physician.
- Report gastric upset or other bothersome GI symptoms to physician.
- Do not breast feed while taking this drug.

NEDOCROMIL SODIUM

(ned′o-cro-mil)

Tilade, Alocril

Classifications: ANTIINFLAMMATORY; MAST CELL STABILIZER; ANTIASTHMATIC

Prototype: Cromolyn sodium

Pregnancy Category: B

AVAILABILITY 1.75 mg aerosol; 2% ophthalmic solution

ACTIONS Inhibits activation of and mediators released from inflammatory cell types associated with asthma (e.g., neutrophils, mast cells, monocytes).

THERAPEUTIC EFFECTS Inhibits release of inflammatory mediators including histamine and prostaglandin D_2. Has no intrinsic bronchodilator, antihistamine, or glucocorticoid effects.

USES Maintenance therapy for patients with mild to moderate asthma. Ocular use for allergic conjunctivitis (see Appendix A-1).

CONTRAINDICATIONS Hypersensitivity to nedocromil; acute bronchospasm, particularly status asthmaticus.

CAUTIOUS USE Pregnancy (category B), lactation. Safety and effectiveness in children <6 y are not established.

ROUTE & DOSAGE

Asthma

Adult: **Inhalation** 2 inhalations q.i.d. at regular intervals, **NOT** for acute asthma attacks
Child: **Inhalation** ≤6 y, 2 inhalations q.i.d.

ADMINISTRATION

Inhalation

- Use correct administration technique to ensure maximum drug efficacy. Review instruction leaflet supplied by manufacturer.
- Reduce dosage in stages, with each lower dose maintained for several weeks of good control prior to further decreasing dose.

ADVERSE EFFECTS (≥1%) **GI:** *Abnormal bitter taste,* nausea, vomiting. **CNS:** Headache, dizziness. **Respiratory:** Sore throat irritation, cough.

INTERACTIONS Drug: No clinically significant interactions established.

PHARMACOKINETICS Absorption: 90% of dose is deposited in throat and swallowed. Less than 7% is absorbed systemically in patients with asthma. **Onset:** 1 wk for therapeutic effect. **Peak:** 10–20 min. **Metabolism:** Does not appear to be metabolized. **Elimination:** 6% excreted in urine in 72 h. **Half-Life:** 2.3 h.

NURSING IMPLICATIONS

Assessment & Drug Effects

- Assess for coughing and bronchospasms induced by nedocromil. These are indications for discontinuation of drug and should be promptly reported.
- Monitor patients for whom systemic or inhaled steroid therapy has been reduced, as nedocromil may not fully substitute for the decrease in dose of steroid.

Patient & Family Education

- Learn to administer the drug properly. Review patient instruction leaflet.
- Do not use it to treat acute bronchospasms because nedocromil is not a bronchodilator.
- Continue regular nedocromil therapy even during symptom-free periods.
- Do not breast feed while taking this drug without consulting physician.

NEFAZODONE

(nef-a-zo′done)
Serzone

Classifications: CENTRAL NERVOUS SYSTEM (CNS) AGENT; PSYCHOTHERAPEUTIC AGENT; ANTIDEPRESSANT; SELECTIVE SEROTONIN REUPTAKE INHIBITOR (SSRI)
Prototype: Fluoxetine HCl
Pregnancy Category: C

AVAILABILITY 50 mg, 100 mg, 150 mg, 200 mg, 250 mg tablets

ACTIONS Antidepressant with a dual mechanism of action. Inhibits neuronal serotonin (5-HT_1) reuptake and also possesses 5-HT_2 antagonist properties. It is unrelated to tricyclic, MAOI, or other antidepressants.

THERAPEUTIC EFFECTS Antidepressant effects with minimal cardiovascular effects, fewer anticholinergic effects, less sedation, and less sexual dysfunction than other antidepressants.

USES Treatment of depression.

CONTRAINDICATIONS Hypersensitivity to nefazodone or alcohol; hepatic disease, hepatitis, jaundice; pregnancy (category C), lactation; mania; severe restlessness, suicidal ideation; surgery, neonates.

CAUTIOUS USE Older adults, women of childbearing age; history of seizure disorders, seizures; renal or hepatic impairment; recent MI, unstable cardiac disease; hypotension; angina, stroke, hypovolemia, dehydration, ECT therapy. Safety and efficacy in children <18 y are not established.

N

ROUTE & DOSAGE

Depression
Adult: **PO** 50–100 mg b.i.d., may need to increase up to 300–600 mg/d in 2–3 divided doses
Geriatric: **PO** Start with 50 mg b.i.d.

ADMINISTRATION

Oral

- Do not give within 14 d of discontinuation of an MAO INHIBITOR.
- Store at 15°–30° C (59°–86° F).

ADVERSE EFFECTS (≥1%) **Body as a Whole:** Anaphylactic reactions, angioedema. **CNS:** *Headache, dizziness, drowsiness,* asthenia, tremor, insomnia, agitation, anxiety. **GI:** Dry mouth, constipation, nausea, liver toxicity. **Special Senses:** Visual disturbances, blurred vision, scotomata. **Endocrine:** Galactorrheas, gynecomastia, serotonin syndrome. **Skin:** Stevens-Johnson syndrome.

INTERACTIONS Drug: May cause confusion, delirium, coma, seizures, or hyperthermia with MAOIS; may increase plasma levels of some BENZODIAZEPINES, including **alprazolam** and **triazolam.** May decrease plasma levels and effects of **propranolol.** May increase levels and toxicity of **buspirone, carbamazepine, cilostazol, digoxin;** reports of QTc prolongation and ventricular arrhythmias with **cisapride, pimozide;** increased risk of rhabdomyolysis with **lovastatin, simvastatin;** may cause **serotonin** syndrome with other SSRIS; increase risk of **ergotamine** toxicity with **dihydroergotamine, ergotamine. Herbal: St. John's wort** may cause **serotonin** syndrome (headache, dizziness, sweating, agitation).

PHARMACOKINETICS Onset: 1 wk. **Peak:** 3–5 wk. **Metabolism:** Metabolized in liver to at least two active metabolites. **Half-Life:** Nefazodone 3.5 h, metabolites 2–33 h.

NURSING IMPLICATIONS

Assessment & Drug Effects

- Monitor for worsening of depression or emergence of suicidal ideation.
- Evaluate concurrent drugs for possible interactions.
- Monitor patients with a history of seizures for increased activity.
- Assess safety, as dizziness and drowsiness are common adverse effects.
- Lab tests: Monitor periodically liver function and CBC during long-term therapy.

Patient & Family Education

- Be aware that significant improvement in mood may not occur for several weeks following initiation of therapy.
- Do not drive or engage in potentially hazardous activities until response to the drug is known.
- Report changes in visual acuity.
- Do not breast feed while taking this drug without consulting physician.

NELFINAVIR MESYLATE

(nel-fin'a-vir)

Viracept

Classifications: ANTIINFECTIVE AGENT; ANTIRETROVIRAL AGENT; PROTEASE INHIBITOR

Prototype: Saquinavir

Pregnancy Category: C

AVAILABILITY 250 mg, 625 mg tablets; 50 mg/g powder

ACTIONS Inhibits HIV-1 protease, which is responsible for the production of HIV-1 viral particles in an infected individual.

THERAPEUTIC EFFECTS Inhibition of the viral protease prevents the cleavage of the viral polypeptide, resulting in the production of an immature, noninfectious virus. Indicated by decreased viral load.

USES Treatment of HIV infection in combination with a nucleoside analog.

CONTRAINDICATIONS Hypersensitivity to nelfinavir; concurrent administration with terfenadine, astemizole, cisapride, amiodarone, quinidine, rifampin, triazolam, or midazolam; lactation.

CAUTIOUS USE Liver function impairment, hemophilia; pregnancy (category C). Safety and effectiveness in children <2 y are not established.

ROUTE & DOSAGE

HIV Infection

Adult: **PO** 750 mg t.i.d. or 1250 mg (2 × 625 mg) b.i.d. with food
Child: **PO** *2–13 y,* 20–30 mg/kg t.i.d. with food (max: 750 mg/dose)

ADMINISTRATION

Oral

- Give with a meal or light snack.
- Oral powder may be mixed with a small amount of water, milk, soy milk, or dietary supplements; liquid should be consumed immediately. Do not mix oral powder in original container nor with acid food or juice (e.g., orange or apple juice, or applesauce).
- Store at 15°–30° C (59°–86° F).

ADVERSE EFFECTS (≥1%) **Body as a Whole:** Allergic reactions, back pain, fever, malaise, pain, asthenia, myalgia, arthralgia. **CNS:** Headache, anxiety, depression, dizziness, insomnia, seizures. **GI:** Abdominal pain, *diarrhea,* nausea, flatulence, anorexia, dyspepsia, <u>GI bleeding</u>, hepatitis, vomiting, pancreatitis, increased liver function tests. **Hematologic:** Anemia, leukopenia, thrombocytopenia. **Respiratory:** Dyspnea, pharyngitis, rhinitis. **Skin:** Rash, pruritus, sweating, urticaria.

INTERACTIONS Drug: Other PROTEASE INHIBITORS, **ketoconazole** may increase nelfinavir levels; **rifabutin, rifampin** may decrease nelfinavir levels; nelfinavir will decrease ORAL CONTRACEPTIVE levels; may increase levels of **atorvastatin, simvastatin;** increase risk of **ergotamine** toxicity with **dihydroergotamine, ergotamine. Herbal: St. John's wort** may decrease antiretroviral activity.

PHARMACOKINETICS Absorption: Food increases the amount of drug absorbed. **Distribution:** >98% protein bound. **Metabolism:** Metabolized in the liver by CYP3A. **Elimination:** Primarily excreted in feces. **Half-Life:** 3.5–5 h.

NURSING IMPLICATIONS

Assessment & Drug Effects

- Monitor hemophiliacs (type A or B) closely for spontaneous bleeding.
- Monitor carefully patients with hepatic impairment for toxic drug effects.

Patient & Family Education

- Drug must be taken exactly as prescribed. Do not alter dose or discontinue drug without consulting physician.
- Use a barrier contraceptive even if using hormonal contraceptives.
- Be aware that diarrhea is a common adverse effect that can usually be controlled by OTC medications.
- Do not breast feed while taking this drug.

NEOMYCIN SULFATE

(nee-oh-mye′sin)

Mycifradin, Myciguent, Neo-Tabs, Neo-fradin

Classifications: ANTIINFECTIVE; AMINOGLYCOSIDE ANTIBIOTIC

Prototype: Gentamicin

Pregnancy Category: D

AVAILABILITY 500 mg tablet; 125 mg/5 mL oral solution; 3.5 mg/g ointment, cream

ACTIONS Aminoglycoside antibiotic obtained from *Streptomyces fradiae;* reported to be the most potent in neuromuscular blocking action and the most toxic of this group.

THERAPEUTIC EFFECTS Active against a wide variety of gram-negative bacteria, including *Citrobacter, Escherichia coli, Enterobacter, Klebsiella, Proteus* (including indole-positive and indole-negative strains), *Pseudomonas aeruginosa,* and *Serratia sp.* Also effective against certain gram-positive organisms, particularly, penicillin-sensitive and some methicillin-resistant strains of *Staphylococcus aureus* (MRSA).

USES Severe diarrhea caused by enteropathogenic *Escherichia coli;* preoperative intestinal antisepsis; to inhibit nitrogen-forming bacteria of GI tract in patients with cirrhosis or hepatic coma and for urinary tract infections caused by susceptible organisms. Also topically for short-term treatment of eye, ear, and skin infections. Available in a variety of creams, ointments, and sprays in combination with other antibiotics and corticosteroids.

CONTRAINDICATIONS Use of oral drug in patients with intestinal obstruction; ulcerative bowel lesions; topical applications over large skin areas; parenteral use in patients with kidney disease or impaired hearing; parkinsonism; myasthenia gravis; pregnancy (category D), lactation.

CAUTIOUS USE Topical otic applications in patients with perforated eardrum, children.

ROUTE & DOSAGE

Intestinal Antisepsis

Adult: **PO** 1 g q1h times 4 doses, then 1 g q4h times 5 doses
Child: **PO** 10.3 mg/kg q4–6h for 3 d

Hepatic Coma

Adult: **PO** 4–12 g/d in 4 divided doses for 5–6 d
Child: **PO** 437.5–1225 mg/m^2 q6h for 5–6 d

Diarrhea
Adult: **PO** 50 mg/kg in 4 divided doses for 2–3 d **IM** 1.3–2.6 mg/kg q6h
Child: **PO** 8.75 mg/kg q6h for 2–3 d

Cutaneous Infections
Adult: **Topical** Apply 1–3 times/d

ADMINISTRATION

Oral

- Preoperative bowel preparation: Saline laxative is generally given immediately before neomycin therapy is initiated.

Topical

- Consult physician about what to use for cleansing skin before each application.
- Make sure ear canal is clean and dry prior to instillation for topical therapy of external ear.

ADVERSE EFFECTS (≥1%) **Body as a Whole:** Neuromuscular blockade with muscular and respiratory paralysis; hypersensitivity reactions. **GI:** Mild laxative effect, diarrhea, nausea, vomiting; prolonged therapy: malabsorption-like syndrome including cyanocobalamin (vitamin B_{12}) deficiency, low serum cholesterol. **Urogenital:** Nephrotoxicity. **Special Senses:** Ototoxicity. **Skin:** *Redness,* scaling, pruritus, dermatitis.

INTERACTIONS Drug: May decrease absorption of **cyanocobalamin.**

PHARMACOKINETICS Absorption: 3% absorbed from GI tract in adults; up to 10% absorbed in neonates. **Peak:** 1–4 h. **Elimination:** 97% excreted unchanged in feces. **Half-Life:** 3 h.

NURSING IMPLICATIONS

Assessment & Drug Effects

- Perform audiometric studies twice weekly in patients with kidney or liver dysfunction receiving extended oral therapy.
- Lab tests: Obtain baseline and daily urinalysis for albumin, casts, and cells; and BUN every other day. Also, serum drug levels (toxic levels reportedly range from 8 to 30 mcg/mL, although individual variations exist).
- Monitor I&O in patients receiving oral or parenteral therapy. Report oliguria or changes in I&O ratio. Inadequate neomycin excretion results in high serum drug levels and risk of nephrotoxicity and ototoxicity.

Patient & Family Education

- Stop treatment and consult your physician if irritation occurs when you are using topical neomycin. Allergic dermatitis is common.
- Report any unusual symptom related to ears or hearing (e.g., tinnitus, roaring sounds, loss of hearing acuity, dizziness).
- Do not exceed prescribed dosage or duration of therapy.
- Do not breast feed while taking this drug.

NEOSTIGMINE BROMIDE (Pr)

(nee-oh-stig'meen)
Prostigmin

NEOSTIGMINE METHYLSULFATE

Prostigmin

Classifications: AUTONOMIC NERVOUS SYSTEM AGENT; CHOLINERGIC (PARASYMPATHOMIMETIC) AGENT; CHOLINESTERASE INHIBITOR
Pregnancy Category: C

AVAILABILITY 15 mg tablets; 1:1000, 1:2000, 1:4000 injection

ACTIONS Produces reversible cholinesterase inhibition or inactivation. Has direct stimulant action on voluntary muscle fibers and possibly on autonomic ganglia and CNS neurons.

THERAPEUTIC EFFECTS Allows intensified and prolonged effect of acetylcholine at cholinergic synapses (basis for use in myasthenia gravis). Also produces generalized cholinergic response including miosis, increased tonus of intestinal and skeletal muscles, constriction of bronchi and ureters, slower pulse rate, and stimulation of salivary and sweat glands.

USES To prevent and treat postoperative abdominal distension and urinary retention; for symptomatic control of and sometimes for differential diagnosis of myasthenia gravis; and to reverse the effects of nondepolarizing muscle relaxants (e.g., tubocurarine).

CONTRAINDICATIONS Hypersensitivity to neostigmine, cholinergics, or bromides; bradycardia, hypotension; mechanical obstruction of intestinal or urinary tract; peritonitis; administration with other cholinergic drugs; pregnancy (category C), lactation.

CAUTIOUS USE Recent ileorectal anastomoses; epilepsy; bronchial asthma; bradycardia, recent coronary occlusion; vagotonia; hyperthyroidism; cardiac arrhythmias; peptic ulcer.

ROUTE & DOSAGE

Diagnosis of Myasthenia Gravis

Adult: **IM** 0.022 mg/kg, may increase to 0.031 mg/kg if first test is inconclusive
Child: **IM** 0.025–0.04 mg/kg

Treatment of Myasthenia Gravis

Adult: **PO** 15–375 mg/d in 3–6 divided doses **IM/IV/SC** 0.5–2.5 mg q1–3h
Child: **PO** 7.5–15 mg t.i.d. or q.i.d. or 0.333 mg/kg or 10 mg/m^2 6 times/d **IM/IV/SC** 0.01–0.04 mg/kg q2–4h
Neonate: **PO** 1–4 mg q2–3h **IM** 0.03 mg/kg q2–4h

Reversal of Nondepolarizing Neuromuscular Blockade

Adult: **IV** 0.5–2.5 mg slowly
Child: **IV** 0.025–0.08 mg/kg
Infant: **IV** 0.025–0.1 mg/kg

Postoperative Distention and Urinary Retention

Adult: **IM/SC** 0.25 mg q4–6h for 2–3 d

ADMINISTRATION

Note: Size of oral dose is considerably larger than that of parenteral dose because drug is poorly absorbed when taken orally (15 mg of oral drug is approximately equivalent to 0.5 mg of parenteral form).

Oral

- Give with food or milk to reduce GI distress.

Intramuscular/Subcutaneous

- Note: 1 mg = 1 mL of the 1:1000 solution; 0.5 mg = 1 mL of the 1:2000 solution; 0.25 mg = 1 mL of the 1:4000 solution.
- Give undiluted.

Intravenous

PREPARE: **Direct:** Give undiluted.
ADMINISTER: **Direct:** Give at a rate of 0.5 mg or a fraction thereof over 1 min.

ADVERSE EFFECTS (≥1%) **Body as a Whole:** Muscle cramps, *fasciculations,* twitching, pallor, fatigability, generalized weakness, paralysis, agitation, fear, death. **CV:** Tightness in chest, bradycardia, hypotension, elevated BP. **GI:** *Nausea,* vomiting, eructation, epigastric discomfort, abdominal cramps, diarrhea, involuntary or difficult defecation. **CNS:** CNS stimulation. **Respiratory:** *Increased salivation* and bronchial secretions, sneezing, cough, dyspnea, diaphoresis, respiratory depression. **Special Senses:** Lacrimation, miosis, blurred vision. **Urogenital:** Difficult micturition.

INTERACTIONS Drug: Succinylcholine decamethonium may prolong phase I block or reverse phase II block; neostigmine antagonizes effects of **tubocurarine; atracurium, vecuronium, pancuronium; procainamide, quinidine, atropine** antagonize effects of neostigmine.

PHARMACOKINETICS Absorption: Poorly absorbed from GI tract (1%–2%). **Onset:** 10–30 min IM or IV; 2–4 h PO. **Peak:** 20–30 min IM or IV; 1–2 h PO. **Distribution:** Not reported to cross placenta or appear in breast milk. **Metabolism:** Hydrolyzed by cholinesterases; also metabolized in liver. **Elimination:** 80% of drug and metabolites excreted in urine within 24 h. **Half-Life:** 50–90 min.

NURSING IMPLICATIONS

Assessment & Drug Effects

- Check pulse before giving drug to bradycardic patients. If below 60/min or other established parameter, consult physician. Atropine will be ordered to restore heart rate.
- Monitor pulse, respiration, and BP during period of dosage adjustment in treatment of myasthenia gravis.
- Report promptly and record accurately the onset of myasthenic symptoms and drug adverse effects in relation to last dose in order to assist physician in determining lowest effective dosage schedule.
- Reduce possible GI (muscarinic) side effects, which occur especially during early therapy, by giving drug with milk or food. Physician may prescribe atropine or other anticholinergic agent to suppress side effects (*note:* these drugs may mask toxic symptoms of neostigmine).
- Note time of muscular weakness onset carefully in myasthenic patients. It may indicate whether patient is in cholinergic or myasthenic crisis: Weakness that appears approximately 1 h after drug administration suggests cholinergic crisis (overdose) and is treated by prompt withdrawal of neostigmine and immediate administration of atropine. Weakness that occurs 3 h or more after drug administration is more likely due to myasthenic crisis (underdose or drug resistance) and is treated by more intensive anticholinesterase therapy.
- Record drug effect and duration of action. S&S of myasthenia gravis relieved by neostigmine include lid ptosis; diplopia; drooping facies; difficulty in chewing, swallowing, breathing, or coughing; and weakness of neck, limbs, and trunk muscles.
- Manifestations of neostigmine overdosage often appear first in muscles of neck and those involved in chewing and swallowing, with muscles of shoulder girdle and upper extremities affected next.
- Monitor respiration, maintain airway or assisted ventilation, and give oxygen as indicated, when used as antidote for tubocurarine or other nondepolarizing neuromuscular blocking agents (usually preceded by atropine). Respiratory assistance is continued until recovery of respiration and neuromuscular transmission is assured.

- Report to physician if patient does not urinate within 1 h after first dose when used to relieve urinary retention.

Patient & Family Education

- Be aware that regulation of dosage interval is extremely difficult; dosage must be adjusted for each patient to deal with unpredictable exacerbations and remissions.
- Be aware that drug therapy is often required both day and night. Larger portions of total dose are given at times of greater fatigue; late afternoon and at mealtimes.
- Keep a diary of "peaks and valleys" of muscle strength.
- Keep an accurate record for physician of your response to drug. Learn how to recognize adverse effects, how to modify dosage regimen according to your changing needs, or how to administer atropine if necessary.
- Be aware that certain factors may require an increase in size or frequency of dose (e.g., physical or emotional stress, infection, menstruation, surgery), whereas remission requires a decrease in dosage.
- Some patients become refractory to neostigmine after prolonged use and require change in dosage or medication.
- Do not breast feed while taking this drug.

NESIRITIDE

(nes-ir′i-tide)

Natrecor

Classifications: CARDIOVASCULAR AGENT; ATRIAL NATRIURETIC PEPTIDE HORMONE

Pregnancy Category: C

AVAILABILITY 1.5 mg vial

ACTIONS Nesiritide is a human B-type natriuretic peptide (hBNP), produced by recombinant DNA, which mimics the actions of human atrial natriuretic hormone (ANH). ANH is secreted by the right atrium when atrial blood pressure increases. Nesiritide, like ANH, inhibits antidiuretic hormone (ADH) by increasing urine sodium loss by the kidney and triggering the formation of a large volume of dilute urine.

THERAPEUTIC EFFECTS Nesiritide binds to a cyclic nucleic acid, which results in smooth muscle cell relaxation. The drug also causes dilation of veins and arteries. It is effective in managing dyspnea at rest in patients with acute congestive heart failure (CHF).

USES Acute treatment of decompensated CHF in patients who have dyspnea at rest or with minimal activity.

CONTRAINDICATIONS Hypersensitivity to nesiritide, patients with a systolic blood pressure <90 mm Hg, cardiogenic shock, patients with low cardiac filling pressures, patients who should not receive vasodilators, such as those with significant valvular stenosis, restrictive or obstructive cardiomyopathy, constrictive pericarditis, pericardial tamponade; pregnancy (category C).

CAUTIOUS USE Lactation, concurrent administration of ACE inhibitors or vasodilators. Safety and efficacy in pediatric patients have not been established.

ROUTE & DOSAGE

Acute Decompensated CHF

Adult: **IV** 2 mcg/kg bolus administered over 60 s, followed by a continuous infusion of 0.01 mcg/kg/min (0.1 mL/kg/hr) (max: 0.03 mcg/kg/min). Monitor blood pressure closely. If hypotension occurs, the dose should be reduced or discontinued. The infusion can subsequently be restarted at a dose that is reduced by 30% (with no bolus administration) after stabilization of hemodynamics.

ADMINISTRATION

Intravenous

PREPARE: **Direct and IV Infusion:** Reconstitute one 1.5 mg vial by adding 5 mL of IV solution removed from a 250 mL bag of selected diluent (i.e., D5W, NS, D5/0.45% NaCl, D5/0.2% NaCl). Rock the vial gently so that all surfaces, including the stopper, contact the diluent ensuring complete reconstitution. Do not shake the vial. Add the entire contents of the vial to the 250 mL IV bag to yield approximately 6 µg/mL. Invert the bag several times to mix completely. Use within 24 h. Prime the IV tubing with 25 mL prior to connecting to the vascular access port.

ADMINISTER: **Direct:** Withdraw the bolus dose from the prepared infusion bag. Determine dose as follows: bolus volume (mL) = (0.33) × (patient weight in kg). Give the bolus dose over 60 sec through an IV port in the tubing. **IV Infusion:** Infuse remainder of IV infusion immediately following the bolus dose. Determine the infusion rate as follows: flow rate (mL/hr) = (0.1) × (patient weight in kg).

INCOMPATIBILITIES **Solution/additive and Y-site: Bumetanide, enalaprilate, ethacrynic acid, furosemide, heparin, hydralazine, insulin.**

- Store at controlled room temperature at 20°–25° C (68°–77° F) or refrigerated.

ADVERSE EFFECTS (≥1%) **Body as a Whole:** Headache, back pain, catheter pain, fever, injection site pain, leg cramps. **CNS:** Insomnia, dizziness, anxiety, confusion, paresthesia, somnolence, tremor. **CV:** *Hypotension,* ventricular tachycardia, ventricular extrasystoles, angina, bradycardia, tachycardia, atrial fibrillation, AV node conduction abnormalities. **GI:** Abdominal pain, nausea, vomiting. **Respiratory:** Cough, hemoptysis, apnea. **Skin:** Sweating, pruritus, rash. **Special Senses:** Amblyopia.

INTERACTIONS Drug: No interaction trials conducted. No clinically significant interactions reported.

PHARMACOKINETICS Onset: 15 min. **Duration:** >60 h depending on dose. **Metabolism/Elimination:** Cleared from the circulation via the following three independent mechanisms, in order of decreasing importance: 1) binding to cell surface clearance receptors with subsequent cellular internalization and lysosomal proteolysis; 2) proteolytic cleavage of the peptide by endopeptidases, such as neutral endopeptidase, which are present on the vascular luminal surface; and 3) renal filtration. **Half-Life:** 18 min.

NURSING IMPLICATIONS

Assessment & Drug Effects

- Monitor hemodynamic parameters (e.g., BP, PCWP, HR, ECG) throughout therapy. Notify physician immediately if systolic BP <90 mm Hg.
- Establish hypotension parameters prior to initiating therapy.
- Reduce the dose or withhold the drug if hypotension occurs during administration. Reinitiate therapy infusion only after hypotension is corrected. Subsequent doses fol-

lowing a hypotensive episode are usually reduced by 30% and given without a prior bolus dose.

- Lab tests: Baseline and periodic serum creatinine.

NETILMICIN SULFATE

(ne-til-mye′sin)

Netromycin

Classifications: ANTIINFECTIVE; AMINOGLYCOSIDE ANTIBIOTIC

Prototype: Gentamicin

Pregnancy Category: D

AVAILABILITY 100 mg/mL injection

ACTIONS Rapid-acting, broad-spectrum, semisynthetic aminoglycoside derivative. Spectrum of activity comparable to that of gentamicin, but netilmicin is also effective against gentamicin-resistant bacteria. Not inactivated by most strains of bacteria resistant to other aminoglycosides.

THERAPEUTIC EFFECTS Bactericidal action primarily against gram-negative organisms including *Citrobacter, Enterobacter, Escherichia coli, Klebsiella, Proteus mirabilis, Pseudomonas aeruginosa, Salmonella, Serratia,* and certain gram-positive bacteria such as *Staphylococcus pyogenes* and *S. faecalis.* Like other aminoglycosides, not effective against most anaerobic bacteria (*Bacteroides* and *Clostridium* species), viruses, or fungi.

USES Short-term treatment of serious or life-threatening infections including septicemia, peritonitis, intraabdominal abscess, lower respiratory tract infections, complicated urinary tract infection, and infections of bones, joints, and skin and its structures. May be administered in conjunction with a beta-lactam antibiotic (e.g., a penicillin or cephalosporin) for synergistic effect pending results of susceptibility testing.

CONTRAINDICATIONS History of hypersensitivity or toxic reaction to netilmicin or other aminoglycosides or to bisulfites or any other ingredient in the formulation; minor infections; pregnancy (category D), lactation.

CAUTIOUS USE Impaired kidney function; premature infants, neonates, older adults; patients with ascites, edema, dehydration; severe burns; cystic fibrosis; fever; anemia; myasthenia gravis, parkinsonism; history of ear disease; infant botulism.

ROUTE & DOSAGE

Note: All doses based on ideal body weight

Moderate to Severe Infections

Adult: **IV/IM** 1.3–2.2 mg/kg q8h or 2–3.25 mg/kg q12h
Child: **IV/IM** *<6 wk,* 2–3.5 mg/kg q12h; *6 wk–12 y,* 1.8–2.7 mg/kg q8h or 2.7–4 mg/kg q12h

Renal Impairment

Cl_{cr} >70 mL/min: Reduce dose by multiplying maintenance dose by 0.85 and administer q8h; 50–69 mL/min: Reduce dose by multiplying maintenance dose by 0.85 and administer q12 h; 25–49 mL/min: Reduce dose by multiplying maintenance dose by 0.85 and administer q24h; <25 mL/min: Reduce dose by multiplying maintenance dose by 0.85 and administer doses based on serum concentrations

Complicated UTI

Adult: **IV/IM** 1.5–2 mg/kg q12h

ADMINISTRATION

Note: Determine doses for obese patient by using ideal body weight. Use manufacturer's guidelines to adjust doses for those with impaired kidney function.

Intramuscular

- Give deep IM into a large muscle.

Intravenous

PREPARE: **Intermittent: Adult,** Dilute a single dose in 50–200 mL of D5W, NS, D5/NS, or RL. **Pediatric,** Dilute to concentration of 2–3 mg/mL.

ADMINISTER: **Intermittent:** Give over 30–120 min or as ordered.

INCOMPATIBILITIES **Solution/additive: Cefepime, furosemide, heparin. Y-site: Allopurinol, amphotericin B cholesteryl complex, furosemide, propofol.**

- Do not use solutions that are discolored or that contain particulate matter.
- Diluted solutions retain potency for up to 72 h when stored in glass containers at 15°–30° C (59°–86° F) or refrigerated.

ADVERSE EFFECTS (≥1%) **CNS:** Headache, lethargy, drowsiness, paresthesias, tremors, muscle twitching, peripheral neuritis, disorientation, seizures, neuromuscular blockade; musculoskeletal weakness or paralysis, respiratory depression or paralysis. **CV:** Palpitation, hypotension. **Special Senses:** Ototoxicity (usually irreversible; eighth cranial nerve auditory branch: tinnitus, hearing loss, ringing, buzzing or fullness in ears; vestibular branch: vertigo, nystagmus, ataxia, nausea, and vomiting), blurred vision. **GI:** Nausea, vomiting, diarrhea, stomatitis, proctitis, enterocolitis. **Hematologic:** Increases in ALT, AST, alkaline phosphatase, bilirubin; anemia, eosinophilia, neutropenia, thrombocytopenia, thrombocytosis, agranulocytosis, leukopenia, leukemoid reaction. **Skin:** Rash, pruritus, induration, and hematoma at injection site. **Urogenital:** Nephrotoxicity, increase in serum creatinine and BUN; decrease in creatinine clearance; hematuria, proteinuria, urinary frequency, oliguria, polyuria. **Body as a Whole:** Fever, edema, arthralgia; pain, **Metabolic:** Hypokalemia.

DIAGNOSTIC TEST INTERFERENCE Concomitant netilmicin-cephalosporin therapy may cause false elevations of ***creatinine*** determinations. Concomitant use of BETA-LACTAMS (cephalosporins, penicillins) may result in falsely low ***aminoglycoside levels*** (mutual inactivation may continue in body fluid specimen unless promptly assayed, or frozen, or treated with beta-lactamase).

INTERACTIONS Drug: ANESTHETICS, SKELETAL MUSCLE RELAXANTS add to neuromuscular blocking effects; **acyclovir, amphotericin B, bacitracin, capreomycin,** CEPHALOSPORINS, **colistin, cisplatin, carboplatin, methoxyflurane, polymyxin B, vancomycin, furosemide, ethacrynic acid** increase risk of ototoxicity or nephrotoxicity or both.

PHARMACOKINETICS Peak: End of IV infusion; 30–60 min IM. **Distribution:** Does not cross blood–brain barrier; accumulates in renal cortex; crosses placenta; distributed into breast milk. **Elimination:** Excreted in urine. **Half-Life:** 2–2.5 h.

NURSING IMPLICATIONS

Assessment & Drug Effects

- Lab tests: Perform C&S tests prior to initiation of therapy. Therapy may begin before test results are available. Evaluate kidney function before and periodically during therapy.

- Monitor high-risk patients closely (i.e., kidney function impairment: older adults, dehydrated patients, burn patients, and patients receiving high doses or prolonged therapy).
- Determine peak serum drug levels by drawing blood 1 h after IM injection or IV infusion begins. To determine trough serum drug levels, draw blood just before next scheduled dose. Desirable peak values: 6–10 mcg/mL; desirable trough values: 0.5–2 mcg/mL. Peak values >16 mcg/mL and trough values >4 mcg/mL are associated with a high potential for toxicity.
- Note: Close monitoring of serum drug concentrations is especially important for patients with fever, edema, severe burns, and anemia. Peak serum drug levels tend to be significantly reduced in these patients.
- Monitor I&O ratio and pattern and report significant changes. Keep patient well hydrated throughout therapy to minimize possibility of chemical irritation of renal tubules and to reduce risk of toxicity.
- Evaluate patients before and during therapy for hearing acuity and vestibular status. Notify physician promptly if patient complains of any hearing loss, tinnitus, vertigo, or ataxia.
- Repeat bacterial susceptibility tests if therapeutic effectiveness is not evident within 3–5 d.
- Watch for S&S of superinfection (see Appendix F), especially of upper respiratory tract. Also suspect overgrowth of opportunistic organisms if patient develops sore rectum, diarrhea, vaginal discharge, sore mouth, fever.

Patient & Family Education

- Report to physician immediately any roaring sounds or ringing in the ears.
- Do not breast feed while taking this drug.

NEVIRAPINE (Pr)

(ne-vir′a-peen)

Viramune

Classifications: ANTIINFECTIVE; ANTIRETROVIRAL AGENT; NONNUCLEOSIDE REVERSE TRANSCRIPTASE INHIBITOR (NNRTI)

Pregnancy Category: C

AVAILABILITY 200 mg tablets

ACTIONS Nonnucleoside reverse transcriptase inhibitor (NNRI) of HIV-1. Binds directly to reverse transcriptase and blocks RNA- and DNA-dependent polymerase activities.

THERAPEUTIC EFFECTS Prevents replication of the HIV-1 virus. Does not inhibit HIV-2 reverse transcriptase and DNA polymerases such as alpha, beta, gamma, and delta polymerases. Resistant strains appear rapidly.

USES In combination with nucleoside analogs for treatment of HIV.

CONTRAINDICATIONS Hypersensitivity to nevirapine; hormonal contraceptives; pregnancy (category C), neonates; lactation.

CAUTIOUS USE Liver or renal disease, hepatitis B or C; CNS disorders.

ROUTE & DOSAGE

HIV

Adult: **PO** 200 mg once daily for first 14 d, then increase to 200 mg b.i.d.

Child: **PO** 120 mg/m^2 q.d. × 14 d, then increase q12h, if tolerated, to 120–200 mg/m^2 q12h (max: 200 mg/dose)

ADMINISTRATION

Oral

- Reinitiate with 200 mg/d for 14 d, then increase to b.i.d. dosing, when dosing is interrupted for >7 d.
- Store at 15°–30° C (59°–86° F) in a tightly closed container.

ADVERSE EFFECTS (≥1%) **Body as a Whole:** Fever, paresthesia, myalgia. **CNS:** Headache. **GI:** Nausea, diarrhea, abdominal pain, hepatitis, increased liver function tests, hepatotoxicity (including fulminant and cholestatic hepatitis, hepatic necrosis, and hepatic failure). **Hematologic:** Anemia, neutropenia. **Skin:** *Rash,* Stevens-Johnson syndrome.

INTERACTIONS Drug: May decrease plasma concentrations of PROTEASE INHIBITORS, ORAL CONTRACEPTIVES; may decrease **methadone** levels inducing opiate withdrawal. **Herbal: St. John's wort** may decrease antiretroviral activity.

PHARMACOKINETICS Absorption: Rapidly absorbed from GI tract. **Peak:** 4h. **Distribution:** 60% protein bound, crosses placenta, distributed into breast milk. **Metabolism:** Metabolized in liver by cytochrome P450-3A (CYP3A). **Elimination:** Excreted primarily in urine. **Half-Life:** 25–40 h.

NURSING IMPLICATIONS

Assessment & Drug Effects

- Lab tests: Obtain baseline and periodic liver and kidney function tests, routine blood chemistry, and CBC.
- Monitor weight, temperature, respiratory status with chest x-ray throughout therapy.
- Monitor carefully, especially during first 6 wk of therapy, for severe rash (with or without fever, blistering, oral lesions, conjunctivitis, swelling, joint aches, or general malaise).
- Withhold drug and notify physician if rash develops or liver function tests are abnormal.

Patient & Family Education

- Learn about common adverse effects.
- Withhold drug and notify physician if severe rash appears.
- Do not drive or engage in potentially hazardous activities until response to drug is known. There is a high potential for drowsiness and fatigue.
- Use or add barrier contraceptive if using hormonal contraceptive.
- Do not breast feed while taking this drug.

NIACIN (VITAMIN B_3, NICOTINIC ACID)

(nye′a-sin)

Niac, Nicobid, Nico-400, Nicolar, Nicotinex, Novoniacin ♣, Tri-B3 ♣

NIACINAMIDE (NICOTINAMIDE)

Classifications: VITAMIN B_3; CARDIOVASCULAR AGENT; ANTILIPEMIC; LIPID-LOWERING AGENT

Pregnancy Category: C

AVAILABILITY 50 mg, 100 mg, 250 mg, 500 mg tablets; 125 mg, 250 mg, 400 mg, 500 mg, 750 mg sustained release tablets, capsules

ACTIONS Water-soluble, heat-stable, B-complex vitamin (B_3) that functions with riboflavin as a control agent in coenzyme system that converts protein, carbohydrate, and fat to energy through oxidation-reduction. Niacinamide, an amide of niacin, is used as an alternative in the prevention and treatment of pellagra.

THERAPEUTIC EFFECTS Produces vasodilation by direct action on vascular smooth muscles. Inhibits hepatic synthesis of VLDL, cholesterol and triglyceride, and, indirectly, LDL. Large doses effectively reduce elevated serum cholesterol and total lipid levels in hypercholesterolemia and hyperlipidemic states.

USES In prophylaxis and treatment of pellagra, usually in combination with other B-complex vitamins, and in deficiency states accompanying carcinoid syndrome, isoniazid therapy, Hartnup's disease, and chronic alcoholism. Also in adjuvant treatment of hyperlipidemia (elevated cholesterol or triglycerides) in patients who do not respond adequately to diet or weight loss. Also as vasodilator in peripheral vascular disorders, Ménière's disease, and labyrinthine syndrome, as well as to counteract LSD toxicity and to distinguish between psychoses of dietary and nondietary origin.

CONTRAINDICATIONS Hypersensitivity to niacin; hepatic impairment; severe hypotension; hemorrhaging or arterial bleeding; active peptic ulcer; pregnancy (category C), lactation, and children <16 y.

CAUTIOUS USE History of gallbladder disease, liver disease, and peptic ulcer; glaucoma; angina; coronary artery disease; diabetes mellitus; predisposition to gout; allergy.

ROUTE & DOSAGE

Niacin Deficiency

Adult: **PO** 10–20 mg/d **IV/IM/SC** 25–100 mg 2–5 times/d

Pellagra

Adult: **PO** 300–500 mg/d in divided doses
Child: **PO** 50–100 mg t.i.d.

Hyperlipidemia

Adult: **PO** 1.5–3 g/d in divided doses, may increase up to 6 g/d if necessary
Child: **PO** 100–250 mg/d in 3 divided doses, may increase by 250 mg/d q2–3 wk as tolerated

ADMINISTRATION

Oral

- Give oral drug with meals to decrease GI distress. Give with cold water (not hot beverage) to facilitate swallowing.
- Ensure that sustained release form is not chewed or crushed. It must be swallowed whole.
- Store at 15°–30° C (59°–86° F) in a light and moisture proof container.

Intravenous

PREPARE: **Intermittent:** Dilute 50–100 mg in 500 mL of NS to yield concentrations of 0.1–0.2 mg/mL.
ADMINISTER: **Intermittent:** Give over 12–24 h.

ADVERSE EFFECTS (≥1%) **CNS:** *Transient headache, tingling of extremities,* syncope. With chronic use: nervousness, panic, toxic amblyopia, proptosis, blurred vision, loss of central vision. **CV:** *Generalized flushing with sensation of warmth,* postural hypotension, vasovagal attacks, arrhythmias (rare). **GI:** *Abnormalities of liver function tests; jaundice, bloating, flatulence, nausea,* vomiting, GI disorders, activation of peptic ulcer, xerostomia. **Skin:** *Increased sebaceous gland activity,* dry skin, skin rash, *pruritus,* keratitis nigricans. **Metabolic:** Hyperuricemia, hyperglycemia, glycosuria, hypoprothrombinemia, hypoalbuminemia.

DIAGNOSTIC TEST INTERFERENCE Niacin causes elevated serum ***bilirubin, uric acid, alkaline phosphatase, AST, ALT, LDH*** levels and may cause ***glucose intolerance.*** Decreases ***serum cholesterol*** 15%–30% and may cause false elevations with certain ***fluorometric methods*** of determining ***urinary catecholamines.*** Niacin may cause false-positive ***urine glucose*** tests using ***copper sulfate reagents,*** e.g., ***Benedict's*** solution.

INTERACTIONS Drug: Potentiates hypotensive effects of ANTIHYPERTENSIVE AGENTS.

PHARMACOKINETICS Absorption: Readily absorbed from GI tract. **Peak:** 20–70 min. **Distribution:** Distributed into breast milk. **Metabolism:** Metabolized in liver. **Elimination:** Excreted primarily in urine. **Half-Life:** 45 min.

NURSING IMPLICATIONS

Assessment & Drug Effects

- Monitor therapeutic effectiveness and record effect of therapy on clinical manifestations of deficiency (fiery red tongue, excessive saliva secretion and infection of oral membranes, nausea, vomiting, diarrhea, confusion). Therapeutic response usually begins within 24 h.
- Lab tests: Obtain baseline and periodic tests of blood glucose and liver function in patients receiving prolonged high dose therapy.
- Monitor diabetics and patients on high doses closely. Hyperglycemia, glycosuria, ketonuria, and increased insulin requirements have been reported.
- Observe patients closely for evidence of liver dysfunction (jaundice, dark urine, light-colored stools, pruritus) and hyperuricemia in patients predisposed to gout (flank, joint, or stomach pain; altered urine excretion pattern).

Patient & Family Education

- Be aware that you may feel warm and flushed in face, neck, and ears within first 2 h after oral ingestion and immediately after parenteral administration and may last several hours. Effects are usually transient and subside as therapy continues.
- Sit or lie down and avoid sudden posture changes if you feel weak or dizzy. Report these symptoms and persistent flushing to your physician. Relief may be obtained by reduction of dosage, increasing subsequent doses in small increments, or by changing to sustained release formulation.
- Be aware that alcohol and large doses of niacin cause increased flushing and sensation of warmth.
- Avoid exposure to direct sunlight until lesions have entirely cleared if you have skin manifestations.
- Do not breast feed while taking this drug.

N

NICARDIPINE HYDROCHLORIDE

(ni-car'di-peen)

Cardene, Cardene IV, Cardene SR

Classifications: CARDIOVASCULAR AGENT; CALCIUM CHANNEL BLOCKER; ANTIHYPERTENSIVE AGENT

Prototype: Nifedipine

Pregnancy Category: C

AVAILABILITY 20 mg, 30 mg capsules; 30 mg, 40 mg, 60 mg sustained release capsules; 2.5 mg/mL injection

ACTIONS Calcium entry blocker that inhibits the transmembrane influx of calcium ions into cardiac muscle and smooth muscle, thus affecting contractility. More selectively affects vascular smooth muscle than cardiac muscle; relaxes coronary vascular smooth muscle with little or no negative inotropic effect.

THERAPEUTIC EFFECTS Significantly decreases systemic vascular resistance. It reduces BP at rest and during isometric and dynamic exercise.

USES Either alone or with beta blockers for chronic, stable (effort-associated) angina; either alone or with other antihypertensives for essential hypertension.

UNLABELED USES CHF, cerebral ischemia, migraine.

CONTRAINDICATIONS Hypersensitivity to nicardipine; advanced aortic stenosis; lactation.

CAUTIOUS USE CHF; renal and hepatic impairment; pregnancy (category C).

N

ROUTE & DOSAGE

Hypertension, Angina

Adult: **PO** 20–40 mg t.i.d. or 30–60 mg SR b.i.d. **IV** Initiation of therapy in a drug-free patient: 5 mg/h initially, increase dose by 2.5 mg/h q15min (or faster) (max: 15 mg/h); for severe hypertension: 4–7.5 mg/h; for postop hypertension: 10–15 mg/h initially, then 1–3 mg/h
Child: **IV** 1–3 mcg/kg/min has been used in children 9 days old to 10 y

Substitute for Oral Nicardipine

Adult: **IV** 20 mg q8h PO = 0.5 mg/h; 30 mg q8h PO = 1.2 mg/h; 40 mg q8h PO = 2.2 mg/h

ADMINISTRATION

Note: To prevent symptoms of withdrawal, do not abruptly discontinue drug.

Oral

- Give on empty stomach. High-fat meals may decrease blood levels.
- Ensure that sustained release form is not chewed or crushed. It must be swallowed whole.
- When converting from IV to oral dose, give first dose of t.i.d. regimen 1 h before discontinuing infusion.

Intravenous

PREPARE: **IV Infusion:** Dilute each 25 mg ampul with 240 mL of D5W or NS to yield 0.1 mg/mL.

ADMINISTER: **IV Infusion:** Usually initiated at 50 mL/h (5 mg/h) with rate increases of 25 mL/h (2.5 mg/h) q5–15 min up to a maximum of 150 mL/h. Infusion is usually slowed to 30 mL/h once the target BP is reached.

INCOMPATIBILITIES **Y-site: Furosemide, heparin, thiopental.**

ADVERSE EFFECTS (≥1%) **CNS:** Dizziness or headache, fatigue, anxiety, depression, parerethesias, insomnia, somnolence, nervousness. **CV:** Pedal edema, hypotension, flushing, palpitations, tachycardia, increased angina. **GI:** Anorexia, nausea, vomiting, dry mouth, constipation, dyspepsia. **Skin:** Rash, pruritus. **Body as a Whole:** Arthralgia or arthritis.

INTERACTIONS Drug: Adenosine prolongs bradycardia. **Amiodarone** may cause sinus arrest and AV block. **Benazepril** blunts increase in heart rate and increase in plasma **norepinephrine** and **aldosterone** seen with nicardipine. BETA BLOCKERS cause hypotension and bradycardia. **Cimetidine** increases levels of nicardipine, resulting in hypotension. Concomitant nicardipine and **cyclosporine** result in significant increase in **cyclosporine** serum concentrations 1–

30 d after initiation of nicardipine therapy; following withdrawal of nicardipine, **cyclosporine** levels decrease. **Magnesium,** when used to retard premature labor, may cause severe hypotension and neuromuscular blockade.

PHARMACOKINETICS Absorption: Immediately 35% of oral dose reaches systemic circulation. **Onset:** 1 min IV; 20 min PO. **Peak:** 0.5–2 h. **Duration:** 3 h IV. **Distribution:** 95% protein bound; distributed in breast milk. **Metabolism:** Rapidly and extensively metabolized in liver; there is an active metabolite that has <1% activity of parent compound. **Elimination:** 35% in feces, 60% in urine; elimination not affected by hemodialysis. **Half-Life:** 8.6 h.

NURSING IMPLICATIONS

Assessment & Drug Effects

- Establish baseline data before treatment is started including BP, pulse, and lab values of liver and kidney function.
- Monitor BP during initiation and titration of dosage carefully. Hypotension with or without an increase in heart rate may occur, especially in patients who are hypertensive or who are already taking antihypertensive medication.
- Avoid too rapid reduction in either systolic or diastolic pressure during parenteral administration.
- Discontinue IV infusion if hypotension or tachycardia develop.
- Observe for large peak and trough differences in BP. Initially, measure BP at peak effect (1–2 h after dosing) and at trough effect (8 h after dosing).

Patient & Family Education

- Record and report any increase in frequency, duration, and severity of angina when initiating or increasing dosage. Keep a record of nitroglycerin use and promptly report any changes in previous anginal pattern. Increased incidence and severity of angina has occurred in some patients using nicardipine.
- Do not change dosage regimen without consulting physician.
- Be aware that abrupt withdrawal may cause an increased frequency and duration of chest pain. This drug must be gradually tapered under medical supervision.
- Rise slowly from a recumbent position; avoid driving or operating potentially dangerous equipment until response to nicardipine is known.
- Notify physician if any of the following occur: Irregular heart beat, shortness of breath, swelling of the feet, pronounced dizziness, nausea, or drop in BP.
- Do not breast feed while taking this drug.

NICOTINE

(nik′o-teen)

Nicotrol NS, Nicotrol Inhaler, Commit

NICOTINE POLACRILEX

Nicorette Gum, Nicorette DS

NICOTINE TRANSDERMAL SYSTEM

Habitrol, Nicoderm, Nicotrol, ProStep

Classifications: CENTRAL NERVOUS SYSTEM AND AUTONOMIC NERVOUS SYSTEM AGENT; SMOKING DETERRENT; CHOLINERGIC (PARASYMPATHOMIMETIC)

Pregnancy Category: X (polacrilex); D (nasal spray, transdermal system)

AVAILABILITY 2 mg, 4 mg gum; 2 mg, 4 mg lozenges; 0.5 mg spray; 4 mg inhaler; 7 mg/d, 14 mg/d, 21 mg/d, 5 mg/d, 10 mg/d, 15 mg/d, 11 mg/d, 22 mg/d transdermal patch.

ACTIONS Ganglionic cholinergic receptor antagonist, which has both adrenergic and cholinergic effects. Include stimulant and depressant effects on the peripheral nervous system and CNS; respiratory stimulation; peripheral vasoconstriction; increased heart rate, contractile force cardiac output, and stroke volume; increased tone and motor activity of GI smooth muscles; increased bronchial secretions (initially); antidiuretic activity. Heavy smokers are tolerant of these effects.
THERAPEUTIC EFFECTS Rationale for use of nicotine is to reduce withdrawal symptoms accompanying cessation of smoking. Success rate appears to be greatest in smokers with high "physical" type of nicotine dependence.

USES In conjunction with a medically supervised behavior modification program, as a temporary and alternate source of nicotine by the nicotine-dependent smoker who is withdrawing from cigarette smoking.

CONTRAINDICATIONS Nonsmokers, immediate post-MI period; life-threatening arrhythmias; active temporomandibular joint disease; severe angina pectoris; women with childbearing potential (unless effective contraception is used). *Nicotine Polacrilex:* pregnancy (category X); *Nicotine Transdermal System:* pregnancy (category D). Safety in children and adolescents is not established.
CAUTIOUS USE Vasospastic disease (e.g., Buerger's disease, Prinzmetal's variant angina), cardiac arrhythmias, hyperthyroidism, type 1 diabetes, pheochromocytoma, esophagitis, oral and pharyngeal inflammation; patient with dentures, denture caps, or partial bridges; hypertension and peptic ulcer disease (active or inactive). During lactation, only if benefit of a smoking cessation program outweighs risks.

ROUTE & DOSAGE

Smoking Cessation

Adult: **PO** Chew 1 piece of gum whenever have urge to smoke, may be repeated as needed (max: 30 pieces of gum/d) **Intranasal** 1 dose = 2 sprays, 1 in each nostril, start with 1–2 doses (2–4 sprays) each hour (max: 5 doses/h, 40 doses/d), may continue for 3 mo **Topical** Apply 1 transdermal patch q24h by the following schedule: ***Habitrol, Nicoderm:*** 21 mg/d × 6 wk, 14 mg/d × 2 wk, 7 mg/d × 2 wk; *weight <45 kg (100 lb), smoke <1/2 pack/d, or have cardiovascular disease,* 14 mg/d × 6 wk, 7 mg/d × 2–4 wk. ***ProStep:*** 22 mg/d × 4–8 wk, 11 mg/d × 2–4 wk; *weight <45 kg (100 lb), smoke <1/2 pack/d, or have cardiovascular disease,* 11 mg/d × 4–8 wk. ***Nicotrol:*** Apply 1 transdermal patch 16 h/d by the following schedule: 15 mg/d × 4–12 wk, 10 mg/d × 2–4 wk, 5 mg/d × 2–4 wk

ADMINISTRATION

Oral

- Note: Most adverse local effects (irritation of tongue, mouth, and throat, jaw-muscle aches, dislike of taste) are transient and subside in a few days. Modification of the chewing technique may help.

Transdermal

- Remove the old patch before applying the next new patch.
- Apply patch to nonhairy, clean, dry skin site; immediately remove from protective container.
- Store at or below 30° C (86° F); patches are sensitive to heat.

ADVERSE EFFECTS (≥1%) **CNS:** *Headache, dizziness, light-headedness,* insomnia, irritability, dependence on nicotine. **CV:** Arrhythmias, tachycardia, palpitations, hypertension. **GI:** Air swallowing, *jaw ache, nausea,* belching, salivation, anorexia, dry mouth, laxative effects, constipation, *indigestion,* diarrhea, dyspepsia, vomiting, sialorrhea, abdominal pain, diarrhea. **Respiratory:** *Sore mouth or throat, cough, hiccups,* hoarseness; injury to mouth, teeth, temporomandibular joint pain, *irritation/tingling of tongue.* **Skin:** *Erythema, pruritus, local edema, rash;* skin reactions may be delayed, occurring after 3 wk of patch use. **Special Senses:** *Runny nose, nasal irritation, throat irritation, watering eyes,* minor epistaxis, nasal ulceration. **Body as a Whole:** Acute overdose/nicotine intoxication (perspiration; severe headache; dizziness; disturbed hearing and vision; mental confusion; severe weakness; fainting; hypotension; dyspnea; weak, rapid, irregular pulse; seizures); death (from respiratory failure secondary to drug-induced respiratory muscle paralysis).

INTERACTIONS Drug: May increase metabolism of **caffeine, theophylline, acetaminophen, insulin, oxazepam, pentazocine propranolol. Food:** Coffee, cola may decrease nicotine absorption from nicotine gum.

PHARMACOKINETICS Absorption: Approximately 90% of the nicotine in a piece of gum is released slowly over 15–30 min; rate of release is controlled by vigor and duration of chewing; readily absorbed from buccal mucosa; transdermal 75%–90% absorbed through skin; 53%–58% of nasal spray is absorbed. **Peak:** Transdermal 8–9 h; nasal spray 4–15 min. **Distribution:** Crosses placenta; distributed into breast milk. **Metabolism:** Metabolized in liver, primarily to cotinine. **Elimination:** Excreted in urine. **Half-Life:** 30–120 min.

NURSING IMPLICATIONS

Assessment & Drug Effects

- Be aware that transient erythema, pruritus, or burning is common with transdermal patch and usually disappears 24 h after patch removal.
- Differentiate cutaneous hypersensitivity (contact sensitization) that does not resolve in 24 h from a transient local reaction. The former is an indication to discontinue the transdermal patch.

Patient & Family Education

- Review carefully specific written instructions packaged with the chewing gum.
- Chew a piece of gum for approximately 30 min to get the full dose of nicotine.
- Chew only one piece of gum at a time. Chewing gum too rapidly can cause excessive buccal absorption and lead to adverse effects: nausea, hiccups, throat irritation.
- Gradually decrease number of pieces of gum chewed in 24 h. Usually, a period of 3 mo is allowed before tapering use of gum.
- Promptly discontinue use of transdermal patch and notify physician if a severe or persistent local or generalized skin reaction occurs.
- Be aware that smoking while using the transdermal nicotine

patch increases the risk of adverse reactions.

- Do not breast feed while taking this drug without consulting physician.

NIFEDIPINE Pr

(nye-fed'i-peen)

Adalat, Adalat CC, Procardia, Procardia XL

Classifications: CARDIOVASCULAR AGENT; CALCIUM CHANNEL BLOCKER; ANTIARRHYTHMIC (CLASS IV); NON-NITRATE VASODILATOR

Pregnancy Category: C

AVAILABILITY 10 mg, 20 mg capsules; 30 mg, 60 mg, 90 mg sustained release tablets

ACTIONS Calcium channel blocking agent that selectively blocks calcium ion influx across cell membranes of cardiac muscle and vascular smooth muscle without changing serum calcium concentrations. Class IV antiarrhythmic.

THERAPEUTIC EFFECTS Reduces myocardial oxygen utilization and supply and relaxes and prevents coronary artery spasm; has little or no effect on SA and AV nodal conduction with therapeutic dosing. Decreases peripheral vascular resistance and increases cardiac output. Vasodilation of both coronary and peripheral vessels is greater than that produced by verapamil or diltiazem and frequently results in reflex tachycardia. Decreased peripheral vascular resistance also leads to a rise in peripheral blood flow, the basis for use of this drug in treatment of Raynaud's phenomenon. Minimal effect on myocardial contractility.

USES Vasospastic "variant" or Prinzmetal's angina and chronic stable angina without vasospasm. Mild to moderate hypertension alone or in combination with a diuretic.

UNLABELED USES Esophageal disorders; vascular headaches; Raynaud's phenomenon; asthma; cardiomyopathy; primary pulmonary hypertension.

CONTRAINDICATIONS Known hypersensitivity to nifedipine. Safety during pregnancy (category C) or in children is not established.

CAUTIOUS USE Concomitant use with hypotensives; CHF; lactation.

ROUTE & DOSAGE

Angina

Adult: **PO** 10–20 mg t.i.d. up to 180 mg/d

Hypertension

Adult: **PO** 10–20 mg t.i.d. up to 180 mg/d or 30–90 mg sustained release once/d

ADMINISTRATION

Oral

- Do not give within the first 1–2 wk following an MI.
- Use only the sustained release form to treat chronic hypertension. Ensure that sustained release form is not chewed or crushed. It must be swallowed whole.
- Discontinue drug gradually, with close medical supervision to prevent severe hypertension and other adverse effects.
- Store at 15°–25° C (59°–77° F); protect from light and moisture.

ADVERSE EFFECTS (≥1%) **Body as a Whole:** Sore throat, weakness, fever, sweating, chills, febrile reaction. **CNS:** *Dizziness, light-headedness,* nervousness, mood changes, weakness, jitteriness, sleep disturbances, blurred vision, retinal ischemia, difficulty in balance, *headache.* **CV:** Hypotension, *facial flushing, heat sensation,* palpitations, *peripheral edema,* MI (rare), prolonged systemic hypotension with overdose. **GI:** Nausea, heartburn, *diarrhea,* constipation, cramps, flatulence, gingival hyperplasia, hepatotoxicity. **Musculoskeletal:** Inflammation, joint stiffness, muscle cramps. **Respiratory:** Nasal congestion, dyspnea, cough, wheezing. **Skin:** Dermatitis, pruritus, urticaria. **Urogenital:** Sexual difficulties, possible male infertility.

DIAGNOSTIC TEST INTERFERENCE Nifedipine may cause mild to moderate increases of ***alkaline phosphatase, CPK, LDH, AST, ALT.***

INTERACTIONS Drug: BETA BLOCKERS may increase likelihood of CHF; may increase risk of **phenytoin** toxicity. **Herbal: Melatonin** may increase blood pressure and heart rate.

PHARMACOKINETICS Absorption: Readily absorbed from GI tract; 45%–75% reaches systemic circulation (first pass metabolism). **Onset:** 10–30 min. **Peak:** 30 min. **Distribution:** Distributed into breast milk. **Metabolism:** Metabolized in liver. **Elimination:** 75%–80% excreted in urine, 15% in feces. **Half-Life:** 2–5 h.

NURSING IMPLICATIONS

Assessment & Drug Effects

- Monitor BP carefully during titration period. Patient may become severely hypotensive, especially if also taking other drugs known to lower BP. Withhold drug and notify physician if systolic BP <90.
- Monitor blood sugar in diabetic patients. Nifedipine has diabetogenic properties.
- Monitor for gingival hyperplasia and report promptly. This is a rare but serious adverse effect (similar to phenytoin-induced hyperplasia).

Patient & Family Education

- Keep a record of nitroglycerin use and promptly report any changes in previous pattern. Occasionally, people develop increased frequency, duration, and severity of angina when they start treatment with this drug or when dosage is increased.
- Be aware that withdrawal symptoms may occur with abrupt discontinuation of the drug (chest pain, increase in anginal episodes, MI, dysrhythmias).
- Inspect gums visually every day. Changes in gingivae may be gradual, and bleeding may be exhibited only with probing.
- Seek prompt treatment for symptoms of gingival hyperplasia (easy bleeding of gingivae and gradual enlarging of gingival mass, especially on buccal side of lower anterior teeth). Drug will be discontinued if gingival hyperplasia occurs.
- Research shows that smoking decreases the efficacy of nifedipine and has direct and adverse effects on the heart in the patient on nifedipine treatment.
- Do not breast feed while taking this drug without consulting physician.

NILUTAMIDE

(ni-lu'ta-mide)

Nilandron

Classifications: ANTINEOPLASTIC AGENT; ANTIANDROGEN

Prototype: Flutamide

Pregnancy Category: C

AVAILABILITY 50 mg tablets

ACTIONS Nonsteroidal with antiandrogen activity.

THERAPEUTIC EFFECTS Blocks the effects of testosterone at the andro-

N

gen receptor sites, thus preventing the normal androgenic response.

USES Use with surgical castration for metastatic prostate cancer.

CONTRAINDICATIONS Severe hepatic impairment; severe respiratory insufficiency; hypersensitivity to nilutamide.

CAUTIOUS USE Pregnancy (category C) and Asian patients relative to interstitial pneumonitis. Safety and effectiveness in children are not established.

ROUTE & DOSAGE

Metastatic Prostate Cancer
Adult: **PO** 300 mg q.d. × 30 d, then reduce to 150 mg q.d.

ADMINISTRATION

Oral
- Give first dose on the day of or day after surgical castration.
- Store below 15°–30° C (59°–86° F) and protect from light.

ADVERSE EFFECTS (≥1%) **Body as a Whole:** *Hot flushes, impotence, decreased libido, malaise,* edema, weight loss, arthritis. **CNS:** Nervousness, paresthesias. **CV:** Angina, heart failure, syncope. **GI:** Diarrhea, GI hemorrhage, melena, dry mouth. **Respiratory:** Cough, interstitial lung disease, rhinitis. **Skin:** Pruritus. **Other:** Alcohol intolerance. **Special Senses:** Cataracts, photophobia.

INTERACTIONS No clinically significant interactions established.

PHARMACOKINETICS Absorption: Rapidly absorbed from GI tract. **Metabolism:** Metabolized in the liver. **Elimination:** Primarily excreted in urine. **Half-Life:** 38–50 h.

NURSING IMPLICATIONS

Assessment & Drug Effects
- Obtain baseline chest x-ray before treatment and periodically thereafter.
- Closely monitor for S&S of pneumonitis; at the first sign of adverse pulmonary effects, withhold drug and notify physician. Abnormal ABGs may indicate need to discontinue drug.
- Lab tests: Monitor liver function before beginning treatment and at 3-mo intervals; if serum transaminases increase >2–3 times upper limit of normal, discontinue treatment.
- Monitor patients taking phenytoin, theophylline, or warfarin closely for toxic levels of these drugs.

Patient & Family Education
- Report following S&S of adverse effects on lungs to physician immediately: Development of chest pain, dyspnea, and cough with fever.
- Report S&S of liver injury to physician: Jaundice, dark urine, fatigue, or signs of GI distress including nausea, vomiting, abdominal pain.
- Use caution when moving from lighted to dark areas because the drug may slow visual adaptation to darkness. Tinted glasses may partially alleviate the problem.

NIMODIPINE
(ni-mo′di-peen)
Nimotop
Classifications: CARDIOVASCULAR AGENT; CALCIUM CHANNEL BLOCKER
Prototype: Nifedipine
Pregnancy Category: C

AVAILABILITY 30 mg capsule

ACTIONS Calcium channel blocking agent that is relatively selective for cerebral arteries compared

with arteries elsewhere in the body. This may be attributed to the drug's high lipid solubility and specific binding to cerebral tissue.
THERAPEUTIC EFFECTS Reduces vascular spasms in cerebral arteries during a stroke.

USES To improve neurologic deficits due to spasm following subarachnoid hemorrhage from ruptured congenital intracranial aneurysms in patients who are in good neurologic condition posticus (e.g., Hunt and Hess Grades I–III).
UNLABELED USES Migraine headaches, ischemic seizures.

CONTRAINDICATIONS None known.
CAUTIOUS USE Hepatic impairment; pregnancy (category C), and lactation. Safety and effectiveness in children are not established.

ROUTE & DOSAGE

Subarachnoid Hemorrhage
Adult: **PO** 60 mg q4h for 21 d, start therapy within 96 h of subarachnoid hemorrhage

ADMINISTRATION

Oral

- Make a hole in both ends of the capsule with an 18-gauge needle and extract the contents into a syringe if patient is unable to swallow. Empty the contents into an enteral (if in use) tube and wash down with 30 mL of NS.
- Store below 40° C (104° F); protect from light.

ADVERSE EFFECTS (≥1%) **CNS:** Headache. **CV:** *Hypotension.* **GI:** Hemorrhage, mild, transient increase in liver function tests.

INTERACTIONS Drug: Hypotensive effects may be increased when nimodipine is combined with other CALCIUM CHANNEL BLOCKERS.

PHARMACOKINETICS Absorption: Readily absorbed from GI tract; approximately 13% reaches systemic circulation (first pass metabolism). **Peak:** 1 h. **Distribution:** Crosses blood–brain barrier; possibly crosses placenta; distributed into breast milk. **Metabolism:** 85% metabolized in liver; 15% metabolized in kidneys. **Elimination:** >50% excreted in urine, 32% in feces. **Half-Life:** 8–9 h.

NURSING IMPLICATIONS

Assessment & Drug Effects

- Take apical pulse prior to administering drug and hold it if pulse is below 60. Notify the physician.
- Establish baseline data before treatment is started: BP, pulse, and laboratory evaluations of liver and kidney function.
- Monitor frequently for adverse drug effects, including hypotension, peripheral edema, tachycardia, or skin rash.
- Monitor frequently for dizziness or lightheadedness in older adult patients; risk of hypotension is increased.

Patient & Family Education

- Report gradual weight gain and evidence of edema (e.g., tight rings on fingers, ankle swelling).
- Keep follow-up appointments for monitoring of progress during therapy.
- Do not breast feed while taking this drug without consulting physician.

NISOLDIPINE

(ni-sol′di-peen)
Nisocor, Sular
Classifications: CARDIOVASCULAR AGENT; CALCIUM CHANNEL BLOCKER; ANTIHYPERTENSIVE
Prototype: Nifedipine
Pregnancy Category: C

N

AVAILABILITY 10 mg, 20 mg, 30 mg, 40 mg sustained release tablets

ACTIONS Structurally similar to nifedipine. Inhibits calcium ion influx across cell membranes of cardiac muscle and vascular smooth muscle, which results in vasodilation, inotropism, and negative chronotropism.

THERAPEUTIC EFFECTS Inhibits vasoconstriction in the peripheral vasculature (10 times as potent than nifedipine). Significantly reduces total peripheral resistance, decreases blood pressure, and increases cardiac output. It is also a potent coronary vasodilator.

USES Hypertension, angina.

UNLABELED USES CHF.

CONTRAINDICATIONS Hypersensitivity to nisoldipine or other calcium blockers; systolic BP <90 mm Hg, advanced aortic stenosis, advanced heart failure, cardiogenic shock, severe hypotension, sick sinus syndrome; pregnancy (category D).

CAUTIOUS USE Liver dysfunction; older adult; paroxysmal atrial fibrillation; digital ischemia, ulceration, or gangrene; nonobstructive hypertrophic cardiomyopathy; Duchenne muscular dystrophy; lactation.

N

ROUTE & DOSAGE

Hypertension, Angina

Adult: **PO** 10–20 mg/d in 2 divided doses (max: 40 mg/d), may need to reduce dose in patients with liver disease (cirrhosis, chronic hepatitis)

ADMINISTRATION

Oral

- Give drug with food to decrease GI distress, but do not give with grapefruit juice or a high fat meal.
- Ensure that sustained release form is not chewed or crushed. It must be swallowed whole.
- Discontinue drug gradually to prevent adverse effects.
- Consider dosage reductions in older adults; initiate therapy at lower doses and follow with gradual increases.
- Store at 15°–30° C (59°–86° F).

ADVERSE EFFECTS (≥1%) **CNS:** Dizziness, anxiety, tremor, weakness, fatigue, *headache*. **CV:** Hypotension, lower extremity edema, palpitations, orthostatic hypotension. **GI:** Abdominal pain, cramps, constipation, dry mouth, diarrhea, nausea. **Skin:** *Flushing,* rash, erythema, urticaria. **Urogenital:** Urinary frequency. **Respiratory:** Pulmonary edema (patients with CHF), wheezing, dyspnea. **Body as a Whole:** Myalgia.

INTERACTIONS Drug: May cause significant increase in **digoxin** level in patients with CHF. BETA BLOCKERS may cause hypotension and bradycardia. **Phenytoin** may significantly decrease nisoldipine levels.

PHARMACOKINETICS Absorption: Rapidly absorbed from GI tract; 4%–8% reaches systemic circulation; absorption not affected by food. **Peak Effect:** 1–3 h. **Duration:** 8–12 h for hypertension, 7–8 h for angina. **Distribution:** 99% protein bound. **Metabolism:** Extensively metabolized in liver. **Elimination:** 70%–75% excreted in urine as metabolites. **Half-Life:** 2–14 h.

NURSING IMPLICATIONS

Assessment & Drug Effects

- Monitor blood pressure carefully during period of drug initiation and with dosage increments.
- Monitor cardiovascular status especially heart rate, frequency of

angina attacks, or worsening heart failure.
- Assess for and report edematous weight gain.
- Monitor digoxin levels closely with concurrent use and watch for S&S of digoxin toxicity (see Appendix F).

Patient & Family Education
- Do not discontinue the drug abruptly.
- Report symptoms of orthostatic hypotension or other bothersome adverse effects to physician.
- Do not drive or engage in potentially hazardous activities until response to drug is known.
- Do not breast feed while taking this drug without consulting physician.

NITAZOXANIDE

(nit-a-zox′-a-nide)
Alinia
Classifications: ANTIINFECTIVE; ANTIPROTOZOAL
Prototype: Metronidazole
Pregnancy Category: B

AVAILABILITY 100 mg/5 mL powder for reconstitution

ACTIONS Antiprotozoal activity believed to be due to interference with an essential enzyme needed for anaerobic energy metabolism in protozoa. Interference with the enzyme may not be the only pathway by which nitazoxanide exhibits antiprotozoal activity.
THERAPEUTIC EFFECTS Inhibits growth of sporozoites and oocysts of *Cryptosporidium parvum* and trophozoites of *Giardia lamblia*.

USES Treatment of diarrhea caused by *Cryptosporidium parvum* and *Giardia lamblia* in children.

CONTRAINDICATIONS Prior hypersensitivity to nitazoxanide.
CAUTIOUS USE Hepatic and biliary disease, renal disease and combined renal and hepatic disease; safety and efficacy in children <1 y or >11 y have not been studied; pregnancy (category B); lactation.

ROUTE & DOSAGE

Diarrhea
Child: **PO** *12–47 mo,* 100 mg (5 mL) q12 h × 3 d; *4–11 y,* 200 mg (10 mL) q12 h × 3 d

ADMINISTRATION

Oral
- Prepare suspension as follows: Tap bottle until powder loosens. Draw up 48 mL of water, add half to bottle, shake to suspend powder, then add remaining 24 mL of water and shake vigorously.
- Give required dose (5 or 10 mL) with food.
- Keep container tightly closed, and shake well before each administration.
- Suspension may be stored for 7 d at 15°–30° C (59°–86° F), after which any unused portion must be discarded.

ADVERSE EFFECTS (≥1%) **CNS:** Headache. **GI:** Abdominal pain, diarrhea, vomiting.

INTERACTIONS Drug: No clinically significant interactions reported.

PHARMACOKINETICS Peak: 1–4 h. **Distribution:** 99% protein bound. **Metabolism:** Rapidly hydrolyzed to an active metabolite, tizoxanide (desacetyl-nitazoxanide). Tizoxanide then undergoes conjugation, primarily by glucuronidation. **Elimination:** Excreted in urine and feces.

N

NURSING IMPLICATIONS

Assessment & Drug Effects

- Monitor for therapeutic effectiveness: No watery stools and ≤2 soft stools with no hematochezia within the past 24 h or no symptoms and no unformed stools within the past 48 h.
- Monitor closely patients with preexisting hepatic or biliary disease for adverse reactions.
- Assess appetite, level of abdominal discomfort and extent of bloating.
- Assess frequency and quantity of diarrhea and monitor total hydration status.
- Weigh daily to aid in assessment of possible fluid loss from diarrhea.

Patient & Family Education

- Note that 5 mL of the oral suspension contains approximately 1.5 g of sucrose.
- Report either no improvement in or worsening of diarrhea and abdominal discomfort.

N

NITROFURANTOIN

(nye-troe-fyoor'an-toyn)

Apo-Nitrofurantoin ♣, Furadantin, Furalan, Furanite, Nephronex ♣, Nitrofan, Novofuran ♣

NITROFURANTOIN MACROCRYSTALS

Macrobid, Macrodantin

Classifications: URINARY TRACT ANTIINFECTIVE; ANTIBIOTIC

Prototype: Trimethoprim

Pregnancy Category: B

AVAILABILITY 25 mg/mL suspension; 25 mg, 50 mg, 100 mg capsules

ACTIONS Synthetic nitrofuran derivative presumed to act by interfering with several bacterial enzyme systems. Highly soluble in urine and reportedly most active in acid urine. Antimicrobial concentrations in urine exceed those in blood.

THERAPEUTIC EFFECTS Active against wide variety of gram-negative and gram-positive micro-organisms, including strains of *Escherichia coli, Staphylococcus aureus, Streptococcus faecalis, enterococci,* and *Klebsiella aerobacter. Pseudomonas aeruginosa* and many strains of *Proteus* are resistant.

USES Pyelonephritis, pyelitis, and cystitis caused by susceptible organisms.

CONTRAINDICATIONS Anuria, oliguria, significant impairment of kidney function (creatinine clearance <40 mL/min); G6PD deficiency; infants <3 mo. Safety during pregnancy (category B), pregnancy at term, or lactation is not established.

CAUTIOUS USE History of asthma, anemia, diabetes, vitamin B deficiency, electrolyte imbalance, debilitating disease.

ROUTE & DOSAGE

Pyelonephritis, Cystitis

Adult: **PO** 50–100 mg q.i.d. or Macrobid 100 mg b.i.d.
Child: **PO** *1 mo–12 y,* 5–7 mg/kg/d in 4 divided doses

Chronic Suppressive Therapy

Adult: **PO** 50–100 mg h.s.
Child: **PO** *1 mo–12 y,* 1 mg/kg/d in 1–2 divided doses

ADMINISTRATION

Oral

- Give with food or milk to minimize gastric irritation.
- Avoid crushing tablets because of the possibility of tooth staining; rather dilute oral suspen-

sion in milk, water, or fruit juice, and rinse mouth thoroughly after taking drug.

ADVERSE EFFECTS (≥1%) **CNS:** Peripheral neuropathy, headache, nystagmus, drowsiness, vertigo. **GI:** *Anorexia, nausea, vomiting,* abdominal pain, diarrhea, cholestatic jaundice, hepatic necrosis. **Hematologic (rare):** Hemolytic or megaloblastic anemia (especially in patients with G6PD deficiency), granulocytosis, eosinophilia. **Body as a Whole:** Angioedema, anaphylaxis, drug fever, arthralgia. **Respiratory:** Allergic pneumonitis, asthmatic attack (patients with history of asthma), pulmonary sensitivity reactions (interstitial pneumonitis or fibrosis). **Skin:** Skin eruptions, pruritus, urticaria, exfoliative dermatitis, transient alopecia. **Urogenital:** Genitourinary superinfections (especially with *Pseudomonas*), crystalluria (older adult patients), dark yellow or brown urine. **Other:** Tooth staining from direct contact with oral suspension and crushed tablets (infants).

DIAGNOSTIC TEST INTERFERENCE Nitrofurantoin metabolite may produce false-positive ***urine glucose*** test results with Benedict's reagent.

INTERACTIONS Drug: ANTACIDS may decrease absorption of nitrofurantoin; **nalidixic acid,** other QUINOLONES may antagonize antimicrobial effects; **probenecid, sulfinpyrazone** increase risk of nitrofurantoin toxicity.

PHARMACOKINETICS Absorption: Readily absorbed from GI tract. **Peak:** Urine: 30 min. **Distribution:** Crosses placenta; distributed into breast milk. **Metabolism:** Partially metabolized in liver. **Elimination:** Primarily excreted in urine. **Half-Life:** 20 min.

NURSING IMPLICATIONS

Assessment & Drug Effects

- Lab tests: Perform C&S prior to therapy; recommended in patients with recurrent infections.
- Monitor I&O. Report oliguria and any change in I&O ratio. Drug should be discontinued if oliguria or anuria develops or creatinine clearance falls below 40 mL/min.
- Be alert to signs of urinary tract superinfections (e.g., milky urine, foul-smelling urine, perineal irritation, dysuria).
- Assess for nausea (which occurs fairly frequently). May be relieved by using macrocrystalline preparation (Macrodantin) or by reducing dosage.
- Watch for acute pulmonary sensitivity reaction, usually within first week of therapy and apparently more common in older adults. May be manifested by mild to severe flu-like syndrome. Eosinophilia generally develops in a few days. Recovery usually occurs rapidly after drug is discontinued.
- With prolonged therapy, monitor for subacute or chronic pulmonary sensitivity reaction, commonly manifested by insidious onset of malaise, cough, dyspnea on exertion, altered ABGs.
- Be alert for and advise the patient to report onset of muscle weakness, tingling, numbness, or other sensations. Peripheral neuropathy can be severe and irreversible. Drug should be withdrawn immediately.

Patient & Family Education

- Be aware that IM injection of nitrofurantoin may be painful (pain may be severe enough to warrant discontinuation of drug by this route).
- Nitrofurantoin may impart a harmless brown color to urine.

- Consult physician regarding fluid intake. Generally, fluids are not forced; however, intake should be adequate.
- Do not breast feed while taking this drug without consulting physician.

NITROFURAZONE

(nye-troe-fyoor′a-zone)

Furacin

Classifications: SKIN AND MUCOUS MEMBRANE AGENT; ANTIINFECTIVE; ANTIBIOTIC

Pregnancy Category: C

AVAILABILITY 0.2% ointment, cream, topical solution

ACTIONS Synthetic nitrofuran related to nitrofurantoin. Acts by inhibiting aerobic and anaerobic cycles in bacterial carbohydrate metabolism.

THERAPEUTIC EFFECTS Bactericidal against most microorganisms causing surface infections, including many that have developed antibiotic resistance. Activity against *Pseudomonas aeruginosa* and certain strains of *Proteus* is limited; has no activity against fungi or viruses.

USES As adjunctive therapy to combat bacterial infection in second- and third-degree burns; to prevent infection of skin grafts and donor sites. Has been used orally in other countries for treatment of late stage of African trypanosomiasis.

CONTRAINDICATIONS Hypersensitivity to nitrofurazone; pregnancy (category C).

CAUTIOUS USE Known or suspected renal impairment; G6PD deficiency; lactation.

ROUTE & DOSAGE

Bacterial Infections Associated with Burns or Skin Grafts

Adult: **Topical** Apply directly to lesion or dressings; reapply dressings or solutions daily for second- or third-degree burns or q4–5d for second-degree burn with minimum exudation

ADMINISTRATION

Topical

- Confine applications to the part of body being treated. With wet dressings: Protect normal skin surrounding the wound with an agent such as sterile petrolatum, petrolatum gauze, or zinc oxide. Consult physician.
- Facilitate dressing removal by flushing the gauze with sterile isotonic saline solution.
- Consult physician regarding procedure for cleaning wound following each dressing removal.
- Preserve in tight, light-resistant container, away from heat.

ADVERSE EFFECTS (≥1%) **Skin:** *Allergic contact dermatitis,* irritation, sensitization, superinfections.

INTERACTIONS No clinically significant interactions established.

PHARMACOKINETICS Not studied.

NURSING IMPLICATIONS

Assessment & Drug Effects

- Withhold drug and notify physician at onset of symptoms of sensitization or allergy (e.g., redness, itching, burning, swelling, rash, failure to heal), and superinfections (e.g., black furry tongue, thrush, malodorous vaginal discharge, anogenital itching, diarrhea).

Patient & Family Education

- Learn appropriate technique for applying medication to skin lesions.
- Do not breast feed while taking this drug without consulting physician.

NITROGLYCERIN (Pr)

(nye-troe-gli'ser-in)

Cellegesic, Deponit, Minitran, Nitro-Bid, Nitro-Bid IV, Nitrocap, Nitrodisc, Nitro-Dur, Nitrogard, Nitrogard-SR, Nitroglyn, Nitrol, Nitrolingual, Nitrong, Nitrong SR, Nitrospan, Nitrostat, Nitrostat I.V., Nitro-T.D., Transderm-Nitro, Tridil

Classifications: CARDIOVASCULAR AGENT; NITRATE VASODILATOR

Pregnancy Category: C

AVAILABILITY 0.5 mg/mL, 5 mg/mL, 10 mg/mL injection; 0.3 mg, 0.4 mg, 0.6 mg sublingual tablets; 0.4 mg/spray translingual spray; 2 mg, 3 mg buccal tablets; 2.5 mg, 6.5 mg, 9 mg, 13 mg sustained-release tablets, capsules; 0.1 mg/h, 0.2 mg/h, 0.3 mg/h, 0.4 mg/h, 0.6 mg/h, 0.8 mg/h transdermal patch; 2% ointment

ACTIONS Organic nitrate and potent vasodilator that relaxes vascular smooth muscle by unknown mechanism, resulting in dose-related dilation of both venous and arterial blood vessels. Promotes peripheral pooling of blood, reduction of peripheral resistance, and decreased venous return to the heart. Both left ventricular preload and afterload are reduced and myocardial oxygen consumption or demand is decreased.

THERAPEUTIC EFFECTS Therapeutic doses may reduce systolic, diastolic, and mean BP; heart rate is usually slightly increased. Produces antianginal, antiischemic, and antihypertensive effects.

USES Prophylaxis, treatment, and management of angina pectoris. IV nitroglycerin is used to control BP in perioperative hypertension, CHF associated with acute MI; to produce controlled hypotension during surgical procedures, and to treat angina pectoris in patients who have not responded to nitrate or beta-blocker therapy.

UNLABELED USES Sublingual and topical to reduce cardiac workload in patients with acute MI and in CHF. Ointment for adjunctive treatment of Raynaud's disease.

CONTRAINDICATIONS Hypersensitivity, idiosyncrasy, or tolerance to nitrates; severe anemia; head trauma, increased ICP; glaucoma (sustained-release forms). Also (IV nitroglycerin): hypotension, uncorrected hypovolemia, constrictive pericarditis, pericardial tamponade; pregnancy (category C), lactation.

CAUTIOUS USE Severe liver or kidney disease, conditions that cause dry mouth, early MI.

ROUTE & DOSAGE

Angina

Adult: **Sublingual** 1–2 sprays (0.4–0.8 mg) or a 0.3–0.6-mg tablet q3–5min as needed (max: 3 doses in 15 min) **PO** 1.3–9 mg q8–12h **IV** Start with 5 mcg/min and titrate q3–5min until desired response **Transdermal Unit** Apply once q24h or leave on for 10–12 h, then remove and have a 10–12 h nitrate free interval **Topical** Apply 1.5–5 cm (1/2–2 in) of ointment q4–6h

Child: **IV** 0.25–0.5 mcg/kg/min, titrate by 0.5–1 mcg/kg/min q3–5 min

ADMINISTRATION

Note: Drug forms appropriate for angina prophylaxis include ointment, transdermal unit, translingual spray, transmucosal tablet, and oral sustained release forms. Drug forms appropriate for acute angina include sublingual tablet, translingual spray, or transmucosal tablet.

Sublingual Tablet

- Give 1 tablet and if pain is not relieved, give additional tablets at 5-min intervals, but not more than 3 tablets in a 15-min period.
- Leave tablets at bedside. Instruct in correct use. Request patient to report all attacks. Count tablets daily.
- Instruct to sit or lie down upon first indication of oncoming anginal pain and to place tablet under tongue or in buccal pouch (hypotensive effect of drug is intensified in the upright position).

N

Sustained-Release Buccal Tablet

- Place tablet between lip and gum above incisors or between cheek and gum allowing slow dissolution over 3–5 h.
- Touching tongue to tablet or drinking hot fluids hastens tablet dissolution, which can lead to decreased duration of medication effect and onset of anginal pain.
- Ensure that tablet is not chewed or swallowed or crushed.

Sustained-Release Tablet or Capsule

- Give on an empty stomach (1 h before or 2 h after meals), with a full glass of water. Ensure it is swallowed whole.
- Be aware that sustained release form helps to prevent anginal attacks; it is not intended for immediate relief of angina.
- Ensure that tablet is not crushed or chewed.

Translingual Spray

- Do not shake canister. Spray preferably on or under tongue. Do not inhale spray.
- Repeat spray if needed q5min for a maximum of 3 metered doses.
- Instruct to wait at least 10 seconds before swallowing.

Transdermal Ointment

- Using dose-determining applicator (paper application patch) supplied with package, squeeze prescribed dose onto this applicator. Using applicator, spread ointment in a thin, uniform layer to premarked 5.5 by 9 cm (2 1/4 by 3 1/2 in.) square. Place patch with ointment side down onto nonhairy skin surface (areas commonly used: chest, abdomen, anterior thigh, forearm). Cover with transparent wrap and secure with tape. Avoid getting ointment on fingers.
- Rotate application sites to prevent dermal inflammation and sensitization. Remove ointment from previously used sites before reapplication.
- Keep ointment container tightly closed and store in cool place.

Transdermal Unit

- Apply transdermal unit (transdermal patch) at the same time each day, preferably to skin site free of hair and not subject to excessive movement. Avoid abraded, irritated, or scarred skin. Clip hair if necessary.
- Change application site each time to prevent skin irritation and sensitization.

Intravenous

Note: Verify correct IV concentration and rate of infusion in infants and children with physician.

- Check to see if patient has transdermal patch or ointment in place before starting IV infusion. The patch (or ointment) is usually removed to prevent overdosage.

- Be aware that when switching from IV to transdermal nitroglycerin, the IV infusion rate is reduced by 50% with simultaneous application of 5 or 10 mg/24 h transdermal patch.

PREPARE: **IV Infusion:** IV nitroglycerin is available in differing concentrations. Be attentive to the dilution, dosage, and directions for administration on each vial or ampul. Note that a number of nitroglycerin preparations are available prediluted. Other forms must be diluted in D5W or NS, usually to concentrations between 25–500 mcg/mL. Use only glass bottles and manufacturer-supplied IV tubing. Withdraw medication into syringe and inject immediately into the IV solution to minimize contact with plastic. Regular IV tubing can absorb 40%–80% of nitroglycerin.

ADMINISTER: **IV Infusion:** Give by continuous infusion regulated exactly by an infusion pump. IV dosage titration requires careful and continuous hemodynamic monitoring.

INCOMPATIBILITIES **Solution/additive: Hydralazine, phenytoin. Y-site: Alteplase.**

- Use only glass containers for storage of reconstituted IV solution. Polyvinyl chloride (PVC) plastic can absorb nitroglycerin and therefore should not be used. Non-polyvinyl-chloride (non-PVC) sets are recommended or provided by manufacturer.

ADVERSE EFFECTS (≥1%) **CNS:** *Headache,* apprehension, blurred vision, weakness, vertigo, dizziness, faintness. **CV:** *Postural hypotension,* palpitations, tachycardia (sometimes with paradoxical bradycardia), increase in angina, syncope, and circulatory collapse. **GI:** Nausea, vomiting, involuntary passing of urine and feces, abdominal pain, dry mouth. **Hematologic:** Methemoglobinemia (high doses). **Skin:** Cutaneous vasodilation with flushing, rash, exfoliative dermatitis, contact dermatitis with transdermal patch; topical allergic reactions with ointment: pruritic eczematous eruptions, anaphylactoid reaction characterized by oral mucosal and conjunctival edema. **Body as a Whole:** Muscle twitching, pallor, perspiration, cold sweat; local sensation in oral cavity at point of dissolution of sublingual forms.

DIAGNOSTIC TEST INTERFERENCE Nitroglycerin may cause increases in determinations of ***urinary catecholamines*** and ***VMA;*** may interfere with the ***Zlatkis-Zak color reaction,*** causing a false report of decreased ***serum cholesterol.***

INTERACTIONS Drug: Alcohol, ANTIHYPERTENSIVE AGENTS compound hypotensive effects; IV nitroglycerin may antagonize **heparin** anticoagulation.

PHARMACOKINETICS Absorption: Significant loss to first pass metabolism after oral dosing. **Onset:** 2 min SL; 3 min PO; 30 min ointment. **Duration:** 30 min SL; 3–5 h PO; 3–6 h ointment. **Distribution:** Widely distributed; not known if distributes to breast milk. **Metabolism:** Extensively metabolized in liver. **Elimination:** Inactive metabolites excreted in urine. **Half-Life:** 1–4 min.

NURSING IMPLICATIONS

Assessment & Drug Effects

- Administer IV nitroglycerin with extreme caution to patients with hypotension or hypovolemia since the IV drug may precipitate a severe hypotensive state.

N

- Monitor patient closely for change in levels of consciousness and for dysrhythmias. IV nitroglycerin solution contains a substantial amount of ethanol as diluent. Ethanol intoxication can develop with high doses of IV nitroglycerin (vomiting, lethargy, coma, breath smells of alcohol). If intoxication occurs, infusion should be stopped promptly; patient recovers immediately with discontinuation of drug administration.
- Be aware that moisture on sublingual tissue is required for dissolution of sublingual tablet. However, because chest pain typically leads to dry mouth, a patient may be unresponsive to sublingual nitroglycerin.
- Assess for headaches. Approximately 50% of all patients experience mild to severe headaches following nitroglycerin. Transient headache usually lasts about 5 min after sublingual administration and seldom longer than 20 min. Assess degree of severity and consult as needed with physician about analgesics and dosage adjustment.
- Supervise ambulation as needed, especially with older adult or debilitated patients. Postural hypotension may occur even with small doses of nitroglycerin. Patients may complain of dizziness or weakness due to postural hypotension.
- Take baseline BP and heart rate with patient in sitting position before initiation of treatment with transdermal preparations.
- One hour after transdermal (ointment or unit) medication has been applied, check BP and pulse again with patient in sitting position. Report measurements to physician.
- Assess for and report blurred vision or dry mouth.
- Assess for and report the following topical reactions. Contact dermatitis from the transdermal patch; pruritus and erythema from the ointment.
- Be aware that local burning or tingling from the sublingual form has no clinical significance.
- Be alert for overdose symptoms: Hypotension, tachycardia; warm, flushed skin becoming cold and cyanotic; headache, palpitations, confusion, nausea, vomiting, moderate fever, and paralysis. Tissue hypoxia leads to coma, convulsions, cardiovascular collapse. Death can occur from asphyxia.

Patient & Family Education

- Sit or lie down upon first indication of oncoming anginal pain.
- Spit out the rest of your sublingual tablet as soon as pain is completely relieved, especially if you are experiencing unpleasant adverse effects such as headache. Relax for 15–20 min after taking tablet to prevent dizziness or faintness.
- Be aware that pain not relieved by 3 sublingual tablets over a 15-min period may indicate acute MI or severe coronary insufficiency. Contact physician immediately or go directly to emergency room.
- Note: Sublingual tablets may be taken prophylactically 5–10 min prior to exercise or other stimulus known to trigger angina (drug effect lasts 30–60 min).
- Keep record for physician of number of angina attacks, amount of medication required for relief of each attack, and possible precipitating factors.
- Be aware that contact with water (swimming, bathing) does not affect your transdermal unit.
- Remove transdermal unit or ointment immediately from skin and notify physician if faintness, diz-

ziness, or flushing occurs following application.

- You can use a sublingual formulation while transdermal unit or ointment is in place.
- Report blurred vision or dry mouth. Both warrant withdrawal of drug.
- Change position slowly and avoid prolonged standing. Dizziness, light-headedness, and syncope (due to postural hypotension) occur most frequently in older adults.
- Do not drink alcohol too soon after taking nitroglycerin. It may cause severe postural hypotension (sharp drop in BP), vertigo, flushing, or pallor if you drink alcohol too soon after taking nitroglycerin.
- Report any increase in frequency, duration, or severity of anginal attack.
- Withdraw gradually after prolonged use to prevent precipitating anginal attack.
- Do not breast feed while taking this drug without consulting physician.

NITROPRUSSIDE SODIUM

(nye-troe-pruss'ide)

Nipride, Nitropress

Classifications: CARDIOVASCULAR AGENT; ANTIHYPERTENSIVE; NONNITRATE VASODILATOR

Prototype: Hydralazine

Pregnancy Category: C

AVAILABILITY 50 mg injection

ACTIONS Potent, rapid-acting hypotensive agent with effects similar to those of nitrates.

THERAPEUTIC EFFECTS Acts directly on vascular smooth muscle to produce peripheral vasodilation, with consequent marked lowering of arterial BP, associated with slight increase in heart rate, mild decrease in cardiac output, and moderate lowering of peripheral vascular resistance.

USES Short-term, rapid reduction of BP in hypertensive crises and for producing controlled hypotension during anesthesia to reduce bleeding.

UNLABELED USES Refractory CHF or acute MI.

CONTRAINDICATIONS Compensatory hypertension, as in atriovenous shunt or coarctation of aorta, and for control of hypotension in patients with inadequate cerebral circulation. Safety during pregnancy (category C) or lactation is not established.

CAUTIOUS USE Hepatic insufficiency, hypothyroidism, severe renal impairment, hyponatremia, older adult patients with low vitamin B_{12} plasma levels or with Leber's optic atrophy.

N

ROUTE & DOSAGE

Hypertensive Crisis

Adult/Child: **IV** 0.5–10 mcg/kg/min (average 3 mcg/kg/min)

ADMINISTRATION

Intravenous

Note: Solutions must be freshly prepared with D5W and used no later than 4 h after reconstitution.

PREPARE: **Continuous:** Dissolve each 50 mg in 2–3 mL of D5W. Further dilute in 250 mL D5W to yield 200 mcg/mL or 500 mL D5W to yield 100 mcg/mL. Following reconstitution, solutions usually have faint brownish tint; if solution is highly colored, do not use it. Promptly wrap container with aluminum foil or other opaque material to protect drug from light.

ADMINISTER: **Continuous:** Administer by infusion pump or similar device that will allow precise measurement of flow rate required to lower BP. Give at the rate required to lower BP but do not exceed the maximum dose of 10 mcg/kg/min.
INCOMPATIBILITIES **Y-site: cisatracurium, haloperidol.**

- Store reconstituted solutions protected from light; stable for 24 h.

ADVERSE EFFECTS (≥1%) **Body as a Whole:** Diaphoresis, apprehension, restlessness, muscle twitching, retrosternal discomfort. Thiocyanate toxicity (profound hypotension, tinnitus, blurred vision, fatigue, metabolic acidosis, pink skin color, absence of reflexes, faint heart sounds, loss of consciousness). **CV:** Profound hypotension, palpitation, increase or transient lowering of pulse rate, bradycardia, tachycardia, ECG changes. **GI:** Nausea, retching, abdominal pain. **Metabolic:** Increase in serum creatinine, fall or rise in total plasma cobalamins. **CNS:** Headache, dizziness. **Special Senses:** Nasal stuffiness. **Other:** Irritation at infusion site.

INTERACTIONS No clinically significant interactions established.

PHARMACOKINETICS Onset: Within 2 min. **Duration:** 1–10 min after infusion is terminated. **Metabolism:** Rapidly converted to cyanogen in erythrocytes and tissue, which is metabolized to thiocyanate in liver. **Elimination:** Excreted in urine primarily as thiocyanate. **Half-Life:** (thiocyanate): 2.7–7 d.

NURSING IMPLICATIONS

Assessment & Drug Effects

- Monitor constantly to titrate IV infusion rate to BP response.
- Relieve adverse effects by slowing IV rate or by stopping drug; minimize them by keeping patient supine.
- Notify physician immediately if BP begins to rise after drug infusion rate is decreased or infusion is discontinued.
- Monitor I&O.
- Lab tests: Monitor blood thiocyanate level in patients receiving prolonged treatment or in patients with severe kidney dysfunction (levels usually are not allowed to exceed 10 mg/dL). Determine plasma cyanogen level following 1 or 2 d of therapy in patients with impaired liver function.

NIZATIDINE

(ni-za'ti-deen)
Axid, Axid AR
Classifications: GASTROINTESTINAL AGENT; ANTISECRETORY (H_2-RECEPTOR ANTAGONIST)
Prototype: Cimetidine
Pregnancy Category: B

AVAILABILITY 75 mg tablets; 150 mg, 300 mg capsules; 15 mg/mL oral solution

ACTIONS Inhibits secretion of gastric acid by reversible, competitive blockage of histamine at the H_2 receptor, particularly those in the gastric parietal cells.
THERAPEUTIC EFFECTS Significantly reduces nocturnal gastric acid secretion for up to 12 h.

USES Active duodenal ulcers; maintenance therapy for duodenal ulcers.

CONTRAINDICATIONS Hypersensitivity to nizatidine; lactation; children <12 y.
CAUTIOUS USE Hypersensitivity to other H_2-receptor antagonists; renal

impairment or renal failure; older adults; pregnancy (category B).

ROUTE & DOSAGE

Active Duodenal Ulcer
Adult: **PO** 150 mg b.i.d. or 300 mg h.s.
Maintenance Therapy
Adult: **PO** 150 mg h.s.

ADMINISTRATION

Oral
- Give drug usually once daily at bedtime. Dose may be divided and given twice daily.
- Administer oral liquid drug using a calibrated measuring device.
- Be aware that antacids consisting of aluminum and magnesium hydroxides with simethicone decrease nizatidine absorption by about 10%. Administer the antacid 2 h after nizatidine.

ADVERSE EFFECTS (≥1%) **CNS:** Somnolence, fatigue. **Skin:** Pruritus, sweating. **Metabolic:** Hyperuricemia.

INTERACTIONS Drug: May decrease absorption of **delavirdine, didanosine, itraconazole, ketoconazole;** ANTACIDS may decrease absorption of nizatidine.

PHARMACOKINETICS Absorption: >90% absorbed from GI tract. **Peak:** 0.5–3 h. **Metabolism:** Metabolized in liver. **Elimination:** 60% excreted in urine unchanged. **Half-Life:** 1–2 h.

NURSING IMPLICATIONS

Assessment & Drug Effects
- Monitor patient for alleviation of symptoms. Most ulcers should heal within 4 wk.
- Monitor cardiac patient's apical pulse because asymptomatic ventricular tachycardia is an adverse effect of the drug.
- Monitor for persistence of ulcer symptoms in patients who continue to smoke during therapy.
- Lab tests: Monitor liver enzyme studies (AST, ALT) and alkaline phosphatase. Nizatidine may cause hepatocellular injury.

Patient & Family Education
- Take medications for the full course of therapy even though symptoms may be relieved.
- Do not take other prescription or OTC medications without consulting physician.
- Stop smoking; smoking adversely affects healing of ulcers and effectiveness of the drug.
- Do not breast feed while taking this drug without consulting physician.

NONOXYNOL-9
(noe-nox'ee-nole)
Conceptrol, Delfen, Emko, Gynol II, Koromex
Classification: SPERMICIDE CONTRACEPTIVE
Pregnancy Category: C

AVAILABILITY 1%, 2%, 2.2%, 3.5%, 4%, 5% gel; 8%, 12.5% foam; 2.27%, 100 mg, 150 mg suppositories

ACTIONS Nonionic surfactant spermicidal incorporated into foams, gels, jelly, or suppositories.
THERAPEUTIC EFFECTS Applied over the cervix, blocks entrance to uterus by sperm, traps and absorbs seminal fluid, then releases the immediately available spermicide. Immobilizes sperm by cell membrane disruption.

USES As barrier contraceptive alone or in conjunction with a vaginal diaphragm or with a condom.

CONTRAINDICATIONS Cystocele, prolapsed uterus, sensitivity or allergy to polyurethane or to nonoxynol-9; vaginitis; history of TSS; pregnancy; immediately after delivery or abortion; during menstruation.

ROUTE & DOSAGE

Contraceptive
Adult: **Topical** Apply or insert 30–60 min before intercourse. Repeat before each intercourse

ADMINISTRATION

Topical
- Apply foams, gels, jelly, cream: Fully load intravaginal applicator and insert about 2/3 of its length [7.5–10 cm (3–4 in.)] into vagina.
- Use with diaphragm: Place 1–3 tsp spermicide formulation in dome prior to insertion. After diaphragm is in place, additional spermicide is recommended. Leave spermicide and diaphragm in place 6 h after intercourse.

ADVERSE EFFECTS (≥1%) **Urogenital:** *Candidiasis;* vaginal irritation and dryness; increase in vaginal infections; menstrual and nonmenstrual Toxic Shock Syndrome (TSS).

INTERACTIONS Drug: intravaginal AZOLE ANTIFUNGALS may inactivate the spermicides.

PHARMACOKINETICS Onset: Spermicidal action is prompt upon contact with sperm; minimal systemic absorption.

NURSING IMPLICATIONS

Patient & Family Education
- Stop using nonoxynol-9 if pregnancy is suspected.
- Report symptoms of vaginal infection to physician: Burning, inflammation, intense vaginal and vulvar itching, cheesy, curd-like discharge, painful intercourse, dysuria. Nonoxynol-9 antifungal properties are weaker than its antibacterial potency, thus vulvovaginal candidiasis frequently occurs.
- Use spermicide before the first and every subsequent act of intercourse.

NOREPINEPHRINE BITARTRATE

(nor-ep-i-nef′rin)
Levarterenol, Levophed, Noradrenaline
Classifications: AUTONOMIC NERVOUS SYSTEM AGENT; ALPHA- AND BETA-ADRENERGIC AGONIST (SYMPATHOMIMETIC)
Prototype: Epinephrine
Pregnancy Category: D

AVAILABILITY 1 mg/mL injection

ACTIONS Direct-acting sympathomimetic amine identical to body catecholamine norepinephrine. Acts directly and predominantly on alpha-adrenergic receptors; little action on beta receptors except in heart ($beta_1$ receptors). Vasoconstriction and cardiac stimulation; also powerful constrictor action on resistance and capacitance blood vessels.
THERAPEUTIC EFFECTS Peripheral vasoconstriction and moderate inotropic stimulation of heart result in increased systolic and diastolic blood pressure, myocardial oxygenation, coronary artery blood flow, and work of heart. Cardiac output varies with systemic BP.

USES To restore BP in certain acute hypotensive states such as shock, sympathectomy, pheochromocytomectomy, spinal anesthesia, poliomyelitis, MI, septicemia, blood transfusion, and drug reactions. Also as adjunct in treatment of cardiac arrest.

CONTRAINDICATIONS Use as sole therapy in hypovolemic states, except as temporary emergency measure; mesenteric or peripheral vascular thrombosis; profound hypoxia or hypercarbia; use during cyclopropane or halothane anesthesia; pregnancy (category D), lactation.
CAUTIOUS USE Hypertension; hyperthyroidism; severe heart disease; older adult patients; within 14 d of MAOI therapy; patients receiving tricyclic antidepressants.

ROUTE & DOSAGE

Hypotension
Adult: **IV** Start with 8–12 mcg/min, titrate to maintenance dose of 2–4 mcg/min
Child: **IV** Start with 2 mcg/min, titrate to maintenance dose of 0.1 mcg/kg/min

ADMINISTRATION

Intravenous

PREPARE: **IV Infusion:** Dilute a 4 mL ampule in 1000 mL of D5W or D5/NS. Do not use solution if discoloration or precipitate is present. Protect from light.
ADMINISTER: **IV Infusion:** Initial rate of infusion is 2–3 mL/min (8–12 mcg/min), then titrated to maintain BP, usually 0.5–1 mL/min (2–4 mcg/min). An infusion pump is used. Usually give at the slowest rate possible required to maintain BP. Constantly monitor flow rate. Check infusion site frequently and immediately report any evidence of extravasation: blanching along course of infused vein (may occur without obvious extravasation), cold, hard swelling around injection site. Antidote for extravasation ischemia: Phentolamine, 5–10 mg in 10–15 mL NS injection, is infiltrated throughout affected area (using syringe with fine hypodermic needle) as soon as possible. If therapy is to be prolonged, change infusion sites at intervals to allow effect of local vasoconstriction to subside. Avoid abrupt withdrawal; when therapy is discontinued, infusion rate is slowed gradually.
INCOMPATIBILITIES **Solution/additive: Aminophylline, amobarbital, whole blood, cephapirin, chlorothiazide, chlorpheniramine, pentobarbital, phenobarbital, phenytoin, secobarbital, sodium bicarbonate, sodium iodide, streptomycin, thiopental. Y-site: Insulin, thiopental.**

N

ADVERSE EFFECTS (≥1%) **Body as a Whole:** Restlessness, anxiety, *tremors,* dizziness, weakness, insomnia, pallor, plasma volume depletion, edema, hemorrhage, intestinal, <u>hepatic</u>, or renal <u>necrosis</u>, retrosternal and pharyngeal pain, profuse sweating. **CV:** Palpitation, hypertension, reflex bradycardia, <u>fatal arrhythmias</u> (large doses), severe hypertension. **GI:** Vomiting. **Metabolic:** Hyperglycemia. **CNS:** Headache, violent headache, <u>cerebral hemorrhage</u>, convulsions. **Respiratory:** Respiratory difficulty. **Skin:** Tissue necrosis at injection site (with extravasation). **Special Senses:** Blurred vision, photophobia.

INTERACTIONS Drug: ALPHA AND BETA BLOCKERS antagonize pressor effects; ERGOT ALKALOIDS, **furazolidone, guanethidine, methyldopa,** TRICYCLIC ANTIDEPRESSANTS may potentiate pressor effects; **halothane, cyclopropane** increase risk of arrhythmias.

PHARMACOKINETICS Onset: Very rapid. **Duration:** 1–2 min after termination of infusion. **Distribution:** Localizes in sympathetic nerve endings; crosses placenta. **Metabolism:** Metabolized in liver and other tissues by catecholamine o-methyl transferase and monoamine oxidase. **Elimination:** Excreted in urine.

NURSING IMPLICATIONS

Assessment & Drug Effects

- Monitor constantly while patient is receiving norepinephrine. Take baseline BP and pulse before start of therapy, then q2min from initiation of drug until stabilization occurs at desired level, then every 5 min during drug administration.
- Adjust flow rate to maintain BP at low normal (usually 80–100 mm Hg systolic) in normotensive patients. In previously hypertensive patients, systolic is generally maintained no higher than 40 mm Hg below preexisting systolic level.
- Observe carefully and record mental status (index of cerebral circulation), skin temperature of extremities, and color (especially of earlobes, lips, nail beds) in addition to vital signs.
- Monitor I&O. Urinary retention and kidney shutdown are possibilities, especially in hypovolemic patients. Urinary output is a sensitive indicator of the degree of renal perfusion. Report decrease in urinary output or change in I&O ratio.
- Be alert to patient's complaints of headache, vomiting, palpitation, arrhythmias, chest pain, photophobia, and blurred vision as possible symptoms of overdosage. Reflex bradycardia may occur as a result of rise in BP.
- Continue to monitor vital signs and observe patient closely after cessation of therapy for clinical sign of circulatory inadequacy.

NORETHINDRONE

(nor-eth-in′drone)

Micronor, Norlutin, Nor-Q.D.

NORETHINDRONE ACETATE

Aygestin ♣, Norlutate ♣

Classifications: HORMONES AND SYNTHETIC SUBSTITUTES; PROGESTIN

Prototype: Progesterone

Pregnancy Category: X

AVAILABILITY 0.35 mg, 5 mg tablets

ACTIONS Synthetic progestational hormone with androgenic, anabolic, and estrogenic properties (acetate form is the most potent anabolic agent). Mechanism for prevention of contraception unclear.

THERAPEUTIC EFFECTS Progestin-only contraceptives alter cervical mucus, exert progestational effect on endometrium, interfere with implantation, and, in some cases, suppress ovulation. May produce excess estrogenic effect.

USES Amenorrhea, abnormal uterine bleeding due to hormonal imbalance in absence of organic pathology; endometriosis. Also alone or in combination with an estrogen for birth control.

CONTRAINDICATIONS Thromboembolic disorders, cerebral vascular or coronary vascular disease; carcinoma of breast, endometrium, or liver; abnormal vaginal bleeding; known or suspected pregnancy (category X), lactation.

ROUTE & DOSAGE

Amenorrhea

Adult: **PO Norethindrone** 5–20 mg on day 5 through day 25 of menstrual cycle; **Acetate** 2.5–10 mg on day 5 through day 25 of menstrual cycle

Endometriosis

Adult: **PO Norethindrone** 10 mg/d for 2 wk; increase by 5 mg/d q2wk up to 30 mg/d, dose may remain at this level for 6–9 mo or until breakthrough bleeding; **Acetate** 5 mg/d for 2 wk, increase by 2.5 mg/d q2wk up to 15 mg/d, dose may remain at this level for 6–9 mo or until breakthrough bleeding

Progestin-Only Contraception

Adult: **PO Norethindrone** 0.35 mg/d starting on day 1 of menstrual flow, then continuing indefinitely

ADMINISTRATION

Oral

- Note: Dosing schedule is based on a 28-day menstrual cycle.
- Use or add a barrier contraceptive when starting the minipill regimen (progestin-only contraception) for the first cycle or for 3 wk to ensure full protection.
- Protect drug from light and from freezing.

ADVERSE EFFECTS (≥1%) **CNS:** Cerebral thrombosis or hemorrhage, depression. **CV:** Hypertension, pulmonary embolism, edema. **GI:** Nausea, vomiting, cholestatic jaundice, abdominal cramps. **Urogenital:** *Breakthrough bleeding,* cervical erosion, changes in menstrual flow, dysmenorrhea, vaginal candidiasis. **Other:** *Weight changes; breast tenderness,* enlargement or secretion.

INTERACTIONS Drug: BARBITURATES, **carbamazepine, fosphenytoin, modafinil, phenytoin, primidone, pioglitazone, rifampin rifabutin, rifapentine, topiramate, troglitazone** can decrease contraceptive effectiveness.

PHARMACOKINETICS Absorption: Readily absorbed from GI tract. **Metabolism:** Metabolized in liver. **Elimination:** Excreted in urine and feces as metabolites.

NURSING IMPLICATIONS

Assessment & Drug Effects

- Monitor for S&S of thrombophlebitis (see Appendix F).
- Withhold drug and notify physician if any of the following occur: Sudden, complete, or partial loss of vision, proptosis, diplopia, or migraine headache.

Patient & Family Education

- Wait at least 3 mo before becoming pregnant after stopping the minipill to prevent birth defects. Use a barrier or nonhormonal method of contraception until pregnancy is desired.
- If you have not taken all your pills and you miss a period, consider the possibility of pregnancy after 45 d from the last menstrual period; stop using progestin-only contraceptive until pregnancy is ruled out.
- If you have taken all your pills and you miss 2 consecutive periods, rule out pregnancy and use a barrier or nonhormonal method of contraception before continuing the regimen.
- Review package insert to ensure you understand how to use norethindrone.
- Promptly report prolonged vaginal bleeding or amenorrhea.
- Learn and do breast self-examination.

- Keep appointments for physical checkups (q6–12mo) while you are taking hormonal birth control.
- Do not breast feed while taking this drug.

NORFLOXACIN

(nor-flox′a-sin)

Chibroxin, Noroxin

Classifications: ANTIINFECTIVE; QUINOLONE ANTIBIOTIC

Prototype: Ciprofloxacin

Pregnancy Category: C

AVAILABILITY 400 mg tablets; 0.3% ophthalmic solution

ACTIONS Potent broad-spectrum antibiotic activity. Alters structure of bacterial DNA gyrase, thus promoting double-stranded DNA breakage, interfering with synthesis of bacterial protein and blocking bacterial survival.

THERAPEUTIC EFFECTS Active against virtually all bacterial urinary tract pathogens including: *Escherichia coli, Klebsiella pneumoniae, Enterobacter cloacae,* indole-positive *Proteus sp, Pseudomonas aeruginosa, Staphylococcus aureus,* group D *Streptococci, Neisseria gonorrhoeae,* and common GI pathogens (e.g., *Salmonella, Shigella*). Generally ineffective against obligate anaerobes. Development of resistance (especially to *P. aeruginosa, K. pneumoniae, Acinetobacter sp,* and *enterococci*) has been reported, but drug has strong activity against many strains of multiple-antibiotic-resistant bacteria.

USES Complicated and uncomplicated urinary tract infection (UTI) caused by susceptible organisms. Conjunctivitis.

UNLABELED USES Gonorrhea, gastroenteritis, and prevention of travelers' diarrhea.

CONTRAINDICATIONS Use in individual with known factors that predispose to seizures; history of hypersensitivity to norfloxacin and other quinolone antiinfectives; pregnancy (category C), lactation. Safety in children is not established.

CAUTIOUS USE Impaired kidney function, adolescents if skeletal growth is complete.

ROUTE & DOSAGE

Urinary Tract Infection
Adult: **PO** 400 mg b.i.d.

Conjunctivitis
Adult: **Ophthalmic** 1–2 drops q.i.d.

Gonorrhea or Gonococcal Urethritis
Adult: **PO** 800 mg once/d

Bacterial Gastroenteritis
Adult: **PO** 400 mg q8–12h

ADMINISTRATION

Oral

- Give 1 h before or 2 h after meals with a full glass of water.
- Administer concomitant antacid at least 2 h after norfloxacin to prevent interference with absorption. Aluminum or magnesium ions in the antacid may bind to and form insoluble complexes with the quinolone in GI tract.
- Store at 40° C (104° F) or less in tightly closed container. Do not freeze.

ADVERSE EFFECTS (≥1%) **Musculoskeletal:** Joint swelling, cartilage erosion in weight-bearing joints, tendonitis. In immunosuppressed adult: acute ankle and hip pain followed by acute pain, tenderness, and swelling of tendon sheath of middle finger of both hands after 4 wk of therapy. **CNS:** *Headache,* dizziness, lightheadedness, fatigue, drowsiness, somnolence, depression, insomnia, seizures. **GI:** *Nausea,* abdominal pain, diarrhea, vomiting, anorexia, dyspepsia, dysphagia, dry mouth, bitter taste, heartburn, flatulence, pruritus ani, increased serum AST, ALT, alkaline phosphatase. **Hematologic:** Leukopenia, neutropenia. **Urogenital:** With high doses: Crystalluria (not associated with renal toxicity), vulvar irritation.

DIAGNOSTIC TEST INTERFERENCE May cause false positive on ***opiate screening tests.***

INTERACTIONS Drug: ANTACIDS, **iron, sucralfate** decrease absorption; **nitrofurantoin** may antagonize antibacterial effects; may increase hypoprothrombinemic effects of **warfarin;** may cause slight increase in **theophylline** levels.

PHARMACOKINETICS Absorption: 30%–40% absorbed from GI tract. **Peak:** 1–2 h. **Distribution:** Renal parenchyma, gallbladder, liver, prostate; crosses placenta; distributed into breast milk. **Metabolism:** Metabolized in liver. **Elimination:** Excreted in urine and feces. **Half-Life:** 3–4 h.

NURSING IMPLICATIONS

Assessment & Drug Effects

- Collect urine specimens for testing before initiating antibiotic.
- Lab tests: Periodic WBC with differential, liver enzymes, and alkaline phosphatase, especially with prolonged use.
- Report to the physician if patient is adequately hydrated, yet I&O ratio and pattern changes are noted, or if condition does not improve within a few days. Dosage may need to be modified.

Patient & Family Education

- Take drug at same times each day.
- Take drug exactly as prescribed. Erratic dosing can encourage emergence of resistant bacteria; underdosing or premature discontinuation of treatment can cause return of UTI symptoms.
- Keep fluid intake high (at least 2500–3000 mL/d if tolerated) to provide adequate urine output and hydration, important in the prevention of crystalluria (rare side effect).
- Do not breast feed while taking this drug without consulting physician.

NORGESTREL

(nor-jess'trel)

Ovrette

Classifications: HORMONES AND SYNTHETIC SUBSTITUTES; PROGESTIN

Prototype: Progesterone

Pregnancy Category: X

AVAILABILITY 0.075 mg tablets

ACTIONS Potent progestational hormone with androgenic, antiestrogenic, and anabolic properties.

THERAPEUTIC EFFECTS Induces and maintains endometrium, preventing uterine bleeding; inhibits production of pituitary gonadotropin, preventing ovulation; and produces thick cervical mucus resistant to passage of sperm.

USES A progestin-only contraceptive (minipill).

CONTRAINDICATIONS Thromboembolic disorders; cerebral vascular or coronary vascular disease; carcinoma of breast, endometrium, or liver; abnormal vaginal bleeding; known or suspected pregnancy (category X), lactation.

ROUTE & DOSAGE

Progestin-Only Contraception
Adult: **PO** 0.075 mg/d starting on day 1 of menstrual flow, then continuing indefinitely

ADMINISTRATION

Oral
- Use a barrier method of contraception, when starting the minipill regimen, for the first cycle or for 3 wk to insure full protection.
- The minipill can be started right after delivery in the nonlactation mother; however, she should be aware of an increased risk of thromboembolic disease during the postpartum period.
- Take the minipill at same time each day, even if menstruating.
- Store at 15°–30° C (59°–86° F) in a tightly closed container.

N

ADVERSE EFFECTS (≥1%) **CNS:** Cerebral thrombosis or hemorrhage, depression. **CV:** Hypertension, pulmonary embolism, edema. **GI:** Nausea, vomiting, cholestatic jaundice, abdominal cramps. **Urogenital:** *Breakthrough bleeding,* cervical erosion, changes in menstrual flow, dysmenorrhea, vaginal candidiasis. **Endocrine:** *Weight changes; breast tenderness,* enlargement, or secretion.

INTERACTIONS No clinically significant interactions established.

PHARMACOKINETICS Absorption: Readily absorbed from GI tract. **Metabolism:** Metabolized in liver. **Elimination:** Excreted in urine and feces as metabolites.

NURSING IMPLICATIONS

Assessment & Drug Effects
- Monitor for S&S of thrombophlebitis (see Appendix F).
- Withhold drug and notify physician if any of the following occur: Sudden complete or partial loss of vision, proptosis, diplopia, or migraine headache.

Patient & Family Education
- Be aware that amount and duration of flow, cycle length, breakthrough bleeding, spotting, and amenorrhea vary greatly with use of the progestin-only contraceptive.
- Wait at least 3 mo before becoming pregnant after stopping the minipill to prevent birth defects. Use a barrier method of contraception until pregnancy is desired.
- If you have not taken all your pills and you miss a period, consider the possibility of pregnancy after 45 d from the last menstrual period; stop using progestin-only contraceptive until pregnancy is ruled out.
- If you have taken all your pills and you miss 2 consecutive periods, rule out pregnancy and use a barrier or nonhormonal method of contraception before continuing the regimen.
- Review package insert to ensure you understand how to use norgestrel.
- Learn and do breast self-examination.
- Do not breast feed while taking this drug.

NORMAL SERUM ALBUMIN, HUMAN (Pr)

(al-byoo'min)

Albuminar, Albutein, Buminate, Plasbumin

Classifications: BLOOD FORMERS, COAGULATORS, AND ANTICOAGULANTS; BLOOD DERIVATIVE; PLASMA VOLUME EXPANDER

Pregnancy Category: C

AVAILABILITY 5%, 25% injection

ACTIONS Obtained by fractionating pooled venous and placental human plasma, which is then sterilized by filtration and heat to minimize possibility of transmitting hepatitis B virus or HIV. Risk of sensitization is reduced because it lacks cellular elements and contains no coagulation factors, Rh factor, or blood group antibodies.

THERAPEUTIC EFFECTS Expands volume of circulating blood by osmotically shifting tissue fluid into general circulation.

USES To restore plasma volume and maintain cardiac output in hypovolemic shock; for prevention and treatment of cerebral edema; as adjunct in exchange transfusion for hyperbilirubinemia and erythroblastosis fetalis; to increase plasma protein level in treatment of hypoproteinemia; and to promote diuresis in refractory edema. Also used for blood dilution prior to or during cardiopulmonary bypass procedures. Has been used as adjunct in treatment of adult respiratory distress syndrome (ARDS).

CONTRAINDICATIONS Severe anemia; cardiac failure, patients with normal or increased intravascular volume. Safety during pregnancy (category C) or lactation is not established.

CAUTIOUS USE Low cardiac reserve, pulmonary disease, absence of albumin deficiency; liver or kidney failure, dehydration, hypertension, restricted sodium intake.

ROUTE & DOSAGE

Emergency Volume Replacement

Adult: **IV** 25 g, may repeat in 15–30 min if necessary (max: 250 g)

Colloidal Volume Replacement (Nonemergency)

Child: **IV** 12.5 g, may repeat in 15–30 min if necessary

Hyperbilirubinemia, Erythroblastosis Fetalis

Child: **IV** 1 g/kg of 25% solution 1–2 h before transfusion

Hypoproteinemia Prophylaxis in Neonates

Child: **IV** 1.4–1.8 mL/kg of 25% solution

ADMINISTRATION

Intravenous

Note: 5% solution = 5 gm/100 mL; 25% solution = 25 gm/mL.

PREPARE: **IV Infusion:** Normal serum albumin, 5%, is infused without further dilution. Normal serum albumin, 25%, may be infused undiluted or diluted in NS or D5W (with sodium restriction).

ADMINISTER: **IV Infusion: Hypovolemic Shock:** Give initially as rapidly as necessary to restore blood volume. As blood volume approaches normal, rate should be reduced to avoid circulatory overload and pulmonary edema. Give 5% albumin at rate not exceeding 2–4 mL/min. Give 25% albumin at a rate not to exceed 1 mL/min. **With Normal Blood Volume:** Give 5% albumin human at a rate not to exceed 5–10 mL/min; give 25% albumin at a rate not to exceed 2 or 3 mL/min. **Children:** Usual rate is 1/4–1/2 the adult rate.

INCOMPATIBILITIES **Solution/additive: verapamil. Y-site: midazolam, vancomycin, verapamil.**

- Store not to exceed 37° C (98.6° F).
- Use solution within 4 h, once container is opened, because it

contains no preservatives or antimicrobials. Discard unused portion.

ADVERSE EFFECTS (≥1%) **Body as a Whole:** Fever, chills, flushing, increased salivation, headache, back pain. **Skin:** Urticaria, rash. **CV:** Circulatory overload, pulmonary edema (with rapid infusion); hypotension, hypertension, dyspnea, tachycardia. **GI:** Nausea, vomiting.

DIAGNOSTIC TEST INTERFERENCE False rise in ***alkaline phosphatase*** when albumin is obtained partially from pooled placental plasma (levels reportedly decline over period of weeks).

INTERACTIONS No clinically significant interactions established.

NURSING IMPLICATIONS

Assessment & Drug Effects

- Monitor BP, pulse and respiration, and IV albumin flow rate. Adjust flow rate as needed to avoid too rapid a rise in BP.
- Lab tests: Monitor dosage of albumin using plasma albumin (normal): 3.5–5 g/dL; total serum protein (normal): 6–8.4 g/dL; Hgb; Hct; and serum electrolytes.
- Observe closely for S&S of circulatory overload and pulmonary edema (see Appendix F). If S&S appear, slow infusion rate just sufficiently to keep vein open, and report immediately to physician.
- Observe for bleeding points that did not bleed at lower BP with injuries or surgery and as BP rises.
- Monitor I&O ratio and pattern. Report changes in urinary output. Increase in colloidal osmotic pressure usually causes diuresis, which may persist 3–20 h.
- Withhold fluids completely during succeeding 8 h, when albumin is given to patients with cerebral edema.

Patient & Family Education

- Report chills, nausea, headache, or back pain to physician immediately.
- Do not breast feed while taking this drug without consulting physician.

NORTRIPTYLINE HYDROCHLORIDE

(nor-trip'ti-leen)

Aventyl, Pamelor

Classifications: CENTRAL NERVOUS SYSTEM AGENT; PSYCHOTHERAPEUTIC; TRICYCLIC ANTIDEPRESSANT

Prototype: Imipramine

Pregnancy Category: D

AVAILABILITY 10 mg, 25 mg, 50 mg, 75 mg capsules; 10 mg/5 mL solution

ACTIONS Secondary amine derivative of amitriptyline. Action mechanism unclear. Tricyclic antidepressant (TCA) with fewer sedative and anticholinergic effects than imipramine.

THERAPEUTIC EFFECTS Mood elevation may be due to its inhibition of reuptake of norepinephrine at the presynaptic membrane.

USES Endogenous depression. Similar in actions, uses, limitations, and interactions to imipramine.

UNLABELED USES Nocturnal enuresis in children.

CONTRAINDICATIONS Acute recovery period after MI; during or within 14 d of MAO inhibitor therapy. Children <12 y, pregnancy (category D), lactation.

CAUTIOUS USE Narrow-angle glaucoma, hyperthyroidism, concurrent administration of thyroid medications, concurrent use with electroshock therapy.

ROUTE & DOSAGE

Antidepressant

Adult: **PO** 25 mg t.i.d. or q.i.d., gradually increased to 100–150 mg/d
Geriatric: **PO** Start with 10–25 mg h.s., increase by 25 mg q3d to 75 mg h.s. (max: 150 mg/d)
Adolescent: **PO** 30–50 mg/d in divided doses
Child 6–12 y: **PO** 10–20 mg/d in 3–4 divided doses

Nocturnal Enuresis

Child: **PO** *6–7 y,* 10 mg/d; *8–11 y,* 10–20 mg/d; *>11 y,* 25–35 mg/d given 30 min before h.s.

ADMINISTRATION

Oral

- Give with food to decrease gastric distress.
- In older adults, total daily dose may be given once a day h.s. (preferred).
- Be aware that Aventyl is a 4% alcohol solution.
- Supervise drug ingestion to be sure patient swallows medication.
- Store at 15°–30° C (59°–86° F) in tightly closed container.

ADVERSE EFFECTS (≥1%) **Body as a Whole:** Tremors, hyperhydrosis. **CV:** *Orthostatic hypotension.* **GI:** Paralytic ileus, *dry mouth.* **Hematologic:** Agranulocytosis (rare). **CNS:** Drowsiness, confusional state (especially in older adults and with high dosage). **Skin:** Photosensitivity reaction. **Special Senses:** Blurred vision. **Urogenital:** *Urinary retention.*

INTERACTIONS Drug: May decrease some antihypertensive response to ANTIHYPERTENSIVES; CNS DEPRESSANTS, **alcohol,** HYPNOTICS, BARBITURATES, SEDATIVES potentiate CNS depression; may increase hypoprothrombinemic effect of ORAL ANTICOAGULANTS; **ethchlorvynol** may cause transient delirium; **levodopa,** SYMPATHOMIMETICS (e.g., **epinephrine, norepinephrine**) pose possibility of sympathetic hyperactivity with hypertension and hyperpyrexia; MAO INHIBITORS pose possibility of severe reactions: toxic psychosis, cardiovascular instability; **methylphenidate** increases plasma TCA levels; THYROID DRUGS may increase possibility of arrhythmias; **cimetidine** may increase plasma TCA levels. **Herbal: Ginkgo** may decrease seizure threshold. **St. John's wort** may cause **serotonin** syndrome (headache, dizziness, sweating, agitation).

PHARMACOKINETICS Absorption: Rapidly absorbed from GI tract. **Peak:** 7–8.5 h. **Duration:** Crosses placenta; distributed in breast milk. **Metabolism:** Metabolized in liver. **Elimination:** Primarily excreted in urine. **Half-Life:** 16–90 h.

N

NURSING IMPLICATIONS

Assessment & Drug Effects

- Be aware that nortriptyline has a narrow therapeutic plasma level range, or "therapeutic window." Drug levels above or below the therapeutic window are associated with decreased rate of response.
- Therapeutic response may not occur for 2 wk or more.
- Monitor BP and pulse rate during adjustment period of TCA therapy. If systolic BP falls more than 20 mm Hg or if there is a sudden increase in pulse rate, withhold medication and notify the physician.
- Notify physician if psychotic signs increase. Because of the small therapeutic window, a substitute TCA may be prescribed rather than an increase in dosage.
- Inspect oral membranes daily if patient is on high doses of TCA.

Urge outpatient to report stomatitis or dry mouth. Sore mouth can be a major cause of poor nutrition and noncompliance. Consult physician about use of a saliva substitute (e.g., VA-Oralube, Moi-Stir).

- Monitor bowel elimination pattern and I&O ratio. Urinary retention and severe constipation are potential problems, especially in older adults. Advise increased fluid intake; consult physician about stool softener.
- Observe patient with history of glaucoma. Symptoms that may signal acute attack (severe headache, eye pain, dilated pupils, halos of light, nausea, vomiting) should be reported promptly.
- Report reduction or alleviation of fine tremors.
- Be aware that alcohol potentiation may increase the danger of overdosage or suicide attempt.

Patient & Family Education

- Be aware that your ability to perform tasks requiring alertness and skill may be impaired.
- Do not use OTC drugs unless physician approves.
- Consult physician about safe amount of alcohol, if any, that can be ingested. Alcohol and nortriptyline both have increased effects when used together and for up to 2 wk after the TCA is discontinued.
- Nortriptyline enhances the effects of barbiturates and other CNS depressants are enhanced.
- Do not breast feed while taking this drug.

NOVOBIOCIN SODIUM

(noe-voe-bye'o-sin)
Albamycin
Classifications: ANTIINFECTIVE; ANTIBIOTIC
Pregnancy Category: C

AVAILABILITY 250 mg capsules

ACTIONS Antibiotic obtained from cultures of *Streptomyces niveus* or *Streptomyces sphaeroides*. Bacteriostatic action appears to involve interference with synthesis of bacterial cell wall and inhibition of bacterial protein and nucleic acid synthesis.
THERAPEUTIC EFFECTS Active in vitro against many gram-positive bacteria including *Staphylococcus aureus, Streptococcus pneumoniae,* Group A *streptococci, viridans streptococci,* and against some gram-positive bacilli. *Enterococci* are usually resistant to novobiocin. Also active against gram-negative bacteria including *Haemophilus influenzae* and *Neisseria gonorrhoeae*. Resistant strains of *S. aureus* may develop rapidly during therapy.

USES Serious infections due to *S. aureus* in patients unresponsive to less toxic antibiotics or not sensitive to other antibiotics.

CONTRAINDICATIONS Neonates; during pregnancy (category C), lactation.
CAUTIOUS USE Liver dysfunction.

ROUTE & DOSAGE

***S. aureus* Infections**
Adult: **PO** 250 mg q6h or 500 mg q12h up to 2 g/d
Child: **PO** 15–45 mg/kg/d in 2–4 divided doses

ADMINISTRATION

Oral

- Give drug at correct time intervals (i.e., q6h or q12h) to ensure effectiveness.
- Schedule the two drugs at least 3 h apart when novobiocin is given concurrently with TETRACYCLINES.

ADVERSE EFFECTS (≥1%) **GI:** *Nausea, vomiting, diarrhea, anorexia, abdominal distress,* jaundice, elevated serum bilirubin. **Hematologic:** Pancytopenia, agranulocytosis, anemia, thrombocytopenia, hemolytic anemia. **Skin:** *Urticaria,* maculopapular dermatitis, Stevens-Johnson syndrome, erythema multiforme, pruritus, eosinophilia. **Body as a Whole:** Dizziness, drowsiness, light-headedness, swollen joints, fever.

DIAGNOSTIC TEST INTERFERENCE A yellow metabolite may appear if serum interferes with ***serum bilirubin*** determinations (***Evelyn-Malloy method***).

INTERACTIONS Drug: TETRACYCLINES may reduce novobiocin effectiveness.

PHARMACOKINETICS Absorption: Readily absorbed from GI tract. **Peak:** 1–4 h. **Distribution:** Highest concentrations in liver, small intestine, and bile; distributed into breast milk. **Elimination:** Excreted primarily in bile and feces.

NURSING IMPLICATIONS

Assessment & Drug Effects

- Report adverse effects promptly; this drug is an extremely potent sensitizing agent.
- Be aware that a yellow metabolite of novobiocin can cause jaundice-like skin coloration. Differentiation of drug-induced effect from frank jaundice will depend on other signs of liver dysfunction (i.e., dark urine, pruritus, elevated serum bilirubin). Advise patient to report symptoms promptly.
- Lab tests: CBC with differential, platelet count, Hct and Hgb, liver function tests at the first sign of an adverse response.
- Inspect skin for signs of thrombocyte dyscrasia: petechiae, ecchymoses, easy bruising. Promptly report these signs or epistaxis or bleeding for unexplained reason.

Patient & Family Education

- Report any reversal in prior evidence of therapeutic response to drug therapy. Drug resistance may develop rapidly.
- Do not stop treatment just because you feel better. Duration of therapy depends on the infection but it will continue about 48 h after your fever is gone or there is no more evidence of the infection.
- Do not change your treatment regimen without consulting physician; sensitivity and adverse effects may occur as well as a loss of therapeutic effects.
- Do not use leftover novobiocin to self-medicate for another infection.
- Report symptoms of superinfections (see Appendix F) immediately because they should receive prompt attention.
- Do not breast feed while taking this drug.

NYSTATIN

(nye-stat'in)

Mycostatin, Nadostine ♣, Nilstat, Nyaderm ♣, Nystex, O-V Statin

Classifications: ANTIINFECTIVE; ANTIFUNGAL ANTIBIOTIC

Prototype: Fluconazole

Pregnancy Category: C

AVAILABILITY 500,000 unit tablets; 100,000 units/mL oral suspension; 200,000 troches; 100,000 units vaginal tablets; 100,000 units/g cream, ointment, powder.

ACTIONS Nontoxic, nonsensitizing antifungal antibiotic produced by *Streptomyces noursei.* Binds to

N

sterols in fungal cell membrane, thereby changing membrane potential and allowing leakage of intracellular components.
THERAPEUTIC EFFECTS Fungistatic and fungicidal activity against a variety of yeasts and fungi; not appreciably active against bacteria, viruses, or protozoa.

USES Local infections of skin and mucous membranes caused by *Candida sp* including *Candida albicans* (e.g., paronychia; cutaneous, oropharyngeal, vulvovaginal, and intestinal candidiasis).

CONTRAINDICATIONS Use of vaginal tablets during pregnancy (category C); vaginal infections caused by *Gardnerella vaginalis* or *Trichomonas sp.*
CAUTIOUS USE Lactation.

ROUTE & DOSAGE

***Candida* Infections**

Adult: **PO** 500,000–1,000,000 U t.i.d.; 1–4 troches 4–5 times/d; Suspension: 400,000–600,000 U q.i.d. **Intravaginal** 1–2 tablets daily for 2 wk
Child: **PO** Suspension: 400,000–600,000 U q.i.d.
Infant: **PO** 100,000–200,000 U q.i.d.

ADMINISTRATION

Oral
- Give reconstituted powder for oral suspension immediately after mixing.
- Rinse mouth with 1–2 tsp using oral suspension. Keep in mouth (swish) as long as possible (at least 2 min), then spit it out. (If you cannot keep the liquid in your mouth or cannot spit, or if you have been told to "swish and swallow," you may swallow the drug.) For children, infants: Apply drug with swab to each side of mouth. Avoid food or drink for 30 min after treatment.

Topical
- Store vaginal tablets in refrigerator below 15° C (59° F).

ADVERSE EFFECTS (≥1%) **GI:** Nausea, vomiting, epigastric distress, diarrhea (especially with high oral doses).

PHARMACOKINETICS Absorption: Poorly absorbed from GI tract. **Elimination:** Excreted in feces.

NURSING IMPLICATIONS

Assessment & Drug Effects
- Monitor oral cavity, especially the tongue, for signs of improvement.
- Avoid occlusive dressings or applications of ointment preparation to moist, dark areas of body because they favor growth of yeast.

Patient & Family Education
- This drug may cause contact dermatitis. Stop using the drug and report to physician if redness, swelling, or irritation develops.
- Take for oral candidiasis (thrush) treatment after meals and at bedtime.
- Dissolve troche in mouth (about 30 min). Do not chew or swallow. Avoid food and drink during period of dissolving and for 30 min after treatment.
- Care of dentures: Remove dentures before each rinse with oral suspension and before use of troche. Remove dentures at night (infection occurs more frequently in person who wears dentures 24 h a day).
- Dust shoes and stockings, as well as feet, with nystatin dusting powder.
- Your physician will probably prescribe cream instead of ointment for intertriginous areas. For

very moist lesions, powder is usually prescribed. Gently clean infected areas with tepid water before each application.

- Be aware that treatment of cutaneous candidal infections is continued for at least 2 wk and discontinued only after two negative tests for Candida.
- Continue medication for vulvovaginal candidiasis during menstruation. In most cases, 2 wk of therapy are sufficient; however, some patients may require longer treatment.
- Use vaginal tablets up to 6 wk before term to prevent thrush in the newborn.
- Do not breast feed while taking this drug without consulting physician.

OCTREOTIDE ACETATE

(oc-tre′o-tide)

Sandostatin, Sandostatin LAR depot

Classifications: HORMONES AND SYNTHETIC SUBSTITUTES; ANTIDIARRHEAL

Pregnancy Category: B

AVAILABILITY 0.05 mg/mL, 0.1 mg/mL, 0.2 mg/mL, 0.5 mg/mL, 1 mg/mL injection; 10 mg/5 mL, 20 mg/5 mL, 30 mg/5 mL depot injection

ACTIONS A long-acting peptide that mimics the natural hormone somatostatin. Suppresses secretion of serotonin, pancreatic peptides, gastrin, vasoactive intestinal peptide, insulin, glucagon, secretin, and motilin.

THERAPEUTIC EFFECTS Stimulates fluid and electrolyte absorption from the GI tract, prolongs intestinal transit time, and also inhibits the growth hormone.

USES Symptomatic treatment of severe diarrhea and flushing episodes associated with metastatic carcinoid tumors. Also watery diarrhea associated with vasoactive intestinal peptide (VIP) tumors.

UNLABELED USES Acromegaly associated with pituitary tumors, fistula drainage, variceal bleeding.

CONTRAINDICATIONS Hypersensitivity to octreotide.

CAUTIOUS USE Cholelithiasis, renal impairment; pregnancy (category B); diabetes, and hypothyroidism. It is not known whether drug is excreted in breast milk.

ROUTE & DOSAGE

Carcinoid Syndrome

Adult: **SC** 100–600 mcg/d in 2–4 divided doses, titrate to response **IM** May switch to depot injection after 2 wk at 20 mg q4wk times 2 mo
Child: **SC** 1–10 mcg/kg/d in 2–4 divided doses, titrate to response

VIPoma

Adult: **SC** 200–300 mcg/d in 2–4 divided doses, titrate to response **IM** May switch to depot injection after 2 wk at 20 mg q4wk times 2 mo
Child: **SC** 1–10 mcg/kg/d in 2–4 divided doses, titrate to response

Acromegaly

Adult: **SC** 50 mcg t.i.d., titrate up to 100 mcg–500 mcg t.i.d. **IM** May switch to depot injection after 2 wk at 20 mg q4wk times at least 3 mo, then reassess

ADMINISTRATION

Subcutaneous/Intramuscular

- Note: Subcutaneous is the preferred route.

O

- Minimize GI side effects by giving injections between meals and at bedtime.
- Avoid multiple injections into the same site. Rotate SC sites on abdomen, hip, and thigh.
- Give deep IM into a large muscle. To reduce local irritation, allow solution to reach room temperature before injection and administer slowly.

Intravenous

PREPARE: **Direct:** Give undiluted. **Intermittent:** Dilute in 50–200 mL D5W.

ADMINISTER: **Direct:** Give a single dose over 3 min. In carcinoid give rapid IV bolus over 60 s. **Intermittent:** Give over 15–30 min.

ADVERSE EFFECTS (≥1%) **CNS:** Headache, fatigue, dizziness. **GI:** *Nausea, diarrhea,* abdominal pain and discomfort. **Metabolic:** Hypoglycemia, hyperglycemia, increased liver transaminases, hypothyroidism (after long-term use). **Body as a Whole:** Flushing, edema, injection site pain.

INTERACTIONS Drug: May decrease **cyclosporine** levels; may alter other drug and nutrient absorption because of alterations in GI motility.

PHARMACOKINETICS Absorption: Rapidly absorbed from SC injection site. **Peak:** 0.4 h. **Duration:** Up to 12 h. **Metabolism:** 68% metabolized in liver. **Elimination:** Excreted in urine. **Half-Life:** 1.5 h.

NURSING IMPLICATIONS

Assessment & Drug Effects

- Lab tests: Periodic blood glucose, liver function tests, and serum electrolytes.
- Monitor for hypoglycemia and hyperglycemia (see Appendix F), because octreotide may alter the balance between insulin, glucagon, and growth hormone.
- Monitor fluid and electrolyte balance, as octreotide stimulates fluid and electrolyte absorption from GI tract.
- Dietary fat absorption may be altered in some clients. Monitor fecal fat and serum carotene to aid in the assessment of possible drug-induced aggravation of fat malabsorption.

Patient & Family Education

- Learn proper technique for SC injection if self-medication is required.
- Note: Preferred sites for SC injections of octreotide are the hip, thigh, and abdomen. Multiple injections at the same SC injection site within short periods of time are not recommended. This is to avoid irritating the area.

OFLOXACIN

(o-flox′a-cin)

Floxin, Floxin Otic, Ocuflox

Classifications: ANTIINFECTIVE; ANTIBIOTIC, QUINOLONE

Prototype: Ciprofloxacin

Pregnancy Category: C

AVAILABILITY 200 mg, 300 mg, 400 mg tablets; 200 mg, 400 mg injection; 0.3% ophthalmic solution; 0.3% otic solution

ACTIONS A fluoroquinolone antibiotic with a broad spectrum of activity against gram-positive and gram-negative aerobic and anaerobic bacteria. Inhibits DNA gyrase, an enzyme necessary for bacterial DNA replication and some aspects of its transcription, repair, recombination, and transposition.

THERAPEUTIC EFFECTS Most effective against gram-negative organisms including *Citrobacter diversus, C. freundii, Enterobacter cloacae, E. aerogenes, Escherichia coli, Klebsiella* species, *Morganella morganii, Proteus* species, *Salmonella* species, *Shigella* species, and *Yersinia enterocolitica*. More potent against *Serratia* species than is norfloxacin, and it is equipotent against *Providencia* species; less active against *Pseudomonas aeruginosa* but more potent against *Xanthomonas maltophilia* than is ciprofloxacin.

USES *Chlamydia trachomatis* infection, uncomplicated gonorrhea, prostatitis, respiratory tract infections, skin and skin structure infections, urinary tract infections due to susceptible bacteria, superficial ocular infections, pelvic inflammatory disease. Otic: otitis externa, otitis media with perforated tympanic membranes.

UNLABELED USES EENT infections, *Helicobacter pylori* infections, *Salmonella* gastroenteritis.

CONTRAINDICATIONS Hypersensitivity to ofloxacin or other quinolone antibacterial agents; tendon pain; sunlight (UV) exposure; viral infection; pregnancy (category C); lactation.

CAUTIOUS USE Renal disease; patients with a history of epilepsy, psychosis, or increased intracranial pressure, cerebrovascular disease, CNS disorders such as seizures, epilepsy, myasthenia gravis; GI disease, colitis, dehydration; syphilis. Safety and effectiveness in children and adolescents <18 y (except for otic preparation) are not established.

ROUTE & DOSAGE

Uncomplicated Gonorrhea
Adult: **PO** 400 mg for 1 dose

Urinary Tract, Respiratory Tract, and Skin and Skin Structure Infections
Adult: **PO** 200–400 mg q12h times 7–10 d **IV** 400 mg q12h times 7 d

Prostatitis
Adult: **PO** 300 mg b.i.d. times 6 wk **IV** 300 mg q12h times 10 d, then switch to **PO** for 6 wk

Superficial Ocular Infections
Adult: **Ophthalmic** Instill 1–2 drops q2–4h for first 2d, then q.i.d. for up to 5 additional d

Otitis Media with Perforation
Adult: **Otic** 10 drops (0.5 mL) q12h for 14 d
Child: **Otic** *≥1 y*, 5 drops (0.25 mL) q12h for 14 d

Otitis Externa
Adult: **Otic** 10 drops (0.5 mL) q12h for 7 d
Child: **Otic** *6 mo–13 y*, 5 drops (0.25 mL) q12h for 7 d

ADMINISTRATION

Oral

- Do not give with meals.
- Avoid administering mineral supplements or vitamins with iron or zinc within 2 h of drug.
- Do not give antacids with magnesium, aluminum, or sucralfate within 4 h before or 2 h after drug.

Instillation

- Do NOT allow tip of dropper for ocular preparation to contact any surface.

Intravenous

PREPARE: **Intermittent:** Withdraw the required dose from a 10 mL

(40 mg/mL) or 20 mL (20 mg/mL) vial and add to 100 mL D5W, NS, D5/NS or other compatible solution. Final concentration may range from 0.4 mg/mL to 4 mg/mL.

ADMINISTER: **Intermittent:** Give a single dose over at least 60 min. Avoid rapid infusion.

INCOMPATIBILITIES **Y-site: Amphotericin B cholesteryl sulfate complex, cefepime, doxorubicin liposome.**

ADVERSE EFFECTS (≥1%) **CNS:** *Headache, dizziness, insomnia,* hallucinations. **GI:** Nausea, vomiting, diarrhea, GI discomfort. **Urogenital:** Pruritus, pain, irritation, burning, vaginitis, vaginal discharge, dysmenorrhea, menorrhagia, dysuria, urinary frequency. **Skin:** Pruritus, rash.

DIAGNOSTIC TEST INTERFERENCE May cause false positive on ***opiate screening tests.***

O

INTERACTIONS Drug: Ofloxacin absorption decreased when it is administered with MAGNESIUM- or ALUMINUM-CONTAINING ANTACIDS. Other CATIONS, including **calcium, iron,** and **zinc,** also appear to interfere with ofloxacin absorption.

PHARMACOKINETICS Absorption: 90%–98% absorbed from GI tract. **Peak:** 1–2 h. **Distribution:** Distributes to most tissues; 50% crosses into CSF with inflamed meninges; 20%–32% protein bound; crosses placenta; distributed into breast milk. **Metabolism:** Slightly metabolized in liver. **Elimination:** 72%–98% excreted in urine within 48 h. **Half-Life:** 5–7.5 h.

NURSING IMPLICATIONS

Assessment & Drug Effects

- Lab tests: Do C&S tests prior to initial dose. Treatment may be implemented pending results.
- Determine history of hypersensitivity reactions to quinolones or other drugs before therapy is started.
- Withhold ofloxacin and notify physician at first sign of a skin rash or other allergic reaction.
- Monitor for seizures, especially in patients with known or suspected CNS disorders. Discontinue ofloxacin and notify physician immediately if seizure occurs.
- Assess for signs and symptoms of superinfection (see Appendix F).

Patient & Family Education

- Drink fluids liberally unless contraindicated.
- Be aware that dizziness or lightheadedness may occur; use appropriate caution.
- Avoid excessive sunlight or artificial ultraviolet light because of the possibility of phototoxicity.
- Do not breast feed while taking this drug.

OLANZAPINE

(o-lan′za-peen)

Zyprexa, Zyprexa Zydis, Zyprexa IntraMuscular

Classifications: CENTRAL NERVOUS SYSTEM (CNS) AGENT; PSYCHOTHERAPEUTIC AGENT; ANTIPSYCHOTIC AGENT; ATYPICAL; SELECTIVE SEROTONIN REUPTAKE INHIBITOR; DOPAMINE-REUPTAKE INHIBITOR

Prototype: Clozapine

Pregnancy Category: C

AVAILABILITY 2.5 mg, 5 mg, 7.5 mg, 10 mg, 15 mg tablets; 10 mg, 15 mg, 20 mg orally-disintegrating tablets; 10 mg powder for injection

ACTIONS Antipsychotic activity is thought to be due to antagonism for both serotonin $5HT_{2A/2C}$ and dopamine D_{1-4} receptors. May inhibit the CNS presynaptic neuronal reuptake of serotonin and dopa-

mine. Antagonism of alfa-adrenergic receptors results in the adverse effect of orthostatic hypotension.
THERAPEUTIC EFFECTS Produces antipsychotic and anticholinergic activity.

USES Management of psychotic disorders, treatment of bipolar disorder, acute agitation (IM).
UNLABELED USES Alzheimer's dementia.

CONTRAINDICATIONS Hypersensitivity to olanzapine; abrupt discontinuation, coma, severe CNS depression, subcutaneous or intramuscular injection of olanzapine; tardive dyskinesia; infants, pregnancy (category C), lactation.
CAUTIOUS USE Known cardiovascular disease, neurological disease, stroke, cerebrovascular disease, Parkinson disease, dementia; history of seizures, conditions that predispose to hypotension (i.e., dehydration, hypovolemia); history of syncope; history of breast cancer; Japanese; diabetes mellitus; prostatic hypertrophy; closed-angle glaucoma; paralytic ileus; urinary retention; hepatic or renal impairment, concurrent use of hepatotoxic drugs, jaundice; predisposition to aspiration pneumonia; may increase risk of stroke in elderly patients with dementia; history of or high risk for suicide. Safety and effectiveness in children <18 y are not established.

ROUTE & DOSAGE

Psychotic Disorders
Adult: **PO** Start with 5–10 mg once/d, may increase by 2.5–5 mg q wk until desired response (usual range 10–15 mg/d, max: 20 mg/d)
Geriatric: **PO** Start with 5 mg once/d

Bipolar Mania
Adult: **PO** Start with 10–15 mg once/d, may increase by 5 mg q24h if needed

Acute Agitation
Adult: **IM** 10 mg, do not repeat more frequently than q2h (max: 30 mg/24h)
Geriatric: **IM** 2.5–5 mg once

ADMINISTRATION

Oral
- Do not push orally disintegrating tablet through blister foil. Peel foil back and remove tablet. Tablet will disintegrate with/without liquid.

ADVERSE EFFECTS (≥1%) **Body as a Whole:** *Weight gain,* fever, back and chest pain, peripheral and lower extremity edema, joint pain, twitching, premenstrual syndrome. **CNS:** *Somnolence, dizziness, headache, agitation, insomnia, nervousness, hostility,* anxiety, personality disorder, akathisia, hypertonia, tremor amnesia, euphoria, stuttering, extrapyramidal symptoms (dystonic events, *parkinsonism, akathisia*), tardive dyskinesia. **CV:** Postural hypotension, hypotension, tachycardia. **Special Senses:** Amblyopia, blepharitis. **GI:** Abdominal pain, constipation, dry mouth, increased appetite, increased salivation, nausea, vomiting, elevated liver function tests. **Metabolic:** Hyperglycemia, diabetes mellitus. **Urogenital:** Premenstrual syndrome, hematuria, urinary incontinence, metrorrhagia. **Respiratory:** Rhinitis, cough, pharyngitis, dyspnea. **Skin:** Rash.

INTERACTIONS Drug: May enhance hypotensive effects of ANTIHYPERTENSIVES. May enhance effects of other CNS ACTIVE DRUGS, **alcohol. Carbamazepine, omeprazole, rif-**

ampin may increase metabolism and clearance of olanzapine. **Fluvoxamine** may inhibit metabolism and clearance of olanzapine. **Herbal: St. John's wort** may cause **serotonin** syndrome (headache, dizziness, sweating, agitation).

PHARMACOKINETICS Absorption: Rapidly absorbed from GI tract, 60% reaches systemic circulation. **Onset:** 15 min IM. **Peak:** 6 h. **Distribution:** 93% protein bound, secreted into breast milk of animals (human secretion unknown). **Metabolism:** Metabolized in liver, primarily by cytochrome P450 1A2 (CYP1A2). **Elimination:** Approximately 57% excreted in urine, 30% in feces. **Half-Life:** 21–54 h.

NURSING IMPLICATIONS

Assessment & Drug Effects

- Monitor diabetics for loss of glycemic control.
- Withhold drug and immediately report S&S of neuroleptic malignant syndrome (see Appendix F); assess for and report S&S of tardive dyskinesia (see Appendix F).
- Lab tests: Periodically monitor ALT, especially in those with hepatic dysfunction or being treated with other potentially hepatotoxic drugs. Periodic blood glucose monitoring.
- Monitor BP and HR periodically. Monitor temperature, especially under conditions such as strenuous exercise, extreme heat, or treatment with other anticholinergic drugs.
- Monitor for seizures, especially in older adults and cognitively impaired persons.

Patient & Family Education

- Carefully monitor blood glucose levels if diabetic.
- Do not drive or engage in potentially hazardous activities until response to drug is known; drug increases risk of orthostatic hypotension and cognitive impairment.
- Learn common adverse effects and possible drug interactions.
- Avoid alcohol and do not take additional medications without informing physician.
- Do not become overheated; avoid conditions leading to dehydration.
- Do not breast feed while taking this drug.

OLMESARTAN MEDOXOMIL

(ol-me-sar'tan)

Benicar

Classifications: CARDIOVASCULAR AGENT; ANGIOTENSIN II RECEPTOR ANTAGONIST

Prototype: Losartan

Pregnancy Category: C (first trimester); D (second & third trimesters)

AVAILABILITY 5 mg, 20 mg, 40 mg tablets

ACTIONS Angiotensin II receptor (type AT1) antagonist acts as a potent vasoconstrictor and primary vasoactive hormone of the renin-angiotensin-aldosterone system.

THERAPEUTIC EFFECTS Selectively blocks the binding of angiotensin II to the AT1 receptors found in many tissues (e.g., vascular smooth muscle, adrenal glands). Antihypertensive effect results from blocking the vasoconstricting and aldosterone-secreting effects of angiotensin II.

USES Treatment of hypertension.

CONTRAINDICATIONS Hypersensitivity to pimecrolimus or components in the cream; Netherton's Syndrome; application to active cutaneous viral infection.

CAUTIOUS USE Infection at topical treatment site; history of untoward effects with topical cyclosporine or tacrolimus; skin papillomas; immunocompromised patients.

ROUTE & DOSAGE

Hypertension
Adult: **PO** 20 mg q.d., may increase to 40 mg q.d. Start with 5–10 mg q.d. if volume depleted

ADMINISTRATION

Oral
- Determine if patient is volume depleted (e.g., patients treated with diuretics) prior to first administration of drug. If volume depletion is suspected, a lower starting dose is recommended.
- Store at 20°–25° C (68°–77° F).

ADVERSE EFFECTS (≥1%) **Body as a Whole:** Back pain, flu-like symptoms. **CNS:** Headache. **CV:** Hypotension (especially if dehydrated). **GI:** Diarrhea. **Metabolic:** Increased CPK, hyperglycemia, hypertriglyceridemia. **Respiratory:** Bronchitis, pharyngitis, rhinitis, sinusitis, upper respiratory infection. **Urogenital:** Hematuria.

INTERACTIONS Drug: May increase hypotensive effect of other ANTIHYPERTENSIVES; may cause hyperkalemia with POTASSIUM-SPARING DIURETICS, POTASSIUM SUPPLEMENTS; increase risk of **lithium** toxicity. **Herbal:** Ephedra, Ma-Huang may antagonize antihypertensive effects.

PHARMACOKINETICS Absorption: Rapidly absorbed, 26% reaches systemic circulation. **Peak:** 1–2 h. **Distribution:** 99% protein bound. **Metabolism:** Not metabolized by CYP 450 system. **Elimination:** 50% excreted in urine, 50% excreted in feces. **Half-Life:** 13 h.

NURSING IMPLICATIONS

Assessment & Drug Effects
- Monitor closely any volume-depleted patient following initial drug doses. If serious hypotension occurs, place patient in supine position and notify physician immediately.
- Monitor BP and HR at drug trough (prior to a scheduled dose). Report hypotension or bradycardia.
- Monitor drug effectiveness, especially in African-Americans, when olmesartan is used as monotherapy.
- Lab tests: Monitor baseline and periodic renal functions; monitor CBC, electrolytes, and liver function with long-term therapy.

Patient & Family Education
- Discontinue drug and notify physician if you experience swelling of the face, tongue, or throat, or if you believe you are pregnant.
- Notify physician of symptoms of hypotension (e.g., dizziness, fainting).
- Do not breast feed while taking this drug without consulting physician.

O

OLOPATADINE HYDROCHLORIDE

(o-lo-pa'ta-deen)
Patanol
Classifications: EYE PREPARATION; OCULAR ANTIHISTAMINE
Prototype: Levocabastine
Pregnancy Category: C

AVAILABILITY 0.1% ophthalmic solution
See Appendix A-1.

OLSALAZINE SODIUM

(ol-sal'a-zeen)

Dipentum

Classifications: GASTROINTESTINAL; MUCOUS MEMBRANE ANTIINFLAMMATORY AGENT

Prototype: Mesalamine

Pregnancy Category: C

AVAILABILITY 250 mg capsules

ACTIONS Converted to 5-aminosalicylic acid (5-ASA) by colonic bacteria. The 5-ASA is absorbed slowly, resulting in a very high local concentration in the colon.

THERAPEUTIC EFFECTS The 5-ASA has antiinflammatory activity in ulcerative colitis.

USES Maintenance therapy in patients with ulcerative colitis.

UNLABELED USES Acute flare-up of ulcerative colitis.

CONTRAINDICATIONS Hypersensitivity to salicylates.

CAUTIOUS USE Patients with preexisting kidney disease; pregnancy (category C). It is not known whether it is excreted in breast milk. Safety and effectiveness in children are not established.

ROUTE & DOSAGE

Ulcerative Colitis
Adult: **PO** 500 mg b.i.d., may increase up to 1.5–3 g/d in 2–4 divided doses

ADMINISTRATION

Oral

- Give with food in two evenly divided doses.

ADVERSE EFFECTS (≥1%) **CNS:** Headache. **GI:** *Diarrhea,* nausea, abdominal pain, indigestion, vomiting, bloating. **Skin:** Rash. **Body as a Whole:** Arthralgia.

PHARMACOKINETICS Absorption: 1%–3% absorbed from GI tract; high colonic concentrations are associated with efficacy. **Metabolism:** Olsalazine, a prodrug, is composed of 2 molecules of 5-ASA, the proposed active antiinflammatory agent, connected by an azo bond; colonic bacterial azo-reductases break the azo bond, thus releasing 2 active molecules of 5-ASA. **Elimination:** Primarily eliminated in feces as 5-ASA. **Half-Life:** At least 6 h.

NURSING IMPLICATIONS

Assessment & Drug Effects

- Monitor kidney function in patients with preexisting renal disease.
- Monitor for S&S of a hypersensitivity reaction (see Appendix F). Withhold olsalazine and notify physician at first sign of an allergic response.

Patient & Family Education

- Report diarrhea, a possible adverse effect, to the physician.

OMALIZUMAB

(o-mal-i-zoo'mab)

Xolair

Classifications: BIOLOGIC RESPONSE MODIFIER; MONOCLONAL ANTIBODY; RESPIRATORY ANTIINFLAMMATORY AGENT

Prototype: Basiliximab

Pregnancy Category: B

AVAILABILITY 150 mg vial

ACTIONS DNA recombinant monoclonal antibody that selectively binds to human IgE. It inhibits binding of IgE to high-affinity IgE receptor on the surface of mast cells and basophils, limiting the release of inflammatory mediators.

THERAPEUTIC EFFECTS Inhibits release of mediators of the allergic response and has an anti-inflammatory action on the respiratory system.

USES Control of moderate to severe allergic asthma.
UNLABELED USES Seasonal allergic rhinitis, food allergies.

CONTRAINDICATIONS Hypersensitivity to omalizumab; severe infections, including chicken pox and other viral infections; acute bronchospasm, status asthmaticus; malignancies; children <12 y.
CAUTIOUS USE Pregnancy (category B), lactation.

ROUTE & DOSAGE

Allergic Asthma
Adult/Adolescent: **SC** 150–375 mg q2–4wk. Dose is based on baseline IgE serum levels

ADMINISTRATION

Subcutaneous

- Reconstitute as follows: 1) Draw 1.4 mL of sterile water for injection into a 3-cc syringe with a 1-inch, 18-gauge needle. 2) Place vial upright on flat surface and inject sterile water. Keep vial upright and gently swirl for about 1 min to wet powder. Do not shake. 3) Gently swirl vial for 5–10 sec q5min to dissolve remaining solids. Some vials may take >20 min to dissolve. Do not use if not completely dissolved by 40 min. 4) Once dissolved, invert vial for 15 sec to allow solution to drain toward stopper. 5) Using a new 3-cc syringe with a 1-inch, 18-gauge needle, insert needle into inverted vial with tip at the very bottom of solution, then withdraw solution. Before removing needle from vial, pull the plunger to end of syringe barrel to remove all solution from inverted vial. 6) Replace 18-gauge needle with a 25-gauge needle for SC injection. 7) Expel air, large bubbles, and any excess solution to obtain the required 1.2 mL dose. A thin layer of small bubbles may remain at top of the solution in syringe.
- Give SC and rotate injection sites. Solution is viscous and takes 5–10 sec to inject.
- Use within 8 h of reconstitution when stored in the vial at 2°–8° C (36°–46° F), or within 4 h of reconstitution when stored at room temperature.

ADVERSE EFFECTS (≥1%) **Body as a Whole:** Anaphylaxis/anaphylactoid reactions, *injection site reactions (bruising, erythema, warmth, burning, stinging, pruritus, hive formation, pain, induration, inflammation),* fatigue, generalized pain. **CNS:** Headache, dizziness. **GI:** *Nausea, vomiting, diarrhea, abdominal pain.* **Hematologic:** Epistaxis, menorrhagia, hematoma, anemia. **Musculoskeletal:** Arthralgia. **Respiratory:** Upper respiratory tract infections, sinusitis, pharyngitis. **Skin:** Rash, pruritus, urticaria, dermatitis. **Special Senses:** Earache.

PHARMACOKINETICS Absorption: Slowly absorbed from SC site; 53%–71% reaches systemic circulation. **Peak:** 7–8 d. **Half-Life:** 22 d.

NURSING IMPLICATIONS

Assessment & Drug Effects

- Monitor for injection site reactions including bruising, redness, warmth, burning, stinging, itching, hive formation, pain, indurations, mass, and inflammation.
- Lab test: Platelet counts if signs of increased tendency to bleed appear.

O

Patient & Family Education

- Do not use this drug for relief of acute bronchospasm or status asthmaticus.
- Promptly report any of the following: bleeding or unusual bruising, difficulty breathing or shortness of breath, skin rash or hives.
- Do not accept a live virus vaccine without consulting physician.
- Do not breast feed while taking this drug without consulting physician.

OMEPRAZOLE Pr

(o-me'pra-zole)

Losec ♣, Prilosec, Prilosec OTC, Zegerid

Classifications: GASTROINTESTINAL AGENT; PROTON PUMP INHIBITOR

Pregnancy Category: C

AVAILABILITY 10 mg, 20 mg, 40 mg capsules; 20 mg powder for oral suspension

O

ACTIONS An antisecretory compound that is a gastric acid pump inhibitor. Suppresses gastric acid secretion by inhibiting the H^+, K^+-ATPase enzyme system [the acid (proton H^+) pump] in the parietal cells.

THERAPEUTIC EFFECTS Suppresses gastric acid secretion relieving gastrointestinal distress and promoting ulcer healing.

USES Duodenal and gastric ulcer. Gastroesophageal reflux disease including severe erosive esophagitis (4 to 8 wk treatment). Long-term treatment of pathologic hypersecretory conditions such as Zollinger-Ellison syndrome, multiple endocrine adenomas, and systemic mastocytosis. In combination with clarithromycin to treat duodenal ulcers associated with *Helicobacter pylori*.

CONTRAINDICATIONS Long-term use for gastroesophageal reflux disease (GERD), duodenal ulcers; proton pump inhibitors (PPIs), hypersensitivity; children <2 y; use of OTC formulation in children <18 y or GI bleeding; pregnancy (category C); use of Zegerid in metabolic alkalosis, hypocalcemia, vomiting, GI bleeding.

CAUTIOUS USE Dysphagia; metabolic or respiratory alkalosis; lactation.

ROUTE & DOSAGE

Gastroesophageal Reflux, Erosive Esophagitis, Duodenal Ulcer

Adult: **PO** 20 mg once/d for 4–8 wk

Gastric Ulcer

Adult: **PO** 20 mg b.i.d. for 4–8 wk

Hypersecretory Disease

Adult: **PO** 60 mg once/d up to 120 mg t.i.d.

Duodenal Ulcer Associated with *H. pylori*

Adult: **PO** 40 mg once/d for 14 d, then 20 mg/d for 14 d, in combination with clarithromycin 500 mg t.i.d. for 14 d

ADMINISTRATION

Oral

- Give before food, preferably breakfast; capsules must be swallowed whole (do not open, chew, or crush).
- Note: Antacids may be administered with omeprazole.

ADVERSE EFFECTS (≥1%) **CNS:** Headache, dizziness, fatigue. **GI:** Diarrhea, abdominal pain, nausea, mild transient increases in liver function tests. **Urogenital:** Hematuria, proteinuria. **Skin:** Rash.

DIAGNOSTIC TEST INTERFERENCE Omeprazole has been reported to significantly impair peak **cortisol**

Common adverse effects in *italic*, life-threatening effects underlined: generic names in **bold**; classifications in SMALL CAPS; ♣ Canadian drug name; Pr Prototype drug

response to exogenous ACTH. This finding is undergoing further investigation.

INTERACTIONS Drug: Concomitant administration of **diazepam** and omeprazole may increase diazepam concentrations. Concomitant administration of **phenytoin** and omeprazole may increase **phenytoin** levels. Concomitant administration of **warfarin** and omeprazole may increase **warfarin** levels.

PHARMACOKINETICS Absorption: Poorly absorbed from GI tract; 30%–40% reaches systemic circulation. **Onset:** 0.5–3.5 h. **Peak:** Peak inhibition of gastric acid secretion: 5 d. **Metabolism:** Metabolized in liver. **Elimination:** 80% excreted in urine, 20% in feces. **Half-Life:** 0.5–1.5 h.

NURSING IMPLICATIONS

Assessment & Drug Effects

- Lab tests: Monitor urinalysis for hematuria and proteinuria. Periodic liver function tests with prolonged use.

Patient & Family Education

- Report any changes in urinary elimination such as pain or discomfort associated with urination, or blood in urine.
- Report severe diarrhea; drug may need to be discontinued.
- Do not breast feed while taking this drug.

ONDANSETRON HYDROCHLORIDE (Pr)

(on-dan'si-tron)

Zofran, Zofran ODT

Classifications: GASTROINTESTINAL AGENT; ANTIEMETIC; 5-HT_3 ANTAGONIST

Pregnancy Category: B

AVAILABILITY 4 mg, 8 mg, 24 mg tablets; 4 mg, 8 mg orally disintegrating tablets; 4 mg/5 mL oral solution; 2 mg/mL injection

ACTIONS Selective serotonin (5-HT_3) receptor antagonist. Serotonin receptors are located centrally in the chemoreceptor trigger zone (CTZ) and peripherally on the vagal nerve terminals. Serotonin is released from the wall of the small intestine and stimulates the vagal efferents through the serotonin receptors and initiates the vomiting reflex.

THERAPEUTIC EFFECTS Prevents nausea and vomiting associated with cancer chemotherapy and anesthesia.

USES Prevention of nausea and vomiting associated with initial and repeated courses of cancer chemotherapy, including high-dose cisplatin; postoperative nausea and vomiting.

UNLABELED USES Treatment of hyperemesis gravidarum

CONTRAINDICATIONS Hypersensitivity to ondansetron.

CAUTIOUS USE Pregnancy (category B), lactation, and children ≤2 y.

ROUTE & DOSAGE

Nausea and Vomiting

Adult: **PO** 8 mg 30 min before chemotherapy, then q8h times 2 more doses
Adult/Child: **IV** *4–18 y,* 0.15 mg/kg or 32 mg infused over 15 min beginning 30 min before start of chemotherapy, followed by 0.15 mg/kg 4 and 8 h after first dose of ondansetron, may also give 8 mg bolus, then 1 mg/h by continuous infusion (max: 32 mg/d), or 32 mg as single dose

O

Child: **PO** >*4 y,* 4 mg 30 min before chemotherapy, then q8h times 2 more doses

Nausea & Vomiting with Highly Emetogenic Chemotherapy

Adult: **PO** Single 24-mg dose 30 min before administration of single-day highly emetogenic chemotherapy

Postoperative Nausea and Vomiting

Adult: **PO** 8–16 mg 1 h preoperatively **IM** 4 mg injected immediately prior to anesthesia induction or once postoperatively if patient experiences nausea/vomiting shortly after surgery **IV** 4 mg by slow IV push, may repeat q8h as needed
Child: **IV** ≥*2 y,* 0.1 mg/kg

Hyperemesis Gravidarum

Adult: **PO/IV** 4–8 mg 2–3 times per day

Hepatic Impairment

Maximum dose 8 mg/day PO/IV in patients with severely impaired liver function according to Child-Pugh criteria

ADMINISTRATION

Oral

- Give tablets 30 min prior to chemotherapy and 1–2 h prior to radiation therapy.
- Do NOT push orally disintegrating tablet through blister foil. Peel foil back and remove tablet. Tablets will disintegrate with/without liquid.

Intravenous

PREPARE: **Direct:** May be given undiluted. **IV Infusion:** Dilute a single does in 50 mL of D5W or NS. May be further diluted in selected IV solution.

ADMINISTER: **Direct:** Give over at least 30 sec, 2–5 min preferred. **IV Infusion:** Give over 15 min. When three separate doses are administered, infuse each over 15 min.

INCOMPATIBILITIES **Solution/additive: Meropenem. Y-site: Acyclovir, allopurinol, aminophylline, amphotericin B, ampicillin, ampicillin/sulbactam, amsacrine, cefepime, cefoperazone, fluorouracil, furosemide, ganciclovir, lorazepam, meropenem, methylprednisolone, piperacillin, sargramostim, sodium bicarbonate, TPN.**

ADVERSE EFFECTS (≥1%) **CNS:** Dizziness and light-headedness, *headache, sedation.* **GI:** *Diarrhea,* constipation, dry mouth, transient increases in liver aminotransferases and bilirubin. **Body as a Whole:** Hypersensitivity reactions.

INTERACTIONS Drug: Rifampin may decrease ondansetron levels.

PHARMACOKINETICS Peak: 1–1.5 h. **Metabolism:** Metabolized in liver. **Elimination:** 44%–60% excreted in urine within 24 h; approximately 25% excreted in feces. **Half-Life:** 3 h.

NURSING IMPLICATIONS

Assessment & Drug Effects

- Monitor fluid and electrolyte status. Diarrhea, which may cause fluid and electrolyte imbalance, is a potential adverse effect of the drug.
- Monitor cardiovascular status, especially in patients with a history of coronary artery disease. Rare cases of tachycardia and angina have been reported.

Patient & Family Education

- Be aware that headache requiring an analgesic for relief is a common adverse effect.

OPIUM, POWDERED OPIUM TINCTURE (LAUDANUM)

(oh'pee-um)

Deodorized Opium Tincture

Classifications: CENTRAL NERVOUS SYSTEM AGENT; NARCOTIC (OPIATE) AGONIST; NARCOTIC ANALGESIC; ANTIDIARRHEAL

Prototype: Morphine

Pregnancy Category: B

Controlled Substance: Schedule II

AVAILABILITY 10%, 2 mg/5 mL liquid

ACTIONS Is obtained from the unripe capsules of *Papaver somniferum* or *Papaver album* and contains several natural alkaloids including morphine, codeine, papaverine.

THERAPEUTIC EFFECTS Antidiarrheal due to inhibition of GI motility and propulsion; leads to prolonged transit of intestinal contents, desiccation of feces, and constipation.

USES Symptomatic treatment of acute diarrhea and to treat severe withdrawal symptoms in neonates born to women addicted to opiates.

CONTRAINDICATIONS Diarrhea caused by poisoning (until poison is completely eliminated); pregnancy (category B), lactation.

CAUTIOUS USE History of opiate agonist dependence; asthma; severe prostatic hypertrophy; hepatic disease.

ROUTE & DOSAGE

Acute Diarrhea

Adult: **PO** 0.6 mL q.i.d. up to 1 mL q.i.d. (max: 6 mL/d)
Child: **PO** 0.005–0.01 mL/kg q3–4h (max: 6 doses/24 h)

Neonatal Withdrawal

Child: **PO** make a 1:25 aqueous dilution, then give 3–6 drops q3–6h as needed or 0.2 mL q3h, may increase by 0.05 mL q3h until withdrawal symptoms are controlled, then gradually decrease dose after withdrawal symptoms have stabilized

ADMINISTRATION

Oral

- Do not confuse this preparation with camphorated opium tincture (paregoric), which contains only 2 mg anhydrous morphine/ 5 mL, thus requiring a higher dose volume than that required for therapeutic dose of Deodorized Opium Tincture.
- Give drug diluted with about one third glass of water to ensure passage of entire dose into stomach.
- Store in tight, light-resistant containers.

ADVERSE EFFECTS (≥1%) **GI:** Nausea and other GI disturbances. **CNS:** Depression of CNS.

INTERACTIONS Drug: Alcohol and other CNS DEPRESSANTS add to CNS effects.

PHARMACOKINETICS Absorption: Variable absorption from GI tract. **Distribution:** Crosses placenta; distributed into breast milk. **Metabolism:** Metabolized in liver. **Elimination:** Excreted in urine.

NURSING IMPLICATIONS

Assessment & Drug Effects

- Withhold medication and report to physician if respirations are 12/min or below or have changed in character and rate.
- Discontinue as soon as diarrhea is controlled; note character and frequency of stools.
- Offer small amounts of fluid frequently but attempt to maintain 3000–4000 mL fluid total in 24 h.

O

- Monitor body weight, I&O ratio and pattern, and temperature. If patient develops fever of 38.8° C (102° F) or above, electrolyte and hydration levels may need to be evaluated. Consult physician.

Patient & Family Education

- Be aware that constipation may be a consequence of antidiarrheal therapy but that normal habit pattern usually is reestablished with resumption of normal dietary intake.
- Note: Addiction is possible with prolonged use or with drug abuse.
- Do not breast feed while taking this drug.

OPRELVEKIN

(o-prel've-kin)

Neumega

Classifications: BLOOD FORMERS, COAGULATORS, AND ANTICOAGULANTS; HEMATOPOIETIC GROWTH FACTOR

Prototype: Epoetin Alfa

Pregnancy Category: C

AVAILABILITY 5 mg injection

ACTIONS Hematopoietic growth factor (interleukin-11) that is produced by recombinant DNA.

THERAPEUTIC EFFECTS Indicated by return of postnadir platelet count toward normal (≥50,000). Increases platelet count in a dose-dependent manner.

USES Prevention of severe thrombocytopenia following myelosuppressive chemotherapy (not effective after myeloablative chemotherapy).

CONTRAINDICATIONS Hypersensitivity to oprelvekin; myeloablative chemotherapy; myeloid malignancies; pregnancy (category C).

CAUTIOUS USE Patients with left ventricular dysfunction, cardiac disease, CHF, history of atrial arrhythmias, or other arrhythmias; electrolyte imbalance, hypokalemia; respiratory disease; papilledema; thromboembolic disorders; older adults; cerebrovascular disease, stroke, TIAs; pleural effusion, pericardial effusion, ascites; increased intracranial pressure, brain tumor, visual disturbances; hepatic or renal dysfunction; lactation.

ROUTE & DOSAGE

Thrombocytopenia

Adult: **SC** 50 mcg/kg once daily starting 6–24 h after completing chemotherapy and continuing until platelet count is ≥50,000 cells/mcL or up to 21 d

Child: **SC** *8 mo–17 y,* 75–100 mcg/kg once daily starting 6–24 h after completing chemotherapy and continuing until platelet count is ≥50,000 cells/mcL or up to 21 d

ADMINISTRATION

Note: Do not use if solution is discolored or if it contains particulate matter.

Subcutaneous

- Reconstitute solution by gently injecting 1 mL of sterile water for injection (without preservative) toward the sides of the vial. Keep needle in vial and gently swirl to dissolve but do not shake solution. Without removing needle, withdraw specified amount of oprelvekin for injection.
- Give as single dose into the abdomen, thigh, hip, or upper arm.
- Discard any unused portion of the vial. It contains no preservatives.
- Use reconstituted solution within 3 h; store at 2°–8° C (36°–46° F) until used.

O

- Store unopened vials at 2°–8° C (36°–46° F). Do not freeze.

ADVERSE EFFECTS (≥1%) **Body as a Whole:** *Edema, neutropenic fever, fever,* asthenia, pain, chills, myalgia, bone pain, dehydration. **CNS:** *Headache, dizziness, insomnia,* nervousness. **CV:** *Tachycardia,* vasodilation, palpitations, syncope, atrial fibrillation/flutter, peripheral edema, capillary leak syndrome. **GI:** *Nausea, vomiting, mucositis, diarrhea,* oral moniliasis, anorexia, constipation, dyspepsia. **Hematologic:** Ecchymosis. **Respiratory:** *Dyspnea, rhinitis, cough, pharyngitis,* pleural effusion, pulmonary edema, exacerbation of preexisting pleural effusion. **Skin:** Alopecia, *rash,* skin discoloration, exfoliative dermatitis. **Special Senses:** Conjunctival injection, amblyopia.

INTERACTIONS Drug: No clinically significant interactions established.

PHARMACOKINETICS Absorption: 80% absorbed from SC injection site. **Onset:** Days 5–9. **Duration:** 7 d after last dose. **Distribution:** Distributes to highly perfused organs. **Elimination:** Excreted in urine. **Half-Life:** 6.9 h.

NURSING IMPLICATIONS

Assessment & Drug Effects

- Lab tests: Monitor platelet counts until adequate recovery; periodically monitor CBC with differential and serum electrolytes.
- Monitor carefully for and immediately report S&S of fluid overload, hypokalemia, and cardiac arrhythmias.
- Monitor persons with preexisting fluid retention carefully (e.g., CHF, pleural effusion, ascites) for worsening of symptoms.

Patient & Family Education

- Review patient information leaflet with special attention to administration directions.
- Report any of the following to the physician: Shortness of breath, edema of arms and/or legs, chest pain, unusual fatigue or weakness, irregular heartbeat, blurred vision.
- Do not breast feed while taking this drug.

ORLISTAT

(or′li-stat)

Xenical

Classifications: GASTROINTESTINAL AGENT; ANORECTANT; NONSYSTEMIC LIPASE INHIBITOR

Prototype: Diethylpropion

Pregnancy Category: B

AVAILABILITY 120 mg capsules

ACTIONS Nonsystemic inhibitor of gastrointestinal lipase. Reduces intestinal absorption of dietary fat by forming inactive enzymes with pancreatic and gastric lipase in the GI tract.

THERAPEUTIC EFFECTS Indicated by weight loss/decreased body mass index (BMI). Reduces the intestinal absorption of dietary fat because at least 95% of orlistat is eliminated in the feces; reduces caloric intake in obese individuals.

USES Weight loss and weight maintenance in patients with BMI ≥30 kg/m^2 or ≥27 kg/m^2 in patients with other risk factors. Reduce risk for weight regain after prior weight loss.

CONTRAINDICATIONS Hypersensitivity to orlistat; malabsorption syndrome; cholestasis; gallbladder disease; hypothyroidism; organic causes of obesity; anorexia ner-

O

vosa, bulimia nervosa; organic causes of obesity, lactation. Safety and efficacy in children <16 y are not established.

CAUTIOUS USE Gastrointestinal diseases including frequent diarrhea; known dietary deficiencies in fat soluble vitamins (i.e., A, D, E); history of calcium oxalate nephrolithiasis or hyperoxaluria; older adults; pregnancy (category B).

ROUTE & DOSAGE

Weight Loss
Adult/Adolescent: **PO** *>16 y,* 120 mg t.i.d. with each main meal containing fat

ADMINISTRATION

Oral

- Give during or up to 1 h after a meal containing fat.
- Omit dose with nonfat-containing meal or if meal is skipped.
- Store at 15°–30° C (59°–86° F). Keep bottle tightly closed; do NOT use after the printed expiration date.

O

ADVERSE EFFECTS (≥1%) **Body as a Whole:** Fatigue. **CNS:** *Headache,* dizziness, anxiety. **CV:** Hypertension, stroke. **GI:** *Oily spotting, flatus with discharge, fecal urgency, fatty/oily stool, oily evacuation, increased defecation,* fecal incontinence, *abdominal pain/discomfort,* nausea, infectious diarrhea, rectal pain/discomfort, tooth disorder, gingival disorder, vomiting. **Skin:** Rash. **Urogenital:** Menstrual irregularity.

INTERACTIONS Drug: Orlistat may increase absorption of **pravastatin;** may decrease absorption of fat soluble VITAMINS (A, D, E, K). Monitor PT/INR inpatients on chronic stable doses of **warfarin.**

PHARMACOKINETICS Absorption: Minimal absorption. **Metabolism:** Metabolized in gastrointestinal wall. **Elimination:** Excreted in feces. **Half-Life:** 1–2 h.

NURSING IMPLICATIONS

Assessment & Drug Effects

- Monitor weight & BMI; closely monitor diabetics for hypoglycemia.
- Coadministered drugs: Monitor PT/INR with warfarin.
- Monitor BP frequently, especially with preexisting hypertension.

Patient & Family Education

- Take a daily multivitamin containing fat-soluble vitamins at least 2 h before/after orlistat.
- Remember common GI adverse effects typically resolve after 4 wk therapy.
- Avoid high fat meals to minimize adverse GI effects. Distribute fat calories over three main meals daily.
- Monitor weight several times weekly. Diabetics: Monitor blood glucose carefully following any weight loss.
- Do not breast feed while taking this drug.

ORPHENADRINE CITRATE

(or-fen′a-dreen)

Banflex, Flexon, Myolin, Norflex

Classifications: SOMATIC NERVOUS SYSTEM AGENT; SKELETAL MUSCLE RELAXANT; CENTRAL-ACTING

Prototype: Cyclobenzaprine

Pregnancy Category: C

AVAILABILITY 100 mg tablets; 100 mg sustained-release tablets; 30 mg/mL injection

ACTIONS Tertiary amine anticholinergic agent and central-acting skeletal muscle relaxant.

THERAPEUTIC EFFECTS Relaxes tense skeletal muscles indirectly, possibly by analgesic action or by atropinelike central action. Has some local anesthetic and antihistaminic activity but less than that of diphenhydramine. Also produces slight euphoria.

USES To relieve muscle spasm discomfort associated with acute musculoskeletal conditions.

CONTRAINDICATIONS Narrow-angle glaucoma; pyloric or duodenal obstruction, stenosing peptic ulcers; prostatic hypertrophy or bladder neck obstruction; myasthenia gravis; cardiospasm (megaloesophagus). Safe use during pregnancy (category C), lactation, or in the pediatric age group is not established. **CAUTIOUS USE** History of tachycardia, cardiac decompensation, arrhythmias, coronary insufficiency.

ROUTE & DOSAGE

Muscle Spasm
Adult: **PO** 100 mg b.i.d. **IM/IV** 60 mg, may repeat in 12 h if needed

ADMINISTRATION

Oral
- Ensure that sustained-release form is not chewed or crushed. It must be swallowed whole.

Intravenous
PREPARE: **Direct:** Give undiluted. Protect from light.
ADMINISTER: **Direct:** Give at a rate of 60 mg (2 mL) over 5 min.

ADVERSE EFFECTS (≥1%) **CNS:** *Drowsiness,* weakness, headache, dizziness; mild CNS stimulation (high doses: restlessness, anxiety, tremors, confusion, hallucinations, agitation, tachycardia, palpitation, syncope). **Special Senses:** Increased ocular tension, dilated pupils, blurred vision. **GI:** *Dry mouth,* nausea, vomiting, abdominal cramps, constipation. **Urogenital:** *Urinary hesitancy* or *retention.* **Body as a Whole:** Hypersensitivity [pruritus, urticaria, rash, <u>anaphylactic reaction</u> (rare)].

INTERACTIONS Drug: Propoxyphene may cause increased confusion, anxiety, and tremors; may worsen schizophrenic symptoms, or increase risk of tardive dyskinesia with **haloperidol;** additive CNS depressant with ANXIOLYTICS, SEDATIVES, HYPNOTICS, **butorphanol, nalbuphine,** OPIATE AGONISTS, **pentazocine, tramadol. Herbal: Valerian, kava kava** POTENTIATE SEDATION.

PHARMACOKINETICS Absorption: Readily absorbed from GI tract. **Peak:** 2 h. **Duration:** 4–6 h. **Distribution:** Rapidly distributed in tissues; crosses placenta. **Metabolism:** Metabolized in liver. **Elimination:** Excreted in urine. **Half-Life:** 14 h.

O

NURSING IMPLICATIONS

Assessment & Drug Effects
- Lab tests: Periodic blood, urine, and liver function studies with prolonged therapy.
- Report complaints of mouth dryness, urinary hesitancy or retention, headache, tremors, GI problems, palpitation, or rapid pulse to physician. Dosage reduction or drug withdrawal is indicated.
- Monitor elimination patterns. Older adults are particularly sensitive to anticholinergic effects (urinary hesitancy, constipation); closely observe.
- Monitor therapeutic drug effect. In the patient with parkinsonism, orphenadrine reduces muscular rigidity but has little effect on tremors. Some reduction in excessive salivation and perspira-

tion may occur, and patient may appear mildly euphoric.

Patient & Family Education

- Relieve mouth dryness by frequent rinsing with clear tepid water, increasing noncaloric fluid intake, sugarless gum, or lemon drops. If these measures fail, a saliva substitute may help.
- Do not drive or engage in potentially hazardous activities until response to drug is known.
- Avoid concomitant use of alcohol and other CNS depressants; these may potentiate depressant effects.
- Do not breast feed while taking this drug without consulting physician.

OSELTAMIVIR PHOSPHATE

(o-sel'tam-i-vir)

Tamiflu

Classifications: ANTIINFECTIVE; ANTIVIRAL AGENT

Prototype: Acyclovir

Pregnancy Category: C

AVAILABILITY 75 mg capsule; 12 mg/mL suspension

ACTIONS Inhibits influenza A and B viral neuroaminidase enzyme, preventing the release of newly formed virus from the surface of the infected cells.

THERAPEUTIC EFFECTS Indicated by relief of flu symptoms. Prevents viral spread across the mucous lining of the respiratory tract. Inhibits replication of the influenza A and B virus.

USES Treatment of uncomplicated acute influenza in adults symptomatic for no more than 2 d.

CONTRAINDICATIONS Hypersensitivity to oseltamivir; pregnancy (category C); children <1 y.

CAUTIOUS USE Renal impairment; lactation. Safety and efficacy in chronic cardiac/respiratory disease are not established.

ROUTE & DOSAGE

Influenza

Adult: **PO** 75 mg b.i.d. times 5 d
Child: **PO** >*1 y* 15 kg, 30 mg b.i.d.; >15–23 kg 45 mg b.i.d.; >23–40 kg, 60 mg b.i.d.; >40 kg, 75 mg b.i.d. × 5 d

Renal Impairment

Cl_{cr} <30 mL/min: 75 mg q.d. times 5 d

ADMINISTRATION

Oral

- Give with food to decrease the risk of GI upset.
- Start within 48 h of onset of flu symptoms.
- Take missed dose as soon as possible unless next dose is due within 2 h.
- Store at 15°–30° C (59°–86° F); protect from moisture, keep dry.

ADVERSE EFFECTS (≥1%) **Body as a Whole:** Fatigue. **CNS:** Dizziness, headache, insomnia, vertigo. **GI:** Nausea, vomiting, diarrhea, abdominal pain. **Respiratory:** Bronchitis, cough.

PHARMACOKINETICS Absorption: Readily absorbed, 75% bioavailable. **Distribution:** 42% protein bound. **Metabolism:** Extensively metabolized to active metabolite oseltamivir carboxylate by liver esterases. **Elimination:** Primarily excreted in urine. **Half-Life:** 1–2 h; oseltamivir carboxylate 6–10 h.

NURSING IMPLICATIONS

Assessment & Drug Effects

- Monitor ambulation in frail and older adult patients due to potential for dizziness and vertigo.

Patient & Family Education

- Do not breast feed while taking this drug.

OXACILLIN SODIUM

(ox-a-sill'in)

Bactocill, Prostaphlin

Classifications: ANTIINFECTIVE; ANTIBIOTIC PENICILLIN; ANTISTAPHYLOCOCCAL PENICILLIN

Prototype: Penicillin G

Pregnancy Category: B

AVAILABILITY 250 mg, 500 mg capsules; 250 mg/5 mL suspension; 250 mg, 500 mg, 1 g, 2 g injection

ACTIONS Semisynthetic, acid-stable, penicillinase-resistant isoxazolyl penicillin.

THERAPEUTIC EFFECTS In common with other isoxazolyl penicillins (cloxacillin, dicloxacillin), it is highly active against most penicillinase-producing *staphylococci,* is less potent than penicillin G against penicillin-sensitive microorganisms, and is generally ineffective against gram-negative bacteria and methicillin-resistant *staphylococci* (MRSA).

USES Primarily, infections caused by penicillinase-producing staphylococci and penicillin-resistant staphylococci. May be used to initiate therapy in suspected staphylococcal infections pending culture and sensitivity test results. As with other penicillins, serum concentrations are enhanced by concurrent use of probenecid.

CONTRAINDICATIONS Hypersensitivity to penicillins or cephalosporins. Safe use during pregnancy (category B) is not established.

CAUTIOUS USE History of or suspected atopy or allergy (hives, eczema, hay fever, asthma); premature infants, neonates, lactation (may cause infant diarrhea).

ROUTE & DOSAGE

***Staphylococcal* Infections**

Adult: **PO** 250–1000 mg q4–6h **IM/IV** 500 mg–2 g q4–6h up to 12 g/d

Child: **PO** 50–100 mg/kg/d in 4 divided doses **IM/IV** 50–150 mg/kg/d divided q4–6h

Neonate: **IV** 50–100 mg/kg/d divided q6–12h

ADMINISTRATION

Note: The total sodium content (including that contributed by buffer) in each gram of oxacillin is approximately 3.1 mEq or 71 mg.

Oral

- Give with a full glass of water on an empty stomach (either 1 h before meals or 2 h after meals). Food reduces absorption.

Intramuscular

- Reconstitute each 250 mg with 1.4 mL sterile water for injection to yield 250 mg/1.5 mL. Shake vial vigorously until drug is completely dissolved. Discard unused portions after 3 d at room temperature or 7 d under refrigeration.
- Administer deep IM to adults by deep intragluteal injection. Follow agency policy for IM site in young children and infants. Rotate injection sites.

Intravascular

Note: Verify correct IV concentration and rate of infusion/injection with physician before IV administration to neonates, infants, children.

PREPARE: **Direct:** Reconstitute each 500 mg or fraction thereof with 5 mL with sterile water for injection or NS to yield 250 mg/

1.5 mL. **Intermittent:** Further dilute in 50–100 mL of D5W, NS, D5/NS, or RL. **Continuous:** Further dilute in up to 1000 mL of compatible IV solutions.

ADMINISTER: **Direct:** Give at a rate of 1 g or fraction thereof over 10 min. **Intermittent:** Give over 15–30 min. **Continuous:** Give over 6 h.

INCOMPATIBILITIES **Solution: additive:** Cytarabine **Y-site: Sodium bicarbonate, verapamil.**

ADVERSE EFFECTS (≥1%) **Body as a Whole:** Thrombophlebitis (IV therapy), superinfections, wheezing, sneezing, fever, <u>anaphylaxis</u>. **GI:** Nausea, vomiting, flatulence, *diarrhea,* hepatocellular dysfunction (elevated AST, ALT, hepatitis). **Hematologic:** Eosinophilia, leukopenia, thrombocytopenia, granulocytopenia, <u>agranulocytosis</u>; neutropenia (reported in children). **Skin:** Pruritus, rash, urticaria. **Urogenital:** Interstitial nephritis, transient hematuria, albuminuria, azotemia (newborns and infants on high doses).

O

DIAGNOSTIC TEST INTERFERENCE Oxacillin in large doses can cause false-positive ***urine protein tests*** using sulfosalicylic acid methods.

PHARMACOKINETICS Absorption: Incompletely and erratically absorbed orally. **Peak:** 30–120 min IM; 15 min IV. **Duration:** 4 h PO; 4–6 h IM. **Distribution:** Distributes into CNS with inflamed meninges; crosses placenta; distributed into breast milk. **Metabolism:** Enters enterohepatic circulation. **Elimination:** Primarily excreted in urine, some in bile. **Half-Life:** 0.5–1 h.

NURSING IMPLICATIONS

Assessment & Drug Effects

- Ask patient prior to first dose about hypersensitivity reactions to penicillins, cephalosporins, and other allergens.
- Lab tests: periodic liver functions, CBC with differential, platelet count, and urinalysis.
- Hepatic dysfunction (possibly a hypersensitivity reaction) has been associated with IV oxacillin; it is reversible with discontinuation of drug. Symptoms may resemble viral hepatitis or general signs of hypersensitivity and should be reported promptly: hives, rash, fever, nausea, vomiting, abdominal discomfort, anorexia, malaise, jaundice (with dark yellow to brown urine, light-colored or clay-colored stools, pruritus).
- Withhold next drug dose and report the onset of hypersensitivity reactions and superinfections (see Appendix F).

Patient & Family Education

- Take oral medication around the clock, do not miss a dose. Take all of the medication prescribed even if you feel better, unless otherwise directed by physician.
- Do not breast feed while taking this drug without consulting physician.

OXALIPLATIN

(ox-a-li-pla'tin)

Eloxatin

Classifications: ANTINEOPLASTIC; ALKYLATING AGENT

Prototype: Cyclophosphamide

Pregnancy Category: D

AVAILABILITY 50 mg, 100 mg vials

ACTIONS Oxaliplatin forms inter- and intra-strand DNA cross-links. These cross-links inhibit DNA replication and transcription. The cytotoxicity of oxaliplatin is cell-cycle nonspecific.

THERAPEUTIC EFFECTS Antitumor activity of oxaliplatin in combination with 5-fluorouracil (5-FU) has antiproliferative activity against colon carcinoma that is greater than either compound alone. In addition it is also used in combination with leucovorin (LV) along with the 5-FU for greater effectiveness.

USES Metastatic cancer of colon and rectum.

CONTRAINDICATIONS History of known allergy to oxaliplatin or other platinum compounds; myelosuppression; pregnancy (category D); lactation. Safety and effectiveness in children are not established.
CAUTIOUS USE Renal impairment, because clearance of ultrafilterable platinum is decreased in mild, moderate, and severe renal impairment; hepatic impairment.

ROUTE & DOSAGE

Metastatic Colon or Rectal Cancer
Adult: **IV** 85 mg/m^2 infused over 120 min once every 2 wk

ADMINISTRATION

Intravenous

- Premedication with an antiemetic is recommended.

PREPARE: **IV Infusion:** NEVER reconstitute with NS or any solution containing chloride. Reconstitute the 50 mg vial or the 100 mg vial by adding 10 mL or 20 mL, respectively, of sterile water for injection or D5W. MUST further dilute in 250–500 mL of D5W for infusion.
ADMINISTER: **IV Infusion:** Do NOT use needles or infusion sets containing aluminum parts. Flush infusion line with D5W before and after administration of any other concomitant medication. Give over 120 min with frequent monitoring of the IV insertion site. Discontinue at the first sign of extravasation and restart IV in a different site.
INCOMPATIBILITIES **Solution/additive:** CHLORIDE-CONTAINING SOLUTIONS, ALKALINE SOLUTIONS, including **sodium bicarbonate, 5-fluorouracil (5-FU) Y-site:** ALKALINE SOLUTIONS, including **sodium bicarbonate, 5-fluorouracil (5-FU).**

- Store reconstituted solution up to 24 h under refrigeration at 2°–8° C (36°–46° F). After final dilution, the IV solution may be stored for 6 h at room temperature [20°–25° C (68°–77° F)] or up to 24 h under refrigeration.

ADVERSE EFFECTS (≥1%) **Body as a Whole:** *Fever, edema, pain,* allergic reaction, arthralgia, rigors. **CNS:** *Fatigue, neuropathy, headache,* dizziness, insomnia. **CV:** Chest pain. **GI:** *Diarrhea, nausea, vomiting, anorexia, stomatitis, constipation, abdominal pain,* reflux, dyspepsia, taste perversion, mucositis, flatulence. **Hematologic:** *Anemia, leukopenia, thrombocytopenia,* neutropenia, thromboembolism. **Metabolic:** Hypokalemia, dehydration. **Respiratory:** *Dyspnea, cough,* rhinitis, pharyngitis, epistaxis, hiccup. **Skin:** Flushing, rash, alopecia, injection site reaction. **Urogenital:** Dysuria.

INTERACTIONS Drug: AMINOGLYCOSIDES, **amphotericin B, vancomycin,** and other **nephrotoxic drugs** may increase risk of renal failure.

PHARMACOKINETICS Distribution: >90% protein bound. **Metabolism:** Rapid and extensive non-enzymatic

O

biotransformation. **Elimination:** Primarily excreted in urine. **Half-Life:** 391 h.

NURSING IMPLICATIONS

Assessment & Drug Effects

- Monitor for S&S of hypersensitivity (e.g., rash, urticaria, erythema, pruritis; rarely, bronchospasm and hypotension). Discontinue drug and notify physician if any of these occur.
- Monitor insertion site. Extravasation may cause local pain and inflammation that may be severe and lead to complications, including necrosis.
- Monitor for S&S of coagulation disorders including GI bleeding, hematuria, and epistaxis.
- Monitor for S&S of peripheral neuropathy (e.g., paresthesia, dysesthesia, hypoesthesia in the hands, feet, perioral area, or throat, jaw spasm, abnormal tongue sensation, dysarthria, eye pain, and chest pressure). Symptoms may be precipitated or exacerbated by exposure to cold temperature or cold objects.
- Lab tests: Before each administration cycle, monitor WBC count with differential, hemoglobin, platelet count, and blood chemistries (including ALT, AST, bilirubin, and creatinine). Monitor baseline and periodic renal functions.
- Do not apply ice to oral mucous membranes (e.g., mucositis prophylaxis) during the infusion of oxaliplatin as cold temperature can exacerbate acute neurological symptoms.

Patient & Family Education

- Use effective methods of contraception while receiving this drug.
- Avoid cold drinks, use of ice, and cover exposed skin prior to exposure to cold temperature or cold objects.
- Do not drive or engage in potentially hazardous activities until response to drug is known.
- Report any of the following to a health care provider: difficulty writing, buttoning, swallowing, walking; numbness, tingling or other unusual sensations in extremities; non-productive cough or shortness of breath; fever, particularly if associated with persistent diarrhea or other evidence of infection.
- Report promptly S&S of a bleeding disorder such as black tarry stool, coke-colored or frankly bloody urine, bleeding from the nose or mucous membranes.
- Do not breast feed while taking this drug without consulting physician.

O

OXAMNIQUINE

(ox-am′ni-kwin)

Vansil

Classifications: ANTIINFECTIVE; ANTHELMINTIC

Prototype: Mebendazole

Pregnancy Category: C

AVAILABILITY 250 mg capsules

ACTIONS Hydroquinone derivative prepared in the presence of *Aspergillus sclerotium*. Mechanism of action not fully explained, but it appears that drug-induced strong contractions and paralysis of worm musculature leads to immobilization of their suckers and dislodgment from their usual residence in mesenteric veins to the liver.

THERAPEUTIC EFFECTS Dislodgment of schistosomes begins about 2 d after single oral dose; movement is not complete until 6 d after treatment with the drug. After treatment, surviving unpaired females return to mesenteric vessels; however, oviposition (egg laying) seems to stop in 24–48 h after drug treatment, reducing egg load and removing principal cause of pathology associated with schistosomal infection.

USES All stages of *Schistosoma mansoni* infection, including acute and chronic phases with hepatosplenic involvement.

CONTRAINDICATIONS Safe use during pregnancy (category C), lactation, or in children is not established. **CAUTIOUS USE** History of convulsant disorders.

ROUTE & DOSAGE

Schistosomiasis
Adult: **PO** 12–15 mg/kg as single dose
Child: **PO** *<30 kg,* 10 mg/kg times 2 doses at 2–8 h intervals

ADMINISTRATION

Oral
- Give on an empty stomach, if possible.
- Administer with food if necessary to reduce GI distress and improve tolerance.
- Store product in tightly closed container at controlled room temperature less than 30° C (86° F).

ADVERSE EFFECTS (≥1%) **CNS:** *Transitory dizziness, drowsiness, headache;* persistent fever (in patients being treated in Egypt); EEG abnormalities, convulsions (rare). **GI:** Anorexia, nausea, vomiting, abdominal pain, elevated liver enzyme concentrations. **Hematologic:** Increased erythrocyte sedimentation rate, reticulocyte count, and increased or decreased leukocyte count. **Skin:** Urticaria. **Urogenital:** Red-orange urine.

INTERACTIONS Food: Rate and extent of absorption are decreased by food.

PHARMACOKINETICS Absorption: Readily absorbed from GI tract. **Peak:** 1–3 h. **Metabolism:** Extensively metabolized in GI mucosa. **Elimination:** Excreted in urine. **Half-Life:** 1–2.5 h.

NURSING IMPLICATIONS

Assessment & Drug Effects
- Supervise ambulation and use other safety precautions because >30% of patients experience dizziness or drowsiness.
- If patient has a history of seizures, the possibility of seizures is increased because of drug action (occurs within hours of drug administration).

Patient & Family Education
- Use caution while driving or performing other tasks requiring alertness because drug can cause dizziness or drowsiness.
- Be aware that drug may change the normal urine color to a harmless orange-red.
- Do not breast feed while taking this drug without consulting physician.

O

OXANDROLONE

(ox-an′dro-lone)
Oxandrin
Classifications: HORMONES & SYNTHETIC SUBSTITUTES; ANDROGEN/ANABOLIC STEROID
Prototype: Testosterone
Pregnancy Category: X
Controlled Substance: Schedule III

AVAILABILITY 2.5 mg tablets

ACTIONS Synthetic steroid with anabolic and androgenic activity. Controls development and maintenance of secondary sexual characteristics. **THERAPEUTIC EFFECTS Androgenic activity:** Responsible for the growth spurt of the adolescent and for growth termination by epiphyseal closure. In males and some females reduces excretion of phosphorus, nitrogen, potassium, sodium, and chloride. Increases erythropoiesis, possibly by stimulating production of renal or extrarenal erythropoietin, and promotes vascularization and darkening of skin. Antagonizes effects of estrogen excess on female breast and endometrium. **Anabolic activity:** Increases protein metabolism and decreases its catabolism. Large doses suppress spermatogenesis, thereby causing testicular atrophy.

USES Adjunctive therapy to promote weight gain, offset protein catabolism associated with prolonged administration of corticosteroids, relieve bone pain accompanying osteoporosis.

CONTRAINDICATIONS Hypersensitivity or toxic reactions to androgens; severe cardiac, hepatic, or renal disease; pregnancy (category X), lactation; possibility of virilization of external genitalia of female fetus; polycythemia; hypercalcemia; known or suspected prostatic or breast cancer in males; benign prostatic hypertrophy with obstruction; patients easily stimulated sexually; older adults, asthenic males who may react adversely to androgenic overstimulation; conditions aggravated by fluid retention; hypertension.

CAUTIOUS USE Cardiac, hepatic, and mild to moderate renal disease, hypercholesterolemia, heart failure, peripheral edema, arteriosclerosis, coronary artery disease, MI; cholestasis; diabetes mellitus; prostatic hypertrophy; prepubertal males, geriatric patients, acute intermittent porphyria.

O

ROUTE & DOSAGE

Weight Gain

Adult: **PO** 2.5 mg b.i.d. to q.i.d. (max: 20 mg/d) for 2–4 wk
Child: **PO** 0.1–0.25 mg/kg/d

ADMINISTRATION

Oral

- Individualize doses; great variations in response exist.
- Store at 15°–30° C (59°–86° F).

ADVERSE EFFECTS (≥1%) **CNS:** Habituation, excitation, insomnia, depression, changes in libido. **Urogenital:** *Males:* Phallic enlargement, increased frequency or persistence of erections, inhibition of testicular function, testicular atrophy, oligospermia, impotence, chronic priapism, epididymitis, bladder irritability; *Females:* Clitoral enlargement, menstrual irregularities. **Hepatic:** Cholestatic jaundice with or without hepatic necrosis and death, hepatocellular neoplasms, peliosis hepatitis (long-term use). **Skin:** Hirsutism and male pattern baldness in females, acne. **Endocrine:** Gynecomastia, deepening of voice in females, premature closure of epiphyses in children, edema, decreased glucose tolerance.

DIAGNOSTIC TEST INTERFERENCE May decrease levels of thyroxine-binding globulin (decreased total T_4 and increased T_3 RU and free T_4).

INTERACTIONS Drug: May increase INR with **warfarin.** May inhibit metabolism of ORAL HYPOGLYCEMIC AGENTS. Concomitant STEROIDS may increase edema. **Herbal: Echinacea** may increase risk of hepatotoxicity.

PHARMACOKINETICS Not studied.

NURSING IMPLICATIONS

Assessment & Drug Effects

- Monitor weight closely throughout therapy.
- Assess for and report development of edema or S&S of jaundice (see Appendix F).
- Lab tests: Monitor periodically liver function, lipid profile, Hct and Hgb, PT and INR, serum electrolytes, and CPK.
- Withhold and notify physician if hypercalcemia develops in breast cancer patient.
- Monitor growth in children closely.

Patient & Family Education

- Women: Report signs of virilization, including acne and changes in menstrual periods.
- Men: Report too frequent or prolonged erections or appearance/worsening of acne.
- Report S&S of jaundice (see Appendix F) or edema.
- Monitor blood glucose for loss of glycemic control if diabetic.
- Do not breast feed while taking this drug.

OXAPROZIN

(ox-a-pro′zin)

Daypro

OXAPROZIN POTASSIUM

Daypro ALTA

Classifications: CENTRAL NERVOUS SYSTEM AGENT; ANALGESIC, NSAID; ANTIPYRETIC

Prototype: Ibuprofen

Pregnancy Category: C

AVAILABILITY 600 mg tablet

ACTIONS Long-acting NSAID agent, which is an effective prostaglandin synthetase inhibitor. Mode of action presumed due to inhibition of prostaglandin E_2 synthesis at site of inflammation.

THERAPEUTIC EFFECTS Antiinflammatory, antipyretic, and analgesic properties.

USES Treatment of osteoarthritis and rheumatoid arthritis.

UNLABELED USES Ankylosing spondylitis, chronic pain, gout, oral surgery pain, temporal arteritis, tendinitis.

CONTRAINDICATIONS Hypersensitivity to oxaprozin or any other NSAID; complete or partial syndrome of nasal polyps; angioedema; pregnancy (category C).

CAUTIOUS USE History of GI bleeding, alcoholism, smoking; history of severe hepatic dysfunction, renal insufficiency; photosensitivity; lactation, older adults. Safety and effectiveness in children are not established.

ROUTE & DOSAGE

Osteoarthritis, Rheumatoid Arthritis

Adult: **PO** 600–1200 mg q.d. (max: 1800 mg/d or 25 mg/kg, whichever is lower)

ADMINISTRATION

Oral

- Give with meals or milk to decrease GI distress.
- Divide doses in those unable to tolerate once-daily dosing.
- Use lower starting doses for those with renal or hepatic dysfunction, advanced age, low body weight, or a predisposition to GI ulceration.

ADVERSE EFFECTS (≥1%) **CNS:** Tinnitus, headache, insomnia, somnolence. **GI:** Diarrhea, abdominal pain, nausea, dyspepsia, flatulence, melena, ulcers, constipation, dry mouth, gastritis. **Skin:** Rash, pruritus. **Urogenital:** Dysuria, urinary frequency.

DIAGNOSTIC TEST INTERFERENCE May cause false-positive reactions for BENZODIAZEPINES with ***urine drug-screening*** tests.

INTERACTIONS Drug: May attenuate the antihypertensive response to DIURETICS. NSAIDS increase the risk of **methotrexate** or **lithium** toxicity. May increase **aspirin** toxicity. **Herbal: Feverfew, garlic, ginger, ginkgo** may increase risk of bleeding.

PHARMACOKINETICS Absorption: Readily absorbed from GI tract. **Peak:** 125 min. **Onset:** 1–6 wk for maximum therapeutic effect. **Distribution:** 99% protein bound. Distributes into synovial fluid, crosses placenta. Distributed into breast milk. **Metabolism:** Metabolized in the liver. **Elimination:** 60% excreted in urine, 30%–35% excreted in feces. **Half-Life:** 40 h.

NURSING IMPLICATIONS

Assessment & Drug Effects

- Monitor for S&S of GI bleeding, especially in patients with a history of inflammation or ulceration of upper GI tract, or those treated chronically with NSAIDS.
- Monitor patients with CHF for increased fluid retention and edema. Report rapid weight increases accompanied by edema.
- Lab tests: Perform baseline and periodic evaluation of Hgb, kidney and liver function. Auditory and ophthalmologic exams are recommended with prolonged or high-dose therapy.

Patient & Family Education

- Be aware that alcoholism and smoking increase risk of GI ulceration.
- Report immediately dark tarry stools, "coffee ground" or bloody emesis, or other GI distress.
- Avoid aspirin or other NSAIDS without explicit permission of physician.
- Be aware of the possibility of photosensitivity, which results in a rash on sun-exposed skin.
- Report immediately to physician ringing in ears, decreased hearing, or blurred vision.
- Do not exceed ordered dose. The goal of therapy is lowest effective dose.
- Do not breast feed while taking this drug without consulting physician.

OXAZEPAM

(ox-a'ze-pam)

Ox-Pam ♣, Serax, Zapex ♣

Classifications: CENTRAL NERVOUS SYSTEM AGENT; ANXIOLYTIC; SEDATIVE-HYPNOTIC; BENZODIAZEPINE

Prototype: Lorazepam

Pregnancy Category: C

Controlled Substance: Schedule IV

AVAILABILITY 10 mg, 15 mg, 30 mg capsules; 15 mg tablets

ACTIONS Benzodiazepine derivative related to lorazepam. Effects are mediated by the inhibitory neurotransmitter GABA. Acts on the thalamic, hypothalamic, and limbic levels of CNS.

THERAPEUTIC EFFECTS Has anxiolytic, sedative, hypnotic, and skeletal muscle relaxant effects.

USES Management of anxiety and tension associated with a wide range of emotional disturbances. Also to control acute withdrawal symptoms in chronic alcoholism.

CONTRAINDICATIONS Hypersensitivity to oxazepam and other ben-

zodiazepines; psychoses, pregnancy (category C), lactation, children <12 y; acute-angle glaucoma, acute alcohol intoxication.
CAUTIOUS USE Older adult and debilitated patients; impaired kidney and liver function; addiction-prone patients; COPD; mental depression.

ROUTE & DOSAGE

Anxiety
Adult: **PO** 10–30 mg t.i.d. or q.i.d.
Acute Alcohol Withdrawal
Adult: **PO** 15–30 mg t.i.d. or q.i.d.

ADMINISTRATION

Oral
- Give with food if GI upset occurs.
- Store in tightly closed container at 15°–30° C (59°–86° F) unless otherwise specified.

ADVERSE EFFECTS (≥1%) **CNS:** *Drowsiness,* dizziness, mental confusion, vertigo, ataxia, headache, lethargy, syncope, tremor, slurred speech, paradoxic reaction (euphoria, excitement). **GI:** Nausea, xerostomia, jaundice. **Skin:** Skin rash, edema. **CV:** Hypotension, edema. **Hematologic:** Leukopenia. **Urogenital:** Altered libido.

INTERACTIONS Drug: Alcohol, CNS DEPRESSANTS, ANTICONVULSANTS potentiate CNS depression; **cimetidine** increases oxazepam plasma levels, increasing its toxicity; may decrease antiparkinsonism effects of **levodopa;** may increase **phenytoin** levels; smoking decreases sedative and antianxiety effects. **Herbal: Kava-kava, valerian** may potentiate sedation.

PHARMACOKINETICS Absorption: Readily absorbed from GI tract. **Peak:** 2–3 h. **Distribution:** Crosses placenta; distributed into breast milk. **Metabolism:** Metabolized in liver. **Elimination:** Primarily excreted in urine, some in feces. **Half-Life:** 2–8 h.

NURSING IMPLICATIONS

Assessment & Drug Effects
- Observe older adult patients closely for signs of overdosage. Report to physician if daytime psychomotor function is depressed.
- Lab tests: Perform liver function and white blood cell counts on a regular planned basis.
- Note: Excessive and prolonged use may cause physical dependence.

Patient & Family Education
- Report promptly any mild paradoxic stimulation of affect and excitement with sleep disturbances that may occur within the first 2 wk of therapy. Dosage reduction is indicated.
- Do not change dose or dose schedule and refrain from using drug to treat a self-diagnosed condition.
- Consult physician before self-medicating with OTC drugs.
- Do not drive or engage in potentially hazardous activities until response to drug is known.
- Do not drink alcoholic beverages while taking oxazepam. The CNS depressant effects of each agent may be intensified.
- Contact physician if you intend to or do become pregnant during therapy about discontinuing the drug.
- Withdraw drug slowly following prolonged therapy to avoid precipitating withdrawal symptoms (seizures, mental confusion, nausea, vomiting, muscle and abdominal cramps, tremulousness, sleep disturbances, unusual irritability, hyperhidrosis).
- Do not breast feed while taking this drug.

OXCARBAZEPINE

(ox-car'ba-ze-peen)

Trileptal

Classifications: CENTRAL NERVOUS SYSTEM AGENT; ANTICONVULSANT

Prototype: Carbamazepine

Pregnancy Category: C

AVAILABILITY 150 mg, 300 mg, 600 mg tablets; 300 mg/5 mL suspension

ACTIONS Structurally related to tricyclic antidepressants (TCAs) but lacks antidepressant properties. Anticonvulsant properties may result from blockage of voltage-sensitive sodium channels, which results in stabilization of hyperexcited neural membranes.

THERAPEUTIC EFFECTS Inhibits repetitive neuronal firing, and decreased propagation of neuronal impulses.

O

USES Monotherapy or adjunctive therapy in the treatment of partial seizures in adults and children age 4–16.

CONTRAINDICATIONS Hypersensitivity to oxcarbazepine; pregnancy (category C), lactation; children <4 y.

CAUTIOUS USE Older adults; renal impairment; children <8 y; infertility, hyponatremia, SIADH, and drugs associated with SIADH as an adverse effect.

ROUTE & DOSAGE

Partial Seizures

Adult: **PO** Start with 300 mg b.i.d. and increase by 600 mg/d q wk to 2400 mg/d in 2 divided doses for monotherapy or 1200 mg/d as adjunctive therapy

Child: **PO** *4–16 y,* Initiate with 8–10 mg/kg/d divided b.i.d. (max: 600 mg/d), gradually increase weekly to target dose (divided b.i.d.) based on weight: *20–29 kg,* 900 mg/d; *29.1–39 kg,* 1200 mg/d; *>39 kg,* 1800 mg/d

Renal Impairment

Cl_{cr} <30 mL/min: Initiate at 1/2 usual starting dose (300 mg b.i.d.)

ADMINISTRATION

Oral

- Initiate therapy at one-half the usual starting dose (300 mg/d) if creatinine clearance <30 mL/min.
- Do not abruptly stop this medication; withdraw drug gradually when discontinued to minimize seizure potential.
- Store preferably at 25° C (77° F), but room temperature permitted. Keep container tightly closed.

ADVERSE EFFECTS (≥1%) **Body as a Whole:** *Fatigue,* asthenia, peripheral edema, generalized edema, chest pain, weight gain. **CV:** Hypotension. **GI:** *Nausea, vomiting, abdominal pain,* diarrhea, dyspepsia, constipation, gastritis, anorexia, dry mouth. **Hematologic:** Lymphadenopathy. **Metabolic:** Hyponatremia. **Musculoskeletal:** Muscle weakness. **CNS:** *Headache, dizziness, somnolence, ataxia, nystagmus, abnormal gait,* insomnia, tremor, nervousness, agitation, abnormal coordination, speech disorder, confusion, abnormal thinking, aggravate convulsions, emotional lability. **Respiratory:** Rhinitis, cough, bronchitis, pharyngitis. **Skin:** Acne, hot flushes, purpura. **Special Senses:** *Diplopia, vertigo, abnormal vision,* abnormal accommodation, taste perversion, ear ache. **Urogenital:** Urinary tract infection, micturition frequency, vaginitis.

INTERACTIONS Drug: Carbamazepine, phenobarbital, phenytoin, valproic acid, verapamil may decrease oxcarbazepine levels; may increase levels of **phenobarbital, phenytoin;** may decrease levels of **felodipine,** ORAL CONTRACEPTIVES. **Herbal: Ginkgo** may decrease anticonvulsant effectiveness.

PHARMACOKINETICS Absorption: Rapidly and completely absorbed from GI tract. **Peak:** Steady-state levels reached in 2–3 d. **Distribution:** 40% protein bound. **Metabolism:** Extensively metabolized in liver to active 10-monohydroxy metabolite (MHD). **Elimination:** 95% excreted in kidneys. **Half-Life:** 2 h, MHD 9 h.

NURSING IMPLICATIONS

Assessment & Drug Effects

- Monitor for and report S&S of: Hyponatremia (e.g., nausea, malaise, headache, lethargy, confusion); CNS impairment (e.g., somnolence, excessive fatigue, cognitive deficits, speech or language problems, incoordination, gait disturbances).
- Monitor phenytoin levels when administered concurrently.
- Lab tests: Periodic serum sodium, T_4 level; when oxcarbazepine is used as adjunctive therapy, closely monitor plasma level of the concomitant antiepileptic drug during titration of the oxcarbazepine dose.

Patient & Family Education

- Notify physician of the following: Dizziness, excess drowsiness, frequent headaches, malaise, double vision, lack of coordination, or persistent nausea.
- Exercise special caution with concurrent use of alcohol or CNS depressants.
- Use caution with potentially hazardous activities and driving until response to drug is known.
- Use or add barrier contraceptive since drug may render hormonal methods ineffective.
- Do not breast feed while taking this drug.

OXICONAZOLE NITRATE

(ox-i-con'a-zole)

Oxistat

Classifications: SKIN AND MUCOUS MEMBRANE AGENT; ANTIFUNGAL

Prototype: Fluconazole

Pregnancy Category: B

AVAILABILITY 1% cream, lotion

ACTIONS Synthetic antifungal agent that presumably works by altering cellular membrane of the fungi, resulting in increased membrane permeability, secondary metabolic effects, and growth inhibition.

THERAPEUTIC EFFECTS Effective against *Trichophyton rubrum, Trichophyton mentagrophytes, Candida albicans, Candida tropicalis.*

USES Topical treatment of tinea pedis, tinea cruris, and tinea corporis due to *Trichophyton rubrum* and *Trichophyton mentagrophytes;* also used for cutaneous candidiasis caused by *Candida albicans* and *Candida tropicalis.*

CONTRAINDICATIONS Hypersensitivity to oxiconazole.

CAUTIOUS USE Pregnancy (category B), lactation.

ROUTE & DOSAGE

Tinea and Other Dermal Infections

Adult: **Topical** Apply to affected area once daily in the evening

O

ADMINISTRATION

Topical

- Apply cream to cover the affected areas once daily (in the evening).
- Treat tinea corporis and tinea cruris for 2 wk; tinea pedis for 1 mo to reduce the possibility of recurrence.
- Store at 15°–30° C (59°–86° F).

ADVERSE EFFECTS (≥1%) **Skin:** Transient burning and stinging, dryness, erythema, pruritus, and local irritation.

INTERACTIONS Drug: No clinically significant interactions established.

PHARMACOKINETICS Absorption: <0.3% is absorbed systemically.

NURSING IMPLICATIONS

Patient & Family Education

- Use only externally. Do not use intravaginally.
- Discontinue drug and contact physician if irritation or sensitivity develops.
- Avoid contact with eyes.
- Contact physician if no improvement is noted after the prescribed treatment period.
- Do not breast feed while using this drug without consulting physician.

O

OXTRIPHYLLINE

(ox-trye'fi-lin)

Choledyl, Choledyl SA, Choline Theophyllinate

Classification: BRONCHODILATOR (RESPIRATORY SMOOTH MUSCLE RELAXANT) XANTHINE

Prototype: Theophylline

Pregnancy Category: C

AVAILABILITY 100 mg, 200 mg tablets; 400 mg, 600 mg sustained-release tablets; 50 mg/5 mL syrup; 100 mg/5 mL elixir

ACTIONS Choline salt of theophylline. Compared to aminophylline, reportedly more stable, more soluble, and more uniformly and predictably absorbed, and produces less gastric irritation.

THERAPEUTIC EFFECTS Relaxes smooth muscle by direct action, particularly of bronchi and pulmonary vessels, and stimulates medullary respiratory center with resulting increase in vital capacity. Also relaxes smooth muscles of biliary and GI tracts. Stimulates myocardium, thereby increasing force of contractions and cardiac output, and stimulates all levels of CNS.

USES As bronchodilator to control asthma or COPD.

CONTRAINDICATIONS Hypersensitivity to xanthines; coronary artery disease; renal or hepatic impairment. Safe use during pregnancy (category C), lactation, or in children <2 y is not established.

CAUTIOUS USE Peptic ulcer; prostatic hypertrophy; diabetes mellitus; glaucoma.

ROUTE & DOSAGE

Asthma, COPD

Adult: **PO** 4.7 mg/kg (usual dose 200 mg) q8h
Child: **PO** *1–9 y*, 6.2 mg/kg q6h; *9–16 y and adult smoker*, 4.7 mg/kg (usual dose 200 mg) q6h

ADMINISTRATION

Oral

- Give on an empty stomach (30 min to 1 h before or 2 h after meals); may be taken after meals and at bedtime to reduce GI distress. Sustained-release tablet permits dosing q12h.

- Ensure that sustained-release form is not chewed or crushed. It must be swallowed whole.
- Protect elixir from light.

ADVERSE EFFECTS (≥1%) **CNS:** Restlessness, dizziness, insomnia, convulsions, *muscle twitching*. **CV:** Palpitation, tachycardia, flushing, hypotension. **GI:** *Nausea,* vomiting, anorexia, epigastric pain, diarrhea, activation of peptic ulcer. **Urogenital:** Transient urinary frequency, kidney irritation. **Body as a Whole:** Urticaria, fever, dehydration.

INTERACTIONS Drug: Increases **lithium** excretion, lowering lithium levels; **cimetidine,** high dose **allopurinol** (600 mg/d), **ciprofloxacin, erythromycin, troleandomycin** can significantly increase theophylline levels.

PHARMACOKINETICS Absorption: Well absorbed from GI tract. **Duration:** 4–8 h; varies with age, smoking, and liver function. **Distribution:** Crosses placenta; distributed into breast milk. **Metabolism:** Extensively metabolized in liver. **Elimination:** Parent drug and metabolites excreted by kidneys. **Half-Life:** 4 h in adults.

NURSING IMPLICATIONS

Note: See theophylline for numerous additional nursing implications.

Assessment & Drug Effects

- Determine patient's tobacco use. Cigarette smoking may alter hepatic microsomal enzyme activity and indicate increase in dosage.
- Use safety precautions with older adults during early therapy; dizziness is a relatively common adverse effect.
- Monitor vital signs and I&O. Improvement in quality of pulse and respiration and diuresis are expected clinical effects.
- Observe and report early signs of possible toxicity: anorexia, nausea, vomiting, dizziness, shakiness, restlessness, abdominal discomfort, irritability, palpitation, tachycardia, marked hypotension, cardiac arrhythmias, seizures.

Patient & Family Education

- Report gastric distress, palpitation, and CNS stimulation (irritability, restlessness, nervousness, insomnia) to physician. Reduction in dosage may be indicated.
- Limit caffeine intake; it may increase incidence of adverse effects.
- Do not take OTC medications, especially cough suppressants, which may cause retention of secretions and CNS depression, without consulting physician.
- Drink adequate fluids (at least 2000 mL/d) to decrease viscosity of airway secretions.
- Do not breast feed while taking this drug without consulting physician.

OXYBUTYNIN CHLORIDE

(ox-i-byoo'ti-nin)

Ditropan, Ditropan XL, Oxytrol

Classifications: AUTONOMIC NERVOUS SYSTEM AGENT; ANTICHOLINERGIC (PARASYMPATHOLYTIC); ANTIMUSCARINIC; ANTISPASMODIC

Prototype: Atropine

Pregnancy Category: B

AVAILABILITY 5 mg tablets; 5 mg, 10 mg sustained-release tablets; 5 mg/5 mL syrup; 3.9 mg/d transdermal patch

ACTIONS Synthetic tertiary amine that exerts direct antispasmodic ac-

tion and inhibits muscarinic effects of acetylcholine on smooth muscle.
THERAPEUTIC EFFECTS Prominent antispasmodic activity.

USES To relieve symptoms associated with voiding in patients with uninhibited neurogenic bladder and reflex neurogenic bladder. Also has been used to relieve pain of bladder spasm following transurethral surgical procedures.

CONTRAINDICATIONS Hypersensitivity of oxybutynin; narrow angle glaucoma, myasthenia gravis, partial or complete GI obstruction, gastric retention, paralytic ileus, intestinal atony (especially older adult or debilitated patients), megacolon, severe colitis, GU obstruction, urinary retention, unstable cardiovascular status.
CAUTIOUS USE Older adults; autonomic neuropathy, hiatus hernia with reflex esophagitis; hepatic or renal dysfunction; urinary infection; hyperthyroidism; CHF, coronary artery disease, hypertension; prostatic hypertrophy; pregnancy (category B), children <18, lactation.

O

ROUTE & DOSAGE

Neurogenic Bladder
Adult: **PO** 5 mg b.i.d. or t.i.d. (max: 20 mg/d) or 5 mg sustained-release q.d., may increase up to 30 mg/d **Topical** Apply 1 patch twice weekly
Geriatric: **PO** 2.5–5 mg b.i.d. (max: 15 mg/d) or 5 mg sustained-release q.d., may increase up to 30 mg/d **Topical** Apply 1 patch twice weekly
Child: **PO** *1–5 y,* 0.2 mg/kg b.i.d.–q.i.d.; *>5 y,* 5 mg b.i.d. (max: 15 mg/d)

ADMINISTRATION

Oral

- Ensure that sustained-release form is not chewed or crushed. It must be swallowed whole.

Topical

- Ensure that old patch is removed prior to application of new patch.

ADVERSE EFFECTS (≥1%) **Body as a Whole:** Severe allergic reactions including urticaria, skin rashes, suppression of lactation, decreased sweating, fever. **CNS:** *Drowsiness,* dizziness, weakness, insomnia, restlessness, psychotic behavior (overdosage). **CV:** Palpitations, tachycardia, flushing. **Special Senses:** Mydriasis, *blurred vision,* cycloplegia, increased ocular tension. **GI:** *Dry mouth,* nausea, vomiting, *constipation,* bloated feeling. **Skin:** *Pruritus at application site,* rash, application site vesicles, erythema. **Urogenital:** Urinary hesitancy or retention, impotence.

PHARMACOKINETICS Absorption: Diffuses across intact skin. **Onset:** 0.5–1 h. **Peak:** 3–6 h. **Duration:** 6–10 h. **PO:** 96 h Transdermal. **Metabolism:** Metabolized in liver. **Elimination:** Excreted primarily in urine. **Half-Life:** 2–5 h

NURSING IMPLICATIONS

Assessment & Drug Effects

- Periodic interruptions of therapy are recommended to determine patient's need for continued treatment. Tolerance has occurred in some patients.
- Keep physician informed of expected responses to drug therapy (e.g., effect on urinary frequency, urgency, urge incontinence, nocturia, completeness of bladder emptying).

- Monitor patients with colostomy or ileostomy closely; abdominal distension and the onset of diarrhea in these patients may be early signs of intestinal obstruction or of toxic megacolon.

Patient & Family Education

- Do not drive or engage in potentially hazardous activities until response to drug is known.
- Exercise caution in hot environments. By suppressing sweating, oxybutynin can cause fever and heat stroke.
- Do not breast feed while taking this drug without consulting physician.

OXYCODONE HYDROCHLORIDE

(ox-i-koe′done)

OxyContin, Percolone, Endocodone, OxyFAST, Roxicodone

Classifications: CENTRAL NERVOUS SYSTEM AGENT; NARCOTIC (OPIATE) AGONIST; ANALGESIC

Prototype: Morphine

Pregnancy Category: B (D for prolonged use or use of high doses at term)

Controlled Substance: Schedule II

AVAILABILITY 5 mg, 15 mg, 30 mg tablets; **OxyContin** 10 mg, 20 mg, 40 mg, 80 mg, 160 mg sustained-release tablets; 5 mg/5 mL, 20 mg/mL oral solution

ACTIONS Semisynthetic derivative of an opium alkaloid with actions qualitatively similar to those of morphine. Most prominent actions involve CNS and organs composed of smooth muscle. Binds with stereo-specific receptors in various sites of CNS to alter both perception of pain and emotional response to pain, but precise mechanism of action not clear. As potent as morphine and 10–12 times more potent than codeine.

THERAPEUTIC EFFECTS Active against moderate to moderately severe pain. Appears to be more effective in relief of acute than long-standing pain.

USES Relief of moderate to moderately severe pain such as may occur with bursitis, dislocations, simple fractures and other injuries, and neuralgia. Relieves postoperative, postextractional, postpartum pain.

CONTRAINDICATIONS Hypersensitivity to oxycodone and principal drugs with which it is combined; during pregnancy (category B); for prolonged use or high doses at term (category D); lactation, and children <6 y.

CAUTIOUS USE Alcoholism; renal or hepatic disease; viral infections; Addison's disease; cardiac arrhythmias; chronic ulcerative colitis; history of drug abuse or dependency; gallbladder disease, acute abdominal conditions; head injury, intracranial lesions; hypothyroidism; prostatic hypertrophy; respiratory disease; urethral stricture; older adult or debilitated patients; peptic ulcer or coagulation abnormalities (combination products containing aspirin).

ROUTE & DOSAGE

Moderate to Severe Pain

Adult: **PO** 5–10 mg q6h prn; OxyContin can be dosed q8h
Child: **PO** *6–12 y,* 1.25 mg q6h prn; *≥12 y,* 2.5 mg q6h prn

ADMINISTRATION

Oral

- Ensure that sustained-release form is not chewed or crushed. It must be swallowed whole.

- Store this DANGEROUS medication in a place inaccessible to children at 15°–30° C (59°–86° F). Protect from light.

ADVERSE EFFECTS (≥1%) **CNS:** Euphoria, dysphoria, light-headedness, dizziness, *sedation*. **GI:** Anorexia, nausea, vomiting, *constipation,* jaundice, hepatotoxicity (combinations containing acetaminophen). **Respiratory:** Shortness of breath, respiratory depression. **Skin:** Pruritus, skin rash. **CV:** Bradycardia. **Body as a Whole:** Unusual bleeding or bruising. **Urogenital:** Dysuria, frequency of urination, urinary retention.

DIAGNOSTIC TEST INTERFERENCE ***Serum amylase*** levels may be elevated because oxycodone causes spasm of sphincter of Oddi. ***Blood glucose determinations:*** false decrease (measured by ***glucose oxidase-peroxidase method***). ***5-HIAA determination:*** false positive with use of ***nitroisonaphthol reagent*** (quantitative test is unaffected).

INTERACTIONS Drug: Alcohol and other CNS DEPRESSANTS add to CNS depressant activity. **Herbal: St. John's wort** may increase sedation.

PHARMACOKINETICS Absorption: Readily absorbed from GI tract. **Onset:** 10–15 min. **Peak:** 30–60 min. **Duration:** 4–5 h. **Distribution:** Crosses placenta; distributed into breast milk. **Metabolism:** Metabolized in liver. **Elimination:** Excreted primarily in urine. **Half-Life:** 3–5 h.

NURSING IMPLICATIONS

Assessment & Drug Effects

- Monitor patient's response closely, especially to sustained-release preparations.
- Consult physician if nausea continues after first few days of therapy.
- Note: Light-headedness, dizziness, sedation, or fainting appear to be more prominent in ambulatory than in nonambulatory patients and may be alleviated if patient lies down.
- Evaluate patient's continued need for oxycodone preparations. Psychic and physical dependence and tolerance may develop with repeated use. The potential for drug abuse is high.
- Lab tests: Check hepatic function and hematologic status periodically in patients on high dosage.
- Be aware that serious overdosage of any oxycodone preparation presents problems associated with a narcotic overdose (respiratory depression, circulatory collapse, extreme somnolence progressing to stupor or coma).

Patient & Family Education

- Do not alter dosage regimen by increasing, decreasing, or shortening intervals between doses. Habit formation and liver damage may result.
- Avoid potentially hazardous activities such as driving a car or operating machinery while using oxycodone preparation.
- Do not drink large amounts of alcoholic beverages while using oxycodone preparations; risk of liver damage is increased.
- Check with physician before taking OTC drugs for colds, stomach distress, allergies, insomnia, or pain.
- Inform surgeon or dentist that you are taking an oxycodone preparation before any surgical procedure is undertaken.
- Do not breast feed while taking this drug.

OXYMETAZOLINE HYDROCHLORIDE

(ox-i-met-az′oh-leen)

Afrin, Dristan Long Lasting, Duramist Plus, Duration, Nafrine ♣, Neo-Synephrine 12 Hour, Nostrilla, Sinex Long Lasting

Classifications: EYE, EAR, NOSE, AND THROAT (EENT) PREPARATION; VASOCONSTRICTOR, DECONGESTANT; SYMPATHOMIMETIC

Prototype: Naphazoline

Pregnancy Category: C

AVAILABILITY 0.025%, 0.05% solution

ACTIONS Sympathomimetic agent that acts directly on alpha receptors of sympathetic nervous system. No effect on beta receptors.

THERAPEUTIC EFFECTS Constricts smaller arterioles in nasal passages and has prolonged decongestant effect.

USES Relief of nasal congestion in a variety of allergic and infectious disorders of the upper respiratory tract; used as nasal tampon to facilitate intranasal examination or before nasal surgery. Also used as adjunct in treatment and prevention of middle ear infection by decreasing congestion of eustachian ostia.

CONTRAINDICATIONS Use in children <2 y. Safe use during pregnancy (category C) or lactation is not established.

CAUTIOUS USE Within 14 d of MAO inhibitors, coronary artery disease, hypertension, hyperthyroidism, diabetes mellitus.

ROUTE & DOSAGE

Nasal Congestion

Adult: **Intranasal** 2–3 drops or 2–3 sprays of 0.05% solution into each nostril b.i.d. for up to 3–5 d

Child: **Intranasal** *2–5 y,* 2–3 drops or 2–3 sprays of 0.025% solution into each nostril b.i.d. for up to 3–5 d; *>6 y,* same as for adult

ADMINISTRATION

Instillation

- Place spray nozzle in nostril without occluding it and tilt head slightly forward prior to instillation of spray; sniff briskly during administration.
- Rinse dropper or spray tip in hot water after each use to prevent contamination of solution by nasal secretions.
- Usually given in the morning and at bedtime. Effects appear within 30 min and last about 6–7 h.

ADVERSE EFFECTS (≥1%) **Special Senses:** *Burning,* stinging, dryness of nasal mucosa, *sneezing.* **Body as a Whole:** Headache, light-headedness, drowsiness, insomnia, palpitations, *rebound congestion.*

INTERACTIONS Drug: No clinically significant interactions established.

PHARMACOKINETICS Onset: 5–10 min. **Duration:** 6–10 h.

NURSING IMPLICATIONS

Assessment & Drug Effects

- Monitor for S&S of excess use. If noted, discuss possibility of rebound congestion.

Patient & Family Education

- Wash hands carefully after handling oxymetazoline. Anisocoria (inequality of pupil size, blurred vision) can develop if eyes are rubbed with contaminated fingers.

- Do not to exceed recommended dosage. Rebound congestion (chemical rhinitis) may occur with prolonged or excessive use.
- Systemic effects can result from swallowing excessive medication.
- Do not breast feed while using this drug without consulting physician.

OXYMETHOLONE

(ox-i-meth'oh-lone)

Anadrol, Anadrol-50, Anapolon ✦

Classifications: HORMONES AND SYNTHETIC SUBSTITUTES; ANDROGEN/ ANABOLIC STEROID

Prototype: Testosterone

Pregnancy Category: X

Controlled Substance: Schedule III

AVAILABILITY 50 mg tablets

ACTIONS Potent steroid with anabolic activity. Mechanism of action in refractory anemias is unclear but may be due to direct stimulation of bone marrow, protein anabolic activity, or to androgenic stimulation of erythropoiesis.

THERAPEUTIC EFFECTS Promotes body tissue building and inhibits tissue-depleting processes; supports nitrogen, potassium, chloride, and phosphorus conservation. Enhances weight gain and combats depression and weakness in debilitating conditions. Stimulates bone growth, aids in bone matrix reconstitution, and may support calcification of metastatic lesions of breast cancer.

USES Aplastic anemia.

UNLABELED USES Osteoporosis, catabolic conditions.

CONTRAINDICATIONS Prostatic hypertrophy with obstruction; pregnancy (category X); prostatic or male breast cancer; cardiac, renal, hepatic decompensation; nephrosis; premature infant; use during lactation is not established.

CAUTIOUS USE Prepubertal males; geriatric male patients; diabetes mellitus; coronary disease; patient taking ACTH, corticosteroids, anticoagulants.

ROUTE & DOSAGE

Aplastic Anemia

Adult/Child: **PO** 1–5 mg/kg/d

ADMINISTRATION

Oral

- A course of therapy for treatment of osteoporosis is 7–21 d.
- For treatment of anemias, a minimum trial period of 3–6 mo is recommended, since response tends to be slow.
- Store at 15°–30° C (59°–86° F). Protect from heat and light.

ADVERSE EFFECTS (≥1%) **Endocrine:** Androgenic in women: Suppression of ovulation, lactation, or menstruation; *hoarseness or deepening of voice* (often irreversible); *hirsutism; oily skin; acne;* clitoral enlargement; regression of breasts; male-pattern baldness (in disseminated breast cancer). Hypoestrogenic effects in women: Flushing, sweating; vaginitis with pruritus, drying, bleeding; menstrual irregularities. Men: prepubertal: premature epiphyseal closure, phallic enlargement, priapism. Postpubertal: testicular atrophy, decreased ejaculatory volume, azoospermia, oligospermia (after prolonged administration or excessive dosage), impotence, epididymitis, gynecomastia. **CV:** *Edema,* skin flush. **GI:** *Nausea, vomiting, anorexia,* diarrhea, jaundice, hepatotoxicity. **Urogenital:** Bladder irritability. **Metabolic:** Hypercalcemia.

INTERACTIONS Drug: May enhance hypoprothrombinemic effects of **warfarin. Herbal: Echinacea** may increase risk of hepatotoxicity.

PHARMACOKINETICS Absorption: Readily absorbed from GI tract. **Metabolism:** Metabolized in liver. **Elimination:** Excreted in urine. **Half-Life:** 9 h.

NURSING IMPLICATIONS

Assessment & Drug Effects

- Monitor patient with a history of seizures closely because an increase in their frequency may be noted.
- Monitor periodically for edema that may develop with or without CHF.
- Monitor for hypercalcemia (see Appendix F), especially in women with breast cancer.
- Lab tests: Periodic serum calcium; periodic liver function tests are especially important for the older adult patient. Drug should be stopped with first sign of liver toxicity (jaundice).

Patient & Family Education

- Monitor blood glucose for loss of glycemic control if diabetic.
- Women: Notify physician of signs of virilization.
- Do not breast feed while taking this drug without consulting physician.

OXYMORPHONE HYDROCHLORIDE

(ox-i-mor'fone)

Numorphan

Classifications: CENTRAL NERVOUS SYSTEM AGENT; NARCOTIC (OPIATE) AGONIST; ANALGESIC

Prototype: Morphine

Pregnancy Category: B (D for prolonged use or high doses at term)

Controlled Substance: Schedule II

AVAILABILITY 1 mg/mL, 1.5 mg/mL injection; 5 mg suppositories

ACTIONS Structurally and pharmacologically related to morphine. Analgesic action of 1 mg is reportedly equivalent to that of 10 mg of morphine.

THERAPEUTIC EFFECTS Produces mild sedation and, unlike morphine, has little antitussive action. In equianalgesic doses, may have less antitussive effect and may cause less constipation than does morphine but causes more nausea, vomiting, and euphoria.

USES Relief of moderate to severe pain, preoperative medication, obstetric analgesia, support of anesthesia, and relief of anxiety in patients with dyspnea associated with acute ventricular failure and pulmonary edema.

CONTRAINDICATIONS Pulmonary edema resulting from chemical respiratory irritants. Safe use during pregnancy [category B (D for prolonged use and high doses)], lactation, or in children <12 y is not established.

ROUTE & DOSAGE

Moderate to Severe Pain

Adult: **SC/IM** 1–1.5 mg q4–6h prn **IV** 0.5 mg q4–6h **PR** 5 mg q4–6h prn

Analgesia during Labor

Adult: **IM** 1–1.5 mg

ADMINISTRATION

Subcutaneous/Intramuscular

- Give undiluted.

Intravenous

PREPARE: **Direct:** Dilute in 5 mL of sterile water or NS.

ADMINISTER: **Direct:** Give at a rate of 0.5 mg over 2–5 min.

- Protect drug from light. Store suppositories in refrigerator 2°–15° C (36°–59° F).

ADVERSE EFFECTS (≥1%) **GI:** *Nausea, vomiting, euphoria.* **CNS:** *Dizziness,* lightheadedness, sedation. **Respiratory:** Respiratory depression (see morphine), apnea, respiratory arrest. **Body as a Whole:** Sweating, coma, shock. **CV:** Cardiac arrest, circulatory depression.

INTERACTIONS Drug: Alcohol and other CNS DEPRESSANTS add to CNS depression.

PHARMACOKINETICS Onset: 5–10 min IV; 10–15 min IM; 15–30 min PR. **Peak:** 1–1.5 h. **Duration:** 3–6 h. **Distribution:** Crosses placenta. **Metabolism:** Metabolized in liver. **Elimination:** Eliminated in urine.

NURSING IMPLICATIONS

O

Assessment & Drug Effects

- Monitor respiratory rate. Withhold drug and notify physician if rate falls below 12 breaths per minute.
- Supervise ambulation and advise patient of possible light-headedness. Older adult and debilitated patients are most susceptible to CNS depressant effects of drug.
- Evaluate patient's continued need for narcotic analgesic. Prolonged use can lead to dependence of morphine type.
- Medication contains sulfite and may precipitate a hypersensitivity reaction in susceptible patient.

Patient & Family Education

- Use caution when walking because of potential for injury from dizziness.
- Do not to consume alcohol while taking oxymorphone.
- Do not breast feed while taking this drug without consulting physician.

OXYTETRACYCLINE

(ox-i-tet-ra-sye′kleen)

Terramycin

OXYTETRACYCLINE HYDROCHLORIDE

Terramycin, Uri-Tet

Classifications: ANTIINFECTIVE; ANTIBIOTIC; TETRACYCLINE

Prototype: Tetracycline

Pregnancy Category: D

AVAILABILITY 250 mg capsules; 50 mg/mL, 125 mg/mL injection

ACTIONS Broad-spectrum antibiotic with actions similar to tetracycline.

THERAPEUTIC EFFECTS Effective against a variety of gram-positive and gram-negative bacteria and against most *Chlamydiae, Mycoplasmas, Rickettsiae,* and certain protozoa (e.g., amebae).

USES Treatment of gonorrhea, Lyme disease, upper and lower respiratory tract infections, Q fever, Rocky Mountain spotted fever, skin and skin structure infections, traveler's diarrhea, and UTIs

CONTRAINDICATIONS Hypersensitivity to tetracyclines; during tooth development [last half of pregnancy (category D)], lactation, infancy, childhood to age 8 y.

CAUTIOUS USE Impaired kidney function.

ROUTE & DOSAGE

Antiinfective

Adult: **PO** 250–500 mg q6–12h **IM** 100 mg q8–12h **IV** 250–500 mg q12h (max: 500 mg q6h)

Common adverse effects in *italic,* life-threatening effects underlined: generic names in **bold**; classifications in SMALL CAPS; ♣ Canadian drug name; ● Prototype drug

Child: **PO** >*8 y*, 25–50 mg/kg/d in 4 divided doses **IM** >*8 y*, 15–25 mg/kg/d in 2–3 divided doses (max: 250 mg/dose) **IV** >*8 y*, 10–20 mg/kg/d in 2 divided doses

ADMINISTRATION

Oral

- Check expiration date. Degradation products of outdated tetracyclines can be highly nephrotoxic.
- Give at least 1 h before or 2 h following meals. Food may interfere with rate and extent of absorption of oral drug. Do **NOT** give with antacids, milk, milk products, or other calcium-containing foods.

Intramuscular

- Note: Commercially available solution contains only 2% lidocaine. Administer by deep IM.
- Do not use IM solution for IV administration.

Intravenous

PREPARE: **Intermittent:** Use only oxytetracycline HCl for IV. Prepare by adding 10 mL of sterile water for injection or D5W to the 250 or 500 mg vial. Further dilute with a minimum of 100 mL D5W, NS, or RL.

ADMINISTER: **Intermittent:** Give slowly over 15–30 min. A slower rate of infusion and a large amount of diluent will reduce vein irritation.

- Store reconstituted solutions in refrigerator at 2°–8° C (36°–46.4° F) for up to 48h.

ADVERSE EFFECTS (≥1%) **GI:** Nausea, vomiting, diarrhea, stomatitis, anorexia, epigastric distress, esophageal ulcers, fatty liver, hepatotoxicity, elevated hepatic enzymes. **Skin:** Skin rash, photosensitivity. **Body as a Whole:** Lightheadedness, dizziness, pseudotumor cerebri, superinfections. **Urogenital:** Renal toxicity. **Hematologic:** Hemolytic anemia, thrombocytopenia. (Also see tetracycline.)

INTERACTIONS Drug: ANTACIDS, **iron, calcium, magnesium, zinc, kaolin and pectin, sodium bicarbonate, bismuth subsalicylate** can significantly decrease oxytetracycline absorption; effects of both **desmopressin** and oxytetracycline antagonized; increases **digoxin** absorption, increasing risk of **digoxin** toxicity; **methoxyflurane** increases risk of renal failure. **Food: Dairy products** significantly decrease oxytetracycline absorption; food may decrease drug absorption.

PHARMACOKINETICS Absorption: About 60% absorbed from GI tract and IM site. **Peak:** 2–4 h. **Distribution:** Appears to concentrate in hepatic system; crosses placenta; distributed into breast milk. **Metabolism:** Partially metabolized. **Elimination:** Excreted in feces and urine. **Half-Life:** 6–10 h.

NURSING IMPLICATIONS

Assessment & Drug Effects

- Monitor for S&S of superinfection (see Appendix F).
- Lab test: Baseline renal function tests. Dosage may need to be reduced in the presence of renal impairment.
- Discontinue drug and notify physician at the first sign of a hypersensitivity response (see Appendix F).

Patient & Family Education

- Discard unused drug when course of therapy has ended.
- Avoid excessive exposure to sunlight because of the possibility of photosensitivity.
- Do not breast feed while taking this drug.

OXYTOCIN INJECTION (Pr)

(ox-i-toe'sin)

Pitocin, Syntocinon, Syntocinon Nasal Spray

Classifications: HORMONES AND SYNTHETIC SUBSTITUTES; OXYTOCIC

Pregnancy Category: X

AVAILABILITY 10 units/mL injection

ACTIONS Synthetic, water-soluble polypeptide consisting of eight amino acids, identical pharmacologically to the oxytocic principle of posterior pituitary.

THERAPEUTIC EFFECTS By direct action on myofibrils, produces phasic contractions characteristic of normal delivery. Promotes milk ejection (letdown) reflex in nursing mother, thereby increasing flow (not volume) of milk; also facilitates flow of milk during period of breast engorgement. Uterine sensitivity to oxytocin increases during gestation period and peaks sharply before parturition. Not used for elective induction of labor.

O

USES To initiate or improve uterine contraction at term only in carefully selected patients and only after cervix is dilated and presentation of fetus has occurred; used to stimulate letdown reflex in nursing mother and to relieve pain from breast engorgement. Uses include management of inevitable, incomplete, or missed abortion; stimulation of uterine contractions during third stage of labor; stimulation to overcome uterine inertia; control of postpartum hemorrhage and promotion of postpartum uterine involution. Also used to induce labor in cases of maternal diabetes, preeclampsia, eclampsia, and erythroblastosis fetalis.

CONTRAINDICATIONS Hypersensitivity to oxytocin; significant cephalopelvic disproportion, unfavorable fetal position or presentations that are undeliverable without conversion before delivery, obstetric emergencies in which benefit-to-risk ratio for mother or fetus favors surgical intervention, fetal distress in which delivery is not imminent, prematurity, placenta previa, prolonged use in severe toxemia or uterine inertia, hypertonic uterine patterns, previous surgery of uterus or cervix including cesarean section, conditions predisposing to thromboplastin or amniotic fluid embolism (dead fetus, abruptio placentae), grand multiparity, invasive cervical carcinoma, primipara >35 y of age, past history of uterine sepsis or of traumatic delivery, intranasal route during labor, simultaneous administration of drug by two routes.

CAUTIOUS USE Concomitant use with cyclopropane anesthesia or vasoconstrictive drugs.

ROUTE & DOSAGE

Antepartum

Adult: **IV** Start at 1 mU/min, may increase by 1 mU/min q15min (max: 20 mU/min)

Postpartum

Adult: **IV** Infuse a total of 10 U at a rate of 20–40 mU/min after delivery

To Promote Milk Ejection

Adult: **Nasal** 1 spray or 1 drop in 1 or both nostrils 2–3 min before nursing or pumping

ADMINISTRATION

Intravenous

PREPARE: **IV Infusion:** When diluting oxytocin for IV infusion, rotate bottle gently to distribute medicine throughout solution. **For**

inducing labor: Add 10 U (1 mL) of oxytocin to 1 L of D5W or NS to yield 10 mU/mL. **For postpartum bleeding:** Add 10–40 U (1–4 mL) of oxytocin to 1 L of D5W or NS to yield 10–40 mU/mL.

ADMINISTER: **IV Infusion:** See ROUTE & DOSAGE for recommended rates (mU/min).

INCOMPATIBILITIES **Solution/additive: Fibrinolysin, warfarin.**

ADVERSE EFFECTS (≥1%) **Body as a Whole:** Fetal trauma from too rapid propulsion through pelvis, fetal death, anaphylactic reactions, postpartum hemorrhage, precordial pain, edema, cyanosis or redness of skin. **CV:** Fetal bradycardia and arrhythmias, maternal cardiac arrhythmias, hypertensive episodes, subarachnoid hemorrhage, increased blood flow, fatal afibrinogenemia, ECG changes, PVCs, cardiovascular spasm and collapse. **GI:** Neonatal jaundice, maternal nausea, vomiting. **Endocrine:** ADH effects leading to severe water intoxication and hyponatremia, hypotension. **CNS:** Fetal intracranial hemorrhage, anxiety. **Respiratory:** Fetal hypoxia, maternal dyspnea. **Urogenital:** Uterine hypertonicity, tetanic contractions, uterine rupture, pelvic hematoma.

INTERACTIONS Drug: VASOCONSTRICTORS cause severe hypertension; **cyclopropane anesthesia** causes hypotension, maternal bradycardia, arrhythmias. **Herbal: Ephedra, ma-huang** may cause hypertension.

PHARMACOKINETICS Absorption: Destroyed in GI tract. **Onset:** Immediately IV; few minutes nasal. **Duration:** 1 h IV; 20 min nasal. **Distribution:** Distributed throughout extracellular fluid; small amount may cross placenta. **Metabolism:** Rapidly destroyed in liver and kidneys. **Elimination:** Small amounts excreted unchanged in urine. **Half-Life:** 3–5 min.

NURSING IMPLICATIONS

Assessment & Drug Effects

- Start flow charts to record maternal BP and other vital signs, I&O ratio, weight, strength, duration, and frequency of contractions, as well as fetal heart tone and rate, before instituting treatment.
- Monitor fetal heart rate and maternal BP and pulse at least q15min during infusion period; evaluate tonus of myometrium during and between contractions and record on flow chart. Report change in rate and rhythm immediately.
- Stop infusion to prevent fetal anoxia, turn patient on her side, and notify physician if contractions are prolonged (occurring at less than 2-min intervals) and if monitor records contractions about 50 mm Hg or if contractions last 90 seconds or longer. Stimulation will wane rapidly within 2–3 min. Oxygen administration may be necessary.
- If local or regional (caudal, spinal) anesthesia is being given to the patient receiving oxytocin, be alert to the possibility of hypertensive crisis (sudden intense occipital headache, palpitation, marked hypertension, stiff neck, nausea, vomiting, sweating, fever, photophobia, dilated pupils, bradycardia or tachycardia, constricting chest pain).
- Monitor I&O during labor. If patient is receiving drug by prolonged IV infusion, watch for symptoms of water intoxication (drowsiness, listlessness, headache, confusion, anuria, weight gain). Report changes in alertness and orientation and changes in I&O ratio (i.e., marked decrease in output with excessive intake).

O

- Check fundus frequently during the first few postpartum hours and several times daily thereafter.
- Incidence of hypersensitivity or allergic reactions is higher when oxytocin is given by IM or IV injection rather than by IV infusion (diluted solution).

Patient & Family Education
- Be aware of purpose and anticipated effect of oxytocin.
- Report sudden, severe headache immediately to healthcare providers.

PACLITAXEL (Pr)

(pac-li-tax'el)
Taxol
Classifications: ANTINEOPLASTIC; TAXANE
Pregnancy Category: X

AVAILABILITY 6 mg/mL injection

ACTIONS Antimicrotubule agent that interferes with microtubule network essential for interphase and mitosis. Induces abnormal spindle formation and multiple asters during mitosis. In addition, normal functioning microtubules are essential for cell shape and organelles present within cells.
THERAPEUTIC EFFECTS Interferes with growth of rapidly dividing cells including cancer cells, and eventually causes cell death. May be used alone or with other chemotherapy agents or radiation therapy.

USES Ovarian cancer, breast cancer, Kaposi's sarcoma, non-small cell lung cancer (NSCLC).
UNLABELED USES Other solid tumors, leukemia, melanoma.

CONTRAINDICATIONS Hypersensitivity to paclitaxel, and patient's with baseline neutropenia of <1500 cells/mm^3; pregnancy (category X), lactation.
CAUTIOUS USE Cardiac arrhythmias; impaired liver function; Safety and efficacy in children are not established.

ROUTE & DOSAGE

Ovarian Cancer, NSCLC
Adult: **IV** 135 mg/m^2 24-h infusion repeated q22d
Breast Cancer
Adult: **IV** 175 mg/m^2 over 3 h q3wk
Solid Tumors, Malignant Melanoma
Adult: **IV** 250 mg/m^2 24-h infusion repeated q3wk
Kaposi's Sarcoma
Adult: **IV** 135 mg/m^2 infused over 3 h q3wk or 100 mg/m^2 infused over 3 h q2wk

ADMINISTRATION

Note: Premedication with dexamethasone, diphenhydramine, and H_2 antagonists (or ephedrine) is recommended to reduce hypersensitivity reactions, and consists of dexamethasone 20 mg PO or IV 14 and 7 h prior to Taxol infusion; diphenhydramine 50 mg IV 30 min prior to Taxol; and cimetidine 300 mg or ranitidine 50 mg IV 30 min before Taxol infusion.

Intravenous
- Follow institutional or standard guidelines for preparation, handling, and disposal of cytotoxic agents.
- Premedicate before using to avoid severe hypersensitivity.
- Do not administer unless neutrophil count is at least 1500/mm^3 and platelet count is at least 100,000/mm^3.

- Reduce dose by 20% if neutrophil count >500 mm^3 or if peripheral neuropathy develops.

PREPARE: **IV Infusion:** Do not use equipment or devices containing polyvinyl chloride (PVC) in preparation of infusion. Dilute to a final concentration of 0.3–1.2 mg/mL in any of the following: D5W, NS, D5/NS, or D5W in Ringer's injection. The prepared solution may be hazy, but this does not indicate a loss of potency.

ADMINISTER: **IV Infusion:** Give a single dose over 24 h every 3 wk. Do not administer subsequent doses unless neutrophil count is at least 1500/mm^3 and platelet count is at least 100,000/mm^3. The prepared solution may be hazy. Administer through IV tubing containing inline (0.22 micron or less) filter. Do not use equipment containing PVC in administration. Use central line if possible. Because tissue necrosis occurs with extravasation, frequently assess patency of a peripheral IV site.

INCOMPATIBILITIES **Solution/additive: PVC bags** and **infusion sets** should be avoided due to leaching of DEHP (plasticizer). Do not mix with any other medications. **Y-site: Amphotericin B, Amphotericin B cholesteryl sulfate complex, chlorpromazine, doxorubicin liposome, hydroxyzine, methylprednisolone, mitoxantrone.**

- Solutions diluted for infusion are stable at room temperature (approximately 25° C/77° F) for up to 27 h.

ADVERSE EFFECTS (≥1%) **CV:** Ventricular tachycardia, ventricular ectopy, *transient bradycardia,* chest pain. **CNS:** Fatigue, headaches, *peripheral neuropathy,* weakness, seizures. **GI:** *Nausea, vomiting,* diarrhea, taste changes, *mucositis,* elevations in serum triglycerides. **Hematologic:** *Neutropenia, anemia, thrombocytopenia*. **Body as a Whole:** *Hypersensitivity reactions (Hypotension, dyspnea with bronchospasm, urticaria, abdominal and extremity pain, diaphoresis, angioedema), myalgias, arthralgias, alopecia.* **Skin:** *Alopecia,* tissue necrosis with extravasation. **Urogenital:** Minor elevations in kidney and liver function tests.

INTERACTIONS Drug: Increased myelosuppression if **cisplatin, doxorubicin** is given before paclitaxel; **ketoconazole** can inhibit metabolism of paclitaxel; additive bradycardia with BETA BLOCKERS, **digoxin, verapamil;** additive risk of bleeding with ANTICOAGULANTS, NSAIDS, PLATELET INHIBITORS (including **aspirin**), THROMBOLYTIC AGENTS.

PHARMACOKINETICS Distribution: Highly protein bound; does not cross CSF. **Metabolism:** Metabolic pathways have yet to be identified. **Elimination:** Only 5%–6% of dose is recovered in urine. Available data suggest that metabolism, biliary excretion, and/or extensive tissue binding account for majority of systemic clearance. **Half-Life:** 1–9 h.

NURSING IMPLICATIONS

Assessment & Drug Effects

- Monitor for hypersensitivity reactions, especially during first and second administrations of the paclitaxel. S&S requiring treatment, but not necessarily discontinuation of the drug, include dyspnea, hypotension, and chest pain. Discontinue immediately and manage symptoms aggressively if angioedema and generalized urticaria develop.
- Monitor vital signs frequently, especially during the first hour of

P

infusion. Bradycardia occurs in approximately 12% of patients, usually during infusion. It does not normally require treatment. Cardiac monitoring is indicated for those with severe conduction abnormalities.

- Lab tests: Monitor hematologic status throughout course of treatment. Severe neutropenia is common but usually of short duration (less than 500/mm^3 for less than 7 d) with the nadir occurring about day 11. Thrombocytopenia occurs less often and is less severe with the nadir around day 8 or 9. The incidence and severity of anemia increase with exposure to paclitaxel.
- Monitor for peripheral neuropathy, the severity of which is dose dependent. Severe symptoms occur primarily with higher than recommended doses.

Patient & Family Education

- Immediately report to physician S&S of paclitaxel hypersensitivity: difficulty breathing, chest pain, palpitations, angioedema (subcutaneous swelling usually around face and neck), and skin rashes or itching.
- Be sure to have periodic blood work as prescribed.
- Avoid aspirin, NSAIDS, and alcohol to minimize GI distress.
- Be aware of high probability of developing hair loss (>80%).
- Do not breast feed while taking this drug.

PALIVIZUMAB

(pal-i-viz'u-mab)
Synagis
Classifications: IMMUNOMODULATOR; IMMUNOGLOBULIN; MONOCLONAL ANTIBODY
Prototype: Basiliximab
Pregnancy Category: C

AVAILABILITY 100 mg vial

ACTIONS Monoclonal antibody ($IgG1_k$ produced by recombinant DNA technology) to the respiratory syncytial virus (RSV).

THERAPEUTIC EFFECTS Provides passive immunity against respiratory syncytial virus. Indicated by prevention of lower respiratory tract infection.

USES Prevention of serious lower respiratory tract infections in children susceptible to RSV.

CONTRAINDICATIONS Hypersensitivity to palivizumab in pediatric patients.

CAUTIOUS USE Hypersensitivity to other immunoglobulin preparations, blood products, or other medications; kidney or liver dysfunction; acute RSV infection. Safety in pregnancy (category C) or lactation is not established.

ROUTE & DOSAGE

RSV
Child: **IM** 15 mg/kg qmo during RSV season

ADMINISTRATION

Intramuscular

- Reconstitute solution by gently injecting 1 mL of sterile water for injection (without preservative) toward the sides of the vial. Gently swirl for 30 s to dissolve (do not shake solution). Allow to stand at room temperature for at least 20 min until solution clears.
- Give IM only into the anterolateral aspect of the thigh. Volumes >1 mL should be divided and given in different sites.
- Use reconstituted solution within 6 h. Discard any unused portion of the vial. It contains no preservatives.

ADVERSE EFFECTS (≥1%) **Body as a Whole:** *Otitis media,* pain, hernia. **GI:** Increased AST, diarrhea, nausea, vomiting, gastroenteritis. **Respiratory:** *URI, rhinitis,* pharyngitis, cough, wheeze, bronchiolitis, asthma, croup, dyspnea, sinusitis, apnea. **Skin:** *Rash.*

INTERACTIONS Drug: No clinically significant interactions established.

PHARMACOKINETICS Half-Life: 20 d.

NURSING IMPLICATIONS

Assessment & Drug Effects

- Lab tests: Periodic monitoring of liver functions may be warranted.
- Monitor carefully for and immediately report S&S of respiratory illness including fever, cough, wheezing, and retractions.
- Assess for and report erythema or indurations at injection site.

Patient & Family Education

- Contact physician if S&S of respiratory illness, vomiting, diarrhea, or redness develop at injection site.
- Do not breast feed while taking this drug without consulting physician.

PALONOSETRON

(pal-o-no'si-tron)
Aloxi
Classifications: GASTROINTESTINAL AGENT; ANTIEMETIC; 5-HT_3 ANTAGONIST
Prototype: Ondansetron
Pregnancy Category: B

AVAILABILITY 0.25 mg/5 mL injection

ACTIONS Selectively blocks serotonin 5-HT_3 receptors found centrally in the chemoreceptor trigger zone (CTZ) in the hypothalamus, and peripherally at vagal nerve endings in the intestines.

THERAPEUTIC EFFECTS Prevents acute chemotherapy-induced nausea and vomiting associated with initial and repeat courses of moderately or highly emetogenic chemotherapy.

USES Prevention of acute and delayed nausea and vomiting associated with highly emetogenic cancer chemotherapy.

CONTRAINDICATIONS Hypersensitivity to palonosetron; safety in patients >65 and children <5 is unknown.

CAUTIOUS USE Pregnancy (category B), lactation.

ROUTE & DOSAGE

Prevention of Chemotherapy-Induced Nausea and Vomiting
Adult: **IV** 0.25 mg infused over 30 sec 30 min prior to chemotherapy; do not repeat for at least 7 d

ADMINISTRATION

Intravenous

PREPARE: **Direct:** Do not dilute and do not mix with other drugs.
ADMINISTER: **Direct:** Give over 30 sec. Flush IV line with NS before and after administration.
INCOMPATIBILITIES Do not mix with other drugs.

- Store at room temperature of 15°–30° C (59°–86° F). Protect from light.

ADVERSE EFFECTS (≥1%) **CNS:** Headache, anxiety, dizziness. **GI:** Constipation, diarrhea, abdominal pain.

INTERACTIONS Drug: May prolong QTc interval; use cautiously with **amiodarone, amoxapine, bretylium, dofetilide, disopyramide, epinephrine, ibutilide, mapro-**

P

tiline, procainamide, quinidine, sotalol, TRICYCLIC ANTIDEPRESSANTS, PHENOTHIAZINES, **haloperidol, pimozide, risperidone, sertindole, ziprasidone, arsenic trioxide, bepridil, cisapride, clarithromycin, cyclobenzaprine, dolasetron, droperidol, erythromycin, flecainide, halofantrine, halothane, pentamidine, probucol, troleandomycin.**

PHARMACOKINETICS Metabolism: Metabolized in liver by CYP2D6. **Elimination:** Primarily renal. **Half-Life:** 40 h.

NURSING IMPLICATIONS

Assessment & Drug Effects

- Monitor closely cardiac status especially in those taking diuretics or otherwise at risk for hypokalemia or hypomagnesemia, with congenital QT syndrome, or patients taking antiarrhythmic or other drugs that lead to QT prolongation.

Patient & Family Education

- Report promptly any of the following: difficulty breathing, wheezing, or shortness of breath; palpitations or chest tightness; skin rash or itching; swelling of the face, tongue, throat, hands, or feet.
- Do not breast feed without consulting physician.

P

PAMIDRONATE DISODIUM

(pa-mi'dro-nate)

Aredia

Classification: BISPHOSPHONATE (REGULATORY, BONE METABOLISM)

Prototype: Etidronate

Pregnancy Category: X

AVAILABILITY 30 mg, 60 mg, 90 mg injection

ACTIONS A bone-resorption inhibitor thought to absorb calcium phosphate crystals in bone. May also inhibit osteoclast activity, thus contributing to inhibition of bone resorption.

THERAPEUTIC EFFECTS Does not inhibit bone formation or mineralization. Reduces bone turnover and, when used in combination with adequate hydration, it increases renal excretion of calcium, and reduces serum calcium concentrations.

USES Hypercalcemia of malignancy and Paget's disease, bone metastases in multiple myeloma.

UNLABELED USES Primary hyperparathyroidism, osteoporosis.

CONTRAINDICATIONS Hypersensitivity to pamidronate; breast cancer, severe renal disease, hypercalcemia, hypercholesterolemia, polycythemia, pregnancy (category X), prostatic cancer, lactation. Safety and effectiveness in children are not established.

CAUTIOUS USE Heart failure, nephrosis or nephrotic syndrome, moderate renal disease; hepatic disease, cholestasis; peripheral edema, prostate hypertrophy; chronic kidney failure.

ROUTE & DOSAGE

Moderate Hypercalcemia of Malignancy (corrected calcium 12–13.5 mg/dL)

Adult: **IV** 15–90 mg infused over 4–24 h, may repeat in 7 d

Severe Hypercalcemia of Malignancy (corrected calcium >13.5 mg/dL)

Adult: **IV** 90 mg infused over 4–24 h, may repeat in 7 d

Paget's Disease, Metastases in Multiple Myeloma

Adult: **IV** 30 mg once daily for 3 days (90 mg total)

ADMINISTRATION

Intravenous

PREPARE: **IV Infusion:** Add 10 mL sterile water for injection to reconstitute the 30, 60, or 90 mg vial to produce concentrations of 3, 6, and 9 mg/1 mL, respectively. Withdraw the recommended dose and further dilute with D5W, NS, or 0.45% NaCl.

ADMINISTER: **IV Infusion: For hypercalcemia of malignancy:** Use 1000 mL of IV solution. **For Paget's disease or osteolytic lesions of multiple myeloma:** Use 500 mL of IV solution.

INCOMPATIBILITIES **Solution/additive:** CALCIUM-CONTAINING SOLUTIONS (including LACTATED RINGER'S).

- Refrigerate reconstituted pamidronate solution at 2°–8° C (36°–46° F); the IV solution may be stored at room temperature. Both are stable for 24 h.

ADVERSE EFFECTS (≥1%) **Body as a Whole:** *Fever with or without rigors* generally occurs within 48 h and subsides within 48 h despite continued therapy; *thrombophlebitis at injection site;* general malaise lasting for several weeks; transient increase in bone pain. **Metabolic:** *Hypocalcemia.* **GI:** Nausea, abdominal pain, *epigastric discomfort.* **CV:** Hypertension. **Skin:** Rash.

INTERACTIONS Drug: Concurrent use of **foscarnet** may further decrease serum levels of ionized calcium.

PHARMACOKINETICS Absorption: 50% of IV dose is retained in body. **Onset:** 24–48 h. **Peak:** 6 d. **Duration:** 2 wk–3 mo. **Distribution:** Accumulates in bone; once deposited, remains bound until bone is remodeled. **Metabolism:** Not metabolized. **Elimination:** 50% excreted in urine unchanged. **Half-Life:** 28 h.

NURSING IMPLICATIONS

Assessment & Drug Effects

- Assess IV injection site for thrombophlebitis.
- Lab tests: Monitor serum calcium and phosphate levels, CBC, and kidney function throughout course of therapy.
- Monitor for S&S of hypocalcemia, hypokalemia, hypomagnesemia, and hypophosphatemia.
- Monitor for seizures especially in those with a preexisting seizure disorder.
- Monitor vital signs. Be aware that drug fever, which may occur with pamidronate use, is self-limiting, usually subsiding in 48 hours even with continued therapy.

Patient & Family Education

- Be aware that transient, self-limiting fever with/without chills may develop.
- Generalized malaise, which may last for several weeks following treatment, is an anticipated adverse effect.
- Report to physician immediately perioral tingling, numbness, and paresthesia. These are signs of hypocalcemia.
- Do not breast feed while taking this drug.

PANCRELIPASE (Pr)

(pan-kre-li'pase)

Cotazym, Cotazym-S, Festal II, Ilozyme, Ku-Zyme-Hp, Pancrease, Ultrase, Viokase

Classifications: ENZYMES; ENZYME REPLACEMENT THERAPY

Pregnancy Category: C

AVAILABILITY Tablets or capsules containing lipase, protease, and amylase

ACTIONS Pancreatic enzyme concentrate of porcine origin standardized for lipase content. Similar to pancreatin but on a weight basis has 12 times the lipolytic activity and at least 4 times the trypsin and amylase content of pancreatin.
THERAPEUTIC EFFECTS Facilitates the hydrolysis of fats into glycerol and fatty acids, starches into dextrins and sugars, and proteins into peptides for easier absorption.

USES Replacement therapy in symptomatic treatment of malabsorption syndrome due to cystic fibrosis and other conditions associated with exocrine pancreatic insufficiency.

CONTRAINDICATIONS History of allergy to hog protein or enzymes; esophageal strictures; pancreatitis; porcine protein hypersensitivity; pregnancy (category C).
CAUTIOUS USE Lactation.

ROUTE & DOSAGE

Pancreatic Insufficiency
Adult: **PO** 1–3 capsules or tablets or 1–2 packets of powder 1–2 h before, during, or 1 h after meals, with an extra dose taken with any food eaten between meals
Child: **PO** 1–2 capsules or tablets 1–2 h before, during, or 1 h after meals, with an extra dose taken with any food eaten between meals

ADMINISTRATION
Oral
- Ensure that enteric-coated preparations are not crushed or chewed.
- Note: For children, powder form may be sprinkled on food.
- Open capsule and sprinkled contents on soft food, which should be swallowed without chewing to prevent mucus membrane irritation. Follow with a full glass of water or juice. Cimetidine, ranitidine, or an antacid may be prescribed to be given before pancrelipase to prevent drug's destruction by gastric pepsin and acid pH.
- Determine dosage in relation to fat content in diet (suggested ratio: 300 mg pancrelipase for each 17 g dietary fat).

ADVERSE EFFECTS (≥1%) **GI:** Anorexia, nausea, vomiting, diarrhea. **Metabolic:** Hyperuricosuria.

INTERACTIONS Drug: Iron absorption may be decreased.

PHARMACOKINETICS Absorption: Not absorbed. **Distribution:** acts locally in GI tract. **Elimination:** Excreted in feces.

NURSING IMPLICATIONS

Assessment & Drug Effects
- Monitor I&O and weight. Note appetite and quality of stools, weight loss, abdominal bloating, polyuria, thirst, hunger, itching. Pancreatic insufficiency is frequently associated with steatorrhea, bulky stools, and insulin-dependent diabetes.

Patient & Family Education
- Learn proper timing of medication in relation to meals.
- Do not breast feed while taking this drug without consulting physician.

PANCURONIUM BROMIDE
(pan-kyoo-roe'nee-um)
Pavulon
Classifications: AUTONOMIC NERVOUS SYSTEM AGENT; SKELETAL MUSCLE RELAXANT, DEPOLARIZING, NONDEPOLARIZING
Prototype: Tubocurarine
Pregnancy Category: C

 Common adverse effects in *italic*, life-threatening effects underlined; generic names in **bold**; classifications in SMALL CAPS; ♣ Canadian drug name; ⊕ Prototype drug

AVAILABILITY 1 mg/mL, 2 mg/mL injection

ACTIONS Synthetic curariform nondepolarizing neuromuscular blocking agent. Similar to tubocurarine chloride, however reported to be approximately five times as potent as tubocurarine but produces little or no histamine release or ganglionic blockade and thus does not cause bronchospasm or hypotension.

THERAPEUTIC EFFECTS Produces skeletal muscle relaxation or paralysis by competing with acetylcholine at cholinergic receptor sites on skeletal muscle endplate and thus blocks nerve impulse transmission. In high doses has direct blocking effect on acetylcholine receptors of heart and may increase heart rate, cardiac output, and arterial pressure.

USES Adjunct to anesthesia to induce skeletal muscle relaxation. Also to facilitate management of patients undergoing mechanical ventilation.

CONTRAINDICATIONS Hypersensitivity to the drug or bromides; tachycardia. Safety during pregnancy (category C) or lactation is not established.

CAUTIOUS USE Debilitated patients; myasthenia gravis; pulmonary, liver or kidney disease; fluid or electrolyte imbalance.

ROUTE & DOSAGE

Skeletal Muscle Relaxation

Adult/Child: **IV** 0.04–0.1 mg/kg initial dose, may give additional doses of 0.01 mg/kg at 30–60 min intervals

ADMINISTRATION

Intravenous

- Plastic syringe may be used for administration, but drug may adsorb to plastic with prolonged storage.
- Use a test dose of 0.02 mg/kg in infants ≥1 mo.

PREPARE: **Direct:** Give undiluted.

ADMINISTER: **Direct:** Give over 30–90 seconds.

INCOMPATIBILITIES **Y-site: Diazepam, thiopental.**

- Refrigerate at 2°–8° C (36°–46° F). Do not freeze.

ADVERSE EFFECTS (≥1%) **CV:** *Increased pulse rate and BP,* ventricular extrasystoles. **Skin:** Transient acneiform rash, burning sensation along course of vein. **Body as a Whole:** Salivation, skeletal muscle weakness, <u>respiratory depression</u>.

DIAGNOSTIC TEST INTERFERENCE Pancuronium may decrease ***serum cholinesterase*** concentrations.

INTERACTIONS Drug: GENERAL ANESTHETICS increase neuromuscular blocking and duration of action; AMINOGLYCOSIDES, **bacitracin, polymyxin B, clindamycin, lidocaine** parenteral **magnesium, quinidine, quinine, trimethaphan, verapamil** increase neuromuscular blockade; DIURETICS may increase or decrease neuromuscular blockade; **lithium** prolongs duration of neuromuscular blockade; NARCOTIC ANALGESICS possibly add to respiratory depression; **succinylcholine** increases onset and depth of neuromuscular blockade; **phenytoin** may cause resistance to or reversal of neuromuscular blockade.

PHARMACOKINETICS Onset: 30–45 s. **Peak:** 2–3 min. **Duration:** 60 min. **Distribution:** Well distributed to tissues and extracellular fluids; crosses placenta in small amounts. **Metabolism:** Small amount metabolized in liver. **Elimination:** Excreted primarily in urine. **Half-Life:** 2 h.

P

NURSING IMPLICATIONS

Assessment & Drug Effects

- Assess cardiovascular and respiratory status continuously.
- Observe patient closely for residual muscle weakness and signs of respiratory distress during recovery period. Monitor BP and vital signs. Peripheral nerve stimulator may be used to assess the effects of pancuronium and to monitor restoration of neuromuscular function.
- Note: Consciousness is not affected by pancuronium. Patient will be awake and alert but unable to speak.

PANTOPRAZOLE SODIUM

(pan-to′pra-zole)

Protonix, Protonix IV

Classifications: GASTROINTESTINAL AGENT; PROTON PUMP INHIBITOR

Prototype: Omeprazole

Pregnancy Category: B

AVAILABILITY 40 mg enteric coated tablets; 40 mg vial

ACTIONS Gastric acid pump inhibitor; belongs to a class of antisecretory compounds. Gastric acid secretion is decreased by inhibiting the H^+, K^+-ATPase enzyme system responsible for acid production.

THERAPEUTIC EFFECTS Specifically, suppresses gastric acid secretion by inhibiting the acid (proton H^+) pump in the parietal cells.

USES Short-term treatment of erosive esophagitis associated with gastroesophageal reflux disease (GERD).

CONTRAINDICATIONS Hypersensitivity to pantoprazole or other proton pump inhibitors (PPIs); severe hepatic insufficiency, cirrhosis.

CAUTIOUS USE Mild to moderate hepatic insufficiency; pregnancy (category B), lactation. Safety and effectiveness in children <18 y are not established.

ROUTE & DOSAGE

Erosive Esophagitis

Adult: **PO** 40 mg q.d. times 8–16 wks **IV** 40 mg q.d. times 7–10 d

ADMINISTRATION

Oral

- Do not crush or break in half. Must be swallowed whole.
- Note: Therapy beyond 16 wks is not recommended.
- Store preferably at 20°–25° C (66°–77° F), but room temperature permitted.

Intravenous

PREPARE: **IV Infusion:** *Two-min infusion:* Reconstitute each 40 mg vial with 10 mL NS. *Fifteen-min infusion:* Reconstitute as for 2-min infusion, then further dilute with 100 mL of D5W, NS, or RL to yield 0.4 mg/mL.

ADMINISTER: **IV Infusion:** Give through a dedicated line or flushed IV line before and after each dose with D5W, NS, or RL. *Two-min infusion:* Give over at least 2 min. *Fifteen-min infusion:* Infuse over 15 min at a rate of 6 mg/min (7 mL/min). Note: Protonix IV packaged with an in-line filter must be used with the provided filter. A newer formulation does not require an in-line filter.

- Reconstituted solution may be stored for up to 2 h at 15–30° C (59–86° F) before further dilution. The diluted 100 mL solution may be stored for up to 22 h.

INCOMPATIBILITIES **Solution/Additive:** Solutions containing **zinc. Y-site: Midazolam.**

ADVERSE EFFECTS (≥1%) **GI:** Diarrhea, flatulence, abdominal pain. **CNS:** Headache, insomnia. **Skin:** Rash.

INTERACTIONS Drug: May decrease absorption of **ampicillin,** IRON SALTS, **itraconazole, ketoconazole;** increases INR with **warfarin.**

PHARMACOKINETICS Absorption: Well absorbed with 77% bioavailability. **Peak:** 2.4 h. **Distribution:** 98% protein bound. **Metabolism:** Metabolized in liver primarily by CYP2C19. **Elimination:** 71% excreted in urine, 18% in feces. **Half-Life:** 1 h.

NURSING IMPLICATIONS

Assessment & Drug Effects

- Monitor for and immediately report S&S of angioedema or a severe skin reaction.
- Lab tests: Urea breath test 4–6 wks after completion of therapy.

Patient & Family Education

- Contact physician promptly if any of the following occur: Peeling, blistering, or loosening of skin; skin rash, hives, or itching; swelling of the face, tongue, or lips; difficulty breathing or swallowing.
- Do not breast feed while taking this drug without consulting physician.

PAPAVERINE HYDROCHLORIDE

(pa-pav′er-een)

Cerespan, Genabid, Pavabid, Pavased, Pavatyme, Paverolan

Classifications: CARDIOVASCULAR AGENT; NONNITRATE VASODILATOR

Prototype: Hydralazine

Pregnancy Category: C

AVAILABILITY 150 mg sustained release capsule; 30 mg/mL injection

ACTIONS Exerts nonspecific direct spasmolytic effect on smooth muscles unrelated to innervation. Action is especially pronounced on coronary, cerebral, pulmonary, and peripheral arteries when spasm is present.

THERAPEUTIC EFFECTS Acts directly on myocardium, depresses conduction and irritability, and prolongs refractory period. Stimulates respiration by action on carotid and aortic body chemoreceptors.

USES Primarily for relief of cerebral and peripheral ischemia associated with arterial spasm and MI complicated by arrhythmias. Also visceral spasm as in ureteral, biliary, and GI colic.

UNLABELED USES Impotence, cardiac bypass surgery.

CONTRAINDICATIONS Parenteral use in complete AV block. Safe during pregnancy (category C) or lactation is not established.

CAUTIOUS USE Glaucoma; myocardial depression; angina pectoris; recent stroke.

ROUTE & DOSAGE

Cerebral and Peripheral Ischemia

Adult: **PO** 100–300 mg 3–5 times/d; 150 mg sustained release q8–12h **IM/IV** 30–120 mg q3h as needed

Child: **IM/IV** 6 mg/kg/24 h divided into 4 doses

Impotence

Adult: **IM** 0.5–37.5 mg injected into the corpus cavernosum of the penis as needed for erection

ADMINISTRATION

Oral

- Give with or following meals; give milk or prescribed antacid to reduce possibility of nausea.

P

- Ensure that sustained release form is not chewed or crushed. Must be swallowed whole.

Intramuscular

- Aspirate carefully before injecting IM to avoid inadvertent entry into blood vessel, and administer slowly.

PREPARE: **Direct:** Give undiluted or diluted in an equal volume of sterile water for injection.

ADMINISTER: **Direct:** Give slowly over 1–2 min. AVOID rapid injection.

ADVERSE EFFECTS (≥1%) **Body as a Whole:** General discomfort, facial flushing, sweating, weakness, coma. **CNS:** Dizziness, drowsiness, headache, sedation. **CV:** Slight rise in BP, paroxysmal tachycardia, transient ventricular ectopic rhythms, AV block, arrhythmias. **GI:** Nausea, anorexia, constipation, diarrhea, abdominal distress, dry mouth and throat, hepatotoxicity (jaundice, eosinophilia, abnormal liver function tests); with rapid IV administration. **Respiratory:** Increased depth of respiration, respiratory depression, fatal apnea. **Skin:** Pruritus, skin rash. **Special Senses:** Diplopia, nystagmus. **Urogenital:** Priapism.

INTERACTIONS Drug: May decrease **levodopa** effectiveness; **morphine** may antagonize smooth muscle relaxation effect of papaverine.

PHARMACOKINETICS Absorption: Readily absorbed from GI tract. **Peak:** 1–2 h. **Duration:** 6 h regular tablets; 12 h sustained release. **Metabolism:** Metabolized in liver. **Elimination:** Excreted in urine chiefly as metabolites. **Half-Life:** 90 min.

NURSING IMPLICATIONS

Assessment & Drug Effects

- Monitor pulse, respiration, and BP in patients receiving drug parenterally. If significant changes are noted, withhold medication and report promptly to physician.
- Lab tests: Perform liver function and blood tests periodically. Hepatotoxicity (thought to be a hypersensitivity reaction) is reversible with prompt drug withdrawal.

Patient & Family Education

- Notify physician if any adverse effect persists or if GI symptoms, jaundice, or skin rash appear. Liver function tests may be indicated.
- Do not drive or engage in potentially hazardous activities until response to drug is known. Alcohol may increase drowsiness and dizziness.
- Do not breast feed while taking this drug without consulting physician.

PARALDEHYDE

(par-al′de-hyde)

Paracetaldehyde, Paral

Classifications: CENTRAL NERVOUS SYSTEM AGENT; ANTICONVULSANT; SEDATIVE-HYPNOTIC; BARBITURATE

Prototype: Phenobarbital

Pregnancy Category: C

Controlled Substance: Schedule IV

AVAILABILITY 1 g/mL liquid

ACTIONS Cyclic ether formed by polymerization of acetaldehyde.

THERAPEUTIC EFFECTS Potent CNS depressant with sedative and hypnotic actions similar to those of alcohol, barbiturates, and chloral hydrate.

USES Sedative and hypnotic in acute agitation due to alcohol withdrawal; used to control convulsions arising from tetanus, eclampsia, Status Epilepticus, and drug poisoning. Has been used rectally to induce basal anesthesia, particularly in children.

CONTRAINDICATIONS Severe hepatic insufficiency; respiratory disease; GI inflammation or ulceration; disulfiram therapy; pregnancy (category C), lactation.

ROUTE & DOSAGE

Hypnotic

Adult: **PO** 10–30 mL prn
Child: **PO** 0.3 mL/kg

Sedative

Adult: **PO** 5–10 mL prn
Child: **PO** 0.15 mL/kg

Seizures Secondary to Tetanus

Adult: **PO** up to 12 mL diluted 1:10 q4h prn

Seizures Secondary to Other Poisons

Adult: **PR** 5–15 mL diluted in 200 mL per rectal tube

Status Epilepticus

Child: **PR** 1 mL/y of age up to 5 mL; may repeat in 1 h if necessary, then change to PO. PO 2–5 mL q2–4h

Alcohol Withdrawal Seizures

Adult: **PO** 5–10 mL q4–6h for 24 h, then q6h prn

ADMINISTRATION

Note: Both oral and rectal doses must be diluted before they are administered.

Oral/Rectal

- Note: On exposure to light, air, and heat, drug liberates acetaldehyde, which oxidizes to acetic acid. Do not use solution if it is colored in any way or smells of acetic acid (vinegar odor).
- Discard unused contents of any container that has been open for more than 24 h. Decomposed paraldehyde is extremely corrosive to tissues and can cause fatal poisoning.
- Do not use plastics for measuring or administering paraldehyde. Contact with plastic materials can decompose paraldehyde to toxic compounds. Draw parenteral preparation into a glass syringe; use rubber catheter for rectal administration.
- Give oral drug well diluted in iced fruit juice or milk to reduce irritation of GI tract and mask odor and taste.
- When given rectally, dilute drug with at least 2 volumes of olive oil or cottonseed oil or dissolved in 200 mL of NS solution to prevent rectal irritation.
- Do not withdraw rapidly after prolonged use; may produce delirium tremens and hallucinations.
- Preserve in tight, light-resistant containers in amounts not exceeding 30 mL and at temperatures not over 25° C (77° F).

ADVERSE EFFECTS (≥1%) **Body as a Whole:** Occasionally confusion and paradoxical excitement. **CNS:** Hangover, dizziness, ataxia. **CV:** Hypotension, dilation and failure of right heart, cardiovascular collapse. **GI:** *Irritation of mucous membrane (oral and rectal routes),* nausea, vomiting, unpleasant taste and odor, toxic hepatitis, bleeding gastritis, liver damage. **Urogenital:** Nephrosis, renal damage. **Metabolic:** Metabolic acidosis, acidosis. **Respiratory:** Rapid labored breathing, respiratory depression, pulmonary hemorrhage and edema. **Skin:** *Erythematous skin rash.*

DIAGNOSTIC TEST INTERFERENCE Chronic use of alcohol (ethanol) and paraldehyde may cause false-positive ***serum ketones (nitroprusside tube dilution method)***

P

and ***urine ketones (Acetest)*** and may interfere with ***urinary steroid (17-OHCS) determinations*** by modification of ***Reddy, Jenkins, Thorn procedure.***

INTERACTIONS Drug: Disulfiram may increase paraldehyde levels; **alcohol** and other CNS DEPRESSANTS add to CNS depressant effects—fatalities reported with **alcohol.**

PHARMACOKINETICS Absorption: Readily absorbed from GI tract. **Onset:** 10–15 min. **Duration:** 6–8 h. **Distribution:** Distributed into CNS; crosses placenta. **Metabolism:** 80%–90% of doses metabolized in liver. **Elimination:** Excreted through lungs (11%–28%) and urine. **Half-Life:** 7.5 h.

NURSING IMPLICATIONS

Assessment & Drug Effects

- Monitor cardiovascular and respiratory status closely.
- Keep the patient turned on side to prevent aspiration since bronchial secretions may be increased. Suctioning may be necessary.
- Be aware that patient's breath will have a characteristic odor for several hours.

P

PAREGORIC (CAMPHORATED OPIUM TINCTURE)

(par-e-gor′ik)

Classifications: GASTROINTESTINAL AGENT; ANTIDIARRHEAL; CENTRAL NERVOUS SYSTEM AGENT; NARCOTIC (OPIATE) AGONIST ANALGESIC

Prototype: Diphenoxylate HCl with atropine sulfate

Pregnancy Category: B (D for prolonged use or high doses at term)

Controlled Substance: Schedule III

AVAILABILITY 2 mg/mL liquid

ACTIONS Contains 2 mg anhydrous morphine, alcohol, benzoic acid, camphor, and anise oil. Pharmacologic activity is due to morphine content.

THERAPEUTIC EFFECTS Increases smooth muscle tone of GI tract, decreases motility and effective propulsive peristalsis while diminishing digestive secretions. Delayed transit of intestinal contents results in desiccation of feces and constipation.

USES Short-term treatment for symptomatic relief of acute diarrhea and abdominal cramps.

CONTRAINDICATIONS Hypersensitivity to opium alkaloids; diarrhea caused by poisons (until eliminated); pregnancy [(category B), with prolonged use or high doses at term (category D)].

CAUTIOUS USE Asthma; liver disease; history of opiate agonist dependence; severe prostatic hypertrophy, lactation.

ROUTE & DOSAGE

Acute Diarrhea

Adult: **PO** 5–10 mL after loose bowel movement, may be administered q2h up to q.i.d. if needed
Child: **PO** 0.25–0.5 mL/kg 1–4 times/d

ADMINISTRATION

Oral

- Give paregoric in sufficient water (2 or 3 swallows) to ensure its passage into the stomach (mixture will appear milky).

ADVERSE EFFECTS (≥1%) **GI:** Anorexia, nausea, vomiting, *constipation,* abdominal pain. **Body as a Whole:** Dizziness, faintness, drowsiness, facial flushing, sweating, physical dependence.

INTERACTIONS Drug: Alcohol and other CNS DEPRESSANTS add to CNS effects.

PHARMACOKINETICS Absorption: Readily absorbed from GI tract. **Duration:** 4–5 h. **Distribution:** Crosses placenta; distributed into breast milk. **Metabolism:** Metabolized in liver. **Elimination:** Excreted in urine. **Half-Life:** 2–3 h.

NURSING IMPLICATIONS

Assessment & Drug Effects

- Paregoric may worsen the course of infection-associated diarrhea by delaying the elimination of pathogens.
- Be aware that adverse effects are primarily due to morphine content. Paregoric abuse results because of the narcotic content of the drug.
- Assess for fluid and electrolyte imbalance until diarrhea has stopped.

Patient & Family Education

- Adhere strictly to prescribed dosage schedule.
- Maintain bed rest if diarrhea is severe with a high level of fluid loss.
- Replace fluids and electrolytes as needed for diarrhea. Drink warm clear liquids and avoid dairy products, concentrated sweets, and cold drinks until diarrhea stops.
- Observe character and frequency of stools. Discontinue drug as soon as diarrhea is controlled. Report promptly to physician if diarrhea persists more than 3 d, if fever is >38.8° C (102° F), abdominal pain develops, or if mucus or blood is passed.
- Understand that constipation is often a consequence of antidiarrheal treatment and a normal elimination pattern is usually established as dietary intake increases.
- Do not breast feed while taking this drug without consulting physician.

PARICALCITOL

(par-i-cal′ci-tol)

Zemplar

Classifications: HORMONES & SYNTHETIC SUBSTITUTES; VITAMIN D ANALOG

Prototype: Calcitriol

Pregnancy Category: C

AVAILABILITY 5 mcg/mL vial

ACTIONS Synthetic Vitamin D analog that reduces parathyroid hormone activity (PTH) levels in chronic kidney failure (CRF) patients.

THERAPEUTIC EFFECTS Lowers serum levels of calcium and phosphate; serum calcium times serum phosphate cross product value may increase. In addition it decreases the parathyroid hormone as well as bone resorption in some patients. Indicated by iPTH levels <1.5–3 times the nonuremic upper limit of normal.

USES Prevention and treatment of secondary hyperparathyroidism associated with CRF.

CONTRAINDICATIONS Hypersensitivity to paricalcitol; hypercalcemia; evidence of Vitamin D toxicity; concurrent administration of phosphate preparations and Vitamin D; pregnancy (category C).

CAUTIOUS USE Lactation; severe liver disease; concurrent administration of digitalis; abnormally low levels of PTH.

ROUTE & DOSAGE

CHF-Associated Secondary Hyperparathyroidism
Adult: **IV** 0.04 mcg/kg–0.1 mcg/kg (max: 24 mcg/kg), no more than every other day during dialysis
Child: **IV** *5–17 y,* 0.04 mcg/kg 3 times/wk during dialysis

ADMINISTRATION

Intravenous

PREPARE: **Direct:** Give undiluted.
ADMINISTER: **Direct:** Give IV bolus dose anytime during dialysis.

- Store at 25° C (77° F). Discard unused portion of a single dose vial.

ADVERSE EFFECTS (≥1%) **Body as a Whole:** Chills, feeling unwell, fever, flu-like symptoms, sepsis, edema. **CNS:** Lightheadedness. **CV:** Palpitations. **GI:** Dry mouth, GI bleeding, *nausea,* vomiting. **Respiratory:** Pneumonia. **Metabolic:** Hypercalcemia.

INTERACTIONS Drug: Hypercalcemia may increase risk of **digoxin** toxicity; may increase **magnesium** absorption and toxicity in renal failure. **Herbal:** Be cautious of **Vitamin D** content in herbal and OTC products.

PHARMACOKINETICS Distribution: >99% protein bound. **Elimination:** Excreted primarily in feces (74%). **Half-Life:** 15 h.

NURSING IMPLICATIONS

Assessment & Drug Effects

- Monitor for S&S of hypercalcemia (see Appendix F).
- Lab tests: Serum calcium and phosphate 2 times a wk during initiation of therapy; then monthly; serum PTH q3mo; periodic serum magnesium, alkaline phosphatase, 24-urinary calcium and phosphate. Increase frequency of lab tests during dosage adjustments.
- Withhold drug and notify physician if hypercalcemia occurs.
- Coadministered drugs: Monitor for digoxin toxicity if serum calcium level is elevated.

Patient & Family Education

- Report immediately any of the following to the physician: Weakness, anorexia, nausea, vomiting, abdominal cramps, diarrhea, muscle or bone pain, or excessive thirst.
- Adhere strictly to dietary regimen of calcium supplementation and phosphorus restriction to ensure successful therapy.
- Avoid excessive use of aluminum-containing compounds such as antacids/vitamins.
- Do not breast feed while taking this drug without consulting physician.

PAROMOMYCIN SULFATE (Pr)

(par-oh-moe-mye'sin)
Humatin
Classifications: ANTIINFECTIVE; AMINOGLYCOSIDE ANTIBIOTIC; AMEBICIDE
Pregnancy Category: C

AVAILABILITY 250 mg tablets

ACTIONS Aminoglycoside antibiotic produced by certain strains of *Streptomyces rimosus* with broad spectrum of antibacterial activity closely paralleling that of kanamycin and neomycin.

THERAPEUTIC EFFECTS Exerts direct bactericidal and amebicidal action, primarily in lumen of GI tract. Ineffective against extraintestinal amebiasis.

USES Acute and chronic intestinal amebiasis and to rid bowel of nitrogen-forming bacteria in patients with hepatic coma; used preoperatively to suppress intestinal flora. Also tapeworm infestation.

CONTRAINDICATIONS Intestinal obstruction; impaired kidney function; pregnancy (category C) and lactation.

CAUTIOUS USE GI ulceration.

ROUTE & DOSAGE

Intestinal Amebiasis

Adult/Child: **PO** 25–35 mg/kg divided in 3 doses for 5–10 d

Hepatic Coma

Adult: **PO** 4 g/d in 2–4 divided doses for 5–6 d

ADMINISTRATION

Oral

- Give after meals to prevent gastric distress.

ADVERSE EFFECTS ($\geq$1%) **CNS:** Headache, vertigo. **GI:** *Diarrhea, abdominal cramps,* steatorrhea, *nausea, vomiting, heartburn,* secondary enterocolitis. **Skin:** Exanthema, rash, pruritus. **Special Senses:** Ototoxicity. **Urogenital:** Nephrotoxicity (in patients with GI inflammation or ulcerations). **Body as a Whole:** Eosinophilia, overgrowth of nonsusceptible organisms.

DIAGNOSTIC TEST INTERFERENCE Prolonged use of paromomycin may cause reduction in ***serum cholesterol.***

INTERACTIONS Drug: May decrease absorption of **cyanocobalamin.**

PHARMACOKINETICS Absorption: Poorly absorbed from intact GI tract. **Elimination:** In feces.

NURSING IMPLICATIONS

Assessment & Drug Effects

- Monitor therapeutic effectiveness. Criterion of cure is absence of amoebae in stool specimens examined at weekly intervals for 6 wk after completion of treatment, and thereafter at monthly intervals for 2 y.
- Monitor for appearance of a superinfection during therapy (see Appendix F).
- Lab test: baseline WBC with differential. Repeat if superfiction is suspected.
- Monitor closely patients with history of GI ulceration for nephrotoxicity and ototoxicity (see Appendix F). Drug absorption can take place through diseased mucosa.

Patient & Family Education

- Do not prepare, process, or serve food until treatment is complete when receiving drug for intestinal amebiasis. Isolation is not required.
- Practice strict personal hygiene, particularly hand washing after defecation and before eating food.
- Do not breast feed while taking this drug.

P

PAROXETINE

(par-ox′e-teen)

Asimia, Paxil, Paxil CR

Classifications: CENTRAL NERVOUS SYSTEM (CNS) AGENT; PSYCHOTHERAPEUTIC AGENT; ANTIDEPRESSANT; SELECTIVE SEROTONIN REUPTAKE INHIBITOR (SSRI)

Prototype: Fluoxetine

Pregnancy Category: C

AVAILABILITY 10 mg, 20 mg, 30 mg, 40 mg tablets; 12.5 mg, 25 mg sustained-release tablets; 10 mg/5 mL suspension

ACTIONS Antidepressant structurally unrelated to other serotonin reuptake inhibitors. Potent and highly selective inhibitor of serotonin reuptake by neurons in CNS.

THERAPEUTIC EFFECTS Efficacious in depression resistant to other antidepressants and in depression complicated by anxiety.

USES Depression, obsessive-compulsive disorders, panic attacks, excessive social anxiety, generalized anxiety, post-traumatic stress disorder (PTSD), premenstrual dysphoric disorder (PMDD).

UNLABELED USES Diabetic neuropathy, myoclonus, bipolar depression in conjunction with lithium, chronic headache, premature ejaculation, fibromyalgia.

CONTRAINDICATIONS Hypersensitivity to paroxetine; concomitant use of MAO inhibitors, pregnancy (category C); alcohol; children or adolescents with major depressive disorder.

CAUTIOUS USE History of mania, suicidal ideation; anorexia nervosa, ECT therapy; seizure disorder, seizures; renal/hepatic impairment, renal failure; history of metabolic disorders; volume-depleted patients, recent MI, unstable cardiac disease; lactation. Safety and efficacy have not been established in children.

P

ROUTE & DOSAGE

Depression

Adult: **PO** 10–50 mg/d (max: 80 mg/d); 25 mg sustained-release q.d. in morning, may increase by 12.5 mg (max: 62.5 mg/d); use lower starting doses for patients with renal or hepatic insufficiency and geriatric patients
Geriatric: **PO** Start with 10 mg/d (12.5 mg/d sustained release), (max: 40 mg/d [50 mg/d sustained release])

Obsessive-Compulsive Disorder

Adult: **PO** 20–60 mg/d

Panic Attacks

Adult: **PO** 40 mg/d

Social Anxiety Disorder

Adult: **PO** 20–60 mg/d

Generalized Anxiety, PTSD

Adult: **PO** Start with 10 mg once daily, may increase by 10 mg/d at weekly intervals if needed to target dose of 40 mg once daily (max: 60 mg/d)
Geriatric: **PO** Start with 10 mg PO once daily, may increase by 10 mg/d at weekly intervals if needed (max: 40 mg/d)

Premenstrual Dysphoric Disorder

Adult: **PO** 12.5 mg once daily (up to 25 mg once daily) throughout the month or daily for 2 wk before menstrual period

ADMINISTRATION

Oral

- Recommended initial dose with older adult, debilitated, or those with severe renal or hepatic impairment is 10 mg/d.
- Ensure that sustained-release form is not chewed or crushed. Must be swallowed whole.
- Be aware that at least 14 d should elapse when switching a patient from/to a MAO inhibitor to/from paroxetine.

ADVERSE EFFECTS (≥1%) **CV:** Postural hypotension. **CNS:** *Headache,* tremor, agitation or nervousness, anxiety, paresthesias, dizziness, insomnia, *sedation.* **GI:** *Nausea,* constipation, vomiting, anorexia, diarrhea, dyspepsia, flatulence, increased appetite, taste aversion, *dry* *mouth*. **Urogenital:** Urinary hesitancy or frequency. **Hepatic:** Isolated reports of elevated liver enzymes. **Special Senses:** Blurred vision. **Skin:** Diaphoresis, rash, pruritus. **Metabolic:** Hyponatremia in older adult.

INTERACTIONS Drug: Activated charcoal reduces absorption of paroxetine. **Cimetidine** increases paroxetine levels. MAO INHIBITORS, **selegiline** may cause an increased vasopressor response leading to hypertensive crisis or death. **Phenytoin** can cause liver enzyme induction resulting in lower paroxetine levels and shorter half-life. **Warfarin** may increase risk of bleeding and **thioridazine** levels, and prolong QTc interval leading to heart block; increase **ergotamine** toxicity with **dihydroergotamine, ergotamine. Herbal: St. John's wort** may cause **serotonin** syndrome (headache, dizziness, sweating, agitation).

PHARMACOKINETICS Absorption: 99% absorbed from GI tract. **Onset:** 2 wk. **Peak:** 5–8 h. **Distribution:** Very lipophilic. 95% protein bound. Distributes into breast milk. **Metabolism:** Extensively metabolized in the liver to inactive metabolites. **Elimination:** Less than 2% is excreted unchanged in urine. Approximately 65% of dose appears in urine as metabolites. Metabolites of paroxetine are also excreted in feces, presumably via bile. **Half-Life:** 24 h.

NURSING IMPLICATIONS

Assessment & Drug Effects

- Monitor for worsening of depression or emergence of suicidal ideation.
- Monitor for adverse effects, which include headache, weakness, sedation, dizziness, insomnia; nausea, constipation, or diarrhea; dry mouth; sweating; male ejaculatory disturbance. These occur in more than 10% of all patients and may result in poor compliance with drug regimen.
- Monitor older adult for fluid and sodium imbalances.
- Monitor those <18 y for suicidal ideation.
- Monitor for significant weight loss.
- Monitor patients with history of mania for reactivation of condition.
- Monitor patients with preexisting cardiovascular disease carefully because paroxetine may adversely affect hemodynamic status.

Patient & Family Education

- Use caution when operating hazardous machinery or equipment until response to drug is known.
- Concurrent use of alcohol may increase risk of adverse CNS effects.
- Adaptation to some adverse effects (especially dizziness and nausea) may occur over a period of 4–6 wk.
- Do not stop drug therapy after improvement in emotional status occurs.
- Notify physician of any distressing adverse effects.
- Do not breast feed while taking this drug without consulting physician.

PEGFILGRASTIM

(peg-fil-gras'tim)

Neulasta

Classifications: BLOOD FORMERS, COAGULATORS, AND ANTICOAGULANTS; HEMATOPOIETIC GROWTH FACTOR

Prototype: Epoetin alfa

Pregnancy Category: C

AVAILABILITY 10 mg/mL injection

ACTIONS Human granulocyte colony-stimulating factor (G-CSF) produced by recombinant DNA technology. Endogenous G-CSF regulates the production of neutrophils within the bone marrow; not species-specific and primarily affects neutrophil proliferation, differentiation and selected end-cell functional activity (including enhanced phagocytic activity, antibody-dependent killing, and the increased expression of some functions associated with cell-surface antigens).

THERAPEUTIC EFFECTS Increases neutrophil proliferation and differentiation within the bone marrow.

USES To decrease the incidence of infection, as manifested by febrile neutropenia, in patients with nonmyeloid malignancies receiving myelosuppressive anticancer drugs associated with a significant incidence of severe neutropenia with fever; to decrease neutropenia associated with bone marrow transplant; to treat chronic neutropenia.

CONTRAINDICATIONS Hypersensitivity to *Escherichia coli*-derived proteins, 14 d before or 24 h after administration of chemotherapy, and myeloid cancers; splenomegaly; ARDS.

CAUTIOUS USE Sickle cell disease; pregnancy (category C), lactation. For use in peripheral blood stem cells (PBSC) mobilization; neutropenic patients with sepsis; leukemia; concurrent lithium therapy.

P

ROUTE & DOSAGE

Neutropenia
Adult: **SC** *>45 kg* 6 mg once per chemotherapy cycle at least 24 h after chemotherapy.

ADMINISTRATION

Subcutaneous & Intravenous

- Do not administer filgrastim 24 h before or after cytotoxic chemotherapy.
- Use only one dose per vial; do not reenter the vial.
- Prior to injection, filgrastim may be allowed to reach room temperature for a maximum of 6 h. Discard any vial left at room temperature for >6 h.

Intravenous

PREPARE: **Intermittent/Continuous:** May dilute with 10–50 mL D5W to yield 15 mcg/mL or greater. If more diluent is used to produce concentrations of 5–15 mcg/mL, 2 mL of 5% human albumin must be added for each 50 mL D5W (prior to adding filgrastim) to prevent adsorption to plastic IV infusion materials.

ADMINISTER: **Intermittent:** Give a single dose over 15–30 min. **Continuous:** Give a single dose over 4–24 h.

- Store refrigerated at 2°–8° C (36°–46° F). Do not freeze. Avoid shaking.

ADVERSE EFFECTS (≥1%) **Body as a Whole:** *Bone pain,* hyperuricemia, *fever.* **Hematologic:** Anemia. **GI:** Nausea, anorexia, increased LFTs. **Body as a Whole:** *Bone pain,* hyperuricemia, *fever.*

INTERACTIONS Drug: Can interfere with activity of CYTOTOXIC AGENTS; do not use 14 d before or <24 h after CYTOTOXIC AGENTS; **lithium** may increase release of neutrophils.

PHARMACOKINETICS Absorption: Readily absorbed from SC site. **Half-Life:** 15–80 h.

NURSING IMPLICATIONS

Assessment & Drug Effects

- Lab tests: Obtain a baseline CBC with differential and platelet count prior to administering drug. Obtain CBC twice weekly during therapy to monitor neutrophil

count and leukocytosis. Monitor Hct and platelet count regularly.
- Discontinue filgrastim if absolute neutrophil count exceeds 10,000/ mm^3 after the chemotherapy-induced nadir. Neutrophil counts should then return to normal.
- Monitor patients with preexisting cardiac conditions closely. MI and arrhythmias have been associated with a small percent of patients receiving filgrastim.
- Monitor temperature q4h. Incidence of infection should be reduced after administration of filgrastim.
- Assess degree of bone pain if present. Consult physician if nonnarcotic analgesics do not provide relief.

Patient & Family Education
- Report bone pain and, if necessary, request analgesics to control pain.
- Note: Proper drug administration and disposal is important. A puncture-resistant container for the disposal of used syringes and needles should be utilized.
- Do not breast feed while taking this drug without consulting physician.

PEGINTERFERON ALFA-2A

(peg-in-ter-fer′on)
Pegasys
Classifications: IMMUNOMODULATOR; INTERFERON
Prototype: Interferon Alfa-2a
Pregnancy Category: C

AVAILABILITY 180 mcg/ml vials; 180 mcg prefilled syringes

ACTIONS Binds to specific cell surface receptors initiating intracellular signaling via a complex cascade leading to rapid activation of gene transcription. Interferon-stimulated genes modulate processes leading to inhibition of viral replication in infected cells, inhibition of cell proliferation, and immunomodulation.
THERAPEUTIC EFFECTS Stimulates production of effector proteins that raises body temperature, and causes reversible decreases in leukocyte and platelet counts. Induces antiviral effects by activation of macrophages, natural killer cells, and T-cells, thus boosting cellular immunity and suppressing hepatic inflammation and replication of hepatitis C virus.

USES Chronic hepatitis C with or without *Ribavirin*.

CONTRAINDICATIONS Hypersensitivity to peginterferon alfa-2a or any of its components; severe immunosuppression (e.g., organ transplant, advanced AIDS); autoimmune thyroid diseases (e.g., Graves' disease, thyroiditis); autoimmune hepatitis; dental work; *E. coli* hypersensitivity, decompensated hepatic disease prior to or during treatment; in neonates and infants because it contains benzyl alcohol; females of childbearing age; lactation; pregnancy (category C); neonates and infants.
CAUTIOUS USE History of neuropsychiatric disorder; alcoholism, substance abuse, bipolar disorder, mania, psychosis; bone marrow suppression; cardiovascular disorders, cardiac arrhythmias, history of MI, cardiac disease, heart failure, uncontrolled hypertension; pulmonary disease, including COPD; thyroid dysfunction; diabetes mellitus, diabetic ketoacidosis; dental disease, older adults; autoimmune disorders; autoimmune hepatitis; ulcerative and hemorrhagic colitis; pancreatitis; pulmonary disorders; HBV or HIV coinfection; retinal disease; renal impairment with creatinine clearance <50

P

mL/min; older adults with possible decreased kidney function; organ transplant recipients; lactation. Safety and efficacy in children <18 y are not established.

ROUTE & DOSAGE

Chronic Hepatitis C

Adult: **SC** 180 mcg once weekly times 48 wk, may decrease to 135 mcg once weekly if not tolerated

Renal Impairment

End stage renal disease: Reduce dose to 135 mcg once weekly

Hepatic Impairment

Reduce dose to 90 mcg once weekly if LFTs progressively increase over baseline

ADMINISTRATION

Subcutaneous

- Give dose on the same day of each week. Administer SC in the abdomen or thigh and rotate injection sites.
- Warm refrigerated vial by rolling in hands for about 1 min. Do not use if particulate matter is visible in the vial or product is discolored. Discard any unused portion.
- Note that manufacturer recommends the following: dose reduction to 135 mcg if neutrophil count <750 cells/mm^3 and with ANC values <500 cells/mm^3, treatment should be suspended until ANC values return to more than 1000 cells/mm^3; dose reduction to 90 mcg if the platelet count is <50,000 cells/mm^3 and discontinuation of therapy if platelet count <25,000 cells/mm^3. Consult physician.
- Store in the refrigerator at 36°–46° F (2°–8° C), do not freeze or shake. Protect from light. Vials are for single use only.

ADVERSE EFFECTS (≥1%) **Body as a Whole:** *Musculoskeletal pain, myalgia, arthralgia, fatigue, inflammation at injection site, flu-like symptoms, rigors, fever,* pain, malaise, asthenia. **CNS:** *Headache, depression,* anxiety, *irritability, insomnia, dizziness,* impaired concentration, impaired memory, suicidal ideation, suicide attempt. **GI:** *Nausea, diarrhea, abdominal pain, anorexia,* dry mouth. **Hematologic:** Thrombocytopenia, *neutropenia.* **Skin:** *Alopecia, pruritus,* dermatitis, sweating, rash.

INTERACTIONS Drug: May increase **theophylline** levels; additive myelosuppression with ANTINEOPLASTICS.

PHARMACOKINETICS Peak: 72–96 h. **Elimination:** 30% excreted in urine. **Half-Life:** 80 h.

NURSING IMPLICATIONS

Assessment & Drug Effects

- Monitor for S&S of hypersensitivity (e.g., angioedema, bronchoconstriction) and, if noted, institute appropriate medical action immediately. Note that transient rashes are not an indication to discontinue treatment.
- Withhold drug and notify physician for any of the following: severe neuropsychiatric events (e.g., psychosis, hallucinations, suicidal ideation, depression, bipolar disorders and mania), severe neutropenia or thrombocytopenia, abdominal pain accompanied by bloody diarrhea and fever, S&S of pancreatitis, new or worsening ophthalmologic disorders, or any other severe adverse event (see CAUTIOUS USE).
- Withhold drug and notify physician for any of the following: Baseline neutrophil counts <1500 cells/mm^3, baseline platelet

counts <90,000 cells/mm or baseline hemoglobin <10 g/dL.

- Note that acceptable baseline limits for therapy include: Platelet count ≥90,000 cells/mm^3 (as low as 75,000 cells/mm^3 in patients with cirrhosis or transition to cirrhosis), absolute neutrophil count (ANC) ≥1500 cells/mm^3; serum creatinine <1.5 × upper limit of normal; TSH and T4 within normal limit. Withhold therapy and notify physician for unacceptable baseline values.
- Monitor respiratory and cardiovascular status; report dyspnea, chest pain, and hypotension immediately; perform baseline and periodic ECG and chest X-ray.
- Lab tests: Baseline and periodic creatinine clearance, uric acid, CBC with differential, platelet count, Hct & Hgb, TSH, ALT, AST, bilirubin, blood glucose; retest CBC with differential, platelet count, Hct & Hgb after 2 wk and other blood chemistries after 4 wk. Serum HCV RNA levels after 24 wk of treatment.
- Baseline and periodic ophthalmology exams are recommended.

Patient & Family Education

- If you miss a drug dose and remember within 2 d of the scheduled dose, take the dose and continue with your regular schedule. If more than 2 d have passed, contact physician for instructions.
- Notify physician immediately for any of the following: severe depression or suicidal thoughts, severe chest pain, difficulty breathing, changes in vision, unusual bleeding or bruising, bloody diarrhea, high fever, severe stomach or lower back pain, severe chest pain, development a new or worsening of a preexisting skin condition.
- Follow up with lab tests; compliance with lab testing is extremely important while taking this drug.
- Do not drive or engage in other potentially hazardous activities until reaction to drug is known.
- Women should use reliable means of contraception while taking this drug and notify physician immediately if they become pregnant.
- Do not breast feed while taking this drug without consulting physician.

PEGINTERFERON ALFA-2B

(peg-in-ter-fer′on)

PEG-Intron

Classifications: IMMUNOMODULATOR; INTERFERON

Prototype: Interferon Alfa-2a

Pregnancy Category: C

AVAILABILITY 100 mcg/mL, 160 mcg/mL, 240 mcg/mL, 300 mcg/mL powder for injection

ACTIONS Binds to specific membrane receptors on the cell surface thereby initiating enzyme induction, suppression of cell proliferation, enhanced phagocytic activity of macrophages, augmentation of specific cytotoxic lymphocytes for target cells, and inhibition of viral replication in virus-infected cells.

THERAPEUTIC EFFECTS Induces antiviral effects by activation of macrophages, natural killer cells, and T-cells, thus boosting cellular immunity and suppressing hepatic inflammation and replication of hepatitis C virus.

USES Chronic hepatitis C.

UNLABELED USES Renal carcinoma.

CONTRAINDICATIONS Hypersensitivity to peginterferon; autoimmune hepatitis; decompensated liver disease; persistently severe or worsening S&S of life-threatening neuro-

P

psychiatric, autoimmune, ischemic, or infectious disorders.

CAUTIOUS USE History of neuropsychiatric disorder; bone marrow suppression; ulcerative and hemorrhagic colitis; pancreatitis; pulmonary disorders; HBV or HIV coinfection; thyroid dysfunction; diabetes mellitus; cardiovascular disease; autoimmune disorders; retinal disease; renal impairment with creatinine clearance <50 mL/min; older adults with possible decreased kidney function; lactation. Safety and efficacy in children are not established.

ROUTE & DOSAGE

Chronic Hepatitis C

Adult: **SC** Based on weight and injected once weekly times 1 y: *37–45 kg*, 40 mcg; *46–56 kg*, 50 mcg; *57–72 kg*, 64 mcg; *73–88 kg*, 80 mcg; *89–106 kg*, 96 mcg; *107–136 kg*, 120 mcg; *137–160 kg*, 150 mcg.

P

ADMINISTRATION

Subcutaneous

- Give dose on the same day of each week.
- Be aware that two Safety Lok™ syringes are provided in the drug package: one for reconstitution and one for injection. Reconstitute with only 0.7 mL of supplied diluent and discard remaining diluent. Enter the vial only once as it does not contain a preservative. Swirl gently to produce a clear, colorless solution. Use solution immediately.
- Serious adverse reactions warrant reduction or discontinuation of dose.
- Store dry vial at 15°–30° C (59°–86° F). If necessary, store reconstituted solution up to 24 h at 2°–8° C (36°–46° F).

ADVERSE EFFECTS (≥1%) **Body as a Whole:** *Musculoskeletal pain, fatigue, inflammation at injection site, flu-like symptoms, rigors, fever, weight loss, viral infection,* pain, malaise, hypertonia. **CNS:** *Headache, depression, anxiety, emotional lability, irritability, insomnia, dizziness.* **GI:** *Nausea, anorexia, diarrhea, abdominal pain,* vomiting, dyspepsia, hepatomegaly. **Endocrine:** Hypothyroidism. **Hematologic:** Thrombocytopenia, neutropenia. **Respiratory:** *Pharyngitis,* sinusitis, cough. **Skin:** *Alopecia, pruritus, dry skin,* sweating, rash, flushing.

INTERACTIONS Drug: May increase **theophylline** levels; additive myelosuppression with ANTINEOPLASTICS; **zidovudine** may increase hematologic toxicity; increase **doxorubicin** toxicity, increase neurotoxicity with **vinblastine; aldesleukin (IL-2)** may potentiate the risk of kidney failure.

PHARMACOKINETICS Peak: 15–44 h. **Duration:** 48–72 h. **Elimination:** 30% excreted in urine. **Half-Life:** 40 h (22–60 h).

NURSING IMPLICATIONS

Assessment & Drug Effects

- Monitor for S&S of hypersensitivity (e.g., angioedema, bronchoconstriction) and, if noted, institute appropriate medical action immediately. Note that transient rashes are not an indication to discontinue treatment.
- Monitor for and report immediately S&S of neuropsychiatric disorders (e.g., psychosis, hallucinations, suicidal ideation, depression).
- Monitor respiratory and cardiovascular status; report dyspnea, chest pain, and hypotension immediately; baseline and periodic ECG and chest X-ray.

- Lab tests: Baseline and periodic creatinine clearance, CBC with differential, platelet count, Hct & Hgb, TSH, ALT, AST, bilirubin, blood glucose; with diabetics or hypertensives. Serum HCV RNA levels are assessed after 24 wk of treatment.
- Withhold drug and notify physician for any of the following: severe neuropsychiatric events, severe neutropenia or thrombocytopenia, abdominal pain accompanied by bloody diarrhea and fever, S&S of pancreatitis, or any other severe adverse event (see CAUTIOUS USE).
- Baseline and periodic ophthalmology exams are recommended.

Patient & Family Education

- Drink fluids liberally while taking this drug, especially during the initial stages of therapy.
- Learn reasons for withholding drug (see ASSESSMENT & DRUG EFFECTS).
- Use effective means of contraception while taking this drug. Women should not become pregnant.
- Follow up with lab tests; compliance with lab testing is extremely important while taking this drug.
- Do not breast feed while taking this drug without consulting physician.

PEGVISOMANT

(peg-vis′o-mant)

Somavert

Classifications: HORMONES & SYNTHETIC SUBSTITUTES; GROWTH HORMONE MODIFIER; GROWTH HORMONE RECEPTOR ANTAGONIST

Pregnancy Category: B

AVAILABILITY 15 mg, 20 mg, 10 g powder for injection

ACTIONS A growth hormone (GH) receptor antagonist that binds to GH receptors on cell surfaces where it blocks the binding of GH and interferes with its action and ability to stimulate production of insulin-like growth factor I (IGF-1).

THERAPEUTIC EFFECTS Produces a significant decrease in the level of serum insulin-like growth factor I (IGF-1), the primary mediator of GH effects on body tissues.

USES Treatment of acromegaly when other treatments have failed or are inappropriate.

CONTRAINDICATIONS Hypersensitivity to pegvisomant; hypersensitivity to latex; lactation.

CAUTIOUS USE Pituitary tumors; diabetes mellitus; hepatic and/or renal impairment; pregnancy (category B); children, and elderly.

ROUTE & DOSAGE

Acromegaly

Adult: **SC** 40 mg loading dose, then 10 mg once daily. Adjust dose in 5 mg increments, up to 30 mg/d, based on serum IGF-I concentrations

ADMINISTRATION

Subcutaneous

- Allow vials to reach room temperature, then reconstitute by adding 1 mL of supplied diluent (sterile water for injection) to the vial. Direct diluent against the glass wall of vial, then mix by gently rolling between palms of hands to dissolve. DO NOT SHAKE. Solution should be clear and colorless. Use within 6 h of reconstitution.
- Inject SC and exercise caution not to inject IV.
- Rotate injection sites and do not use any site more than once every 1–2 mo.

P

■ Store vials of powder at 2°–8° C (36°–46° F).

ADVERSE EFFECTS (≥1%) **Body as a Whole:** Asthenia, flu-like syndrome, infection, injection site reactions, back pain, paresthesias, peripheral edema. **CNS:** Dizziness. **CV:** Angina, chest pain, hypertension, MI. **GI:** Elevated liver function tests, diarrhea, nausea, vomiting. **Metabolic:** Hypercholesterolemia, hypoglycemia, and low titer non-neutralizing antigrowth hormone antibodies. **Musculoskeletal:** Arthralgia. **Respiratory:** Sinusitis.

DIAGNOSTIC TEST INTERFERENCE Similar to growth hormone and may cross-react with ***growth hormone assays.*** Do not use these assays to monitor pegvisomant therapy.

INTERACTIONS Drug: OPIATE AGONISTS may lead to higher **pegvisomant** dosing requirements; may need to decrease doses of **insulin,** ORAL ANTIDIABETIC AGENTS.

PHARMACOKINETICS Absorption: 57% absorbed from SC injection site. **Peak:** 33–77 h. **Half-Life:** 6 d.

NURSING IMPLICATIONS

Assessment & Drug Effects

- Montior CV status with baseline and periodic BP measurements.
- Monitor diabetics for loss of glycemic control.
- Withhold drug and notify physician for significant elevation in AST/ALT or S&S of hepatitis.
- Lab tests: IGF-1 levels 4–6 wk after initiation of therapy or any dose adjustment, then q6mo after IGF-1 levels have normalized; periodic LFTs and lipid profile; frequent blood glucose monitoring, especially if diabetic.

Patient & Family Education

- Report promptly any of the following: chest pain or tightness, signs of infection (e.g., fever, chills, flu-like symptoms).
- Discontinue drug and notify physician immediately if jaundice appears.
- Do not drive or engage in other hazardous activities until reaction to drug is known.
- Do not breast feed without consulting physician.

PEMETREXED

(pe-me-trex′ed)
Alimta
Classifications: ANTINEOPLASTIC AGENT; ANTIMETABOLITE
Prototype: Fluorouracil
Pregnancy Category: D

AVAILABILITY 500 mg powder for injection

ACTIONS Suppresses tumor growth by inhibiting both DNA synthesis and folate metabolism at multiple target enzymes.
THERAPEUTIC EFFECTS Appears to arrest the cell cycle, thus inhibiting tumor growth. Some data suggest that pemetrexed may increase the effects of radiation therapy in cells sensitive to the drug.

USES Treatment of malignant pleural mesothelioma that is unresectable or in patients that are not surgery candidates in combination with cisplatin; treatment of locally advanced or metastatic non-small cell lung cancer (NSCLC).
UNLABELED USES Has been used investigationally in other solid tumors, including bladder, breast, colorectal, gastric, head and neck, pancreatic, and renal cell cancers.

CONTRAINDICATIONS Mannitol hypersensitivity; creatinine clearance is <45 mL/min, renal failure, moderate or severe renal impairment; dental work; active infection; IM injections; vaccines; children <18 y; pregnancy (category D); lactation.
CAUTIOUS USE Anemia, thrombocytopenia, neutropenia, dental disease; older adults; hepatic disease, hypoalbuminemia, hypovolemia, dehydration, ascites, pleural effusion.

ROUTE & DOSAGE

Malignant Mesothelioma, Non-Small Cell Lung Cancer

Adult: **IV** 500 mg/m^2 on day 1 of each 21-d cycle

Renal Impairment

Not recommended if Cl_{cr} <45 mL/min

ADMINISTRATION

Intravenous

Pre-/posttreatment with folic acid, vitamin B_{12}, and dexamethasone are needed to reduce hematologic and gastrointestinal toxicity, and the possibility of severe cutaneous reactions from pemetrexed.

PREPARE: **IV Infusion:** Reconstitute each 500-mg vial with 20 mL of preservative-free NS. Do not use any other diluent. Swirl gently to dissolve. Each vial will contain 25 mg/mL. Withdraw the needed amount of reconstituted solution and add to 100 mL of preservative-free NS. Discard any unused portion.

ADMINISTER: **IV Infusion:** Do NOT give a bolus dose. Infuse over 10 min.

INCOMPATIBILITIES **Solution/additive:** Solutions containing **calcium, Lactated Ringer's. Y-site: Amphotericin B, cefazolin, cefotaxime, cefotetan, cefoxitin, ceftazidime, chlorpromazine, ciprofloxacin, dobutamine, doxorubicin, doxycycline, droperidol, gemcitabine, gentamicin, irinotecan, metronidazole, minocycline, mitoxantrone, nalbuphine, ondansetron, prochlorperazine, tobramycin, topotecan.**

- Store unopened single-use vials at room temperature between 15°–30° C (59°–86° F). The reconstituted drug is stable for up to 24 h at 2°–8° C (36°–46° F) or at 25° C (77° F).

ADVERSE EFFECTS (≥1%) **Body as a Whole:** *Fatigue, fever,* hypersensitivity reaction, edema, myalgia, arthralgia. **CNS:** Neuropathy, *mood alteration, depression.* **CV:** Chest pain, thromboembolism. **GI:** *Nausea, vomiting, constipation, anorexia, stomatitis, diarrhea,* dehydration, dysphagia, esophagitis, odynophagia, increased LFTs. **Hematologic:** *Neutropenia, leukopenia, anemia, thrombocytopenia.* **Respiratory:** *Dyspnea.* **Skin:** *Rash, desquamation,* alopecia. **Urogenital:** *Increases serum creatinine,* renal failure.

INTERACTIONS Drug: Increased risk of renal toxicity with other nephrotoxic drugs **(acyclovir, adefovir, amphotericin B,** AMINOGLYCOSIDES, **carboplatin, cidofovir, cisplatin, cyclosporine, foscarnet, ganciclovir, sirolimus, tacrolimus, vancomycin);** NSAIDS may increase risk of renal toxicity in patients with preexisting renal insufficiency; may cause additive risk of bleeding with ANTICOAGULANTS, PLATELET INHIBITORS, **aspirin,** THROMBOLYTIC AGENTS.

PHARMACOKINETICS Metabolism: Not extensively metabolized. **Elimination:** Primarily excreted in urine. **Half-Life:** 3.5 h.

P

NURSING IMPLICATIONS

Assessment & Drug Effects

- Withhold drug and notify physician if the absolute neutrophil count (ANC) is <1500 cells/mm^3 or the platelet count is less than at least 100,000 cells/mm^3, or if the Cl_{cr} is < 45 mL/min.
- Lab tests: Baseline and periodic CBC with differential; monitor for nadir and recovery before each dose (on day 8 and 15, respectively, of each cycle); periodic LFTs, serum creatinine and BUN.
- Notify physician for S&S of neuropathy (paresthesia) or thromboembolism.

Patient & Family Education

- Report promptly any of the following to physician: symptoms of anemia (e.g., chest pain, unusual weakness or tiredness, fainting spells, lightheadedness, shortness of breath); symptoms of poor blood clotting (e.g., bruising; red spots on skin; black, tarry stools; blood in urine); symptoms of infection (e.g., fever or chills, cough, sore throat, pain or difficulty passing urine); symptoms of liver problems (e.g., yellowing of skin).
- Do not take nonsteroidal antiinflammatory drugs (NSAIDS) without first consulting the physician.
- Do not breast feed while taking this drug.

PEMIROLAST POTASSIUM

(pem-ir'o-last po-tass'i-um)
Alamast
Classifications: EAR, EYE, NOSE AND THROAT PREPARATION; ANTIHISTAMINE; OCULAR
Prototype: Levocabastine
Pregnancy Category: C

AVAILABILITY 0.1% solution

See Appendix A-1.

PEMOLINE

(pem'oh-leen)
Cylert
Classifications: CENTRAL NERVOUS SYSTEM AGENT; CEREBRAL STIMULANT
Prototype: Amphetamine
Pregnancy Category: B
Controlled Substance: Schedule IV

AVAILABILITY 18.75 mg, 37.5 mg, 75 mg tablets; 37.5 mg chewable tablets

ACTIONS Action qualitatively similar to those of amphetamine but with weak sympathomimetic activity.
THERAPEUTIC EFFECTS Capable of producing increased motor activity, mental alertness, diminished sense of fatigue, and mild euphoria. Also thought to have anorexigenic effect.

USES Adjunctive therapy to other remedial measures (psychologic, educational, social) in minimal brain dysfunction [attention deficit disorder (ADD)] in carefully selected children.
UNLABELED USES Mild stimulant for geriatric patients.

CONTRAINDICATIONS Known hypersensitivity to pemoline; children <6 y. Safety during pregnancy (category B) or lactation is not established.
CAUTIOUS USE Impaired hepatic and kidney function; history of drug abuse; psychosis; emotional instability.

ROUTE & DOSAGE

Attention Deficit Disorder
Child: **PO** >6 y, 37.5 mg/d, may be increased by 18.75 mg at weekly intervals (max: 112.5 mg/d)

ADMINISTRATION

Oral

- Give in morning to provide maximal effectiveness and to avoid insomnia.

ADVERSE EFFECTS (≥1%) **Body as a Whole:** Malaise, irritability, fatigue, dyskinetic movements, hallucinations, excitement, agitation, restlessness. **CNS:** *Insomnia,* mild depression, dizziness, headache, drowsiness, convulsions, nervousness. **CV:** Tachycardia. **GI:** *Anorexia,* abdominal discomfort, liver failure, nausea, diarrhea, elevated AST, ALT, and alkaline phosphatase (after several months of therapy); jaundice. **Skin:** Skin rash. **Special Senses:** Dyskinetic movements of eyes.

INTERACTIONS Drug: MONOAMINE OXIDASE INHIBITORS (e.g., **selegiline, Parnate**) should be stopped 14 d before **sertraline** is started because of serious problems with other SEROTONIN-REUPTAKE INHIBITORS (shivering, nausea, diplopia, confusion, anxiety). **Tolbutamide** and **diazepam** clearance may be reduced. Use cautiously with other centrally acting CNS drugs. **Herbal: St. John's wort** may cause serotonin syndrome.

PHARMACOKINETICS Absorption: Readily absorbed from GI tract. **Onset:** 2–3 wk. **Peak:** 2–4 h. **Duration:** 8 h. **Metabolism:** Metabolized in liver. **Elimination:** Excreted in urine. **Half-Life:** 9–14 h.

NURSING IMPLICATIONS

Assessment & Drug Effects

- Monitor therapeutic effectiveness. Drug should be withdrawn if substantial clinical benefit is not seen following 3 wk of therapy.
- Note: Insomnia and anorexia (most frequent adverse effects) appear to be dose-related.
- Monitor weight and height (growth rate) throughout therapy. Anorexia is often accompanied by weight loss.
- Be aware that careful clinical evaluation and supervision of patient are essential.
- Lab tests: Obtain baseline and biweekly liver function studies for patients receiving long-term therapy. Discontinue pemoline if significantly abnormal liver functions are noted.

Patient & Family Education

- Report to physician immediately any sign of liver malfunction such as dark urine, jaundice, loss of appetite.
- Avoid potentially hazardous activities until the resonse to drug is known.
- Significant benefits of drug therapy may not be evident until third week of drug administration.
- Be aware that pemoline can produce tolerance and physical and psychologic dependence.

P

PENBUTOLOL

(pen-bu'tol-ol)

Levatol

Classifications: AUTONOMIC NERVOUS SYSTEM AGENT; BETA-ADRENERGIC ANTAGONIST (BLOCKING AGENT, SYMPATHOLYTIC); ANTIHYPERTENSIVE

Prototype: Propranolol

Pregnancy Category: C

AVAILABILITY 20 mg tablets

ACTIONS Synthetic $beta_1$- and $beta_2$-adrenergic blocking agent which competes with epinephrine and norepinephrine for available beta receptor sites.

THERAPEUTIC EFFECTS Lowers both supine and standing BP in hypertensive patients. Hypotensive effect is associated with decreased cardiac output, suppressed renin activity, as well as beta blockage.

USES Mild to moderate hypertension. May be used alone or with other antihypertensive agents.

CONTRAINDICATIONS Clients with cardiogenic shock, sinus bradycardia, second and third degree AV block; bronchial asthma; hypersensitivity to the drug.
CAUTIOUS USE Cardiac failure; chronic bronchitis, emphysema; diabetes; pregnancy (category C), lactation. Safety and effectiveness in children is not established.

ROUTE & DOSAGE

Hypertension
Adult: **PO** 10–20 mg once/d, may increase to 40–80 mg/d if needed

P

ADMINISTRATION

Oral
- Discontinue by reducing the dose gradually over 1 to 2 wk.

ADVERSE EFFECTS (≥1%) **CNS:** Dizziness, fatigue, *headache,* insomnia. **CV:** AV block, bradycardia. **GI:** Nausea, diarrhea, dyspepsia. **Respiratory:** Cough, dyspnea. **Urogenital:** Impotence.

INTERACTIONS Drug: DIURETICS and other HYPOTENSIVE AGENTS increase hypotensive effect; effects of **albuterol, metaproterenol, terbutaline, pirbuterol,** and penbutolol are antagonized; NSAIDS blunt hypotensive effect; decreases hypoglycemic effect of **glyburide; amiodarone** increases risk of bradycardia and sinus arrest.

PHARMACOKINETICS Absorption: Readily absorbed from GI tract. **Peak:** 2–3 h. **Duration:** 20 h. **Metabolism:** Metabolized in liver. **Elimination:** Excreted in urine. **Half-Life:** 5 h.

NURSING IMPLICATIONS

Assessment & Drug Effects
- Take apical pulse before administering drug. If pulse is below 60, or other established parameter, hold the drug and contact physician.
- Take a BP reading before giving drug, if BP is not stabilized. If systolic pressure is ≤90 mm Hg, hold drug and contact physician.
- Check BP near end of dosage interval or before administration of next dose to evaluate effectiveness.
- Monitor therapeutic effectiveness. Full effectiveness of the drug may not be seen for 4–6 wk.
- Watch for S&S of bronchial constriction. Report promptly and withhold drug.
- Monitor diabetics for loss of glycemic control. Drug suppresses clinical signs of hypoglycemia (e.g., BP changes, increased pulse rate) and may prolong hypoglycemic state.
- Monitor carefully for exacerbation of angina during drug withdrawal.

Patient & Family Education
- Do not discontinue the drug without physician's advice because of the possible exacerbation of ischemic heart disease.
- If diabetic, report persistent S&S of hypoglycemia (see Appendix F) to physician (diabetics).
- Avoid driving or other potentially hazardous activities until response to drug is known.
- Make position changes slowly and avoid prolonged standing. Notify physician if dizziness and light-headedness persist.

- Comply with and do not alter established regimen (i.e., do not omit, increase, or decrease dosage or change dosage interval).
- Avoid prolonged exposure of extremities to cold.
- Avoid excesses of alcohol. Heavy alcohol consumption (i.e., >60 mL [2 oz]/d) may elevate arterial pressure; therefore, to maintain treatment effectiveness, either avoid alcohol or drink moderately (<60 mL/d). Consult physician.
- Do not breast feed while taking this drug without consulting physician.

PENCICLOVIR

(pen-cy'clo-vir)
Denavir
Classifications: ANTIINFECTIVE; ANTIVIRAL
Prototype: Acyclovir
Pregnancy Category: B

AVAILABILITY 10 mg/g cream

ACTIONS Antiviral agent active against herpes simplex virus type 1 (HSV-1) and type 2 (HSV-2).
THERAPEUTIC EFFECTS HSV-1 and HSV-2 infected cells phosphorylate penciclovir utilizing viral thymidine kinase. Resulting form of penciclovir competes with viral DNA, thus inhibiting both viral DNA synthesis and replication.

USES Treatment of recurrent herpes labialis (cold sores).

CONTRAINDICATIONS Hypersensitivity to penciclovir, lactation.
CAUTIOUS USE Pregnancy (category B). Safety and efficacy in children have not been established. Safety in immunocompromised patients is not established.

ROUTE & DOSAGE

Cold Sores
Adult: **Topical** Apply q2h while awake times 4 d

ADMINISTRATION

Topical
- Apply as soon as possible after developing lesion.
- Do not apply to mucous membranes or near the eyes.
- Store at or below 30° C (86° F). Do not freeze.

ADVERSE EFFECTS (≥1%) **CNS:** Headache. **Skin:** Erythema.

INTERACTIONS Drug: No clinically significant interactions established.

PHARMACOKINETICS Absorption: Minimally absorbed from cold sore.

NURSING IMPLICATIONS

Assessment & Drug Effects
- Monitor the extent of lesions and treatment effectiveness.

Patient & Family Education
- Wash hands before and after application. Avoid contact of drug with eyes.
- Apply sunscreen to lips; may minimize recurrence of lesions.
- Do not breast feed while taking this drug.

PENICILLAMINE

(pen-i-sill'a-meen)
Cuprimine, Depen
Classification: CHELATING AGENT
Pregnancy Category: D

AVAILABILITY 150 mg, 250 mg capsules; 250 mg tablets

ACTIONS Thiol compound prepared by hydrolysis of penicillin but lacking antibacterial activity. Also combines chemically with cystine to form a soluble disulfide complex that prevents stone formation and may even dissolve existing cystic stones. Mechanism of action in rheumatoid arthritis not known but appears to be related to inhibition of collagen formation. Cross-sensitivity between penicillin and penicillamine can occur.

THERAPEUTIC EFFECTS Forms stable soluble chelate with copper, zinc, iron, lead, mercury, and possibly other heavy metals and promotes their excretion in urine. With Wilson's disease, therapeutic effectiveness is indicated by improvement in psychiatric and neurologic symptoms, visual symptoms, and liver function. In some patients, neurologic symptoms become more prominent during initial therapy and then subside. With rheumatoid arthritis, improvement in grip strength, decrease in stiffness following immobility, reduction of pain, decrease in sedimentation rate and rheumatoid factor.

P

USES To promote renal excretion of excess copper in Wilson's disease (hepatolenticular degeneration). Active rheumatoid arthritis in patients who have failed to respond to conventional therapy. Cystinuria.

UNLABELED USES Scleroderma, primary biliary cirrhosis, porphyria catenae tarda, lead poisoning.

CONTRAINDICATIONS Hypersensitivity to penicillamine or to any penicillin; history of penicillamine-related aplastic anemia or agranulocytosis; patients with rheumatoid arthritis who have renal insufficiency or who are pregnant; pregnancy (category D), lactation; concomitant administration with drugs that can cause severe hematologic or renal reactions (e.g., antimalarials, gold salts, immunosuppressants, oxyphenbutazone, phenylbutazone).

CAUTIOUS USE Allergy-prone individuals.

ROUTE & DOSAGE

Wilson's Disease

Adult: **PO** 250 mg q.i.d., with 3 doses 1 h a.c. and the last dose at least 2 h after the last meal
Child: **PO** 20 mg/kg/d in 2–4 divided doses (max: 1 g/d)

Cystinuria

Adult: **PO** 250–500 mg q.i.d., with doses adjusted to limit urinary excretion of cystine to 100–200 mg/d
Child: **PO** 30 mg/kg/d in 4 divided doses with doses adjusted to limit urinary excretion of cystine to 100–200 mg/d

Rheumatoid Arthritis

Adult: **PO** 125–250 mg/d; may increase at 1–3 mo intervals up to 1–1.5 g/d
Child: **PO** 3 mg/kg/d (≤250 mg/d) times 3 mo, then 6 mg/kg/d (≤500 mg/d) in 2 divided doses times 3 mo (max: of 10 mg/kg/d [≤1.5 g/d] in 3–4 divided doses)

Lead Poisoning

Child: **PO** 30–40 mg/kg/d in 3–4 divided doses (max: 1.5 g/d); initiate at 25% target dose, gradually increase to full dose over 2–3 wk

ADMINISTRATION

Oral

- Give on empty stomach (60 min before or 2 h after meals) to avoid absorption of metals in foods by penicillamine.
- Give contents in 15–30 mL of chilled fruit juice or pureed fruit

(e.g., applesauce) if patient cannot swallow capsules or tablets.

ADVERSE EFFECTS (≥1%) **Body as a Whole:** Fever, arthralgia, lymphadenopathy, thyroiditis, SLE-like syndrome, thrombophlebitis, hyperpyrexia, myasthenia gravis syndrome, tingling of feet, weakness. **GI:** *Anorexia, nausea, vomiting,* epigastric pain, diarrhea, oral lesions, *reduction or loss of taste perception (particularly salt and sweet), metallic taste,* activation of peptic ulcer, pancreatitis. **Urogenital:** Membranous glomerulopathy, *proteinuria,* hematuria. **Hematologic:** Thrombocytopenia, leukopenia, agranulocytosis, thrombotic thrombocytopenic purpura, hemolytic anemia, aplastic anemia. **Metabolic:** Pyridoxine deficiency. **Skin:** *Generalized pruritus, urticaria,* mammary hyperplasia, alveolitis, skin friability, excessive skin wrinkling, *early and late occurring rashes,* pemphigus-like rash, alopecia. **Special Senses:** Tinnitus, optic neuritis, ptosis.

INTERACTIONS Drug: ANTIMALARIALS, CYTOTOXICS, **gold** therapy may potentiate hematologic and renal adverse effects; **iron** may decrease penicillamine absorption.

PHARMACOKINETICS Absorption: Readily absorbed from GI tract. **Peak:** 1 h. **Distribution:** Crosses placenta. **Metabolism:** Metabolized in liver. **Elimination:** Excreted in urine and feces.

NURSING IMPLICATIONS

Assessment & Drug Effects

- Lab tests: Check WBC with differential, direct platelet counts, Hgb, and urinalyses prior to initiation of therapy and every 3 d during the first month of therapy, then every 2 wk thereafter. Perform liver function tests and eye examinations before start of therapy and at least twice yearly thereafter.
- Withhold drug and contact physician if the patient with rheumatoid arthritis develops proteinuria >1 g (some clinicians accept >2 g) or if platelet count drops to <100,000/mm^3, or platelet count falls below 3500–4000/mm^3, or neutropenia occurs.

Patient & Family Education

- Note: Clinical evidence of therapeutic effectiveness may not be apparent until 1–3 mo of drug therapy.
- Take exactly as prescribed. Allergic reactions occur in about one third of patients receiving penicillamine. Temporary interruptions of therapy increase possibility of sensitivity reactions.
- Take temperature nightly during first few months of therapy. Fever is a possible early sign of allergy.
- Observe skin over pressure sites: knees, elbows, shoulder blades, toes, buttocks. Penicillamine increases skin friability.
- Report unusual bruising or bleeding, sore mouth or throat, fever, skin rash, or any other unusual symptoms to physician.
- Do not breast feed while taking this drug.

P

PENICILLIN G BENZATHINE

(pen-i-sill′in)

Bicillin, Bicillin L-A, Permapen

Classifications: ANTIINFECTIVE; BETA-LACTAM ANTIBIOTIC; NATURAL PENICILLIN

Prototype: Penicillin G potassium

Pregnancy Category: B

AVAILABILITY 300,000 units/mL, 600,000 units/mL, 1,200,000 units/2 mL, 2,400,000 units/4 mL injection

ACTIONS Acid-stable, penicillinase-sensitive, long-acting form of penicillin G. Absorbed slowly in body because of extremely low water solubility. Produces lower blood concentrations than other penicillin G compounds but has the longest duration of antimicrobial activity of all other available parenteral or repository penicillins.

THERAPEUTIC EFFECTS Effective against many strains of *Staphylococcus aureus*, gram-positive cocci, gram-negative cocci. Also effective against gram-positive bacilli and gram-negative bacilli.

USES Infections highly susceptible to penicillin G, such as *Streptococcal, Pneumococcal,* and *Staphylococcal* infections, venereal disease such as syphilis (including early, late, and congenital forms), and nonvenereal diseases (e.g., yaws, bejel, and pinta). Also used in prophylaxis of rheumatic fever.

CONTRAINDICATIONS Hypersensitivity to penicillins or cephalosporins; lactation; pregnancy (category B).

CAUTIOUS USE History of or suspected allergy (eczema, hives, hay fever, asthma).

ROUTE & DOSAGE

Mild to Moderate Infections

Adult: **IM** 1,200,000 U once/d
Child: **IM** >27 kg: 900,000 U once/d; <27 kg: 300,000–600,000 U once/d

Syphilis

Adult: **IM** <1 y duration: 2,400,000 U as single dose; >1 y duration: 2,400,000 U/wk for 3 wk
Child: **IM** Congenital: 50,000 U/kg as single dose

Prophylaxis for Rheumatic Fever

Adult: **IM** 1,200,000 U q4wk
Child: **IM** 1,200,000 U q3–4wk

ADMINISTRATION

Intramuscular

- Do not confuse Penicillin G benzathine with preparations containing procaine penicillin G (e.g., Bicillin C-R).
- Make IM injection deep into upper outer quadrant of buttock. In infants and small children, the preferred site is the midlateral aspect of the thigh.
- Shake multiple-dose vial vigorously before withdrawing desired IM dose. Shake prepared cartridge unit vigorously before injecting drug.
- Select IM site with care. Injection into or near a major peripheral nerve can result in nerve damage. Inadvertent IV administration has resulted in arterial occlusion and cardiac arrest.
- Make injections at a slow steady rate to prevent needle blockage.
- Store at 15°–30° C (59°–86° F).

ADVERSE EFFECTS (≥1%) **Body as a Whole:** *Local pain,* tenderness, and fever associated with IM injection, chills, fever, wheezing, <u>anaphylaxis</u>, neuropathy, <u>nephrotoxicity</u>; superinfections, Jarisch-Herxheimer reaction in patients with syphilis. **Skin:** Pruritus, urticaria and other skin eruptions. **Hematologic:** Eosinophilia, hemolytic anemia and other blood abnormalities. Also see penicillin G.

INTERACTIONS Drug: Probenecid decreases renal elimination; may decrease efficacy of ORAL CONTRACEPTIVES.

PHARMACOKINETICS Absorption: Slowly absorbed from IM site. **Peak:** 12–24 h. **Duration:** 26 d. **Dis-**

tribution: Crosses placenta; distributed into breast milk. **Metabolism:** Hydrolyzed to penicillin in body. **Elimination:** Excreted slowly by kidneys.

NURSING IMPLICATIONS

Note: See penicillin G potassium for numerous additional nursing implications.

Assessment & Drug Effects

- Determine history of hypersensitivity reactions to penicillins, cephalosporins, or other allergens prior to initiation of drug therapy.
- Lab tests: Perform C&S tests prior to initiation of therapy and periodically thereafter. Perform periodic renal function tests.

Patient & Family Education

- Report immediately to physician the onset of an allergic reaction. There is great risk of severe and prolonged reactions because drug is absorbed so slowly.
- Do not breast feed while taking this drug.

PENICILLIN G POTASSIUM Pr

(pen-i-sill'in)

Megacillin ✦, Pentids, Pfizerpen

PENICILLIN G SODIUM

Classifications: ANTIINFECTIVE; BETA-LACTAM ANTIBIOTIC; NATURAL PENICILLIN

Pregnancy Category: B

AVAILABILITY 1,000,000 units, 5,000,000 units, 10,000,000 units, 20,000,000 units vials; 1,000,000 units/50 mL, 2,000,000 units/50 mL 3,000,000 units/50 mL injection

ACTIONS Acid-labile, penicillinase-sensitive, natural penicillin derived from cultures of *Penicillium notatum* or related molds. Antimicrobial spectrum is relatively narrow compared to that of the semisynthetic penicillins. Bactericidal at therapeutic serum levels; bacteriostatic at lower concentrations. Acts by interfering with synthesis of mucopeptides essential to formation and integrity of bacterial cell wall. Action is inhibited by penicillinase; therefore, penicillin G is ineffective against many strains of *Staphylococcus aureus.*

THERAPEUTIC EFFECTS Highly active against gram-positive cocci (e.g., non-penicillinase-producing *Staphylococcus, Streptococcus* groups A, C, G, H, L, M, and *Streptococcus pneumoniae*); and gram-negative cocci *(Neisseria gonorrhoeae, N. meningitidis).* Also effective against gram-positive bacilli *(Bacillus anthracis, Clostridium* species including gas gangrene and tetanus, and certain species of *Corynebacterium, Erysipelothrix,* and *Listeria);* gram-negative bacilli *(Fusobacterium, Pasteurella, Streptobacillus,* and *Bacteroides species).* Parenteral penicillin G is effective against some strains of *Salmonella* and *Shigella* and spirochetes *(Treponema pallidum, T. pertenue, Leptospira).*

USES Moderate to severe systemic infections caused by penicillin-sensitive microorganisms: actinomycosis, anthrax, diphtheria (carrier state), empyema, erysipelas, gas gangrene, gonorrheal infections, leptospirosis, mastoiditis, meningitis, acute osteomyelitis, otitis media, pinta, pneumonia, rat-bite fever, sinus infections; certain staphylococcal infections; streptococcal infections, including scarlet fever; syphilis (all stages), tetanus, urinary tract infections, Vincent's gingivostomatitis, yaws. Also used as prophylaxis in patients with rheumatic or congenital heart dis-

P

ease. Since oral preparations are absorbed erratically and thus must be given in comparatively high doses, this route is generally used only for mild or stabilized infections or long-term prophylaxis.

CONTRAINDICATIONS Hypersensitivity to any of the penicillins or cephalosporins; administration of oral drug to patients with severe infections; nausea, vomiting, hypermotility, gastric dilatation; cardiospasm. Use of penicillin G sodium in patients on sodium restriction. Safety during pregnancy (category B) or lactation is not established.

CAUTIOUS USE History of or suspected allergy (asthma, eczema, hay fever, hives); history of allergy to cephalosporins; kidney or liver dysfunction, myasthenia gravis, epilepsy, neonates, young infants. Use during lactation may lead to sensitization of infants.

ROUTE & DOSAGE

Moderate to Severe Infections

Adult: **PO** 1.6–3.2 million U divided q6h **IV/IM** 1.2–24 million U divided q4h
Child: **PO** 25,000–100,000 U/kg divided q6h **IV/IM** 25,000–300,000 U/kg divided q4h

Meningococcal Meningitis

Adult: **IM** 1–2 million U q 2 h **IV** 200,000–300,000/kg/d divided q 2–4 h or 2 million to 3 million units/d by continuous infusion
Child: **IV** 25,000–300,000 U/kg divided q4h

ADMINISTRATION

Note: Check whether physician has prescribed penicillin G potassium or sodium.

Oral

- Give on an empty stomach, at least 1 h before or 2 h after meals to reduce possibility of drug destruction by gastric acid and delay in absorption by food.
- Give with a full glass of water. Instruct patient to avoid acidic or carbonated beverages 1 h before and after taking oral penicillin G.
- Store tablets at 15°–30° C (59°–86° F) in tightly closed containers. Avoid excessive heat. Store oral suspensions and syrups in refrigerator and discard unused portions after 14 d.

Intramuscular

- Do not use the 20,000,000 unit dosage form for IM injection.
- Reconstitute for IM: Loosen powder by shaking bottle before adding diluent (sterile water for injection or sterile NS). Keep the total volume to be injected small. Solutions containing up to 100,000 units/mL cause the least discomfort. Adding 10 mL diluent to the 1,000,000 unit vial = 100,000 units/mL. Shake well to dissolve.
- Select IM site carefully. IM injection is made deep into a large muscle mass. Inject slowly. Rotate injection sites.

Intravenous

PREPARE: **Intermittent/Continuous:** Reconstitute as for IM injection then withdraw the required dose and add to 100–1000 mL of D5W or NS IV solution, depending on length of each infusion.

ADMINISTER: **Intermittent/Continuous:** Give intermittent infusion over at least 1 h and continuous infusion at a rate required to infuse the daily dose in 24 h. With high doses, IV penicillin G should be administered slowly to avoid electrolyte imbalance from potassium or sodium content.

Physician will often prescribe specific flow rate.

INCOMPATIBILITIES **Solution/additive: Dextran 40, fat emulsion, aminophylline, amphotericin B, cephalothin, chlorpromazine, dopamine, hydroxyzine, metaraminol,** TETRACYCLINES, **pentobarbital, prochlorperazine, promazine, sodium bicarbonate, thiopental, metoclopramide.**

- Store dry powder (for parenteral use) at room temperature. After reconstitution (initial dilution), store solutions for 1 wk under refrigeration. Intravenous infusion solutions containing penicillin G are stable at room temperature for at least 24 h.

ADVERSE EFFECTS (≥1%) **Body as a Whole:** Coughing, sneezing, feeling of uneasiness; systemic anaphylaxis, fever, widespread increase in capillary permeability and vasodilation with resulting edema (mouth, tongue, pharynx, larynx), laryngospasm, malaise, serum sickness (fever, malaise, pruritus, urticaria, lymphadenopathy, arthralgia, angioedema of face and extremities, neuritis prostration, eosinophilia), SLE-like syndrome, Injection site reactions (pain, inflammation, abscess, phlebitis), superinfections (especially with *Candida* and gram-negative bacteria), neuromuscular irritability (twitching, lethargy, confusion, stupor, hyperreflexia, multifocal myoclonus, localized or generalized seizures, coma). **CV:** Hypotension, circulatory collapse, cardiac arrhythmias, cardiac arrest. **GI:** Vomiting, diarrhea, severe abdominal cramps, nausea, epigastric distress, diarrhea, flatulence, dark discoloration of tongue, sore mouth or tongue. **Urogenital:** Interstitial nephritis, Loeffler's syndrome, vasculitis. **Hematologic:** Hemolytic anemia, thrombocytopenia. **Metabolic:** Hyperkalemia (penicillin G potassium); hypokalemia, alkalosis, hypernatremia, CHF (penicillin G sodium). **Respiratory:** Bronchospasm, asthma. **Skin:** Itchy palms or axilla, pruritus, *urticaria,* flushed skin, *delayed skin rashes* ranging from urticaria to exfoliative dermatitis, Stevens-Johnson syndrome, fixed-drug eruptions, contact dermatitis.

DIAGNOSTIC TEST INTERFERENCE ***Blood grouping and compatibility tests:*** possible interference associated with penicillin doses greater than 20 million units daily. ***Urine glucose:*** massive doses of penicillin may cause false-positive test results with ***Benedict's solution*** and possibly ***Clinitest*** but not with ***glucose oxidase methods*** e.g., ***Clinistix, Diastix, TesTape.*** ***Urine protein:*** massive doses of penicillin can produce false-positive results when turbidity measures are used (e.g., ***acetic acid*** and ***heat, sulfo-salicylic acid***); ***Ames reagent*** reportedly not affected. ***Urinary PSP excretion tests:*** false decrease in urinary excretion of PSP. ***Urinary steroids:*** large IV doses of penicillin may interfere with accurate measurement of ***urinary 17-OHCS*** (***Glenn-Nelson technique*** not affected).

INTERACTIONS Drug: Probenecid decreases renal elimination; penicillin G may decrease efficacy of ORAL CONTRACEPTIVES; **colestipol** decreases penicillin absorption; POTASSIUM-SPARING DIURETICS may cause hyperkalemia with penicillin G potassium. **Food:** Food increases breakdown in stomach.

PHARMACOKINETICS Absorption: 15%–30% of PO dose absorbed; very acid labile. **Peak:** 30–60 min

P

PO; 15–30 min IM. **Distribution:** Widely distributed; good CSF concentrations with inflamed meninges; crosses placenta; distributed in breast milk. **Metabolism:** 16%–30% metabolized. **Elimination:** 60% excreted in urine within 6 h. **Half-Life:** 0.4–0.9 h.

NURSING IMPLICATIONS

Assessment & Drug Effects

- Obtain an exact history of patient's previous exposure and sensitivity to penicillins and cephalosporins and other allergic reactions of any kind prior to treatment with penicillin.
- Hypersensitivity reactions are more likely to occur with parenteral penicillin but may also occur with the oral drug. Skin rash is the most common type allergic reaction and should be reported promptly to physician.
- Lab tests: Perform C&S tests prior to initiation of therapy; treatment may be started before results are known. Evaluate renal, hepatic, and hematologic systems at regular intervals in patients on high-dose therapy. Additionally, check electrolyte balance periodically in patients receiving high parenteral doses.
- Observe all patients closely for at least 30 min following administration of parenteral penicillin. The rapid appearance of a red flare or wheal at the IM or IV injection site is a possible sign of sensitivity. Also suspect an allergic reaction if patient becomes irritable, has nausea and vomiting, breathing difficulty, or sudden fever. Report any of the foregoing to physician immediately.
- Be aware that reactions to penicillin may be rapid in onset or may not appear for days or weeks. Symptoms usually disappear fairly quickly once drug is stopped, but in some patients may persist for 5 d or more and require hospitalization for treatment.
- Allergy to penicillin is unpredictable. It has occurred in patients with a negative history of penicillin allergy and also in patients with no known prior contact with penicillin (sensitization may have occurred from penicillin used commercially in foods and beverages).
- Be alert for neuromuscular irritability in patients receiving parenteral penicillin in excess of 20 million U/d who have renal insufficiency, hyponatremia, or underlying CNS disease, notably myasthenia gravis or epilepsy. Seizure precautions are indicated. Symptoms usually begin with twitching, especially of face and extremities.
- Monitor I&O, particularly in patients receiving high parenteral doses. Report oliguria, hematuria, and changes in I&O ratio. Consult physician regarding optimum fluid intake. Dehydration increases the concentration of drug in kidneys and can cause renal irritation and damage.
- Observe closely for signs of toxicity: Neonates, young infants, the older adult, and patients with impaired kidney function receiving high-dose penicillin therapy. Urinary excretion of penicillin is significantly delayed in these patients.
- Observe patients on high-dose therapy closely for evidence of bleeding, and bleeding time should be monitored. (In high doses, penicillin interferes with platelet aggregation.)

Patient & Family Education

- Understand that hypersensitivity reaction may be delayed. Report skin rashes, itching, fever, malaise, and other signs of a delayed reaction to physician immediately (see ADVERSE EFFECTS).

- Penicillin is to be taken around the clock (i.e., t.i.d. means q8h, q.i.d. means q6h, etc.). Do not miss any doses and continue taking medication until it is all gone, unless otherwise directed by the physician.
- Measure liquid dosage form with specially marked measuring device; household teaspoons vary in size and measure.
- Notify physician if following symptoms appear when taking penicillin for treatment of syphilis (i.e., Jarisch-Herxheimer reaction occurs 8–24 h after treatment): Headache, chills, fever, myalgia, arthralgia, malaise, and worsening of syphilitic skin lesions. Reaction is usually self-limiting. Check with physician if symptoms do not improve within a few days or get worse.
- Report S&S of superinfection (see Appendix F).
- Understand importance of medical follow-up; present evidence suggests that glomerulonephritis, a possible complication of streptococcal infection, may not be prevented by penicillin.
- Do not breast feed while taking this drug without consulting physician.

PENICILLIN G PROCAINE

(pen-i-sill'in)

Crysticillin A.S., Pfizerpen-AS, Procaine Benzylpenicillin, Wycillin

Classifications: ANTIINFECTIVE; BETA-LACTAM ANTIBIOTIC; NATURAL PENICILLIN

Prototype: Penicillin G potassium

Pregnancy Category: B

AVAILABILITY 600,000 units/1 mL, 1,200,000 units/2 mL, 2,400,000 units/4 mL injection

ACTIONS Long-acting form of penicillin G. The procaine salt has low solubility and thus creates a tissue depot from which penicillin is slowly absorbed. Onset of action is slower and produces lower serum concentrations than equivalent doses of penicillin G potassium, but has longer duration of action.

THERAPEUTIC EFFECTS Same actions and antibacterial activity as for penicillin G potassium and is similarly inactivated by penicillinase and gastric acid.

USES Moderately severe infections due to penicillin G-sensitive microorganisms that are susceptible to low but prolonged serum penicillin concentrations. Commonly, uncomplicated *Pneumococcal* pneumonia, 1 day treatment of uncomplicated gonorrheal infections, and all stages of syphilis. May be used concomitantly with penicillin G or probenecid when more rapid action and higher blood levels are indicated.

CONTRAINDICATIONS History of hypersensitivity to any of the penicillins, cephalosporins, or to procaine or any other "caine-type" local anesthetic; neonates; pregnancy (category B), lactation.

CAUTIOUS USE History of or suspected allergy.

ROUTE & DOSAGE

Moderate to Severe Infections

Adult: **IM** 600,000–1,200,000 U once/d

Child: **IM** 300,000 U once/d

Pneumococcal Pneumonia

Adult: **IM** 600,000 U q12h

Uncomplicated Gonorrhea

Adult: **IM** 4,800,000 U divided between 2 different injection sites

P

at one visit preceded by 1 g of probenecid 30 min before injections

Syphilis

Adult: **IM** Primary, secondary, latent: 600,000 U/d for 8 d; late latent, tertiary, neurosyphilis: 600,000 U/d for 10–15 d
Child: **IM** 500,000–1,000,000 U/m^2 once/d

ADMINISTRATION

Intramuscular

- Shake multiple-dose vial thoroughly before withdrawing medication to ensure uniform suspension of drug.
- Use 20-gauge needle to avoid clogging.
- Give IM deep into upper outer quadrant of gluteus muscle; in infants and small children midlateral aspect of thigh is generally preferred. Select IM site carefully. Accidental injection into or near major peripheral nerves and blood vessels can cause neurovascular damage.
- Aspirate carefully before injecting drug to avoid entry into a blood vessel. Inadvertent IV administration reportedly has resulted in pulmonary infarcts and death.
- Inject drug at a slow, but steady rate to prevent needle blockage. Give in two sites if the dose is very large. Rotate injection sites.

ADVERSE EFFECTS (≥1%) **Body as a Whole:** Procaine toxicity [e.g., mental disturbances (anxiety, confusion, depression, combativeness, hallucinations), expressed fear of impending death, weakness, dizziness, headache, tinnitus, unusual tastes, palpitation, changes in pulse rate and BP, seizures]. Also see Penicillin G.

INTERACTIONS Drug: Probenecid decreases renal elimination; may decrease efficacy of ORAL CONTRACEPTIVES.

PHARMACOKINETICS Absorption: Slowly absorbed from IM site. **Peak:** 1–3 h. **Duration:** 15–20 h. **Distribution:** Crosses placenta; distributed into breast milk. **Metabolism:** Hydrolyzed to penicillin in body. **Elimination:** Excreted by kidneys within 24–36 h.

NURSING IMPLICATIONS

Assessment & Drug Effects

- Obtain an exact history of patient's previous exposure and sensitivity to penicillins, cephalosporins, and to procaine, and other allergic reactions of any kind prior to treatment.
- Test patient by injecting 0.1 mL of 1%–2% procaine hydrochloride intradermally if sensitivity is suspected. Appearance of a wheal, flare, or eruption indicates procaine sensitivity.
- Be alert to the possibility of a transient toxic reaction to procaine, particularly when large single doses are administered. The reaction manifested by mental disturbance and other symptoms (see ADVERSE EFFECTS) occurs almost immediately and usually subsides after 15–30 min.

Patient & Family Education

- Report any skin reaction at the site of injection.
- Report onset of rash, itching, fever, chills or other symptoms of an allergic reaction to physician.
- Do not breast feed while taking this drug.

PENICILLIN V

PENICILLIN V POTASSIUM

(pen-i-sill'in)

Apo-Pen-VK ♣, Beepen VK, Betapen-VK, Ledercillin VK, Nadopen-V ♣, Novopen-VK ♣, Penicillin VK, Pen-V, Pen-Vee K, Robicillin VK, V-Cillin K, Veetids

Classifications: ANTIINFECTIVE; BETA-LACTAM ANTIBIOTIC; NATURAL PENICILLIN

Prototype: Penicillin G potassium

Pregnancy Category: B

AVAILABILITY 250 mg, 500 mg tablets; 125 mg/5 mL, 250 mg/5 mL suspension

ACTIONS Acid-stable analog of Penicillin G with which it shares actions; it is bactericidal, and is inactivated by penicillinase.

THERAPEUTIC EFFECTS Less active than penicillin G against gonococci and other gram-negative microorganisms.

USES Mild to moderate infections caused by susceptible *Streptococci, Pneumococci,* and *Staphylococci*. Also Vincent's infection and as prophylaxis in rheumatic fever.

CONTRAINDICATIONS Hypersensitivity to any penicillin or cephalosporin or beta-lactamase inhibitors; pregnancy (category B), lactation.

CAUTIOUS USE History of or suspected allergy (hay fever, asthma, hives, eczema); cystic fibrosis; renal impairment, hepatic impairment; children <12 y, newborns.

ROUTE & DOSAGE

Mild to Moderate Infections

Adult: **PO** 125–500 mg q6h

Child: **PO** *<12 y,* 15–50 mg/kg/d in 3–6 divided doses

Endocarditis Prophylaxis

Adult: **PO** 2 g 30–60 min before procedure, then 500 mg q6h for 8 doses

Child: **PO** *<30 kg,* 1 g 30–60 min before procedure, then 250 mg q6h for 8 doses

ADMINISTRATION

Oral

- Give after a meal rather than on an empty stomach; drug may be better absorbed and result in higher blood levels.
- Do not coadminister with neomycin if both drugs are being used; malabsorption of penicillin V may result.
- Shake well before pouring. Following reconstitution, oral solution is stable for 14 d under refrigeration.

ADVERSE EFFECTS (≥1%) **Body as a Whole:** Nausea, vomiting, *diarrhea,* epigastric distress. *Hypersensitivity reactions* (e.g., flushing, pruritus, urticaria or other skin eruptions, eosinophilia, anaphylaxis; hemolytic anemia, leukopenia, thrombocytopenia, neuropathy, superinfections).

INTERACTIONS Drug: Probenecid decreases renal elimination; may decrease efficacy of ORAL CONTRACEPTIVES; **colestipol** decreases absorption. **Food:** Food increases breakdown in stomach.

PHARMACOKINETICS Absorption: 60%–73% absorbed from GI tract. **Peak:** 30–60 min. **Duration:** 6 h. **Distribution:** Highest levels in kidneys; crosses placenta; distributed into breast milk. **Elimination:** Excreted in urine. **Half-Life:** 30 min.

NURSING IMPLICATIONS

Note: See penicillin G potassium for numerous additional nursing implications.

Assessment & Drug Effects

- Obtain careful history concerning hypersensitivity reactions to penicillins, cephalosporins, and other allergens before therapy begins.
- Lab tests: Perform C&S tests prior to initiation and at regular intervals throughout therapy. Evaluate renal, hepatic, and hematologic systems at regular intervals in patients receiving prolonged therapy.

Patient & Family Education

- Take penicillin V around the clock at specific intervals to maintain a constant blood level.
- Do not miss any doses and continue taking medication until it is all gone unless otherwise directed by the physician.
- Discontinue medication and promptly report to physician the onset of hypersensitivity reactions and superinfections (see Appendix F).
- Use specially marked measuring device to ensure accurate doses of oral liquid preparation.
- Do not breast feed while taking this drug.

P

PENTAMIDINE ISOETHIONATE

(pen-tam'i-deen)

Nebupent, Pentacarinat ✦, Pentam 300

Classifications: ANTIINFECTIVE; ANTIPROTOZOAL

Pregnancy Category: C

AVAILABILITY 300 mg injection; 300 mg aerosol

ACTIONS Aromatic diamide antiprotozoal drug. Action mechanism is unclear, but drug appears to block parasite reproduction by interfering with nucleotide (DNA, RNA), phospholipid, and protein synthesis. Effective against the *Sporozoan* parasite, *Pneumocystis carinii*. Pentamidine also has trypanosomicidal and leishmanicidal activity, but required doses for these conditions are quite toxic.

THERAPEUTIC EFFECTS The parasite, *Pneumocystis carinii,* rarely causes infection in the general population, but if the patient is immunocompromised (e.g., AIDS) it can be fatal.

USE *P. carinii* pneumonia (PCP).

UNLABELED USES African trypanosomiasis and visceral leishmaniasis. (Drug supplied for the latter uses is through the Centers for Disease Control and Prevention, Atlanta, GA.)

CONTRAINDICATIONS Pregnancy (category C) and lactation.

CAUTIOUS USE Hypertension, hypotension; hyperglycemia; hypoglycemia; hypocalcemia; blood dyscrasias; liver or kidney dysfunction; diabetes mellitus.

ROUTE & DOSAGE

Treatment of *Pneumocystis carinii* Pneumonia

Adult/Child: **IM/IV** 4 mg/kg once/d for 14–21 d; infuse IV over 60 min

Prophylaxis of *Pneumocystis carinii* Pneumonia

Adult: **Inhaled** 300 mg per nebulizer q4wk

ADMINISTRATION

Inhaled

- Reconstitute contents of one vial in 6 mL sterile water (not saline) and administer using nebulizer.
- Do not mix with any other drug.

Intramuscular

- Dissolve contents of 1 vial (300 mg) in 3 mL sterile water for injection.

- Give deep IM into a large muscle.
- The IM injection is painful and frequently causes local reactions (pain, indurations, swelling). Select alternate sites for daily doses and institute local treatment if indicated.

Intravenous

PREPARE: **IV Infusion:** Dissolve contents of 1 vial in 3–5 mL sterile water for injection or D5W. Further dilute in 50–250 mL of D5W.

ADMINISTER: **IV Infusion:** Give over 60 min.

INCOMPATIBILITIES **Y-site: Aldesleukin,** CEPHALOSPORINS, **foscarnet, fluconazole.**

- Note: IV solutions are stable at room temperature for up to 24 h. Protect solution from light.

ADVERSE EFFECTS (≥1%) **CNS:** Confusion, hallucinations, neuralgia, dizziness, sweating. **CV:** Sudden, severe hypotension, cardiac arrhythmias, ventricular tachycardia, phlebitis. **GI:** Anorexia, nausea, vomiting, pancreatitis, unpleasant taste. **Urogenital:** Acute kidney failure. **Hematologic:** Leukopenia, thrombocytopenia, anemia. **Metabolic:** Hypoglycemia, hypocalcemia, *hyperkalemia*. **Respiratory:** *Cough, bronchospasm,* laryngitis, shortness of breath, chest pain, pneumothorax. **Skin:** Stevens-Johnson syndrome, facial flush (with IV injection), *local reactions at injection site.*

INTERACTIONS Drug: AMINOGLYCOSIDES, **amphotericin B, cidofovir, cisplatin, ganciclovir, cyclosporine, vancomycin,** other nephrotoxic drugs increase risk of nephrotoxicity.

PHARMACOKINETICS Absorption: Readily absorbed after IM injection. **Distribution:** Leaves bloodstream rapidly to bind extensively to body tissues. **Elimination:** 50%–66% excreted in urine within 6 h; small amounts found in urine for as long as 6–8 wk. **Half-Life:** 6.5–13.2 h.

NURSING IMPLICATIONS

Assessment & Drug Effects

- Monitor BP closely. Sudden severe hypotension may develop after a single dose. Place patient in supine position while receiving the drug. Monitor BP and HR continuously during the infusion, every half hour for 2 h thereafter, and then every 4 h until BP stabilizes.
- Lab tests: Monitor periodically serum electrolytes, renal function, CBC with differential, platelet count, and blood glucose.
- Measure and record I&O ratio and pattern and check patient's pulse (to detect arrhythmia) at least twice daily.
- Be alert and report promptly S&S of impending kidney dysfunction (e.g., changed I&O ratio, oliguria, edema). Dosage adjustment is indicated in renal failure.
- Characteristics of pneumonia in the immunocompromised patient include constant fever, scanty (if any) sputum, dyspnea, tachypnea, and cyanosis.
- Monitor temperature changes and institute measures to lower the temperature as indicated. Fever is a constant symptom in *P. carinii* pneumonia, but may be rapidly elevated (as high as 40° C [104° F]) shortly after drug infusion.

Patient & Family Education

- Report promptly to physician increasing respiratory difficulty.
- Monitor blood glucose for loss of glycemic control if diabetic.
- Report any unusual bruising or bleeding. Avoid using aspirin or other NSAIDs.

- Increase fluid intake (if not contraindicated) to 2–3 quarts (liters) per day.
- Do not breast feed while taking this drug without consulting physician.

PENTAZOCINE HYDROCHLORIDE

(pen-taz'oh-seen)

Talwin, Talwin NX

Classifications: CENTRAL NERVOUS SYSTEM AGENT; NARCOTIC (OPIATE) AGONIST-ANTAGONIST; ANALGESIC

Prototype: Pentazocine

Pregnancy Category: C

Controlled Substance: Schedule IV

AVAILABILITY 30 mg/mL injection

ACTIONS Synthetic analgesic with analgesic potency approximately one third that of morphine and somewhat greater than codeine. In general, adverse reactions are qualitatively similar to those of morphine. Unlike morphine, large doses may increase BP and heart rate.

THERAPEUTIC EFFECTS Effective for moderate to severe pain relief. Acts as weak narcotic antagonist and has sedative properties.

USES Relief of moderate to severe pain; also used for preoperative analgesia or sedation, and as supplement to surgical anesthesia.

CONTRAINDICATIONS Head injury, increased intracranial pressure; emotionally unstable patients, or history of drug abuse. Safety during pregnancy (other than labor) (category C), lactation, or in children <12 y is not established.

CAUTIOUS USE Impaired kidney or liver function; respiratory depression; biliary surgery; patients with MI who have nausea and vomiting.

ROUTE & DOSAGE

Moderate to Severe Pain (Excluding Patients in Labor)

Adult: **PO** 50–100 mg q3–4h (max: 600 mg/d) **IM/IV/SC** 30 mg q3–4h (max: 360 mg/d)
Geriatric: **PO** 50 mg q4h. **IM** 30 mg q4h

Women in Labor

Adult: **IM** 20–30 mg; 20 mg may be repeated 1 or 2 times at 2–3 h intervals

ADMINISTRATION

Subcutaneous/Intramuscular

- IM is preferred to SC route when frequent injections over an extended period are required.
- Observe injection sites daily for signs of irritation or inflammation.

Intravenous

PREPARE: **Direct:** Give undiluted or diluted with 1 mL sterile water for injection for each 5 mg.
ADMINISTER: **Direct:** Give slowly at a rate of 5 mg over 60 seconds.
INCOMPATIBILITIES **Solution/additive: Aminophylline,** BARBITURATES, **sodium bicarbonate, glycopyrrolate, heparin, nafcillin. Y-site: Glycopyrrolate, heparin, nafcillin.**

ADVERSE EFFECTS (≥1%) **Body as a Whole:** Flushing, allergic reactions, shock. **CNS:** *Drowsiness,* sweating, *dizziness, light-headedness, euphoria,* psychotomimetic effects, confusion, anxiety, hallucinations, disturbed dreams, bizarre thoughts, euphoria and other mood alterations. **CV:** Hypertension, palpitation, tachycardia. **GI:** *Nausea, vomiting,* constipation, dry mouth, alterations of taste. **Urogenital:** Urinary retention. **Respiratory:** Respiratory depression. **Skin:** Injection-site reactions (induration, nodule formation, sloughing, sclerosis, cutaneous depression), rash, pruritus. **Special Senses:** Visual disturbances.

INTERACTIONS Drug: Alcohol and other CNS DEPRESSANTS add to CNS depression; NARCOTIC ANALGESICS may precipitate narcotic withdrawal syndrome.

PHARMACOKINETICS Absorption: Readily absorbed from GI tract; 20% reaches systemic circulation (first pass metabolism). **Onset:** 15–30 min PO, IM, SC; 2–3 min IV. **Peak:** 1–3 h PO, IM; 15 min IV. **Duration:** 3 h PO, IM; 1 h IV. **Distribution:** Crosses placenta. **Metabolism:** Extensively metabolized in liver. **Elimination:** Excreted primarily in urine; small amount in feces. **Half-Life:** 2–3 h.

NURSING IMPLICATIONS

Assessment & Drug Effects

- Monitor therapeutic effect. Tolerance to analgesic effect sometimes occurs. Psychologic and physical dependence have been reported in patients with history of drug abuse, but rarely in patients without such history. Addiction liability matches that of codeine.
- Be aware that pentazocine may produce acute withdrawal symptoms in some patients who have been receiving opioids on a regular basis.

Patient & Family Education

- Avoid driving and other potentially hazardous activities until response to drug is known.
- Do not discontinue drug abruptly following extended use; may result in chills, abdominal and muscle cramps, yawning, runny nose, tearing, itching, restlessness, anxiety, drug-seeking behavior.
- Do not breast feed while taking this drug without consulting physician.

PENTOBARBITAL

(pen-toe-bar'bi-tal)
Nembutal

PENTOBARBITAL SODIUM

Nembutal Sodium, Novopentobarb ♣

Classifications: CENTRAL NERVOUS SYSTEM AGENT; ANXIOLYTIC; SEDATIVE-HYPNOTIC; BARBITURATE
Prototype: Secobarbital
Pregnancy Category: D
Controlled Substance: Schedule II

AVAILABILITY 50 mg, 100 mg capsules; 20 mg/5 mL liquid; 30 mg, 60 mg, 120 mg, 200 mg suppositories; 50 mg/mL injection

ACTIONS Short-acting barbiturate. Potent respiratory depressant. Initially, barbiturates suppress REM sleep, but with chronic therapy REM sleep returns to normal. Has no analgesic properties, and small doses may increase reaction to painful stimuli.

THERAPEUTIC EFFECTS Effective as a sedative and hypnotic. CNS depression may range from mild sedation to coma, depending on dosage, route of administration, degree of nervous system excitability, and drug tolerance.

USES Sedative or hypnotic for preanesthetic medication, induction of general anesthesia, adjunct in manipulative or diagnostic procedures, and emergency control of acute convulsions.

CONTRAINDICATIONS Pregnancy (category D) or lactation. History of sensitivity to barbiturates; parturition, fetal immaturity, uncontrolled pain. Use of sterile injection containing polyethylene glycol vehicle in patients with renal insufficiency. **CAUTIOUS USE** Pregnant women with toxemia or history of bleeding.

ROUTE & DOSAGE

Sedative
Adult: **PO** 20–30 mg b.i.d. to q.i.d.
Child: **PO** 2–6 mg/kg/d in 3 divided doses (max: 100 mg/d)

Preoperative Sedation
Adult: **PO** 150–200 mg in 2 divided doses **IM** 150–200 mg in 2 divided doses **IV** 100 mg; may increase to 500 mg if necessary

Hypnotic
Adult: **PO** 120–200 mg. **IM** 150–200 mg
Child: **PO** 30–120 mg. **IM** 2–6 mg/kg (max: 100 mg)

P

ADMINISTRATION

Note: Do not give within 14 d of starting/stopping a MAO inhibitor.

Intramuscular

- Do not use parenteral solutions that appear cloudy or in which a precipitate has formed.
- Make IM injections deep into large muscle mass, preferably upper outer quadrant of buttock. Aspirate needle carefully before injecting it to prevent inadvertent entry into blood vessel. Inject no more than 5 mL (250 mg) in any one site because of possible tissue irritation.

Intravenous

- Use IV route ONLY when other routes are not feasible.

PREPARE: **Direct:** Give undiluted or diluted (preferred) with sterile water, D5W, NS, or other compatible IV solutions.

ADMINISTER: **Direct:** Give slowly. Do not exceed rate of 50 mg/min.

INCOMPATIBILITIES **Solution/additive: Chlorpheniramine, codeine, ephedrine, hydrocortisone, hydroxyzine, inulin, levorphanol, methadone, norepinephrine,** TETRACYCLINES, **penicillin G, pentazocine, phenytoin, promazine, promethazine, sodium bicarbonate, streptomycin, succinylcholine, triflubromazine, vancomycin, cimetidine, benzquinamide, butorphanol, chlorpromazine, dimenhydrinate, diphenhydramine, droperidol, fentanyl, glycopyrrolate, meperidine, midazolam, morphine, nalbuphine, perphenazine, prochlorperazine, ranitidine. Y-site: Cimetidine, butorphanol, glycopyrrolate, midazolam, nalbuphine, perphenazine, ranitidine.**

- Take extreme care to avoid extravasation. Necrosis may result because parenteral solution is highly alkaline.
- Do not use cloudy or precipitated solution.

ADVERSE EFFECTS (≥1%) **Body as a Whole:** Drowsiness, lethargy, hangover, paradoxical excitement in the older adult patient. **CV:** Hypotension with rapid IV. **Respiratory:** With rapid IV (respiratory depression, laryngospasm, bronchospasm, apnea).

INTERACTIONS Drug: Phenmetrazine antagonizes effects of pentobarbital; CNS DEPRESSANTS, **alcohol,** SEDATIVES add to CNS depression; MAO INHIBITORS cause excessive CNS depression; **methoxyflurane** creates risk of nephrotoxicity.

Herbal: Kava-kava, valerian may potentiate sedation.

PHARMACOKINETICS Onset: 15–30 min PO; 10–15 min IM; 1 min IV. **Duration:** 1–4 h PO; 15 min IV. **Distribution:** Crosses placenta. **Metabolism:** Metabolized primarily in liver. **Elimination:** Excreted in urine. **Half-Life:** 4–50 h.

NURSING IMPLICATIONS

Assessment & Drug Effects

- Monitor BP, pulse, and respiration q3–5min during IV administration. Observe patient closely; maintain airway. Have equipment for artificial respiration immediately available.
- Observe patient closely for adverse effects for at least 30 min after IM administration of hypnotic dose.

Patient & Family Education

- Exercise caution when driving or operating machinery for the remainder of day after taking drug.
- Avoid alcohol and other CNS depressants for 24 h after receiving this drug.

PENTOXIFYLLINE

(pen-tox-i'fi-leen)

Trental

Classifications: BLOOD FORMERS, COAGULATORS, AND ANTICOAGULANTS; HEMORRHEOLOGIC AGENT; ANTIPLATELET AGENT

Pregnancy Category: C

AVAILABILITY 400 mg tablets; 400 mg sustained release tablets

ACTIONS Useful in restoration of blood flow through nutritive capillary microcirculation that has been compromised by structural and flow dynamic changes in cerebral and peripheral vascular disorders. Action mechanism unclear, but drug action interrupts the vicious cycle of tissue hypoxia, sludging and stasis of capillary blood flow, microthrombotic activity, reduced oxygen delivery to ischemic cells.

THERAPEUTIC EFFECTS Decreased blood viscosity and improved blood flow, with consequent reduction of tissue hypoxia. Resultant increased blood flow to the extremities reduces pain and paresthesia of intermittent claudication; further, psychopathologic conditions associated with cerebral hypoxia are improved.

USES Intermittent claudication associated with occlusive peripheral vascular disease; diabetic angiopathies.

UNLABELED USES To improve psychopathologic symptoms in patient with cerebrovascular insufficiency and to reduce incidence of stroke in the patient with recurrent TIAs.

CONTRAINDICATIONS Intolerance to pentoxifylline or to methylxanthines (caffeine and theophylline). Safety in pregnancy (category C), lactation, or in children <18 y is not established.

CAUTIOUS USE Angina, hypotension, arrhythmias, cerebrovascular disease.

ROUTE & DOSAGE

Intermittent Claudication

Adult: **PO** 400 mg t.i.d. with meals

ADMINISTRATION

Oral

- Give on an empty stomach or with food; be consistent with time of day and relationship to food in establishing the daily regimen.
- Store tablets at 15°–30° C (59°–86° F).

ADVERSE EFFECTS (≥1%) **Body as a Whole:** Fever, flushing, convulsions, somnolence, loss of consciousness. **CNS:** Agitation, nervousness, *dizziness,* drowsiness, headache, insomnia, tremor, confusion. **CV:** Angina, chest pain, dyspnea, arrhythmias, palpitations, hypotension, edema, flushing. **Eye:** Blurred vision, conjunctivitis, scotomas. **GI:** Abdominal discomfort, belching, flatus, bloating, diarrhea, *dyspepsia, nausea, vomiting.* **Skin:** Brittle fingernails, pruritus, rash, urticaria. **Other:** Earache, unpleasant taste, excessive salivation, leukopenia, malaise, sore throat, swollen neck glands, weight change.

INTERACTIONS Drug: Ciprofloxacin, cimetidine may increase levels and toxicity

PHARMACOKINETICS Absorption: Readily absorbed from GI tract; 10%–50% reaches systemic circulation (first pass metabolism). **Peak:** 2–4 h. **Distribution:** Distributed into breast milk. **Metabolism:** Metabolized in liver and erythrocytes. **Elimination:** Excreted primarily in urine. **Half-Life:** 0.4–0.8 h.

P

NURSING IMPLICATIONS

Assessment & Drug Effects

- Monitor therapeutic effectiveness which is indicated by relief from pain and cramping in calf muscles, buttocks, thighs, and feet during exercise and improves walking performance (time and duration).
- Monitor BP if patient is also on antihypertensive treatment. Drug may slightly decrease an already stabilized BP, necessitating a reduced dose of the hypotensive drug.

Patient & Family Education

- Consult physician to determine CV status and capacity before reestablishing walking as exercise.
- Pay particular attention to care of the feet because of arterial insufficiency (diminished perfusion to feet).
- Be aware that bleeding and prolonged PT/INR associated with this treatment have been reported. Report promptly unexplained bleeding, easy bruising, nose bleed, pinpoint rash to physician.
- Avoid driving or working with hazardous machinery until drug response has stabilized because of potential for tiredness, blurred vision, dizziness.
- Do not breast feed while taking this drug without consulting physician.

PERGOLIDE

(per'go-lide)
Permax
Classifications: AUTONOMIC NERVOUS SYSTEM AGENT; ANTICHOLINERGIC (PARASYMPATHOLYTIC); ANTIPARKINSON AGENT
Prototype: Levodopa
Pregnancy Category: B

AVAILABILITY 0.05 mg, 0.25 mg, 1 mg tablets

ACTIONS Potent dopamine receptor agonist at both D_1- and D_2-dopamine receptor sites. Parkinsonism involves an excess of acetylcholine and a deficiency of dopamine neurotransmitters in the basal ganglia. The reduced tonic stimulation of dopaminergic D_2 receptors located on intrastriatal cholinergic neurons is most likely the cause of parkinsonian symptoms.

THERAPEUTIC EFFECTS Thought that stimulation of the D_2-dopamine receptor alleviates the majority of parkinsonian symptoms.

USES Adjunct to levodopa/carbidopa for the treatment of Parkinson's disease.
UNLABELED USES Acromegaly, hyperprolactinemia.

CONTRAINDICATIONS Hypersensitivity to pergolide or other ergot derivatives; history of hallucinations, history of hypotension; lactation.
CAUTIOUS USE Cardiac dysrhythmias, pregnancy (category B); pericarditis, pericardial effusion, valvular heart disease; retroperitoneal fibrosis. Safety and efficacy in children are not established.

ROUTE & DOSAGE

Parkinson's Disease

Adult: **PO** Initiate with 0.05 mg daily for 2 d, then increase by 0.1 or 0.15 mg/d every 3 d for the next 12 d, then dose may be increased by 0.25 mg every third day until the desired therapeutic response is achieved; give in divided doses t.i.d. (max: 5 mg/d)

Acromegaly

Adult: **PO** 0.1–1.5 mg once/d

Hyperprolactinemia

Adult: **PO** 0.025–0.6 mg once/d

ADMINISTRATION

Oral

- Note that dosage increases should occur no more than every 3 d with Parkinson's disease.

ADVERSE EFFECTS (≥1%) **CNS:** *Confusion, anxiety, light-headedness, headache,* transient somnolence (may fall asleep without warning), hallucinations, nightmares. **CV:** Ventricular arrhythmias, PVCs, edema, *orthostatic hypotension.* **GI:** *Nausea, vomiting,* constipation. **Body as a Whole:** Rhinitis, withdrawal symptoms (hallucinations, confusion, paranoid ideations, worsening of parkinsonian symptoms). **Skin:** Rash.

DIAGNOSTIC TEST INTERFERENCE Suppresses ***prolactin*** levels.

INTERACTIONS Drug: Addition of pergolide to **levodopa** therapy has produced an increased incidence of dyskinesias in patients with Parkinson's disease; **haloperidol,** PHENOTHIAZINES can antagonize therapeutic effects.

PHARMACOKINETICS Absorption: Readily absorbed from GI tract; extensive first-pass metabolism. **Onset:** Prolactin levels decrease within 15–30 min. **Peak:** Prolactin nadir in 15 h. **Duration:** 22–24 h. **Distribution:** 90% protein bound; crosses placenta; distributed into breast milk. **Metabolism:** Metabolized in liver. **Elimination:** 55% excreted in urine within 48 h; 40%–50% excreted in feces. **Half-Life:** 27 h.

NURSING IMPLICATIONS

Assessment & Drug Effects

- Monitor carefully for orthostatic hypotension and syncope when initiating therapy.
- Assess neurologic status; concurrent levodopa and pergolide may increase incidence of dyskinesias. If this occurs, levodopa may need to be reduced.
- Monitor patients with cardiac arrhythmias carefully, as drug may induce certain arrhythmias in persons at risk.

Patient & Family Education

- Note: May fall asleep without warning.
- Learn ways to reduce risk of orthostatic hypertension. Make position changes slowly and in stages.

P

- Understand all potential adverse effects including hallucinations.
- Report worsening neurologic status to physician.
- Do not discontinue drug abruptly.
- Do not breast feed while taking this drug.

PERINDOPRIL ERBUMINE

(per-in′do-pril)

Aceon

Classifications: CARDIOVASCULAR AGENT; ANGIOTENSIN-CONVERTING ENZYME INHIBITOR; ANTIHYPERTENSIVE

Prototype: Captopril

Pregnancy Category: C (first trimester); D (second and third trimesters)

AVAILABILITY 2 mg, 4 mg, 8 mg tablets

ACTIONS Angiotensin-converting enzyme (ACE) inhibitor. ACE catalyzes the conversion of angiotensin I to angiotensin II, a vasoconstrictor substance. Therefore, angiotensin II levels are decreased by perindopril, thus decreasing vasopressor activity and aldosterone secretion.

THERAPEUTIC EFFECTS Lowers BP by inhibition of ACE. Reduced aldosterone is associated with potassium-sparing effect. In addition, decreases systemic vascular resistance (afterload) and pulmonary capillary wedge pressure (PCWP), a measure of preload, and improves cardiac output as well as activity tolerance.

USES Hypertension, CHF

CONTRAINDICATIONS Hypersensitivity to perindopril or any other ACE inhibitor; history of angioedema induced by an ACE inhibitor, pregnancy [category C (first trimester), category D (second and third trimester)]; patients with hypertrophic cardiomyopathy, renal artery stenosis.

CAUTIOUS USE Renal insufficiency, volume-depleted patients, severe liver dysfunction; autoimmune diseases, immunosuppressant drug therapy; hyperkalemia or potassium-sparing diuretics; older adult; surgery; neutropenia; lactation; febrile illness.

ROUTE & DOSAGE

Hypertension, CHF

Adult: **PO** 4 mg once daily, may be increased to 8 mg daily in 1 or 2 divided doses (max:16 mg/d)

Renal Impairment

Cl_{cr} May need to use lower doses in patients with mild to moderate impairment

ADMINISTRATION

Oral

- Manufacturer recommends an initial dose of 2–4 mg in 1 or 2 divided doses if concurrently ordered diuretic cannot be discontinued 2–3 days before beginning perinodopril. Consult physician.
- Give on an empty stomach 1 h before meals.
- Dosage adjustments are generally made at intervals of at least 1 wk.
- Store at 20°–25° C (68°–77° F) and protect from moisture.

ADVERSE EFFECTS (≥1%) **CNS:** Dizziness, light-headedness (in the absence of postural hypotension), headache, mood and sleep disorders, fatigue. **CV:** Palpitations. **Endocrine:** Hyperkalemia. **GI:** Nausea, vomiting, epigastric pain, diarrhea, taste disturbances, dyspepsia. **Urogenital:** Proteinuria, impotence, sexual dysfunction. **Special Senses:** Dry eyes, blurred vision. **Body as a Whole:** *Cough,* angioedema, pruritus, muscle cramps, sinusitis, hypertonia, fever. **Skin:** Rash.

INTERACTIONS Drug: POTASSIUM-SPARING DIURETICS **(amiloride, spironolactone, triamterene)** may increase the risk of hyperkalemia. POTASSIUM SUPPLEMENTS increase the risk of hyperkalemia. **Food:** Food can decrease drug absorption 35%.

PHARMACOKINETICS Absorption: Readily absorbed from GI tract, absorption significantly decreased when taken with food. **Peak:** Perindopril: 1 h; perindoprilat: 3–7 h. **Duration:** 24 h. **Metabolism:** Hydrolyzed in the liver to its active form, perindoprilat. **Elimination:** Primarily excreted in urine. **Half-Life: Perindopril:** 0.8–1 h, **perindoprilat:** 30–120 h.

NURSING IMPLICATIONS

Assessment & Drug Effects

- Monitor BR and HR carefully following initial dose for several hours until stable, especially in patients using concurrent diuretics, on salt restriction, or volume depleted.
- Place patient immediately in a supine position if excess hypotension develops.
- Lab tests: Monitor serum potassium, serum sodium, BUN and creatinine, ALT, blood glucose, lipid profile, and WBC with differential periodically.
- Monitor kidney function in patients with CHF closely.
- Monitor serum lithium levels and assess for S&S of lithium toxicity frequently when used concurrently; increased caution is needed when diuretic therapy is also used.

Patient & Family Education

- Discontinue drug and immediately report S&S of angioedema (i.e., swelling) of face or extremities to physician. Seek emergency help for swelling of the tongue or any other signs of potential airway obstruction.
- Be aware that light-headedness can occur, especially during early therapy; excess fluid loss of any kind (e.g., vomiting, diarrhea) will increase risk of hypotension and syncope.
- Avoid using potassium supplements unless specifically directed to do so by physician.
- Report S&S of infection (e.g., sore throat, fever) promptly to physician.
- Do not breast feed while taking this drug without consulting physician.

PERMETHRIN Pr

(per-meth'rin)

Nix, Elimite, Acticin

Classifications: SKIN AND MUCOUS MEMBRANE AGENT; PEDICULICIDE

Pregnancy Category: B

AVAILABILITY 5% cream; 1% liquid

ACTIONS Pediculicidal and ovicidal activity against *Pediculus humanus* var. *capitis* (head louse). Inhibits sodium ion influx through nerve cell membrane channels, resulting in delayed repolarization of the action potential and paralysis of the pest.

THERAPEUTIC EFFECTS It prevents burrowing into host's skin. Since lice are completely dependent on blood for survival, they die within 24–48 h. Also active against ticks, mites, and fleas.

USES *Pediculosis capitis.*

CONTRAINDICATIONS Hypersensitivity to pyrethrins, chrysanthemums, sulfites, or other preservatives or dyes; acute inflammation of the scalp; lactation.

CAUTIOUS USE Children <2 y (liquid); pregnancy (category B).

ROUTE & DOSAGE

Head Lice

Adult/Child: **Topical** >2 y, Apply sufficient volume to clean wet hair to saturate the hair and scalp; leave on 10 min, then rinse hair thoroughly

ADMINISTRATION

Topical

- Saturate scalp as well as hair with the lotion; this is not a shampoo.
- Hair should be washed with regular shampoo before treatment with permethrin, thoroughly rinsed and dried.
- Shake lotion well before application. One container holds enough for at least one treatment, but two containers may be necessary if patient has long hair.
- Rinse hair and scalp thoroughly and dry with a clean towel following 10 min exposure to the medication. Head lice are usually eliminated with one treatment.
- Store drug away from heat at 15°–25° C (59°–77° F) and direct light. Avoid freezing.

ADVERSE EFFECTS (≥1%) **Skin:** *pruritus, transient tingling,* burning, stinging, numbness; erythema, edema, rash.

INTERACTIONS Drug: No clinically significant interactions established.

PHARMACOKINETICS Absorption: <2% of amount applied is absorbed through intact skin. **Metabolism:** Rapidly hydrolyzed to inactive metabolites. **Elimination:** Excreted primarily in urine.

NURSING IMPLICATIONS

Assessment & Drug Effects

- Do not attempt therapy if patient is known to be sensitive to any pyrethrin or pyrethroid. Stop treatment if a reaction occurs.

Patient & Family Education

- When hair is dry, comb with a fine-tooth comb (furnished with medication) to remove dead lice and remaining nits or nit shells.
- Be aware that drug remains on hair shaft up to 14 d; therefore, recurrence of infestation rarely occurs (<1%).
- Inspect hair shafts daily for at least 1 wk to determine drug effectiveness. Contact physician if live lice are observed after 7 d. A renewed prescription for a second treatment may be ordered. Signs of inadequate treatment: Itching, redness of skin, skin abrasion, infected scalp areas.
- Resume regular shampooing after treatment; residual deposit of drug on hair is not reduced.
- Be aware that drug is usually irritating to the eyes and mucosa. Flush well with water if medicine accidentally gets into eyes.

PERPHENAZINE

(per-fen'a-zeen)

Phenazine, Trilafon

Classifications: CENTRAL NERVOUS SYSTEM AGENT; PSYCHOTHERAPEUTIC; PHENOTHIAZINE ANTIPSYCHOTIC; ANTIEMETIC

Prototype: Chlorpromazine

Pregnancy Category: C

AVAILABILITY 2 mg, 4 mg, 6 mg, 8 mg, 16 mg, tablets; 16 mg/5 mL liquid; 5 mg/mL injection

ACTIONS Affects all parts of CNS similar to chlorpromazine, particularly the hypothalamus. Antipsychotic effect: Antagonizes the neurotransmitter dopamine by action on dopamine receptors in the brain. Antiemetic action results from direct blockade of dopamine in the chemoreceptor trigger zone (CTZ) in the medulla.

THERAPEUTIC EFFECTS Has antipychotic and antiemetic properties. Produces less sedation and hypotension, greater antiemetic effects, higher incidence of extrapyramidal effects, and lower levels of anticholinergic adverse effects than chlorpromazine.

USES Psychotic disorders, symptomatic control of severe nausea and vomiting, acute conditions such as violent retching during surgery, and intractable hiccups.

CONTRAINDICATIONS Hypersensitivity to perphenazine and other phenothiazines; preexisting liver damage; suspected or established subcortical brain damage, comatose states; bone marrow depression. Safety during pregnancy (category C), lactation, or in children <12 y is not established.

CAUTIOUS USE Previously diagnosed breast cancer; liver or kidney dysfunction; cardiovascular disorders; alcohol withdrawal, epilepsy, psychic depression, patients with suicidal tendency; glaucoma; history of intestinal or GU obstruction; geriatric or debilitated patients; patients who will be exposed to extremes of heat or cold, or to phosphorous insecticides.

ROUTE & DOSAGE

Psychotic Disorders

Adult: **PO** 4–16 mg b.i.d. to q.i.d.; 8–32 mg sustained release b.i.d. (max: 64 mg/d) **IM** 5 mg q6h (max: 15–30 mg/d) **IV** Dilute to 0.5 mg/mL in NS, administer at not more than 1 mg q1–2min or 5 mg by slow infusion
Child: **PO** 4 mg b.i.d. to q.i.d.; 8 mg sustained release b.i.d. (max:16 mg/d) **IM/IV** Same as adult

Dementia Behavior

Geriatric: **PO** 2–4 mg 1–2 times/d, may increase q4–7d (max: 32 mg/d)

Nausea

Adult: **PO** 8–16 mg b.i.d. to q.i.d. **IM** 5 mg q6h (max:15 mg/d)

ADMINISTRATION

Oral

- Ensure that sustained release form is not chewed or crushed. Must be swallowed whole.
- Dilute oral concentrate before administration: Dilute each 5 mL (16 mg) to 60 mL water, milk, saline solution, 7-Up, or other compatible carbonated beverages. Do not use liquids that cause color changes or precipitate.

Intramuscular

- Give deep IM into a large muscle with patient in recumbent position. Advise patient to continue lying down for at least 1 h after injection. Injection may be painful. Observe daily for signs of inflammation.

Intravenous

PREPARE: **Direct:** Dilute each 5 mg in 9 mL NS.
ADMINISTER: **Direct:** Give at a rate of 0.5 mg (1 mL) over 60 seconds.
INCOMPATIBILITIES **Solution/additive: Midazolam, pentobarbital, thiethylperazine. Y-site: Cefoperazone, midazolam, pentobarbital.**

- Do not use precipitated or darkened parenteral solution; however,

P

slight yellowing does not alter potency or therapeutic effects.
- Protect solutions from light.

ADVERSE EFFECTS (≥1%) **CNS:** *Extrapyramidal effects (dystonic reactions, akathisia, parkinsonian syndrome, tardive dyskinesia), sedation,* convulsions. **CV:** *Orthostatic hypotension,* tachycardia, bradycardia. **Special Senses:** Mydriasis, blurred vision, corneal and lenticular deposits. **GI:** Constipation, *dry mouth,* increased appetite, adynamic ileus, Abnormal liver function tests, cholestatic jaundice. **Urogenital:** *Urinary retention,* gynecomastia, menstrual irregularities, inhibited ejaculation. **Hematologic:** Agranulocytosis, thrombocytopenic purpura, aplastic or hemolytic anemia. **Body as a Whole:** Photosensitivity, itching, erythema, urticaria, angioneurotic edema, drug fever, anaphylactoid reaction, pain at injection site, sterile abscess. Nasal congestion, decreased sweating. **Metabolic:** Hyperprolactinemia, galactorrhea, weight gain.

P

DIAGNOSTIC TEST INTERFERENCE Perphenazine may cause falsely abnormal ***thyroid function*** tests because of elevations of ***thyroid globulin.***

INTERACTIONS Drug: Alcohol and other CNS DEPRESSANTS enhance CNS depression; ANTACIDS, ANTIDIARRHEALS may decrease absorption of phenothiazines; ANTICHOLINERGIC AGENTS add to anticholinergic effects including fecal impaction and paralytic ileus; BARBITURATES, ANESTHETICS increase hypotension and excitation. **Herbal: Kava-kava** increased risk and severity of dystonic reactions.

PHARMACOKINETICS Absorption: Poorly absorbed from GI tract; 20% reaches systemic circulation. **Onset:** 10 min IM. **Peak:** 1–2 h IM; 4–8 h PO. **Duration:** 6–12 h. **Distribution:** Crosses placenta. **Metabolism:** Metabolized in liver with some metabolism in GI tract. **Elimination:** Excreted in urine and feces. **Half-Life:** 9.5 h.

NURSING IMPLICATIONS

Assessment & Drug Effects

- Establish baseline BP before initiation of drug therapy and check it at regular intervals, especially during early therapy.
- Monitor BP and pulse continuously during IV administration. Keep patient supine until assured that vital signs are stable. Observe older adult patients carefully for hypotension and extrapyramidal reactions.
- Report restlessness, weakness of extremities, dystonic reactions (spasms of neck and shoulder muscles, rigidity of back, difficulty swallowing or talking); motor restlessness (akathisia: inability to be still); and parkinsonian syndrome (tremors, shuffling gait, drooling, slow speech). A high incidence of extrapyramidal effects accompanies use of perphenazine, particularly with high doses and parenteral administration.
- Withhold medication and report IMMEDIATELY to physician S&S of irreversible tardive dyskinesia (i.e., fine, wormlike movements or rapid protrusions of the tongue, chewing motions, lip smacking). Patients on long-term therapy are high risk. Teach patients and responsible family members about symptoms because early reporting is essential.
- Lab tests: Obtain differential blood cell counts and liver; and kidney function studies.

- ECG and ophthalmologic examination are recommended prior to initiation and periodically during therapy.
- Suspect hypersensitivity, withhold drug, and report to physician if jaundice appears between weeks 2 and 4.
- Monitor I&O ratio and bowel elimination pattern.
- Be alert to potential for altered tolerance to environmental temperature changes. Be cautious with external heat devices. Conditioned avoidance behavior may be depressed, and a severe burn could result.

Patient & Family Education

- Make all position changes slowly and in stages, particularly from recumbent to upright posture, and to lie down or sit down if light-headedness or dizziness occurs.
- Do not drive or engage in potentially hazardous activities until response to drug is known. Drug may produce hypotension (dizziness, light-headedness), and sedation especially during early therapy.
- Discontinue drug and report to physician immediately if jaundice appears between weeks 2 and 4.
- Avoid long exposure to sunlight and to sunlamps. Photosensitivity results in skin color changes from brown to blue-gray.
- Adhere to dosage regimen strictly. Contact physician before changing it for any reason.
- Discontinue gradually over a period of several weeks following prolonged therapy.
- Avoid OTC drugs unless physician prescribes them.
- Be aware that perphenazine may discolor urine reddish brown.
- Do not breast feed while taking this drug without consulting physician.

PHENAZOPYRIDINE HYDROCHLORIDE

(fen-az-oh-peer′i-deen)

Azo-Standard, Baridium, Geridium, Phenazo ♣, Phenazodine, Pyridiate, Pyridium, Pyronium ♣, Urodine, Urogesic

Classification: URINARY TRACT ANALGESIC

Pregnancy Category: B

AVAILABILITY 95 mg, 97.2 mg, 100 mg, 150 mg, 200 mg tablets

ACTIONS Azo dye. Precise mechanism of action not known.
THERAPEUTIC EFFECTS Local anesthetic action on urinary tract mucosa which imparts little or no antibacterial activity.

USES Symptomatic relief of pain, burning, frequency, and urgency arising from irritation of urinary tract mucosa, as from infection, trauma, surgery, or instrumentation.

CONTRAINDICATIONS Renal insufficiency, glomerulonephritis, pyelonephritis during pregnancy (category B); severe hepatitis.
CAUTIOUS USE GI disturbances; glucose-6-phosphate dehydrogenase deficiency, lactation.

ROUTE & DOSAGE

Cystitis
Adult: **PO** 200 mg t.i.d.
Child: **PO** 12 mg/kg/d in 3 divided doses

ADMINISTRATION

Oral

- Give with or after meals.

ADVERSE EFFECTS (≥1%) **Body as a Whole:** Headache, vertigo. **GI:** Mild

P

GI disturbances. **Urogenital:** Kidney stones, transient acute kidney failure. **Metabolic:** Methemoglobinemia, hemolytic anemia. **Skin:** Skin pigmentation. **Special Senses:** May stain soft contact lenses.

DIAGNOSTIC TEST INTERFERENCE Phenazopyridine may interfere with any urinary test that is based on color reactions or spectrometry: ***bromsulphalein*** and ***phenolsulfonphthalein*** excretion tests; urinary ***glucose*** test using ***Clinistix*** or ***TesTape*** (***copper-reduction methods*** such as ***Clinitest*** and ***Benedict's test*** reportedly not affected); ***bilirubin*** using "foam test" or ***Ictotest; ketones*** using ***nitroprusside*** (e.g., ***Acetest, Ketostix,*** or ***Gerhardt ferric chloride***); ***urinary protein*** using ***Albustix, Albutest,*** or ***nitric acid ring test;*** urinary ***steroids; urobilinogen; assays*** for ***porphyrins.***

INTERACTIONS Drug: No clinically significant interactions established.

P

PHARMACOKINETICS Absorption: Readily absorbed from GI tract. **Distribution:** Crosses placenta in trace amounts. **Metabolism:** Metabolized in liver and other tissues. **Elimination:** Primarily excreted in urine.

NURSING IMPLICATIONS

Assessment & Drug Effects

- Lab tests: Obtain periodic blood work and kidney function tests in patients on prolonged therapy or with impaired kidney function.

Patient & Family Education

- Be aware that drug will impart an orange to red color to urine and may stain fabric.
- Discontinue drug report to physician immediately the appearance of yellowish tinge to skin or sclerae may indicate drug accumulation due to renal impairment.
- Discontinue drug when pain and discomfort are relieved (usually 3–15 d). Keep physician informed.
- Do not breast feed while taking this drug without consulting physician.

PHENELZINE SULFATE (Pr)

(fen′el-zeen)

Nardil

Classifications: CENTRAL NERVOUS SYSTEM AGENT; PSYCHOTHERAPEUTIC; ANTIDEPRESSANT; MONOAMINE OXIDASE (MAO) INHIBITOR

Pregnancy Category: C

AVAILABILITY 15 mg tablets

ACTIONS Potent hydrazine (monoamine oxidase) MAO inhibitor. Precise mode of action is not known. Antidepressant and diverse effects believed to be due to irreversible inhibition of MAO, thereby permitting increased concentrations of endogenous epinephrine, norepinephrine, serotonin, and dopamine within presynaptic neurons and at receptor sites. Also thought to inhibit hepatic microsomal drug-metabolizing enzymes; thus it may intensify and prolong the effects of many drugs.

THERAPEUTIC EFFECTS Antidepressant utilization of the drug is limited to individuals who do not respond well to other classes of antidepressants. Termination of drug action depends on regeneration of MAO, which occurs 2–3 wk after discontinuation of therapy.

USES Management of endogenous depression, depressive phase of manic-depressive psychosis, and severe exogenous (reactive) depression not responsive to more commonly used therapy.

CONTRAINDICATIONS Hypersensitivity to MAO inhibitors; pheochromocytoma; hyperthyroidism; CHF, cardiovascular or cerebrovascular disease; impaired kidney function, hypernatremia; atonic colitis; glaucoma; history of frequent or severe headaches; history of liver disease, abnormal liver function tests; older adult or debilitated patients; paranoid schizophrenia. Safety during pregnancy (category C), lactation, or in children <6 y of age is not established.

CAUTIOUS USE Epilepsy; pyloric stenosis; diabetes; depression accompanying alcoholism or drug addiction; manic-depressive states; agitated patients; suicidal tendencies; chronic brain syndromes; history of angina pectoris.

ROUTE & DOSAGE

Depression

Adult: **PO** 15 mg t.i.d., rapidly increase to at least 60 mg/d, may need up to 90 mg/d

ADMINISTRATION

Oral

- Discontinue at least 10 d before elective surgery to allow time for recovery from MAO before anesthetics are given.
- Avoid rapid withdrawal of MAO inhibitors, particularly after high dosage, since a rebound effect may occur (e.g., headache, excitability, hallucinations, and possibly depression).
- Store in tightly covered containers away from heat and light.

ADVERSE EFFECTS (≥1%) **Body as a Whole:** Dizziness or vertigo, headache, *orthostatic hypotension,* drowsiness or *insomnia,* weakness, fatigue, edema, tremors, twitching, akathisia, ataxia, hyperreflexia, faintness, hyperactivity, marked agitation, anxiety, seizures, trismus, opisthotonos, respiratory depression, coma. **CNS:** Mania, hypomania, confusion, memory impairment, delirium, hallucinations, euphoria, acute anxiety reaction, toxic precipitation of schizophrenia, convulsions, peripheral neuropathy. **CV:** Hypertensive crisis (intense occipital headache, palpitation, marked hypertension, stiff neck, nausea, vomiting, sweating, fever, photophobia, dilated pupils, bradycardia or tachycardia, constricting chest pain, intracranial bleeding), hypotension or hypertension, circulatory collapse. **GI:** *Constipation, dry mouth, nausea,* vomiting, *anorexia,* weight gain. **Hematologic:** Normocytic and normochromic anemia, leukopenia. **Skin:** Hyperhidrosis, skin rash, photosensitivity. **Special Senses:** Blurred vision.

DIAGNOSTIC TEST INTERFERENCE

Phenelzine may cause a slight false increase in ***serum bilirubin.***

INTERACTIONS Drug: TRICYCLIC ANTIDEPRESSANTS may cause hyperpyrexia, seizures; **fluoxetine, sertraline, paroxetine** may cause hyperthermia, diaphoresis, tremors, seizures, delirium; SYMPATHOMIMETIC AGENTS (e.g., **amphetamine, phenylephrine, phenylpropanolamine**), **guanethidine** and **reserpine** may cause hypertensive crisis; CNS DEPRESSANTS have additive CNS depressive effects; OPIATE ANALGESICS (especially **meperidine**) may cause hypertensive crisis and circulatory collapse; **buspirone,** hypertension; GENERAL ANESTHETICS, prolonged hypotensive and CNS depressant effects; hypertension, headache, hyperexcitability reported with **dopamine, methyldopa, levodopa, tryptophan; metrizamide**

P

may increase risk of seizures; HYPOTENSIVE AGENTS and DIURETICS have additive hypotensive effects. **Food:** Aged meats or aged cheeses, protein extracts, sour cream, alcohol, anchovies, liver, sausages, overripe figs, bananas, avocados, chocolate, soy sauce, bean curd, natural yogurt, fava beans—**tyramine**-containing foods—may precipitate hypertensive crisis. **Herbal: Ginseng, ephedra, ma huang, St. John's wort** may cause hypertensive crisis.

PHARMACOKINETICS Absorption: Readily absorbed from GI tract. **Onset:** 2 wk. **Metabolism:** Rapidly metabolized. **Elimination:** 79% of metabolites excreted in urine in 96 h.

NURSING IMPLICATIONS

Assessment & Drug Effects

- Evaluate patient's BP in standing and recumbent positions. Prior to initiation of treatment.
- Lab tests: Perform baseline CBC and liver function tests. Also perform periodic CBC and liver function tests during prolonged or high-dose therapy.
- Monitor BP and pulse between doses when titrating initial dosages. Observe closely for evidence of adverse drug effects. Thereafter, monitor at regular intervals throughout therapy.
- Report immediately if hypomania (exaggeration of motility, feelings, and ideas) occurs as depression improves. This reaction may also appear at higher than recommended doses or with long-term therapy.
- Observe for and report therapeutic effectiveness of drug: Improvement in sleep pattern, appetite, physical activity, interest in self and surroundings, as well as lessening of anxiety and bodily complaints.
- Observe patient with diabetes closely for S&S of hypoglycemia (see Appendix F). Patients on prolonged therapy should be checked periodically for altered color perception, changes in fundi or visual fields. Changes in red-green vision may be the first indication of eye damage.

Patient & Family Education

- Drug is usually discontinued if no therapeutic response occurs after 3 or 4 wk. Maximum antidepressant effects generally appear in 2–6 wk and persist several weeks after drug withdrawal.
- Avoid self-medication. OTC preparations containing dextromethorphan, sympathomimetic agents, or antihistamines (e.g., cough, cold, and hay fever remedies, appetite suppressants) can precipitate severe hypertensive reactions if taken during therapy or within 2–3 wk after discontinuation of an MAO inhibitor.
- Report immediately to physician the onset of headache and palpitation, prodromal symptoms of hypertensive crisis or any other unusual effects which may indicate need to discontinue therapy.
- Do not consume foods and beverages containing tyramine or tryptophan or drugs containing pressor agent. These can cause severe hypertensive reactions. Get a list from your care provider.
- Avoid drinking excessive caffeine beverages (e.g., coffee, tea, cocoa, or cola).
- Discuss with physician wearing elastic stockings and elevating legs when sitting to minimize hypotensive effects of drug.
- Make position changes slowly, especially from recumbent to upright posture, and dangle legs over bed a few minutes before rising to

P

walk. Avoid standing still for prolonged periods. Also avoid hot showers and baths (resulting vasodilatation may potentiate hypotension); lie down immediately if feeling light-headed or faint.

- Check weight 2 or 3 times per week and report unusual gain.
- Report jaundice. Hepatotoxicity is believed to be a hypersensitivity reaction unrelated to dosage or duration of therapy.
- Avoid overexertion while taking this drug. MAO inhibitors may suppress anginal pain that would otherwise serve as a warning sign of myocardial ischemia.
- Do not breast feed while taking this drug without consulting physician.

PHENOBARBITAL (Pr)

(fee-noe-bar'bi-tal)

Barbital, Luminal, Solfoton

PHENOBARBITAL SODIUM

Luminal Sodium

Classifications: CENTRAL NERVOUS SYSTEM AGENT; ANTICONVULSANT; SEDATIVE-HYPNOTIC; BARBITURATE

Pregnancy Category: D

Controlled Substance: Schedule IV

AVAILABILITY 15 mg, 16 mg, 16.2 mg, 30 mg, 60 mg, 90 mg, 100 mg tablets; 16 mg capsules; 15 mg/5 mL, 20 mg/5 mL liquid; 30 mg/mL, 60 mg/mL, 65 mg/mL, 130 mg/mL injection

ACTIONS Long-acting barbiturate. Sedative and hypnotic effects of barbiturates appear to be due primarily to interference with impulse transmission of cerebral cortex by inhibition of reticular activating system. CNS depression may range from mild sedation to coma, depending on dosage, route of administration, degree of nervous system excitability, and drug tolerance. Initially, barbiturates suppress REM sleep, but with chronic therapy REM sleep returns to normal.

THERAPEUTIC EFFECTS Produces sedative and hypnotic effects with no analgesic properties, and small doses may increase reaction to painful stimuli. Phenobarbital limits spread of seizure activity by increasing threshold for motor cortex stimuli. Barbiturates are habit forming.

USES Long-term management of tonic-clonic (grand mal) seizures and partial seizures; status epilepticus, eclampsia, febrile convulsions in young children. Also used as a sedative in anxiety or tension states; in pediatrics as preoperative and postoperative sedation and to treat pylorospasm in infants.

UNLABELED USES Treatment and prevention of hyperbilirubinemia in neonates and in the management of chronic cholestasis; benzodiazepine withdrawal.

CONTRAINDICATIONS Sensitivity to barbiturates; manifest hepatic or familial history of porphyria; severe respiratory or kidney disease; history of previous addiction to sedative hypnotics; uncontrolled pain; pregnancy (particularly early pregnancy) (category D), lactation; sustained release formulation for children <12 y of age.

CAUTIOUS USE Impaired liver, kidney, cardiac, or respiratory function; history of allergies; older adult or debilitated patients; patients with fever; hyperthyroidism; diabetes mellitus or severe anemia; during labor and delivery; patient with borderline hypoadrenal function.

P

ROUTE & DOSAGE

Anticonvulsant

Adult: **PO** 100–300 mg/d **IV/IM** 200–600 mg up to 20 mg/kg
Child: **PO/IV** 3–8 mg/kg or 125 $mg/m^2/d$
Neonate: **PO/IV** 3–4 mg/kg/d (max: 5 mg/kg/d)

Status Epilepticus

Adult/Child: **IV** 15–18 mg/kg in single or divided doses (max: 20 mg/kg)
Neonate: **IV** 15–20 mg/kg in single or divided doses

Sedative

Adult: **PO** 30–120 mg/d **IV/IM** 100–200 mg/d
Child: **PO** 6 mg/kg/d or 180 mg/m^2 in 3 divided doses **IV/IM** 16–100 mg/d (1–3 mg/kg)

ADMINISTRATION

Oral

- Make sure patient actually swallows pill and does not "cheek" it.
- Give crushed and mixed with a fluid or with food if patient cannot swallow pill. Do not permit patient to swallow dry crushed drug.

Intramuscular

- Give IM deep into large muscle mass; do not exceed 5 mL at any one site.

Intravenous

Note: Verify correct IV concentration and rate of infusion for neonates, infants, children with physician. Use IV route ONLY if other routes are not feasible.

PREPARE: **Direct:** Slowly add at least 10 mL of sterile water for injection to ampule. Rotate ampule to dissolve (may take several minutes). If solution not clear in 5 min or if a precipitate remains, discard.

ADMINISTER: **Direct:** Give 60 mg or fraction thereof over at least 60 sec. Give within 30 min after preparation.

INCOMPATIBILITIES **Solution/additive: Benzquinamide, cephalothin, chlorpromazine, codeine phosphate, ephedrine, hydralazine, hydrocortisone sodium succinate, hydroxyzine, insulin, levorphanol, meperidine, methadone, morphine, norepinephrine,** TETRACYCLINES, **procaine, prochlorperazine, promazine, promethazine, ranitidine, streptomycin, vancomycin. Y-site: Amphotericin B cholesteryl complex, hydromorphone, TPN with albumin.**

- Be aware that extravasation of IV phenobarbital may cause necrotic tissue changes that necessitate skin grafting. Check injection site frequently.

ADVERSE EFFECTS (≥1%)

Body as a Whole: Myalgia, neuralgia, <u>CNS depression, coma, and death</u>. **CNS:** *Somnolence,* nightmares, insomnia, "hangover," headache, anxiety, thinking abnormalities, dizziness, nystagmus, irritability, paradoxic excitement and exacerbation of hyperkinetic behavior (in children); confusion or depression or marked excitement (older adult or debilitated patients); ataxia. **CV:** Bradycardia, syncope, hypotension. **GI:** Nausea, vomiting, constipation, diarrhea, epigastric pain, liver damage. **Hematologic:** Megaloblastic anemia, <u>agranulocytosis</u>, thrombocytopenia. **Metabolic:** Hypocalcemia, osteomalacia, rickets. **Musculoskeletal:** Folic acid deficiency, vitamin D deficiency. **Respiratory:** <u>Respiratory depression</u>. **Skin:** Mild maculopapular, morbilliform rash; erythema multiforme, <u>Stevens-</u>

Johnson syndrome, exfoliative dermatitis (rare).

DIAGNOSTIC TEST INTERFERENCE BARBITURATES may affect ***bromsulphalein*** retention tests (by enhancing liver uptake and excretion of dye) and increase ***serum phosphatase.***

INTERACTIONS Drug: Alcohol, CNS DEPRESSANTS compound CNS depression; phenobarbital may decrease absorption and increase metabolism of ORAL ANTICOAGULANTS; increases metabolism of CORTICOSTEROIDS, ORAL CONTRACEPTIVES, ANTICONVULSANTS, **digitoxin,** possibly decreasing their effects; ANTIDEPRESSANTS potentiate adverse effects of phenobarbital; **griseofulvin** decreases absorption of phenobarbital. **Herbal: Kava-kava, valerian** may potentiate sedation.

PHARMACOKINETICS Absorption: 70%–90% absorbed slowly from GI tract. **Peak:** 8–12 h PO; 30 min IV. **Duration:** 4–6 h IV. **Distribution:** 20%–45% protein bound; crosses placenta; enters breast milk. **Metabolism:** Oxidized in liver to inactivated metabolites. **Elimination:** Excreted in urine. **Half-Life:** 2–6 d.

NURSING IMPLICATIONS

Assessment & Drug Effects

- Observe patients receiving large doses closely for at least 30 min to ensure that sedation is not excessive.
- Keep patient under constant observation when drug is administered IV, and record vital signs at least every hour or more often if indicated.
- Lab tests: Obtain liver function and hematology tests and determinations of serum folate and vitamin D levels during prolonged therapy.
- Monitor serum drug levels. Serum concentrations >50 mcg/mL may cause coma. Therapeutic serum concentrations of 15–40 mcg/mL produce anticonvulsant activity in most patients. These values are usually attained after 2 or 3 wk of therapy with a dose of 100–200 mg/d.
- Expect barbiturates to produce restlessness when given to patients in pain because these drugs do not have analgesic action.
- Be prepared for paradoxical responses and report promptly in older adult or debilitated patient and children (i.e., irritability, marked excitement [inappropriate tearfulness and aggression in children], depression, and confusion).
- Monitor for drug interactions. Barbiturates increase the metabolism of many drugs, leading to decreased pharmacologic effects of those drugs. Whenever a barbiturate is added to an established regimen of another drug, observe for changes in effectiveness of the first drug at least during early phase of barbiturate use.
- Monitor for and report chronic toxicity symptoms (e.g., ataxia, slurred speech, irritability, poor judgment, slight dysarthria, nystagmus on vertical gaze, confusion, insomnia, somatic complaints).

Patient & Family Education

- Be aware that anticonvulsant therapy may cause drowsiness during first few weeks of treatment, but this usually diminishes with continued use.
- Avoid potentially hazardous activities requiring mental alertness until response to drug is known.
- Do not consume alcohol in any amount when taking a barbiturate; it may severely impair judgment and abilities.

- Increase vitamin D-fortified foods (e.g., milk products) because drug increases vitamin D metabolism. A vitamin D supplement may be prescribed.
- Maintain adequate dietary folate intake: fresh vegetables (especially green leafy), fresh fruits, whole grains, liver. Long-term therapy may result in nutritional folate (B_9) deficiency. A supplement of folic acid may be prescribed.
- Adhere to drug regimen (i.e., do not change intervals between doses or increase or decrease doses) without contacting physician.
- Do not stop taking drug abruptly because of danger of withdrawal symptoms (8–12 h after last dose), which can be fatal.
- Report to physician the onset of fever, sore throat or mouth, malaise, easy bruising or bleeding, petechiae, jaundice, rash when on prolonged therapy.
- Avoid pregnancy when receiving barbiturates. Use or add barrier device to hormonal contraceptive when taking prolonged therapy.
- Do not breast feed while taking this drug.

P

PHENOXYBENZAMINE HYDROCHLORIDE

(fen-ox-ee-ben'za-meen)

Dibenzyline

Classifications: AUTONOMIC NERVOUS SYSTEM AGENT; ALPHA-ADRENERGIC ANTAGONIST (BLOCKING AGENT), SYMPATHOLYTIC; ANTIHYPERTENSIVE AGENT

Prototype: Prazosin

Pregnancy Category: C

AVAILABILITY 10 mg capsules

ACTIONS Long-acting alpha-adrenergic blocking agent. Apparently produces noncompetitive blockade of alpha-adrenergic receptor sites at postganglionic synapse. Alpha-receptor sites are thus unable to react to endogenous or exogenous sympathomimetic agents.

THERAPEUTIC EFFECTS Blocks excitatory effects of epinephrine, including vasoconstriction, but does not affect adrenergic cardiac inhibitory actions. It produces a "chemical sympathectomy" and it can maintain it. Causes orthostatic hypotension in both normotensive and hypertensive patients.

USES Management of pheochromocytoma.

UNLABELED USES To improve circulation in peripheral vasospastic conditions such as Raynaud's acrocyanosis and frostbite sequelae, for adjunctive treatment of shock, hypertensive crisis.

CONTRAINDICATIONS Instances when fall in BP would be dangerous; compensated congestive heart failure; pregnancy (category C), lactation.

CAUTIOUS USE Marked cerebral or coronary arteriosclerosis, CHF; renal insufficiency; respiratory infections.

ROUTE & DOSAGE

Management of Pheochromocytoma

Adult: **PO** 5–10 mg b.i.d., may increase by 10 mg/d at 4-d intervals to desired response (usual range 20–60 mg/d in 2–3 divided doses)

Child: **PO** 0.2 mg/kg/d in 1–2 divided doses, may increase by 0.2 mg/kg/d at 4 d intervals to desired response (usual range 0.4–1.2 mg/kg/d)

ADMINISTRATION

Oral

- Give with milk or in divided doses to reduce gastric irritation.
- Preserve in airtight containers protected from light.

ADVERSE EFFECTS (≥1%) **Body as a Whole:** *Dizziness,* fainting, drowsiness, sedation, tiredness, weakness, lethargy, confusion, headache, shock. **CNS:** CNS stimulation (large doses). **CV:** *Postural hypotension, tachycardia,* palpitation. **GI:** Dry mouth. **Urogenital:** Inhibition of ejaculation. **Respiratory:** *Nasal congestion.* **Skin:** Allergic contact dermatitis. **Special Senses:** *Miosis,* drooping of eyelids.

INTERACTIONS Drug: inhibits effects of **methoxamine, norepinephrine, phenylephrine;** additive hypotensive effects with ANTIHYPERTENSIVES.

PHARMACOKINETICS Absorption: Variably absorbed (approximately 30%) from GI tract. **Onset:** 2 h. **Peak:** 4–6 h. **Duration:** 3–4 d. **Distribution:** Accumulates in adipose tissue. **Elimination:** 80% excreted in urine and bile within 24 h. **Half-Life:** 24 h.

NURSING IMPLICATIONS

Assessment & Drug Effects

- Monitor BP and note pulse quality, rate, and rhythm in recumbent and standing positions during period of dosage adjustment. Observe patient closely for at least 4 d from one dosage increment to the next; hypotension and tachycardia are most likely to occur in standing position.
- Drug has cumulative action, thus onset of therapeutic effects may not occur until after 2 wk of therapy, and full therapeutic effects may not be apparent for several more weeks.

Patient & Family Education

- Make position changes slowly, particularly from reclining to upright posture, and dangle legs and exercise ankles and feet for a few minutes before standing.
- Be aware that light headedness, dizziness, and palpitations usually disappear with continued therapy but may reappear under conditions that promote vasodilation, such as strenuous exercise or ingestion of a large meal or alcohol.
- Pupil constriction, nasal stuffiness, and inhibition of ejaculation generally decrease with continued therapy.
- Do not take OTC medications for coughs, colds, or allergy without approval of physician. Many contain agents that cause BP elevation.
- Do not breast feed while taking this drug.

PHENSUXIMIDE

(fen-sux'i-mide)

Milontin

Classifications: CENTRAL NERVOUS SYSTEM AGENT; ANTICONVULSANT SUCCINIMIDE

Prototype: Ethosuximide

Pregnancy Category: D

AVAILABILITY 500 mg capsules

ACTIONS Succinimide derivative reportedly less potent and less effective than other drugs of this class. Reduces the frequency of epileptiform attacks.

THERAPEUTIC EFFECTS Apparently depresses the motor cortex and elevates the threshold of CNS sensitivity to seizure activity, thus lessening the incidence of seizure activity.

USES Management of petit mal epilepsy (absence seizures) and with other anticonvulsants when other forms of epilepsy coexist with petit mal.

CONTRAINDICATIONS Intermittent porphyria; liver or kidney disease; pregnancy (category D), lactation.

ROUTE & DOSAGE

Absence Seizures

Adult/Child: **PO** 0.5–1 g b.i.d. or t.i.d.

ADMINISTRATION

Oral

- Give consistently with respect to time of day.

ADVERSE EFFECTS (≥1%) **Body as a Whole:** *Drowsiness, dizziness, ataxia,* muscle weakness, flushing, periorbital edema, **GI:** *Anorexia, nausea, vomiting.* **Urogenital:** Reversible nephropathy. **Hematologic:** Granulocytopenia. **Skin:** Alopecia, pruritus, skin rash.

INTERACTIONS Drug: Carbamazepine decreases phensuximide levels; **isoniazid** significantly increases phensuximide levels; levels of both **phenobarbital** and phensuximide may be altered with increased seizure frequency.

PHARMACOKINETICS Absorption: Readily absorbed from GI tract. **Peak:** 1–4 h. **Metabolism:** Metabolized in liver. **Elimination:** Excreted slowly in urine; small amounts excreted in bile and feces. **Half-Life:** 5–12 h.

NURSING IMPLICATIONS

Assessment & Drug Effects

- Monitor weight, especially in children, since anorexic effects of drug might cause weight loss.
- Lab tests: Perform baseline and periodic liver and kidney function tests. Perform periodic blood tests, especially with long-term therapy.

Patient & Family Education

- Report onset of skin rash or other unusual symptoms to physician.
- Be aware that phensuximide may color urine pink, red, or red-brown.
- Do not use OTC drugs unless the physician approves; loss of seizure control can be induced by ingredients in some popular OTC drugs.
- Do not drive or engage in potentially hazardous activities until response to drug is known.
- Do not breast feed while taking this drug.

PHENTERMINE HYDROCHLORIDE

(phen-ter'meen)

Ionamin, Fastin, Zantryl, Adipex-P, Obe-Nix-30

Classifications: GASTROINTESTINAL AGENT; ANOREXIANT

Prototype: Diethylpropion

Pregnancy Category: C

Controlled Substance: Schedule IV

AVAILABILITY 8 mg, 30 mg, 37.5 mg tablets; 15 mg, 18.75 mg, 30 mg, 37.5 mg capsules

ACTIONS Sympathetic amine with pharmacological similarity to amphetamine. Actions include CNS stimulation and blood pressure elevation.

THERAPEUTIC EFFECTS Appetite suppression or metabolic effects along with diet adjustment result in weight loss in obese individuals.

USES Short term (8–12 wks) adjunct for weight loss.

CONTRAINDICATIONS History of hypertension, moderate-to-severe hypertension, advanced arteriosclerosis, cardiovascular disease; hyperthyroidism; known hypersensitivity to sympathetic amines; agitated states; history of drug abuse; during or within 14 d of administration of MAOI; concurrent administration of serotonin reuptake inhibitors (SSRIs); valvular heart disease; glaucoma; pregnancy (category C), lactation, or children <16 y.

CAUTIOUS USE Mild hypertension, diabetes mellitus.

ROUTE & DOSAGE

Obesity

Adult: **PO** 8 mg t.i.d. 30 min before meals or 15–37.5 mg q.d. before breakfast or 10–14 h before retiring

ADMINISTRATION

Oral

- Ensure that at least 14 days have elapsed between the first dose of phentermine and the last dose of a MAO inhibitor.
- Give 30 minutes before meals.
- Do not administer if a SSRI is currently prescribed.
- Store in a tight container.

ADVERSE EFFECTS (≥1%) **Body as a Whole:** Hypersensitivity (urticaria, rash, erythema, burning sensation), chest pain, excessive sweating, clamminess, chills, flushing, fever, myalgia. **CV:** Palpitations, tachycardia, arrhythmias, hypertension or hypotension, syncope, precordial pain, pulmonary hypertension. **GI:** Dry mouth, altered taste, nausea, vomiting, abdominal pain, diarrhea, constipation, stomach pain. **Endocrine:** Gynecomastia. **Hematologic:** Bone marrow suppression, agranulocytosis, leukopenia. **Musculoskeletal:** Muscle pain. **CNS:** Overstimulation, nervousness, restlessness, dizziness, insomnia, weakness, fatigue, malaise, anxiety, euphoria, drowsiness, depression, agitation, dysphoria, tremor, dyskinesia, dysarthria, confusion, incoordination, headache, change in libido. **Skin:** Hair loss, ecchymosis. **Special Senses:** Mydriasis, blurred vision. **Urogenital:** Dysuria, polyuria, urinary frequency, impotence, menstrual upset.

INTERACTIONS Drug: MAO INHIBITORS, **furazolidone** may increase pressor response resulting in hypertensive crisis. TRICYCLIC ANTIDEPRESSANTS may decrease anorectic response. May decrease hypotensive effects of **guanethidine.**

PHARMACOKINETICS Absorption: Absorbed from the small intestine. **Duration:** 4–14 h. **Elimination:** Excreted primarily in urine. **Half-Life:** 19–24 h.

NURSING IMPLICATIONS

Assessment & Drug Effects

- Assess for tolerance to the anorectic effect of the drug. Withhold drug and report to physician when this occurs.
- Lab tests: Periodic CBC with differential and blood glucose.
- Monitor periodic cardiovascular status, including BP, exercise tolerance, peripheral edema.
- Monitor weight at least 3 times/wk.

Patient & Family Education

- Do not take this drug late in the evening because it could cause insomnia.
- Report immediately any of the following: Shortness of breath, chest pains, dizziness or fainting, swelling of the extremities.
- Tolerance to the appetite suppression effects of the drug usually develops in a few weeks. Notify

P

physician, but do not increase the drug dose.

- Weigh yourself at least 3 times/wk at the same time of day with the same amount of clothing.
- Do not breast feed while taking this drug.

PHENTOLAMINE MESYLATE

(fen-tole'a-meen)

Regitine, Rogitine ✦

Classifications: AUTONOMIC NERVOUS SYSTEM AGENT; ALPHA-ADRENERGIC ANTAGONIST (BLOCKING AGENT), SYMPATHOLYTIC

Prototype: Prazosin

Pregnancy Category: C

AVAILABILITY 5 mg injection

ACTIONS Alpha-adrenergic blocking agent structurally related to tolazoline but with more potent blocking effects. Competitively blocks alpha-adrenergic receptors, but action is transient and incomplete. Prevents hypertension resulting from elevated levels of circulating epinephrine or norepinephrine.

THERAPEUTIC EFFECTS Causes vasodilation and decreases general vascular resistance and pulmonary arterial pressure, primarily by direct action on vascular smooth muscle. Through stimulation of beta-adrenergic receptors, produces positive inotropic and chronotropic cardiac effects and increases cardiac output.

USES Diagnosis of pheochromocytoma and to prevent or control hypertensive episodes prior to or during pheochromocytomectomy.

UNLABELED USES Prevention of dermal necrosis and sloughing following IV administration or extravasation of norepinephrine.

CONTRAINDICATIONS MI (previous or present), coronary artery disease. Safety during pregnancy (category C) or lactation is not established.

CAUTIOUS USE Gastritis, peptic ulcer.

ROUTE & DOSAGE

To Prevent Hypertensive Episode During Surgery

Adult: **IV/IM** 2–5 mg as needed
Child: **IV/IM** 1 mg or 0.1 mg/kg (max: 5 mg/dose)

To Test for Pheochromocytoma

Adult: **IV/IM** 5 mg
Child: **IV/IM** 0.1 mg/kg

To Prevent Necrosis from Norepinephrine Infusions

Adult: **IV** 10 mg added to each liter of IV fluid containing norepinephrine

To Treat Catecholamine Extravasation

Adult/Child: **Intradermal** 5–10 mg diluted in 10 mL of normal saline injected into affected area within 12 h of extravasation
Neonate: **Intradermal** 2.5–5 mg diluted in 10 mL of normal saline injected into affected area within 12 h of extravasation (max: dose 0.1 mg/kg or 2.5 mg total)

ADMINISTRATION

Note: Place patient in supine position when receiving drug parenterally. Monitor BP and pulse q2min until stabilized.

Intramuscular

- Reconstitute 5 mg vial with 1 mL of sterile water for injection.

Intravenous

PREPARE: **Direct:** Reconstitute as for IM. May be further diluted with up to 10 mL of sterile water. Use immediately.

ADMINISTER: **Direct:** Give a single dose over 60 sec.

ADVERSE EFFECTS (≥1%) **Body as a Whole:** Weakness, dizziness, flushing, *orthostatic hypotension*. **GI:** *Abdominal pain, nausea, vomiting, diarrhea, exacerbation of peptic ulcer.* **CV:** *Acute and prolonged hypotension, tachycardia, anginal pain,* cardiac arrhythmias, MI, cerebrovascular spasm, shock-like state. **Special Senses:** Nasal stuffiness, conjunctival infection.

INTERACTIONS Drug: may antagonize BP raising effects of **epinephrine, ephedrine.**

PHARMACOKINETICS Peak: 2 min IV; 15–20 min IM. **Duration:** 10–15 min IV; 3–4 h IM. **Elimination:** Excreted in urine. **Half-Life:** 19 min.

NURSING IMPLICATIONS

Assessment & Drug Effects

- Test for pheochromocytoma: (1) Withhold medications not deemed absolutely essential for at least 24 h, preferably 48–72 h; antihypertensive agents withheld until BP returns to pretreatment level (rauwolfia drugs withdrawn at least 4 wk prior to testing). (2) Keep patient at rest in supine position throughout test, preferably in quiet darkened room. (3) Take BP q10min for at least 30 min; when BP stabilizes, (4) IV administration: Record BP immediately after injection and at 30-second intervals for first 3 min; then at 1-min intervals for next 7 min. IM administration: BP determinations at 5-min intervals for 30–45 min.

Patient & Family Education

- Avoid sudden changes in position, particularly from reclining to upright posture and dangle legs and exercise ankles and toes for a few minutes before standing to walk.
- Lie down or sit down in head-low position immediately if lightheaded or dizzy.

PHENYLEPHRINE HYDROCHLORIDE

(fen-ill-ef′rin)

AK-Dilate Ophthalmic, Alconefrin, Isopto Frin, Mydfrin, Neo-Synephrine, Nostril, Prefrin Liquifilm, Rhinall, Sinarest Nasal, Sinex, Vacon

Classifications: AUTONOMIC NERVOUS SYSTEM AGENT; ALPHA-ADRENERGIC AGONIST; EYE AND NOSE PREPARATION; MYDRIATIC; DECONGESTANT

Prototype: Methoxamine

Pregnancy Category: C

AVAILABILITY 10 mg chewable tablet; 0.125%, 0.16%, 0.5%, 1% nasal solution; 0.12%, 2.5%, 10% ophthalmic solution; 10 mg/mL injection

ACTIONS Potent, synthetic, direct-acting sympathomimetic with strong alpha-adrenergic and weak beta-adrenergic cardiac stimulant actions.

THERAPEUTIC EFFECTS Produces little or no CNS stimulation. Elevates systolic and diastolic pressures through arteriolar constriction; also constricts capacitance vessels and increases venous return to heart. Rise in BP causes reflex bradycardia. Topical applications to eye produce vasoconstriction and prompt mydriasis of short duration, usually without causing cycloplegia. Reduces intraocular pressure by increasing outflow and decreasing rate of aqueous humor secretion. Nasal decongestant action qualitatively similar to that of epinephrine but more potent and has longer duration of action.

USES Parenterally to maintain BP during anesthesia, to treat vascular failure in shock, and to overcome paroxysmal supraventricular tachycardia. Used topically for rhinitis of common cold, allergic rhinitis, and sinusitis; in selected patients with wide-angle glaucoma; as mydriatic for ophthalmoscopic examination or surgery, and for relief of uveitis.

CONTRAINDICATIONS Severe coronary disease, severe hypertension, ventricular tachycardia; narrow-angle glaucoma (ophthalmic preparations); pregnancy (category C), lactation.

CAUTIOUS USE Hyperthyroidism; diabetes mellitus; myocardial disease, cerebral arteriosclerosis, bradycardia; older adult patients; 21 d before or following termination of MAO inhibitor therapy. **Ophthalmic solution (10%):** Cardiovascular disease; diabetes mellitus; hypertension; aneurysms; infants.

ROUTE & DOSAGE

Hypotension

Adult: **IM/SC** 1–10 mg (initial dose not to exceed 5 mg) q10–15min as needed **IV** 0.1–0.18 mg/min until BP stabilizes; then 0.04–0.06 mg/min for maintenance

Ophthalmoscopy

See Appendix A

Vasoconstrictor

Adult: **Ophthalmic** See Appendix A-1 **Intranasal** Small amount of nasal jelly placed into each nostril q3–4h as needed or 2–3 drops or sprays of 0.25%–0.5% solution q3–4h as needed
Child: **Intranasal** *<6 y,* 2–3 drops or sprays of 0.125% solution q3–4h as needed; *6–12 y,* 2–3 drops or sprays of 0.25% solution q3–4h as needed

ADMINISTRATION

Instillation

- Nasal preparations: Instruct patient to blow nose gently (with both nostrils open) to clear nasal passages before administration of medication.
- Instillation (drops): Tilt head back while sitting or standing up, or lie on bed and hang head over side. Stay in position a few minutes to permit medication to spread through nose. (Spray): With head upright, squeeze bottle quickly and firmly to produce 1 or 2 sprays into each nostril; wait 3–5 min, blow nose, and repeat dose. (Jelly): Place in each nostril and sniff it well back into nose.
- Clean tips and droppers of nasal solution dispensers with hot water after use to prevent contamination of solution. Droppers of ophthalmic solution bottles should not touch any surface including the eye.
- Ophthalmic preparations: To avoid excessive systemic absorption, apply pressure to lacrimal sac during and for 1–2 min after instillation of drops.

Subcutaneous/Intramuscular

- Give undiluted.

Intravenous

PREPARE: **Direct:** Dilute each 1 mg in 9 mL of sterile water. **IV Infusion:** Further dilute each 10 mg in 500 mL D5W or NS (concentration: 0.2 mg/mL).

ADMINISTER: **Direct:** Give a single dose over 60 sec. **IV Infusion:** Titrate to maintain BP.

INCOMPATIBILITIES **Y-site: Thiopental.**

- Protect from exposure to air, strong light, or heat, any of which can cause solutions to change color to brown, form a precipitate, and lose potency.

ADVERSE EFFECTS (≥1%) **Special Senses:** *Transient stinging,* lacrimation, brow ache, headache, blurred vision, allergy (pigmentary deposits on lids, conjunctiva, and cornea with prolonged use), increased sensitivity to light. *Rebound nasal congestion* (hyperemia and edema of mucosa), *nasal burning,* stinging, dryness, *sneezing.* **CV:** Palpitation, tachycardia, bradycardia (over dosage), extrasystoles, hypertension. **Body as a Whole:** Trembling, sweating, pallor, sense of fullness in head, tingling of extremities, sleeplessness, dizziness, light-headedness, weakness, restlessness, anxiety, precordial pain, *tremor,* <u>severe visceral or peripheral vasoconstriction</u>, necrosis if IV infiltrates.

INTERACTIONS Drug: ERGOT ALKALOIDS, **guanethidine, reserpine,** TRICYCLIC ANTIDEPRESSANTS increase pressor effects of phenylephrine; **halothane, digoxin** increase risk of arrhythmias; MAO INHIBITORS cause hypertensive crisis; **oxytocin** causes persistent hypertension; ALPHA BLOCKERS, BETA BLOCKERS antagonize effects of phenylephrine.

PHARMACOKINETICS Onset: Immediate IV; 10–15 min IM/SC. **Duration:** 15–20 min IV; 30–120 min IM/SC; 3–6 h topical. **Metabolism:** Metabolized in liver and tissues by monoamine oxidase.

NURSING IMPLICATIONS

Assessment & Drug Effects

- Monitor pulse, BP, and central venous pressure (q2–5min) during IV administration.
- Control flow rate and dosage to prevent excessive dosage. IV overdoses can induce ventricular dysrhythmias.
- Observe for congestion or rebound miosis after topical administration to eye.

Patient & Family Education

- Be aware that instillation of 2.5%–10% strength ophthalmic solution can cause burning and stinging.
- Do not exceed recommended dosage regardless of formulation.
- Inform the physician if no relief is experienced from preparation in 5 d.
- Be aware that systemic absorption from nasal and conjunctival membranes can occur, though infrequently (see ADVERSE EFFECTS). Discontinue drug and report to the physician if adverse effects occur.
- Wear sunglasses in bright light because after instillation of ophthalmic drops, pupils will be large and eyes may be more sensitive to light than usual. Stop medication and notify physician if sensitivity persists beyond 12 h after drug has been discontinued.
- Be aware that some ophthalmic solutions may stain contact lenses.
- Do not breast feed while taking this drug.

PHENYTOIN (Pr)

(fen′i-toy-in)

Dilantin-125, Dilantin-30 Pediatric, Dilantin Infatab

PHENYTOIN SODIUM EXTENDED

Dilantin Kapseals

PHENYTOIN SODIUM PROMPT

Dilantin

Classifications: CENTRAL NERVOUS SYSTEM AGENT; ANTICONVULSANT; HYDANTOIN

Pregnancy Category: D

AVAILABILITY 100 mg prompt release capsule; 30 mg, 100 mg sustained release capsule; 50 mg chewable tablet; 125 mg/5 mL suspension; 50 mg/mL injection

ACTIONS Hydantoin derivative chemically related to phenobarbital. Precise mechanism of anticonvulsant action is not known, but drug use is accompanied by reduced voltage, frequency, and spread of electrical discharges within the motor cortex. Class IB antiarrhythmic properties similar to those of lidocaine and tocainide (also class IB agents). Has class IB antiarrhythmic properties.

THERAPEUTIC EFFECTS Inhibits seizure activity. In abnormal tissue causes slight increase in AV conduction velocity depressed by digitalis glycoside; prolongs effective refractory period, suppresses ventricular pacemaker automaticity, and may slow conduction or cause complete block in abnormal ventricular fibers.

USES To control tonic-clonic (grand mal) seizures, psychomotor and nonepileptic seizures (e.g., Reye's syndrome, after head trauma). Also used to prevent or treat seizures occurring during or after neurosurgery. Is not effective for absence seizures.

UNLABELED USES Antiarrhythmic agent (phenytoin IV) especially in treatment of digitalis-induced arrhythmias; treatment of trigeminal neuralgia (tic douloureux).

CONTRAINDICATIONS Hypersensitivity to hydantoin products; rash; seizures due to hypoglycemia; sinus bradycardia, complete or incomplete heart block; Adams-Stokes syndrome; pregnancy (category D), lactation.

CAUTIOUS USE Impaired liver or kidney function; alcoholism; blood dyscrasias; hypotension, heart block, bradycardia, severe myocardial insufficiency, impending or frank heart failure; older adult, debilitated, gravely ill patients; pancreatic adenoma; diabetes mellitus, hyperglycemia; respiratory depression; acute intermittent porphyria.

ROUTE & DOSAGE

Anticonvulsant

Adult: **PO** 15–18 mg/kg or 1 g loading dose, then 300 mg/d in 1–3 divided doses, may be gradually increased by 100 mg/wk until seizures are controlled **IV** 15–18 mg/kg or 1 g loading dose, then 100 mg t.i.d.

Child: **PO/IV** 15–20 mg/kg loading dose, then 5 mg/kg or 250 mg/m^2 in 2–3 divided doses

ADMINISTRATION

Oral

- Ensure that sustained release form is not chewed or crushed. Must be swallowed whole.
- Do not give within 2–3 h of antacid ingestion.
- Shake suspension vigorously before pouring to ensure uniform distribution of drug.
- Note: Prompt release capsules and chewable tablets are not intended for once-a-day dosage since drug is too quickly bioavailable and can therefore lead to toxic serum levels.
- Use sustained release capsules ONLY for once-a-day dosage regimens.

Intravenous

Note: Verify correct rate of IV injection for administration to infants or children with physician.

- Inspect solution prior to use. May use a slightly yellowed injectable solution safely. Precipitation may be caused by refrigeration, but slow warming to room temperature restores clarity.

PREPARE: **Direct:** Give undiluted. Use only when clear without precipitate.

ADMINISTER: **Direct:** Give 50 mg or fraction thereof over 1 min (25 mg/min in older adult or when used as antiarrhythmic). Follow with an injection of sterile saline through the same in-place catheter or needle. Do not use solutions containing dextrose.

INCOMPATIBILITIES **Solution/additive: 5% dextrose, amikacin, aminophylline, bretylium, cephapirin, codeine phosphate, dobutamine, hydromorphone, insulin, levorphanol, lidocaine, lincomycin, meperidine, metaraminol, methadone, morphine, nitroglycerin, norepinephrine, pentobarbital, procaine, secobarbital, streptomycin, sufentanil. Y-site: Amikacin, amphotericin B cholesteryl complex, bretylium, ciprofloxacin, clindamycin, diltiazem, dobutamine, enalaprilat, lidocaine, heparin, hydromorphone, potassium chloride, propofol, sufentanil, theophylline, TPN, vitamin B complex with C.**

- Observe injection site frequently during administration to prevent infiltration. Local soft tissue irritation may be serious, leading to erosion of tissues.

ADVERSE EFFECTS (≥1%) **CNS:** Usually dose-related: Nystagmus, *drowsiness,* ataxia, dizziness, mental confusion, tremors, insomnia, headache, seizures. **CV:** Bradycardia, hypotension, <u>cardiovascular collapse</u>, ventricular fibrillation, phlebitis. **Special Senses:** Photophobia, conjunctivitis, diplopia, blurred vision. **GI:** *Gingival hyperplasia,* nausea, vomiting, constipation, epigastric pain, dysphagia, loss of taste, weight loss, hepatitis, liver necrosis. **Hematologic:** Thrombocytopenia, leukopenia, leukocytosis, <u>agranulocytosis</u>, pancytopenia, eosinophilia; megaloblastic, hemolytic, or <u>aplastic anemias</u>. **Metabolic:** Fever, hyperglycemia, glycosuria, weight gain, edema, transient increase in serum thyrotropic (TSH) level, osteomalacia or rickets associated with hypocalcemia and elevated alkaline phosphatase activity. **Skin:** Alopecia, hirsutism (especially in young female); rash: scarlatiniform, maculopapular, urticaria, morbilliform; <u>bullous, exfoliative, or purpuric dermatitis; Stevens-Johnson syndrome, toxic epidermal necrolysis</u>, keratosis, neonatal hemorrhage. **Urogenital:** Acute renal failure, Peyronie's disease. **Respiratory:** Acute pneumonitis, pulmonary fibrosis. **Body as a Whole:** Periarteritis nodosum, acute systemic lupus erythematosus, craniofacial abnormalities (with enlargement of lips); lymphadenopathy.

DIAGNOSTIC TEST INTERFERENCE Phenytoin (HYDANTOINS) may produce lower than normal values for ***dexamethasone*** or ***metyrapone*** tests; may increase serum levels of ***glucose, BSP,*** and ***alkaline phosphatase*** and may decrease ***PBI*** and ***urinary steroid*** levels.

INTERACTIONS Drug: Alcohol decreases phenytoin effects; OTHER ANTICONVULSANTS may increase or decrease phenytoin levels; phenytoin may decrease absorption and increase metabolism of ORAL ANTICOAGULANTS; phenytoin increases metabolism of CORTICOSTEROIDS, ORAL CONTRACEPTIVES, and **nisoldipine,** thus decreasing their effectiveness; **amiodarone, chloramphenicol, omeprazole,** and **ticlopidine** increase phenytoin levels; ANTITUBERCULOSIS AGENTS decrease phenytoin levels. **Food: Folic acid, calcium,** and **vitamin D** absorption may be decreased by phenytoin; phenytoin absorption may be decreased by enteral nutrition supplements. **Herbal: Ginkgo** may decrease anticonvulsant effectiveness.

PHARMACOKINETICS Absorption: Completely absorbed from GI tract. **Peak:** 1.5–3 h prompt release; 4–12 h sustained release. **Distribution:** 95% protein bound; crosses placenta; small amount in breast milk. **Metabolism:** Oxidized in liver to inactive metabolites. **Elimination:** Metabolites excreted by kidneys. **Half-Life:** 22 h.

NURSING IMPLICATIONS

Assessment & Drug Effects

- Continuously monitor vital signs and symptoms during IV infusion and for an hour afterward. Watch for respiratory depression. Constant observation and a cardiac monitor are necessary with older adults or patients with cardiac disease. Margin between toxic and therapeutic IV doses is relatively small.
- Be aware of therapeutic serum concentration: 10–20 mcg/mL; toxic level: 30–50 mcg/mL; lethal level: 100 mcg/mL. Steady-state therapeutic levels are not achieved for at least 7–10 d.
- Lab tests: Periodic serum phenytoin concentration; CBC with differential, platelet count, and Hct and Hgb; serum glucose, serum calcium, and serum magnesium; and liver funtion tests.
- Observe patient closely for neurologic adverse effects following IV administration. Have on hand oxygen, atropine, vasopressor, assisted ventilation, seizure precaution equipment (mouth gag, nonmetal airway, suction apparatus).
- Be aware that gingival hyperplasia appears most commonly in children and adolescents and never occurs in patients without teeth.
- Make sure patients on prolonged therapy have adequate intake of vitamin D-containing foods and sufficient exposure to sunlight.
- Monitor diabetics for loss of glycemic control.
- Check periodically for decrease in serum calcium levels. Particularly susceptible: patients receiving other anticonvulsants concurrently, as well as those who are inactive, have limited exposure to sun, or whose dietary intake is inadequate.
- Observe for symptoms of folic acid deficiency: neuropathy, mental dysfunction.
- Be alert to symptoms of hypomagnesemia (see Appendix F); neuromuscular symptoms: tetany, positive Chvostek's and Trousseau's signs, seizures, tremors, ataxia, vertigo, nystagmus, muscular fasciculations.

Patient & Family Education

- Be aware that drug may make urine pink or red to red-brown.
- Report symptoms of fatigue, dry skin, deepening voice when receiving long-term therapy because phenytoin can unmask a low thyroid reserve.
- Do not alter prescribed drug regimen. Stopping drug abruptly may precipitate seizures and status epilepticus.
- Do not to request/accept change in drug brand when refilling prescription without consulting physician.
- Understand the effects of alcohol: Alcohol intake may increase phenytoin serum levels, leading to phenytoin toxicity.
- Discontinue drug immediately if a measles-like skin rash or jaundice appears and notify physician.
- Be aware that influenza vaccine during phenytoin treatment may increase seizure activity. Under-

P

stand that a change in dose may be necessary.

- Do not breast feed while taking this drug.

PHYSOSTIGMINE SALICYLATE

(fi-zoe-stig′meen)

Antilirium

Classifications: AUTONOMIC NERVOUS SYSTEM AGENT; CHOLINERGIC (PARASYMPATHOMIMETIC); CHOLINESTERASE INHIBITOR

Prototype: Neostigmine

Pregnancy Category: C

AVAILABILITY 1 mg/mL injection

ACTIONS Reversible anticholinesterase and tertiary amine. Chief effect is increasing concentration of acetylcholine at cholinergic transmission sites which prolongs and exaggerates its action.

THERAPEUTIC EFFECTS Similar to neostigmine in actions and adverse effects, but produces greater secretion of glands, constriction of pupils, and effect on BP and less action on skeletal muscle. Also has direct blocking action on autonomic ganglia. Parenteral physostigmine can produce transient decrease in manic symptoms as well as precipitate mental depression.

USES To reverse CNS and cardiac effects of tricyclic antidepressant overdose, to reverse CNS toxic effects of atropine, scopolamine, and similar anticholinergic drugs, and to antagonize CNS depressant effects of diazepam. **Orphan Drug:** For hereditary ataxias.

CONTRAINDICATIONS Asthma; diabetes mellitus; gangrene, cardiovascular disease; mechanical obstruction of intestinal or urogenital tract; any vagotonic state; secondary glaucoma; inflammatory disease of iris or ciliary body; concomitant use with choline esters (e.g., methacholine, bethanechol) or depolarizing neuromuscular blocking agents (e.g., decamethonium, succinylcholine). Safety during pregnancy (category C) or lactation is not established.

CAUTIOUS USE Epilepsy; Parkinsonism; bradycardia; hyperthyroidism; peptic ulcer; hypotension.

ROUTE & DOSAGE

Reversal of Anticholinergic Effects

Adult: **IM/IV** 0.5–3 mg (IV not faster than 1 mg/min), repeat as needed

Child: **IV** 0.01–0.03 mg/kg, may repeat q15–20 min (max: total dose of 2 mg)

ADMINISTRATION

Intramuscular/Intravenous

- Give undiluted.
- Use only clear, colorless solutions. Red-tinted solution indicates oxidation, and such solutions should be discarded.

Intravenous

Note: Verify correct rate of IV injection for infants or children with physician.

PREPARE: **Direct:** Give undiluted.

ADMINISTER: **Direct:** Give at a slow rate, no more than 1 mg/min. Rapid administration and overdosage can cause a cholinergic crisis.

ADVERSE EFFECTS (≥1%) **Body as a Whole:** *Sweating,* cholinergic crisis (acute toxicity), hyperactivity, respiratory distress, convulsions. **CNS:** Restlessness, hallucinations, twitching, tremors, *sweating,*

P

weakness, ataxia, convulsions, collapse. **GI:** *Nausea, vomiting, epigastric pain, diarrhea, salivation.* **Urogenital:** Involuntary urination or defecation. **Special Senses:** Miosis, *lacrimation,* rhinorrhea. **Respiratory:** Dyspnea, bronchospasm, respiratory paralysis, pulmonary edema. **Cardiovascular:** Irregular pulse, palpitation, bradycardia, rise in BP.

INTERACTIONS Drug: Antagonizes effects of **echothiophate, isoflurophate.**

PHARMACOKINETICS Absorption: Readily absorbed from mucous membranes, muscle, subcutaneous tissue; 10%–12% absorbed from GI tract. **Onset:** 3–8 min IM/IV. **Duration:** 0.5–5 h IM/IV. **Distribution:** Crosses blood-brain barrier. **Metabolism:** Metabolized in plasma by cholinesterase. **Elimination:** Excretion not fully understood; small amounts excreted in urine. **Half-Life:** 15–40 min.

P

NURSING IMPLICATIONS

Assessment & Drug Effects

- Monitor vital signs and state of consciousness closely in patients receiving drug for atropine poisoning. Since physostigmine is usually rapidly eliminated, patient can lapse into delirium and coma within 1 to 2 h; repeat doses may be required.
- Monitor closely for adverse effects related to CNS and for signs of sensitivity to physostigmine. Have atropine sulfate readily available for clinical emergency.
- Discontinue parenteral or oral drug if following symptoms arise: Excessive salivation, emesis, frequent urination, or diarrhea.
- Eliminate excessive sweating or nausea with dose reduction.

PHYTONADIONE (VITAMIN K_1)

(fye-toe-na-dye'one)

AquaMEPHYTON, Konakion, Mephyton, Phylloquinone

Classifications: HORMONES AND SYNTHETIC SUBSTITUTES; VITAMIN; ANTIDOTE

Pregnancy Category: C

AVAILABILITY 5 mg tablets; 2 mg/mL, 10 mg/mL injection

ACTIONS Fat-soluble naphthoquinone derivative chemically identical to and with similar activity as naturally occurring vitamin K. Vitamin K is essential for hepatic biosynthesis of blood clotting Factors II, VII, IX, and X.

THERAPEUTIC EFFECTS Promotes liver synthesis of clotting factors by unknown mechanism. Does not reverse anticoagulant action of heparin. Reportedly demonstrates wide margin of safety when used in newborns.

USES Drug of choice as antidote for overdosage of coumarin and indandione oral anticoagulants. Also reverses hypoprothrombinemia secondary to administration of oral antibiotics, quinidine, quinine, salicylates, sulfonamides, excessive vitamin A, and secondary to inadequate absorption and synthesis of vitamin K (as in obstructive jaundice, biliary fistula, ulcerative colitis, intestinal resection, prolonged hyperalimentation). Also prophylaxis of and therapy for neonatal hemorrhagic disease.

CONTRAINDICATIONS Hypersensitivity to AquaMEPHYTON; severe liver disease.

CAUTIOUS USE Pregnancy (category C); lactation. Effect on fertility and teratogenic potential is not known.

ROUTE & DOSAGE

Anticoagulant Overdose

Adult: **PO/SC/IM** 2.5–10 mg; rarely up to 50 mg/d, may repeat parenteral dose after 6–8 h if needed or PO dose after 12–24 h

IV Emergency only: 10–15 mg at a rate of ≤1 mg/min, may be repeated in 4 h if bleeding continues

Hemorrhagic Disease of Newborns

Infant: **IM/SC** 0.5–1 mg immediately after delivery, may repeat in 6–8 h if necessary

Other Prothrombin Deficiencies

Adult: **IM/SC** 2–25 mg
Child: **IM/SC** 5–10 mg
Infant: **IM/SC** 1 mg

ADMINISTRATION

Intramuscular

Note: Konakion, which contains a phenol preservative, is intended ONLY for IM use. AquaMEPHYTON may be given SC, IM, or IV as prescribed.

- Give IM injection in adults and older children in upper outer quadrant of buttocks. For infants and young children, anterolateral aspect of thigh or deltoid region is preferred.
- Aspirate carefully to avoid intravascular injection.
- Apply gentle pressure to site following injection. Swelling (internal bleeding) and pain sometimes occur with SC or IM administration.

Intravenous

Note: Reserve IV route only for emergencies.

PREPARE: **Direct:** Dilute a single dose in 10 mL D5W, NS, or D5/NS.

ADMINISTER: **Direct:** Give solution immediately after dilution at a rate not to exceed 1 mg/min.

INCOMPATIBILITIES **Solution/additive: Ranitidine Y-site: Dobutamine.**

- Protect infusion solution from light by wrapping container with aluminum foil or other opaque material.
- Discard unused solution and contents in open ampul.

ADVERSE EFFECTS (≥1%) **Body as a Whole:** Hypersensitivity or anaphylaxis-like reaction: facial flushing, cramp-like pains, convulsive movements, chills, fever, diaphoresis, weakness, dizziness, shock, cardiac arrest. **CNS:** Headache (after oral dose), brain damage, death. **GI:** Gastric upset. **Hematologic:** Paradoxic hypoprothrombinemia (patients with severe liver disease), severe hemolytic anemia. **Metabolic:** Hyperbilirubinemia, kernicterus. **Respiratory:** Bronchospasm, dyspnea, sensation of chest constriction, respiratory arrest. **Skin:** Pain at injection site, hematoma, and nodule formation, erythematous skin eruptions (with repeated injections). **Special Senses:** Peculiar taste sensation.

DIAGNOSTIC TEST INTERFERENCE Falsely elevated ***urine steroids*** (by modifications of ***Reddy, Jenkins, Thorn procedure***).

INTERACTIONS Drug: Antagonizes effects of **warfarin, cholestyramine, colestipol, mineral oil** decrease absorption of oral phytonadione.

PHARMACOKINETICS Absorption: Readily absorbed from intestinal

P

lymph only if bile is present. **Onset:** 6–12 h PO; 1–2 h IM/SC; 15 min IV. **Peak:** Hemorrhage usually controlled within 3–8 h; normal prothrombin time may be obtained in 12–14 h after administration. **Distribution:** Concentrates briefly in liver after absorption; crosses placenta; distributed into breast milk. **Metabolism:** Rapidly metabolized in liver. **Elimination:** Excreted in urine and bile.

NURSING IMPLICATIONS

Assessment & Drug Effects

- Monitor patient constantly. Severe reactions, including fatalities, have occurred during and immediately after IV injection (see ADVERSE EFFECTS).
- Lab tests: Baseline and frequent PT/INR.
- Frequency, dose, and therapy duration are guided by PT/INR clinical response.
- Monitor therpeutic effectiveness which is indicated by shortened PT, INR, bleeding, and clotting times, as well as decreased hemorrhagic tendencies.
- Be aware that patients on large doses may develop temporary resistance to coumarin-type anticoagulants. If oral anticoagulant is reinstituted, larger than former doses may be needed. Some patients may require change to heparin.

Patient & Family Education

- Maintain consistency in diet and avoid significant increases in daily intake of vitamin K-rich foods when drug regimen is stabilized. Know sources rich in vitamin K: Asparagus, broccoli, cabbage, lettuce, turnip greens, pork or beef liver, green tea, spinach, watercress, and tomatoes.

PILOCARPINE HYDROCHLORIDE Pr

PILOCARPINE NITRATE

(pye-loe-kar′peen)

Adsorbocarpine, Isopto Carpine, Minims Pilocarpine ✦, Miocarpine ✦, Ocusert, Pilo, Pilocar, Salagen

Classifications: EYE PREPARATION; MIOTIC (ANTIGLAUCOMA AGENT); AUTONOMIC NERVOUS SYSTEM AGENT; DIRECT-ACTING CHOLINERGIC (PARASYMPATHOMIMETIC)

Pregnancy Category: C

AVAILABILITY 0.25%, 0.5%, 1%, 2%, 3%, 4%, 5%, 6%, 8%, 10% ophthalmic solution; 4% ophthalmic gel; 20 mcg/h, 40 mcg/h ocular insert; 5 mg tablets

ACTIONS Tertiary amine that acts directly on cholinergic receptor sites, thus mimicking acetylcholine. Induces miosis, spasm of accommodation, and fall in intraocular pressure (IOP) that may be preceded by a transitory rise.

THERAPEUTIC EFFECTS Decrease in IOP results from stimulation of ciliary and papillary sphincter muscles, which pull iris away from filtration angle, thus facilitating outflow of aqueous humor. Also decreases production of aqueous humor.

USES Open-angle and angle-closure glaucomas; to reduce IOP and to protect the lens during surgery and laser iridotomy; to counteract effects of mydriatics and cycloplegics following surgery or ophthalmoscopic examination; to treat xerostomia.

CONTRAINDICATIONS Secondary glaucoma, acute iritis, acute inflammatory disease of anterior segment of eye; pregnancy (category C), lactation.

CAUTIOUS USE Bronchial asthma; hypertension. **Ocular therapeutic system:** Not used in acute infectious conjunctivitis, keratitis, retinal detachment, or when intense miosis is required.

ROUTE & DOSAGE

Acute Glaucoma

Adult/Child: **Ophthalmic** 1 drop of 1%–2% solution in affected eye q5–10min for 3–6 doses, then 1 drop q1–3h until IOP is reduced

Chronic Glaucoma

Adult/Child: **Ophthalmic** 1 drop of 0.5%–4% solution in affected eye q4–12h or 1 ocular system (Ocusert) q7d

Miotic

Adult/Child: **Ophthalmic** 1 drop of 1% solution in affected eye

Xerostomia

Adult: **PO** 5 mg t.i.d., may increase up to 10 mg t.i.d.

ADMINISTRATION

Instillation

- Note: During acute phase, physician may prescribe instillation of drug into unaffected eye to prevent bilateral attack of acute glaucoma.
- Apply gentle digital pressure to periphery of nasolacrimal drainage system for 1–2 min immediately after instillation of drops to prevent delivery of drug to nasal mucosa and general circulation.

ADVERSE EFFECTS (≥1%) **CNS:** Oral (asthenia, headaches, dizziness, chills). **Special Senses:** Ciliary spasm with brow ache, twitching of eyelids, eye pain with change in eye focus, miosis, *diminished vision in poorly illuminated areas,* blurred vision, reduced visual acuity, sensitivity, contact allergy, lacrimation, follicular conjunctivitis, conjunctival irritation, cataract, <u>retinal detachment</u>. **GI:** *Nausea,* vomiting, abdominal cramps, diarrhea, epigastric distress, *salivation*. **Respiratory:** Bronchospasm, rhinitis. **CV:** Tachycardia. **Body as a Whole:** Tremors, *increased sweating,* urinary frequency.

INTERACTIONS Drug: The actions of pilocarpine and **carbachol** are additive when used concomitantly. Oral form may cause conduction disturbances with BETA BLOCKERS. Antagonizes the effects of concurrent ANTICHOLINERGIC DRUGS (e.g., **atropine, ipratropium**). **Food:** high-fat meal decreases absorption of pilocarpine.

PHARMACOKINETICS Absorption: Topical penetrates cornea rapidly; readily absorbed from GI tract. **Onset:** Miosis 10–30 min; IOP reduction 60 min; salivary stimulation 20 min. **Peak:** Miosis 30 min; IOP reduction 75 min; salivary stimulation 60 min. **Duration:** Miosis 4–8 h; IOP reduction 4–14 h (7 d with Ocusert); salivary stimulation 3–5 h. **Metabolism:** Inactivated at neuronal synapses and in plasma. **Elimination:** Excreted in urine. **Half-Life:** 0.76–1.35 h.

NURSING IMPLICATIONS

Assessment & Drug Effects

- Be aware that hourly tonometric tests may be done during early treatment because drug may cause an initial transitory increase in IOP.
- Monitor changes in visual acuity.
- Monitor for adverse effects. Brow pain and myopia tend to be more prominent in younger patients and generally disappear with continued use of drug.

Patient & Family Education

- Understand that therapy for glaucoma is prolonged and that adherence to established regimen is crucial to prevent blindness.
- Do not drive or engage in potentially hazardous activities until vision clears. Drug causes blurred vision and difficulty in focusing.
- Discontinue medication if symptoms of irritation or sensitization persist and report to physician.
- Do not breast feed while taking this drug without consulting physician.

Ocular Therapeutic System (Ocusert)

- Review information/directions about inserting the ocular system included in the drug package with health care provider. Demonstrate to establish ability to adjust, insert, and remove the system.
- Unit is placed in the eye cul-de-sac, where it remains for a week. Slow release of drug provides a nonfluctuating concentration of pilocarpine in the ciliary body and iris.
- Induced myopia, miosis, and spasm of accommodation are less than that produced by eyedrops. However, since transient blurring and dimness of vision may occur following Ocusert insertion, have patient do so at bedtime; myopia will be at a stable level in the a.m.
- Several hours after Ocusert insertion, induced myopia decreases to a low base level that persists for the life of the therapeutic system.
- Notify physician if following symptoms do not subside: Conjunctival irritation with mild erythema and increase in mucus secretion; generally accompany early use of Ocusert.
- Wash system with cool tap water before replacing it into cul-de-sac if it contacts an unclean surface.
- If retention of the system is a problem, the superior conjunctival cul-de-sac may be a preferred site for insertion. This location is also preferred during sleep.
- To change placement: Ocusert may be transferred from the lower conjunctival sac to the superior sac by closing eyelids, rolling the eye toward the nose and, with gentle digital pressure through the closed eyelid, directly moving the system. Avoid moving it over the colored part of the eye.
- Remove system and replace with a new one if an unexpected increase in drug action occurs (sudden miosis, ciliary spasm, decreased visual acuity).

PIMECROLIMUS

(pim-e-cro-lim′us)
Elidel
Classification: IMMUNOSUPPRESSANT
Prototype: Cyclosporine
Pregnancy Category: C

AVAILABILITY 1% cream

ACTIONS Pimecrolimus selectively inhibits the inflammatory action of skin cells by blocking T-cell activation and cytokine release. It appears to inhibit the production of IL-2, IL-4, IL-10, and interferon gamma in T-cells. It also prevents release of inflammatory cytokines and mediators from mast cells after activation by antigen and IgE.

THERAPEUTIC EFFECTS Topically applied to the skin, pimecrolimus produces significant antiinflammatory activity without evidence of skin atrophy. (Topical steroids can cause skin atrophy along with their antiinflammatory activity).

USES Short-term intermittent mild to moderate atopic dermatitis.

CONTRAINDICATIONS Hypersensitivity to pimecrolimus or components in the cream; Netherton's syndrome; application to active cutaneous viral infection.
CAUTIOUS USE Infection at topical treatment sites; history of untoward effects with topical cyclosporine or tacrolimus; skin papillomas; immunocompromised patients.

ROUTE & DOSAGE

Atopic Dermatitis
Adult: **Topical** Apply thin layer to affected skin b.i.d.

ADMINISTRATION

Topical

- Do not apply to any skin surface that appears to be infected.

ADVERSE EFFECTS (≥1%) **Body as a Whole:** Flu-like symptoms, infections, fever. **CNS:** Headache. **GI:** Gastroenteritis, abdominal pain, nausea, vomiting, diarrhea, constipation. **Respiratory:** Sore throat, *upper respiratory infection, cough,* nasal congestion, asthma exacerbation, rhinitis, epistaxis. **Skin:** *Burning,* irritation, pruritus, skin infection, impetigo, folliculitis, skin papilloma, Herpes simplex dermatitis, urticaria, acne. **Special Senses:** Ear infection, earache, conjunctivitis.

INTERACTIONS Drug: No clinically significant interactions established.

PHARMACOKINETICS Absorption: Minimal absorption through intact skin. **Metabolism:** No evidence of skin-mediated metabolism, metabolized in liver by CYP 3A. **Elimination:** Primarily excreted in feces.

NURSING IMPLICATIONS

Assessment & Drug Effects

- Assess for and report persistent skin irritation that develops following application of the cream and lasts for more than 1 wk.

Patient & Family Education

- Minimize exposure of treated area to natural or artificial sunlight.
- Stop topical application once signs of dermatitis have disappeared. Resume application at the first sign of recurrence.
- Wash hand thoroughly after application if hands are not the treatment sites.
- Report any significant skin irritation that results from application of the cream.

PIMOZIDE

(pi'moe-zide)

Orap

Classifications: CENTRAL NERVOUS SYSTEM AGENT; PSYCHOTHERAPEUTIC; ANTIPSYCHOTIC; BUTYROPHENONE
Prototype: Haloperidol
Pregnancy Category: C

AVAILABILITY 2 mg tablet

ACTIONS Potent central dopamine antagonist that alters release and turnover of central dopamine stores; has no effect on turnover of norepinephrine.
THERAPEUTIC EFFECTS Blockade of CNS dopaminergic receptors results in suppression of the motor and phonic tics that characterize Tourette's disorder. Produces less sedation and fewer extrapyramidal reactions than haloperidol; lowers seizure threshold.

USES To suppress severe motor and phonic tics in patient with Tourette's disorder who has failed to respond satisfactorily to standard treatment (e.g., haloperidol).

P

CONTRAINDICATIONS Treatment of simple tics other than those associated with Tourette's disorder; drug-induced tics; history of cardiac dysrhythmias and conditions marked by prolonged QT syndrome, patient taking drugs that may prolong QT interval (e.g., quinidine); severe toxic CNS depression. Safety in children <12 y, during pregnancy (category C), or lactation is not established.

CAUTIOUS USE Kidney and liver dysfunction; patients receiving anticonvulsant therapy.

ROUTE & DOSAGE

Tourette's Disorder

Adult: **PO** 1–2 mg/d in divided doses, gradually increase dose q.o.d. up to 0.2 mg/kg/d or 7–16 mg/d in divided doses whichever is less (max: 0.2 mg/kg/d or 10 mg/d)

ADMINISTRATION

Oral

- Increase drug dose gradually, usually over 1–3 wk, until maintenance dose is reached.
- Follow regimen prescribed by physician for withdrawal: Usually slow, gradual changes over a period of days or weeks (drug has a long half-life). Sudden withdrawal may cause reemergence of original symptoms (motor and phonic tics) and of neuromuscular adverse effects of the drug.

ADVERSE EFFECTS (≥1%) **Body as a Whole:** *Akathisia,* speech disorder, *torticollis, tremor,* handwriting changes, *akinesia,* fainting, hyperpyrexia, tardive dyskinesia, *rigidity, oculogyric crisis,* hyperreflexia; seizures, neuroleptic malignant syndrome; *extrapyramidal dysfunction,* hyperthermia, autonomic dysfunction; diaphoresis, weight changes, asthenia, chest pain, periorbital edema. **CNS:** Headache, *sedation, drowsiness,* insomnia, seizures, stupor. **CV:** Prolongation of QT interval, inverted or flattened T wave, appearance of U wave, labile blood pressure. **Urogenital:** Loss of libido, impotence, nocturia, urinary frequency, amenorrhea, dysmenorrhea, mild glactorrhea, urinary retention, acute renal failure. **Respiratory:** Dyspnea, respiratory failure. **Skin:** Sweating, skin irritation. **Special Senses:** Visual disturbances, photosensitivity, decreased accommodation, blurred vision, cataracts. **GI:** Increased salivation, nausea, vomiting, diarrhea, anorexia, abdominal cramps, constipation.

INTERACTIONS Drug: Alcohol and other CNS DEPRESSANTS increase CNS depression; ANTICHOLINERGIC AGENTS (e.g., TRICYCLIC ANTIDEPRESSANTS, **atropine**) increase anticholinergic effects; PHENOTHIAZINES, TRICYCLIC ANTIDEPRESSANTS, ANTIARRHYTHMICS, MACROLIDE ANTIBIOTICS, AZOLE ANTIFUNGALS **(itraconazole, ketoconazole, fluconazole)**, PROTEASE INHIBITORS, **nefazodone, sertraline, zileuton** increase risk of arrhythmias and heart block; pimozide antagonizes effects of ANTICONVULSANTS—there is loss of seizure control. **Food: Grapefruit juice** may inhibit metabolism of pimozide.

PHARMACOKINETICS Absorption: Slowly and variably absorbed from GI tract (40%–50% absorbed). **Peak:** 6–8 h. **Metabolism:** Metabolized in liver to 2 major metabolites by CYP3A4. **Elimination:** 80%–85% excreted in urine, 15–20% in feces. **Half-Life:** 55 h.

NURSING IMPLICATIONS

Note: See haloperidol for additional nursing implications.

Assessment & Drug Effects

- Obtain ECG baseline data at beginning of therapy and check periodically, especially during dosage adjustments.
- Notify physician immediately for widening or prolongation of the QT interval, which suggests developing cardiotoxicity (QT interval [QRS complex and T wave] representing both ventricular depolarization and repolarization).
- Risk of tardive dyskinesia appears to be greatest in women, older adults, and those on high-dose therapy.
- Be aware that extrapyramidal reactions often appear within the first few days of therapy, are dose-related, and usually occur when dose is high.
- Be aware that anticholinergic effects (dry mouth, constipation) may increase as dose is increased.

Patient & Family Education

- Adhere to established drug regimen (i.e., do not change dose or intervals and discontinue only with physician's guidance).
- Use measures to relieve dry mouth (frequent rinsing with water, saliva substitute, increased fluid intake) and constipation (increased dietary fiber, drink 6–8 glasses of water daily).
- Do not drive or engage in potentially hazardous activities because drug-caused hand tremors, drowsiness, and blurred vision may impair alertness and abilities.
- Pseudoparkinsonism symptoms are usually mild and reversible with dose adjustment.
- Be alert to the earliest symptom of tardive dyskinesia ("flycatching"—an involuntary movement of the tongue), and report promptly to the physician.
- Return to physician for periodic assessments of therapy benefit and cardiac status.
- Understand dangers of ingesting alcohol to prevent augmenting CNS depressant effects of pimozide.
- Do not breast feed while taking this drug without consulting physician.

PINDOLOL

(pin'doe-lole)

Visken

Classifications: BETA-ADRENERGIC ANTAGONIST (BLOCKING AGENT); SYMPATHOLYTIC; ANTIHYPERTENSIVE

Prototype: Propranolol

Pregnancy Category: B

AVAILABILITY 5 mg, 10 mg tablets

ACTIONS Nonselective beta-adrenergic blocking agent. Possesses slight intrinsic sympathomimetic activity (ISA) or partial beta agonist effect in therapeutic dose ranges. Hypotensive mechanism is similar to that of propranolol. It competitively blocks beta-adrenergic receptors primarily in myocardium, and beta receptors within bronchial and smooth muscle.

THERAPEUTIC EFFECTS Exerts vasodilator as well as hypotensive effects. Has negative chronotropic and inotropic properties and slows conduction in AV node. Does not consistently affect cardiac output, resting heart rate, or renin release; it does, however, decrease peripheral vascular resistance.

USES Management of hypertension concurrently with a thiazide diuretic or as single agent. Used in patient who has failed to respond to diet, exercise, and weight reduction.

UNLABELED USES Stress and exercise-induced chronic stable angina pectoris.

CONTRAINDICATIONS Bronchospastic diseases; severe bradycardia, cardiogenic shock, cardiac failure. Safety in pregnancy (category B), lactation, or children is not established.

CAUTIOUS USE Nonallergic bronchospasm; CHF; diabetes mellitus; hyperthyroidism; impaired liver and kidney function.

ROUTE & DOSAGE

Hypertension

Adult: **PO** 5 mg b.i.d., may increase by 10 mg/d q2–3wk if needed up (max: 60 mg/d in 2–3 divided doses)

Geriatric: **PO** Start with 5 mg q.d.

Angina Pectoris

Adult: **PO** 15–40 mg/d in 3–4 divided doses

P

ADMINISTRATION

Oral

- Give drug at same time of day each day with respect to time of food intake for most predictable results.
- Withdraw or discontinue treatment gradually over a period of 1–2 wk.

ADVERSE EFFECTS (≥1%) **CNS:** *Fatigue,* dizziness, insomnia, drowsiness, confusion, fainting, decreased libido. **CV:** *Bradycardia,* hypotension, CHF. **GI:** Nausea, *diarrhea, constipation,* flatulence. **Respiratory:** Bronchospasm, pulmonary edema, dyspnea. **Body as a Whole:** Back or joint pain. Sensitivity reactions seen as antinuclear antibodies (ANA) (10%–30% of patients). **Hematologic:** Agranulocytosis. **Urogenital:** Impotence. **Metabolic:** Hypoglycemia (may mask symptoms of a hypoglycemic reaction).

INTERACTIONS Drug: DIURETICS and other HYPOTENSIVE AGENTS increase hypotensive effect; effects of **albuterol, metaproterenol, terbutaline, pirbuterol** and pindolol antagonized; NSAIDS blunt hypotensive effect; decreases hypoglycemic effect of **glyburide; amiodarone** increases risk of bradycardia and sinus arrest.

PHARMACOKINETICS Absorption: Rapidly absorbed from GI tract; 50%–95% reaches systemic circulation (first pass metabolism). **Onset:** 3 h. **Peak:** 1–2 h. **Duration:** 24 h. **Distribution:** Distributed into breast milk. **Metabolism:** 40%–60% metabolized in liver. **Elimination:** Excreted in urine. **Half-Life:** 3–4 h.

NURSING IMPLICATIONS

Assessment & Drug Effects

- Monitor HR and BP. Report bradycardia and hypotension. Dosage adjustment may be indicated.
- Note: Hypotensive effect may begin within 7 d but is not at maximum therapeutically until about 2 wk after beginning of treatment.
- Lab test: Periodic CBC with differential, kidney function tests, and blood glucose.

Patient & Family Education

- Pindolol masks the dizziness and sweating symptoms of hypoglycemia. Monitor blood glucose for loss of glycemic control.
- Adhere to the prescribed drug regimen; if a change is desired, consult physician first. Abrupt withdrawal of drug might precipitate a thyroid crisis in a patient with hyperthyroidism, and angina in the patient with ischemic heart disease, leading to an MI.

- Do not breast feed while taking this drug without consulting physician.

PIOGLITAZONE HYDROCHLORIDE

(pi-o-glit'a-zone)

Actos

Classifications: HORMONES AND SYNTHETIC SUBSTITUTES; ANTIDIABETIC; THIAZOLIDINEDIONE

Prototype: Rosiglitazone Maleate

Pregnancy Category: C

AVAILABILITY 15 mg, 30 mg, 45 mg tablets

ACTIONS Results in insulin sensitivity by affecting insulin receptors. Decreases hepatic glucose output and increases insulin-dependent muscle glucose uptake in skeletal muscle and adipose tissue.

THERAPEUTIC EFFECTS Improves glycemic control in noninsulin dependent diabetic (type 2) patients by enhancing insulin sensitivity of cells without stimulating pancreatic insulin secretion. Indicated by improved blood glucose levels and decreased HbA_{1C}.

USES Adjunct to diet in the treatment of type 2 diabetes mellitus.

CONTRAINDICATIONS Hypersensitivity to pioglitazone, troglitazone, rosiglitazone, englitazone; type 1 diabetes, or treatment of DKA; active liver disease or ALT levels >2.5 times normal limit; pregnancy (category C), lactation.

CAUTIOUS USE Liver dysfunction; cardiovascular disease (New York Heart Association [NYHA]) Class III and Class IV (e.g., CHF); hypertension, edema; renal impairment; older adults. Safety and efficacy in children <18 y are not established.

ROUTE & DOSAGE

Type 2 Diabetes Mellitus

Adult: **PO** 15–30 mg once daily (max: 45 mg q.d.)

ADMINISTRATION

Oral

- Give without regard to food.
- Do not initiate therapy if baseline serum ALT >2.5 times normal.
- Store at 15°–30° C (59°–86° F) in tightly closed container; protect from humidity and moisture.

ADVERSE EFFECTS (≥1%) **Body as a Whole:** Headache, myalgia, edema. **CV:** Edema, fluid retention, exacerbation of heart failure. **GI:** Tooth disorder. **Respiratory:** *Upper respiratory tract infection,* sinusitis, pharyngitis. **Metabolic:** Hypoglycemia, mild anemia.

INTERACTIONS Drug: Pioglitazone may decrease serum levels of ORAL CONTRACEPTIVES; **ketoconazole** may increase serum levels of **pioglitazone. Herbal: Garlic, ginseng** may potentiate hypoglycemic effects.

PHARMACOKINETICS Absorption: Rapidly absorbed. **Peak:** 2 h; steady state concentrations within 7 d. **Duration:** 24 h. **Distribution:** >99% protein bound. **Metabolism:** Metabolized in liver to active metabolites. **Elimination:** Primarily excreted in bile and feces. **Half-Life:** 16–24 h.

NURSING IMPLICATIONS

Assessment & Drug Effects

- Monitor for S&S hypoglycemia (possible when insulin/sulfonylureas are coadministered).
- Monitor closely for S&S of CHF or exacerbation of symptoms with preexisting CHF.
- Lab tests: Baseline serum ALT, then q2mo for first y, then period-

P

ically (more often if elevated); periodic HbA_{1c}, Hgb and Hct, and lipid profile.

- Discontinue drug if ALT >3 times ULN or patient has jaundice.
- Monitor weight and notify physician of development of edema.

Patient & Family Education

- Be aware that resumed ovulation is possible in nonovulating premenopausal women.
- Use or add barrier contraceptive if using hormonal contraception.
- Report immediately to physician: Unexplained anorexia, nausea, vomiting, abdominal pain, fatigue, dark urine; or S&S of fluid retention such as weight gain, edema, or activity intolerance.
- Combination therapy: May need adjustment of other antidiabetic drugs to avoid hypoglycemia.
- Learn of and adhere strictly to guideliness for liver function tests. Be sure to have blood tests for liver function every 2 mo for first y; then periodically.
- Do not breast feed while taking this drug.

P

PIPECURONIUM BROMIDE

(pi-pe-cu-ron'i-um)

Arduan

Classifications: AUTONOMIC NERVOUS SYSTEM AGENT; NONDEPOLARIZING SKELETAL MUSCLE RELAXANT

Prototype: Tubocurarine

Pregnancy Category: C

AVAILABILITY 10 mg injection

ACTIONS Nondepolarizing neuromuscular blocking agent. Appears to lack vagolytic or autonomic activity and results in minimal cardiovascular effects.

THERAPEUTIC EFFECTS Drug of choice in coronary artery bypass surgery and patients with coronary artery disease because it does not appear to cause tachycardia or elevated blood pressure as observed with other neuromuscular blocking agents.

USES Adjunct to general anesthesia, and to provide skeletal muscle relaxation during surgery. Should only be used for procedures expected to last ≥90 min.

UNLABELED USES Skeletal muscle relaxation for endotracheal intubation.

CONTRAINDICATIONS Hypersensitivity to pipecuronium or bromide.

CAUTIOUS USE Patients with myasthenia gravis; renal failure; hepatic insufficiency; amyotrophic lateral sclerosis (ALS); burn patients; children and infants; pregnancy (category C), lactation.

ROUTE & DOSAGE

Adjunct for General Anesthesia

Adult/Child: **IV** 85 to 100 mcg/kg, ideal body weight, given as rapid bolus over 5–10 s or may give over 1 min if desired **IV Maintenance** Smaller supplemental doses (usually 5–25 mcg/kg) may be given to maintain muscle relaxation during long surgical procedures

Renal Impairment

Cl_{cr} Dose based on ideal body weight: <80 mL/min: 70 mcg/kg; <60 mL/min: 55 mcg/kg; <40 mL/min: 50 mcg/kg

ADMINISTRATION

Intravenous

PREPARE: **Direct:** Reconstitute 10 mg vial with 10 mL of sterile water for injection, bacteriostatic water for injection (not for use in newborns), D5W, NS, D5/NS, or RL. Do not dilute into or administer from large-volume IV solutions. Refrigerate when reconstituted and use within 24 h.

ADMINISTER: **Direct:** Give a single dose over 10–15 sec.

ADVERSE EFFECTS (≥1%) **CV:** Bradycardia, hypotension. **Musculoskeletal:** Prolonged duration of action resulting in muscle weakness to paralysis resulting in respiratory insufficiency or apnea.

INTERACTIONS Drug: Capreomycin may increase the action of neuromuscular blocking agents. **Enflurane, isoflurane** may prolong the pipecuronium-induced neuromuscular blockade. Dose reductions of pipecuronium may be needed.

PHARMACOKINETICS Onset: 2–3 min. **Peak:** 3–6 min. **Duration:** Dose dependent: 50–70 mcg/kg lasts approximately 1 h. Concomitant anesthetic agents will also affect duration of action. **Distribution:** Approximately 32% protein bound (animal studies). **Metabolism:** Partially metabolized in the liver. It is unknown if metabolites have any pharmacologic activity. **Elimination:** Excreted by the kidneys. About 56% of the dose is excreted in the urine within 24 h. **Half-Life:** 137–161 min.

NURSING IMPLICATIONS

Assessment & Drug Effects

- Monitor hemodynamic status; clinically significant bradycardia, hypotension, and hypertension have occurred in a small percentage (<3%) of patients.
- Use a peripheral nerve stimulator to monitor drug response.

PIPERACILLIN SODIUM

(pi-per'a-sill-in)

Pipracil

Classifications: ANTIINFECTIVE; BETA-LACTAM ANTIBIOTIC; ANTIPSEUDOMONAL PENICILLIN

Prototype: Mezlocillin

Pregnancy Category: B

AVAILABILITY 2 g, 3 g, 4 g injection

ACTIONS Action is similar to that of other penicillins. Interference with bacterial cell wall synthesis promotes loss of membrane integrity and leads to death of the organism.

THERAPEUTIC EFFECTS Extended-spectrum parenteral penicillin with antibiotic activity against most gram-negative and many gram-positive anaerobic and aerobic organisms including members of *Clostridium, Bacteroides, Klebsiella, Enterobacter, Pseudomonas, Proteus,* and *Serratia* species and the anaerobic and aerobic cocci. Less active than penicillin G against *Pneumococci* and group A *Streptococci* but comparable to ampicillin against *Enterococci*. Penicillinase-producing *Staphylococci* are resistant to piperacillin.

USES Susceptible organisms that cause gynecologic, skin and skin structure, gonococcal, and streptococcal infections; lower respiratory tract, intraabdominal, and bone and joint infections; septicemia, urinary tract infections. Also prophylactically prior to and during surgery and as empiric antiinfective therapy in granulocytopenic patients.

CONTRAINDICATIONS Hypersensitivity to penicillins, cephalosporins, or other drugs. Safety in children <12 y, pregnancy (category B), lactation.

P

CAUTIOUS USE Liver and kidney dysfunction; hypersensitivity to cephalosporins.

ROUTE & DOSAGE

Uncomplicated Urinary Tract Infection

Adult: **IV/IM** 8–16 g/d divided q6–8h

Mild to Moderate Infections

Child: **IV** 200–300 mg/kg/d divided q4–6h (max: 24 g/d)
Neonate: **IV** 150–200 mg/kg/d divided q6–8h

Moderate to Severe Infections

Adult: **IV/IM** 4 g q6h (150–200 mg/kg/d)
Geriatric: **IV** 2–4 g q6–8h. **IM** 1–2 g q8–12h

Life-threatening Infection, *Pseudomonas* Infections

Adult: **IV/IM** 3 g q4h (max: 24 g/d)

Uncomplicated Gonococcal Infections

Adult: **IM** 2 g with 1 g probenecid given 30 min before piperacillin

ADMINISTRATION

Note: Patients undergoing hemodialysis usually receive a maximum dosage of 2 g piperacillin q8h and an additional 1 g dose after each dialysis period. Doses and frequency are usually modified if creatinine clearance is <40 mL/min.

Intramuscular

- Limit IM injections to 2 g/site. Use the gluteal muscle, preferably. Use deltoid muscle only if well developed.
- Diluents for reconstitution include sterile or bacteriostatic water for injection, bacteriostatic NaCl injection, and sterile lidocaine HCl injection 0.5%–1.0% without epinephrine for IM. When reconstituted, solution contains 1 g/2.5 mL.

Intravenous

Note: Verify correct IV concentration and rate of infusion for administration to neonates, infants, or children with physician.

PREPARE: **Direct:** (Not preferred): Reconstitute by diluting 1 g with 5 mL sterile water or NS for injection. Shake well until dissolved. **Intermittent:** (Preferred): Further dilute with 50–100 mL NS or D5W.

ADMINISTER: **Direct:** (Not preferred): Give over 3–5 min. Avoid rapid injection. **Intermittent:** (Preferred): Give over 30 min.

INCOMPATIBILITIES **Solution/additive:** AMINOGLYCOSIDES. **Y-site:** AMINOGLYCOSIDES, **amphotericin B cholesteryl complex, cisatracurium, filgrastim, fluconazole, gemcitabine, ondansetron, sargramostim, vinorelbine.**

ADVERSE EFFECTS (≥1%) **Body as a Whole:** Coughing, sneezing, feeling of uneasiness; systemic anaphylaxis, fever, widespread increase in capillary permeability and vasodilation with resulting edema (mouth, tongue, pharynx, larynx), laryngospasm, malaise, serum sickness (fever, malaise, pruritus, urticaria, lymphadenopathy, arthralgia, angioedema of face and extremities, neuritis prostration, eosinophilia), SLE-like syndrome, Injection site reactions (pain, inflammation, abscess, phlebitis), superinfections (especially with *Candida* and gram-negative bacteria), neuromuscular irritability (twitching, lethargy, confusion, stupor, hyperreflexia, multifocal myoclonus, localized or generalized seizures, coma). **CV:** Hypotension, circulatory collapse, cardiac arrhythmias, cardiac arrest. **GI:** Vomiting, diarrhea, severe abdominal cramps, nausea, epigastric distress, diarrhea, flatulence, dark discoloration of tongue, sore mouth or tongue. **Urogenital:** Interstitial nephritis, Loeffler's syndrome, vasculitis. **Hematologic:** Hemolytic anemia, thrombocytopenia. **Metabolic:** Hyperkalemia (penicillin G potassium); hypokalemia, alkalosis, hypernatremia, CHF (penicillin G sodium). **Respiratory:** Bronchospasm, asthma. **Skin:** Itchy palms or axilla, pruritus, *urticaria*, flushed skin, *delayed skin rashes* ranging from urticaria to exfoliative dermatitis, Stevens-Johnson syndrome, fixed-drug eruptions, contact dermatitis.

INTERACTIONS Drug: May increase risk of bleeding with ANTICOAGULANTS; **probenecid** decreases elimination of piperacillin.

PHARMACOKINETICS Peak: 45 min IM; 5 min IV. **Distribution:** Widely distributed with highest concentrations in urine and bile; adequate CSF penetration with inflamed meninges; crosses placenta; distributed into breast milk. **Metabolism:** Slightly metabolized in liver. **Elimination:** Primarily excreted in urine, partly in bile. **Half-Life:** 0.6–1.35 h.

NURSING IMPLICATIONS

Assessment & Drug Effects

- Obtain history of hypersensitivity to penicillins, cephalosporins, or other drugs prior to administration.
- Lab tests: C&S prior to first dose of the drug; start drug pending results. Periodic CBC with differential, platelet count, Hgb and Hct, and serum electrolytes.
- Monitor for hypersensitivity response; discontinue drug and notify physician if allergic response noted.
- Lab tests: Periodic CBC with differential, platelet count, Hgb and Hct, and serum electrolytes.
- Monitor for hemorrhagic manifestations because high doses may induce coagulation abnormalities.

Patient & Family Education

- Report significant, unexplained diarrhea.
- Withhold drug and report to physician if signs of an allergic reaction develop (e.g., itching, rash, hives).
- Do not breast feed while taking this drug without consulting physician.

PIPERACILLIN/TAZOBACTAM

(pi-per'a-cil-lin/taz-o-bac'tam)
Zosyn
Classifications: ANTIINFECTIVE; BETA-LACTAM ANTIBIOTIC; ANTIPSEUDOMONAL PENICILLIN
Prototype: Mezlocillin
Pregnancy Category: B

P

AVAILABILITY 2 g, 3 g, 4 g injection

ACTIONS Antibacterial combination product consisting of the semisynthetic piperacillin and the beta-lactamase inhibitor tazobactam. Tazobactam component does not decrease the activity of the piperacillin component against susceptible organisms.

THERAPEUTIC EFFECTS Tazobactam is an inhibitor of a wide variety of bacterial beta–lactamases. It has little antibacterial activity itself; however, in combination with piperacillin, it extends the spectrum of bacteria that are susceptible to piperacillin. Two-drug combination has antibiotic activity against an extremely broad spectrum of gram-positive, gram-negative, and anaerobic bacteria.

USES Treatment of moderate to severe appendicitis, uncomplicated and complicated skin and skin structure infections, endometritis, pelvic inflammatory disease, or nosocomial or community-acquired pneumonia caused by piperacillin-resistant, piperacillin/tazobactam-susceptible, beta-lactamase-producing bacteria.

CONTRAINDICATIONS Hypersensitivity to piperacillin, tazobactam, penicillins, cephalosporins, or beta-lactamase inhibitors such as clavulanic acid and sulbactam.
CAUTIOUS USE Kidney failure; pregnancy (category B), lactation.

ROUTE & DOSAGE

Moderate to Severe Infections
Adult: **IV** 3.375 g q6h, infused over 30 min, for 7–10 d
Child: **IV** *<6 mo,* 150–300 mg piperacillin/kg/d divided q6–8h; *≥6 mo,* 240 mg piperacillin component/kg/d divided q8h

Nosocomial Pneumonia
Adult: **IV** 4.5 g q6h, infused over 30 min, for 7–10 d

Renal Insufficiency
Cl_{cr} 20–40 mL/min: 2.25 g q6h; <20 mL/min: 2.25 g q8h

ADMINISTRATION

Note: Verify correct IV concentration and rate of infusion for administration to infants or children with physician.

Intravenous
For hemodialysis patients, the maximum dose is 2.25 g q8h; give one extra 0.75g dose after each dialysis period.
PREPARE: **Intermittent:** Reconstitute powder with 5 mL of diluent (e.g., D5W, NS); shake well until dissolved. Further dilute to at least 50 mL of selected diluent. Use single-dose vials immediately after reconstitution.
ADMINISTER: **Intermittent:** Give over at least 30 min.
INCOMPATIBILITIES **Solution/additive: Aminoglycosides, lactated ringers, albumin, blood products, solutions containing sodium bicarbonate. Y-site: Acyclovir, aminoglycosides, amphotericin B, amphotericin B cholesteryl complex, chlorpromazine, cisplatin, dacarbazine, daunorubicin, doxorubicin, doxycycline, droperidol, famotidine, ganciclovir, gemcitabine, hydroxyzine, idarubicin, minocycline, mitomycin, mitoxantrone, nalbuphine, prochlorperazine, promethazine, vancomycin.**

ADVERSE EFFECTS (≥1%) **CNS:** Headache, insomnia, fever. **GI:** Diarrhea, constipation, nausea, vomiting, dyspepsia, <u>pseudomembranous colitis</u>. **Skin:** Rash, pruritus, hypersensitivity reactions.

INTERACTIONS **Drug:** May increase risk of bleeding with ANTICOAGULANTS; **probenecid** decreases elimination of piperacillin.

PHARMACOKINETICS **Distribution:** Distributes into many tissues, including lung, blister fluid, and bile; crosses placenta; distributed into breast milk. **Metabolism:** Metabolized in liver. **Elimination:** Piperacillin and tazobactam are excreted in urine. **Half-Life:** 0.7–1.2 h.

NURSING IMPLICATIONS

Assessment & Drug Effects
- Obtain history of hypersensitivity to penicillins, cephalosporins, or other drugs prior to administration.

- Lab tests: C&S prior to first dose of the drug; start drug pending results. Monitor hematologic status with prolonged therapy (Hct and Hgb, CBC with differential and platelet count).
- Monitor patient carefully during the first 30 min after initiation of the infusion for signs of hypersensitivity (See Appendix F).

Patient & Family Education
- Report rash, itching, or other signs of hypersensitivity immediately.
- Report loose stools or diarrhea as these may indicate pseudomembranous colitis.
- Do not breast feed while taking this drug without consulting physician.

PIRBUTEROL ACETATE

(pir-bu'ter-ol)
Maxair
Classifications: AUTONOMIC NERVOUS SYSTEM AGENT; BETA-ADRENERGIC AGONIST (SYMPATHOMIMETIC); BRONCHODILATOR
Prototype: Albuterol
Pregnancy Category: C

AVAILABILITY 0.2 mg aerosol

ACTIONS Exhibits preferential effect on beta$_2$-adrenergic receptors compared with isoproterenol and, consequently, a lengthened duration of action. Stimulation of beta$_2$-adrenoreceptors relaxes bronchospasm and increases ciliary motion. Activates adenyl cyclase, the enzyme that catalyzes the conversion of ATP to cyclic adenosine monophosphate (cAMP).
THERAPEUTIC EFFECTS Increased cAMP is associated with relaxation of bronchial smooth muscle and inhibition of the release of histamine and other mediators of hypersensitivity from mast cells.

USES Prevention and reversal of bronchospasm associated with asthma.

CONTRAINDICATIONS Hypersensitivity to pirbuterol or any other adrenergic agent such as epinephrine, albuterol, or isoproterenol. Pregnancy (category C), lactation.
CAUTIOUS USE Heart disease, irregular heartbeat; high blood pressure, history of stroke or seizures; diabetes; Parkinson's disease; thyroid disease; prostate disease; glaucoma. Safety and effectiveness in children <12 y not established.

ROUTE & DOSAGE

Asthma
Adult/Child: **Inhaled** >*12 y,* 2 inhalations (0.4 mg) q6h (max: 12 inhalations/d)

ADMINISTRATION

Inhalation
- Shake inhaler canister well immediately before using.
- Direct patient to exhale deeply, loosely close lips around mouthpiece, then inhale slowly and deeply through mouthpiece while pressing top of canister.
- Store at 15°–30° C (59°–86° F).

ADVERSE EFFECTS (≥1%) **CNS:** Nervousness, headache, dizziness, tremor. **CV:** Palpitations, tachycardia. **GI:** Dry mouth, nausea, glossitis, abdominal pain, cramps, anorexia, diarrhea, stomatitis. **Other:** Cough, tolerance.

INTERACTIONS **Drug:** **Epinephrine** and other SYMPATHOMIMETIC BRONCHODILATORS may have additive effects. BETA BLOCKERS may antagonize the effects.

P

PHARMACOKINETICS Onset: 5 min. **Peak:** 30 min. **Duration:** 3–4 h. **Metabolism:** Metabolized in liver. **Elimination:** Eliminated by kidneys. **Half-Life:** 2–3 h.

NURSING IMPLICATIONS

Assessment & Drug Effects

- Monitor arterial blood gases and pulmonary functions periodically.
- Monitor vital signs. Report tachycardia, palpitations, and hypertension or hypotension.

Patient & Family Education

- Learn proper technique for using the inhaler.
- Report palpitations, chest pain, nervousness, tremors, or other bothersome adverse effects promptly to physician.
- Contact physician immediately if symptoms of asthma worsen or you do not respond to the usual dose.
- Adhere rigidly to dosing directions and contact physician if breathing difficulty persists.
- Do not breast feed while taking this drug.

P

PIROXICAM

(peer-ox′i-kam)

Feldene

Classifications: CENTRAL NERVOUS SYSTEM AGENT; ANTIPYRETIC; ANALGESIC; NSAID

Prototype: Ibuprofen

Pregnancy Category: C

AVAILABILITY 10 mg, 20 mg capsules

ACTIONS Nonsteroidal antiinflammatory agent. Exact mechanism of action unclear. Strongly inhibits enzyme cyclooxygenase, biogenic catalyst of prostaglandin synthesis.

THERAPEUTIC EFFECTS Drug-induced reduction in prostaglandin levels is associated with decreased inflammatory processes in bone-joint disease, and with possible interference with platelet aggregation.

USES Acute and long-term relief of mild to moderate pain and for symptomatic treatment of osteoarthritis and rheumatoid arthritis.

UNLABELED USES Acute and chronic relief of mild to moderate pain.

CONTRAINDICATIONS Hemophilia; syndrome (bronchospasm, nasal polyps, angioedema) precipitated by aspirin or other NSAID; active peptic ulcer, GI bleeding. Safety in children, during pregnancy (category C), or lactation is not established.

CAUTIOUS USE History of upper GI disease including ulcerative colitis; kidney dysfunction; compromised cardiac function; hypertension or other conditions predisposing to fluid retention; coagulation disorders.

ROUTE & DOSAGE

Arthritis, Pain

Adult: **PO** 10–20 mg 1–2 times/d

ADMINISTRATION

Oral

- Give at the same time every day.
- Give capsule with food or fluid to help reduce GI irritation.
- Give older adults (>70 y) 1/2 of the usual adult dose.
- Make dose adjustments on basis of clinical response at intervals of weeks rather than days in order to prevent over dosage.
- Store in tightly closed container at 15°–30° C (59°–86° F) unless otherwise directed.

ADVERSE EFFECTS (≥1%) **CNS:** Somnolence, dizziness, vertigo, depression, insomnia, nervousness. **CV:** Peripheral edema, hypertension, worsening of CHF, exacerbation of angina. **Special Senses:** Tinnitus, hearing loss, blurred vision, reduced visual acuity, changes in color vision, scotomas, corneal deposits, retinal disturbances. **GI:** *Nausea, vomiting, dyspepsia,* GI bleeding, diarrhea, constipation, flatulence, dry mouth, peptic ulceration, anorexia, jaundice, hepatitis. **Hematologic:** Anemia, decreases in Hgb, Hct; leukopenia, eosinophilia, aplastic anemia; thrombocytopenia, *prolonged bleeding time.* **Skin:** Urticaria, erythema multiforme, maculopapular, vesiculobullous rash; photosensitivity, sweating, Stevens-Johnson syndrome, bruising, dermatitis. **Body as a Whole:** Allergic rhinitis, angioedema, fever, palpitations, syncope, muscle cramps, fever, hypersensitivity reactions. **Metabolic:** Hypoglycemia, hyperglycemia, hyperkalemia, weight gain. **Urogenital:** Dysuria, acute kidney failure, papillary necrosis, hematuria, proteinuria, nephrotic syndrome. **Respiratory:** Bronchospasm, dyspnea.

INTERACTIONS Drug: ORAL ANTICOAGULANTS, **heparin** may prolong bleeding time; may increase **lithium** toxicity; **alcohol, aspirin** increase risk of GI hemorrhage. **Herbal: Feverfew, garlic, ginger, ginkgo** may increase bleeding potential.

PHARMACOKINETICS Absorption: Well absorbed from GI tract. **Onset:** 1 h analgesia; 7 d for rheumatoid arthritis. **Peak:** 3–5 h analgesia; 2–4 wk antirheumatic. **Duration:** 48–72 h analgesia. **Distribution:** Small amount distributed into breast milk. **Metabolism:** Extensively metabolized in liver. **Elimination:** Excreted primarily in urine, some in bile (<5%). **Half-Life:** 30–86 h.

NURSING IMPLICATIONS

Assessment & Drug Effects

- Wait at least 7 d to evaluate antirheumatic effect.
- Clinical evidence of benefits from drug therapy include pain relief in motion and in rest, reduction in night pain, stiffness, and swelling; increased ROM (range of motion) in all joints.
- Be aware that adverse effects may not appear for 7–10 d after start of therapy (except for an allergic reaction).
- Lab tests: Periodic BUN, ALT, AST, CBC, Hgb and Hct in patient (especially the older adult) receiving drug for an extended period.

Patient & Family Education

- If a dose is missed, take drug when missed dose is discovered if it is 6–8 h before the next scheduled dose. Otherwise, omit dose and reestablish regimen at next scheduled hour.
- Do not self-dose with aspirin or other OTC drug without physician's advice.
- Do not increase dosage beyond prescribed regimen. Understand that long half-life of drug may cause delayed therapeutic effect. Higher than recommended doses are associated with increased incidence of GI irritation and peptic ulcer.
- Incidence of GI bleeding with this drug is relatively high. Report symptoms of GI bleeding (e.g., dark, tarry stools, coffee-colored emesis) or severe gastric pain promptly to physician.
- Be alert to symptoms of drug-induced anemia: Profound fatigue,

skin and mucous membrane pallor, lethargy.

- Avoid alcohol since it may increase the risk of GI bleeding.
- Be alert to signs of hypoprothrombinemia including bruises, pinpoint rash, unexplained bleeding, nose bleed, blood in urine, when piroxicam is taken concomitantly with an anticoagulant.
- Do not drive or engage in potentially hazardous activities until response to drug is known.
- Drink at least 6–8 full glasses of water daily and report signs of renal insufficiency (see Appendix F) to physician because most of drug is excreted by kidneys and impaired kidney function increases danger of toxicity.
- Do not breast feed while taking this drug without consulting physician.

PLASMA PROTEIN FRACTION

(plas'ma)

Plasmanate, Plasma-Plex, Plasmatein, PPF, Protenate

Classifications: BLOOD FORMERS, COAGULATORS, AND ANTICOAGULANTS; PLASMA VOLUME EXPANDER

Prototype: Normal serum albumin, human

Pregnancy Category: C

AVAILABILITY 5% injection

ACTIONS Oncotic action approximately equivalent to that of human plasma; does not provide coagulation factors or gamma globulins.

THERAPEUTIC EFFECTS Heat-treated to minimize hazard of transmitting serum hepatitis; risk of sensitization is reduced because it lacks cellular elements. Does not require cross matching.

USES Emergency treatment of hypovolemic shock due to burns, trauma, surgery, infections; temporary measure in treatment of blood loss when whole blood is not available; to replenish plasma protein in patients with hypoproteinemia (if sodium restriction is not a problem).

CONTRAINDICATIONS Severe anemia; cardiac failure; patients undergoing cardiopulmonary bypass surgery; pregnancy (category C).

CAUTIOUS USE Patients with low cardiac reserve; absence of albumin deficiency; liver or kidney failure.

ROUTE & DOSAGE

Plasma Volume Expansion

Adult: **IV** 250–500 mL at a maximum rate of 10 mL/min

Child: **IV** 6.6–33 mL/kg at a rate of 5–10 mL/min

Hypoproteinemia

Adult: **IV** 1–1.5 L/d infused at a rate not to exceed 5–8 mL/min

ADMINISTRATION

Intravenous

- Do not use solutions that show a sediment or appear turbid.
- Do not use solutions that have been frozen.

PREPARE: **IV Infusion:** Give undiluted. Once container is opened, solution should be used within 4 h because it contains no preservatives. Discard unused portions.

ADMINISTER: **IV Infusion:** Rate of infusion and volume of total dose will depend on patient's age, diagnosis, degree of venous and pulmonary congestion, Hct, and Hgb determinations. As with any oncotically active solution, infusion rate should be relatively slow. Range may vary from 1–10 mL/min.

ADVERSE EFFECTS (≥1%) **GI:** Nausea, vomiting, hypersalivation, headache. **Body as a Whole:** Tingling, chills, fever, cyanosis, chest tightness, backache, urticaria, erythema, shock (systemic anaphylaxis), circulatory overload, pulmonary edema.

INTERACTIONS Drug: No clinically significant interactions established.

PHARMACOKINETICS Not studied.

NURSING IMPLICATIONS

Assessment & Drug Effects

- Monitor vital signs (BP and pulse). Frequency depends on patient's condition. Flow rate adjustments are made according to clinical response and BP. Slow or stop infusion if patient suddenly becomes hypotensive.
- Report a widening pulse pressure (difference between systolic and diastolic); it correlates with increase in cardiac output.
- Report changes in I&O ratio and pattern.
- Observe patient closely during and after infusion for signs of hypervolemia or circulatory overload (see Appendix F). Report these symptoms immediately to physician.
- Make careful observations of patient who has had either injury or surgery in order to detect bleeding points that failed to bleed at lower BP.

PLICAMYCIN

(plik-a-mi'cin)

Mithracin, Mithramycin

Classifications: ANTINEOPLASTIC; ANTIBIOTIC

Prototype: Doxorubicin

Pregnancy Category: C

AVAILABILITY 2500 mcg injection

ACTIONS Cytotoxic antibiotic produced by *Streptomyces plicatus,* with minimal immunosuppressive activity. Complexes with DNA, thus inhibiting DNA-directed RNA synthesis.

THERAPEUTIC EFFECTS May lower serum calcium levels by unclear mechanism. Appears to block hypercalcemic action of vitamin D, and may inhibit parathyroid hormone effect on osteoclasts. Interferes with synthesis of various clotting factors. High toxicity with low therapeutic index limits clinical use.

USES To treat hospitalized patients with hypercalcemia or hypercalciuria associated with advanced neoplasms and to treat testicular malignancy.

CONTRAINDICATIONS Bleeding and coagulation disorders, myelosuppression; electrolyte imbalance (especially hypocalcemia, hypokalemia, hypophosphatemia); pregnancy (category C), lactation.

CAUTIOUS USE Patients with prior abdominal or mediastinal radiology; liver or renal impairment.

P

ROUTE & DOSAGE

Neoplasia

Adult: **IV** 25–30 mcg/kg once/d for 8–10 d or until toxicity necessitates discontinuing (max: 30 mcg/kg/d for 10 d)

Malignant Hypercalcemia

Adult: **IV** 25 mcg/kg once/d for 3–4 d, may repeat after 1 wk

ADMINISTRATION

Intravenous

- Base drug dose on ideal body weight when edema, ascites, or hydrothorax is present.

PREPARE: **IV Infusion:** Dilute each 2.5 mg with 4.9 mL of sterile water to yield 500 mcg/mL. Withdraw the calculated dose and further dilute in 1000 mL of D5W or D5/NS.

ADMINISTER: **IV Infusion:** Give at a rate of 4–6 h per liter. Regulate IV flow rate carefully (established by physician); GI adverse effects increase when rate is too fast. Terminate infusion immediately if extravasation occurs. Apply moderate heat to disperse the drug and to minimize tissue irritation.

INCOMPATIBILITIES **Y-site: Cefepime.**

- Discard unused portions of reconstituted solution and prepare new ones daily. ■ Refrigerate unreconstituted vials at 2°–8° C (36°–46° F).

ADVERSE EFFECTS (≥1%) **CNS:** Drowsiness, irritability, dizziness, weakness, headache, mental depression. **GI:** *Stomatitis, anorexia, nausea, vomiting, diarrhea,* widespread intestinal hemorrhage. **Hematologic:** Thrombocytopenia, <u>bleeding and coagulation disorders</u> (dose related), leukopenia (mild). **Body as a Whole:** Fever, marked facial flushing, hemoptysis, abnormal liver and renal function tests. **Skin:** Nonspecific or acneiform skin rash, phlebitis. **Metabolic:** Hypophosphatemia, hypokalemia, hypocalciuria.

INTERACTIONS Drug: Concomitant administration of **vitamin D** may enhance hypercalcemia.

PHARMACOKINETICS Distribution: Crosses blood–brain barrier; appears to localize in areas of bone active resorption. **Elimination:** Excreted in urine.

NURSING IMPLICATIONS

Assessment & Drug Effects

- Note: Therapy is usually interrupted if leukocyte count is <4000/mm^3, if platelet count is <150,000/mm^3, or if PT is >4 seconds higher than control (normal: 12–14 seconds).
- Establish flow chart at beginning of therapy, permitting continuous record of weight and I&O ratio and pattern.
- Lab tests: Perform frequent assessments of liver and hematologic (platelet count, bleeding and prothrombin times) and kidney function throughout therapy and for several days after last dose; periodic serum electrolytes.
- Report marked facial flushing. It is often an early symptom or thrombocytopenia, which frequently is evidenced by a single or persistent episode of epistaxis or hematemesis; may be rapid in onset during or after a course of treatment.
- Inspect skin daily for signs of purpura. Report hemoptysis immediately, which may occur because of bleeding into metastasis.
- Note: Rebound hypercalcemia (normal: 9–10.6 mg/dL) following plicamycin-induced hypocalcemia may persist 2–4 d (see Appendix F).
- Monitor I&O ratio to assure adequate fluid intake; the hypercalcemia patient may be dehydrated.
- Monitor for S&S of adverse effects on the GI mucosal cells (hematemesis, melena) that will necessitate stopping drug use.
- Check patient's bowel function daily to prevent high fecal impaction due to diminished peristalsis.
- Consult physician about dietary calcium intake and coordinate dietary planning with dietitian, patient, and family.

Patient & Family Education

- Use a reliable form of birth control during and for several months following completion of treatment with plicamycin.
- Report easy bruising or bleeding immediately to your physician.

PODOPHYLLUM RESIN (Podophyllin)

(pode-oh-fill'um)

Podo-ben, Podofin

PODOFILOX

Condylox

Classifications: SKIN AND MUCOUS MEMBRANE AGENT; KERATOLYTIC AGENT

Pregnancy Category: X

AVAILABILITY **Podophyllum** 25% liquid **Podofilox** 0.5% gel, solution

ACTIONS Potent cytotoxic and keratolytic agent with caustic action, derived from rhizomes and roots of *Podophyllum peltatum* (mandrake, May apple). Directly affects epithelial cell metabolism, causing degeneration and arrest of mitosis.

THERAPEUTIC EFFECTS Slow disruption of cells and tissue erosion as a result of its caustic action. Selectively affects embryonic and tumor cells more than adult cells.

USES Benign growths including external genital and perianal warts, papillomas, fibroids.

CONTRAINDICATIONS Birthmarks, moles, or warts with hair growth from them; cervical, urethral, oral warts; normal skin and mucous membranes peripheral to treated areas; pregnancy (category X), lactation; diabetes mellitus; patient with poor circulation; irritated, friable, or bleeding skin; application of drug over large area.

ROUTE & DOSAGE

Condylomata Acuminata

Adult: **Topical** Use 10% solution and repeat 1–2 times/wk for up to 4 applications

Verruca Vulgaris (Common Wart)

Adult: **Topical** Apply 0.5% solution q12h for up to 4 wks

Multiple Superficial Epitheliomatosis, Keratoses

Adult: **Topical** Apply 0.5% solution or gel daily for several days

ADMINISTRATION

Note: Use 10%–25% solution for areas <10 cm^2 or 5% solution for areas of 10–20 cm^2, anal, or genital warts; apply drug to dry surface, allowing area to dry between drops, wash off after 1–4h.

Topical

- Avoid podophyllum resin contact with eyes or similar mucosal surfaces; if it occurs, flush thoroughly with lukewarm water for 15 min and remove film precipitated by the water.
- Avoid application of drug to normal tissue. If it occurs, remove with alcohol. Protect surfaces surrounding area to be treated with a layer of petrolatum or flexible collodion.
- Remove drug thoroughly with soap and water after each treatment of accessible tissue surface.
- Apply a protective coat of talcum powder after treatment and drying of anogenital area.
- Remove drug with alcohol, if application causes extreme pain, pruritus, or swelling.
- Store in a tight, light-resistant container; avoid exposure to excessive heat.

ADVERSE EFFECTS (≥1%) **Body as a Whole:** Severe systemic toxicity (sometimes fatal), sensorimotor neuropathy (reversible), symptomatic orthostatic hypotension, paresthesias and weakness of extremities, stocking-glove sensory loss, absent ankle reflexes, decreased response to

P

painful stimuli. **CNS:** Lethargy, mental confusion, disorientation, delirium, agitation, seizures, progressive stupor, polyneuritis, pyrexia, coma, visual and auditory hallucinations, acute psychotic reaction, ataxia, hypotonia, areflexia, increased CSF protein, paralytic ileus. **CV:** Sinus tachycardia. **Hematologic:** Bone marrow suppression similar to that caused by antineoplastic drug toxicity, leukopenia, thrombocytopenia. **GI:** *Nausea, vomiting, diarrhea, abdominal pain,* hepatotoxicity, increased serum concentrations of LDH, AST, and alkaline phosphatase. **Urogenital:** Renal failure, urinary retention. **Respiratory:** Decreased respirations, apnea, hyperventilation.

INTERACTIONS No clinically significant interactions established.

PHARMACOKINETICS Not studied.

NURSING IMPLICATIONS

Assessment & Drug Effects

- Warts become blanched, then necrotic within 24–48 h. Sloughing begins after about 72 h with no scarring. Frequently, a mild topical antiinfective agent, with or without a dressing, is applied until the healing is complete.
- Monitor neurologic status. Sensorimotor polyneuropathy, if it occurs, appears about 2 wk after application of drug, worsens for 3 mo, and may persist for up to 9 mo. Cerebral effects may persist for 7–10 d; ataxia, hypotonia, and areflexia improve more slowly than effects on sensorium.

Patient & Family Education

- Learn proper technique of treatment if self-administered as treatment of verruca vulgaris (common wart). Also be fully aware of the need to report treatment failure to physician.
- Be aware that as with any STD, the patient's sex partner should be examined.
- Systemic toxicity may be severe and serious and is associated with application of drug to large areas, to tissue that is friable, bleeding, or recently biopsied, or for prolonged time. Toxicity may occur within hours of application. There are significant dangers from overuse or misuse of this drug.
- Learn symptoms of toxicity and report any that appear promptly to physician. (see ADVERSE EFFECTS.)
- Do not breast feed while taking this drug.

POLYCARBOPHIL

(pol-i-kar'boe-fil)

FiberCon, Mitrolan, Equalactin, FiberNorm

Classifications: GASTROINTESTINAL AGENT; BULK LAXATIVE; ANTIDIARRHEAL

Prototype: Psyllium

Pregnancy Category: C

AVAILABILITY 500 mg, 625 mg tablets; 500 mg, 625 mg chewable tablets

ACTIONS Hydrophilic agent which absorbs free water in intestinal tract and opposes dehydrating forces of bowel by forming a gelatinous mass.

THERAPEUTIC EFFECTS Restores more normal moisture level and motility in the lower GI tract; produces well-formed stool and reduces diarrhea.

USES Constipation or diarrhea associated with acute bowel syndrome, diverticulosis, irritable bowel and in patients who should not strain during defecation. Also choleretic diarrhea, diarrhea caused by small-bowel surgery or vagotomy, and disease of terminal ileum.

CONTRAINDICATIONS Partial or complete GI obstruction; fecal impaction; dysphagia; acute abdominal pain; rectal bleeding; undiagnosed abdominal pain, or other symptoms symptomatic of appendicitis; poisonings; before radiologic bowel examination; bowel surgery. Safety in children <3 y is not established.
CAUTIOUS USE Pregnancy (category C), lactation.

ROUTE & DOSAGE

Constipation or Diarrhea
Adult: **PO** 1 g q.i.d. prn (max: 6 g/d)
Child: **PO** *3–6 y,* 500 mg b.i.d. prn (max: 1.5 g/d); *6–12 y,* 500 mg t.i.d. prn (max: 3 g/d)

ADMINISTRATION

Oral

- Chewable tablets should be chewed well before swallowing.
- Give each dose with a full glass (240 mL [8 oz]) of water or other liquid.
- Repeat dose every 30 min up to the maximum dose in 24 h with severe diarrhea.
- Store at 15°–30° C (59°–86° F) in tightly closed container unless otherwise directed.

ADVERSE EFFECTS (≥1%) **GI:** Esophageal blockage, intestinal impaction, *abdominal fullness.* **Metabolic:** Low serum potassium, elevated blood glucose levels (with extended use). **Respiratory:** Asthma. **Skin:** Skin rash.

INTERACTIONS Drug: May decrease absorption and clinical effects of ANTIBIOTICS, **warfarin, digoxin, nitrofurantoin,** SALICYLATES.

PHARMACOKINETICS Absorption: Not absorbed from GI tract. **Onset:** 12–24 h. **Peak:** 1–3 d.

NURSING IMPLICATIONS

Assessment & Drug Effects

- Determine duration and severity of diarrhea in order to anticipate signs of fluid-electrolyte losses.
- Monitor and record number and consistency of stools per day, presence and location of abdominal discomfort (i.e., tenderness, distension), and bowel sounds.
- Monitor and record I&O ratio and pattern. Dehydration is indicated if output is <30 mL/h.
- Inspect oral cavity for dryness, and be alert to systemic signs of dehydration (e.g., thirst and fever). Dehydration from an episode of diarrhea appears rapidly in young children and older adults.

Patient & Family Education

- Consult physician if sudden changes in bowel habit persist more than 1 wk, action is minimal or ineffective for 1 wk, or if there is no antidiarrheal action within 2 d.
- Be aware that extended use of this drug may cause dependence for normal bowel function.
- Do not discontinue polycarbophil unless physician advises if also taking an oral anticoagulant, digoxin, salicylates, or nitrofurantoin.
- Do not breast feed while taking this drug without consulting physician.

P

POLYMYXIN B SULFATE

(pol-i-mix'in)
Aerosporin
Classifications: ANTIINFECTIVE; ANTIBIOTIC
Pregnancy Category: B

AVAILABILITY 500,000 unit injection; 500,000 unit ophthalmic solution

ACTIONS Antibiotic derived from strains of *Bacillus polymyxa.* Binds to lipid phosphates in bacterial membranes and, through cationic detergent action, changes permeability to permit leakage of cytoplasm.
THERAPEUTIC EFFECTS Bactericidal against susceptible gram negative organisms, particularly most strains of *Escherichia coli, Haemophilus influenzae, Enterobacter aerogenes,* and *Klebsiella pneumoniae.* Most species of *Proteus* and *Neisseria* are resistant, as are all gram-positive organisms and fungi.

USES Topically and in combination with other antiinfectives or corticosteroids for various superficial infections of eye, ear, mucous membrane, and skin. Concurrent systemic antiinfective therapy may be required for treatment of intraocular infection and severe progressive corneal ulcer. Used parenterally only in hospitalized patients for treatment of severe acute infections of urinary tract, bloodstream, and meninges; and in combination with Neosporin for continuous bladder irrigation to prevent bacteremia associated with use of indwelling catheter.

CONTRAINDICATIONS Hypersensitivity to polymyxin antibiotics; concurrent and sequential use of other nephrotoxic and neurotoxic drugs; concurrent use of skeletal muscle relaxants, ether, or sodium citrate. Safety during pregnancy (category B) or children <2 months is not established.
CAUTIOUS USE Impaired kidney function; myasthenia gravis; lactation.

ROUTE & DOSAGE

Infections
Adult: **IV** 15,000–25,000 U/kg/d divided q12h **IM** 25,000–30,000 U/kg/d divided q4–6h **GU** 1 mL/L NS q24h **Topical** 1–2 drops in eye q1h
Child: **IV** 15,000–25,000 U/kg/d divided q12h **IM** 25,000–30,000 U/kg/d divided q4–6h

ADMINISTRATION

Intramuscular
- Routine administration by IM routes not recommended because it causes intense discomfort, along the peripheral nerve distribution, 40–60 min after IM injection.
- Make IM injection in adults deep into upper outer quadrant of buttock. Select IM site carefully to avoid injection into nerves or blood vessels. Rotate injection sites. Follow agency policy for IM site used in children.

Intravenous
PREPARE: **Intermittent:** Reconstitute by dissolving 500,000 U in 5 mL sterile water for injection or NS to yield 100,000 U/mL. Withdraw a single dose and then further dilute in 300–500 mL of D5W.
ADMINISTER: **Intermittent:** Infuse over period of 60–90 min. Inspect injection site for signs of phlebitis and irritation.
INCOMPATIBILITIES **Solution/additive: Amphotericin B, cephalothin, chloramphenicol, chlorothiazide, heparin, magnesium sulfate, prednisolone,**

sodium phosphate, tetracycline.

- Protect unreconstituted product and reconstituted solution from light and freezing. Store in refrigerator at 2°–8° C (36°–46° F). Parenteral solutions are stable for 1 wk when refrigerated. Discard unused portion after 72 h.

ADVERSE EFFECTS (≥1%) **Body as a Whole:** Irritability, facial flushing, ataxia, circumoral, lingual, and peripheral paresthesias (stocking-glove distribution); severe pain (IM site), thrombophlebitis (IV site), superinfections, electrolyte disturbances (prolonged use; also reported in patients with acute leukemia); local irritation and burning (topical use), <u>anaphylactoid reactions</u> (rare). **CNS:** Drowsiness, dizziness, vertigo, convulsions, coma; <u>neuromuscular blockade (generalized muscle weakness, respiratory depression or arrest)</u>; meningeal irritation, increased protein and cell count in cerebrospinal fluid, fever, headache, stiff neck (intrathecal use). **Special Senses:** Blurred vision, nystagmus, slurred speech, dysphagia, ototoxicity (vestibular and auditory) with high doses. **GI:** GI disturbances. **Urogenital:** Albuminuria, cylindruria, azotemia, hematuria.

INTERACTIONS Drug: ANESTHETICS and NEUROMUSCULAR BLOCKING AGENTS may prolong skeletal muscle relaxation. AMINOGLYCOSIDES and **amphotericin B** have additive nephrotoxic potential.

PHARMACOKINETICS Absorption: Not absorbed from GI tract. **Peak:** 2 h IM. **Distribution:** Widely distributed except to CSF, synovial fluid, and eye; does not cross placenta. **Metabolism:** Unknown. **Elimination:** 60% Excreted unchanged in urine. **Half-Life:** 4.3–6 h.

NURSING IMPLICATIONS

Assessment & Drug Effects

- Lab tests: Obtain C&S tests prior to first dose and periodically thereafter to determine continuing sensitivity of causative organisms. Perform baseline serum electrolytes and kidney function tests before parenteral therapy. Frequent monitoring of kidney function and serum drug levels is advised during therapy. Monitor electrolytes at regular intervals during prolonged therapy.
- Review electrolyte results. Patients with low serum calcium and low intracellular potassium are particularly prone to develop neuromuscular blockade.
- Inspect tongue every day. Assess for S&S of superinfection (see Appendix F). Polymyxin therapy supports growth of opportunistic organisms. Report symptoms promptly.
- Monitor I&O. Maintain fluid intake sufficient to maintain daily urinary output of at least 1500 mL. Some degree of renal toxicity usually occurs within first 3 or 4 d of therapy even with therapeutic doses. Consult physician.
- Withhold drug and report findings to physician for any of the following: Decreases in urine output (change in I&O ratio), proteinuria, cellular casts, rising BUN, serum creatinine, or serum drug levels (not associated with dosage increase). All can be interpreted as signs of nephrotoxicity.
- Nephrotoxicity is generally reversible, but it may progress even after drug is discontinued. Therefore, close monitoring of kidney function is essential, even following termination of therapy.
- Be alert for respiratory arrest after the first dose and also as long as 45 d after initiation of therapy. It

P

occurs most commonly in patients with kidney failure and high plasma drug levels and is often preceded by dyspnea and restlessness.

Patient & Family Education

- Report to physician immediately any muscle weakness, shortness of breath, dyspnea, depressed respiration. These symptoms are rapidly reversible if drug is withdrawn.
- Stop drug administration immediately and report to physician if you experience eyelid irritation, itching, and burning with ophthalmic drops.
- Report promptly to physician transient neurologic disturbances (burning or prickling sensations, numbness, dizziness). All occur commonly and usually respond to dosage reduction.
- Report promptly to physician the onset of stiff neck and headache (possible symptoms of neurotoxic reactions, including neuromuscular blockade). This response is usually associated with high serum drug levels or nephrotoxicity.
- Report promptly S&S of superinfection (see Appendix F).
- Do not breast feed while taking this drug without consulting physician.

POLYTHIAZIDE

(pol-i-thye'a-zide)

Renese

Classifications: ELECTROLYTIC AND WATER BALANCE AGENT; THIAZIDE DIURETIC

Prototype: Hydrochlorothiazide

Pregnancy Category: D

AVAILABILITY 1 mg, 2 mg, 4 mg

ACTIONS Benzothiadiazine (thiazide) derivative. Diuretic action is associated with drug interference with transport of sodium ions across renal tubular epithelium. Enhances excretion of sodium, chloride, potassium, bicarbonates and water.

THERAPEUTIC EFFECTS Reduces edema and results in a hypotensive action.

USES Primary agent in antihypertensive treatment and adjunctively in the management of edema associated with CHF, renal pathology, and hepatic cirrhosis.

CONTRAINDICATIONS Hypersensitivity to other thiazides or sulfonamides; anuria; pregnancy (category D), lactation.

CAUTIOUS USE Kidney and liver dysfunction; SLE; gout; diabetes mellitus.

ROUTE & DOSAGE

Edema

Adult: **PO** 1–4 mg/d or q.o.d.

Hypertension

Adult: **PO** 2–4 mg/d
Child: **PO** 0.02–0.08 mg/kg/d

ADMINISTRATION

Oral

- Give drug early in morning after eating (to reduce gastric irritation) and to prevent interrupted sleep because of diuresis.
- Store drug in tightly closed container.

ADVERSE EFFECTS (≥1%) **Hematologic:** <u>Agranulocytosis</u>, vascular thrombosis. **Metabolic:** *Hyperuricemia, hypokalemia, hyperglycemia.* **Body as a Whole:** Orthostatic hypotension, hepatic encephalopathy, photosensitivity.

INTERACTIONS Drug: Amphotericin B, CORTICOSTEROIDS increase hypokalemic effects; may antagonize hypoglycemic effects of **insulin,** SULFONYLUREAS; **cholestyramine, colestipol** decrease thiazide absorption; intensifies hypoglycemic and hypotensive effects of **diazoxide.** Increased **potassium** and **magnesium** loss may cause **digoxin** toxicity; decreases **lithium** excretion, increasing its toxicity; NSAIDS may attenuate diuresis and increase risk of NSAID-induced kidney failure.

PHARMACOKINETICS Onset: 2 h. **Peak:** 6 h. **Duration:** 24–48 h. **Distribution:** Distributed throughout extracellular tissue; concentrates in kidney; crosses placenta; distributed into breast milk. **Metabolism:** Does not appear to be metabolized. **Elimination:** Excreted in urine.

NURSING IMPLICATIONS

Assessment & Drug Effects

- Older adult patients may be more sensitive to the average adult therapeutic dose. Excessive diuresis may induce sudden hypotension and serious electrolyte imbalance.
- Be aware that antihypertensive effects may be noted in 3–4 d; maximal effects may require 3–4 wk. Effects persist for at least 1 wk after drug is discontinued.
- Lab tests: Periodic serum electrolytes and blood glucose.
- Monitor for S&S of hypokalemia and hyperglycemia (see Appendix F).

Patient & Family Education

- Change position slowly and in stages, particularly from lying down to upright positions; avoid hot baths or showers, extended exposure to sunlight, and standing still.
- Include specific sources of potassium in daily diet such as a banana (about 370 mg potassium) and at least 180 mL (6 oz) orange juice (about 330 mg potassium).
- Monitor blood glucose for loss of glycemic control of diabetic.
- Be aware of the possibility of photosensitivity reaction and notify physician if it occurs. Thiazide-related photosensitivity is considered a photoallergy and occurs 10–14 d after initial sun exposure. Use sunscreen lotion with a high SPF (12–15).
- Avoid OTC drugs unless approved by the physician. Many preparations contain both potassium and sodium and if misused can induce electrolyte adverse effects.
- Do not breast feed while taking this drug.

PORACTANT ALPHA

(por-act′ant)

Curosurf

Classification: LUNG SURFACTANT

Prototype: Beractant

Pregnancy Category: Not applicable

AVAILABILITY 120 mg/1.5 mL, 240 mg/3 mL vials

ACTIONS Lung surfactant obtained from minced porcine lungs. Endogenous pulmonary surfactant lowers the surface tension on alveoli surfaces during respiration, and stabilizes the alveoli against collapse at resting pressures.

THERAPEUTIC EFFECTS Alleviates respiratory distress syndrome (RDS) in premature infants caused by deficiency of surfactant.

USES Treatment (rescue) of respiratory distress syndrome in premature infants.

CONTRAINDICATIONS Hypersensitivity to porcine products or poractant alpha.

CAUTIOUS USE Infants born >3 wk after ruptured membranes; intraventricular hemorrhage of grade III or IV; major congenital malformations; nosocomial infection; pretreatment of hypothermia or acidosis due to increased risk of intracranial hemorrhage.

ROUTE & DOSAGE

Respiratory Distress Syndrome
Adult: **Intratracheal** 2.5 mL/kg birth weight, may repeat with 1.25 mL/kg q12h times 2 more doses if needed

ADMINISTRATION

Note: Correction of acidosis, hypotension, anemia, hypoglycemia and hypothermia is recommended prior to administration of poractant alfa.

Intratracheal

- Warm vial slowly to room temperature; gently turn upside down to form uniform suspension, but do NOT shake.
- Withdraw slowly the entire contents of a vial (concentration equals 80 mg/mL) into a 3 or 5 mL syringe through a large gauge (>20 gauge) needle.
- Attach a 5 French catheter, precut to 8 cm, to the syringe.
- Fill the catheter with poractant alfa and discard excess through the catheter so that only the total dose to be given remains in the syringe.
- Refer to specific instruction provided by manufacturer for proper dosing technique. Follow instructions carefully regarding installation of drug and ventilation of infant. Note that catheter tip should not extend beyond distal tip of endotracheal tube.
- Store refrigerated at 2°–8° C (36°–46° F) and protect from light. Do not shake vials. Do not warm to room temperature and return to refrigeration more than once.

ADVERSE EFFECTS (≥1%) **CV:** Bradycardia, hypotension. **Respiratory:** Intratracheal tube blockage, oxygen desaturation.

PHARMACOKINETICS Not studied.

NURSING IMPLICATIONS

Assessment & Drug Effects

- Stop administration of poractant alfa and take appropriate measures if any of the following occur: Transient episodes of bradycardia, decreased oxygen saturation, reflux of poractant alfa into endotracheal tube, or airway obstruction. Dosing may resume after stabilization.
- Do not suction airway for 1 h after poractant alfa instillation unless there is significant airway obstruction.

POTASSIUM CHLORIDE

(poe-tass′ee-um)

Apo-K ♣, K-10, Kalium Durules ♣, Kaochlor, Kaochlor-20 Concentrate, Kaon-Cl, Kato, Kay Ciel, KCl 5% and 20%, K-Long ♣, Klor, Klor-10%, Klor-Con, Kloride, Klorvess, Klotrix, K-Dur, K-Lyte/Cl, K-tab, Micro-K Extentabs, Novolente K ♣, Roychlor 10% and 20% ♣, Rum-K, SK-Potassium Chloride, Slo-Pot ♣, Slow-K

POTASSIUM GLUCONATE

Kaon, Kaylixir, K-G Elixir, Potassium Rougier ♣, Royonate ♣

Classifications: ELECTROLYTIC AND WATER BALANCE AGENT; REPLACEMENT SOLUTION

Pregnancy Category: A

AVAILABILITY Chloride 6.7 mEq, 8 mEq, 10 mEq, 20 mEq sustained release tablets; 500 mg, 595 mg tablets; 20 mEq, 25 mEq, 50 mEq effervescent tablets; 20 mEq/15 mL, 40 mEq/15 mL, 45 mEq/15 mL liquid; 15 mEq, 20 mEq, 25 mEq powder; 2 mEq/mL injection; 10 mEq, 20 mEq, 30 mEq, 40 mEq, 60 mEq, 90 mEq vials **Gluconate** 20 mEq/15 mL liquid

ACTIONS Principal intracellular cation; essential for maintenance of intracellular isotonicity, transmission of nerve impulses, contraction of cardiac, skeletal, and smooth muscles, maintenance of normal kidney function, and for enzyme activity. Plays a prominent role in both formation and correction of imbalances in acid–base metabolism.

THERAPEUTIC EFFECTS Given special importance as therapeutic agents but are also dangerous if improperly prescribed and administered. Utilized for treatment of hypokalemia.

USES To prevent and treat potassium deficit secondary to diuretic or corticosteroid therapy. Also indicated when potassium is depleted by severe vomiting, diarrhea; intestinal drainage, fistulas, or malabsorption; prolonged diuresis, diabetic acidosis. Effective in the treatment of hypokalemic alkalosis (chloride, not the gluconate).

CONTRAINDICATIONS Severe renal impairment; severe hemolytic reactions; untreated Addison's disease; crush syndrome; early postoperative oliguria (except during GI drainage); adynamic ileus; acute dehydration; heat cramps, hyperkalemia, patients receiving potassium-sparing diuretics, digitalis intoxication with AV conduction disturbance.

CAUTIOUS USE Cardiac or kidney disease; systemic acidosis; slow-release potassium preparations in presence of delayed GI transit or Meckel's diverticulum; extensive tissue breakdown (such as severe burns); pregnancy (category A); lactation.

ROUTE & DOSAGE

Hypokalemia

Adult: **PO** 10–100 mEq/d in divided doses **IV** 10–40 mEq/h diluted to at least 10–20 mEq/100 mL of solution (max: 200–400 mEq/d, monitor higher doses carefully)

Child: **PO** 1–3 mEq/kg/d in divided doses; sustained release tablets not recommended in children **IV** Up to 3 mEq/kg/24 h at a rate <0.02 mEq/kg/min

ADMINISTRATION

Oral

- Give while patient is sitting up or standing (never in recumbent position) to prevent drug–induced esophagitis. Some patients find it difficult to swallow the large sized KCl tablet.
- Do not crush or allow to chew any potassium salt tablets. Observe to make sure patient does not suck tablet (oral ulcerations have been reported if tablet is allowed to dissolve in mouth).
- Swallow whole tablet with a large glass of water or fruit juice (if allowed) to wash drug down and to start esophageal peristalsis.
- Follow directions for diluting various liquid forms of KCl exactly. In general, dilute each 20 mEq potassium in at least 90 mL water or juice and allowed to completely before administration.

P

- Dilute liquid forms as directed before giving it through nasogastric tube.

Intravenous

PREPARE: **IV Infusion:** Add desired amount to 100–1000 mL IV solution (compatible with all standard solutions). Usual maximum is 80 mEq/1000 mL, however, 40 mEq/L is preferred to lessen irritation to veins. Note: **NEVER** add KCl to an IV bag/bottle which is hanging. After adding KCl invert bag/bottle several times to ensure even distribution.

ADMINISTER: **IV Infusion:** KCl is **never** given IV push or in concentrated amounts by any route. Infuse at rate not to exceed 10 mEq/h. Adult patients with severe potassium depletion may be able to tolerate 20 mEq/h. Too rapid infusion may cause fatal hyperkalemia.

- Take extreme care to prevent extravasation and infiltration. At first sign, discontinue infusion and select another site.

INCOMPATIBILITIES **Solution/additive: Amphotericin B, dobutamine (potassium phosphate only). Y-site: Amphotericin B cholesteryl complex, diazepam, ergotamine, methylprednisolone, phenytoin, promethazine.**

P

ADVERSE EFFECTS (≥1%) **GI:** *Nausea, vomiting,* diarrhea, abdominal distension. **Body as a Whole:** Pain, mental confusion, irritability, listlessness, paresthesias of extremities, muscle weakness and heaviness of limbs, difficulty in swallowing, flaccid paralysis. **Urogenital:** Oliguria, anuria. **Hematologic:** Hyperkalemia. **Respiratory:** Respiratory distress. **CV:** Hypotension, bradycardia; cardiac depression, arrhythmias, or arrest; altered sensitivity to digitalis glycosides. *ECG changes in hyperkalemia:* Tenting (peaking) of T wave (especially in right precordial leads), lowering of R with deepening of S waves and depression of RST; prolonged P-R interval, widened QRS complex, decreased amplitude and disappearance of P waves, prolonged Q-T interval, signs of right and left bundle block, deterioration of QRS contour and finally ventricular fibrillation and death.

INTERACTIONS Drug: POTASSIUM-SPARING DIURETICS, ANGIOTENSIN-CONVERTING ENZYME (ACE) INHIBITORS may cause hyperkalemia.

PHARMACOKINETICS Absorption: Readily absorbed from upper GI tract. **Elimination:** 90% excreted in urine, 10% in feces.

NURSING IMPLICATIONS

Assessment & Drug Effects

- Monitor I&O ratio and pattern in patients receiving the parenteral drug. If oliguria occurs, stop infusion promptly and notify physician.
- Lab test: Frequent serum electrolytes are warranted.
- Monitor for and report signs of GI ulceration (esophageal or epigastric pain or hematemesis).
- Monitor patients receiving parenteral potassium closely with cardiac monitor. Irregular heartbeat is usually the earliest clinical indication of hyperkalemia.
- Be alert for potassium intoxication (hyperkalemia, see S&S, Appendix F); may result from any therapeutic dosage, and the patient may be asymptomatic.
- The risk of hyperkalemia with potassium supplement increases (1) in older adults because of decremental changes in kidney function associated with aging, (2) when dietary

intake of potassium suddenly increases, and (3) when kidney function is significantly compromised.

Patient & Family Education

- Do not be alarmed when the tablet carcass appears in your stool. The sustained release tablet (e.g., Slow-K) utilizes a wax matrix as carrier for KCl crystals that passes through the digestive system.
- Learn about sources of potassium with special reference to foods and OTC drugs.
- Avoid licorice; large amounts can cause both hypokalemia and sodium retention.
- Do not use any salt substitute unless it is specifically ordered by the physician. These contain a substantial amount of potassium and electrolytes other than sodium.
- Do not self-prescribe laxatives. Chronic laxative use has been associated with diarrhea–induced potassium loss.
- Notify physician of persistent vomiting because losses of potassium can occur.
- Report continuing signs of potassium deficit to physician: Weakness, fatigue, polyuria, polydipsia.
- Advise dentist or new physician that a potassium drug has been prescribed as long-term maintenance therapy.
- Do not open foil-wrapped powders and tablets before use.
- Do not breast feed while taking this drug without consulting physician.

POTASSIUM IODIDE

(poe-tass′ee-um)

Pima, SSKI, Thyro-Block ♣

Classifications: EXPECTORANT; ANTITHYROID AGENT

Prototype: Guaifenesin

Pregnancy Category: D

AVAILABILITY 325 mg/5 mL syrup; 1 g/mL solution

ACTIONS Pharmacologic use primarily related to iodide portion of molecule. Exact mechanism not clear but believed to increase secretion of respiratory fluids by direct action on bronchial tissue, thereby decreasing mucus viscosity. If patient is euthyroid, excess iodide ions causes minimal change in thyroid gland mass. Conversely, when the thyroid gland is hyperplastic, excess iodide ions temporarily inhibits secretion of thyroid hormone, fosters accumulation in thyroid follicles, and decreases vascularity of gland.

THERAPEUTIC EFFECTS Return of thyrotoxic symptoms may occur after 10–14 d of continuous treatment; consequently potassium iodide administration for hyperthyroidism is limited to short-term therapy. As an expectorant, the iodine ion portion of the molecule increases mucous secretion formation in the bronchi, and decreases viscosity of the mucous.

P

USES To facilitate bronchial drainage and cough in emphysema, asthma, chronic bronchitis, bronchiectasis, and respiratory tract allergies characterized by difficult-to-raise sputum. Also used alone for hyperthyroidism or in conjunction with antithyroid drugs and propranolol in treatment of thyrotoxic crisis; in immediate preoperative period for thyroidectomy to decrease vascularity, fragility, and size of thyroid gland and for treatment of persistent or recurring hyperthyroidism that occurs in Graves' disease patients. Used as a radiation protectant in patients receiving radioactive iodine and to shield the thyroid gland from radiation in the wake of a serious nuclear plant accident. (Use as an expectorant has been largely replaced by other agents.)

CONTRAINDICATIONS Hypersensitivity or idiosyncrasy to iodine; hyperthyroidism; hyperkalemia; acute bronchitis. Safety during pregnancy (category D), lactation, or in children <1 y is not established.

CAUTIOUS USE Renal impairment; cardiac disease; pulmonary tuberculosis; Addison's disease.

ROUTE & DOSAGE

To Reduce Thyroid Vascularity

Adult/Child: **PO** 50–250 mg t.i.d. for 10–14 d before surgery

Expectorant

Adult: **PO** 300–650 mg p.c. b.i.d. or t.i.d.
Child: **PO** 60–250 mg p.c. b.i.d. or t.i.d.

Thyroid Blocking in Radiation Emergency

Adult: **PO** 130 mg/d for 10 d
Child: **PO** *<1 y,* 65 mg/d for 10 d; *>1 y,* 130 mg/d for 10 d

P

ADMINISTRATION

Oral

- Give with meals in a full glass (240 mL) of water or fruit juice and at bedtime with food or juice to disguise salty taste and minimize gastric distress.
- Avoid giving KI with milk; absorption of the drug may be decreased by dairy products.
- Adhere strictly to schedule and accurate dose measurements when iodide is administered to prepare thyroid gland for surgery, particularly at end of treatment period when possibility of "escape" (from iodide) effect on thyroid gland increases.
- Place container in warm water and gently agitating to dissolve if crystals are noted in the solution.
- Discard any solution that has turned a brownish yellow on standing, especially if exposed to light (caused by liberated trace of free iodine).
- Store in airtight, light-resistant container.

ADVERSE EFFECTS (≥1%) **GI:** Diarrhea, nausea, vomiting, stomach pain, nonspecific small bowel lesions (associated with enteric coated tablets). **Body as a Whole:** Angioneurotic edema, cutaneous and mucosal hemorrhage, fever, arthralgias, lymph node enlargement, eosinophilia, paresthesias, periorbital edema, weakness. *Iodine poisoning (iodism):* Metallic taste, stomatitis, salivation, coryza, sneezing; swollen and tender salivary glands (sialadenitis), frontal headache, vomiting (blue vomitus if stomach contained starches, otherwise yellow vomitus), bloody diarrhea. **Metabolic:** Hyperthyroid adenoma, goiter, hypothyroidism, collagen disease–like syndromes. **CV:** Irregular heartbeat. **CNS:** Mental confusion. **Skin:** Acneiform skin lesions (prolonged use), flare-up of adolescent acne. **Respiratory:** Productive cough, pulmonary edema.

DIAGNOSTIC TEST INTERFERENCE Potassium iodide may alter ***thyroid function*** test results and may interfere with ***urinary 17-OHCS*** determinations.

INTERACTIONS Drug: ANTITHYROID DRUGS, **lithium** may potentiate hypothyroid and goitrogenic actions; POTASSIUM-SPARING DIURETICS, POTASSIUM SUPPLEMENTS, ACE INHIBITORS increase risk of hyperkalemia.

PHARMACOKINETICS Absorption: Adequately absorbed from GI tract.

Distribution: Crosses placenta. **Elimination:** Cleared from plasma by renal excretion or thyroid uptake.

NURSING IMPLICATIONS

Assessment & Drug Effects

- Lab tests: Determine serum potassium levels before and periodically during therapy.
- Keep physician informed about characteristics of sputum: quantity, consistency, color.

Patient & Family Education

- Report to physician promptly the occurrence of GI bleeding, abdominal pain, distension, nausea, or vomiting.
- Report clinical S&S of iodism (see ADVERSE EFFECTS). Usually, symptoms will subside with dose reduction and lengthened intervals between doses.
- Avoid foods rich in iodine if iodism develops: Seafood, fish liver oils, and iodized salt.
- Be aware that sudden withdrawal following prolonged use may precipitate thyroid storm.
- Do not use OTC drugs without consulting physician. Many preparations contain iodides and could augment prescribed dose [e.g., cough syrups, gargles, asthma medication, salt substitutes, cod liver oil, multiple vitamins (often suspended in iodide solutions)].
- Be aware that optimum hydration is the best expectorant when taking KI as an expectorant. Increase daily fluid intake.
- Do not breast feed while taking this drug without consulting physician.

PRALIDOXIME CHLORIDE

(pra-li-dox'eem)

2-PAM, Protopam Chloride

Classification: ANTIDOTE

Pregnancy Category: C

AVAILABILITY 600 mg, 1 g injection

ACTIONS Reactivates cholinesterase inhibited by phosphate esters by displacing the enzyme from its receptor sites; the free enzyme then can resume its function of degrading accumulated acetylcholine, thereby restoring normal neuromuscular transmission.

THERAPEUTIC EFFECTS Less effective against carbamate anticholinesterases (ambenonium, neostigmine, pyridostigmine). More active against effects of anticholinesterases at skeletal neuromuscular junction than at autonomic effector sites or in CNS respiratory center; therefore, atropine must be given concomitantly to block effects of acetylcholine and its accumulation in these sites.

USES As antidote in treatment of poisoning by organophosphate insecticides and pesticides with anticholinesterase activity (e.g., parathion, TEPP, sarin) and to control overdosage by anticholinesterase drugs used in treatment of myasthenia gravis (cholinergic crisis).

UNLABELED USES To reverse toxicity of echothiophate ophthalmic solution.

CONTRAINDICATIONS Use in poisoning by carbamate insecticide Sevin, inorganic phosphates, or organophosphates having no anticholinesterase activity; asthma, peptic ulcer, severe cardiac disease, patients receiving aminophylline, theophylline, morphine, succinylcholine, reserpine, or phenothiazines; pregnancy (category C).

CAUTIOUS USE Myasthenia gravis; renal insufficiency; concomitant use of barbiturates in organophosphorous poisoning; lactation, children.

ROUTE & DOSAGE

Organophosphate Poisoning

Adult: **IV** 1–2 g in 100 mL NS infused over 15–30 min; or 1–2 g as 5% solution in sterile water over not less than 5 min, may repeat after 1 h if muscle weakness not relieved **IM/SC** 1–2 g if IV route is not feasible
Child: **IV** 20–40 mg/kg as for adult

Anticholinesterase Overdose in Myasthenia Gravis

Adult: **IV** 1–2 g in 100 mL NS infused over 15–30 min, followed by increments of 250 mg q5min prn

ADMINISTRATION

Subcutaneous/Intramuscular

- Give only if unable to give IV; NOT preferred routes.
- Reconstitute as for direct IV injection (see below).

Intravenous

PREPARE: **Direct:** Reconstitute 1-g vial by adding 20 mL NS to yield 50 mg/mL (a 5% solution). If pulmonary edema is present, give without further dilution. **IV Infusion:** Preferred method is to further dilute in 100 mL NS.

ADMINISTER: **Direct:** In pulmonary edema, 1 g or fraction thereof over 5 min; do not exceed 200 mg/min. **IV Infusion:** Give over 15–30 min (preferred).

- Stop infusion and reduce rate if hypertension occurs.

ADVERSE EFFECTS (≥1%) **CNS:** Dizziness, headache, drowsiness. **GI:** Nausea. **Special Senses:** Blurred vision, diplopia, impaired accommodation. **CV:** Tachycardia, hypertension (dose-related). **Body as a Whole:** Hyperventilation, muscular weakness, laryngospasm, muscle rigidity.

INTERACTIONS Drug: May potentiate the effects of BARBITURATES.

PHARMACOKINETICS Peak: 5–15 min IV; 10–20 min IM. **Distribution:** Distributed throughout extracellular fluids; crosses blood–brain barrier slowly if at all. **Metabolism:** Probably metabolized in liver. **Elimination:** Rapidly excreted in urine. **Half-Life:** 0.8–2.7 h.

NURSING IMPLICATIONS

Assessment & Drug Effects

- Monitor BP, vital signs, and I&O. Report oliguria or changes in I&O ratio.
- Monitor closely. It is difficult to differentiate toxic effects of organophosphates or atropine from toxic effects of pralidoxime.
- Be alert for and report immediately: Reduction in muscle strength, onset of muscle twitching, changes in respiratory pattern, altered level of consciousness, increases or changes in heart rate and rhythm.
- Observe necessary safety precautions with unconscious patient because excitement and manic behavior reportedly may occur following recovery of consciousness.
- Keep patient under close observation for 48–72 h, particularly when poison was ingested, because of likelihood of continued absorption of organophosphate from lower bowel.
- In patients with myasthenia gravis, overdosage with pralidoxime may convert cholinergic crisis into myasthenic crisis.

PRAMIPEXOLE DIHYDROCHLORIDE

(pra-mi-pex'ole)

Mirapex

Classifications: AUTONOMIC NERVOUS SYSTEM AGENT; ANTICHOLINERGIC (PARASYMPATHOMIMETIC); ANTIPARKINSONISM AGENT

Prototype: Dopamine

Pregnancy Category: C

AVAILABILITY 0.125 mg, 0.25 mg, 1 mg, 1.5 mg tablets

ACTIONS Nonergot dopamine receptor agonist structurally similar to ropinirole for treatment of Parkinson's disease. Exhibits high affinity for the D_2 subfamily of dopamine receptors in the brain and higher binding affinity to D_3 than to D_2 or D_4 dopamine receptor subtypes. Precise mechanism of action and treatment for Parkinson's disease is not known.

THERAPEUTIC EFFECTS Increases level of dopamine in the brain, since it binds to the dopamine receptors. Effectiveness is indicated by improved control of neuromuscular functioning.

USES Treatment of idiopathic Parkinson's disease.

CONTRAINDICATIONS Hypersensitivity to pramipexole or ropinirole; lactation; pregnancy (category C).

CAUTIOUS USE Renal and liver function impairment; concomitant use of CNS depressants. Safety and efficacy in children are not established.

ROUTE & DOSAGE

Parkinson's Disease

Adult: **PO** Start with 0.125 mg t.i.d. times 1 wk, then 0.25 mg t.i.d. times 1 wk, continue to increase by 0.25 mg/dose t.i.d. qwk to a target dose of 1.5 mg t.i.d.

Renal Impairment

Cl_{cr} 35–60 mL/min: same titration schedule dosed b.i.d. (max: 1.5 mg b.i.d.); 15–35 mL/min: same titration schedule dosed q.d. (max: 1.5 mg q.d.)

ADMINISTRATION

Oral

- Titrate dose increments gradually with at least 5–7 d between increases.
- Reduce doses for creatinine clearance >60 mL/min.
- Give with food if nausea develops.

ADVERSE EFFECTS (≥1%) **Body as a Whole:** *Asthenia,* general edema, malaise, fever, decreased weight. **CNS:** *Dizziness, somnolence, sudden sleep attacks, insomnia, hallucinations, dyskinesia, extrapyramidal syndrome,* headache, confusion, amnesia, hypesthesia, dystonia, akathisia, myoclonus, peripheral edema. **CV:** *Postural hypotension,* chest pain. **GI:** *Nausea, constipation,* anorexia, dysphagia, dry mouth. **Respiratory:** Dyspnea, rhinitis. **Urogenital:** Decreased libido, impotence, urinary frequency or incontinence. **Special Senses:** Vision abnormalities.

INTERACTIONS Drug: Cimetidine decreases clearance; BUTYROPHENONES, **metoclopramide**, PHENOTHIAZINES may antagonize effects.

PHARMACOKINETICS Absorption: Rapidly absorbed from GI tract >90% bioavailability. **Peak:** 2 h. **Distribution:** 15% protein bound. **Metabolism:** Minimally metabolized in the liver. **Elimination:** Primarily excreted in urine. **Half-Life:** 8–12 h.

P

NURSING IMPLICATIONS

Assessment & Drug Effects

- Monitor for S&S of orthostatic hypotension, especially when the dosage is increased.
- Monitor cardiac status, especially in those with significant orthostatic hypotension.
- Lab tests: Monitor BUN and creatinine periodically; monitor CPK with complaints of muscle pain.
- Monitor for and report signs of tardive dyskinesia (see Appendix F).

Patient & Family Education

- Hallucinations are an adverse effect of this drug and occur more often in older adults.
- Make position changes slowly especially from a lying or sitting to standing.
- Use caution with potentially dangerous activities until response to drug is known; drowsiness is a common adverse effect.
- Avoid alcohol and use extra caution if taking other prescribed CNS depressants; both may exaggerate drowsiness, dizziness, and orthostatic hypotension.
- Do not abruptly stop taking this drug. It should be discontinued over a period of 1 wk.
- Do not breast feed while taking this drug.

PRAMOXINE HYDROCHLORIDE

(pra-mox'een)

Fleet Relief Anesthetic Hemorrhoidal, Prax, ProctoFoam, Tronolane, Tronothane ♣

Classifications: CENTRAL NERVOUS SYSTEM AGENT; LOCAL ANESTHETIC (MUCOSAL); ANTIPRURITIC

Prototype: Procaine

Pregnancy Category: C

AVAILABILITY 1% cream, gel, lotion, spray

ACTIONS Differs chemically from the amide- or ester-type anesthetics; therefore, it can be used in patients sensitive to these classes of drugs.

THERAPEUTIC EFFECTS Produces anesthesia by blocking conduction and propagation of sensory nerve impulses in skin and mucous membranes. Potency matches that of benzocaine as a topical anesthetic. Does not abolish gag reflex.

USES To relieve pain caused by minor burns and wounds; for temporary relief of pruritus secondary to dermatoses, hemorrhoids, and anal fissures; and to facilitate sigmoidoscopic examination.

CONTRAINDICATIONS Application to large areas of skin; prolonged use; preparation for laryngopharyngeal examination, bronchoscopy, or gastroscopy. Safety in children <2 y or during pregnancy (category C) is not established.

CAUTIOUS USE Extensive skin disorders; lactation.

ROUTE & DOSAGE

Relief of Minor Pain and Itching

Adult/Child: **Topical** >*2 y,* Apply t.i.d. or q.i.d.

ADMINISTRATION

Topical

- Clean thoroughly and dry rectal area before use for temporary relief of hemorrhoidal pain and itching.
- Administer rectal preparations in the morning and evening and after bowel movement or as directed by physician.
- Apply lotion or cream to affected surfaces with a gloved hand. Wash

hands thoroughly before and after treatment.
- Do not apply to eyes or nasal membranes.

ADVERSE EFFECTS (≥1%) **Skin:** Burning, stinging, sensitization.

INTERACTIONS No clinically significant interactions established.

PHARMACOKINETICS Onset: 3–5 min. **Duration:** Up to 5 h.

NURSING IMPLICATIONS

Patient & Family Education
- Drug is usually discontinued if condition being treated does not improve within 2–3 wk or if it worsens, or if rash or condition not present before treatment appears, or if treated area becomes inflamed or infected.
- Discontinue and consult physician if rectal bleeding and pain occur during hemorrhoid treatment.
- Do not breast feed while taking this drug without consulting physician.

PRAVASTATIN

(pra-vah-stat′in)
Pravachol
Classifications: CARDIOVASCULAR AGENT; ANTILIPEMIC; HMG-CoA REDUCTASE INHIBITOR (STATIN)
Prototype: Lovastatin
Pregnancy Category: X

AVAILABILITY 10 mg, 20 mg, 40 mg, 80 mg tablets

ACTIONS Competitively inhibits 3-hydroxy-3-methylglutaryl-coenzyme A (HMG-CoA) reductase, the enzyme that catalyzes cholesterol biosynthesis. HMG-CoA reductase inhibitors (statins) increase serum HDL cholesterol levels and decrease serum LDL cholesterol, VLDL cholesterol, and plasma triglyceride levels.
THERAPEUTIC EFFECTS It is effective in reducing total and LDL cholesterol in various forms of hypercholesterolemia.

USES Hypercholesterolemia (alone or in combination with bile acid sequestrants) and familial hypercholesterolemia.

CONTRAINDICATIONS Hypersensitivity to pravastatin; active liver disease or unexplained elevated liver function test; pregnancy (category X), lactation. Safety and efficacy in children <8 y are not established.
CAUTIOUS USE Alcoholics, history of liver disease; renal impairment.

ROUTE & DOSAGE

Hyperlipidemia
Adult: **PO** 10–80 mg q.d.
Child: **PO** *8–13 y,* 20 mg q.d.

ADMINISTRATION

Oral
- Give without regard to meals.
- Give in the evening.

ADVERSE EFFECTS (≥1%) **GI:** Nausea, diarrhea, abdominal pain, vomiting, constipation, flatulence, heartburn, transient elevations in serum liver transaminase levels. **Other:** Fatigue, rhinitis, cough, transient elevations in CPK.

INTERACTIONS Drug: May increase PT when administered with **warfarin**.

PHARMACOKINETICS Absorption: Poorly absorbed from GI tract; 17% reaches systemic circulation. **Onset:** 2 wk. **Peak:** 4 wk. **Distribution:** 43%–55% protein bound; does not cross blood–brain barrier; crosses placenta; distributed into

P

breast milk. **Metabolism:** Extensive first-pass metabolism in liver; has no active metabolites. **Elimination:** 20% of dose excreted in urine, 71% in feces. **Half-Life:** 1.8–2.6 h.

NURSING IMPLICATIONS

Assessment & Drug Effects

- Lab tests: Perform liver function tests at start of therapy and then at 12 wk. If normal at 12 wk, may change to semiannual monitoring. Monitor cholesterol levels throughout therapy.
- Monitor coagulation studies with patients receiving concurrent warfarin therapy. PT may be prolonged.
- Monitor CPK levels if patient experiences unexplained muscle pain.

Patient & Family Education

- Report unexplained muscle pain, tenderness, or weakness, especially if accompanied by malaise or fever, to physician promptly.
- Report signs of bleeding to physician promptly when taking concomitant warfarin therapy.
- Do not breast feed while taking this drug.

P

PRAZIQUANTEL

(pray-zi-kwon'tel)
Biltricide
Classifications: ANTIINFECTIVE; ANTHELMINTIC
Prototype: Mebendazole
Pregnancy Category: B

AVAILABILITY 600 mg tablets

ACTIONS Synthetic agent with broad-spectrum anthelmintic activity against all developmental stages of schistosomes and other trematodes (flukes) and against cestodes (tapeworm). Increases permeability of parasite cell membrane to calcium. Leads to immobilization of their suckers and dislodgment from their residence in blood vessel walls.

THERAPEUTIC EFFECTS Active against all developmental stages of schistosomes, including cercaria (free-swimming larvae). Activity against other trematodes (flukes) not fully understood; activity against cestodes (tapeworms) not clear but may be similar to that against schistosomes.

USES All stages of schistosomiasis (bilharziasis) caused by all schistosoma species pathogenic to humans. Other trematode infections caused by Chinese liver fluke.

UNLABELED USES Lung, sheep liver, and intestinal flukes and tapeworm infections.

CONTRAINDICATIONS Hypersensitivity to drug; ocular cysticercosis. Safety in children <4 y is not established; use during pregnancy (category B) only when clearly needed. Women should not breast feed on day of praziquantel therapy or for 72 h after last dose of drug.

ROUTE & DOSAGE

Schistosomiasis

Adult/Child: **PO** >4 y, 60 mg/kg in 3 equally divided doses at 4–6 h intervals on the same day, may repeat in 2–3 mo after exposure

Other Trematodes

Adult/Child: **PO** >4 y, 75 mg/kg in 3 equally divided doses at 4–6 h intervals on the same day

Cestodiasis (Adult or Intestinal Stage)

Adult: **PO** 10–20 mg/kg as single dose

Cestodiasis (Larval or Tissue Stage)

Adult: **PO** 50 mg/kg in 3 divided doses/d for 14 d

ADMINISTRATION

Oral

- Give dose with food and fluids. Tablets can be broken into quarters but should NOT be chewed.
- Advise patient to take sufficient fluid to wash down the medication. Tablets are soluble in water; gagging or vomiting because of bitter taste may result if tablets are retained in the mouth.
- Treatment for cestodiasis (tapeworm) is followed by gentle purgation 2 h after drug administration to facilitate rapid removal of tapeworms and ova.
- Store tablets in tight containers at <30° C (86° F).

ADVERSE EFFECTS (≥1%) **CNS:** *Dizziness, headache, malaise,* drowsiness, lassitude, CSF reaction syndrome (exacerbation of neurologic signs and symptoms such as seizures, increased CSF protein concentration, increased anticysticercal IgG levels, hyperthermia, intracranial hypertension) in patient treated for cerebral cysticercosis. **GI:** *Abdominal pain or discomfort with or without nausea;* vomiting, anorexia, diarrhea. **Hepatic:** *Increased AST, ALT (slight).* **Skin:** Pruritus, urticaria. **Body as a Whole:** Fever, sweating, symptoms of host-mediated immunologic response to antigen release from worms (fever, eosinophilia).

DIAGNOSTIC TEST INTERFERENCE Be mindful that selected drugs may interfere with stool studies for ova and parasites: ***iron, bismuth, oil*** (***mineral*** or ***castor***), ***Metamucil*** (if ingested within 1 wk of test), ***barium, antibiotics, antiamebic*** and ***antimalarial drugs,*** and ***gallbladder dye*** (if administered within 3 wk of test).

INTERACTIONS Drug: Phenytoin can lead to therapeutic failure.

PHARMACOKINETICS Absorption: Rapidly absorbed, 80% reaches systemic circulation. **Peak:** 1–3 h. **Distribution:** Enters cerebrospinal fluid. **Metabolism:** Extensively metabolized to inactive metabolites. **Elimination:** Excreted primarily in urine. **Half-Life:** 0.8–1.5 h.

NURSING IMPLICATIONS

Assessment & Drug Effects

- Patient is reexamined in 2 or 3 mo to ensure complete eradication of the infections.

Patient & Family Education

- Do not drive or operate other hazardous machinery on day of treatment or the following day because of potential drug-induced dizziness and drowsiness.
- Usually, all schistosomal worms are dead 7 d following treatment.
- Contact physician if you develop a sustained headache or high fever.
- Do not breast feed while taking this drug without consulting physician (see CONTRAINDICATIONS).

PRAZOSIN HYDROCHLORIDE (Pr)

(pra′zoe-sin)

Minipress

Classifications: AUTONOMIC NERVOUS SYSTEM AGENT; ALPHA-ADRENERGIC ANTAGONIST (BLOCKING AGENT, SYMPATHOLYTIC); CARDIOVASCULAR AGENT; ANTIHYPERTENSIVE; VASODILATOR

Pregnancy Category: C

AVAILABILITY 1 mg, 2 mg, 5 mg capsules

ACTIONS Selective inhibition of $alpha_1$-adrenoceptors; produces vasodilation in both resistance (arterioles) and capacitance (veins) vessels with the result that both peripheral vascular resistance and blood pressure are reduced.

THERAPEUTIC EFFECTS Lowers blood pressure in supine and standing positions with most pronounced effect on diastolic pressure. Minor effect on heart rate and cardiac output in the supine position and does not increase plasma renin activity. Tolerance to antihypertensive effect rarely occurs. Effective when used concomitantly with a beta-adrenergic blocking agent and a thiazide diuretic. Infrequently used in monotherapy because of tendency to support sodium and water retention resulting in increased plasma volume.

USES Treatment of hypertension.

UNLABELED USES Severe refractory congestive heart failure, Raynaud's disease or phenomenon, ergotamine-induced peripheral ischemia, pheochromocytoma, benign prostatic hypertrophy.

CONTRAINDICATIONS Safety during pregnancy (category C) or lactation is not established.

CAUTIOUS USE Chronic kidney failure; hypertensive patient with cerebral thrombosis; men with sickle cell trait.

ROUTE & DOSAGE

Hypertension

Adult: **PO** Start with 1 mg h.s., then 1 mg b.i.d. or t.i.d., may increase to 20 mg/d in divided doses

Child: **PO** Start with 5 mcg/kg q6h, gradually increase to 25 mcg/kg q6h (max: 15 mg or 0.4 mg/kg/d)

ADMINISTRATION

Oral

- Give initial dose at bedtime to reduce possibility of adverse effects such as postural hypotension and syncope. However, if first dose is taken during the day, advise patient not to drive a car for about 4 h after ingestion of drug.
- Give drug with food to reduce incidence of faintness and dizziness; food may delay absorption but does not affect extent of absorption.
- Store in tightly closed container away from strong light. Do not freeze.

ADVERSE EFFECTS (≥1%) **CNS:** *Dizziness, headache, drowsiness,* nervousness, vertigo, depression, paresthesia, insomnia. **CV:** Edema, dyspnea, syncope *first-dose phenomenon,* postural hypotension, *palpitations,* tachycardia, angina. **Special Senses:** Blurred vision, tinnitus, reddened sclerae. **GI:** Dry mouth, *nausea,* vomiting, diarrhea, constipation, abdominal discomfort, pain. **Urogenital:** Urinary frequency, incontinence, priapism (especially in men with sickle cell anemia), impotence. **Skin:** Rash, pruritus, alopecia, lichen planus. **Body as a Whole:** Diaphoresis, epistaxis, nasal congestion, arthralgia, transient leukopenia, increased serum uric acid, and BUN.

INTERACTIONS Drug: DIURETICS and other HYPOTENSIVE AGENTS increase hypotensive effects.

PHARMACOKINETICS Absorption: Approximately 60% of oral dose reaches the systemic circulation. **Onset:** 2 h. **Peak:** 2–4 h. **Duration:** <24 h. **Distribution:** Widely distributed, including into breast milk. **Metabolism:** Extensively metabolized in liver. **Elimination:** 6%–10%

excreted in urine, the rest in bile and feces. **Half-Life:** 2–4 h.

NURSING IMPLICATIONS

Assessment & Drug Effects

- Be alert for first-dose phenomenon (rare adverse effect: 0.15% of patients); characterized by a precipitous decline in BP, bradycardia, and consciousness disturbances (syncope) within 90–120 min after the initial dose of prazosin. Recovery is usually within several hours. Preexisting low plasma volume (from diuretic therapy or salt restriction), beta-adrenergic therapy, and recent stroke appear to increase the risk of this phenomenon.
- Monitor blood pressure. If it falls precipitously with first dose, notify physician promptly.
- Full therapeutic effect may not be achieved until 4–6 wk of therapy.

Patient & Family Education

- Avoid situations that would result in injury if you should faint, particularly during early phase of treatment. In most cases, effect does not recur after initial period of therapy; however, it may occur during acute febrile episodes, when drug dose is increased, or when another antihypertensive drug is added to the medication regimen.
- Make position and direction changes slowly and in stages. Dangle legs and move ankles a minute or so before standing when arising in the morning or after a nap.
- Lie down immediately if you experience light-headedness, dizziness, a sense of impending loss of consciousness, or blurred vision. Attempting to stand or walk may result in a fall.
- Do not drive or engage in other potentially hazardous activities until response to drug is known.
- Take drug at same time(s) each day. Keep a daily record noting BP and time taken, when medication was taken, which arm was used, position (i.e., standing, sitting), and time of day. Take this record to physician for reference at checkup appointment.
- Report priapism or impotence. A change in the drug regimen usually reverses these difficulties. Since acute episodes of priapism followed by impotence spontaneously occur in men with sickle cell anemia, another antihypertensive should be selected. In these patients, drug-induced priapism is frequently irreversible.
- Do not take OTC medications, especially those that may contain an adrenergic agent (e.g., remedies for coughs, colds, allergy), without consulting physician.
- Be aware that adverse effects usually disappear with continuation of therapy, but dosage reduction may be necessary.
- Do not breast feed while taking this drug without consulting physician.

PREDNISOLONE

(pred-niss'oh-lone)

Delta-Cortef, Prelone

PREDNISOLONE ACETATE

Econopred, Key-Pred, Pred Forte, Predcor

PREDNISOLONE SODIUM PHOSPHATE

AK-Pred, Hydeltrasol, Inflamase, Inflamase Forte, Inflamase Mild, Pred Mild

P

PREDNISOLONE TEBUTATE

Hydeltra-T.B.A., Prednisol TBA

Classifications: HORMONES AND SYNTHETIC SUBSTITUTES; ADRENAL CORTICOSTEROID; GLUCOCORTICOID

Prototype: Prednisone

Pregnancy Category: C

AVAILABILITY **Prednisolone** 5 mg tablet; 5 mg/5 mL, 15 mg/5 mL syrup, 0.12%, 0.125%, 1% ophthalmic suspension **Acetate** 25 mg/mL, 50 mg/mL injection **Sodium Phosphate** 5 mg/5 mL liquid; 20 mg/mL injection; 0.125%, 1% ophthalmic solution **Tebuate** 20 mg/mL injection

ACTIONS Analog of hydrocortisone with 3–5 times greater potency. Mineralocorticoid properties are minimal, and potential for sodium and water retention as well as potassium loss is reduced.

THERAPEUTIC EFFECTS Effective as an anti-inflammatory agent.

USES Principally as an antiinflammatory and immunosuppressant agent.

CONTRAINDICATIONS Safety during pregnancy (category C) or lactation is not established.

ROUTE & DOSAGE

Antiinflammatory

Adult: **PO** 5–60 mg/d in single or divided doses **IM** Acetate/Phosphate: 6–60 mg/d; Tebutate: 2–60 mg qwk **IV** Phosphate: 4–60 mg/d **Ophthalmic** See Appendix A-1

Child: **PO** 0.14–2 mg/kg/d in single or divided doses **IM** Acetate/Phosphate: 0.04–0.25 mg/kg 1–2 times/d **IV** Phosphate: 0.04–0.25 mg/kg 1–2 times/d

ADMINISTRATION

Oral

- Give with meals to reduce gastric irritation. If distress continues, consult physician about possible adjunctive antacid therapy.

Alternate-Day Therapy (ADT) for Patient on Long-term Therapy

- With ADT, the 48-h requirement for steroids is administered as a single dose every other morning.
- Be aware that ADT minimizes adverse effects associated with long-term treatment while maintaining the desired therapeutic effect.
- See **prednisone** for numerous additional nursing implications.

Intramuscular

Note: Verify that drug supplied is appropriate for the ordered route. Prednisolone acetate is for IM use.

- Give deep IM into a large muscle.

Intravenous

PREPARE: **Direct:** May be given undiluted. **IV Infusion:** May be added to 50–1000 mL of D5W or NS.

ADMINISTER: **Direct:** Give at a rate of 10 mg or fraction thereof over 60 s. **IV Infusion:** Do not exceed 10 mg/min.

INCOMPATIBILITIES **Solution/additive: Calcium gluceptate, metaraminol, methotrexate, polymyxin B.**

ADVERSE EFFECTS (≥1%) **Endocrine:** Hirsutism (occasional), adverse effects on growth and development of the individual and on sperm. **Special Senses:** Perforation of cornea (with topical drug). **Body as a Whole:** Sensitivity to heat; fat embolism, hypotension and shock-like reactions. **CNS:** Insomnia. **GI:** Gastric irritation or ulceration. **Skin:** Ecchymotic skin lesions; vasomotor symptoms. Also see prednisone.

INTERACTIONS Drug: BARBITURATES, **phenytoin, rifampin** increase steroid metabolism, therefore may need increased doses of prednisolone; **amphotericin B,** DIURETICS add to **potassium** loss; **ambenonium, neostigmine, pyridostigmine** may cause severe muscle weakness in patients with myasthenia gravis; VACCINES, TOXOIDS may inhibit antibody response.

PHARMACOKINETICS Absorption: Readily absorbed from GI tract. **Peak:** 1–2 h. **Duration:** 1–1.5 d. **Distribution:** Crosses placenta; distributed into breast milk. **Metabolism:** Metabolized in liver. **Elimination:** HPA suppression: 24–36 h; Excreted in urine. **Half-Life:** 3.5 h.

NURSING IMPLICATIONS

Assessment & Drug Effects

- Be alert to subclinical signs of lack of improvement such as continued drainage, low-grade fever, and interrupted healing. In diseases caused by microorganisms, infection may be masked, activated, or enhanced by corticosteroids. Observe and report exacerbation of symptoms after short period of therapeutic response.
- Be aware that temporary local discomfort may follow injection of prednisolone into bursa or joint.

Patient & Family Education

- Adhere to established dosage regimen (i.e., do not increase, decrease, or omit doses or change dose intervals).
- Report gastric distress or any sign of peptic ulcer.
- Do not breast feed while taking this drug without consulting physician.

PREDNISONE (Pr)

(pred′ni-sone)

Apo-Prednisone ✦, Deltasone, Meticorten, Orasone, Panasol, Prednicen-M, Sterapred, Winpred ✦

Classifications: HORMONES AND SYNTHETIC SUBSTITUTES; ADRENAL CORTICOSTEROID; GLUCOCORTICOID

Pregnancy Category: C

AVAILABILITY 1 mg, 2.5 mg, 5 mg, 10 mg, 20 mg, 50 mg tablets; 5 mg/5 mL, 5 mg/mL solution

ACTIONS Immediate-acting synthetic analog of hydrocortisone. Effect depends on biotransformation to prednisolone, a conversion that may be impaired in patient with liver dysfunction. Less mineralocorticoid activity than hydrocortisone, but sodium retention and potassium depletion can occur.

THERAPEUTIC EFFECTS Has antiinflammatory properties.

USES May be used as a single agent or conjunctively with antineoplastics in cancer therapy; also used in treatment of myasthenia gravis and inflammatory conditions and as an immunosuppressant.

CONTRAINDICATIONS Systemic fungal infections and known hypersensitivity.

CAUTIOUS USE Patients with infections; nonspecific ulcerative colitis; diverticulitis; active or latent peptic ulcer; renal insufficiency; hypertension; osteoporosis; myasthenia gravis. Safety during pregnancy (category C) or lactation is not established.

ROUTE & DOSAGE

Antiinflammatory

Adult: **PO** 5–60 mg/d in single or divided doses

P

Child: **PO** 0.1–0.15 mg/kg/d in single or divided doses

Acute Asthma

Child: **PO** <*1 y*, 1–2 mg/kg/d times 3–5 d or 10 mg q12h; *1–4 y*, 20 mg q12h; *5–13 y*, 30 mg q12h; >*13 y*, 40 mg q12h times 3–5 d

ADMINISTRATION

Oral

- Crush tablet and give with fluid of patient's choice if unable to swallow whole.
- Give at mealtimes or with a snack to reduce gastric irritation.
- Dose adjustment may be required if patient is subjected to severe stress (serious infection, surgery, or injury) or if a remission or disease exacerbation occurs.
- Do not abruptly stop drug. Reduce dose gradually by scheduled decrements (various regimens) to prevent withdrawal symptoms and permit adrenals to recover from drug-induced partial atrophy.

Alternate-Day Therapy (ADT) for Patient on Long-term Therapy

- With ADT, the 48-h requirement for steroids is administered as a single dose every other morning.
- Be aware that ADT minimizes adverse effects associated with long-term treatment while maintaining the desired therapeutic effect.
- See **prednisone** for numerous additional nursing implications.

ADVERSE EFFECTS (≥1%) **CNS:** Euphoria, headache, insomnia, confusion, psychosis. **CV:** CHF, edema. **GI:** Nausea, vomiting, peptic ulcer. **Musculoskeletal:** Muscle weakness, delayed wound healing, muscle wasting, osteoporosis, aseptic necrosis of bone, spontaneous fractures. **Endocrine:** Cushingoid features, growth suppression in children, carbohydrate intolerance, hyperglycemia. **Special Senses:** Cataracts. **Hematologic:** Leukocytosis. **Metabolic:** Hypokalemia.

INTERACTIONS Drug: BARBITURATES, **phenytoin, rifampin** increase steroid metabolism—increased doses of prednisone may be needed; **amphotericin B,** DIURETICS increase **potassium** loss; **ambenonium, neostigmine, pyridostigmine** may cause severe muscle weakness in patients with myasthenia gravis; may inhibit antibody response to VACCINES, TOXOIDS.

PHARMACOKINETICS Absorption: Readily absorbed from GI tract. **Peak:** 1–2 h. **Duration:** 1–1.5 d. **Distribution:** Crosses placenta; distributed into breast milk. **Metabolism:** Metabolized in liver. **Elimination:** Hypothalamus-pituitary axis suppression: 24–36 h; Excreted in urine. **Half-Life:** 3.5 h.

NURSING IMPLICATIONS

Assessment & Drug Effects

- Establish baseline and continuing data regarding BP, I&O ratio and pattern, weight, and sleep pattern. Start flow chart as reference for planning individualized pharmacotherapeutic patient care.
- Check and record BP during dose stabilization period at least 2 times daily. Report an ascending pattern.
- Monitor patient for evidence of HPA axis suppression during long-term therapy by determining plasma cortisol levels at weekly intervals.
- Lab tests: Obtain fasting blood glucose, serum electrolytes, and routine laboratory studies at regular intervals during long-term steroid therapy.

- Be aware that older adult patients and patients with low serum albumin are especially susceptible to adverse effects because of excess circulating free glucocorticoids.
- Be alert to signs of hypocalcemia (see Appendix F). Patients with hypocalcemia have increased requirements for pyridoxine (vitamin B_6), vitamins C and D, and folates.
- Be alert to possibility of masked infection and delayed healing (antiinflammatory and immunosuppressive actions). Prednisone suppresses early classic signs of inflammation. When patient is on an extended therapy regimen, incidence of oral *Candida* infection is high. Inspect mouth daily for symptoms: white patches, black furry tongue, painful membranes and tongue.
- Monitor bone density. Compression and spontaneous fractures of long bones and vertebrae present hazards, particularly in long-term corticosteroid treatment of rheumatoid arthritis or diabetes, in immobilized patients, and older adults.
- Be aware of previous history of psychotic tendencies. Watch for changes in mood and behavior, emotional stability, sleep pattern, or psychomotor activity, especially with long-term therapy, that may signal onset of recurrence. Report symptoms to physician.
- If a patient is receiving aspirin concomitantly with a corticosteroid, salicylism may be induced when the corticosteroid dosage is decreased or discontinued.
- Be aware that long-term corticosteroid therapy is ordinarily not interrupted when patient undergoes major surgery, but dosage may be increased.
- Monitor for withdrawal syndrome (e.g., myalgia, fever, arthralgia, malaise) and hypocorticism (e.g., anorexia, vomiting, nausea, fatigue, dizziness, hypotension, hypoglycemia, myalgia, arthralgia) with abrupt discontinuation of corticosteroids after long-term therapy.

Patient & Family Education

- Take drug as prescribed and do not alter dosing regimen or stop medication without consulting physician.
- Be aware that a slight weight gain with improved appetite is expected, but after dosage is stabilized, a sudden slow but steady weight increase [2 kg (5 lb) per wk] should be reported to physician.
- Avoid or minimize alcohol and caffeine may contribute to steroid-ulcer development in long-term therapy.
- Report symptoms of GI distress to physician and do not self-medicate to find relief.
- Do not use aspirin or other OTC drugs unless they are prescribed specifically by the physician.
- Report slow healing, any vague feeling of being sick, or return of pretreatment symptoms.
- Be fastidious about personal hygiene; give special attention to foot care, and be particularly cautious about bruising or abrading the skin.
- Report persistent backache or chest pain (possible symptoms of vertebral or rib fracture) that may occur with long-term therapy.
- Tell dentist or new physician about prednisone therapy.
- Carry medical information at all times. It needs to indicate medical diagnosis, medication(s), physician's name(s), address(es), and telephone number(s).
- Do not breast feed while taking this drug without consulting physician.

PRIMAQUINE PHOSPHATE

(prim'a-kween)
Primaquine
Classifications: ANTIINFECTIVE; ANTIMALARIAL
Prototype: Chloroquine
Pregnancy Category: C

AVAILABILITY 26.3 mg tablets; 5 g, 25 g, 100 g, 500 g powder

ACTIONS Acts on primary exoerythrocytic forms of *Plasmodium vivax* and *Plasmodium falciparum* by an incompletely known mechanism. Destroys late tissue forms of *P. vivax* and thus effects radical cure (prevents relapse).
THERAPEUTIC EFFECTS Gametocidal activity against all species of plasmodia that infect man; interrupts transmission of malaria.

USES To prevent relapse ("radical" or "clinical" cure) of *P. vivax* and *P. ovale* malarias and to prevent attacks after departure from areas where *P. vivax* and *P. ovale* malarias are endemic. With clindamycin for the treatment of *Pneumocystis carinii* pneumonia (PCP) in AIDS.

CONTRAINDICATIONS Rheumatoid arthritis; lupus erythematosus (SLE); hemolytic drugs, concomitant or recent use of agents capable of bone marrow depression (e.g., quinacrine; patients with G6PD deficiency). NADH methemoglobin reductase deficiency; pregnancy (category C), lactation.

ROUTE & DOSAGE

Malaria Relapse Prevention
Adult: **PO** 15 mg once/d for 14 d concomitantly or consecutively with chloroquine or hydroxychloroquine on first 3 d of acute attack
Child: **PO** 0.3 mg/kg once/d for 14 d concomitantly or consecutively with chloroquine or hydroxychloroquine on first 3 d of acute attack

Malaria Prophylaxis
Adult: **PO** 15 mg once/d for 14 d beginning immediately after leaving malarious area
Child: **PO** 0.3 mg/kg once/d for 14 d beginning immediately after leaving malarious area

ADMINISTRATION

Oral
- Give drug at mealtime or with an antacid (prescribed); may prevent or relieve gastric irritation. Notify physician if GI symptoms persist.
- Store in tight, light-resistant containers.

ADVERSE EFFECTS (≥1%) **Hematologic:** Hematologic reactions including granulocytopenia and acute hemolytic anemia in patients with G6PD deficiency, moderate leukocytosis or leukopenia, anemia, granulocytopenia, agranulocytosis. **GI:** Nausea, vomiting, epigastric distress, abdominal cramps. **Skin:** Pruritus. **Metabolic:** Methemoglobinemia (cyanosis). **Body as a Whole:** Headache, confusion, mental depression. **Special Senses:** Disturbances of visual accommodation. **CV:** Hypertension, arrhythmias (rare).

INTERACTIONS Drug: Toxicity of both **quinacrine** and primaquine increased.

PHARMACOKINETICS Absorption: Readily absorbed from GI tract. **Peak:** 6 h. **Metabolism:** Rapidly metabolized in liver to active metabolites. **Elimination:** Excreted in urine. **Half-Life:** 3.7–9.6 h.

NURSING IMPLICATIONS

Assessment & Drug Effects

- Be aware drug may precipitate acute hemolytic anemia in patients with G6PD deficiency, an inherited error of metabolism carried on the X chromosome, present in about 10% of American black males and certain white ethnic groups: Sardinians, Sephardic Jews, Greeks, and Iranians. Whites manifest more intense expression of hemolytic reaction than do blacks. Screen for prior to initiation of therapy.
- Lab tests: Perform repeated hematologic studies (particularly blood cell counts and Hgb) and urinalyses during therapy.

Patient & Family Education

- Examine urine after each voiding and to report to physician darkening of urine, red-tinged urine, and decrease in urine volume. Also report chills, fever, precordial pain, cyanosis (all suggest a hemolytic reaction). Sudden reductions in hemoglobin or erythrocyte count suggest an impending hemolytic reaction.
- Do not breast feed while taking this drug.

PRIMIDONE

(pri′mi-done)

Apo-Primidone ♣, Mysoline

Classifications: CENTRAL NERVOUS SYSTEM AGENT; BARBITURATE, ANTICONVULSANT

Prototype: Phenobarbital

Pregnancy Category: D

AVAILABILITY 50 mg, 250 mg tablets; 250 mg/5 mL suspension

ACTIONS Closely related chemically to barbiturates and with similar mechanism of action. Converted in body to phenobarbital. Impairs vitamin D, calcium, folic acid, and vitamin B_{12} metabolism and utilization.

THERAPEUTIC EFFECTS Antiepileptic properties result from raising the seizure threshold and changing seizure patterns.

USES Alone or concomitantly with other anticonvulsant agents in the prophylactic management of complex partial (psychomotor) and generalized tonic-clonic (grand mal) seizures.

UNLABELED USES Essential tremor.

CONTRAINDICATIONS Hypersensitivity to barbiturates, porphyria. Safety during pregnancy (category D) or lactation is not established.

CAUTIOUS USE Chronic lung disease; liver or kidney disease; hyperactive children.

ROUTE & DOSAGE

Seizures

Adult/Child: **PO** ≥*8 y*, 250 mg/d, increased by 250 mg/wk (max: 2 g in 2–4 divided doses)
Child: **PO** <*8 y*, 125 mg/d, increased by 125 mg/wk (max: 2 g in 2–4 divided doses)

ADMINISTRATION

Oral

- Give whole or crush with fluid of patient's choice.
- Give with food if drug causes GI distress.
- Note: Transition from another anticonvulsant to primidone normally requires at least 21 wks.

ADVERSE EFFECTS (≥1%) **CNS:** *Drowsiness, sedation, vertigo, ataxia, headache,* excitement (children), confusion, unusual fatigue, hyperirritability, emotional disturbances, acute psychoses (usually patients with psychomotor epilepsy). **Special Senses:** Diplopia, nystagmus, swelling of eyelids. **GI:** *Nausea, vomiting, anorexia.* **Hematologic:** Leukopenia, thrombocytopenia, eosinophilia, decreased serum folate levels, megaloblastic anemia (rare). **Skin:** Alopecia, maculopapular or morbilliform rash, edema, lupus erythematosus-like syndrome. **Urogenital:** Impotence. **Body as a Whole:** Lymphadenopathy, osteomalacia.

INTERACTIONS Drug: Alcohol, CNS DEPRESSANTS compound CNS depression; **phenobarbital** may decrease absorption and increase metabolism of ORAL ANTICOAGULANTS; increases metabolism of CORTICOSTEROIDS, ORAL CONTRACEPTIVES, ANTICONVULSANTS, **digitoxin,** possibly decreasing their effects; ANTIDEPRESSANTS potentiate adverse effects of primidone; **griseofulvin** decreases absorption of primidone. **Herbal: Kava-kava, valerian** may potentiate sedation.

PHARMACOKINETICS Absorption: Approximately 60%–80% absorbed from GI tract. **Peak:** 4 h. **Distribution:** Distributed into breast milk. **Metabolism:** Metabolized in liver to phenobarbital and PEMA. **Elimination:** Excreted in urine. **Half-Life:** Primidone 3–24 h, PEMA 24–48 h; phenobarbital 72–144 h.

NURSING IMPLICATIONS

Assessment & Drug Effects

- Lab tests: Perform baseline and periodic CBC, complete blood chemistry (q6mo), and primidone blood levels. (Therapeutic blood level for primidone: 5–10 mcg/mL.)
- Monitor primidone plasma levels (concentrations of primidone >10 mcg/mL are usually associated with significant ataxia and lethargy).
- Therapeutic response may not be evident for several weeks.
- Observe for S&S of folic acid deficiency: Mental dysfunction, psychiatric disorders, neuropathy, megaloblastic anemia. Determine serum folate levels if indicated.
- Be aware that presence of unusual drowsiness in breast fed newborns of primidone-treated mothers is an indication to discontinue breast feeding.

Patient & Family Education

- Avoid driving and other potentially hazardous activities during beginning of treatment because drowsiness, dizziness, and ataxia may be severe. Symptoms tend to disappear with continued therapy; if they persist, dosage reduction or drug withdrawal may be necessary.
- Avoid alcohol and other CNS depressants unless otherwise directed by physician.
- Do not take OTC medications unless approved by physician.
- Pregnant women should receive prophylactic vitamin K therapy for 1 mo prior to and during delivery to prevent neonatal hemorrhage.
- Withdraw primidone gradually to avoid precipitating status epilepticus.
- Carry medical information at all times. It needs to indicate medical diagnosis, medication(s), physician's name(s), address(es), and telephone number(s).
- Do not breast feed while taking this drug without consulting physician.

PROBENECID

(proe-ben'e-sid)

Benemid, Benuryl ✦, Probalan, SK-Probenecid

Classifications: ANTIGOUT AGENT; SULFONAMIDE; URICOSURIC AGENT

Prototype: Colchicine

Pregnancy Category: B

AVAILABILITY 0.5 g tablet

ACTIONS Sulfonamide-derivative renal tubular blocking agent. In sufficiently high doses, competitively inhibits renal tubular reabsorption of uric acid, thereby promoting its excretion and reducing serum urate levels.

THERAPEUTIC EFFECTS Prevents formation of new tophaceous deposits and causes gradual shrinking of old tophi by preventing uric acid build-up in the serum and tissues. As an additive to penicillin, it increases the serum concentration of the antibiotic, and also prolongs the serum concentration of the penicillins.

USES Hyperuricemia in chronic gouty arthritis and tophaceous gout.

UNLABELED USES Adjuvant to therapy with penicillin G and penicillin analogs to elevate and prolong plasma concentrations of these antibiotics; to promote uric acid excretion in hyperuricemia secondary to administration of thiazides and related diuretics, furosemide, ethacrynic acid, pyrazinamide.

CONTRAINDICATIONS Blood dyscrasias; uric acid kidney stones; during or within 2–3 wk of acute gouty attack; over excretion of uric acid (>1000 mg/d); patients with creatinine clearance <50 mg/min; use with penicillin in presence of known renal impairment; use for hyperuricemia secondary to cancer chemotherapy. Safety during pregnancy (category B), lactation, or in children <2 y is not established.

CAUTIOUS USE History of peptic ulcer.

ROUTE & DOSAGE

Gout

Adult: **PO** 250 mg b.i.d. for 1 wk, then 500 mg b.i.d. (max: 3 g/d)

Adjunct for Penicillin or Cephalosporin Therapy

Adult: **PO** 500 mg q.i.d. or 1 g with single dose therapy (e.g., gonorrhea)

Child: **PO** *2–14 y* or *<50 kg,* 25–40 mg/kg/d in 4 divided doses

ADMINISTRATION

Oral

- Therapy is usually not initiated during an acute gouty attack. Consult physician.
- Minimize GI adverse effects by giving after meals, with food, milk, or antacid (prescribed). If symptoms persist, dosage reduction may be required.
- Give with a full glass of water if not contraindicated.
- Be aware that physician may prescribe concurrent prophylactic doses of colchicine for first 3–6 mo of therapy because frequency of acute gouty attacks may increase during first 6–12 mo of therapy.

ADVERSE EFFECTS (≥1%) **Body as a Whole:** Flushing, dizziness, fever, anaphylaxis. **CNS:** *Headache.* **GI:** *Nausea, vomiting, anorexia,* sore gums, <u>hepatic necrosis (rare)</u>. **Urogenital:** Urinary frequency. **Hematologic:** Anemia, <u>hemolytic anemia (possibly related to G6PD deficiency), aplastic anemia (rare)</u>. **Musculoskeletal:** Exacerbations of gout, uric acid kidney stones. **Skin:** Dermatitis, pruritus. **Respiratory:** <u>Respiratory depression</u>.

DIAGNOSTIC TEST INTERFERENCE False-positive results ***urine glucose*** tests are possible with ***Benedict's solution*** or ***Clinitest*** (***glucose oxidase methods*** not affected, e.g., ***Clinistix, TesTape***).

INTERACTIONS Drug: SALICYLATES may decrease uricosuric activity;

may decrease **methotrexate** elimination, causing increased toxicity; decreases **nitrofurantoin** efficacy and increases its toxicity.

PHARMACOKINETICS Absorption: Readily absorbed from GI tract. **Onset:** 30 min. **Peak:** 2–4 h. **Duration:** 8 h. **Distribution:** Crosses placenta. **Metabolism:** Metabolized in liver. **Elimination:** Excreted in urine. **Half-Life:** 4–17 h.

NURSING IMPLICATIONS

Assessment & Drug Effects

- Decrease daily dosage with caution by 0.5 g q6mo to lowest effective dosage that maintains stable serum urate levels when gouty attacks have been absent for 6 mo or more and serum urate levels are controlled.
- Lab tests: Periodic serum urate levels, Hct and Hgb, and urinalysis. Determine acid–base balance periodically when urinary alkalinizers are used. Some physicians prescribe acetazolamide at bedtime to keep urine alkaline and dilute throughout night.
- Patients taking sulfonylureas may require dosage adjustment. Probenecid enhances hypoglycemic actions of these drugs (see DIAGNOSTIC TEST INTERFERENCES).
- Expect urate tophaceous deposits to decrease in size. Classic locations are in cartilage of ear pinna and big toe, but they can occur in bursae, tendons, skin, kidneys, and other tissues.

Patient & Family Education

- Drink fluid liberally (approximately 3000 mL/d) to maintain daily urinary output of at least 2000 mL or more. This is important because increased uric acid excretion promoted by drug predisposes to renal calculi.
- Physician may advise restriction of high-purine foods during early therapy until uric acid level stabilizes. Foods high in purine include organ meats (sweetbreads, liver, kidney), meat extracts, meat soups, gravy, anchovies, and sardines. Moderate amounts are present in other meats, fish, seafood, asparagus, spinach, peas, dried legumes, wild game.
- Avoid alcohol because it may increase serum urate levels.
- Do not stop taking drug without consulting physician. Irregular dosage schedule may sharply elevate serum urate level and precipitate acute gout.
- Be aware that lifelong therapy is usually required in patients with symptomatic hyperuricemia. Keep scheduled appointments with physician and for kidney function and hematology lab work.
- Report symptoms of hypersensitivity to physician. Discontinuation of drug is indicated.
- Do not take aspirin or other OTC medications without consulting physician. If a mild analgesic is required, acetaminophen is usually allowed.
- Do not breast feed while taking this drug without consulting physician.

PROCAINAMIDE HYDROCHLORIDE (Pr)

(proe-kane-a′mide)

Procan, Procanbid, Pronestyl, Pronestyl SR

Classifications: CARDIOVASCULAR AGENT; ANTIARRHYTHMIC, CLASS IA

Pregnancy Category: C

AVAILABILITY 250 mg, 375 mg, 500 mg tablets, capsules; 250 mg, 500 mg, 750 mg, 1000 mg sustained release tablets; 100 mg/mL, 500 mg/mL injection

ACTIONS Amide analog of procaine hydrochloride with cardiac actions similar to those of quinine. Class IA antiarrhythmic agent. Depresses excitability of myocardium to electrical stimulation, reduces conduction velocity in atria, ventricles, and His-Purkinje system. Increases duration of refractory period, especially in the atria.

THERAPEUTIC EFFECTS Produces slight change in contractility of cardiac muscle and cardiac output; suppresses automaticity of His-Purkinje ventricular muscle. Produces peripheral vasodilation and hypotension, especially with IV use.

USES Prophylactically to maintain normal sinus rhythm following conversion of atrial flutter or fibrillation by other methods. Also to prevent recurrence of paroxysmal atrial fibrillation and tachycardia, paroxysmal AV junctional rhythm, ventricular tachycardia, ventricular and atrial premature contractions. Also cardiac arrhythmias associated with surgery and anesthesia.

UNLABELED USES Malignant hyperthermia.

CONTRAINDICATIONS Myasthenia gravis; hypersensitivity to procainamide or procaine; blood dyscrasias; complete AV block, second and third degree AV block unassisted by pacemaker.

CAUTIOUS USE Patient who has undergone electrical conversion to sinus rhythm; hypotension, cardiac enlargement, CHF, MI, coronary occlusion, ventricular dysrhythmia from digitalis intoxication; hepatic or renal insufficiency; electrolyte imbalance; bronchial asthma; history of SLE. Safety during pregnancy (category C) or lactation is not established.

ROUTE & DOSAGE

Arrhythmias

Adult: **PO** 1 g followed by 250–500 mg q3h or 500 mg–1 g q6h sustained release (b.i.d. for Procanbid) **IM** 0.5–1 g q4–6h until able to take PO **IV** 100 mg q5min at a rate of 25–50 mg/min until arrhythmia is controlled or 1 g given, then 2–6 mg/min
Child: **PO** 40–60 mg/kg/d divided q4–6h **IV** 3–6 mg/kg q 10–30 min (max: 100 mg/dose), then 0.02–0.08 mg/kg/min

ADMINISTRATION

Oral

- Give first PO dose at least 4 h after last IV dose
- Give oral preparation on empty stomach, 1 h before or 2 h after meals, with a full glass of water to enhance absorption. If drug causes gastric distress, give with food.
- Crush immediate release (but NOT sustained release) tablet if patient is unable to swallow it whole.
- Swallow sustained release tablet whole. It has a wax matrix that is not absorbed but appears in the stool.

Intramuscular

- Assess procainamide blood levels if more than three IM injections are required.

Intravenous

- Use IV route for emergency situations.

PREPARE: **Direct:** When given direct IV, dilute each 100 mg with 5–10 mL of D5W or sterile water for injection. **IV Infusion:** When given by IV infusion, add 1 g of procainamide to 250–500 mL of D5W solution to yield 4 mg/mL in 250 mL or 2 mg/mL in 500 mL.

P

ADMINISTER: **Direct:** Usual rate 20 mg/min. Faster rates (up to 50 mg/min) should be used with caution. **IV Infusion:** 2–6 mg/min.

INCOMPATIBILITIES **Solution/additive: Bretylium, esmolol, ethacrynate, milrinone. Y-site: Inamrinone (amrinone).**

- Control IV administration over several hours by assessment of procainamide plasma levels.
- Use an infusion pump with constant monitoring. Keep patient in supine position. Be alert to signs of too rapid administration of drug (speed shock: irregular pulse, tight feeling in chest, flushed face, headache, loss of consciousness, shock, cardiac arrest).
- Store solution for up to 24 h at room temperature and for 7 d under refrigeration at 2°–8° C (36°–46° F). Slight yellowing does not alter drug potency, but discard solution if it is markedly discolored or precipitated.

P

ADVERSE EFFECTS (≥1%) **CNS:** Dizziness, psychosis. **CV:** Severe hypotension, pericarditis, ventricular fibrillation, AV block, tachycardia, flushing. **GI:** Bitter taste, nausea, vomiting, diarrhea, anorexia, (all mostly PO). **Hematologic:** Agranulocytosis with repeated use; thrombocytopenia. **Body as a Whole:** Fever, muscle and joint pain, angioneurotic edema, myalgia, *SLE-like syndrome (50% of patients on large doses for 1 y):* Polyarthralgias, pleuritic pain, pleural effusion. **Skin:** Maculopapular rash, pruritus. erythema, skin rash.

DIAGNOSTIC TEST INTERFERENCE Procainamide increases the plasma levels of ***alkaline phosphatase, bilirubin, lactic dehydrogenase*** and ***AST.*** It may also alter results of the ***edrophonium test.***

INTERACTIONS Drug: Other ANTIARRHYTHMICS add to therapeutic and toxic effects; ANTICHOLINERGIC AGENTS compound anticholinergic effects; ANTIHYPERTENSIVES add to hypotensive effects; **cimetidine** may increase procainamide and NAPA levels with increase in toxicity.

PHARMACOKINETICS Absorption: 75%–95% absorbed from GI tract. **Peak:** 15–60 min IM; 30–60 min PO. **Duration:** 3 h; 8 h with sustained release. **Distribution:** Distributed to CSF, liver, spleen, kidney, brain, and heart; crosses placenta; distributed into breast milk. **Metabolism:** Metabolized in liver to *N*-acetylprocainamide (NAPA), an active metabolite (30%–60% metabolized to NAPA). **Elimination:** Excreted in urine. **Half-Life:** 3 h procainamide, 6 h NAPA.

NURSING IMPLICATIONS

Assessment & Drug Effects

- Check apical radial pulses before each dose during period of adjustment to the oral route.
- Patients with severe heart, liver, or kidney disease and hypotension are at particular risk for adverse effects.
- Monitor the patient's ECG and BP continuously during IV drug administration.
- Discontinue IV drug temporarily when (1) arrhythmia is interrupted, (2) severe toxic effects are present, (3) QRS complex is excessively widened (greater than 50%), (4) PR interval is prolonged, or (5) BP drops 15 mm Hg or more. Obtain rhythm strip and notify physician.
- Ventricular dysrhythmias are usually abolished within a few minutes after IV dose and within an hour after PO or IM administration.

- Report promptly complaints of chest pain, dyspnea, and anxiety. Digitalization may have preceded procainamide in patients with atrial arrhythmias. Cardiotonic glycosides may induce sufficient increase in atrial contraction to dislodge atrial mural emboli, with subsequent pulmonary embolism.
- Therapeutic procainamide blood levels are reached in approximately 24 h if kidney function is normal but are delayed in presence of renal impairment.

Patient & Family Education

- Keep a record of weekly weight. Notify physician if weight gain of 1 kg (2 lb) or more is accompanied by local edema.
- Record and report date, time, and duration of fibrillation episodes when taking maintenance doses: Light-headedness, giddiness, weakness, or faintness.
- Keep a record of pulse rates. Report to physician changes in rate or quality.
- Report to physician signs of reduced procainamide control: Weakness, irregular pulse, unexplained fatigability, anxiety.
- Do not double dose or change an interval because a previous dose was missed. Take procainamide at evenly spaced intervals around the clock unless otherwise prescribed.
- Do not breast feed while taking this drug without consulting physician.

PROCAINE HYDROCHLORIDE

(proe'kane)

Novocain

Classifications: CENTRAL NERVOUS SYSTEM AGENT; LOCAL ANESTHETIC (ESTER-TYPE)

Pregnancy Category: C

AVAILABILITY 1%, 2%, 10% injection

ACTIONS Decreases sodium flux into nerve cell, thus depressing initial depolarization and preventing propagation and conduction of the nerve impulse.

THERAPEUTIC EFFECTS Local anesthetic action produces loss of sensation and motor activity in circumscribed areas of the body close to the injection or application site.

USES Spinal anesthesia and epidural and peripheral nerve block by injection and infiltration methods.

CONTRAINDICATIONS Known hypersensitivity to procaine or to other drugs of similar chemical structure, to PABA, and to parabens; generalized septicemia, inflammation, or sepsis at proposed injection site; cerebrospinal diseases (e.g., meningitis, syphilis); heart block, hypotension, hypertension; bowel pathology, GI hemorrhage. Safety during early pregnancy (category C) or lactation is not established.

CAUTIOUS USE Debilitated, older adults, or acutely ill patients; obstetric delivery; increased intraabdominal pressure; known drug allergies and sensitivities, dysrhythmias; shock.

ROUTE & DOSAGE

Spinal Anesthesia

Adult: **SC** 10% solution diluted with NS at 1 mL/5 s

Infiltration Anesthesia/Peripheral Nerve Block

Adult: **SC** 0.25%–0.5% solution

ADMINISTRATION

Subcutaneous

- Reconstitute solution: To prepare 60 mL of a 0.5% solution (5 mg/

P

mL), dilute 30 mL of 1%-solution with 30 mL sterile distilled water. Add 0.5–1 mL epinephrine 1:1000/ 100 mL anesthetic solution for vasoconstrictive effect (1:200,000–1:100,000).

- Do not use solutions that are cloudy, discolored, or that contain crystals. Discard unused portion of solutions not containing a preservative. Avoid use of solution with preservative for spinal, epidural, or caudal block.
- Inject slowly with frequent aspirations to avoid inadvertent intravascular administration, which can lead to a systemic reaction.

INCOMPATIBILITIES **Solution/additive: Aminophylline, amobarbital, chlorothiazide, magnesium sulfate, phenobarbital, phenytoin, secobarbital, sodium bicarbonate.**

ADVERSE EFFECTS (≥1%) **CNS:** Anxiety, nervousness, dizziness, circumoral paresthesia, tremors, drowsiness, sedation, convulsions, respiratory arrest. With spinal anesthesia: postspinal headache, arachnoiditis, palsies, spinal nerve paralysis, meningism. **Special Senses:** Tinnitus, blurred vision. **CV:** Myocardial depression, arrhythmias including bradycardia (also fetal bradycardia); hypotension. **GI:** Nausea, vomiting. **Skin:** Cutaneous lesions of delayed onset, urticaria, pruritus, angioneurotic edema, sweating, syncope, anaphylactoid reaction. **Urogenital:** Urinary retention, fecal or urinary incontinence, loss of perineal sensation and sexual function, slowing of labor and increased incidence of forceps delivery (all with caudal or epidural anesthesia).

INTERACTIONS Drug: May antagonize effects of SULFONAMIDES; increased risk of hypotension with MAOIS, ANTIHYPERTENSIVES.

PHARMACOKINETICS Absorption: Rapidly absorbed from injection site. **Onset:** 2–5 min. **Duration:** 1 h. **Metabolism:** Hydrolyzed by plasma pseudocholinesterases. **Elimination:** 80% of metabolites excreted in urine. **Half-Life:** 7.7 min.

NURSING IMPLICATIONS

Assessment & Drug Effects

- Be aware that reactions during dental procedure are usually mild, transient, and produced by epinephrine added to local anesthetic (e.g., headache, palpitation, tachycardia, hypertension, dizziness).
- Use procaine with epinephrine with caution in body areas with limited blood supply (e.g., fingers, toes, ears, nose). If used, inspect particular area for evidence of reduced perfusion (vasospasm): Pale, cold, sensitive skin.
- Hypotension is the most important complication of spinal anesthesia. Risk period is during first 30 min after induction and is intensified by changes in position that promote decreased venous return, or by preexisting hypertension, pregnancy, old age, or hypovolemia.

Patient & Family Education

- Understand that that there will be temporary loss of sensation in the area of the injection.
- Do not consume hot liquids or foods until sensation returns when drug used for dental procedure.

PROCARBAZINE HYDROCHLORIDE

(proe-kar′ba-zeen)

Matulane, Natulan ✦

Classifications: ANTINEOPLASTIC; ANTIMETABOLITE

Prototype: Fluorouracil

Pregnancy Category: D

P

AVAILABILITY 50 mg capsules

ACTIONS Hydrazine derivative with antimetabolite properties; cell cycle-specific for the S phase of cell division. Precise mechanism of action unknown. Suppresses mitosis at interphase, and causes chromatin derangement.

THERAPEUTIC EFFECTS Highly toxic to rapidly proliferating tissue. Has immunosuppressive properties and exhibits MAO inhibition activity. May delay myelosuppression. Reportedly does not affect survival time but may produce remissions of at least 1 mo duration.

USES Adjunct in palliative treatment of Hodgkin's disease.

UNLABELED USES Solid tumors.

CONTRAINDICATIONS Myelosuppression; alcohol ingestion; foods high in tyramine content; sympathomimetic drugs. MAO inhibitors should be discontinued 14 d prior to therapy; tricyclic antidepressants, 7 d before therapy. Safety during pregnancy (category D) or lactation is not established.

CAUTIOUS USE Concomitant administration with CNS depressants; hepatic or renal impairment; following radiation or chemotherapy before at least 1 mo has elapsed; hepatic and renal impairment; infection; diabetes mellitus.

ROUTE & DOSAGE

Adjunct for Hodgkin's Disease

Adult: **PO** 2–4 mg/kg/d in single or divided doses for 1 wk, then 4–6 mg/kg/d until WBC <4000/mm^3 or platelets are <100,000/mm^3 or maximum response obtained; drug is then discontinued until bone marrow recovery is satisfactory; treatment is started again at 1–2 mg/kg/d

Child: **PO** 50 mg/m^2/d in single or divided doses for 1 wk, then 100 mg/m^2/d until WBC is <4000/mm^3 or platelets are <100,000/mm^3 or maximum response obtained; drug is then discontinued until bone marrow recovery is satisfactory; treatment is started again at 50 mg/m^2/d

ADMINISTRATION

Oral

- Do not give if WBC count <4000/mm^3 or platelet count <100,000/mm^3. Consult physician.
- Store at 15°–30° C (59°–86° F). Protect from freezing, moisture, and light.

ADVERSE EFFECTS (≥1%) **CNS:** Myalgia, arthralgia, paresthesias, weakness, fatigue, lethargy, drowsiness, neuropathies, mental depression, acute psychosis, hallucinations, dizziness, headache, ataxia, nervousness, insomnia, coma, confusion, seizures. **GI:** *Severe nausea and vomiting,* anorexia, stomatitis, dry mouth, dysphagia, diarrhea, constipation, jaundice, ascites. **Hematologic:** Bone marrow suppression (leukopenia, anemia, thrombocytopenia), hemolysis, bleeding tendencies. **Skin:** Dermatitis, pruritus, herpes, hyperpigmentation, flushing, alopecia. **Respiratory:** *Pleural effusion, cough,* hoarseness. **CV:** Hypotension, tachycardia. **Body as a Whole:** Chills, fever, sweating, photosensitivity; intercurrent infections. **Urogenital:** Gynecomastia, depressed spermatogenesis, atrophy of testes.

DIAGNOSTIC TEST INTERFERENCE Procarbazine may enhance the effects of **CNS depressants.** A disulfiram-like reaction may occur following ingestion of ***alcohol.***

INTERACTIONS Drug: Alcohol, PHENOTHIAZINES, and other CNS DEPRESSANTS add to CNS depression; TRICYCLIC ANTIDEPRESSANTS, MAO INHIBITORS, SYMPATHOMIMETICS, **ephedrine, phenylpropanolamine** may precipitate hypertensive crisis, hyperpyrexia; seizures, or death. **Food: Tyramine**-containing foods may precipitate hypertensive crisis [see **phenelzine sulfate** (MAO INHIBITOR)].

PHARMACOKINETICS Absorption: Readily absorbed from GI tract. **Peak:** 1 h. **Distribution:** Widely distributed with high concentrations in liver, kidneys, intestinal wall, and skin. **Metabolism:** Metabolized in liver. **Elimination:** Excreted in urine. **Half-Life:** 1 h.

NURSING IMPLICATIONS

Assessment & Drug Effects

- Start flow sheet and record baseline BP, weight, temperature, pulse, and I&O ratio and pattern.
- Lab tests: Determine hematologic status (Hgb, Hct, WBC, differential, reticulocyte, and platelet counts) initially and at least q3–4d. Hepatic and renal studies (transaminase, alkaline phosphatase, BUN, urinalysis) are also indicated initially and at least weekly during therapy.
- Protect patient from exposure to infection and trauma when nadir of leukopenia ($<4000/mm^3$) is approached. Note and report changes in voiding pattern, hematuria, and dysuria (possible signs of urinary tract infection). Monitor I&O ratio and temperature closely.
- Withhold drug and notify physician of any of the following: CNS S&S (e.g., paresthesias, neuropathies, confusion); leukopenia (WBC count $<4000/mm^3$; thrombocytopenia (platelet count $<100,000/mm^3$); hypersensitivity reaction, the first small ulceration or persistent spot of soreness in oral cavity, diarrhea, and bleeding.
- Monitor for and report any of the following: chills, fever, weakness, shortness of breath, productive cough. Drug will be discontinued.
- Assess for signs of liver dysfunction: Jaundice (yellow skin, sclerae, and soft palate), frothy or dark urine, clay-colored stools.
- Tolerance to nausea and vomiting (most common adverse effects) usually develops by end of first week of treatment. Doses are kept at a minimum during this time. If vomiting persists, therapy will be interrupted.

Patient & Family Education

- Avoid OTC nose drops, cough medicines, and antiobesity preparations containing sympathomimetic drugs (e.g., ephedrine, amphetamine, epinephrine) and tricyclic antidepressants because they may cause hypertensive crises since procarbazine has MAO inhibitory activity. Do not to use OTC preparations without physician's approval.
- Report to physician any sign of impending infection.
- Do not eat foods high in tyramine content (e.g., aged cheese, beer, wine).
- Avoid alcohol; ingestion of any form of alcohol may precipitate a disulfiram-type reaction (see Appendix F).
- Report to physician immediately signs of hemorrhagic tendencies: Bleeding into skin and mucosa, epistaxis, hemoptysis, hematemesis, hematuria, melena, ecchymoses, petechiae. Bone marrow depression often occurs 2–8 wk after start of therapy.
- Avoid excessive exposure to the sun because of potential photosensitivity reaction: Cover as much

skin area as possible with clothing, and use sunscreen lotion (SPF >12) on all exposed skin surfaces.
- Use caution while driving or performing hazardous tasks until response to drug is known since drowsiness, dizziness, and blurred vision are possible adverse effects.
- Use contraceptive measures during procarbazine therapy.
- Do not breast feed while taking this drug without consulting physician.

PROCHLORPERAZINE (Pr)

(proe-klor-per′a-zeen)
Compazine

PROCHLORPERAZINE EDISYLATE

Compazine

PROCHLORPERAZINE MALEATE

Compazine, Stemetil ♣

Classifications: PSYCHOTHERAPEUTIC; ANTIPSYCHOTIC PHENOTHIAZINE; GASTROINTESTINAL AGENT; ANTIEMETIC
Pregnancy Category: C

AVAILABILITY 5 mg, 10 mg, 25 mg tablets; 10 mg, 15 mg, 30 mg sustained release capsule; 2.5 mg, 5 mg, 25 mg suppositories; 5 mg/mL injection **Edisylate** 5 mg/5 mL syrup, 5 mg/mL injection

ACTIONS Phenothiazine derivative similar to chlorpromazine. Mechanism that produces strong antipsychotic effects is unclear, but thought to be related to blockade of postsynaptic dopamine receptors in the brain. Action on the hypothalamus and reticular formation results in sedative effects. Antiemetic effect is produced by suppression of the chemoreceptor trigger zone (CTZ).

THERAPEUTIC EFFECTS Inhibits dopamine reuptake; may be basis for moderate extrapyramidal symptoms. Greater extrapyramidal effects and antiemetic potency but fewer sedative, hypotensive, and anticholinergic effects than chlorpromazine.

USES Management of manifestations of psychotic disorders, of excessive anxiety, tension, and agitation, and to control severe nausea and vomiting.

CONTRAINDICATIONS Hypersensitivity to phenothiazines; bone marrow depression; comatose or severely depressed states; children <9 kg (20 lb) or 2 y of age; pediatric surgery; short-term vomiting in children or vomiting of unknown etiology; Reye's syndrome or other encephalopathies; history of dyskinetic reactions or epilepsy; pregnancy (category C), lactation.
CAUTIOUS USE Patient with previously diagnosed breast cancer, children with acute illness or dehydration.

ROUTE & DOSAGE

Severe Nausea, Vomiting, Anxiety, Psychotic Disorders

Adult: **PO** 5–10 mg t.i.d. or q.i.d.; sustained release: 10–15 mg q12h **IM** 5–10 mg q3–4h up to 40 mg/d **IV** 2.5–10 mg q6–8h (max: 40 mg/d) **PR** 25 mg b.i.d.
Child: **PO** 2.5 mg 1–3 times/d or 5 mg b.i.d. (max: 15 mg/d) **IM** 0.13 mg/kg q3–4h **PR** 2.5 mg b.i.d. or t.i.d. up to 20–25 mg/d

ADMINISTRATION

Oral
- Dosages for older adults, emaciated patients and children should be increased slowly.

P

- Ensure that sustained release form is not chewed or crushed. Must be swallowed whole.
- Do not give oral concentrate to children.
- Avoid skin contact with oral concentrate or injection solution because of possibility of contact dermatitis.

Intramuscular
- Do not inject drug SC.
- Make injection deep into the upper outer quadrant of the buttock in adults. Follow agency policy regarding IM injection site for children.

Intravenous

PREPARE: **Direct:** Dilute each 5 mg (1 mL) in 4 mL of NS or other compatible solution to yield 1 mg/mL. **IV Infusion:** Dilute in 50–100 mL of D5W, NS, D5/0.45% NaCl, RL or other compatible solution.

ADMINISTER: **Direct:** Do not exceed 10 mg for a single dose. Do not give a bolus dose. Give at a maximum rate of 5 mg/min. **IV Infusion:** Give over 15–30 min. Do not exceed direct IV rate.

INCOMPATIBILITIES **Solution/additive: Aminophylline, amphotericin B, ampicillin, calcium gluceptate, calcium gluconate, cephalothin, chloramphenicol, chlorothiazide, dimenhydrinate, furosemide, hydrocortisone, ketorolac, methohexital, midazolam, morphine, penicillin G sodium, pentobarbital, phenobarbital, sodium bicarbonate, dimenhydrinate, hydromorphone, thiopental. Y-site: Aldesleukin, allopurinol, amifostine, amphotericin B cholesteryl complex, aztreonam, cefepime, etoposide, fludarabine, foscarnet, filgrastim, piperacillin-tazobactam.**

- Discard markedly discolored solutions; slight yellowing does not appear to alter potency.

ADVERSE EFFECTS (≥1%) **CNS:** *Drowsiness,* dizziness, *extrapyramidal reactions (akathisia, dystonia or parkinsonism),* persistent tardive dyskinesia, acute catatonia. **CV:** Hypotension. **GI:** Cholestatic jaundice. **Skin:** Contact dermatitis, photosensitivity. **Endocrine:** Galactorrhea, amenorrhea. **Special Senses:** Blurred vision. **Hematologic:** Leukopenia, agranulocytosis.

INTERACTIONS Drug: Alcohol, CNS DEPRESSANTS increase CNS depression; ANTACIDS, ANTIDIARRHEALS decrease absorption, therefore, administer 2 h apart; **phenobarbital** increases metabolism of prochlorperazine; GENERAL ANESTHETICS increase excitation and hypotension; antagonizes antihypertensive action of **guanethidine; phenylpropanolamine** poses possibility of sudden death; TRICYCLIC ANTIDEPRESSANTS intensify hypotensive and anticholinergic effects; decreases seizure threshold—ANTICONVULSANT dosage may need to be increased. **Herbal: Kava-kava** may increase risk and severity of dystonic reactions.

PHARMACOKINETICS Absorption: Readily absorbed from GI tract. **Onset:** 30–40 min PO; 60 min PR; 10–20 min IM. **Duration:** 3–4 h PO; 10–12 h sustained release PO; 3–4 h PR; up to 12 h IM. **Distribution:** Crosses placenta; distributed into breast milk. **Metabolism:** Metabolized in liver. **Elimination:** Excreted in urine.

NURSING IMPLICATIONS

Assessment & Drug Effects
- Positioned nauseated patients who have received prochlorperazine carefully to prevent aspiration of

Common adverse effects in *italic*, life-threatening effects underlined: generic names in **bold**; classifications in SMALL CAPS; ♣ Canadian drug name; ⓟ Prototype drug

P

vomitus; may have depressed cough reflex.
- Most older adult and emaciated patients and children, especially those with dehydration or acute illness, appear to be particularly susceptible to extrapyramidal effects. Be alert to onset of symptoms: Early in therapy watch for pseudoparkinson's and acute dyskinesia. After 1–2 mo, be alert to akathisia.
- Keep in mind that the antiemetic effect may mask toxicity of other drugs or make it difficult to diagnose conditions with a primary symptom of nausea, such as intestinal obstruction and increased intracranial pressure.
- Lab tests: Periodic CBC with differential in long-term therapy.
- Be alert to signs of high core temperature: Red, dry, hot skin; full bounding pulse; dilated pupils; dyspnea; confusion; temperature over 40.6° C (105° F); elevated BP. Exposure to high environmental temperature, to sun's rays, or to a high fever associated with serious illness places this patient at risk for heat stroke. Inform physician and institute measures to reduce body temperature rapidly.

Patient & Family Education
- Take drug only as prescribed and do not alter dose or schedule. Consult physician before stopping the medication.
- Avoid hazardous activities such as driving a car until response to drug is known because drug may impair mental and physical abilities, especially during first few days of therapy.
- Be aware that drug may color urine reddish brown. It also may cause the sun-exposed skin to turn gray-blue.
- Protect skin from direct sun's rays and use a sunscreen lotion (SPF >12) to prevent photosensitivity reaction.
- Withhold dose and report to the physician if the following symptoms persist more than a few hours: Tremor, involuntary twitching, exaggerated restlessness. Other reportable symptoms include light-colored stools, changes in vision, sore throat, fever, rash.
- Do not breast feed while taking this drug.

PROCYCLIDINE HYDROCHLORIDE

(proe-sye'kli-deen)

Kemadrin, Procyclid ✦

Classifications: AUTONOMIC NERVOUS SYSTEM AGENT; ANTICHOLINERGIC (PARASYMPATHOLYTIC); ANTIMUSCARINIC; ANTISPASMODIC; ANTIPARKINSONISM AGENT

Prototype: Atropine

Pregnancy Category: C

AVAILABILITY 5 mg tablets

ACTIONS Centrally acting synthetic anticholinergic agent with actions similar to those of atropine. Selectively blocks muscarinic responses to acetylcholine (ACh), whether excitatory or inhibitory.

THERAPEUTIC EFFECTS Diminishes the characteristic tremor of parkinsonism.

USES To relieve symptoms of parkinsonism syndrome (postencephalitic, arteriosclerotic, and idiopathic), and drug-induced extrapyramidal symptoms.

CONTRAINDICATIONS Angle-closure glaucoma. Safety during pregnancy (category C), lactation, or in children is not established.

CAUTIOUS USE Hypotension; mental disorders; tachycardia; prostatic hypertrophy.

ROUTE & DOSAGE

Parkinsonism Symptoms

Adult: **PO** 2.5 mg t.i.d. p.c., may be gradually increased to 5 mg t.i.d. if tolerated with an additional 5 mg h.s. (max: 45–60 mg/d)
Geriatric: **PO** Start with 2.5 mg 1–2 times/d

ADMINISTRATION

Oral

- Minimize adverse effects by administration of drug during or after meals.
- Store at 15°–30° C (59°–86° F) in tightly closed containers unless otherwise directed.

ADVERSE EFFECTS (≥1%) **Body as a Whole:** Flushing of skin, decreased sweating, headache, lightheadedness, dizziness, feeling of muscle weakness. **Special Senses:** Blurred vision, mydriasis, photophobia. **CV:** Palpitation, tachycardia, *hypotension*. **GI:** *Dry mouth,* nausea, vomiting, epigastric distress, constipation, paralytic ileus, acute suppurative parotitis. **Urogenital:** Urinary retention. **Skin:** Skin eruptions (occasionally). **CNS:** Mental confusion, psychotic-like symptoms.

INTERACTIONS Drug: Additive adverse effects with ANTICHOLINERGIC AGENTS.

PHARMACOKINETICS Onset: 35–40 min. **Duration:** 4–6 h.

NURSING IMPLICATIONS

Assessment & Drug Effects

- Monitor heart rate and rhythm and BP. Report palpitations, tachycardia, paradoxical bradycardia, or decreasing BP. Dosage adjustment or discontinuation of drug may be indicated.
- Monitor therapeutic effectiveness. Generally more effective in controlling rigidity than tremors. Tremors may temporarily appear to be exaggerated as rigidity is relieved, especially in patients with severe spasticity.
- Observe for and report symptoms of mental confusion, disorientation, agitation, and psychotic-like symptoms, particularly in older adult patients who have low BP, to physician.
- Check for constipation and abdominal distention and provide information for preventing constipation.

Patient & Family Education

- Void before taking drug if urinary hesitancy or retention is a problem.
- Avoid potentially hazardous activities until response to drug is known because drug may cause blurred vision and dizziness.
- Relieve dry mouth by rinsing frequently with water, chewing sugarless gum or sucking hard candy, or increasing noncaloric fluid intake. If these measures fail, a saliva substitute, available OTC, may help (e.g., Orex, Xero-Lube).
- Avoid alcohol and do not to take other CNS depressants unless otherwise advised by physician.
- Do not breast feed while taking this drug without consulting physician.

PROGESTERONE (Pr)

(proe-jess′ter-one)

Crinone Gel, Gesterol 50, Progestaject, Progestasert, Prometrium

Classifications: HORMONES AND SYNTHETIC SUBSTITUTES; PROGESTIN

Pregnancy Category: X

AVAILABILITY 100 mg capsules; 50 mg/mL injection; 8% gel

ACTIONS Steroid hormone synthesized and released by testes, ovary, adrenal cortex, and placenta. Estrogenic, anabolic, and androgenic activity. Physiologic precursor to estrogens, androgens, and adrenocortical steroids. Transforms endometrium from proliferative to secretory state; suppresses pituitary gonadotropin secretion, thereby blocking follicular maturation and ovulation. Acting with estrogen, promotes mammary gland development without causing lactation and increases body temperature 1° F at time of ovulation.

THERAPEUTIC EFFECTS Relaxes estrogen-primed myometrium and prohibits spontaneous contraction of uterus. Sudden drop in blood levels of progestin (and estradiol) causes "withdrawal bleeding" from endometrium. Intrauterine placement of progesterone (intrauterine progesterone contraceptive system) hypothetically inhibits sperm survival, and suppresses endometrial proliferation (antiestrogenic effect).

USES Secondary amenorrhea, functional uterine bleeding, endometriosis, and premenstrual syndrome. As an intrauterine agent (Progestasert) and in combination with estrogens provides fertility control. Largely supplanted by new progestins, which have longer action and oral effectiveness. Treatment of infertile women with progesterone deficiency.

CONTRAINDICATIONS Hypersensitivity to progestins, known or suspected breast or genital malignancy; use as a pregnancy test; thrombophlebitis, thromboembolic disorders; cerebral apoplexy (or its history); severely impaired liver function or disease; undiagnosed vaginal bleeding, missed abortion; use during first 4 mo of pregnancy (category X), lactation. *Progestasert:* Pregnancy or suspicion of pregnancy. *Prometrium* (oral): Patients with peanut allergy.

CAUTIOUS USE Anemia; diabetes mellitus; history of psychic depression; persons susceptible to acute intermittent porphyria or with conditions that may be aggravated by fluid retention (asthma, seizure disorders, cardiac or kidney function, migraine); impaired liver function; previous ectopic pregnancy; presence or history of salpingitis; venereal disease; unresolved abnormal Pap smear; genital bleeding of unknown etiology; previous pelvic surgery.

ROUTE & DOSAGE

Amenorrhea

Adult: **IM** 5–10 mg for 6–8 consecutive days **PO** 400 mg h.s. times 10 d

Uterine Bleeding

Adult: **IM** 5–10 mg/d for 6 d

Premenstrual Syndrome

Adult: **PR** 200–400 mg/d

Intrauterine Contraceptive

Adult: **Intrauterine** Insert in uterus for 1 y

ADMINISTRATION

Intramuscular

- Immerse vial in warm water momentarily to redissolve crystals (if present) and to facilitate aspiration of drug into syringe.
- Inject deeply IM. Injection site may be irritated. Inspect IM sites carefully and rotate areas systematically.
- Do not give oral capsules, which contain peanut oil, to patients allergic to peanuts.
- Store drug at 15°–30° C (59°–86° F) unless otherwise specified by

P

manufacturer. Protect from freezing and light.

ADVERSE EFFECTS (≥1%) **CNS:** Migraine headache, *dizziness,* lethargy, mental depression, somnolence, insomnia. **CV:** Thromboembolic disorder, pulmonary embolism. **Special Senses:** Change in vision, proptosis, diplopia, papilledema, retinal vascular lesions. **GI:** Hepatic disease, cholestatic jaundice; *nausea,* vomiting, *abdominal cramps.* **Urogenital:** Vaginal candidiasis, chloasma, cervical erosion and changes in secretions, *breakthrough bleeding,* dysmenorrhea, amenorrhea, pruritus vulvae. **Metabolic:** Hyperglycemia, decreased libido, transient increase in sodium and chloride excretion, pyrexia. **Skin:** *Acne,* pruritus, allergic rash, photosensitivity, urticaria, hirsutism, alopecia. **Body as a Whole:** *Edema, weight changes;* pain at injection site; fatigue. **Endocrine:** Gynecomastia, galactorrhea.

P

DIAGNOSTIC TEST INTERFERENCE PROGESTINS may decrease levels of ***urinary pregnanediol*** and increase levels of ***serum alkaline phosphatase, plasma amino acids, urinary nitrogen,*** and ***coagulation factors VII, VIII, IX,*** and ***X.*** They also decrease ***glucose tolerance*** (may cause false-positive ***urine glucose tests***) and lower ***HDL*** (high-density lipoprotein) levels.

INTERACTIONS Drug: BARBITURATES, **carbamazepine, phenytoin, rifampin** may alter contraceptive effectiveness; **ketoconazole** may inhibit progesterone metabolism; may antagonize effects of **bromocriptine.**

PHARMACOKINETICS Absorption: Rapid absorption from IM site; PO peaks at 3 h. **Metabolism:** Extensively metabolized in liver. **Elimination:** Excreted primarily in urine; excreted in breast milk. **Half-Life:** 5 min.

NURSING IMPLICATIONS

Assessment & Drug Effects

- Record baseline data for comparative value about patient's weight, BP, and pulse at onset of progestin therapy. Report deviations promptly.
- Lab tests: Periodic liver function tests, blood glucose, and serum electrolytes.
- Monitor for and report immediately S&S of thrombophlebitis or thromboembolic disease.
- Be alert for S&S of acute intermittent porphyria in susceptible patients (e.g., severe, colicky abdominal pain, vomiting, distention, diarrhea, constipation).

Patient & Family Education

- Avoid exposure to UV light and prolonged periods of time in the sun. Photosensitivity severity is related to both time of exposure and dose. A phototoxic drug reaction usually looks like an exaggerated sunburn and occurs within 5–18 h after exposure to sun and is maximal by 36–72 h.
- Use sunscreen lotion (SPF >12) that contains paraaminobenzoic acid (PABA) on exposed skin surfaces whenever outdoors, even on dark days.
- Inform physician promptly if any of the following occur: Sudden severe headache or vomiting, dizziness or fainting, numbness in an arm or leg, pain in calves accompanied by swelling, warmth, and redness; acute chest pain or dyspnea.
- Report to physician promptly unexplained sudden or gradual, par-

tial or complete loss of vision, ptosis, or diplopia.
- Monitor for loss of glycemic control if diabetic.
- Notify physician if you become or suspect pregnancy. Learn the potential risk to the fetus from exposure to progestin.
- Do not breast feed while taking this drug.

Intrauterine Progesterone Contraceptive System (Progestasert)
- Use another method of birth control (foam or condom) during the first 2 mo of Progestasert use.
- Regular cyclic pattern of ovulation continues while Progestasert is in place.
- Be prepared for heavier and longer menstrual periods during Progestasert use. Consult physician if increased menstrual bleeding continues.
- Check Progestasert threads frequently during first few months and after menstruation (times when expulsion is most likely to occur). If you cannot feel threads, return to physician for an examination and prescription for another method of birth control.
- Do not pull on threads for any reason. If the IUD is partially expelled, it should be removed; however, do not try to remove it yourself nor allow your partner to attempt to do so.
- Consult physician if a period is missed and pregnancy is suspected. Remove the device during pregnancy.
- Report to the physician for immediate treatment if you experience fever, acute pelvic pain and tenderness, unusual bleeding, or severe cramping. These are symptoms that indicate infection.

PROMAZINE HYDROCHLORIDE

(proe′ma-zeen)
Prozine-50, Sparine
Classifications: CENTRAL NERVOUS SYSTEM AGENT; PSYCHOTHERAPEUTIC; ANTIPSYCHOTIC; PHENOTHIAZINE
Prototype: Chlorpromazine
Pregnancy Category: C

AVAILABILITY 25 mg, 50 mg tablets; 25 mg/mL, 50 mg/mL injection

ACTIONS Derivative of phenothiazine. Compared with chlorpromazine has weak antipsychotic activity and extrapyramidal effects occur less frequently. Thought to block the postsynaptic dopamine receptors in the brain, with a higher affinity for D_1 over D_2 dopamine receptors.
THERAPEUTIC EFFECTS Antipsychotic drugs are sometimes called neuroleptics (or tranquilizers) because they tend to reduce initiative and interest in the environment, decrease displays of emotions or affect, suppress spontaneous movements and complex behavior, and decrease psychotic symptoms.

USES Manifestations of psychotic disorders and for reducing agitation and paranoia associated with alcohol withdrawal.

CONTRAINDICATIONS Hypersensitivity to phenothiazines; myelosuppression; CNS depression; children <12 y of age, Reye's syndrome. Safety during pregnancy (category C) or lactation is not established.
CAUTIOUS USE Prostatic hypertrophy; cardiovascular or liver disease; paralytic ileus; xerostomia; angle closure glaucoma; persons exposed to extremes in temperature or to organophosphorous insecticides; convulsive disorders.

P

ROUTE & DOSAGE

Psychotic Disorders

Adult: **PO/IM** 10–200 mg q4–6h up to 1000 mg/d
Adolescent: **PO/IM** >12 y, 10–25 mg q4–6h

Dementia Behavior

Geriatric: **PO/IM** Start with 25 mg 1–2 times/d, may increase q4–7d in divided doses (max: 500 mg/d)

ADMINISTRATION

Oral

- Use oral route whenever possible. Reserve parenteral administration for acutely disturbed or uncooperative patients or those who cannot tolerate oral preparation.
- Give 1 h before or 2 h after antacid; absorption is inhibited by antacids.
- Dilute the concentrate immediately before administration with fruit juice, chocolate-flavored drinks, carbonated drinks, or soup (for best taste, 10 mL of diluent for each 25 mg of drug). Avoid coffee or tea ingestion at or near medication times. Explain dosage and dilution to patient if drug is to be self-administered.
- Avoid contact of liquid preparations with skin.

Intramuscular

- Make IM injection deep into upper outer quadrant of buttock. Carefully aspirate before injecting drug slowly. Tissue irritation can occur if given SC. Intraarterial injection can cause arterial or arteriolar spasm and consequent impairment of local circulation. Rotate injection sites.
- Store at 15°–30° C (59°–86° F) in light-resistant container unless otherwise directed.

ADVERSE EFFECTS (≥1%) **Body as a Whole:** *Drowsiness, orthostatic hypotension,* syncope. **Special Senses:** Blurred vision, photosensitivity. **GI:** Constipation, xerostomia. **CNS:** Extrapyramidal effects, tardive dyskinesia, epileptic seizures in susceptible individuals, leukopenia, <u>agranulocytosis</u> (rare). **CV:** Hypotension, sinus tachycardia.

INTERACTIONS Drug: Alcohol, CNS DEPRESSANTS increases CNS depression; **phenobarbital** increases metabolism; GENERAL ANESTHETICS increase excitation and hypotension; antagonizes antihypertensive action of **guanethidine; phenylpropanolamine** poses possibility of sudden death; TRICYCLIC ANTIDEPRESSANTS intensify hypotensive and anticholinergic effects; ANTICONVULSANTS decrease seizure threshold—may need to increase anticonvulsant dose. **Herbal: Kava-kava** may increase risk and severity of dystonic reactions.

PHARMACOKINETICS Absorption: Variable, absorbed from GI tract. **Metabolism:** Metabolized in liver.

NURSING IMPLICATIONS

Assessment & Drug Effects

- Monitor BP and pulse before administration and between doses. Keep patient recumbent for about 1 h after IM dose is given because incidence of postural hypotension and drowsiness is particularly high after parenteral administration.
- Encourage adequate fluid intake as prophylaxis for constipation and xerostomia. The depressed patient may not seek help for either symptom or for urinary retention.
- Report symptoms suggesting agranulocytosis promptly (see Appendix F).

P

Patient & Family Education

- Make position changes slowly, particularly from lying down to upright positions. Dizziness or faintness may occur on arising.
- Avoid alcohol during therapy.
- Do not spill oral solutions on hands or clothing; wash exposed skin well with soap and water. Drug may cause contact dermatitis.
- Be aware that promazine may color urine pink to red to reddish brown.
- Do not take OTC drugs without physician approval.
- Do not breast feed while taking this drug without consulting physician.

PROMETHAZINE HYDROCHLORIDE

(proe-meth'a-zeen)

Histantil ♣, Pentazine, Phenazine, Phencen, Phenergan, Phenoject-50, Prometh, Prorex, Prothazine, V-Gan

Classifications: GASTROINTESTINAL AGENT; ANTIEMETIC; ANTIVERTIGO AGENT; PHENOTHIAZINE

Prototype: Prochlorperazine

Pregnancy Category: C

AVAILABILITY 12.5 mg, 25 mg, 50 mg tablets; 6.25 mg/5 mL, 25 mg/5 mL syrup; 12.5 mg, 25 mg, 50 mg suppositories; 25 mg/mL, 50 mg/mL injection

ACTIONS Long-acting derivative of phenothiazine with marked antihistamine activity and prominent sedative, amnesic, antiemetic, and anti-motion-sickness actions. Unlike other phenothiazine derivatives, relatively free of extrapyramidal adverse effects; however, in high doses it carries same potential for toxicity.

THERAPEUTIC EFFECTS In common with other antihistamines, exerts antiserotonin, anticholinergic, and local anesthetic action. Antiemetic action thought to be due to depression of CTZ in medulla.

USES Symptomatic relief of various allergic conditions, to ameliorate and prevent reactions to blood and plasma, and in prophylaxis and treatment of motion sickness, nausea, and vomiting. Preoperative, postoperative, and obstetric sedation and as adjunct to analgesics for control of pain.

CONTRAINDICATIONS Hypersensitivity to phenothiazines; narrow-angle glaucoma; stenosing peptic ulcer, pyloroduodenal obstruction; prostatic hypertrophy; bladder neck obstruction; epilepsy; bone marrow depression; comatose or severely depressed states; pregnancy (category C), lactation, newborn or premature infants, acutely ill or dehydrated children; children <2 y; Reye's syndrome, encephalopathy, hepatic diseases.

CAUTIOUS USE Impaired liver function; cardiovascular disease; asthma; acute or chronic respiratory impairment (particularly in children); hypertension; older adult or debilitated patients; children >2 y.

ROUTE & DOSAGE

Motion Sickness

Adult: **PO/PR/IM/IV** 25 mg b.i.d.
Child: **PO/PR/IM/IV** 12.5–25 mg b.i.d.

Nausea

Adult: **PO/PR/IM/IV** 12.5–25 mg q4–6h prn
Child: **PO/PR/IM/IV** 0.25–0.5 mg/kg q4–6h prn

Allergies

Adult: **PO/PR/IM/IV** 12.5 mg q.i.d. or 25 mg h.s.

Child: **PO/PR/IM/IV** 6.25–12.5 mg q.i.d. or 25 mg h.s.

Sedation

Adult: **PO/PR/IM/IV** 25–50 mg preoperatively or h.s.

Child: **PO/PR/IM/IV** 12.5–25 mg preoperatively or h.s.

ADMINISTRATION

Oral

- Give with food, milk, or a full glass of water may minimize GI distress.
- Tablets may be crushed and mixed with water or food before swallowing.
- Oral doses for allergy are generally prescribed before meals and on retiring or as single dose at bedtime.

Intramuscular

- Give IM injection deep into large muscle mass. Aspirate carefully before injecting drug. Intraarterial injection can cause arterial or arteriolar spasm, with resultant gangrene. Subcutaneous injection (also contraindicated) can cause chemical irritation and necrosis. Rotate injection sites and observe daily.

Intravenous

PREPARE: **Direct:** Concentrations of 25 mg/mL or less may be given undiluted. Dilute more concentrated preparations in NS to yield no more than 25 mg/mL (e.g., diluting the 50 mg/mL concentration in 9 mL yields 5mg/mL). ▪ Inspect parenteral drug before preparation. Discard if it is darkened or contains precipitate.

ADMINISTER: **Direct:** Give each 25 mg over at least 1 min.

INCOMPATIBILITIES **Solution/additive: Aminophylline, carbenicillin, cefotetan, chloramphenicol, chlorothiazide, heparin, hydrocortisone, methicillin, methohexital, penicillin G sodium, pentobarbital, phenobarbital, thiopental, diatrizoate, dimenhydrinate, iodipamide, iothalamate, nalbuphine. Y-site: Aldesleukin, allopurinol, amphotericin B cholesteryl complex, cefepime, cefoperazone, cefotetan, doxorubicin liposome, foscarnet, heparin, methotrexate.**

- Store at 15°–30° C (59°–86° F) in tight, light-resistant container unless otherwise directed.

ADVERSE EFFECTS (≥1%) **Body as a Whole:** Deep sleep, coma, convulsions, cardiorespiratory symptoms, extrapyramidal reactions, nightmares (in children), CNS stimulation, abnormal movements. **Respiratory:** Irregular respirations, <u>respiratory depression</u>. **CNS:** Sedation *drowsiness,* confusion, dizziness, disturbed coordination, restlessness, tremors. **CV:** Transient mild hypotension or hypertension. **GI:** Anorexia, nausea, vomiting, constipation. **Hematologic:** Leukopenia, <u>agranulocytosis</u>. **Special Senses:** *Blurred vision, dry mouth,* nose, or throat. **Skin:** Photosensitivity. **Urogenital:** Urinary retention.

DIAGNOSTIC TEST INTERFERENCE Promethazine may interfere with ***blood grouping in ABO system*** and may produce false results with ***urinary pregnancy tests*** (***Gravindex, false-positive; Prepurex*** and ***Dap tests,*** false-negative). Promethazine can cause significant alterations of ***flare response*** in ***intradermal allergen tests*** if performed within 4 d of patient's receiving promethazine.

INTERACTIONS Drug: Alcohol and other CNS DEPRESSANTS add to CNS depression and anticholinergic effects.

PHARMACOKINETICS Absorption: Readily absorbed from GI tract. **Onset:** 20 min PO/PR/IM; 5 min IV. **Duration:** 2–8 h. **Distribution:** Crosses placenta. **Metabolism:** Metabolized in liver. **Elimination:** Slowly excreted in urine and feces.

NURSING IMPLICATIONS

Assessment & Drug Effects

- Supervise ambulation. Promethazine sometimes produces marked sedation and dizziness.
- Be aware that antiemetic action may mask symptoms of unrecognized disease and signs of drug overdosage as well as dizziness, vertigo, or tinnitus associated with toxic doses of aspirin or other ototoxic drugs.
- Patients in pain may develop involuntary (athetoid) movements of upper extremities following parenteral administration. These symptoms usually disappear after pain is controlled.
- Monitor respiratory function in patients with respiratory problems, particularly children. Drug may suppress cough reflex and cause thickening of bronchial secretions.

Patient & Family Education

- For motion sickness: Take initial dose 30–60 min before anticipated travel and repeat at 8–12 h intervals if necessary. For duration of journey, repeat dose on arising and again at evening meal.
- Do not drive or engage in other potentially hazardous activities requiring mental alertness and normal reaction time until response to drug is known.
- Avoid sunlamps or prolonged exposure to sunlight. Use sunscreen lotion during initial drug therapy.
- Do not take OTC medications without physician's approval.
- Avoid alcohol and other CNS depressants.
- Relieve dry mouth by frequent rinses with water or by increasing noncaloric fluid intake (if allowed), chewing sugarless gum, or sucking hard candy. If these measures fail, add a saliva substitute (e.g., Moi-Stir, Orex, Xero-Lube).
- Do not breast feed while taking this drug.

PROPAFANONE

(pro-pa′fan-one)

Rythmol

Classifications: CARDIOVASCULAR AGENT; ANTIARRHYTHMIC CLASS IC

Prototype: Flecainide

Pregnancy Category: C

AVAILABILITY 150 mg, 225 mg, 300 mg tablets

ACTIONS Class IC antiarrhythmic drug with a direct stabilizing action on myocardial membranes. Reduces spontaneous automaticity.

THERAPEUTIC EFFECTS Appropriate dose and concentration decreases rate of single and multiple PVCs. In addition, suppresses ventricular tachycardia. Exerts a negative inotropic effect on the myocardium.

USES Ventricular arrhythmias.

UNLABELED USES Atrial tachyarrhythmias, reentrant arrhythmias, Wolff-Parkinson-White syndrome.

CONTRAINDICATIONS Uncontrolled CHF, cardiogenic shock, sinoatrial, AV or intraventricular disorders (e.g., sick sinus node syndrome, AV block) without a pacemaker; bradycardia, marked hypotension; bronchospastic disorders; electrolyte imbalances; hypersensitivity to propafanone; nonlife-

P

threatening arrhythmias; chronic bronchitis, emphysema; lactation.
CAUTIOUS USE CHF, AV block; hepatic/renal impairment; older adult patients; pregnancy (category C). Safety and efficacy in children are not established.

ROUTE & DOSAGE

Ventricular Arrhythmias
Adult: **PO** Initiate with 150 mg q8h, may be increased at 3–4 d intervals (max: 300 mg q8h)

ADMINISTRATION
- Dosage increments gradually are usually made with older adults or those with previous extensive myocardial damage.
- Significant dose reduction is warranted with severe liver dysfunction. Consult physician.
- Store at 15°–30° C (59°–86° F).

ADVERSE EFFECTS (≥1%) **CNS:** *Blurred vision, dizziness,* paresthesias, fatigue, somnolence, vertigo, headache. **CV:** Arrhythmias, ventricular tachycardia, hypotension, bundle branch block, AV block, <u>complete heart block</u>, sinus arrest, CHF. **Hematologic:** Leukopenia, granulocytopenia (both rare). **GI:** Nausea, abdominal discomfort, constipation, vomiting, dry mouth, *taste alterations,* cholestatic hepatitis. **Skin:** Rash.

INTERACTIONS Drug: Amiodarone, quinidine increases the levels and toxicity of propafenone. May increase levels and toxicity of TRICYCLIC ANTIDEPRESSANTS, **cyclosporine, digoxin,** BETA BLOCKERS, **theophylline,** and **warfarin** may increase levels of both **propafenone** and **diltiazem. Phenobarbital** decreases levels of propafenone.

PHARMACOKINETICS Absorption: Readily absorbed from GI tract. **Peak:** 3.5 h. **Distribution:** 97% protein bound, highest concentrations in the lung. Crosses placenta, distributed into breast milk. **Metabolism:** Extensively metabolized in the liver. **Elimination:** 18.5%–38% of dose excreted in urine as metabolites. **Half-Life:** 5–8 h.

NURSING IMPLICATIONS

Assessment & Drug Effects
- Monitor cardiovascular status frequently (e.g., ECG, Holter monitor) to determine effectiveness of drug and development of new or worsened arrhythmias.
- Monitor patients with preexisting CHF closely for worsening of this condition. Monitor for digoxin toxicity with concurrent use, because drug may increase serum digoxin levels.
- Report development of second- or third-degree AV block or significant widening of the QRS complex. Dosage adjustment may be warranted.

Patient & Family Education
- Report to physician any of following: Chest pain, palpitations, blurred or abnormal vision, dyspnea, or signs and symptoms of infection.
- Be aware when taking concurrent warfarin of possible increase in plasma levels that increase bleeding risk. Report unusual bleeding or bruising.
- Monitor radial pulse daily and report decreased heart rate or development of an abnormal heartbeat.
- Be aware of possibility of dizziness and need for caution with walking, especially in older adult or debilitated patients.
- Do not breast feed while taking this drug.

PROPANTHELINE BROMIDE

(proe-pan'the-leen)

Pro-Banthine, Propanthel ♣

Classifications: ANTISPASMODIC; ANTICHOLINERGIC; ANTIMUSCARINIC AGENT

Prototype: Atropine

Pregnancy Category: C

AVAILABILITY 7.5 mg, 15 mg tablets

ACTIONS Similar to atropine in peripheral effects. Has potent antimuscarinic activity and ganglionic blocking action. Very high doses block neurotransmission at myoneural junction.

THERAPEUTIC EFFECTS Decreases motility (smooth muscle tone) in the GI, biliary, and urinary tracts. Results in antispasmodic action.

USES Adjunct in treatment of peptic ulcer, irritable bowel syndrome, pancreatitis, ureteral and urinary bladder spasm. Also used prior to radiologic diagnostic procedures to reduce duodenal motility.

CONTRAINDICATIONS Pregnancy (category C), lactation; narrow angle glaucoma; tachycardia, MI; paralytic ileus, GI obstructive disease; myasthenia gravis. Safety in children is not established.

CAUTIOUS USE CAD, CHF, cardiac arrhythmias; liver disease, ulcerative colitis, hiatus hernia, esophagitis; kidney disease; prostatic hypertrophy; glaucoma; debilitated patients; hyperthyroidism; autonomic neuropathy; brain damage; Down's syndrome; spastic disorders.

ROUTE & DOSAGE

Irritable Bowel Syndrome

Adult: **PO** 15 mg 30 min a.c. and 30 mg h.s. (max: 120 mg/d)

Geriatric: **PO** 7.5 mg 2–3 times/d a.c. (max: 90 mg/d)

ADMINISTRATION

Oral

- Give 30–60 min before meals and at bedtime. Advise not to chew tablet; drug is bitter.
- Give at least 1 h before or 1 h after an antacid (or antidiarrheal agent).
- Store dry powder and tablets at 15°–30° C (59°–86° F); protect from freezing and moisture.

ADVERSE EFFECTS (≥1%) **GI:** *Constipation, dry mouth.* **Special Senses:** Blurred vision, mydriasis, increased intraocular pressure. **CNS:** Drowsiness. **Urogenital:** Decreased sexual activity, difficult urination.

INTERACTIONS **Drug:** Decreased absorption of **ketoconazole;** ORAL POTASSIUM may increase risk of GI ulcers; **Food:** Food significantly decreases absorption.

PHARMACOKINETICS **Absorption:** Incompletely absorbed from GI tract. **Onset:** 30–45 min. **Duration:** 4–6 h. **Metabolism:** 50% metabolized in GI tract before absorption; 50% metabolized in liver. **Elimination:** Excreted primarily in urine; some excreted in bile. **Half-Life:** 9 h.

NURSING IMPLICATIONS

Assessment & Drug Effects

- Assess bowel sounds, especially in presence of ulcerative colitis, since paralytic ileus may develop, predisposing to toxic megacolon.
- Be aware that older adult or debilitated patients may respond to a usual dose with agitation, excitement, confusion, drowsiness. Stop drug and report to physician if these symptoms are observed.
- Check BP, heart sounds and rhythm periodically in patients with cardiac disease.

P

Patient & Family Education

- Void just prior to each dose to minimize risk of urinary hesitancy or retention. Record daily urinary volume and report problems to physician.
- Relieve dry mouth by rinsing with water frequently, chewing sugar-free gum or sucking hard candy.
- Maintain adequate fluid and high-fiber food intake to prevent constipation.
- Make all position changes slowly and lie down immediately if faintness, weakness, or palpitations occur. Report symptoms to physician.
- Do not drive or engage in potentially hazardous activities until response to drug is known.
- Do not breast feed while taking this drug.

PROPOFOL

(pro′po-fol)

Diprivan

Classifications: CENTRAL NERVOUS SYSTEM AGENT, GENERAL ANESTHESIA; SEDATIVE-HYPNOTIC

Prototype: Thiopental

Pregnancy Category: B

AVAILABILITY 10 mg/mL injection

ACTIONS Sedative-hypnotic used in the induction and maintenance of anesthesia or sedation.

THERAPEUTIC EFFECTS Rapid onset (40 s) and minimal excitation during induction of anesthesia.

USES Induction or maintenance of anesthesia as part of a balanced anesthesia technique; conscious sedation in mechanically ventilated patients.

CONTRAINDICATIONS Hypersensitivity to propofol or propofol emulsion, which contain soybean oil and egg phosphatide; obstetrical procedures; patients with increased intracranial pressure or impaired cerebral circulation; pregnancy (category B), lactation. Do not use for conscious sedation in children <3 y.

CAUTIOUS USE Patients with severe cardiac or respiratory disorders or history of epilepsy or seizures.

ROUTE & DOSAGE

Induction of Anesthesia

Adult: **IV** 2–2.5 mg/kg q10s until induction onset

Geriatric: **IV** 1–1.5 mg/kg q10s until induction onset

Child: **IV** ≥*3 y,* 2.5–3.5 mg/kg over 20–30 s

Maintenance of Anesthesia

Adult: **IV** 100–200 mcg/kg/min

Geriatric: **IV** 50–100 mcg/kg/min

Child: **IV** ≥*3 y,* 125–300 mcg/kg/min

Conscious Sedation

Adult: **IV** 5 mcg/kg/min for at least 5 min, may increase by 5–10 mcg/kg/min q5–10 min until desired level of sedation is achieved (may need maintenance rate of 5–50 mcg/kg/min)

ADMINISTRATION

- Use strict aseptic technique to prepare propofol for injection; drug emulsion supports rapid growth of microorganisms.
- Inspect ampuls and vials for particulate matter and discoloration. Discard if either is noted.
- Shake well before use. Inspect for separation of the emulsion. Do not use if there is evidence of separation of phases of the emulsion.

Intravenous

PREPARE: **IV Infusion:** Give undiluted or diluted in D5W to a concentration not less than 2 mg/mL. Must draw up into a sterile syringe immediately after ampules or vials are opened. Begin drug administration immediately and completed within 6 h.

ADMINISTER: **IV Infusion:** Use syringe or volumetric pump to control rate. Determine rate by weight. Administer immediately after spiking the vial. Complete infusion within 6 h.

INCOMPATIBILITIES **Y-site: Amikacin, amphotericin B, atracurium, bretylium, calcium chloride, ciprofloxacin, diazepam, digoxin, doxorubicin, gentamicin, methotrexate, methylprednisolone, metoclopramide, minocycline, mitoxantrone, netilmicin, phenytoin, tobramycin, verapamil.**

- Store unopened between 4° C (40° F) and 22° C (72° F). Refrigeration is not recommended. Protect from light.

ADVERSE EFFECTS (≥1%) **CNS:** Headache, dizziness, *twitching, bucking, jerking, thrashing, clonic/myoclonic movements.* **Special Senses:** Decreased intraocular pressure. **CV:** Hypotension, ventricular asystole (rare). **GI:** Vomiting, abdominal cramping. **Respiratory:** Cough, hiccups, apnea. **Other:** Pain at injection site.

DIAGNOSTIC TEST INTERFERENCE Propofol produces a temporary reduction in ***serum cortisol levels.*** However, propofol does not seem to inhibit adrenal responsiveness to ***ACTH.***

INTERACTIONS Drug: Concurrent continuous infusions of propofol and **alfentanil** produce higher plasma levels of **alfentanil** than expected. CNS DEPRESSANTS cause additive CNS depression.

PHARMACOKINETICS Onset: 9–36 s. **Duration:** 6–10 min. **Distribution:** Highly lipophilic, crosses placenta, excreted in breast milk. **Metabolism:** Extensively metabolized in the liver. **Elimination:** Approximately 88% of the dose is recovered in the urine as metabolites. **Half-Life:** 5–12 h.

NURSING IMPLICATIONS

Assessment & Drug Effects

- Monitor hemodynamic status and assess for dose-related hypotension.
- Take seizure precautions. Tonic-clonic seizures have occurred following general anesthesia with propafol.
- Be alert to the potential for drug induced excitation (e.g., twitching, tremor, hyperclonus) and take appropriate safety measures.
- Provide comfort measures; pain at the injection site is quite common especially when small veins are used.

P

PROPOXYPHENE HYDROCHLORIDE

(proe-pox′i-feen)

Darvon 642 ♣, Novopropoxyn ♣

PROPOXYPHENE NAPSYLATE

Darvon-N

Classifications: CENTRAL NERVOUS SYSTEM AGENT; NARCOTIC (OPIATE) AGONIST, ANALGESIC
Prototype: Morphine
Pregnancy Category: C (D for prolonged use)
Controlled Substance: Schedule IV

AVAILABILITY **Napsylate** 100 mg tablets **Hydrochloride** 65 mg capsules

ACTIONS Centrally acting opioid structurally related to methadone. Analgesic potency about 1/2–2/3 that of codeine. Unlike codeine, propoxyphene has little or no antitussive effect.

THERAPEUTIC EFFECTS Potent analgesic. Note that excessive doses or use with alcohol have resulted in death.

USES Relief of mild to moderate pain.

UNLABELED USES To suppress narcotic withdrawal symptoms.

CONTRAINDICATIONS Hypersensitivity to drug; suicidal individuals; alcoholism; dependence on opiates; lactation. Safety during pregnancy [category C (D for prolonged use)] or in children is not established.

CAUTIOUS USE Kidney or liver disease.

P

ROUTE & DOSAGE

Mild to Moderate Pain

Adult: **PO** 65 mg HCl or 100 mg napsylate q4h prn (max: 390 mg HCl/d, 600 mg napsylate/d)

ADMINISTRATION

Note: 100 mg napsylate = 65 mg HCl

- Empty capsules and mix contents with water or food if unable to swallow capsule whole.
- Be aware that absorption may be delayed by presence of food in stomach.
- Store at 15°–30° C (59°–86° F).

ADVERSE EFFECTS (≥1%) **CNS:** Dizziness, light-headedness, *drowsiness,* sedation, unusual fatigue or weakness, restlessness, tremor, euphoria, dysphoria, headache, paradoxic excitement, mental confusion, toxic psychosis, <u>coma</u>, convulsions. **GI:** Nausea, vomiting, abdominal pain, constipation, liver dysfunction. **Special Senses:** Minor visual disturbances, pinpoint pupils (dilate with advancing hypoxia). **Skin:** Skin eruptions (hypersensitivity). **Metabolic:** Hypoglycemia (patients with impaired kidney function), acidosis, nephrogenic diabetes insipidus. **Respiratory:** <u>Respiratory depression</u>, pulmonary edema. **CV:** <u>Circulatory collapse</u>, ECG abnormalities.

INTERACTIONS **Drug:** **Alcohol** and other CNS DEPRESSANTS add to CNS depression, also fatalities reported with alcohol use; may increase hypoprothrombinemic effects of **warfarin;** may increase **carbamazepine** toxicity through decreased metabolism; **orphenadrine** increases CNS stimulation, anxiety, tremors, confusion. **Herbal:** **St. John's wort** may increase sedation.

PHARMACOKINETICS **Absorption:** Readily absorbed from upper part of small intestine. **Onset:** 15–60 min. **Peak:** 2–3 h. **Duration:** 4–6 h. **Distribution:** Crosses placenta; distributed into breast milk. **Metabolism:** Metabolized in liver. **Elimination:** Excreted in urine. **Half-Life:** 6–12 h, 30–36 h for metabolite.

NURSING IMPLICATIONS

Assessment & Drug Effects

- Evaluate need for drug since abuse potential is high.
- Monitor CNS effects, respiratory status and therapeutic effectiveness.
- Overdose: Prompt action required; fatalities occur commonly within first hour following overdosage.

Patient & Family Education

- Do not drive or engage in potentially hazardous activities until response to drug is known.
- Do not exceed recommended dose; do not use alcohol and other CNS depressants with propoxyphene.
- Lie down if dizziness, light-headedness, drowsiness, nausea, or vomiting occur while ambulating.
- Be aware that tolerance and physical or psychic dependence of the morphine type can occur with excessive use.
- Do not breast feed while taking this drug.

PROPRANOLOL HYDROCHLORIDE Pr

(proe-pran′oh-lole)

Apo-Propranolol ♣, Detensol ♣, Inderal, Inderal LA, InnoPran XL, Novopranol ♣

Classifications: AUTONOMIC NERVOUS SYSTEM AGENT; BETA-ADRENERGIC ANTAGONIST; ANTIHYPERTENSIVE AGENT; ANTIARRHYTHMIC, CLASS II

Pregnancy Category: C

AVAILABILITY 10 mg, 20 mg, 40 mg, 60 mg, 80 mg, 90 mg tablets; 60 mg, 80 mg, 120 mg, 160 mg sustained-release capsules; 80 mg, 120 mg delayed-release capsules; 4 mg/mL, 8 mg/mL, 80 mg/mL solution; 1 mg/mL injection

ACTIONS Nonselective beta-blocker of both cardiac and bronchial adrenoreceptors which competes with epinephrine and norepinephrine for available beta-receptor sites. In higher doses, exerts direct quinidine-like effects, which depresses cardiac function including contractility and arrhythmias. Lowers both supine and standing blood pressures in hypertensive patients. Mechanism of antimigraine action unknown but thought to be related to inhibition of cerebral vasodilation and arteriolar spasms.

THERAPEUTIC EFFECTS Blocks cardiac effects of beta-adrenergic stimulation; as a result, reduces heart rate, myocardial irritability (Class II antiarrhythmic) and force of contraction, depresses automaticity of sinus node and ectopic pacemaker, and decreases AV and intraventricular conduction velocity. Hypotensive effect is associated with decreased cardiac output, suppressed renin activity, as well as beta-blockade. Also decreases platelet aggregability.

USES Management of cardiac arrhythmias, myocardial infarction, tachyarrhythmias associated with digitalis intoxication, anesthesia, and thyrotoxicosis, hypertrophic subaortic stenosis, angina pectoris due to coronary atherosclerosis, pheochromocytoma, hereditary essential tremor; also treatment of hypertension alone, but generally with a thiazide or other antihypertensives.

UNLABELED USES Anxiety states, migraine prophylaxis, essential tremors, schizophrenia, tardive dyskinesia, acute panic symptoms (e.g., stage fright), recurrent GI bleeding in cirrhotic patients, treatment of aggression and rage.

CONTRAINDICATIONS Greater than first-degree heart block; CHF, right ventricular failure secondary to pulmonary hypertension; ventricular dysfunction; sinus bradycardia, cardiogenic shock, significant aortic or mitral valvular disease; bronchial asthma or bronchospasm, severe COPD, pulmonary edema, allergic rhinitis during pollen season; concurrent use with adrenergic-augmenting psychotropic drugs or within 2 wk of MAO inhibition therapy; abrupt discontinuation; major depression; peripheral vascular disease, Raynaud's disease; pregnancy (category C).

CAUTIOUS USE Peripheral arterial insufficiency; history of systemic insect sting reaction; patients prone to nonallergenic bronchospasm (e.g., chronic bronchitis, emphysema); major surgery; cerebrovascular disease, stroke; renal or hepatic disease; pheochromocytoma, vasospastic angina; older adults; diabetes mellitus; patients prone to hypoglycemia; hyperthyroidism, thyrotoxicosis; surgery; myasthenia gravis; Wolff-Parkinson-White syndrome; lactation.

ROUTE & DOSAGE

Hypertension
Adult: **PO** 40 mg b.i.d., usually need 160–480 mg/d in divided doses; **InnoPran XL** dose 80 mg q hs, may increase to 120 mg hs
Child: **PO** 1 mg/kg/d in 2 divided doses (1–5 mg/kg/d)
Neonate: **PO** 0.25 mg/kg q6–8h (max: 5 mg/kg/d) **IV** 0.01 mg/kg slow IV push over 10 min q6–8h prn (max: 0.15 mg/kg q6–8h)

Angina
Adult: **PO** 10–20 mg b.i.d. or t.i.d., may need 160–320 mg/d in divided doses

Arrhythmias
Adult: **PO** 10–30 mg t.i.d. or q.i.d. **IV** 0.5–3 mg q4h prn
Child: **PO** 1–4 mg/kg/d in 4 divided doses (max: 16 mg/kg/d) **IV** 10–20 mcg/kg/min over 10 min

Acute MI
Adult: **PO** 180–240 mg/d in divided doses

Migraine Prophylaxis
Adult: **PO** 80 mg/d in divided doses, may need 160–240 mg/d

ADMINISTRATION

- Do not give within 2 wks of a MAO inhibitor.
- Note that InnoPran XL should be given hs.
- Be consistent with regard to giving with food or on an empty stomach to minimize variations in absorption.
- Take apical pulse and BP before administering drug. Withhold drug if heart rate <60 bpm or systolic BP <90 mm Hg. Consult physician for parameters.
- Ensure that sustained release form is not chewed or crushed. Must be swallowed whole.
- Reduce dosage gradually over a period of 1–2 wk and monitor patient closely when discontinued.

Intravenous

Note: Verify correct IV concentration and rate of infusion for neonates with physician.

PREPARE: **Direct:** Give undiluted or dilute each 1 mg in 10 mL of D5W. **Intermittent:** Dilute a single dose in 50 mL of NS.

ADMINISTER: **Direct:** Give each 1 mg over 1 min. **Intermittent:** Give each dose over 15–20 min.

INCOMPATIBILITIES **Y-site: Amphotericin B cholesteryl complex, diazoxide.**

- Store at 15°–30° C (59°–86° F) in tightly closed, light-resistant containers.

ADVERSE EFFECTS (≥1%) **Body as a Whole:** Fever; pharyngitis; respiratory distress, weight gain, LE-like reaction, cold extremities, leg fatigue, arthralgia, anaphylactic/anaphylactoid reactions. **Urogenital:** Impotence or decreased libido. **Skin:** Erythematous, psoriasis-like eruptions; pruritus, Stevens-Johnson syndrome, toxic epidermal necrolysis, erythema multiforme, exfoliative dermatitis, urticaria. Reversible alopecia, hyperkeratoses of scalp, palms, feet; nail changes, dry skin. **CNS:** Drug-induced psychosis, sleep disturbances, depression, *confusion,* agitation, giddiness, light-headedness, *fatigue,* vertigo, syncope, weakness, *drowsiness,* insomnia, vivid dreams, visual hallucinations, delusions, reversible organic brain syndrome. **CV:** Palpitation, profound *bradycardia,* AV heart block, cardiac standstill, hypotension, angina pectoris, tachyarrhythmia, acute CHF, peripheral arterial insufficiency resembling Raynaud's disease, myotonia, paresthesia of *hands.* **Special Senses:** Dry eyes (gritty sensation), visual disturbances, conjunctivitis, tinnitus, hearing loss, nasal stuffiness. **GI:** Dry mouth, cheilostomatitis, nausea, vomiting, heartburn, diarrhea, constipation, flatulence, abdominal cramps, mesenteric arterial thrombosis, ischemic colitis, pancreatitis. **Hematologic:** Transient eosinophilia, thrombocytopenic or nonthrombocytopenic purpura, agranulocytosis. **Metabolic:** Hypoglycemia, hyperglycemia, hypocalcemia (patients with hyperthyroidism). **Respiratory:** Dyspnea, laryngospasm, bronchospasm.

DIAGNOSTIC TEST INTERFERENCE
BETA-ADRENERGIC BLOCKERS may produce false-negative test results in exercise tolerance ECG tests, and elevations in ***serum potassium, peripheral platelet count, serum uric acid, serum transaminase, alkaline phosphatase, lactate dehydrogenase, serum creatinine, BUN,*** and an increase or decrease in ***blood glucose*** levels in diabetic patients.

INTERACTIONS Drug: PHENOTHIAZINES have additive hypotensive effects. BETA-ADRENERGIC AGONISTS (e.g., **albuterol**) antagonize effects. **Atropine** and TRICYCLIC ANTIDEPRESSANTS block bradycardia. DIURETICS and other HYPOTENSIVE AGENTS increase hypotension. High doses of **tubocurarine** may potentiate neuromuscular blockade. **Cimetidine** decreases clearance, increases effects. ANTACIDS may decrease absorption.

PHARMACOKINETICS Absorption: Completely absorbed from GI tract but undergoes extensive first-pass metabolism. **Peak:** 60–90 min immediate release; 6 h sustained release; 5 min IV. **Distribution:** Widely distributed including CNS, placenta, and breast milk. **Metabolism:** Almost completely metabolized in liver. **Elimination:** 90%–95% excreted in urine as metabolites; 1%-4% excreted in feces. **Half-Life:** 2.3 h.

NURSING IMPLICATIONS

Assessment & Drug Effects

- Obtain careful medical history to rule out allergies, asthma, and obstructive pulmonary disease. Propranolol can cause bronchiolar constriction even in normal subjects.
- Monitor apical pulse, respiration, BP, and circulation to extremities closely throughout period of dosage adjustment. Consult physician for acceptable parameters.
- Evaluate adequate control or dosage interval for patients being treated for hypertension by checking blood pressure near end of dosage interval or before administration of next dose.
- Be aware that adverse reactions occur most frequently following IV administration soon after therapy is initiated; however, incidence is also high following oral use in the older adult and in patients with impaired kidney func-

P

tion. Reactions may or may not be dose related.

- Lab tests: Obtain periodic hematologic, kidney, liver, and cardiac functions when propranolol is given for prolonged periods.
- Monitor I&O ratio and daily weight as significant indexes for detecting fluid retention and developing heart failure.
- Consult physician regarding allowable salt intake. Drug plasma volume may increase with consequent risk of CHF if dietary sodium is not restricted in patients not receiving concomitant diuretic therapy.
- Fasting for more than 12 h may induce hypoglycemic effects fostered by propranolol.
- If patient complains of cold, painful, or tender feet or hands, examine carefully for evidence of impaired circulation. Peripheral pulses may still be present even though circulation is impaired. Caution patient to avoid prolonged exposure of extremities to cold.

P

Patient & Family Education

- Learn usual pulse rate and take radial pulse before each dose. Report to physician if pulse is below the established parameter or becomes irregular.
- Be aware that propranolol suppresses clinical signs of hypoglycemia (e.g., BP changes, increased pulse rate) and may prolong hypoglycemia.
- Understand importance of compliance. Do not alter established regimen (i.e., do not omit, increase, or decrease dosage or change dosage interval).
- Do not discontinue abruptly; can precipitate withdrawal syndrome (e.g., tremulousness, sweating, severe headache, malaise, palpitation, rebound hypertension, MI, and life-threatening arrhythmias in patients with angina pectoris).
- Be aware that drug may cause mild hypotension (experienced as dizziness or lightheadedness) in normotensive patients on prolonged therapy. Make position changes slowly and avoid prolonged standing. Notify physician if symptoms persist.
- Do not drive or engage in potentially hazardous activities until response to drug is known.
- Consult physician before self-medicating with OTC drugs.
- Inform dentist, surgeon, or ophthalmologist that you are taking propranolol (drug lowers normal and elevated intraocular pressure).
- Do not breast feed while taking this drug without consulting physician.

PROPYLTHIOURACIL (PTU) Pr

(proe-pill-thye-oh-yoor'a-sill)

Propyl-Thyracil ♣

Classifications: HORMONES AND SYNTHETIC SUBSTITUTES; ANTITHYROID AGENT

Pregnancy Category: D

AVAILABILITY 50 mg tablets

ACTIONS Interferes with use of iodine and blocks synthesis of thyroxine (T_4) and triiodothyronine (T_3). Does not interfere with release and utilization of stored thyroid hormone; thus antithyroid action is delayed days and weeks until preformed T_3 and T_4 are degraded.

THERAPEUTIC EFFECTS Drug-induced hormone reduction results in compensatory release of thyrotropin (TSH), which causes marked hyperplasia and vascularization of thyroid gland. With good adherence to drug regimen, chemical euthyroidism can be achieved 6–12 wk after start of therapy.

USES Hyperthyroidism, iodine-induced thyrotoxicosis, and hyperthyroidism associated with thyroiditis; to establish euthyroidism prior to surgery or radioactive iodine treatment; palliative control of toxic nodular goiter.

CONTRAINDICATIONS Last trimester of pregnancy (category D), lactation; concurrent administration of sulfonamides or coal tar derivatives such as aminopyrine or antipyrine.
CAUTIOUS USE Infection; concomitant administration of anticoagulants or other drugs known to cause agranulocytosis; bone marrow depression; impaired liver function.

ROUTE & DOSAGE

Hyperthyroidism
Adult: **PO** 300–450 mg/d divided q8h, may need 600–1200 mg/d initially
Geriatric: **PO** 150–300 mg/d divided q8h
Child: **PO** *6–10 y,* 50–150 mg/d; *>10 y,* 150–300 mg/d or 150 mg/m^2/d
Neonates: **PO** 5–10 mg/kg/d

Thyrotoxic Crisis
Adult: **PO** 200 mg q4–6h until full control achieved

ADMINISTRATION

- Give at the same time each day with relation to meals. Food may alter drug response by changing absorption rate.
- If drug is being used to improve thyroid state before radioactive iodine (RAI) treatment, discontinued 3 or 4 d before treatment to prevent uptake interference. PTU therapy may be resumed if necessary 3–5 d after the RAI administration.
- Store drug at 15°–30° C (59°–86° F) in light resistant container.

ADVERSE EFFECTS (≥1%) **CNS:** Paresthesias, headache, vertigo, drowsiness, neuritis. **GI:** Nausea, vomiting, diarrhea, dyspepsia, loss of taste, sialoadenitis, hepatitis. **Hematologic:** Myelosuppression, lymphadenopathy, periarteritis, hypoprothrombinemia, thrombocytopenia, leukopenia, agranulocytosis. **Metabolic:** Hypothyroidism (goitrogenic): Enlarged thyroid, reduced GI motility, periorbital edema, puffy hands and feet, bradycardia, cool and pale skin, worsening of ophthalmopathy, sleepiness, fatigue, mental depression, dizziness, vertigo, sensitivity to cold, paresthesias, nocturnal muscle cramps, changes in menstrual periods, unusual weight gain. **Skin:** Skin rash, urticaria, pruritus, hyperpigmentation, lightening of hair color, abnormal hair loss. **Body as a Whole:** Drug fever, lupus-like syndrome, arthralgia, myalgia, hypersensitivity vasculitis.

DIAGNOSTIC TEST INTERFERENCE Propylthiouracil may elevate ***prothrombin time*** and serum ***alkaline phosphatase, AST, ALT*** levels.

INTERACTIONS Drug: Amiodarone, potassium iodide, sodium iodide, THYROID HORMONES can reverse efficacy.

PHARMACOKINETICS Absorption: Rapidly absorbed from GI tract. **Peak:** 1–1.5 h. **Distribution:** Appears to concentrate in thyroid gland; crosses placenta; some distribution into breast milk. **Metabolism:** Rapidly metabolized to inactive metabolites. **Elimination:** 35% excreted in urine within 24 h. **Half-Life:** 1–2 h.

P

NURSING IMPLICATIONS

Assessment & Drug Effects

- Be aware that about 10% of patients with hyperthyroidism have leukopenia <4000 cells/mm^3 and relative granulopenia.
- Observe for signs of clinical response to PTU (usually within 2 or 3 wk): Significant weight gain, reduced pulse rate, reduced serum T_4.
- Lab tests: Baseline and periodic T_3 and T_4; periodic CBC with differential and platelet count.
- Satisfactory euthyroid state may be delayed for several months when thyroid gland is greatly enlarged.
- Be alert to signs of hypoprothrombinemia: Ecchymoses, purpura, petechiae, unexplained bleeding. Warn ambulatory patients to report these signs promptly.
- Be alert for important diagnostic signs of excess dosage: Contraction of a muscle bundle when pricked, mental depression, hard and nonpitting edema, and need for high thermostat setting and extra blankets in winter (cold intolerance).
- Monitor for urticaria (occurs in 3%–7% of patients during weeks 2–8 of treatment). Report severe rash.

Patient & Family Education

- Note that PTU treatment may be reinstituted if surgery fails to produce normal thyroid gland function.
- Be aware that thyroid hormone may be given concomitantly with PTU throughout pregnancy to prevent hypothyroidism in mother with little effect on fetus.
- Report severe skin rash or swelling of cervical lymph nodes. Therapy may be discontinued.
- Report to physician sore throat, fever, and rash immediately (most apt to occur in first few months of treatment). Drug will be discontinued and hematologic studies initiated.
- Avoid use of OTC drugs for asthma, or cough treatment without checking with the physician. Iodides sometimes included in such preparations are contraindicated.
- Learn how to take pulse accurately and check daily. Report to physician continued tachycardia.
- Report diarrhea, fever, irritability, listlessness, vomiting, weakness; these are signs of inadequate therapy or thyrotoxicosis.
- Chart weight 2 or 3 times weekly; clinical response is monitored through changes in weight and pulse.
- Continue monitoring and recording weight and pulse rate while in remission. Report onset of tremor, anxiety state, gradual ascending pulse rate, and loss of weight to physician (signs of hormone deficiency).
- Do not alter drug regimen (e.g., increase, decrease, omit doses, change dosage intervals).
- Check with physician about use of iodized salt and inclusion of seafood in the diet.
- Do not breast feed while taking this drug.

PROTAMINE SULFATE

(proe′ta-meen)

Protamine Sulfate

Classification: ANTIDOTE

Pregnancy Category: C

AVAILABILITY 10 mg/mL injection

ACTIONS Purified mixture of simple, low-molecular-weight proteins obtained from sperm or testes of suitable fish species. Anticoagulant effect when used alone.

P

THERAPEUTIC EFFECTS Because protamine is strongly basic, it combines with strongly acidic heparin to produce a stable complex; thus anticoagulant effect of both drugs is neutralized.

USES Antidote for heparin calcium or heparin sodium overdosage (after heparin has been discontinued).
UNLABELED USES Antidote for heparin administration during extracorporeal circulation.

CONTRAINDICATIONS Hemorrhage not induced by heparin overdosage; pregnancy (category C).
CAUTIOUS USE Cardiovascular disease; history of allergy to fish; vasectomized or infertile males; lactation; patients who have received protamine-containing insulin.

ROUTE & DOSAGE

Antidote for Heparin Overdose
Adult/Child: **IV** 1 mg for every 100 units of heparin to be neutralized (max: 100 mg in a 2 h period), give the first 25–50 mg by slow direct IV and the rest over 2–3 h

ADMINISTRATION

Note: Titrate dose carefully to prevent excess anticoagulation because protamine has a longer halflife than heparin and also has some anticoagulant effect of its own.

Intravenous
Note: Verify correct IV concentration and rate of infusion for infants or children with physician.

PREPARE: **Direct:** Reconstitute each 50 mg with 5 mL of sterile water for injection. Shake until dissolved. **Continuous:** Further dilute in 50 mL or more of NS or D5W.

ADMINISTER: **Direct:** Give each 50 mg or fraction thereof slowly over 10–15 min. NEVER give more than 50 mg in any 10 min period or 100 mg in any 2 h period. **Continuous:** Do not exceed direct rate. Give over 2–3 h or longer as determined by coagulation studies.
INCOMPATIBILITIES **Solution/additive:** RADIOCONTRAST MATERIALS.

- Store protamine sulfate injection at 2°–8° C (36°–46° F); protamine powder for injection and reconstituted solution at 15°–30° C (59°–86° F). Solutions are stable for 72 h at this temperature.

ADVERSE EFFECTS (≥1%) **CV:** *Abrupt drop in BP* (with rapid IV infusion), bradycardia. **Body as a Whole:** Urticaria, <u>angioedema</u>, pulmonary edema, <u>anaphylaxis</u>, dyspnea, lassitude; transient flushing and feeling of warmth. **GI:** Nausea, vomiting. **Hematologic:** Protamine overdose or "heparin rebound" (hyperheparinemia).

INTERACTIONS No clinically significant interactions established.

PHARMACOKINETICS Onset: 5 min. **Duration:** 2 h.

NURSING IMPLICATIONS

Assessment & Drug Effects
- Do not use protamine if only minor bleeding occurs during heparin therapy because withdrawal of heparin will usually correct minor bleeding within a few hours.
- Monitor BP and pulse q15–30min, or more often if indicated. Continue for at least 2–3 h after each dose, or longer as dictated by patient's condition. Be prepared to treat patient for shock as well as hemorrhage.
- Lab tests: Monitor effect of protamine in neutralizing heparin by

P

aPTT or ACT values. Coagulation tests are usually performed 5–15 min after administration of protamine, and again in 2–8 h if desirable.

- Observe patients undergoing extracorporeal dialysis or patients who have had cardiac surgery carefully for bleeding (heparin rebound). Even with apparent adequate neutralization of heparin by protamine, bleeding may occur 30 min to 18 h after surgery. Monitor vital signs closely. Additional protamine may be required in these patients.

PROTRIPTYLINE HYDROCHLORIDE

(proe-trip'te-leen)

Triptil ✦, **Vivactil**

Classifications: CENTRAL NERVOUS SYSTEM AGENT; PSYCHOTHERAPEUTIC; TRICYCLIC ANTIDEPRESSANT

Prototype: Imipramine

Pregnancy Category: C

AVAILABILITY 5 mg, 10 mg tablets

ACTIONS Tricyclic antidepressant (TCA) with more rapid onset of action than imipramine. Has little if any sedative properties characteristic of most other TCAs, but causes tachycardia, CNS stimulation, and strong anticholinergic activity. Orthostatic hypotension occurs frequently with usage.

THERAPEUTIC EFFECTS TCAs potentiate both norepinephrine and serotonin in CNS by blocking their reuptake by presynaptic neurons. Effective in the treatment of mentally depressed individuals particularly those who are withdrawn.

USES Symptomatic treatment of endogenous depression in patients under close medical supervision. Particularly effective for depression manifested by psychomotor retardation, apathy, and fatigue.

CONTRAINDICATIONS Use in children; concurrent use of MAOIS; during acute recovery phase following MI; pregnancy (category C).

CAUTIOUS USE Hepatic, cardiovascular, or kidney dysfunction; diabetes mellitus; hyperthyroidism; patients with insomnia; lactation.

ROUTE & DOSAGE

Antidepressant

Adult: **PO** 15–40 mg/d in 3–4 divided doses (max: 60 mg/d)
Adolescent: **PO** 15 mg/d in divided doses

ADMINISTRATION

- Give whole or crush and mix with fluid or food.
- Give dosage increases in the morning dose to prevent sleep interference and because this TCA has psychic energizing action.
- Give last dose of day no later than midafternoon; insomnia rather than drowsiness is a frequent adverse effect.
- Store at 15°–30° C (59°–86° F) in tightly closed container.

ADVERSE EFFECTS (≥1%) **Body as a Whole:** Photosensitivity, edema (general or of face and tongue). **GI:** *Xerostomia, constipation,* paralytic ileus. **Special Senses:** Blurred vision. **Urogenital:** *Urinary retention.* **CNS:** Insomnia, headache, confusion. **CV:** Change in heat or cold tolerance; *orthostatic hypotension, tachycardia.*

INTERACTIONS Drug: May decrease some response to ANTIHYPERTENSIVES; CNS DEPRESSANTS, **alcohol,** HYPNOTICS, BARBITURATES, SEDATIVES potentiate CNS depression; ORAL ANTICOAGU-

LANTS may increase hypoprothrombinemic effects; **ethchlorvynol** causes transient delirium; **levodopa** SYMPATHOMIMETICS (e.g., **epinephrine, norepinephrine**) increases possibility of sympathetic hyperactivity with hypertension and hyperpyrexia; MAO INHIBITORS present possibility of severe reactions—toxic psychosis, cardiovascular instability; **methylphenidate** increases plasma TCA levels; THYROID DRUGS may increase possibility of arrhythmias; **cimetidine** may increase plasma TCA levels. **Herbal: Ginkgo** may decrease seizure threshold; **St. John's wort** may cause **serotonin** syndrome (headache, dizziness, sweating, agitation).

PHARMACOKINETICS Absorption: Rapidly absorbed from GI tract. **Peak Levels:** 24–30 h. **Distribution:** Crosses placenta; distributed into breast milk. **Metabolism:** Metabolized in liver. **Elimination:** Primarily excreted in urine. **Half-Life:** 54–98 h.

NURSING IMPLICATIONS

Assessment & Drug Effects

- Monitor therapeutic effectiveness. Onset of initial effect characterized by increased activity and energy is fairly rapid, usually within 1 wk after therapy is initiated. Maximum effect may not occur for 2 wk or more.
- Monitor vital signs closely and CV system responses during early therapy, particularly in patients with cardiovascular disorders and older adults receiving daily doses in excess of 20 mg. Withhold drug and inform physician if BP falls more than 20 mm Hg or if there is a sudden increase in pulse rate.
- Lab tests: Obtain periodic liver function and blood cell counts in patients receiving large doses for prolonged periods or in combination with other drugs.
- Monitor I&O ratio and question patient about bowel regularity during early therapy and when patient is on large doses.
- Assess and advise physician as indicated for prominent anticholinergic effects (xerostomia, blurred vision, constipation, paralytic ileus, urinary retention, delayed micturition).
- Assess condition of oral membranes frequently; institute symptomatic treatment if necessary. Xerostomia can interfere with appetite, fluid intake, and integrity of tooth surfaces.
- Supervise patient closely during early treatment period. Suicide is an inherent risk with any depressed patient and may remain until there is significant improvement.
- Bear in mind that the potentiation of TCA effects may increase the danger of overdosage or suicide attempt (especially in patients who use excessive amounts of alcohol).

Patient & Family Education

- Consult physician about safe amount of alcohol, if any, that can be taken. Actions of both alcohol and protriptyline are potentiated when used together for up to 2 wk after the TCA is discontinued.
- Stop or to reduce smoking; smoking reduces TCAs effectiveness. Apparent treatment failure may be due to the nicotine effect.
- Consult physician before taking any OTC medications.
- Be aware that effects of barbiturates and other CNS depressants are enhanced by TCAs.
- Avoid potentially hazardous activities requiring alertness and skill until response to drug is known.
- Avoid exposure to the sun without protecting skin with sunscreen lo-

tion (SPF >12). Photosensitivity reactions may occur.

- Do not breast feed while taking this drug without consulting physician.

PSEUDOEPHEDRINE HYDROCHLORIDE

(soo-doe-e-fed'rin)

Cenafed, Decongestant Syrup, Dorcol Children's Decongestant, Eltor ✦, Eltor 120 ✦, Halofed, Novafed, PediaCare, Pseudofrin ✦, Robidrine ✦, Sudafed, Sudrin

Classifications: AUTONOMIC NERVOUS SYSTEM AGENT; ALPHA- AND BETA-ADRENERGIC AGONIST (SYMPATHOMIMETIC); DECONGESTANT

Prototype: Epinephrine

Pregnancy Category: C

AVAILABILITY 30 mg, 60 mg tablets; 120 mg, 240 mg sustained release tablets; 15 mg/5 mL, 30 mg/5 mL liquid; 7.5 mg/0.8 mL drops

ACTIONS Sympathomimetic amine that, like ephedrine, produces decongestion of respiratory tract mucosa by stimulating the sympathetic nerve endings including alpha-, beta-1 and beta-2 receptors. Unlike ephedrine, also acts directly on smooth muscle and constricts renal and vertebral arteries. Has fewer adverse effects, less pressor action, and longer duration of effects than ephedrine.

THERAPEUTIC EFFECTS Effective as a nasal decongestant.

USES Symptomatic relief of nasal congestion associated with rhinitis, coryza, and sinusitis and for eustachian tube congestion.

CONTRAINDICATIONS Hypersensitivity to sympathomimetic amines; severe hypertension; coronary artery disease; use within 14 d of MAOIS; glaucoma; hyperthyroidism; prostatic hypertrophy. Safety during pregnancy (category C), lactation, or in children <6 y is not established.

CAUTIOUS USE Hypertension, heart disease.

ROUTE & DOSAGE

Nasal Congestion

Adult: **PO** 60 mg q4–6h or 120 mg sustained release q12h
Geriatric: **PO** 30–60 mg q6h prn
Child: **PO** *2–6 y,* 15 mg q4–6h (max: 60 mg/d); *6–11 y,* 30 mg q4–6h (max: 120 mg/d)

ADMINISTRATION

Oral

- Ensure that sustained release form is not chewed or crushed. Must be swallowed whole.

ADVERSE EFFECTS (≥1%) **Body as a Whole:** *Transient stimulation,* tremulousness, difficulty in voiding. **CV:** Arrhythmias, palpitation, *tachycardia.* **CNS:** *Nervousness,* dizziness, headache, sleeplessness, numbness of extremities. **GI:** Anorexia, dry mouth, nausea, vomiting.

INTERACTIONS Drug: Other SYMPATHOMIMETICS increase pressor effects and toxicity; MAO INHIBITORS may precipitate hypertensive crisis; BETA BLOCKERS may increase pressor effects; may decrease antihypertensive effects of **guanethidine, methyldopa, reserpine.**

PHARMACOKINETICS Absorption: Readily absorbed from GI tract. **Onset:** 15–30 min. **Duration:** 4–6 h (8–12 h sustained release). **Distribution:** Crosses placenta; distributed into breast milk. **Metabolism:** Partially metabolized in liver. **Elimination:** Excreted in urine.

NURSING IMPLICATIONS

Assessment & Drug Effects

- Monitor HR and BP, especially in those with a history of cardiac disease. Report tachycardia or hypertension.

Patient & Family Education

- Avoid taking it within 2 h of bedtime because drug may act as a stimulant.
- Discontinue medication and consult physician if extreme restlessness or signs of sensitivity occur.
- Consult physician before concomitant use of OTC medications; many contain ephedrine or other sympathomimetic amines and might intensify action of pseudoephedrine.
- Do not breast feed while taking this drug without consulting physician.

PSYLLIUM HYDROPHILIC MUCILLOID (Pr)

(sill′ I-um)

Hydrocil, Instant, Karasil ♣, Konsyl, Metamucil, Modane Bulk, Perdiem Plain, Reguloid, Serutan, Siblin, Syllact, V-Lax

Classifications: GASTROINTESTINAL AGENT; BULK LAXATIVE

Pregnancy Category: C

AVAILABILITY 3.4 g/dose powder; 2.5 g, 3.4 g, 4.03 g/teaspoon granules

ACTIONS Highly refined colloid of psyllium seed (*Plantago ovata*) with equal amount of dextrose added as dispersing agent.

THERAPEUTIC EFFECTS Bulk-producing laxative that promotes peristalsis and natural elimination.

USES Chronic atonic or spastic constipation and constipation associated with rectal disorders or anorectal surgery.

CONTRAINDICATIONS Esophageal and intestinal obstruction, nausea, vomiting, fecal impaction, undiagnosed abdominal pain, appendicitis; children <2 y.

CAUTIOUS USE Diabetics; pregnancy (category C), lactation.

ROUTE & DOSAGE

Constipation or Diarrhea

Adult: **PO** 1–2 rounded tsp or 1 packet 1–3 times/d prn

Child: **PO** >6 y, 1 tsp in water h.s.

ADMINISTRATION

Oral

- Fill an 8-oz (240-mL) water glass with cool water, milk, fruit juice, or other liquid; sprinkle powder into liquid; stir briskly; and give immediately (if effervescent form is used, add liquid to powder). Granules should not be chewed.
- Follow each dose with an additional glass of liquid to obtain best results.
- Exercise caution with older adult patient who may aspirate the drug.

ADVERSE EFFECTS (≥1%) **Hematologic:** Eosinophilia. **GI:** Nausea and vomiting, diarrhea (with excessive use); GI tract strictures when drug used in dry form, abdominal cramps.

INTERACTIONS Drug: Psyllium may decrease absorption and clinical effects of ANTIBIOTICS, **warfarin, digoxin, nitrofurantoin,** SALICYLATES.

PHARMACOKINETICS Absorption: Not absorbed from GI tract. **Onset:** 12–24 h. **Peak:** 1–3 d.

P

NURSING IMPLICATIONS

Assessment & Drug Effects

- Report promptly to physician if patient complains of retrosternal pain after taking the drug. Drug may be lodged as a gelatinous mass (because of poor mixing) in the esophagus.
- Monitor therapeutic effectiveness. When psyllium is used as either a bulk laxative or to treat diarrhea, the expected effect is formed stools. Laxative effect usually occurs within 12–24 h. Administration for 2 or 3 d may be needed to establish regularity.
- Assess for complaints of abdominal fullness. Smaller, more frequent doses spaced throughout the day may be indicated to relieve discomfort of abdominal fullness.
- Monitor warfarin and digoxin levels closely if either is given concurrently.

Patient & Family Education

- Note sugar and sodium content of preparation if on low-sodium or low-calorie diet. Some preparations contain natural sugars, whereas others contain artificial sweeteners.
- Understand that drug works to relieve both diarrhea and constipation by restoring a more normal moisture level to stool.
- Be aware that drug may reduce appetite if it is taken before meals.
- Do not breast feed while taking this drug without consulting physician.

P

PYRANTEL PAMOATE

(pi-ran′tel)

Antiminth, Pin-Rid

Classifications: ANTIINFECTIVE; ANTHELMINTIC

Prototype: Mebendazole

Pregnancy Category: C

AVAILABILITY 180 mg capsules; 50 mg/mL suspension

ACTIONS Exerts selective depolarizing neuromuscular blocking action, which results in spastic paralysis of worm; also inhibits cholinesterase.

THERAPEUTIC EFFECTS Evacuation of worms from intestines.

USES *Enterobius vermicularis* (pinworm) and *Ascaris lumbricoides* (roundworm) infestations.

UNLABELED USES Hookworm infestations; trichostrongylosis.

CONTRAINDICATIONS Safety during pregnancy (category C), lactation, or in children <2 y is not established.

CAUTIOUS USE Liver dysfunction; malnutrition; dehydration; anemia.

ROUTE & DOSAGE

Pinworm or Roundworm

Adult/Child: **PO** 11 mg/kg as a single dose (max: 1 g)

ADMINISTRATION

Oral

- Shake suspension well before pouring it to ensure accurate dosage.
- Give with milk or fruit juices and without regard to prior ingestion of food or time of day.
- Store below 30° C (86° F). Protect from light.

ADVERSE EFFECTS (≥1%) **CNS:** Dizziness, headache, drowsiness, insomnia. **GI:** Anorexia, *nausea,* vomiting, abdominal distention, diarrhea, *tenesmus,* transient elevation of AST. **Skin:** Skin rashes.

INTERACTIONS Drug: Piperazine and pyrantel may be mutually antagonistic.

PHARMACOKINETICS Absorption: Poorly absorbed from GI tract. **Peak:** 1–3 h. **Metabolism:** Metabolized in liver. **Elimination:** >50% excreted in feces, 7% in urine.

NURSING IMPLICATIONS

Assessment & Drug Effects

- Lab tests: Monitor baseline and periodic AST/ALT in individuals with known liver dysfunction.

Patient & Family Education

- Do not drive or engage in other potentially hazardous activities until response to drug is known.
- Do not breast feed while taking this drug without consulting physician.

PYRAZINAMIDE

(peer-a-zin'a-mide)

PZA, Tebrazid ♣

Classifications: ANTIINFECTIVE; ANTITUBERCULOSIS AGENT

Prototype: Isoniazid

Pregnancy Category: C

AVAILABILITY 500 mg tablets

ACTIONS Pyrazinoic acid amide, analog of nicotinamide which is bacteriostatic against *Mycobacterium tuberculosis.* When employed alone, resistance may develop in 6–7 wk; therefore, administration with other effective agents is recommended. Appears to interfere with renal capacity to concentrate and excrete uric acid. Thus it may cause hyperuricemia.

THERAPEUTIC EFFECTS Bacteriostatic against *Mycobacterium tuberculosis.* Not used as sole agent against TB infection.

USES Short-term therapy of advanced tuberculosis before surgery and to treat patients unresponsive to primary agents (e.g., isoniazid, streptomycin).

CONTRAINDICATIONS Severe liver damage, pregnancy (category C), and lactation.

CAUTIOUS USE Presence or family history of gout or diabetes mellitus; impaired kidney function; history of peptic ulcer; acute intermittent porphyria.

ROUTE & DOSAGE

Tuberculosis

Adult: **PO** 15–35 mg/kg/d in 3–4 divided doses (max: 2 g/d)
Child: **PO** 20–40 mg/kg/d divided q12–24h (max: 2 g/d)

ADMINISTRATION

Oral

- Discontinue drug if hepatic reactions (jaundice, pruritus, icteric sclerae, yellow skin) or hyperuricemia with acute gout (severe pain in great toe and other joints) occur.
- Store at 15°–30° C (59°–86° F) in tightly closed container.

ADVERSE EFFECTS (≥1%) **Body as a Whole:** *Active gout,* arthralgia, lymphadenopathy. **Urogenital:** Difficulty in urination. **CNS:** Headache. **Skin:** Urticaria. **Hematologic:** Hemolytic anemia, decreased plasma prothrombin. **GI:** Splenomegaly, <u>fatal hemoptysis</u>, aggravation of peptic ulcer, *hepatotoxicity, abnormal liver function tests.* **Metabolic:** *Rise in serum uric acid.*

DIAGNOSTIC TEST INTERFERENCE Pyrazinamide may produce a temporary decrease in ***17-ketoster-***

oids and an increase in ***protein-bound iodine.***

INTERACTIONS Drug: Increase in liver toxicity (including fatal hepatoxicity in when treating latent TB) with **rifampin.**

PHARMACOKINETICS Absorption: Readily absorbed from GI tract. **Peak:** 2 h. **Distribution:** Crosses blood–brain barrier. **Metabolism:** Metabolized in liver. **Elimination:** Excreted slowly in urine. **Half-Life:** 9–10 h.

NURSING IMPLICATIONS

Assessment & Drug Effect

- Observe and supervise closely. Patients should receive at least one other effective antituberculosis agent concurrently.
- Examine patients at regular intervals and question about possible signs of toxicity: Liver enlargement or tenderness, jaundice, fever, anorexia, malaise, impaired vascular integrity (ecchymoses, petechiae, abnormal bleeding).
- Hepatic reactions appear to occur more frequently in patients receiving high doses.
- Lab tests: Obtain liver function tests (especially AST, ALT, serum bilirubin) prior to and at 2–4 wk intervals during therapy. Blood uric acid determinations are advised before, during, and following therapy.

Patient & Family Education

- Report to physician onset of difficulty in voiding. Keep fluid intake at 2000 mL/d if possible.
- Monitor blood glucose (diabetics) for possible loss of glycemic control.
- Do not breast feed while taking this drug without consulting physician.

P

PYRETHRINS

(peer′e-thrins)

A-200 Pyrinate, Barc, Blue, Pyrinate, Pyrinyl, R & C, RID, TISIT, Triple X

Classifications: SKIN AND MUCOUS MEMBRANE AGENT; ANTIINFECTIVE; PEDICULICIDE

Prototype: Permethrin

Pregnancy Category: C

AVAILABILITY 0.18%, 0.2%, 0.3% liquid; 0.3% gel; 0.3% shampoo

ACTIONS Pediculicide solution comprised of pyrethrins and piperonyl butoxide in deodorized kerosene. Acts as a contact poison affecting the parasite's nervous system, causing paralysis and death.

THERAPEUTIC EFFECTS Controls head lice, pubic (crab) lice, and body lice and their eggs (nits).

USES External treatment of *Pediculus humanus* infestations.

CONTRAINDICATIONS Sensitivity to solution components; skin infections and abrasions; pregnancy (category C), lactation.

CAUTIOUS USE Ragweed-sensitized patient, infants, children.

ROUTE & DOSAGE

***Pediculus humanus* Infestations**

Adult: **Topical** See nursing implications for appropriate application

ADMINISTRATION

Topical

- Apply enough solution to completely wet infested area, including hair. Allow to remain on area for 10 min.

- Wash and rinse with large amounts of warm water.
- Use fine-toothed comb to remove lice and eggs from hair.
- Shampoo hair to restore body and luster.
- Repeat treatment once in 24 h if necessary.
- Repeat treatment in 7–10 d to kill newly hatched lice.
- Do not apply to eyebrows or eyelashes without consulting physician.
- Flush eyes with copious amounts of warm water if accidental contact occurs.

ADVERSE EFFECTS (≥1%) **Body as a Whole:** Irritation with repeated use.

INTERACTIONS No clinically significant interactions established.

PHARMACOKINETICS Not studied.

NURSING IMPLICATIONS

Patient & Family Education

- Do not swallow, inhale, or allow pyrethrins to contact mucosal surfaces or the eyes.
- Discontinue use and consult physician if treated area becomes irritated.
- Examine each family member carefully; if infested, treat immediately to prevent spread or reinfestation of previously treated patient.
- Dry clean, boil, or otherwise treat contaminated clothing. Sterilize (soak in pyrethrins) comb and brushes used by patient.
- Do not share combs, brushes, or other headgear with another person.
- Do not breast feed while taking this drug without consulting physician.

PYRIDOSTIGMINE BROMIDE

(peer-id-oh-stig′meen)

Mestinon

Classifications: AUTONOMIC NERVOUS SYSTEM AGENT; CHOLINERGIC (PARASYMPATHOMIMETIC); CHOLINESTERASE INHIBITOR

Prototype: Neostigmine

Pregnancy Category: C

AVAILABILITY 60 mg/5 ml syrup; 60 mg tablet; 180 mg extended-release tablet 5 mg/mL injection

ACTIONS Analog of neostigmine; indirect-acting cholinergic that inhibits cholinesterase activity. Drug facilitates transmission of impulses across myoneural junctions by blocking destruction of acetylcholine. Has fewer adverse effects and longer duration of action than neostigmine.

THERAPEUTIC EFFECTS Direct stimulant action on voluntary muscle fibers and possibly on autonomic ganglia and CNS neurons. Produces increased tone in skeletal muscles.

USES Myasthenia gravis and as an antagonist to nondepolarizing skeletal muscle relaxants (e.g., curariform drugs).

CONTRAINDICATIONS Hypersensitivity to anticholinesterase agents or to bromides. Mechanical obstruction of urinary or intestinal tract; bradycardia, hypotension; pregnancy (category C), and lactation.

CAUTIOUS USE Bronchial asthma; epilepsy; vagotonia; hyperthyroidism; peptic ulcer; cardiac dysrhythmias.

ROUTE & DOSAGE

Myasthenia Gravis

Adult: **PO** 60 mg–1.5 g/d spaced according to requirements

and response of individual patient; sustained release: 180–540 mg 1–2 times/d at intervals of at least 6 h **IM/IV** Approximately 1/30th of PO dose
Child: **PO** 7 mg/kg/d divided into 5–6 doses
Neonates: **PO** 5 mg q4–6h. **IM/IV** 0.05–0.15 mg/kg q4–6h

Reversal of Muscle Relaxants

Adult: **IV** 10–20 mg immediately preceded by IV atropine

ADMINISTRATION

Oral

- Give with food or fluid.
- Ensure that sustained release form is not chewed or crushed. Must be swallowed whole.
- Note: A syrup is available. Some patients may not like it because it is sweet; try to make it more palatable by giving it over ice chips. The syrup formulation contains 5% alcohol.

Intramuscular

- Note: Parenteral dose is about 1/30 the oral adult dose.
- Give deep IM into a large muscle.

Intravenous

PREPARE: **Direct:** Give undiluted. Do NOT add to IV solutions.
ADMINISTER: **Direct:** Give at a rate of 0.5 mg over 1 min for myasthenia gravis; 5 mg over 1 min for reversal of muscle relaxants.

- Store at 15°–30° C (59°–86° F). Protect from light and moisture.

ADVERSE EFFECTS (≥1%) **Skin:** Acneiform rash. **Hematologic:** Thrombophlebitis (following IV administration). **GI:** *Nausea, vomiting, diarrhea.* **Special Senses:** *Miosis.* **Body as a Whole:** *Excessive salivation and sweating,* weakness, fasciculation. **Respiratory:** Increased bronchial secretion, bronchoconstriction. **CV:** Bradycardia, hypotension.

INTERACTIONS Drug: Atropine NONDEPOLARIZING MUSCLE RELAXANTS antagonize effects of pyridostigmine.

PHARMACOKINETICS Absorption: Poorly absorbed from GI tract. **Onset:** 30–45 min PO; 15 min IM; 2–5 min IV. **Duration:** 3–6 h. **Distribution:** Crosses placenta. **Metabolism:** Metabolized in liver and in serum and tissue by cholinesterases. **Elimination:** Excreted in urine.

NURSING IMPLICATIONS

Assessment & Drug Effects

- Report increasing muscular weakness, cramps, or fasciculations. Failure of patient to show improvement may reflect either underdosage or overdosage.
- Observe patient closely if atropine is used to abolish GI adverse effects or other muscarinic adverse effects because it may mask signs of overdosage (cholinergic crisis): Increasing muscle weakness, which through involvement of respiratory muscles can lead to death.
- Monitor vital signs frequently, especially respiratory rate.
- Observe for signs of cholinergic reactions (see Appendix F), particularly when drug is administered IV.
- Observe neonates of myasthenic mothers, who have received pyridostigmine, closely for difficulty in breathing, swallowing, or sucking.
- Observe patient continuously when used as muscle relaxant antagonist. Airway and respiratory assistance must be maintained until full recovery of voluntary respiration and neuromuscular transmission is assured. Com-

plete recovery usually occurs within 30 min.

Patient & Family Education

- Be aware that duration of drug action may vary with physical and emotional stress, as well as with severity of disease.
- Report onset of rash to physician. Drug may be discontinued.
- Sustained release tablets may become mottled in appearance; this does not affect their potency.
- Do not breast feed while taking this drug without consulting physician.

PYRIDOXINE HYDROCHLORIDE (VITAMIN B_6)

(peer-i-dox'een)

Beesix, hexaBetalin, NesTrex

Classifications: HORMONES AND SYNTHETIC SUBSTITUTES; VITAMIN

Pregnancy Category: A (C if >RDA)

AVAILABILITY 25 mg, 50 mg, 100 mg, 250 mg, 500 mg tablets; 100 mg/mL injection

ACTIONS Water-soluble complex of three closely related compounds with B_6 activity. Considered essential to human nutrition, although a deficiency syndrome is not well defined. Converted in body to pyridoxal, a coenzyme that functions in protein, fat, and carbohydrate metabolism and in facilitating release of glycogen from liver and muscle. In protein metabolism, participates in many enzymatic transformations of amino acids and conversion of tryptophan to niacin and serotonin. Aids in energy transformation in brain and nerve cells, and is thought to stimulate heme production.

THERAPEUTIC EFFECTS Evaluated by improvement of B_6 deficiency manifestations: Nausea, vomiting, skin lesions resembling those of riboflavin and niacin deficiency (seborrhea-like lesions about eyes, nose, and mouth, glossitis, stomatitis), edema, CNS symptoms (depression, irritability, peripheral neuritis, convulsions), hypochromic microcytic anemia.

USES Prophylaxis and treatment of pyridoxine deficiency, as seen with inadequate dietary intake, drug-induced deficiency (e.g., isoniazid, oral contraceptives), and inborn errors of metabolism (vitamin B_6-dependent convulsions or anemia). Also to prevent chloramphenicol-induced optic neuritis, to treat acute toxicity caused by overdosage of cycloserine, hydralzine, isoniazid (INH); alcoholic polyneuritis; sideroblastic anemia associated with high serum iron concentration. Has been used for management of many other conditions ranging from nausea and vomiting in radiation sickness and pregnancy to suppression of postpartum lactation.

CONTRAINDICATIONS Safety of large doses in pregnancy [category A (C if >RDA)] or lactation is not established.

ROUTE & DOSAGE

Dietary Deficiency

Adult: **PO/IM/IV** 2.5–10 mg/d times 3 wk, then may reduce to 2.5–5 mg/d

Child: **PO** 5–25 mg/d times 3 wk, then 1.5–2.5 mg/d

Pyridoxine Deficiency Syndrome

Adult: **PO/IM/IV** Initial dose up to 600 mg/d may be required; **PO/IM/IV Maintenance Dose:** Up to 50 mg/d

P

Isoniazid-induced Deficiency
Adult: **PO/IM/IV** 100–200 mg/d times 3 wk, then 25–100 mg/d
Child: **PO** 10–50 mg/d times 3 wk, then 1–2 mg/kg/d

Pyridoxine-dependent Seizures
Neonate/Infant: **PO/IM/IV** 50–100 mg/d

ADMINISTRATION

Oral
- Ensure that sustained release and enteric forms are not chewed or crushed. Must be swallowed whole.

Intramuscular
- Give deep IM into a large muscle.

Intravenous

PREPARE: **Direct:** Give undiluted. **Continuous:** May be added to most standard IV solutions.
ADMINISTER: **Direct:** Give at a rate of 50 mg or fraction thereof over 60 seconds. **Continuous:** Give according to ordered rate for infusion.

- Store at 15°–30° C (59°–86° F) in tight, light-resistant containers. Avoid freezing.

ADVERSE EFFECTS (≥1%) **Body as a Whole:** Paresthesias, slight flushing or feeling of warmth, temporary burning or stinging pain in injection site. **CNS:** Somnolence seizures (particularly following large parenteral doses). **Metabolic:** Low folic acid levels.

INTERACTIONS Drug: Isoniazid, cycloserine, penicillamine, hydralazine and ORAL CONTRACEPTIVES, may increase pyridoxine requirements; may reverse or antagonize therapeutic effects of **levodopa.**

PHARMACOKINETICS Absorption: Readily absorbed from GI tract. **Distribution:** Stored in liver; crosses placenta. **Metabolism:** Metabolized in liver. **Elimination:** Excreted in urine.

NURSING IMPLICATIONS

Assessment & Drug Effects
- Monitor neurologic status to determine therapeutic effect in deficiency states.
- Record a complete dietary history so poor eating habits can be identified and corrected (a single vitamin deficiency is rare; patient can be expected to have multiple vitamin deficiencies).
- Lab tests: Periodic Hct and Hgb, and serum iron.

Patient & Family Education
- Learn rich dietary sources of vitamin B_6: Yeast, wheat germ, whole grain cereals, muscle and glandular meats (especially liver), legumes, green vegetables, bananas.
- Do not self-medicate with vitamin combinations (OTC) without first consulting physician.
- Do not breast feed while taking this drug without consulting physician.

PYRIMETHAMINE

(peer-i-meth′a-meen)
Daraprim
Classifications: ANTIINFECTIVE; ANTIMALARIAL
Prototype: Chloroquine
Pregnancy Category: C

AVAILABILITY 25 mg tablets

ACTIONS Long-acting folic acid antagonist chemically related to metabolite of chloroguanide. Selectively inhibits action of dehydrofolic reductate in parasites with resulting blockade of folic acid metabolism.

Common adverse effects in *italic*, life-threatening effects underlined: generic names in **bold**; classifications in SMALL CAPS; ♣ Canadian drug name; ⓟ Prototype drug

THERAPEUTIC EFFECTS No gametocidal activity but prevents development of fertilized gametes in the mosquito and thus helps to prevent transmission of malaria. Exhibits little value as single agent in treatment of acute primary malarial attack because action against blood-borne schizonts is slow in onset. Cross-resistance with chloroguanide may occur.

USES Prophylaxis of malaria due to susceptible strains of plasmodia. May be used conjointly with fast-acting antimalarial (e.g., chloroquine, quinacrine, quinine) to initiate transmission control and suppressive cure. Used with a sulfonamide to provide synergistic action in treatment of toxoplasmosis.

CONTRAINDICATIONS Chloroguanide-resistant malaria; hypersensitivity to sulfonamides; megaloblastic anemia caused by folate deficiency; lactation; children <2 mo; pregnancy (category C).
CAUTIOUS USE Patients with convulsive disorders receiving high doses of an anticonvulsant (e.g., phenytoin).

ROUTE & DOSAGE

Malaria Chemoprophylaxis

Adult: **PO** 25 mg once/wk
Child: **PO** *<4 y,* 6.25 mg once/wk; *4–10 y,* 12.5 mg once/wk; *>10 y,* 25 mg once/wk

Toxoplasmosis

Adult: **PO** 50–75 mg/d with a sulfonamide for 1–3 wk, then decrease dose by half and continue for 1 mo
Child: **PO** 1 mg/kg/d divided into 2 doses with a sulfonamide for 1–3 wk, then decrease to 0.5 mg/kg/d for 1 mo (max: 25 mg/d)

ADMINISTRATION

Oral

- Minimize GI distress by giving with meals. If symptoms persist, dosage reduction may be necessary.
- Give on same day each week for malaria prophylaxis. Begin when individual enters malarious area and continue for 10 wk after leaving the area.

ADVERSE EFFECTS (≥1%) **GI:** Anorexia, vomiting, atrophic glossitis, abdominal cramps, diarrhea. **Skin:** Skin rashes. **Hematologic:** *Folic acid deficiency (megaloblastic anemia, leukopenia, thrombocytopenia, pancytopenia,* diarrhea). **CNS:** CNS stimulation including convulsions, respiratory failure.

INTERACTIONS Drug: Folic acid, *para*-aminobenzoic acid (PABA) may decrease effectiveness against toxoplasmosis.

PHARMACOKINETICS Absorption: Readily absorbed from GI tract. **Peak:** 2 h. **Distribution:** Concentrates in kidneys, lungs, liver, and spleen; distributed into breast milk. **Elimination:** Excreted slowly in urine; excretion may extend over 30 d or longer. **Half-Life:** 54–148 h.

NURSING IMPLICATIONS

Assessment & Drug Effects

- Monitor patient response closely. Dosages required for treatment of toxoplasmosis approach toxic levels.
- Lab tests: Perform blood counts, including platelets, twice weekly during therapy.
- Withhold drug and notify physician if hematologic abnormalities appear.

Patient & Family Education

- Be aware that folic acid deficiency may occur with long-term use of pyrimethamine. Report to physician weakness, and pallor (from

P

anemia), ulcerations of oral mucosa, superinfections, glossitis; GI disturbances such as diarrhea and poor fat absorption, fever. Folate (folinic acid) replacement may be prescribed. Increase food sources of folates (if allowed) in diet.
- Do not breast feed while taking this drug.

QUAZEPAM
(qua'ze-pam)
Doral
Classifications: CENTRAL NERVOUS SYSTEM AGENT; BENZODIAZEPINE; ANXIOLYTIC; SEDATIVE-HYPNOTIC
Prototype: Lorazepam
Pregnancy Category: X
Controlled Substance: Schedule IV

AVAILABILITY 7.5 mg, 15 mg tablets

ACTIONS Believed to potentiate gamma-aminobutyric acid (GABA) neuronal inhibition in the limbic, neocortical, and mesencephalic reticular systems.
THERAPEUTIC EFFECTS Significantly decreases sleep latency and total wake time and significantly increases sleep time. REM sleep is essentially unchanged. No transient sleep disturbance such as "rebound insomnia" was observed after withdrawal of the drug.

USES Insomnia characterized by difficulty in falling asleep, frequent nocturnal awakenings, or early morning awakenings.

CONTRAINDICATIONS Hypersensitivity to quazepam or benzodiazepines; sleep apnea; pregnancy (category X), lactation.
CAUTIOUS USE Impaired liver and kidney function. Safety and effectiveness in children <18 y are not established.

ROUTE & DOSAGE

Insomnia
Adult: **PO** 7.5–15 mg h.s.

ADMINISTRATION

Oral
- Initial dose is usually 15 mg but can often be effectively reduced after several nights of therapy.
- Use lowest effective dose in older adults as soon as possible.

ADVERSE EFFECTS (≥1%) **CNS:** *Drowsiness, headache*, fatigue, dizziness, dry mouth. **GI:** Dyspepsia.

INTERACTIONS Drug: Alcohol, CNS DEPRESSANTS, ANTICONVULSANTS potentiate CNS depression; **cimetidine** increases quazepam plasma levels, increasing its toxicity; may decrease antiparkinsonism effects of **levodopa;** may increase **phenytoin** levels; **smoking** decreases sedative effects of quazepam. **Herbal: Kava-kava, valerian** may potentiate sedation.

PHARMACOKINETICS Absorption: Readily absorbed from GI tract. **Onset:** 30 min. **Peak:** 2 h. **Distribution:** Crosses placenta; distributed into breast milk. **Metabolism:** Metabolized in liver to active metabolites. **Elimination:** Excreted in urine and feces. **Half-Life:** 39 h.

NURSING IMPLICATIONS

Assessment & Drug Effects
- Monitor for respiratory depression in patients with chronic respiratory insufficiency.
- Monitor for suicidal tendencies in previously depressed clients.
- Daytime drowsiness is more likely to occur in older adult clients.

Patient & Family Education

- Inform physician about any alcohol consumption and prescription or nonprescription medication that you take. Avoid alcohol use since it potentiates CNS depressant effects.
- Inform physician immediately if you become pregnant. This drug causes birth defects.
- Do not drive or engage in potentially hazardous activities until response to drug is known.
- Do not increase the dose of this drug; inform physician if the drug no longer works.
- This drug may cause daytime sedation, even for several days after drug is discontinued.
- Do not breast feed while taking this drug.

QUETIAPINE FUMARATE

(Ce-ti-a′peen)

Seroquel

Classifications: CENTRAL NERVOUS SYSTEM (CNS) AGENT; PSYCHOTHERAPEUTIC AGENT; ANTIPSYCHOTIC, ATYPICAL

Prototype: Clozapine

Pregnancy Category: C

AVAILABILITY 25 mg, 100 mg, 200 mg tablets

ACTIONS Antagonizes multiple neurotransmitter receptors in the brain including serotonin (5-HT_{1A} and 5-HT_2) as well as dopamine D_1 and D_2 receptors. Mechanism of action is unknown, however, antipsychotic properties thought to be related to antagonized responses. Antagonizes histamine H_1 receptors resulting in possible somnolence, and adrenergic $alpha_1$ and $alpha_2$ receptors which may lead to orthostatic hypotension.

THERAPEUTIC EFFECTS Indicated by a reduction in psychotic behavior.

USES Management of psychotic disorders, management of bipolar disorder.

UNLABELED USES Management of agitation and dementia.

CONTRAINDICATIONS Hypersensitivity to quetiapine; pregnancy (category C), lactation; alcohol use. Safety and efficacy in children have not been established.

CAUTIOUS USE Liver function impairment, older adults, cardiovascular disease (history of MI or ischemic heart disease, heart failure, arrhythmias, CVA, hypotension, dehydration, treatment with antihypertensives; history of seizures or suicide; breast cancer; Alzheimer's, Parkinson's disease; concurrent use of centrally acting drugs; patient at risk for aspiration pneumonia; debilitated patients; cerebrovascular disease.

ROUTE & DOSAGE

Psychosis, Acute Mania

Adult: **PO** Initiate with 25 mg b.i.d., may increase by 25–50 mg b.i.d. to t.i.d. on the second or third day as tolerated to a target dose of 300–400 mg/d divided b.i.d. to t.i.d., may adjust dose by 25–50 mg b.i.d. q.d. as needed (max: 800 mg/d)

Geriatric: **PO** Initiate with 25 mg b.i.d., titrate more slowly than adult patients, target range 150–200 mg/day in divided doses

Agitation, Dementia

Geriatric: **PO** Initiate with 25 mg b.i.d., may increase by 25–50 mg b.i.d. q 2–7 d if needed (max: 200 mg/d)

ADMINISTRATION

Oral

- Titrate dose over 4 d usually to a target range of 300–400 mg/d.

Make further dose adjustments of 25–50 mg 2 times/d at intervals of at least 2 d.

- Retitrate to desired dose when patient has been off the drug for >1 wk.
- Follow recommended lower doses and slower titration for the older adults, the debilitated, and those with hepatic impairment or a predisposition to hypotension.
- Store at 15°–30° C (59°–86° F).

ADVERSE EFFECTS (≥1%) **Body as a Whole:** Asthenia, fever, hypertonia, dysarthria, flu syndrome, weight gain, peripheral edema. **CNS:** *Dizziness, headache, somnolence.* **CV:** Postural hypotension, tachycardia, palpitations. **GI:** Dry mouth, dyspepsia, abdominal pain, constipation, anorexia. **Metabolic:** hyperglycemia, diabetes mellitus. **Respiratory:** Rhinitis, pharyngitis, cough, dyspnea. **Skin:** Rash, sweating. **Hematologic:** Leukopenia.

INTERACTIONS Drug: BARBITURATES, **carbamazepine, phenytoin, rifampin, thioridazine** may increase clearance of quetiapine. Quetiapine may potentiate the cognitive and motor effects of **alcohol,** enhance the effects of ANTIHYPERTENSIVE AGENTS, antagonize the effects of **levodopa** and DOPAMINE AGONISTS. **Ketoconazole, itraconazole, fluconazole, erythromycin** may decrease clearance of quetiapine. **Herbal: St. John's wort** may cause **serotonin** syndrome (headache, dizziness, sweating, agitation).

PHARMACOKINETICS Absorption: Rapidly and completely absorbed from GI tract. **Peak:** 1.5 h. **Distribution:** 83% protein bound. **Metabolism:** Extensively metabolized in the liver by CYP3A4. **Elimination:** 73% excreted in urine, 20% in feces. **Half-Life:** 6 h.

NURSING IMPLICATIONS

Assessment & Drug Effects

- Monitor diabetics for loss of glycemic control.
- Reassess need for continued treatment periodically.
- Withhold the drug and immediately report S&S of tardive dyskinesia or neuroleptic malignant syndrome (see Appendix F).
- Lab tests: Periodically monitor liver function, lipid profile, thyroid function, blood glucose, CBC with differential.
- Monitor ECG periodically, especially in those with known cardiovascular disease.
- Perform baseline cataract exam when therapy is started and at 6 mo intervals thereafter.
- Monitor patients with a history of seizures for lowering of the seizure threshold.

Patient & Family Education

- Carefully monitor blood glucose levels if diabetic.
- Exercise caution with potentially dangerous activities requiring alertness, especially during the first week of drug therapy or during dose increments.
- Make position changes slowly, especially when changing from lying or sitting to standing to avoid dizziness, palpitations, and fainting.
- Avoid alcohol consumption and activities that may cause overheating and dehydration.
- Inform physician immediately if you become pregnant.
- Do not breast feed while taking this drug.

QUINAPRIL HYDROCHLORIDE

(quin′a-pril)

Accupril

Classifications: CARDIOVASCULAR AGENT; ANGIOTENSIN-CONVERTING ENZYME (ACE) INHIBITOR

Prototype: Captopril

Pregnancy Category: D

AVAILABILITY 5 mg, 10 mg, 20 mg, 40 mg tablets

ACTIONS Potent, long-acting second-generation ACE inhibitor that lowers BP by interrupting the conversion sequences initiated by renin to form angiotensin II; a vasoconstrictor. Inhibition of ACE also decreases circulating aldosterone, a secretory response to angiotensin II stimulation. Reduces pulmonary capillary wedge pressure, systemic vascular resistance, and mean arterial pressure, with concurrent increases in cardiac output, cardiac index, and stroke volume.

THERAPEUTIC EFFECTS Lowers BP by producing vasodilation. Effective in the treatment of CHF because improves cardiac indicators.

USES Mild to moderate hypertension, CHF.

CONTRAINDICATIONS Hypersensitivity to quinapril or other ACE inhibitors; pregnancy (category D), lactation.

CAUTIOUS USE Renal insufficiency, autoimmune disease, volume-depleted patients, renal artery stenosis, neutropenia.

ROUTE & DOSAGE

Hypertension, CHF

Adult: **PO** 10–20 mg q.d., may increase up to 80 mg/d in 1–2 divided doses

Geriatric: **PO** Start with 2.5–5 mg q.d.

ADMINISTRATION

Oral

- Discontinue diuretics 2–3 d before initiation of quinapril. Do NOT exceed initial dose of 5 mg if diuretics cannot be discontinued.
- Store at 15°–30° C (59°–86° F) and protect from moisture.

ADVERSE EFFECTS (≥1%) **CV:** Edema, hypotension. **CNS:** Dizziness, fatigue, headache. **GI:** Nausea, vomiting, diarrhea. **Hematologic:** Eosinophilia, neutropenia. **Metabolic:** Hyperkalemia, proteinuria. **Respiratory:** Cough. **Body as a Whole:** Angioedema, myalgia.

DIAGNOSTIC TEST INTERFERENCE May increase ***BUN*** or ***serum creatinine.***

INTERACTIONS Drug: POTASSIUM-SPARING DIURETICS may increase risk of hyperkalemia. May elevate serum **lithium** levels, resulting in **lithium** toxicity.

PHARMACOKINETICS Absorption: Rapidly absorbed from GI tract. **Onset:** 1 h. **Peak:** 2–4 h. **Duration:** Up to 24 h. **Distribution:** 97% bound to plasma proteins; crosses placenta; not known if distributed into breast milk. **Metabolism:** Extensively metabolized in liver to its active metabolite, quinaprilat. **Elimination:** 50%–60% excreted in urine, primarily as quinaprilat; 30% excreted in feces. **Half-Life:** 2 h.

NURSING IMPLICATIONS

Assessment & Drug Effects

- Monitor BP at time of peak effectiveness, 2–4 h after dosing, and at end of dosing interval just before next dose.

Q

- Report diminished antihypertensive effect toward end of dosing interval. Inadequate trough response may indicate need to divide daily dose.
- Monitor for first-dose hypotension, especially in salt- or volume-depleted clients.
- Lab tests: Monitor BUN and serum creatinine periodically. Increases may necessitate dose reduction or discontinuation of drug. Monitor serum potassium values.
- Observe for S&S of hyperkalemia (see Appendix F).

Patient & Family Education

- Discontinue quinapril and report S&S of angioedema (e.g., swelling of face or extremities, difficulty breathing or swallowing) to physician.
- Maintain adequate fluid intake and avoid potassium supplements or salt substitutes unless specifically prescribed by physician.
- Note: A high-fat meal may lessen drug's absorption.
- Do not breast feed while taking this drug.

Q

QUINIDINE SULFATE

(kwin'i-deen sul-fate)

Apo-Quinidine ♣, Novoquinidin ♣, Quinidex Extentabs, Quinora

QUINIDINE GLUCONATE

Quinaglute Duratabs

QUINIDINE POLYGALACTURONATE

Cardioquin

Classifications: CARDIOVASCULAR AGENT; ANTIARRHYTHMIC CLASS IA

Prototype: Procainamide

Pregnancy Category: C

AVAILABILITY **Quinidine sulfate** 200 mg, 300 mg tablets; 300 mg sustained release tablets **Quinidine gluconate** 324 mg sustained release tablets; 80 mg/mL injection **Quinidine polygalacturonate** 275 mg tablets

ACTIONS Dextro-isomer of quinine and alkaloid of *Cinchona*. Class I-A antiarrhythmic. Cardiac actions similar to those of procainamide. Depresses myocardial excitability, contractility, automaticity, and conduction velocity, and prolongs effective refractory period. Anticholinergic action blocks vagal stimulation of AV node, thus tending to increase ventricular rate, particularly in larger doses.

THERAPEUTIC EFFECTS Depresses myocardial excitability, conduction velocity, and irregularity of nerve impulse conduction.

USES Premature atrial, AV junctional, and ventricular contraction; paroxysmal atrial tachycardia, chronic ventricular tachycardia (when not associated with complete heart block); maintenance therapy after electrical conversion of atrial fibrillation or flutter.

UNLABELED USES Quinidine gluconate for severe malaria.

CONTRAINDICATIONS Hypersensitivity or idiosyncrasy to quinine or *Cinchona* derivatives; pregnancy (category C), lactation. Thrombocytopenic purpura resulting from prior use of quinidine; intraventricular conduction defects, complete AV block, ectopic impulses and rhythms due to escape mechanisms; thyrotoxicosis; acute rheumatic fever; subacute bacterial endocarditis, extensive myocardial damage, frank CHF, hypotensive states; myasthenia gravis; digitalis intoxication.

CAUTIOUS USE Incomplete heart block; impaired kidney or liver function; bronchial asthma or other respiratory disorders; myasthenia gravis; potassium imbalance.

ROUTE & DOSAGE

Ectopic Beats
Sulfate
Adult: **PO:** 200–300 mg t.i.d. or q.i.d.
Child: **PO** 6 mg/kg 5 times/d

Ventricular Arrhythmias
Sulfate
Adult: **PO** 400–600 mg q2–3h until arrhythmia terminates, then 200–300 mg 3–4 times/d

Atrial Fibrillation or Flutter
Sulfate
Adult: **PO** 200 mg q2–3h for 5–8 doses until sinus rhythm restored or toxicity occurs (max: 3–4 g), then 200–300 mg t.i.d. or q.i.d.

Polygalacturonate
Adult: **PO** 275–825 mg q3–4h for 4 or more doses until arrhythmia terminates, then 137.5–275 mg b.i.d. or t.i.d.

Acute Tachycardia
Gluconate
Adult: **PO** 324–660 mg q8–12h **IM** 600 mg, then 400 mg q2h prn **IV** 200–750 mg at a rate of 16 mg/min

ADMINISTRATION

Note: Sulfate contains 83% anhydrous quinidine base; polygalacturonate, 80%; and gluconate, 62%. Examine parenteral solution before preparation; use only if clear and colorless.

Oral

- Note: Test dose is used by some physicians to determine idiosyncrasy before establishing full dosage schedule.
- Take with a full glass of water on an empty stomach for optimum absorption (i.e., 1 h before or 2 h after meals). Administer drug with food if GI symptoms occur (nausea, vomiting, diarrhea are most common).
- Reserve sustained release tablets for maintenance and prophylactic therapy.
- Adjust dosage to maintain plasma concentration between 2–5 mcg/mL. Levels of 8 mcg/mL or more are associated with myocardial toxicity.
- Store in tight, light-resistant containers away from excessive heat.

Intramuscular

- Aspirate carefully before injection to avoid inadvertent entry into blood vessel.

Intravenous

PREPARE: **IV Infusion:** Dilute 800 mg (10 mL) in at least 40 mL D5W to yield a maximum concentration of 16 mg/mL.

ADMINISTER: **IV Infusion:** Give via infusion pump at a rate not to exceed 16 mg (1 mL)/min.

INCOMPATIBILITIES **Solution/additive: Amiodarone, atracurium. Y-site: Furosemide, heparin in dextrose.**

- Use supine position during drug administration; severe hypotension is most likely to occur in patients receiving drug via IV. ▪ Protect IV solutions from light and heat to prevent brownish discoloration and possibly precipitation.

ADVERSE EFFECTS (≥1%) **CNS:** Headache, fever, tremors, apprehension, delirium, syncope with sudden loss of consciousness, seizures. **CV:** Hypotension, CHF, widened QRS complex, bradycardia, heart block, atrial flutter, ventricular flutter, fibrillation or tachycardia; quinidine syncope, torsades de pointes. **Special Senses:** Mydriasis, blurred vision, disturbed color perception, reduced visual field, photophobia, diplopia, night blindness, scotomas, optic neuritis, disturbed hearing (tinnitus, auditory acuity). **GI:** *Nausea, vomiting, diarrhea, abdominal pain*, hepatic dysfunction. **Hematologic:** Acute hemolytic anemia (especially in patients with G6PD deficiency), hypoprothrombinemia, leukopenia. Thrombocytopenia, agranulocytosis (both rare). **Body as a Whole:** Cinchonism (nausea, vomiting, headache, dizziness, fever, tremors, vertigo, tinnitus, visual disturbances), angioedema, acute asthma, respiratory depression, vascular collapse. **Skin:** Rash, urticaria, cutaneous flushing with intense pruritus, photosensitivity. **Metabolic:** SLE, hypokalemia.

INTERACTIONS Drug: May increase **digoxin** levels by 50%; **amiodarone** may increase quinidine levels, thus increasing its risk of heart block; other ANTIARRHYTHMICS, PHENOTHIAZINES, **reserpine** add to cardiac depressant effects; ANTICHOLINERGIC AGENTS add to vagolytic effects; CHOLINERGIC AGENTS may antagonize cardiac effects; ANTICONVULSANTS, BARBITURATES, **rifampin** increase the metabolism of quinidine, thus decreasing its efficacy; CARBONIC ANHYDRASE INHIBITORS, **sodium bicarbonate,** CHRONIC ANTACIDS decrease renal elimination of quinidine, thus increasing its toxicity; **verapamil** causes significant hypotension; may increase hypoprothrombinemic effects of **warfarin. Diltiazem** may increase levels and decrease elimination of quinidine.

PHARMACOKINETICS Absorption: Almost completely absorbed from GI tract. **Onset:** 1–3 h. **Peak:** 0.5–1 h. **Duration:** 6–8 h. **Distribution:** Widely distributed to most body tissues except the brain; crosses placenta; distributed into breast milk. **Metabolism:** Metabolized in liver. **Elimination:** >95% excreted in urine, <5% in feces. **Half-Life:** 6–8 h.

NURSING IMPLICATIONS

Assessment & Drug Effects

- Observe cardiac monitor and report immediately the following indications for stopping quinidine: (1) sinus rhythm, (2) widening QRS complex in excess of 25% (i.e., >0.12 seconds), (3) changes in QT interval or refractory period, (4) disappearance of P waves, (5) sudden onset of or increase in ectopic ventricular beats (extrasystoles, PVCs), (6) decrease in heart rate to 120 bpm. Also report immediately any worsening of minor side effects.
- Continuous monitoring of ECG and BP is required. Observe patient closely (check sensorium and be alert for any sign of toxicity); determine plasma quinidine concentrations frequently when large doses (more than 2 g/d) are used or when quinidine is given parenterally (i.e., quinidine gluconate).
- Observe patient closely following each parenteral dose. Amount of subsequent dose is gauged by response to preceding dose.
- Monitor vital signs q1–2h or more often as needed during acute treatment. Count apical pulse for a full minute. Report any change in pulse rate, rhythm, or quality or any fall in BP.
- Severe hypotension is most likely to occur in patients receiving high oral doses or parenteral quinidine (i.e., quinidine gluconate).
- Be aware: Reversion to sinus rhythm in long-standing fibrillation or when fibrillation is complicated by CHF involves some risk

Q

of embolization from dislodgment of atrial mural emboli.
- Quinidine can cause unpredictable rhythm abnormalities in the digitalized heart. Patients with atrial flutter or fibrillation may be pretreated with digitalis (until ventricular rate is 100 bpm) to increase AV nodal block and thus reduce possibility of paradoxic tachycardia.
- Lab tests: Periodic blood counts, serum electrolyte determinations, and kidney and liver function during long-term therapy.
- Monitor I&O. Diarrhea occurs commonly during early therapy; most patients become tolerant to this side effect. Evaluate serum electrolytes, acid-base, and fluid balance when symptoms become severe; dosage adjustment may be required.

Patient & Family Education
- Report feeling of faintness to physician. "Quinidine syncope" is caused by quinidine-induced changes in ventricular rhythm resulting in decreased cardiac output and syncope.
- Note: Hypersensitivity reactions usually appear 3–20 d after drug is started. Fever occurs commonly and may or may not be accompanied by other symptoms. Inform physician if these S&S occur.
- Eat a balanced diet with no excesses in fruit or fruit juices, milk, or a vegetarian diet. A diet high in alkaline ash foods (vegetables, citrus fruit, milk) may prolong half-life of quinidine by decreasing its excretion and increasing danger of toxicity.
- Do not self-medicate with OTC drugs without advice from physician.
- Do not increase, decrease, skip, or discontinue doses without consulting physician.
- Notify physician immediately of disturbances in vision, ringing in ears, sense of breathlessness, onset of palpitations, and unpleasant sensation in chest. Be sure to note the time of occurrence and duration of chest symptoms.
- Do not breast feed while taking this drug.

QUININE SULFATE
(kwye'nine)
Novoquinine ♣, Quinamm, Quiphile
Classifications: ANTIINFECTIVE; ANTIMALARIAL
Prototype: Chloroquine
Pregnancy Category: X

AVAILABILITY 200 mg, 260 mg, 325 mg capsules; 260 mg tablets

ACTIONS Chief alkaloid from bark of cinchona tree. Exact mechanism of antimalarial action uncertain. Inhibits protein synthesis and depresses many enzyme systems in malaria parasite. Has schizonticidal action and is gametocidal with *Plasmodium vivax* and *Plasmodium malariae* but not *Plasmodium falciparum*. Resembles salicylates in analgesic and antipyretic properties and exerts curare-like skeletal muscle relaxant effect. Also has oxytocic action and hypoprothrombinemic effect. Qualitatively similar to quinidine in cardiovascular effects. Generally replaced by less toxic and more effective agents in treatment of malaria.

THERAPEUTIC EFFECTS Effective against *Plasmodium vivax* and *Plasmodium malariae* but not *Plasmodium falciparum*. Generally replaced by less toxic and more effective agents in treatment of malaria.

Q

USES Chloroquine-resistant falciparum malaria and in combination with other antimalarials for radical cure of relapsing vivax malaria; also relief of nocturnal recumbency leg cramps.

CONTRAINDICATIONS Tinnitus, optic neuritis; myasthenia gravis; G6PD deficiency; pregnancy (category X), avoid use during lactation.
CAUTIOUS USE Cardiac arrhythmias. Same precautions as for quinidine sulfate when used in patients with cardiovascular conditions.

ROUTE & DOSAGE

Acute Malaria

Adult: **PO** 650 mg q8h for 3 d
Child: **PO** 25 mg/kg/d in three divided doses q8h for 3 d

Malaria Chemoprophylaxis

Adult: **PO** 325 mg b.i.d. for 6 wk

Nocturnal Leg Cramps

Adult: **PO** 260–300 mg h.s.

ADMINISTRATION

Oral

- Give with or after meals or a snack to minimize gastric irritation. Quinine has potent local irritant effect on gastric mucosa. Do not crush capsule; drug is not only irritating but also extremely bitter.
- Store in tight, light-resistant containers.

ADVERSE EFFECTS (≥1%) **Body as a Whole:** Cinchonism (Tinnitus, decreased auditory acuity, dizziness, vertigo, headache, visual impairment, *nausea, vomiting, diarrhea,* fever); hypersensitivity (Cutaneous flushing, visual impairment, pruritus, skin rash, fever, gastric distress, dyspnea, tinnitus); hypothermia, coma. **CNS:** Confusion, excitement, apprehension, syncope, delirium, convulsions, blackwater fever (extensive intravascular hemolysis with renal failure), death. **CV:** Angina, hypotension, tachycardia, cardiovascular collapse. **Hematologic:** Leukopenia, thrombocytopenia, agranulocytosis, hypoprothrombinemia, hemolytic anemia. **Respiratory:** Decrease respiration.

DIAGNOSTIC TEST INTERFERENCE Quinine may interfere with determinations of ***urinary catecholamines*** (***Sobel*** and ***Henry modification procedure***) and ***urinary steroids (17-hydroxycorticosteroids)*** (modification of ***Reddy, Jenkins, Thorn*** method).

INTERACTIONS Drug: May increase **digoxin** levels; ANTICHOLINERGIC AGENTS add to vagolytic effects; CHOLINERGIC AGENTS may antagonize cardiac effects; ANTICONVULSANTS, BARBITURATES, **rifampin** increase the metabolism of quinine, thus decreasing its efficacy; CARBONIC ANHYDRASE INHIBITORS, **sodium bicarbonate,** CHRONIC ANTACIDS decrease renal elimination of quinine, thus increasing its toxicity; **warfarin** may increase hypoprothrombinemic effects.

PHARMACOKINETICS Absorption: Well absorbed from GI tract. **Peak:** 1–3 h. **Duration:** 6–8 h. **Distribution:** Widely distributed to most body tissues except the brain; crosses placenta; distributed into breast milk. **Metabolism:** Metabolized in liver. **Elimination:** >95% excreted in urine, <5% in feces. **Half-Life:** 8–21 h.

NURSING IMPLICATIONS

Assessment & Drug Effects

- Be alert for S&S of rising plasma concentration of quinine marked by tinnitus and hearing impairment, which usually do not occur until concentration is 10 mcg/mL or more.

- Follow the same precautions with quinine as are used with quinidine in patients with atrial fibrillation; quinine may produce cardiotoxicity in these patients.

Patient & Family Education

- Learn possible adverse reactions and report onset of any unusual symptom promptly to physician.
- Do not breast feed while taking this drug.

QUINUPRISTIN/DALFOPRISTIN

(quin-u-pris'tin/dal'fo-pris-tin)

Synercid

Classifications: ANTIINFECTIVE; ANTIBIOTIC, STREPTOGRAMIN

Pregnancy Category: B

AVAILABILITY 500 mg vial (150 mg quinupristin/350 mg dalfopristin)

ACTIONS Streptogramin (cyclic macrolide) antibiotic that is produced by various streptomyces bacteria. Active against gram-positive pathogens including Vancomycin Resistant *Enterococcus faecium* (VREF), as well as some gram-negative anaerobes.

THERAPEUTIC EFFECTS Indicated by clinical improvement in S&S of infection. Effective against VREF resistant organisms and Methicillin Resistant *Staphylococcus aureus* (MRSA), and *Streptococcus pneumoniae*. Synercid is not effective against *Pseudomonas aeruginosa*, *Enterobacteriaceae* or Vancomycin resistant *Enterococcus raecalis*.

USES Serious or life-threatening infections associated with Vancomycin resistant *Enterococcus faecium* (VREF) bacteremia; complicated skin and skin structure infections caused by *Staphylococcus aureus* or *Streptococcus pyogenes*.

CONTRAINDICATIONS Hypersensitivity to quinupristin/dalfopristin or pristinamycin; lactation.

CAUTIOUS USE Renal or hepatic dysfunction; pregnancy (category B).

ROUTE & DOSAGE

Vancomycin Resistant *Enterococcus faecium*

Adult: **IV** 7.5 mg/kg infused over 60 min q 8 h

Complicated skin and skin structure infections

Adult: **IV** 7.5 mg/kg infused over 60 min q 12 h times 7 d

ADMINISTRATION

Intravenous

PREPARE: **Intermittent:** Reconstitute a single vial by adding 5 mL D5W or sterile water for injection to yield 100 mg/mL. Gently swirl to dissolve but do NOT shake. Allow solution to clear. Withdraw the required dose and further dilute by adding to 100 mL (central line) or 250–500 mL (peripheral site) of D5W.

ADMINISTER: **Intermittent:** Flush line before & after with D5W. Do NOT use saline. Administer over 1 h.

INCOMPATIBILITIES **Solution/additive: Saline solutions** and **Lactated Ringers** solution (flush lines with D5W before infusing other drugs). **Y-site:** Any drugs diluted in **saline; acyclovir, aminophylline, amphotericin B, cefotaxime, ceftazidime, ceftizoxime, dobutamine, dopamine, erythromycin lactobionate, digoxin, furosemide, gentamicin, imipenem-cilastatin, insulin, meropenem, metronidazole, piperacillin,**

Q

piperacillin-tazobactam, ticarcillin-clavulanate.

- Refrigerate unopened vials. After reconstitution solution is stable for 5 h at room temperature and 54 h refrigerated.

ADVERSE EFFECTS (≥1%) **Body as a Whole:** Headache, pain, *myalgia, arthralgia*. **GI:** Nausea, diarrhea, vomiting. **Skin:** Rash, pruritus. **Other:** *Inflammation, pain, or edema at infusion site, other infusion site reactions*, thrombophlebitis.

INTERACTIONS Drug: Inhibits metabolism of **cyclosporine, midazolam, nifedipine, and terfenadine;** may also increase levels of **astemizole,** PROTEASE INHIBITORS, **vincristine, vinblastine, docetaxel, paclitaxel, diazepam, cisapride, tacrolimus, carbamazepine, quinidine, lidocaine, disopyramide** due to inhibition of CYP3A4 metabolism.

PHARMACOKINETICS Distribution: Moderately protein bound. **Metabolism:** Metabolized to several active metabolites. **Elimination:** Primarily excreted in feces (75%–77%). **Half-Life:** 3 h quinupristin, 1 h dalfopristin.

R

NURSING IMPLICATIONS

Assessment & Drug Effects

- Monitor for S&S of infusion site irritation; change infusion site if irritation is apparent.
- Monitor for cutaneous reaction (e.g., pruritus/erythema of neck, face, upper body).
- Lab tests: C&S from site of infection prior to initiating therapy; WBC with differential; and liver function (especially with preexisting hepatic insufficiency).

Patient & Family Education

- Report burning, itching, or pain at infusion site to physician.
- Report any sensation of swelling of face and tongue; difficulty swallowing.
- Do not breast feed while taking this drug.

RABEPRAZOLE SODIUM

(rab-e-pra′zole)

AcipHex

Classifications: GASTROINTESTINAL AGENT; PROTON PUMP INHIBITOR

Prototype: Omeprazole

Pregnancy Category: B

AVAILABILITY 20 mg tablets

ACTIONS Gastric proton pump inhibitor that specifically suppresses gastric acid secretion by inhibiting the H^+, K^+-ATPase enzyme system (the acid [proton H^+] pump) in the parietal cells of the stomach.

THERAPEUTIC EFFECTS Indicated by a negative urea breath test for *H. pylori* with preexisting gastric ulcer; also by elimination of S&S with GERD or peptic ulcers. Produces an antisecretory effect on the hydrogen ion (H^+) in the parietal cells. It does not exhibit H_2-histamine receptor antagonist properties.

USES Healing and maintenance of healing of erosive or ulcerative gastroesophageal reflux disease (GERD); healing of duodenal ulcers; treatment of hypersecretory conditions.

CONTRAINDICATIONS Hypersensitivity to rabeprazole, lansoprazole, or omeprazole or proton pump inhibitors (PPIs) hypersensitivity; lactation.

CAUTIOUS USE Pregnancy (category B); severe hepatic impairment; mild to moderate hepatic disease; Japanese. Safety & efficacy in children <18 are not established.

ROUTE & DOSAGE

Healing of Erosive GERD

Adult: **PO** 20 mg q.d. × 48 wk, may continue up to 16 wk if needed

Maintenance Therapy for GERD

Adult: **PO** 20 mg q.d.

Healing Duodenal Ulcer

Adult: **PO** 20 mg q.d. × 4 wk

Hypersecretory Disease

Adult: **PO** 60 mg q.d. in 1–2 divided doses (max: 100 mg q.d. or 60 mg b.i.d.)

ADMINISTRATION

Oral

- Adjust dose as needed with preexisting liver disease.
- Store at 15°–30° C (59°–86° F).

ADVERSE EFFECTS (≥1%) **Body as a Whole:** Headache. **Skin:** (Rare) Stevens-Johnson syndrome, toxic epidermal necrolysis, erythema multiforme.

INTERACTIONS Drug: Rabeprazole sodium may decrease absorption of **ketoconazole**; may increase **digoxin** levels.

PHARMACOKINETICS Absorption: 52% bioavailability. **Distribution:** 96% protein bound. **Metabolism:** Metabolized in liver by CYP3A and CYP2C19. **Elimination:** Excreted primarily in urine. **Half-Life:** 1–2 h.

NURSING IMPLICATIONS

Assessment & Drug Effects

- Lab tests: Routine serum chemistry; serum gastrin in long-term therapy.
- Coadministered drugs: Monitor for changes in digoxin blood level.

Patient & Family Education

- Report diarrhea, skin rash, other bothersome adverse effects to physician.
- Do not breast feed while taking this drug.

RALOXIFENE HYDROCHLORIDE

(ra-lox′i-feen)

Evista

Classifications: HORMONE AND SYNTHETIC SUBSTITUTE; SELECTIVE ESTROGEN RECEPTOR ANTAGONIST/AGONIST

Prototype: Tamoxifen

Pregnancy Category: X

AVAILABILITY 60 mg tablets

ACTIONS Tamoxifen analog that exhibits selective estrogen receptor antagonist activity on uterus and breast tissue. Prevents tissue proliferation in both sites. Decreases bone resorption and increases bone density. Decreases serum total cholesterol and LDL cholesterol without lowering HDL cholesterol or triglycerides.

THERAPEUTIC EFFECTS Indicated by increased bone mineral density, lowers serum total cholesterol and LDL cholesterol.

USES Prevention and treatment of osteoporosis in postmenopausal women.

CONTRAINDICATIONS Active thromboembolic event; hypersensitivity to raloxifene; pregnancy (category X), lactation, children.

CAUTIOUS USE Concurrent use of raloxifene and estrogen hormone replacement therapy and lipid-lowering agents.

R

ROUTE & DOSAGE

Prevention or Treatment of Osteoporosis
Adult: **PO** 60 mg q.d.

ADMINISTRATION

Oral
- Discontinue 72 h before and during prolonged immobilization.
- Store at 15°–30° C (59°–86° F) in a tightly closed container and protect from light.

ADVERSE EFFECTS (≥1%) **Body as a Whole:** Infection, flu-like syndrome, leg cramps, fever, arthralgia, myalgia, arthritis. **CNS:** Migraine headache, depression, insomnia. **CV:** *Hot flashes*, chest pain, peripheral edema, decreased serum cholesterol. **GI:** Nausea, dyspepsia, vomiting, flatulence, GI disorder, gastroenteritis, weight gain. **Respiratory:** Sinusitis, pharyngitis, cough, pneumonia, laryngitis. **Skin:** Rash, sweating. **Urogenital:** Vaginitis, UTI, cystitis, leukorrhea, endometrial disorder, breast pain, vaginal bleeding.

INTERACTIONS Drug: Concomitant use of ESTROGENS not recommended; absorption reduced by **cholestyramine.**

PHARMACOKINETICS Absorption: 60% absorbed, absolute bioavailability 2%. **Metabolism:** Extensive first-pass metabolism in liver. **Elimination:** Excreted primarily in feces. **Half-Life:** 27.7–32.5 h.

NURSING IMPLICATIONS

Assessment & Drug Effects
- Lab tests: Periodically monitor bone density, liver function, and plasma lipids; with concurrent oral anticoagulants, carefully monitor PT and INR.
- Monitor carefully for and immediately report S&S of thromboembolic events.
- Do not give drug concurrently with cholestyramine; however, if unavoidable, space the two drugs as widely as possible.

Patient & Family Education
- Contact physician immediately if unexplained calf pain or tenderness occurs.
- Avoid prolonged restriction of movement during travel.
- Drug does not prevent and may induce hot flashes.
- Do not take drug with other estrogen-containing drugs.
- Tell prescriber if you are taking drugs to lower your cholesterol.
- Do not breast feed while taking this drug.

RAMIPRIL
(ram'i-pril)
Altace
Classifications: CARDIOVASCULAR AGENT; ANGIOTENSIN-CONVERTING ENZYME (ACE) INHIBITOR
Prototype: Captopril
Pregnancy Category: D

AVAILABILITY 1.25 mg, 2.5 mg, 5 mg, 10 mg capsules

ACTIONS Reduces peripheral vascular resistance by inhibiting the formation of angiotensin II, a potent vasoconstrictor.

THERAPEUTIC EFFECTS Lowers BP. Inhibition of ACE also decreases serum aldosterone levels; reduces peripheral arterial resistance (afterload) and improves cardiac output as well as exercise tolerance.

USES Mild to moderate hypertension, CHF.

R

CONTRAINDICATIONS Hypersensitivity to ramipril or any other ACE inhibitor, patients with history of angioneurotic edema; pregnancy (category D), lactation.

CAUTIOUS USE Impaired kidney or liver function, surgery or anesthesia. Safety and effectiveness in children are not established.

ROUTE & DOSAGE

Hypertension, CHF

Adult: **PO** 2.5–5 mg q.d., may increase up to 20 mg/d in 1–2 divided doses

ADMINISTRATION

Oral

- Discontinue diuretics 2–3 d before initiation of drug. Limit initial dose to 1.25 mg if diuretics cannot be discontinued.
- Store at 15°–30° C (59°–86° F) and protect from moisture.

ADVERSE EFFECTS (≥1%) **CNS:** Dizziness, fatigue, headache. **GI:** Nausea, vomiting, diarrhea, eructation. **Metabolic:** Hyperkalemia, hyponatremia. **Skin:** erythema, pruritus. **Body as a Whole:** Angioedema. **Respiratory:** Cough.

INTERACTIONS Drug: POTASSIUM-SPARING DIURETICS may increase risk of hyperkalemia. May, elevate, serum **lithium** levels, resulting in lithium toxicity. NSAIDS may attenuate antihypertensive effects.

PHARMACOKINETICS Absorption: 60% absorbed from GI tract. **Onset:** 2 h. **Peak:** 6–8 h. **Duration:** Up to 24 h. **Distribution:** Crosses placenta; not known if distributed into breast milk. **Metabolism:** Rapidly metabolized in liver to its active metabolite, ramiprilat. **Elimination:** 40%–60% excreted in urine, 40% in feces. **Half-Life:** 2–3 h.

NURSING IMPLICATIONS

Assessment & Drug Effects

- Monitor BP at time of peak effectiveness, 3–6 h after dosing and at end of dosing interval just before next dose.
- Report diminished antihypertensive effect.
- Monitor for first-dose hypotension, especially in salt- or volume-depleted persons.
- Lab tests: Monitor BUN and serum creatinine periodically. Increases may necessitate dose reduction or discontinuation of drug. Monitor serum potassium values.
- Observe for S&S of hyperkalemia (see Appendix F).

Patient & Family Education

- Discontinue drug and report S&S of angioedema to physician (e.g., swelling of face or extremities, difficulty breathing or swallowing).
- Maintain adequate fluid intake and avoid potassium supplements or salt substitutes unless specifically prescribed by the physician.
- Do not breast feed while taking this drug.

RANITIDINE HYDROCHLORIDE

(ra-nye'te-deen)

Zantac, Zantac EFFERdose, Zantac GELdose, Zantac-75

Classifications: GASTROINTESTINAL AGENT; ANTISECRETORY (H_2-RECEPTOR ANTAGONIST)

Prototype: Cimetidine

Pregnancy Category: B

AVAILABILITY 75 mg, 150 mg, 300 mg tablets; 25 mg, 150 mg effervescent tablets; 150 mg, 300 mg capsules; 15 mg/mL syrup; 0.5 mg/mL, 25 mg/mL injection

ACTIONS Potent anti-ulcer drug that competitively and reversibly inhibits histamine action at H_2-receptor sites on parietal cells, thus blocking gastric acid secretion. Indirectly reduces pepsin secretion but appears to have minimal effect on fasting and postprandial serum gastrin concentrations or secretion of gastric intrinsic factor or mucus.

THERAPEUTIC EFFECTS Blocks daytime and nocturnal basal gastric acid secretion stimulated by histamine and reduces gastric acid release in response to food, pentagastrin, and insulin. Shown to inhibit 50% of the stimulated gastric acid secretion.

USES Short-term treatment of active duodenal ulcer; maintenance therapy for duodenal ulcer patient after healing of acute ulcer; treatment of gastroesophageal reflux disease; short-term treatment of active, benign gastric ulcer; treatment of pathologic GI hypersecretory conditions (e.g., Zollinger-Ellison syndrome, systemic mastocytosis, and postoperative hypersecretion); heartburn.

CONTRAINDICATIONS Hypersensitivity to ranitidine; acute porphyria; OTC administration in children <12 y.

CAUTIOUS USE Hypersensitivity to H_2-blockers; hepatic and renal dysfunction; renal failure; PKU; pregnancy (category B), infants <1 mo, lactation.

ROUTE & DOSAGE

Duodenal Ulcer, Gastric Ulcer, Gastroesophageal Reflux

Adult: **PO** 150 mg b.i.d. or 300 mg h.s. **IV** 50 mg q6–8h; 150–300 mg/24 h by continuous infusion
Child: **PO** 4–5 mg/kg/d divided q8–12h (max: 6 mg/kg/d or 300 mg/d) **IM/IV** 2–4 mg/kg/d divided q6–8h; 0.1–0.125 mg/kg/h by continuous infusion
Infant: **PO** <2 wk, 2 mg/kg/d divided q12h **IV** 1.5 mg/kg/d divided q12h or 0.04 mg/kg/h by continuous infusion

Duodenal Ulcer, Maintenance Therapy

Adult: **PO** 150 mg h.s.

Pathologic Hypersecretory Conditions

Adult: **PO** 150 mg b.i.d. up to 6.3 g/d **IV** 50 mg q6–8h

Heartburn

Adult: **PO** 75–150 mg b.i.d.

ADMINISTRATION

Oral

- Give with or without food; simultaneous administration does not appear to reduce absorption or serum concentrations.
- Administer adjunctive antacid treatment 2 h before or after drug.
- Store tablets in light-resistant, tightly capped container at 15°–30° C (59°–86° F) in a dry place.

Intramuscular

- Note: Does not need to be diluted.

Intravenous

Note: Verify correct IV concentration and rate of infusion for infants and children with physician.

PREPARE: **Direct:** Dilute 50 mg NS, D5W, RL, or other compatible IV solution to a total volume of 20 mL. **Intermittent:** Dilute 50 mg in 50–100 mL of NS, D5W, RL, or other compatible IV solution. **Continuous:** Dilute total daily dose in 250 mL of NS, D5W, RL, or other compatible IV solution. Final concentration should be ≤2.5 mg/mL.

ADMINISTER: **Direct:** Give at a rate of 4 mL/min or 20 mL over not less than 5 min. **Intermittent:** Give over 15–30 min. **Continuous:** Give over 24 h.

INCOMPATIBILITIES **Solution/additive: Amphotericin B, atracurium, cefamandole, cefazolin, cefoxitin, ceftazidime, cefuroxime, clindamycin, chlorpromazine, diazepam, ethacrynic acid, hydroxyzine, methotrimeprazine, midazolam, nalbuphine, pentobarbital, phenobarbital, phytonadione** OPIUM ALKALOIDS, **phenobarbital. Y-site: Amphotericin B cholesteryl complex, methotrimeprazine, midazolam,** OPIUM ALKALOIDS, **phenobarbital.**

- Schedule dose to coincide with end of treatment if patient is having hemodialysis.

ADVERSE EFFECTS (≥1%) **CNS:** Headache, malaise, dizziness, somnolence, insomnia, vertigo, mental confusion, agitation, depression, hallucinations in older adults. **CV:** Bradycardia (with rapid IV push). **GI:** Constipation, nausea, abdominal pain, diarrhea. **Skin:** Rash. **Hematologic:** Reversible decrease in WBC count, thrombocytopenia. **Body as a Whole:** Hypersensitivity reactions, anaphylaxis (rare).

DIAGNOSTIC TEST INTERFERENCE Ranitidine may produce slight elevations in ***serum creatinine*** (without concurrent increase in ***BUN***); (rare) increases in ***AST, ALT, alkaline phosphatase, LDH,*** and total ***bilirubin.*** Produces false-positive tests for ***urine protein*** with ***Multistix*** (use ***sulfosalicylic acid*** instead).

INTERACTIONS Drug: may reduce absorption of **cefpodoxime, cefuroxime, delavirdine, ketoconazole, itraconazole.**

PHARMACOKINETICS Absorption: Incompletely absorbed from GI tract (50% reaches systemic circulation). **Peak:** 2–3 h PO. **Duration:** 8–12 h. **Distribution:** Distributed into breast milk. **Metabolism:** Metabolized in liver. **Elimination:** Excreted in urine, with some excreted in feces. **Half-Life:** 2–3 h.

NURSING IMPLICATIONS

Assessment & Drug Effects

- Potential toxicity results from decreased clearance (elimination) and therefore prolonged action; greatest in the older adult patients or those with hepatic or renal dysfunction.
- Lab tests: Periodic liver functions. Monitor creatinine clearance if renal dysfunction is present or suspected. When clearance is <50 mL/min, manufacturer recommends reduction of the dose to 150 mg once q24h with cautious and gradual reduction of the interval to q12h or less, if necessary.
- Be alert for early signs of hepatotoxicity (though low and thought to be a hypersensitivity reaction): jaundice (dark urine, pruritus, yellow sclera and skin), elevated transaminases (especially ALT) and LDH.
- Long-term therapy may lead to vitamin B_{12} deficiency.

Patient & Family Education

- Note: Long duration of action provides ulcer pain relief that is maintained through the night as well as the day.
- Be aware that even if symptomatic relief is provided by ranitidine, this should not be interpreted as absence of gastric malignancy. Follow-up examinations will be scheduled after therapy is discontinued.

- Adhere to scheduled periodic laboratory checkups during ranitidine treatment.
- Do not supplement therapy with OTC remedies for gastric distress or pain without physician's advice (e.g., Mylanta II reduces ranitidine absorption).
- Do not smoke; research shows smoking decreases ranitidine efficacy and adversely affects ulcer healing.
- Do not breast feed while taking this drug without consulting physician.

RASBURICASE

(ras-bur'i-case)
Elitek
Classifications: ANTIGOUT AGENT; ANTIMETABOLITE
Prototype: Colchicine
Pregnancy Category: C

AVAILABILITY 1.5 mg/vial powder for injection

ACTIONS A recombinant urate-oxidase enzyme produced by DNA technology from *Aspergillus flavus*. In humans, uric acid is the final step in the catabolic pathway of purines. Rasburicase catalyzes enzymatic oxidation of uric acid, thus it is only active at the end of the purine catabolic pathway.

THERAPEUTIC EFFECTS Used to manage plasma uric acid levels in pediatric patients with leukemia, lymphoma, and solid tumor malignancies who are receiving anticancer therapy that results in tumor lysis, and therefore elevates plasma uric acid.

USES Initial management of increased uric acid levels secondary to tumor lysis.

CONTRAINDICATIONS Deficiency in glucose-6-phosphate dehydrogenase (G6PD); history of anaphylaxis or hypersensitivity reactions; hypersensitivity to rasburicase; hemolytic reactions or methemoglobinemia reactions to rasburicase; pregnancy (category C), lactation, children <1 mo.

CAUTIOUS USE Patients at risk for G6PD deficiency (e.g., African or Mediterranean ancestry). Safety and efficacy in adults and elderly are unknown.

ROUTE & DOSAGE

Hyperuricemia
Child: **IV** *>1 mo*, 0.15–0.2 mg/kg once/d starting 4–24 h before chemotherapy × 5 d

ADMINISTRATION

Intravenous

PREPARE: **IV Infusion:** Reconstitute each 1.5 mg vial of ELITEK with 1 mL of the provided diluent and mix by swirling very gently. **Do not shake.** Discard if particulate matter is visible or if product is discolored after reconstitution. Remove the predetermined dose from the reconstituted vials and inject enough NS into an infusion bag to achieve a final total volume of 50 mL.

ADMINISTER: **IV Infusion:** Give over 30 min. **DO NOT GIVE BOLUS DOSE.** Infuse through an **unfiltered** line used for no other medications. If a separate line is not possible, flush the line with at least 15 mL of saline solution before/after infusion of rasburicase.

- Immediately discontinue IV infusion and institute emergency measures for S&S of anaphylaxis including chest pain, dyspnea, hypotension, and/or urticaria.

INCOMPATIBILITIES **Solution/additive/Y-site:** Do not mix or infuse with other drugs.

ADVERSE EFFECTS (≥1%) **Body as a Whole:** *Fever,* sepsis, severe hypersensitivity reactions including anaphylaxis. **CNS:** *Headache.* **GI:** *Mucositis, vomiting, nausea, diarrhea, abdominal pain.* **Hematologic:** Neutropenia. **Skin:** *Rash.*

DIAGNOSTIC TEST INTERFERENCE May give false elevations for ***uric acid*** if blood sample is left at room temperature.

INTERACTIONS Drug: No clinically significant interactions established.

PHARMACOKINETICS Half-Life: 18 h.

NURSING IMPLICATIONS

Assessment & Drug Effects

- Lab tests: Patients at higher risk for G6PD deficiency (e.g., patients of African or Mediterranean ancestry) should be screened prior to starting therapy as this deficiency is a contraindication for this drug.
- Lab test special instructions: Blood for uric acid anaylsis must be collected into prechilled tubes containing heparin anticoagulant and **immediately immersed in an ice water bath.** Plasma samples must be prepared by centrifugation in a precooled centrifuge (4° C) and plasma must be maintained in an ice water bath and analyzed for uric acid within 4 h of collection.
- Monitor closely for S&S of hypersensitivity and be prepared to institute emergency measures for anaphylaxis.
- Monitor cardiovascular, respiratory, neurologic, and renal status throughout therapy.

Patient & Family Education

- Report immediately any distressing S&S to physician.

REMIFENTANIL HYDROCHLORIDE

(rem-i-fent'a-nil)

Ultiva

Classifications: CENTRAL NERVOUS SYSTEM AGENT; ANALGESIC; NARCOTIC (OPIATE) AGONIST; GENERAL ANESTHESIA

Prototype: Morphine

Pregnancy Category: C

AVAILABILITY 1 mg/mL injection

ACTIONS Synthetic, potent narcotic agonist analgesic similar to fentanyl. Rapidly metabolized, therefore respiratory depression is of shorter duration than fentanyl analogs when discontinued.

THERAPEUTIC EFFECTS Used as the analgesic component of an anesthesia regime.

USES Analgesic during induction and maintenance of general anesthesia, as the analgesic component of monitored anesthesia care.

CONTRAINDICATIONS Hypersensitivity to fentanyl analogs, epidural or intrathecal administration.

CAUTIOUS USE Pregnancy (category C), lactation; head injuries, increased intracranial pressure; older adults, debilitated, poor-risk patients; COPD, other respiratory problems, bradyarrhythmia. Safety in labor and delivery has not been demonstrated. Safety and efficacy in children <2 y are not established.

ROUTE & DOSAGE

Adjunct to Anesthesia

Adult/Child: **IV** >2 y, 0.025–2 mcg/kg/min or 1 mcg/kg injected over 30–60 s

R

ADMINISTRATION

Note: See manufacturer's guidelines for reconstitution information and infusion rates.

Intravenous

- Reduce starting doses by 50% for patients >65 y. Base doses on ideal body weight for obese patients (>30% over ideal body weight).
- Clear IV tubing completely of the drug following discontinuation of remifentanil infusion to ensure that inadvertent administration of the drug will not occur at a later time.
- Reconstituted solution is stable for 24 h at room temperature. Store vials of powder at 2°–25° C (36°–77° F).

ADVERSE EFFECTS (≥1%) **Body as a Whole:** Muscle rigidity, shivering. **CNS:** Dizziness, headache. **CV:** Hypotension, hypertension, bradycardia. **GI:** *Nausea*, vomiting. **Respiratory:** Respiratory depression, apnea. **Skin:** Pruritus.

INTERACTIONS Drug: Alcohol and other CNS DEPRESSANTS potentiate effects; MAO INHIBITORS may precipitate hypertensive crisis.

PHARMACOKINETICS Duration: 12 min. **Distribution:** 70% protein bound. **Metabolism:** Hydrolyzed by nonspecific esterases in the blood and tissues. **Elimination:** Excreted in urine. **Half-Life:** 3–10 min.

NURSING IMPLICATIONS

Assessment & Drug Effects

- Monitor vital signs during postoperative period; observe for and immediately report any S&S of respiratory distress or respiratory depression, or skeletal and thoracic muscle rigidity and weakness.
- Monitor for adequate postoperative analgesia.

REPAGLINIDE (Pr)

(rep-a-gli'nide)

Prandin, GlucoNorm ♣

Classifications: HORMONES & SYNTHETIC SUBSTITUTES; ANTIDIABETIC AGENT; MEGLITINIDE

Pregnancy Category: C

AVAILABILITY 0.5 mg, 1 mg, 2 mg tablets

ACTIONS Oral hypoglycemic agent that lowers blood glucose levels by stimulating release of insulin from the pancreatic islets.

THERAPEUTIC EFFECTS Significantly reduces postprandial blood glucose in type 2 diabetes [preprandial blood glucose between 80 and 120 mg/dL and HbA_{1c} (glycosylated Hgb <7%)]. Minimal effects on fasting blood glucose were observed.

USES Adjunct to diet and exercise in type 2 diabetes. May also be used in combination with metformin.

CONTRAINDICATIONS Hypersensitivity to repaglinide; insulin-dependent diabetes, diabetic ketoacidosis, hypoglycemia; severe renal dysfunction; pregnancy (category C), lactation.

CAUTIOUS USE Hypoglycemia; loss of glycemic control due to secondary failure; hepatic impairment; older adults, surgery, fever, systemic infection, trauma. No studies have been done in children.

ROUTE & DOSAGE

Type 2 Diabetes

Adult: **PO** 0.5–4 mg 15–30 min before meals (2–4 doses/d depending on meal pattern; max: 16 mg/d)

R

ADMINISTRATION

Oral

- Give within 30 min of beginning a meal.
- Store at 15°–30° C (59°–86° F) in a tightly closed container and protect from moisture.

ADVERSE EFFECTS (≥1%) **Body as a Whole:** Arthralgia, back pain, paresthesia, allergy. **CNS:** Headache. **CV:** Chest pain, angina. **GI:** Nausea, diarrhea, constipation, vomiting, dyspepsia. **Respiratory:** URI, sinusitis, rhinitis, bronchitis. **Metabolic:** *Hypoglycemia.*

INTERACTIONS Drug: Erythromycin, ketoconazole may inhibit metabolism and potentiate hypoglycemia; BARBITURATES, **carbamazepine, rifabutin, rifampin, rifapentine, pioglitazone** may induce metabolism and cause hyperglycemia; **gemfibrozil** may increase risk of hypoglycemia and duration of action. **Herbal: Ginseng, garlic** may increase hypoglycemic effects.

PHARMACOKINETICS Absorption: Rapidly absorbed from GI tract, 56% bioavailability. **Peak:** 1 h. **Distribution:** 98% protein bound. **Metabolism:** Metabolized in liver by cytochrome P450 3A4. **Elimination:** 90% excreted in feces. **Half-Life:** 1 h.

NURSING IMPLICATIONS

Assessment & Drug Effects

- Lab tests: Frequent FBS and postprandial blood glucose monitoring and HbA_{1c} q3mo to determine effective dose.
- Monitor carefully for S&S of hypoglycemia especially during the 1-wk period following transfer from a longer-acting sulfonylurea such as chlorpropamide.

Patient & Family Education

- Take only with meals to lessen the chance of hypoglycemia. If a meal is skipped, skip a dose; if a meal is added, add a dose.
- Start repaglinide the morning after the other agent is stopped when changing from another oral hypoglycemia drug.
- Be alert for S&S of hyperglycemia or hypoglycemia (see Appendix F); report poor blood glucose control to physician.
- Do not breast feed while taking this drug.

RESERPINE (Pr)

(re-ser'peen)

Serpalan, Sk-Reserpine

Classifications: CARDIOVASCULAR AGENT; RAUWOLFIA ALKALOID; ANTIHYPERTENSIVE

Pregnancy Category: D

AVAILABILITY 0.1 mg, 0.25 mg tablets

ACTIONS Principal alkaloid of *Rauwolfia serpentina.* Interferes with binding of serotonin at receptor sites, decreases synthesis of norepinephrine by depleting dopamine (its precursor), and competitively inhibits their reuptake in storage granules. Depletes norepinephrine and serotonin in CNS, peripheral nervous system, heart, and other organs and tissues.

THERAPEUTIC EFFECTS Sympathetic inhibition seen in small but persistent decrease in BP, frequently associated with bradycardia, and reduced cardiac output. Central effect results in tranquilization and sedation similar to that produced by chlorpromazine.

USES Mild essential hypertension and as adjunctive therapy with other antihypertensive agents in the more severe forms of hypertension. Also used in agitated psychotic states, primarily in patients intolerant to phenothiazine or patients who also require antihypertensive medication.

UNLABELED USES Reduce vasospastic attacks in Raynaud's phenomenon and other peripheral vascular disorders, and for short-term symptomatic treatment of thyrotoxicosis.

CONTRAINDICATIONS Hypersensitivity to rauwolfia alkaloids; history of mental depression; acute peptic ulcer, ulcerative colitis; patients receiving electroconvulsive therapy; within 7–14 days of MAO inhibitor therapy. Safe use during pregnancy (category D) or lactation is not established.

CAUTIOUS USE Renal insufficiency; cardiac arrhythmias; cardiac damage; cerebrovascular accident; epilepsy; bronchitis, asthma; older adults, debilitated patients; gallstones; obesity; chronic sinusitis; parkinsonism; pheochromocytoma.

ROUTE & DOSAGE

Hypertension

Adult: **PO** 0.5 mg/d initially, reduced to 0.1–0.25 mg/d
Geriatric: **PO** Start with 0.05 mg q.d., increase by 0.05 mg per wk

ADMINISTRATION

Oral

- Give with meals or with milk or other food to minimize possibility of gastric irritation (drug increases gastric secretions).
- Store in tight, light-resistant containers, preferably at 15°–30° C (59°–86° F), unless otherwise directed by manufacturer.

ADVERSE EFFECTS (≥1%) **CNS:** *Drowsiness*, sedation, *lethargy*, mental depression, nervousness, anxiety, nightmares, increased dreaming, headache, dizziness, increased appetite, dull sensorium; prolonged use of large doses: CNS stimulation (parkinsonian syndrome): tremors, muscle rigidity; <u>respiratory depression</u>, convulsions, hypothermia. **CV:** Bradycardia, *edema*, orthostatic hypotension, increased AV conduction time (prolonged therapy); angina-like symptoms, arrhythmias, CHF (rare). **Special Senses:** *Nasal congestion,* epistaxis, lacrimation, blurred vision; miosis, ptosis, conjunctival congestion (acute toxicity). **GI:** Dry mouth or excessive salivation, nausea, vomiting, abdominal cramps, diarrhea, reactivation of peptic ulcer (hypersecretion), heartburn, biliary colic. **Hematologic:** Thrombocytopenic purpura, anemia, prolonged BT. **Body as a Whole:** Hypersensitivity (Pruritus, rash, asthma), Muscle aches, dysuria, fixed-drug eruptions. **Urogenital:** Menstrual irregularities, breast engorgement, galactorrhea, gynecomastia, feminization (males), impaired sexual function, impotence.

DIAGNOSTIC TEST INTERFERENCE Possibility of elevated ***blood glucose*** values; however, it is also reported that reserpine may decrease thiazide-induced hyperglycemia. Increase in ***serum prolactin*** with chronic administration of ***rauwolfia*** alkaloids; overdoses may cause initial increase in excretion of ***urinary catecholamines;*** decreases with chronic administration. Large doses may cause initial rise in ***urinary 5 HIAA*** excretion. Initial IM doses may increase ***urinary VMA*** excretion followed by decrease by end of third day of therapy (with oral or parenteral administration). Possible interference with ***urinary steroid*** colorimetric determinations: ***17-OHCS*** and ***17-KS.***

INTERACTIONS Drug: Diuretics, other HYPOTENSIVE AGENTS compound hypotensive effects; CARDIAC GLYCOSIDES **(digoxin)** may increase risk of arrhythmias; MAO INHIBITORS may cause excitation and hypertension; CNS DEPRESSANTS compound depression; may decrease response to **levodopa. Herbal: St. John's wort** may antagonize hypotensive effects.

PHARMACOKINETICS Peak: 2 h. **Distribution:** Widely distributed, especially to adipose tissue; crosses blood–brain barrier and placenta; distributed in breast milk. **Metabolism:** Extensively metabolized to inactive compounds. **Elimination:** Slowly excreted, 60% in feces within 96 h and 10% in urine. **Half-Life:** 4.5 and 11.3 h.

NURSING IMPLICATIONS

Assessment & Drug Effects

- Assess vital signs at intervals prescribed by physician. Compare readings with baseline data and keep physician informed. (Note: Drop in BP may be accompanied by bradycardia.)
- Lab tests: Periodic CBC with differential, platelet count, serum electrolytes, and plasma glucose.
- Supervise ambulation as indicated; postural hypotension occurs rarely with usual PO doses but is not uncommon in patients receiving large parenteral doses.
- Monitor I&O, especially in patients with impaired kidney function. Report changes in I&O ratio and pattern.
- Full therapeutic effect of oral drug for hypertension may not occur until 2–3 wk of therapy, and effects may persist for as long as 4–6 wk after drug is discontinued.
- Take special precautions with older adult and obese patients (half-life is reportedly prolonged in obese patients). Anticipate increased incidence of adverse effects.
- Be aware that mental depression is a serious adverse effect and may be severe. It occurs most commonly in high dosage regimens (e.g., 0.5–1 mg/d or more) and may not appear until 2–8 mo of therapy and may last for several months after drug is withdrawn.

Patient & Family Education

- Take drug at the same time each day, do not to skip or double doses, and do not to stop therapy without advice of physician.
- Do not drive or engage in potentially hazardous activities until response to drug is known.
- Learn about possible adverse effects and report promptly to physician.
- Report the following possible beginning symptoms of depression: early morning insomnia, anorexia, inability to concentrate, despondency, self-deprecation, attitude of detachment, mood swings, or impotence. Hospitalization may be necessary.
- Make position changes slowly, particularly from recumbent to upright posture, and lie down or sit down (head-low position) if patient feels faint. Do not take hot showers or hot tub baths, and do not to stand still for prolonged periods. Report symptoms of dizziness or lightheadedness to physician.
- Check for edema and record weight daily to help make a distinction between weight gain from edema and that from increased appetite. Consult physician about gain of 1–2 kg (3–5 lb) in 1 wk.
- Do not take OTC medications without consulting physician or pharmacist (many preparations for coughs and colds contain

R

adrenergic agents that affect the actions of rauwolfia alkaloids).

- Do not breast feed while taking this drug without consulting physician.

RESPIRATORY SYNCYTIAL VIRUS IMMUNE GLOBULIN (RSV-IVIG)

(res-pir'a-tory sin-cy'ti-al)

RespiGam

Classifications: BIOLOGIC RESPONSE MODIFIER; IMMUNOGLOBULIN

Prototype: Immune Globulin

Pregnancy Category: C

AVAILABILITY 2500 mg/50 mL vial

ACTIONS Contains IgG immune globulin antibodies from human plasma.

THERAPEUTIC EFFECTS The preparation contains large amounts of RSV-neutralizing antibodies. Recipients should be high-risk premature infants and children.

USES Prevention of serious lower respiratory tract infection caused by RSV in children <24 mo with bronchopulmonary dysplasia or history of premature birth; hypervolemia.

CONTRAINDICATIONS Previous severe reaction to RespiGam or other human immunoglobulin preparation, selective IgA deficiency, congenital heart disease, hepatic disease, pregnancy (category C).

CAUTIOUS USE Immunodeficiency, AIDS, CHF, renal failure.

ROUTE & DOSAGE

RSV

Child/Infant/Neonate: **IV** 750 mg/kg infused at 1.5 mL/kg/h for first 15 min, then 3 mL/kg/h for next 15 min, then 6 mL/kg/h for rest of infusion, may repeat monthly as needed

ADMINISTRATION

Intravenous

PREPARE: **IV Infusion:** Give undiluted.

ADMINISTER: **IV Infusion:** Do not shake vial; infuse vial contents undiluted through a separate IV line if possible; if "piggyback" must be used, see manufacturer's directions. DO NOT EXCEED IV INFUSION RATES given in Route & Dosage table! Use a constant infusion pump.

INCOMPATIBILITIES **Solution/additive or Y-site:** Do not mix with other drugs.

- Store vials at 2°–8° C (35°–46° F). Begin infusion within 6 h after vial is entered and complete within 12 h.

ADVERSE EFFECTS (≥1%) **Body as a Whole:** Fever, pyrexia, fluid overload. **CV:** Tachycardia, hypertension. **GI:** Vomiting, diarrhea, gastroenteritis. **Respiratory:** Respiratory distress, wheezing, rales, hypoxia, hypoxemia, tachypnea. **Skin:** Injection site inflammation.

INTERACTIONS Drug: May interfere with immune response to LIVE VIRUS VACCINES (mumps, rubella, measles), may need to repeat vaccine if given within 10 mo of **RespiGam.**

PHARMACOKINETICS Half-Life: 22–28 d.

NURSING IMPLICATIONS

Assessment & Drug Effects

- Monitor closely during and after each IV rate change.
- Assess vital signs and respiratory status prior to infusion, during and after each rate change, and at 30-min intervals until 30 min after

R

infusion is completed, and periodically thereafter for 24 h.
- Slow infusion immediately if S&S of fluid overload appear and report to physician.
- Lab tests: Monitor routine blood chemistry, serum electrolytes, blood gases, osmolality.
- Monitor for aseptic meningitis syndrome, which may begin up to 2 d after infusion.

Patient & Family Education
- Be aware of the possibility of aseptic meningitis syndrome; learn S&S to report (headache, drowsiness, fever, photophobia, painful eye movements, muscle rigidity, nausea, vomiting).

RETEPLASE RECOMBINANT
(re′te-plase)
Retavase
Classifications: BLOOD FORMERS, COAGULATORS, AND ANTICOAGULANTS; THROMBOLYTIC ENZYME
Prototype: Alteplase
Pregnancy Category: C

AVAILABILITY 10.8 IU vials

ACTIONS DNA recombinant human tissue-type plasminogen activator (TPA) that acts as a catalyst in the cleavage of plasminogen to plasmin.
THERAPEUTIC EFFECTS Forms plasmin; responsible for degrading the fibrin matrix of the clot, and thus has antithrombolytic properties.

USES Thrombolysis management of acute MI to reduce the incidence of CHF and mortality.

CONTRAINDICATIONS Active internal bleeding, history of CVA, recent neurologic surgery or trauma, intercranial neoplasm, or aneurysm, bleeding disorders, severe uncontrolled hypertension.

CAUTIOUS USE Pregnancy (category C), lactation; any condition in which bleeding constitutes a significant hazard (i.e., severe hepatic or renal disease, CVA, hypertension, acute pancreatitis, septic thrombophlebitis). Safety and efficacy in children are not established.

ROUTE & DOSAGE

Thrombolysis During Acute MI
Adult: **IV** 10 U injected over 2 min. Repeat dose in 30 min (20 U total)

ADMINISTRATION
Intravenous
PREPARE: **Direct:** Reconstitute using only the diluent, syringe, needle, and dispensing pin provided with reteplase. Withdraw diluent with syringe provided. Remove needle from syringe, replace with dispensing pin and transfer diluent to vial of reteplase. Leave pin and syringe in place in vial and swirl to dissolve. Do NOT shake. When completely dissolved, remove 10 mL solution, replace dispensing pin with a 20-gauge needle.
ADMINISTER: **Direct:** Flush IV line before & after with 30 mL NS or D5W and do NOT give any other drug simultaneously through the same IV line. Give a single dose evenly over 2 min.
INCOMPATIBILITIES **Solution/additive: Heparin. Y-site: Heparin.**
- Store drug kit unopened at 2°–25° C (36°–77° F).

ADVERSE EFFECTS (≥1%) **Hematologic:** *Hemorrhage* (including *intracranial*, GI, genitourinary), anemia. **CV:** Reperfusion arrhythmias.

DIAGNOSTIC TEST INTERFERENCE Causes decreases in plasminogen and fibrinogen, making coagulation and fibrinolytic tests unreliable.

R

INTERACTIONS Drug: Aspirin, abciximab, dipyridamole, heparin may increase risk of bleeding.

PHARMACOKINETICS Elimination: Excreted in urine. **Half-Life:** 13–16 min.

NURSING IMPLICATIONS

Assessment & Drug Effects

- Discontinue concomitant heparin immediately if serious bleeding not controllable by local pressure occurs and, if not already given, withhold the second reteplase bolus.
- Monitor carefully all potential bleeding sites; monitor for S&S of internal hemorrhage (e.g., GI, GU, intracranial, retroperitoneal, pulmonary).
- Monitor carefully cardiac status for arrhythmias associated with reperfusion.
- Avoid invasive procedures, arterial and venous punctures, IM injections, and nonessential handling of the patient during reteplase therapy.

Patient & Family Education

- Report changes in consciousness or signs of bleeding to physician immediately.

R

RHo(D) IMMUNE GLOBULIN

(row)

BayRho-D Full Dose, RhoGAM, WinRho SDF

RHo(D) IMMUNE GLOBULIN MICRO-DOSE

BayRho-D Mini Dose, MICRhoGAM

Classifications: BIOLOGIC RESPONSE MODIFIER; IMMUNOGLOBULIN

Prototype: Immune Globulin

Pregnancy Category: C

AVAILABILITY BayRho-D 15–18% solution in single dose vial **RhoGAM, MICRhoGAM** 5% solution in prefilled syringes **WinRho SDF** 120 mcg, 300 mcg, 1000 mcg vials

ACTIONS Sterile nonpyrogenic gamma globulin solution containing immunoglobulins (IgG) of at least 90% IgG, which provides passive immunity by suppressing active antibody response and formation of anti-Rh_0(D) (isoimmunization) in Rh-negative (Rh_0[D]-negative) individuals previously exposed to Rh-positive (Rh_0[D]-positive, D^u-positive) blood.

THERAPEUTIC EFFECTS Effective for exposure in Rh-negative women when Rh-positive fetal RBCs enter maternal circulation during third stage of labor, fetal-maternal hemorrhage (as early as second trimester), amniocentesis, or other trauma during pregnancy, termination of pregnancy, and following transfusion with Rh-positive RBC, whole blood, or components (platelets, WBC) prepared from Rh-positive blood.

USES To prevent isoimmunization in Rh-negative individuals exposed to Rh-positive RBC (see above). Rh_0(D) immune globulin microdose is for use only after spontaneous or induced abortion or termination of ectopic pregnancy up to and including 12 wk of gestation.

CONTRAINDICATIONS Rh_0(D)-positive patient; person previously immunized against Rh_0(D) factor, hypersensitivity for thimerosal (in commercial preparations), severe immune globulin hypersensitivity, bleeding disorders; pregnancy (category C), neonates, pediatric clients.

CAUTIOUS USE Idiopathic thrombocytopenia purpura (ITP), IgA deficiency.

ROUTE & DOSAGE

Note: Only WinRho SDF can be given IV. BayRho-E and RhoGAM are available in regular and mini-dose vials

Antepartum Prophylaxis

Adult: **IM/IV** 1 vial or 300 mcg at approximately 28 wk; followed by 1 vial of mini-dose or 120 mcg within 72 h of delivery if infant is Rh-positive

Postpartum Prophylaxis

Adult: **IM/IV** 1 vial or 300 mcg within 72 h of delivery if infant is Rh-positive

Following Amniocentesis, Miscarriage, Abortion, Ectopic Pregnancy

Adult: **IM** 1 vial of the microdose, preferably within 3 h but at least within 72 h

Transfusion Accident

Adult: **IM/IV** 1 vial or 300 mcg for each volume of RBCs infused divided by 15, given within at least 72 h of accident

ADMINISTRATION

Note: Each vial of Rh_0(D) immune globulin contains enough anti-Rh_0(D) to suppress the immunizing potential of 15 mL Rh-positive packed RBC. Each vial of microdose contains enough anti-Rh_0(D) to suppress the immune response to 2.5 mL of Rh-positive packed RBC.

Intramuscular

- Make sure that lot numbers of drug used for the cross-match and the drug to be administered are the same.
- Administer Rh_0(D) immune globulin via IM to the mother only; not to the infant.
- Use the deltoid muscle. Give in divided doses at different sites, all at once or at intervals, as long as the entire dose is given within 72 h after delivery or termination of pregnancy.
- Reconstitute with 1.25 mL of NS (using the same method to dissolve as for IV). Give immediately after reconstitution.
- Keep epinephrine immediately available; systemic allergic reactions sometimes occur.

Intravenous

Note: 5 IU equals 1 mcg.

PREPARE: **Direct:** Reconstitute each vial with 2.5 ml NS (provided by manufacturer). Direct stream of diluent to side of vial, swirl to dissolve, do not shake. Concentration of reconstituted vials: 600 IU yields 240 IU/mL and 1500 IU vial yields 600 IU/mL.

ADMINISTER: **Direct:** Give a single dose over 3–5 min.

- Refrigerate commercially prepared solutions, although may remain stable up to 30 d at room temperature according to manufacturers. Discard solutions that have been frozen. Store powder at 2°–8° C (36°–46° F) unless otherwise directed; avoid freezing.

ADVERSE EFFECTS (≥1%) **Body as a Whole:** Injection site irritation, slight fever, myalgia, lethargy.

INTERACTIONS Drug: May interfere with immune response to LIVE VIRUS VACCINE; should delay use of LIVE VIRUS VACCINES for 3 mo after administration of **Rh_0(D) immune globulin.**

PHARMACOKINETICS Peak: 2 h IV, 5–10 d IM. **Half-Life:** 25 d.

NURSING IMPLICATIONS

Assessment & Drug Effects

- Obtain history of systemic allergic reactions to human immune globulin preparations prior to drug administration.
- Send sample of newborn's cord blood to laboratory for crossmatch and typing immediately after delivery and before administration of Rh_0(D) immune globulin. Confirm that mother is Rh_0(D) and D^u-negative. Infant must be Rh-positive.

Patient & Family Education

- Be aware that administration of Rh_0(D) immune globulin (antibody) prevents hemolytic disease of the newborn in a subsequent pregnancy.

RIBAVIRIN

(rye-ba-vye′rin)

Virazole, Rebetol, Copegus, Ribasphere

Classifications: ANTIINFECTIVE; ANTIVIRAL AGENT

Prototype: Acyclovir

Pregnancy Category: X

AVAILABILITY 6 g/100 mL vial; 200 mg tablets; 200 mg capsules; 40 mg/mL oral solution

ACTIONS Synthetic nucleoside with broad-spectrum antiviral activity against DNA and RNA viruses. Exact mode of action is not fully understood but believed to involve multiple mechanisms including selective interference with viral ribonucleic protein synthesis. It does not influence interferon synthesis.

THERAPEUTIC EFFECTS Active against many RNA and DNA viruses, including respiratory syncytial virus (RSV), influenza A and B, parainfluenza, measles, mumps, Lassa fever, enterovirus 72 (formerly called hepatitis A), yellow fever, HIV, herpes simplex virus (HSV-1 and HSV-2), and vaccinia. Immune responses appear to depend on cellular drug concentrations. Low concentrations seem to stimulate immune responses while high concentrations appear to inhibit those responses. Generally not active against poliovirus and coxsackie viruses. Unlike other antiviral agents, virus resistance to ribavirin does not appear to develop.

USES Aerosol treatment of carefully selected hospitalized infants and young children with severe lower respiratory tract infection caused by respiratory syncytial virus (RSV). Oral used in combination with interferon-alfa to treat hepatitis C.

UNLABELED USES Prophylaxis and treatment of influenza A and B, pneumonia caused by adenovirus; Lassa fever, measles, HSV-1, HSV-2, hepatitis A, herpes zoster, and for carefully selected patients with AIDS and AIDS-related complex (ARC).

CONTRAINDICATIONS Mild RSV infections of lower respiratory tract; infants requiring simultaneous assisted ventilation; severe cardiovascular disease, congestive heart failure, angina, unstable cardiac disease; pancreatitis, prolonged or multiple courses of ribavirin inhalation therapy; autoimmune hepatitis; renal failure, or Cl_{cr} <50 mL/min; pregnancy (category X), lactation; hemoglobinopathy, thalassemia major, sickle cell disease.

CAUTIOUS USE COPD, asthma; anemia; history of MI, cardiac arrhythmias; older adults, decreased renal, hepatic, or cardiac function; respiratory depression.

ROUTE & DOSAGE

RSV

Child: **Inhalation** 20 mg via SPAG nebulizer administered over 12–18 h/d for a minimum of 3 d (max: 7 d)

Hepatitis C
(in combination with interferon-alfa)

Adult: **PO** *>75 kg,* 600 mg b.i.d. for 24–48 wk; *<75 kg,* 400 mg in a.m., 600 mg in p.m. for 24–48 wk.
Child: **PO** *>3 y and >75 kg,* 600 mg b.i.d.; *62–75 kg,* 400 mg in a.m., 600 mg in p.m.; *50–61 kg,* 400 mg b.i.d.; *37–49 kg,* 200 mg in a.m. and 400 mg in p.m.; *25–36 kg,* 200 mg b.i.d. for 24–48 wk.

Renal Impairment

Cl_{cr} <50 mL/min oral ribavirin should not be used

ADMINISTRATION

Note: Aerosol solution is prepared with either sterile water for injection or sterile water for inhalation, without preservatives or any other added substance. See manufacturer's package insert for preparation directions. Inspect solution for discoloration or presence of particulate matter. Discard discolored or cloudy solutions.

Inhalation

- Administer only by SPAG-2 aerosol generator, following manufacturer's directions.
- Caution: Ribavirin has demonstrated teratogenicity in animals. Advise pregnant healthcare personnel of the potential teratogenic risks associated with exposure during ribavirin administration to patients.
- Do not give other aerosol medication concomitantly with ribavirin.
- Discard solution in the SPAG-2 reservoir at least q24h and whenever liquid level is low before fresh reconstituted solution is added.
- Store unopened vial in a dry place at 15°–25° C (59°–78° F) unless otherwise directed.
- Following reconstitution, store solution at 20°–30° C (68°–86° F) for 24 h.

ADVERSE EFFECTS (≥1%) **CV:** Hypotension (faintness, light-headedness, unusual fatigue), MI, cardiac arrest. **Special Senses:** Conjunctivitis, erythema of eyelids. **Hematologic:** Reticulocytosis, hemolytic anemia. **Respiratory:** Deterioration of respiratory function, dyspnea, apnea, chest soreness, bacterial pneumonia, ventilator dependence. **GI:** Transient increases in AST, ALT, bilirubin; abdominal cramps, jaundice.

INTERACTIONS Drug: Ribavirin may antagonize the antiviral effects of **zidovudine** against HIV.

PHARMACOKINETICS Absorption: Rapidly absorbed orally (44%) and systemically from lungs. **Peak:** Inhaled 60–90 min. PO 1.7–3 h. **Distribution:** Crosses placenta; distributed into breast milk. **Metabolism:** Metabolized in cells to an active metabolite. **Elimination:** 85% excreted in urine, 15% in feces. **Half-Life:** 24 h in plasma, 16–40 d in RBCs.

NURSING IMPLICATIONS

Assessment & Drug Effects

- Obtain specimens for rapid diagnosis of RSV infection before therapy is initiated or at least during the first 24 h of ribavirin therapy. Do not continue therapy without laboratory confirmation of RSV infection.
- Treatment efficacy in RSV infections appears greatest if initiated within the first 3 d.

- Monitor respiratory function and fluid status closely during therapy. Note baseline rate and character of respirations and pulse. Observe for signs of labored breathing: dyspnea, apnea; rapid, shallow respirations, intercostal and substernal retraction, nasal flaring, limited excursion of lungs, cyanosis. Auscultate lungs for abnormal breath sounds.
- Observe patients requiring simultaneous assisted ventilation closely for S&S of worsening pulmonary function. Check equipment carefully every 2 h, including endotracheal tube, for malfunction. Precipitation of ribavirin and accumulation of fluid in tubing can obstruct the apparatus and cause inadequate ventilation and gas exchange.
- Consult physician about management of fluid and food intake and keep an accurate record of I&O.

RIBOFLAVIN (VITAMIN B_2)

(rye'bo-flay-vin)

Riboflavin (Vitamin B_2)

Classifications: HORMONE AND SYNTHETIC SUBSTITUTE; VITAMIN

Pregnancy Category: A (C if >RDA)

AVAILABILITY 50 mg, 100 mg tablets

ACTIONS Water-soluble vitamin and component of the flavoprotein enzymes, which work together with a wide variety of proteins to catalyze many cellular respiratory reactions by which the body derives its energy.

THERAPEUTIC EFFECTS Evaluated by improvement of clinical manifestations of deficiency: digestive disturbances, headache, burning sensation of skin (especially "burning" feet), cracking at corners of mouth (cheilosis), glossitis, seborrheic dermatitis (often at angle of nose and anogenital region) and other skin lesions, mental depression, corneal vascularization (with photophobia, burning and itchy eyes, lacrimation, roughness of eyelids), anemia, neuropathy.

USES To prevent riboflavin deficiency and to treat ariboflavinosis; also to treat microcytic anemia and as a supplement to other B vitamins in treatment of pellagra and beri-beri.

CONTRAINDICATIONS None.

CAUTIOUS USE Pregnancy [(category A); (category C if >RDA)].

ROUTE & DOSAGE

Nutritional Supplement

Adult: **PO** 5–10 mg/d
Child: **PO** 1–4 mg/d

Nutritional Deficiency

Adult: **PO** 5–30 mg/d in divided doses
Child: **PO** 3–10 mg/d

ADMINISTRATION

Oral

- Give with food to enhance absorption.
- Store in airtight containers protected from light.

ADVERSE EFFECTS (≥1%) **Urogenital:** May discolor urine bright yellow.

DIAGNOSTIC TEST INTERFERENCE In large doses, riboflavin may produce yellow-green fluorescence in ***urine*** and thus cause false elevations in certain ***fluorometric determinations*** of ***urinary catecholamines.***

INTERACTIONS Drug: No clinically significant interactions established.

PHARMACOKINETICS Absorption: Readily absorbed from GI tract. **Distribution:** Little is stored; excess amounts are excreted in urine. **Elimination:** Excreted in urine. **Half-Life:** 66–84 min.

NURSING IMPLICATIONS

Assessment & Drug Effects

- Collaborate with physician, dietitian, patient, and responsible family member in planning for diet. A complete dietary history is an essential part of vitamin replacement so that poor eating habits can be identified and corrected. Deficiency in one vitamin is usually associated with other vitamin deficiencies.

Patient & Family Education

- Be aware that large doses may cause an intense yellow discoloration of urine.
- Note: Rich dietary sources of riboflavin are found in liver, kidney, beef, pork, heart, eggs, milk and milk products, yeast, whole-grain cereals, vitamin A-enriched breakfast cereals, green vegetables, and mushrooms.

RIFABUTIN

(rif-a-bu′tin)

Ansamycin, Mycobutin

Classifications: ANTIINFECTIVE; ANTITUBERCULOSIS AGENT

Prototype: Isoniazid

Pregnancy Category: B

AVAILABILITY 150 mg capsules

ACTIONS Semisynthetic bacteriostatic antibiotic. Mode of action may be to inhibit DNA-dependent RNA polymerase (an enzyme) in susceptible bacterial cells but not in human cells.

THERAPEUTIC EFFECTS Effective against, *Mycobacterium, avium, complex* (MAC) (or *M. avium-intracellulare*) and many strains of *M. tuberculosis*.

USES The prevention of disseminated *Mycobacterium avium* complex (MAC) disease in patients with advanced HIV infection.

CONTRAINDICATIONS Hypersensitivity to rifabutin or any other rifamycins; lactation.

CAUTIOUS USE Pregnancy (category B).

ROUTE & DOSAGE

Prevention of MAC

Adult: **PO** 300 mg q.d., may give 150 mg b.i.d. if nausea is a problem
Child: **PO** 75 mg q.d.

ADMINISTRATION

Oral

- Give as usual dose of 300 mg/d or in two divided doses of 150 mg with food if needed to reduce GI upset.
- Store at room temperature, 15°–30° C (59°–86° F), unless otherwise directed.

ADVERSE EFFECTS (≥1%) **CNS:** *Headache,* **GI:** *Abdominal pain, dyspepsia, nausea, taste perversion, increased liver enzymes.* **Hematologic:** Thrombocytopenia, eosinophilia, leukopenia, neutropenia. **Skin:** Rash. **Other:** *Turns urine, feces, saliva, sputum, perspiration, and tears orange. Soft contact lenses may be permanently discolored.*

INTERACTIONS Drug: May decrease levels of BENZODIAZEPINES, BETA BLOCK-

R

ERS, **clofibrate, dapsone,** NARCOTICS, ANTICOAGULANTS, CORTICOSTEROIDS, **cyclosporine, quinidine,** ORAL CONTRACEPTIVES, PROGESTINS, SULFONYLUREAS, **ketoconazole, fluconazole,** BARBITURATES, **theophylline,** and ANTICONVULSANTS, resulting in therapeutic failure.

PHARMACOKINETICS Absorption: 12%–20% of oral dose reaches the systemic circulation. **Peak:** 2–3 h. **Distribution:** 85% protein bound. Widely distributed, high concentrations in the lungs, liver, spleen, eyes, and kidney. Crosses placenta, distributed into breast milk. **Metabolism:** Metabolized in the liver. Causes induction of hepatic enzymes. **Elimination:** Approximately 53% of dose is excreted in urine as metabolites, 30% is excreted in feces. **Half-Life:** 16–96 h (average 45 h).

NURSING IMPLICATIONS

Assessment & Drug Effects

- Monitor patients for S&S of active TB. Report immediately.
- Lab tests: Monitor periodic blood work for neutropenia and thrombocytopenia.
- Evaluate patients on concurrent oral hypoglycemic therapy for loss of glycemic control.
- Review patient's complete drug regimen because dosage adjustment of a significant number of drugs may be needed when rifabutin is added to regimen.

Patient & Family Education

- Learn S&S of TB and MAC (e.g., persistent fever, progressive weight loss, anorexia, night sweats, diarrhea) and notify physician if any of these develop.
- Notify physician of following: Muscle or joint pain, eye pain or other discomfort, chest pain with dyspnea, rash, or a flu-like syndrome.
- Be aware that urine, feces, saliva, sputum, perspiration, tears, and skin may be colored brown-orange. Soft contact lens may be permanently discolored.
- Rifabutin may reduce the activity of a wide variety of drugs. Provide a complete and accurate list of concurrent drugs to the physician for evaluation.
- Do not breast feed while taking this drug.

RIFAMPIN (Pr)

(rif′am-pin)

Rifadin, Rimactane, Rofact ♣

Classifications: ANTIINFECTIVE; ANTIBIOTIC; ANTITUBERCULOSIS AGENT

Pregnancy Category: C

AVAILABILITY 150 mg, 300 mg capsules; 600 mg injection

ACTIONS Semisynthetic derivative of rifamycin B, an antibiotic derived from *Streptococcus mediterranei,* with bacteriostatic and bactericidal actions. Inhibits DNA-dependent RNA polymerase activity in susceptible bacterial cells, thereby suppressing RNA synthesis.

THERAPEUTIC EFFECTS Active against *Mycobacterium tuberculosis, M. leprae, Neisseria meningitidis,* and a wide range of gram-negative and gram-positive organisms. It is used in conjunction with other antitubercular agents to treat tuberculosis because resistant strains emerge rapidly when it is employed alone.

USES Primarily as adjuvant with other antituberculosis agents in initial treatment and retreatment of clinical tuberculosis; as short-term therapy to eliminate meningococci from nasopharynx of asymptomatic carriers of *N. meningitidis* when risk of meningococcal meningitis is high.

UNLABELED USES Chemoprophylaxis in contacts of patients with *Haemophilus influenzae* type B infection; alone or in combination with dapsone and other antiinfectives in treatment of leprosy (especially dapsone-resistant leprosy). Also infections caused by susceptible gram-negative and gram-positive bacteria that fail to respond to other antiinfectives; in combination with erythromycin or tetracycline for treatment of Legionnaire's disease.

CONTRAINDICATIONS Hypersensitivity to rifampin; obstructive biliary disease; meningococcal disease; intermittent rifampin therapy; lactation. Safe use during pregnancy (category C) or in children <5 y is not established.

CAUTIOUS USE Hepatic disease; history of alcoholism; concomitant use of other hepatotoxic agents.

ROUTE & DOSAGE

Pulmonary Tuberculosis

Adult: **PO/IV** 600 mg once/d in conjunction with other antituberculosis agents
Child: **PO** 10–20 mg/kg/d (max: 600 mg/d)

Meningococcal Carriers

Adult: **PO** 600 mg b.i.d. for 2 consecutive d
Child: **PO** 10–20 mg/kg b.i.d. for 2 consecutive d (max: 600 mg/d)

Prophylaxis for *H. influenzae* Type B

Adult: **PO** 600 mg/d for 4 d
Child: **PO** 10–20 mg/kg/d for 4 d (max: 600 mg/d)

Dapsone-Sensitive Multibacillary Leprosy

Adult: **PO** 600 mg once/mo with clofazimine and dapsone for a minimum of 2 y

ADMINISTRATION

Oral

- Give 1 h before or 2 h after a meal. Peak serum levels are delayed and may be slightly lower when given with food; capsule contents may be emptied into fluid or mixed with food.
- Note: An oral suspension can be prepared from capsules for use with pediatric patients. Consult pharmacist for directions.
- Keep a desiccant in bottle containing capsules to prevent moisture causing instability.

Intravenous

PREPARE: **IV Infusion:** Dilute by adding 10 mL of sterile water for injection to each 600-mg vial to yield 60 mg/mL. Swirl to dissolve. Withdraw the ordered dose and further dilute in 500 mL (preferred) of D5W. If necessary, 100 mL of D5W may be used.

ADMINISTER: **IV Infusion:** Infuse 500 mL solution over 3 h and 100 mL solution over 30 min. Note: A less concentrated solution infused over a longer period is preferred.

INCOMPATIBILITIES **Solution/additive: Minocycline. Y-site: Diltiazem.**

- Use diluted solution within 4 h of preparation.

ADVERSE EFFECTS (≥1%) **CNS:** Fatigue, drowsiness, headache, ataxia, confusion, dizziness, inability to concentrate, generalized numbness, pain in extremities, muscular weakness. **Special Senses:** Visual disturbances, transient low-frequency hearing loss, conjunctivitis. **GI:** *Heartburn, epigastric distress, nausea, vomiting, anorexia, flatulence, cramps, diarrhea,* pseudomembranous colitis, *transient elevations in liver function tests* (bilirubin, BSP, alkaline phosphatase, ALT, AST), pancreatitis. **Hematologic:** Thrombocytopenia, transient leukopenia, anemia, including hemolytic anemia. **Body as a Whole:** Hypersensitivity (fever, pruritus, urticaria, skin eruptions, soreness of mouth and tongue, eosinophilia, hemolysis), flu-like syndrome. **Urogenital:** Hemoglobinuria, hematuria, acute renal failure, light-chain proteinuria, menstrual disorders, hepatorenal syndrome, (with intermittent therapy). **Respiratory:** Hemoptysis. **Other:** Increasing lethargy, liver enlargement and tenderness, jaundice, brownish-red or orange discoloration of skin, sweat, saliva, tears, and feces; unconsciousness.

DIAGNOSTIC TEST INTERFERENCE Rifampin interferes with contrast media used for ***gallbladder study;*** therefore, test should precede daily dose of rifampin. May also cause retention of ***BSP.*** Inhibits standard assays for ***serum folate*** and ***vitamin*** B_{12}.

INTERACTIONS Drug: Alcohol, isoniazid, pyrazinamide increase risk of hepatotoxicity (including fatal hepatotoxicity when used for latent TB); ***p*-aminosalicylic acid (PAS)** decreases concentrations of rifampin; decreases concentrations of **alfentanil, alosetron, alprazolam, amprenavir,** BARBITURATES, BENZODIAZEPINES, **carbamazepine, atovaquone, cevimeline, chloramphenicol, clofibrate,** CORTICOSTEROIDS, **cyclosporine, dapsone, delavirdine, diazepam, digoxin, diltiazem, disopyramide, estazolam, estramustine, fentanyl, fosphenytoin, fluconazole galantamine, indinavir, itraconazole, ketoconazole, lamotrigine, levobupivacaine, lopinavir, methadone, metoprolol, mexiletine, midazolam, nelfinavir,** ORAL SULFONYLUREAS, ORAL CONTRACEPTIVES, **phenytoin,** PROGESTINS, **propafenone, propranolol, quinidine, quinine, ritonavir, sirolimus, theophylline,** THYROID HORMONES, **tocainide, tramadol, verapamil, warfarin, zaleplon,** and **zonisamide,** leading to potential therapeutic failure.

PHARMACOKINETICS Absorption: Readily absorbed from GI tract. **Peak:** 2–4 h. **Distribution:** Widely distributed, including CSF; crosses placenta; distributed into breast milk. **Metabolism:** Metabolized in liver to active and inactive metabolites; is enterohepatically cycled. **Elimination:** Up to 30% excreted in urine, 60%–65% in feces. **Half-Life:** 3 h.

NURSING IMPLICATIONS

Assessment & Drug Effects

- Lab tests: Periodic liver function tests are advised. Closely monitor patients with hepatic disease.
- Check prothrombin time daily or as necessary to establish and maintain required anticoagulant activity when patient is also receiving an anticoagulant.

Patient & Family Education

- Do not interrupt prescribed dosage regimen. Hepatorenal reaction with flu-like syndrome has occurred when therapy has been resumed following interruption.
- Be aware that drug may impart a harmless red-orange color to urine, feces, sputum, sweat, and

tears. Soft contact lenses may be permanently stained.
- Report onset of jaundice, hypersensitivity reactions, and persistence of GI adverse effects to physician.
- Use or add barrier contraceptive if using hormonal contraception. Concomitant use of rifampin and oral contraceptives leads to decreased effectiveness of the contraceptive and to menstrual disturbances (spotting, breakthrough bleeding).
- Keep drug out of reach of children.
- Do not breast feed while taking this drug.

RIFAPENTINE

(rif'a-pen-teen)
Priftin
Classifications: ANTIINFECTIVE; ANTIBIOTIC; ANTITUBERCULOSIS AGENT
Prototype: Isoniazid
Pregnancy Category: C

AVAILABILITY 150 mg tablets

ACTIONS Rifamycin derivative similar to rifampin. Inhibits DNA-dependent RNA polymerase activity in susceptible bacterial cells, thereby suppressing RNA synthesis.
THERAPEUTIC EFFECTS Indicated by improvement in clinical S&S (e.g., fever, cough, pleuritic pain, fatigue) and on chest x-ray. Inhibits the growth of *Mycobacterium tuberculosis*. Used in conjunction with other antitubercular agents because resistant strains emerge rapidly when employed alone.

USES Pulmonary tuberculosis in conjunction with at least one other antitubercular agent.

CONTRAINDICATIONS Hypersensitivity to any rifamycins (e.g., rifampin, rifabutin, rifapentine); pregnancy (category C); lactation.
CAUTIOUS USE Patients with abnormal liver function tests or hepatic disease; HIV disease or concurrent use of protease inhibitors. Safety and efficacy in children <12 y are not established.

ROUTE & DOSAGE

Tuberculosis: Short-Course Therapy
Adult: **PO** 600 mg twice weekly (at least 72 h apart) times 2 mo, then 600 mg once weekly times 4 mo

ADMINISTRATION

Oral
- Give with an interval of NO LESS than 72 h between doses.
- Give with food to minimize GI upset.
- Store at 15°–30° C (59°–86° F) in a tightly closed container and protect from excess moisture.

ADVERSE EFFECTS (≥1%) **CNS:** Headache, dizziness. **CV:** Hypertension. **GI:** Increased liver function tests (ALT, AST), anorexia, nausea, vomiting, dyspepsia, diarrhea. **GU:** *Hyperuricemia*, pyuria, proteinuria, hematuria, urinary casts. **Hematologic:** Neutropenia, lymphopenia, anemia, leukopenia, thrombocytosis. **Respiratory:** Hemoptysis. **Skin:** Rash, pruritus, acne. **Body as a Whole:** Arthralgia, pain.

INTERACTIONS Drug: Decreased levels of **indinavir** and possibly other PROTEASE INHIBITORS; increased metabolism and decreased activity of ORAL CONTRACEPTIVES, **phenytoin, disopyramide, mexiletine, quinidine, tocainide, warfarin, fluconazole, itraconazole, ketocon-**

R

azole, diazepam, BETA BLOCKERS, CALCIUM CHANNEL BLOCKERS, CORTICOSTEROIDS, **haloperidol,** SULFONYLUREAS, **cyclosporine, tacrolimus, levothyroxine,** NARCOTIC ANALGESICS, **quinine,** REVERSE TRANSCRIPTASE INHIBITORS, TRICYCLIC ANTIDEPRESSANTS, **sildenafil, theophylline.**

PHARMACOKINETICS Absorption: Approximately 70% absorbed. **Peak:** 5–6 h. **Distribution:** 97.7% protein bound. **Metabolism:** Hydrolyzed by esterase enzyme to active metabolite in liver; inducer of cytochromes P450 3A4 and 2C8/9. **Elimination:** 70% excreted in feces, 17% in urine. **Half-Life:** 13.3 h.

NURSING IMPLICATIONS

Assessment & Drug Effects

- Lab tests: Sputum smear and culture, CBC, baseline liver functions (especially serum transaminases) to rule out preexisting hepatic disease and serum creatinine and BUN.
- Monitor carefully for S&S of toxicity with concurrent use of oral anticoagulants, digitalis preparations, or anticonvulsants.

R

Patient & Family Education

- Follow strict adherence to the prescribed dosing schedule to prevent emergence of resistant strains of tuberculosis.
- Be aware that food may be useful in preventing GI upset.
- Report immediately any of the following to the physician: fever, weakness, nausea or vomiting, loss of appetite, dark urine or yellowing of eyes or skin, pain or swelling of the joints, severe or persistent diarrhea.
- Use or add barrier contraceptive if using hormonal contraception.
- Do not breast feed while taking this drug.

RIFAXIMIN

(ri-fax′i-min)

Xifaxan

Classifications: ANTIINFECTIVE; RIFAMYCIN ANTIBIOTIC

Prototype: Rifampin

Pregnancy Category: C

AVAILABILITY 200 mg tablets

ACTIONS A rifamycin antibiotic structurally related to rifampin. Its spectrum of activity includes gram-positive and gram-negative aerobes and anaerobes.

THERAPEUTIC EFFECTS Coverage against gram-positive cocci is better than its coverage against *Enterobacteriaceae*. Inhibits *E. coli* RNA synthesis. Unlike other rifamycin antibiotics, rifaximin is largely unabsorbed by the GI tract in subjects with intact and damaged intestinal mucosa.

USES Treatment of traveler's diarrhea cause by noninvasive strains of *E. coli*.

CONTRAINDICATIONS Hypersensitivity to rifaximin, other rifamycin antimicrobial agents or to any of its components; ulcerative intestinal disease; dysentery; children <12 y; pregnancy (category C); lactation.

CAUTIOUS USE Diarrhea with fever and/or blood in the stool, or diarrhea due to organisms other than *E. coli;* worsening diarrhea or diarrhea persisting for >24–48 h.

ROUTE & DOSAGE

Traveler's Diarrhea

Adult: **PO** 200 mg t.i.d. for 3 d

ADMINISTRATION

Oral

- May be given without regard to food.
- Store at 15°–30° C (59°–86° F).

ADVERSE EFFECTS (≥1%) **Body as a Whole:** Fever. **CNS:** Headache. **GI:** *Flatulence,* abdominal pain, rectal tenesmus, defecation urgency, nausea, constipation, vomiting.

PHARMACOKINETICS Absorption: <0.4% absorbed orally. **Peak:** 1.21 h. **Elimination:** Eliminated in feces. **Half-Life:** 5.85 h.

NURSING IMPLICATIONS

Assessment & Drug Effects

- Withhold drug and notify physician if symptoms worsen or last >48 h after starting drug; an alternative treatment should be considered.
- Report promptly the appearance of blood in the stool.

Patient & Family Education

- Report promptly any of the following: fever; difficulty breathing; skin rash, itching, or hives; worsening diarrhea during or after treatment or blood in the stool.
- Do not breast feed while taking this drug without consulting physician.

RILUZOLE

(ri-lu′zole)

Rilutek

Classifications: CENTRAL NERVOUS SYSTEM AGENT; ANTI-AMYOTROPHIC LATERAL SCLEROSIS (ALS) AGENT

Pregnancy Category: C

AVAILABILITY 50 mg tablets

ACTIONS Glutamate antagonist used for treating amyotrophic lateral sclerosis (ALS). Inhibits the presynaptic release of glutamic acid in the CNS.

THERAPEUTIC EFFECTS Effectiveness based on hypothesis that pathogenesis of ALS is related to injury of motor neurons by glutamate. Also protects neurons against the excitotoxicity of glutamic acid.

USES Treatment of ALS, may extend survival or time to tracheostomy.

CONTRAINDICATIONS Hypersensitivity to riluzole; lactation.

CAUTIOUS USE Hepatic dysfunction, renal impairment; hypertension, history of other CNS disorders, pregnancy (category C). Safety and efficacy in children are not established.

ROUTE & DOSAGE

ALS

Adult: **PO** 50 mg q12h at least 1 h before or 2 h after meals

ADMINISTRATION

Oral

- Give at same time daily and at least 1 h before or 2 h after a meal. Do not give before/after a high-fat meal.
- Store at room temperature; protect from bright light.

ADVERSE EFFECTS (≥1%) **Body as a Whole:** *Asthenia,* headache, back pain, malaise, arthralgia, weight loss, peripheral edema, flu-like syndrome. **CNS:** Hypertonia, depression, dizziness, dry mouth, insomnia, somnolence, circumoral paresthesia. **CV:** Hypertension, tachycardia, phlebitis, palpitation. **GI:** Abdominal pain, *nausea,* vomiting, dyspepsia, anorexia, diarrhea, flatulence, stomatitis. **Respiratory:** *Decreased lung function,* rhinitis, increased cough, apnea, bronchitis, dysphagia, dyspnea. **Skin:** Pruritus, eczema, alopecia, exfoliative dermatitis (rare). **Urogenital:** UTI.

INTERACTIONS Drug: BARBITURATES, **carbamazepine** may increase risk of hepatotoxicity.

PHARMACOKINETICS Absorption: Well absorbed from GI tract, 60% reaches systemic circulation. **Peak:** Steady-state levels by day 5. **Distribution:** 96% protein bound. **Metabolism:** Metabolized in liver by cytochrome P4501A2 (CYP1A2). **Elimination:** 90% eliminated in urine. **Half-Life:** 12 h.

NURSING IMPLICATIONS

Assessment & Drug Effects

- Lab tests: Monitor periodically Hct and Hgb, routine blood chemistries, and alkaline phosphatase. If febrile illness develops, monitor WBC count. Monitor liver function before and during course of therapy; evaluate ALT/SGPT every month for first 3 mo, every 3 mo for remainder of first year, and periodically thereafter.
- Withhold drug and notify physician if liver enzymes are elevated.

Patient & Family Education

- Do not increase dose. There is no increased benefit from daily doses >50 mg q12h.
- Report any febrile illness to physician.
- Do not drive or engage in potentially hazardous activities until response to drug is known.
- Learn common adverse effects and possible adverse interaction with alcohol.
- Do not breast feed while taking this drug.

RIMANTADINE

(ri-man′ta-deen)
Flumadine
Classifications: ANTIINFECTIVE; ANTIVIRAL
Prototype: Acyclovir
Pregnancy Category: C

AVAILABILITY 100 mg tablets; 50 mg/5 mL syrup

ACTIONS Antiviral agent for treatment and prophylaxis of influenza A infections. Thought to exert an inhibitory effect early in the viral replication cycle, probably by interfering with the viral uncoating procedure of the influenza A virus.
THERAPEUTIC EFFECTS Inhibits synthesis of both viral RNA and viral protein, thus preventing or interrupting influenza A infections.

USES Prophylaxis and treatment of influenza A in adults and prophylaxis of influenza A in children.

CONTRAINDICATIONS Hypersensitivity to rimantadine and amantadine; pregnancy (category C), lactation, children <1 y.
CAUTIOUS USE History of seizures. Safety and efficacy in treatment of symptomatic influenza infection in children are not established.

ROUTE & DOSAGE

Prophylaxis of Influenza A

Adult/Child: **PO** >*10 y,* 100 mg b.i.d., reduce to 100 mg daily in older adults or patients with liver disease
Child: **PO** <*10 y,* 5 mg/kg once daily (max: 150 mg/d)

Treatment of Influenza A

Adult: **PO** 100 mg b.i.d., reduce to 100 mg daily in older adults or patients with liver disease, initiate as soon as possible and preferably within 48 h of onset of symptoms and continue for about 7 d

ADMINISTRATION

Oral

- Store at 15°–30° C (59°–86° F).

ADVERSE EFFECTS (≥1%) **CNS:** Nervousness, dizziness, headache, sleep disturbances, fatigue or malaise, drowsiness, anticholinergic effects. **GI:** Nausea, vomiting, diarrhea, dyspepsia, dry mouth, anorexia, abdominal pain.

INTERACTIONS Drug: No clinically significant interactions established.

PHARMACOKINETICS Absorption: Readily absorbed from GI tract. **Peak:** Serum levels 3.2–4.3 h. **Distribution:** Concentrates in respiratory secretions. **Metabolism:** Extensively metabolized in liver. **Elimination:** Excreted by kidneys. **Half-Life:** 20–36 h.

NURSING IMPLICATIONS

Assessment & Drug Effects

- Monitor carefully for seizure activity in patients with a history of seizures. Seizures are an indication to discontinue the drug.
- Monitor cardiac, respiratory, and neurologic status while on drug. Report palpitations, hypertension, dyspnea, or pedal edema.

Patient & Family Education

- Report bothersome adverse effects to physician; especially hallucinations, palpitations, difficulty breathing, and swelling of legs.
- Use caution with hazardous activities until reaction to drug is known.
- Do not breast feed while taking this drug.

RIMEXOLONE

(rim-ex′o-lone)

Vexol

Classifications: HORMONE AND SYNTHETIC SUBSTITUTE; OPHTHALMIC CORTICOSTEROID; ANTIINFLAMMATORY AGENT

Prototype: Hydrocortisone

Pregnancy Category: C

AVAILABILITY 1% suspension

See Appendix A-1.

RISEDRONATE SODIUM

(ri-se-dron′ate)

Actonel

Classifications: BISPHOSPHONATE; REGULATOR, BONE METABOLISM

Prototype: Etidronate Disodium

Pregnancy Category: C

AVAILABILITY 5 mg, 30 mg tablets

ACTIONS Diphosphate preparation with primary action on bone. Mechanism of action not fully understood. Lowers serum alkaline phosphatase, presumably by decreasing release of phosphate from bone and increasing excretion of parathyroid hormone.

THERAPEUTIC EFFECTS Indicated by decreased bone and joint pain and improved bone density. Slows rate of bone resorption and new bone formation in pagetic bone lesions and in normal remodeling process. One thousand times more potent than etidronate.

USES Paget's disease, prevention and treatment of postmenopausal osteoporosis and steroid-induced osteoporosis.

CONTRAINDICATIONS Hypersensitivity to risedronate or other bisphosphonates; hypocalcemia, vitamin D deficiency; lactation; severe renal impairment (creatinine clearance <30 mL/min); pregnancy (category C).

CAUTIOUS USE Renal impairment; CHF; hyperphosphatemia; hepatic disease; fever related to infection or other causes. Safety and efficacy in children are not established.

ROUTE & DOSAGE

Paget's Disease

Adult: **PO** 30 mg q.d. at least 30 min before the first food or drink of the day times 2 mo, may repeat after 2 mo rest if necessary

Prevention & Treatment of Osteoporosis

Adult: **PO** 5 mg q.d. 30 min before first food or drink

ADMINISTRATION

Oral

- Give on an empty stomach (before first food or drink of the day) with at least 6–8 oz plain water.
- Note: Patient should be upright. Maintain upright position and empty stomach for at least 30 min after administration.
- Space calcium supplements and antacids as far as possible from risedronate.
- Store at 15°–30° C (59°–86° F) in a tightly closed container and protect from light.

ADVERSE EFFECTS (≥1%) **Body as a Whole:** Flu-like syndrome, asthenia, arthralgia, bone pain, leg cramps, myasthenia. **CNS:** Headache, dizziness. **CV:** Chest pain, peripheral edema. **GI:** *Diarrhea,* abdominal pain, nausea, constipation, belching, colitis. **Respiratory:** Bronchitis, sinusitis. **Skin:** Rash. **Special Senses:** Amblyopia, tinnitus, dry eyes.

DIAGNOSTIC TEST INTERFERENCE May interfere with the use of bone-imaging agents.

INTERACTIONS Drug: Calcium, ANTACIDS significantly decrease absorption.

PHARMACOKINETICS Absorption: Minimally absorbed from GI tract, bioavailability 0.63%. **Peak:** 1 h. **Distribution:** Approximately 60% of dose is distributed to bone. **Metabolism:** Not metabolized. **Elimination:** Excreted in urine; unabsorbed drug excreted in feces. **Half-Life:** 220 h.

NURSING IMPLICATIONS

Assessment & Drug Effects

- Lab tests: Baseline and periodic serum calcium, phosphorus, and alkaline phosphatase.
- Monitor carefully for and immediately report S&S of GI bleeding and hypocalcemia.

Patient & Family Education

- Learn administration guidelines regarding upright position, empty stomach, and spacing relative to calcium supplements and antacids must be strictly followed.
- Report any of the following to physician: eye irritation, significant GI upset, or flu-like symptoms.
- Do not breast feed while taking this drug.

RISPERIDONE

(ris-per'i-done)

Risperdal, Risperdal M-TAB, Risperdal Consta

Classifications: CENTRAL NERVOUS SYSTEM (CNS) AGENT; ANTIPSYCHOTIC; ATYPICAL

Prototype: Clozapine

Pregnancy Category: C

AVAILABILITY 0.25 mg, 0.5 mg, 1 mg, 2 mg, 3 mg, 4 mg tablets; 0.5 mg, 1 mg, 2 mg quick-dissolving tablets; 1 mg/mL solution; 25 mg, 37.5 mg, 50 mg injection

ACTIONS Mechanism is not well understood. Interferes with binding of dopamine to D_2-interlimbic region of the brain, serotonin (5-HT_2) receptors, and alpha-adrenergic receptors in the occipital cortex. It has low to moderate affinity for the other serotonin (5-HT) receptors and no affinity to nondopaminergic sites (e.g., cholinergic, muscarinic, or beta-adrenergic receptors).

THERAPEUTIC EFFECTS Effective in controlling symptoms of schizophrenia as well as other psychotic symptoms.

USES Reduction or elimination of psychotic symptoms in schizophrenia and related psychoses; treatment of bipolar disorder. Seems to improve negative symptoms such as apathy, blunted affect, and emotional withdrawal.

UNLABELED USES Management of patients with dementia-related psychotic symptoms. Adjunctive treatment of behavioral disturbances in patients with mental retardation.

CONTRAINDICATIONS Hypersensitivity to risperidone; QT prolongation, Reye's syndrome, brain tumor, severe CNS depression, head trauma; suicidal ideation, tardive dyskinesia; sunlight (UV) exposure, tanning beds; pregnancy (category C), lactation, children <15 y.

CAUTIOUS USE Older adults; arrhythmias, hypotension, breast cancer, blood dyscrasia, cardiac disorders, cerebrovascular disease, hypotension, dehydration, diabetes mellitus, diabetic ketoacidosis, hyperglycemia, hypokalemia, hypomagnesemia, hyponatremia, MI, obesity, orthostatic hypotension, mild or moderate CNS depression, coma; GI obstruction, dysphagia; electrolyte imbalance, ethanol intoxication, heart failure, renal or hepatic dysfunction; seizure disorder, seizures, stroke, Parkinson's disease.

ROUTE & DOSAGE

Psychosis

Adult: **PO** 1–6 mg b.i.d., start with 1 mg b.i.d., increase by 1 mg b.i.d. daily to an initial target dose of 3 mg b.i.d. (max: 8 mg/d) **IM** 25 mg once q2wk (max: 50 mg)

Geriatric: **PO** Start with 0.5 mg b.i.d. and increase by 0.5 mg b.i.d. daily to an initial target of 1.5 mg b.i.d. (max: 4 mg/d) **IM** 25 mg once q2wk (max: 25 mg)

Bipolar Disorder

Adult: **PO** 2–3 mg once daily for up to 3 wk

Geriatric: **PO** Start with 0.5 mg b.i.d. and increase by 0.5 mg b.i.d. daily to an initial target of 1.5 mg b.i.d. (max: 4 mg/d). May convert to once daily dosing after stabilized in b.i.d. 2–3 d

Dementia-Related Psychotic Symptoms

Geriatric: **PO** Start with 0.5 mg b.i.d., increase by 0.5 mg b.i.d. daily to an initial target of 1 mg b.i.d. (max: 2 mg/d)

Renal Impairment

Cl_{cr} <30 mL/min: Start with 0.5 mg b.i.d., increase by 0.5 mg b.i.d. daily to an initial target of 1.5 mg b.i.d., may increase by 0.5 mg b.i.d. at weekly intervals (max: 6 mg/d)

ADMINISTRATION

Oral

- Note that quick-dissolving tablets dissolve rapidly when placed on tongue.
- Do not exceed increases/decreases of 1 mg b.i.d. in normal populations or 0.5 mg b.i.d. in older adults or the debilitated during dosage adjustments.

- Make further increases at 1-wk or longer intervals after the target dose of 3 mg b.i.d. in normal populations and 1.5 mg b.i.d. in older adults or the debilitated are reached.
- Store at 15°–30° C (59°–86° F).

Intramuscular

- Reconstitute the 25, 37.5, or 50 mg vial using the supplied 2 mL prefilled syringe. Shake vigorously for at least 10 sec to produce a uniform, thick, milky suspension. If 2 min or more pass before injection, shake vial again.
- Give deep IM into the upper-outer quadrant of the gluteal muscle with the supplied needle; do not substitute. Follow the manufacturer's instructions for use of the SmartSite Needle-Free Vial Access Device and Needle-Pro device.
- Store unopened vials at 2°–8° C (36°–46° F). Protect from light.

ADVERSE EFFECTS (≥1%) **Body as a Whole:** Orthostatic hypotension with initial doses, sweating, weakness, fatigue. **CNS:** *Sedation, drowsiness, headache,* transient blurred vision, *insomnia,* disinhibition, *agitation,* anxiety, increased dream activity, dizziness, catatonia, *extrapyramidal symptoms* (akathisia, dystonia, pseudoparkinsonism), especially with doses >10 mg/d, <u>neuroleptic malignant syndrome</u> (rare), increased risk of stroke in elderly. **CV:** Prolonged QTc interval, tachycardia. **GI:** Dry mouth, dyspepsia, nausea, vomiting, diarrhea, constipation, abdominal pain, elevated liver function tests (AST, ALT). **Endocrine:** Galactorrhea. **Metabolic:** Hyperglycemia, diabetes mellitus. **Respiratory:** Rhinitis, cough, dyspnea. **Skin:** Photosensitivity. **Urogenital:** Urinary retention, menorrhagia, decreased sexual desire, erectile dysfunction, sexual dysfunction male and female.

DIAGNOSTIC TEST INTERFERENCE Liver function tests (AST, ALT) are elevated.

INTERACTIONS Drug: Risperidone may enhance the effects of certain ANTIHYPERTENSIVE AGENTS. May antagonize the antiparkinson effects of **bromocriptine, cabergoline, levodopa, pergolide, pramipexole, ropinirole. Carbamazepine** may decrease risperidone levels. **Clozapine** may increase risperidone levels. **Cisapride** may cause dysrhythmias.

PHARMACOKINETICS Absorption: Rapidly absorbed; not affected by food. **Onset:** Therapeutic effect 1–2 wk. **Peak:** 1–2 h. **Distribution:** 0.7 L/kg; in animal studies, risperidone has been found in breast milk. **Metabolism:** Metabolized primarily in liver by cytochrome P450 with an active metabolite, 9-hydroxyrisperidone. **Elimination:** 70% excreted in urine; 14% in feces. **Half-Life:** 20 h for slow metabolizers, 30 h for fast metabolizers.

NURSING IMPLICATIONS

Assessment & Drug Effects

- Monitor diabetics for loss of glycemic control.
- Reassess patients periodically and maintain on the lowest effective drug dose.
- Monitor closely neurologic status of older adults.
- Monitor cardiovascular status closely; assess for orthostatic hypotension, especially during initial dosage titration.
- Monitor closely those at risk for seizures.
- Assess degree of cognitive and motor impairment, and assess for environmental hazards.
- Lab tests: Monitor periodically blood glucose, serum electrolytes, liver function, and complete blood counts.

Patient & Family Education

- Carefully monitor blood glucose levels if diabetic.
- Do not engage in potentially hazardous activities until the response to drug is known.
- Be aware of the risk of orthostatic hypotension.
- Learn adverse effects and report to physician those that are bothersome.
- Wear sunscreen and protective clothing to avoid photosensitivity.
- Notify physician if you intend to or become pregnant.
- Do not breast feed while taking this drug.

RITODRINE HYDROCHLORIDE

(ri'toe-dreen)
Yutopar
Classifications: AUTONOMIC NERVOUS SYSTEM AGENT; BETA-ADRENERGIC AGONIST
Prototype: Isoproterenol
Pregnancy Category: C

AVAILABILITY 10 mg/mL, 15 mg/mL, 0.3 mg/mL injection

ACTIONS Preferentially stimulates $beta_2$-receptors in uterine smooth muscle, reducing intensity and frequency of uterine contractions and lengthening gestation period. (Actions may be eliminated by beta-adrenergic antagonists.) Transitory cardiovascular effects include increased cardiac output, increased maternal and fetal heart rates, and widening of maternal pulse pressure ($beta_1$ stimulation).

THERAPEUTIC EFFECTS $Beta_2$-adrenergic agonist clinically effective in preventing or delaying preterm labor (tocolytic effect). Uterine contractions will decrease in frequency and intensity during treatment.

USES To manage premature labor in selected patients.

CONTRAINDICATIONS Mild to moderate preeclampsia or eclampsia, intrauterine infection, cervix dilated 4 cm or more (in a single pregnancy); pregnancy (category C); hypertension; diabetes mellitus; prior to 20th wk or after 36th wk of pregnancy or if continuation of pregnancy would be hazardous to mother and fetus (e.g., antepartum hemorrhage, eclampsia, intrauterine fetal death, maternal cardiac disease, pulmonary hypertension, maternal hyperthyroidism, severe diabetes mellitus). Also hypovolemia, cardiac arrhythmias associated with tachycardia or digitalis intoxication, uncontrolled hypertension; thyrotoxicosis; bronchial asthma being treated with betamimetics or steroids; lactation.

CAUTIOUS USE Concomitant use of potassium-depleting diuretics, cardiac disease.

ROUTE & DOSAGE

Premature Labor
Adult: **PO** Start 30 min before terminating infusion, 10 mg q2h for first 24 h, then 10–20 mg q4–6h (max: 120 mg/d) **IV** 50–100 mcg/min, may increase by 50 mcg/min q10min until uterine relaxation is achieved, may continue for up to 12 h after contractions have ceased

ADMINISTRATION

Note: IV solution should be clear. Discard if cloudy or a precipitate is present.

Intravenous

PREPARE: **IV Infusion:** Add 150 mg ritodrine to 500 mL D5W or NS solution to yield 0.3 mg/mL (300 mcg/mL).

ADMINISTER: **IV Infusion:** Begin at 50 mcg/min and increase by 50 mcg q10 min until desired response. Monitor IV infusion flow rate to prevent circulation overload. Use a microdrip and infusion pump.

- Place patient in left lateral recumbent position throughout the infusion period to reduce risk of hypotension.
- Store drug below 30° C (86° F). Do not freeze.

ADVERSE EFFECTS (≥1%) **Body as a Whole:** erythema, *nervousness,* restlessness, anxiety, malaise, *anaphylactic shock,* sweating, chills, drowsiness, weakness, myotonic and muscular dystrophies. **CNS:** Tremor, headache. **CV:** *Altered maternal and fetal heart rates and maternal BP* (dose related), *palpitations,* arrhythmias, chest pain, pulmonary edema. **Endocrine:** *Temporary hyperglycemia.* **GI:** Nausea, vomiting, epigastric distress, ileus, bloating, constipation, diarrhea. **Urogenital:** Glycosuria. **Respiratory:** Dyspnea, hyperventilation. **Skin:** Rash.

R

DIAGNOSTIC TEST INTERFERENCE Ritodrine (IV route) may produce an increase in ***serum*** levels of ***glucose, insulin,*** and ***free fatty acids,*** and a decrease in ***serum potassium.*** It temporarily elevates results of ***glucose tolerance test.***

INTERACTIONS Drug: CORTICOSTEROIDS may precipitate pulmonary edema; BETA AGONISTS add to cardiovascular adverse effects; effects of both ritodrine and BETA BLOCKERS antagonized.

PHARMACOKINETICS Absorption: 30% absorbed from GI tract. **Peak:** 30–60 min. **Distribution:** Crosses placenta. **Metabolism:** Metabolized in liver. **Elimination:** Excreted in urine. **Half-Life:** 1.7–2.6 h.

NURSING IMPLICATIONS

Assessment & Drug Effects

- Monitor continuously for pronounced dose-related adverse effects to maternal and fetal heart rates and maternal BP while infusion is running.
- Be alert to S&S of pulmonary edema (see Appendix F).

Patient & Family Education

- Report immediately any of the following: palpitations, chest pain, dizziness, respiratory distress, weakness, tremors, sweating or chills.
- Do not breast feed while taking this drug.

RITONAVIR

(ri-ton′a-vir)

Norvir

Classifications: ANTIINFECTIVE; ANTIVIRAL AGENT; PROTEASE INHIBITOR

Prototype: Saquinavir

Pregnancy Category: B

AVAILABILITY 100 mg capsules; 80 mg/mL solution

ACTIONS HIV protease is an enzyme required to produce the polyprotein procurers of functional proteins in infectious HIV. Protease inhibitors prevent cleavage of the viral polyproteins, resulting in the formation of immature noninfectious virus particles.

THERAPEUTIC EFFECTS Protease inhibitor of both HIV-1 and HIV-2 resulting in the formation of noninfectious viral particles.

USES Alone or in combination with other antiretroviral agents or protease inhibitors for treatment of HIV infection.

CONTRAINDICATIONS Hypersensitivity to ritonavir; antimicrobial resistance to protease inhibitors; pancreatitis; lactation. Safety and efficacy in children <2 y are not established.

CAUTIOUS USE Pregnancy (category B); hepatic diseases, hepatic insufficiency, liver enzyme abnormalities, or hepatitis, jaundice, advanced HIV disease; diabetes mellitus, diabetic ketoacidosis, hyperglycemia, hyperlipidemia, hypertriglyceridemia; hemophilia A or B, renal insufficiency, concurrent administration with HMG-CoA reductase inhibitors.

ROUTE & DOSAGE

HIV
Adult: **PO** 600 mg b.i.d. 1 h before or 2 h after meal (may take with a light snack)
Child: **PO** *2–16 y,* 400 mg/m² b.i.d. (max: 600 mg b.i.d.), start with 250 mg/m² b.i.d., increase by 50 mg/m² q2–3d

ADMINISTRATION

Oral

- Give preferably with food; oral solution may be mixed with chocolate milk within 1 h of dosing to improve taste.
- Do not give concurrently with any of the following drugs: alprazolam, amiodarone, astemizole, bepridil, bupropion, cisapride, clozapine, clorazepate, diazepam, dihydroergotamine, ergotamine, encainide, estazolam, flecainide, flurazepam, meperidine, midazolam, piroxicam, propafenone, propoxyphene, quinidine, rifabutin, triazolam, zolpidem.
- Store refrigerated at 2°–8° C (36°–46° F). Protect from light in tightly closed container.

ADVERSE EFFECTS (≥1%) **Body as a Whole:** Myalgia, allergic reaction, bronchitis, cough, rhinitis, taste alterations, visual disturbances, dysuria, hyperglycemia, diabetes. **CNS:** *Asthenia,* fatigue, headache, fever, malaise, circumoral or peripheral paresthesia, insomnia, dizziness, somnolence, abnormal thinking, amnesia, agitation, anxiety, confusion, convulsions, aphasia, ataxia, diplopia, emotional lability, euphoria, hallucinations, decreased libido, nervousness, neuralgia, neuropathy, peripheral neuropathy, paralysis, tremor, vertigo. **CV:** Palpitations, vasodilation, hypotension, postural hypotension, syncope, tachycardia. **Hematologic:** Anemia, thrombocytopenia, lymphadenopathy. **GI:** *Nausea, diarrhea, vomiting,* abdominal pain, dyspepsia, stomatitis, anorexia, dry mouth, constipation, flatulence, cholecystitis, cholestasis, abnormal liver function tests, hepatitis. **Skin:** Rash, sweating, acne, contact dermatitis, pruritus, urticaria, skin ulceration, dry skin.

INTERACTIONS Drug: Carbamazepine, dexamethasone, phenobarbital, phenytoin, rifabutin, rifampin, smoking can decrease ritonavir levels. **Ritonavir** may increase serum levels and toxicity of **clarithromycin,** especially in patients with renal insufficiency (reduce **clarithromycin** dose in patients with Cl_{cr} <60 ml/min); **desipramine; saquinavir, amiodarone, astemizole, bepridil, bupropion, cisapride, clozapine, dihydroergotamine, flecainide, meperidine, pimozide, piroxicam, propoxyphene, quinidine, rifabutin, trazodone. Ritonavir** decreases levels of ORAL CONTRACEPTIVES, **theophylline;** may increase **ergotamine** toxicity with **dihydroergotamine, ergotamine;** may increase systemic steroid exposure with **fluticasone.** Liquid formulation may cause disulfiram-like reaction with **alcohol** or **metronidazole.** See the complete prescribing information for a comprehensive table of potential, but not studied, drug interactions. **Herbal: St. John's wort** may decrease antiretroviral activity.

PHARMACOKINETICS Absorption: Rapidly absorbed from GI tract. **Peak:** 2–4 h. **Distribution:** 98%–99% protein bound. **Metabolism:** Metabolized in liver by cytochrome P4503A4 (CYP3A4). **Elimination:** Excreted primarily in feces (>80%).

NURSING IMPLICATIONS

Assessment & Drug Effects

- Lab tests: Monitor periodically CBC with differential and platelet count, liver function, kidney function, serum albumin, lipid profile, CPK, serum amylase, electrolytes, blood glucose HbA1c, and alkaline phosphatase.
- Withhold drug and notify physician in the presence of abnormal liver function.
- Assess for S&S of GI distress, peripheral neuropathy, and other potential adverse effects.

Patient & Family Education

- Learn potential adverse reactions and drug interactions; report to physician use of any OTC or prescription drugs.
- Do not breast feed while taking this drug.
- Take this drug exactly as prescribed. Do not skip doses. Take at same time each day.

R

RITUXIMAB

(rit-ux'i-mab)

Rituxan

Classifications: ANTINEOPLASTIC AGENT; IMMUNOMODULATOR

Prototype: Basiliximab

Pregnancy Category: C

AVAILABILITY 10 mg/mL injection

ACTIONS Genetically engineered monoclonal antibody that binds with the CD20 antigen on the surface of normal and malignant B lymphocytes.

THERAPEUTIC EFFECTS Administration of drug results in a rapid and sustained depletion of circulating and tissue-based (e.g., thymus, spleen) B lymphocytes in non-Hodgkin's lymphoma.

USES Relapsed or refractory CD20 positive, B-cell non-Hodgkin's lymphoma.

CONTRAINDICATIONS Hypersensitivity to murine proteins, rituximab, or abciximab; angina, cardiac arrhythmias, cardiac disease; pulmonary disease, chronic lymphocytic leukemia (CLL), lymphoma, severe hypotension; oliguria, rising serum creatinine; viral hepatitis B (HBV), vaccination; pregnancy (category C), lactation, children.

CAUTIOUS USE Prior exposure to murine-based monoclonal antibodies; history of allergies; asthma and other pulmonary disease (increased risk of bronchospasm); respiratory insufficiency; CAD; thrombocytopenia; history of cardiac arrhythmias; hypertension, renal impairment. Safety and efficacy in children are not established.

ROUTE & DOSAGE

Non-Hodgkin's Lymphoma

Adult: **IV** 375 mg/m^2 infused at 50 mg/h, may increase infusion rate q30min (max: 400 mg/h if tolerated), repeat dose on days 8, 15, and 22 (total of 4 doses)

ADMINISTRATION

Intravenous

PREPARE: **IV Infusion:** Dilute ordered dose to 1–4 mg/mL by adding to an infusion bag of NS or D5W. Examples: 500 mg in 400 mL yields 1 mg/mL; 500 mg in 75 mL yields 4 mg/mL. Gently invert bag to mix. Discard unused portion left in vial.

ADMINISTER: **IV Infusion:** Infuse first dose at a rate of 50 mg/h; may increase rate at 50 mg/h increments q30min to maximum rate of 400 mg/h. For subsequent doses, infuse at a rate of 100 mg/h and increase by 100 mg/h increments q30min up to maximum rate of 400 mg/h.

- Slow or stop infusion if S&S of hypersensitivity appear (see Appendix F).

- Store unopened vials at 2°–8° C (36°–46° F) and protect from light.

ADVERSE EFFECTS (≥1%) **Body as a Whole:** Angioedema, *fatigue,* asthenia, night sweats, *fever, chills,* myalgia. **CNS:** Headache, dizziness, depression. **CV:** Hypotension, tachycardia, peripheral edema. **GI:** *Nausea,* vomiting, throat irritation, anorexia, abdominal pain, hepatitis B reactivation with <u>fulminant hepatitis, hepatic failure, and death</u>. **Hematologic:** <u>Leukopenia, thrombocytopenia, anemia, neutropenia</u>. **Respiratory:** Bronchospasm, dyspnea, rhinitis. **Skin:** Pruritus, rash urticaria. **Other:** Infusion-related reactions: *Fever, chills, rigors, pruritus, urticaria, pain, flushing,* chest pain, hypotension, hypertension, dyspnea; <u>fatal infusion-related reactions</u> have been reported.

INTERACTIONS Drug: ANTIHYPERTENSIVE AGENTS should be stopped 12 h prior to rituximab to avoid excessive hypotension; **cisplatin** may cause additive nephrotoxicity.

PHARMACOKINETICS Duration: 6–12 mo. **Half-Life:** 60–174 h (increases with multiple infusions).

NURSING IMPLICATIONS

Assessment & Drug Effects

- Lab tests: CBC with differential, peripheral CD20+ B lymphocytes.
- Monitor carefully BP and ECG status during infusion and immediately report S&S of hypersensitivity (e.g., fever, chills, urticaria, pruritus, hypotension, bronchospasms; see Appendix F for others).

Patient & Family Education

- Do not take antihypertensive medication within 12 h of rituximab infusions.
- Note: Use effective contraception during and for up to 12 mo following rituximab therapy.
- Report any of the following experienced during infusion: itching, difficulty breathing, tightness in throat, dizziness, headache, nausea.
- Do not breast feed while taking this drug.

R

RIVASTIGMINE TARTRATE

(ri-vas′tig-meen)

Exelon

Classifications: AUTONOMIC NERVOUS SYSTEM AGENT; CHOLINERGIC (PARASYMPATHOMIMETIC); CHOLINESTERASE INHIBITOR

Prototype: Neostigmine Bromide

Pregnancy Category: B

AVAILABILITY 2 mg/mL solution

ACTIONS Inhibits acetylcholinesterase G_1 form of this enzyme.

THERAPEUTIC EFFECTS The G_1 form of acetylcholinesterase is found in higher levels in the brains of patients with Alzheimer's disease. Rivastigmine inhibits acetylcholinesterase more specifically in the brain (hippocampus and cortex) than the heart or skeletal muscle.

USES Treatment of mild to moderate dementia of the Alzheimer's type.

CONTRAINDICATIONS Hypersensitivity to rivastigmine or carbamate derivatives; lactation.
CAUTIOUS USE History of toxicity to cholinesterase inhibitors (e.g. tacrine); diabetes mellitus, cardiovascular/pulmonary disease; GI disorders including intestinal obstruction/peptic ulcer disease; concurrent use of other cholinergic agents, or anticholinergic agents; urogenital tract obstruction; Parkinson disease; pregnancy (category B); hepatic or renal insufficiency; concurrent use of NSAIDs.

ROUTE & DOSAGE

Alzheimer's Dementia

Adult/Geriatric: **PO** Start with 1.5 mg b.i.d with food, may increase by 1.5 mg b.i.d. q 2 wks if tolerated, target dose 3–6 mg b.i.d. (max: 12 mg b.i.d.) [if discontinued for a few doses, restart at ≤ last dose, if treatment is interrupted for several days, reinitiate with 1.5 mg b.i.d. and titrate q2wk as above]

ADMINISTRATION

Oral
- Give both capsules and liquid with food.
- Give liquid form undiluted or mixed with water, juice, or soda (do not mix with other liquids). Stir completely to dissolve. Ensure that entire mixture is swallowed.
- Discontinue drug for several days if significant anorexia, nausea, or vomiting occur. When adverse effects subside, restart at same or lower dose level (see ROUTE & DOSAGE).
- Store capsules and oral solution below 25° C (77° F). Ensure that bottle of liquid is in an UPRIGHT position.

ADVERSE EFFECTS (≥1%) **Body as a Whole:** Asthenia, increased sweating, syncope, fatigue, malaise, flu-like syndrome. **CV:** Hypertension. **GI:** *Nausea, vomiting, anorexia*, dyspepsia, *diarrhea, abdominal pain*, constipation, flatulence, eructation. **Metabolic:** Weight loss. **CNS:** *Dizziness, headache*, somnolence, tremor, insomnia, confusion, depression, anxiety, hallucination, aggressive reaction. **Respiratory:** Rhinitis.

INTERACTIONS Drug: May exaggerate muscle relations with **succinylcholine** and other NEUROMUSCULAR BLOCKING AGENTS, may attenuate effects of ANTICHOLINERGIC AGENTS.

PHARMACOKINETICS Absorption: Well absorbed, 40% reaches systemic circulation. **Peak:** 1 h. **Duration:** 10 h. **Distribution:** Crosses blood-brain barrier with CSF peak concentrations in 1.4–2.6 h, 40% protein bound. **Metabolism:** Metabolized by cholinesterase-mediated hydrolysis. **Elimination:** Excreted in urine. **Half-Life:** 1.5 h.

NURSING IMPLICATIONS

Assessment & Drug Effects
- Monitor cognitive function and ability to perform ADLs.

- Monitor for and report S&S of GI distress: Anorexia, weight loss, nausea and vomiting.
- Lab tests: Periodic ECG, serum electrolytes, Hgb & Hct, urinalysis, blood glucose HbA_{1C}, especially with long-term therapy.
- Monitor ambulation as dizziness is a common adverse effect.
- Monitor diabetics for loss of glycemic control.

Patient & Family Education

- Review instruction sheet provided with liquid form of the drug.
- Monitor weight at least weekly.
- Report any of the following to the physician: Loss of appetite, weight loss, significant nausea and/or vomiting.
- Supervise activity since there is a high potential for dizziness.
- Do not breast feed while taking this drug.

RIZATRIPTAN BENZOATE

(ri-za-trip'tan ben'zo-ate)

Maxalt, Maxalt-MLT

Classifications: AUTONOMIC NERVOUS SYSTEM AGENT; ADRENERGIC ANTAGONIST (SYMPATHOLYTIC); SEROTONIN $5\text{-}HT_{1B/1D}$ RECEPTOR AGONIST

Prototype: Sumatriptan

Pregnancy Category: C

AVAILABILITY 5 mg, 10 mg tablets; 5 mg, 10 mg disintegrating tablets

ACTIONS Selective ($5HT_{1B/1D}$) receptor agonist. The agonist effects at $5HT_{1B/1D}$ reverse the vasodilation of cranial blood vessels associated with a migraine.

THERAPEUTIC EFFECTS Activation of the $5HT_{1B/1D}$ receptors reduces the pain pathways associated with the migraine headache as well as reversing vasodilation of cranial blood vessels.

USES Acute migraine headaches with or without aura.

CONTRAINDICATIONS Hypersensitivity to rizatriptan; CAD; Prinzmetal's angina (potential for vasospasm); risk factors for CAD such as hypertension, hypercholesterolemia, obesity, diabetes, smoking, and strong family history; concurrent administration with ergotamine drugs or sumatriptan; concurrent administration with MAOIS; basilar or hemiplegic migraine.

CAUTIOUS USE Hypersensitivity to sumatriptan; renal or hepatic impairment; pregnancy (category C), lactation; hypertension; asthmatic patients. Safety and effectiveness in patients <18 y are not established.

ROUTE & DOSAGE

Acute Migraine

Adult: **PO** 5–10 mg, may repeat in 2 h if necessary (max: 30 mg/24 h); 5 mg with concurrent propranolol (max: 15 mg/24 h)

ADMINISTRATION

Oral

- Give any time after symptoms of migraine appear. If symptoms return, a second tablet may be given but no sooner than 2 h after the first.
- Do not exceed 30 mg (three doses) in any 24 h period.
- Do not give within 24 h of an ergot-containing drug or another $5\text{-}HT_1$ agonist.
- Store at 15°–30° C (59°–86° F) and protect from light and moisture.

ADVERSE EFFECTS (≥1%) **Body as a Whole:** Asthenia, fatigue, pain,

R

pressure sensation, paresthesias, throat pressure, warm/cold sensations. **CNS:** Somnolence, dizziness, headache, hypesthesia, decreased mental acuity, euphoria, tremor. **CV:** Coronary artery vasospasm, transient myocardial ischemia, MI, ventricular tachycardia, ventricular fibrillation, chest pain/tightness/heaviness, palpitations. **GI:** Dry mouth, nausea, vomiting, diarrhea. **Respiratory:** Dyspnea. **Skin:** Flushing. **Endocrine:** Hot flashes.

INTERACTIONS Drug: Propranolol may increase concentrations of rizatriptan, use smaller rizatriptan doses; **dihydroergotamine, methysergide,** other 5-HT1 AGONISTS may cause prolonged vasospastic reactions; SSRIS have rarely caused weakness, hyperreflexia, and incoordination; MAOIS should not be used with 5-HT1 agonists. **Herbal: Gingko, ginseng, echinacea, St. John's wort** may increase triptan toxicity.

PHARMACOKINETICS Absorption: 45% of oral dose reaches systemic circulation. **Peak:** 1–1.5 h for oral tabs; 1.6–2.5 h for orally disintegrating tablets. **Metabolism:** Metabolized via oxidative deamination by monoamine oxidase A. **Elimination:** Excreted primarily in urine (82%). **Half-Life:** 2–3 h.

R

NURSING IMPLICATIONS

Assessment & Drug Effects

- Monitor cardiovascular status carefully following first dose in patients at risk for CAD (e.g., postmenopausal women, men over 40 years old, persons with known CAD risk factors) or coronary artery vasospasms.
- ECG is recommended following first administration of rizatriptan to someone with known CAD risk factors.
- Report immediately to physician: chest pain or tightness in chest or throat that is severe or does not quickly resolve.
- Monitor periodically cardiovascular status with continued rizatriptan use.

Patient & Family Education

- Do not exceed 30 mg (three doses) in 24 h.
- Allow orally disintegrating tablets to dissolve on tongue; no liquid is needed.
- Contact physician immediately if any of the following develop following rizatriptan use: symptoms of angina (e.g., severe and/or persistent pain or tightness in chest or throat), hypersensitivity (e.g., wheezing, facial swelling, skin rash, or hives), abdominal pain.
- Report any other adverse effects (e.g., tingling, flushing, dizziness) at next physician visit.
- Do not breast feed while taking this drug without consulting physician.

ROPINIROLE HYDROCHLORIDE

(ro-pi'ni-role)

Requip

Classifications: AUTONOMIC NERVOUS SYSTEM AGENT; ANTICHOLINERGIC (PARASYMPATHOMIMETIC); ANTIPARKINSONISM AGENT

Prototype: Levodopa

Pregnancy Category: C

AVAILABILITY 0.25 gm, 0.5 mg, 1 mg, 2 mg, 5 mg tablets

ACTIONS Nonergot dopamine receptor agonist structurally similar to pramipexole, for treatment of Parkinson's disease. It has high affinity for the D_2 subfamily of dopamine receptors and higher binding affin-

ity to D_3 than to D_2 or D_4 receptor subtypes. The precise mechanism of action is not known.
THERAPEUTIC EFFECTS Indicated by improvement in Parkinson's disease.

USES Idiopathic Parkinson's disease.

CONTRAINDICATIONS Hypersensitivity to ropinirole or pramipexole; lactation, pregnancy (category C).
CAUTIOUS USE Renal and hepatic impairment; concomitant use of CNS depressants. Safety and efficacy in children are not established.

ROUTE & DOSAGE

Parkinson's Disease
Adult: **PO** Start with 0.25 mg t.i.d., may titrate up by 0.25 mg/dose t.i.d. qwk to a target dose of 1 mg t.i.d.; if response is still not satisfactory, may continue to increase by 1.5 mg/d q wk to a dose of 9 mg/d, and then by ≤3 mg/d weekly (max: dose of 24 mg/d)

ADMINISTRATION

Oral
- Give with food to reduce occurrence of nausea.
- Titrate dose as needed at weekly intervals (see ROUTE & DOSAGE).
- Discontinue drug gradually over 7 d by decreasing from t.i.d. to b.i.d. dosing for 4 d, and then to q.d. dosing for 3 d.
- Note: Lower initial and maintenance doses with moderate-to-severe renal impairment.
- Store at 15°–30° C (59°–86° F).

ADVERSE EFFECTS (≥1%) **Body as a Whole:** Increased sweating, dry mouth, flushing, asthenia, *fatigue,* pain, edema, malaise, *viral infection,* UTI, impotence. **CNS:** *Dizziness, somnolence, sudden sleep attacks*, hallucinations, confusion, amnesia, hypesthesia, yawning, hyperkinesia, impaired concentration, vertigo. **CV:** *Syncope,* chest pain, orthostatic symptoms, hypertension, palpitations, atrial fibrillation, extrasystoles, hypotension, tachycardia, peripheral edema, peripheral ischemia. **GI:** *Nausea, vomiting, dyspepsia,* abdominal pain, anorexia, flatulence. **Respiratory:** Pharyngitis, rhinitis, sinusitis, bronchitis, dyspnea. **Special Senses:** Abnormal vision, xerophthalmia, eye abnormality.

INTERACTIONS Drug: Ropinirole levels may be increased by ESTROGENS, QUINOLONE ANTIBIOTICS, **cimetidine, diltiazem, erythromycin, fluvoxamine, mexiletine, tacrine;** effects may be antagonized by PHENOTHIAZINES, BUTYROPHENONES, **metoclopramide.**

PHARMACOKINETICS Absorption: Rapidly absorbed from GI tract; 55% bioavailability. **Peak:** 1–2 h. **Distribution:** 30%–40% protein bound. **Metabolism:** Metabolized in the liver by CYP1A2. **Elimination:** Primarily excreted in urine. **Half-Life:** 6 h.

NURSING IMPLICATIONS

Assessment & Drug Effects
- Lab test: Periodically monitor BUN and creatinine, hepatic function.
- Schedule periodic eye exams and chest x-rays during long-term use.
- Monitor carefully for orthostatic hypotension, especially during dose escalation.

Patient & Family Education
- Be aware that hallucinations are a possible adverse effect and occur more often in older adults.

- Make position changes slowly, especially after long periods of lying or sitting. Postural hypotension is common, especially during early treatment.
- Exercise caution with hazardous activities requiring alertness since drowsiness and sedation are common adverse effects. Effects are additive with alcohol or other CNS depressants.
- Immediately notify physician if you become pregnant.
- Do not breast feed while taking this drug.

ROPIVACAINE HYDROCHLORIDE

(ro-piv'i-cane)

Naropin

Classifications: CENTRAL NERVOUS SYSTEM AGENT; LOCAL ANESTHETIC (ESTER-TYPE)

Prototype: Procaine HCl

Pregnancy Category: B

AVAILABILITY 2 mg/mL, 5 mg/mL, 7.5 mg/mL, 10 mg/mL injection

ACTIONS Blocks the generation and conduction of nerve impulses, probably by increasing the threshold for electrical excitability.

THERAPEUTIC EFFECTS Local anesthetic action produces loss of sensation and motor activity in areas of the body close to the injection site.

USES Local and regional anesthesia, postoperative pain management, anesthesia/pain management for obstetric procedures.

CONTRAINDICATIONS Hypersensitivity to ropivacaine or any local anesthetic of the amide type; generalized septicemia, inflammation or sepsis at the proposed injection site; cerebral spinal diseases (e.g., meningitis); heart block, hypotension, hypertension, GI hemorrhage.

CAUTIOUS USE Pregnancy (category B), lactation, debilitated, older adult, or acutely ill patients; arrhythmias, shock.

ROUTE & DOSAGE

Surgical Anesthesia

Adult: **Epidural** 25–200 mg (0.5–1% solution) **Nerve block** 5–250 mg (0.5%, 0.75% solution)

Labor Pain

Adult: **Epidural** 20–40 mg (0.2% solution)

Postoperative Pain Management

Adult: **Epidural** 12–20 mg/h (0.2% solution) **Infiltration** 2–200 mg (0.2–0.5% solution)

ADMINISTRATION

Intrathecal

- Avoid rapid injection of large volumes of ropivacaine. Incremental doses should always be used to achieve the smallest effective dose and concentration.
- Use an infusion concentration of 2 mg/mL (0.2%) for postoperative analgesia.
- Do not use disinfecting agents containing heavy metal ions (e.g., mercury, copper, zinc, etc.) on skin insertion site or to clean the ropivacaine container top.
- Discard continuous infusions solution after 24 h; it contains no preservatives.
- Store unopened at 20°–25° C (68°–77° F).

ADVERSE EFFECTS (≥1%) **Body as a Whole:** Pain, fever, rigors, hypoesthesia. **CNS:** Paresthesia, headache, dizziness, anxiety. **CV:** *Hypotension,* bradycardia, hypertension, tachycardia, chest pain, fetal bradycardia. **GI:** Nausea. **Skin:** Pruritus. **Urogenital:** Urinary retention, oliguria. **Hematologic:** Anemia.

INTERACTIONS Drug: Additive adverse effects with other LOCAL ANESTHETICS.

PHARMACOKINETICS Onset: 1–30 min (average 10–20 min) depending on dose/route of administration. **Duration:** 0.5–8 h depending on dose/route of administration. **Distribution:** 94% protein bound. **Metabolism:** Metabolized in the liver by CYP1A. **Elimination:** Excreted in urine. **Half-Life:** 1.8–4.2 h.

NURSING IMPLICATIONS

Assessment & Drug Effects

- Monitor carefully cardiovascular and respiratory status throughout treatment period. Assess for hypotension and bradycardia.
- Report immediately S&S of CNS stimulation or CNS depression.

Patient & Family Education

- Report any of the following to physician immediately: restlessness, anxiety, tinnitus, blurred vision, tremors.
- Do not breast feed without consulting physician.

ROSIGLITAZONE MALEATE (Pr)

(ros-i-glit′a-zone)

Avandia

Classifications: HORMONES AND SYNTHETIC SUBSTITUTES; ANTIDIABETIC; THIAZOLIDINEDIONES

Pregnancy Category: C

AVAILABILITY 2 mg, 4 mg, 8 mg tablets

ACTIONS Antidiabetic agent that lowers blood sugar levels by improving target cell response to insulin in Type 2 diabetics. It reduces cellular insulin resistance and decreases hepatic glucose output (gluconeogenesis).

THERAPEUTIC EFFECTS Reduces hyperglycemia and hyperlipidemia, thus improving hyperinsulinemia without stimulating pancreatic insulin secretion. Indicated by decreased HbA_{1C}.

USES Adjunct to diet in the treatment of Type 2 diabetes. May also be used in combination with metformin.

CONTRAINDICATIONS Hypersensitivity to rosiglitazone; pregnancy (category C), lactation; active hepatic disease or ALT >2.5 times normal.

CAUTIOUS USE As monotherapy in Type 1 diabetes mellitus or diabetic ketoacidosis; cardiovascular disease, particularly hypertensive patients with New York Heart Association Class III and IV cardiac status (e.g. CHF); hepatic impairment. Safety & efficacy in children <18 y are not established.

ROUTE & DOSAGE

Type 2 Diabetes Mellitus

Adult: **PO** start at 4 mg q.d. or 2 mg b.i.d., may increase after 12 wk (max: 8 mg/d in 1–2 divided doses)

ADMINISTRATION

Oral

- Do not initiate therapy if baseline serum ALT >2.5.
- Store at 15°–30° C (59°–86° F) in tight, light-resistant container.

ADVERSE EFFECTS (≥1%) **Body as a Whole:** Edema, anemia, headache, back pain, fatigue. **CV:** edema, fluid retention, exacerbation of heart failure. **GI:** Diarrhea. **Respiratory:** Upper respiratory tract infection, sinusitis. **Other:** Hyperglycemia.

INTERACTIONS Drug: Insulin may increase risk of heart failure or edema; enhance hypoglycemia with ORAL ANTIDIABETIC AGENTS, **ketoconazole. Herbal: Garlic, ginseng** may potentiate hypoglycemic effects.

PHARMACOKINETICS Absorption: 99% absorbed from GI tract. **Peak:** 1 h, food delays time to peak by 1.75 h. **Duration:** >24 h. **Distribution:** >99% protein bound. **Metabolism:** Extensively metabolized in liver by CYP2C8 to inactive metabolites. **Elimination:** 64% excreted in urine, 23% excreted in feces. **Half-Life:** 3–4 h. Moderate to severe liver disease increases serum concentrations and increases half-life by 2 h.

NURSING IMPLICATIONS

Assessment & Drug Effects

- Monitor for S&S of hypoglycemia (possible when insulin/sulfonylureas are coadministered).
- Monitor for S&S of CHF or exacerbation of symptoms with preexisting CHF.
- Lab tests: Liver function and serum ALT at baseline, then q2mo for first year; then periodically (more often when elevated); periodic HbA_{1C}, Hgb & Hct, and lipid profile.
- Withhold drug and notify physician if ALT >3 times normal or patient jaundiced.
- Monitor weight and notify physician of development of edema.

Patient & Family Education

- Have blood tested for liver function every 2 months for first year; then periodically.
- Be aware that resumed ovulation is possible in nonovulating premenopausal women.
- Use or add barrier contraceptive if using hormonal contraception.
- Report immediately to physician: S&S of liver dysfunction such as unexplained anorexia, nausea, vomiting, abdominal pain, fatigue, dark urine; or S&S of fluid retention such as weight gain, edema, or activity intolerance.
- Combination therapy: May need adjustment of other antidiabetic drugs to avoid hypoglycemia.
- Do not breast feed while taking this drug.

ROSUVASTATIN

(ro-su-va-sta'ten)

Crestor

Classifications: CARDIOVASCULAR AGENT; ANTILIPEMIC; HMG-CoA REDUCTASE INHIBITOR (STATIN)

Prototype: Lovastatin

Pregnancy Category: X

AVAILABILITY 5 mg, 10 mg, 20 mg, 40 mg tablets

ACTIONS Rosuvastatin is a potent inhibitor of HMG-CoA reductase, an enzyme that catalyzes the conversion of HMG-CoA to mevalonic acid, an early and rate-limiting step in cholesterol biosynthesis. Interference with this enzyme's activity reduces the quantity of mevalonic acid, a precursor of cholesterol.

THERAPEUTIC EFFECTS Reduces total cholesterol and LDL cholesterol, and also lowers plasma triglycerides and apolipoprotein B while increasing HDL.

USES Adjunct to diet for the reduction of LDL cholesterol and triglycerides in patients with primary hypercholesterolemia and mixed dyslipidemia.

CONTRAINDICATIONS Hypersensitivity to any component of the product, active liver disease, pregnancy (category X), women of child-bearing potential not using appropriate contraceptive measures, lactation.
CAUTIOUS USE Concomitant use of cyclosporine and gemfibrozil, excessive alcohol use or history of liver disease, renal impairment, advanced age, hypothyroidism.

ROUTE & DOSAGE

Hyperlipidemia
Adult: **PO** 10 mg once daily (5–40 mg/d), max dose 40 mg/d. If taking cyclosporine, start with 5 mg/d (max: 5 mg/d). If taking gemfibrozil, start with 5 mg/d (max: 10 mg/d)

Renal Impairment
Cl_{cr} <30 mL/min: 5 mg once daily (max: 10 mg/d)

ADMINISTRATION

Oral
- May give any time of day without regard to food.
- Store at or below 30° C (86° F).

ADVERSE EFFECTS (≥1%) **Body as a Whole:** Asthenia, back pain, flu syndrome, chest pain, infection, pain, peripheral edema. **CNS:** Headache, dizziness, insomnia, hypertonia, paresthesia, depression, anxiety, vertigo, neuralgia. **CV:** Hypertension, angina, vasodilatation, palpitations. **GI:** Diarrhea, dyspepsia, nausea, abdominal pain, constipation, gastroenteritis, vomiting, flatulence, gastritis. **Endocrine:** Diabetes. **Hematologic:** Anemia, ecchymosis. **Musculoskeletal:** Myalgia, arthritis, arthralgia. **Respiratory:** Pharyngitis, rhinitis, sinusitis, bronchitis, increased cough, dyspnea, pneumonia, asthma. **Skin:** Rash, pruritus. **Urogenital:** UTI.

INTERACTIONS Drug: Cyclosporine, gemfibrozil, niacin, may increase risk of rhabdomyolysis; ANTACIDS may decrease rosuvastatin absorption; may cause increase in INR with **warfarin.**

PHARMACOKINETICS Absorption: Well absorbed. **Peak:** 3–5 h. **Metabolism:** Limited metabolism in the liver (not CYP 3A4). **Elimination:** Eliminated primarily in feces (90%). **Half-Life:** 20 h.

NURSING IMPLICATIONS

Assessment & Drug Effects
- Monitor for and report promptly S&S of myopathy (e.g., skeletal muscle pain).
- Withhold drug and notify physician if CPK levels are markedly elevated (≥10×ULN) or if myopathy is diagnosed or suspected.
- Lab tests: CPK levels for S&S of myopathy; periodic LFTs; more frequent INR values with concomitant warfarin therapy.
- Monitor CV status, especially with a known history of hypertension or heart disease.
- Monitor diabetics for loss of glycemic control.

Patient & Family Education
- Do not take antacids within 2 h of taking this drug.
- Do not breast feed while taking this drug.
- Females should use reliable means of contraception while taking this drug to prevent pregnancy.

SALMETEROL XINAFOATE

(sal-me′ter-ol xin′a-fo-ate)

Serevent

Classifications: AUTONOMIC NERVOUS SYSTEM AGENT; BETA-ADRENERGIC AGONIST (SYMPATHOMIMETIC); BRONCHODILATOR; RESPIRATORY SMOOTH MUSCLE RELAXANT

Prototype: Albuterol

Pregnancy Category: C

AVAILABILITY 25 mcg aerosol; 50 mcg powder diskus for inhalation

ACTIONS Long-acting $beta_2$-adrenoreceptor agonist and an analog of albuterol. Stimulation of $beta_2$-adrenoreceptors relaxes bronchospasm and increases ciliary motility, thus facilitating expectoration. Inhibits the release of mediators (i.e., histamine) from mast cells, macrophages, and eosinophils.

THERAPEUTIC EFFECTS Relaxes bronchospasm and increases ciliary motility, thus facilitating expectoration of pulmonary secretions. Salmeterol also decreases airway reaction to allergens.

USES Maintenance therapy for asthma or bronchospasm. Prevention of exercise-induced bronchospasm. Do not use to treat acute bronchospasm.

CONTRAINDICATIONS Hypersensitivity to salmeterol; primary treatment of status asthmaticus; pregnancy (category C), lactation; safety and efficacy in children <4 y not established.

CAUTIOUS USE Cardiovascular disorders, cardiac arrhythmias, hypertension; history of seizures or thyrotoxicosis; liver and renal impairment, older adults, diabetes mellitus, sensitivity to other beta-adrenergic agonists; women in labor.

ROUTE & DOSAGE

Asthma or Bronchospasm

Adult/Child: ≥4 y **Inhalation** 2 inhalations of aerosol (42 mcg) or 1 powder diskus (50 mcg) b.i.d. approximately 12 h apart

Prevention of Exercise-Induced Bronchospasm

Adult/Child: ≥4 y **Inhaled** 2 inhalations of aerosol (42 mcg) or 1 powder diskus (50 mcg) 30–60 min before exercise

ADMINISTRATION

Inhalation

- Do not use to relieve symptoms of acute asthma.
- Shake canister well before using; close lips tightly around the mouthpiece, and patient inhales deeply during each actuation.
- Store at room temperature, 15°–30° C (59°–86° F).

ADVERSE EFFECTS (≥1%) **CNS:** Dizziness, headache, tremor. **CV:** Palpitations, sinus tachycardia. **Respiratory:** Respiratory arrest (rare). **Skin:** Rash. **Body as a Whole:** Tolerance (tachyphylaxis).

INTERACTIONS Drug: Effects antagonized by BETA BLOCKERS.

PHARMACOKINETICS Onset: 10–20 min. **Peak:** Effect 2 h. **Duration:** Up to 12 h. **Distribution:** 94%–95% protein bound. **Metabolism:** Dissociates in solution; salmeterol base and xinafoate salt are metabolized, absorbed, distributed, and excreted independently; salmeterol is extensively metabolized by hydroxylation. **Elimination:** Eliminated primarily in feces. **Half-Life:** 3–4 h.

NURSING IMPLICATIONS

Assessment & Drug Effects

- Withhold drug and notify physician immediately if bronchospasms occur following its use.
- Monitor cardiovascular status; report tachycardia.
- Monitor liver enzymes periodically with long-term therapy.

Patient & Family Education

- Notify physician immediately of worsening asthma or failure to respond to the usual dose of salmeterol.
- Do not use an additional dose prior to exercise if taking twice-daily doses of salmeterol.
- Take the preexercise dose 30–60 min before exercise and wait 12 h before an additional dose.
- Do not breast feed while taking this drug.

SALSALATE

(sal′sal-ate)

Artha-G, Disalcid, Mono-Gesic, Salflex, Salsitab

Classifications: CENTRAL NERVOUS SYSTEM AGENT; ANALGESIC; SALICYLATE; ANTIPYRETIC

Prototype: Aspirin

Pregnancy Category: C

AVAILABILITY 500 mg capsules; 500 mg, 750 mg tablets

ACTIONS Action similar to those of other salicylates. Clinical studies suggest that salsalate does not produce significant gastric irritation, and it has not been associated with reactions causing asthmatic attacks in susceptible individuals. Unlike aspirin, it does not appear to inhibit platelet aggregation. Salsalate lowers body temperature by causing vasodilation of peripheral vessels. Its antiinflammatory and analgesic activity may be mediated through inhibition of the prostaglandin synthetase enzyme complex.

THERAPEUTIC EFFECTS Analgesic, antipyretic, antiinflammatory and antirheumatic effects.

USES Symptomatic treatment, rheumatoid arthritis, osteoarthritis, and related rheumatic disorders.

CONTRAINDICATIONS Hypersensitivity to salicylates or NSAIDS, especially patients with history of asthma, nasal polyposis, or chronic urticaria; chronic renal insufficiency; peptic ulcer; children <12 y; hemophilia; chicken pox, influenza, tinnitus.

CAUTIOUS USE Liver function impairment; pregnancy (category C), lactation.

ROUTE & DOSAGE

Arthritis

Adult: **PO** 325–3000 mg/d in divided doses (max: 4 g/d)

ADMINISTRATION

Oral

- Give with a full glass of water or food or milk to reduce GI adverse effects.

ADVERSE EFFECTS (≥1%) **GI:** Nausea, dyspepsia, heartburn, vomiting, diarrhea. **Special Senses:** Tinnitus, hearing loss (reversible). **Body as a Whole:** Vertigo, flushing, headache, confusion, hyperventilation, sweating. **CNS:** Drowsiness.

INTERACTIONS Drug: Aminosalicylic acid increases risk of salicylate toxicity. **Ammonium chloride** and other ACIDIFYING AGENTS decrease renal elimination and increase risk of salicylate toxicity. ANTICOAGULANTS increase risk of bleeding. ORAL HYPOGLYCEMIC AGENTS increase hypoglycemic activity with salsalate doses >2 g/d. CARBONIC ANHYDRASE INHIBITORS enhance salicylate toxicity. CORTICOSTEROIDS add to ulcerogenic effects. **Methotrexate** toxicity is increased. Low doses of salicylates may antagonize uricosuric effects of **probenecid** and **sulfinpyrazone. Herbal: Feverfew, garlic, ginger, ginkgo** may increase bleeding potential.

PHARMACOKINETICS Absorption: Readily absorbed from small intestine. **Peak:** 1.5–4 h. **Metabolism:** Hydrolyzed in liver, GI mucosa, plasma, whole blood, and other tissues. **Elimination:** Excreted in urine. **Half-Life:** 1 h.

NURSING IMPLICATIONS

Assessment & Drug Effects

- Symptom relief is gradual (may require 3–4 d to establish steady-state salicylate level).
- Monitor for adverse GI effects, especially in patient with a history of peptic ulcer disease.

Patient & Family Education

- Do not to take another salicylate (e.g., aspirin) while on salsalate therapy.
- Monitor blood glucose for loss of glycemic control in diabetes; drug may induce hypoglycemia when used with sulfonylureas.
- Report tinnitus, hearing loss, vertigo, rash, or nausea.
- Do not breast feed while taking this drug without consulting physician.

S

SAQUINAVIR MESYLATE Pr

(sa-quin'a-vir mes'y-late)

Fortovase, Invirase

Classifications: ANTIRETROVIRAL AGENT; PROTEASE INHIBITOR

Pregnancy Category: B

AVAILABILITY Invirase 200 mg capsules; **Fortovase** 200 mg soft gel capsules

ACTIONS Synthetic peptide that inhibits the activity of HIV protease and prevents the cleavage of viral polyproteins essential for the maturation of HIV.

THERAPEUTIC EFFECTS Indicated by reduced viral load (decreased number of RNA copies), and increased number of T helper CD4 cells.

USES Advanced HIV infection, usually in combination with zidovudine or zalcitabine.

CONTRAINDICATIONS Significant hypersensitivity to saquinavir; concurrent administration with lovastatin, simvastatin, antimicrobial resistance to other protease inhibitors, monotherapy, lactation.

CAUTIOUS USE Hepatic insufficiency; hepatitis B or C; diabetes mellitus, diabetic ketoacidosis, hemophilia A or B, pregnancy (category B). Safety and effectiveness in HIV-infected children <16 y are not established.

ROUTE & DOSAGE

Note: Invirase and Fortovase are NOT bioequivalent and CANNOT be interchanged.

HIV

Adult: **PO** Invirase 600 mg (3 × 200 mg) t.i.d. taken 2 h after a full meal; Fortovase 1200 mg (6 × 200 mg) t.i.d. with meals; or 1000 mg b.i.d. with ritonavir 100 mg b.i.d.

ADMINISTRATION

Oral

- Give with or up to 2 h after a full meal to ensure adequate absorption and bioavailability.

- Do not administer to anyone taking rifampin or rifabutin because these drugs significantly decrease the plasma level of saquinavir.
- Store Invirase at 15°–30° C (59°–86° F) in tightly closed bottle. Store Fortovase in refrigerator. Capsules are stable for 3 mo at room temperature ≤25° C (≤77° F).

ADVERSE EFFECTS (≥1%) **CNS:** Headache, paresthesia, numbness, dizziness, peripheral neuropathy, ataxia, confusion, convulsions, hyperreflexia, hyporeflexia, tremor, agitation, amnesia, anxiety, depression, excessive dreaming, hallucinations, euphoria, irritability, lethargy, somnolence. **CV:** Chest pain, hypertension, hypotension, syncope. **Endocrine:** Dehydration, hyperglycemia, diabetes, weight changes. **Hematologic:** Anemia, splenomegaly, thrombocytopenia, pancytopenia. **GI:** *Nausea, diarrhea, abdominal discomfort,* dyspepsia, mucosal damage, change in appetite, dry mouth. **Skin:** Rash, pruritus, acne, erythema, seborrhea, hair changes, photosensitivity, skin ulceration, dry skin. **Body as a Whole:** Myalgia, allergic reaction. **Respiratory:** Bronchitis, cough, dyspnea, epistaxis, hemoptysis, laryngitis, rhinitis. **Special Senses:** Xerophthalmia, ear ache, taste alterations, tinnitus, visual disturbances.

INTERACTIONS Drug: Rifampin, rifabutin significantly decrease **saquinavir** levels. **Phenobarbital, phenytoin, dexamethasone, carbamazepine** may also reduce **saquinavir** levels. **Saquinavir** levels may be increased by **delavirdine, ketoconazole, ritonavir, clarithromycin, indinavir.** May increase serum levels of **cisapride, triazolam, midazolam,** ERGOT DERIVATIVES, **nelfinavir, sildenafil.** May significantly increase **simvastatin** levels and toxicity; may increase risk of **ergotamine** toxicity of **dihydroergotamine, ergotamine. Herbal: St. John's wort** may decrease antiretroviral activity.

PHARMACOKINETICS Absorption: Rapidly absorbed from GI tract; only 4% reaches systemic circulation; food significantly reduces absorption. **Distribution:** 98% protein bound. **Metabolism:** Metabolized in liver by cytochrome P450. **Elimination:** Excreted primarily in feces (>70%).

NURSING IMPLICATIONS

Assessment & Drug Effects

- Lab tests: Monitor serum electrolytes, CBC with differential, liver function, blood glucose and HbA_{1C}, CPK, and serum amylase prior to initiating therapy and periodically thereafter.
- Monitor for and report S&S of peripheral neuropathy.
- Assess for buccal mucosa ulceration or other distressing GI S&S.
- Monitor weight periodically.
- Monitor for toxicity if any of the following drugs is used concomitantly: calcium channel blockers, clindamycin, dapsone, quinidine, triazolam, or simvastatin.

Patient & Family Education

- Take drug within 2 h of a full meal.
- Be aware of all drugs which should not be taken concurrently with saquinavir.
- Be aware that saquinavir is not a cure for HIV infection and that its long-term effects are unknown.
- Report any distressing adverse effects to physician.
- Do not breast feed while taking this drug.

SARGRAMOSTIM (GM-CSF)

(sar-gra′mos-tim)

Leukine, Leukine Liquid, Prokine

Classifications: BLOOD FORMERS, COAGULATORS AND ANTICOAGULANTS; HEMATOPOIETIC GROWTH FACTOR

Prototype: Epoetin alfa

Pregnancy Category: C

AVAILABILITY 250 mcg, 500 mcg injection

ACTIONS Recombinant human granulocyte macrophage colony stimulating factor (GM-CSF) produced by recombinant DNA technology in a yeast. GM-CSF is a hematopoietic growth factor that stimulates proliferation and differentiation of hematopoietic progenitor cells in the granulocyte-macrophage pathways.

THERAPEUTIC EFFECTS Increases the cytotoxicity of monocytes to certain neoplastic cell lines and activates polymorphonuclear neutrophils (PMNs) to inhibit the growth of tumor cells.

USES Myeloid reconstitution after autologous bone marrow transplantation for patients with non-Hodgkin's lymphoma (NHL), acute lymphoblastic leukemia (ALL), and Hodgkin's disease; mobilization of peripheral blood stem cells (PBSCs) for autologous transplantation.

UNLABELED USES To increase WBC counts in AIDS patients; to decrease leukopenia secondary to myelosuppressive chemotherapy; to correct neutropenia in aplastic anemia and in liver and kidney transplantations.

CONTRAINDICATIONS Excessive leukemic myeloid blasts in bone marrow or blood; known hypersensitivity to GM-CSF or yeast products.

CAUTIOUS USE History of cardiac arrhythmias, preexisting cardiac disease, hypoxia, CHF, pulmonary infiltrates; kidney and liver dysfunction; pregnancy (category C), lactation. Safety and efficacy in children are not established; however, adverse side effects have been comparable to those in adults.

ROUTE & DOSAGE

Autologous Bone Marrow Transplant

Adult: **IV** 250 mcg/m²/d infused over 2 h for 21 d, begin 2–4 h after bone marrow transfusion and not less than 24 h after last dose of chemotherapy or 12 h after last radiation therapy

Child: **IV/SC** 250 mcg/m²/d times 21 d, begin 2–4 h after bone marrow infusion or not less than 24 h after chemotherapy

Neutropenia

Adult/Child: **SC** 3–15 mcg/kg/d

ADMINISTRATION

Note: Do not give within 24 h preceding or following chemotherapy or within 12 h preceding or following radiotherapy.

Subcutaneous

- Reconstitute each 250 or 500 mcg vial with 1 mL of sterile water for injection (without preservative). Direct sterile water against side of vial and swirl gently. Avoid excessive or vigorous agitation. Do not shake. Use without further dilution for SC injection.

Intravenous

Note: Verify correct IV concentration and rate of infusion administration in infants and children with physician.

PREPARE: **IV Infusion:** Reconstitute as for SC, then further dilute reconstituted solution with NS. If the final concentration is <1 mcg/mL, add albumin (human) to NS before addition of sargramostim. Use 1 mg albumin per 1 mL of NS to give a final concentration of 0.1% albumin. Administer as soon as possible and within 6 h of reconstitution or dilution for IV infusion. Discard after 6 h. Sargramostim vials are single-dose vials, do not reenter or reuse. Discard unused portion.

ADMINISTER: **IV Infusion:** Give over 2 h. Do not use an in-line membrane filter.

INCOMPATIBILITIES **Solution/additive: Hydrocortisone, hydroxyzine, haloperidol. Y-site: Acyclovir, amphotericin B, ampicillin, ampicillin/sulbactam, amsacrine, cefonicid, cefoperazone, chlorpromazine, ganciclovir, haloperidol, hydrocortisone, hydromorphone, hydroxyzine, idarubicin, imipenem/cilastatin, lorazepam, methylprednisolone, mitomycin, morphine, nalbuphine, ondansetron, piperacillin, sodium bicarbonate, tobramycin.**

- Interrupt administration and reduce the dose by 50% if absolute neutrophil count exceeds 20,000/mm^3 or if platelet count exceeds 500,000/mm^3. Notify physician.
- Reduce the IV rate 50% if patient experiences dyspnea during administration. Discontinue infusion if respiratory symptoms worsen. Notify physician.

- Refrigerate the sterile powder, the reconstituted solution, and store diluted solution at 2°–8° C (36°–46° F). Do not freeze or shake.

ADVERSE EFFECTS (≥1%) **CNS:** Lethargy, malaise, headache, fatigue. **CV:** Abnormal ST segment depression, supraventricular arrhythmias, edema, *hypotension, tachycardia,* pericardial effusion, pericarditis. **Hematologic:** Anemia, *thrombocytopenia.* **GI:** Nausea, vomiting, diarrhea, anorexia. **Body as a Whole:** *Bone pain, myalgia, arthralgias,* weight gain, hyperuricemia, *fever.* **Respiratory:** Pleural effusion. **Skin:** *Rash, pruritus.* **Other:** *First-dose reaction* (some or all of the following symptoms: hypotension, tachycardia, fever, rigors, flushing, nausea, vomiting, diaphoresis, back pain, leg spasms, and dyspnea).

INTERACTIONS Drug: CORTICOSTEROIDS should be used cautiously with sargramostim because the myeloproliferative effects may be potentiated. **Lithium** should be used with caution with sargramostim because it may potentiate the myeloproliferative effects.

PHARMACOKINETICS Absorption: Readily absorbed from SC site. **Onset:** 3–6 h. **Peak:** 1–2 h. **Duration:** 5–10 d SC. **Elimination:** Probably excreted in urine. **Half-Life:** 80–150 min.

NURSING IMPLICATIONS

Assessment & Drug Effects

- Lab tests: Obtain a CBC and platelet count prior to initiation of therapy. Monitor biweekly CBC with differential during therapy. Monitor kidney and liver function biweekly in patients with kidney or liver dysfunction prior to the initiation of therapy.
- Discontinue treatment if WBC 50,000/mm^3. Notify the physician.
- Occasional transient supraventricular arrhythmias have occurred during administration, particularly in those with a history of cardiac arrhythmias. Arrhythmias are reversed with discontinuation of drug.

S

- Give special attention to respiratory symptoms (dyspnea) during and immediately following infusion, especially in patients with preexisting pulmonary disease.
- Use drug with caution in patients with preexisting fluid retention, pulmonary infiltrates, or CHF. Peripheral edema, pleural or pericardial effusion has occurred after administration. It is reversible with dose reduction.
- Notify physician of any severe adverse reaction immediately.
- Discontinue therapy and notify physician if disease progression is detected. Potentially, drug can act as a growth factor for myeloid malignancies.

Patient & Family Education

- Notify nurse or physician immediately of any adverse effect (e.g., dyspnea, palpitations, peripheral edema, bone or muscle pain) during or after drug administration.
- Do not breast feed while taking this drug without consulting physician.

SCOPOLAMINE

(skoe-pol'a-meen)

Transderm-Scop, Transderm-V ✦

SCOPOLAMINE HYDROBROMIDE

Hyoscine, Isopto-Hyoscine, Murocoll, Triptone

Classifications: AUTONOMIC NERVOUS SYSTEM AGENT; ANTICHOLINERGIC (PARASYMPATHOLYTIC); ANTIMUSCARINIC; ANTISPASMODIC

Prototype: Atropine

Pregnancy Category: C

AVAILABILITY **Scopolamine** 0.4 mg tablets 1.5 mg transdermal patch **Scopolamine HBr** 0.4 mg tablets 0.3 mg/mL, 0.4 mg/mL, 0.86 mg/mL, 1 mg/mL injection 0.25% ophthalmic solution

ACTIONS Alkaloid of belladonna with peripheral actions resembling those of atropine. In contrast to atropine, produces CNS depression with marked sedative and tranquilizing effects, and is less effective in preventing reflex bradycardia during anesthesia. More potent in mydriatic and cycloplegic actions and in inhibiting secretions of salivary, bronchial, and sweat glands, but has less prominent effect on heart, intestines, and bronchial muscles.

THERAPEUTIC EFFECTS More potent than atropine in mydriatic and cycloplegic actions. Produces CNS depression with marked sedative and tranquilizing effects for use in anesthesia. Used as a preanesthetic agent to control bronchial, nasal, pharyngeal and salivary secretions.

USES In obstetrics with morphine to produce amnesia and sedation ("twilight sleep") and as preanesthetic medication. To control spasticity (and drooling) in postencephalitic parkinsonism, paralysis agitans, and other spastic states, as prophylactic agent for motion sickness and as mydriatic and cycloplegic in ophthalmology. Therapeutic system (Transderm-Scop) is used to prevent nausea and vomiting associated with motion sickness.

CONTRAINDICATIONS Asthma; hepatitis; toxemia of pregnancy; hypersensitivity to anticholinergic drugs; hypersensitive to belladonna or barbiturates; narrow angle glaucoma; GI or urogenital obstructive diseases; myasthenia gravis; pregnancy (category C), lactation.

CAUTIOUS USE Coronary heart disease, CHF, cardiac arrhythmias, tachycardia, hypertension; patients over 40 y, pyloric obstruction, urinary bladder neck obstruction, angle-closure glaucoma, thyrotoxicosis, liver disease; paralytic ileus; hiatal hernia, ulcerative colitis, gastric ulcer; older adults, parkinsonism; COPD, asthma or allergies; hyperthyroidism; brain damage, spastic paralysis; tartrazine or sulfite sensitivity.

ROUTE & DOSAGE

Preanesthetic

Adult: **PO** 0.5–1 mg **IM/SC/IV** 0.3–0.6 mg
Child: **PO/IM/SC/IV** 0.006 mg/kg

Motion Sickness

Adult: **PO** 0.25–0.6 mg 1 h before anticipated travel **Topical** 1 patch q72h starting 12 h before anticipated travel
Child: **PO** 0.006 mg/kg 1 h before anticipated travel

Refraction

Adult: **Ophthalmic** 1–2 drops in eye 1 h before refraction

Uveitis

Adult: **Ophthalmic** 1–2 drops in eye up to q.i.d.

ADMINISTRATION

Instillation

- Minimize possibility of systemic absorption by applying pressure against lacrimal sac during and for 1 or 2 min following instillation of eye drops.

Transdermal

- Apply transdermal disc system (Transderm-Scop, a Controlled-Release System) to dry surface behind the ear.
- Replace with another disc on another site behind the ear if disc system becomes dislodged.

Subcutaneous or Intramuscular

- Give undiluted.

Intravenous

PREPARE: **Direct:** Dilute required dose in 10 mL of sterile water for injection.

ADMINISTER: **Direct:** Give a single dose over 1 min.

- Preserve in tight, light-resistant containers.

ADVERSE EFFECTS (≥1%) **Body as a Whole:** Fatigue, dizziness, *drowsiness,* disorientation, restlessness, hallucinations, toxic psychosis. **GI:** *Dry mouth and throat, constipation.* **Urogenital:** Urinary retention. **CV:** Decreased heart rate. **Special Senses:** Dilated pupils, photophobia, blurred vision, *local irritation,* follicular conjunctivitis. **Respiratory:** <u>Depressed respiration</u>. **Skin:** Local irritation from patch adhesive, rash.

INTERACTIONS Drug: Amantadine, ANTIHISTAMINES, TRICYCLIC ANTIDEPRESSANTS, **quinidine, disopyramide, procainamide** add to anticholinergic effects; decreases **levodopa** effects; **methotrimeprazine** may precipitate extrapyramidal effects; decreases antipsychotic effects (decreased absorption) of PHENOTHIAZINES.

PHARMACOKINETICS Absorption: Readily absorbed from GI tract and percutaneously. **Peak:** 20–60 min. **Duration:** 5–7 d. **Distribution:** Crosses placenta; distributed to CNS. **Metabolism:** Metabolized in liver. **Elimination:** Excreted in urine.

NURSING IMPLICATIONS

Assessment & Drug Effects

- Observe patient closely; some patients manifest excitement, delirium, and disorientation shortly after drug is administered until sedative effect takes hold.

S

- Use of side rails is advisable, particularly for older adults, because of amnesic effect of scopolamine.
- In the presence of pain, scopolamine may cause delirium, restlessness, and excitement unless given with an analgesic.
- Be aware that tolerance may develop with prolonged use.
- Terminate ophthalmic use if local irritation, edema, or conjunctivitis occur.

Patient & Family Education

- Vision may blur when used as mydriatic or cycloplegic; do not drive or engage in potentially hazardous activities until vision clears.
- Place disc on skin site the night before an expected trip or anticipated motion for best therapeutic effect.
- Wash hands carefully after handling scopolamine. Anisocoria (unequal size of pupils, blurred vision can develop by rubbing eye with drug-contaminated finger).

SECOBARBITAL SODIUM (Pr)

(see-koe-bar'bi-tal)

Seconal Sodium

Classifications: CENTRAL NERVOUS SYSTEM AGENT; SEDATIVE-HYPNOTIC; BARBITURATE; ANXIOLYTIC

Pregnancy Category: D

Controlled Substance: Schedule II

AVAILABILITY 100 mg capsules

ACTIONS Short-acting barbiturate with CNS depressant effects as well as mood alteration from excitation to mild sedation, hypnosis, and deep coma. Depresses the sensory cortex, decreases motor activity, alters cerebellar function and produces drowsiness, sedation and hypnosis.

THERAPEUTIC EFFECTS Alters cerebellar function and produces drowsiness, sedation and hypnosis.

USES Hypnotic for simple insomnia and preoperatively to provide basal hypnosis for general, spinal, or regional anesthesia.

CONTRAINDICATIONS History of sensitivity to barbiturates; porphyria; severe liver function; severe respiratory disease; nephritic syndrome; pregnancy (category D), parturition, fetal immaturity; uncontrolled pain. Use of sterile injection containing polyethylene glycol vehicle in patients with renal insufficiency.

CAUTIOUS USE Pregnant women with toxemia or history of bleeding; labor and delivery, lactation; liver or kidney function impairment, older adult, debilitated individuals; children.

ROUTE & DOSAGE

Sedative

Adult: **PO** 100–300 mg/d in 3 divided doses
Child: **PO** 4–6 mg/kg/d in 3 divided doses

Preoperative Sedative

Adult: **PO** 100–300 mg 1–2 h before surgery
Child: **PO** 50–100 mg 1–2 h before surgery

Hypnotic

Adult: **PO** 100–200 mg

ADMINISTRATION

Oral

- Give hypnotic dose only after patient retires for the evening.
- Crush and mix with a fluid or with food if patient cannot swallow pill.

ADVERSE EFFECTS (≥1%) **CNS:** Drowsiness, lethargy, hangover, paradoxical excitement in the older adult patient. **Respiratory:** Respiratory depression, laryngospasm.

INTERACTIONS Drug: Phenmetrazine antagonizes effects of secobarbital; CNS DEPRESSANTS, **alcohol,** SEDATIVES compound CNS depression; MAO INHIBITORS cause excessive CNS depression; **methoxyflurane** increases risk of nephrotoxicity. **Herbal: Kava-kava, valerian** may potentiate sedation.

PHARMACOKINETICS Absorption: 90% absorbed from GI tract. **Onset:** 15–30 min. **Duration:** 1–4 h. **Distribution:** Crosses placenta; distributed into breast milk. **Metabolism:** Metabolized in liver. **Elimination:** Excreted in urine. **Half-Life:** 30 h.

NURSING IMPLICATIONS

Assessment & Drug Effects

- Be alert to unexpected responses and report promptly. Older adult or debilitated patients and children sometimes have paradoxical response to barbiturate therapy (i.e., irritability, marked excitement as inappropriate tearfulness and aggression in children, depression, and confusion). Protect older adult patients from falling, irrational behavior, and effects of depression (anorexia, social withdrawal).
- Patient may become irritable, and uncooperative after a subhypnotic dose of a short-acting barbiturate (uncommon response).
- Be aware that barbiturates do not have analgesic action, and may produce restlessness when given to patients in pain.
- Long-term therapy may result in nutritional folate (B_9) and vitamin D deficiency.
- Lab tests: Obtain liver function and hematology tests, serum folate and vitamin D levels during prolonged therapy.
- Observe closely for changes in established drug regimen effectiveness whenever a barbiturate is added, at least during early phase of barbiturate use. Barbiturates increase the metabolism of many drugs, leading to decreased pharmacologic effects of those drugs.
- Be alert for acute toxicity (intoxication) characterized by profound CNS depression, respiratory depression that may progress to Cheyne-Stokes respirations, hypoventilation, cyanosis, cold clammy skin, hypothermia, constricted pupils (but may be dilated in severe intoxication), shock, oliguria, tachycardia, hypotension, respiration arrest, circulatory collapse, and death.

Patient & Family Education

- Do not drive or engage in potentially hazardous activities until response to drug is established.
- Store barbiturates in a safe place; not on the bedside table or other readily accessible places. It is possible to forget having taken the drug, and in half-wakened conditions take more and accidentally overdose.
- Barbiturates are reportedly teratogenic. Do not become pregnant. Use or add barrier contraception if using hormonal contraceptives.
- Report onset of fever, sore throat or mouth, malaise, easy bruising or bleeding, petechiae, jaundice, rash to physician during prolonged therapy.
- Do not consume alcohol in any amount when taking a barbiturate. It may severely impair judgment and abilities.
- Do not breast feed while taking this drug without consulting physician.

SELEGILINE HYDROCHLORIDE (L-Deprenyl)

(se-leg'i-leen)

Carbex, Eldepryl

Classifications: AUTONOMIC NERVOUS SYSTEM AGENT; ANTICHOLINERGIC (PARASYMPATHOLYTIC); ANTIPARKINSONISM AGENT

Prototype: Levodopa (L-dopa)

Pregnancy Category: C

AVAILABILITY 5 mg tablets, capsules

ACTIONS Mechanism of action is not fully understood. Increase in dopaminergic activity is thought to be primarily due to selective inhibition of MAO type B activity. Although MAOs are widely distributed throughout the body, most of the MAO in the brain is type B.

THERAPEUTIC EFFECTS Control of parkinsonism due to increased dopaminergic activity by interfering with dopamine reuptake at the synapse of neurons as well as its inhibition of MAO type B dopaminergic activity in the brain.

USES Adjunctive therapy of Parkinson's disease for patients being treated with levodopa and carbidopa who exhibit deterioration in the quality of their response to therapy.

CONTRAINDICATIONS Hypersensitivity to selegiline; concomitant use with meperidine and other opioids; lactation.

CAUTIOUS USE Hypertension and pregnancy (category C). Safety and efficacy in children are not established.

ROUTE & DOSAGE

Parkinson's Disease

Adult: **PO** 5 mg b.i.d. with breakfast and lunch (doses >10 mg/d are associated with increased risk of toxicity due to MAO inhibition)

Geriatric: **PO** Start with 5 mg qa.m.

ADMINISTRATION

Oral

- Do not give daily doses exceeding 10 mg/d.
- Note: Concurrent levodopa and carbidopa doses are usually reduced 10%–30% after 2–3 d of selegiline therapy.
- Do not use concurrently with opioids (especially meperidine).
- Store at 15°–30° C (59°–86° F).

ADVERSE EFFECTS (≥1%) **CNS:** Sleep disturbances, psychosis, agitation, confusion, dyskinesia, dizziness, hallucinations, dystonia, akathisia. **CV:** Hypotension. **GI:** Anorexia, *nausea,* vomiting, abdominal pain, constipation, diarrhea.

INTERACTIONS Drug: TRICYCLIC ANTIDEPRESSANTS may cause hyperpyrexia, seizures; **fluoxetine, sertraline, paroxetine** may cause hyperthermia, diaphoresis, tremors, seizures, delirium; SYMPATHOMIMETIC AGENTS (e.g., **amphetamine, phenylephrine, phenylpropanolamine**), **guanethidine,** and **reserpine** may cause hypertensive crisis; CNS DEPRESSANTS have additive CNS depressive effects; OPIATE ANALGESICS (especially **meperidine**) may cause hypertensive crisis and circulatory collapse; **buspirone,** hypertension; GENERAL ANESTHETICS—prolonged hypotensive and CNS depressant effects; hypertension, headache, hyperexcitability reported with **dopamine, methyldopa, levodopa, tryptophan; metrizamide** may increase risk of seizures; HYPOTENSIVE AGENTS and DIURETICS have additive hypotensive effects. **Food:** Aged meats or aged cheeses, protein extracts, sour cream, alcohol, anchovies, liver, sausages, overripe figs, bananas, avocados, chocolate, soy sauce, bean curd, natural yogurt, fava beans—**tyramine**-containing foods—may precipitate hypertensive crisis (less frequent with usual doses of **selegiline** than with other MAOIS. **Herbal: Ginseng, ephedra, ma huang, St. John's wort** may cause hypertensive crisis.

PHARMACOKINETICS Absorption: Rapidly absorbed; 73% reaches systemic circulation. **Onset:** 1 h. **Duration:** 1–3 d. **Distribution:** Crosses placenta; not known if distributed into breast milk. **Metabolism:** Metabolized in liver to *N*-desmethyldeprenyl-amphetamine, and methamphetamine. **Elimination:** Excreted in urine. **Half-Life:** 15 min (metabolites 2–20 h).

NURSING IMPLICATIONS

Assessment & Drug Effects

- Monitor vital signs, particularly during period of dosage adjustment. Report alterations in BP or pulse. Indications for discontinuation of the drug include orthostatic hypotension, hypertension, and arrhythmias.
- Monitor all patients closely for behavior changes (e.g., hallucinations, confusion, depression, delusions).

Patient & Family Education

- Do not exceed the prescribed drug dose.
- Report symptoms of MAO inhibitor-induced hypertension (e.g., severe headache, palpitations, neck stiffness, nausea, vomiting) immediately to physician.
- Do not drive or engage in potentially hazardous activities until response to drug is known.
- Make positional changes slowly and in stages. Orthostatic hypotension is possible as well as dizziness, light-headedness, and fainting.
- Do not breast feed while taking this drug without consulting physician.

SELENIUM SULFIDE

(se-lee′nee-um)

Exsel, Selsun, Selsun Blue

Classifications: SKIN AND MUCOUS MEMBRANE AGENT; ANTIINFECTIVE; ANTIBIOTIC; ANTIFUNGAL

Pregnancy Category: C

AVAILABILITY 1% lotion, shampoo

ACTIONS Has antibacterial and mild antifungal activity, although mechanism of action and causal relationships is not established. Absorption of selenium sulfide into epithelial tissue cells is followed by degradation of compound to selenium and sulfide ions. Selenium ions block enzyme systems involved in epithelial cell growth. As a result, rate of turnover in cells with normal or higher than normal turnover rates is reduced.

THERAPEUTIC EFFECTS Active against *Pityrosporum ovale,* a yeast-like fungus found in the normal flora of the scalp. Also decreases rate of growth of the epithelial cells of the scalp and other epithelial layers of cells in the body. Utilized in treatment of seborrheic dermatitis and tinea versicolor.

USES Itching and flaking of the scalp associated with dandruff, seborrheic dermatitis of the scalp, and tinea versicolor.

CONTRAINDICATIONS Application to damaged or inflamed skin surfaces; as treatment of tinea versicolor during pregnancy. Use during pregnancy (category C) as antiseborrheic only when clearly needed; kidney failure or biliary tract obstruction, GI malfunction; Wilson's disease.
CAUTIOUS USE Prolonged skin contact; use in genital area or skin folds.

ROUTE & DOSAGE

Dandruff Control, Seborrheic Dermatitis

Adult/Child: **Topical** Massage 5–10 mL of a 1%–2.5% solution into wet scalp and leave on for 2–3 min, rinse thoroughly, then repeat application and rinse well again (initially, shampoo 2 times/wk for 2 wk, then decrease to once q1–4wk prn)

Tinea Versicolor

Adult/Child: **Topical** Apply a 2.5% solution to affected area with a small amount of water to form a lather, leave on for 10 min, then rinse thoroughly, repeat once/d for 7 d

ADMINISTRATION

Topical

- Wash hands thoroughly after application of selenium sulfide to affected areas. Remove jewelry before treatment; drug will damage it.
- Rinse genital areas and skin folds well with water and dry thoroughly after treatment for tinea versicolor to prevent irritation.
- Store at 15°–30° C (59°–86° F) in tight container; protected from heat. Avoid freezing.

ADVERSE EFFECTS (≥1%) **Skin:** *Skin irritation (stinging),* rebound oiliness of scalp, hair discoloration, diffuse hair loss (reversible), systemic toxicity (if applied to abraded, infected skin).

INTERACTIONS Drug: No clinically significant interactions established.

PHARMACOKINETICS Absorption: No percutaneous absorption if skin is intact.

NURSING IMPLICATIONS

Assessment & Drug Effects

- Monitor therapeutic effectiveness.

Patient & Family Education

- Rinse thoroughly with water if lotion contacts eyes in order to prevent chemical conjunctivitis.
- Do not use drug more frequently than required to maintain control of dandruff.
- Hair loss is reversible, usually within 2–3 wk after treatment is discontinued.
- Discontinue use if skin is irritated or treatment fails. Systemic toxicity may result from application of lotion to damaged skin (percutaneous absorption) or from prolonged use (overdosage). Toxicity symptoms include: Tremors, anorexia, occasional vomiting, lethargy, weakness, severe perspiration, garlicky breath, lower abdominal pain. Symptoms disappear 10–12 d after treatment is stopped.

SENNA (SENNOSIDES)

(sen′na)

Black-Draught, Gentlax B, Senexon, Senokot, Senolax

Classifications: GASTROINTESTINAL AGENT; STIMULANT LAXATIVE

Prototype: Bisacodyl

Pregnancy Category: C

AVAILABILITY 8.6 mg, 15 mg, 25 mg tablets; 8.6 mg/5 mL, 15 mg/5 mL syrup

ACTIONS Prepared from dried leaflet of *Cassia acutifolia* or *Cassia angustifolia*. Similar to *cascara sagrada* but with more potent action. Senna glycosides are converted in colon to active aglycone, which stimulates peristalsis. Concentrate is purified and standardized for uniform action and is claimed to produce less colic than crude form.

THERAPEUTIC EFFECTS Peristalsis stimulated by conversion of drug to active chemical.

USES Acute constipation and preoperative and preradiographic bowel evacuation.

CONTRAINDICATIONS Hypersensitivity; appendicitis, fecal impaction, irritable colon, nausea, vomiting, undiagnosed abdominal pain, intestinal obstruction; pregnancy (category C), lactation; children <2 y.

CAUTIOUS USE Diabetes mellitus; fluid and electrolyte imbalances.

ROUTE & DOSAGE

Constipation

Adult: **PO Standard Senna Concentrate** 1–2 tablets or 1/2–1 tsp h.s. (max: 4 tablets or 2 tsp b.i.d.); **Syrup, Liquid** 10–15 mL at h.s.

Child: **PO Standard Senna Concentrate** *>27 kg,* 1 tablet or 1/2 tsp h.s.; **Syrup, Liquid** *1 mo–1 y,* 1.25–2.5 mL h.s.; *1–5 y,* 2.5–5 mL h.s.; *5–15 y,* 5–10 mL h.s.

ADMINISTRATION

Oral

- Give at bedtime, generally.
- Avoid exposing drug to excessive heat; protect fluid extracts from light.

ADVERSE EFFECTS (≥1%) **GI:** Abdominal cramps, flatulence, nausea, watery diarrhea, excessive loss of water and electrolytes, weight loss, melanotic segmentation of colonic mucosa (reversible).

PHARMACOKINETICS Onset: 6–10 h; may take up to 24 h. **Metabolism:** Metabolized in liver. **Elimination:** Excreted in feces.

NURSING IMPLICATIONS

Assessment & Drug Effects

- Reduce dose in patients who experience considerable abdominal cramping.

Patient & Family Education

- Be aware that drug may alter urine and feces color; yellowish brown (acid), reddish brown (alkaline).
- Continued use may lead to dependence. Consult physician if constipation persists.
- See bisacodyl for additional nursing implications.
- Do not breast feed while taking this drug.

SERTACONAZOLE NITRATE

(ser-ta-con′a-zole)

Ertaczo

Classifications: ANTIINFECTIVE; ANTIBIOTIC; AZOLE ANTIFUNGAL

Prototype: Fluconazole

Pregnancy Category: C

AVAILABILITY 2% cream in 15 g and 30 g tubes

ACTIONS Antifungal that belongs to the azole class of antifungals. While the exact mechanism of action of azole antifungals is not known, it is believed that they act primarily by inhibiting the cytochrome P450-dependent synthesis of ergosterol, a key component of the cell membrane of fungi resulting in fungal cell injury.

S

THERAPEUTIC EFFECTS Active against the following organisms: *Trichophyton rubrum, Trichophyton mentagrophytes,* and *Epidermophyton floccosum.*

USES Treatment of tinea pedis in immunocompetent patients.

CONTRAINDICATIONS Onychomycosis; children <12 y; pregnancy (category C).
CAUTIOUS USE History of hypersensitivity to azole antifungals; lactation.

ROUTE & DOSAGE

Tinea Pedis
Adult/Child: **Topical** >*12 y* Apply thin layer to affected area twice daily for 4 wk

ADMINISTRATION

Topical
- Cleanse the affected area and dry thoroughly before application.
- Apply a thin layer of the cream to affected area between the toes and the immediately surrounding healthy skin. Gently rub into the skin.
- Store at 15°–30° C (57°–86° F).

ADVERSE EFFECTS (≥1%) **Skin:** Contact dermatitis, dry skin, burning, application site reaction, skin tenderness.

PHARMACOKINETICS Absorption: Negligible absorption through intact skin.

NURSING IMPLICATIONS

Assessment & Drug Effects
- Monitor for clinical improvement, which should be seen about 2 wk after initiating treatment.

Patient & Family Education
- Report any of the following: severe skin irritation, redness, burning, blistering, or itching.
- Do not stop using this medication prematurely. Athlete's foot takes about 4 wk to clear completely.
- Nursing mothers should ensure that this topical cream does not accidentally get on the breast.

SERTRALINE HYDROCHLORIDE

(ser'tra-leen)
Zoloft
Classifications: CENTRAL NERVOUS SYSTEM (CNS) AGENT; PSYCHOTHERAPEUTIC AGENT; ANTIDEPRESSANT; SELECTIVE SEROTONIN REUPTAKE INHIBITOR (SSRI)
Prototype: Fluoxetine
Pregnancy Category: C

AVAILABILITY 25 mg, 50 mg, 100 mg tablets; 20 mg/mL liquid

ACTIONS Potent inhibitor of serotonin (5HT) reuptake in the brain, and chemically unrelated to TCA, tetracyclic or other available antidepressants. Chronic administration of sertraline results in down regulation of norepinephrine, a reaction found with other effective antidepressants. Sertraline does not inhibit MAO.
THERAPEUTIC EFFECTS Treats depression, obsessive-compulsive disorder, anxiety, and panic disorder.

USES Major depression, obsessive-compulsive disorder, panic disorder, social anxiety disorder, premenstrual dysphoric disorder, generalized anxiety, post-traumatic stress disorder.

CONTRAINDICATIONS Patients taking MAO inhibitors or within 14 d of discontinuing MAO inhibitor; antabuse; suicidal ideation, hyponatremia; mania or hypomania, pregnancy (category C); third trimester of pregnancy.

CAUTIOUS USE Seizure disorders, major affective disorders, suicidal patients; liver dysfunction, renal impairment; abrupt discontinuation; anorexia nervosa, recent history of MI or unstable cardiac disease, dehydration; diabetes mellitus; older adults; ECT therapy, seizure disorder, seizures. Unknown if sertraline is excreted in breast milk. Safety and effectiveness in children <6 y are not established.

ROUTE & DOSAGE

Depression, Anxiety

Adult: **PO** Begin with 50 mg/d, gradually increase every few weeks according to response (range: 50–200 mg)
Geriatric: **PO** Start with 25 mg/d

Premenstrual Dysphoric Disorder

Adult: **PO** Begin with 50 mg/d for first cycle, may titrate up to 150 mg/d

Obsessive-Compulsive Disorder

Adult: **PO** Begin with 50 mg/d, may titrate at weekly intervals up to 200 mg/d
Child: **PO** *6–12 y,* Begin with 25 mg/d, may increase by 50 mg/wk, as tolerated and needed, up to 200 mg/d

ADMINISTRATION

Oral

- Give in the morning or evening.
- Do not give concurrently with a MAO inhibitor or within 14 d of discontinuing an MAOI.

ADVERSE EFFECTS (≥1%) **CV:** Palpitations, chest pain, hypertension, hypotension, edema, syncope, tachycardia. **CNS:** *Agitation, insomnia, headache, dizziness, somnolence, fatigue,* ataxia, incoordination, vertigo, abnormal dreams, aggressive behavior, delusions, hallucinations, emotional lability, paranoia, suicidal ideation, depersonalization. **Endocrine:** Gynecomastia, male sexual dysfunction. **GI:** Nausea, vomiting, diarrhea, constipation, indigestion, anorexia, flatulence, abdominal pain, dry mouth. **Special Senses:** Exophthalmos, blurred vision, dry eyes, diplopia, photophobia, tearing, conjunctivitis, mydriasis. **Skin:** Rash, urticaria, acne, alopecia. **Respiratory:** Rhinitis, pharyngitis, cough, dyspnea, bronchospasm. **Body as a Whole:** Myalgia, arthralgia, muscle weakness. **Metabolic:** Hyponatremia in older adults.

DIAGNOSTIC TEST INTERFERENCE May cause asymptomatic elevations in ***liver function tests.*** Slight decrease in ***uric acid.***

INTERACTIONS Drug: MAOIS (e.g., **selegiline, phenelzine**) should be stopped 14 d before sertraline is started because of serious problems with other SEROTONIN REUPTAKE INHIBITORS (shivering, nausea, diplopia, confusion, anxiety). **Sertraline may increase levels and toxicity of diazepam, pimozide, tolbutamide.** Use cautiously with other centrally acting CNS drugs; increase risk of **ergotamine** toxicity with **dihydroergotamine, ergotamine. Herbal: St. John's wort** may cause **serotonin** syndrome (headache, dizziness, sweating, agitation).

PHARMACOKINETICS Absorption: Slowly absorbed from GI tract. **Onset:** 2–4 wk. **Distribution:** 99% protein bound; not known if distributed into breast milk. **Metabolism:** Extensive first-pass metabolism in liver to inactive metabolites. **Elimi-**

nation: 40%–45% excreted in urine, 40%–45% in feces. **Half-Life:** 24 h.

NURSING IMPLICATIONS

Assessment & Drug Effects

- Supervise patients at risk for suicide closely during initial therapy.
- Monitor for worsening of depression or emergence of suicidal ideation.
- Monitor older adults for fluid and sodium imbalances.
- Monitor patients with a history of a seizure disorder closely.
- Lab tests: Monitor PT and INR with patients receiving concurrent warfarin therapy.

Patient & Family Education

- Report diarrhea, nausea, dyspepsia, insomnia, drowsiness, dizziness, or persistent headache to physician.
- Report signs of bleeding promptly to physician when taking concomitant warfarin.
- Do not breast feed while taking this drug without consulting physician.

SEVELAMER HYDROCHLORIDE (Pr)

(se-vel′a-mer)

Renagel

Classifications: ELECTROLYTE AND WATER BALANCE AGENT; PHOSPHATE BINDER

Pregnancy Category: C

AVAILABILITY 403 mg capsules; 400 mg, 800 mg tablets

ACTIONS Polymer that binds intestinal phosphate; interacts with phosphate by way of ion-exchange and hydrogen binding. Advantageously, does not contain aluminum or calcium acetate in treating hyperphosphatemia in End Stage Kidney Failure.

THERAPEUTIC EFFECTS Indicated by a serum phosphate level ≤6.0 mg/dL.

USES Reduction of serum phosphorus in patients with end-stage kidney disease.

CONTRAINDICATIONS Hypophosphatemia; hypersensitivity to sevelamer HCl; bowel obstruction; pregnancy (category C), lactation. Safety and efficacy in children <18 y are not established.

CAUTIOUS USE GI motility disorders, dysphagia, GI surgery patients; vitamin deficiencies (especially Vitamins D, E, K and folic acid).

ROUTE & DOSAGE

Hyperphosphatemia

Adult: **PO** 2 capsules or tablets t.i.d. for serum phosphorus >6 and <7.5 mg/dL; 3 capsules or tablets t.i.d. for serum phosphorus >7.5 and <9 mg/dL; 4 capsules or tablets t.i.d. for serum phosphorus ≥9 mg/dL

ADMINISTRATION

Oral

- Give with meals; do not open or chew capsule.
- Give other oral medications 1 h before or 3 h after Renagel.
- Discard capsules after printed expiration date.
- Store at 15°–30° C (59°–86° F); protect from moisture.

ADVERSE EFFECTS (≥1%) **Body as a Whole:** Headache, infection, pain. **CV:** Hypertension, hypotension, thrombosis. **GI:** Diarrhea, dyspepsia, vomiting, nausea, constipation, flatulence. **Respiratory:** Increased cough.

INTERACTIONS Drug: No clinically significant interactions established.

PHARMACOKINETICS Absorption: No systemic absorption.

NURSING IMPLICATIONS

Assessment & Drug Effects

- Lab tests: Obtain frequent serum phosphate levels.

Patient & Family Education

- Do not use capsules after printed expiration date.
- Take daily multivitamin supplement approved by physician.
- Do not breast feed while taking this drug.

SIBUTRAMINE HYDROCHLORIDE MONOHYDRATE

(si-bu′tra-meen)

Meridia

Classifications: CENTRAL NERVOUS SYSTEM AGENT; SELECTIVE SEROTONIN REUPTAKE INHIBITOR (SSRI); NOREPINEPHRINE REUPTAKE INHIBITOR

Prototype: Fluoxetine

Pregnancy Category: C

Controlled Substance: Schedule IV

AVAILABILITY 5 mg, 10 mg, 15 mg capsules

ACTIONS Inhibits reuptake of serotonin ($5HT_3$), monoamine reuptake, as well as norepinephrine and dopamine reuptake, by blocking their receptors.

THERAPEUTIC EFFECTS Appetite suppression via the mechanism of Meridia. Indicated by a loss of at least 4 lb during the first 4 wk of therapy.

USES Management of obesity, including weight loss and maintenance of weight loss, in patients with BMI of at least 30 kg/m^2 or BMI of at least 27 kg/m^2 and other risk factors (hypertension, diabetes, dyslipidemia).

CONTRAINDICATIONS Anorexia nervosa; arrhythmias; concurrent administration with other serotonin reuptake inhibitors (e.g., fluoxetine), MAOIS, lithium, tryptophan; severe hepatic or renal impairment; CHF, stroke, CAD; uncontrolled or poorly controlled hypertension; pregnancy (category C).

CAUTIOUS USE History of hypertension; older adults; narrow-angle glaucoma; seizures; lactation. Safety and efficacy in patients <16 y are not established.

ROUTE & DOSAGE

Weight Loss

Adult: **PO** 10 mg once daily, preferably in morning, may be increased to 15 mg if inadequate weight loss (<4 lb) in 4 wk

ADMINISTRATION

Oral

- Note: Doses above 15 mg/d are not recommended.
- Allow at least 2 wks to elapse between discontinuing an MAOIS and starting sibutramine.
- Store at 15°–30° C (59°–86° F) in a tightly closed container; protect from light.

ADVERSE EFFECTS (≥1%) **Body as a Whole:** Back pain, flu-like syndrome, asthenia, arthralgia. **CNS:** *Headache,* insomnia, migraine headache, dizziness, nervousness, anxiety, depression, paresthesias, seizures (rare). **CV:** Increase in BP, tachycardia, vasodilation, palpitations. **GI:** *Dry mouth,* anorexia, constipation, abdominal pain, increased appetite, nausea, dyspepsia, taste

S

perversion. **Respiratory:** Rhinitis, pharyngitis, sinusitis, cough. **Skin:** Rash, sweating. **Urogenital:** Dysmenorrhea, UTI.

INTERACTIONS Drug: DECONGESTANTS, COUGH AND ALLERGY MEDICATIONS may cause additional increase in BP; MAOIS, ERGOT DERIVATIVES, **sumatriptan, naratriptan, rizatriptan, zolmitriptan, dextromethorphan, meperidine, pentazocine, fentanyl, lithium;** SSRIS may predispose to **serotonin** syndrome (see Appendix F); **ketoconazole, erythromycin** may inhibit metabolism of sibutramine. **Herbal: St. John's wort** may cause **serotonin** syndrome (headache, dizziness, sweating, agitation).

PHARMACOKINETICS Absorption: Rapidly absorbed from GI tract. **Peak:** 1.2 h. **Distribution:** 97% protein bound; concentrates in liver and kidneys. **Metabolism:** Metabolized in liver by cytochrome P450 3A4 to 2 active metabolites. **Elimination:** Excreted primarily in kidneys. **Half-Life:** 14–16 h (active metabolites).

NURSING IMPLICATIONS

Assessment & Drug Effects

- Monitor weight changes carefully to determine therapeutic effect.
- Lab tests: Periodic liver function, bilirubin, alkaline phosphatases, lipid profile.
- Monitor BR and HR regularly; report sustained increases in BP or HR immediately.
- Monitor for and immediately report S&S of serotonin syndrome (see Appendix F).
- Monitor persons with narrow-angle glaucoma closely for worsening intraocular pressure.

Patient & Family Education

- Notify physician if any of the following develop: Rash, hives, or other S&S of an allergic reaction; signs of hyperstimulation such as restlessness, shivering, profuse sweating, irritability, and tremor.
- Take in the morning; causes less interference with sleep.
- Check with physician before taking any OTC cough, cold, allergy, or weight-loss drugs.
- Maintain strict adherence to prescribed antihypertensives.
- Inform physician of all drugs being taken. Serious adverse effects may be experienced with concomitant use of some drugs used to treat depression.
- Do not breast feed while taking this drug without consulting physician.

SILDENAFIL CITRATE (Pr)

(sil-den'a-fil ci'trate)

Viagra

Classifications: IMPOTENCE AGENT; PHOSPHODIESTERASE (PDE) INHIBITOR

Pregnancy Category: B

AVAILABILITY 25 mg, 50 mg, 100 mg tablets

ACTIONS Oral treatment for erectile dysfunction, whether organic or psychogenic in origin.

THERAPEUTIC EFFECTS Enhances vasodilation effect of nitric oxide in the corpus cavernosus of the penis, thus sustaining an erection.

USES Erectile dysfunction.

CONTRAINDICATIONS Hypersensitivity to sildenafil; concurrent administration of organic nitrates and nitroglycerin; pregnancy (category B); lactation. Not recommended for women or children.

CAUTIOUS USE CAD, heart failure, MI, cardiac arrhythmias, stroke within 6 mo of starting drug; hypotension and hypertension; risk factors for CVA; aortic stenosis; anatomic deformity of the penis; sickle cell anemia, polycythemia; multiple myeloma; leukemia; active bleeding or a peptic ulcer; GERD, hiatal hernia; coagulopathy; retinitis pigmentosa; hepatic disease, hepatitis, cirrhosis; severe renal impairment (Cl_{cr} <30 mL/min); older adults; concurrent use with other medicines for penile dysfunction.

ROUTE & DOSAGE

Erectile Dysfunction

Adult: **PO** 50 mg 0.5–4 h before sexual activity (dose range: 25 to 100 mg once/d); max dose: 25 mg/d with itraconazole or ketoconazole; max dose: 25 mg/48 h with ritonavir

Geriatric: **PO** 25 mg approximately 1 h before sexual activity

Hepatic or Severe Renal Impairment

25 mg approximately 1 h before sexual activity

ADMINISTRATION

Oral

- Give 1 h prior to sexual activity (effective range is 0.5–4 h).
- Do not give within 24 h of taking any medication with nitrates (i.e., nitroglycerine).
- Do not give more than once a day.
- Store at 15°–30° C (59°–86° F) in a tightly closed container; protect from light.

ADVERSE EFFECTS (≥1%) **Body as a Whole:** Face edema, photosensitivity, shock, asthenia, pain, chills, fall, allergic reaction, arthritis, myalgia. **CNS:** *Headache,* dizziness, migraine, syncope, cerebral thrombosis, ataxia, neuralgia, paresthesias, tremor, vertigo, depression, insomnia, somnolence, abnormal dreams. **CV:** Flushing, chest pain, MI, angina, AV block, tachycardia, palpitation, hypotension, postural hypotension, cardiac arrest, sudden cardiac death, heart failure, cardiomyopathy, abnormal ECG, edema. **GI:** Dyspepsia, diarrhea, abdominal pain, vomiting, colitis, dysphagia, gastritis, gastroenteritis, esophagitis, stomatitis, dry mouth, abnormal liver function tests, thirst. **Respiratory:** Nasal congestion, asthma, dyspnea, laryngitis, pharyngitis, sinusitis, bronchitis, cough. **Skin:** Rash, urticaria, pruritus, sweating, exfoliative dermatitis. **Urogenital:** UTI. **Special Senses:** Abnormal vision (color changes, photosensitivity, blurred vision). **Hematologic:** Anemia, leukopenia. **Metabolic:** Gout, hyperglycemia, hyperuricemia, hypoglycemia, hypernatremia.

INTERACTIONS Drug: NITRATES increase risk of serious hypotension; if used within 4 h of **doxazosin, prazosin, terazosin, tamsulosin; cimetidine, erythromycin, ketoconazole, itraconazole,** PROTEASE INHIBITORS increase sildenafil levels; **rifampin** can decrease sildenafil levels.

PHARMACOKINETICS Absorption: Rapidly absorbed from GI tract. **Peak:** 30–120 min. **Distribution:** 96% protein bound. **Metabolism:** Metabolized in liver by cytochromes P450 3A4 (primary) and 2C9 (minor). **Elimination:** 80% excreted in feces, 12% in urine. **Half-Life:** 4 h.

NURSING IMPLICATIONS

Assessment & Drug Effects

- Monitor carefully for and immediately report S&S of cardiac distress.

Patient & Family Education

- Do not take sildenafil within 4 h of taking doxazosin, prazosin, terazosin, or tamsulosin.
- Consuming a high-fat meal before taking drug may cause delay in drug action.
- Report to physician: Headaches, flushing, chest pain, indigestion, blurred vision, sensitivity to light, changes in color vision.

SILVER SULFADIAZINE

(sul-fa-dye′a-zeen)

Silvadene

Classifications: ANTIINFECTIVE; SULFONAMIDE

Prototype: Sulfisoxazole

Pregnancy Category: C

AVAILABILITY 10 mg/g cream

ACTIONS Produced by reaction of silver nitrate with sulfadiazine. Mechanism of action differs from that of either component. Silver salt is released slowly and exerts bactericidal effect only on bacterial cell membrane and wall, rather than by inhibiting folic acid synthesis; antibacterial activity is not inhibited by *p*-aminobenzoic acid (PABA). Contact with sodium chloride in body tissues and fluids results in slow release of sulfadiazine, which may be systemically absorbed from application site.

THERAPEUTIC EFFECTS Broad antimicrobial activity including many gram-negative and gram-positive bacteria and yeast.

USES Prevention and treatment of sepsis in second- and third-degree burns.

CONTRAINDICATIONS Hypersensitivity to other sulfonamides; G6PD deficiency; pregnancy (category C), pregnant women at term, lactation, premature infants and neonates <2 mo.

CAUTIOUS USE Impaired kidney or liver function; impaired respiratory function.

ROUTE & DOSAGE

Burn Wound Treatment

Adult/Child: **Topical** Apply 1% cream 1–2 times/d to thickness of approximately 1.5 mm (1/16 in)

ADMINISTRATION

Topical

- Do not use if cream darkens; it is water soluble and white.
- Apply with sterile, gloved hands to cleansed, debrided burned areas. Reapply cream to areas where it has been removed by patient activity; cover burn wounds with medication at all times.
- Bathe patient daily (in whirlpool or shower or in bed) as aid to debridement. Reapply drug.
- Note: Dressings are not required but may be used if necessary. Drug does not stain clothing.
- Store at room temperature away from heat.

ADVERSE EFFECTS (≥1%) **Body as a Whole:** Pain (occasionally), burning, itching, rash, reversible leukopenia. Potential for toxicity as for other sulfonamides if applied to extensive areas of the body surface.

INTERACTIONS Drug: PROTEOLYTIC ENZYMES are inactivated by silver in cream.

PHARMACOKINETICS Absorption: Not absorbed through intact skin, however, approximately 10% could be absorbed when applied to second- or third-degree burns. **Distribu-**

S

tion: Distributed into most body tissues. **Metabolism:** Metabolized in the liver. **Elimination:** Excreted in urine.

NURSING IMPLICATIONS

Assessment & Drug Effects

- Observe for and report hypersensitivity reaction: Rash, itching, or burning sensation in unburned areas.
- Lab tests: Obtain serum sulfa concentrations, urinalysis, and kidney function tests when drug is applied to extensive areas. Significant quantities of drug may be absorbed.
- Observe patient for reactions attributed to sulfonamides.
- Note: Analgesic may be required. Occasionally, pain is experienced on application; intensity and duration depend on depth of burn.
- Continue treatment until satisfactory healing or burn site is ready for grafting, unless adverse reactions occur.

Patient & Family Education

- Do not breast feed while taking this drug.

SIMVASTATIN

(sim-vah-sta′-tin)

Zocor

Classifications: CARDIOVASCULAR AGENT; ANTILIPEMIC; HMG-CoA REDUCTASE INHIBITOR (STATIN)

Prototype: Lovastatin

Pregnancy Category: X

AVAILABILITY 5 mg, 10 mg, 20 mg, 40 mg, 80 mg tablets

ACTIONS Inhibitor of 3-hydroxy-3-methylglutaryl coenzyme A (HMG-CoA) reductase; similar in action to lovastatin but more potent. HMG-CoA reductase inhibitors increase HDL cholesterol, and decrease LDL cholesterol, and total cholesterol synthesis.

THERAPEUTIC EFFECTS Indicated by decreased serum triglycerides, decreased LDL, cholesterol, and modest increases in HDL cholesterol.

USES Hypercholesterolemia (alone or in combination with bile acid sequestrants), familial hypercholesterolemia. Reduces risk of coronary death and nonfatal MI.

CONTRAINDICATIONS Hypersensitivity to simvastatin; active liver disease; pregnancy (category X), lactation.

CAUTIOUS USE Homozygous familial hypercholesterolemia, history of liver disease, alcoholics. Safety and effectiveness in children and adolescents are not established.

ROUTE & DOSAGE

Hypercholesterolemia

Adult: **PO** 5–40 mg q.d. (max: 80 mg q.d.)

ADMINISTRATION

Oral

- Adjust dosage usually at 4-wk intervals.
- Give in the evening.
- Store at 15°–30° C (59°–86° F).

ADVERSE EFFECTS (≥1%) **CV:** Angina. **CNS:** Dizziness, headache, vertigo, asthenia, fatigue, insomnia. **GI:** Nausea, diarrhea, vomiting, abdominal pain, constipation, flatulence, heartburn, transient elevations in liver transaminases, transient elevations in CPK. **Body as a Whole:** Fatigue. **Respiratory:** Rhinitis, cough.

INTERACTIONS Drug: May increase PT when administered with **war-**

farin; cyclosporine, gemfibrozil, fenofibrate, clofibrate, antilipemic doses of **niacin, fluconazole, itraconazole, ketoconazole, miconazole, nefazodone, nelfinavir, ritonavir, saquinavir, sildenafil, tacrolimus** may increase serum levels and increase risk of myopathy, rhabdomyolysis and acute kidney failure. **Food: Grapefruit juice** may increase risk of myopathy, rhabdomyolysis.

PHARMACOKINETICS Absorption: Rapidly absorbed from GI tract. **Onset:** 2 wk. **Peak:** 4–6 wk. **Distribution:** 95% protein bound; achieves high liver concentrations; crosses placenta. **Metabolism:** Extensive first-pass metabolism in liver to its active metabolite. **Elimination:** 13% excreted in urine, 60% in bile and feces.

NURSING IMPLICATIONS

Assessment & Drug Effects

- Lab tests: Obtain baseline and periodic (q6mo) liver function during the first year and yearly thereafter. Monitor cholesterol levels throughout therapy.
- Monitor coagulation studies with patients receiving concurrent warfarin therapy. PT may be prolonged.
- Assess for and report unexplained muscle pain. Determine CPK level at onset of muscle pain.

Patient & Family Education

- Report unexplained muscle pain, tenderness, or weakness, especially if accompanied by malaise or fever, to physician.
- Report signs of bleeding to physician promptly when taking concurrent warfarin.
- Moderate intake of grapefruit juice while taking this medication.
- Do not breast feed while taking this drug.

SIROLIMUS

(sir-o-li′mus)

Rapamune

Classifications: IMMUNOMODULATOR; IMMUNOSUPPRESSANT

Prototype: Cyclosporine

Pregnancy Category: C

AVAILABILITY 1 mg tablets; 1 mg/mL oral solution

ACTIONS Macrolide antibiotic structurally related to tacrolimus with immunosuppressive activity. Active in reducing a transplant rejection by inhibiting the response of helper T-lymphocytes and B-lymphocytes to cytokinesis ([interleukin] IL-2, IL-4 and IL-5).

THERAPEUTIC EFFECTS Inhibits antibody production and acute transplant rejection reaction in autoimmune disorders [e.g., systemic lupus erythematosus (SLE)]. Indicated by nonrejection of transplanted organ.

USES Prophylaxis of kidney transplant rejection.

UNLABELED USES Treatment of psoriasis.

CONTRAINDICATIONS Hypersensitivity to sirolimus; lung or liver transplant patients; soya lecithin (soy fatty acids) hypersensitivity; lymphoma, neoplastic disease; children <13 y; females of childbearing age; pregnancy (category C); lactation.

CAUTIOUS USE Hypersensitivity to or concurrent administration with tacrolimus; impaired renal function; concurrent use of aminoglycosides, and amphotericin B; renal transplant patients; dialysis patients, UV exposure, retransplant patients, multiorgan transplant recipients, African-American transplant patients; viral or bacterial infection; hypertriglyceridemia, hyperlipidemia, diabetic patients, atrial fibrillation, CHF, hypervolemia, palpitations; mild to moderate hepatic disease; coronary artery disease; myelosuppression; liver disease.

ROUTE & DOSAGE

Kidney Transplant

Adult: **PO** 6 mg loading dose immediately after transplant, then 2 mg/d. Doses will need to be much higher (up to 40 mg/d) if not on cyclosporine
Adolescent: **PO** *≥13 y and <40 kg,* 3 mg/m^2 loading dose immediately after transplant, then 1 mg/m^2/d. Doses will need to be much higher (up to 40 mg/d) if not on cyclosporine

Hepatic Impairment

Reduce maintenance dose by 33%

ADMINISTRATION

Oral

- Give 4 h after oral cyclosporine.
- Add prescribed amount of sirolimus to a glass containing ≥2 oz (60 mL) of water or orange juice (do not use any other type of liquid). Stir vigorously and administer immediately. Refill glass with ≥4 oz (120 mL) of water or orange juice. Stir vigorously and administer immediately.
- Give consistently with respect to amount and type of food.
- Refrigerate; protect from light; use multidose bottles within 1 mo of opening.

ADVERSE EFFECTS (≥1%) **Body as a Whole:** *Asthenia, back pain, chest pain, fever, pain, arthralgia;* flu-like syndrome; generalized edema; infection; lymphocele; malaise; sepsis, arthrosis, bone necrosis, leg cramps, myalgia, osteoporosis, tetany, abscess, ascites, cellulitis, chills, face edema, hernia, pelvic pain, peritonitis. **CNS:** *Insomnia, tremor, headache,* anxiety, confusion, depression, dizziness, emotional lability, hypertonia, hyperesthesia, hypotonia, neuropathy, paresthesia, somnolence. **CV:** *Hypertension,* atrial fibrillation, CHF, hypervolemia, hypotension, palpitation, peripheral vascular disorder, postural hypotension, syncope, tachycardia, thrombophlebitis, thrombosis, vasodilation. **GI:** *Constipation, diarrhea, dyspepsia, nausea, vomiting, abdominal pain,* anorexia, dysphagia, eructation, esophagitis, flatulence, gastritis, gastroenteritis, gingivitis, gum hyperplasia, ileus, mouth ulceration, oral moniliasis, stomatitis, abnormal liver function tests. **Hematologic:** *Anemia, thrombocytopenia,* leukopenia, hemorrhage, ecchymosis, leukocytosis, lymphadenopathy, polycythemia, thrombotic, thrombocytopenic purpura. **Metabolic:** *Edema, hypercholesterolemia, hyperkalemia, hyperlipidemia, hypokalemia, hypophosphatemia, peripheral edema, weight gain,* Cushing's syndrome, diabetes, acidosis, hypercalcemia, hyperglycemia, hyperphosphatemia, hypocalcemia, hypoglycemia, hypomagnesemia, hyponatremia; increased LDH, alkaline phosphatase, BUN, creatine phosphokinase, ALT, or AST; weight loss. **Respiratory:** *Dyspnea, pharyngitis, upper respiratory tract infection,* asthma, atelectasis, bronchitis, cough, epistaxis, hypoxia, lung edema, pleural effusion, pneumonia, rhinitis, sinusitis. **Skin:** *Acne, rash,* fungal dermatitis, hirsutism, pruritus, skin hypertrophy, skin ulcer, sweating. **Urogenital:** *UTI,* albuminuria, bladder pain, dysuria, hematuria, hydronephrosis, impotence, kidney pain, nocturia, renal tubular necrosis, oliguria, pyuria, scrotal edema, incontinence, urinary retention, glycosuria. **Special Senses:** Abnormal vision, cataract, conjunctivitis, deafness, ear pain, otitis media, tinnitus.

INTERACTIONS Drug: Sirolimus concentrations increased by **clarithromycin, cyclosporine, diltiazem, erythromycin, ketoconazole, itraconazole, telithromycin;** sirolimus concentrations decreased by **rifabutin, rifampin;** VACCINES may be less effective with sirolimus; **tacrolimus** increases mortality, hepatic artery thrombosis, and graft loss. **Food: Grapefruit juice** significantly decreases absorption of sirolimus.

PHARMACOKINETICS Absorption: Rapidly absorbed with 14% bioavailability. **Peak:** 2 h. **Distribution:** 92% protein bound, distributes in high concentrations to heart, intestines, kidneys, liver, lungs, muscle, spleen, and testes. **Metabolism:** Metabolized in liver by CYP3A4. **Elimination:** 91% excreted in feces, 2.2% in urine. **Half-Life:** 62 h.

NURSING IMPLICATIONS

Assessment & Drug Effects

- Monitor for S&S of graft rejection.
- Control hyperlipidemia prior to initiating drug.
- Draw trough whole-blood sirolimus levels 1 h before a scheduled dose.
- Lab tests: Obtain periodic lipid profile, CBC with differential, fasting plasma glucose, blood chemistry, BUN, and creatinine (especially with other drugs known to cause renal impairment).

Patient & Family Education

- Avoid grapefruit juice within 2 h of taking sirolimus.
- Limit exposure to sunlight (UV exposure).
- Note: Decreased effectiveness possible for vaccines during therapy.
- Use or add barrier contraceptive before, during, and for 12 wk after discontinuing therapy.
- Do not breast feed while taking this drug.

S

SODIUM BICARBONATE ($NAHCO_3$)

(sod'i-um bi-car'bon-ate)

Sodium Bicarbonate

Classifications: GASTROINTESTINAL AGENT; ANTACID; FLUID AND ELECTROLYTE BALANCE AGENT

Pregnancy Category: C

AVAILABILITY 325 mg, 520 mg, 650 mg tablets; 4.2%, 5%, 7.5%, 8.4% injection

ACTIONS Short-acting, potent systemic antacid. Rapidly neutralizes gastric acid to form sodium chloride, carbon dioxide, and water. After absorption of sodium bicarbonate, plasma alkali reserve is increased and excess sodium and bicarbonate ions are excreted in urine, thus rendering urine less acid. Not suitable for treatment of peptic ulcer because it is short-acting, high in sodium, and may cause gastric distention, systemic alkalosis, and possibly acid-rebound.

THERAPEUTIC EFFECTS Short-acting, potent systemic antacid; rapidly neutralizes gastric acid or systemic acidosis.

USES Systemic alkalinizer to correct metabolic acidosis (as occurs in diabetes mellitus, shock, cardiac arrest, or vascular collapse), to minimize uric acid crystallization associated with uricosuric agents, to increase the solubility of sulfonamides, and to enhance renal excretion of barbiturate and salicylate overdosage. Commonly used as home remedy for relief of occasional heartburn, indigestion, or sour stomach. Used topically as paste, bath, or soak to relieve itching and minor skin irritations such as sunburn, insect bites, prickly heat, poison ivy, sumac, or oak. Sterile solutions are used to buffer acidic parenteral solutions to prevent acidosis. Also as a buffering agent in many commercial products (e.g., mouthwashes, douches, enemas, ophthalmic solutions).

CONTRAINDICATIONS Prolonged therapy with sodium bicarbonate; patients losing chloride (as from vomiting, GI suction, diuresis); heart disease, hypertension; renal insufficiency; peptic ulcer; pregnancy (category C).

CAUTIOUS USE Edema, sodium-retaining disorders; lactation; older adult patients.

ROUTE & DOSAGE

Antacid

Adult: **PO** 0.3–2 g 1–4 times/d or 1/2 tsp of powder in glass of water

Urinary Alkalinizer

Adult: **PO** 4 g initially, then 1–2 g q4h
Child: **PO** 84–840 mg/kg/d in divided doses

Cardiac Arrest

Adult: **IV** 1 mEq/kg of a 7.5% or 8.4% solution initially, then 0.5 mEq/kg q10 min depending on arterial blood gas determinations (8.4% solutions contain 50 mEq/ 50 mL), give over 1–2 min
Child: **IV** 0.5–1 mEq/kg of a 4.2% solution q10 min depending on arterial blood gas determinations, give over 1–2 min

Metabolic Acidosis

Adult: **IV** 2–5 mEq/kg by IV infusion over 4–8 h
Infant: **IV** 2–3 mEq/kg/d of a 4.2% solution over 4–8 h

ADMINISTRATION

Oral

- Do not add oral preparation to calcium-containing solutions.

Topical

- Use manufacturer's directions: Bath or soak, 1/2 cup or more into tub of warm water; Footsoak, 4 tbsp/L(qt) warm water; soak 5–10 min; Paste, 3 parts sodium bicarbonate to 1 part water
- Note: Solutions in water slowly decompose, decomposition is accelerated by agitating or warming the solution.

Intravenous

PREPARE: **IV Infusion:** May give 4.2% (0.5 mEq/mL) and 5% (0.595 mEq/mL) $NaHCO_3$ solutions undiluted. Dilute 7.5% (0.892 mEq/mL) and 8.4% (1 mEq/mL) solutions with compatible IV solutions. Dilute to at least 4.2% for infants and children.

ADMINISTER: **IV Infusion:** Give a bolus dose only in emergency situations. Usually, the rate is 2–5 mEq/kg over 4–8 h; do not exceed 50 mEq/h. Stop infusion immediately if extravasation occurs. Severe tissue damage has followed tissue infiltration.

INCOMPATIBILITIES **Solution/additive: Alcohol 5%, lactated Ringer's, amoxicillin, ascorbic acid, bupivacaine, carboplatin, carmustine, cisplatin, codeine, corticotropin, dobutamine, dopamine, epinephrine, etidocaine, glycopyrrolate, hydromorphone, imipenem-cilastatin, insulin,**

S

isoproterenol, labetalol, levorphanol, lidocaine, magnesium sulfate, meperidine, mepivacaine, meropenem, methadone, methicillin, metoclopramide, morphine, norepinephrine, oxytetracycline, pentazocine, pentobarbital, phenobarbital, procaine, secobarbital, streptomycin, succinylcholine, tetracycline, thiopental, vancomycin, vitamin B complex with C. Y-site: Allopurinol, amiodarone, amphotericin B cholesteryl complex, calcium chloride, diltiazem, doxorubicin liposome, idarubicin, imipenem/cilastatin, inamrinone, leucovorin, midazolam, nalbuphine, ondansetron, oxacillin, sargramostim, verapamil, vincristine, vindesine, vinorelbine.

- Store in airtight containers.
- Note expiration date.

ADVERSE EFFECTS (≥1%) **GI:** *Belching, gastric distention,* flatulence. **Metabolic:** Metabolic alkalosis; electrolyte imbalance: sodium overload (pulmonary edema), hypocalcemia (tetany), hypokalemia, milk-alkali syndrome, dehydration. **Other:** Rapid IV in neonates (Hypernatremia, reduction in CSF pressure, <u>intracranial hemorrhage</u>). **Skin:** Severe tissue damage following extravasation of IV solution. **Urogenital:** Renal calculi or crystals, impaired kidney function.

DIAGNOSTIC TEST INTERFERENCE Small increase in ***blood lactate*** levels (following IV infusion of sodium bicarbonate); false-positive ***urinary protein*** determinations (using ***ames reagent, sulfacetic acid,*** heat and ***acetic acid*** or ***nitric acid ring method***); elevated ***urinary urobilinogen*** levels (***urobilinogen*** excretion increases in alkaline urine).

INTERACTIONS Drug: May decrease absorption of **ketoconazole;** may decrease elimination of **dextroamphetamine, ephedrine, pseudoephedrine, quinidine;** may increase elimination of **chlorpropamide, lithium,** SALICYLATES, TETRACYCLINES.

PHARMACOKINETICS Absorption: Readily absorbed from GI tract. **Onset:** 15 min. **Duration:** 1–2 h. **Elimination:** Excreted in urine within 3–4 h.

NURSING IMPLICATIONS

Assessment & Drug Effects

- Be aware that long-term use of oral preparation with milk or calcium can cause milk-alkali syndrome: Anorexia, nausea, vomiting, headache, mental confusion, hypercalcemia, hypophosphatemia, soft tissue calcification, renal and ureteral calculi, renal insufficiency, metabolic alkalosis.
- Lab tests: Urinary alkalinization: Monitor urinary pH as a guide to dosage (pH testing with nitrazine paper may be done at intervals throughout the day and dosage adjustments made accordingly).
- Lab tests: Metabolic acidosis: Monitor patient closely by observations of clinical condition; measurements of acid-base status (blood pH, Po_2, Pco_2, HCO_3^-, and other electrolytes, are usually made several times daily during acute period). Observe for signs of alkalosis (over treatment) (see Appendix F).
- Observe for and report S&S of improvement or reversal of metabolic acidosis (see Appendix F).

Patient & Family Education

- Do not use sodium bicarbonate as antacid. A nonabsorbable OTC alternative for repeated use is safer.

- Do not take antacids longer than 2 wk except under advice and supervision of a physician. Self-medication with routine doses of sodium bicarbonate or soda mints may cause sodium retention and alkalosis, especially when kidney function is impaired.
- Be aware that commonly used OTC antacid products contain sodium bicarbonate: Alka-Seltzer, Bromo-Seltzer, Gaviscon.
- Do not breast feed while taking this drug without consulting physician.

SODIUM CHLORIDE 20%

(sod′i-um)

Sodium Chloride 20%

Classification: ABORTIFACIENT

Pregnancy Category: X

AVAILABILITY 20% solution

ACTIONS Hypertonic saline instillation into the amniotic sac induces abortion and fetal death. Mechanism is unclear, but abortifacient activity may be a response to prostaglandins released by hypertonic NaCl-damaged decidual cells.

THERAPEUTIC EFFECTS Uterine contractions induced by the saline solution are sufficient to cause evacuation of fetus and placenta; however, in 25%–40% of the patients, abortion may be incomplete.

USES To induce abortion late in the second trimester of pregnancy. Oxytocin may be used as an adjunct (concurrent) uterine stimulant.

CONTRAINDICATIONS Pregnancy (category X) of less than 15 wk or more than 24 wk; prior uterine surgery (including cervix), pelvic adhesions; sickle cell disease, diabetes mellitus; increased intraamniotic pressure (as in contracting or hypertonic uterus); poor health, blood disorders, coagulation factor deficiencies.

CAUTIOUS USE Malignant hypertension, cardiovascular and kidney disease, thrombocytopenia, fibrinolytic defects.

ROUTE & DOSAGE

Abortion Induction

Adult: **Instillation** Intraamniotic with 20% solution in volumes equal to amount of amniotic fluid removed (max: 200–250 mL) administered slowly over 20–30 min; repeat in 48 h if uterine contractility, cervical effacement, or cervical dilation is inadequate or if labor has not begun

ADMINISTRATION

Instillation

- Prepare skin as for surgery prior to procedure. Withdraw about 1 mL of amniotic fluid by transabdominal tap to confirm location of needle (amniotic fluid has pH 7.4 and ability to fern). If blood is present or if no amniotic fluid is withdrawn, needle is repositioned. Some clinicians then remove all amniotic fluid (30–250 mL); others wait until NaCl instillation.
- Instill NaCl through 3-way stopcock with needle and polyethylene catheter inserted into amniotic cavity.
- Administer IV infusion of dilute solution of oxytocin within 1–2 h after hypertonic solution instillation and after uterine response to the solution has ceased at rate, 20–100 mU/min. Oxytocin action as an adjunctive uterine stimulant shortens the abortifacient-abortion interval.

S

- Be prepared to treat extraamniotic injection: Stop procedure promptly. Start IV infusion of D5W; additional support for hypernatremic shock.

ADVERSE EFFECTS (≥1%) **Hematologic:** (Within 12–24 h of instillation) Coagulation changes; increased plasma volume, fibrin levels, thrombin, prothrombin, and partial thromboplastin times; mild self-limiting form of disseminated intravascular coagulation. **Metabolic:** Ascites, hypervolemia, circulation failure, uterine necrosis, severe electrolyte disturbances. **Urogenital:** Cervical lacerations and perforation, uterine rupture, retained placenta, hemorrhagic fever, infection, sepsis. **Respiratory:** Pulmonary embolism. **Body as a Whole:** Fever, flushing, cortical necrosis of kidneys.

INTERACTIONS Drug: Indomethacin may delay onset time of abortion; **terbutaline, ritodrine** inhibit uterine activity induced by hypertonic **NaCl.**

PHARMACOKINETICS Absorption: Some drug diffuses into maternal blood. **Onset:** Within 51 h. **Distribution:** Sodium concentration in amniotic fluid must be at least 2.2 mEq/mL to induce abortion; most of drug concentrates in decidua and fetal part of placenta.

NURSING IMPLICATIONS

Assessment & Drug Effects

- Observe patient for at least 30 min after instillation procedure. Be available for complaints and to check vital signs: temperature, pulse rate, BP.
- Note: Intraamniotic instillation is a painless procedure. No anesthetic or sedative is needed or given so that patient is able to report early signs of extraamniotic injection including mental confusion, hypotension, severe headache, vague distress, extreme nervousness, pain, sensation of heat, thirst, fingertip numbness, dry mouth, salty taste, tinnitus.
- Suspect accidental intraperitoneal, intravascular, or myometrial injection if patient begins vomiting. Cardiovascular collapse, seizures, and maternal death may follow.

Patient & Family Education

- Drink at least 2 L water on day of procedure to promote NaCl excretion.
- Return promptly to treatment center with onset of labor, signs of rupture of fetal membrane, vaginal bleeding, fever, or any other untoward symptom.
- Return to physician for evaluation and treatment if labor has not begun within 48 h of hypertonic saline instillation.

SODIUM FERRIC GLUCONATE COMPLEX

(so′di-um fer′ric glu′co-nate)

Ferrlecit

Classifications: BLOOD FORMERS, COAGULATORS AND ANTICOAGULANTS; IRON PREPARATION

Prototype: Ferrous Sulfate

Pregnancy Category: B

AVAILABILITY 62.5 mg elemental iron/5 mL ampule

ACTIONS Stable iron complex used to restore iron loss in chronic kidney failure patients. The use of erythropoietin therapy, and blood loss through hemodialysis requires iron replacement.

THERAPEUTIC EFFECTS The ferric ion combines with transferrin and is transported to bone marrow where it is incorporated into hemoglobin. Indicated by improved Hgb and Hct, iron saturation, serum ferritin levels.

USES Treatment of iron deficiency in patients on chronic hemodialysis and receiving erythropoietin therapy.

CONTRAINDICATIONS All anemias not related to iron deficiency; hypersensitivity to sodium ferric gluconate complex; hemochromatosis, hemosiderosis; hemolytic anemia.
CAUTIOUS USE Active or suspected infection; pregnancy (category B), lactation; older adults. Safety and efficacy in children <18 y are not established.

ROUTE & DOSAGE

Iron Deficiency in Dialysis Patients
Adult: **IV** 125 mg infused over 1 h

ADMINISTRATION

Intravenous

PREPARE: **IV Infusion:** Dilute 10 mL of Ferrlecit in 100 mL of NS. Use immediately after dilution.
ADMINISTER: **IV Infusion:** Give over NOT LESS than 60 min. Never administer at a rate greater than 2.1 mg/min.
INCOMPATIBILITIES **Solution/additive:** Do not mix with any other medications or add to parenteral nutrition solutions.

- Store unopened ampules at 20°–25° C (68°–77° F).

ADVERSE EFFECTS (≥1%) **Body as a Whole:** Hypersensitivity reaction (cardiovascular collapse, cardiac arrest, bronchospasm, oral/pharyngeal edema, dyspnea, angioedema, urticaria, pruritus). **CV:** Flushing, hypotension.

PHARMACOKINETICS Not studied.

NURSING IMPLICATIONS

Assessment & Drug Effects
- Monitor closely for S&S of severe hypersensitivity (see Appendix F) during IV administration.
- Monitor vital signs periodically during IV administration (transient hypotension possible especially during dialysis).
- Stop infusion immediately and notify physician if hypersensitivity is suspected.
- Lab tests: Periodic Hgb, Hct, Fe saturation, serum ferritin.

Patient & Family Education
- Report to physician immediately: Difficulty breathing, itching, flushing, rash, weakness, light-headedness, pain, or any other discomfort during infusion.
- Do not breast feed while taking this drug without consulting physician.

SODIUM FLUORIDE

(sod'i-um)
Fluorinse, Fluoritab, Flura-Drops, Karidium, Pediaflor, Point-Two, Thera-Flur-N
Classifications: ELECTROLYTE AND WATER BALANCE AGENT; DENTAL PROPHYLACTIC
Pregnancy Category: C

AVAILABILITY 0.25 mg, 0.5 mg, 1 mg tablets; 0.125 mg, 0.25 mg, 0.5 mg drops; 0.2 mg/mL solution; 0.02%, 0.04%, 0.09%, 2% rinse; 0.5%, 1.2% gel

ACTIONS Source of the fluorine ion, a trace element. Incorporates into developing tooth enamel, hardens surfaces, and increases resistance to cariogenic microbial processes. Topical application reduces acid production by bacteria in dental plaque and promotes

S

remineralization of acid-damaged enamel. Application to exposed root surfaces supports formation of insoluble materials within dentinal tubules, thereby blocking transport of offending stimuli. Arrests rapid dental decay associated with drug-, radiation-, or age-related xerostomia. One of the few agents known that stimulates osteoblastic activity, leading to increased bone mass.
THERAPEUTIC EFFECTS Topical application reduces acid production by bacteria in dental plaque and promotes remineralization of enamel.

USES When fluoride ion concentration in drinking water is 0.7 ppm or less, to prevent periodontal disease and dental caries, to treat dental cervical hypersensitivity, and to control dental caries associated with xerostomia.
UNLABELED USES Adjunctive treatment of osteoporosis; management of bone lesions in multiple myeloma; to reduce bone pain in patient with metastatic prostatic carcinoma; to stabilize progression of hearing loss in a limited number of patients with otosclerosis.

CONTRAINDICATIONS When daily intake of fluoride from drinking water exceeds 0.7 ppm; low-sodium or sodium-free diets; hypersensitivity to fluoride; gels or dental rinses by children <6 y, 1 mg tablet or rinse in children <3 y, or 1 mg rinse in children <6 y, pregnancy (category C).

S

ROUTE & DOSAGE

Prevent Periodontal Disease (Drinking Water Concentration <0.3 ppm)
Child: **PO** *Birth–2 y,* 0.25 mg/d; *2–3 y,* 0.5 mg/d; *3–13 y,* 1 mg/d

Prevent Periodontal Disease (Drinking Water Concentration 0.3–0.7 ppm)
Child: **PO** *Birth–2 y,* 0.125 mg/d; *2–3 y,* 0.25 mg/d; *3–13 y,* 0.5 mg/d

Prevent Dental Caries
Child: **Topical** *6–12 y,* 5 mL of 0.2% solution daily; *>12 y,* 10 mL of 0.2% solution daily

Desensitization of Exposed Root Surfaces
Child: **Topical** 0.2% rinsing solution once nightly after brushing and flossing

ADMINISTRATION

Oral

- Avoid giving sodium fluoride with milk or dairy products. Calcium from these products combines with fluorine, decreasing its absorption.
- Give drops preferably after meals. Give undiluted or mixed with fluids or foods.
- Dissolve tablets in the mouth or chew before swallowing. Administer at bedtime (after brushing the teeth).

Topical

- Apply all fluorine preparations after thoroughly brushing and flossing; preferably at bedtime.
- Do not swallow topical or rinse preparations.
- If patient's mouth is sore, the neutral preparation (Thera-Flur N) is better tolerated.
- Use as treatment for dental cervical hypersensitivity: thoroughly brush teeth; then swish PO solution around and between teeth for 1 min; expectorate. If gel is used, apply a few drops to toothbrush and brush gently onto affected surfaces.
- Apply Gel-drops with applicators supplied by the dentist. Spread gel

on inner surfaces of applicators, which are placed over lower and upper teeth at the same time. User bites down lightly for 6 min, then removes applicators and rinses mouth thoroughly. Applicators are cleaned with cold water.

- Store all forms in tight plastic or paraffin-lined glass containers (sodium fluoride reacts with ordinary glass at a slow but appreciable rate) at 15°–30° C (59°–86° F). Avoid freezing.

ADVERSE EFFECTS (≥1%) **Skin:** Rash, atopic dermatitis, urticaria, stomatitis. **Body as a Whole:** GI and respiratory allergic reactions, salty or soapy taste, dehydration, thirst, excessive salivation, muscle weakness, tremors, <u>shock, death from cardiac and respiratory failure</u>. **Musculoskeletal:** Dental fluorosis (brown or white mottling of tooth enamel), osseous fluorosis (patchy mineralization and possible decrease in bone strength).

INTERACTIONS Drug: Aluminum, calcium, magnesium-containing products may decrease **fluoride** absorption.

PHARMACOKINETICS Absorption: Readily absorbed from GI tract. **Distribution:** Fluoride is stored in bones and teeth; crosses placenta; distributed into breast milk. **Elimination:** Rapidly excreted, primarily in urine with small amounts in feces.

NURSING IMPLICATIONS

Assessment & Drug Effect

- Monitor therapeutic effectiveness.

Patient & Family Education

- Do not eat, drink, or rinse mouth for at least 30 min after using the rinsing solution.
- Do not exceed recommended dosage. If mottling of teeth occurs, notify dentist.
- Apply sodium fluoride gel or solution used in orthodontic treatment regimen immediately before attachment or reattachment of the tooth-encircling bands.
- To be effective, fluorine supplementation must be consistent and continuous from infancy until 12–14 y.
- Consult dentist about continuing fluoride therapy if you move or there is a change in water supply (mottling may occur if drinking water has fluorine content >1.5 ppm).
- Do not breast feed while taking or using this drug without consulting physician.

SODIUM OXYBATE (GHB)

(sod'i-um ox'y-bate)

Xyrem

Classifications: CENTRAL NERVOUS SYSTEM AGENT; CNS DEPRESSANT

Pregnancy Category: B

Controlled Substance: Schedule III

AVAILABILITY 500 mg/mL solution

ACTIONS CNS depressant; the precise mechanism by which sodium oxybate produces anticataplexy in narcolepsy is unknown. Sodium oxybate is GHB, a known drug of abuse.

THERAPEUTIC EFFECTS Produces anticataplectic effects in narcolepsy and decreases the number of cataplexy events in individuals with narcolepsy.

USES Treatment of cataplexy in patients with narcolepsy.

CONTRAINDICATIONS Alcohol or sedative hypnotics or other CNS depressants; patients being treated with sedative hypnotic agents; psychosis; patients with succinic semialdehyde dehydrogenase deficiency;

S

compromised respiratory drive, severe depression, or suicide tendencies; lactation; children <16 y.

CAUTIOUS USE Hepatic dysfunction; compromised respiratory function; sleep disorders; history of seizures; heart failure, hypertension, impaired renal function; previous history of depressive illness or suicide attempt; elderly; sleepwalking; pregnancy (category B).

ROUTE & DOSAGE

Cataplexy

Adult: **PO** Start with 2.25 g given at bedtime while in bed and repeated 2.5–4 h later. Dose may be increased by 1.5 g/d every 2 wk to a max of 9 g/d in 2 divided doses

Hepatic Impairment

Reduce dose by 50% in patients with hepatic impairment

ADMINISTRATION

Oral

- Give at bedtime at least 2–3 h after the evening meal.
- Dilute each dose with 2 oz (60 mL) of water in the dosing cups provided.
- Instruct patient to remain in bed after taking sodium oxybate.
- Discard any diluted dose that has not been used within 24 h.
- Store at 15°–30° C (59°–86° F).

ADVERSE EFFECTS (≥1%) **Body as a Whole:** *Pain, infection,* flu-like syndrome, asthenia, allergic reactions, chills. **CNS:** Confusion, depression, sleepwalking, *headache, dizziness, somnolence,* nervousness, abnormal dreams, insomnia, agitation, ataxia, convulsion, stupor, tremor. **CV:** Hypertension. **GI:** *Nausea,* diarrhea, vomiting, dyspepsia, abdominal pain, anorexia, constipation. **Metabolic:** Increased alkaline phosphatase, edema, hypercholesteremia, hypocalcemia, weight gain. **Respiratory:** *Pharyngitis,* rhinitis, sinusitis **Skin:** Increased sweating, acne, alopecia, rash. **Special Senses:** Amblyopia, tinnitus. **Urogenital:** Urinary incontinence, dysmenorrhea, albuminuria, cystitis, hematuria, metrorrhagia, urinary frequency.

INTERACTIONS Drug: Alcohol, SEDATIVE-HYPNOTICS, other CNS DEPRESSANTS may increase CNS depressant effects. **Food: High fat meal** will significantly reduce absorption.

PHARMACOKINETICS Absorption: Incompletely absorbed, 25% reaches systemic circulation. **Peak:** 0.05–1.25 h. **Metabolism:** Oxidized in the Kreb's cycle to carbon dioxide and water. **Elimination:** Primarily eliminated as carbon dioxide in respiration. **Half-Life:** 0.5–1 h.

NURSING IMPLICATIONS

Assessment & Drug Effects

- Monitor for and report immediately any of the following: seizure, respiratory depression, or decreased level of consciousness.
- Monitor closely patients with hepatic insufficiency for adverse events.
- Monitor for and report excessive weight gain and development of edema.
- Lab tests: Perform baseline LFTs; monitor periodically serum electrolytes and lipid profile.

Patient & Family Education

- Do not take sodium oxybate at any time other than at night, immediately before bedtime.
- Be consistent with timing of the evening meal and take this drug at least 2–3 h after eating.

- Prepare both doses prior to bedtime. After ingesting each dose remain in bed.
- Do not consume alcohol or use other sedative hypnotic drugs with sodium oxybate.
- Do not drive or engage in potentially hazardous activities until reaction to drug is known.
- Do not breast feed while taking this drug without consulting physician.

SODIUM POLYSTYRENE SULFONATE

(pol-ee-stye'reen)

Kayexalate, SPS Suspension

Classifications: ELECTROLYTE AND WATER BALANCE AGENT; CATION EXCHANGE

Pregnancy Category: C

AVAILABILITY 15 g/60 mL suspension; 100 mg/g powder

ACTIONS Sulfonic cation-exchange resin that removes potassium from body by exchanging sodium ion for potassium, particularly in large intestine; potassium-containing resin is then excreted. Small amounts of other cations such as calcium and magnesium may be lost during treatment.

THERAPEUTIC EFFECTS Removes potassium from body by exchanging sodium ion for potassium through the large intestine.

USES Hyperkalemia.

CONTRAINDICATIONS Patients with hypokalemia; hypersensitivity to Kayexalate.

CAUTIOUS USE Older adults; acute or chronic kidney failure; patients receiving digitalis preparations; patients who cannot tolerate even a small increase in sodium load (e.g., CHF, severe hypertension, and marked edema); pregnancy (category C), lactation.

ROUTE & DOSAGE

Hyperkalemia

Adult: **PO** 15 g suspended in 70% sorbitol or 20–100 mL of other fluid 1–4 times/d **PR** 30–50 g/100 mL 70% sorbitol q6h as warm emulsion high into sigmoid colon

Child: **PO** Calculate appropriate amount on exchange rate of 1 mEq of potassium per gram of resin and suspend in 70% sorbitol or other appropriate solution (Usual dose: 1 g/kg q6h) **PR** 1 g/kg q2–6h

ADMINISTRATION

Oral

- Give as a suspension in a small quantity of water or in syrup. Usual amount of fluid ranges from 20–100 mL or approximately 3–4 mL/g of drug.

Rectal

- Use warm fluid (as prescribed) to prepare the emulsion for enema.
- Administer at body temperature and introduce by gravity, keeping suspension particles in solution by stirring. Flush suspension with 50–100 mL of fluid; then clamp tube and leave it in place.
- Urge patient to retain enema at least 30–60 min but as long as several hours if possible.
- Irrigate colon (after enema solution has been expelled) with 1 or 2 quarts flushing solution (nonsodium containing). Drain returns constantly through a Y-tube connection.
- Store remainder of prepared solution for 24 h; then discard.

S

ADVERSE EFFECTS (≥1%) **GI:** *Constipation, fecal impaction (in older adults);* anorexia, gastric irritation, nausea, vomiting, diarrhea (with sorbitol emulsions). **Metabolic:** Sodium retention, hypocalcemia, hypokalemia, hypomagnesemia.

INTERACTIONS Drug: ANTACIDS, LAXATIVES containing **calcium** or **magnesium** may decrease potassium exchange capability of the resin.

PHARMACOKINETICS Absorption: Not absorbed systemically. **Onset:** Several hours to days. **Metabolism:** Not metabolized. **Elimination:** Excreted in feces.

NURSING IMPLICATIONS

Assessment & Drug Effects

- Lab tests: Determine serum potassium levels daily throughout therapy. Monitor acid–base balance, electrolytes, and minerals in patients receiving repeated doses.
- Serum potassium levels do not always reflect intracellular potassium deficiency. Observe patient closely for early clinical signs of severe hypokalemia (see Appendix F). ECGs are also recommended.
- Consult physician about restricting sodium content from dietary and other sources since drug contains approximately 100 mg (4.1 mEq) of sodium per gram (1 tsp, 15 mEq sodium).

Patient & Family Education

- Check bowel function daily. Usually, a mild laxative is prescribed to prevent constipation (common adverse effect). Older adult patients are particularly prone to fecal impaction.

SOLIFENACIN SUCCINATE

(sol-i-fen′a-sin)

VESIcare

Classifications: AUTONOMIC NERVOUS SYSTEM AGENT; ANTICHOLINERGIC; PARASYMPATHOLYTIC; ANTIMUSCARINIC; ANTISPASMODIC

Prototype: Atropine

Pregnancy Category: C

AVAILABILITY 5 mg, 10 mg tablets

ACTIONS Solifenacin is a selective muscarinic antagonist that depresses both voluntary and involuntary bladder contractions caused by detrusor overactivity.

THERAPEUTIC EFFECTS Solifenacin improves the volume of urine per void and reduces the frequency of incontinent and urgency episodes.

USES Treatment of overactive bladder (OAB) with symptoms of urinary incontinence, urgency, and frequency.

CONTRAINDICATIONS Hypersensitivity to solifenacin or any component of its formulations; severe hepatic impairment; pregnancy (category C); gastric retention; uncontrolled narrow-angle glaucoma; urinary retention; toxic megacolon; GI obstruction; ileus; GERD.

CAUTIOUS USE Bladder outflow obstruction; concurrent use of ketoconazole or other potent CYP3A4 inhibitors; obstructive disorders; decreased GI motility; hepatic impairment; history of QT prolongation or concurrent use of medications known to prolong the QT interval; controlled narrow-angle glaucoma; renal impairment; renal disease; renal failure; mild to moderate hepatic impairment; older adults.

ROUTE & DOSAGE

Overactive Bladder

Adult: **PO** 5 mg once daily; may be increased to 10 mg once daily if tolerated (max of 5 mg/d if taking drugs that inhibit CYP3A4—see Interactions, Drug)

Adjustment for Hepatic Impairment

If moderate hepatic impairment, does not exceed 5 mg/d. If severe hepatic impairment, do not use.

Adjustment for Renal Impairment

Cl_{cr} <30 mL/min: max dose 5 mg/d

ADMINISTRATION

Oral

- Tablets should be swallowed whole.
- Store at 15–30° C (59–86° F).

ADVERSE EFFECTS (≥1%) **Body as a Whole:** Edema, fatigue. **CNS:** Dizziness, depression. **CV:** Hypertension. **GI:** *Dry mouth, constipation,* nausea, vomiting, dyspepsia, upper abdominal pain. **Respiratory:** Cough. **Special Senses:** Blurred vision, dry eyes. **Urogenital:** Urinary tract infection, urinary retention.

INTERACTIONS Drug: CYP3A4 INHIBITORS (e.g., **clarithromycin, delavirdine, diltiazem, efavirenz, erythromycin, fluconazole, fluvoxamine, itraconazole, nefazodone, norfloxacin, omeprazole,** PROTEASE INHIBITORS, **quinine, verapamil, troleandomycin, voriconazole, zafirlukast**) may increase levels and toxicity (max dose 5 mg/d); **amantadine, amoxapine, bupropion, clozapine, cyclobenzaprine, diphenhydramine, disopyramide, maprotiline, olanzapine, orphenadrine,** PHENOTHIAZINES, TRICYCLIC ANTIDEPRESSANTS have additive anticholinergic adverse effects. **Food: Grapefruit juice** may increase solifenacin levels and toxicity.

PHARMACOKINETICS Absorption: 90% absorbed from GI tract. **Peak:** 3–8 h. **Metabolism:** Extensively metabolized in the liver by CYP3A4. **Elimination:** Primarily excreted in urine, 22% excreted in feces. **Half-Life:** 45–68 h.

NURSING IMPLICATIONS

Assessment & Drug Effects

- Monitor ECG in patients with a known history of QT prolongation or patients taking medications that prolong the QT interval.

Patient & Family Education

- Stop taking this drug and report to physician if urinary retention occurs.
- Report promptly any of the following: blurred vision or difficulty focusing vision, palpitations, confusion, or severe dizziness.
- Report to physician problems with bowel elimination, especially constipation lasting 3 or more days.
- Exercise caution in hot environments, as the risk of heat prostration increases with this drug.
- Do not breast feed while taking this drug without consulting physician.

S

SOMATREM

(soe′ma-trem)

Protropin

Classifications: HORMONE AND SYNTHETIC SUBSTITUTE; GROWTH HORMONE

Prototype: Somatropin

Pregnancy Category: C

AVAILABILITY 5 mg (approximately 15 IU), 10 mg (approximately 30 IU) vials

ACTIONS Biosynthetic product of recombinant DNA technology. Contains exact sequence of 191 amino acids in pituitary-derived human growth hormone (GH) plus an amino terminal methionyl group not found in natural GH. In presence of GH deficiency, promotes skeletal growth at epiphyseal plates of long bones by increasing levels of the mediator somatomedin-C and by increasing synthesis of protein, chondroitin sulfate, and collagen. Increases number and size of muscle cells. May induce GH antibody formation (IgG), but effect of antibodies on endogenous GH activity is unknown.

THERAPEUTIC EFFECTS Therapeutically equivalent to natural GH (somatropin) of pituitary origin. Affects metabolism and growth of most body tissues including red cell mass, with possible exception of eye and brain.

USES Long-term treatment of children with growth failure due to deficiency of endogenous GH.

CONTRAINDICATIONS Patient with closed epiphyses; underlying progressive intracranial tumor; pregnancy (category C).

CAUTIOUS USE Diabetes mellitus or family history of the disease; concomitant use of glucocorticoids; concomitant or prior use of thyroid or androgens in prepubertal male; hypothyroidism. Patient with known sensitivity to benzyl alcohol; lactation.

S

ROUTE & DOSAGE

Growth Hormone Deficiency

Child: **IM/SC** Doses up to 0.1 mg/kg (0.2 U/kg) 3 times/wk with a minimum of 48 h between doses, may be increased in older children if epiphyses have not closed

ADMINISTRATION

Intramuscular/Subcutaneous

- Reconstitute each vial (containing 5 mL lyophilized powder) with 1–5 mL bacteriostatic water for injection, aiming stream of water against vial wall. Swirl vial gently to mix contents. Do not shake.
- Note: pH of reconstituted solution is about 7.8.
- Do not use if reconstituted solution is cloudy or has crystals immediately after reconstitution or refrigeration.
- Reconstitute with sterile water for injection, USP, when administering to newborns; benzyl alcohol is the preservative in bacteriostatic water for injection and may be toxic to this age group.
- Use disposable syringe small enough to administer prescribed doses with accuracy and needle long enough to ensure injection into muscle layer.
- Discard unused reconstituted solution within 7 d.
- Store lyophilized powder and reconstituted solution at 2°–8° C (36°–46° F). Do not freeze. Expiration dates are on labels.

ADVERSE EFFECTS (≥1%) **Body as a Whole:** Allergic reactions, peripheral edema, headache, myalgia, weakness, organ enlargement, acromegalic features in children. **CV:** Hypertension, atherosclerosis. **Metabolic:** Glucose intolerance, ACTH deficiency, hypothyroidism, diabetes. **Other:** Recurrent intracranial tumor growth, persistent antibodies to GH; pain, swelling at injection site.

DIAGNOSTIC TEST INTERFERENCE Somatrem may reduce ***glucose tolerance, serum T_4 (thyroxin) concentration, RAI uptake,*** and ***thyroxine-binding capacity.***

INTERACTIONS Drug: ANABOLIC STEROIDS, **thyroid hormone,** ANDROGENS, ESTROGENS may accelerate epiphyseal closure; **ACTH,** CORTICOSTEROIDS may inhibit growth response to somatrem.

PHARMACOKINETICS Metabolism: Metabolized in liver. **Elimination:** Excreted in urine. **Half-Life:** 3–5 h with chronic administration.

NURSING IMPLICATIONS

Assessment & Drug Effects

- Assess bone age annually in all patients and especially those also receiving thyroid, androgen, or estrogen replacement therapy, since concurrent use of these agents may precipitate early epiphyseal closure. Urge parent to take child for growth assessment on appointed annual dates.
- Evaluate thyroid status at regular intervals. Untreated hypothyroidism may interfere with response to drug.
- Observe diabetics or those with family history of diabetes closely. Check blood or urine glucose and HbA_{1C} regularly to recognize glucose intolerance.

Patient & Family Education

- Be aware that first year growth of 17.5 cm (7 in) with somatrem has been reported, but average expectations are 7.5–12.5 cm (3–5 in), slightly less in second year, and after that, normal growth rate. Also, subcutaneous fat diminishes but returns to pretreatment level later.
- Record accurate height measurements at regular intervals and report to physician if rate is less than expected.
- Report child's complaints of hip or knee pain or a limp. Slipped capital femoral epiphysis may occur in patients with endocrine disorders.

SOMATROPIN ⓟ

(soe-ma-troe'pin)

Bio-Tropin, Genotropin, Humatrope, Norditropin, Norditropin NordiFlex, Nutropin, Nutropin AQ, Nutropin AQ Pen, Serostim, Saizen, Zorptive

Classifications: HORMONES & SYNTHETIC SUBSTITUTES; GROWTH HORMONE

Pregnancy Category: B, C (brand dependent)

AVAILABILITY 1.5 mg, 4 mg, 5 mg, 5.8 mg, 6 mg, 8 mg, 10 mg injection; 5 mg/1.5 mL, 15 mg/1.5 mL prefilled syringe

ACTIONS New recombinant growth hormone with the natural sequence of 191 amino acids characteristic of endogenous growth hormone (GH). Differs from somatrem by absence of an extra methionyl group in its structure. Somatropin appears to be less likely to produce serum antibodies to endogenous GH than somatrem.

THERAPEUTIC EFFECTS Induces growth responses similar to those produced in children treated with somatrem or with GH obtained from human pituitary glands.

USES Growth failure due to GH deficiency; replacement therapy prior to epiphyseal closure in patients with idiopathic GH deficiency; GH deficiency secondary to intracranial tumors or panhypopituitarism; inadequate GH secretion; short stature in girls with Turner's syndrome; AIDS wasting syndrome; short bowel syndrome.

CONTRAINDICATIONS Patient with closed epiphyses; underlying progressive intracranial tumor, cresol hypersensitivity, glycerin hypersensitivity; diabetic retinopathy; during chemotherapy, radiation therapy, active neoplastic disease; Prader-Willi syndrome; untreated hypothyroidism, obesity; pregnancy (category B or category C depending on the brand).

CAUTIOUS USE Diabetes mellitus or family history of the disease; lactation; concomitant or prior use of thyroid or androgens in prepubertal male; hypothyroidism; surgery, trauma; neonates with benzyl alcohol hypersensitivity; neonates.

ROUTE & DOSAGE

Note: Dosing will vary with specific products

Growth Hormone Deficiency

Adult: **SC Humatrope** 0.006 mg/kg (0.018 IU/kg) q.d., may increase (max: 0.0125 mg/kg/d [0.0375 IU/kg/d]); **Nutropin, Nutropin AQ** 0.006 mg/kg q.d. (max: *<35 y,* 0.025 mg/kg/d; *>35 y,* 0.0125 mg/kg/d)

Child: **SC Genotropin** 0.16–0.24 mg/kg/wk divided into 6–7 q.d. doses; **Humatrope** 0.18 mg/kg/wk (0.54 IU/kg/wk) divided into equal doses given on either 3 alternate days or 6 times/wk; **Norditropin** 0.024–0.034 mg/kg/d 6–7 times/wk; **Nutropin, Nutropin AQ** 0.3 mg/kg/wk (0.9 IU/kg/wk) divided into 6–7 q.d. doses

Inadequate Growth Hormone Secretion

Child: **SC Nutropin** 0.3 mg/kg every week

AIDS Wasting or Cachexia

Adult: **SC Serostim** *>55 kg,* 6 mg qh.s.; *45–55 kg,* 5 mg qh.s.; *35–45 kg,* 4 mg qh.s.; *<35 kg,* 0.1 mg/kg qh.s.

Short Bowel Syndrome

Adult: **SC Zorptive** 0.1 mg/kg once daily for 4 wk (max: 8 mg/d)

ADMINISTRATION

Subcutaneous

- Reconstitute each brand following it's manufacturer's instructions (vary from brand to brand).
- Read and carefully follow directions for use supplied with the Nutropin AQ Pen™ Cartridge if this is the product being used.
- Rotate injection sites; abdomen and thighs are preferred sites. Do not use buttocks until the child has been walking for a year or more and the muscle is adequately developed.
- Store lyophilized powder at 2°–8° C (36°–46° F). After reconstitution, most preparations are stable for at least 14 d under refrigeration. DO NOT FREEZE.

ADVERSE EFFECTS (≥1%) **Body as a Whole:** Pain, swelling at injection site; myalgia. Fatalities reported in patients with Prader-Willi syndrome and one or more of severe obesity, history of respiratory impairment or sleep apnea, or unidentified respiratory infection, especially male patients. **Metabolic:** *Hypercalciuria;* over saturation of bile with cholesterol, hyperglycemia, ketosis. **Endocrine:** High circulating GH antibodies with resulting treatment failure, accelerated growth of intracranial tumor.

INTERACTIONS Drug: ANABOLIC STEROIDS, **thyroid hormone,** ANDROGENS, ESTROGENS may accelerate epiphyseal closure; **ACTH,** CORTICOSTEROIDS may inhibit growth response to somatropin.

PHARMACOKINETICS Metabolism: Metabolized in liver. **Elimination:** Excreted in urine. **Half-Life:** 15–50 min.

NURSING IMPLICATIONS

Assessment & Drug Effects

- Assess bone age annually in all patients and especially those also receiving concurrent thyroid or androgen treatment, since these drugs may precipitate early epiphyseal closure. Urge parent to take child for bone age assessment on appointed annual dates.

- Lab test: Periodic serum and urine calcium and plasma glucose.
- Hypercalciuria, a frequent adverse effect in the first 2–3 mo of therapy, may be symptomless; however, it may be accompanied by renal calculi, with these reportable symptoms: flank pain and colic, GI symptoms, urinary frequency, chills, fever, hematuria.
- Test for circulating GH antibodies (antisomatropin antibodies) in patients who respond initially but later fail to respond to therapy.
- Observe diabetics or those with family history of diabetes closely. Obtain regular urine for glycosuria or fasting blood glucose and HbA_{1C}.
- Examine patients with GH deficiency secondary to intracranial lesion frequently for progression or recurrence of underlying disease.

Patient & Family Education

- Be aware that during first 6 mo of successful treatment, linear growth rates may be increased 8–16 cm or more per year (average about 7 cm/y or approximately 3 in.). Additionally, SC fat diminishes but returns to pretreatment value later.
- Record accurate height measurements at regular intervals and report to physician if rate is less than expected.
- In general, growth response to somatropin is inversely proportional to duration of treatment.
- Discontinue treatment when patient has reached satisfactory adult height, when epiphyses have fused, or when patient fails to exhibit growth response.

SOTALOL

(so-ta'lol)

Betapace, Betapace AF

Classifications: AUTONOMIC NERVOUS SYSTEM AGENT; BETA-ADRENERGIC ANTAGONIST (BLOCKING AGENT, SYMPATHOLYTIC); CARDIOVASCULAR AGENT; ANTIARRHYTHMIC CLASS III

Prototype: Amiodarone

Pregnancy Category: B

AVAILABILITY **Betapace** 80 mg, 120 mg, 160 mg, 240 mg tablets. **Betapace AF** 80 mg, 120 mg, 160 mg tablets

ACTIONS Has both class II and class III antiarrhythmic properties. Slows heart rate, decreases AV nodal conduction, and increases AV nodal refractoriness.

THERAPEUTIC EFFECTS Produces significant reductions in both systolic and diastolic blood pressure. Antiarrhythmic properties are effective in controlling ventricular arrhythmias as well as atrial fibrillation/flutter.

USES Treatment of life-threatening ventricular arrhythmias (sustained ventricular tachycardia) and maintenance of normal sinus rhythm in patients with atrial fibrillation/flutter.

UNLABELED USES Hypertension, angina.

CONTRAINDICATIONS Hypersensitivity to sotalol; bronchial asthma, sinus bradycardia, sick sinus syndrome; second and third degree heart block, long QT syndrome, cardiogenic shock, uncontrolled CHF; chronic bronchitis, emphysema; hypokalemia <4 mEq/L; creatinine clearance of <40 mL/min; lactation.

S

CAUTIOUS USE CHF, electrolyte disturbances, recent MI, diabetes, sick sinus rhythm, renal impairment; pregnancy (category B); concomitant use of drugs which prolong the QT segment, and antiarrhythmic drugs; excessive diarrhea, or profuse sweating.

ROUTE & DOSAGE

Ventricular Arrhythmias (Betapace)

Adult: **PO** Initial dose of 80 mg b.i.d. or 160 mg q.d. taken prior to meals, may increase every 3–4 d in 40–160 mg increments (most patients respond to 240–320 mg/d in 2 or 3 divided doses, doses >640 mg/d have not been studied)

Renal Impairment

Cl_{cr} >60 mL/min: q12h; 30–60 mL/min: q24h; 10–30 mL/min: q36–48h; <10 mL/min: Individualize carefully

Atrial Fibrillation/flutter (Betapace AF)

Adult: **PO** Initial dose of 80 mg b.i.d., may increase every 3–4 d (max: 240 mg/d in 1–2 divided doses)

Renal Impairment

Cl_{cr} >60 mL/min: q12h; 40–60 mL/min: q24h; <40 mL/min contraindicated

ADMINISTRATION

Oral

- Give on an empty stomach 1 h before or 2 h after meals. Do not give with milk or milk products.
- Initiate and increase doses only under close supervision, preferably in a hospital with cardiac rhythm monitoring and frequent assessment.
- Use smallest effective dose for patients with nonallergic bronchospasms.
- Do not discontinue drug abruptly. Gradually reduce dose over 1–2 wk.
- Store at room temperature, 15°–30° C (59°–86° F).

ADVERSE EFFECTS (≥1%) **CV:** AV block, hypotension, aggravation of CHF, although the incidence of heart failure may be lower than for other beta-blockers, <u>life-threatening ventricular arrhythmias, including polymorphous ventricular tachycardia or torsades de pointes</u>, *bradycardia, dyspnea, chest pain, palpitation,* bleeding (<2%). **CNS:** Headache, *fatigue, dizziness,* weakness, lethargy, depression, lassitude. **GI:** Nausea, vomiting, diarrhea, dyspepsia, dry mouth. **Urogenital:** Impotence, decreased libido. **Metabolic:** Hyperglycemia. **Special Senses:** Visual disturbances. **Respiratory:** Respiratory complaints. **Skin:** Rash.

INTERACTIONS Drug: Antagonizes the effects of BETA AGONISTS. **Amiodarone** may lead to symptomatic bradycardia and sinus arrest. **Astemizole** may prolong QT interval leading to arrhythmias. The hypoglycemic effects of ORAL HYPOGLYCEMIC AGENTS may be potentiated. May cause resistance to **epinephrine** in anaphylactic reactions. Should be used with caution with other ANTIARRHYTHMIC AGENTS. **Food:** absorption of **sotalol** may be reduced by food, especially **milk** and MILK PRODUCTS.

PHARMACOKINETICS Absorption: Slowly and completely absorbed from GI tract. Negligible first-pass metabolism. Absorption of sotalol may be reduced by food, especially milk and milk products. **Peak:** 2–3 h. **Duration:** 24 h. **Distri-**

bution: Drug is hydrophilic and will enter the CSF slowly (about 10%). Crosses placental barrier. Distributed in breast milk. Not appreciably protein bound. **Metabolism:** Does not undergo significant hepatic enzyme metabolism and no active metabolites have been identified. **Elimination:** Excreted by glomerular filtration in the urine with 75% of the drug excreted unchanged within 72 h. **Half-Life:** 7–18 h.

NURSING IMPLICATIONS

Assessment & Drug Effects

- Monitor ECG for initial baseline and periodically thereafter (especially when doses are increased) because proarrhythmic events most often occur within 7 d of initiating therapy or increasing dose.
- Lab test: Baseline serum electrolytes. Correct electrolyte imbalances of hypokalemia or hypomagnesemia prior to initiating therapy.
- Monitor cardiac status carefully, including ECG, throughout therapy. Exercise special caution when sotalol is used concurrently with other antiarrhythmics, digoxin, or calcium channel blockers.
- Monitor patients with bronchospastic disease (e.g., bronchitis, emphysema) carefully for inhibition of bronchodilation.
- Monitor diabetics for loss of glycemic control. Beta blockage reduces the release of endogenous insulin in response to hyperglycemia and may blunt symptoms of acute hypoglycemia (e.g., tachycardia, BP changes).

Patient & Family Education

- Be aware of risk for hypotension and syncope, especially with concurrent treatment with catecholamine-depleting drugs (e.g., reserpine, guanethidine).
- Take radial pulse daily and report marked bradycardia (pulse below 60 or other established parameter) to physician.
- Type 2 diabetics are at increased risk for hyperglycemia. All diabetics are at risk of possible masking of symptoms of hypoglycemia.
- Do not abruptly discontinue drug because of the risk of exacerbation of angina, arrhythmias, and possible myocardial infarction.
- Do not breast feed while taking this drug.

SPARFLOXACIN

(spar-flox'a-sin)

Zagam

Classifications: ANTIINFECTIVE; QUINOLONE

Prototype: Ciprofloxacin

Pregnancy Category: C

AVAILABILITY 200 mg tablets

ACTIONS Synthetic quinolone that is a broad-spectrum bactericidal agent. Inhibits DNA-gyrase, an enzyme necessary for bacterial DNA replication and some aspects of transcription, repair, recombination, and transposition.

THERAPEUTIC EFFECTS Effective against many gram-positive and gram-negative organisms. Indicated by negative cultures and resolution of S&S of infection.

USES Treatment of community-acquired pneumonia, acute exacerbations of chronic bronchitis caused by susceptible bacteria.

CONTRAINDICATIONS History of hypersensitivity or photosensitivity reactions; patients with known QT_c prolongation, antiarrhythmic agents that prolong the QT_C interval (e.g., Class 1A and Class III); exposure to sun while taking sparfloxacin; pregnancy (category C), lactation; hypokalemia, significant bradycardia, CHF, myocardial ischemia, and atrial fibrillation.

CAUTIOUS USE History of seizures; kidney dysfunction with Cl_{cr} <50 mL/min; severe cerebral arteriosclerosis. Safety and effectiveness in children <18 y are not established.

ROUTE & DOSAGE

Community-Acquired Pneumonia, Bronchitis

Adult: **PO** 400 mg day 1, then 200 mg q.d. day 2–10

Renal Impairment

Cl_{cr} <50 mL/min: 400 mg day 1, then 200 mg q48h day 2–10

ADMINISTRATION

Oral

- Do not give drug within 4 h of drugs containing aluminum, magnesium, iron, zinc, calcium, or sucralfate.
- Store at 20°–25° C (68°–77° F) in a tightly closed container.

ADVERSE EFFECTS (≥1%) **CNS:** Headache, dizziness, insomnia, somnolence. **CV:** Prolonged QT_C interval on ECG. **GI:** Pseudomembranous colitis, diarrhea, nausea, dyspepsia, abdominal pain, taste perversion, vomiting, flatulence, dry mouth. **Skin:** *Phototoxicity* (burning, redness, swelling, blisters, rash, itching, dermatitis), pruritus, rash. **Urogenital:** Vaginal moniliasis.

DIAGNOSTIC TEST INTERFERENCE May cause false positive on ***opiate screening tests.***

INTERACTIONS Drug: MAGNESIUM- or ALUMINUM-CONTAINING ANTACIDS decrease absorption; torsades de pointes arrhythmias in patients on **disopyramide, amiodarone, quinidine, procainamide, sotalol, bepridil.**

PHARMACOKINETICS Absorption: Rapidly absorbed from GI tract. 92% bioavailability. **Peak:** 3–6 h. **Distribution:** 45% protein bound. Penetrates lower respiratory tract tissues. Crosses placenta, distributed into breast milk. **Metabolism:** Metabolized in the liver. Does not utilize Cyt P450 enzymes. **Elimination:** Excreted in urine. **Half-Life:** 20 h (16–30 h).

NURSING IMPLICATIONS

Assessment & Drug Effects

- Lab tests: Obtain C&S prior to beginning therapy and periodically during therapy.
- Do not give sparfloxacin to persons with proarrhythmic conditions such as hypokalemia, CHF, atrial fibrillation, etc.
- Discontinue therapy and notify physician immediately if any of the following occur: Skin rash or other signs of a hypersensitivity reaction (see Appendix F); skin eruption following sun exposure; symptoms of colitis such as persistent diarrhea; joint pain, inflammation, or other signs of rupture of a tendon; CNS symptoms such as seizures, restlessness, anxiety, confusion, hallucinations, depression, suicidal ideation.
- Monitor those at risk for seizures carefully.

Patient & Family Education

- Learn important indications for discontinuing drug and immediately notifying physician.

- Drink fluids liberally while taking sparfloxacin.
- Allow a minimum of 4 h between drug and any of the following: Aluminum or magnesium antacids, iron and calcium supplements, multivitamins with zinc, or sucralfate.
- Avoid all exposure to direct or indirect sunlight or artificial UV light during treatment and for 5 d after therapy. If brief sunlight exposure is necessary, cover as much skin surface as possible with clothing. Discontinue drug at first sign of phototoxicity (e.g., burning skin, redness, swelling, itching) and notify physician.

SPECTINOMYCIN HYDROCHLORIDE

(spek-ti-noe-mye'sin)

Trobicin

Classifications: ANTIINFECTIVE; ANTIBIOTIC

Pregnancy Category: B

AVAILABILITY 400 mg injection

ACTIONS Antibiotic produced by *Streptomyces spectabilis*. Action is usually bacteriostatic. Variable activity against a wide variety of gram-negative and gram-positive organisms.

THERAPEUTIC EFFECTS Inhibits majority of *Neisseria gonorrhoeae* strains; effective for urethral and anorectal infections, but not pharyngeal. Not active against syphilis or chlamydial and mycoplasmal infections.

USES Only for treatment of uncomplicated gonorrhea in patients sensitized or resistant to penicillin or other effective drugs approved by US Centers for Disease Control.

UNLABELED USES Disseminated gonococcal infections caused by penicillinase-producing strains of *N. gonorrhoeae* (PPNG) and sexually transmitted epididymoorchitis.

CONTRAINDICATIONS Safety during pregnancy (category B), lactation, and in infants and children is not established.

CAUTIOUS USE History of allergies.

ROUTE & DOSAGE

Uncomplicated Gonorrhea

Adult: **IM** 2 g as single dose

Child: **IM** 40 mg/kg as single dose

Disseminated Gonorrhea

Adult: **IM** 2 g q12h

ADMINISTRATION

Intramuscular

- Give IM injection deep into upper outer quadrant of gluteus. No more than 5 mL should be injected into single site (using 20-gauge needle). Injection may be painful.
- Reconstitute with supplied diluent (bacteriostatic water for injection with 0.9% benzyl alcohol). Shake vial vigorously immediately after adding diluent and before withdrawing drug.
- Use solution within 24 h of reconstitution.
- Store at 15°–30° C (59°–86° F) unless otherwise directed.

ADVERSE EFFECTS (≥1%) **Skin:** *Pain and soreness at injection site,* urticaria, pruritus, transient rash. **Body as a Whole:** Headache, dizziness, chills, fever, insomnia, nervousness. **GI:** Nausea, vomiting. **Metabolic:** Decrease in Hgb, Hct, Cl_{cr}, elevated serum alkaline phosphatase, ALT, BUN.

S

INTERACTIONS Drug: No clinically significant interactions established.

PHARMACOKINETICS Absorption: Readily absorbed from IM site. **Peak:** 1 hr. **Metabolism:** Metabolized in liver. **Elimination:** Excreted in urine. **Half-Life:** 1.2–2.8 h.

NURSING IMPLICATIONS

Assessment & Drug Effects

- Observe patient for 45–60 min after injection. Systemic anaphylaxis has been reported (apprehension, pruritus, hypertension, abdominal pain, collapse).
- Obtain serologic tests for syphilis at time of diagnosis in patients with gonorrhea and again after 3 mo.
- Monitor clinical effectiveness of drug to detect antibiotic resistance.
- Culture all gonococcal infection sites 3–7 d after spectinomycin therapy is completed to verify eradication of infection.
- Lab tests: Monitor Hgb and Hct when multiple doses are required.

Patient & Family Education

- Notify sexual partners of their risk of infection.
- Refrain from sexual intercourse until infection is resolved.
- Do not breast feed while taking this drug without consulting physician.

S

SPIRONOLACTONE Pr

(speer-on-oh-lak′tone)

Aldactone, Novospiroton ♣

Classifications: ELECTROLYTIC AND WATER BALANCE AGENT; POTASSIUM-SPARING DIURETIC

Pregnancy Category: D

AVAILABILITY 25 mg, 50 mg, 100 mg tablets

ACTIONS Steroidal compound and specific pharmacologic antagonist of aldosterone. Presumably acts by competing with aldosterone for cellular receptor sites in distal renal tubule. Promotes sodium and chloride excretion without concomitant loss of potassium. Diuretic effect reportedly not associated with hyperuricemia or hyperglycemia. Activity depends on presence of endogenous or exogenous aldosterone.

THERAPEUTIC EFFECTS A diuretic agent that promotes sodium and chloride excretion without concomitant loss of potassium. Lowers systolic and diastolic pressures in hypertensive patients.

USES Clinical conditions associated with augmented aldosterone production, as in essential hypertension, refractory edema due to CHF, hepatic cirrhosis, nephrotic syndrome, and idiopathic edema. May be used to potentiate actions of other diuretics and antihypertensive agents or for its potassium-sparing effect. Also used for treatment of (and as presumptive test for) primary aldosteronism.

UNLABELED USES Hirsutism in women with polycystic ovary syndrome or idiopathic hirsutism; adjunct in treatment of myasthenia gravis and familial periodic paralysis.

CONTRAINDICATIONS Anuria, acute renal insufficiency; progressing impairment of kidney function, hyperkalemia; pregnancy (category D), lactation.

CAUTIOUS USE BUN of 40 mg/dL or greater, liver disease.

ROUTE & DOSAGE

Edema

Adult: **PO** 25–200 mg/d in divided doses, continued for at least 5 d (dose adjusted to optimal response; if no response, a thiazide or loop diuretic may be added)
Child: **PO** 3.3 mg/kg/d in single or divided doses, continued for at least 5 d (dose adjusted to optimal response)
Neonate: **PO** 1–3 mg/kg/d divided q12–24h

Hypertension

Adult: **PO** 25–100 mg/d in single or divided doses, continued for at least 2 wk (dose adjusted to optimal response)

Primary Aldosteronism: Diagnosis

Adult: **PO** Short Test: 400 mg/d for 4 d; long test: 400 mg/d for 3–4 wk

Primary Aldosteronism: Treatment

Adult: **PO** 100–400 mg/d in divided doses

ADMINISTRATION

Oral

- Give with food to enhance absorption.
- Crush tablets and give with fluid of patient's choice if unable to swallow whole.
- Store in tight, light-resistant containers. Suspension is stable for 1 mo under refrigeration.

ADVERSE EFFECTS (≥1%) **CNS:** Lethargy, mental confusion, fatigue (with rapid weight loss), headache, drowsiness, ataxia. **Endocrine:** Gynecomastia (both sexes), inability to achieve or maintain erection, androgenic effects (hirsutism, irregular menses, deepening of voice); parathyroid changes, decreased glucose tolerance, SLE. **GI:** Abdominal cramps, nausea, vomiting, anorexia, diarrhea. **Skin:** Maculopapular or erythematous rash, urticaria. **Metabolic:** Fluid and electrolyte imbalance (particularly hyperkalemia and hyponatremia); elevated BUN, mild acidosis, hyperuricemia, gout. **Body as a Whole:** Drug fever. **Hematologic:** Agranulocytosis. **CV:** Hypertension (post-sympathectomy patient).

DIAGNOSTIC TEST INTERFERENCE May produce marked increases in ***plasma cortisol*** determinations by ***Mattingly fluorometric*** method; these may persist for several days after termination of drug (spironolactone metabolite produces fluorescence). There is the possibility of false elevations in measurements of ***digoxin serum levels*** by ***RIA*** procedures.

INTERACTIONS Drug: Combinations of spironolactone and acidifying doses of **ammonium chloride** may produce systemic acidosis; use these combinations with caution. Diuretic effect of spironolactone may be antagonized by **aspirin** and other SALICYLATES. **Digoxin** should be monitored for decreased effect of CARDIAC GLYCOSIDE. Hyperkalemia may result with POTASSIUM SUPPLEMENTS, ACE INHIBITORS, ARBS, **heparin** may decrease **lithium** clearance resulting in increased tenacity; may alter anticoagulant response in **warfarin. Food: Salt substitutes** may increase risk of hyperkalemia.

PHARMACOKINETICS Absorption: Approximately 73% absorbed from GI tract. **Onset:** Gradual. **Peak:** 2–3 d; maximum effect may take up to 2 wk. **Duration:** 2–3 d or more. **Distribution:** Crosses placenta, distributed into breast milk. **Metabolism:** Me-

S

tabolized in liver and kidneys to active metabolites. **Elimination:** 40%–57% excreted in urine, 35%–40% in bile. **Half-Life:** 1.3–2.4 h parent compound, 18–23 h metabolites.

NURSING IMPLICATIONS

Assessment & Drug Effects

- Check blood pressure before initiation of therapy and at regular intervals throughout therapy.
- Lab tests: Monitor serum electrolytes (sodium and potassium) especially during early therapy; monitor digoxin level when used concurrently.
- Assess for signs of fluid and electrolyte imbalance, and signs of digoxin toxicity.
- Monitor daily I&O and check for edema. Report lack of diuretic response or development of edema; both may indicate tolerance to drug.
- Weigh patient under standard conditions before therapy begins and daily throughout therapy. Weight is a useful index of need for dosage adjustment. For patients with ascites, physician may want measurements of abdominal girth.
- Observe for and report immediately the onset of mental changes, lethargy, or stupor in patients with liver disease.
- Adverse reactions are generally reversible with discontinuation of drug. Gynecomastia appears to be related to dosage level and duration of therapy; it may persist in some after drug is stopped.

Patient & Family Education

- Be aware that the maximal diuretic effect may not occur until third day of therapy and that diuresis may continue for 2–3 d after drug is withdrawn.
- Report signs of hyponatremia or hyperkalemia (see Appendix F), most likely to occur in patients with severe cirrhosis.
- Avoid replacing fluid losses with large amounts of free water (can result in dilutional hyponatremia).
- Weigh 2–3 times each week. Report gains/loss of ≥5 lbs.
- Do not drive or engage in potentially hazardous activities until response to the drug is known.
- Avoid excessive intake of high-potassium foods and salt substitutes.
- Do not breast feed while taking this drug.

STANOZOLOL

(stan-oh'zoe-lole)

Winstrol

Classifications: HORMONES AND SYNTHETIC SUBSTITUTES; ANDROGEN/ANABOLIC STEROID

Prototype: Testosterone

Pregnancy Category: X

Controlled Substance: Schedule III

AVAILABILITY 2 mg tablets

ACTIONS Synthetic steroid with relatively strong anabolic and weak androgenic activity, similar to those for testosterone.

THERAPEUTIC EFFECTS Increases protein metabolism and decreases catabolism through anabolic action. Can cause testicular atrophy. Androgenic activity controls secondary sex characteristics, adolescent growth spurts, as well as stimulation of renal production of erythropoietin.

USES Primarily to increase hemoglobin in selected cases of aplastic anemia, prophylaxis to decrease the frequency and severity of hereditary angioedema.

CONTRAINDICATIONS Male patients with carcinoma of the breast or with known or suspected carcinoma of the prostate; carcinoma of the breast in females with hypercalcemia; androgenic anabolic steroids may stimulate osteolytic resorption of bone; nephrosis, or the nephrotic phase of nephritis; pregnancy (category X)—use may be fatal; lactation. **CAUTIOUS USE** Diabetic patients; bleeding disorders, concurrent administration of anticoagulants; hepatic impairment; hypercholesterolemia.

ROUTE & DOSAGE

Anemia
Adult: **PO** 2 mg t.i.d.; *young women,* 2 mg 1–2 times/d
Child: **PO** <6 y, 1 mg b.i.d.; *6–12 y,* 2 mg t.i.d.

ADMINISTRATION

Oral

- Give just before or with meals to reduce incidence of gastric distress.
- Note: Smaller dose for young women is given to prevent virilizing effects of the drug. Notify physician if such effects appear (early sign: change of voice).

ADVERSE EFFECTS (≥1%) **CNS:** Excitation, insomnia. **CV:** Skin flushing and vascularization. **GI:** Nausea, vomiting, anorexia, diarrhea, gastric pain, jaundice. **Hematologic:** Leukopenia. **Metabolic:** Hypercalcemia, hypercholesterolemia, *sodium and water retention (especially in older adults) with edema.* **Renal:** Renal calculi (especially in the immobilized patient), bladder irritability. **Urogenital:** *Increased libido.* **Skin:** *Acne,* injection site irritation and sloughing. **Body as a Whole:** Hypersensitivity to testosterone, anaphylactoid reactions (rare). **Hematologic:** precipitation of acute intermittent porphyria. **Endocrine:** Female–Suppression of ovulation, lactation, or menstruation; hoarseness or deepening of voice (often irreversible); hirsutism; oily skin; clitoral enlargement; regression of breasts; male-pattern baldness (in disseminated breast cancer); flushing, sweating; vaginitis with pruritus, drying, bleeding; menstrual irregularities. Male–*Prepubertal:* premature epiphyseal closure, phallic enlargement, priapism. *Postpubertal:* Testicular atrophy, decreased ejaculatory volume, azoospermia, oligospermia (after prolonged administration or excessive dosage), impotence, epididymitis, priapism, *gynecomastia.*

INTERACTIONS Drug: Prolongs action of **succinylcholine** and possibly other NEUROMUSCULAR BLOCKING AGENTS due to inhibition of plasma pseudocholinesterase. Increases **theophylline** concentrations twofold. **Cimetidine** increases concentration of **tacrine** by 64%. May deplete **iron** stores; may increase risk of bleeding with ORAL ANTICOAGULANTS. **Herbal: Echinacea** may increase risk of hepatotoxicity.

PHARMACOKINETICS Metabolism: Metabolized in liver. See testosterone.

NURSING IMPLICATIONS

Assessment & Drug Effects

- Lab tests: Monitor Hct and Hgb periodically to determine efficacy of drug. Periodic serum electrolytes and lipid profile.
- Check with physician concerning restricted salt intake.
- Be alert to symptoms of hypercalcemia (see Appendix F).

Patient & Family Education

- Use with high-calorie, high-protein diet unless contraindicated.
- Drug does not enhance athletic ability.
- Do not breast feed while taking this drug.

S

STAVUDINE (D4T)

(sta′vu-deen)

Zerit

Classifications: ANTIINFECTIVE; ANTIVIRAL

Prototype: Zidovudine (AZT)

Pregnancy Category: C

AVAILABILITY 15 mg, 20 mg, 30 mg, 40 mg capsules; 1 mg/mL solution

ACTIONS Synthetic analog of thymidine (a major nucleoside in DNA) with antiviral action against HIV, the causative agent of AIDS. Phosphorylated to stavudine triphosphate by endogenous thymidine kinase. Appears to act by being incorporated into the growing DNA chains by viral transcriptase, thus terminating viral replication.

THERAPEUTIC EFFECTS Inhibits the replication of HIV in human cells. Useful in patients with advanced disease, who are intolerant of other viral agents.

USES Treatment of adults with advanced HIV infection who are intolerant of other antiretroviral agents (zidovudine, didanosine, zalcitabine) or who have deteriorated on the other agents.

S

CONTRAINDICATIONS Hypersensitivity to stavudine; pregnancy (category C), lactation.

CAUTIOUS USE Previous hypersensitivity to zidovudine, didanosine, or zalcitabine; folic acid or B_{12} deficiency; liver and renal insufficiency; peripheral neuropathy; history of pancreatitis.

ROUTE & DOSAGE

Advanced HIV Infection

Adult: **PO** *<60 kg,* 30 mg q12h; *≥60 kg,* 40 mg q12h

Child: **PO** *<30 kg,* give 2 mg/kg/d in 2 divided doses; *≥30 kg,* same as adult

Renal Impairment

Cl_{cr} 25–50 mL/min: Reduce dose by 50% (also in patients with peripheral neuropathy)

ADMINISTRATION

Oral

- Adhere strictly to 12-h interval between doses.
- Reconstitute powder by adding 202 mL of water to the container. Shake vigorously. Yields 200 mL of 1 mg/mL solution.
- Store at room temperature, 15°–30° C (59°–86° F).

ADVERSE EFFECTS (≥1%) **CNS:** *Peripheral neuropathy*, paresthesias. **GI:** *Anorexia, nausea, vomiting, diarrhea,* cramping, pancreatitis, abdominal pain, elevated liver function tests, abdominal pain. **Body as a Whole:** *Headache,* chills/fever, *myalgia*. **Hematologic:** Anemia, neutropenia. **Skin:** *Rash*. **Metabolic:** Lactic acidosis in pregnant women.

INTERACTIONS Drug: Didanosine may increase risk of pancreatitis and hepatotoxicity; **probenecid** can decrease elimination.

PHARMACOKINETICS Absorption: Readily absorbed from GI tract; 82% reaches systemic circulation. **Peak:** Effect 6 wk. **Distribution:** Distributes into CSF; excreted in breast milk of animals. **Metabolism:** Metabolized in liver; in addition to hepatic metabolism, some investigators suggest that degradation and salvage by other pyrimidine pathways may contribute to elimination; intracellularly, stavudine is phosphorylated by cellular enzymes to its active triphosphate form. **Elimina-**

tion: Excreted primarily in urine. **Half-Life:** 1–1.6 h.

NURSING IMPLICATIONS

Assessment & Drug Effects

- Monitor for peripheral neuropathy and report numbness, tingling, or pain, which may indicate a need to interrupt stavudine.
- Lab tests: Monitor liver enzymes, CBC with differential, PT and INR, and kidney function periodically.
- Monitor for development of opportunistic infection.

Patient & Family Education

- Take drug exactly as prescribed.
- Report to physician any adverse drug effects that are bothersome.
- Report symptoms of peripheral neuropathy to physician immediately.
- Do not breast feed while taking this drug.

STREPTOKINASE

(strep-toe-kye′nase)

Kabikinase, Streptase

Classifications: BLOOD FORMERS, COAGULATORS, AND ANTICOAGULANTS; THROMBOLYTIC ENZYME

Prototype: Alteplase

Pregnancy Category: C

AVAILABILITY 250,000 IU, 750,000 IU, 1,500,000 IU vials

ACTIONS Derivative of the beta-hemolytic streptococci. Promotes thrombolysis by activating the conversion of plasminogen to plasmin, the enzyme that degrades fibrin, fibrinogen, and other procoagulant proteins into soluble fragments. Decreases blood and plasma viscosity and erythrocyte aggregation tendency, thus increasing perfusion of collateral blood vessels.

THERAPEUTIC EFFECTS Promotes thrombolysis. The fibrinolytic activity of streptokinase is effective both outside and within the formed thrombus/embolus.

USES Acute extensive deep venous thrombosis, acute arterial thrombosis or embolism, acute pulmonary embolus, coronary artery thrombosis, MI, and arteriovenous cannula occlusion.

CONTRAINDICATIONS Active internal bleeding; very recent cardiopulmonary resuscitation; recent (within 2 mo) intraspinal, intracranial, intraarterial procedures; intracranial neoplasm; CVA, severe uncontrolled hypertension; history of allergic response to SK, recent streptococcal infection; obstetrical delivery; diabetic hemorrhagic retinopathy; ulcerative colitis, diverticulitis; any condition in which bleeding presents a hazard or would be difficult to manage because of location; pregnancy (category C). Safety and efficacy in children are not established.

CAUTIOUS USE Patient with preexisting hemostatic deficits; conditions accompanied by risk of cerebral embolism; septic thrombophlebitis; uremia; liver failure; lactation.

ROUTE & DOSAGE

Coronary Artery Thrombosis, MI

Adult: **IV** 1.5 million IU infused over 60 min **Intracoronary** 15,000–20,000 IU bolus, followed by 2000–4000 IU/min for 60 min

Deep Vein Thrombosis, Pulmonary Embolism, Arterial Embolism

Adult: **IV** 250,000 IU over 30 min loading dose, then 100,000 IU/h for 48–72 h

Occluded Cannula
Adult: **IV** 250,000 IU in 2 mL over 25–35 min; clamp for 2 h, then aspirate cannula

ADMINISTRATION

Intravenous

PREPARE: **IV Infusion:** *All uses except cannula occlusion*—Reconstitute with 5 mL NS (preferred) or 5 mL D5W. Roll or tilt vial to dissolve; avoid shaking to prevent foaming or increase in flocculation. Further dilute by carefully adding an additional 40 mL to the vial, avoiding shaking or agitation of the solution. If necessary, may be further diluted in 45 mL increments to approximately 500 mL. Slight flocculation does not interfere with drug action; discard solution with large amount of flocculent.

ADMINISTER: **IV Infusion:** Start IV infusion as soon as possible after the thrombotic event; thrombi more than 7 d old respond poorly to SK therapy. Give at rate specified under Route & Dosage for specific indication (e.g., 1.5 million IU over 60 min for coronary artery thrombosis). Observe infusion site frequently. If phlebitis occurs, it can usually be controlled by diluting the infusion solution.

- Store unopened vials at 15°–30° C (59°–86° F).
- Store reconstituted solution at 2°–4° C (36°–39° F). Discard after 24 h.

ADVERSE EFFECTS (≥1%) **Body as a Whole:** *Allergic reactions* (bronchospasm, periorbital swelling, angioneurotic edema, anaphylaxis); urticaria, itching, headache, musculoskeletal pain, flushing, nausea, pyrexia. **Hematologic:** Phlebitis, *bleeding or oozing at sites of percutaneous trauma;* prolonged systemic hypocoagulability; spontaneous bleeding (GI, urogenital, retroperitoneal). **CV:** Unstable blood pressure; reperfusion atrial or ventricular dysrhythmias.

DIAGNOSTIC TEST INTERFERENCE Streptokinase promotes increases in ***TT, APTT,*** and ***PT.***

INTERACTIONS Drug: ANTICOAGULANTS increase risk of bleeding; **aminocaproic acid** reverses the action of streptokinase.

PHARMACOKINETICS Metabolism: Rapidly cleared from circulation by antibodies. **Elimination:** Does not cross placenta, but antibodies do. **Half-Life:** 83 min.

NURSING IMPLICATIONS

Assessment & Drug Effects

- Lab tests: Discontinue heparin and obtain baseline control levels for TT, aPTT, PT, INR, Hct, and platelet count prior to treatment. Treatment is delayed until TT and aPTT are less than 2 times the normal control level. During treatment with SK, TT is generally kept at about 2 times or more baseline value and checked q3–4h.
- Protect patient from invasive procedures: IM injections are contraindicated. Also prevent undue manipulation during thrombolytic therapy to prevent bruising. Spontaneous bleeding occurs about twice as often with SK as with heparin.
- Monitor for excessive bleeding q15min for the first hour of therapy, q30min for second to eighth hour, then q8h.
- Be aware that patient is at risk for postthrombolytic bleeding

for 2–4 d after intracoronary SK treatment. Continue monitoring vital signs until laboratory tests confirm anticoagulant control.

- Report signs of potential serious bleeding; gum bleeding, epistaxis, hematoma, spontaneous ecchymoses, oozing at catheter site, increased pulse, pain from internal bleeding. SK infusion should be interrupted, then resumed when bleeding stops.
- Report promptly symptoms of a major allergic reaction; therapy will be discontinued and emergency treatment instituted. Minor symptoms (e.g., itching, nausea) respond to concurrent antihistamine or corticosteroid treatment or both without interruption of SK administration.
- Check cardiac monitor frequently. Be alert to changes in cardiac rhythm, especially during intracoronary instillation. Dysrhythmias signal need to stop therapy at once.
- Monitor BP. Mild changes can be expected, but report substantial changes (greater than ±25 mm Hg). Therapy may be discontinued.
- Check patient's temperature during treatment. A slight elevation, 0.8° C (1.5° F), perhaps with chills, occurs in about one third of the patients. Higher elevations may be treated with acetaminophen.
- Avoid giving aspirin because of its antiplatelet action if an analgesic-antipyretic is indicated.

Patient & Family Education

- Report immediately to physician symptoms of hypersensitivity (e.g., labored, difficult breathing; hives; itching skin).

STREPTOMYCIN SULFATE

(strep-toe-mye'sin)

Streptomycin

Classifications: ANTIINFECTIVE; AMINOGLYCOSIDE ANTIBIOTIC; ANTITUBERCULOSIS AGENT

Prototype: Gentamicin

Pregnancy Category: C

AVAILABILITY 400 mg/mL, 1 g injection

ACTIONS Aminoglycoside antibiotic derived from *Streptomyces griseus,* with bactericidal and bacteriostatic actions. Most commonly used concurrently with other antimicrobial agents because of rapid emergence of resistant strains when used alone.

THERAPEUTIC EFFECTS Active against a variety of gram-positive, gram-negative, and acid-fast organisms. Reportedly, it is the least nephrotoxic of the aminoglycosides.

USES Only in combination with other antitubercular drugs in treatment of all forms of active tuberculosis caused by susceptible organisms. Used alone or in conjunction with tetracycline for tularemia, plague, and brucellosis. Also used with other antibiotics in treatment of subacute bacterial endocarditis due to *Enterococci* and *Streptococci* (viridans group) and *Haemophilus influenzae* and in treatment of peritonitis, respiratory tract infections, granuloma inguinale, and chancroid when other drugs have failed.

CONTRAINDICATIONS History of toxic reaction or hypersensitivity to aminoglycosides; labyrinthine disease; myasthenia gravis; concurrent or sequential use of other neurotoxic or nephrotoxic agents; pregnancy (category C); lactation.

S

CAUTIOUS USE Impaired kidney function (given in reduced dosages); use in older adults and in prematures, neonates, and children.

ROUTE & DOSAGE

Tuberculosis
Adult: **IM** 15 mg/kg up to 1 g/d as single dose
Geriatric: **IM** 10 mg/kg (max: 750 mg/d)
Child: **IM** 20–40 mg/kg/d up to 1 g/d as single dose
Infant: **IM** 10–15 mg/kg q12h
Neonate: **IM** 10–20 mg/kg q24h

Tularemia
Adult: **IM** 1–2 g/d in 1–2 divided doses for 7–10 d
Child: **IM** 20–40 mg/kg/d divided q6–12h

Plague
Adult: **IM** 2 g/d in 2–4 divided doses
Child: **IM** 30 mg/kg/d divided q8–12

ADMINISTRATION

Intramuscular

- Give IM deep into large muscle mass to minimize possibility of irritation. Injections are painful.
- Avoid direct contact with drug; sensitization can occur. Use gloves during preparation of drug.
- Use commercially prepared IM solution undiluted; intended only for IM injection (contains a preservative, and therefore is not suitable for other routes).
- Store ampules at room temperature. Protect from light; exposure to light may slightly darken solution, with no apparent loss of potency.

ADVERSE EFFECTS (≥1%) **CNS:** Paresthesias (peripheral, facial). **Body as a Whole:** Hypersensitivity angioedema, drug fever, enlarged lymph nodes, anaphylactic shock, headache, inability to concentrate, lassitude, muscular weakness, *pain and irritation at IM site,* superinfections, neuromuscular blockade, arachnoiditis. **GI:** Stomatitis, hepatotoxicity. **Hematologic:** Blood dyscrasias (leukopenia, neutropenia, pancytopenia, hemolytic or aplastic anemia, eosinophilia). **Special Senses:** *Labyrinthine damage,* auditory damage, optic nerve toxicity (scotomas). **Urogenital:** Nephrotoxicity. **CNS:** Encephalopathy, CNS depression syndrome in infants (stupor, flaccidity, coma, paralysis, cardiac arrest). **Respiratory:** Respiratory depression. **Skin:** Skin rashes, pruritus, exfoliative dermatitis.

DIAGNOSTIC TEST INTERFERENCE Streptomycin reportedly produces false-positive ***urinary glucose*** tests using ***copper sulfate methods (Benedict's solution, Clinitest)*** but not with ***glucose oxidase methods*** (e.g., ***Clinistix, Tes-Tape***). False increases in protein content in ***urine*** and ***CSF*** using ***Folin-Ciocalteau reaction*** and decreased ***BUN*** readings with ***Berthelot reaction*** may occur from test interferences. ***C&S*** tests may be affected if patient is taking salts such as sodium and potassium chloride, sodium sulfate and tartrate, ammonium acetate, calcium and magnesium ions.

INTERACTIONS Drug: May potentiate anticoagulant effects of **warfarin;** additive nephrotoxicity with **acyclovir, amphotericin B,** AMINOGLYCOSIDES, **carboplatin, cidofovir, cisplatin, cyclosporine, foscarnet, ganciclovir,** SALICYLATES, **tacrolimus, vancomycin.**

PHARMACOKINETICS Peak: 1–2 h. **Distribution:** Diffuses into most body tissues and extracellular fluids; crosses placenta; distributed into breast milk. **Elimination:** Excreted in urine. **Half-Life:** 2–3 h adults, 4–10 h newborns.

NURSING IMPLICATIONS

Assessment & Drug Effects

- Lab tests: Obtain C&S tests prior to and periodically during course of therapy. In patients with impaired kidney function, frequent determinations of serum drug concentrations and periodic kidney and liver function tests are advised (serum concentrations should not exceed 25 mcg/mL in these patients).
- Be alert for and report immediately symptoms of ototoxicity (see Appendix F). Symptoms are most likely to occur in patients with impaired kidney function, patients receiving high doses (1.8–2 g/d) or other ototoxic or neurotoxic drugs, and older adults. Irreversible damage may occur if drug is not discontinued promptly.
- Early damage to vestibular portion of eighth cranial nerve (higher incidence than auditory toxicity) is initially manifested by moderately severe headache, nausea, vomiting, vertigo in upright position, difficulty in reading, unsteadiness, and positive Romberg sign.
- Be aware that auditory nerve damage is usually preceded by vestibular symptoms and high-pitched tinnitus, roaring noises, impaired hearing (especially to high-pitched sounds), sense of fullness in ears. Audiometric test should be done if these symptoms appear, and drug should be discontinued. Hearing loss can be permanent if damage is extensive. Tinnitus may persist several days to weeks after drug is stopped.
- Monitor I&O. Report oliguria or changes in I&O ratio (possible signs of diminishing kidney function). Sufficient fluids to maintain urinary output of 1500 mL/24 h are generally advised. Consult physician.

Patient & Family Education

- Report any unusual symptoms. Review adverse reactions with physician periodically, especially with prolonged therapy.
- Be aware of possibility of ototoxicity and its symptoms (see Appendix F).
- Report to physician immediately any of the following: Nausea, vomiting, vertigo, incoordination, tinnitus, fullness in ears, impaired hearing.
- Do not breast feed while taking this drug.

STREPTOZOCIN

(strep-toe-zoe′sin)

Zanosar

Classifications: ANTINEOPLASTIC; ALKYLATING AGENT; ANTIBIOTIC

Prototype: Cyclophosphamide

Pregnancy Category: C

AVAILABILITY 1 g injection

ACTIONS Similar to other nitrosourea antineoplastics (e.g., carmustine) but with weaker alkylating effects. In general, this drug is highly toxic and has a low therapeutic index; thus a clinically effective response is likely to be accompanied by some evidence of toxicity. Inhibits DNA synthesis in both bacterial and mammalian cells and prevents progression of cells into mitosis, affecting all phases of the cell cycle (cell-cycle nonspecific). Appears to have minimal effects on RNA or protein synthesis. Delays repair of DNA damaged by nitrosourea-induced alkylation. Unlike other nitrosoureas, has markedly

S

significant specificity for pancreatic beta and exocrine cells.

THERAPEUTIC EFFECTS Functional islet cell tumors produce and secrete a variety of hormones including glucagon, insulin, calcitonin, serotonin, and others. Successful therapy with streptozocin (alone or in combination) produces a biochemical response evidenced by decreased secretion of hormones as well as measurable tumor regression. Thus, serial fasting insulin levels during treatment indicate response to this drug.

USES Metastatic functional and nonfunctional islet cell carcinoma of pancreas, as single agent or in combination with fluorouracil.

UNLABELED USES A variety of other malignant neoplasms including metastatic carcinoid tumor or carcinoid syndrome, refractory advanced Hodgkin's disease, and metastatic colorectal cancer.

CONTRAINDICATIONS Liver and kidney dysfunction. Pregnancy (category C), lactation. Safety in children is not established.

CAUTIOUS USE Renal impairment; patients with history of hypoglycemia; hepatic impairment.

S

ROUTE & DOSAGE

Islet Cell Carcinoma of Pancreas

Adult: **IV** 500 mg/m^2/d for 5 consecutive days q6wk or 1 g/m^2/wk for 2 wk, then increase to 1.5 g/m^2/wk, infuse dose over 15 min to 6 h

ADMINISTRATION

Intravenous

- Use only under constant supervision by physician experienced in therapy with cytotoxic agents and only when the benefit to risk ratio is fully and thoroughly understood by patient and family.
- Wear gloves to protect against topical exposure, which may pose a carcinogen hazard, when handling streptozocin. If solution or powder comes in contact with skin or mucosa, promptly flush the area thoroughly with soap and water.

PREPARE: **IV Infusion:** Reconstitute with 9.5 mL D5W or NS, to yield 100 mg/mL. Solution will be pale gold. May be further diluted with up to 250 mL of the original diluent. Protect reconstituted solution and vials of drug from light.

ADMINISTER: **IV Infusion:** Give over 15–60 min. Inspect injection site frequently for signs of extravasation (patient complaints of stinging or burning at site, swelling around site, no blood return or questionable blood return). If extravasation occurs, area requires immediate attention to prevent necrosis. Remove needle, apply ice, and contact physician regarding further treatment to infiltrated tissue.

INCOMPATIBILITIES **Y-site: Allopurinol, aztreonam, cefepime, piperacillin/tazobactam.**

- Note: An antiemetic given routinely every 4 or 6 h and prophylactically 30 min before a treatment may provide sufficient control to maintain the treatment regimen (even if it reduces but not completely eliminates nausea and vomiting).
- Discard reconstituted solutions after 12 h (contains no preservative and not intended for multidose use).

ADVERSE EFFECTS (≥1%) **CNS:** Confusion, lethargy, depression. **GI:** *Nausea, vomiting,* diarrhea, transient increase in AST, ALT, or alkaline phosphatase; hypoalbuminemia. **Hematologic:** *Mild* to moderate myelosuppression *(leukopenia, thrombocytopenia, anemia)*. **Metabolic:** Glucose tolerance abnormalities (moderate and reversible); glycosuria without hyperglycemia, insulin shock (rare). **Urogenital:** Nephrotoxicity: azotemia, anuria, proteinuria, hypophosphatemia, hyperchloremia; *Fanconi-like syndrome* (proximal renal tubular reabsorption defects, alkaline pH of urine, glucosuria, acetonuria, aminoaciduria): Hypokalemia, hypocalcemia. **Other:** Local necrosis following extravasation.

INTERACTIONS Drug: MYELOSUPPRESSIVE AGENTS add to hematologic toxicity; nephrotoxic agents (e.g., AMINOGLYCOSIDES, **vancomycin, amphotericin B, cisplatin**) increase risk of nephrotoxicity; **phenytoin** may reduce cytotoxic effect on pancreatic beta cells.

PHARMACOKINETICS Absorption: Undetectable in plasma within 3 h. **Distribution:** Metabolite enters CSF. **Metabolism:** Metabolized in liver and kidneys. **Elimination:** 70%–80% of dose excreted in urine, 1% in feces, and 5% in expired air. **Half-Life:** 35–40 min.

NURSING IMPLICATIONS

Assessment & Drug Effects

- Lab tests: Perform CBC at least weekly, and liver function tests prior to each course of therapy. Dosage adjustment or discontinuation may be required if there is evidence of decreased liver or bone marrow function. Obtain serial urinalyses and determinations of BUN, creatinine clearance, and serum electrolytes prior to and weekly during therapy, then for 4 wk after termination of therapy.
- Ensure that repeat courses of streptozocin treatment are not given until patient's liver, kidney, and hematologic functions are within acceptable limits. Platelet and leukocyte nadirs generally occur 1–2 wk after beginning therapy.
- Report evidence of drug-induced declining kidney function promptly; changes are dose related and cumulative.
- Be alert to early laboratory evidence of kidney dysfunction: Hypophosphatemia, mild proteinurea, and changes in I&O ratio and pattern.
- Mild adverse renal effects may be reversible following discontinuation of streptozocin, but nephrotoxicity may be irreversible, severe, or fatal.
- Be alert to symptoms of sepsis and superinfections (leukopenia) or increased tendency to bleed (thrombocytopenia). Myelosuppression is severe in 10%–20% of patients and may be cumulative and more severe if patient has had prior exposure to radiation or to other antineoplastics.
- Monitor for S&S of superinfection (see Appendix F).
- Monitor and record temperature pattern to promptly recognize impending sepsis.

Patient & Family Education

- Inspect site at weekly intervals and report changes in tissue appearance if extravasation occurred during IV infusion.
- Report symptoms of hypoglycemia (see Appendix F) even though this drug has minimal, if any, diabetogenic action.
- Drink fluids liberally (2000–3000 mL/d). Hydration may protect against drug toxicity effects.

S

- Report S&S of nephrotoxicity (see Appendix F).
- Do not take aspirin without consulting physician.
- Report to physician promptly any signs of bleeding: Hematuria, epistaxis, ecchymoses, petechial.
- Report symptoms that suggest anemia: Shortness of breath, pale mucous membranes and nail beds, exhaustion, rapid pulse.
- Do not breast feed while taking this drug.

SUCCINYLCHOLINE CHLORIDE (Pr)

(suk-sin-ill-koe'leen)

Anectine, Quelicin, Sucostrin

Classifications: AUTONOMIC NERVOUS SYSTEM AGENT; DEPOLARIZING SKELETAL MUSCLE RELAXANT

Pregnancy Category: C

AVAILABILITY 20 mg/mL, 50 mg/mL, 100 mg/mL injection; 500 mg, 1 g vials

ACTIONS Synthetic, ultrashort-acting depolarizing neuromuscular blocking agent with high affinity for acetylcholine (ACh) receptor sites.

THERAPEUTIC EFFECTS Initial transient contractions and fasciculations are followed by sustained flaccid skeletal muscle paralysis produced by state of accommodation that develops in adjacent excitable muscle membranes. Rapidly hydrolyzed by plasma pseudocholinesterase.

USES To produce skeletal muscle relaxation as adjunct to anesthesia; to facilitate intubation and endoscopy, to increase pulmonary compliance in assisted or controlled respiration, and to reduce intensity of muscle contractions in pharmacologically induced or electroshock convulsions.

CONTRAINDICATIONS Hypersensitivity to succinylcholine; family history of malignant hyperthermia. Safety in pregnancy (category C) is not established.

CAUTIOUS USE During delivery by cesarean section; lactation; kidney, liver, pulmonary, metabolic, or cardiovascular disorders; dehydration, electrolyte imbalance, patients taking digitalis, severe burns or trauma, fractures, spinal cord injuries, degenerative or dystrophic neuromuscular diseases, low plasma pseudocholinesterase levels (recessive genetic trait, but often associated with severe liver disease, severe anemia, dehydration, marked changes in body temperature, exposure to neurotoxic insecticides, certain drugs); collagen diseases, porphyria, intraocular surgery, glaucoma.

ROUTE & DOSAGE

Surgical and Anesthetic Procedures

Adult: **IV** 0.3–1.1 mg/kg administered over 10–30 s, may give additional doses prn **IM** 2.5–4 mg/kg up to 150 mg

Child: **IV** 1–2 mg/kg administered over 10–30 s, may give additional doses prn **IM** 2.5–4 mg/kg up to 150 mg

Prolonged Muscle Relaxation

Adult: **IV** 0.5–10 mg/min by continuous infusion

ADMINISTRATION

Intramuscular

- Give IM injections deeply, preferably high into deltoid muscle.

Intravenous

- Use only freshly prepared solutions; succinylcholine hydrolyzes rapidly with consequent loss of potency.
- Give initial small test dose (0.1 mg/kg) to determine individual drug sensitivity and recovery time.

PREPARE: **Direct:** Give undiluted. **Intermittent/Continuous:** Dilute 1 g in 500–1000 mL of D5W or NS.

ADMINISTER: **Direct:** Give a bolus dose over 30 sec. **Intermittent/Continuous:** Preferred. Give at a rate of 0.5–10 mg/min. Do not exceed 10 mg/min.

INCOMPATIBILITIES **Solution/additive: Sodium bicarbonate, thiopental.**

- Note: Expiration date and storage before and after reconstitution; varies with the manufacturer.

ADVERSE EFFECTS (≥1%) **CNS:** *Muscle fasciculations,* profound and prolonged muscle relaxation, muscle pain. **CV:** *Bradycardia,* tachycardia, hypotension, hypertension, arrhythmias, sinus arrest. **Respiratory:** Respiratory depression, bronchospasm, hypoxia, apnea. **Body as a Whole:** Malignant hyperthermia, increased IOP, excessive salivation, enlarged salivary glands. **Metabolic:** Myoglobinemia, hyperkalemia. **GI:** Decreased tone and motility of GI tract (large doses).

INTERACTIONS Drug: Aminoglycosides, colistin, cyclophosphamide, cyclopropane, echothiophate iodide, halothane, lidocaine, MAGNESIUM SALTS, **methotrimeprazine,** NARCOTIC ANALGESICS, ORGANOPHOSPHAMIDE INSECTICIDES, MAO INHIBITORS, PHENOTHIAZINES, **procaine, procainamide, quinidine, quinine, propranolol** may prolong neuromuscular blockade; DIGITALIS GLYCOSIDES may increase risk of cardiac arrhythmias.

PHARMACOKINETICS Onset: 0.5–1 min IV; 2–3 min IM. **Duration:** 2–3 min IV; 10–30 min IM. **Distribution:** Crosses placenta in small amounts. **Metabolism:** Metabolized in plasma by pseudocholinesterases. **Elimination:** Excreted in urine.

NURSING IMPLICATIONS

Assessment & Drug Effects

- Lab tests: Obtain baseline serum electrolytes. Electrolyte imbalance (particularly potassium, calcium, magnesium) can potentiate effects of neuromuscular blocking agents.
- Be aware that transient apnea usually occurs at time of maximal drug effect (1–2 min); spontaneous respiration should return in a few seconds or, at most, 3 or 4 min.
- Have immediately available: Facilities for emergency endotracheal intubation, artificial respiration, and assisted or controlled respiration with oxygen.
- Monitor vital signs and keep airway clear of secretions.

Patient & Family Education

- Patient may experience postprocedural muscle stiffness and pain (caused by initial fasciculations following injection) for as long as 24–30 h.
- Be aware that hoarseness and sore throat are common even when pharyngeal airway has not been used.
- Report residual muscle weakness to physician.

S

SUCRALFATE

(soo-kral'fate)

Carafate, Sulcrate ♣

Classifications: GASTROINTESTINAL AGENT; ANTIULCER

Pregnancy Category: B

AVAILABILITY 1 g tablets; 1 g/10 mL suspension

ACTIONS A complex of aluminum hydroxide and sulfated sucrose structurally related to heparin that lacks its anticoagulant activity. Action is chemically unlike any other drug used for antiulcer therapy. Following oral administration, sucralfate and gastric acid react to form a viscous, adhesive, paste-like substance that resists further reaction with acid. This "paste" adheres to the GI mucosa with a major portion binding electrostatically to the positively charged protein molecules in the damaged mucosa of an ulcer crater or an acute gastric erosion caused by alcohol or other drugs.

THERAPEUTIC EFFECTS Absorbs bile, inhibits the enzyme pepsin, and blocks back diffusion of H^+ ions. These actions plus adherence of the paste-like complex protect damaged mucosa against further destruction from ulcerogenic secretions and drugs.

USES Short-term (up to 8 wk) treatment of duodenal ulcer.

UNLABELED USES Short-term treatment of gastric ulcer, aspirin-induced erosions, suspension for chemotherapy-induced mucositis.

CONTRAINDICATIONS Pregnancy (category B). Safety and efficacy in children are not established.

CAUTIOUS USE Chronic kidney failure or dialysis due to aluminum accumulation; lactation.

ROUTE & DOSAGE

Duodenal Ulcer

Adult: **PO** 1 g q.i.d. 1 h a.c. and h.s. **PO Maintenance** 1 g b.i.d.

ADMINISTRATION

Oral

- Use drug solubilized in an appropriate diluent by a pharmacist when given through nasogastric tube.
- Administer antacids prescribed for pain relief 30 min before or after sucralfate.
- Separate administration of QUINOLONES, digoxin, phenytoin, tetracycline from that of sucralfate by 2 h to prevent sucralfate from binding to these compounds in the intestinal tract and reducing their bioavailability.
- Store in tight container at room temperature, 15°–30° C (59°–86° F). Stable for 2 y after manufacture.

ADVERSE EFFECTS (≥1%) **GI:** Nausea, gastric discomfort, *constipation,* diarrhea.

INTERACTIONS Drug: May decrease absorption of QUINOLONES (e.g., **ciprofloxacin, norfloxacin**), **digoxin, phenytoin, tetracycline.**

PHARMACOKINETICS Absorption: Minimally absorbed from GI tract (<5%). **Duration:** Up to 6 h (depends on contact time with ulcer crater). **Elimination:** 90% Excreted in feces.

NURSING IMPLICATIONS

Assessment & Drug Effects

- Be aware of drug interactions and schedule other medications accordingly.

Patient & Family Education

- Although healing has occurred within the first 2 wk of therapy, treatment is usually continued 4–8 wk.
- Be aware that constipation is a drug-related problem. Follow these measures unless contraindicated: Increase water intake to 8–10 glasses per day; increase physical exercise, increase dietary bulk. Consult physician: a suppository or bulk laxative (e.g., Metamucil) may be prescribed.
- Do not breast feed while taking this drug without consulting physician.

SUFENTANIL CITRATE

(soo-fen'ta-nil)

Sufenta

Classifications: CENTRAL NERVOUS SYSTEM AGENT; NARCOTIC (OPIATE) AGONIST ANALGESIC; GENERAL ANESTHETIC

Prototype: Morphine

Pregnancy Category: C

Controlled Substance: Schedule II

AVAILABILITY 50 mcg/mL injection

ACTIONS Synthetic opioid related to fentanyl with similar pharmacologic actions, but about 7 times more potent. Onset of action and recovery from anesthesia occur more rapidly with sufentanil than with fentanyl. In common with other opiate agonists, sufentanil can cause respiratory depression and suppression of cough reflex.

THERAPEUTIC EFFECTS Effective agent for analgesia as a supplement or a primary anesthesia.

USES Analgesic supplement in maintenance of balanced general anesthesia and also as a primary anesthetic.

CONTRAINDICATIONS Pregnancy (category C), lactation.

CAUTIOUS USE Pulmonary disease, reduced respiratory reserve; impaired liver or kidney function.

ROUTE & DOSAGE

Adjunct to General Anesthesia

Adult: **IV** 1–8 mcg/kg, depending on duration of surgery, may give additional doses of 10–25 mcg if needed

As Primary Anesthetic

Adult: **IV** 1–30 mcg/kg administered with 100% oxygen and a muscle relaxant, may give additional doses of 10–25 mcg if needed

Child: **IV** *<12 y,* 10–25 mcg/kg administered with 100% oxygen and a muscle relaxant, may give additional doses of 25–50 mcg up to 1–2 mcg/kg/dose if needed

ADMINISTRATION

Intravenous

- Administer only by qualified personnel, specifically trained in the use of IV anesthesia and in the management of respiratory depression.
- Have available a narcotic antagonist (e.g., naloxone) to reverse respiratory depression.

PREPARE: **Direct:** Examine solution for particulate matter and discoloration (solution should be clear) before administration. Give undiluted.

ADMINISTER: **Direct:** Give a bolus dose over 3–5 sec. **Epidural:** Give by slow injection and closely monitor respirations after each injection.

INCOMPATIBILITIES **Solution/additive: Diazepam, lorazepam,**

phenobarbital, phenytoin, sodium bicarbonate. Y-site: Lorazepam, phenytoin, thiopental.

- Store at 15°–30° C (59°–86° F) unless otherwise directed; protect from light.

ADVERSE EFFECTS (≥1%) **CV:** Bradycardia, tachycardia, hypotension, hypertension, arrhythmias. **GI:** Nausea, vomiting, constipation. **Respiratory:** Bronchospasm, respiratory depression, apnea. **Body as a Whole:** *Skeletal muscle rigidity (especially of trunk),* chills, *itching,* spasms of sphincter of Oddi, urinary retention.

INTERACTIONS Drug: BETA-ADRENERGIC ANTAGONISTS increase incidence of bradycardia; **alcohol** and other CNS DEPRESSANTS such as BARBITURATES, TRANQUILIZERS, OPIATES and INHALATION GENERAL ANESTHETICS add to CNS depression; **cimetidine** increases risk of respiratory depression.

PHARMACOKINETICS Onset: 1.5–3 min. **Duration:** 40 min. **Distribution:** Crosses blood–brain barrier. **Metabolism:** Metabolized in liver and small intestine. **Elimination:** Excreted in urine and feces. **Half-Life:** 2–3 h.

S

NURSING IMPLICATIONS

Assessment & Drug Effects

- Monitor vital signs. Observe for skeletal muscle rigidity, especially of chest wall, and respiratory depression, particularly in older adults, and in patients who are obese, debilitated, or who have received high doses.
- Bear in mind that if naloxone is given to reverse respiratory depression, the duration of sufentanil-induced respiratory depression may exceed the duration of naloxone.

Patient & Family Education

- Avoid activities which require mental alertness for at least 24 h after receiving this drug.

SULFACETAMIDE SODIUM

(sul-fa-see'ta-mide)

AK-Sulf, Bleph 10, Cetamide, Isopto Cetamide, Ophthacet, Sebizon, Sodium Sulamyd, Sulf-10

SULFACETAMIDE SODIUM/ SULFUR

Sulfacet, Rosula

Classifications: ANTIINFECTIVE; SULFONAMIDE ANTIBIOTIC
Prototype: Sulfisoxazole
Pregnancy Category: C

AVAILABILITY Sulfacetamide 10% lotion; 1%, 10%, 15%, 30% solution; 10% ointment **Sulfacetamide/ Sulfur** 10%/5% gel, lotion

ACTIONS Highly soluble sulfonamide that exerts bacteriostatic effect by interfering with bacterial utilization of PABA, thereby inhibiting folic acid biosynthesis required for bacterial growth.

THERAPEUTIC EFFECTS Effective against a wide range of gram-positive and gram-negative microorganisms.

USES Ophthalmic preparations are used for conjunctivitis, corneal ulcers, and other superficial ocular infections and as adjunct to systemic sulfonamide therapy for trachoma. The topical lotion is used for scaly dermatoses, seborrheic dermatitis, seborrhea sicca, and other bacterial skin infections.

CONTRAINDICATIONS Hypersensitivity to sulfonamides or to any ingredients in the formulation. Pregnancy (category C).

CAUTIOUS USE Application of lotion to denuded or debrided skin; lactation.

ROUTE & DOSAGE

Conjunctivitis

Adult: **Ophthalmic** 1–3 drops of 10%, 15%, or 30% solution into lower conjunctival sac q2–3h, may increase interval as patient responds or use 1.5–2.5 cm (1/2–1 in) of 10% ointment q6h and at h.s.

Seborrhea, Rosacea

Adult: **Topical** Apply thin film to affected area 1–3 times per day

ADMINISTRATION

Instillation

- Be aware that ophthalmic preparations and skin lotion are not interchangeable.
- Check strength of medication prescribed.
- See patient instructions for instilling eye drops.
- Discard darkened solutions; results when left standing for a long time.
- Store at 8°–15° C (46°–59° F) in tightly closed containers unless otherwise directed.

ADVERSE EFFECTS (≥1%) **Special Senses:** *Temporary stinging or burning sensation,* retardation of corneal healing associated with long-term use of ophthalmic ointment. **Body as a Whole:** Hypersensitivity reactions (Stevens-Johnson syndrome, lupus-like syndrome), superinfections with nonsusceptible organisms.

INTERACTIONS Drug: Tetracaine and other LOCAL ANESTHETICS DERIVED FROM PABA may antagonize the antibacterial effects of sulfonamides; SILVER PREPARATIONS may precipitate sulfacetamide from solution.

PHARMACOKINETICS Absorption: Minimal systemic absorption, but may be enough to cause sensitization. **Metabolism:** Metabolized in liver to inactive metabolites. **Elimination:** Excreted in urine.

NURSING IMPLICATIONS

Assessment & Drug Effects

- Discontinue if symptoms of hypersensitivity appear (erythema, skin rash, pruritus, urticaria).

Patient & Family Education

- Wash hands thoroughly with soap and running water (before and after instillation).
- Examine eye medication; discard if cloudy or dark in color.
- Avoid contaminating any part of eye dropper that is inserted in bottle.
- Tilt head back, pull down lower lid. At the same time, look up while drop is being instilled into conjunctival sac. Immediately apply gentle pressure just below the eyelid and next to nose for 1 min. Close eyes gently, so as not to squeeze out medication.
- Report purulent eye discharge to physician. Sulfacetamide sodium is inactivated by purulent exudates.

SULFADIAZINE

(sul-fa-dye'a-zeen)

Microsulfon

Classifications: ANTIINFECTIVE; SULFONAMIDE ANTIBIOTIC

Prototype: Sulfisoxazole

Pregnancy Category: B

AVAILABILITY 500 mg tablets

ACTIONS Short-acting sulfonamide, slightly less soluble than sulfisoxazole. Exerts bacteriostatic effect by interfering with bacterial utilization of PABA, thereby inhibiting folic acid biosynthesis required for bacterial growth.

THERAPEUTIC EFFECTS Effective against a wide range of gram-positive and gram-negative microorganisms.

USES Used in combination with pyrimethamine for treatment of cerebral toxoplasmosis and chloroquine-resistant malaria.

CONTRAINDICATIONS Hypersensitivity to sulfonamides or to any ingredients in the formulation; pregnancy (category C).

CAUTIOUS USE Application of lotion to denuded or debrided skin; lactation.

ROUTE & DOSAGE

Mild to Moderate Infections

Adult: **PO Loading Dose** 2–4 g loading dose **PO Maintenance Dose** 2–4 g/d in 4–6 divided doses
Child: **PO Loading Dose** *>2 mo,* 75 mg/kg **PO Maintenance Dose** 150 mg/kg/d in 4–6 divided doses (max: 6 g/d)

Rheumatic Fever Prophylaxis

Adult: **PO** *<30 kg,* 500 mg/d; *>30 kg,* 1 g/d

Toxoplasmosis

Adult: **PO** 2–8 g/d divided q6h
Child: **PO** *>2 mo,* 100–200 mg/kg/d divided q6h
Neonate: **PO** 50 mg/kg q12h times 12 mo

ADMINISTRATION

Oral

- Maintain sufficient fluid intake to produce urinary output of at least 1500 mL/24 h for children between 3000 and 4000 mL/24 h for adults. Concomitant administration of urinary alkalinizer may be prescribed to reduce possibility of crystalluria and stone formation.
- Store in tight, light-resistant containers.

ADVERSE EFFECTS (≥1%) **CNS:** Headache, peripheral neuritis, peripheral neuropathy, tinnitus, hearing loss, vertigo, insomnia, drowsiness, mental depression, acute psychosis, ataxia, convulsions, kernicterus (newborns). **GI:** *Nausea, vomiting, diarrhea,* abdominal pains, hepatitis, jaundice, pancreatitis, stomatitis. **Hematologic:** Acute hemolytic anemia (especially in patients with G6PD deficiency), <u>aplastic anemia</u>, methemoglobinemia, <u>agranulocytosis</u>, thrombocytopenia, leukopenia, eosinophilia, hypoprothrombinemia. **Body as a Whole:** Headache, *fever,* chills, arthralgia, malaise, allergic myocarditis, serum sickness, <u>anaphylactoid reactions</u>, lymphadenopathy, local reaction following IM injection, fixed drug eruptions, diuresis, overgrowth of nonsusceptible organisms, LE phenomenon. **Skin:** Pruritus, urticaria, rash, erythema multiforme including <u>*Stevens-Johnson syndrome, exfoliative dermatitis,*</u> alopecia, photosensitivity, vascular lesions. **Urogenital:** *Crystalluria,* hematuria, proteinuria, anuria, toxic nephrosis, reduction in sperm count. **Metabolic:** Goiter, hypoglycemia. **Special Senses:** Conjunctivitis, conjunctival or scleral infection, retardation of corneal healing (ophthalmic ointment).

INTERACTIONS Drug: PABA-CONTAINING LOCAL ANESTHETICS may antagonize sulfa's effects; ORAL ANTICOAGULANTS potentiate hypoprothrombinemia; may potentiate SULFONYLUREA-induced hypoglycemia. May decrease concentrations of **cyclosporine;** may increase levels of **phenytoin.**

PHARMACOKINETICS Absorption: Readily absorbed from GI tract. **Peak:** 3–6 h. **Distribution:** Distributed to most tissues, including CSF; crosses placenta. **Metabolism:** Metabolized in liver. **Elimination:** Excreted in urine.

NURSING IMPLICATIONS

Assessment & Drug Effects

- Lab tests: Baseline and periodic urine C&S to determine drug effectiveness; with long-term therapy, CBC, Hct and Hgb.
- Monitor hydration status.

Patient & Family Education

- Take drug exactly as prescribed. Do not alter schedule or dose; take total amount prescribed unless physician changes the regimen.
- Drink fluids liberally unless otherwise directed.
- Report early signs of blood dyscrasias (sore throat, pallor, fever) promptly to the physician.
- Do not breast feed while taking this drug without consulting physician.

SULFAMETHOXAZOLE

(sul-fa-meth-ox'a-zole)

Sulfamethoxazole

Classifications: ANTIINFECTIVE; ANTIBIOTIC, SULFONAMIDE

Prototype: Sulfisoxazole

Pregnancy Category: B

AVAILABILITY 500 mg tablets

ACTIONS Intermediate-acting sulfonamide antibiotic closely related to sulfisoxazole. Intestinal absorption and urinary excretion is slow, therefore, it is rarely used due to the potential of excessive blood level.

THERAPEUTIC EFFECTS Sulfonamides exert their bacteriostatic action by interfering with folic acid synthesis required for bacterial growth.

USES Acute, recurrent, or chronic urinary tract infections, lymphogranuloma venereum, and other infections caused by susceptible organisms.

CONTRAINDICATIONS Hypersensitivity to sulfonamides; use in treatment of group A beta-hemolytic *Streptococcal* infections; infants <2 mo of age; advanced kidney or liver disease; intestinal or urinary obstruction.

CAUTIOUS USE Impaired kidney or liver function; severe allergy; bronchial asthma; blood dyscrasias, patients with G6PD deficiency; pregnancy (category C).

ROUTE & DOSAGE

Mild to Moderate Infections

Adult: **PO Loading Dose** 2 g **PO Maintenance Dose** 1 g q8–12h
Child: **PO Loading Dose** *>2 mo,* 50–60 mg/kg **PO Maintenance Dose** 25–30 mg/kg q12h (max: 75 mg/kg/d)

ADMINISTRATION

Oral

- Give with fluid of patient's choice; tablet may be crushed.
- Maintain sufficient fluid intake to produce urinary output of at least 1500 mL/24 h for children and between 3000 and 4000 mL/24 h for adults. Concomitant administration of urinary alkalinizer may be prescribed to reduce possibility of crystalluria and stone formation.
- Store 15°–30° C (59°–86° F) in tight, light-resistant containers. Do not freeze.

ADVERSE EFFECTS (≥1%) **CNS:** Headache, peripheral neuritis, peripheral neuropathy, tinnitus, hear-

S

ing loss, vertigo, insomnia, drowsiness, mental depression, acute psychosis, ataxia, convulsions, kernicterus (newborns). **GI:** *Nausea, vomiting, diarrhea,* abdominal pains, hepatitis, jaundice, pancreatitis, stomatitis. **Hematologic:** Acute hemolytic anemia (especially in patients with G6PD deficiency), aplastic anemia, methemoglobinemia, agranulocytosis, thrombocytopenia, leukopenia, eosinophilia, hypoprothrombinemia. **Body as a Whole:** Headache, *fever,* chills, arthralgia, malaise, allergic myocarditis, serum sickness, anaphylactoid reactions, lymphadenopathy, local reaction following IM injection, fixed drug eruptions, diuresis, overgrowth of nonsusceptible organisms, LE phenomenon. **Skin:** Pruritus, urticaria, rash, erythema multiforme including *Stevens-Johnson syndrome, exfoliative dermatitis,* alopecia, photosensitivity, vascular lesions. **Urogenital:** *Crystalluria,* hematuria, proteinuria, anuria, toxic nephrosis, reduction in sperm count. **Metabolic:** Goiter, hypoglycemia. **Special Senses:** Conjunctivitis, conjunctival or scleral infection, retardation of corneal healing (ophthalmic ointment).

INTERACTIONS Drug: PABA-CONTAINING LOCAL ANESTHETICS may antagonize sulfa's effects; ORAL ANTICOAGULANTS potentiate hypoprothrombinemia; may potentiate SULFONYLUREA-induced hypoglycemia, may decrease concentrations of **cyclosporine;** may increase levels of **phenytoin.**

PHARMACOKINETICS Absorption: Incompletely absorbed from GI tract. **Peak:** 3–4 h. **Distribution:** Distributed to most tissues, including CSF; crosses placenta. **Metabolism:** Metabolized in liver. **Elimination:** Excreted in urine. **Half-Life:** 7–12 h.

NURSING IMPLICATIONS

Assessment & Drug Effects

- Lab tests: Baseline and periodic urine C&S to determine drug effectiveness; with long-term therapy, CBC, Hct and Hgb.
- Monitor hydration status.

Patient & Family Education

- Take drug exactly as prescribed. Do not alter schedule or dose; take total amount prescribed unless physician changes the regimen.
- Drink fluids liberally unless otherwise directed.
- Report early signs of blood dyscrasias (sore throat, pallor, fever) promptly to the physician.

SULFASALAZINE

(sul-fa-sal′a-zeen)

Azulfidine, PMS Sulfasalazine ✤, PMS Sulfasalazine E.C. ✤, Salazopyrin ✤, SAS Enteric-500 ✤, S.A.S.-500 ✤

Classifications: GASTROINTESTINAL AGENT; MUCOUS MEMBRANE AGENT; ANTIINFLAMMATORY; SULFONAMIDE

Prototype: Mesalamine

Pregnancy Category: B (D if near term)

AVAILABILITY 500 mg tablets; 500 mg sustained release tablets

ACTIONS Locally acting sulfonamide. Believed to be converted by intestinal microflora to sulfapyridine (provides antibacterial action) and 5-aminosalicylic acid (5-ASA) or mesalamine, which may exert an antiinflammatory effect. Other proposed mechanisms of action include inhibition of prostaglandins known to cause diarrhea and affect mucosal transport, and interference with absorption of fluids and electrolytes from colon.

THERAPEUTIC EFFECTS Reduces *Clostridium* and *Escherichia coli* in the stools. Antiinflammatory and immunomodulatory properties are effective in controlling the S&S of ulcerative colitis and rheumatoid arthritis.

USES Ulcerative colitis and relatively mild regional enteritis; rheumatoid arthritis.

UNLABELED USES Granulomatous colitis, Crohn's disease, scleroderma.

CONTRAINDICATIONS Sensitivity to sulfasalazine, other sulfonamides and salicylates; agranulocytosis; children <2 y; intestinal and urinary tract obstruction; pregnancy (category B, category D near term); porphyria.

CAUTIOUS USE Severe allergy, or bronchial asthma; blood dyscrasias; hepatic or renal impairment; older adults; lactation; children <6 y.

ROUTE & DOSAGE

Ulcerative Colitis, Rheumatoid Arthritis

Adult: **PO** 1–2 g/d in 4 divided doses, may increase up to 8 g/d if needed

Child: **PO** 40–50 mg/kg/d in 4 divided doses (max: 75 mg/kg/d)

Juvenile Rheumatoid Arthritis

Child: **PO** 10 mg/kg/d, increase weekly by 10 mg/kg/d (usual dose: 15–25 mg/kg q12h [max: 2 g/d])

ADMINISTRATION

Oral

- Give after eating to provide longer intestine transit time.
- Do not crush or chew sustained release tablets; must be swallowed whole.
- Use evenly divided doses over each 24-h period; do not exceed 8-h intervals between doses.
- Consult physician if GI intolerance occurs after first few doses. Symptoms are probably due to irritation of stomach mucosa and may be relieved by spacing total daily dose more evenly over 24 h or by administration of enteric-coated tablets.
- Store at 15°–30° C (59°–86° F) in tight, light-resistant containers.

ADVERSE EFFECTS (≥1%) **Body as a Whole:** *Nausea, vomiting, bloody diarrhea; anorexia,* arthralgia, rash, anemia, oligospermia (reversible), blood dyscrasias, liver injury, infectious mononucleosis–like reaction, *allergic reactions.*

INTERACTIONS Drug: Iron, ANTIBIOTICS may alter absorption of sulfasalazine.

PHARMACOKINETICS Absorption: 10%–15% absorbed from GI tract unchanged; remaining drug is hydrolyzed in colon to sulfapyridine (most of which is absorbed) and 5-aminosalicylic acid (30% of which is absorbed). **Peak:** 1.5–6 h sulfasalazine; 6–24 h sulfapyridine. **Distribution:** Crosses placenta; distributed into breast milk. **Metabolism:** Metabolized in intestines and liver. **Elimination:** All metabolites are excreted in urine. **Half-Life:** 5–10 h.

NURSING IMPLICATIONS

Assessment & Drug Effects

- Monitor for GI distress. GI symptoms that develop after a few days of therapy may indicate need for dosage adjustment. If symptoms persist, physician may withhold drug for 5–7 d and restart it at a lower dosage level.

- Be aware that adverse reactions generally occur within a few days to 12 wk after start of therapy; most likely to occur in patients receiving high doses (4 g or more).
- Lab tests: Measure RBC folate in patients on high doses (more than 2 g/d); a daily supplement may be prescribed.

Patient & Family Education

- Examine stools and report to physician if enteric-coated tablets have passed intact in feces. Some patients lack enzymes capable of dissolving coating; conventional tablet will be ordered.
- Be aware that drug may color alkaline urine and skin orange-yellow.
- Remain under close medical supervision. Relapses occur in about 40% of patients after initial satisfactory response. Response to therapy and duration of treatment are governed by endoscopic examinations.
- Do not breast feed while taking this drug without consulting physician.

S

SULFINPYRAZONE

(sul-fin-peer'a-zone)

Antazone ✤, Anturan ✤, Anturane, Apo-Sulfinpyrazone ✤, Novopyrazone ✤

Classification: ANTIGOUT AGENT
Prototype: Colchicine
Pregnancy Category: C

AVAILABILITY 100 mg tablets; 200 mg capsules

ACTIONS Potent renal tubular blocking agent of uric acid in the kidney that lowers serum blood level. Like all uricosurics, low doses may inhibit tubular secretion of uric acid and cause urate retention. Inhibits release of adenosine diphosphate and 5-hydroxytryptophan, and thus decreases platelet adhesiveness and increases platelet survival time; has no effect on prothrombin or blood clotting time.

THERAPEUTIC EFFECTS Promotes urinary excretion of uric acid and reduces serum urate levels by competitively inhibiting tubular reabsorption of uric acid in the kidney.

USES Maintenance therapy in chronic gouty arthritis and tophaceous gout.

UNLABELED USES Drug-induced hyperuricemia, to decrease platelet aggregation and increase their survival in prevention of TIAs and stroke.

CONTRAINDICATIONS Known hypersensitivity to phenylbutazone, or pyrazoline derivatives; active peptic ulcer; concurrent administration of salicylates; blood dyscrasias; patients with creatinine clearance less than 50 mg/min, treatment of hyperuricemia secondary to neoplastic disease or cancer chemotherapy.

CAUTIOUS USE Impaired kidney function; history of healed peptic ulcer; use in conjunction with sulfonamides and sulfonylureas; pregnancy (category C), lactation.

ROUTE & DOSAGE

Gout

Adult: **PO** 100–200 mg b.i.d. for 1 wk, then increase to 200–400 mg b.i.d., may reduce to 200 mg/d after serum urate levels are controlled (max: 800 mg/d)

Inhibition of Platelet Aggregation

Adult: **PO** 200 mg t.i.d. or q.i.d.

ADMINISTRATION

Oral

- Give with meals, milk, or antacid (prescribed) to prevent local drug irritant effect. Severity and frequency of symptoms increase with dosage. Persistence of GI symptoms may require discontinuation of drug.
- Ensure fluid intake sufficient to support urinary output of at least 2000–3000 mL/d during early therapy (consult physician). Also alkalinize urine (e.g., with large doses vitamin C) to increase solubility of uric acid and minimize risk of uric acid stones.

ADVERSE EFFECTS (≥1%) **GI:** *Nausea,* vomiting, diarrhea, *epigastric pain, blood loss, reactivation or aggravation of peptic ulcer,* jaundice. **CNS:** Ataxia, dizziness, vertigo, convulsions, coma. **Special Senses:** Tinnitus. **Body as a Whole:** Edema, labored respirations, hypersensitivity, reactions (skin rashes, fever). **Urogenital:** Precipitation of acute gout, urolithiasis, renal colic.

DIAGNOSTIC TEST INTERFERENCE Sulfinpyrazone decreases urinary excretion of ***aminohippuric acid*** and ***phenolsulfonphthalein.***

INTERACTIONS Drug: May decrease efficacy of **nitrofurantoin** for UTI and increase its systemic toxicity. May displace SULFONYLUREAS from protein binding and increase risk of hypoglycemia; may augment prothrombin time increased by **warfarin; cholestyramine** decreases absorption of sulfinpyrazone; **aspirin** may inhibit uricosuric effects of sulfinpyrazone.

PHARMACOKINETICS Absorption: Readily absorbed from GI tract. **Peak:** 1–2 h. **Duration:** 4–6 h; may persist up to 10 h. **Metabolism:** Metabolized in liver to active and inactive metabolites. **Elimination:** Slowly excreted in urine; 5% excreted in feces. **Half-Life:** 3 h.

NURSING IMPLICATIONS

Assessment & Drug Effects

- Monitor therapy using serum urate levels (lower to about 6 mg/dL) to reduce joint changes, tophi formation, and frequency of acute attacks and to improve kidney function.
- Lab tests: Obtain periodic blood cell counts during prolonged therapy. Also kidney function, particularly with renal impairment. Monitor PT and INR with concurrent warfarin use.
- Frequency of acute gouty attacks may increase during first 6–12 mo of therapy, even when serum urate levels appear to be controlled. Concurrent prophylactic doses of colchicine may be prescribed during first 3–6 mo of treatment to prevent or lessen severity of attacks.

Patient & Family Education

- Remain under close medical supervision; therapy is continued indefinitely.
- Do not experiment with dosage; subtherapeutic doses may enhance urate retention and large doses may increase risk of toxicity.
- Continue medication without interruption even during acute gouty attack. Contact physician for concomitant treatment with full therapeutic doses of colchicine or other antiinflammatory agent.
- Avoid aspirin-containing medications. If an analgesic is required (in patients with normal kidney

S

function), acetaminophen is generally recommended.
- Do not breast feed while taking this drug without consulting physician.

SULFISOXAZOLE (Pr)

(sul-fi-sox'a-zole)

Gantrisin

Classifications: ANTIINFECTIVE; SULFONAMIDE

Pregnancy Category: B (D if near term)

AVAILABILITY 500 mg tablets

ACTIONS Short-acting derivative of sulfanilamide. Bacteriostatic action believed to be by competitive inhibition of *p*-aminobenzoic acid (PABA), thereby interfering with folic acid biosynthesis required for bacterial growth.

THERAPEUTIC EFFECTS Exhibits broad antimicrobial spectrum against both gram-positive and gram-negative organisms.

USES Acute, recurrent, and chronic urinary tract infections and chancroid; adjunctive therapy in trachoma, chloroquine-resistant strains of malaria, acute otitis media due to *Haemophilus influenzae,* and meningococcal and *H. influenzae* meningitis. Ophthalmic preparations used in treatment of conjunctivitis, corneal ulcer, and other superficial eye infections and as adjunct to systemic sulfonamide therapy for trachoma. Topical vaginal preparation used for *H. vaginalis* vaginitis.

CONTRAINDICATIONS History of hypersensitivity to sulfonamides, salicylates, or chemically related drugs; use in treatment of group A beta-hemolytic streptococcal infections; infants <2 mo of age (except in treatment of congenital toxoplasmosis); porphyria; advanced kidney or liver disease; intestinal and urinary obstruction; pregnancy (category B, category D if near term), lactation.

CAUTIOUS USE Impaired kidney or liver function; severe allergy; bronchial asthma; blood dyscrasias; patients with G6PD deficiency.

ROUTE & DOSAGE

Infection by Susceptible Organisms

Adult: **PO** 2–4 g initially, followed by 4–8 g/d in 4–6 divided doses **Vaginal** 1 applicator full 1–2 times/d

Child: **PO** *>2 mo,* 75 mg/kg initially, followed by 150 mg/kg/d in 4–6 divided doses (max: 6 g/d)

ADMINISTRATION

Oral

- Give with full glass of water or other fluid; tablet may be crushed.
- Store at 15°–30° C (59°–86° F) in tight, light-resistant containers.

ADVERSE EFFECTS (≥1%) **CNS:** Headache, peripheral neuritis, peripheral neuropathy, tinnitus, hearing loss, vertigo, insomnia, drowsiness, mental depression, acute psychosis, ataxia, convulsions, kernicterus (newborns). **GI:** *Nausea, vomiting, diarrhea,* abdominal pains, hepatitis, jaundice, pancreatitis, stomatitis. **Hematologic:** Acute hemolytic anemia (especially in patients with G6PD deficiency), <u>aplastic anemia</u>, methemoglobinemia, <u>agranulocytosis</u>, thrombocytopenia, leukopenia, eosinophilia, hypoprothrombinemia. **Body as a Whole:** Headache, *fever,* chills, arthralgia, malaise, allergic myocarditis, serum

S

sickness, anaphylactoid reactions, lymphadenopathy, local reaction following IM injection, fixed drug eruptions, diuresis, overgrowth of nonsusceptible organisms, LE phenomenon. **Skin:** Pruritus, urticaria, rash, erythema multiforme including *Stevens-Johnson syndrome exfoliative, dermatitis,* alopecia, photosensitivity, vascular lesions. **Urogenital:** *Crystalluria,* hematuria, proteinuria, anuria, toxic nephrosis, reduction in sperm count. **Metabolic:** Goiter, hypoglycemia. **Special Senses:** Conjunctivitis, conjunctival or scleral infection, retardation of corneal healing (ophthalmic ointment).

DIAGNOSTIC TEST INTERFERENCE Sulfonamides may interfere with ***BSP*** retention and ***PSP*** excretion tests and may affect results of ***thyroid function*** tests (***I-131*** may be decreased for about 7 d). Large doses of sulfonamides reportedly may produce false-positive ***urine glucose*** determinations with ***copper reduction methods*** (e.g., ***Benedict's*** and ***Clinitest***). SULFONAMIDES may produce false-positive results for ***urinary protein*** (with ***sulfosalicylic acid test***) and may interfere with ***urine urobilinogen*** determinations using ***Ehrlich's reagent*** or ***Urobilistix.*** Follow-up cultures are unreliable unless PABA is added to culture medium.

INTERACTIONS Drug: PABA-CONTAINING LOCAL ANESTHETICS may antagonize sulfa's effects; ORAL ANTICOAGULANTS potentiate hypoprothrombinemia; may potentiate SULFONYLUREA-induced hypoglycemia; may decrease concentrations of **cyclosporine;** may increase levels of **phenytoin**.

PHARMACOKINETICS Absorption: Readily absorbed from GI tract. **Peak:** 2–4 h. **Distribution:** Distributed in extracellular space; crosses blood–brain barrier and placenta; detected in breast milk. **Metabolism:** Metabolized in liver. **Elimination:** 95% excreted in urine in 24 h. **Half-Life:** 4.6–7.8 h.

NURSING IMPLICATIONS

Assessment & Drug Effects

- Lab tests: Obtain a specimen for C&S prior to initiation of therapy. Perform frequent kidney function tests and urinalyses; complete blood counts and liver function tests, especially during regimens longer than 2 wk.
- Monitor I&O. Report oliguria and changes in I&O ratio. Fluid intake should be adequate to support urinary output of at least 1500 mL/d to prevent crystalluria and stone formation.
- Check urine pH daily with Nitrazine paper or Labstix; fall in urinary pH (more acidic) increases risk of crystalluria.
- Report increasing urine acidity. If urine is highly acidic, physician may prescribe a urinary alkalinizer.
- Monitor temperature. Sudden appearance of fever may signify sensitization (serum sickness) or hemolytic anemia (frequent in patients with G6PD deficiency, which is most common among black males and Mediterranean ethnic groups). Reactions generally develop within 10 d. Agranulocytosis may develop after 10 d–6 wk of therapy.
- Report early manifestations of blood dyscrasias or hypersensitivity reactions immediately (fever with sore throat, malaise, unusual fatigue, joint pains, pallor, bleeding tendencies, rash, jaundice).
- Be alert for skin lesions, papular or vesiculobullous lesions, especially on sun-exposed areas,

S

Stevens-Johnson syndrome (severe erythema multiforme) may be preceded by high fever, severe headache, stomatitis, conjunctivitis, rhinitis, urticaria, balanitis (inflammation of penis or clitoris). Termination of drug therapy is indicated.

- Observe diabetic patients receiving oral hypoglycemic agents closely for hypoglycemic reactions. Obtain blood glucose and HbA1c levels before and shortly after initiation of therapy.

Patient & Family Education

- Do not take OTC medications without consulting physician. Many analgesic mixtures contain aspirin in combination with *p*-aminobenzoic acid; avoid to prevent crystallization in urine.
- Use or add barrier contraceptives if using hormonal contraceptives, which may be unreliable while taking this drug.
- Avoid exposure to ultraviolet light and excessive sunlight to prevent photosensitivity reaction during therapy and for several months after treatment is discontinued.
- Inform dentist or new physician that you are taking a sulfonamide.
- Do not breast feed while taking this drug.

S

SULINDAC

(sul-in′dak)
Clinoril
Classifications: CENTRAL NERVOUS SYSTEM AGENT; ANALGESIC, ANTIPYRETIC; NONSTEROIDAL ANTIINFLAMMATORY DRUG (NSAID)
Prototype: Ibuprofen
Pregnancy Category: B (D in third trimester)

AVAILABILITY 150 mg, 200 mg tablets

ACTIONS Acetic acid derivative structurally and pharmacologically related to indomethacin. Exact mechanism of antiinflammatory action not known but thought to result from inhibition of prostaglandin synthesis. Comparable to aspirin in antiinflammatory activity with longer half-life, lower incidence of GI intolerance and tinnitus, and less effect on bleeding time and platelet function. May prolong bleeding time, but prothrombin time, whole blood clotting time, and platelet count are not affected.

THERAPEUTIC EFFECTS Exhibits antiinflammatory, analgesic, and antipyretic properties.

USES Acute and long-term symptomatic treatment of osteoarthritis, rheumatoid arthritis, ankylosing spondylitis; acute painful shoulder (acute subacromial bursitis or supraspinatus tendinitis); acute gouty arthritis.

CONTRAINDICATIONS Hypersensitivity to sulindac; hypersensitivity to aspirin (patients with "aspirin triad": acute asthma, rhinitis, nasal polyps) or to other NSAIDS; significant kidney or liver dysfunction; pregnancy (category B; category D in third trimester), lactation. Safety in children is not established.

CAUTIOUS USE History of upper GI tract disorders; compromised cardiac function, hypertension, hemophilia or other bleeding tendencies.

ROUTE & DOSAGE

Arthritis, Ankylosing Spondylitis, Acute Gouty Arthritis

Adult: **PO** 150–200 mg b.i.d. (max: 400 mg/d)

ADMINISTRATION

Oral

- Crush and give mixed with liquid or food if patient cannot swallow tablet.
- Administer with food, milk, or antacid (if prescribed) to reduce possibility of GI upset. Note: Food retards absorption and delays and lowers peak concentrations.

ADVERSE EFFECTS (≥1%) **CNS:** Drowsiness, *dizziness, headache,* anxiety, nervousness. **CV:** Palpitation, peripheral edema, CHF, (patients with marginal cardiac function). **Special Senses:** Blurred vision, amblyopia, vertigo, tinnitus, decreased hearing. **GI:** *Abdominal pain, dyspepsia, nausea, vomiting, constipation,* diarrhea, ulceration, flatulence, anorexia; stomatitis, sore or dry mucous membranes, dry mouth; GI bleeding, gastritis. **Hematologic:** Prolonged bleeding time, aplastic anemia, thrombocytopenia, leukopenia, eosinophilia. **Body as a Whole:** Angioneurotic edema, fever, chills, anaphylaxis. **Skin:** Stevens-Johnson syndrome, toxic epidermal necrolysis syndrome, rash, pruritus. **Urogenital:** Renal impairment.

DIAGNOSTIC TEST INTERFERENCE Abnormalities in ***liver function tests*** may occur.

INTERACTIONS Drug: **Heparin,** ORAL ANTICOAGULANTS may prolong bleeding time; may increase **lithium** toxicity; **aspirin,** other NSAIDS add to ulcerogenic effects; may increase **methotrexate** toxicity; **dimethylsulfoxide (DMSO)** may decrease effects of sulindac. **Herbal: Feverfew, garlic, ginger, ginkgo** may increase bleeding potential.

PHARMACOKINETICS Absorption: 90% absorbed from GI tract. **Peak:** 2 h without food, 3–4 h with food. **Duration:** 10–12 h. **Distribution:** Minimal passage across placenta; distributed into breast milk. **Metabolism:** Metabolized in liver to active sulfide metabolite. **Elimination:** 75% excreted in urine, 25% in feces. **Half-Life:** 7.8 h sulindac, 16.4 h sulfide metabolite.

NURSING IMPLICATIONS

Assessment & Drug Effects

- Lab tests: Obtain baseline and periodic evaluations of Hgb, kidney and liver function.
- Schedule auditory and ophthalmic examinations in patients receiving prolonged or high-dose therapy.
- Recommend an ophthalmoscopic examination if patient has eye complaints.

Patient & Family Education

- Do not drive or engage in potentially hazardous activities until response to drug is known.
- Report any incidence of unexplained bleeding or bruising immediately to physician (e.g., bleeding gums, black and tarry stools, coffee-colored emesis).
- Report onset of skin rash, itching, hives, jaundice, swelling of feet or hands, sore throat or mouth, shortness of breath, or night cough to physician.
- Be aware that adverse GI effects are relatively common. Report abdominal pain, nausea, dyspepsia, diarrhea, or constipation.
- Note: Initial effect may take up to 7 d; peak effect is usually experienced in 2–3 wk (relief of joint pain and stiffness, reduction in joint swelling, increase in

grip strength, and improved mobility).

- Avoid alcohol and aspirin as they may increase risk of GI ulceration and bleeding tendencies.
- Inform dentist or surgeon of drug regimen because bleeding time may be prolonged.
- Do not breast feed while taking this drug.

SUMATRIPTAN Ⓟ

(sum-a-trip'tan)

Imitrex

Classifications: AUTONOMIC NERVOUS SYSTEM AGENT; 5-HT_1 SEROTONIN AGONIST

Pregnancy Category: C

AVAILABILITY 25 mg, 50 mg tablets; 12 mg/mL injection; 5 mg, 20 mg nasal spray

ACTIONS Selective agonist for a serotonin receptor (probably 5-HT_{1D}) that causes vasoconstriction of cranial carotid arteries. This does not result in decreased arterial blood pressure or total peripheral resistance.

THERAPEUTIC EFFECTS Causes vasoconstriction of cranial carotid arteries, thus relieving the migraine headache. Also relieves photophobia, phonophobia, nausea and vomiting associated with migraine attacks.

USES Treatment of acute migraine attacks with or without aura, cluster headache.

CONTRAINDICATIONS Hypersensitivity to sumatriptan; IV use; coronary artery disease (CAD); risk factors for CAD such as hypertension, hypercholesterolemia, obesity, diabetes, smoking, and strong family history; concurrent use with ergotamine drugs; concurrent use of oral sumatriptan with MAO INHIBITORS; basilar or hemiplegic migraine.

CAUTIOUS USE Impaired liver or kidney function; concurrent use of subcutaneous sumatriptan and MAO INHIBITORS; pregnancy (category C), lactation. Safety and effectiveness in children are not established.

ROUTE & DOSAGE

Migraine or Cluster Headache

Adult: **SC** 6 mg any time after onset of migraine. If headache returns, may repeat with 6 mg SC at least 1 h after first injection (max: 12 mg/24 h) **PO** 25 mg × 1 dose, if headache returns may repeat once after 2 h (max: 100 mg) **Intranasal** 5, 10, or 20 mg in one nostril. If headache returns, may repeat once after 2 h (max: 40 mg/24 h)

ADMINISTRATION

Note: Do not give within 24 h of an ergot-containing drug.

Oral

- Give any time after symptoms of migraine appear.
- A second tablet may be given if symptoms return but no sooner than 2 h after the first tablet.
- Do not exceed 100 mg in a single oral dose or 300 mg/d.

Intranasal

- Note: A single dose is one spray into ONE nostril.

Subcutaneous

- A second injection may be given 1 h or longer following first injection if initial relief is not obtained or if migraine returns.

S

- Be aware that if adverse effects are dose limiting, a lower dose may be effective.
- Store all forms at room temperature, 15°–30° C (59°–86° F). Protect from light.

ADVERSE EFFECTS (≥1%) **CV:** Chest pressure and tightness, hypotension or hypertension, hypertensive crisis, syncope, peripheral cyanosis, thromboembolism, heart block, sinus bradycardia, atrial fibrillation, ventricular fibrillation, ventricular tachycardia, <u>coronary artery vasospasm</u>, angina, transient myocardial ischemia, <u>MI, cardiac arrest</u>. **CNS:** *Tingling, warming sensation, pressure, numbness,* headache, *dizziness, vertigo,* drowsiness, sedation, seizure, CNS hemorrhage, subarachnoid hemorrhage, stroke. **Body as a Whole:** Dizziness, lightheadedness, myalgia, or muscle cramps, *pain on injection,* weakness, flushing and a sensation of warmth or burning after injection. **GI:** Abdominal pain, cramping, diarrhea, nausea, vomiting.

INTERACTIONS Drug: Dihydroergotamine, ERGO ALKALOIDS may cause vasospasm and a slight elevation in blood pressure. MAO INHIBITORS increase sumatriptan levels and toxicity (especially the oral form); do not use concurrently or within 2 wk of stopping MAO INHIBITORS. **Herbal: Gingko, ginseng, echinacea, St. John's wort** may increase triptan toxicity.

PHARMACOKINETICS Onset: 10–30 min after SC administration. **Duration:** 1–2 h. **Distribution:** Widely distributed, 10%–20% protein bound. May be excreted in breast milk. **Metabolism:** Hepatically metabolized to inactive metabolite. **Elimination:** 57% excreted in urine, 38% excreted in feces. **Half-Life:** 2 h.

NURSING IMPLICATIONS

Assessment & Drug Effects

- Monitor cardiovascular status carefully following first dose in patients at relatively high risk for coronary artery disease (e.g., postmenopausal women, men over 40 years old, persons with known CAD risk factors) or who have coronary artery vasospasms.
- Report to physician immediately chest pain or tightness in chest or throat that is severe or does not quickly resolve following a dose of sumatriptan.
- Monitor therapeutic effectiveness. Pain relief usually begins within 10 min of injection, with complete relief in approximately 65% of all patients within 2 h.

Patient & Family Education

- Review patient information leaflet provided by the manufacturer carefully.
- Learn correct use of autoinjector for self-administration of SC dose.
- Pain or redness at injection site is common but usually disappears in less than 1 h.
- Notify physician immediately if symptoms of severe angina (e.g., severe or persistent pain or tightness in chest, back, neck, or throat) or hypersensitivity (e.g., wheezing, facial swelling, skin rash, or hives) occur.
- Do not take any other serotonin receptor agonist (Axert, Maxalt, Zomig, Amerge) within 24 h of taking sumatriptan.
- Check with physician before taking any new OTC or prescription drugs.
- Report any other adverse effects (e.g., tingling, flushing, dizziness) at next physician visit.
- Do not breast feed while taking this drug without consulting physician.

TACRINE

(tac'rine)

Cognex

Classifications: AUTONOMIC NERVOUS SYSTEM AGENT; CHOLINERGIC (PARASYMPATHOMIMETIC); CHOLINESTERASE INHIBITOR

Prototype: Neostigmine

Pregnancy Category: C

AVAILABILITY 10 mg, 20 mg, 30 mg, 40 mg capsules

ACTIONS Cholinesterase inhibitor, presumably elevates acetylcholine in the cerebral cortex by slowing degradation of acetylcholine release by the remaining intact neurons. Balance pathologic changes in neurons that result in deficiency of acetylcholine in early stages of Alzheimer's disease.

THERAPEUTIC EFFECTS Slows manifestations of Alzheimer's disease.

USE Improvement of memory in mild to moderate Alzheimer's dementia.

UNLABELED USES HIV infection (severe dementia), tardive dyskinesia, acute anticholinergic syndrome with possible advantage over physostigmine.

CONTRAINDICATIONS Hypersensitivity to tacrine; patients who develop jaundice while taking tacrine.

CAUTIOUS USE Anesthesia, sick sinus rhythm, bradycardia; history of ulcers, GI bleeding, abnormal liver function; patients with asthma, hypotension, hyperthyroidism, urinary tract obstruction, intestinal obstruction; pregnancy (category C), lactation. Safety and efficacy in children are not established.

ROUTE & DOSAGE

Alzheimer's Disease

Adult: **PO** 10 mg q.i.d. (taken between meals if tolerated), increase in 40 mg/d increments not sooner than q6wk (max: 160 mg/d)

Hepatic Impairment

Dose-related hepatotoxic effects have been observed, use with caution or not at all in patients with history of past or current liver disease

ADMINISTRATION

Oral

- Give at least 1 h before meals; bioavailability reduced 30%–40% when taken with food. Effectiveness depends on administration at regular intervals.
- Titrate dose upward as long as serum transaminase (ALT) levels remain less than or equal to 3 times upper limit of normal (ULN).
- Reduce daily dose by 40 mg/d when ALT exceeds 3 times but is less than or equal to 5 times ULN. Resume titration when ALT returns to normal.
- Stop treatment if ALT exceeds 5 times ULN.
- Store at room temperature, 15°–30° C (59°–86° F), away from moisture.

ADVERSE EFFECTS (≥1%) **CNS:** Agitation, dizziness and confusion, ataxia, insomnia, somnolence, hallucinations. **GI:** Nausea, *vomiting,* belching, *diarrhea,* abdominal discomfort, anorexia, *hepatotoxicity.* **Skin:** Purpura. **Urogenital:** Excessive micturition and incontinence with UTI infections. **Body as a Whole:** Diaphoresis.

INTERACTIONS Drug: Prolongs action of **succinylcholine** and possibly other NEUROMUSCULAR BLOCK-

ING AGENTS due to inhibition of plasma pseudocholinesterase. Increases **theophylline** concentrations two-fold. **Cimetidine** increases concentration of tacrine by 64%. **Herbal: Echinacea** may increase risk of hepatotoxicity.

PHARMACOKINETICS Absorption: Approximately 17% absorbed from GI tract. Food decreases rate and extent of absorption by 30–40%. **Onset:** 30–90 min. **Peak:** 2 h. Steady state in 24–36 h. **Distribution:** Penetrates blood–brain barrier. Protein binding is 55%. **Metabolism:** Metabolized in the liver by cytochrome P-450 system. At least three hydroxylated metabolites have been identified that may be biologically active. Females have lower activity in cytochrome P-450 isoenzymes so plasma levels are approximately 50% higher than men with same dose. **Elimination:** Less than 3% of dose recovered in urine in 24 h. **Half-Life:** 3.5 h.

NURSING IMPLICATIONS

Assessment & Drug Effects

- Monitor for clinical improvement (defined as a 4-point improvement in Alzheimer's Disease Assessment Scale/Cognitive Subscale). Improvement has been observed after 1–4 wk; may take 6 mo for maximum benefit.
- Lab tests: Monitor serum transaminase (ALT) levels according to following schedule: Every 2 wk for first 16 wk, then monthly for 2 mo, then every 3 mo thereafter; resume weekly monitoring for 6 wk with each dose increase; continue weekly monitoring if ALT remains more than 2 times normal; if therapy is interrupted more than 4 wk then restarted, resume full ALT monitoring schedule.
- Monitor I&O because tacrine may cause bladder outflow obstruction.
- Monitor for seizure activity and take appropriate precautions.
- Monitor patients with history of angle-closure glaucoma for a worsening of this condition.
- Monitor for GI distress and bleeding, especially in patients with a history of peptic ulcer disease or on concurrent NSAID therapy.
- Supervise ambulation because dizziness occurs in more than 10% of patients.
- Monitor cardiovascular status including periodic ECG monitoring. Assess for fluid retention and worsening of CHF.
- Monitor periodically for development of drug-induced diabetes.

Patient & Family Education

- Be aware of adverse effects related to initiation of therapy or dosage increases (e.g., nausea, vomiting, diarrhea) as well as delayed effects (e.g., rash, GI bleeding, jaundice). Report adverse effects to the physician.
- Do not discontinue or reduce dosage of 80 mg/d or more abruptly because it may precipitate acute deterioration of cognitive function.
- Make sure to have regular follow-up and liver function tests.
- Tacrine may induce seizures, vertigo, and syncope. Use appropriate precautions.
- Understand that tacrine therapy is not a cure and will become ineffective at some point as the disease progresses.

TACROLIMUS

(tac-rol'i-mus)

Prograf, Protopic

Classification: IMMUNOSUPPRESSANT
Prototype: Cyclosporine
Pregnancy Category: C

T

AVAILABILITY 0.5 mg, 1 mg, 5 mg capsules; 5 mg/mL injection; 0.1%, 0.03% ointment

ACTIONS Macrolide antibiotic produced by a soil fungus with immunosuppressant activity more marked than that of cyclosporine. Inhibits helper T-lymphocytes by selectively inhibiting secretion of interleukin-2, interleukin-3, and interleukin-gamma; thus reduces transplant rejection.
THERAPEUTIC EFFECTS Inhibits antibody production (thus subduing immune response) by creating an imbalance in favor of suppressor T-lymphocytes.

USES Liver rejection prophylaxis; rejection prophylaxis for other organ transplants (kidney, heart, bone marrow, pancreas, small bowel), moderate to severe atopic dermatitis (e.g., eczema).
UNLABELED USES Acute organ transplant rejection, severe plaque-type psoriasis.

CONTRAINDICATIONS Hypersensitivity to tacrolimus or castor oil; pregnancy (category C), lactation.
CAUTIOUS USE Renal or hepatic insufficiency, hyperkalemia, diabetes mellitus, gout, history of seizures, hypertension.

T

ROUTE & DOSAGE

Rejection Prophylaxis
Adult: **PO** 0.15–0.3 mg/kg/d in 2 divided doses q12h, start no sooner than 6 h after transplant; give first oral dose 8–12 h after discontinuing IV therapy **IV** 0.05–0.1 mg/kg/d as continuous IV infusion, start no sooner than 6 h after transplant, continue until patient can take oral therapy
Child: **PO** Same as adult but start with upper end of dosage range **IV** Same as adult but start with upper end of dosage range

Atopic Dermatitis
Adult: **Topical** Apply thin layer to affected area b.i.d., continue for 1 wk after clearing of symptoms
Child: **Topical** *2–15 y,* Apply thin layer of 0.03% ointment to affected area b.i.d., continue for 1 wk after clearing of symptoms

Severe Plaque-Type Psoriasis
Adult: **PO** Start with 0.05 mg/kg/d, increase to 0.1 mg/kg/d at week 3 and to 0.15 mg/kg/d at week 6 if necessary

ADMINISTRATION

Oral
- Discontinue cyclosporine at least 24 h before the first dose of tacrolimus.
- Convert patient from IV to oral therapy as soon as possible.
- Give first oral dose 8–12 h after discontinuing IV infusion.

Topical
- Ensure that skin is clean and completely dry before application.
- Apply a thin layer to the affected area and rub in gently and completely.
- Do not apply occlusive dressing over the site.

Intravenous

PREPARE: **IV Infusion:** Dilute 5 mg/mL ampuls with NS or D5W to a concentration of 0.004–0.02 mg/mL, or less for pediatric patients.
ADMINISTER: **IV Infusion:** Give as continuous IV.
INCOMPATIBILITIES **Y-site: Phenytoin.**

- Store ampuls between 5° and 25° C (41° and 77° F); store capsules at room temperature, 15°–30° C (59°–86° F). ▪ Store the diluted infusion in glass or polyethylene containers and discard after 24 h.

ADVERSE EFFECTS (≥1%) **CNS:** *Headache, tremors, insomnia, paresthesia, hyperesthesia* and/or sensations of warmth, circumoral numbness. **CV:** *Mild to moderate hypertension.* **Endocrine:** Hirsutism, *hyperglycemia, hyperkalemia, hypokalemia, hypomagnesemia,* hyperuricemia, decreased serum cholesterol. **GI:** *Nausea, abdominal pain, gas,* appetite changes, *vomiting, anorexia, constipation,* diarrhea, ascites. **Hematologic:** *Anemia, leukocytosis, thrombocytopenia purpura.* **Urogenital:** UTI, oliguria, nephrotoxicity. **Respiratory:** *Pleural effusion, atelectasis, dyspnea.* **Special Senses:** Blurred vision, photophobia. **Skin:** *Flushing, rash, pruritus, skin irritation,* alopecia, erythema, folliculitis, hyperesthesia, exfoliative dermatitis, hirsutism, photosensitivity, skin discoloration, skin ulcer, sweating. **Body as a Whole:** *Pain, fever, peripheral edema.*

INTERACTIONS Drug: Use with **cyclosporine** increases risk of nephrotoxicity. **Erythromycin, metoclopramide** may increase tacrolimus levels; **caspofungin, rifampin** may decrease levels. NSAIDS may lead to oliguria or anuria.

PHARMACOKINETICS Absorption: Erratic and incompletely absorbed from GI tract; absolute bioavailability approximately 14–25%; absorption reduced by food. **Peak:** PO 1–4 h. **Duration:** IV 12 h. **Distribution:** Within plasma, tacrolimus is found primarily in lipoprotein-deficient fraction; 75%–97% protein bound, mainly to albumin and alpha$_1$-acid glycoprotein; distributed into red blood cells; blood:plasma ratio reported >4; animal studies have demonstrated high concentrations of tacrolimus in lung, kidney, heart, and spleen, and similar tissue profile is to be expected in humans; distributed into breast milk. **Metabolism:** Extensively metabolized in liver. **Elimination:** Metabolites excreted primarily in bile. **Half-Life:** 8.7–11.3 h.

NURSING IMPLICATIONS

Assessment & Drug Effects

- Lab tests: Monitor serum electrolytes, blood glucose, uric acid, BUN, and creatinine clearance periodically.
- Monitor kidney function closely; report elevated serum creatinine or decreased urinary output.
- Monitor for neurotoxicity, and report tremors, changes in mental status, or other signs of toxicity.
- Monitor cardiovascular status and report hypertension.

Patient & Family Education

- Learn complete dosing instructions.
- Be aware of potential adverse effects.
- Minimize exposure to natural or artificial sunlight while using the ointment.
- Notify physician of S&S of neurotoxicity.
- Do not breast feed while taking this drug.

TADALAFIL

(ta-dal'a-fil)
Cialis
Classifications: IMPOTENCE AGENT; PHOSPHODIESTERASE (PDE) INHIBITOR; VASODILATOR
Prototype: Sildenafil
Pregnancy Category: B

AVAILABILITY 5 mg, 10 mg, 20 mg tablets

ACTIONS Tadalafil is a selective phosphodiesterase (PDE) type 5 inhibitor. PDE type 5 is responsible for degradation of cyclic GMP in the corpus cavernosum of the penis. Cyclic GMP causes smooth muscle relaxation in the corpus cavernosum, thereby allowing inflow of blood into the penis.

THERAPEUTIC EFFECTS Tadalafil promotes sustained erection only in the presence of sexual stimulation.

USES Treatment of erectile dysfunction.

CONTRAINDICATIONS Hypersensitivity to tadalafil, vardenafil, or sildenafil; concurrent administration of nitrates, nitroglycerin, or any alpha-adrenergic antagonist (other than 0.4 mg qd tamsulosin); MI within last 90 d; Class 2 or greater heart failure within last 6 mo; unstable angina or angina during intercourse; uncontrolled cardiac arrhythmias; hypotension, uncontrolled hypertension; CVA within last 6 mo; left ventricular outflow obstruction, aortic stenosis; not recommended for women, pregnancy (category B), or children; lactation.

CAUTIOUS USE CAD, risk factors for CVA; renal insufficiency; hepatic impairment, hepatic disease; anatomic deformity of the penis; sickle cell anemia; multiple myeloma; leukemia; active bleeding or a peptic ulcer; hiatal hernia, GERD; sickle cell disease; retinitis pigmentosa; hepatitis, cirrhosis; severe renal impairment; older adults; concurrent use with other medicines for penile dysfunction.

ROUTE & DOSAGE

Erectile Dysfunction

Adult: **PO** 10 mg prior to anticipated sexual activity. May increase to max dose 20 mg/d or reduce to 5 mg/d if needed. If taking ritonavir, itraconazole, ketoconazole, or voriconazole, max dose 10 mg q72h

Hepatic Impairment

Mild to Moderate Impairment: max 10 mg/d; not recommended with severe hepatic impairment

Renal Impairment

Cl_{cr} 30–50 ml/min: start at 5 mg once daily (max: 10 mg q48h); <30 mL/min: max dose 5 mg

ADMINISTRATION

Oral

- Take approximately 1 h before expected intercourse, but preferably not after a heavy or high-fat meal.
- Store at 15°–30° C (59°–86° F).

ADVERSE EFFECTS (≥1%) **Body as a Whole:** Flushing, back pain, asthenia, facial edema, fatigue, pain. **CNS:** *Headache,* dizziness, insomnia, somnolence, vertigo, hypesthesia, paresthesia. **CV:** Angina, chest pain, hypertension, hypotension, MI, orthostatic hypotension, palpitations, syncope, sinus tachycardia. **GI:** Dyspepsia, nausea, vomiting, abdominal pain, abnormal liver function tests, diarrhea, loose stools, dysphagia, esophagitis, gastritis, GERD, xerostomia. **Metabolic:** Increased GGTP. **Musculoskeletal:** Arthralgia, myalgia, neck pain. **Respiratory:** Nasal congestion, dyspnea, epistaxis, pharyngitis. **Skin:** Rash, pruritus, sweating. **Special Senses:** Blurred vision, changes in color vision, conjunctivitis, eye pain, lacrimation, swelling of eyelids. **Urogenital:** Spontaneous penile erection.

INTERACTIONS Drug: May potentiate hypotensive effects of ETHANOL, NITRATES, **alfuzosin, doxazosin, prazosin, tamsulosin** (doses >0.4 mg/d), **terazosin; erythromycin** (and other MACROLIDES), **indinavir, intraconazole, ketoconazole,** PROTEASE INHIBITORS, **ritonavir, saquinavir, voriconazole** may increase levels and toxicity of tadalafil; **barbiturates, bosentan, carbamazepine, dexamethasone, fosphenytoin, nevirapine, rifampin phenytoin, rifabutin, troglitazone** may reduce level and effectiveness of tadalafil. **Food: Grapefruit juice** may increase levels and toxicity of tadalafil.

PHARMACOKINETICS Absorption: Rapidly absorbed, 15% reaches systemic circulation. **Onset:** 30–45 min. **Peak:** 2 h. **Duration:** Up to 36 h. **Metabolism:** Metabolized in liver by CYP3A4. **Elimination:** Excreted in feces (61%) and urine (39%). **Half-Life:** 17.5 h.

NURSING IMPLICATIONS

Assessment & Drug Effects

- Monitor CV status and report angina or other S&S of cardiac dysfunction.
- Lab tests: Baseline and periodic LFTs.

Patient & Family Education

- Do not take more than once per day.
- Note: With moderate renal insufficiency, the maximum recommended dose is 10 mg not more than once in every 48 h.
- Moderate use of alcohol when taking this drug.
- Do not take this drug without consulting physician if you are taking drugs called "alpha blockers" or "nitrates" or any other drugs for high blood pressure, chest pain, or enlarged prostate.
- Report promptly any of the following: palpitations, chest pain, back pain, difficulty breathing, or shortness of breath; dizziness or fainting; changes in vision; swollen eyelids; muscle aches; painful or prolonged erection (lasting longer than 4 h); skin rash, or itching.

TAMOXIFEN CITRATE (Pr)

(ta-mox'i-fen)

Nolvadex, Nolvadex-D ♣, Tamofen ♣

Classifications: ANTINEOPLASTIC AGENT; HORMONES & SYNTHETIC SUBSTITUTES; ANTIESTROGEN

Pregnancy Category: D

AVAILABILITY 10 mg, 20 mg tablets

ACTIONS Nonsteroidal gonad-stimulating drug with potent antiestrogenic activity. Competes with estradiol at estrogen receptor sites in target tissues such as breast, uterus, vagina, anterior pituitary, tumor with high concentration of estrogen receptors.

THERAPEUTIC EFFECTS Tamoxifen-receptor complexes move into the cell nucleus, decreasing DNA synthesis and estrogen responses. Ovulation may be induced by stimulation of the release of hypothalamic gonadotropic-releasing factor.

USES Palliative treatment of advanced breast cancer in postmenopausal women, adjunctively with surgery in the treatment of breast carcinoma with positive lymph nodes.

UNLABELED USES Investigationally to stimulate ovulation in selected anovulatory women desiring pregnancy.

T

CONTRAINDICATIONS Anticoagulant therapy, pregnancy (category D), especially during first trimester; preexisting endometrial hyperplasia; intramuscular injections if platelets <50,000/mm^3; history of thromboembolic disease; lactation; children.
CAUTIOUS USE Vision disturbances; cataracts, visual disturbance; leukopenia, bone marrow suppression; thrombocytopenia; hypercalcemia; hypercholesterolemia, lipid protein abnormalities.

ROUTE & DOSAGE

Breast Carcinoma
Adult: **PO** 10–20 mg 1–2 times/d (morning and evening)
Stimulation of Ovulation
Adult: **PO** 5–40 mg b.i.d. for 4 d

ADMINISTRATION

Oral
- With severe adverse effects, a simple reduction in dosage gives sufficient relief without losing control of disease. Consult physician.
- Store at 15°–30° C (59°–86° F); protect from light.

ADVERSE EFFECTS (≥1%) **Body as a Whole:** Increased bone pain, and transient local disease flair; loss of hair, weight gain, shortness of breath, photosensitivity, *hot flashes.* **CNS:** Depression, light-headedness, dizziness, headache, mental confusion, sleepiness. **CV:** Thrombosis, pulmonary embolism, increased risk of stroke. **GI:** *Nausea and vomiting (about 25% of patients),* distaste for food, anorexia. **Hematologic:** Leukopenia, thrombocytopenia. **Metabolic:** Hypercalcemia. **Skin:** Skin rash or dryness. **Special Senses:** Retinopathy, decreased visual acuity, blurred vision. **Urogenital:** Changes in menstrual period, milk production and leaking from breasts, vaginal discharge and bleeding, pruritus vulvae.

DIAGNOSTIC TEST INTERFERENCE Tamoxifen may produce transient increase in ***serum calcium.***

INTERACTIONS Drug: May enhance hypoprothrombinemic effects of **warfarin;** may increase risk of thromboembolic events with CYTOTOXIC AGENTS; **bromocriptine** may elevate tamoxifen levels, SSRI ANTIDEPRESSANTS may decrease effectiveness of tamoxifen.

PHARMACOKINETICS Absorption: Slowly absorbed from GI tract. **Peak:** 3–6 h. **Metabolism:** Metabolized in liver, enterohepatically cycled. **Elimination:** Excreted primarily in feces. **Half-Life:** 7 d.

NURSING IMPLICATIONS

Assessment & Drug Effects
- Monitor therapeutic effectiveness. An objective response may require 4–10 wk of therapy, longer if there is bone metastasis.
- Administer analgesics for pain relief as necessitated by bone and tumor pain or local disease flair. Reassure patient that this discomfort frequently signals a good tumor response.
- Be aware that local swelling and marked erythema over preexisting lesions or the development of new lesions may signal soft-tissue disease response to tamoxifen. These symptoms rapidly subside.
- Lab tests: Assess CBC, including platelet counts, periodically. Transient leukopenia and thrombocytopenia (50,000–100,000/mm^3) without hemorrhagic tendency have been reported. Monitor serum calcium periodically.

Patient & Family Education

- Do not change established dose schedule.
- Report to physician occurrence of marked weakness, sleepiness, mental confusion, edema, dyspnea, blurred vision.
- Understand the possibility of drug-induced menstrual irregularities before starting treatment.
- Avoid prolonged sun exposure, especially if skin is unprotected. Apply sunscreen lotions (SPF 12 or greater) to all exposed skin surfaces.
- Avoid OTC drugs unless specifically prescribed by the physician; particularly OTC pain medicines.
- Report onset of tenderness or redness in an extremity.
- Do not breast feed while taking this drug without consulting physician.

TAMSULOSIN HYDROCHLORIDE

(tam′su-lo-sin)

Flomax

Classifications: AUTONOMIC NERVOUS SYSTEM AGENT; ALPHA-ADRENERGIC ANTAGONIST (SYMPATHOLYTIC AGENT)

Prototype: Prazosin HCl

Pregnancy Category: B

AVAILABILITY 0.4 mg capsules

ACTIONS Antagonist of the $alpha_{1A}$-adrenergic receptors located in the prostate. Symptoms related to benign prostatic hypertrophy (BPH) are related to bladder outlet obstruction.

THERAPEUTIC EFFECTS Blockage of $alpha_{1A}$-adrenergic receptors can cause smooth muscles in the bladder outlet and the prostate gland to relax, resulting in improvement in urinary blood flow and a reduction in symptoms of BPH. Indicated by improved voiding.

USE Benign prostatic hypertrophy.

CONTRAINDICATIONS Hypersensitivity to tamsulosin; in conjunction with another $alpha_{1A}$-adrenergic blocking agent; lactation, pediatric patients.

CAUTIOUS USE Pregnancy (category B); history of syncope, hypotension.

ROUTE & DOSAGE

Benign Prostatic Hypertrophy

Adult: **PO** 0.4 mg q.d. 30 min after a meal, may increase up to 0.8 mg q.d.

ADMINISTRATION

Oral

- Give 30 min after the same meal each day.
- Instruct to swallow capsules whole; not to crush, chew, or open.
- If dose is interrupted for several days, reinitiate at the lowest dose, 0.4 mg.
- Store at 20°–25° C (68°–77° F).

ADVERSE EFFECTS (≥1%) **Body as a Whole:** Asthenia, back or chest pain. **CNS:** *Headache, dizziness,* insomnia. **CV:** *Orthostatic hypotension (especially with first dose).* **GI:** Diarrhea, nausea. **Respiratory:** *Rhinitis,* pharyngitis, increased cough, sinusitis. **Urogenital:** Decreased libido, *abnormal ejaculation.* **Special Senses:** Amblyopia.

INTERACTIONS Drug: Cimetidine may decrease clearance of **tamsulosin.**

PHARMACOKINETICS Absorption: Rapidly absorbed from GI tract. >90% bioavailability. **Peak:** 4–5 h fasting, 6–7 h fed. **Distribution:** Widely distributed in body tissues, including kidney and prostate. **Metabolism:** Metabolized in the liver. **Elimination:** 76% excreted in urine. **Half-Life:** 14–15 h.

NURSING IMPLICATIONS

Assessment & Drug Effects

- Monitor for signs of orthostatic hypotension; take BP lying down, then upon standing. Report a systolic pressure drop of ≥15 mm Hg or a HR ≥15 beats upon standing.
- Monitor patients on warfarin therapy closely.

Patient & Family Education

- Make position changes slowly to minimize orthostatic hypotension.
- Report dizziness, vertigo, or fainting to physician. Exercise caution with hazardous activities until response to drug is known.
- Be aware that concurrent use of cimetidine may increase the orthostatic hypotension adverse effect.

TAZAROTENE

(ta-zar′o-teen)

Avage, Tazorac

Classifications: SKIN AND MUCOUS MEMBRANE AGENT; ANTIACNE; RETINOID

Prototype: Isotretinoin

Pregnancy Category: X

AVAILABILITY 0.05%, 0.1% gel, cream

ACTIONS Retinoid prodrug that blocks epidermal cell proliferation and hyperplasia. Mechanism of action in acne is not known.

THERAPEUTIC EFFECTS Suppresses inflammation present in the epidermis of psoriasis patients. Indicated by improvement in acne or psoriasis; effective in treatment of mild to moderate acne.

USES Topical treatment of plaque psoriasis on up to 20% of the body, mild to moderate acne, facial fine wrinkling, mottled hypo- and hyperpigmentation (blotchy skin discoloration), and benign facial lentigines.

CONTRAINDICATIONS Hypersensitivity to tazarotene; pregnancy (category X), women who are or may become pregnant.

CAUTIOUS USE Concurrent administration with drugs that are photosensitizers (e.g., thiazide diuretics, tetracyclines). Lactation. Safety and efficacy in children <12 y are not established.

ROUTE & DOSAGE

Plaque Psoriasis

Adult: **Topical** Apply thin film to affected area once daily in evening

Acne

Adult: **Topical** After cleansing and drying face, apply thin film to acne lesions once daily in evening

Fine Wrinkles

Adult: **Topical** Apply thin film of cream to affected area once daily

ADMINISTRATION

Topical

- Dry skin completely before application of a thin film of medication.
- Apply medication to no more than 20% of body surface in those with psoriasis.
- Apply only to affected areas; avoid contact with eyes and mucous membranes.

ADVERSE EFFECTS (≥1%) **Skin:** *Pruritus, burning/stinging, erythema, worsening of psoriasis, irritation, skin pain,* rash, desquamation of skin, irritant contact dermatitis, inflammation, fissuring, bleeding, dry skin, sunburn.

T

INTERACTIONS Drug: Increased risk of photosensitivity reactions with QUINOLONES (especially **sparfloxacin**), PHENOTHIAZINES, SULFONAMIDES, SULFONYLUREAS, TETRACYCLINES, THIAZIDE DIURETICS.

PHARMACOKINETICS Absorption: Rapidly absorbed through skin. **Distribution:** Active metabolite >99% protein bound; crosses placenta, distributed into breast milk. **Metabolism:** Undergoes esterase hydrolysis to active metabolite AGN 190299. **Elimination:** Eliminated in both urine and feces. **Half-Life:** 18 h.

NURSING IMPLICATIONS

Assessment & Drug Effects

- Monitor for photosensitivity in those concurrently using any of the following: thiazides, tetracyclines, fluoroquinolones, phenothiazines, sulfonamides.

Patient & Family Education

- Understand fully the risk of serious fetal harm. Use reliable forms of effective contraception. Discontinue treatment and notify physician if pregnancy occurs.
- Alert: Immediately rinse thoroughly with water if contact with eyes occurs.
- Avoid all unnecessary exposure to sunlight or artificial UV light. If brief exposure is necessary, cover as much skin surface as possible and use sunscreens (minimum SPF 15).
- Do not apply to sunburned skin.
- Discontinue medication and notify physician if any of the following occur: pruritus, burning, skin redness, excessive peeling, worsening of psoriasis.
- Limit application of topicals with strong skin-drying effects to skin areas being treated with tazarotene.
- Do not breast feed while using this drug without consulting physician.

TEGASEROD MESYLATE

(teg-a-se′rod mes′y-late)

Zelnorm

Classifications: GASTROINTESTINAL AGENT; SEROTONIN 5-HT_4 RECEPTOR AGONIST

Pregnancy Category: B

AVAILABILITY 2 mg, 6 mg tablets

ACTIONS A serotonin 5-HT_4 receptor agonist that triggers the peristaltic reflex by activating 5-HT_4 receptors thereby normalizing impaired GI motility.

THERAPEUTIC EFFECTS Significantly decreases gastric lag time, accelerates gastric emptying, reduces small bowel transit time and accelerates colonic transit time; thus, it increases the number of bowel movements and facilitates stool formation.

USES Short term treatment of Irritable Bowel Syndrome (IBS) in women whose primary symptom is constipation, chronic idiopathic constipation in males and females <65 y.

UNLABELED USES IBS in men; diabetic gastroparesis.

CONTRAINDICATIONS Hypersensitivity to tegaserod; severe hepatic or renal dysfunction; cirrhosis; renal failure; bowel obstruction; symptomatic gall bladder disease, abdominal pain, colitis, GI bleeding; renal failure; syncope; hypotension; patients who are currently or frequently experiencing diarrhea; lactation; children <18 y.

CAUTIOUS USE Mild to moderate hepatic and renal impairment; MI, cardiac disease; history of ovarian cysts; patients in whom increased

T

diarrhea could have negative effects; pregnancy (category B).

ROUTE & DOSAGE

Irritable Bowel Syndrome
Adult: **PO** 6 mg b.i.d. before meals for 4–6 wk. May extend therapy an additional 4–6 wk if needed and responding

Chronic Constipation
Adult: **PO** 2–6 mg b.i.d.

ADMINISTRATION

Oral

- Give drug just prior to a meal with a full glass of water.
- Determine duration of therapy prior to drug administration as manufacturer states maximum duration of therapy should be 12 wk.
- Do not initiate therapy with patients experiencing frequent diarrhea. Report to physician.
- Store at 15°–30° C (59°–86° F).

ADVERSE EFFECTS (≥1%) **Body as a Whole:** Leg pain. **CNS:** *Headache,* dizziness, migraine. **GI:** *Abdominal pain,* diarrhea, nausea, flatulence. **Musculoskeletal:** Back pain, arthropathy.

INTERACTIONS Food: Food significantly decreases the bioavailability of tegaserod.

PHARMACOKINETICS Absorption: Poorly absorbed, 10% bioavailability on an empty stomach. **Peak:** 1 h. **Distribution:** 99% protein bound to alpha-1 glycoprotein. **Metabolism:** Presystemic hydrolysis in stomach to an inactive metabolite. Glucuronidation in liver of remaining drug. **Elimination:** 2/3 excreted in feces, 1/3 excreted in urine. **Half-Life:** 11 h.

NURSING IMPLICATIONS

Assessment & Drug Effects

- Lab tests: Monitor baseline and periodic LFTs and renal functions.
- Monitor symptom relief. Report lack of symptom relief or frequent diarrhea.
- Monitor cardiovascular status especially with preexisting CV disease.

Patient & Family Education

- Report no relief of symptoms after 4 wk of therapy as manufacturer recommends discontinuation of therapy in this case.
- Do not breast feed while taking this drug.
- Notify physician if you experience new or worsening abdominal pain unlike your typical IBS symptoms.

TELITHROMYCIN

(tel-i-thro-my'sin)
Ketek, Ketek Pak
Classifications: ANTIINFECTIVES; ANTIBIOTIC, MACROLIDE; KETOLIDE
Prototype: Erythromycin
Pregnancy Category: C

AVAILABILITY 400 mg tablets

ACTIONS Telithromycin concentrates in phagocytes where it works against intracellular respiratory pathogens.
THERAPEUTIC EFFECTS Its broad spectrum of activity is effective against respiratory pathogens, including erythromycin- and penicillin-resistant pneumococci.

USES Treatment of acute bacterial sinusitis, acute bacterial exacerbations of chronic bronchitis (AECB), and mild to moderate community-acquired pneumonia due to susceptible bacteria.

CONTRAINDICATIONS Congenital QT prolongation, ongoing proarrhythmic conditions such as hypokalemia, hypomagnesemia, significant bradycardia, concurrent administration of Class IA or Class III antiarrhythmic drugs; macrolide antibiotic hypersensitivity; myasthenia gravis, unless no other therapeutic option is available; pregnancy (category C); severe renal impairment or renal failure; concurrent administration with cisapride, pimozide, or terfenadine; viral infections. Safety and efficacy in children <18 y are not established.

CAUTIOUS USE History of GI disease; hepatic disease; history of hepatitis or jaundice; lactation.

ROUTE & DOSAGE

Acute Exacerbations of Chronic Bronchitis, Acute Maxillary Sinusitis

Adult: **PO** 800 mg once daily for 5 d

Community-Acquired Pneumonia

Adult: **PO** 800 mg once daily for 7–10 d

ADMINISTRATION

Oral

- Do not administer concurrently with simvastatin, lovastatin, atorvastatin, Class 1A (e.g., quinidine, procainamide) or Class III (e.g., dofetilide) antiarrhythmic agents. See drug interactions for other prohibited drug combinations.
- Store at 15°–30° C (59°–86° F). Keep container tightly closed. Protect from light.

ADVERSE EFFECTS (≥1%) **CNS:** Headache, dizziness. **CV:** Potential to cause QTc prolongation. **GI:** *Diarrhea,* nausea, vomiting, loose stools, dysgeusia. **Metabolic:** Elevated LFTs. **Musculoskeletal:** May exacerbate myasthenia gravis. **Special Senses:** Blurred vision, diplopia, difficulty focusing.

INTERACTIONS Drug: Cisapride, pimozide may cause life-threatening arrhythmias; may increase concentrations of **atorvastatin, lovastatin, simvastatin, midazolam,** other BENZODIAZEPINES; **rifampin** decreases telithromycin levels; ERGOT DERIVATIVES **(ergotamine, dihydroergotamine)** may cause severe peripheral vasospasm; **theophylline** may exacerbate adverse GI effects.

PHARMACOKINETICS Absorption: 57% bioavailable. **Peak:** 1 h. **Metabolism:** 50% metabolized in liver by CYP3A4, 50% metabolized by CYP-independent mechanisms. **Elimination:** Excreted in urine and feces. **Half-Life:** 10 h.

NURSING IMPLICATIONS

Assessment & Drug Effects

- Monitor ECG in patients at risk for QTc interval prolongation (i.e., bradycardia).
- Withhold drug and notify physician for S&S of QTc interval prolongation such as dizziness or fainting; liver dysfunction.
- Lab tests: baseline LFTs, BUN and creatinine, serum potassium.

Patient & Family Education

- Stop taking drug and notify physician for episodes of dizziness or fainting; jaundice (yellow color of the skin and/or eyes).
- Exercise caution when engaging in potentially hazardous activities; visual disturbances (e.g., blurred vision, difficulty focusing, double vision) are potential side effects of this drug. If visual problems occur, avoid quick changes in viewing between close and distant objects.
- Do not breast feed while taking this drug without consulting physician.

T

TELMISARTAN

(tel-mi-sar'tan)
Micardis
Classifications: CARDIOVASCULAR AGENT; ANTIHYPERTENSIVE; ANGIOTENSIN II RECEPTOR ANTAGONIST
Prototype: Losartan potassium
Pregnancy Category: C (D in second and third trimester)

AVAILABILITY 40 mg, 80 mg tablets

ACTIONS Angiotensin II receptor (type AT_1) antagonist. Selectively blocks the binding of angiotensin II to the AT_1 receptors in many tissues (e.g., vascular smooth muscles, adrenal glands).

THERAPEUTIC EFFECTS Blocks the vasoconstricting and aldosterone-secreting effects of angiotensin II, thus resulting in an antihypertensive effect. Indicated by a reduction in BP.

USES Treatment of hypertension.

CONTRAINDICATIONS Hypersensitivity to telmisartan or other angiotensin receptor antagonists (e.g., losartan, eprosartan, etc.); pregnancy [(category C) first trimester, (category D) second and third trimester], lactation.

CAUTIOUS USE Coronary artery disease (CAD); hypertropic cardiomyopathy; CHF; oliguria; hypotension; renal artery stenosis; older adult patients; biliary obstruction; liver dysfunction; renal impairment. Safety and efficacy in children <18 y are not established.

ROUTE & DOSAGE

Hypertension
Adult: **PO** 40 mg q.d., may increase to 80 mg/d

ADMINISTRATION

Oral

- Do not remove tablets from blister pack until immediately before administration.
- Correct volume depletion prior to initial dose.
- Store at 15°–30° C (59°–86° F).

ADVERSE EFFECTS (≥1%) **Body as a Whole:** Back pain, flu-like syndrome, myalgia, headache, fatigue. **CNS:** Dizziness. **CV:** Hypotension, hypertension, chest pain, peripheral edema. **GI:** Diarrhea, dyspepsia, abdominal pain, nausea. **Respiratory:** Sinusitis, pharyngitis.

INTERACTIONS Drug: Telmisartan may increase **digoxin** levels.

PHARMACOKINETICS Absorption: Absorption is dose dependent, 42% of 40 mg dose is absorbed. **Peak:** 0.5–1 h. **Distribution:** >99% protein bound. **Metabolism:** Minimally metabolized. **Elimination:** Primarily excreted in feces as unchanged drug. **Half-Life:** 24 h.

NURSING IMPLICATIONS

Assessment & Drug Effects

- Monitor BP carefully after initial dose; and periodically thereafter. Monitor more frequently with preexisting biliary obstructive disorders or hepatic insufficiency.
- Monitor dialysis patients closely for orthostatic hypotension.
- Lab tests: Periodic Hgb, creatinine clearance, liver enzymes.
- Monitor concomitant digoxin levels throughout therapy.

Patient & Family Education

- Report pregnancy to physician immediately.
- Allow between 2–4 wk for maximum therapeutic response.
- Do not breast feed while taking this drug.

TEMAZEPAM

(te-maz′e-pam)

Restoril

Classifications: CENTRAL NERVOUS SYSTEM AGENT; ANXIOLYTIC; SEDATIVE-HYPNOTIC; BENZODIAZEPINE

Prototype: Lorazepam

Pregnancy Category: X

Controlled Substance: Schedule IV

AVAILABILITY 7.5 mg, 15 mg, 30 mg capsules

ACTIONS Benzodiazepine derivative with hypnotic, anxiolytic, sedative effects. Principal effect is significant improvement in sleep parameters.

THERAPEUTIC EFFECTS Reduces night awakenings and early morning awakenings; increases total sleep times, absence of rebound effects. Minimal change in REM sleep.

USES To relieve insomnia associated with frequent nocturnal awakenings or early morning awakenings.

CONTRAINDICATIONS Pregnancy (category X); safety in children <8 y is not established; narrow-angle glaucoma; psychoses.

CAUTIOUS USE Severely depressed patient or one with suicidal ideation; history of drug abuse or dependence, acute intoxication; liver or kidney dysfunction; older adult patients; sleep apnea; lactation.

ROUTE & DOSAGE

Insomnia

Adult: **PO** 7.5–30 mg h.s.
Geriatric: **PO** 7.5 mg h.s.

ADMINISTRATION

Oral

- Give 20–30 min before patient retires.
- Store at 15°–30° C (59°–86° F) in tight container unless otherwise specified by manufacturer.

ADVERSE EFFECTS (≥1%) **CNS:** *Drowsiness,* dizziness, lethargy, confusion, headache, euphoria, relaxed feeling, weakness. **GI:** Anorexia, diarrhea. **CV:** Palpitations.

INTERACTIONS Drug: Alcohol, CNS DEPRESSANTS, ANTICONVULSANTS potentiate CNS depression; **cimetidine** increases temazepam plasma levels, thus increasing its toxicity; may decrease antiparkinsonism effects of **levodopa;** may increase **phenytoin** levels; smoking decreases sedative effects. **Herbal: Kava-kava, valerian** may potentiate sedation.

PHARMACOKINETICS Absorption: Readily absorbed from GI tract. **Onset:** 30–50 min. **Peak:** 2–3 h. **Duration:** 10–12 h. **Distribution:** Crosses placenta; distributed into breast milk. **Metabolism:** Metabolized in liver to oxazepam. **Elimination:** Excreted in urine. **Half-Life:** 8–24 h.

NURSING IMPLICATIONS

Assessment & Drug Effects

- Be alert to signs of paradoxical reaction (excitement, hyperactivity, and disorientation) in older adults. Psychoactive drugs are the most frequent cause of acute confusion in this age group.
- CNS adverse effects are more apt to occur in the patient with hypoalbuminemia, liver disease, and in older adults. Report promptly incidence of bradycardia, drowsiness, dizziness, clumsiness, lack of coordination. Supervise ambulation, especially at night.
- Lab tests: Obtain liver and kidney function tests during long-term use.
- Be alert to S&S of overdose: Weakness, bradycardia, somno-

lence, confusion, slurred speech, ataxia, coma with reduced or absent reflexes, hypertension, and respiratory depression.

Patient & Family Education

- Be aware that improvement in sleep will not occur until after 2–3 doses of drug.
- Notify physician if dreams or nightmares interfere with rest. An alternate drug or reduced dose may be prescribed.
- Be aware that difficulty getting to sleep may continue. Drug effect is evidenced by the increased amount of rest once asleep.
- Consult physician if insomnia continues in spite of medication.
- Do not smoke after medication is taken.
- Do not use OTC drugs (especially for insomnia) without advice of physician.
- Consult physician before discontinuing drug especially after long-term use. Gradual reduction of dose may be necessary to avoid withdrawal symptoms.
- Avoid use of alcohol and other CNS depressants.
- Do not drive or engage in other potentially hazardous activities until response to drug is known. This drug may depress psychomotor skills and cause sedation.
- Do not breast feed while taking this drug without consulting physician. Distribution in the breast milk may cause sedation and possibly feeding problems and weight loss in the infant.

T

TEMOZOLOMIDE

(tem-o-zol′o-mide)

Temodar

Classifications: ANTINEOPLASTIC; ALKYLATING AGENT

Prototype: Cyclophosphamide

Pregnancy Category: D

AVAILABILITY 5 mg, 20 mg, 100 mg, 250 mg capsules

ACTIONS Cytotoxic agent with alkylating properties structurally similar to dacarbazine. Effects are cell cycle nonspecific.

THERAPEUTIC EFFECTS Interferes with purine (e.g. guanine) metabolism and thus protein synthesis in rapidly proliferating cells. Effectiveness is indicated by objective evidence of tumor regression.

USES Adult patients with refractory anaplastic astrocytoma.

CONTRAINDICATIONS Hypersensitivity to temozolomide, DTIC, or dacarbazine; pregnancy (category D), lactation.

CAUTIOUS USE Bacterial or viral infection; older adults; severe hepatic or renal impairment; myelosuppression; prior radiotherapy or chemotherapy. Safety and efficacy in children are not established.

ROUTE & DOSAGE

Astrocytoma

Adult: **PO** 150 mg/m^2 q.d. times 5 consecutive d per 28 d treatment cycle; subsequent doses are based on absolute neutrophil count on day 21 or at least 48 h before next scheduled cycle (see prescribing information for dosage adjustments based on neutrophil count)

ADMINISTRATION

Oral

- Give consistently with regard to food.
- Do not administer unless absolute neutrophil count >1500 per microliter and platelet count >100,000 per microliter.
- Do not open capsules. Avoid inhalation or contact with skin or mu-

cous membranes, if accidentally opened/damaged.
- Store at room temperature, 15°–30° C (59°–86° F).

ADVERSE EFFECTS (≥1%) **Body as a Whole:** *Headache, fatigue, asthenia, fever,* back pain, myalgia, weight gain; viral infection. **CNS:** *Convulsions, hemiparesis, dizziness, abnormal coordination, amnesia, insomnia,* paresthesia, somnolence, paresis, ataxia, dysphasia, abnormal gait, confusion, anxiety, depression. **CV:** *Peripheral edema.* **GI:** *Nausea, vomiting, constipation, diarrhea,* abdominal pain, anorexia. **Hematologic:** Anemia, *neutropenia, thrombocytopenia,* leukopenia. **Respiratory:** Upper respiratory tract infection, pharyngitis, sinusitis, cough. **Skin:** Rash, pruritus. **Metabolic:** Adrenal hypercorticism. **Urogenital:** Urinary incontinence. **Special Senses:** Diplopia, abnormal vision.

INTERACTIONS Drug: Valproic acid may decrease **temozolomide** levels.

PHARMACOKINETICS Absorption: Rapidly absorbed. **Peak:** 1 h. **Metabolism:** Spontaneously metabolized to active metabolite MTIC. **Elimination:** Excreted primarily in urine. **Half-Life:** 1.8 h.

NURSING IMPLICATIONS

Assessment & Drug Effects
- Monitor for S&S of toxicity: Infection, bleeding episodes, jaundice, rash, CNS disturbances.
- Lab tests: CBC with differential on day 22 and weekly until absolute neutrophil count (ANC) >1500 per microliter and platelet count >100,000 per microliter; periodic liver function tests & routine serum chemistry, including serum calcium.

Patient & Family Education
- Take consistently with respect to meals.
- Report to physician signs of infection, bleeding, discoloration of skin or skin rash, dizziness, lack of balance, or other bothersome side effects promptly.
- Exercise caution with hazardous activities until response to drug is known.
- Use effective methods of contraception; avoid pregnancy.
- Do not breast feed while taking this drug.

TENECTEPLASE RECOMBINANT
(ten-ect′e-plase)
TNKase
Classifications: BLOOD FORMERS, COAGULATORS, AND ANTICOAGULANTS; THROMBOLYTIC ENZYME
Prototype: Alteplase
Pregnancy Category: C

AVAILABILITY 50 mg vial

ACTIONS Tenecteplase (TNK-tPA) is a third generation thrombolytic agent with advantages over alteplase: Longer half-life, more rapid thrombolysis, greater fibrin specificity. Also, rate of noncerebral bleeding is less than in alteplase.
THERAPEUTIC EFFECTS Effective in producing thrombolysis of a clot involved in a myocardial infarction.

USES Reduction of mortality associated with acute myocardial infarction (AMI).

CONTRAINDICATIONS Active internal bleeding; history of CVA; intracranial or intraspinal surgery with 2 mo; intracranial neoplasm; arteriovenous malformation, or aneurysm; known bleeding diathesis; severe uncontrolled hypertension.

CAUTIOUS USE Recent major surgery, previous puncture of compressible vessels, CVA, recent GI or GU bleeding, recent trauma; hypertension, mitral valve stenosis, acute pericarditis, bacterial endocarditis; severe liver or kidney disease; hemorrhagic ophthalmic conditions; septic thrombophlebitis or occluded, infected AV cannula; advanced age; concurrent administration of oral anticoagulants, recent administration of GP IIb/IIIa inhibitors, condition involving bleeding. Pregnancy (category C), lactation. Safety and efficacy in children are not established.

ROUTE & DOSAGE

Acute Myocardial Infarction

Adult: **IV** Infuse dose over 5 sec, *<60 kg,* 30 mg; *60–70 kg,* 35 mg; *70–80 kg,* 40 mg; *80–90 kg,* 45 mg; *>90 kg,* 50 mg

ADMINISTRATION

Intravenous

PREPARE: **Direct:** Read and follow instructions supplied with TwinPak™ Dual Cannula Device. Withdraw 10 mL of sterile water for injection from the supplied vial; inject entire contents into the TNKase vial directing the diluent stream into the powder. Gently swirl until dissolved but do not shake. The resulting solution contains 5 mg/mL. Withdraw the appropriate dose and discard any unused solution. Follow directions supplied with TwinPak™ for proper handling of syringe.

ADMINISTER: **Direct:** Dextrose-containing IV line must be flushed before and after bolus with NS. Give as a single bolus dose over 5 s. The total dose given should not exceed 50 mg.

- Store unopened TwinPak™ at ≤30° C (86° F) or under refrigeration at 2°–8° C (36°–46° F).

ADVERSE EFFECTS (≥1%) **Hematologic:** Major bleeding, *hematoma,* GI bleed, bleeding at puncture site, hematuria, pharyngeal, epistaxis.

DIAGNOSTIC TEST INTERFERENCE Unreliable results for ***coagulation test I*** and measures of ***fibrinolytic activity.***

PHARMACOKINETICS Metabolism: Metabolized in liver. **Half-Life:** 90–130 min.

NURSING IMPLICATIONS

Assessment & Drug Effects

- Avoid IM injections and unnecessary handling or invasive procedures for the first few hours after treatment.
- Monitor for S&S of bleeding. Should bleeding occur, discontinue concomitant heparin and antiplatelet therapy; notify physician.
- Monitor cardiovascular and neurologic status closely. Persons at increased risk for life-threatening cardiac events include those with: A high potential for bleeding, recent surgery, severe hypertension, mitral stenosis and atrial fibrillation, anticoagulant therapy, and advanced age.
- Lab tests: Baseline and 1 h after administration of drug determine cardiac enzymes, circulating myoglobin, cardiac troponin-1, creatine kinase-MB; Hgb & Hct postinfusion.
- Coagulation parameters may not predict bleeding episodes.

Patient & Family Education

- Notify physician of the following immediately: A sudden, severe headache; any sign of bleeding; signs or symptoms of hypersensitivity (see Appendix F).

- Stay as still as possible and do not attempt to get out of bed until directed to do so.

TENOFOVIR DISOPROXIL FUMARATE

(ten-o-fo′vir di-so-prox′il fum′a-rate)

Viread

Classifications: ANTIINFECTIVE; ANTIRETROVIRAL AGENT; NUCLEOSIDE REVERSE TRANSCRIPTASE INHIBITOR (NRTI)

Prototype: Zidovudine

Pregnancy Category: B

AVAILABILITY 300 mg tablets

ACTIONS Tenofovir is a potent inhibitor of retroviruses, including HIV-1. It may be active against nucleoside-resistant HIV strains.

THERAPEUTIC EFFECTS The active form of tenofovir persists in HIV-infected cells for prolonged periods, thus, it results in sustained inhibition of HIV replication. It reduces the viral load (plasma HIV-RNA), and CD4 counts. It reduces the viral load (plasma HIV-RNA) of the patient.

USES In combination with other antiretrovirals for the treatment of HIV.

CONTRAINDICATIONS Hypersensitivity to tenofovir; hepatitis; lactic acidosis; concurrent administration of nephrotoxic agents, renal failure; lactation.

CAUTIOUS USE Hepatic dysfunction, alcoholism; renal impairment; obesity; children, pregnancy (category B).

ROUTE & DOSAGE

HIV Infection

Adult: **PO** 300 mg once daily with meal

Renal Insufficiency

Clcr <50 mL/min use not recommended until more data are known

ADMINISTRATION

Oral

- Give at the same time each day with a meal.
- Give 2 h before or 1 h after didanosine (if ordered concurrently).
- Store at room temperature; excursions to 15°–30° C (59°–80° F) are permitted.

ADVERSE EFFECTS (≥1%) **Body as a Whole:** Asthenia. **CNS:** Headache. **GI:** *Nausea,* vomiting, diarrhea, flatulence, abdominal pain, anorexia. **Hematologic:** Neutropenia. **Metabolic:** Increased *creatine kinase,* AST, ALT, serum amylase, triglycerides, serum glucose.

INTERACTIONS Drug: May increase **didanosine** toxicity; **acyclovir, amphotericin B, cidofovir, foscarnet, ganciclovir, probenecid, valacyclovir, valganciclovir** may increase tenofovir toxicity by decreasing its renal elimination. **Food:** Food increases absorption.

PHARMACOKINETICS Absorption: Bioavailability 25% fasting, 40% with high fat meal. **Peak:** 1 h. **Distribution:** <7% protein bound. **Metabolism:** Not metabolized by CYP450 enzyme system. **Elimination:** Renally eliminated. **Half-Life:** 11–14 h.

NURSING IMPLICATIONS

Assessment & Drug Effects

- Lab tests: Monitor baseline and periodic renal function and LFTs;

monitor periodically serum electrolytes, and ABGs if lactic acidosis is suspected.

- Monitor for S&S of bone abnormalities (e.g., bone pain, stress fractures).
- Monitor closely patients receiving other nephrotoxic agents for changes in serum creatinine and phosphorus. Withhold drug and notify physician for creatinine clearance <60 mL/min.
- Withhold drug and notify physician if patient develops clinical or lab findings suggestive of lactic acidosis or pronounced hepatotoxicity (e.g., hepatomegaly and steatosis even in the absence of marked transaminase elevations).

Patient & Family Education

- Take this drug exactly as prescribed. Do not miss any doses. If you miss a dose, take it as soon as possible and then take your next dose at its regular time. If it is almost time for your next dose, do not take the missed dose. Wait and take the next dose at the regular time. Do not double the next dose.
- Report any of the following to physician: unexplained anorexia, nausea, vomiting, abdominal pain, fatigue, dark urine.
- Do not breast feed while taking this drug.

T

TERAZOSIN

(ter-ay'zoe-sin)

Hytrin

Classifications: AUTONOMIC NERVOUS SYSTEM AGENT; ALPHA-ADRENERGIC ANTAGONIST (SYMPATHOLYTIC, BLOCKING AGENT); ANTIHYPERTENSIVE

Prototype: Prazosin

Pregnancy Category: C

AVAILABILITY 1 mg, 2 mg, 5 mg, 10 mg capsules

ACTIONS Quinazoline antihypertensive and vasodilator chemically similar to prazosin. Selectively blocks alpha$_1$-adrenergic receptors in vascular smooth muscle producing relaxation that leads to reduction of peripheral vascular resistance and lowered BP. Vasodilation is accompanied by minimal reflex increase in heart rate.

THERAPEUTIC EFFECTS Antihypertensive drug therapy reserved for patient who has failed to respond to diet, exercise, weight reduction, and other drug therapy. Effective when used with a beta-adrenergic blocking agent and a thiazide diuretic.

USES To treat hypertension alone or in combination with other antihypertensive agents (beta-adrenergic blocking agents, diuretics). To treat benign prostatic hypertrophy.

UNLABELED USES Urinary outflow obstruction.

CONTRAINDICATIONS Hypersensitivity. Safety during pregnancy (category C) or in children is not established.

CAUTIOUS USE Patients with BPH; prostate cancer; history of hypotensive episodes; lactation.

ROUTE & DOSAGE

Hypertension, Benign Prostatic Hypertrophy, Urinary Obstruction

Adult: **PO** Start with 1 mg h.s., then 1–5 mg/d (max: 20 mg/d)

ADMINISTRATION

Oral

- Give initial dose at bedtime to reduce the potential for severe hypotensive effect, which may occur with first few doses. After the initial dose, give any time of day.
- Store at 15°–30° C (59°–86° F) in tightly closed container away

from heat and strong light. Do not freeze.

ADVERSE EFFECTS (≥1%) **CNS:** *Asthenia (weakness), dizziness, headache,* drowsiness, weakness. **CV:** Postural hypotension, palpitation, *first-dose phenomenon (syncope).* **Special Senses:** Blurred vision. **GI:** Nausea. **Body as a Whole:** Weight gain, pain in extremities, peripheral edema. **Respiratory:** Nasal congestion, sinusitis, dyspnea, **Urogenital:** Impotence.

INTERACTIONS Drug: Antihypertensive effects may be attenuated by NSAIDS.

PHARMACOKINETICS Absorption: Readily absorbed from GI tract. **Peak:** 1–2 h. **Metabolism:** Metabolized in liver. **Elimination:** 60% excreted in feces, 40% in urine. **Half-Life:** 9–12 h.

NURSING IMPLICATIONS

Assessment & Drug Effects

- Be alert for possible first-dose phenomenon (precipitous decline in BP with consciousness disturbance). This is rare; occurs within 90–120 min of initial dose.
- Monitor BP at end of dosing interval (just before next dose) to determine level of antihypertensive control. Check BP also 2–3 h after the dose to determine if maximum and minimal responses are similar.
- Be aware that drug-induced decrease in BP appears to be more position dependent (i.e., greater in the erect position) during the first few hours after dosing than at end of 24 h.
- A greatly diminished hypotensive response at end of 24 h indicates need for change in dosage (increased dose or twice daily regimen). Report to physician.

Patient & Family Education

- Avoid situations that would result in injury should syncope (loss of consciousness) occur after first dose. If faintness develops, lie down promptly.
- Make position changes slowly (i.e., change in direction or from recumbent to upright posture). Dangle legs and move ankles a minute or so before standing when arising. Orthostatic hypotension (greatest shortly after dosing) can pose a problem with ambulation.
- Do not drive or engage in potentially hazardous activities for at least 12 h after first dose, after dosage increase, or when treatment is resumed after interruption of therapy. Twelve hours should be sufficient time for serious adverse effects (syncope, orthostatic hypotension, light-headedness, dizziness) to appear if they are going to do so.
- Monitor weight: Report sudden gain of more than 0.5–1 kg (1–2 lb) accompanied by edema in extremities to physician. Dose adjustment may be indicated.
- Do not alter established drug regimen. Consult physician if drug is omitted for several days. Drug will be started with the initial dosing regimen.
- Keep scheduled appointments for assessment of BP control and other clinically significant tests.
- Keep a daily record noting BP and time taken, which arm was used, position (i.e., standing, sitting), and time when medication was taken. Take this record to physician for reference at checkup appointment.
- Do not take OTC medications, particularly those that may contain an adrenergic agent (e.g., remedies for coughs, colds, allergy) without first consulting physician.
- Do not breast feed while taking this drug without consulting physician.

TERBINAFINE HYDROCHLORIDE

(ter-bin'a-feen)

Lamisil, Lamisil DermaGel

Classifications: ANTIINFECTIVE; ANTIBIOTIC; ANTIFUNGAL

Prototype: Fluconazole

Pregnancy Category: B

AVAILABILITY 250 mg tablets; 1% cream; 1.12% gel

ACTIONS Synthetic antifungal agent that inhibits sterol biosynthesis in fungi and ultimately causes fungal cell death.

THERAPEUTIC EFFECTS Ergosterol, the principal sterol in the fungal cell membrane, becomes depleted and interferes with cell membrane function, thus producing the antifungicidal effect.

USES Topical treatment of superficial mycoses such as interdigital tinea pedis, tinea cruris, and tinea corporis due to *Epidermophyton floccosum, Trichophyton mentagrophytes,* or *T. rubrum;* oral treatment of onychomycosis due to tinea unguium.

CONTRAINDICATIONS Hypersensitivity to terbinafine; lactation.

CAUTIOUS USE Pregnancy (category B). Safety and efficacy in children <12 y are not established.

T

ROUTE & DOSAGE

Tinea Pedis, Tinea Cruris, or Tinea Corporis

Adult: **Topical** Apply q.d. or b.i.d. to affected and immediately surrounding areas until clinical signs and symptoms are significantly improved (1–7 wk)

Onychomycosis

Adult: **PO** 250 mg q.d. times 6 wk for fingernails or times 12 wk for toenails

ADMINISTRATION

Topical

- Apply externally. Avoid application to mucous membranes and avoid contact with eyes.
- Do not use occlusive dressings unless specifically directed to do so by physician.
- Store at 15°–30° C (59°–86° F).

ADVERSE EFFECTS (≥1%) **Skin:** Pruritus, local burning, dryness, rash, vesiculation, redness, contact dermatitis at application site. **CNS:** *Headache.* **GI:** Diarrhea, dyspepsia, abdominal pain, liver test abnormalities, liver failure (rare). **Hematologic:** Neutropenia (rare). **Special Senses:** Taste disturbances.

INTERACTIONS Drug: May increase **theophylline** levels; may decrease **cyclosporine** levels; **rifampin** may decrease **terbinafine** levels.

PHARMACOKINETICS Absorption: 70% PO; approximately 3.5% of topical dose is absorbed systemically. **Elimination:** Excreted in urine. **Half-Life:** 36 h.

NURSING IMPLICATIONS

Patient & Family Education

- Learn correct technique for application of cream.
- Notify physician if drug causes increased skin irritation or sensitivity.
- Be aware that medication must be used for full treatment time to be effective.
- Do not breast feed while taking this drug.

TERBUTALINE SULFATE

(ter-byoo'te-leen)

Brethaire, Brethine, Bricanyl

Classifications: AUTONOMIC NERVOUS SYSTEM AGENT; BETA-ADRENERGIC AGONIST; BRONCHODILATOR

Prototype: Albuterol

Pregnancy Category: B

AVAILABILITY 2.5 mg, 5 mg tablets; 0.2 mg aerosol; 1 mg/mL injection

ACTIONS Synthetic adrenergic stimulant with selective $beta_2$- and negligible $beta_1$-agonist (cardiac) activity. Exerts preferential effect on $beta_2$ receptors in bronchial smooth muscles, inhibits histamine release from mast cells, and increases ciliary motility.

THERAPEUTIC EFFECTS Relieves bronchospasm in chronic obstructive pulmonary disease (COPD) and significantly increases vital capacity. Promotes relaxation of vascular smooth muscle, contraction of GI and urinary sphincters, increase in renin, pancreatic beta-cell secretion, and serum HDL-cholesterol concentration. Increases uterine relaxation (thereby preventing or abolishing high intrauterine pressure).

USES Orally or subcutaneously as a bronchodilator in bronchial asthma and for reversible airway obstruction associated with bronchitis and emphysema.

UNLABELED USES To delay delivery in preterm labor.

CONTRAINDICATIONS Known hypersensitivity to sympathomimetic amines; severe hypertension and coronary artery disease; tachycardia with digitalis intoxication; within 14 d of MAO inhibitor therapy; angle-closure glaucoma. Used only after evaluation of risk-benefit ratio in pregnancy (category B) and lactation.

CAUTIOUS USE Angina, stroke, hypertension; diabetes mellitus; thyrotoxicosis; history of seizure disorders; cardiac arrhythmias; older adults; kidney and liver dysfunction.

ROUTE & DOSAGE

Bronchodilator

Adult: **PO** 2.5–5 mg t.i.d. at 6 h intervals (max: 15 mg/d) **SC** 0.25 mg q15–30min up to 0.5 mg in 4 h **Inhaled** 2 inhalations separated by 60 s q4–6h

Adolescent: **PO** *12–15 y,* 2.5 mg t.i.d. at 6 h intervals (max: 7.5 mg/d) **SC** 0.25 mg q15–30min up to 0.5 mg in 4 h **Inhaled** 2 inhalations separated by 60 s q4–6h

Child: **PO** *<12 y,* 0.05 mg/kg q8h, gradually increase up to 0.15 mg/kg q8h (max: 5 mg/d) **SC** 0.005–0.01 mg/kg (max: 0.4 mg) q15–20min times 2 doses

Premature Labor

Adult: **PO** 2.5 mg q4–6h

ADMINISTRATION

Oral

- Give with fluid of patient's choice; tablets may be crushed.
- Be certain about recommended doses: PO preparation, 2.5 mg; SC, 0.25 mg. A decimal point error can be fatal.
- Give with food if GI symptoms occur.

Subcutaneous

- Give SC injection into lateral deltoid area.
- Store all forms at 15°–30° C (59°–86° F); protect from light. Do not freeze.

ADVERSE EFFECTS (≥1%) **CNS:** *Nervousness, tremor,* headache, *light-*

T

headedness, drowsiness, fatigue, seizures. **CV:** *Tachycardia,* hypotension or hypertension, *palpitation,* maternal and fetal tachycardia. **GI:** Nausea, vomiting. **Body as a Whole:** Sweating, muscle cramps.

DIAGNOSTIC TEST INTERFERENCE Terbutaline may increase ***blood glucose*** and free ***fatty acids.***

INTERACTIONS Drug: Epinephrine, other SYMPATHOMIMETIC BRONCHODILATORS may add to effects; MAO INHIBITORS, TRICYCLIC ANTIDEPRESSANTS potentiate action on vascular system; effects of both BETA-ADRENERGIC BLOCKERS and terbutaline antagonized.

PHARMACOKINETICS Absorption: 33%–50% absorbed from GI tract. **Onset:** 30 min PO; <15 min SC; 5–30 min inhaled. **Peak:** 2–3 h PO; 30–60 min SC; 1–2 h inhaled. **Duration:** 4–8 h PO; 1.5–4 h SC; 3–4 h inhaled. **Distribution:** Distributed into breast milk. **Metabolism:** Metabolized in liver. **Elimination:** Excreted primarily in urine, 3% in feces. **Half-Life:** 3–4 h.

NURSING IMPLICATIONS

Assessment & Drug Effects

- Assess vital signs: Baseline pulse and BP and before each dose. If significantly altered from baseline level, consult physician. Cardiovascular adverse effects are more apt to occur when drug is given by SC route or it is used by a patient with cardiac arrhythmia.
- Most adverse effects are transient, however, rapid heart rate may persist for a relatively long time.
- Be aware that onset and degree of effect and incidence and severity of adverse effects of SC formulation resemble those of epinephrine.
- Aerosolized drug produces minimal cardiac stimulation or tremors.
- Be aware that muscle tremor is a fairly common adverse effect that appears to subside with continued use.
- Monitor for symptoms of hypoglycemia in neonates born of a mother who used terbutaline during pregnancy.
- Monitor patient being treated for premature labor for CV S&S for 12 h after drug is discontinued. Report tachycardia promptly.
- Monitor I&O ratio. Fluid restriction may be necessary. Consult physician.

Patient & Family Education

- Adhere to established dosage regimen (i.e., do not change dose intervals or omit, increase, or decrease the dose).
- Inhalator therapy: Review instructions for use of inhalator (included in the package).
- Learn how to take your own pulse and the limits of change that indicate need to notify the physician.
- Consult physician if breathing difficulty is not relieved or if it becomes worse within 30 min after an oral dose.
- Keep appointments with physician for evaluation of continued drug effectiveness and clinical condition. Terbutaline appears to have a short clinical period for sustained effectiveness.
- Consult physician if symptomatic relief wanes; tolerance can develop with chronic use. Usually, a substitute agent will be prescribed.
- Do not self-dose this drug, particularly during long-term therapy. In the face of waning response, increasing the dose will not improve the clinical condition and may cause overdosage. Understand that decreasing relief with

continued treatment indicates need for another bronchodilator, not an increase in dose.
- Do not puncture container, use or store it near heat or open flame, or expose to temperatures above 49° C (120° F), which may cause bursting. Contents of the aerosol (inhalator) are under pressure.
- Do not use any other aerosol bronchodilator while being treated with aerosol terbutaline. Do not self-medicate with an OTC aerosol.
- Do not use OTC drugs without physician approval. Many cold and allergy remedies, for example, contain a sympathomimetic agent that when combined with terbutaline may cause harmful adverse effects.
- Do not breast feed while taking/using this drug.

TERCONAZOLE

(ter-con'a-zole)

Terazol-7, Terazol-3

Classifications: ANTIINFECTIVE; ANTIFUNGAL

Prototype: Fluconazole

Pregnancy Category: C

AVAILABILITY 0.4%, 0.8% vaginal cream; 80 mg vaginal suppositories

ACTIONS Exact mechanism of action is uncertain; however, it may exert its antifungal activity by disruption of normal fungal cell membrane permeability.

THERAPEUTIC EFFECTS Exhibits fungicidal activity against *Candida albicans.*

USES Local treatment of vulvovaginal candidiasis.

CONTRAINDICATIONS Hypersensitivity to terconazole; lactation.

CAUTIOUS USE Pregnancy (category C). Safety and efficacy in children are not established.

ROUTE & DOSAGE

Candidiasis

Adult: **Intravaginal** One suppository (2.5 g) q.h.s. times 3 d; one applicator full of 0.4% cream q.h.s. times 7 d; one applicator full of 0.8% cream q.h.s. times 3 d

ADMINISTRATION

Intravaginal
- Insert applicator high into the vagina (except during pregnancy).
- Wash applicator before and after each use.
- Store away from direct heat and light.

ADVERSE EFFECTS (≥1%) **CNS:** *Headache.* **Urogenital:** Vaginal itching, burning, irritation. **Body as a Whole:** Rash, flu-like syndrome (fever, chills, headache, hypotension).

INTERACTIONS Drug: May inactivate **nonoxynol-9** spermicides.

PHARMACOKINETICS Absorption: Slow minimal absorption from vagina. **Onset:** Within 3 d. **Metabolism:** Metabolized in liver. **Elimination:** Half eliminated in urine, half in feces. **Half-Life:** 4–11 h.

NURSING IMPLICATIONS

Assessment & Drug Effects
- Do not use if patient has a history of allergic reaction to other antifungal agents, such as miconazole.
- Monitor for sensitization and irritation; these may indicate need to discontinue drug.

Patient & Family Education
- Use correct application technique.
- Learn potential adverse reactions, including sensitization and allergic response.

T

- Be aware that terconazole may interact with diaphragms and latex condoms; avoid concurrent use within 72 h.
- Refrain from sexual intercourse while using terconazole.
- Wear only cotton underwear; change daily.
- Do not breast feed while using this drug.

TERIPARATIDE

(ter-i-par'a-tide)

Forteo

Classifications: HORMONES & SYNTHETIC SUBSTITUTES; PARATHYROID HORMONE AGONIST

Pregnancy Category: C

AVAILABILITY 750 mcg/3 mL injection

ACTIONS Parathyroid hormone (PTH) is the primary regulator of calcium and phosphate metabolism in bone and kidney. Actions of PTH include regulation of bone metabolism, renal reabsorption of calcium and phosphate, and intestinal calcium absorption. The biological actions of PTH and teriparatide are similar in bone and the kidneys.

THERAPEUTIC EFFECTS Stimulates new bone formation by preferential stimulation of osteoblastic activity over osteoclastic activity; improves bone microarchitecture, and increases bone mass and strength by stimulating new bone formation.

USES Treatment of osteoporosis in postmenopausal women at high risk for fracture; increase bone mass in men with primary or hypogonadal osteoporosis who are at high risk for fracture.

CONTRAINDICATIONS Use >2 y; hypersensitivity to teriparatide; osteosarcoma; Paget's disease; unexplained elevations of alkaline phosphatase; bone metastases or a history of skeletal malignancies; metabolic bone diseases other than osteoporosis; preexisting hypercalcemia; prior history of radiation therapy involving the skeleton; pediatric patients or young adults with open epiphyses; lactation; pregnancy (category C).

CAUTIOUS USE Active or recent urolithiasis, hypercalciuria; hypotension; concurrent use of digitalis; hepatic, renal, and cardiac disease.

ROUTE & DOSAGE

Osteoporosis

Adult: **SC** 20 mcg q.d.

ADMINISTRATION

Subcutaneous

- Do not administer to anyone with hypercalcemia. Consult physician.
- Rotate SC injection sites.

ADVERSE EFFECTS (≥1%) **Body as a Whole:** *Pain,* asthenia, neck pain. **CNS:** Headache, dizziness, depression, insomnia, vertigo. **CV:** Hypertension, angina, syncope. **GI:** Nausea, constipation, dyspepsia, vomiting. **Metabolic:** *Transient increase in calcium levels,* increase in serum uric acid, antibodies to teriparatide after 12 mo therapy. **Musculoskeletal:** *Arthralgia,* leg cramps. **Respiratory:** Rhinitis, cough, pharyngitis, dyspnea, pneumonia. **Skin:** Rash, sweating.

INTERACTIONS Drug: May increase risk of **digoxin** toxicity.

PHARMACOKINETICS Absorption: Extensively absorbed from SC site. **Onset:** 2 h for calcium concentration increase. **Peak:** Max. calcium concentrations 4–6 h. **Duration:** 16–24 h.

Metabolism: Parathyroid hormone is metabolized non-specific enzymes. **Elimination:** Primarily excreted in urine. **Half-Life:** 1 h SC.

NURSING IMPLICATIONS

Assessment & Drug Effects

- Monitor cardiovascular status including BP and subjective reports of angina.
- Lab tests: Monitor periodically serum calcium, alkaline phosphatase, uric acid and bone density levels.
- Concurrent drugs: Monitor closely for digoxin toxicity with concurrent use.

Patient & Family Education

- Report unexplained leg cramps and bone pain.
- Learn correct technique for SC injection.

TESTOLACTONE

(tess-toe-lak'tone)

Teslac

Classifications: ANTINEOPLASTIC; HORMONE; ANABOLIC STEROID

Pregnancy Category: C

Controlled Substance: Schedule III

AVAILABILITY 50 mg tablets

ACTIONS Chemotherapeutic agent with chemical configuration similar to certain androgens but devoid of androgenic activity (virilization) in therapeutic doses. Exact mechanism of antineoplastic action unknown.

THERAPEUTIC EFFECTS In breast cancer, effect may result from depression of ovarian function by inhibition of synthesis of pituitary gonadotropin. Indicated by decrease in size of tumor; more than 50% of nonosseous lesions decrease in size even though all bone lesions remain static.

USES Adjunctive treatment in palliation of breast carcinoma in postmenopausal women when hormone therapy is indicated. Also effective in women diagnosed before menopause in whom ovarian function has been subsequently terminated.

CONTRAINDICATIONS Premenopausal women; breast cancer in males. Pregnancy (category C), lactation.

CAUTIOUS USE Hypercalcemia; cardiorenal disease.

ROUTE & DOSAGE

Adjunctive Therapy for Breast Cancer

Adult: **PO** 250 mg q.i.d.

ADMINISTRATION

Oral

- Note: If anticoagulants are concurrently ordered, dose is usually reduced when testolactone is initiated.
- Store at 15°–30° C (59°–86° F) unless otherwise directed. Protect from freezing.

ADVERSE EFFECTS (≥1%) **CNS:** Paresthesias. **Endocrine:** Deepening of the voice, acne, facial hair growth, clitoral enlargement. **GI:** Glossitis, anorexia; nausea, vomiting. **CV:** Hypertension, edema in extremities.

DIAGNOSTIC TEST INTERFERENCE ***Urinary 17-OHCS*** determinations may be elevated.

INTERACTIONS Drug: May enhance hypoprothrombinemic effects of ORAL ANTICOAGULANTS.

PHARMACOKINETICS Absorption: Readily absorbed from GI tract. **Metabolism:** Metabolized in liver. **Elimination:** Excreted in urine.

NURSING IMPLICATIONS

Assessment & Drug Effects

- Monitor therapeutic effectiveness. Clinical response usually occurs in 6–12 wk.
- Lab tests: Check plasma calcium levels periodically (normal serum calcium: 8.5–10.6 mg/dL).
- Monitor PT and INR carefully with concurrent anticoagulant therapy.
- Report S&S that suggest impending hypercalcemia (see Appendix F).
- Monitor I&O ratio and pattern.
- Encourage patient mobility if feasible; if not, assist with passive exercises.

Patient & Family Education

- Drug treatment is usually continued for a minimum of 3 mo to evaluate response (unless there is active progression of the disease).
- Be aware that hypercalcemia represents active remission of bone metastasis; if it occurs, appropriate therapy is instituted.
- Do not breast feed while taking this drug.

TESTOSTERONE (Pr)

(tess-toss′ter-one)

Androderm, AndroGel, Striant, Testoderm, Testoderm TTS, Testopel, Testim

TESTOSTERONE CYPIONATE

Andro-Cyp, Andronate, Depo-Testosterone, Depotest, Duratest

TESTOSTERONE ENANTHATE

Delatest, Delatestryl, Malogex ✦, Testone L.A., Testrin PA, and others

Classifications: HORMONES AND SYNTHETIC SUBSTITUTES; ANDROGEN/ANABOLIC STEROID; ANTINEOPLASTIC
Pregnancy Category: X
Controlled Substance: Schedule III

AVAILABILITY **Testosterone** 75 mg implantable pellets; 2.5 mg/24 h, 4 mg/24 h, 5 mg/24 h, 6 mg/24 h, transdermal patch; 1% gel; 2.5 g, 5 g gel packets; 30 mg buccal patch **Testosterone Cypionate** 100 mg/mL, 200 mg/mL injection **Testosterone Enanthate** 100 mg/mL, 200 mg/mL injection

ACTIONS Synthetic steroid compound with both androgenic and anabolic activity (1:1). Controls development and maintenance of secondary sexual characteristics. **Androgenic activity:** Responsible for the growth spurt of the adolescent and for growth termination by epiphyseal closure. In males and some females, reduces excretion of phosphorus, nitrogen, potassium, sodium, and chloride. Increases erythropoiesis, possibly by stimulating production of renal or extrarenal erythropoietin, and promotes vascularization and darkening of skin. **Anabolic activity:** Increases protein metabolism and decreases its catabolism. Large doses suppress spermatogenesis, thereby causing testicular atrophy.

THERAPEUTIC EFFECTS Antagonizes effects of estrogen excess on female breast and endometrium. Responsible for the growth spurt of the adolescent male and onset of puberty.

USES Androgen replacement therapy, delayed puberty (male), palliation of female mammary cancer (1–5 y postmenopausal), and to treat postpartum breast engorgement. Available in fixed combination with estrogens in many preparations.

CONTRAINDICATIONS Hypersensitivity or toxic reactions to androgens; serious cardiac, liver, or kidney disease; hypercalcemia; known or suspected prostatic or breast cancer in male; benign prostatic hypertrophy with obstruction; patients easily stimulated sexually; older adults; asthenic males who may react adversely to androgenic overstimulation; conditions aggravated by fluid retention; hypertension. Pregnancy (category X), possibility of virilization of external genitalia of female fetus, lactation.

CAUTIOUS USE Cardiac, liver, and kidney disease; prepubertal males, geriatric patients, acute intermittent porphyria.

ROUTE & DOSAGE

Male Hypogonadism

Adult: **IM Cypionate, Enanthate** 50–400 mg q2–4wk **Topical** Start with 6 mg/d system applied daily, if scrotal area inadequate, use 4 mg/d system; **Androderm** Apply to torso; **AndroGel** Apply one packet to upper arms, shoulders, or abdomen once daily; **Striant** Apply one patch to the gum region just above the incisor tooth q12h

Delayed Puberty

Adult: **IM Cypionate, Enanthate** 50–200 mg q2–4wk

Metastatic Breast Cancer

Adult: **IM Cypionate, Enanthate** 200–400 mg q2–4wk

ADMINISTRATION

Buccal

- Apply buccal patch to gum just above the incisor tooth.

Transdermal

- Apply transdermal system on clean, dry scrotal skin. Dry shave scrotal hair for optimal skin contact. Do not use chemical depilatories. Wear patch for 22–24 h.
- Apply Androderm patches to abdomen, back, thigh, or upper arm. Alternate application site q24h with ≥7 d between same site.
- Store at 15°–30° C (59°–86° F).

Intramuscular

- Give IM injections deep into gluteal musculature.
- Store IM formulations prepared in oil at room temperature. Warming and shaking vial will redisperse precipitated crystals.

ADVERSE EFFECTS (≥1%) **CNS:** Excitation, insomnia. **CV:** Skin flushing and vascularization. **GI:** Nausea, vomiting, anorexia, diarrhea, gastric pain, jaundice. **Hematologic:** Leukopenia. **Metabolic:** Hypercalcemia, hypercholesterolemia, *sodium and water retention (especially in older adults) with edema*. **Renal:** Renal calculi (especially in the immobilized patient), bladder irritability. **Urogenital:** *Increased libido*. **Skin:** *Acne,* injection site irritation and sloughing. **Body as a Whole:** Hypersensitivity to testosterone, <u>anaphylactoid reactions</u> (rare). **Hematologic:** Precipitation of acute intermittent porphyria. **Endocrine:** Female—suppression of ovulation, lactation, or menstruation; hoarseness or deepening of voice (often irreversible); hirsutism; oily skin; clitoral enlargement; regression of breasts; male-pattern baldness (in disseminated breast cancer); flushing, sweating; vaginitis with pruritus, drying, bleeding; menstrual irregularities. Male—prepubertal-premature epiphyseal closure, phallic enlargement, priapism. Postpubertal—testicular atrophy, decreased ejaculatory volume, azoospermia, oligospermia (after prolonged administration or excessive dosage), impotence, epididymitis, priapism, *gynecomastia*.

DIAGNOSTIC TEST INTERFERENCE Testosterone alters ***glucose tolerance*** tests; decreases ***thyroxine-***

binding globulin concentration (resulting in decreased ***total T_4*** serum levels and increased ***resin of T_3*** and ***T_4***). Increases ***creatinine*** and ***creatinine*** excretion (lasting up to 2 wk after therapy is discontinued) and alters response to ***metyrapone test.*** It suppresses ***clotting factors II, V, VII, X*** and decreases excretion of ***17-ketosteroids.*** May increase or decrease ***serum cholesterol.***

INTERACTIONS Drug: ORAL ANTICOAGULANTS may potentiate hypoprothrombinemia. May decrease **insulin** requirements. **Herbal: Echinacea** may increase risk of hepatotoxicity.

PHARMACOKINETICS Absorption: **Cypionate** and **enanthate** are slowly absorbed from lipid tissue. **Duration:** 2–4 wk **cypionate** and **enanthate. Distribution:** 98% bound to sex hormone-binding globulin. **Metabolism:** Primarily metabolized in liver. **Elimination:** 90% excreted in urine, 6% in feces. **Half-Life:** 10–100 min.

NURSING IMPLICATIONS

Assessment & Drug Effects

- Therapeutic response from testosterone therapy is slow; breast cancer, usually apparent within 3 mo after regimen begins. Terminate therapy if signs of disease progression appear.
- Check I&O and weigh patient daily during dose adjustment period. Weight gain (due to sodium and water retention) suggests need for decreased dosage. When dosage is stabilized, urge patient to check weight at least twice weekly and to report increases, particularly if accompanied by edema in dependent areas. Dose adjustment and diuretic therapy may be started.
- Lab tests: Periodic serum cholesterol, serum electrolytes as well as liver function tests throughout therapy.
- Monitor serum calcium closely. Androgenic therapy is usually terminated if serum calcium rises above 14 mg/dL.
- Report S&S of hypercalcemia (see Appendix F) promptly. The immobilized patient is particularly prone to develop hypercalcemia, which indicates progression of bone metastasis in patients with metastatic breast cancer. Treatment includes withdrawing testosterone and checking calcium, phosphate, and BUN levels daily.
- Instruct diabetic to report sweating, tremor, anxiety, vertigo. Testosterone-induced anabolic action enhances hypoglycemia (hyperinsulinism). Dosage adjustment of antidiabetic agent may be required.
- Observe patients on concomitant anticoagulant treatment for signs of overdosage (e.g., ecchymoses, petechiae). Report promptly to physician; anticoagulant dose may need to be reduced.
- Monitor prepubertal or adolescent males throughout therapy to avoid precocious sexual development and premature epiphyseal closure. Skeletal stimulation may continue 6 mo beyond termination of therapy.

Patient & Family Education

- Review directions for application of transdermal patches.
- Report soreness at injection site, because postinjection furunculosis may be an associated adverse reaction.
- Report priapism (sustained and often painful erections occurring especially in early replacement therapy), reduced ejaculatory volume, and gynecomastia to

physician. Symptoms indicate necessity for temporary withdrawal or discontinuation of testosterone therapy.

- Notify physician promptly if pregnancy is suspected or planned. Masculinization of the fetus is most likely to occur if testosterone (androgen) therapy is provided during first trimester of pregnancy.
- Androgens may cause virilism in women at dosage required to treat carcinoma. Report increase in libido (early sign of toxicity), growth of facial hair, deepening of voice, male-pattern baldness. The onset of hoarseness can easily be overlooked unless its significance as an early and possibly irreversible sign of virilism is appreciated. Reevaluation of treatment plan is indicated.

TETRACAINE HYDROCHLORIDE

(tet′ra-kane)

Pontocaine

Classifications: CENTRAL NERVOUS SYSTEM AGENT; LOCAL ANESTHETIC (ESTER TYPE)

Prototype: Procaine HCl

Pregnancy Category: C

AVAILABILITY 1%, 0.2%, 0.3% injection; 20 mg powder; 2% solution; 1%, 2% cream; 2% gel; 1% ointment; 0.5% ophthalmic solution

ACTIONS Local anesthetic that depresses the initial depolarization phase of the action potential, thus preventing propagation and conduction of the nerve impulse. Local anesthetic approximately 10 times more potent and toxic than procaine.

THERAPEUTIC EFFECTS Indicated by loss of sensation and motor activity in circumscribed body areas close to injection or application site.

USES Spinal anesthesia (high, low, saddle block) and topically to produce surface anesthesia. **Eye:** To anesthetize conjunctiva and cornea prior to superficial procedures (including tonometry, gonioscopy, removal of foreign bodies or sutures, corneal scraping). **Nose and Throat:** To abolish laryngeal and esophageal reflexes prior to bronchoscopy, esophagoscopy. **Skin:** To relieve pruritus, pain, burning.

CONTRAINDICATIONS Older adult and debilitated patients; prolonged use of ophthalmic preparations; known hypersensitivity to tetracaine or other local anesthetics of ester type (e.g., procaine, chloroprocaine, cocaine) or to PABA or its derivatives; infection at application or injection site.

CAUTIOUS USE Shock; cachexia, cardiac decompensation; lactation. Safety during pregnancy (category C) or in children is not established.

ROUTE & DOSAGE

Local Anesthesia

Adult: **Topical** Before procedure, 1–2 drops of 0.5% solution or 1.25–2.5 cm of ointment in lower conjunctival fornix or 0.5% solution or ointment to nose or throat **Spinal** 1% solution diluted with equal volume of 10% dextrose injected in subarachnoid space

ADMINISTRATION

Topical

- Avoid use of solutions that are cloudy, discolored, or crystallized.
- When tetracaine is used on mucosa of larynx, trachea, or esophagus, the manufacturer recommends adding 0.06 mL of a 0.1% epinephrine solution to each mL

tetracaine solution to slow absorption of the anesthetic.

- Store ophthalmic solution and ointment at 15°–30° C (59°–86° F); refrigerate topical. Avoid freezing. Use tight, light-resistant containers.

ADVERSE EFFECTS (≥1%) **Body as a Whole:** Anaphylactic reactions, convulsions, faintness, syncope. **CNS:** Postspinal headache, headache, spinal nerve paralysis, anxiety, nervousness, seizures. **CV:** Bradycardia, arrhythmias, hypotension. **Special Senses:** Stinging; corneal erosion, retardation or prevention of healing of corneal abrasion, transient pitting and sloughing of corneal surface, dry corneal epithelium; dry mucous membranes, prolonged depression of cough reflex.

INTERACTIONS Drug: May antagonize effects of SULFONAMIDES.

PHARMACOKINETICS Onset: 1 min eye; 3 min mucosal surface; 3 min spinal. **Duration:** Up to 15 min eye; 30–60 min mucosal surface; 1.5–3 h spinal. **Metabolism:** Metabolized in liver and plasma. **Elimination:** Excreted in urine.

NURSING IMPLICATIONS

Assessment & Drug Effects

- Recovery from anesthesia to the pharyngeal area is complete when patient has feeling in the hard and soft palates and when muscles in the faucial (tonsillar) pillars contract with stimulation.
- Do not give food or liquids until these normal pharyngeal responses are present (usually about 1 h after anesthetic administration). The first small amount of liquid (water) should be given under supervision of care provider.
- Be aware that increased blood concentration of the drug may result from excess application of tetracaine to the skin (to relieve pruritus or burning), application to debrided or infected skin surfaces, or too rapid injection rate.
- High blood concentrations of tetracaine can lead to adverse systemic effects involving CNS and CV systems: Convulsions, respiratory arrest, dysrhythmias, cardiac arrest.

Patient & Family Education

- Do not use ophthalmic drug longer than prescribed period. Prolonged use to eye surface may cause corneal epithelial erosions and retard healing of corneal surface.
- Natural barriers to eye infection and injury are removed by the anesthesia. Do not rub eye after drug instillation until anesthetic effect has dissipated (evidenced by return of blink reflex). Patching for temporary protection of the corneal epithelium may be ordered.
- Wash or disinfect hands before and after self-administration of solutions or ointment.

TETRACYCLINE HYDROCHLORIDE (Pr)

(tet-ra-sye'kleen)

Achromycin, Achromycin V, Nor-Tet, Novotetra ♣, Panmycin, Robitet, SK-Tetracycline, Sumycin, Tetracap, Tetracyn, Tetralan, Tetram, Topicycline

Classifications: ANTIINFECTIVE; ANTIBIOTIC; TETRACYCLINE

Pregnancy Category: D

AVAILABILITY 100 mg, 250 mg, 500 mg capsules; 250 mg, 500 mg tablets; 125 mg/mL suspension; 2.2 mg/mL topical solution; 3% ointment

ACTIONS Broad spectrum antibiotic derived from *Streptomyces aureofaciens* or produced semisynthetically from oxytetracycline. Tetracyclines usually are bacteriostatic but may be bactericidal in high concentrations. Exerts antiacne action by suppressing growth of *Propionibacterium acnes* within sebaceous follicles, thereby reducing free fatty acid content in sebum. Free fatty acids are thought to be produced by breakdown of triglycerides by lipases liberated from *P. acne* and are believed to be largely responsible for inflammatory skin lesions (papules, pustules, cysts) and comedones of acne. Evidence suggests that topical tetracycline may be as effective as the oral preparation for treatment of mild to moderate acne; moderate to severe acne may require oral and topical tetracycline.

THERAPEUTIC EFFECTS Effective against a variety of gram-positive and gram-negative bacteria and against most *chlamydiae, mycoplasmas, rickettsiae,* and certain protozoa (e.g., amebae). Exerts antiacne action by suppressing growth of *Propionibacterium acnes* within sebaceous follicles.

USES Chlamydial infections (e.g., lymphogranuloma venereum, psittacosis, trachoma, inclusion conjunctivitis, nongonococcal urethritis); mycoplasmal infections (e.g., *Mycoplasma pneumoniae*); rickettsial infections (e.g., Q fever, Rocky Mt spotted fever, typhus); spirochetal infections: relapsing fever *(Borrelia),* leptospirosis, syphilis (penicillin-hypersensitive patients); amebiases; uncommon gram-negative bacterial infections (e.g., brucellosis, shigellosis, cholera, gonorrhea [penicillin-hypersensitive patients], granuloma inguinale, tularemia); gram-positive infections (e.g., tetanus). Also used orally and topically (solution) for inflammatory acne vulgaris; topical ointment is used for superficial skin infections. See tetracycline HCl, ophthalmic, for ophthalmic uses.

UNLABELED USES Actinomycosis, acute exacerbations of chronic bronchitis; Lyme disease; pericardial effusion (metastatic); acute PID; sexually transmitted epididymoorchitis; with quinine for multidrug-resistant strains of *Plasmodium falciparum* malaria; antiinfective prophylaxis for rape victims; recurrent cystic thyroid nodules; melioidosis; and as fluorescence test for malignancy.

CONTRAINDICATIONS Hypersensitivity to tetracyclines or to any ingredient in the formulation; severe renal or hepatic impairment, common bile duct obstruction. Use during tooth development (last half of pregnancy [category D]), during infancy and childhood to the 8th year, or lactation. Safety of topical tetracycline preparations in children <11 y is not established.

CAUTIOUS USE History of kidney or liver dysfunction; myasthenia gravis; history of allergy, asthma, hay fever, urticaria; undernourished patients.

ROUTE & DOSAGE

Systemic Infection

Adult: **PO** 250–500 mg b.i.d.–q.i.d. (1–2 g/d) **IM** 250 mg once/d or 300 mg/d in 2–3 divided doses
Child: **PO** *>8 y,* 25–50 mg/kg/d in 2–4 divided doses **IM** *>8 y,* 15–25 mg/kg/d in 2–3 divided doses (max: 250 mg/injection)

Acne

Adult/Child: **PO** *>8 y,* 500–1000 mg/d in 4 divided doses **Topical** Apply to cleansed areas twice daily

ADMINISTRATION

Oral

- Give with a full glass of water on an empty stomach at least 1 h before or 2 h after meals (food, milk, and milk products can reduce absorption by 50% or more).
- Do not give immediately before bed.
- Give with food if patient is having GI symptoms (e.g., nausea, vomiting, anorexia); do not give with foods high in calcium such as milk or milk products.
- Shake suspension well before pouring to ensure uniform distribution of drug. Use calibrated liquid measure to dispense.
- Consult physician about ordering the oral suspension formulation if patient cannot swallow pills.
- Check expiration date for all tetracyclines. Fanconi-like syndrome (renal tubular dysfunction) and also an LE-like syndrome have been attributed to outdated tetracycline preparations.
- Tetracycline decomposes with age, exposure to light, and when improperly stored under conditions of extreme humidity, heat, or cold. The resultant product may be toxic.
- Store at 15°–30° C (59°–86° F) in tightly covered container in dry place. Protect from light.

Intramuscular

- Ask patient if he is allergic to any of the "caine" local anesthetics. (Tetracycline for IM use contains 40 mg procaine HCl per vial.)
- Reconstitute powder by adding 2 mL sterile water for injection or NS injection to 100- or 250-mg vial.
- Give injection deep into body of a relatively large muscle mass (e.g., gluteus maximus or midlateral thigh). Alternate injection sites and observe daily for irritation and swelling.
- Forewarn patient that IM administration may cause local irritation and is extremely painful.
- Store solution at room temperature. Discard after 24 h (directions may vary with manufacturer).

ADVERSE EFFECTS ($\geq$1%) **CNS:** Headache, intracranial hypertension (rare). **Special Senses:** Pigmentation of conjunctiva due to drug deposit. **GI:** Reported mostly for oral administration, but also may occur with parenteral tetracycline (*nausea, vomiting,* epigastric distress, heartburn, *diarrhea,* bulky loose stools, steatorrhea, *abdominal discomfort, flatulence,* dry mouth); dysphagia, retrosternal pain, esophagitis, esophageal ulceration with oral administration, abnormally high liver function test values, decrease in serum cholesterol, <u>fatty degeneration of liver (jaundice, increasing nitrogen retention [azotemia], hyperphosphatemia, acidosis, irreversible shock)</u>; foul-smelling stools or vaginal discharge, stomatitis, glossitis; black hairy tongue (lingua nigra), diarrhea: staphylococcal enterocolitis. **Body as a Whole:** Drug fever, angioedema, serum sickness, <u>anaphylaxis</u>. **Urogenital:** Particularly in patients with kidney disease; increase in BUN/serum creatinine, renal impairment even with therapeutic doses; <u>Fanconi-like syndrome (outdated tetracycline)</u> (characterized by polyuria, polydipsia, nausea, vomiting, glycosuria, proteinuria acidosis, aminoaciduria); vulvovaginitis, pruritus vulvae or ani (possibly hypersensitivity). **Skin:** Dermatitis, *phototoxicity:* discoloration of nails, onycholysis (loosening of nails); cheilosis; fixed drug eruptions particularly on genitalia; thrombocytopenic purpura; Urticaria, rash, <u>exfoliative dermatitis</u>; With topical applications: skin irritation, dry scaly skin, transient stinging or burning sensation, slight yellowing of skin at application site, acute contact dermatitis. **Other:** Pancreatitis, local reactions: pain and irritation (IM site), Jarisch-Herxheimer reaction (see Nursing Implications).

DIAGNOSTIC TEST INTERFERENCE Tetracyclines may cause false increases in ***urinary catecholamines*** (by ***fluorometric methods***), and false decreases in ***urinary urobilinogen.*** Parenteral TETRACYCLINES containing ***ascorbic acid*** reportedly may produce false-positive ***urinary glucose*** determinations by ***copper reduction methods*** (e.g., ***Benedict's reagent, Clinitest***); TETRACYCLINES may cause false-negative results with ***glucose oxidase methods*** (e.g., ***Clinistix, TesTape***).

INTERACTIONS Drug: ANTACIDS, **calcium**, and **magnesium** bind tetracycline in gut and decrease absorption. ORAL ANTICOAGULANTS potentiate hypoprothrombinemia. ANTIDIARRHEAL AGENTS with **kaolin** and pectin may decrease absorption. Effectiveness of ORAL CONTRACEPTIVES decreased. **Methoxyflurane** may produce fatal nephrotoxicity. **Food:** Dairy products and iron supplements decrease tetracycline absorption.

PHARMACOKINETICS Absorption: 75%–80% of dose absorbed orally. **Peak:** 2–4 h. **Distribution:** Widely distributed, preferentially binds to rapid growing tissues; crosses placenta; enters breast milk. **Metabolism:** Not metabolized; enterohepatic cycling. **Elimination:** 50%–60% excreted in urine within 72 h. **Half-Life:** 6–12 h.

NURSING IMPLICATIONS

Assessment & Drug Effects

- Lab tests: Obtain baseline and periodic C&S tests to confirm susceptibility of infecting organism to tetracycline. Also, preform initial and periodic kidney, liver, and hematopoietic function tests, particularly during high-dose, long-term therapy. Determine serum tetracycline levels in patients at-risk for hepatotoxicity (sometimes associated with pancreatitis and occurs most frequently in patients receiving other hepatotoxic drugs or with history of renal or hepatic impairment).
- Report GI symptoms (e.g., nausea, vomiting, diarrhea) to physician. These are generally dose-dependent, occurring mostly with oral forms in patients receiving 2 g/d or more and during prolonged therapy. Frequently, symptoms are controlled by reducing dosage or administering with compatible foods.
- Be alert to evidence of superinfections (see Appendix F). Regularly inspect tongue and mucous membrane of mouth for candidiasis (thrush). Suspect superinfection if patient complains of irritation or soreness of mouth, tongue, throat, vagina, or anus, or persistent itching of any area, diarrhea, or foul-smelling excreta or discharge.
- Withhold drug and notify physician if superinfection develops. Superinfections occur most frequently in patients receiving prolonged therapy, the debilitated, or those who have diabetes, leukemia, systemic LE, or lymphoma. Women taking oral contraceptives reportedly are more susceptible to vaginal candidiasis.
- Obtain follow-up cultures from all gonococcal infection sites 3–7 d after completion of tetracycline therapy to verify eradication of infection.

T

- Monitor I&O in patients receiving parenteral tetracycline. Report oliguria or any changes in appearance of urine or in I&O.

Patient & Family Education

- Report onset of diarrhea to physician. It is important to determine whether diarrhea is due to irritating drug effect or superinfections or pseudomembranous colitis (caused by overgrowth of toxin-producing bacteria: *Clostridium difficile*) (see Appendix F). The latter two conditions can be **LIFE THREATENING** and require immediate withdrawal of tetracycline and prompt initiation of symptomatic and supportive therapy.
- Reduce incidence of superinfection (see Appendix F) by meticulous care of mouth, skin, and perineal area. Rinse mouth of food debris after eating; floss daily and use a soft-bristled toothbrush. Wash hands several times a day, particularly after each bowel movement and before eating.
- Avoid direct exposure to sunlight during and for several days after therapy is terminated to reduce possibility of photosensitivity reaction (appearing like an exaggerated sunburn, it begins a few minutes to hours following sun exposure, often with tingling, burning sensation).
- Report onset of severe headache or visual disturbances immediately. These are possible symptoms of increased intracranial pressure and necessitate prompt withdrawal of tetracycline to prevent irreversible loss of vision.
- Note: Tetracycline therapy for brucellosis or spirochetal infections may cause a Jarisch-Herxheimer reaction. The reaction is usually mild and appears abruptly within 6–24 h after initiation of therapy. It is manifested by malaise, fever, chills, headache, adenopathy, leukocytosis, exacerbation of skin lesions, arthralgia, transient hypotension. Treatment is symptomatic; recovery generally occurs within 24 h.
- Report immediately sudden onset of painful or difficult swallowing (dysphagia) to physician. Esophagitis and esophageal ulceration have been associated with bedtime administration of tetracycline capsules or tablets with insufficient fluid, particularly to patients with hiatal hernia or esophageal problems.
- Do not allow topical medication to contact eyes, nose, or mouth. Be aware that tetracycline may stain clothing.
- Clean affected skin area with soap and water; rinse and dry well before application of topical drug.
- Report a worsening infection or stinging and burning sensation with topical applications to physician if pronounced.
- Skin treated with topical drug will exhibit bright yellow to green fluorescence under ultraviolet light and "black light."
- Be aware that topicycline contains a sulfite that can cause an allergic reaction (itching, wheezing, anaphylaxis) in susceptible persons (e.g., asthmatics or allergic individuals).
- Response to acne therapy usually requires 2–8 wk, maximal results may not be apparent for up to 12 wk.
- Do not breast feed while taking/using this drug.

TETRAHYDROZOLINE HYDROCHLORIDE

(tet-ra-hye-drozz'a-leen)

Collyrium, Mallazine, Murine Plus, Optigene, Soothe, Tyzine, Visine

Classifications: EYE, EAR, NOSE, AND THROAT PREPARATION; VASOCONSTRICTOR; DECONGESTANT

Prototype: Naphazoline

Pregnancy Category: C

AVAILABILITY 0.05% ophthalmic solution; 0.05%, 0.1% nasal solution

ACTIONS Related to naphazoline but shares more marked alpha-adrenergic than beta-adrenergic activity; large doses cause CNS depression rather than the stimulation produced by other sympathomimetic amines.

THERAPEUTIC EFFECTS Ophthalmic solution is effective for allergic reactions of the eye; nasal solution is antiinflammatory and also decreases allergic congestion.

USES Symptomatic relief of minor eye irritation and allergies and for nasopharyngeal congestion of allergic or inflammatory origin.

CONTRAINDICATIONS Hypersensitivity to any component; use of ophthalmic preparation in glaucoma or other serious eye diseases; use within 14 d of MAO inhibitor therapy. Use in children <2 y; use of 0.1% or higher strengths in children <6 y. Safety during pregnancy (category C) is not established.

CAUTIOUS USE Hypertension; cardiovascular disease; hyperthyroidism; diabetes mellitus; young children; lactation.

ROUTE & DOSAGE

Decongestant

Adult: **Ophthalmic** See Appendix A-1. **Nasal** 2–4 drops of 0.1% solution or spray in each nostril q3h prn

Child: **Nasal** *2–6 y,* 2–4 drops of 0.05% solution or spray in each nostril q3h prn; *≥ 6 y,* same as adult

ADMINISTRATION

Instillation

- Make sure interval between doses is at least 4–6 h since drug action lasts 4–8 h.
- Place patient in upright position when using nasal spray. (If patient is reclining, a stream rather than a spray may be ejected, with consequent overdosage.)
- Use lateral, head-low position to administer nasal drops.

ADVERSE EFFECTS (≥1%) **Special Senses:** *Transient stinging,* irritation, *sneezing,* dryness, headache, tremors, drowsiness, light-headedness, insomnia, palpitation. **Body as a Whole:** With overdose: marked drowsiness, sweating, coma, hypotension, shock, bradycardia.

INTERACTIONS Drug: No clinically significant interactions established.

PHARMACOKINETICS Absorption: May be absorbed from nasal mucosa. **Duration:** 4–8 h.

NURSING IMPLICATIONS

Patient & Family Education

- Discontinue medication and consult physician if relief is not obtained within 48 h or if symptoms persist or increase.
- Do not exceed recommended dosage. Rebound congestion and rhi-

T

nitis may occur with frequent or prolonged use of nasal preparation.

- Do not breast feed while using this drug without consulting physician.

THALIDOMIDE

(tha-lid'o-mide)

Thalomid

Classifications: IMMUNOSUPPRESSANT; TUMOR NECROSIS FACTOR MODIFIER

Pregnancy Category: X

AVAILABILITY 50 mg capsules

ACTIONS Mechanism of action in inducing immunosuppression is unknown, however, drug has several antiinflammatory and immunologic actions. Antiinflammatory effects may be due to its inhibition of neutrophil chemotaxis and decrease of monocyte phagocytosis. Immunosuppressive effect may result from suppression of excessive tumor necrosis factor-alpha (TNF-alpha) production. Also, reduces helper T cells and increases suppressor T cells.

THERAPEUTIC EFFECTS Antiinflammatory and immunosuppressive actions. Indicated by control of cutaneous manifestations of erythema nodosum leprosum.

USES Acute and maintenance treatment of cutaneous manifestations of moderate to severe erythema nodosum leprosum. Refractory Crohn's disease.

UNLABELED USES Stimulate appetite in patients with HIV-associated cachexia, lupus, multiple myeloma.

CONTRAINDICATIONS Hypersensitivity to thalidomide; peripheral neuropathy. Pregnancy (category X), lactation, children <12 y.

CAUTIOUS USE Liver and kidney disease; CHF or hypertension; constipation or other GI disorders; neurologic disorders or history of neuritis.

ROUTE & DOSAGE

Erythema Nodosum Leprosum

Adult: **PO** 100–300 mg q.d. (max: 400 mg/d) times at least 2 wk
Child: **PO** *11–17 y,* 100 mg q.d.

Refractory Crohn's Disease

Adult: **PO** 50–100 mg q.d. (doses up to 300 mg studied)

ADMINISTRATION

Oral

- Give at bedtime and at least 1 h after the evening meal.
- Give this drug only to persons who understand and have signed the required consent form.
- Verify, prior to administration, that this drug was prescribed and dispensed only by persons registered by the STEPS (System for Thalidomide Education and Prescribing Safety) program.
- Store at 15°–30° C (59°–86° F); protect from light.

ADVERSE EFFECTS (≥1%) **Body as a Whole:** Asthenia, back pain, chills, facial edema, *fever,* malaise, pain. **CNS:** Drowsiness, *somnolence,* peripheral neuropathy (possibly irreversible), *dizziness,* orthostatic hypotension, headache, agitation, insomnia, nervousness, paresthesia, tremor, vertigo, seizures. **CV:** Bradycardia, peripheral edema, hyperlipidemia. **GI:** Abdominal pain, anorexia, constipation, *diarrhea,* dry mouth, flatulence, abnormal liver function tests, nausea, oral moniliasis. **Hematologic:** Neutropenia, anemia, *leukopenia,* lymphadenopathy. **Respiratory:** Pharyngitis, rhinitis, sinusitis. **Skin:** *Rash,* acne, nail disorder, fungal dermatitis, pruritus, sweating, toxic epiderma necrolysis. **Body as a Whole:** Hypersensitivity reaction (rash, fever, tachycardia, hypotension), HIV viral load increase, infection. **Urogenital:** Teratogenicity, albuminuria, hematuria, impotence.

INTERACTIONS Drug: Enhances sedation associated with BARBITURATES, **alcohol, chlorpromazine, reserpine.**

PHARMACOKINETICS Absorption: Slowly absorbed from GI tract. **Peak:** 2.9–5.7 h. **Distribution:** Crosses placenta; present in ejaculate in males. **Metabolism:** Does not appear to be hepatically metabolized. **Half-Life:** 6–7.5 h.

NURSING IMPLICATIONS

Assessment & Drug Effects

- Lab tests: Monitor WBC with differential prior to therapy and periodically thereafter.
- Monitor carefully for and immediately report S&S of peripheral neuropathy. Discontinue drug and notify prescriber if peripheral neuropathy is suspected.

Patient & Family Education

- Do not share this medication with anyone else under any circumstances.
- Use effective methods of birth control (both women and men); starting 1 mo before, during, and 1 mo following discontinuation of thalidomide therapy. Men MUST use condoms when engaging in sexual activity.
- Exercise caution while driving or engaging in potentially hazardous activities because drug may cause dizziness.
- Report pain, numbness, or tingling in the hands or feet to physician immediately.
- Do not breast feed while taking this drug.

THEOPHYLLINE (Pr)

(thee-off′i-lin)

Bronkodyl, Elixophyllin, Lanophyllin, PMS Theophylline ✦, Pulmopylline ✦, Quibron-T, Respbid, Slo-Bid, Slo-Phyllin, Somophyllin, Somophyllin-12 ✦, Theo-Dur, Theo-24, Theolair, Theophylline Ethylenediamine, Theospan-SR, Uni-Dur, Uniphyl

Classifications: BRONCHODILATOR (RESPIRATORY SMOOTH MUSCLE RELAXANT); XANTHINE

Pregnancy Category: C

AVAILABILITY 100 mg, 125 mg, 200 mg, 250 mg, 300 mg tablets; 100 mg, 200 mg capsules; 80 mg/15 mL, 150 mg/15 mL liquid; 100 mg, 200 mg, 250 mg, 300 mg, 450 mg, 500 mg, 600 mg sustained-release tablets; 50 mg, 75 mg, 100 mg, 125 mg, 200 mg, 250 mg, 260 mg, 300 mg sustained-release capsules; 200 mg, 400 mg, 800 mg injection

ACTIONS Xanthine derivative that relaxes smooth muscle by direct action, particularly of bronchi and pulmonary vessels, and stimulates medullary respiratory center with resulting increase in vital capacity. Also relaxes smooth muscles of biliary and GI tracts. Stimulates myocardium, thereby increasing force of contractions and cardiac output, and stimulates all levels of CNS, but to a lesser degree than caffeine.

THERAPEUTIC EFFECTS Effective for relief of bronchospasm in asth-

T

matics, chronic bronchitis, and emphysema.

USES Prophylaxis and symptomatic relief of bronchial asthma, as well as bronchospasm associated with chronic bronchitis and emphysema. Also used for emergency treatment of paroxysmal cardiac dyspnea and edema of CHF.

UNLABELED USES Treatment of apnea and bradycardia of prematures and to reduce severe bronchospasm associated with cystic fibrosis and acute descending respiratory infection. Theophylline sodium glycinate is a mixture of sodium theophylline and aminoacetic (glycine). Contains 45%–47% theophylline. Similar actions, uses, adverse reactions, and precautions as other theophylline derivatives but claimed to produce less gastric irritation.

CONTRAINDICATIONS Hypersensitivity to xanthines; coronary artery disease or angina pectoris when myocardial stimulation might be harmful; severe renal or liver impairment. Safety during pregnancy (category C) or lactation is not established.

CAUTIOUS USE Children; compromised cardiac or circulatory function, hypertension; hyperthyroidism; peptic ulcer; prostatic hypertrophy; glaucoma; diabetes mellitus; older adults and neonates.

T

ROUTE & DOSAGE

Bronchospasm

Adult/Child: **PO/IV Loading Dose** 5 mg/kg
Adult: **PO/IV Maintenance Dose*** *Nonsmoker,* 0.4 mg/kg/h (*IV by continuous infusion, PO divided q6h [immediate release] or q8–12h [sustained release]); *Smoker,* 0.6 mg/kg/h; *with CHF or cirrhosis,* 0.2 mg/kg/h
Child: **PO/IV Maintenance Dose*** *1–9 y,* 0.8 mg/kg/h; *10–12 y,* 0.6 mg/kg/h
Infant: **PO/IV Maintenance Dose*** *2–6 mo,* 0.4 mg/kg/h; *6–11 mo,* 0.7 mg/kg/h
Neonate: **PO/IV Maintenance Dose*** 0.13 mg/kg/h

ADMINISTRATION

Note: All doses based on ideal body weight.

Oral

- Wait 4–6 h after the last IV dose, when switching from IV to oral dosing.
- Give with a full glass of water and after meals to minimize gastric irritation.
- Give sustained-release forms and enteric-coated tablets whole. Chewable tablets must be chewed thoroughly before swallowing. Sustained-release granules from capsules can be taken on an empty stomach or mixed with applesauce or water.
- Note: Timing of dose is critical. Be certain patient understands necessity to adhere to the correct intervals between doses.

Intravenous

- Give *prediluted solutions* at a rate not to exceed 20 mg/min.

PREPARE: **IV Infusion:** Give IV theophylline ethylenediamine solution with a concentration of 25 mg/mL undiluted by direct IV or diluted (preferred) in up to 200 mL of D5W.

ADMINISTER: **IV Infusion:** Give at a rate not to exceed 20 mg/min.

INCOMPATIBILITIES **Solution/additive: Amikacin, ascorbic acid, bleomycin,** CEPHALOSPORINS, **chlorpromazine, clindamycin, codeine phosphate, dimenhydrinate, dobutamine, dopa-**

mine, doxapram, doxorubicin, epinephrine, hydralazine, hydroxyzine, insulin, isoproterenol, levorphanol, meperidine, methadone, methylprednisolone, morphine, nafcillin, norepinephrine, oxytetracycline, papaverine, penicillin G, pentazocine, procaine, prochlorperazine, promazine, promethazine, tetracycline, verapamil, vitamin B complex with C. Y-site: Amiodarone, codeine phosphate, clindamycin, PHENOTHIAZINES **(chlorpromazine, prochlorperazine), epinephrine, dobutamine, dopamine, levorphanol, meperidine, methadone, morphine, norepinephrine, phenytoin, verapamil.**

ADVERSE EFFECTS (≥1%) **CNS:** Stimulation (Irritability, restlessness, insomnia, dizziness, headache, tremor, hyperexcitability, muscle twitching, drug-induced seizures). **CV:** Palpitation, *tachycardia,* extrasystoles, flushing, marked hypotension, circulatory failure. **GI:** *Nausea,* vomiting, anorexia, epigastric or abdominal pain, diarrhea, activation of peptic ulcer. **Urogenital:** Transient urinary frequency, albuminuria, kidney irritation. **Respiratory:** Tachypnea, respiratory arrest. **Body as a Whole:** Fever, dehydration.

DIAGNOSTIC TEST INTERFERENCE False-positive elevations of ***serum uric acid*** (***Bittner*** or colorimetric methods). ***Probenecid*** may cause false high serum theophylline readings, and spectrophotometric methods of determining ***serum theophylline*** are affected by a furosemide, sulfathiazole, phenylbutazone, probenecid, theobromine.

INTERACTIONS Drug: Increases **lithium** excretion, lowering lithium levels; **cimetidine,** high-dose **allopurinol** (600 mg/d), **tacrine,** QUINOLONES, MACROLIDE ANTIBIOTICS, and **zileuton** can significantly increase theophylline levels. **Herbal: St. John's wort** may decrease theophylline efficacy.

PHARMACOKINETICS Absorption: Most products are 100% absorbed from GI tract. **Peak:** IV 30 min; uncoated tablet 1 h; sustained release 4–6 h. **Duration:** 4–8 h; varies with age, smoking, and liver function. **Distribution:** Crosses placenta. **Metabolism:** Extensively metabolized in liver. **Elimination:** Parent drug and metabolites excreted by kidneys; excreted in breast milk.

NURSING IMPLICATIONS

Assessment & Drug Effects

- Lab tests: Monitor plasma level of theophylline. Be aware that therapeutic plasma level ranges from 10–20 mcg/mL (a narrow therapeutic range). Levels exceeding 20 mcg/mL are associated with toxicity.
- Monitor drug levels in heavy smokers closely. Cigarette smoking induces hepatic microsomal enzyme activity, decreasing serum half-life and increasing body clearance of theophylline. An increase of dosage from 50%–100% is usual in heavy smokers.
- Monitor plasma drug level closely in patients with heart failure, kidney or liver dysfunction, alcoholism, high fever. Plasma clearance of xanthines may be reduced.
- Take necessary safety precautions and forewarn older adult patients of possible dizziness during early therapy.
- Monitor vital signs. Improvement in respiratory status is the expected outcome.

T

- Observe and report early signs of possible toxicity: Anorexia, nausea, vomiting, dizziness, shakiness, restlessness, abdominal discomfort, irritability, palpitation, tachycardia, marked hypotension, cardiac arrhythmias, seizures.
- Monitor for tachycardia which may be worse in patients with severe cardiac disease. Conversely, theophylline toxicity may be masked in patients with tachycardia.
- Monitor patients on sustained release preparations for S&S of overdosage. Continued slow absorption leads to high plasma concentrations for a prolonged period.
- Note: Neonates of mothers using this drug have exhibited slight tachycardia, jitteriness, and apnea.
- Monitor CLOSELY for adverse effects in infants <6 mo and prematures; theophylline metabolism is prolonged as is the half-life in this age group.

Patient & Family Education

- Take medication at the same time every day.
- Avoid charcoal-broiled foods (high in polycyclic carbon content); may increase theophylline elimination and reduce the half-life as much as 50%.
- Limit caffeine intake because it may increase incidence of adverse effects.
- Cigarette smoking may significantly lower theophylline plasma concentration.
- Be aware that a low-carbohydrate, high-protein diet increases theophylline elimination, and a high-carbohydrate, low-protein diet decreases it.
- Drink fluids liberally (2000–3000 mL/d) if not contraindicated to decrease viscosity of airway secretions.
- Avoid self-dosing with OTC medications, especially cough suppressants, which may cause retention of secretions and CNS depression.
- Do not breast feed while taking this drug without consulting physician. Since theophylline is distributed into breast milk, it may be advisable to nurse the infant just before taking the drug.

THIABENDAZOLE

(thye-a-ben'da-zole)
Mintezol
Classifications: ANTIINFECTIVE; ANTHELMINTIC
Prototype: Mebendazole
Pregnancy Category: C

AVAILABILITY 500 mg chewable tablets; 500 mg/5 mL suspension

ACTIONS Structurally related to mebendazole. Precise mechanism of action is not clear, however, it has a wide spectrum of anthelmintic activity. Inhibits helminth-specific enzyme fumarate reductase.
THERAPEUTIC EFFECTS Suppresses production of eggs or larvae by some parasites and may inhibit subsequent development of eggs or larvae passed in feces. Demonstrates antiinflammatory, antipyretic, and analgesic effects.

USES Enterobiasis (pinworm infestation), ascariasis (roundworm), strongyloidiasis (threadworm), cutaneous larva migrans (creeping eruption), and hookworm infestations caused by *Ancyclostoma duodenale* or *Necator americanus*. Used during invasive stage of trichinosis to relieve symptoms and for mixed helminthic infestations.

CONTRAINDICATIONS Safety during pregnancy (category C) or lactation is not established.
CAUTIOUS USE Liver or kidney dysfunction; when vomiting can be dan-

T

gerous, severe dehydration or malnutrition; anemia; children weighing <15 kg.

ROUTE & DOSAGE

Enterobiasis, Ascariasis, Strongyloidiasis, Hookworm

Adult: **PO** *<70 kg,* 25 mg/kg b.i.d. times 2 d; *>70 kg,* 1.5 g b.i.d. (max: 3 g/d) times 2 d
Child: **PO** *14–70 kg,* 25 mg/kg b.i.d. times 2 d

ADMINISTRATION

Oral

- Give after meals. Chewable tablets must be chewed thoroughly before swallowing.
- Shake suspension well before pouring.

ADVERSE EFFECTS (≥1%) **CNS:** Weariness, *dizziness,* drowsiness, headache. **CV:** Hypotension, bradycardia. **GI:** *Anorexia, nausea, vomiting,* epigastric distress, jaundice, cholestasis, parenchymal liver damage, diarrhea, perianal rash. **Urogenital:** Malodor of urine, crystalluria, hematuria, nephrotoxicity, enuresis. **Metabolic:** Transient rise in AST, transient leukopenia, hypersensitivity, hyperglycemia. **Skin:** Pruritus.

PHARMACOKINETICS Absorption: Readily absorbed from GI tract. **Peak:** 1–2 h. **Metabolism:** Metabolized in liver. **Elimination:** >90% excreted in urine; 5% in feces.

NURSING IMPLICATIONS

Assessment & Drug Effects

- Provide supportive treatment prior to therapy if patient is anemic, dehydrated, or malnourished.
- Adverse effects generally occur 3–4 h after administration, are mild, and last for 2–8 h. Incidence tends to be related to dose and duration of treatment.
- Discontinued immediately with S&S of hypersensitivity: Fever, facial flush, chills, conjunctival infection, skin rashes, or erythema multiforme (including Stevens-Johnson syndrome), which can be fatal.

Patient & Family Education

- Do not drive or engage in potentially hazardous activities until response to drug is known. CNS adverse effects occur frequently.
- Do not breast feed while taking this drug without consulting physician.

THIAMINE HYDROCHLORIDE (VITAMIN B_1)

(thye'a-min)

Betalins, Bewon, Biamine

Classification: VITAMIN B

Pregnancy Category: A

AVAILABILITY 50 mg, 100 mg, 250 mg tablets; 20 mg enteric-coated tablet; 100 mg/mL injection

ACTIONS Water-soluble B_1 vitamin and member of B-complex group used for thiamine replacement therapy.

THERAPEUTIC EFFECTS Functions as an essential coenzyme in carbohydrate metabolism. Also has role in conversion of tryptophan to nicotinamide. Effectiveness is evidenced by improvement of clinical manifestations of thiamine deficiency: Anorexia, gastric distress, depression, irritability, insomnia, palpitations, tachycardia, loss of memory, paresthesias, muscle weakness and pain, elevated blood pyruvic acid level (diagnostic test

T

for thiamine deficiency), and elevated lactic acid level.

USES Treatment and prophylaxis of beriberi, to correct anorexia due to thiamine deficiency states, and in treatment of neuritis associated with pregnancy, pellagra, and alcoholism, including Wernicke-Korsakoff syndrome. Therapy generally includes other members of vitamin B complex, since thiamine deficiency rarely occurs alone. Severe deficiency is characterized by ophthalmoplegia, polyneuropathy, muscle wasting ("dry" beriberi), edema, serous effusions, and CHF ("wet" beriberi).

CONTRAINDICATIONS None

ROUTE & DOSAGE

Thiamine Deficiency
Adult: **IV/IM** 50–100 mg t.i.d.
Child: **IV/IM** 10–25 mg t.i.d.

Beriberi
Adult: **IV/IM** 10–500 mg t.i.d. for 2 wk
Child: **IV/IM** 10–50 mg t.i.d.

Dietary Supplement
Adult: **PO** 15–30 mg/d
Child: **PO** 10–50 mg/d

ADMINISTRATION

Oral
- Do not crush or chew enteric-coated tablets. These must be swallowed whole.

Intramuscular
- Give deep IM into a large muscle; may be painful. Rotate sites and apply cold compresses to area if necessary for relief of discomfort.

Intravenous
Note: Intradermal test dose is recommended prior to administration in suspected thiamine sensitivity. Deaths have occurred following IV use.

PREPARE: **Direct:** Give undiluted. **IV Infusion:** Diluted in 1000 mL of most IV solutions.
ADMINISTER: **Direct:** Give at a rate of 100 mg over 5 min. **IV Infusion:** Give at the ordered rate.
INCOMPATIBILITIES **Solution/additive: Amobarbital, diazepam, erythromycin, furosemide, phenobarbital.**
- Preserve in tight, light-resistant, nonmetallic containers. Thiamine is unstable in alkaline solutions (e.g., solutions of acetates, barbiturates, bicarbonates, carbonates, citrates) and neutral solutions.

ADVERSE EFFECTS (≥1%) **Body as a Whole:** Feeling of warmth, weakness, sweating, restlessness, tightness of throat, angioneurotic edema, anaphylaxis. **Respiratory:** Cyanosis, pulmonary edema. **CV:** Cardiovascular collapse, slight fall in BP following rapid IV administration. **GI:** GI hemorrhage, nausea. **Skin:** Urticaria, pruritus.

INTERACTIONS Drug: No clinically significant interactions established.

PHARMACOKINETICS Absorption: Limited absorption from GI tract. **Distribution:** Widely distributed, including into breast milk. **Elimination:** Excreted in urine.

NURSING IMPLICATIONS

Assessment & Drug Effects
- Record patient's dietary history carefully as an essential part of vitamin replacement therapy. Collaborate with physician, dietitian, patient, and responsible family member in developing a diet teaching plan that can be sustained by patient.

T

- Note: Body requirement of thiamine is directly proportional to carbohydrate intake and metabolic rate; requirement increases when diet consists predominantly of carbohydrates. Total absence of dietary thiamine produce deficiency state in about 3 wk.

Patient & Family Education

- Food–drug relationships: Learn about rich dietary sources of thiamine (e.g., yeast, pork, beef, liver, wheat and other whole grains, nutrient-added breakfast cereals, fresh vegetables, especially peas and dried beans).

THIETHYLPERAZINE MALEATE

(thye-eth-il-per'a-zeen)

Torecan

Classifications: GASTROINTESTINAL AGENT; ANTIEMETIC

Prototype: Prochlorperazine

Pregnancy Category: X

AVAILABILITY 10 mg tablets; 5 mg/mL injection

ACTIONS Piperazine phenothiazine derivative similar to prochlorperazine. Reportedly higher ratio of antiemetic action to tranquilizing action than other phenothiazines. Acts directly on chemoreceptor trigger zone as well as the vomiting center of the brain.

THERAPEUTIC EFFECTS Effectively controls nausea and vomiting because it is centrally acting.

USES To control nausea and vomiting.

UNLABELED USES Treatment of vertigo.

CONTRAINDICATIONS Hypersensitivity to phenothiazines; CNS depression or comatose states; IV administration; pregnancy (category X). Safety in children <12 y, lactation, or following intracardiac or intracranial surgery is not established.

CAUTIOUS USE Kidney or liver disease.

ROUTE & DOSAGE

Nausea and Vomiting

Adult: **PO/PR/IM** 10 mg 1–3 times/d

ADMINISTRATION

Intramuscular

- Examine parenteral solution and administer only if it is clear and colorless.
- Note: Patient should be recumbent when drug is being administered IM. Postural hypotension (manifested by weakness, lightheadedness, faintness) and drowsiness may occur, particularly after initial injection. Advise patient to remain in bed for about 1 h or longer, if indicated, and supervise ambulation.
- Give IM deep into large muscle mass and aspirate hypodermic carefully before injecting drug to avoid inadvertent entry into a blood vessel. IV administration is specifically CONTRAINDICATED because it can cause severe hypotension.
- Store at 15°–30° C (59°–86° F) away from heat, in light-resistant containers. Store suppositories below 25° C (77° F).

ADVERSE EFFECTS (≥1%) **CNS:** *Drowsiness,* dizziness, headache, restlessness, fever, orthostatic hypotension, extrapyramidal symptoms including convulsions. **Special Senses:** *Dry mouth and nose,* blurred vision, tinnitus, sialorrhea with altered taste sensations. **GI:** Cholestatic jaundice.

T

INTERACTIONS Drug: Additive adverse effects with other PHENOTHIAZINES; additive CNS depression with **alcohol,** ANXIOLYTICS, SEDATIVE-HYPNOTICS; may increase **phenytoin** levels; may decrease effectiveness of **bromocriptine, cabergoline.**

PHARMACOKINETICS Onset: 1 h PO, PR; 30 min IM.

NURSING IMPLICATIONS

Assessment & Drug Effects

- Patients who have received drug preoperatively may manifest restlessness or depression during anesthesia recovery.
- Report immediately onset of extrapyramidal effects: Gait disturbances, difficulty in speaking, muscle spasms, torticollis, deviations in eye movements. Reduction in dosage or discontinuation of medication is indicated.

Patient & Family Education

- Do not drive or engage in potentially hazardous activities until response to drug is known.
- Do not breast feed while taking this drug without consulting physician.

THIMEROSAL

(thye-mer'oh-sal)

Mersol, Merthiolate

Classifications: SKIN AND MUCOUS MEMBRANE AGENT; ANTIINFECTIVE

Pregnancy Category: C

AVAILABILITY 1:1000 solution, tincture, spray

ACTIONS Topical organic mercurial with sustained bacteriostatic and fungistatic activity. Ineffective against spore-forming organisms.

THERAPEUTIC EFFECTS Utilized as a topical antiseptic because it is both a bacteriostatic and fungistatic agent.

USES First-aid treatment of contaminated wounds, in antisepsis of intact skin, before surgery, and in pustular dermatosis; as antifungal agent in athlete's foot for wound irrigations. Ophthalmic preparation is used to treat conjunctivitis and corneal ulcer and for prevention of infection following removal of foreign bodies. Used as preservative in most solutions sold for cleaning, wetting, soaking, and storage of contact lenses; also used as preservative for biologic and pharmaceutical products.

CONTRAINDICATIONS History of sensitivity to thio or mercurial compounds; prolonged use; pregnancy (category C).

CAUTIOUS USE Lactation.

ROUTE & DOSAGE

Antiseptic

Adult: **Topical** 1:1000 solution, apply locally 1–3 times/d

ADMINISTRATION

Topical

- Clean before applying antiseptic for first-aid treatment.
- Do not apply bandage or other occlusive dressing until tincture application has completely dried in order to prevent skin irritation.
- Store in tightly covered, light-resistant containers. Avoid exposure to excessive heat.

ADVERSE EFFECTS (≥1%) **Skin:** Itching erythema, papular or vesicular eruptions. **Body as a Whole:** Mercury poisoning with prolonged use (metallic taste, salivation, stomatitis, lethargy, peripheral neuropathy).

INTERACTIONS Drug: No clinically significant interactions established.

PHARMACOKINETICS Absorption: May have mercury absorption with prolonged use over large areas.

NURSING IMPLICATIONS

Assessment & Drug Effects

- Be aware that Aqueous Merthiolate contains thimerosal and borate (0.14%). Both are toxic if absorbed systemically.

THIOGUANINE (TG, 6-THIOGUANINE)

(thye-oh-gwah'neen)

Lanvis ♣

Classifications: ANTINEOPLASTIC; ANTIMETABOLITE

Prototype: Fluorouracil

Pregnancy Category: D

AVAILABILITY 40 mg tablets

ACTIONS Antimetabolite and purine antagonist with immunosuppressive activity. Highly toxic. Drug is incorporated into the DNA and RNA of human bone marrow cells.

THERAPEUTIC EFFECTS Delays myelosuppression; has potential mutagenic and carcinogenic properties. Normally accompanied by evidence of toxicity.

USES In combination with other antineoplastics for remission induction in acute myelogenous leukemia and as treatment of chronic myelogenous leukemia. Has little advantage over mercaptopurine.

CONTRAINDICATIONS Patients with prior resistance to this drug. Pregnancy (category D), lactation.

ROUTE & DOSAGE

Leukemia

Adult: **PO** 2 mg/kg/d, may increase to 3 mg/kg/d if no response after 4 wk

ADMINISTRATION

Oral

- Withhold drug and notify physician if toxicity develops. There is no known antagonist; prompt discontinuation of the drug is essential to avoid irreversible myelosuppression from toxicity.
- Store at 15°–30° C (59°–86° F) in airtight container.

ADVERSE EFFECTS (≥1%) **Hematologic:** <u>Leukopenia, thrombocytopenia,</u> anemia. **GI:** Jaundice, nausea, vomiting, anorexia, stomatitis, diarrhea. **Urogenital:** *Hyperuricemia.*

INTERACTIONS Drug: Severe hepatotoxicity with **busulfan;** may decrease immune response to VACCINES; increase risk of bleeding with ANTICOAGULANTS; NSAIDS, SALICYLATES; PLATELET INHIBITORS, THROMBOLYTIC AGENTS; effects may be reversed by **filgrastim, sargramostim.**

PHARMACOKINETICS Absorption: Variable and incomplete absorption from GI tract. **Peak:** 8 h. **Distribution:** Crosses placenta. **Metabolism:** Metabolized in liver. **Elimination:** Excreted in urine. **Half-Life:** 11 h.

NURSING IMPLICATIONS

Assessment & Drug Effects

- Lab tests: Monitor blood counts weekly (CBC with differential and platelet count).
- Determine hematologic parameters for withholding drug.
- Monitor I&O ratio and report oliguria.

- Observe patient's skin and sclera for jaundice. It should be reported promptly as a symptom of toxicity; drug will be discontinued promptly.
- Expect that the drop in leukocyte count may be slow over a period of 2–4 wk. Treatment is interrupted if there is a rapid fall within a few days.

Patient & Family Education

- Maintenance doses are continued throughout remissions.
- Do not breast feed while taking this drug.

THIOPENTAL SODIUM (Pr)

(thye-oh-pen'tal)

Pentothal

Classifications: CENTRAL NERVOUS SYSTEM AGENT; GENERAL ANESTHETIC; SEDATIVE-HYPNOTIC; BARBITURATE

Pregnancy Category: C

Controlled Substance: Schedule III

AVAILABILITY 20 mg/mL, 25 mg/mL injection

ACTIONS Ultrashort-acting barbiturate; induces brief general anesthesia without analgesia by depression of CNS. Loss of consciousness is rapid. Reduction in cardiac output and peripheral vasodilation frequently accompany anesthesia. Rapid redistribution of agent out of brain reduces anesthesia level and increases reflex airway hyperactivity to mechanical stimulation. Muscle relaxation is slight, and reflexes are poorly controlled.

THERAPEUTIC EFFECTS Since analgesia is slight, thiopental is seldom used alone except for brief minor procedures. It does not act as an analgesic when given as an analgesic.

USES To induce hypnosis and anesthesia prior to or as supplement to other anesthetic agents or as sole agent for brief (15-min) operative procedures. Also used as an anticonvulsant and sedative-hypnotic and for narcoanalysis and narcosynthesis in psychiatric disorders.

CONTRAINDICATIONS Hypersensitivity to barbiturates; history of paradoxic excitation; absence of suitable veins for IV administration; status asthmaticus; acute intermittent or other hepatic porphyrias. Safety during pregnancy (category C), lactation, or children is not established.

CAUTIOUS USE Coronary artery disease, hypotension, shock; conditions that may potentiate or prolong hypnotic effect including excessive premedication, liver or kidney dysfunction, myxedema, Addison's disease, severe anemia, increased BUN; increased intracranial pressure; myasthenia gravis; asthma and other respiratory diseases.

ROUTE & DOSAGE

Induction

Adult: **IV Test Dose** 25–75 mg, then 50–75 mg at 20–40 s intervals, an additional 50 mg may be given if needed
Child: **IV** 3–5 mg/kg initially, followed by 1 mg/kg if needed
Infant: **IV** 5–8 mg/kg
Neonate: **IV** 3–4 mg/kg

Convulsions

Adult: **IV** 75–125 mg
Child: **IV** 2–3 mg/kg

Narcoanalysis

Adult: **IV** 100 mg/min until confusion occurs

ADMINISTRATION

Note: Verify correct IV concentration and rate of infusion to neonates, infants, children with physician.

Intravenous

Test dose: May be given to assess unusual sensitivity to drug. Following administration, observe patient for at least 1 min for unexpected deep anesthesia or respiratory depression.

PREPARE: **Direct:** Reconstitute each 500 mg of powder by adding at least 20 mL of sterile water for injection to yield a 2.5% solution (25 mg/1 mL). Add 20 mL of reconstituted solution to at least 100 mL of NS or D5W. Prepare solution freshly and use promptly. If a precipitate is present, discard solution. Unused portions should be discarded within 24 h.

ADMINISTER: **Direct:** Infuse each 25 mg over 1 min or more. Do not infuse solution with a concentration <2.5% (concentration <2% causes hemolysis).

INCOMPATIBILITIES **Solution/additive:** DEXTROSE RINGER'S COMBINATIONS, **Ringer's lactate, 10% dextrose, amikacin, benzquinamide, cephapirin, chlorpromazine, codeine phosphate, dimenhydrinate, diphenhydramine, doxapram, ephedrine, fibrinolysin, glycopyrrolate, hydromorphone, insulin, levorphanol, meperidine, metaraminol, methadone, morphine, norepinephrine, penicillin G, prochlorperazine, promazine, promethazine, sodium bicarbonate, succinylcholine, tetracycline.** **Y-site: Alfentanil, ascorbic acid, atracurium, atropine, cisatracurium, diltiazem, dobutamine, dopamine, ephedrine, epinephrine, furosemide, hydromorphone, labetalol, lidocaine, lorazepam, midazolam, morphine, nicardipine, norepinephrine, pancuronium, phenylephrine, succinylcholine, sufentanil, vecuronium.**

- Consult physician if intraarterial injection or extravasation occurs. The site will require particular attention to prevent arteritis, neuritis, and skin slough. An intraarterial injection usually causes extreme pain before patient loses consciousness.

- Store at 15°–30° C (59°–86° F). Avoid excessive heat; protect from freezing.

ADVERSE EFFECTS (≥1%) **CNS:** Headache, retrograde amnesia, emergence delirium, prolonged somnolence and recovery. **CV:** Myocardial depression, arrhythmias, circulatory depression. **GI:** Nausea, vomiting, regurgitation of gastric contents, rectal irritation, cramping, rectal bleeding, diarrhea. **Respiratory:** Respiratory depression with apnea; hiccups, sneezing, coughing, bronchospasm, laryngospasm. **Body as a Whole:** Hypersensitivity reactions, anaphylaxis (rare), hypothermia, thrombosis and sloughing (with extravasation); salivation, shivering, skeletal muscle hyperactivity.

DIAGNOSTIC TEST INTERFERENCE ***Thiopental*** may cause decrease in ***I^{123} and I^{131} thyroidal uptake*** test results.

INTERACTIONS Drug: CNS DEPRESSANTS potentiate CNS and respiratory depression. PHENOTHIAZINES increase risk of hypotension. **Probenecid** may prolong anesthesia. **Herbal: Kava-kava, valerian** may potentiate sedation.

PHARMACOKINETICS Onset: 30–60 s. **Duration:** 10–30 min. **Distribution:** Distributed into muscle and liver; crosses placenta. **Metabolism:** Metabolized in liver. **Elimination:** Excreted in urine. **Half-Life:** 12 min.

T

NURSING IMPLICATIONS

Assessment & Drug Effects

- Monitor vital signs q3–5min before, during, and after anesthetic administration until recovery and into postoperative period, if necessary.
- Report increases in pulse rate or drop in blood pressure. Hypovolemia, cranial trauma, or premedication with opioids increases potential for apnea and symptoms of myocardial depression (decreased cardiac output and arterial pressure).
- Shivering, excitement, muscle twitching may develop during recovery period if patient is in pain.

Patient & Family Education

- Onset of drug effect is rapid, with loss of consciousness within 30–60 s.

THIORIDAZINE HYDROCHLORIDE

(thye-or-rid'a-zeen)

Mellaril, Novoridazine ♣

Classifications: CENTRAL NERVOUS SYSTEM AGENT; PSYCHOTHERAPEUTIC; PHENOTHIAZINE ANTIPSYCHOTIC

Prototype: Chlorpromazine

Pregnancy Category: C

AVAILABILITY 10 mg, 15 mg, 25 mg, 50 mg, 100 mg, 150 mg, 200 mg tablets; 30 mg/mL, 100 mg/mL solution; 25 mg/5 mL suspension

ACTIONS Phenothiazine similar to chlorpromazine. Rarely produces extrapyramidal effects. Has weak antiemetic but strong anticholinergic and alpha-adrenergic agonist activity and potent sedative action.

THERAPEUTIC EFFECTS Effective in reducing excitement, hypermotility, abnormal initiative, affective tension, and agitation by inhibiting psychomotor functions. Also effective as an antipsychotic agent, and for behavioral disorders in children.

USES Management of nonpsychotic behavioral disturbances of senility, manifestations of psychotic disorders, alcohol withdrawal; symptomatic treatment of organic brain disease. Short-term treatment of moderate to marked depression and for management of hyperkinetic behavior syndrome (attention deficit disorder).

CONTRAINDICATIONS Hypersensitivity to phenothiazines. Severe CNS depression; CV disease; children <2 y. Safety during pregnancy (category C) or lactation is not established.

CAUTIOUS USE Premature ventricular contractions; previously diagnosed breast cancer; patients exposed to extremes in heat or to organophosphorus insecticides; respiratory disorders.

ROUTE & DOSAGE

Psychotic Disorders

Adult: **PO** 50–100 mg t.i.d., may increase up to 800 mg/d as needed or tolerated
Geriatric: **PO** 10 mg t.i.d., may increase up to 200 mg/d
Child: **PO** *>2 y,* 0.5–3 mg/kg/d in divided doses; if hospitalized, may start at 25 mg t.i.d.

Moderate to Marked Depression

Adult: **PO** 25 mg t.i.d., may increase up to 200 mg/d in divided doses

Dementia Behavior

Geriatric: **PO** 10–25 mg 1–2 times/d, may increase q4–7d (max: 400 mg/d in divided doses)

ADMINISTRATION

Oral

- Give with fluid of patient's choice; tablet may be crushed.
- Schedule phenothiazine at least 1 h before or 1 h after an antacid or antidiarrheal medication.
- Dilute liquid concentrate just prior to administration with 1/2 glass of fruit juice, milk, water, carbonated beverage, or soup.
- Add increases in dose to the first dose of the day to prevent sleep disturbance.
- Store at 15°–30° C (59°–86° F) in tightly covered, light-resistant containers unless otherwise indicated.

ADVERSE EFFECTS (≥1%) **CNS:** *Sedation,* dizziness, drowsiness, lethargy, extrapyramidal syndrome, nocturnal confusion, hyperactivity. **Special Senses:** Nasal congestion, blurred vision, pigmentary retinopathy. **GI:** Xerostomia, *constipation,* paralytic ileus. **Urogenital:** Amenorrhea, breast engorgement, gynecomastia, galactorrhea, *urinary retention.* **CV:** Ventricular dysrhythmias, hypotension, prolonged QTc interval.

INTERACTIONS Drug: Alcohol, ANXIOLYTICS, SEDATIVE-HYPNOTICS, other CNS DEPRESSANTS add to CNS depression; additive adverse effects with other PHENOTHIAZINES; **amiodarone, amoxapine, arsenic trioxide, astemizole, bepridil, cisapride, clarithromycin, daunorubicin, diltiazem, disopyramide, dofetilide, dolasetron, doxorubicin, encainide, erythromycin, flecainide, fluoxetine, fluvoxamine gatifloxacin, grepafloxacin, haloperidol, ibutilide, indapamide, local anesthetics, maprotiline, moxifloxacin, octreotide, paroxetine, pentamidine, pimozide, procainamide, probucol, quinidine, risperidone, sotalol, sertraline, sparfloxacin, terfenadine, terodiline, tocainide, tricyclic antidepressants, venlafaxine, verapamil, ziprasidone** can prolong QTc interval resulting in arrhythmias. **Herbal: Kava-kava** may increase risk and severity of dystonic reactions.

PHARMACOKINETICS Absorption: Well absorbed from GI tract. **Onset:** Days to weeks. **Distribution:** Crosses placenta; distributed into breast milk. **Metabolism:** Metabolized in liver. **Elimination:** Excreted in urine. **Half-Life:** 26–36 h.

NURSING IMPLICATIONS

Assessment & Drug Effects

- Orthostatic hypotension may occur in early therapy. Female patients appear to be more susceptible than males.
- Be aware that patients may be unable to adjust to extremes of temperature because drug effects heat regulatory center in the hypothalamus. Patient may complain of being cold even at average room temperature; older adults are particularly susceptible.
- Monitor I&O ratio and bowel elimination pattern. Check for abdominal distension and pain. Encourage adequate fluid intake as prophylaxis for constipation and xerostomia. The depressed patient may not seek help for either symptom or for urinary retention.
- Lab tests: Obtain periodic CBC and liver function tests during therapy.
- Supervise patient closely during early course of therapy. Suicide is an inherent risk with any depressed patient and may remain

T

a problem until there is significant clinical improvement.

Patient & Family Education

- Exercise care not to spill drug on skin because of danger of contact dermatitis. Wash skin well in soap and water if liquid drug is spilled.
- Take drug as prescribed and do not alter dosing regimen or stop medication without consulting physician.
- Avoid alcohol during phenothiazine therapy. Concomitant use enhances CNS depression effects.
- Be aware that marked drowsiness generally subsides with continued therapy or reduction in dosage.
- Do not drive or engage in potentially hazardous activities until response to drug is known.
- Make position changes slowly, particularly from lying down to upright posture; dangle legs a few minutes before standing.
- Vasodilation produced by hot showers or baths or by long exposure to environmental heat may accentuate hypotensive effect.
- Do not apply heating pad or hot water bottles to the body for external heat. Because of depressed conditioned avoidance behaviors, a severe burn may result.
- Report the onset of any change in visual acuity, brownish coloring of vision, or impairment of night vision to physician. Symptoms suggest pigmentary retinopathy (observed primarily in patients receiving extremely high doses). An ophthalmic consultation may be indicated.
- Note: Thioridazine may color urine pink-red to reddish brown.
- Do not use any OTC drugs unless approved by the physician.
- Do not breast feed while taking this drug without consulting physician.

T

THIOTEPA

(thye-oh-tep'a)
Thioplex, TSPA
Classifications: ANTINEOPLASTIC; ALKYLATING AGENT
Prototype: Cyclophosphamide
Pregnancy Category: D

AVAILABILITY 15 mg injection

ACTIONS Cell cycle nonspecific alkylating agent that selectively reacts with DNA phosphate groups to produce chromosome cross-linkage and consequent blocking of nucleoprotein synthesis.
THERAPEUTIC EFFECTS Nonvesicant, highly toxic hematopoietic agent. Myelosuppression is cumulative and unpredictable and may be delayed. Has some immunosuppressive activity.

USES To produce remissions in malignant lymphomas, including Hodgkin's disease, and adenocarcinoma of breast and ovary. Also in chronic granulocytic and lymphocytic leukemia, superficial papillary carcinoma of urinary bladder, bronchogenic carcinoma, and in malignant effusions secondary to neoplastic disease of serosal cavities.
UNLABELED USES Prevention of pterygium recurrences following postoperative beta-irradiation; leukemia, malignant meningeal neoplasms.

CONTRAINDICATIONS Hypersensitivity to drug; acute leukemia; pregnancy (category D), lactation.
CAUTIOUS USE Chronic lymphocytic leukemia; myelosuppression produced by radiation; with other antineoplastics; bone marrow invasion by tumor cells; impaired kidney or liver function.

ROUTE & DOSAGE

Malignant Lymphomas

Adult: **IV** 0.3–0.4 mg/kg q1–4wk **Intratumor** 0.6–0.8 mg/kg directly into tumor q1–4wk **Intracavitary** 0.6–0.8 mg/kg instilled through same tubing used for paracentesis at intervals of at least 1 wk **Intravesicular** 60 mg in 30–60 mL of distilled water instilled into bladder to be retained for 2 h once/wk for 4 wk **Intrathecal** 1–10 mg/m_2 1–2 times/wk

ADMINISTRATION

Intravenous

- Use only under constant supervision by physicians experienced in therapy with cytotoxic agents.
- Avoid exposure of skin and respiratory tract to particles of thiotepa during solution preparation.

PREPARE: **Direct:** Reconstitute each 15 mg vial with 1.5 mL sterile water for injection (supplied) to yield 10 mg/mL. Further dilute with 50–100 mL NS. Filter solution through a 0.22 micron filter to eliminate haze. Use immediately.
ADMINISTER: **Direct:** Give 60 mg or fraction thereof over 1 min.
INCOMPATIBILITIES **Solution/additive: Cisplatin Y-site: Cisplatin, filgrastim, minocycline, vinorelbine.**

- Store powder for injection and reconstituted solutions at 2°–8° C (35°–46° F); protect from light. Solutions reconstituted with sterile water only are stable for 8 h under refrigeration.

ADVERSE EFFECTS (≥1%) **GI:** Anorexia, nausea, vomiting, stomatitis, ulceration of intestinal mucosa. **Hematologic:** Leukopenia, thrombocytopenia, anemia, pancytopenia. **Skin:** Hives, rash, pruritus. **Urogenital:** Amenorrhea, interference with spermatogenesis. **Body as a Whole:** Headache, febrile reactions, pain and weeping of injection site, hyperuricemia, slowed or lessened response in heavily irradiated area, sensation of throat tightness. **Other:** Reported with intravesical administration (lower abdominal pain, hematuria, hemorrhagic chemical cystitis, vesical irritability).

INTERACTIONS Drug: May prolong muscle paralysis with **mivacurium;** ANTICOAGULANTS, NSAIDS, SALICYLATES, ANTIPLATELET AGENTS may increase risk of bleeding.

PHARMACOKINETICS Absorption: Rapidly cleared from plasma. **Onset:** Gradual response over several wk. **Metabolism:** Metabolized in liver. **Elimination:** 60% of IV dose excreted in urine within 24–72 h.

NURSING IMPLICATIONS

Assessment & Drug Effects

- Monitor closely because most patients will manifest some evidence of toxicity.
- Be aware that because of cumulative effects, maximum myelosuppression may be delayed 3–4 wk after termination of therapy.
- Discontinue therapy (per manufacturer) if leukocyte count falls to 3000/mm^3 or below or if platelet count falls below 150,000/mm^3.
- Lab tests: Determine Hgb level, WBC with differential, and thrombocyte (i.e., platelet) counts at least weekly during therapy and for at least 3 wk after therapy is discontinued.
- Monitor leukocyte and thrombocyte counts as indicators for

T

adaptations in nursing and drug regimens.

Patient & Family Education
- Be aware of possibility of amenorrhea (usually reversible in 6–8 mo).
- Report onset of fever, bleeding, a cold or illness, no matter how mild to physician; medical supervision may be necessary.
- Do not breast feed while taking this drug.

THIOTHIXENE HYDROCHLORIDE

(thye-oh-thix'een)
Navane
Classifications: CENTRAL NERVOUS SYSTEM AGENT; PSYCHOTHERAPEUTIC; PHENOTHIAZINE ANTIPSYCHOTIC
Prototype: Chlorpromazine
Pregnancy Category: C

AVAILABILITY 1 mg, 2 mg, 5 mg, 10 mg, 20 mg capsules; 5 mg/mL solution

ACTIONS Xanthene derivative chemically and pharmacologically similar to chlorprothixene and the piperazine phenothiazines. Mechanism of antipsychotic effects is unclear; thought to be related to blockade of postsynaptic dopamine receptors in the brain.
THERAPEUTIC EFFECTS Possesses antipsychotic, sedative, adrenolytic, antiemetic, and weak anticholinergic activity.

USES Manifestations of psychotic disorders.
UNLABELED USES Antidepressant.

CONTRAINDICATIONS Hypersensitivity to thioxanthenes and phenothiazines; children <12 y; comatose states; CNS depression; circulatory collapse; blood dyscrasias. Safety during pregnancy (category C) or lactation is not established.
CAUTIOUS USE History of convulsive disorders; alcohol withdrawal; glaucoma; prostatic hypertrophy; cardiovascular disease; patients who might be exposed to organophosphorus insecticides or to extreme heat; concomitant use of atropine or related drugs or ototoxic medications (especially ototoxic antibiotics); previously diagnosed breast cancer.

ROUTE & DOSAGE

Psychotic Disorders
Adult: **PO** 2 mg t.i.d., may increase up to 15 mg/d as needed or tolerated (max: 60 mg/d) **IM** 4 mg b.i.d. to q.i.d. (max: 30 mg/d)
Dementia Behavior
Geriatric: **PO** 1–2 mg 1–2 times/d, may increase q4–7d (max: of 30 mg/d in divided doses)

ADMINISTRATION

Oral
- Avoid contact between oral concentrate and skin or clothing to prevent contact dermatitis. If concentrate spills, wash skin promptly with water.
- Give oral concentrate (contains 7% alcohol) diluted in a cupful of water, fruit juice, carbonated beverage, milk, or soup.
- Empty capsule and give with water or mix with food; useful if patient unable or unwilling to swallow the capsule.

Intramuscular
- Give IM injection deep into upper outer quadrant of buttock. Aspirate

T

carefully before injection. Rotate injection sites.

- Do not permit access to more than one dose of medication if patient has suicidal tendency; supervise ingestion to prevent hoarding.
- Store at 15°–30° C (59°–86° F) in light-resistant containers unless otherwise indicated.

ADVERSE EFFECTS (≥1%) **CNS:** *Drowsiness,* insomnia, dizziness, cerebral edema, convulsions, *extrapyramidal symptoms (dose related),* paradoxical exaggeration of psychotic symptoms; sudden death, neuroleptic malignant syndrome, tardive dyskinesia, depressed cough reflex. **GI:** Xerostomia, constipation. **CV:** Tachycardia, *orthostatic hypotension* (especially with IM). **Urogenital:** Impotence, gynecomastia, galactorrhea, amenorrhea. **Skin:** Rash, contact dermatitis, photosensitivity. **Special Senses:** Blurred vision, pigmentary retinopathy. **Metabolic:** Decreased serum uric acid levels.

INTERACTIONS Drug: Alcohol, ANXIOLYTICS, SEDATIVE-HYPNOTICS, other CNS DEPRESSANTS add to CNS depression; additive adverse effects with other PHENOTHIAZINES; **Herbal: Kava-kava** may increase risk and severity of dystonic reactions.

PHARMACOKINETICS Absorption: Slowly absorbed from GI tract. **Onset:** Days to weeks PO; 1–6 h IM. **Duration:** Up to 12 h. **Distribution:** May remain in body for several weeks; crosses placenta. **Metabolism:** Metabolized in liver. **Elimination:** Excreted in bile and feces. **Half-Life:** 34 h.

NURSING IMPLICATIONS

Assessment & Drug Effects

- Monitor for therapeutic response. Although therapeutic response can be observed 1–6 h following IM injection, it may be days or several weeks before there is a response with oral drug.
- Keep patient recumbent for at least 1 h following IM because of possibility of orthostatic hypotension. Check BP periodically.
- Monitor BP for excessive hypotensive response when thiothixene is added to drug regimen of patient on hypertensive treatment until therapy is stabilized.
- Monitor response when patient is changed from IM to PO forms (capsules, concentrate). Dosage adjustment may be necessary.
- Monitor infants delivered from mothers who have received thiothixene. Hyperreflexia has been reported.
- Lab tests: Periodic blood chemistry and liver function tests with prolonged therapy.
- Report extrapyramidal effects (pseudoparkinsonism, akathisia, dystonia) to physician; dose adjustment or short-term therapy with an antiparkinsonism agent may provide relief.
- Be alert to first symptoms of tardive dyskinesia (see Appendix F). Discontinue drug immediately and inform physician.

Patient & Family Education

- Make position changes slowly, particularly from lying down to upright because of danger of light-headedness; sit a few minutes before walking.
- Do not drive or engage in potentially hazardous activities until response to drug is known.
- Avoid alcohol and other depressants during therapy.
- Take drug as prescribed; do not alter dosing regimen or stop medication without consulting physi-

T

cian. Abrupt discontinuation can cause delirium.

- Do not use any OTC drugs without approval of physician.
- Note: Hyperhidrosis, while an uncomfortable adverse effect, does not indicate need to terminate therapy.
- Avoid excessive exposure to sunlight to prevent a photosensitivity reaction. If sun exposure is expected, protect skin with sunscreen lotion (SPF 12 or above).
- Do not breast feed while taking this drug without consulting physician.
- Schedule periodic eye exams and report blurred vision to physician.

THROMBIN

(throm'bin)

Thrombinar, Thrombostat

Classifications: BLOOD FORMERS, COAGULATORS, AND ANTICOAGULANTS; HEMOSTATIC

Prototype: Aminocaproic acid

Pregnancy Category: C

AVAILABILITY 1,000, 5,000, 10,000, 20,000, 50,000 unit vials

ACTIONS Sterile plasma protein prepared from prothrombin of bovine origin. Induces clotting of whole blood or fibrinogen solution without addition of other substances.

THERAPEUTIC EFFECTS Facilitates conversion of fibrinogen to fibrin resulting in clotting of whole blood.

USES When oozing of blood from capillaries and small venules is accessible, as in dental extraction, plastic surgery, grafting procedures, and epistaxis; also to shorten bleeding time at puncture sites in heparinized patient (i.e., following hemodialysis).

CONTRAINDICATIONS Known hypersensitivity to any of drug components or to material of bovine origin; parenteral use; entry or infiltration into large blood vessels.

CAUTIOUS USE Pregnancy (category C).

ROUTE & DOSAGE

Oozing Blood

Adult: **Topical** 100–2000 NIH U/mL, depending on extent of bleeding, may be used as solution, in dry form, by mixing thrombin with blood plasma to form a fibrin "glue," or in conjunction with absorbable gelatin sponge

ADMINISTRATION

Topical

- Ensure that sponge recipient area is free of blood before applying thrombin.
- Prepare solutions in sterile distilled water or isotonic saline.
- Use solutions within a few hours of preparation. If several hours are to elapse between time of preparation and use, solution should be refrigerated, or preferably frozen, and used within 48 h.
- Store lyophilized preparation at 2°–8° C (36°–46° F).

ADVERSE EFFECTS (≥1%) **Body as a Whole:** Sensitivity, allergic and febrile reactions, intravascular clotting and death when thrombin is allowed to enter large blood vessels.

INTERACTIONS Drug: No clinically significant interactions established.

PHARMACOKINETICS Not applicable

THYROID

(thye'roid)

Armour Thyroid, Thyrar

Classifications: HORMONE AND SYNTHETIC SUBSTITUTE; THYROID AGENT

Prototype: Levothyroxine sodium

Pregnancy Category: A

AVAILABILITY 15 mg (1/4 grain), 30 mg (1/2 grain), 60 mg (1 grain), 90 mg (1 1/2 grain), 120 mg (2 grain), 180 mg (3 grain), 240 mg (4 grain), 300 mg (5 grain) tablets

ACTIONS Preparation of desiccated animal thyroid gland containing active thyroid hormones, *l*-thyroxine (T_4) and *l*-triiodothyronine (T_3). Action mechanism unknown; T_4 is largely converted to T_3, which exerts the principal effects.

THERAPEUTIC EFFECTS Influences growth and maturation of various tissues (including skeletal and CNS) at critical periods. Promotes a generalized increase in metabolic rate of body tissues. Indicated by diuresis, accompanied by loss of weight and puffiness, followed by sense of well-being, increased pulse rate, increased pulse pressure, increased appetite, increased psychomotor activity, loss of constipation, normalization of skin texture and hair, and increased T_3 and T_4 serum levels.

USES Replacement or substitution therapy in primary hypothyroidism (cretinism, myxedema, simple goiter, deficiency states in pregnancy and older adults) and secondary hypothyroidism caused by surgery, excess radiation, or antithyroid drug therapy. May be given as adjunct to antithyroid agents when it is desirable to limit release of thyrotropic hormones and to prevent goitrogenesis and hypothyroidism.

CONTRAINDICATIONS Thyrotoxicosis; acute MI uncomplicated by hypothyroidism, cardiovascular disease; morphologic hypogonadism; nephrosis; uncorrected hypoadrenalism.

CAUTIOUS USE Angina pectoris, hypertension, older adults who may have occult cardiac disease; renal insufficiency; concomitant administration of catecholamines; diabetes mellitus; hyperthyroidism (history of); malabsorption states; pregnancy (category A), lactation.

ROUTE & DOSAGE

Mild to Moderate Hypothyroidism

Adult: **PO** 60 mg/d, may increase q30d to 60–180 mg/d

Severe Hypothyroidism

Adult: **PO** 15 mg/d, increased q2wk to 60 mg/d, then may increase q30d if needed

Child: **PO** 15 mg/d, may increase by 15 mg q2wk if needed

ADMINISTRATION

Oral

- Give as a single dose, preferably on an empty stomach.
- Initiate dosage generally at low level and systematically increase in small increments to desired maintenance dose.
- Store in dark bottle to minimize spontaneous deiodination. Keep desiccated thyroid dry.

ADVERSE EFFECTS (≥1%) **Endocrine:** Hyperthyroidism, thyroid storm (high temperature [as high as 41° C (106° F)], tachycardia, vomiting, shock, coma). **Special Senses:** Staring expression in eyes. **CV:** CHF, angina, cardiac arrhythmias, palpitation, tachycardia. **Body as a Whole:** Weight loss, tremors, headache, nervousness, fever, insomnia, warm and moist skin, heat intolerance, leg cramps, menstrual irregularities, shock, changes in appetite. **GI:** Diarrhea or abdominal cramps. **Metabolic:** Hyperglycemia (usually offset by increased tissue oxidation of sugar).

DIAGNOSTIC TEST INTERFERENCE Thyroid increases ***basal metabolic rate;*** may increase ***blood glucose levels, creatine phosphokinase, AST, LDH, PBI.*** It may decrease ***serum uric acid, cholesterol, thyroid-stimulating hormone (TSH), iodine 131*** uptake. Many medications may produce false results in ***thyroid function tests.***

INTERACTIONS Drug: ORAL ANTICOAGULANTS potentiate hypoprothrombinemia; may increase requirements for **insulin,** SULFONYLUREAS; **epinephrine** may precipitate coronary insufficiency; **cholestyramine** may decrease thyroid absorption.

PHARMACOKINETICS Absorption: Variably absorbed from GI tract. **Peak:** 1–3 wk. **Distribution:** Does not readily cross placenta; minimal amounts in breast milk. **Metabolism:** Deiodination in thyroid gland. **Elimination:** Excreted in urine and feces. **Half-Life:** T_3, 1–2 d; T_4, 6–7 d.

T

NURSING IMPLICATIONS

Assessment & Drug Effects

- Observe patient carefully during initial treatment for untoward reactions such as angina, palpitations, cardiac pain.
- Be alert for symptoms of overdosage (see ADVERSE EFFECTS) that may occur 1–3 wk after therapy is started. If they develop, interrupt treatment for several days and restart with reduced dosage.
- Monitor response until regimen is stabilized to prevent iatrogenic hyperthyroidism. In drug-induced hyperthyroidism, there may also be increased bone loss. Such a patient is vulnerable to pathologic fractures.
- Monitor vital signs: Pulse rate is an important clue to drug effectiveness. Assess pulse before each dose during period of dosage adjustment. Consult physician if rate is 100 or more or if there has been a marked change in rate or rhythm.
- Lab tests: Monitor thyroid function q3mo during dose adjustment period. Monitor prothrombin time closely if patient is receiving concurrent anticoagulant therapy. A decrease in requirement usually develops within 1–4 wk after starting treatment with thyroid.
- Be aware that toxic effects of thyroid develop slowly and disappear gradually. T_4 effects require up to 3–6 wk to dissipate; T_3 effects last 6–14 d after drug withdrawal.

Patient & Family Education

- Adhere to established dosage regimen; do not change dose intervals without approval of the physician.
- Be aware that replacement therapy for hypothyroidism is lifelong; continued follow-up care is important.
- Do not change brands of thyroid unless physician approves. Hormone content varies among brands.
- Monitor pulse rate and report increases greater than parameter set by physician.
- Report onset of chest pain or other signs of aggravated CV disease (dyspnea, tachycardia) to physician promptly.
- Report evidence of any unexplained bleeding to physician when taking concomitant anticoagulant.

- Use serial height and weight measurement to monitor growth in juvenile undergoing treatment.
- Do not breast feed while taking this drug without consulting physician.

TIAGABINE HYDROCHLORIDE

(ti-a'ga-been)

Gabitril Filmtabs

Classifications: CENTRAL NERVOUS SYSTEM AGENT; ANTICONVULSANT; GABA INHIBITOR

Prototype: Valproic acid sodium (Sodium valproate)

Pregnancy Category: C

AVAILABILITY 2 mg, 4 mg, 12 mg, 16 mg, 20 mg tablets

ACTIONS GABA inhibitor for the treatment of partial epilepsy. Potent and selective inhibitor of GABA uptake into presynaptic neurons; allows more GABA to bind to the surfaces of postsynaptic neurons in the CNS.

THERAPEUTIC EFFECTS Effectiveness indicated by reduction in seizure activity.

USES Adjunctive therapy for partial seizures.

CONTRAINDICATIONS Hypersensitivity to tiagabine; pregnancy (category C).

CAUTIOUS USE Liver function impairment; lactation; history of spike and wave discharge on EEG; status epilepticus.

ROUTE & DOSAGE

Seizures

Adult: **PO** Start with 4 mg q.d., may increase dose by 4–8 mg/d qwk (max: 56 mg/d in 2–4 divided doses)

Adolescent: **PO** *12–18 y,* Start with 4 mg q.d., after 2 wk may increase dose by 4–8 mg/d qwk (max: 32 mg/d in 2–4 divided doses)

ADMINISTRATION

Oral

- Give with food.
- Make dosage increases, when needed, at weekly intervals.
- Store at 15°–30° C (59°–86° F) in a tightly closed container and protect from light.

ADVERSE EFFECTS (≥1%) **Body as a Whole:** Infection, flu-like syndrome, pain, myasthenia, allergic reactions, chills, malaise, arthralgia. **CNS:** *Dizziness, asthenia, tremor, somnolence, nervousness,* difficulty concentrating, ataxia, depression, insomnia, abnormal gait, hostility, confusion, speech disorder, difficulty with memory, paresthesias, emotional lability, agitation, dysarthria, euphoria, hallucinations, hyperkinesia, hypertonia, hypotonia, myoclonus, twitching, vertigo. **CV:** Vasodilation, hypertension, palpitations, tachycardia, syncope, edema, peripheral edema. **GI:** Abdominal pain, diarrhea, nausea, vomiting, increased appetite, mouth ulcers. **Respiratory:** Pharyngitis, cough, bronchitis, dyspnea, epistaxis, pneumonia. **Skin:** Rash, pruritus, alopecia, dry skin, sweating, ecchymoses. **Special Senses:** Amblyopia, nystagmus, tinnitus. **Urogenital:** Dysmenorrhea, dysuria, metrorrhagia, incontinence, vaginitis, UTI.

INTERACTIONS Drug: Carbamazepine, phenytoin, phenobarbital decrease levels of tiagabine. **Herbal: Ginkgo** may decrease anticonvulsant effectiveness.

PHARMACOKINETICS Absorption: Rapidly absorbed; 90% bioavailabil-

T

ity. **Peak:** 45 min. **Distribution:** 96% protein bound. **Metabolism:** Metabolized in liver, probably by cytochrome P450 3A isoform. **Elimination:** 25% excreted in urine, 63% excreted in feces. **Half-Life:** 7–9 h (4–7 h with other enzyme-inducing drugs).

NURSING IMPLICATIONS

Assessment & Drug Effects

- Lab tests: Measure plasma levels of tiagabine before and after changes are made in the drug regimen.
- Be aware that concurrent use of other anticonvulsants may decrease effectiveness of tiagabine or increase the potential for adverse effects.
- Monitor carefully for S&S of CNS depression.

Patient & Family Education

- Do not stop taking drug abruptly; may cause sudden onset of seizures.
- Exercise caution while engaging in potentially hazardous activities because drug may cause dizziness.
- Use caution when taking other prescription or OTC drugs that can cause drowsiness.
- Report any of the following to the physician: Rash or hives; red, peeling skin; dizziness; drowsiness; depression; GI distress; nervousness or tremors; difficulty concentrating or talking.
- Do not breast feed while taking this drug without consulting physician.

TICARCILLIN DISODIUM

(ti-car-sill'in)

Ticar

Classifications: ANTIINFECTIVE; ANTIBIOTIC; ANTIPSEUDOMONAL PENICILLIN

Prototype: Mezlocillin

Pregnancy Category: C

AVAILABILITY 1 g, 3 g, 6 g injection

ACTIONS Semisynthetic injectable penicillin that is bactericidal against gram-positive and gram-negative organisms.

THERAPEUTIC EFFECTS Susceptible organisms include *Pseudomonas aeruginosa, Escherichia coli, Proteus mirabilis, Proteus vulgaris, Enterobacter species, Haemophilus influenzae, Staphylococcus pneumoniae.*

USES Primarily for gram-negative bacterial infections, bacterial septicemia, skin and soft-tissue infections, acute and chronic respiratory infections, genitourinary tract infection by susceptible organisms, intraabdominal infections and infections of the female pelvis and reproductive system.

CONTRAINDICATIONS History of allergic reaction to any penicillin.

CAUTIOUS USE Allergy to cephalosporins; pregnancy (category C), lactation; renal impairment.

ROUTE & DOSAGE

Urinary Tract Infections

Adult: **IM/IV** 200 mg/kg/d in 4 divided doses or 1–2 g q6h
Child: **IM/IV** 50–200 mg/kg/d in 4 divided doses

Systemic Infections

Adult: **IM/IV** 15–40 g/d in 6 divided doses (max: 40 g/d)
Child: **IM/IV** 250–500 mg/kg/d in 6 divided doses (max: 40 g/d)
Neonate: **IV** 150–300 mg/kg/d divided q6–12h

ADMINISTRATION

Intramuscular

- Do not exceed 2 g/per injection.
- Reconstitute each 1 g of ticarcillin with 2 mL of sterile water for injection or NS injection and use promptly. Resulting concentration is 1 g/2.6 mL.

Intravenous

Note: Verify correct IV concentration and rate of infusion for administration to neonates, infants, children with physician.

PREPARE: **Direct:** Reconstitute each 1 g of ticarcillin with 4 mL of sterile water for injection. Further dilute with at least 20 mL of D5W, NS, or other compatible IV solution. **Intermittent:** May dilute further in 50–100 mL of additional compatible IV solution.

ADMINISTER: **Direct:** Give slowly at a rate of 1 g over 5 min or longer. **Intermittent:** Give 1 g over 30–120 min.

INCOMPATIBILITIES **Solution/additive:** AMINOGLYCOSIDES, **amphotericin b, bleomycin, chloramphenicol, cytarabine, doxapram, lincomycin,** TETRACYCLINES, **vitamin B complex with C. Y-site:** AMINOGLYCOSIDES, **amphotericin B cholesteryl complex, fluconazole, promethazine, vancomycin.**

- Do not use solutions refrigerated longer than 72 h for multidose purposes. ▪ Store dry powder at 15°–30° C (59°–86° F) or below.

ADVERSE EFFECTS (≥1%) **Body as a Whole:** Hypersensitivity reactions, pain, burning, swelling at injection site; phlebitis, thrombophlebitis; superinfections. **CNS:** Headache, blurred vision, mental deterioration, convulsions, hallucinations, seizures, giddiness, neuromuscular hyperirritability. **GI:** *Diarrhea, nausea,* vomiting, disturbances of taste or smell, stomatitis, flatulence. **Hematologic:** Eosinophilia, thrombocytopenia, leukopenia, neutropenia, hemolytic anemia. **Metabolic:** Hypernatremia, transient increases in serum AST, ALT, BUN, and alkaline phosphatase; increases in serum LDH, bilirubin, and creatinine and decreased serum uric acid.

PHARMACOKINETICS Peak: 1–2 h IM. **Distribution:** Low concentrations in CSF unless meninges are inflamed; crosses placenta; distributed into breast milk. **Elimination:** 80%–90% excreted unchanged in urine within 24 h. **Half-Life:** 67 min.

NURSING IMPLICATIONS

Assessment & Drug Effects

- Obtain baseline C&S tests before initiating therapy; drug may be started pending results.
- Be aware that serious and sometimes fatal anaphylactoid reactions have been reported in patients with penicillin hypersensitivity or history of sensitivity to multiple allergens.
- Assess IV access site frequently for vein irritation and phlebitis.
- Discontinue ticarcillin if bleeding manifestations occur (some patients on high doses may develop hemorrhagic manifestations associated with abnormalities of coagulation).
- Lab tests: Monitor kidney and liver functions, CBC, platelet counts, and serum electrolytes during prolonged treatment.
- Monitor cardiac status because of the high sodium content in drug.
- Monitor for and report for hypokalemia (see Appendix F).

Patient & Family Education

- Report urticaria, rashes, or pruritus to physician immediately.
- Report frequent loose stools, diarrhea, or other possible signs of pseudomembranous colitis (see Appendix F) to physician.
- Do not breast feed while taking this drug without consulting physician.

TICARCILLIN DISODIUM/ CLAVULANATE POTASSIUM

(tye-kar-sill′in/clav-yoo′la-nate)

Timentin

Classifications: ANTIINFECTIVE; ANTIBIOTIC; ANTIPSEUDOMONAL PENICILLIN

Prototype: Mezlocillin

Pregnancy Category: B

AVAILABILITY 3.1 g injection

ACTIONS Injectable extended-spectrum penicillin and fixed combination of ticarcillin disodium with the potassium salt of clavulanic acid, a beta-lactamase inhibitor produced by fermentation of *Streptomyces clavuligerus*. Used alone, clavulanic acid antibacterial activity is weak but in combination with ticarcillin prevents degradation by beta-lactamase and extends ticarcillin spectrum of activity against many strains of beta-lactamase-producing bacteria (synergistic effect). Synergism between the two drugs does not occur against organisms susceptible to ticarcillin alone.

THERAPEUTIC EFFECTS Susceptible strains of organisms include beta-lactamase strains of *Klebsiella sp, Escherichia coli, Staphylococcus aureus, Pseudomonas aeruginosa, Haemophilus influenzae, Citrobacter sp, Enterobacter cloacae, Serratia marcescens.*

T

USES Infections of lower respiratory tract and urinary tract and skin and skin structures, infections of bone and joint, and septicemia caused by susceptible organisms. Also mixed infections and as presumptive therapy before identification of causative organism.

CONTRAINDICATIONS Hypersensitivity to penicillins or to cephalosporins. Safety during pregnancy (category B) is not established.

CAUTIOUS USE Lactation; renal impairment.

ROUTE & DOSAGE

Moderate to Severe Infections

Adult: **IV** *>60 kg,* 3.1 g q4–6h
Child: **IV** *>3 mo,* 200–300 mg/kg/d divided q4–6h (based on ticarcillin)
Infant: **IV** *<3 mo,* 200–300 mg/kg/d divided q6–8h (based on ticarcillin)

ADMINISTRATION

Intravenous

Note: Verify correct IV concentration and rate of infusion for administration to infants and children with physician.

PREPARE: **Intermittent:** Reconstitute by adding to 3.1 g of powder 13 mL sterile water for injection or NS injection to yield 200 mg/mL ticarcillin with 6.7 mg/mL clavulanic acid. Shake until dissolved. Further dilute with NS, D5W, or RL. Do not use if discoloration or particulate matter is present.

ADMINISTER: **Intermittent:** Give over 30 min.

INCOMPATIBILITIES **Solution/additive:** AMINOGLYCOSIDES, **doxapram. Y-site:** AMINOGLYCOSIDES, **amphotericin B cholesteryl complex, vancomycin.**

■ Store vial with sterile powder at 21°–24° C (69°–75° F) or colder. If exposed to higher temperature, powder will darken, indicating degradation of clavulanate potassium and loss of potency. Discard vial. See package insert for information about storage and stability of reconstituted and diluted IV solutions of drug.

ADVERSE EFFECTS (≥1%) **Body as a Whole:** Hypersensitivity reactions, pain, burning, swelling at injection site; phlebitis, thrombophlebitis; superinfections. **CNS:** Headache, blurred vision, mental deterioration, convulsions, hallucinations, seizures, giddiness, neuromuscular hyperirritability. **GI:** *Diarrhea, nausea,* vomiting, disturbances of taste or smell, stomatitis, flatulence. **Hematologic:** Eosinophilia, thrombocytopenia, leukopenia, neutropenia, hemolytic anemia. **Metabolic:** Hypernatremia, transient increases in serum AST, ALT, BUN, and alkaline phosphatase; increases in serum LDH, bilirubin, and creatinine and decreased serum uric acid.

DIAGNOSTIC TEST INTERFERENCE May interfere with test methods used to determine ***urinary proteins*** except for tests for urinary protein that use ***bromphenol blue. Positive direct antiglobulin (Coombs') test*** results, apparently caused by clavulanic acid, have been reported. This test may interfere with ***transfusion cross-matching procedures.***

INTERACTIONS Drugs: May increase risk of bleeding with ANTICOAGULANTS; **probenecid** decreases elimination of ticarcillin.

PHARMACOKINETICS Distribution: Widely distributed with highest concentrations in urine and bile; crosses placenta; distributed into breast milk. **Metabolism:** Slightly metabolized in liver. **Elimination:** Excreted in urine. **Half-Life:** 1.1–1.2 h ticarcillin, 1.1–1.5 h clavulanate.

NURSING IMPLICATIONS

Assessment & Drug Effects

- Lab tests: Obtain baseline C&S tests before initiating therapy; drug may be started pending results. Monitor kidney and liver functions, CBC, platelet count, and serum electrolytes during prolonger treatment.
- Be aware that serious and sometimes fatal anaphylactoid reactions have been reported in patient with penicillin hypersensitivity or history of sensitivity to multiple allergens. Reported incidence is low with this combination drug.
- Monitor cardiac status because of high sodium content of drug.
- Overdose symptoms: This drug may cause neuromuscular hyperirritability or seizures.

Patient & Family Education

- Report urticaria, rashes, or pruritus to physician immediately.
- Report frequent loose stools, diarrhea, or other possible signs of pseudomembranous colitis (see Appendix F) to physician.
- Do not breast feed while taking this drug without consulting physician.

TICLOPIDINE Pr

(ti-clo′pi-deen)

Ticlid

Classifications: BLOOD FORMERS, COAGULATORS, AND ANTICOAGULANTS; ANTIPLATELET AGENT

Pregnancy Category: B

AVAILABILITY 250 mg tablets

ACTIONS Platelet aggregation inhibitor that interferes with platelet membrane functioning and therefore platelet interactions.

THERAPEUTIC EFFECTS Prevents release of platelet constituents and prolongs bleeding time.

USES Reduction of the risk of thrombotic stroke in patients intolerant to aspirin.

T

UNLABELED USES Prevention of venous thromboembolic disorders; maintenance of bypass graft patency and of vascular access sites in hemodialysis patients; improvement of exercise performance in patients with ischemic heart disease and intermittent claudication; prevention of postoperative deep venous thrombosis (DVT).

CONTRAINDICATIONS Hypersensitivity to ticlopidine; hematopoietic disease, pathologic bleeding; severe liver impairment.

CAUTIOUS USE Hepatic function impairment, renal impairment; patients at risk for bleeding from trauma, surgery, or a bleeding disorder; GI bleeding; pregnancy (category B). It is not known if ticlopidine is excreted in breast milk. Safety and effectiveness in patients <18 y are not established.

ROUTE & DOSAGE

Stroke Prevention
Adult: **PO** 250 mg b.i.d. with food

ADMINISTRATION

Oral

- Give with food or just after eating to minimize GI irritation.
- Discontinue anticoagulants or fibrinolytic drugs before ticlopidine administration.
- Store at 15°–30° C (59°–86° F).

ADVERSE EFFECTS (≥1%) **CNS:** Dizziness. **GI:** Nausea, vomiting, abdominal cramps; dyspepsia, flatulence, anorexia; abnormal liver function tests (few cases of hepatotoxicity reported). **Hematologic:** Neutropenia (resolves in 1–3 wk), thrombocytopenia, leukopenia, agranulocytosis (usually within first 3 mo), and pancytopenia; hemorrhage (ecchymosis, epistaxis, menorrhagia, GI bleeding), thrombotic thrombocytopenia purpura (usually within first month). **Skin:** Urticaria, maculopapular rash, erythema nodosum (generally occur within the first 3 mo of therapy, with most occurring within the first 3–6 wk).

DIAGNOSTIC TEST INTERFERENCE Increases ***total serum cholesterol*** by 8%–10% within 4 wk of beginning therapy. ***Lipoprotein ratios*** remain unchanged. Elevates ***alkaline phosphatase*** and ***serum transaminases.***

INTERACTIONS Drug: ANTACIDS decrease bioavailability of ticlopidine. ANTICOAGULANTS increase risk of bleeding. **Cimetidine** decreases clearance of ticlopidine. CORTICOSTEROIDS counteract increased bleeding time associated with ticlopidine. May decrease **cyclosporine** levels (one case report). Increases **theophylline** half-life by 42%, possibly increasing **theophylline** serum levels. May increase **phenytoin** levels. **Food:** Food may increase bioavailability of ticlopidine.

PHARMACOKINETICS Absorption: 90% absorbed from GI tract; increased absorption when taken with food. **Onset:** Antiplatelet activity, 24–48 h; maximal effect at 3–5 d. **Peak:** Peak serum levels at 2 h. **Duration:** Bleeding times return to baseline within 4–10 d. **Distribution:** 90% bound to plasma proteins. **Metabolism:** Rapidly and extensively metabolized in liver. **Elimination:** Only 1% excreted unchanged; 60% of metabolites excreted in urine, 23% in feces. **Half-Life:** 12.6 h; terminal half-life is 4–5 d with repeated dosing.

NURSING IMPLICATIONS

Assessment & Drug Effects

- Lab tests: Monitor platelet count and bleeding time periodically.

Monitor CBC with differentials q2wk from second week to end of third month of therapy and thereafter if S&S of infection develop.
- Report promptly laboratory values indicative of neutropenia, thrombocytopenia, or agranulocytosis.
- Monitor for signs of bleeding (e.g., ecchymosis, epistaxis, hematuria, GI bleeding).

Patient & Family Education
- Report promptly to physician any of the following: Nausea, diarrhea, rash, sore throat, or other signs of infection, signs of bleeding, or signs of cholestasis (e.g., yellow skin or sclera, dark urine or clay-colored stools).
- Understand risk of GI bleeding; do not take aspirin along with ticlopidine.
- Do not take antacids within 2 h of ticlopidine.
- Keep appointments for regularly scheduled blood tests.

TILUDRONATE DISODIUM

(til-u′dro-nate)
Skelid
Classification: REGULATOR, BONE METABOLISM (BISPHOSPHONATE)
Prototype: Etidronate disodium
Pregnancy Category: C

AVAILABILITY 240 mg tablets

ACTIONS Mechanism of action of this diphosphate is to inhibit osteoclastic activity, which leads to resorption of the bone matrix.

THERAPEUTIC EFFECTS Acts primarily by inhibiting normal or abnormal bone resorption, thus reducing bone formation. Effectiveness indicated by decreasing levels of alkaline phosphatase.

USE Treatment of Paget's disease.

CONTRAINDICATIONS Hypersensitivity to diphosphonates (e.g., alendronate, etidronate, pamidronate, tiludronate); severe kidney failure (Cl_{cr} <30 mL/min).

CAUTIOUS USE Hypocalcemia, active UGI problems (e.g., gastritis, dysphagia, ulcer, esophageal disease); CHF. Pregnancy (category C), lactation. Safety and efficacy in children are not established.

ROUTE & DOSAGE

Paget's Disease
Adult: **PO** 400 mg/d with 6–8 oz of water times 3 mo

ADMINISTRATION

Oral
- Give with 6–8 oz of plain water 2 h before or after food.
- Do not give within 2 h of drugs containing calcium, aspirin, or indomethacin. Give aluminum- or magnesium-containing antacids no sooner than 2 h after tiludronate.
- Store in manufacturer's packaging at 15°–30° C (59°–86° F).

ADVERSE EFFECTS (≥1%) **Body as a Whole:** *Pain,* flu-like syndrome, edema. **CNS:** Headache, dizziness, paresthesias. **CV:** Chest pain. **GI:** *Nausea, diarrhea,* dyspepsia, vomiting, flatulence. **Special Senses:** Cataract, conjunctivitis, glaucoma. **Respiratory:** Rhinitis, sinusitis, coughing, pharyngitis. **Skin:** Rash. **Metabolic:** Hyperparathyroidism, vitamin D deficiency, **Musculoskeletal:** Arthralgia, arthrosis.

INTERACTIONS Drug: Absorption decreased by CALCIUM, ALUMINUM- or MAGNESIUM-CONTAINING ANTACIDS, **aspirin.** Absorption increased by **indomethacin.**

PHARMACOKINETICS Absorption: Poorly absorbed from GI tract.

T

Steady-State: 30 d. **Metabolism:** Not metabolized. **Elimination:** Primarily excreted in urine. **Half-Life:** 150 h.

NURSING IMPLICATIONS

Assessment & Drug Effects

- Monitor for S&S of upper GI dysfunction or ulceration.
- Lab tests: Periodic serum calcium and serum phosphate.

Patient & Family Education

- Do not remove tablets from foil strips until time to be taken.
- Wait at least 2 h after taking tiludronate to take aluminum- and magnesium-containing antacids.
- Consult physician to determine appropriate daily intake of vitamin D and calcium.
- Do not breast feed while taking this drug without consulting physician.

TIMOLOL MALEATE

(tye'moe-lole)

Betimol, Blocadren, Istalol, Timoptic, Timoptic XE

Classifications: AUTONOMIC NERVOUS SYSTEM AGENT; BETA-ADRENERGIC ANTAGONIST (SYMPATHOLYTIC); EYE PREPARATION; MIOTIC

Prototype: Propranolol

Pregnancy Category: C

AVAILABILITY 5 mg, 10 mg, 20 mg tablets; 0.25%, 0.5% ophthalmic solution or gel

ACTIONS Nonselective beta-adrenergic blocking agent similar to propranolol. Demonstrates antihypertensive, antiarrhythmic, and antianginal properties, and suppresses plasma renin activity. When applied topically, lowers elevated and normal intraocular pressure (IOP) by unknown mechanism but appears to act by reducing formation of aqueous humor and possibly by increasing outflow. In contrast to pilocarpine and other miotics, timolol does not constrict pupil and therefore does not cause night blindness, and it does not affect accommodation or visual acuity.

THERAPEUTIC EFFECTS Topically, lowers elevated and normal intraocular pressure (IOP). Orally, therapeutically useful for mild hypertension and migraine headaches.

USES Topically (ophthalmic solution) to reduce elevated IOP in chronic, open-angle glaucoma, aphakic glaucoma, secondary glaucoma, and ocular hypertension. May be used alone or in conjunction with epinephrine, pilocarpine, or a carbonic anhydrase inhibitor such as acetazolamide. Oral preparation is used as monotherapy or in combination with a thiazide diuretic to prevent reinfarction after MI and to treat mild hypertension.

UNLABELED USES Prophylactic management of stable, uncomplicated angina pectoris and migraine headaches.

CONTRAINDICATIONS Bronchospasm; severe COPD; bronchial asthma; heart failure; pregnancy (category C), lactation, abrupt discontinuation, acute bronchospasm, AV block, bradycardia, cardiogenic shock, acute pulmonary edema, compromised left ventricular dysfunction, Raynaud's disease. Safety in children is not established.

CAUTIOUS USE Bronchitis, patients subject to bronchospasm, asthma; sinus bradycardia, greater than first-degree heart block, heart failure; hepatic disease; vasospastic angina, peripheral vascular disease; pheochromocytoma; thyrotoxicosis, hyperthyroidism; right ventricular failure secondary to pulmonary hypertension, COPD; stroke, cerebrovascular disease; depression; older adults; psoriasis; myasthenia gravis; concomitant use with adrenergic augmenting drugs, e.g., MAO inhibitors.

ROUTE & DOSAGE

Glaucoma
See Appendix A-1.
Hypertension
Adult: **PO** 10 mg b.i.d., may increase to 60 mg/d in 2 divided doses
Angina
Adult: **PO** 15–45 mg in 3 divided doses

ADMINISTRATION

Oral
- Give with fluid of patient's choice; tablet may be crushed.
- Make dosage increases for hypertension at weekly intervals..

ADVERSE EFFECTS (≥1%) **CNS:** Fatigue, lethargy, weakness, somnolence, anxiety, headache, dizziness, confusion, psychic dissociation, depression. **CV:** Palpitation, bradycardia, hypotension, syncope, AV conduction disturbances, CHF, aggravation of peripheral vascular insufficiency. **Special Senses:** *Eye irritation* including conjunctivitis, blepharitis, keratitis, superficial punctate keratopathy. **GI:** Anorexia, dyspepsia, nausea. **Skin:** Rash, urticaria. **Respiratory:** Difficulty in breathing, bronchospasm. **Body as a Whole:** Fever. **Metabolic:** Hypoglycemia, hypokalemia.

INTERACTIONS Drug: ANTIHYPERTENSIVE AGENTS, DIURETICS potentiate hypotensive effects; NSAIDS may antagonize hypotensive effects.

PHARMACOKINETICS Absorption: 90% absorbed from GI tract; 50% reaches systemic circulation; some systemic absorption from topical application. **Peak:** 1–2 h PO; 1–5 h topical. **Distribution:** Distributed into breast milk. **Metabolism:** 80% metabolized in liver to inactive metabolites. **Elimination:** Excreted in urine.

NURSING IMPLICATIONS

Assessment & Drug Effects
- Check pulse before administering timolol, topical or oral. If there are extremes (rate or rhythm), withhold medication and call the physician.
- Assess pulse rate and BP at regular intervals and more aften in patients with severe heart disease.
- Note: Some patients develop tolerance during long-term therapy.

Patient & Family Education
- Be aware that drug may cause slight reduction in resting heart rate. Learn how to assess pulse rate and report significant changes. Consult physician for parameters.
- Do not stop drug abruptly; angina may be exacerbated. Dosage is reduced over a period of 1–2 wk.
- Report difficulty in breathing promptly to physician. Drug withdrawal may be indicated.
- Do not breast feed while taking this drug without consulting physician.

T

TINIDAZOLE
(tin′i-da-zole)
Tindamax
Classifications: ANTIINFECTIVE; AZOLE ANTIBIOTIC; ANTIPROTOZOAL; AMEBICIDE
Prototype: Metronidazole
Pregnancy Category: First trimester D, second and third trimesters C

AVAILABILITY 250 mg, 500 mg tablets

ACTIONS Made from cell extracts of *Trichomonas*. The free radicals generated as a result of this process may be responsible for its antiprotozoal activity; however, the mechanism of action is unknown.

THERAPEUTIC EFFECTS Demonstrates activity against infections caused by the following protozoa: *Trichomonas vaginalis*, *Giardia duodenalis* (also termed *G. lamblia*), and *Entamoeba histolytica*.

USES Treatment of trichomoniasis, giardiasis, amebiasis, and amebic liver abscess.

CONTRAINDICATIONS First trimester of pregnancy (category D), second and third trimesters pregnancy (category C); known hypersensitivity to tinidazole or other azole antibiotics (e.g., metronidazole); lactation within 72 h of tinidazole use; children <3 y.

CAUTIOUS USE CNS diseases, liver dysfunction, alcoholism, ethanol intoxication; hematologic disease; neurologic disease; bone marrow depression; dialysis; candidiasis.

ROUTE & DOSAGE

Giardiasis

Adult: **PO** 2 g as single dose with food
Child: **PO** ≥*3 y* 50 mg/kg (up to 2 g) as single dose with food

Intestinal Amebiasis

Adult: **PO** 2 g once daily for 3 d
Child: **PO** ≥*3 y* 50 mg/kg/d (up to 2 g/d) once daily for 3 d

Amebic Liver Abscess

Adult: **PO** 2 g once daily for 3–5 d
Child: **PO** ≥*3 y* 50 mg/kg/d (up to 2 g/d) once daily for 3–5 d

Trichomoniasis

Adult: **PO** 2 g as single dose

ADMINISTRATION

Oral

- Give with food to minimize GI distress; may be crushed in artificial cherry syrup if tablets cannot be swallowed whole.
- If given on a dialysis day, add a 50% dose of tinidazole at the end of hemodialysis.
- Separate the dosing of cholestyramine and tinidazole by 2–4 h when used concurrently.
- Do not give within 2 wk of the last dose of disulfiram.
- Store at 15°–30° C (59°–86° F). Protect from light.

ADVERSE EFFECTS (≥1%) **Body as a Whole:** Weakness, fatigue, malaise. **CNS:** Dizziness, headache. **GI:** Metallic/bitter taste, nausea, anorexia, dyspepsia, cramps, epigastric discomfort, vomiting, constipation.

INTERACTIONS Drug: May increase INR with **warfarin; alcohol** may cause abdominal cramps, nausea, vomiting, headache, flushing; psychotic reactions with **disulfiram;** may increase the half-life of **fosphenytoin, phenytoin;** may increase levels and toxicity of **lithium, fluorouracil, cyclosporine, tacrolimus; cholestyramine** may decrease absorption of tinidazole.

PHARMACOKINETICS Peak: 2 h. **Distribution:** Crosses blood–brain barrier, placenta and is excreted in breast milk. **Metabolism:** Metabolized in the liver by CYP3A4. **Elimination:** Primarily excreted in urine. **Half-Life:** 12–14 h.

NURSING IMPLICATIONS

Assessment & Drug Effects

- Withhold drug and notify physician for S&S of CNS dysfunction (e.g., seizures, numbness or paresthesia of extremities). Drug should be discontinued if abnormal neurologic signs appear.

- Lab tests: baseline LTFs; CBC with differential, if retreatment is required.
- Monitor INR/PT frequently with concomitant oral anticoagulants. Continue monitoring for at least 8 d after discontinuation of tinidazole.
- Monitor serum lithium levels with concurrent use.
- Monitor for phenytoin toxicity with concurrent IV phenytoin.

Patient & Family Education

- Stop taking the drug and report promptly: convulsions, numbness, tingling, pain, or weakness in the hands or feet; dizziness or unsteadiness; fever.
- Harmless urine discoloration may occur while taking this drug.
- Do not breast feed while taking this drug. Wait at least 3 d after the last dose to resume breast-feeding.

TINZAPARIN SODIUM

(tinz'a-par-in)

Innohep

Classifications: BLOOD FORMERS, COAGULATORS, AND ANTICOAGULANTS; LOW MOLECULAR WEIGHT HEPARIN

Prototype: Enoxaparin

Pregnancy Category: B

AVAILABILITY 40,000 anti-Xa IU/2 mL vials

See Appendix A-2.

TIOCONAZOLE

(ti-o-con'a-zole)

Vagistat-1

Classifications: ANTIINFECTIVE; ANTIFUNGAL

Prototype: Fluconazole

Pregnancy Category: C

AVAILABILITY 6.5% vaginal ointment

ACTIONS Broad-spectrum antifungal agent that inhibits growth of human pathogenic yeasts.

THERAPEUTIC EFFECTS Effective against *Candida albicans,* other species of *Candida,* and *Torulopsis glabrata.*

USES Local treatment of vulvovaginal candidiasis.

CONTRAINDICATIONS Hypersensitivity to tioconazole or other imidazole antifungal agents; lactation.

CAUTIOUS USE Pregnancy (category C), diabetes mellitus. Safety and efficacy in children are not established.

ROUTE & DOSAGE

Candidiasis

Adult: **Intravaginal** One applicator full h.s. times 1 d

ADMINISTRATION

Instillation

- Insert applicator high into the vagina (except during pregnancy).
- Wash applicator before and after each use.
- Store away from direct heat and light.

ADVERSE EFFECTS (≥1%) **Urogenital:** Mild erythema, burning, discomfort, rash, itching.

INTERACTIONS Drug: May inactivate spermicidal effects of **nonoxynol-9.**

PHARMACOKINETICS Absorption: Minimal absorption from vagina.

NURSING IMPLICATIONS

Assessment & Drug Effects

- Do not use for patient with a history of allergic reaction to other

T

antifungal agents, such as miconazole.
- Monitor for sensitization and irritation; these may be an indication to discontinue drug.

Patient & Family Education
- Learn correct application technique.
- Understand potential adverse reactions, including sensitization and allergic response.
- Tioconazole may interact with diaphragms and latex condoms; avoid concurrent use within 72 h.
- Refrain from sexual intercourse while using tioconazole.
- Wear only cotton underwear; change daily.
- Do not breast feed while using this drug.

TIOTROPIUM BROMIDE

(ti-o-tro′pi-um)
Spiriva
Classifications: AUTONOMIC NERVOUS SYSTEM AGENT; ANTICHOLINERGIC; PARASYMPATHOLYTIC; ANTIMUSCARINIC; ANTISPASMODIC
Prototype: Atropine
Pregnancy Category: C

AVAILABILITY 18 mcg capsules with powder for inhalation

ACTIONS A long-acting, antispasmodic agent. In the bronchial airways, it exhibits inhibition of muscarinic receptors of the smooth muscle resulting in bronchodilation. The drug effect can last up to 24 h.
THERAPEUTIC EFFECTS Bronchodilation after inhalation of tiotropium is predominantly a site-specific effect.

USES Maintenance treatment of bronchospasm associated with chronic obstructive pulmonary disease (COPD).

CONTRAINDICATIONS Hypersensitivity to tiotropium, atropine, or ipratropium; pregnancy (category C); children <18 y.
CAUTIOUS USE Decreased renal function; BPH, urinary bladder neck obstruction; narrow-angle glaucoma; older adults; lactation.

ROUTE & DOSAGE

COPD
Adult: **Inhaled** Inhale the contents of one capsule once daily using hand inhaler device provided.

ADMINISTRATION

Inhalation
- Place capsule in HandiHaler® and press button to puncture. Instruct patient to exhale deeply then put the mouthpiece to the lips and breathe in the dose deeply and slowly; remove HandiHaler® and hold breath for at least 10 sec, and then exhale slowly; rinse mouth with water to minimize dry mouth.
- Ensure that drug does not contact the eyes.
- Store at 15°–30° C (59°–86° F).

ADVERSE EFFECTS (≥1%) **Body as a Whole:** Nonspecific chest pain, dependent edema, infection, moniliasis, flu-like syndrome, cough, allergic reactions. **CNS:** Dysphonia, paresthesia, depression. **GI:** Abdominal pain, constipation, *dry mouth,* dyspepsia, vomiting, reflux, stomatitis. **Metabolic:** Hypercholesterolemia, hyperglycemia. **Musculoskeletal:** Myalgia, skeletal pain. **Respiratory:** Epistaxis, pharyngitis, rhinitis, laryngitis, *sinusitis, upper respiratory tract infection.* **Skin:** Rash. **Special Senses:** Cataract. **Urogenital:** Urinary tract infection.

INTERACTIONS Drug: May cause additive anticholinergic effects

Common adverse effects in *italic*, life-threatening effects underlined: generic names in **bold**; classifications in SMALL CAPS; ♣ Canadian drug name; ⓟ Prototype drug

with other ANTICHOLINERGIC AGENTS.

PHARMACOKINETICS Absorption: 19.5% absorbed from the lungs. **Peak:** 5 min. **Metabolism:** <25% of dose is metabolized in liver by CYP2D6 and 3A4. **Elimination:** 14% of dose excreted in urine; remaining is excreted in feces as nonabsorbed drug. **Half-Life:** 5–6 d.

NURSING IMPLICATIONS

Assessment & Drug Effects

- Withhold drug and notify physician if S&S of angioedema occurs.
- Monitor for anticholinergic effects (e.g., tachycardia, urinary retention).

Patient & Family Education

- Do not allow powdered medication to contact the eyes, as this may cause blurring of vision and pupil dilation.
- Tiotropium bromide is intended as a once-daily maintenance treatment. It is not useful for treatment of acute episodes of bronchospasm (i.e., rescue therapy).
- Withhold drug and notify physician if swelling around the face, mouth, or neck occurs.
- Report any of the following: constipation, increased heart rate, blurred vision, urinary difficulty.
- Do not breast feed while taking this drug without consulting physician.

TIROFIBAN HYDROCHLORIDE

(tir-o-fi'ban)

Aggrastat

Classifications: BLOOD FORMERS, COAGULATORS, AND ANTICOAGULANTS; ANTIPLATELET AGENT; GLYCOPROTEIN IIB/IIIA RECEPTOR INHIBITOR

Prototype: Abciximab

Pregnancy Category: B

AVAILABILITY 250 mcg/mL, 50 mcg/mL injection

ACTIONS Antiplatelet agent that binds to the glycoprotein IIb/IIIa receptor of platelets.

THERAPEUTIC EFFECTS Inhibits platelet aggregation. Effectiveness indicated by minimizing thrombotic events during treatment of acute coronary syndrome.

USES Acute coronary syndromes (unstable angina, MI).

CONTRAINDICATIONS Active internal bleeding within 30 d; acute pericarditis; aortic dissection; concurrent use with another glycoprotein IIb/IIIa receptor inhibitor (e.g., eptifibatide, abciximab); history of aneurysm or AV malformation; history of intracranial hemorrhage or neoplasm; hypersensitivity to tirofiban; major surgery or trauma within 3 d; stroke within 30 d; history of hemorrhagic stroke; thrombocytopenia following administration of tirofiban; pregnancy (category B); lactation.

CAUTIOUS USE Concomitant use with thrombolytic agents or drugs that cause hemolysis; hemorrhagic retinopathy; platelet count <150,000 mm^3; severe renal insufficiency. Safety and efficacy in children <18 y are unknown.

ROUTE & DOSAGE

Acute Coronary Syndromes

Adult: **IV Loading Dose** 0.4 mcg/kg/min times 30 min **IV Maintenance Dose** 0.1 mcg/kg/min for 12–24 h after angioplasty or arteriectomy

Renal Impairment

Cl_{cr} <30 mL/min: Reduce rate of infusion 50%

ADMINISTRATION

Intravenous

PREPARE: **IV Infusion:** Withdraw 100 mL from a 500-mL bag of NS or D5W and replace with 100 mL of tirofiban HCl injection. If a 250-mL IV bag is used, withdraw 50 mL of IV solution and replace with 50 mL of tirofiban injection. Either preparation yields 50 mcg/mL. Mix well before infusing. Note: Commercially premixed IV tirofiban solutions are available.
ADMINISTER: **IV Infusion:** An initial loading dose of 0.4 mcg/kg/min for 30 min is usually followed by a maintenance infusion of 0.1 mcg/kg/min.

■ Discard unused IV solution 24 h following start of infusion. ■ Store unopened containers at 15°–30° C (59°–86° F). Do not freeze and protect from light.

ADVERSE EFFECTS (≥1%) **Body as a Whole:** Edema, swelling, pelvic pain, vasovagal reaction, leg pain. **CNS:** Dizziness. **CV:** Bradycardia, <u>coronary artery dissection</u>. **GI:** GI bleeding. **Hematologic:** *Bleeding* (<u>major bleeding</u>), anemia, thrombocytopenia. **Skin:** Sweating.

INTERACTIONS Drug: Increased risk of bleeding with ANTICOAGULANTS, NSAIDS, SALICYLATES, ANTIPLATELET AGENTS. **Herbal: Feverfew, garlic, ginger, ginkgo, horse chestnut** may increase risk of bleeding.

PHARMACOKINETICS Duration: 4–8 h after stopping infusion. **Distribution:** 65% protein bound. **Metabolism:** Minimally metabolized. **Elimination:** 65% excreted in urine, 25% in feces. **Half-Life:** 2 h.

NURSING IMPLICATIONS

Assessment & Drug Effects

- Lab tests: Monitor platelet count, Hgb and Hct before treatment, (within 6 h of infusing loading dose), and frequently throughout treatment; monitor aPTT, INR, and ACT.
- Withhold drug and notify physician if thrombocytopenia (platelets <100,000) is confirmed.
- Monitor carefully for and immediately report S&S of internal or external bleeding.
- Wait at least 3–4 h after heparin is stopped and until ACT <180 s and aPPT <45 s before removing the femoral catheter sheath.
- Minimize unnecessary invasive procedures and devices to reduce the risk of bleeding.

Patient & Family Education

- Report unexplained pelvic or abdominal pain.

TIZANIDINE HYDROCHLORIDE

(ti-zan′i-deen)
Zanaflex
Classifications: AUTONOMIC NERVOUS SYSTEM AGENT; SKELETAL MUSCLE RELAXANT, CENTRAL-ACTING
Prototype: Cyclobenzaprine
Pregnancy Category: C

AVAILABILITY 4 mg tablets; 2 mg, 4 mg, 6 mg capsules

ACTIONS Centrally-acting alpha-adrenergic agonist that reduces spasticity by increasing presynaptic inhibition of motor neurons. No effect on skeletal muscle fibers, the neuromuscular junction, or monosynaptic spinal reflexes. Greatest effect on polysynaptic afferent reflex activity at the spinal cord level.

THERAPEUTIC EFFECTS Site of action is the spinal cord; reduces skeletal muscle spasm. Effectiveness indicated by decreased muscle tone.

USES Acute and intermittent management of increased muscle tone associated with spasticity.

CONTRAINDICATIONS Hypersensitivity to tizanidine; lactation. Safety in labor and delivery is unknown.
CAUTIOUS USE Patients with hepatic impairment, renal insufficiency (Cl_{cr} <25 mL/min); concurrent use of antihypertensive therapy; women taking oral contraceptives; pregnancy (category C); older adults because of renal impairment. Safety and efficacy in children are not established.

ROUTE & DOSAGE

Spasticity
Adult: **PO** Start with 4 mg and gradually increase to 8 mg q6–8h prn (max: 3 doses or 36 mg/24 h)

Renal Impairment
Cl_{cr} <25 mL/min: Use lower dose

ADMINISTRATION

Oral

- Make dose increments gradually in 2- to 4-mg steps.
- Store at 15°–30° C (59°–86° F).

ADVERSE EFFECTS (≥1%) **Body as a Whole:** *Asthenia (tiredness),* flu-like syndrome, fever, myasthenia, back pain, infection. **CNS:** *Somnolence, dizziness,* dyskinesia, nervousness, depression, anxiety, paresthesia. **CV:** *Hypotension, bradycardia.* **GI:** *Dry mouth,* constipation, abnormal liver function tests, vomiting, abdominal pain, diarrhea, dyspepsia. **Respiratory:** Pharyngitis, rhinitis. **Skin:** Rash, sweating, skin ulcer. **Urogenital:** *UTI,* urinary frequency. **Special Senses:** Speech disorder, blurred vision.

INTERACTIONS Drug: ORAL CONTRACEPTIVES decrease clearance of **tizanidine. Alcohol** will increase peak levels and decrease clearance of tizanidine. **Herbal: Kava-kava, valerian** may potentiate sedation.

PHARMACOKINETICS Absorption: Rapidly absorbed from GI tract; 40% bioavailability. **Peak:** 1–2 h. **Duration:** 3–6 h. **Distribution:** Crosses placenta, distributed into breast milk. **Metabolism:** Metabolized in the liver. **Elimination:** 60% excreted in urine, 20% in feces. **Half-Life:** 2.5 h.

NURSING IMPLICATIONS

Assessment & Drug Effects

- Lab tests: Monitor liver function tests (AST, ALT) during the first 6 mo of treatment (baseline, 1, 3, and 6 mo) and periodically thereafter.
- Monitor cardiovascular status and report orthostatic hypotension or bradycardia.
- Monitor closely older adults, those with renal impairment, and women taking oral contraceptives for adverse effects because drug clearance is reduced.

Patient & Family Education

- Exercise caution with potentially hazardous activities requiring alertness since sedation is a common adverse effect. Effects are additive with alcohol or other CNS depressants.
- Make position changes slowly because of the risk of orthostatic hypotension.
- Report unusual sensory experiences; hallucinations and delusions have occurred with tizanidine use.
- Do not breast feed while taking this drug.

T

TOBRAMYCIN SULFATE

(toe-bra-mye'sin)

Nebcin, Tobrex, TOBI, Tomycine

Classifications: ANTIINFECTIVE; AMINOGLYCOSIDE ANTIBIOTIC

Prototype: Gentamicin sulfate

Pregnancy Category: D

AVAILABILITY 10 mg/mL, 40 mg/mL injection; 300 mg/5 mL inhalation solution; 0.3% ophthalmic solution; 3 mg/g ophthalmic ointment

ACTIONS Broad-spectrum, aminoglycoside antibiotic derived from *Streptomyces tenebrarius*. Closely related to gentamicin in spectrum of antibacterial activity and pharmacologic properties. Reportedly causes less nephrotoxicity than gentamicin, but incidence of ototoxicity is similar. Cross-allergenicity and some cross-resistance among aminoglycosides have been demonstrated.

THERAPEUTIC EFFECTS Exhibits greater antibiotic activity against *Pseudomonas aeruginosa* than other aminoglycosides.

USES Treatment of severe infections caused by susceptible organisms.

CONTRAINDICATIONS History of hypersensitivity to tobramycin and other aminoglycoside antibiotics. Safety during pregnancy (category D) or lactation is not established.

CAUTIOUS USE Impaired kidney function; premature and neonatal infants; concurrent use with other neurotoxic or nephrotoxic agents or potent diuretics

ROUTE & DOSAGE

Moderate to Severe Infections

Adult: **IV** 3 mg/kg/d divided q8h up to 5 mg/kg/d infused over 20–60 min **IM** 3 mg/kg/d divided q8h up to 5 mg/kg/d **Topical** 1–2 drops in affected eye q1–4h
Child: **IM/IV** <5 *y*, 2.5 mg/kg q8h **IV** ≥5 *y*, 3 mg/kg/d divided q8h up to 5 mg/kg/d infused over 20–60 min **IM** ≥5 *y*, 3 mg/kg/d divided q8h up to 5 mg/kg/d
Neonate: **IM/IV** 2.5 mg/kg q12–24h

Cystic Fibrosis

Adult/Child: **IM/IV** 2.5–3.5 mg/kg q6–8h **Nebulized** 300 mg inhaled b.i.d. times 28 d, may repeat after 28 d drug-free period

ADMINISTRATION

Note: All doses based on ideal body weight.

Instillation

- Wash hands before and after instillation of eye medication. Apply gentle finger pressure to lacrimal sac (under inside of eyelid) for 1 min after drug has been instilled in eye.

Intramuscular

- Give deep IM into a large muscle. Rotate injection sites.

Intravenous

Note: Verify correct IV concentration and rate of infusion to neonates, infants, or children with physician.

PREPARE: **Intermittent:** Dilute each dose in 50–100 mL or more of D5W, NS or D5/NS. Final concentration should not exceed 1 mg/mL.

ADMINISTER: **Intermittent:** Infuse diluted solution over 20–60 min. *INCOMPATIBILITIES* **Solution/additive: Alcohol 5% in dextrose,** CEPHALOSPORINS, PENICILLINS, **clindamycin, heparin. Y-site: Allopurinol, amphotericin B cholesteryl complex,** CEPHALOSPORINS, **clindamycin, penicillins, heparin hetastarch, indomethacin, propofol, sargramostim.**

- Store at 15°–30° C (59°–86° F) prior to reconstitution. After reconstitution, solution may be refrigerated and used within 96 h. If kept at room temperature, use within 24 h.

ADVERSE EFFECTS (≥1%) **CNS:** Neurotoxicity (including ototoxicity), *nephrotoxicity,* increased AST, ALT, LDH, serum bilirubin; anemia, fever, rash, pruritus, urticaria, nausea, vomiting, headache, lethargy, superinfections; hypersensitivity. **Special Senses:** *Burning, stinging of eye after drug instillation;* lid itching and edema.

INTERACTIONS Drug: ANESTHETICS, SKELETAL MUSCLE RELAXANTS add to neuromuscular blocking effects; **acyclovir, amphotericin B, bacitracin, capreomycin,** CEPHALOSPORINS, **colistin, cisplatin, carboplatin, methoxyflurane, polymyxin B, vancomycin, furosemide, ethacrynic acid** increased risk of ototoxicity, nephrotoxicity.

PHARMACOKINETICS Peak: 30–90 min IM. **Duration:** Up to 8 h. **Distribution:** Crosses placenta; accumulates in renal cortex. **Elimination:** Excreted in urine. **Half-Life:** 2–3 h in adults.

NURSING IMPLICATIONS

Assessment & Drug Effects

- Weigh patient before treatment for calculation of dosage.
- Obtain bacterial C&S tests prior to and during therapy.
- Observe patient receiving tobramycin closely because of the high potential for toxicity, even in conventional doses.
- Lab tests: Baseline and periodic kidney function; monitor serum drug concentrations to minimize rise of toxicity. Prolonged peak serum concentrations >10 mcg/mL or trough concentrations >2 mcg/mL are not recommended.
- Monitor auditory, and vestibular functions closely, particularly in patients with known or suspected renal impairment and patients receiving high doses.
- Be aware that drug-induced auditory changes are irreversible (partial or total); usually bilateral. In cochlear damage, patient may be asymptomatic, and partial or bilateral deafness may continue to develop even after therapy discontinued.
- Evidence of renal insufficiency, ototoxicity (see Appendix F), or vestibular damage indicates need for dosage adjustment or withdrawal of drug.
- Monitor I&O. Report oliguria, changes in I&O ratio, and cloudy or frothy urine (may indicate proteinuria). Keep patient well hydrated to prevent chemical irritation in renal tubules; older adults are especially susceptible to renal toxicity.
- Monitor patient with neuromuscular disorder (e.g., myasthenia gravis) for muscular weakness. Observe ambulation and assist if necessary.
- Be aware that prolonged use of ophthalmic solution may encourage superinfection with nonsusceptible organisms including fungi.
- Report overdose symptoms for eye medication: Increased lacri-

T

mation, keratitis, edema and itching of eyelids.

Patient & Family Education

- Report symptoms of superinfections (see Appendix F) to physician. Prompt treatment with an antibiotic or antifungal medication may be necessary.
- Report S&S of hearing loss, tinnitus, or vertigo to physician.
- Do not breast feed while taking this drug without consulting physician.

TOCAINIDE HYDROCHLORIDE

(toe-kay'nide)
Tonocard
Classifications: CARDIOVASCULAR AGENT; ANTIARRHYTHMIC (CLASS IB)
Prototype: Lidocaine
Pregnancy Category: C

AVAILABILITY 400 mg, 600 mg tablets

ACTIONS Antiarrhythmic agent (class IB) and analog of lidocaine, with similar electrophysiologic characteristics and hemodynamic properties. Effective orally. Suppresses PVCs and may have particular use in arrhythmias associated with a prolonged QT interval that do not respond to quinidine-like antiarrhythmics (Class IA). Decreases action potential duration in Purkinje fibers and slightly decreases resting membrane potential. QRS and QT intervals do not change.

THERAPEUTIC EFFECTS Antiarrhythmic action results from shortening the effective refractory periods of atria, AV node, and ventricles without affecting AV conduction.

USES Refractory ventricular arrhythmia. To increase effectiveness, it may be combined with a class IA antiarrhythmic (e.g., quinidine, disopyramide) or with propranolol. Also used to prevent ventricular tachyarrhythmia after acute MI.

CONTRAINDICATIONS Hypersensitivity to tocainide and to local anesthetics of the amide type; second- or third-degree AV block (in absence of artificial ventricular pacemaker); hypokalemia; myasthenia gravis; pregnancy (category C), lactation. Safety in children is not established.

CAUTIOUS USE Multiple drug therapy; known heart failure patient with minimum cardiac reserve; kidney or liver disease.

ROUTE & DOSAGE

Ventricular Arrhythmias
Adult: **PO** 1.2–1.8 g/d in 3 divided doses, may increase up to 2.4 g/d

ADMINISTRATION

Oral

- Give with food to decrease GI distress. This also protects against high peak concentration and toxicity because absorption rate is slowed.

ADVERSE EFFECTS (≥1%) **CNS:** *Tremors, dizziness, light-headedness, visual disturbances, vertigo, tinnitus,* hearing loss, ataxia, paresthesia, confusion. **CV:** Exacerbation of arrhythmias, complete heart block, sinus node slowing (in patient with preexisting conduction system disease); hypotension, palpitations, bradycardia, chest pain, left ventricular failure, PVCs, hot flashes. **GI:** Nausea, vomiting, anorexia, abdominal pain, diarrhea, hepatitis (rare), metallic or menthol taste. **Respiratory:** Pulmonary fibrosis, edema, embolism and alveolitis; pneumonia, dyspnea, hiccups. **Body as a Whole:** Alopecia, sweating, night sweats, tiredness/drowsiness, sleepiness, hot/cold feelings, claudication, cold extremities, leg cramps. **Hematologic:** Leukopenia, agranulocytosis, thrombocytopenia, hypoplastic anemia. **Urogenital:** Urinary retention, polyuria.

INTERACTIONS Drug: Lidocaine may increase risk of CNS toxicity, including seizures. BETA BLOCKERS may lead to paranoia and additive cardiac depressant effects; **cimetidine** decreases **tocainide** bioavailability; **rifampin** decreases **tocainide** levels.

PHARMACOKINETICS Absorption: Rapidly and completely absorbed from GI tract. **Peak:** 0.5–2 h. **Distribution:** Not fully known; does distribute into CNS. **Metabolism:** Metabolized in liver. **Steady-State:** 70 h. **Elimination:** 70%–80% excreted in urine within 72 h. **Half-Life:** 10–17 h.

NURSING IMPLICATIONS

Assessment & Drug Effects

- Effective serum concentration is 3.5–10 mcg/mL.
- Monitor plasma level when steady-state drug level is attained, especially if patient has kidney or liver dysfunction.
- Lab tests: Baseline serum potassium, liver and kidney functions. Monitor blood counts during first 6 mo of treatment; abnormal counts usually stabilize within 1 mo after withdrawal of treatment.
- Correct preexisting hypokalemia prior to initiating drug therapy.
- Be aware that onset of tremors is good clinical indicator that maximum dose is being approached.
- Monitor I&O ratio and pattern. Report symptoms of kidney dysfunction. Drug elimination is significantly decreased in patient with kidney or liver dysfunction.
- Anticipate and report evidence of blood dyscrasia (see Appendix F).

Patient & Family Education

- Understand significance of irregular pulse and when and how to check it.
- Do not drive or engage in potentially hazardous activities until response to drug is known.
- Report symptomatic bradycardia to physician. Dose adjustment or withdrawal will follow.
- Report chest pain, exertional dyspnea, wheezing, and cough even if no fever is present promptly to physician. Pulmonary fibrosis is a serious adverse effect and should be ruled out. Drug is discontinued if pulmonary symptoms persist or if pulmonary disorder is diagnosed.
- Do not breast feed while taking this drug.

TOLAZAMIDE

(tole-az′a-mide)

Tolinase

Classifications: HORMONE AND SYNTHETIC SUBSTITUTE; SULFONYLUREA ANTIDIABETIC

Prototype: Glyburide

Pregnancy Category: C

AVAILABILITY 100 mg, 250 mg, 500 mg tablets

ACTIONS Orally effective sulfonylurea hypoglycemic structurally and pharmacologically related to tolbutamide but about 5 times more potent. Lowers blood glucose primarily by stimulating pancreatic beta cells to secrete insulin.

THERAPEUTIC EFFECTS Antidiabetic action is a result of stimulation of the pancreas to secrete more insulin in the presence of blood sugar. As with other sulfonyl-

T

ureas, ineffective in the absence of functioning beta cells.

USES Mild to moderately severe type 2 diabetes mellitus that cannot be controlled by diet and weight reduction and that is uncomplicated by acidosis, ketosis, coma. Effective in primary or secondary failures to other sulfonylurea

CONTRAINDICATIONS Known sensitivity to sulfonylureas and to sulfonamides; type 1 diabetes complicated by ketoacidosis; infection; trauma; pregnancy (category C). Safety in lactation or children is not established.

ROUTE & DOSAGE

Type 2 Diabetes Mellitus
Adult: **PO** 100 mg–1 g q.d. to b.i.d. a.c., may adjust dose by 100–250 mg/d at weekly intervals (max: 1 g/d)

ADMINISTRATION

Oral
- Give in the morning with or before meals.
- Divide dose of more than 500 mg and give b.i.d.
- Crush tablet if patient is unable to swallow it whole. Be sure to give with an allowable fluid, not dry.
- Store at 15°–30° C (59°–86° F) in a tightly closed container unless otherwise directed. Keep drug out of the reach of children.

ADVERSE EFFECTS (≥1%) **GI:** Nausea, vomiting, cholestatic jaundice. **Metabolic:** Hypoglycemia. **CNS:** Vertigo. **Skin:** Photosensitivity. **Hematologic:** Agranulocytosis.

INTERACTIONS Drug: Alcohol elicits disulfiram-type reaction in some patients; ORAL ANTICOAGULANTS, **chloramphenicol, clofibrate, phenylbutazone,** MAO INHIBITORS, SALICYLATES, **probenecid,** SULFONAMIDES may potentiate hypoglycemic actions; THIAZIDES may antagonize hypoglycemic effects; **cimetidine** may increase tolazamide levels, causing hypoglycemia. **Herbal: Garlic, ginseng** may potentiate hypoglycemic effects.

PHARMACOKINETICS Absorption: Slowly absorbed from GI tract. **Onset:** 60 min. **Peak:** 4–6 h. **Duration:** 10–15 h (up to 20 h in some patients). **Distribution:** Distributed in highest concentrations in liver, kidneys, and intestines; crosses placenta; distributed into breast milk. **Metabolism:** Metabolized extensively in liver. **Elimination:** 85% excreted in urine, 15% in feces. **Half-Life:** 7 h.

NURSING IMPLICATIONS

Assessment & Drug Effects
- Be aware that reduction of dose frequently alleviates most mild to moderately severe hypoglycemic symptoms.
- Observe patients with a history of ketoacidosis or coma closely, especially during the early adjustment period.

Patient & Family Education
- Check blood glucose and urine daily for sugar and acetone. Important to continue close medical supervision for first 6 wk of treatment.
- Be aware that doses >1000 mg/d rarely provide improvement in diabetic control.
- Do not take OTC preparations unless approved or prescribed by physician.
- Understand that alcohol can precipitate a disulfiram-type reaction.
- Do not breast feed while taking this drug without consulting physician.

TOLBUTAMIDE

(tole-byoo'ta-mide)

Mobenol ♣, Novobutamide ♣, Orinase

TOLBUTAMIDE SODIUM

Orinase Diagnostic

Classifications: HORMONES AND SYNTHETIC SUBSTITUTES; SULFONYLUREA ANTIDIABETIC

Prototype: Glyburide

Pregnancy Category: C

AVAILABILITY 500 mg tablets; 1 g vial

ACTIONS Short-acting sulfonylurea compound chemically related to sulfonamides, but without antiinfective activity. Lowers blood glucose concentration by stimulating pancreatic beta cells to synthesize and release insulin. No action demonstrated if functional beta cells are absent. Responsiveness to blood glucose–lowering effects with long-term therapy may decline in some patients. Alternatively, patient who has become poorly responsive to other sulfonylureas may be responsive to tolbutamide.

THERAPEUTIC EFFECTS Lowers blood glucose concentration by stimulating pancreatic beta cells to synthesize and release insulin.

USES Management of mild to moderately severe, stable type 2 diabetes that is not controlled by diet and weight reduction alone. Also used in treatment of patients who are unresponsive to other sulfonylureas and adjunctively with insulin to stabilize certain cases of labile diabetes. Used as diagnostic agent to rule out pancreatic islet cell adenoma or diabetes.

CONTRAINDICATIONS Hypersensitivity to sulfonylureas or to sulfonamides; history of repeated episodes of diabetic ketoacidosis (with or without coma); type 1 diabetes as sole therapy; diabetic coma; severe stress, infection, trauma, or major surgery; severe renal insufficiency, liver or endocrine disease. Safety during pregnancy (category C) or use in children is not established.

CAUTIOUS USE Cardiac, thyroid, pituitary, or adrenal dysfunction; lactation; history of peptic ulcer; alcoholism; older adults, debilitated, malnourished, or uncooperative patient.

ROUTE & DOSAGE

Type 2 Diabetes

Adult: **PO** 250 mg to 3 g/d in 1–2 divided doses

Diagnosis of Functioning Insulinoma

Adult: **IV** 1 g over 2–3 min

ADMINISTRATION

Oral

- Give total dose before breakfast but preferably in divided doses after meals.
- Crush tablet and give with full glass of water if patient desires.
- Do not give at bedtime because of danger of nocturnal hypoglycemia, unless specifically prescribed.
- Discontinue at least 2 wk before the expected delivery date to prevent prolonged severe hypoglycemia (4–10 d) in the neonate if used during pregnancy.
- Store below 40° C (104° F), preferably between 15°–30° C (59°–86° F) in well-closed container. Avoid freezing.

ADVERSE EFFECTS (≥1%) **GI:** Nausea, epigastric fullness, heartburn, anorexia, constipation, diarrhea,

T

cholestatic jaundice (rare). **Hematologic:** Agranulocytosis, thrombocytopenia, leukopenia, hemolytic anemia, aplastic anemia, pancytopenia. **Metabolic:** Hepatic porphyria, disulfiram-like reactions, SIADH, hypoglycemia without loss of consciousness or neurologic symptoms (unusual fatigue, tremulousness, hunger, drowsiness, GI distress, sweating, anxiety, headache) severe hypoglycemia (visual disturbances, ataxia, paresthesias, confusion, tachycardia, seizures, coma). **Skin:** Allergic skin reactions: pruritus, erythema, urticaria, morbilliform or maculopapular eruptions; porphyria cutanea tarda, photosensitivity. **Special Senses:** Taste alterations. **CNS:** Headache.

DIAGNOSTIC TEST INTERFERENCE The SULFONYLUREAS may produce abnormal ***thyroid function test*** results and reduced ***RAI uptake*** (after long-term administration). A tolbutamide metabolite may cause false-positive ***urinary protein*** values when turbidity procedures are used (such as heat and ***acetic acid*** or ***sulfosalicylic acid***); ***Ames reagent*** strips reportedly not affected.

INTERACTIONS Drug: Phenylbutazone increases hypoglycemic effects; THIAZIDE DIURETICS may attenuate hypoglycemic effects; **alcohol** may produce disulfiram reaction; BETA BLOCKERS may mask symptoms of a hypoglycemic reaction. **Herbal: Garlic, ginseng** may potentiate hypoglycemic effects.

PHARMACOKINETICS Absorption: Readily absorbed from GI tract. **Peak:** 3–5 h. **Distribution:** Distributed into extracellular fluids. **Metabolism:** Principally metabolized in liver. **Elimination:** 75%–85% excreted in urine; some elimination in feces. **Half-Life:** 7 h.

NURSING IMPLICATIONS

Assessment & Drug Effects

- Supervise closely during initial period of therapy until dosage is established. One or 2 wk of therapy may be required before full therapeutic effect is achieved.
- Give low initial dose before breakfast to older adults, who may be hyperresponsive to oral antidiabetic therapy. If blood and urine glucose tests are negative during first 24 h of therapy, initial dose may be continued on a daily basis.
- Monitor closely during adjustment period, watching for S&S of impending hypoglycemia (see Appendix F). Detection of a hypoglycemic reaction in a diabetic patient also receiving a beta blocker, especially older adults, is difficult.
- Evaluate nondefinitive vague complaints; hypoglycemic symptoms may be especially vague in older adults. Observe patient carefully, especially 2–3 h after eating, check urine for sugar and ketone bodies and capillary blood glucose.
- Lab tests: Baseline liver and kidney function tests; periodic HbA_{1C}, serum electrolytes, CBC with differential, and platelet counts.
- Report repetitive complaints of headache and weakness a few hours after eating; may signal incipient hypoglycemia.
- Be aware that pruritus and rash, frequently reported adverse effects, may clear spontaneously; if these persist, drug will be discontinued.

Patient & Family Education

- Understand need to inform physician promptly of symptoms of hyperglycemia and ketoacidosis: Flushed, dry skin, weight loss, fatigue, Kussmaul respiration, double or blurred vision, soft eyeballs, irritability, fruity-smelling breath, abdominal cramps, nausea, vomiting, diarrhea, dyspnea, polydipsia, polyphagia, polyuria, headache, hypotension, weak and rapid pulse, positive ketonuria and glycosuria.

- Hypoglycemia is frequently caused by overdosage of hypoglycemic drug, inadequate or irregular food intake, nausea, vomiting, diarrhea, and added exercise without caloric supplement or dose adjustment. Its occurrence indicates need for immediate reevaluation of patient's diet, medication regimen, and compliance. It is most likely to appear in patients >50 y of age.
- Report any illness promptly. Physician may want to evaluate need for insulin.
- Do not self-medicate with OTC drugs unless approved or prescribed by physician.
- Be aware that alcohol, even in moderate amounts, can precipitate a disulfiram-type reaction (see Appendix F). A hypoglycemic response after ingesting alcohol requires emergency treatment.
- Protect exposed skin areas from the sun with a sunscreen lotion (SPF 12–15) because of potential photosensitivity (especially in the alcoholic).
- Weigh at least weekly and report a progressive gain, especially if edema is present. These signs indicate the necessity to discontinue tolbutamide.
- Be alert to added danger of loss of control (hyperglycemia) when a drug that affects the hypoglycemic action of sulfonylureas (see DRUG INTERACTIONS) is withdrawn or added to the tolbutamide regimen. Monitor blood glucose carefully.
- Use or add barrier contraceptive if using hormonal contraceptives.
- Carry medical identification at all times. It needs to indicate medical diagnosis, medication(s) and doses, patient and physician's names, addresses, and telephone numbers.
- Do not breast feed while taking this drug without consulting physician.
- Potential for hypoglycemia in breast fed infants presents the necessity to decide whether to discontinue breast feeding or temporarily transfer to insulin (if diet alone is inadequate for blood sugar control).

TOLCAPONE (Pr)

(tol′ca-pone)

Tasmar

Classifications: AUTONOMIC NERVOUS SYSTEM AGENT; ANTICHOLINERGIC (PARASYMPATHOLYTIC); CATECHOLAMINE-O-METHYLTRANSFERASE (COMT) INHIBITOR

Pregnancy Category: C

AVAILABILITY 100 mg, 200 mg tablets

ACTIONS Selective inhibitor of catecholamine-O-methyltransferase (COMT). COMT is the enzyme responsible for metabolizing levodopa.

THERAPEUTIC EFFECTS Concurrent administration of tolcapone and levodopa increases the amount of levodopa available to control Parkinson's disease by increasing dopaminergic brain stimulation.

USES Idiopathic Parkinson's disease as adjunct to levodopa/carbidopa.

CONTRAINDICATIONS Hypersensitivity to tolcapone; liver disease; pregnancy (category C).

CAUTIOUS USE History of hypersensitivity to other COMT inhibitors (e.g., entacapone, nitecapone); lactation.

ROUTE & DOSAGE

Parkinson's Disease

Adult: **PO** 100 mg t.i.d. (max: 200 mg t.i.d.)

ADMINISTRATION

Oral

- Give with food if GI upset occurs.
- Give only in conjunction with levodopa/carbidopa therapy.
- Note: Doses >100 mg t.i.d. are not recommended with moderate to severe liver impairment.
- Store at 20°–25° C (68°–77° F) in a tightly closed container.

ADVERSE EFFECTS (≥1%) **Body as a Whole:** Muscle cramps, orthostatic complaints, fatigue, falling, balance difficulties, hyperkinesia, stiffness, arthritis, hypokinesia. **CNS:** *Dyskinesia, sleep disorder, dystonia, excessive dreaming,* somnolence, confusion, dizziness, headache, hallucination, syncope, paresthesias. **CV:** Chest pain, hypotension. **GI:** *Nausea,* anorexia, diarrhea, vomiting, constipation, <u>fulminant liver failure, severe hepatocellular injury</u>, dry mouth, abdominal pain, dyspepsia, flatulence. **Respiratory:** URI, dyspnea, sinus congestion. **Skin:** Sweating. **Urogenital:** UTI, urine discoloration, micturition disorder.

T

INTERACTIONS Drug: Will increase **levodopa** levels when taken simultaneously; CNS DEPRESSANTS may cause additive sedation; do not give with non-selective MAOIS **(isocarboxazid, phenelzine, or tranylcypromine furazolidone, linezolid, procarbazine).**

PHARMACOKINETICS Absorption: Rapidly absorbed from GI tract, bioavailability 65%; food decreases bioavailability. **Peak:** 2 h. **Distribution:** >99% protein bound. **Metabolism:** Extensively metabolized by COMT and glucuronidation. **Elimination:** 60% excreted in urine, 40% in feces; clearance is reduced by 50% in patients with moderate cirrhotic liver disease. **Half-Life:** 2–3 h.

NURSING IMPLICATIONS

Assessment & Drug Effects

- Lab tests: Monitor liver functions monthly for first 3 mo, every 6 wk for the next 3 mo, and periodically thereafter.
- Monitor PT and INR carefully when given concurrently with warfarin.
- Monitor carefully for and immediately report S&S of hepatic impairment (e.g., jaundice, dark urine).

Patient & Family Education

- Do not engage in hazardous activities until response to drug is known. Avoid use of alcohol or sedative drugs while on tolcapone.
- Rise slowly from a sitting or lying position to avoid a rapid drop in BP with possible weakness or fainting.
- Nausea is a common possible adverse effect especially at the beginning of therapy.
- Do not suddenly stop taking this drug. Doses must be gradually reduced over time.
- Notify physician promptly about any of following: Increased loss of muscle control, fainting, yellowing of skin or eyes, darkening of urine, severe diarrhea, hallucinations.
- Do not breast feed while taking this drug without consulting physician.

TOLMETIN SODIUM

(tole′met-in)

Tolectin, Tolectin DS

Classifications: CENTRAL NERVOUS SYSTEM AGENT; ANALGESIC; NSAID; ANTIPYRETIC

Prototype: Ibuprofen

Pregnancy Category: B (D in third trimester)

AVAILABILITY 200 mg, 600 mg tablets; 400 mg capsules

ACTIONS Related to indomethacin. Exact mode of antiinflammatory action not known. Inhibition of platelet aggregation is less than that produced by equal therapeutic doses of aspirin. Comparable to aspirin and indomethacin in antirheumatic activity, but incidence of GI symptoms and tinnitus is less than in aspirin-treated patients, and CNS effects are less than in patients receiving indomethacin.

THERAPEUTIC EFFECTS Possesses analgesic, antiinflammatory, and antipyretic activity.

USES In acute flares and management of chronic rheumatoid arthritis. May be used alone or in combination with gold or corticosteroids.

CONTRAINDICATIONS History of intolerance or hypersensitivity to tolmetin, aspirin, and other NSAIDS; active peptic ulcer, patients with asthma, nasal polyps, rhinitis, "aspirin triad", in patients with functional class IV rheumatoid arthritis (severely incapacitated, bedridden, or confined to a wheelchair). Safety during pregnancy (category B, category D in third trimester), lactation, or children <2 y is not established.

CAUTIOUS USE History of upper GI tract disease; impaired kidney function; compromised cardiac function.

ROUTE & DOSAGE

Arthritis

Adult: **PO** 400 mg t.i.d. (max: 2 g/d)

Child: **PO** ≥2 y, 20 mg/kg/d in 3–4 divided doses (max: 30 mg/kg/d)

ADMINISTRATION

Oral

- Schedule treatment (preferred) to include a morning dose (on arising) and a bedtime dose.
- Give with fluid of patient's choice; crush tablet or empty capsule to mix with water or food if patient cannot swallow tablet/capsule.
- Store at 15°–30° C (59°–86° F) in tightly capped and light-resistant container unless otherwise instructed.

ADVERSE EFFECTS (≥1%) **CNS:** *Headache, dizziness, vertigo, lightheadedness,* mood elevation or depression, tension, nervousness, weakness, drowsiness, insomnia, tinnitus. **CV:** Mild edema (about 7% patients), sodium and water retention, mild to moderate hypertension. **GI:** Epigastric or abdominal pain, dyspepsia, *nausea,* vomiting, heartburn, constipation, peptic ulcer, GI bleeding. **Hematologic:** Transient and small decreases in hemoglobin and hematocrit, purpura, petechiae, granulocytopenia, leukopenia. **Urogenital:** Hematuria, proteinuria, increased BUN. **Skin:** Toxic epidermal necrolysis, morbilliform eruptions, urticaria, pruritus. **Body as a Whole:** Anaphylaxis (especially after drug is discontinued and then reinstituted).

DIAGNOSTIC TEST INTERFERENCE Tolmetin prolongs ***bleeding time,*** inhibits ***platelet aggregation,*** elevates ***BUN, alkaline phosphatase,*** and ***AST*** levels; may decrease ***hemoglobin*** and ***hematocrit*** values. Metabolites may produce false-positive results for ***proteinuria*** (with tests that rely on acid precipitation, e.g., ***sulfosalicylic acid***).

INTERACTIONS Drug: ORAL ANTICOAGULANTS, **heparin** may prolong bleeding time; may increase **lithium** toxicity; **aspirin,** other NSAIDS add to ulcerogenic effects; may increase **methotrexate** toxicity. **Herbal: Feverfew, garlic, ginger, ginkgo** may increase bleeding potential.

PHARMACOKINETICS Absorption: Rapidly absorbed from GI tract. **Peak:** 30–60 min. **Distribution:** Crosses blood–brain barrier and placenta; distributed into breast milk. **Metabolism:** Metabolized in liver. **Elimination:** Excreted in urine. **Half-Life:** 60–90 min.

NURSING IMPLICATIONS

Assessment & Drug Effects

- Monitor therapeutic effect. Therapeutic response for rheumatoid arthritis or osteoarthritis generally occurs within 1 wk with progressive improvement in succeeding week: Reduced joint pain and swelling, reduction in duration of morning stiffness, improved functional capacity (increase in grip strength, delayed onset of fatigue).
- Monitor patients with kidney damage closely. Evaluate I&O ratio and encourage patient to increase fluid intake to at least 8 full glasses per day.
- Lab tests: Obtain periodic kidney function tests (routine urinalysis, creatinine clearance, and serum creatinine) for patient on long-term therapy.
- Check self-medicating habits of the patient. Sodium bicarbonate alkalinizes the urine, which increases urinary excretion of tolmetin and may reduce degree and duration of effectiveness.

Patient & Family Education

- Take drug with meals or milk if GI disturbances occur. Notify physician if symptoms persist; dosage reduction may be necessary, or antacid added.
- Monitor weight and report an increase >2 kg (4 lb)/wk with impaired kidney or cardiac function; check for swelling in ankles, tibiae, hands, and feet.
- Inform surgeon or dentist before treatment if you are taking tolmetin because of possible enhanced bleeding.
- Report promptly signs of abnormal bleeding (ecchymosis, epistaxis, melena, petechiae), itching, skin rash, persistent headache, edema.
- Avoid potentially hazardous activities until response to drug is known because dizziness and drowsiness are common adverse effects.
- Do not breast feed while taking this drug without consulting physician.

TOLNAFTATE

(tole-naf'tate)

Aftate, Pitrex ✦, Tinactin

Classifications: SKIN AND MUCOUS MEMBRANE AGENT; ANTIINFECTIVE; ANTIFUNGAL ANTIBIOTIC

Prototype: Fluconazole

Pregnancy Category: C

AVAILABILITY 1% cream, solution, gel, powder, spray

ACTIONS Synthetic topical antifungal agent. Action mechanism not clear, but has been shown that tolnaftate distorts hyphae and stunts mycelial growth on susceptible fungi.

THERAPEUTIC EFFECTS Fungistatic or fungicidal to *Microsporum,* specifically *M. gypseum, M. canis, M. audouinii, M. japonicum, Trichophyton, T. rubrum, T. schoenleinii, T. tonsurans,* and *Epidermophyton floccosum,* but ineffective against *Candida albicans, Cryptococcus neoformans, Aspergillus fumigatus,* bacteria, protozoa, and viruses.

USES Tinea pedis (athlete's foot), tinea cruris (jock itch), tinea corporis (body ringworm); also tinea capitis and tinea unguium if infection is superficial, plantar or palmar lesions adjunctively with keratolytic agents, and tinea versicolor (caused by *Malassezia furfur*).

CONTRAINDICATIONS Skin irritations prior to therapy, nail and scalp infections. Safety during pregnancy (category C), lactation, or by children <2 y is not established.

CAUTIOUS USE Excoriated skin.

ROUTE & DOSAGE

Tinea Infestations

Adult/Child: **Topical** Apply 0.5–1 cm (1/4–1/2 in) of cream or 3 drops of solution b.i.d. in morning and evening; powder may be used prophylactically in normally moist areas

ADMINISTRATION

Topical

- Cleanse site thoroughly with water and dry completely before applying. Massage thin layer gently into skin. Make sure area is not wet from excess drug after application.
- Shake aerosol powder container well before use.
- Note: Cream and powder are not recommended for nail or scalp infection.
- Use liquids (solutions) for scalp infection or to treat hairy areas.
- Store cream, gel, powder, and topical solution in light-resistant containers at 15°–30° C (59°–86° F); store aerosol container at 2°–30° C (38°–86° F). Avoid freezing and exposure to light.

ADVERSE EFFECTS (≥1%) **Skin:** Local irritation, stinging of skin from aerosol formulation.

INTERACTIONS Drug: No clinically significant interactions established.

PHARMACOKINETICS Not studied.

NURSING IMPLICATIONS

Patient & Family Education

- Expect relief from pruritus, soreness, and burning within 24–72 h after start of treatment.
- Continue treatment for 2–3 wk after disappearance of all symptoms to prevent recurrence.
- Return to physician for reevaluation in absence of improvement within 4 wk.
- Note: If skin has thickened as a result of the infection, desired clinical response may be delayed for 4–6 wk.
- Avoid contact with eyes of all drug forms.
- Place container in warm water to liquefy contents if solution solidifies. Potency is unaffected.
- Do not breast feed while using this drug without consulting physician.

TOLTERODINE TARTRATE

(tol-ter'o-deen tar'trate)
Detrol, Detrol LA
Classifications: AUTONOMIC NERVOUS SYSTEM AGENT; ANTICHOLINERGIC AGENT; ANTIMUSCARINIC AGENT; MUSCARINIC RECEPTOR ANTAGONIST
Prototype: Atropine
Pregnancy Category: C

AVAILABILITY 1 mg, 2 mg tablets; 2 mg, 4 mg sustained release

ACTIONS Selective muscarinic urinary bladder receptor antagonist.
THERAPEUTIC EFFECTS Reduces urinary incontinence, urgency, and frequency. Controls urinary bladder incontinence by controlling contractions.

USES Overactive bladder (urinary frequency, urgency, urge incontinence).

CONTRAINDICATIONS Gastric retention; hypersensitivity to tolterodine; uncontrolled narrow-angle glaucoma; urinary retention; pregnancy (category C).
CAUTIOUS USE Lactation; cardiovascular disease; liver disease; controlled narrow-angle glaucoma; obstructive GI disease; obstructive uropathy; paralytic ileus or intestinal atony; renal impairment; ulcerative colitis.

T

ROUTE & DOSAGE

Overactive Bladder

Adult: **PO** 2 mg b.i.d. or 4 mg sustained release q.d.

Hepatic Impairment

May decrease to 1 mg b.i.d. or 2 mg sustained release q.d. in those with significantly reduced liver function or taking drugs that inhibit cytochrome P450 3A4 (see ADMINISTRATION)

ADMINISTRATION

Oral

- Do not crush or chew sustained release tablets. These must be swallowed whole.
- Do not give doses >1 mg b.i.d. to those with significantly reduced liver function or concurrently receiving macrolide antibiotics, azole antifungal agents, or other cytochrome P450 3A4 inhibitors.
- Store at 20°–25° C (68°–77° F) in a tightly closed container.

ADVERSE EFFECTS (≥1%) **Body as a Whole:** Back pain, fatigue, flu-like syndrome, falls, arthralgia, weight gain. **CNS:** Headache, paresthesias, vertigo, dizziness, nervousness, somnolence. **CV:** Chest pain, hypertension. **GI:** *Dry mouth,* dyspepsia, constipation, abdominal pain, diarrhea, flatulence, nausea, vomiting. **Urogenital:** Dysuria, micturition frequency, urinary retention, UTI. **Respiratory:** Bronchitis, cough, pharyngitis, rhinitis, sinusitis, URI. **Skin:** Pruritus, rash, erythema, dry skin. **Special Senses:** Dry eyes, vision abnormalities.

INTERACTIONS Drug: Additive anticholinergic effects with **amantadine, amoxapine, bupropion, clozapine, cyclobenzaprine, disopyramide, maprotiline, olanzapine, orphenadrine,** SEDATING H_1-BLOCKERS, PHENOTHIAZINES, TRICYCLIC ANTIDEPRESSANTS. **Food: Grapefruit juice** may increase **tolterodine** levels in some patients.

PHARMACOKINETICS Absorption: 77% absorbed, significantly decreased with food. **Peak:** 1–2 h. **Distribution:** 96% protein bound. **Metabolism:** Metabolized in liver by cytochrome P450 2D6 enzymes to active metabolite. **Elimination:** 77% excreted in urine, 17% in feces. **Half-Life:** 1.9–3.7 h.

NURSING IMPLICATIONS

Assessment & Drug Effects

- Monitor intraocular pressure more frequently with glaucoma patients.
- Monitor vital signs carefully (HR and BP), especially in those with cardiovascular disease.

Patient & Family Education

- Notify physician promptly if you experience eye pain, rapid heartbeat, difficulty breathing, skin rash or hives, confusion, or incoordination.
- Report blurred vision, sensitivity to light, and dry mouth (all common adverse effects) to physician if bothersome.
- Avoid the use of alcohol or OTC antihistamines.
- Do not breast feed while taking this drug without consulting physician.

TOPIRAMATE

(to-pir'a-mate)

Topamax

Classifications: CENTRAL NERVOUS SYSTEM AGENT; ANTICONVULSANT

Pregnancy Category: C

AVAILABILITY 25 mg, 100 mg, 200 mg tablets; 15 mg, 25 mg, 50 mg capsules

ACTIONS Sulfamate-substituted monosaccharide with a broad spectrum of anticonvulsant activity. Its precise mechanism of action is unknown. Exhibits sodium channel-blocking action, as well as enhancing the ability of GABA to induce a flux of chloride ions into the neurons, thus potentiating the activity of this inhibitory neurotransmitter (GABA).

THERAPEUTIC EFFECTS Indicated by a decrease in seizure activity. Effectively controls partial onset seizures in adults and children by inhibiting GABA.

USES Adjunctive therapy for partial-onset seizures in adults and children age 2–16 y; migraine prophylaxis.

CONTRAINDICATIONS Hypersensitivity to topiramate; epilepsy, pregnancy (category C). Effect on labor and delivery is unknown.

CAUTIOUS USE Moderate and severe renal impairment, hepatic impairment; lactation. While topiramate has been studied in patients 2–17 y of age, safety and effectiveness in younger children are not established.

ROUTE & DOSAGE

Partial-Onset Seizures

Adult: **PO** Initiate with 25 mg b.i.d., increase by 50 mg/wk to efficacy **PO Maintenance Dose** 200–400 mg/d divided b.i.d. (max: 1600 mg/d)

Child: **PO** *2–16 y,* Initiate with 1–3 mg/kg h.s. × 1 wk, then increase by 1–3 mg/kg/d in 2 divided doses q1–2wk to a target range of 5–9 mg/kg/d

Migraine Prophylaxis

Adult: **PO** Initiate with 25 mg b.i.d., increase by 25 mg/wk to 200 mg/d or max tolerated dose

Renal Impairment

Cl_{cr} <70 mL/min: decrease dose by 50%

ADMINISTRATION

Oral

- Make dosage increments of 50 mg at weekly intervals to the recommended dose, usually 400 mg/d.
- Do not break tablets unless absolutely necessary because of bitter taste.

T

- Store at 15°–30° C (59°–86° F) in a tightly closed container. Protect from light and moisture.

ADVERSE EFFECTS (≥1%) **Body as a Whole:** *Fatigue, speech problems,* weight loss; decreased sweating and hyperthermia in children. **CNS:** *Somnolence, dizziness, ataxia, psychomotor slowing, confusion, nystagmus, paresthesia, memory difficulty, difficulty concentrating, nervousness,* depression, anxiety, tremor. **GI:** Anorexia. **Special Senses:** Angle closure glaucoma (rare).

INTERACTIONS Drug: Increased CNS depression with **alcohol** and other CNS DEPRESSANTS; may increase **phenytoin** concentrations; may decrease ORAL CONTRACEPTIVE, **valproate** concentrations; may increase risk of kidney stone formation with other CARBONIC ANHYDRASE INHIBITORS. **Carbamazepine, phenytoin, valproate** may decrease topiramate concentrations. **Herbal: Ginkgo** may decrease anticonvulsant effectiveness.

PHARMACOKINETICS Absorption: Rapidly absorbed from GI tract; 80% bioavailability. **Peak:** 2 h. **Distribution:** 13%–17% protein bound. **Metabolism:** Minimally metabolized in the liver. **Elimination:** Excreted primarily in urine. **Half-Life:** 21 h.

T

NURSING IMPLICATIONS

Assessment & Drug Effects

- Monitor mental status and report significant cognitive impairment.
- Lab tests: Periodically monitor CBC with Hgb and Hct.

Patient & Family Education

- Do not stop drug abruptly; discontinue gradually to minimize seizures.
- To minimize risk of kidney stones, drink at least 6–8 full glasses of water each day.
- Exercise caution with potentially hazardous activities. Sedation is common, especially with concurrent use of alcohol or other CNS depressants.
- Use or add barrier contraceptive if using hormonal contraceptives.
- Be aware that psychomotor slowing and speech/language problems may develop while on topiramate therapy.
- Report adverse effects that interfere with activities of daily living.
- Do not breast feed while taking this drug without consulting physician.

TOPOTECAN HYDROCHLORIDE Pr

(toe-po-tee'can)

Hycamtin

Classifications: ANTINEOPLASTIC, CAMPTOTHECIN AGENT; TOPOISOMERASE I INHIBITOR

Pregnancy Category: D

AVAILABILITY 4 mg vials

ACTIONS Antitumor mechanism is related to inhibition of activity of topoisomerase I, an enzyme required for DNA replication. Topoisomerase I is essential for the relaxation of supercoiled double-stranded DNA, which enables replication and transcription to proceed. Topotecan binds to the DNA-topoisomerase I complex.

THERAPEUTIC EFFECTS Permits uncoiling but prevents recoiling of the two strands of DNA, resulting in a permanent break in the DNA strands.

USE Metastatic ovarian cancer.

CONTRAINDICATIONS Previous hypersensitivity to topotecan, irinotecan, or other camptothecin analogs; acute infection; pregnancy (category D), lactation.

CAUTIOUS USE Myelosuppression; history of bleeding disorders; previous cytotoxic or radiation therapy.

ROUTE & DOSAGE

Metastatic Ovarian Cancer

Adult: **IV** 1.5 mg/m^2 daily for 5 d starting on day 1 of a 21 d course. Four courses of therapy recommended. Subsequent doses can be adjusted by 0.25 mg/m^2 depending on toxicity

ADMINISTRATION

Intravenous

- Initiate therapy only if baseline neutrophil count ≥1500/mm^3 and platelet count ≥100,000/mm^3. Do not give subsequent doses until neutrophils >1000/mm^3, platelets ≥100,000/mm^3, and Hgb = 9.0 mg/dL. ■ Note: Dosage adjustments to 0.75 mg/m^2 are recommended with moderate renal impairment.

PREPARE: **IV Infusion:** Reconstitute each 4-mg vial with 4 mL sterile water for injection to yield 1 mg/mL. Withdraw the required dose and inject into 50–100 mL of NS or D5W. If skin contacts drug during preparation, wash immediately with soap and water.

ADMINISTER: **IV Infusion:** Give over 30 min immediately after preparation.

- Store vials at 20°–25° C (68°–77° F); protect from light. Reconstituted vials are stable for 24 h.

ADVERSE EFFECTS (≥1%) **Body as a Whole:** *Asthenia, fever, fatigue.* **GI:** *Nausea, vomiting, diarrhea, constipation, abdominal pain, stomatitis, anorexia,* transient elevations in liver function tests. **Hematologic:** *Leukopenia, neutropenia, anemia, thrombocytopenia.* **Respiratory:** *Dyspnea.* **Skin:** *Alopecia.*

INTERACTIONS Drug: Increased risk of bleeding with ANTICOAGULANTS, NSAIDS, SALICYLATES, ANTIPLATELET AGENTS.

PHARMACOKINETICS Distribution: 35% bound to plasma proteins. **Metabolism:** Undergoes pH-dependent hydrolysis. **Elimination:** Approximately 30% excreted in urine. **Half-Life:** 2–3 h.

NURSING IMPLICATIONS

Assessment & Drug Effects

- Lab tests: Obtain CBC counts with differential frequently; periodically monitor ALT.
- Assess for GI distress, respiratory distress, neurosensory symptoms, and S&S of infection throughout therapy.

Patient & Family Education

- Learn common adverse effects and measures to control or minimize when possible. Immediately report any distressing adverse effects to physician.
- Avoid pregnancy during therapy.
- Do not breast feed while taking this drug.

TOREMIFENE CITRATE

(tor-em'i-feen ci'trate)

Fareston

Classifications: ANTINEOPLASTIC; HORMONES AND SYNTHETIC SUBSTITUTES; ANTIESTROGEN

Prototype: Tamoxifen

Pregnancy Category: D

AVAILABILITY 60 mg tablets

ACTIONS Nonsteroidal antiestrogen chemical derivative of tamox-

T

ifen. Antitumor activity thought to be due to ability to compete with estrogen for binding sites in the cancer cells.
THERAPEUTIC EFFECTS Depresses tumor growth.

USES Metastatic breast cancer in postmenopausal women who are estrogen receptor positive.

CONTRAINDICATIONS Hypersensitivity to toremifene; pregnancy (category D).
CAUTIOUS USE Preexisting endometrial hyperplasia; bone metastases (may result in hypercalcemia); geriatric patients; leukopenia and thrombocytopenia; liver disease; history of thrombolytic disease; lactation.

ROUTE & DOSAGE

Breast Cancer
Adult: **PO** 60 mg q.d.

ADMINISTRATION

Oral
- Withhold drug and notify physician if severe hypercalcemia develops.
- Store at 15°–30° C (59°–86° F) in a tightly closed container and protect from light.

ADVERSE EFFECTS (≥1%) **Body as a Whole:** *Hot flashes, sweating,* edema. **CNS:** Dizziness. **GI:** *Nausea,* vomiting, abnormal liver function tests. **Respiratory:** <u>Pulmonary embolism</u>. **Urogenital:** *Vaginal discharge,* vaginal bleeding. **Special Senses:** Cataracts, dry eyes, corneal keratopathy.

INTERACTIONS Drug: THIAZIDE DIURETICS increase risk of hypercalcemia; increased PT on **warfarin; carbamazepine, phenobarbital, phenytoin** may increase toremifene metabolism.

PHARMACOKINETICS Absorption: Rapidly absorbed from GI tract. **Peak:** 3 h. **Distribution:** >99% protein bound; crosses placenta. **Metabolism:** Metabolized in liver by cytochrome P450 3A4. **Elimination:** Excreted primarily in feces. **Half-Life:** 5 d.

NURSING IMPLICATIONS

Assessment & Drug Effects
- Lab tests: Periodically monitor CBC with differential, serum calcium, liver and kidney functions.
- Monitor patients carefully with bone metastases or those on drugs that decrease calcium excretion (e.g., thiazide diuretics) for S&S of hypercalcemia (see Appendix F).
- Monitor PT and INR carefully when given concurrently with warfarin.

Patient & Family Education
- Report to physician promptly any of the following: Unexplained weakness or fatigue, musculoskeletal pain or calf pain and tenderness, sudden chest pain, vaginal bleeding.
- Schedule periodic eye exams with long-term therapy.
- Do not breast feed while taking this drug without consulting physician.

TORSEMIDE

(tor′se-mide)
Demadex
Classifications: ELECTROLYTE AND WATER BALANCE AGENT; LOOP DIURETIC
Prototype: Furosemide
Pregnancy Category: B

AVAILABILITY 5 mg, 10 mg, 20 mg, 100 mg tablets; 10 mg/mL injection

ACTIONS Long-acting potent sulfonamide "loop" diuretic that inhibits reabsorption of sodium and chloride primarily in the Loop of Henle and also in the proximal and distal renal tubules. Binds to the sodium/potassium/chloride carrier in the Loop of Henle and in the renal tubules. Lower potassium-wasting effects than furosemide and a longer half-life.

THERAPEUTIC EFFECTS Long-acting potent sulfonamide "Loop" diuretic and antihypertensive agent.

USES Management of edema associated with CHF, chronic kidney failure, hepatic cirrhosis; hypertension.

CONTRAINDICATIONS Hypersensitivity to torsemide or sulfonamides; anuria, fluid and electrolyte depletion states; hepatic coma; pregnancy (category B).

CAUTIOUS USE Renal impairment; concurrent use of other ototoxic drugs; gout or hyperuricemia; diabetes mellitus or history of pancreatitis; liver disease; hearing impairment; lactation.

ROUTE & DOSAGE

CHF, Chronic Kidney Failure

Adult: **PO/IV** 10–20 mg once daily, may increase up to 200 mg/d as needed

Hepatic Cirrhosis

Adult: **PO/IV** 5–10 mg once daily administered with an aldosterone antagonist or potassium-sparing diuretic, may increase up to 40 mg/d as needed

Hypertension

Adult: **PO/IV** 5 mg once daily, may increase to 10 mg/d if no response after 4–6 wk

ADMINISTRATION

Note: With hepatic cirrhosis, use an aldosterone antagonist concomitantly to prevent hypokalemia and metabolic alkalosis.

Oral

- Be aware that oral and IV doses are therapeutically equivalent; patients may be switched between the two forms with no change in dosage.

Intravenous

PREPARE: **Direct:** Given undiluted.
ADMINISTER: **Direct:** Give slowly over 2 min.

- Store at 15°–30° C (59°–86° F).

ADVERSE EFFECTS (≥1%) **CNS:** Headache, dizziness, fatigue, insomnia. **CV:** Orthostatic hypotension. **Endocrine:** *Hypokalemia,* hyponatremia, hyperuricemia. **GI:** Nausea, diarrhea. **Skin:** Rash, pruritus. **Body as a Whole:** Muscle cramps, rhinitis.

INTERACTIONS Drug: NSAIDS may reduce diuretic effects. Also see furosemide for potential drug interactions such as increased risk of **digoxin** toxicity due to hypokalemia, prolonged neuromuscular blockade with NEUROMUSCULAR BLOCKING AGENTS, and decreased **lithium** elimination with increased toxicity.

PHARMACOKINETICS Absorption: Readily absorbed from GI tract. **Onset:** IV 10 min; PO 60 min. **Peak:** IV within 60 min; PO 60–120 min. **Duration:** 6–8 h. **Metabolism:** Metabolized in liver by cytochrome P450 system. **Elimination:** 80% excreted in bile; 20% excreted in urine. **Half-Life:** 210 min.

NURSING IMPLICATIONS

Assessment & Drug Effects

- Monitor BP often and assess for orthostatic hypotension; periodi-

T

cally assess weight as an index of fluid retention.
- Lab tests: Monitor serum electrolytes, uric acid, blood glucose, BUN, and creatinine periodically throughout the course of therapy.
- Monitor coagulation parameters and lithium levels in patients on concurrent anticoagulant and/or lithium therapy.

Patient & Family Education
- Check weight at least weekly and report abrupt gains or losses to physician.
- Understand the risk of orthostatic hypotension.
- Report symptoms of hypokalemia (see Appendix F) or hearing loss immediately to physician.
- Monitor blood glucose for loss of glycemic control if diabetic.
- Do not breast feed while taking this drug without consulting physician.

TRAMADOL HYDROCHLORIDE

(tra′ma-dol)

Ultram, Zydol ✦

Classifications: CENTRAL NERVOUS SYSTEM (CNS) AGENT; ANALGESIC; NARCOTIC (OPIATE) AGONIST

Prototype: Morphine sulfate

Pregnancy Category: C

AVAILABILITY 50 mg tablets

ACTIONS Centrally acting opiate receptor agonist that inhibits the uptake of norepinephrine and serotonin, suggesting both opioid and nonopioid mechanisms of pain relief. May produce opioid-like effects, but causes less respiratory depression than morphine.

THERAPEUTIC EFFECTS Effective agent for control of moderate to moderately severe pain.

USES Management of moderate to moderately severe pain.

CONTRAINDICATIONS Hypersensitivity to tramadol or other opioid analgesics; patients on MAO inhibitors; patients acutely intoxicated with alcohol, hypnotics, centrally acting analgesics, opioids, or psychotropic drugs; substance abuse; patients on obstetric preoperative medication; abrupt discontinuation; alcohol intoxication; pregnancy (category C); lactation; children <16 y.

CAUTIOUS USE Debilitated patients; chronic respiratory disorders; respiratory depression; older adults; liver disease; renal impairment; myxedema, hypothyroidism, or hypoadrenalism; GI disease; acute abdominal conditions; increased ICP or head injury, increased intracranial pressure; history of seizures; patients >75 y.

ROUTE & DOSAGE

Pain

Adult: **PO** 50–100 mg q4–6h prn (max: 400 mg/d), may start with 25 mg/d if not well tolerated, and increase by 25 mg q3d up to 200 mg/d

Geriatric: **PO** 50–100 mg q4–6h prn (max: 300 mg/d), may start with 25 mg/d if not well tolerated, and increase by 25 mg q3d up to 200 mg/d

Renal Impairment

Cl_{cr} <30 mL/min: decrease to 50–100 mg q12h

Hepatic Impairment

Cirrhosis decrease to 50–100 mg q12h

ADMINISTRATION

Oral
- Note: Dosage reduction is recommended for patients with renal insufficiency and hepatic impairment.
- Store at 15°–30° C (59°–86° F).

ADVERSE EFFECTS (≥1%) **CNS:** Drowsiness, *dizziness, vertigo, fatigue, headache, somnolence,* restlessness, euphoria, confusion, anxiety, coordination disturbance, sleep disturbances, seizures. **CV:** Palpitations, vasodilation. **GI:** *Nausea, constipation,* vomiting, xerostomia, dyspepsia, diarrhea, abdominal pain, anorexia, flatulence. **Body as a Whole:** Sweating, anaphylactic reaction (even with first dose), withdrawal syndrome (anxiety, sweating, nausea, tremors, diarrhea, piloerection, panic attacks, paresthesia, hallucinations) with abrupt discontinuation. **Skin:** Rash. **Special Senses:** Visual disturbances. **Urogenital:** Urinary retention/frequency, menopausal symptoms.

DIAGNOSTIC TEST INTERFERENCE Increased ***creatinine, liver enzymes;*** decreased ***hemoglobin; proteinuria.***

INTERACTIONS Drug: Carbamazepine significantly decreases tramadol levels (may need up to twice usual dose). Tramadol may increase adverse effects of MAO INHIBITORS. TRICYCLIC ANTIDEPRESSANTS, **cyclobenzaprine,** PHENOTHIAZINES, SELECTIVE SEROTONIN-REUPTAKE INHIBITORS (SSRIS), MAO INHIBITORS may enhance seizure risk with tramadol. May increase CNS adverse effects when used with other CNS DEPRESSANTS. **Herbal: St. John's wort** may increase sedation.

PHARMACOKINETICS Absorption: Rapidly absorbed from GI tract; 75% reaches systemic circulation. **Onset:** 30–60 min. **Peak:** 2 h. **Duration:** 3–7 h. **Distribution:** Approximately 20% bound to plasma proteins; probably crosses blood–brain barrier; crosses placenta; 0.1% excreted into breast milk. **Metabolism:** Metabolized extensively in liver by cytochrome P450 system. **Elimination:** Excreted primarily in urine. **Half-Life:** 6–7 h.

NURSING IMPLICATIONS

Assessment & Drug Effects

- Assess for level of pain relief and administer prn dose as needed but not to exceed the recommended total daily dose.
- Monitor vital signs and assess for orthostatic hypotension or signs of CNS depression.
- Discontinue drug and notify physician if S&S of hypersensitivity occur.
- Assess bowel and bladder function; report urinary frequency or retention.
- Use seizure precautions for patients who have a history of seizures or who are concurrently using drugs that lower the seizure threshold.
- Monitor ambulation and take appropriate safety precautions.

Patient & Family Education

- Exercise caution with potentially hazardous activities until response to drug is known.
- Understand potential adverse effects and report problems with bowel and bladder function, CNS impairment, and any other bothersome adverse effects to physician.
- Do not breast feed while taking this drug.

TRANDOLAPRIL

(tran-do'la-pril)

Mavik

Classifications: CARDIOVASCULAR AGENT; ANGIOTENSIN-CONVERTING ENZYME INHIBITOR; ANTIHYPERTENSIVE

Prototype: Captopril

Pregnancy Category: C first trimester (D in second and third trimester)

AVAILABILITY 1 mg, 2 mg, 4 mg tablets

ACTIONS Inhibits ACE and interrupts conversion sequences initiated by renin which leads to the formation of angiotensin II from angiotensin I. Angiotensin II is a potent endogenous vasoconstrictor. Peripheral vascular resistance is lowered by vasodilation. Therefore inhibition of ACE leads to vasodilation and also to decreased circulating aldosterone. Decreased aldosterone leads to diuresis and a slight increase in serum potassium. All of these factors produce the antihypertensive effect of the drug.

THERAPEUTIC EFFECTS Lowers blood pressure by specific inhibition of ACE. Unlike other ACE inhibitors, all racial groups respond to trandolapril, including low-renin hypertensives.

USES Treatment of hypertension, alone or in combination with other antihypertensive agents.

UNLABELED USES CHF.

CONTRAINDICATIONS Hypersensitivity to trandolapril; history of angioedema related to previous treatment with an ACE inhibitor; pregnancy (category C, first trimester; category D, second and third trimesters), lactation.

CAUTIOUS USE Renal impairment, hepatic insufficiency; patients prone to hypotension (e.g., CHF, ischemic heart disease, aortic stenosis, CVA, dehydration); SLE, scleroderma. Safety and effectiveness in children <18 y are not established.

ROUTE & DOSAGE

Note: Discontinue diuretics 2–3 d before starting trandolapril.

Hypertension

Adult: **PO** 1 mg in nonblack patients, 2 mg in black patients once daily, may increase weekly to 2–4 mg once daily (max: 8 mg/d)

Renal Impairment

Cl_{cr} <30 mL/min: start with 0.5 mg once daily

Hepatic Impairment

Hepatic cirrhosis: start with 0.5 mg once daily

ADMINISTRATION

Oral

- Note: If concurrently ordered diuretic cannot be discontinued 2–3d before beginning trandolapril therapy, reduce initial dose to 0.5 mg.
- Make dosage adjustments generally at intervals of at least 1 wk.
- Store at 15°–30° C (59°–86° F).

ADVERSE EFFECTS (≥1%) **Body as a Whole:** Fatigue, angioedema. **CNS:** Dizziness, headache. **CV:** Hypotension. **GI:** Diarrhea. **Respiratory:** Cough. **Skin:** Rash, pruritus. **Metabolic:** Hyperkalemia.

INTERACTIONS Drug: DIURETICS may enhance hypotensive effects. POTASSIUM-SPARING DIURETICS (amiloride, spironolactone, triamterene), POTASSIUM SUPPLEMENTS, POTASSIUM-CONTAINING SALT SUBSTITUTES may increase risk of hyperkalemia. May increase serum levels and toxicity of **lithium.**

PHARMACOKINETICS Absorption: Rapidly absorbed from GI tract and converted to active form, trandolaprilat, in liver; 70% of dose reaches systemic circulation as trandolaprilat. **Peak:** 4–10 h. **Distribution:** 80% protein bound; crosses placenta, secreted into breast milk of animals (human secretion unknown). **Metabolism:** Metabolized in liver to active metabolite, trandolaprilat. **Elimination:** 33% excreted in urine, 66% in feces. **Half-Life:** 6 h trandolapril, 10 h trandolaprilat.

NURSING IMPLICATIONS

Assessment & Drug Effects

- Monitor BP carefully for 1–3 h following initial dose, especially in patients using concurrent diuretics, on salt restriction, or volume depleted.
- Lab tests: Monitor BP and cardiac status; serum potassium, sodium, creatinine, and ALT/SGTP; and WBC with differential periodically.
- Monitor serum lithium levels frequently with concurrent use and assess for S&S of lithium toxicity; increase caution when diuretic therapy is also used.

Patient & Family Education

- Discontinue drug and immediately report S&S of angioedema of face or extremities to physician. Advise to seek emergency help for swelling of the tongue or any other sign of potential airway obstruction.
- Be aware that light-headedness can occur, especially during early therapy. Excess fluid loss of any kind will increase risk of hypotension and syncope.
- Do not breast feed while taking this drug.

TRANYLCYPROMINE SULFATE

(tran-ill-sip′roe-meen)

Parnate

Classifications: CENTRAL NERVOUS SYSTEM AGENT; PSYCHOTHERAPEUTIC; ANTIDEPRESSANT; MAO INHIBITOR

Prototype: Phenelzine

Pregnancy Category: C

AVAILABILITY 10 mg tablets

ACTIONS Potent nonhydrazine MAO inhibitor structurally similar to amphetamine. Actions and toxicity similar to those of hydrazine MAO inhibitors but also has rapid and direct amphetamine-like CNS stimulatory action, is less likely to cause hepatotoxicity and does not produce prolonged MAO inhibition (reversible binding).

THERAPEUTIC EFFECTS Drug of last choice for severe depression unresponsive to other MAO inhibitors.

USES Severe depression.

CONTRAINDICATIONS Pregnancy (category C); patients >60 y; confirmed or suspected cerebrovascular defect, cardiovascular disease, hypertension, pheochromocytoma, history of severe or recurrent headaches; lactation.

ROUTE & DOSAGE

Severe Depression

Adult: **PO** 30 mg/d in 2 divided doses (20 mg in a.m., 10 mg in p.m.), may increase by 10 mg/d at 3 wk intervals (max: 60 mg/d)

ADMINISTRATION

Oral

- Crush tablet and give with fluid or mix with food if patient cannot swallow pill.
- Note: Usually not given in the evening because of possibility of insomnia.

ADVERSE EFFECTS (≥1%) **CNS:** Vertigo, dizziness, tremors, muscle twitching, headache, blurred vision. **CV:** *Orthostatic hypotension,* arrhythmias, <u>hypertensive crisis</u>. **GI:** Dry mouth, anorexia, constipation, diarrhea, abdominal discomfort. **Skin:** Rash. **Urogenital:** Impotence. **Body as a Whole:** Peripheral edema, sweating.

INTERACTIONS Drug: TRICYCLIC ANTIDEPRESSANTS, **fluoxetine,** AMPHETAMINES, **ephedrine, phenylpropanolamine, reserpine, guanethi-**

T

dine, buspirone, methyldopa, dopamine, levodopa, tryptophan may precipitate hypertensive crisis, headache, or hyperexcitability; **alcohol** and other CNS DEPRESSANTS add to CNS depressant effects; **meperidine** can cause fatal cardiovascular collapse; ANESTHETICS exaggerate hypotensive and CNS depressant effects; **metrizamide** increases risk of seizures; DIURETICS and other ANTIHYPERTENSIVE AGENTS add to hypotensive effects. **Food: Tyramine**-containing foods may precipitate hypertensive crisis (e.g., aged cheeses, processed cheeses, sour cream, wine, champagne, beer, pickled herring, anchovies, caviar, shrimp, liver, dry sausage, figs, raisins, overripe bananas or avocados, chocolate, soy sauce, bean curd, yeast extracts, yogurt, papaya products, meat tenderizers, broad beans). **Herbal: Ginseng, ephedra, ma huang, St. John's wort** may lead to hypertensive crisis; **ginseng** may lead to manic episodes.

PHARMACOKINETICS Absorption: Completely absorbed from GI tract. **Onset:** 10 d. **Metabolism:** Rapidly metabolized in liver to active metabolite. **Elimination:** Primarily excreted in urine. **Half-Life:** 2.5 h (but may take 120 h for urinary tryptamine levels to return to normal).

T

NURSING IMPLICATIONS

Assessment & Drug Effects

- Monitor BP closely. Incidence of severe hypertensive reactions appears to be greater with tranylcypromine than with other MAO inhibitors.
- Expect therapeutic response within 3 d, but full antidepressant effects may not be obtained until 2–3 wk of drug therapy.

Patient & Family Education

- Do not eat tyramine-containing foods (see FOOD–DRUG INTERACTIONS).
- Be aware that excessive use of caffeine-containing beverages (chocolate, coffee, tea, cola) can contribute to development of rapid heartbeat, arrhythmias, and hypertension.
- Make position changes slowly, particularly from recumbent to upright posture.
- Avoid potentially hazardous activities until response to drug is known.
- Avoid alcohol or other CNS depressants because of their possible additive effects.
- Do not breast feed while taking this drug.

TRASTUZUMAB

(tra-stu'zu-mab)

Herceptin

Classifications: IMMUNOSUPPRESSANT; MONOCLONAL ANTIBODY; ANTI-HER

Pregnancy Category: B

AVAILABILITY 440 mg vial

ACTIONS Recombinant DNA monoclonal antibody (I_gG_1 kappa) that selectively binds to the human epidermal growth factor receptor-2 protein (HER_2).

THERAPEUTIC EFFECTS Inhibits growth of human tumor cells that over express HER_2 proteins.

USES Metastatic breast cancer in those whose tumors over express the HER_2 protein.

CONTRAINDICATIONS Concurrent administration of anthracycline or radiation; lactation during and for 6

mo following administration of trastuzumab.

CAUTIOUS USE Preexisting cardiac dysfunction; previous administration of cardiotoxic therapy (e.g., anthracycline or radiation); pregnancy (category B); older adults; hypersensitivity to benzyl alcohol (preservative in bacteriostatic water).

ROUTE & DOSAGE

Metastatic Breast Cancer
Adult: **IV Loading Dose** 4 mg/kg **IV Maintenance Dose** 2 mg/kg qwk

ADMINISTRATION

Intravenous

PREPARE: **IV Infusion:** Reconstitute each vial with 20 mL of supplied diluent (bacteriostatic water) to produce a multidose vial containing 21 mg/mL. Note: For patients with a hypersensitivity to benzyl alcohol, reconstitute with sterile water for injection; this solution must be used immediately with any unused portion discarded. Withdraw the ordered dose and add to a 250-mL of NS and invert bag to mix. Do not give or mix with dextrose solutions.

ADMINISTER: **IV Infusion:** Infuse loading dose (4 mg/kg) over 90 min; infuse subsequent doses (2 mg/kg) over 30 min. Do not give IV push or as a bolus dose.

INCOMPATIBILITIES **Solution/additive:** Dextrose solution; do not mix or coadminister with other drugs.

- Store unopened vials and reconstituted vials at 2°–8° C (36°–46° F). Discard reconstituted vials 28 days after reconstitution.

ADVERSE EFFECTS (≥1%) **Body as a Whole:** *Pain, asthenia, fever, chills,* flu syndrome, allergic reaction, bone pain, arthralgia, hypersensitivity (anaphylaxis, urticaria, bronchospasm, angioedema, or hypotension), increased incidence of infections, infusion reaction (*chills, fever,* nausea, vomiting, pain, rigors, headache, dizziness, dyspnea, hypotension, rash). **CNS:** *Headache, insomnia, dizziness, paresthesias,* depression, peripheral neuritis, neuropathy. **CV:** CHF, cardiac dysfunction (dyspnea, cough, paroxysmal nocturnal dyspnea, peripheral edema, S3 gallop, reduced ejection fraction), tachycardia, edema. **GI:** *Diarrhea, abdominal pain, nausea, vomiting,* anorexia. **Hematologic:** *Anemia, leukopenia.* **Respiratory:** *Cough, dyspnea,* rhinitis, pharyngitis, sinusitis. **Skin:** *Rash,* herpes simplex, acne.

INTERACTIONS Drug: Paclitaxel may increase trastuzumab levels and toxicity.

PHARMACOKINETICS Half-Life: 5.8 d.

NURSING IMPLICATIONS

Assessment & Drug Effects

- Lab tests: Periodically monitor CBC with differential, platelet count, and Hgb and Hct.
- Monitor for chills and fever during the first IV infusion; these adverse events usually respond to prompt treatment without the need to discontinue the infusion. Notify physician immediately.
- Monitor carefully cardiovascular status at baseline and throughout course of therapy, assessing for S&S of heart failure (e.g., dyspnea, increased cough, PND, edema, S3 gallop). Those with preexisting cardiac dysfunction are at high risk for cardiotoxicity.

Patient & Family Education

- Report promptly any unusual symptoms (e.g., chills, nausea, fever) during infusion.
- Report promptly any of the following: Shortness of breath, swelling of feet or legs, persistent cough, difficulty sleeping, loss of appetite, abdominal bloating.
- Do not breast feed during and for 6 mo following administration of trastuzumab.

TRAVAPROST

(tra′-va-prost)

Travatan

Classifications: EYE PREPARATION; PROSTAGLANDIN

Prototype: Latanoprost

Pregnancy Category: C

AVAILABILITY 0.004% solution

See Appendix A-1.

TRAZODONE HYDROCHLORIDE

(tray′zoe-done)

Desyrel, Desyrel Dividose

Classifications: CENTRAL NERVOUS SYSTEM (CNS) AGENT; PSYCHOTHERAPEUTIC AGENT; ANTIDEPRESSANT

Prototype: Imipramine

Pregnancy Category: C

AVAILABILITY 50 mg, 100 mg, 150 mg, 300 mg tablets

ACTIONS Centrally acting triazolopyridine derivative antidepressant chemically and structurally unrelated to tricyclic, tetracyclic, or other antidepressants. Potentiates serotonin effects by selectively blocking its reuptake at presynaptic membranes in CNS. Does not stimulate CNS and causes fewer anticholinergic genitourinary and neurologic effects as compared with other antidepressants. Produces varying degrees of sedation in normal and mentally depressed patient.

THERAPEUTIC EFFECTS Increases total sleep time, decreases number and duration of awakenings in depressed patient, and decreases REM sleep. Has anxiolytic effect in severely depressed patient.

USES Both inpatient and outpatient with major depression with or without prominent anxiety.

UNLABELED USES Adjunctive treatment of alcohol dependence, anxiety neuroses, drug-induced dyskinesias.

CONTRAINDICATIONS Initial recovery phase of MI; ventricular ectopy; electroshock therapy. Safety during pregnancy (category C) or in children <8 y is not established.

CAUTIOUS USE Patient with suicidal ideation; bipolar disorder, older adults; cardiac arrhythmias or disease; hepatic disease, renal impairment; lactation.

ROUTE & DOSAGE

Depression

Adult: **PO** 150 mg/d in divided doses, may increase by 50 mg/d q3–4d (max: 400–600 mg/d)
Geriatric: **PO** 25–50 mg h.s., may increase q3–7d to usual range of 75–150 mg/d
Child: **PO** *6–18 y,* 1.5–2 mg/kg/d in divided doses, increase q3–4d prn (max: 6 mg/kg/d)

ADMINISTRATION

Oral

- Give drug with food; increases amount of absorption by 20% and appears to decrease incidence of dizziness or light-headedness. Maintain the same schedule for food-drug intake throughout treat-

ment period to prevent variations in serum concentration.
- Store in tightly closed, light-resistant container at 15°–30° C (59°–86° F).

ADVERSE EFFECTS (≥1%) **CNS:** *Drowsiness,* light-headedness, tiredness, dizziness, insomnia, headache, agitation, impaired memory and speech, disorientation. **CV:** *Hypotension (including orthostatic hypotension),* hypertension, syncope, shortness of breath, chest pain, tachycardia, palpitations, bradycardia, PVCs, ventricular tachycardia (short episodes of 3–4 beats). **Special Senses:** Nasal and sinus congestion, blurred vision, eye irritation, sweating or clamminess, tinnitus. **GI:** *Dry mouth,* anorexia, constipation, abdominal distress, nausea, vomiting, dysgeusia, flatulence, diarrhea. **Urogenital:** Hematuria, increased frequency, delayed urine flow, early or absent menses, male priapism, ejaculation inhibition. **Hematologic:** Anemia. **Musculoskeletal:** Skeletal aches and pains, muscle twitches. **Skin:** Skin eruptions, rash, pruritus, acne, photosensitivity. **Body as a Whole:** Weight gain or loss.

INTERACTIONS Drug: ANTIHYPERTENSIVE AGENTS may potentiate hypotensive effects; **alcohol** and other CNS DEPRESSANTS add to depressant effects; may increase **digoxin** or **phenytoin** levels; MAO INHIBITORS may precipitate hypertensive crisis; **ketoconazole, indinavir, ritonavir** may increase levels and toxicity.

PHARMACOKINETICS Absorption: Readily absorbed from GI tract. **Onset:** 1–2 wk. **Peak:** 1–2 h. **Distribution:** Distributed into breast milk. **Metabolism:** Metabolized in liver. **Elimination:** 75% excreted in urine, 25% in feces. **Half-Life:** 5–9 h.

NURSING IMPLICATIONS

Assessment & Drug Effects

- Monitor pulse rate and regularity before administration if patient has preexisting cardiac disease.
- Note: Adverse effects generally are mild and tend to decrease and disappear after the first few weeks of treatment.
- Observe patient's level of activity. If it appears to be increasing toward sleeplessness and agitation with changes in reality orientation, report to physician. Manic episodes have been reported.
- Check patient for symptoms of hypotension. If orthostatic hypotension is troublesome, suggest measures to reduce danger of falling and help patient to tolerate the effects. Discuss with physician; reduction of dose or discontinuation of the drug may be prescribed.
- Male patient should report inappropriate or prolonged penile erections. The drug may be discontinued.
- Be aware that overdose is characterized by an extension of common adverse effects: Vomiting, lethargy, drowsiness, and exaggerated anticholinergic effects. Seizures or arrhythmias are unusual.

Patient & Family Education

- Expect therapeutic response to begin in 1 wk; may require 2–4 wk to reach maximum levels. Adhere to regimen.
- Do not alter dose or intervals between doses.
- Consult physician if drowsiness becomes a distressing adverse effect. Dose regimen may be changed so that largest dose is at bedtime.
- Limit or abstain from alcohol use. The depressant effects of CNS depressants and alcohol may be potentiated by this drug.

T

- Do not self-medicate with OTC drugs for colds, allergy, or insomnia treatment without advice of physician. Many of these drugs contain CNS depressants.
- Keep follow-up appointments to permit dose adjustment or discontinuation, as indicated.
- Alert dentist, surgeon, or emergency personnel that drug is being used. Trazodone is discontinued as long as possible prior to elective surgery.
- Do not breast feed while taking this drug without consulting physician.

TREPROSTINIL SODIUM

(tre-pros'tin-il)

Remodulin

Classifications: PROSTAGLANDIN; ANTIHYPERTENSIVE; ANTIPLATELET AGENT

Prototype: Dinoprostone

Pregnancy Category: B

AVAILABILITY 1 mg/mL, 2.5 mg/mL, 5 mg/mL, 10 mg/mL injection

ACTIONS Causes direct vasodilation of the pulmonary and systemic arterial vascular beds, and inhibition of platelet aggregation. The vasodilatory effects reduce right and left ventricular afterload, and increase cardiac output and stroke volume. Also improves dyspnea, fatigue, and signs and symptoms of pulmonary arterial hypertension (PAH).

THERAPEUTIC EFFECTS Vasodilation of the arteries in the pulmonary system results in lowering of pulmonary arterial hypertension (PAH).

USES Treatment of pulmonary arterial hypertension (PAH) in patients with severe heart failure.

UNLABELED USES Severe intermittent claudication

T

CONTRAINDICATIONS Severe hepatic insufficiency; hypersensitivity to treprostinil.

CAUTIOUS USE Mild or moderate hepatic insufficiency; bleeding disorders; concurrent use of anticoagulants, NSAIDS, hypotensive drugs (e.g., diuretics, antihypertensive agents, etc.); lactation, pregnancy (category B); elderly. Safety and efficacy in children <16 y not established.

ROUTE & DOSAGE

Pulmonary Arterial Hypertension

Adult: **SC** *>16 y* 1.25 ng/kg/min. If dose is not tolerated, reduce to 0.625 ng/kg/min. Then increase rate by no more than 1.25 ng/kg/min/wk for first 4 wk, then by 2.5 ng/kg/min/wk until achieve desired response. There is little experience with doses >40 ng/kg/min

Transition from Epoprostenol to Treprostinil

Adult: **SC** *>16 y* While still receiving IV epoprostenol, initiate a dose of SC treprostinil no greater than one-half of the current epoprostenol dose (generally ≤5 ng/kg/min). Maintain treprostinil at this dose for at least 6 h. During this time, reduce the epoprostenol dose in no greater than 2 ng/kg/min decrements, based on appearance of prostacyclin-related signs and symptoms. Continue to increase treprostinil dose by no more than one-half of the current dose and maintain for 6 h while reducing epoprostenol dose by no greater than 2 ng/kg/min decrements until epoprostenol is discontinued.

ADMINISTRATION

Subcutaneous

- Initiate therapy only in a setting with adequate personnel and equipment for physiological monitoring and emergency.
- Administer Remodulin undiluted.
- Avoid abrupt withdrawal or sudden large reductions in dosage as these may lead to worsening of PAH symptom.
- Note that in patients with mild-to-moderate hepatic insufficiency, the initial dose of should be 0.625 ng/kg/min ideal body weight and should be increased cautiously.
- Store at 15°–25° C (59°–77° F).

ADVERSE EFFECTS (≥1%) **Body as a Whole:** *Jaw pain,* flushing, syncope. **CNS:** *Headache,* dizziness. **CV:** *Vasodilation,* edema, hypotension. **GI:** *Diarrhea, nausea, vomiting.* **Skin:** *Rash,* pruritus. **Other:** *Infusion site reactions (erythema, hematoma, induration, pruritus, rash, injection site pain).*

INTERACTIONS Drug: NSAIDS, ANTICOAGULANTS may increase risk of bleeding; ANTIHYPERTENSIVE AGENTS, DIURETICS, VASODILATORS may exacerbate hypotension; **ephedrine, pseudoephedrine** may antagonize antihypertensive effects. **Herbal: Ephedra, ma huang** may antagonize antihypertensive effects.

PHARMACOKINETICS Absorption: Completely absorbed from SC site. **Onset:** Steady state reached in 10 h. **Metabolism:** Extensively metabolized in liver by unknown enzyme system. **Elimination:** 79% excreted in urine, 13% excreted in feces. **Half-Life:** 2–4 h.

NURSING IMPLICATIONS

Assessment & Drug Effects

- Monitor for therapeutic effectiveness indicated by less dyspnea and fatigue, increased activity tolerance, and improved hemodynamic parameters.
- Monitor for and report symptoms of excessive response to the drug including: headache, nausea, emesis, restlessness, anxiety and infusion site pain or reaction (e.g., erythema, induration or rash). If these occur, the rate of SC infusion should be slowed.
- Monitor BP closely, especially if taking concurrent antihypertensive drugs (e.g., diuretics, vasodilators).
- Lab tests: Baseline and periodic LFTs and renal function tests. Monitor periodically coagulation parameters (more often if on concurrent anticoagulation therapy).

Patient & Family Education

- Note: Therapy with this drug may be needed for prolonged periods, possibly years.
- Report any of the following: headache, nausea, vomiting, restlessness, anxiety and infusion site pain.
- Do not breast feed while taking this drug without consulting the physician.

TRETINOIN

(tret′i-noyn)

Avita, Renova, Retin-A, Retin-A Micro, Retinoic Acid, Vesanoid, Vitamin A Acid

Classifications: SKIN AND MUCOUS MEMBRANE AGENT; ANTIACNE (RETINOID); ANTIPSORIATIC

Prototype: Isotretinoin

Pregnancy Category: B

AVAILABILITY 0.025%, 0.05%, 0.1% cream; 0.025%, 0.01% gel; 0.05% liquid; 10 mg capsules

ACTIONS Contact irritant containing retinoic acid and vitamin A

T

acid. Reverses retention hyperkeratosis and comedo formation, primary events in acne pathology. Exact mechanism of action unknown. Suggested that keratinocytes in the sebaceous follicle become less adherent and turnover of follicular epithelial cells is increased; two processes that promote easy extrusion of the comedo and prevent it from reformation. Also increases permeability of skin and supports conversion of follicular epithelium into a less sturdy, and almost fragile condition.

THERAPEUTIC EFFECTS Early treatment and control of acne vulgaris grades I–III.

USES Topical treatment of acne vulgaris grades I–III, especially during early stages when number of comedones is greatest; adjunctively in management of associated comedones and in treatment of flat warts; oral for remission induction treatment of acute promyelocytic leukemia; cream as adjunctive therapy for mitigation of fine wrinkles.

UNLABELED USES Psoriasis, senile keratosis, ichthyosis vulgaris, keratosis palmaris and plantaris, basal cell carcinoma, photodamaged skin (photoaging), and other skin conditions. **Orphan drug:** For squamous metaplasia of conjunctiva or cornea with mucous deficiency and keratinization.

CONTRAINDICATIONS Eczema; exposure to sunlight or ultraviolet rays (as with sunlamp), sunburn; pregnancy (category B).

CAUTIOUS USE Patient in an occupation necessitating considerable sun exposure or weather extremes; lactation.

ROUTE & DOSAGE

Acne

Adult: **Topical** Apply once/d h.s.

Acute Promyelocytic Leukemia

Adult: **PO** 45 mg/m^2/d

Antiwrinkle Cream

Adult: **Topical** (0.05% cream) Apply to face once daily h.s.

ADMINISTRATION

Topical

- Wait long enough for recovery if patient has been using a desquamative agent before starting treatment.
- Cleanse using a mild bland soap, and thoroughly dry areas being treated before applying drug. Avoid use of medicated, drying, or abrasive soaps and cleansers.
- Wash hands before and after treatment. Apply lightly over affected areas. Do not apply to nonaffected skin area.
- Avoid contact of drug with eyes, mouth, angles of nose, open wounds, mucous membranes.
- Store gel and liquid formulations below 30° C (86° F) and solution below 27° C (80° F).

ADVERSE EFFECTS (≥1%) **Body as a Whole: Note**–Listed adverse effects occur primarily with oral administration; only skin effects with topical administration. *Bone pain, malaise, shivering, hemorrhage, peripheral edema, pain, chest discomfort, weight gain or loss,* DIC. **CNS:** *Dizziness, paresthesias, anxiety, insomnia, depression, headache, fever, weakness, fatigue,* cerebral hemorrhage, intracranial hypertension, hallucinations. **CV:** *Arrhythmias, flushing, hypotension, hypertension,* CHF. **Special Senses:** Visual disturbances, ocular disturbances, change in visual acuity, earache. **GI:** *Nausea, vomiting, abdominal pain, diarrhea, constipation, dyspepsia, GI hemorrhage*. **Respiratory:** *Dyspnea, respiratory insufficiency, pneumonia, rales, pleural effusion, wheezing*. **Skin:** Local inflammatory reactions, transient stinging or warmth on site, *redness, scaling, severe erythema,* blistering, crusting and peeling, temporary hypopigmentation or hyperpigmentation, *increased sweating*. **Urogenital:** Renal insufficiency, dysuria, acute kidney failure.

INTERACTIONS Drug: TOPICAL ACNE MEDICATIONS (including **sulfur, resorcinol, benzoyl peroxide,** and **salicylic acid**) may increase inflammation and peeling; topical products containing **alcohol** or **menthol** may cause stinging.

PHARMACOKINETICS Absorption: Minimally absorbed from intact skin, Topical; 60% absorbed, PO. **Elimination:** About 0.1% of topical dose is excreted in urine within 24 h; 63% excreted in urine and 31% in feces, PO. **Half-Life:** 45 min, Topical; 2–2.5 h, PO.

NURSING IMPLICATIONS

Assessment & Drug Effects

- Be aware that treatment to dark-skinned individuals may cause unsightly postinflammatory hyperpigmentation; that is reversible with termination of drug treatment.
- Clinical response should be evident in 2–3 wk; complete and satisfactory response (in 75% of the patients) may require 3–4 mo. Once achieved, control is maintained by less frequent applications or a change in formulation or dosage.

Patient & Family Education

- Be aware that erythema and desquamation during the first 1–3 wk of treatment do not represent exacerbation of the skin problem but a probable response to the drug from deep previously unseen lesions.
- As treatment is continued, lesions gradually disappear, leaving an inflammatory background; scaling and redness decrease after 8–10 wk of therapy.
- Wash face no more often than 2–3 times daily.
- Do not use topical preparations with high concentrations of alcohol, astringents, spices or lime, perfumes and shaving lotions during treatment period.
- Be aware that drug is not curative; relapses commonly occur within 3–6 wk after treatment has been discontinued.
- Remove nonmedicated cosmetics thoroughly before drug is applied.
- Avoid exposure to sun; when cannot be avoided, use a SPF 15 or higher sunscreen.
- Do not self-medicate with additional acne treatment because of danger of drug interactions.
- Do not breast feed while using or taking this drug without consulting physician.

T

TRIAMCINOLONE

(trye-am-sin′oh-lone)

Aristocort, Atolone, Kenacort, Kenalog-E

TRIAMCINOLONE ACETONIDE

Azmacort, Cenocort A_2, Kenalog, Nasacort HFA, Triam-A, Triamonide, Tri-kort, Trilog, Tri-Nasal

TRIAMCINOLONE DIACETATE

Amcort, Aristocort Forte, Articulose LA, Cenocort Forte, Kenacort, Triam-Forte, Trilone, Tristoject

TRIAMCINOLONE HEXACETONIDE

Aristospan

Classifications: HORMONES & SYNTHETIC SUBSTITUTES; ADRENAL CORTICOSTEROID; GLUCOCORTICOID; ANTI-INFLAMMATORY

Prototype: Prednisone

Pregnancy Category: C

AVAILABILITY **Triamcinolone** 4 mg, 8 mg tablets; 4 mg/5 mL syrup **Triamcinolone acetonide** 3 mg/mL, 10 mg/mL, 40 mg/mL injection; 100 mcg aerosol; 55 mcg inhaler; 55 mcg spray; 0.5 mg/mL nasal spray; 0.025%, 0.1%, 0.5% cream, ointment, lotion; 10.3% topical spray **Triamcinolone diacetate** 25 mg/mL, 40 mg/mL injection **Triamcinolone hexacetonide** 5 mg/mL, 20 mg/mL injection.

ACTIONS Immediate acting synthetic fluorinated adrenal corticosteroid with glucocorticoid and antirheumatic activity 7–13 times more potent than that of hydrocortisone. Possesses minimal sodium and water retention properties in therapeutic doses.

THERAPEUTIC EFFECTS Antiinflammatory and immunosuppressant drug that is effective in the treatment of bronchial asthma.

USES An inflammatory or immunosuppressant agent. Orally inhaled: bronchial asthma in patient who has not responded to conventional inhalation treatment. Therapeutic doses do not appear to suppress HPA (hypothalamic-pituitary-adrenal) axis.

CONTRAINDICATIONS Safety during pregnancy (category C), lactation, or in children <6 y is not established. Kidney dysfunction; glaucoma. Also see hydrocortisone.

CAUTIOUS USE Coagulopathy, hemophilia, diabetes mellitus, GI disease; congestive heart failure; herpes infection; infection; inflammatory bowel disease; myasthenia gravis; MI; ocular exposure, ocular infection; osteoporosis; peptic ulcer disease; PVD; skin abrasion.

ROUTE & DOSAGE

Inflammation, Immunosuppression

Adult: **PO/IM/SC** 4–48 mg/d in divided doses **Intraarticular/Intradermal** 4–48 mg/d **Inhaled** 2–4 inhalations q.i.d. **Topical** See Appendix A

Child: **PO/IM/SC** 3.3–50 mg/m^2/d in divided doses **Intraarticular/Intradermal** 3.3–50 mg/m^2/d

Acetonide

Adult: **IM** 60 mg, may repeat with 20–100 mg q6wk **Intradermal** 1 mg per injection site (max: 30 mg total) **Intraarticular** 2.5–4.0 mg **Inhalation** See Appendix A

Child: **IM** *6–12 y,* 0.03–0.2 mg q1–7d **Inhalation** See Appendix A

Diacetate

Adult: **PO** 4–48 mg/d in 1–4 divided doses **IM** 40 mg once/wk **Intradermal** 5–48 mg (max: 75 mg/wk), may repeat q1–2wk if needed **Intraarticular** 2–40 mg q1–8wk

Child: **PO** 0.117–1.66 mg/kg/d

Hexacetonide

Adult: **Intralesional** Up to 0.5 mg/in^2 of skin **Intraarticular** 2–20 mg q3–4wk

ADMINISTRATION

Oral

- Give with fluid of patient's choice; tablet may be crushed.

Subcutaneous/Intramuscular

- Do not give triamcinolone injection IV.
- See hydrocortisone for additional administration information.
- Store at 15°–30° C (59°–86° F). Protect from light.

ADVERSE EFFECTS (≥1%) **CNS:** Euphoria, headache, insomnia, confusion, psychosis. **CV:** CHF, edema. **GI:** Nausea, vomiting, peptic ulcer. **Musculoskeletal:** Muscle weakness, delayed wound healing, muscle wasting, osteoporosis, aseptic necrosis of bone, spontaneous fractures. **Endocrine:** Cushingoid features, growth suppression in children, carbohydrate intolerance, hyperglycemia. **Special Senses:** Cataracts. **Hematologic:** Leukocytosis. **Metabolic:** Hypokalemia. **Skin:** Burning, itching, folliculitis, hypertrichosis, hypopigmentation.

INTERACTIONS Drug: BARBITURATES, **phenytoin, rifampin** increase steroid metabolism—may need increased doses of triamcinolone; **amphotericin B,** DIURETICS add to potassium loss; **ambenonium, neostigmine, pyridostigmine** may cause severe muscle weakness in patients with myasthenia gravis; may inhibit antibody response to VACCINES, TOXOIDS.

PHARMACOKINETICS Absorption: Readily absorbed from all routes. **Onset:** 24–48 h PO, IM. **Peak:** 1–2 h PO; 8–10 h IM. **Duration:** 2.25 d PO; 1–6 wk IM. **Metabolism:** Metabolized in liver. **Elimination:** Excreted in urine. **Half-Life:** 2–5 h; HPA suppression, 18–36 h.

NURSING IMPLICATIONS

Assessment & Drug Effects

- Discuss adequate diet with dietitian, patient, and physician to counter natriuresis, negative nitrogen balance, with weight loss in most patients (along with headache, fatigue, and dizziness) and sodium retention with weight gain and moon facies in others. High-protein, high-potassium diet is often needed.
- Lab tests: Periodic serum electrolytes and blood glucose.
- Discontinue occlusive dressing and start appropriate antimicrobial treatment if a local infection develops at site of application. Consult physician.
- Report symptoms of hypercortisolism or Cushing's syndrome (see Appendix F), hyperglycemia (see Appendix F), and glucosuria (e.g., polyuria). These may arise from systemic absorption after topical application, especially in children and if used over extensive areas for prolonged periods or if occlusive dressings are used.

Patient & Family Education

- Be aware that postural hypotension may accompany sodium loss and weight loss.
- Adhere to drug regimen; do not increase or decrease established regimen and do not discontinue abruptly.
- Do not breast feed while using or taking this drug without consulting physician.

T

TRIAMTERENE

(trye-am′ter-een)

Dyrenium

Classifications: FLUID AND WATER BALANCE AGENT; POTASSIUM-SPARING DIURETIC

Prototype: Spironolactone

Pregnancy Category: B

AVAILABILITY 50 mg, 100 mg capsules

ACTIONS Structurally related to folic acid. Like spironolactone has weak diuretic action and a potassium-sparing effect. Promotes excretion of sodium, chloride (to lesser extent), and carbonate. Unlike spironolactone, blocks potassium excretion by direct action on distal renal tubule rather than by inhibiting aldosterone. Decreased glomerular filtration rate and elevated BUN are associated with daily administration.

THERAPEUTIC EFFECTS Weak diuretic action and a potassium-sparing effect.

USES Adjunct in the management of edema associated with CHF, hepatic cirrhosis, nephrotic syndrome, idiopathic edema, steroid-induced edema, and edema due to secondary hyperaldosteronism. Also alone or in conjunction with a thiazide or loop diuretic in patients with hypertension because of its potassium-sparing activity.

CONTRAINDICATIONS Hypersensitivity to drug; anuria, severe or progressive kidney disease or dysfunction; severe liver disease; elevated serum potassium. Safety during pregnancy (category B) or lactation is not established.

CAUTIOUS USE Impaired kidney or liver function; history of gouty arthritis; diabetes mellitus, history of kidney stones.

ROUTE & DOSAGE

Edema

Adult: **PO** 100 mg b.i.d. (max: 300 mg/d), may be able to decrease to 100 mg/d or q.o.d.
Geriatric: **PO** 50 mg/d (max: 100 mg/d in 1–2 divided doses)
Child: **PO** 2–4 mg/kg/d in divided doses or q.o.d. (max: 300 mg/d)

ADMINISTRATION

Oral

- Empty capsule and give with fluid or mix with food, if patient cannot swallow capsule.
- Give drug with or after meals to prevent or minimize nausea.
- Schedule doses to prevent interruption of sleep from diuresis (e.g., with or after breakfast if a single dose is taken, or no later than 6 p.m. if more than one dose is prescribed). Consult physician.
- Withdraw drug gradually in patients on prolonged or high-dose therapy in order to prevent rebound increased urinary excretion of potassium.
- Store in tight, light-resistant containers at 15°–30° C (59°–86° F) unless otherwise directed.

ADVERSE EFFECTS (≥1%) **GI:** Diarrhea, nausea, vomiting, and other GI disturbances. **CNS:** Dizziness, headache, dry mouth, <u>anaphylaxis</u>, weakness, muscle cramps. **Skin:** Pruritus, rash, photosensitivity. **CV:** Hypotension (large doses). **Metabolic:** *Hyperkalemia* and other electrolyte imbalances, elevated BUN, elevated uric acid (patients predisposed to gouty arthritis), hyperchloremic acidosis. **Hematologic:** Blood dyscrasias: granulocytopenia, eosinophilia, megaloblastic anemia in patients with reduced folic acid stores (e.g., hepatic cirrhosis).

DIAGNOSTIC TEST INTERFERENCE Pale blue fluorescence in urine interferes with ***fluorometric assay*** of ***quinidine*** and ***lactic dehydrogenase activity.*** Triamterene may cause increases in ***blood glucose*** levels (diabetic patients), ***BUN, se-***

rum potassium, magnesium, and ***uric acid*** and ***urinary calcium excretion.***

INTERACTIONS Drug: May increase **lithium** levels, thus increasing its toxicity; **indomethacin** may decrease renal elimination of triamterene; ANGIOTENSIN-CONVERTING ENZYME (ACE) INHIBITORS, other POTASSIUM-SPARING DIURETICS may cause hyperkalemia.

PHARMACOKINETICS Absorption: Rapidly but variably absorbed from GI tract. **Onset:** 2–4 h. **Duration:** 7–9 h. **Metabolism:** Metabolized in liver to active and inactive metabolites. **Elimination:** Excreted in urine. **Half-Life:** 100–150 min.

NURSING IMPLICATIONS

Assessment & Drug Effects

- Monitor BP during periods of dosage adjustment. Hypotensive reactions, although rare, have been reported. Take care with ambulation, particularly for older adults.
- Weigh patient under standard conditions, prior to drug initiation and daily during therapy.
- Diuretic response usually occurs on first day of therapy; maximum effect may not occur for several days.
- Monitor and report oliguria and unusual changes in I&O ratio. Consult physician regarding allowable fluid intake.
- Be alert for S&S of kidney stone formation; reported in patients taking high doses or who have low urine volume and increased urine acidity.
- Lab tests: Obtain baseline and periodic determinations of serum potassium and other electrolytes. Obtain periodic kidney function (BUN, serum creatinine) in patients with known or suspected renal insufficiency. Obtain periodic blood studies in patients on prolonged therapy or with cirrhosis since both are prone to develop megaloblastic anemia.
- Observe for S&S of hyperkalemia (see Appendix F), particularly in patients with renal insufficiency, on high-dose or prolonged therapy, older adults, and those with diabetes.
- Do not give to a diabetic patient unless blood glucose is controlled because triamterene may increase blood glucose. Monitor patients closely.

Patient & Family Education

- Do not take potassium supplements, potassium-rich diet, and salt substitutes; unlike most diuretics, triamterene promotes potassium retention.
- Do not restrict salt; there is a possibility of low-salt syndrome (hyponatremia). Consult physician.
- Report overpowering fatigue or weakness, malaise, fever, sore throat, or mouth (possible symptoms of granulocytopenia) and unusual bleeding or bruising (thrombocytopenia) to physician.
- Be aware that drug may cause photosensitivity; avoid exposure to sun and sunlamps.
- Drug may impart a harmless pale blue fluorescence to urine.
- Do not breast feed while taking this drug without consulting physician.

T

TRIAZOLAM

(trye-ay'zoe-lam)

Halcion

Classifications: CENTRAL NERVOUS SYSTEM AGENT; BENZODIAZEPINE; ANXIOLYTIC; SEDATIVE-HYPNOTIC

Prototype: Lorazepam

Pregnancy Category: X

Controlled Substance: Schedule IV

AVAILABILITY 0.125 mg, 0.25 mg tablets

ACTIONS Benzodiazepine derivative with hypnotic effects with fewer residual daytime effects. Its blockade of cortical and limbic arousal results in hypnotic activity.
THERAPEUTIC EFFECTS Drug-induced effects on sleep include decreased sleep latency and number of nocturnal awakenings, decreased total nocturnal wake time, and increased duration of sleep.

USES Short-term management of insomnia characterized by difficulty in falling asleep, frequent wakeful periods. Following long-term use, tolerance or adaptation may develop.

CONTRAINDICATIONS Hypersensitivity to triazolam and benzodiazepines; pregnancy (category X), lactation; concurrent administration with the following medications which impair cytochrome P450 3A (e.g. ketoconazole, itraconazole, and nefazodone.
CAUTIOUS USE Depression; older adults and debilitated patients; patients with suicidal tendency; impaired kidney or liver function; chronic pulmonary insufficiency; sleep apnea.

ROUTE & DOSAGE

Insomnia
Adult: **PO** 0.125–0.25 mg h.s. (max: 0.5 mg/d)
Geriatric: **PO** 0.0625–0.125 mg h.s.

ADMINISTRATION

Oral
- Give immediately before bed; onset of drug action is rapid.
- Do not exceed recommended doses.
- Store at 15°–30° C (59°–86° F).

ADVERSE EFFECTS (≥1%) **CNS:** *Drowsiness,* light-headedness, headache, dizziness, ataxia, visual disturbances, confusional states, *memory impairment, "rebound insomnia," anterograde amnesia,* paradoxical reactions, minor changes in EEG patterns. **GI:** Nausea, vomiting, constipation.

INTERACTIONS Drug: Alcohol, CNS DEPRESSANTS, ANTICONVULSANTS, **nefazodone,** BENZODIAZEPINES potentiate CNS depression; **cimetidine** increases triazolam plasma levels, thus increasing its toxicity; may decrease antiparkinsonism effects of **levodopa**. **Herbal: Kava-kava, valerian** may potentiate sedation.

PHARMACOKINETICS Absorption: Readily absorbed from GI tract. **Onset:** 15–30 min. **Peak:** 1–2 h. **Duration:** 6–8 h. **Distribution:** Crosses placenta; distributed into breast milk. **Metabolism:** Metabolized in liver to active metabolites. **Elimination:** Excreted in urine. **Half-Life:** 2–3 h.

NURSING IMPLICATIONS

Assessment & Drug Effects
- Be aware that signs of developing tolerance or adaptation (with long-term use) include increased daytime anxiety, increased wakefulness during last one third of the night.
- Lab tests: Obtain periodic blood counts, urinalysis, and blood chemistries during long-term use.
- Do not use with addiction-prone patients (drug addicts, alcoholics) unless careful surveillance by health personnel is available. Habituation and dependence can occur.
- Evaluate smoking habit. As with other benzodiazepines, smoking may decrease hypnotic effects.

- Monitor for symptoms of overdosage: Slurred speech, somnolence, confusion, impaired coordination, and coma.

Patient & Family Education

- Do not drive or engage in potentially hazardous activities until response to drug is known.
- Avoid use of alcohol or other CNS depressants while on this drug; they may increase sedative effects.
- Do not stop taking drug suddenly, especially if you are subject to seizures. Withdrawal symptoms may occur and range from mild dysphoria to more serious symptoms (e.g., tremors, abdominal and muscle cramps, convulsions). Consult physician for schedule to discontinue therapy.
- Do not increase dose without physician's advice because of toxic potential of drug.
- Do not breast feed while taking this drug.

TRICHLORMETHIAZIDE

(trye-klor-meth-eye'a-zide)

Diurese, Metahydrin, Naqua, Niazide, Trichlorex

Classifications: FLUID AND WATER BALANCE AGENT; THIAZIDE DIURETIC; ANTIHYPERTENSIVE

Prototype: Hydrochlorothiazide

Pregnancy Category: B

AVAILABILITY 2 mg, 4 mg tablets

ACTIONS Benzothiadiazine (thiazide) derivative. Similar to hydrochlorothiazide. Diuretic effect associated with drug interference with transport of sodium ions across renal tubular epithelium, which enhances excretion of sodium, chloride, potassium, bicarbonate, and water. Site of drug action is the cortical dilution segment of the nephron.

THERAPEUTIC EFFECTS Loss of fluid and sodium results in antihypertensive effect.

USES To treat hypertension as sole agent or to enhance the effects of another antihypertensive when given in combination. Also to treat edema associated with CHF, renal decompensation, and hepatic cirrhosis.

CONTRAINDICATIONS Anuria; hypersensitivity to thiazides, sulfonamides; pregnancy (category B), lactation.

CAUTIOUS USE History of allergy; kidney and liver disease; gout; diabetes mellitus.

ROUTE & DOSAGE

Edema

Adult: **PO** 1–4 mg 1–2 times/d

Hypertension

Adult: **PO** 2–4 mg/d in 1–2 divided doses

Child: **PO** 0.07 mg/kg/d in 1–2 divided doses

ADMINISTRATION

Oral

- Give early in a.m. after breakfast to reduce gastric irritation and prevent interruption of sleep because of diuresis. If 2 doses are ordered, schedule second dose no later than 3 p.m.
- Store in tightly closed container at 15°–30° C (59°–86° F) unless otherwise instructed.

ADVERSE EFFECTS (≥1%) **CNS:** Mood changes, unusual tiredness or weakness, dizziness, light-headedness, paresthesias. **CV:** Irregular heartbeat, weak pulse, orthostatic hypotension, vasculitis. **GI:** Dry mouth, increased thirst, nausea, vomiting, anorexia, diarrhea, pan-

T

creatitis, jaundice. **Hematologic:** Agranulocytosis, thrombocytopenia, aplastic anemia, leukopenia. **Metabolic:** *Hyperglycemia,* glycosuria, *hyperuricemia, hypokalemia,* exacerbation of gout, SLE. **Body as a Whole:** Hypersensitivity reactions, muscle spasm. **Skin:** Photosensitivity. **Special Senses:** Blurred vision, yellow vision (xanthopsia).

INTERACTIONS Drug: Amphotericin B, CORTICOSTEROIDS increase hypokalemic effects; may antagonize hypoglycemic effects of SULFONYLUREAS, **insulin; cholestyramine, colestipol** decrease thiazide absorption; intensifies hypoglycemic and hypotensive effects of **diazoxide;** increased **potassium** and **magnesium** loss with **digoxin**—may cause **digoxin** toxicity; decreases **lithium** excretion, thus increasing its toxicity; NSAIDS may attenuate diuresis—risk of NSAID-induced kidney failure increased.

PHARMACOKINETICS Onset: 2 h. **Peak:** 6 h. **Duration:** 24 h. **Distribution:** Crosses placenta; distributed into breast milk. **Elimination:** Excreted in urine.

NURSING IMPLICATIONS

Assessment & Drug Effects

- Monitor BP and I&O ratio during first phase of antihypertensive therapy. Report a sudden fall in BP, which may initiate severe postural hypotension and potentially dangerous perfusion problems, especially in the extremities.
- Note: Antihypertensive effects may be noted in 3–4 d; maximal effects may require 3–4 wk.
- Monitor older adult patients closely; they may be more sensitive to average adult dose.
- Lab tests: Periodic serum electrolytes, blood glucose, CBC with differential, and platelet count.
- Monitor patient for S&S of hypokalemia (see Appendix F) and report promptly. Hypokalemia is rarely severe in most patients even on long-term therapy, but older adults are especially susceptible.
- Monitor diabetics for loss of glycemic control or early signs of hyperglycemia (e.g., drowsiness, polyuria, anorexia, polydipsia).

Patient & Family Education

- Eat a balanced diet (usually includes potassium-rich foods such as fruits and fruit juices) to prevent onset of hypokalemia.
- Avoid OTC drugs unless approved by the physician. Many preparations contain both potassium and sodium and misused can induce electrolyte imbalance adverse effects.
- Maintain prescribed dosage regimen, do not skip, reduce, or double doses or change dose intervals.
- Do not breast feed while taking this drug.

TRIFLUOPERAZINE HYDROCHLORIDE

(trye-floo-oh-per'a-zeen)

Novoflurazine ✦, Solazine ✦, Stelazine, Terfluzine ✦

Classifications: CENTRAL NERVOUS SYSTEM AGENT; PSYCHOTHERAPEUTIC; ANTIPSYCHOTIC PHENOTHIAZINE

Prototype: Chlorpromazine

Pregnancy Category: C

AVAILABILITY 1 mg, 2 mg, 5 mg, 10 mg tablets; 10 mg/mL liquid; 2 mg/mL injection

ACTIONS Phenothiazine similar to chlorpromazine. Produces less sedative, cardiovascular, and anticholinergic effects and more prominent antiemetic and extrapyramidal effects than other phenothiazines.

Antipsychotic effects thought related to blockade of postsynaptic dopamine receptors in the brain.
THERAPEUTIC EFFECTS Indicated by increase in mental and physical activity. Strong antipsychotic drug with more prolonged pharmacologic effects than that of chlorpromazine.

USES Management of manifestations of psychotic disorders; "possibly effective" control of excessive anxiety and tension associated with neuroses or somatic conditions.

CONTRAINDICATIONS Hypersensitivity to phenothiazines; comatose states; CNS depression; blood dyscrasias; children <6 y; bone marrow depression; preexisting liver disease; pregnancy (category C), lactation.
CAUTIOUS USE Previously detected breast cancer; compromised respiratory function; seizure disorders.

ROUTE & DOSAGE

Psychotic Disorders
Adult: **PO** 1–2 mg b.i.d., may increase up to 20 mg/d in hospitalized patients **IM** 1–2 mg q4–6h (max: 10 mg/d)
Child: **PO** *6–12 y,* 1 mg 1–2 times/d, may increase up to 15 mg/d in hospitalized patients **IM** *6–12 y,* 1 mg 1–2 times/d, may increase up to 15 mg/d

Dementia Behavior
Geriatric: **PO** 0.5–1 mg 1–2 times/d, may increase q4–7d (max: 40 mg in divided doses) **IM** 1 mg q4–6h (max: 6 mg/d)

ADMINISTRATION

Oral
- Separate antacid and phenothiazine doses by at least 2 h.
- Dilute oral concentrate just before administration with about 60–120 mL suitable diluent (e.g., water, fruit juices, carbonated beverage, milk, soups, puddings). Avoid coffee or tea near time of taking oral preparation. Explain dosage and dilution to patient if drug is to be self-administered.
- Crush tablet and give with fluid or mix with food if patient will not or cannot swallow pill.
- Monitor ingestion of tablet to ensure that patient does not hoard medication.

Intramuscular
- Give IM injection deep into upper outer quadrant of buttock.
- Note: Slight yellow discoloration of injectable drug reportedly does not alter potency. If color is markedly changed, discard solution.
- Wash hands if undiluted concentrate is spilled on skin to prevent contact dermatosis.
- Store in light-resistant container at 15°–30° C (59°–86° F) unless otherwise directed.

ADVERSE EFFECTS (≥1%) **CNS:** *Drowsiness,* insomnia, dizziness, agitation, *extrapyramidal effects,* neuroleptic malignant syndrome. **Special Senses:** Nasal congestion, *dry mouth,* blurred vision, pigmentary retinopathy. **Hematologic:** Agranulocytosis. **Skin:** Photosensitivity, skin rash, sweating. **GI:** Constipation. **CV:** Tachycardia, *hypotension.* **Respiratory:** Depressed cough reflex. **Endocrine:** Gynecomastia, galactorrhea.

INTERACTIONS Drug: Alcohol and other CNS DEPRESSANTS add to CNS depression. **Herbal: Kava-kava** may increase risk and severity of dystonic reactions.

PHARMACOKINETICS Absorption: Well absorbed from GI tract. **Onset:** Rapid onset. **Peak:** 2–3 h. **Duration:** Up to 12 h. **Metabolism:** Metabolized in liver. **Elimination:** Excreted in bile and feces.

NURSING IMPLICATIONS

Assessment & Drug Effects

- Monitor HR and BP. Hypotension is a common adverse effect.
- Hypotension and extrapyramidal effects (especially akathisia and dystonia) are most likely to occur in patients receiving high doses or parenteral administration and in older adults. Withhold drug and notify physician if patient has dysphagia, neck muscle spasm, or if tongue protrusion occurs.
- Monitor I&O ratio and bowel elimination pattern. Check for abdominal distention and pain. Encourage adequate fluid intake as prophylaxis for constipation and xerostomia. The depressed patient may not seek help for either symptom or for urinary retention.
- Be aware that since trifluoperazine potentiates analgesics, its use may reduce amount of narcotic required in painful long-term illness such as cancer.
- Agitation, jitteriness, and sometimes insomnia may simulate original neurotic or psychotic symptoms. These adverse effects may disappear spontaneously.
- Expect maximum therapeutic response within 2–3 wk after initiation of therapy.

Patient & Family Education

- Take drug as prescribed; do not alter dosing regimen or stop medication without consulting physician.
- Consult physician about use of any OTC drugs during therapy.
- Do not take alcohol and other depressants during therapy.
- Avoid potentially hazardous activities such as driving or operating machinery, until response to drug is known. Drowsiness and dizziness may be prominent during this time.
- Cover as much skin surface as possible with clothing when you must be in direct sunlight. Use a SPF >12 sunscreen on exposed skin.
- Urine may be discolored or reddish brown and this is harmless.
- Do not breast feed while taking this drug.

TRIFLURIDINE

(trye-flure'i-deen)

Viroptic

Classifications: ANTIINFECTIVE; ANTIVIRAL

Prototype: Acyclovir

Pregnancy Category: C

AVAILABILITY 1% ophthalmic solution

ACTIONS Pyrimidine nucleoside whose mechanism of antiviral action is not completely known but appears to involve inhibition of viral DNA synthesis and viral replication.

THERAPEUTIC EFFECTS Active against herpes simplex virus (HSV) types 1 and 2, vaccinia virus, and certain strains of *Adenovirus*. Not effective against bacteria, fungi, or *Chlamydia*.

USES Topically to eyes for treatment of primary keratoconjunctivitis and recurring epithelial keratitis caused by herpes simplex virus types 1 and 2. Also for other herpetic ophthalmic infections including stromal keratitis, uveitis, and for infections caused by vaccinia and *Adenovirus*, but clinical effectiveness has not been established.

CONTRAINDICATIONS Safety during pregnancy (category C) or lactation is not established.

CAUTIOUS USE Dry eye syndrome.

ROUTE & DOSAGE

Viral Infections of Eye

Adult: **Ophthalmic** 1 drop 1% ophthalmic solution into affected eye q2h during waking hours until healing (reepithelialization) has occurred (max: 9 drops/d); when healing appears to be complete, dosage reduced to 1 drop q4h during waking hours for an additional 7 d (max: 5 drops/d); continuous administration beyond 21 d not recommended

ADMINISTRATION

Instillation

- Wait several minutes between applications when used concurrently with other eye drops.
- Store refrigerated at 2°–8° C (36°–46° F) unless otherwise directed.

ADVERSE EFFECTS (≥1%) **Special Senses:** Mild transient burning or stinging, mild irritation of conjunctiva or cornea, photophobia, edema of eyelids and cornea, punctal occlusion, superficial punctate keratopathy, epithelial keratopathy, stromal edema, keratitis sicca, hyperemia, increased intraocular pressure.

INTERACTIONS Drug: No clinically significant interactions established.

PHARMACOKINETICS Absorption: Following topical application to eye, trifluridine penetrates cornea and aqueous humor (inflammation enhances penetration). Systemic absorption does not appear to be significant.

NURSING IMPLICATIONS

Assessment & Drug Effects

- Expect epithelial eye infections to respond to therapy within 2–7 d, with complete healing occurring in 1–2 wk.

Patient & Family Education

- Inform physician of progress and keep follow-up appointments. Herpetic eye infections have a tendency to recur and can lead to corneal damage if not adequately treated.
- Do not breast feed while taking this drug without consulting physician.

TRIHEXYPHENIDYL HYDROCHLORIDE

(trye-hex-ee-fen′i-dill)

Aparkane ♣, Apo-Trihex ♣, Novohexidyl ♣, Trihexy

Classifications: AUTONOMIC NERVOUS SYSTEM AGENT; ANTICHOLINERGIC (PARASYMPATHOLYTIC); ANTIPARKINSONISM AGENT; ANTI-MUSCARINIC; ANTISPASMODIC

Prototype: Atropine

Pregnancy Category: C

AVAILABILITY 2 mg, 5 mg tablets; 5 mg sustained release capsules; 2 mg/5 mL elixir

ACTIONS Synthetic tertiary amine anticholinergic agent similar to atropine. Thought to act by blocking excess of acetylcholine at certain cerebral synaptic sites. Relaxes smooth muscle by direct effect and by atropinelike blocking action on the parasympathetic nervous system.

THERAPEUTIC EFFECTS Anticholinergic agent diminishes the characteristic tremor of Parkinson's disease. Antispasmodic action appears to be one-half that of atropine.

USES Symptomatic treatment of all forms of parkinsonism (arteriosclerotic, idiopathic, postencephalitic). Also to prevent or control drug-induced extrapyramidal disorders.

T

UNLABELED USES Huntington's chorea, spasmodic torticollis.

CONTRAINDICATIONS Narrow-angle glaucoma. Safety during pregnancy (category C), lactation, or in children is not established.

CAUTIOUS USE History of drug hypersensitivities; arteriosclerosis; hypertension; cardiac disease, kidney or liver disorders; obstructive diseases of GI or genitourinary tracts; older adults with prostatic hypertrophy.

ROUTE & DOSAGE

Parkinsonism

Adult: **PO** 1 mg day 1, 2 mg day 2, then increase by 2 mg q3–5d up to 6–10 mg/d in 3 or more divided doses (max: 15 mg/d)

Extrapyramidal Effects

Adult: **PO** 5–15 mg/d in divided doses

ADMINISTRATION

Oral

- Give before or after meals, depending on how patient reacts. Older adults and patients prone to excessive salivation (e.g., postencephalitic parkinsonism) may prefer to take drug after meals. If drug causes excessive mouth dryness, it may be better given before meals, unless it causes nausea.
- Once stabilized on conventional dosage forms, patient may be switched to sustained-release capsules to permit once- or twice-a-day dosing.
- Do not crush or chew sustained-release capsules. These must be swallowed whole.
- Store at 15°–30° C (59°–86° F) in tight container unless otherwise directed.

ADVERSE EFFECTS (≥1%) **GI:** *Dry mouth, nausea,* constipation. **Special Senses:** *Blurred vision,* mydriasis, photophobia, angle-closure glaucoma. **Urogenital:** Urinary hesitancy or retention. **CNS:** *Dizziness, nervousness,* insomnia, drowsiness, confusion, agitation, delirium, psychotic manifestations, euphoria. **CV:** Tachycardia, palpitations, hypotension, orthostatic hypotension. **Body as a Whole:** Hypersensitivity reactions.

INTERACTIONS Drug: Reduces therapeutic effects of **chlorpromazine, haloperidol,** PHENOTHIAZINES; increases bioavailability of **digoxin;** MAO INHIBITORS potentiate actions of trihexyphenidyl.

PHARMACOKINETICS Absorption: Readily absorbed from GI tract. **Onset:** Within 1 h. **Peak:** 2–3 h. **Duration:** 6–12 h. **Elimination:** Excreted in urine.

NURSING IMPLICATIONS

Assessment & Drug Effects

- Be aware that incidence and severity of adverse effects are usually dose related and may be minimized by dosage reduction. Older adults appear more sensitive to usual adult doses.
- Monitor vital signs. Pulse is a particularly sensitive indicator of response to drug. Report tachycardia, palpitations, paradoxical bradycardia, or fall in BP.
- Assess for and report severe CNS stimulation (see ADVERSE EFFECTS) that occurs with high doses, and in patients with arteriosclerosis, or those with history of hypersensitivity to other drugs.
- In patients with severe rigidity, tremors may appear to be accentuated during therapy as rigidity diminishes.

- Monitor daily I&O if patient develops urinary hesitancy or retention. Voiding before taking drug may relieve problem.
- Check for abdominal distention and bowel sounds if constipation is a problem.
- Monitor intraocular pressure at regular intervals.
- Provide close follow-up care. Tolerance may develop, necessitating dosage adjustment or use of combination therapy. Patients ≥60 y frequently develop sensitivity to drug action.

Patient & Family Education
- Learn measures to relieve drug-induced dry mouth; rinse mouth frequently with water and suck ice chips, sugarless gum, or hard candy. Maintain adequate total daily fluid intake.
- Avoid excessive heat because drug suppresses perspiration and, therefore, heat loss.
- Do not to engage in potentially hazardous activities requiring alertness and skill. Drug causes dizziness, drowsiness, and blurred vision. Help walking may be indicated.
- Do not breast feed while taking this drug without consulting physician.

TRIMETHAPHAN CAMSYLATE

(trye-meth'a-fan)
Arfonad
Classifications: CARDIOVASCULAR AGENT; NONNITRATE VASODILATOR; ANTIHYPERTENSIVE
Prototype: Hydralazine
Pregnancy Category: X

AVAILABILITY 50 mg/mL injection

ACTIONS Potent, short-acting ganglionic blocking agent. Blocks transmission in both adrenergic and cholinergic ganglia by competing with acetylcholine for receptor sites on postganglionic membranes. Adrenergic blockade results in vasodilation, improved peripheral blood flow, and thus decrease in BP.
THERAPEUTIC EFFECTS Direct peripheral vasodilation action produces marked hypotension. BP is significantly lower in head-up position because venous dilation and peripheral pooling reduce cardiac output.

USES To produce controlled hypotension for certain surgical procedures (e.g., neurologic, ophthalmic, and plastic surgery) and for short-term treatment of hypertensive crises associated with pulmonary edema.
UNLABELED USES Acute dissecting aneurysm of aorta and ischemic heart disease.

CONTRAINDICATIONS Anemia, hypovolemia, shock; asphyxia, respiratory insufficiency; glaucoma; pregnancy (category X), lactation.
CAUTIOUS USE History of allergy; older adults and debilitated patients, children; cardiac disease, arteriosclerosis; liver or kidney disease; degenerative CNS disease; Addison's disease; diabetes mellitus; patients receiving steroids, antihypertensives, anesthetics (especially spinal), and diuretics.

ROUTE & DOSAGE

Controlled Hypotension, Short-Term Treatment of Hypertensive Crisis

Adult: **IV** Dilute 500 mg in 500 mL of 5% dextrose, infuse at 0.5–1 mg/min with gradual increase until BP control is achieved
Child: **IV** 50–150 mcg/kg/min at a rate of 0.3–6 mg/min

T

ADMINISTRATION

Intravenous

PREPARE: **IV Infusion:** Dilute one 10 mL ampule (500 mg) in 500 mL of D5W, NS, or RL to yield 1 mg/mL.

ADMINISTER: **IV Infusion:** Start at 3–4 mL (3–4 mg)/min and then adjust to maintain desired effect. IV flow rate is usually prescribed by physician to maintain desired BP level. Rate of infusion should be monitored constantly. Individuals vary considerably in response to drug.

INCOMPATIBILITIES **Solution/additive: Tubocurarine.**

■ Use of an infusion pump, microdrip regulator, or similar device is recommended for precise measurement of flow rate. ■ Terminate infusion gradually while BP is closely monitored. It is stopped before wound closure in surgery to allow BP to return to normal.

■ Stable when refrigerated, avoid freezing. Diluted solution (500 mg/500 mL) is stable at room temperature for 24 h. Store at 15°–30° C (59°–86° F).

ADVERSE EFFECTS (≥1%) **CV:** Tachycardia or decrease in heart rate, orthostatic hypotension, angina. **GI:** Nausea, vomiting, anorexia. **Skin:** Urticaria, pruritus, histamine-like reaction along course of vein. **Urogenital:** Atony of urinary bladder or GI tract, urinary retention. **Special Senses:** Cycloplegia, mydriasis. **Body as a Whole:** Dry mouth, suppression of perspiration, restlessness, extreme weakness. **Respiratory:** <u>Respiratory depression, respiratory arrest (following large doses)</u>.

DIAGNOSTIC TEST INTERFERENCE Trimethaphan may decrease ***serum potassium*** and may prevent elevation of ***blood glucose*** that usually occurs during postoperative period.

INTERACTIONS Drug: DIURETICS, ANESTHETICS, **procainamide** add to hypotensive effects.

PHARMACOKINETICS Onset: Immediate. **Duration:** 10 min. **Distribution:** Crosses placenta. **Metabolism:** Metabolized by pseudocholinesterases in plasma. **Elimination:** Excreted in urine.

NURSING IMPLICATIONS

Assessment & Drug Effects

- Assess vital signs prior to initiation of therapy as a baseline for comparison during drug administration.
- Observe continuously while receiving infusion. Check BP q2min until stabilized at desired level, then q5min for duration of treatment. Monitor pulse and respiration closely.
- Intensity of hypotensive effect is largely dependent on positioning. Decrease in BP is most marked in sitting or standing position.
- Continue to monitor vital signs at regular intervals after completion of treatment. Since BP returns to pretreatment level within 10 min after the infusion is terminated, an oral antihypertensive is usually initiated as soon as desired BP level has been achieved.
- Monitor I&O. Ganglionic blockade may reduce renal blood flow initially as well as voiding contractions and urge to void. Check lower abdomen for bladder distension.
- Notify physician promptly if BP fails to respond. Some patients become refractory to trimethaphan (tachyphylaxis) within 48 h after initiation of therapy.

T

TRIMETHOBENZAMIDE HYDROCHLORIDE

(trye-meth-oh-ben′za-mide)
Arrestin, Ticon, Tigan, T-Gen
Classifications: GASTROINTESTINAL AGENT; ANTIEMETIC
Prototype: Prochlorperazine
Pregnancy Category: C

AVAILABILITY 100 mg, 250 mg, 300 mg capsules; 100 mg, 200 mg suppositories; 100 mg/mL injection

ACTIONS Structurally related to ethanolamine antihistamines, but in therapeutic doses antihistamine activity is weak. Sedative and antiemetic actions; less effective than phenothiazine antiemetics but produces fewer adverse effects. Must be used with other agents when vomiting is severe. Primary locus of action is thought to be the chemoreceptor trigger zone (CTZ) in medulla.

THERAPEUTIC EFFECTS Less effective than phenothiazine antiemetics but produces fewer adverse effects.

USES Control of nausea and vomiting.

CONTRAINDICATIONS Uncomplicated vomiting in viral illness; parenteral use in children; rectal administration in prematures and newborns; known sensitivity to benzocaine (in suppository) or to similar local anesthetics. Safety during pregnancy (category C) or lactation is not established.

CAUTIOUS USE Patients who have recently received other centrally acting drugs; in presence of high fever, dehydration, electrolyte imbalance.

ROUTE & DOSAGE

Nausea and Vomiting

Adult: **PO** 250–300 mg t.i.d. or q.i.d. **Rectal/IM** 200 mg t.i.d. or q.i.d.

Child: **PO/Rectal** *15–45 kg,* 100–200 mg t.i.d. or q.i.d. **Rectal** *<15 kg,* 100 mg t.i.d. or q.i.d.

ADMINISTRATION

Oral

- Empty capsule and give with water or mix with food if patient cannot swallow capsule.

Intramuscular

- Give IM deep into upper outer quadrant of buttock.
- Minimize possibility of irritation and pain by avoiding escape of solution along needle track. Use Z-track technique. Rotate injection sites.

ADVERSE EFFECTS (≥1%) **Body as a Whole:** Hypersensitivity reactions (including allergic skin eruptions), muscle cramps, pain, stinging, burning, redness, irritation at IM site; local irritation following rectal administration. **CNS:** Pseudoparkinsonism. **CV:** Hypotension. **GI:** Diarrhea, exaggeration of nausea, acute hepatitis, jaundice.

INTERACTIONS Drug: Alcohol and other CNS DEPRESSANTS add to depressant activity; BELLADONNA ALKALOIDS may intensify anticholinergic effects; PHENOTHIAZINES may precipitate extrapyramidal syndrome.

PHARMACOKINETICS Onset: 10–40 min PO; 15 min IM. **Duration:** 3–4 h PO; 2–3 h IM. **Elimination:** 30–50% of dose excreted unchanged in urine within 48–72 h.

NURSING IMPLICATIONS

Assessment & Drug Effects

- Monitor BP. Hypotension may occur particularly in surgical patients receiving drug parenterally.
- Report promptly and stop drug therapy if an acute febrile illness accompanies or begins during therapy.

- Antiemetic effect of drug may obscure diagnoses of GI or other pathologic conditions or signs of toxicity from other drugs.

Patient & Family Education

- Report promptly to physician onset of rash or other signs of hypersensitivity (see Appendix F). Discontinue drug immediately.
- Do not drive or engage in potentially hazardous activities until response to drug is known.
- Do not drink alcohol or alcoholic beverages during therapy with this drug.
- Do not breast feed while taking this drug without consulting physician.

TRIMETHOPRIM Pr

(trye-meth'oh-prim)

Primsol, Proloprim, Trimpex

Classifications: ANTIINFECTIVE; URINARY TRACT

Pregnancy Category: C

AVAILABILITY 100 mg, 200 mg tablets; 50 mg/5 mL liquid

ACTIONS Antiinfective and folic acid antagonist with slow bactericidal action. Binding and interference with cell growth is 1000 times stronger in bacterial than in mammalian cells. Most pathogens causing urinary tract infection (UTI) are in normal vaginal and fecal flora.

THERAPEUTIC EFFECTS Effective against most common UTI pathogens, including *Escherichia coli, Enterobacter species, Klebsiella pneumoniae, Proteus mirabilis,* most strains of *Haemophilus influenzae, Streptococcus pneumoniae, Streptococcus pyogenes, Staphylococcus* organisms (including *S. saprophyticus*). Not effective against *Bacteroides, Lactobacillus* species, *Chlamydia* or *Pneumocystis carinii, Pseudomonas aeruginosa*. Resistant strains of *Enterobacteriaceae* (*E. coli* and *Klebsiella* and *Proteus* species) may develop during therapy.

USES Initial episodes of acute uncomplicated UTIs, acute otitis media in children.

UNLABELED USES Treatment and prophylaxis of chronic and recurrent UTI in both men and women; treatment in conjunction with dapsone of initial episodes of *Pneumocystis carinii* pneumonia; treatment of travelers' diarrhea.

CONTRAINDICATIONS Megaloblastic anemia secondary to folate deficiency; creatinine clearance <15 mL/min, impaired kidney or liver function; possible folate deficiency; pregnancy (category C), lactation, or in children with fragile X chromosome associated with mental retardation. Safety in infants <2 mo and efficacy in children <12 y is not established.

ROUTE & DOSAGE

Urinary Tract Infection

Adult: **PO** 100 mg b.i.d. or 200 mg once/d

Child: **PO** 2–3 mg/kg q12h times 10 d

Acute Otitis Media

Child: **PO** *>6 mo,* 10 mg/kg divided q12 h times 10 d

Travelers' Diarrhea

Adult: **PO** 200 mg b.i.d.

ADMINISTRATION

Oral

- Give with 240 mL (8 oz) of fluid if not contraindicated.
- Store at 15°–30° C (59°–86° F) in dry, light-protected place.

ADVERSE EFFECTS (≥1%) **GI:** Epigastric discomfort, nausea, vomiting, glossitis, abnormal taste sensation. **Hematologic:** Neutropenia, *megaloblastic anemia,* methemoglobinemia, leukopenia, thrombocytopenia (rare). **Skin:** *Rash, pruritus,* exfoliative dermatitis, photosensitivity. **Body as a Whole:** Fever. **Metabolic:** Increased serum transaminases (ALT, AST), bilirubin, creatinine, BUN.

DIAGNOSTIC TEST INTERFERENCE Interferes with serum ***methotrexate assays*** that use a competitive binding protein technique with a bacterial dihydrofolate reductase as the binding protein. May cause falsely elevated ***creatinine*** values when ***Jaffe reaction*** is used.

INTERACTIONS Drug: May inhibit **phenytoin** metabolism causing increased levels.

PHARMACOKINETICS Absorption: Almost completely absorbed from GI tract. **Peak:** 1–4 h. **Distribution:** Widely distributed, including lung, saliva, middle ear fluid, bile, bone, CSF; crosses placenta; appears in breast milk. **Metabolism:** Metabolized in liver. **Elimination:** 80% excreted in urine unchanged. **Half-Life:** 8–11 h.

NURSING IMPLICATIONS

Assessment & Drug Effects

- Lab tests: Obtain C&S tests before trimethoprim therapy is initiated; therapy may be started before results are received. Obtain periodic urine cultures, BUN, creatinine clearance, CBC, Hgb, and Hct. Follow-up cultures may be ordered at end of treatment to verify elimination of causative organism.
- Reinforce necessity to adhere to established drug regimen. Recurrent infection after terminating prophylactic treatment of UTI may occur even after 6 mo of therapy.
- Assess urinary pattern during treatment. Altered pattern (frequency, urgency, nocturia, retention, polyuria) may reflect emerging drug resistance, necessitating change of drug regimen. Periodically check for bladder distention.
- Be alert for toxic effects on bone marrow, particularly in older adults, malnourished, alcoholic, pregnant, or debilitated patients. Recognize and report signs of infection or anemia.
- Drug-induced rash, a common adverse effect, is usually maculopapular, pruritic, or morbilliform and appears 7–14 d after start of therapy with daily doses of 200 mg or less.
- Watch for overdose symptoms: Nausea, vomiting, diarrhea, mental depression, confusion, facial swelling, elevated serum transaminases.

Patient & Family Education

- Take all prescribed medication; uncomplicated UTIs usually respond to treatment.
- Drink fluids liberally (2000–3000 mL/d, if not contraindicated) to help flush out urinary bacteria.
- Take urinary analgesic for pain and discomfort with voiding before full drug effects are experienced. Report pain and hematuria to physician immediately.
- Do not postpone voiding even though increases in fluid intake may cause more frequent urination.
- Do not use douches or sprays during treatment periods; practice careful perineal hygiene to prevent reinfection.
- Report to physician promptly any symptoms of a hematologic disorder (fever, sore throat, pallor, purpura, ecchymosis).
- Consult physician if severe traveler's diarrhea does not respond to

T

3–5 d therapy (i.e., persistence of symptoms of severe nausea, abdominal pain, diarrhea with mucus or blood, and dehydration).
- Do not breast feed while taking this drug.

TRIMETHOPRIM-SULFAMETHOXAZOLE (TMP-SMZ)

(tri-meth′o-prim-sul-fa-meth′ox-a-zole)

Bactrim, Co-Trimoxazole, Septra

Classifications: ANTIINFECTIVE; URINARY TRACT AGENT; SULFONAMIDE

Prototype: Trimethoprim

Pregnancy Category: C

AVAILABILITY 80 mg trimethoprim/400 mg sulfamethoxazole, 160 mg trimethoprim/800 mg sulfamethoxazole tablets; 40 mg trimethoprim/200 mg sulfamethoxazole/5 ml suspension; 16 mg trimethoprim/80 mg sulfamethoxazole/5 ml, 80 mg trimethoprim/400 mg sulfamethoxazole/5 ml injection

ACTIONS Fixed combination of sulfamethoxazole (SMZ), an intermediate acting antiinfective sulfonamide, and trimethoprim (TMP), a synthetic antiinfective. Both components of the combination are synthetic folate antagonist antiinfectives. Mechanism of action is principally enzyme inhibition, which prevents bacterial synthesis of essential nucleic acids and proteins.

THERAPEUTIC EFFECTS Effective against *Pneumocystis carinii pneumonitis, Shigellosis enteritis,* and severe complicated UTIs due to most strains of the *Enterobacteriaceae.* Bacterial resistance to the combined drugs develops more slowly than to either of the drugs alone.

USES *Pneumocystis carinii pneumonitis, Shigellosis* enteritis, and severe complicated UTIs due to most strains of the *Enterobacteriaceae.* Also children with acute otitis media due to susceptible strains of *Haemophilus influenzae,* and acute episodes of chronic bronchitis in adults.

UNLABELED USES Isosporiasis; prevention of traveler's diarrhea; cholera; treatment of infections caused by *Nocardia, Legionella micdadei,* and *Legionella pneumophila* and genital ulcers caused by *Haemophilus ducreyi;* prophylaxis for *P. carinii* pneumonia in neutropenic patients.

CONTRAINDICATIONS Hypersensitivity to TMP, SMZ, sulfonamides, or bisulfites; group A beta-hemolytic streptococcal pharyngitis; megaloblastic anemia due to folate deficiency; creatinine clearance <15 mL/min; pregnancy (category C), lactation. Not recommended for infants <2 mo.

CAUTIOUS USE Impaired kidney or liver function; possible folate deficiency; severe allergy or bronchial asthma; G6PD deficiency, hypersensitivity to sulfonamide derivative drugs (e.g., acetazolamide, thiazides, tolbutamide).

ROUTE & DOSAGE

Systemic Infections

Adult: **PO** 160 mg TMP/800 mg SMZ (1 double strength [DS] tablet) q12h **IV** 8–10 mg/kg/d TMP divided q6–12h infused over 60–90 min

Child: **PO** *>2 mo & <40 kg,* 4 mg/kg/d TMP q12h; *>40 kg,* 160 mg TMP/800 mg SMZ (1 DS tablet) q12h **IV** *>2 mo,* 8–10 mg/kg/d TMP divided q6–12h infused over 60–90 min

Pneumocystis carinii Pneumonia

Adult: **IV** 20 mg/kg/d TMP divided q6h infused over 60–90 min

Prophylaxis for *Pneumocystis carinii* Pneumonia

Adult: **PO** 160 mg TMP/800 mg SMZ q24h
Child: **PO** 150 mg/m^2 TMP/750 mg/m^2 SMZ b.i.d. 3 consecutive d/wk (max: 320 mg TMP/d)

Renal Impairment

Cl_{cr} 10–30 mL/min: reduce dose by 50%; <10 mL/min: reduce dose by 75%. For all indications

ADMINISTRATION

Oral

- Give with a full glass of desired fluid.
- Maintain adequate fluid intake (at least 1500 mL/d) during therapy.

Intravenous

PREPARE: **Intermittent:** Add contents of 5-mL ampul to 125 mL D5W. Use within 6 h. If less fluid is desired, dilute in 75 or 100 mL and use within 2 h or 4 h, respectively. Do not refrigerate.

ADMINISTER: **Intermittent:** Give over 60–90 min. Avoid bolus or rapid injection. Do not mix other drugs or solutions with IV infusion. Discard solution if cloudy or if crystallization appears after mixing.

INCOMPATIBILITIES **Solution/additive:** Stability in **dextrose** and **normal saline** is concentration dependent; **fluconazole, verapamil. Y-site: Fluconazole, foscarnet, midazolam, vinorelbine.**

- Store at 15°–30° C (59°–86° F) in dry place protected from light. Avoid freezing.

ADVERSE EFFECTS (≥1%) **Skin:** *Mild to moderate rashes (including fixed drug eruptions),* toxic epidermal necrolysis. **GI:** *Nausea, vomiting,* diarrhea, *anorexia,* hepatitis, pseudomembranous enterocolitis, stomatitis, glossitis, abdominal pain. **Urogenital:** Kidney failure, oliguria, anuria, crystalluria. **Hematologic:** Agranulocytosis (rare), aplastic anemia (rare), megaloblastic anemia, hypoprothrombinemia, thrombocytopenia (rare). **Body as a Whole:** Weakness, arthralgia, myalgia, photosensitivity, allergic myocarditis.

DIAGNOSTIC TEST INTERFERENCE May elevate levels of serum creatinine, transaminase, bilirubin, alkaline phosphatase.

INTERACTIONS Drug: May enhance hypoprothrombinemic effects of ORAL ANTICOAGULANTS; may increase **methotrexate** toxicity.

PHARMACOKINETICS Absorption: Readily absorbed from GI tract. **Peak:** 1–4 h PO. **Distribution:** Widely distributed, including CNS; crosses placenta; distributed into breast milk. **Metabolism:** Metabolized in liver. **Elimination:** Excreted in urine. **Half-Life:** 8–10 h TMP, 10–13 h SMZ.

NURSING IMPLICATIONS

Assessment & Drug Effects

- Be aware that IV Septra contains sodium metabisulfite, which produces allergic-type reactions in susceptible patients: Hives, itching, wheezing, anaphylaxis. Susceptibility (low in general population) is seen most frequently in asthmatics or atopic nonasthmatic persons.
- Lab tests: Baseline and followup urinalysis; CBC with differential,

platelet count, BUN and creatinine clearance with prolonged therapy.
- Monitor coagulation tests and prothrombin times in patient also receiving warfarin. Change in warfarin dosage may be indicated.
- Monitor I&O volume and pattern. Report significant changes to forestall renal calculi formation. Also report failure of treatment (i.e., continued UTI symptoms).
- Older adult patients are at risk for severe adverse reactions, especially if liver or kidney function is compromised or if certain other drugs are given. Most frequently observed: Thrombocytopenia (with concurrent thiazide diuretics); severe decrease in platelets (with or without purpura); bone marrow suppression; severe skin reactions.
- Be alert for overdose symptoms (no extensive experience has been reported): Nausea, vomiting, anorexia, headache, dizziness, mental depression, confusion, and bone marrow depression.

Patient & Family Education
- Report immediately to physician if rash appears. Other reportable symptoms are sore throat, fever, purpura, jaundice; all are early signs of serious reactions.
- Monitor for and report fixed eruptions to physician. This drug can cause fixed eruptions at the same sites each time the drug is administered. Every contact with drug may not result in eruptions; therefore, patient may overlook the relationship.
- Drink 2.5–3 liters (1 liter is approximately equal to 1 quart) daily, unless otherwise directed.
- Do not breast feed while taking this drug.

TRIMETREXATE
(tri-me-trex′ate)
Neutrexin
Classifications: ANTINEOPLASTIC; ANTIMETABOLITE
Prototype: Methotrexate
Pregnancy Category: D

AVAILABILITY 25 mg injection

ACTIONS Antimetabolite and folic acid antagonist. Blocks folinic acid (active form of folic acid) participation in nucleic acid synthesis, thereby interfering with miotic process. Acts as a dihydrofolate reductase (DHFR) inhibitor in a similar manner to methotrexate.
THERAPEUTIC EFFECTS Disrupts DNA, RNA, and protein synthesis, with consequent cell death.

USES Used with concurrent leucovorin administration, as an alternate therapy for moderate-to-severe *Pneumocystis carinii* pneumonia (PCP) in immunocompromised patients, including AIDS patients.
UNLABELED USES Advanced non-small cell lung cancer, metastatic cancer of the head and neck, metastatic colorectal adenocarcinoma, pancreatic carcinoma.

CONTRAINDICATIONS Hypersensitivity to trimetrexate, leucovorin, or methotrexate; profound myelosuppression; pregnancy (category D), lactation.
CAUTIOUS USE Seizures; mild myelosuppression; severe kidney or liver dysfunction; hypoalbuminemia or hypoproteinemia; concomitant use of myelosuppressive, hepatotoxic, or renal toxic drugs; previous radiation of bone marrow or extensive chemotherapy with

myelotoxic agents. Safety and efficacy in children <18 y are not established.

ROUTE & DOSAGE

***Pneumocystis carinii* Pneumonia**

Adult: **PO** 60 mg/m²/d prepared as the IV solution has been given orally to AIDS patients with PCP. **IV** 45 mg/m² once daily by IV infusion over 60–90 min with concurrent leucovorin 20 mg/m² q6h (IV or PO, trimetrexate times 21 d and leucovorin times 24 d).

ADMINISTRATION

Intravenous

PREPARE: **IV Infusion:** Reconstitute 25 mg with 2 mL of D5W or sterile water for injection to yield 12.5 mg/mL. Allow 30 s for complete dissolution. Manufacturer recommends filtering (0.22 micron) reconstituted solution prior to dilution. Further dilute with 10–100 mL of D5W to a final concentration of 0.25–2 mg/mL.

ADMINISTER: **IV Infusion:** Give over 60–90 min. Flush IV line with at least 10 mL of D5W before and after administering trimetrexate.

INCOMPATIBILITIES **Solution/additive & Y-site:** CHLORIDE-CONTAINING SOLUTIONS (including **sodium chloride**), **foscarnet, indomethacin.**

- Wash with soap and water immediately if drug contacts skin.
- Store reconstituted solution at room temperature or refrigerated for 24 h.

ADVERSE EFFECTS (≥1%) **Hematologic:** Myelosuppression, granulocytopenia, thrombocytopenia. **GI:** *Nausea, vomiting, stomatitis.* **Skin:** Erythematous rash with post-eruption hyperpigmentation. **Metabolic:** Mild transient elevations in serum creatinine and liver function tests.

DIAGNOSTIC TEST INTERFERENCE Mild increases in ***serum creatinine*** and ***liver function tests.***

INTERACTIONS Drug: Cimetidine, erythromycin, fluconazole (and other AZOLE ANTIFUNGAL AGENTS) may increase trimetrexate levels and toxicity. **Rifabutin, rifampin** may decrease trimetrexate levels. **Zidovudine** may cause additive hematologic toxicity.

PHARMACOKINETICS Absorption: Approximately 44% absorbed from GI tract. **Onset:** 3 d. **Distribution:** Very low CSF concentrations; distributes into lung tissue; 98% protein bound. **Metabolism:** Extensively metabolized in liver. **Elimination:** Excreted in urine and feces. **Half-Life:** 15–17 h.

NURSING IMPLICATIONS

Assessment & Drug Effects

- Lab tests: Monitor complete blood count at least twice a week during therapy. Myelosuppression nadir occurs around day 8. Monitor kidney and liver functions; impaired functioning may indicate need for dosage reduction.

Patient & Family Education

- Learn potential adverse effects and report those that are bothersome.
- Understand that myelosuppression is the primary dose-limiting adverse effect.
- Do not breast feed while taking this drug.

T

TRIMIPRAMINE MALEATE

(tri-mip′ra-meen)

Surmontil

Classifications: CENTRAL NERVOUS SYSTEM AGENT; PSYCHOTHERAPEUTIC; TRICYCLIC ANTIDEPRESSANT

Prototype: Imipramine

Pregnancy Category: C

AVAILABILITY 25 mg, 50 mg, 100 mg capsules

ACTIONS Tricyclic antidepressant (TCA) pharmacologically similar to imipramine. Moderate anticholinergic and strong sedative effects; useful in depression associated with anxiety and sleep disturbances. Recent studies suggest strong, active H_2-receptor antagonism is a characteristic of TCAs.

THERAPEUTIC EFFECTS More effective in alleviation of endogenous depression than other depressive states.

USES Treatment of major depression.

UNLABELED USES Peptic ulcer disease.

CONTRAINDICATIONS Prostatic hypertrophy; during recovery period after MI. Safety during pregnancy (category C) or lactation is not established.

CAUTIOUS USE Schizophrenia, electroshock therapy, suicidal tendency; cardiovascular, liver, thyroid, kidney disease.

T

ROUTE & DOSAGE

Depression

Adult: **PO** 75–100 mg/d in divided doses, may increase gradually up to 300 mg/d if needed **PO Maintenance Dose** Usually 50–150 mg/d

Geriatric: **PO** 25 mg h.s., may increase q3d (max: 100 mg/d)

ADMINISTRATION

Oral

- Give with food to decrease gastric distress.
- Store in tightly closed container at 15°–30° C (59°–86° F) unless otherwise specified.

ADVERSE EFFECTS (≥1%) **CNS:** Seizures, tremor, confusion, *sedation.* **Special Senses:** Blurred vision. **CV:** Tachycardia, *orthostatic hypotension,* hypertension. **GI:** *Xerostomia, constipation,* paralytic ileus. **Urogenital:** *Urinary retention.* **Skin:** Photosensitivity, sweating.

INTERACTIONS Drug: May decrease some antihypertensive response to ANTIHYPERTENSIVES; CNS DEPRESSANTS, **alcohol,** HYPNOTICS, BARBITURATES, SEDATIVES potentiate CNS depression; may increase hypoprothrombinemic effect of ORAL ANTICOAGULANTS; **ethchlorvynol** may cause transient delirium; with **levodopa**, SYMPATHOMIMETICS (e.g., **epinephrine, norepinephrine**), possibility of sympathetic hyperactivity with hypertension and hyperpyrexia; with MAO INHIBITORS, possibility of severe reactions, toxic psychosis, cardiovascular instability; **methylphenidate increases plasma TCA levels;** THYROID AGENTS may increase possibility of arrhythmias; **cimetidine** may increase plasma TCA levels. **Herbal: Ginkgo** may decrease seizure threshold; **St. John's wort** may cause **serotonin** syndrome.

PHARMACOKINETICS Absorption: Rapidly absorbed from GI tract. **Peak:** 2 h. **Metabolism:** Metabolized in liver. **Elimination:** Excreted in urine and feces. **Half-Life:** 9.1 h.

NURSING IMPLICATIONS

Assessment & Drug Effects

- Assess vital signs (BP and pulse rate) during adjustment period of

tricyclic antidepressant (TCA) therapy. If BP falls more than 20 mm Hg or if there is a sudden increase in pulse rate, withhold medication and notify physician.
- Orthostatic hypotension may be sufficiently severe to require protective assistance when patient is ambulating. Instruct patient to change position from recumbency to standing slowly and in stages.
- Report signs of liver dysfunction: Yellow skin and sclerae, light-colored stools, pruritus, abdominal discomfort.
- Report fine tremors, a distressing extrapyramidal adverse effect, to physician.
- Monitor bowel elimination pattern and I&O ratio. Severe constipation and urinary retention are potential problems, especially in older adults. Advise increased fluid intake to at least 1500 mL/d (if allowed).
- Monitor patient carefully during initial drug therapy when therapeutic "lag period" may foster noncompliance.
- Inspect oral membranes daily with high-dose therapy. Urge outpatient to report symptoms of stomatitis or xerostomia.
- Regulate environmental temperature and patient's clothing carefully; drug may cause intolerance to heat or cold.
- Excessive alcohol may potentiate TCA effects and increase the danger of overdosage or suicide attempt.

Patient & Family Education
- Be aware that your ability to perform tasks requiring alertness and skill may be impaired.
- Do not use OTC drugs unless approved by physician.
- Understand that the actions of both alcohol and trimipramine are increased when used together during therapy and for up to 2 wk after the TCA is discontinued. Consult physician about safe amounts of alcohol, if any, that can be taken.
- Be aware that the effects of barbiturates and other CNS depressants may also be enhanced by trimipramine.
- Expect that therapeutic response will be delayed because TCAs have a "lag period" of 2–4 wk. Increased dosage does not shorten period but rather increases incidence of adverse reactions. Keep physician advised and do not interrupt therapy.
- Do not breast feed while taking this drug without consulting physician.

TRIOXSALEN
(trye-ox′sa-len)
Trisoralen
Classifications: SKIN AND MUCOUS MEMBRANE AGENT; PSORALEN
Prototype: Methoxsalen
Pregnancy Category: C

AVAILABILITY 5 mg tablets

ACTIONS Systemic psoralen derivative structurally and pharmacologically related to methoxsalen but produces less intense melanogenic and erythremic responses. Produces resistance to solar damage in persons particularly susceptible to painful reactions with exposure to sunlight.
THERAPEUTIC EFFECTS Accelerates pigmentation only when followed by exposure of skin to sunlight or ultraviolet irradiation, and may reach equivalence of a full summer of sun exposure.

USES In conjunction with controlled exposure to ultraviolet light or sunlight to repigment vitiliginous

T

skin, to improve tolerance to sunlight in patients with albinism, and to enhance pigmentation.

CONTRAINDICATIONS Idiosyncratic reactions to psoralen compounds; melanoma or history of melanoma; invasive squamous cell carcinomas; aphakia (increased risk of retinal damage because of the absence of lenses); history of light sensitive diseases (porphyria, lupus, xeroderma pigmentosum, albinism); concomitant use with any preparation having internal or external photosensitizing capacity; cardiac disease. Safety during pregnancy (category C), lactation, or in children is not established. **CAUTIOUS USE** Basal cell carcinoma; hepatic insufficiency.

ROUTE & DOSAGE

Repigment Vitiliginous Skin
Adult: **PO** 10 mg/d as single dose 2–4 h before controlled exposure to ultraviolet-A (UVA) or sunlight

ADMINISTRATION

Oral
- Give with milk or after a meal to reduce gastric distress.
- Note: If trioxsalen is used to increase tolerance of skin to sunlight, treatment is usually continued no longer than 14 d, with dosage not exceeding 140 mg.
- Store in tightly closed, light-resistant container at 15°–30° C (59°–86° F).

ADVERSE EFFECTS (≥1%) **Skin:** Severe edema and erythema, painful blisters, burning and peeling of skin. **GI:** GI distress, nausea, vomiting. **CNS:** Nervousness, vertigo, mental depression or excitation.

INTERACTIONS Drug: Coal tar, griseofulvin, SULFONAMIDES, PHENOTHIAZINES, THIAZIDES may increase photosensitivity reactions.

PHARMACOKINETICS Not well studied in humans.

NURSING IMPLICATIONS

Assessment & Drug Effects
- Expect that repigmentation of idiopathic vitiligo may begin a few weeks after start of treatment, but significant effects require 6–9 mo of therapy.
- Note: Drug is discontinued if repigmentation is not apparent after 3 mo of treatment.

Patient & Family Education
- Maintain pigmentation by periodic exposure to sunlight.
- Avoid the following: Figs, limes, parsley, parsnips, mustard, carrots, celery. Concomitant ingestion of furocoumarin-containing foods may intensify adverse reactions.
- Adhere to dosage and exposure time prescribed by physician. Severe burning may occur with overdosage.
- Do not breast feed while taking this drug without consulting physician.

TRIPELENNAMINE HYDROCHLORIDE

(tri-pel-enn'a-meen)
PBZ-SR, Pelamine, Pyribenzamine ♣
Classification: ANTIHISTAMINE (H_1-RECEPTOR ANTAGONIST)
Prototype: Diphenhydramine
Pregnancy Category: B

AVAILABILITY 25 mg, 50 mg tablets; 100 mg sustained-release tablets

ACTIONS Antihistamine with mild CNS depressant effects and relatively high incidence of GI side effects. Antagonizes histamine action (i.e., increased capillary permeability, edema formation, itching, and constriction of respiratory, GI, and vascular smooth muscle). Does not inhibit gastric secretion.

THERAPEUTIC EFFECTS Has antihistamine, antitussive, anticholinergic, and local anesthetic action.

USES To relieve symptoms of various allergic conditions, to ameliorate reactions to blood or plasma, and in anaphylaxis as adjunct to epinephrine and other standard measures after acute symptoms have been controlled. Also to provide oral mucous membrane analgesia in young children with herpetic gingiva-stomatitis.

CONTRAINDICATIONS Narrow-angle glaucoma; symptomatic prostatic hypertrophy; bladder neck obstruction; GI obstruction or stenosis; lower respiratory tract symptoms, including asthma; within 14 d of MAO inhibitor therapy. Safety during pregnancy (category B), lactation, or in neonates and prematures is not established.

CAUTIOUS USE History of asthma; convulsive disorders; increased intraocular pressure; hyperthyroidism; cardiovascular disease; hypertension; diabetes mellitus.

ROUTE & DOSAGE

Allergic Conditions

Adult: **PO** 25–50 mg q4–6h or 100 mg sustained-release q8–12h (max: 600 mg/d)
Child: **PO** 5 mg/kg/d in 4–6 divided doses (max: 300 mg/d)

ADMINISTRATION

Oral

- Give with or immediately after meals or food or with a glass of milk or water to lessen GI adverse effects.
- Do not use sustained-release formulation (100 mg) with children of any age.
- Do not crush, break, or chew sustained-release tablets. These must be swallowed whole.
- Store in tight, light-resistant containers.

ADVERSE EFFECTS (≥1%) **Respiratory:** Thickened bronchial secretions, wheezing, sensation of chest tightness. **Special Senses:** Blurred vision, diplopia. **Urogenital:** Urinary hesitancy or retention; dysuria. **CV:** Palpitation, tachycardia, mild hypotension or hypertension, <u>cardiovascular collapse</u>. **CNS:** *Drowsiness,* dizziness, tinnitus, vertigo, fatigue, headache; disturbed coordination, tingling, tremors, euphoria, nervousness, restlessness, insomnia, hallucinations, excitement. **GI:** *Epigastric distress, anorexia, nausea, vomiting, constipation* or diarrhea, *dry mouth, nose,* and *throat.* **Hematologic:** Leukopenia, hemolytic anemia. **Skin:** Skin rash, urticaria, photosensitivity. **Body as a Whole:** <u>Anaphylactic shock</u>, fever, ataxia, athetosis, convulsions, <u>coma</u>.

INTERACTIONS Drug: Alcohol and other CNS DEPRESSANTS add to CNS depression; MAO INHIBITORS may intensify anticholinergic effects.

PHARMACOKINETICS Absorption: Readily absorbed from GI tract. **Onset:** 15–30 min. **Peak:** 2–3 h. **Duration:** 4–6 h (up to 8 h with sustained-release). **Distribution:** Crosses placenta; distributed into breast milk. **Metabolism:** Metabolized in liver. **Elimination:** Excreted in urine.

NURSING IMPLICATIONS

Assessment & Drug Effects

- Assist older adults during ambulation; dizziness, sedation, and hy-

potension are more likely to occur in this age group.
- Lab tests: Obtain periodic blood cell counts during long-term therapy with antihistamines.

Patient & Family Education
- Void just before taking drug if urinary hesitancy is a problem.
- Do not drive or engage in potentially hazardous activities until response to drug is known. Mild to moderate drowsiness, blurred vision, and dizziness occur in some patients.
- Be aware that the effects of antihistamines may be augmented by concomitant use of alcohol or other CNS depressants.
- Do not take OTC preparations without consulting physician.
- Discontinue antihistamines within 4 d before skin testing procedure for allergy because drug may interfere with reactions and obscure test results.
- Do not breast feed while taking this drug without consulting physician.

TRIPTORELIN PAMOATE
(trip-tor'e-lyn)
Trelstar Depot
Classifications: HORMONE AND SYNTHETIC SUBSTITUTE; GONADOTROPIN-RELEASING HORMONE ANALOG
Prototype: Leuprolide Acetate
Pregnancy Category: X

AVAILABILITY 3.75 mg injection

ACTIONS Synthetic luteinizing releasing hormone agonist (LHRH or GnRH) with greater potency than naturally occurring luteinizing hormone.
THERAPEUTIC EFFECTS Potent inhibitor of gonadotropin secretion. In men, the level of serum testosterone is equivalent to a surgically castrated man.

USES Palliative treatment of advanced prostate cancer.

CONTRAINDICATIONS Hypersensitivity to triptorelin, other LHRH agonists, or LHRH; pregnancy (category X), lactation.
CAUTIOUS USE Prostatic carcinoma; patients with impending spinal cord compression or severe urogenital disorder; premenstrual syndrome; renal insufficiency.

ROUTE & DOSAGE

Prostate Cancer
Adult: **IM** 3.75 mg q mo

ADMINISTRATION

Intramuscular
- Give deep into a large muscle.

ADVERSE EFFECTS (≥1%) **Body as a Whole:** *Hot flushes,* pain, leg pain, fatigue. **CV:** Hypertension. **GI:** Diarrhea, vomiting. **Hematologic:** Anemia. **Musculoskeletal:** Skeletal pain. **CNS:** Headache, dizziness, insomnia, impotence, emotional lability. **Skin:** Pruritus. **Urogenital:** Urinary retention, UTI. **Other:** Pain at injection site.

DIAGNOSTIC TEST INTERFERENCE May interfere with tests for ***pituitary-gonadal function.***

PHARMACOKINETICS Peak: 1–3 h. **Duration:** 1 mo. **Metabolism:** Unknown. **Elimination:** Eliminated by liver and kidneys. **Half-Life:** 3 h.

NURSING IMPLICATIONS

Assessment & Drug Effects
- Monitor for S&S of disease flare, especially during the first 1–2 wks of therapy: Increased bone pain,

blood in urine, urinary obstruction, or symptoms of spinal compression.

- Lab tests: Periodic serum testosterone, PSA, acid phosphatase levels; urinary and serum calcium; urinary calcium/creatinine ratio; lipid profile in those at risk for atherosclerosis.

Patient & Family Education

- Disease flare (see ASSESSMENT & DRUG EFFECTS) is a common, temporary adverse effect of therapy; however, symptoms may become serious enough to report to the physician.
- Notify physician promptly of the following: S&S of an allergic reaction (itching, hives, swelling of face, arms, or legs; tingling in mouth or throat, tightness in chest or trouble breathing); weakness or loss of muscle control; rapid weight gain.

TROLEANDOMYCIN

(troe-lee-an-doe-mye'sin)

Tao

Classifications: ANTIINFECTIVE; MACROLIDE ANTIBIOTIC

Prototype: Erythromycin

Pregnancy Category: C

AVAILABILITY 250 mg capsules

ACTIONS Derivative of oleandomycin, a macrolide antibiotic prepared from cultures of *Streptomyces antibioticus*. Chemically related to erythromycin and has similar range of antibacterial activity, but reportedly less effective; has high potential for toxicity.

THERAPEUTIC EFFECTS Effective against susceptible strains of pneumococci and group A beta-hemolytic streptococci. Cross-sensitivity with erythromycin reported.

USES Acute, severe infections of upper respiratory tract caused by susceptible strains of pneumococci and group A beta-hemolytic streptococci.

CONTRAINDICATIONS History of hypersensitivity to any of the macrolide antibiotics; bacteriemia; patients receiving astemizide, cisapride, or pimozide; use for prophylaxis or for minor infections; pregnancy (category C); porphyria.

CAUTIOUS USE Impaired liver function; lactation.

ROUTE & DOSAGE

Upper Respiratory Tract Infections

Adult: **PO** 250–500 mg q6h

Child: **PO** 6.6–11 mg/kg (125–250 mg) q6h

ADMINISTRATION

Oral

- Give on an empty stomach (1 h before or 2 h after meals).
- Give in evenly spaced intervals throughout the day, preferably around the clock, in order to maintain effective blood levels.

ADVERSE EFFECTS (≥1%) **GI:** *Abdominal cramps and discomfort, nausea,* vomiting, diarrhea, cholestatic jaundice. **Body as a Whole:** Allergic reactions (urticaria, skin rash, <u>anaphylaxis</u>); superinfections.

DIAGNOSTIC TEST INTERFERENCE Troleandomycin may cause false elevations of ***urinary 17-ketosteroids (Drekter),*** and ***17-hydroxycorticosteroids (Porter-Silver method).***

INTERACTIONS Drug: May increase levels of **carbamazepine,** CYCLOSPO-

RINES, and **theophylline** and their toxicity; ORAL CONTRACEPTIVES may cause cholestatic jaundice; **warfarin** may increase **prothrombin time (PT); ergotamine** may induce ischemia and peripheral vasospasm.

PHARMACOKINETICS Absorption: Incompletely absorbed from GI tract. **Peak:** 2 h. **Distribution:** Distributed throughout body fluids; diffusion into CSF is poor unless meninges are inflamed. **Metabolism:** Metabolized in liver. **Elimination:** Excreted in bile and urine.

NURSING IMPLICATIONS

Assessment & Drug Effects

- Lab tests: Obtain periodic liver function tests in patients receiving drug longer than 10 d or in repeated courses.
- Some patients develop an allergic type of hepatitis with right upper quadrant pain, fever, nausea, vomiting, jaundice, eosinophilia, and leukocytosis. Liver changes are reversible if drug is discontinued immediately.
- Be aware that superinfections are most likely to occur in patients on prolonged or repeated therapy. Withdraw if symptoms present (see Appendix F), and start appropriate therapy.

Patient & Family Education

- Report signs of jaundice: Clay-colored stools, pruritus, yellow sclerae.
- Do not stop drug before full course of therapy is completed. Do not interrupt and then restart therapy or increase or decrease dose or interval.
- Do not breast feed while taking this drug without consulting physician.

TROMETHAMINE

(troe-meth'a-meen)

Tham, Tham-E

Classifications: FLUID AND ELECTROLYTIC BALANCE AGENT; SYSTEMIC ALKALINIZER

Pregnancy Category: C

AVAILABILITY 18 g/500 mL injection

ACTIONS Sodium-free organic amine that acts as a proton acceptor in the body buffering system, thus preventing or correcting acidosis. As a weak base, it combines with hydrogen ions from carbonic, lactic, pyruvic, and other metabolic acids, and penetrates the cell membrane to combine with intracellular acid.

THERAPEUTIC EFFECTS Acts as a weak osmotic diuretic increasing urine pH and excretion of fixed acids, CO_2, and electrolytes. Used to correct or prevent metabolic acidosis. May be preferable to sodium bicarbonate in treatment of severe metabolic acidosis when sodium or CO_2 elimination is restricted.

USES To prevent or correct metabolic acidosis associated with cardiac bypass surgery and cardiac arrest and to correct excess acidity of stored blood [preserved with acid citrate dextrose (CD)] and used in cardiac bypass surgery. (Stored blood has a pH range of 6.8–6.22.)

UNLABELED USES Metabolic acidosis of status asthmaticus and neonatal respiratory distress syndrome.

CONTRAINDICATIONS Anuria, uremia; chronic respiratory acidosis; pregnancy (category C), children, neonates.

CAUTIOUS USE Renal impairment; >1 d of therapy.

ROUTE & DOSAGE

Note: Dosage may be estimated from buffer base deficit of extracellular fluid using the following formula as a guide: mL of 0.3-M tromethamine solution = body weight (kg) × base deficit (mEq/L)

Metabolic Acidosis Associated with Cardiac Arrest

Adult: **IV** 3.5–6 mL/kg (126–216 mg/kg) of a 0.3-M solution into large peripheral vein; if chest is open, 55–165 mL (2–6 g) 0.3-M solution into ventricular cavity

Systemic Acidosis During Cardiac Bypass Surgery

Adult: **IV** 9 mL/kg or approximately 500 mL (18 g) 0.3-M solution; a single dose of up to 1000 mL (36 g) may be necessary in severe acidosis

Excess Acidity of ACD Priming Blood

Adult: **IV** 14–70 mL (0.5–2.5 g) 0.3-M solution added to each 500 mL blood

ADMINISTRATION

Intravenous

PREPARE: **IV Infusion:** Maximum allowable concentration is 0.3 M. Available premixed as a 0.3-M solution or may be prepared by adding 36 g to 1 L of sterile water.

ADMINISTER: **IV Infusion:** Give undiluted by slow IV infusion or added to pump-oxygenator blood or other priming fluid. Give over a period of no less than 1 h.

- Observe entry site carefully. Perivascular infiltration of the highly alkaline solution may lead to vasospasm, necrosis, and tissue sloughing. Stop infusion if extravasation occurs. ▪ Treat extravasation with a procaine and hyaluronidase infiltration to reduce vasospasm and to dilute tromethamine remaining in tissues. If necessary, local infiltration of an alpha-adrenergic blocking agent (e.g., phentolamine) into the area may be ordered.

- Discard solution 24 h after reconstitution; solution is highly alkaline and can erode glass. ▪ Store drug (available as solution or powder) away from extreme heat. Do not freeze.

ADVERSE EFFECTS (≥1%) **Body as a Whole:** *Local irritation,* tissue inflammation, *chemical phlebitis,* extravasation. **Respiratory:** <u>Respiratory depression</u>. **Metabolic:** Transient decrease in blood glucose, hypervolemia, hyperkalemia (with depressed kidney function).

PHARMACOKINETICS Metabolism: No appreciable metabolism. **Elimination:** Rapidly and preferentially excreted by kidneys; 75% excreted within 8 h.

NURSING IMPLICATIONS

Assessment & Drug Effects

- Watch for signs of hypoxia (see Appendix F). Hypoxia and hypoventilation may result from drug-induced reduction of CO_2 tension (a potent stimulus to breathing), particularly if respiratory acidosis is also present.
- Drug-induced hypoxia is a particular risk when concomitant use of other respiratory depressants or with COPD or impaired kidney function.
- Lab tests: Monitor blood pH, Pco_2, Po_2, bicarbonate, glucose, and electrolytes before, during, and after treatment. Dosage is controlled

T

to raise blood pH to normal limits (arterial: 7.35–7.45) and to correct acid–base imbalance.

- Monitor ECG and serum potassium if drug is given to patient with impaired kidney function (reduced drug elimination). Since hyperkalemia is often associated with metabolic acidosis, be alert to early signs (see Appendix F).
- Be alert for overdose symptoms (from total drug or too rapid administration): Alkalosis, overhydration, prolonged hypoglycemia, solute overload.

TROPICAMIDE

(troe-pik′a-mide)

Mydriacyl, Tropicacyl

Classifications: EYE PREPARATION; MYDRIATIC; CYCLOPLEGIC

Prototype: Homatropine

Pregnancy Category: C

AVAILABILITY 0.5%, 1% ophthalmic solution

See Appendix A-1.

TROSPIUM CHLORIDE

(tro-spi′um)

Sanctura

Classifications: AUTONOMIC NERVOUS SYSTEM AGENT; ANTISPASMODIC; ANTICHOLINERGIC (PARASYMPATHOLYTIC) AGENT; ANTIMUSCARINIC AGENT

Prototype: Atropine

Pregnancy Category: C

AVAILABILITY 20 mg tablets

ACTIONS Antagonizes the effect of acetylcholine on muscarinic receptors in smooth muscle. Its parasympatholytic action reduces the tonus of the smooth muscle of the bladder.

THERAPEUTIC EFFECTS Trospium decreases urinary frequency, urgency, and urge incontinence in patients with overactive bladders.

USES Treatment of overactive (neurogenic) bladder with symptoms of urgency, frequency, and urge urinary incontinence.

CONTRAINDICATIONS Hypersensitivity to trospium; patients with or at risk for urinary retention; uncontrolled narrow-angle glaucoma; gastric tension, GI obstruction, ileus, pyloric stenosis, toxic megacolon, severe ulcerative colitis; pregnancy (category C). Safety and effectiveness in children have not been established.

CAUTIOUS USE Significant bladder obstruction, BPH; ulcerative colitis, GERD, intestinal atony; myasthenia gravis, autonomic neuropathy; moderate or severe hepatic dysfunction; severe renal insufficiency, renal failure; glaucoma; older adults; lactation.

ROUTE & DOSAGE

Overactive Bladder

Adult: **PO** 20 mg twice daily on empty stomach
Geriatric: **PO** 20 mg twice daily on empty stomach, may decrease to 20 mg once daily at bedtime if anticholinergic adverse effects are intolerable

Renal Impairment

Cl_{cr} < 30 mL/min: reduce dose to 20 mg once daily at bedtime.

ADMINISTRATION

Oral

- Give at least 1 h before meals or on an empty stomach.
- Store at 20°–25° C (66°–77° F).

ADVERSE EFFECTS (≥1%) **Body as a Whole:** Fatigue. **CNS:** Headache. **GI:** *Dry mouth, constipation,* abdominal pain, dyspepsia, flatulence. **Special Senses:** Dry eyes. **Urogenital:** Urinary retention.

INTERACTIONS Drug: Increased anticholinergic adverse effects with ANTICHOLINERGIC AGENTS.

PHARMACOKINETICS Absorption: <10% absorbed orally. **Peak:** 5–6 h. **Elimination:** Primarily excreted in feces (unabsorbed dose), renal tubular secretion of absorbed dose. **Half-Life:** 20 h.

NURSING IMPLICATIONS

Assessment & Drug Effects

- Monitor bowel and bladder function. Report urinary hesitancy or significant constipation.
- Withhold drug and notify physician if urinary retention develops.
- Monitor for and report worsening of GI symptoms in those with GERD.
- Frequent monitoring of IOP is required in those with controlled narrow-angle glaucoma.

Patient & Family Education

- Report promptly any of the following: signs of an allergic reaction, (e.g., itching or hives), blurred vision or difficulty focusing, confusion, dizziness, difficulty passing urine.
- Moderate intake of tea, coffee, caffeinated sodas, and alcohol to minimize side effects of this drug.
- Avoid situations in which overheating is likely, as drug may impair sweating, which is a normal cooling mechanism.
- Do not engage in hazardous activities until response to the drug is known.
- Do not breast feed while taking this drug without consulting physician.

TUBOCURARINE CHLORIDE (Pr)

(too-boe-kyoo-ar'een)

Tubocurarine Chloride

Classifications: AUTONOMIC NERVOUS SYSTEM AGENT; NONDEPOLARIZING SKELETAL MUSCLE RELAXANT

Pregnancy Category: C

AVAILABILITY 3 mg/mL injection

ACTIONS Curare alkaloid that is a nondepolarizing neuromuscular blocking agent extracted from the plant *Chondodendron tomentosum.* Produces skeletal muscle relaxation or paralysis by competing with acetylcholine at cholinergic receptor sites on skeletal muscle endplate and thus blocks nerve impulse transmission. Also has histamine-releasing and ganglionic blocking properties.

THERAPEUTIC EFFECTS Blocks nerve impulse transmission to skeletal muscles, thus producing relaxation or paralysis of skeletal muscles. Utilized with general anesthesia and as an adjunct to mechanical ventilation.

USES To induce skeletal muscle relaxation as adjunct to general anesthesia, to facilitate management of mechanical ventilation, to reduce intensity of muscle contractions in tetanus and in pharmacologically or electrically induced convulsions, to treat spastic states in children, and for diagnosis of myasthenia gravis when conventional tests have been inconclusive.

CONTRAINDICATIONS Hypersensitivity to curare preparations; when histamine release is a hazard; hyperthermia; electrolyte imbalance; acidosis; neuromuscular disease; kidney disease. Safety during pregnancy (category C) or lactation is not established.

CAUTIOUS USE Impaired cardiovascular, kidney, liver, pulmonary, or endocrine function; hypotension; carcinomatosis; thyroid disorders; collagen diseases; porphyria; familial periodic paralysis; history of allergies; myasthenia gravis; older adults or debilitated patients.

ROUTE & DOSAGE

Adjunct to General Anesthesia
Adult: **IV** 6–9 mg followed by 3–4.5 mg in 3–5 min if necessary
Child: **IV** 0.2–0.5 mg/kg followed by 0.04–0.1 mg/kg prn to maintain paralysis
Neonate: **IV** *<1 mo,* 0.3 mg/kg followed by 0.1 mg/kg prn to maintain paralysis

Electroshock
Adult: **IV** 0.165 mg/kg administered slowly IV

Diagnosis of Myasthenia Gravis
Adult: **IV** 0.004–0.033 mg/kg

ADMINISTRATION

Note: Verify correct IV dilution and rate of IV injection for neonates, infants, children with physician.

Intravenous

PREPARE: **IV Infusion:** May be given undiluted (3 mg/mL).
ADMINISTER: **IV Infusion:** Give bolus dose over 60–90 s.
INCOMPATIBILITIES **Solution/additive:** BARBITURATES, **sodium bicarbonate; trimethaphan.**

- Do not use solutions of drug if more than faintly discolored.
- Do not mix in same syringe with solutions that have a high pH such as barbiturates and sodium bicarbonate.

ADVERSE EFFECTS (≥1%) **Body as a Whole:** Slight dizziness, feeling of warmth, malignant hyperthermia, hypersensitivity reactions. **Musculoskeletal:** Profound and prolonged muscle weakness and flaccidity. **Respiratory:** Respiratory depression, hypoxia, apnea, increased bronchial and salivary secretions, bronchospasm. **GI:** Decreased GI motility. **CV:** *Hypotension,* circulatory collapse.

INTERACTIONS Drug: SKELETAL MUSCLE RELAXANTS, INHALED ANESTHETICS, AMINOGLYCOSIDES, **polymyxin B, clindamycin, quinidine, quinine, procainamide,** DIURETICS, **amphotericin B** may potentiate neuromuscular blockade.

PHARMACOKINETICS Peak: 2–5 min. **Duration:** 20–30 min if used alone. **Metabolism:** Demethylated in liver. **Elimination:** 33%–75% excreted in urine within 24 h; 11% excreted in bile; crosses placenta. **Half-Life:** 1–3 h.

NURSING IMPLICATIONS

Assessment & Drug Effects

- Lab tests: Obtain baseline kidney function and determinations of serum electrolytes. Electrolyte imbalance (particularly potassium and magnesium) can potentiate the effects of nondepolarizing neuromuscular blocking agents.
- Monitor BP, vital signs, and airway until assured of patient's recovery from drug effects. Ganglionic blockade (hypotension) and histamine liberation (increased salivation, bronchospasm) and neuromuscular blockade (respiratory depression) are known effects of tubocurarine.
- Be aware that selective muscle paralysis following drug administration occurs in the following sequence: Jaw muscles, levator eyelid muscles and other muscles of head

and neck, limbs, intercostals and diaphragm, abdomen, trunk. Facial and diaphragm muscles are first to recover, followed in order by legs, arms, shoulder girdle, trunk, larynx, hands, feet, pharynx. Muscle function is usually restored within 90 min.

- Measure and record I&O ratio during day of drug administration. Renal dysfunction will prolong drug action. Peristaltic action may be suppressed. Check for bowel sounds.

Patient & Family Education

- Note: Tubocurarine is retained in the body long after effects of neuromuscular blockade appear to have dissipated. Report residual muscle weakness to physician.

UNOPROSTONE ISOPROPYL

(un-o-pros′tone iso′propyl)

Rescula

Classifications: PROSTAGLANDIN; EYE PREPARATION; MIOTIC (ANTIGLAUCOMA AGENT)

Prototype: Latanoprost

Pregnancy Category: C

AVAILABILITY 0.15% ophthalmic solution

See Appendix A-1.

UREA

(yoor-ee′a)

Aquacare, Carbamide, Carmol, Nutraplus, Ureacin, Ureaphil

Classifications: ELECTROLYTIC AND WATER BALANCE AGENT; OSMOTIC DIURETIC; OXYTOCIC

Prototype: Mannitol

Pregnancy Category: C

AVAILABILITY 40 g/150 mL injection; 10%, 20%, 40% cream; 10%, 25% lotion

ACTIONS When present in high concentrations in blood, induces diuresis by elevating osmotic pressure of glomerular filtrate, with subsequent decrease in sodium and water reabsorption and promotion of chloride and potassium excretion.

THERAPEUTIC EFFECTS Volume and rate of urine flow is increased. Increased blood toxicity results in transudation of fluid from tissue, including brain, cerebrospinal, and intraocular fluid into the blood. When used as an abortifacient, urea (in dextrose) is injected into amniotic sac, followed by IV oxytocin at a rate of about 400 mU/min or prostaglandin F_2.

USES To reduce or prevent intracranial pressure (cerebral edema) and intraocular pressure and to prevent acute kidney failure during prolonged surgery or trauma. Also transabdominally for aborting second trimester of pregnancy. Topical preparation promotes hydration and removal of excess keratin in dry skin and hyperkeratotic conditions.

UNLABELED USES Severe migraine attacks; acute sickle cell crisis.

CONTRAINDICATIONS Severely impaired liver or kidney function; CHF; active intracranial bleeding; marked dehydration; IV injection into lower extremities, especially in older adult patients; topical use for viral skin diseases or impaired circulation. (Contraindications for intraamniotic urea: impaired kidney function, frank liver failure, active intracranial bleeding; marked dehydration, diabetes mellitus, sickle cell anemia).

CAUTIOUS USE Safe use in pregnancy (category C), lactation, or in children is not established. Use on face or broken skin.

ROUTE & DOSAGE

Reduction of Intracranial or Intraocular Pressure, Diuresis

Adult: **IV** 1–1.5 g/kg of 30% solution infused slowly over 1–2.5 h at a rate not to exceed 4 mL/min (max: 120 g/24 h)
Child: **IV** *>2 y,* 0.5–1.5 g/kg of 30% solution infused slowly over 1–2.5 h at a rate not to exceed 4 mL/min; *<2 y,* 0.1–0.5 g/kg of 30% solution infused slowly over 1–2.5 h at a rate not to exceed 4 mL/min

Hydration of Dry Skin

Adult: **Topical** Apply 2–40% cream or lotion to affected area 1–3 times/d

Second-Trimester Abortion

Adult: **Intraamniotic** Instill 40–50% urea solution in 5% dextrose in volumes equal to amount of amniotic fluid removed (max: 200–250 mL)

ADMINISTRATION

Topical

- Prepare fresh solution for each patient; discard unused portion. Urea may be reconstituted with 5% or 10% dextrose injection or 10% invert sugar in water.
- Action of topical preparation is enhanced by applying it to skin that is still moist following washing or bathing.

Intravenous

PREPARE: **IV Infusion:** Reconstitute (for 30%) by adding 105 mL D5W, 10% dextrose, or 10% invert sugar to a 40 g vial; yields 135 mL of 30% solution containing 300 mg urea/mL. Reconstituted solution should be used immediately. Discard unused portions.

ADMINISTER: **IV Infusion:** Give (30% solution) at a rate no greater than 4 mL/min. Infusion flow rate will be prescribed by physician. Rapid administration may be associated with increased capillary bleeding and hemolysis.

- Use extreme care to avoid extravasation; thrombosis and tissue necrosis can occur. Urea has the potential for causing tissue damage because of its osmotic properties. Inspect injection site frequently. If extravasation is suspected, discontinue the IV line STAT. Institute local treatment (according to institution protocol or physician's instructions); elevate body part even if extravasation is minor.

ADVERSE EFFECTS (≥1%) **CNS:** Somnolence (prolonged use in patients with kidney dysfunction), *headache,* acute psychosis, confusion, disorientation, nervousness. **CV:** Tachycardia, hypotension, syncope. **GI:** *Nausea, vomiting,* increased thirst. **Metabolic:** Fluid and electrolyte imbalance, dehydration. **Special Senses:** Intraocular hemorrhage (rapid IV). **Skin:** Skin rash, pain, irritation, sloughing, venous thrombosis, chemical phlebitis at injection site. **Body as a Whole:** Hyperthermia. **Hematologic:** Hemolysis (rapid IV).

INTERACTIONS Drug: May increase rate of **lithium** excretion, decreasing its effectiveness.

PHARMACOKINETICS Peak: 1–2 h. **Duration:** 3–10 h for diuresis and intracranial pressure reduction; 5–6 h for intraocular pressure. **Distribution:** 10% of intraamniotic instillation diffuses into maternal blood; distributed widely; good ocular penetration; crosses placenta; distributed into breast milk. **Elimina-**

tion: Excreted in urine; 50% may be reabsorbed. **Half-Life:** 1 h.

NURSING IMPLICATIONS

Assessment & Drug Effects

- Monitor I&O. If diuresis does not occur within 6–12 h following administration or if BUN exceeds 75 mg/dL, withhold drug and notify physician so that kidney function may be evaluated.
- Monitor vital signs and mental status; promptly report any changes.
- Observe postoperative patients closely for signs of hemorrhage. Urea reportedly may increase prothrombin time and promote internal oozing at suture sites.
- Withhold oral fluids and consult physician for hydration parameters if patient complains of a headache.
- Lab tests: Serum electrolytes and urinary sodium q12h. Frequent kidney function studies are advised, particularly in patients suspected of having kidney dysfunction.
- Watch for S&S of hyponatremia, hypokalemia, dehydration, or transient overhydration (due to hyperosmotic activity) (see Appendix F).
- Monitor for complaints of lower abdominal pain following intraamniotic instillation. If patient complains of lower abdominal pain, it may be that drug is going into abdomen rather than into the amniotic sac.
- See mannitol for additional nursing implications.

Patient & Family Education

- Drink fluids to hasten excretion of urea. However, if a headache develops, stop drinking because the fluid intake may be counteracting the effects of the drug. Alert physician.
- Do not breast feed while taking this drug without consulting physician.

UROKINASE

(yoor-oh-kin′ase)

Abbokinase, Open-Cath

Classifications: BLOOD FORMERS, COAGULATORS, AND ANTICOAGULANTS; THROMBOLYTIC ENZYME

Prototype: Alteplase

Pregnancy Category: B

AVAILABILITY 250,000 IU vial; 5,000 IU/mL vials

ACTIONS Enzyme produced by kidneys and isolated from human kidney tissue cultures. Promotes thrombolysis by acting directly on the endogenous fibrinolytic system to convert plasminogen to the enzyme plasmin.

THERAPEUTIC EFFECTS The formation of plasmin is an action that occurs within as well as on the surface of a thrombus or embolus; plasmin has direct fibrinolytic action on a clot. Urokinase also has an anticoagulant effect because its action leads to high plasma levels of fibrin and fibrinogen degradation products. Its most effective action is on fresh, recently formed thrombi.

USES Lysis of acute massive pulmonary emboli and peripheral emboli and restoration of patency in occluded IV catheters (including central venous catheter); acute MI, retinal vessel occlusion, lysis of clot-occluded arteriovenous cannulas, and various other conditions associated with thromboembolization phenomenon.

CONTRAINDICATIONS Pregnancy (category B), lactation, and in children; active internal bleeding; very recent CPR; recent (within two months) intraspinal, intracranial, or intraarterial procedures; intracranial neoplasm, CVA, severe uncontrolled

U

hypertension; history of allergic response to thrombolytic agent, recent streptococcal infection; obstetrical delivery; diabetic hemorrhagic retinopathy; ulcerative colitis, diverticulitis; any condition in which bleeding presents a hazard or would be difficult to manage because of location.

CAUTIOUS USE Patient with preexisting hemostatic deficits, conditions accompanied by risk of cerebral embolism, septic thrombophlebitis; uremia, hepatic failure.

ROUTE & DOSAGE

Pulmonary Embolus

Adult: **IV** 4400 IU/kg diluted in 0.9% NaCl or 5% dextrose infused over 10 min, followed by continuous infusion of 4400 IU/kg/h for 12 h

Occluded Coronary Artery

Adult: **IV** Precede urokinase with bolus of heparin (2500–10,000 U IV), then instill urokinase 6000 IU/min for periods up to 2 h, continue until artery is maximally opened (usually 15–30 min using about 500,000 IU)

Central Venous Catheter Clearance

Adult: **IV** Instill 5000 IU/mL solution into catheter port, after 5 min attempt to aspirate urokinase and clot, if no success after 30 min, cap port and wait 30–60 min and try again (instruct patient to exhale and hold breath any time catheter is disconnected from syringe or IV tubing and avoid excessive pressure of instillation to prevent rupture of catheter or forcing clot into circulation)

U

ADMINISTRATION

Intravenous

- Reconstitute immediately before use.

PREPARE: **Direct: For IV Catheter Clearance** – Use Abbokinase Open-Cath without dilution or add 1 mL of initially reconstituted Abbokinase (50,000 IU/mL) to 9 mL sterile water for injection to yield 5000 IU/mL. **IV Infusion: For Pulmonary Embolism** – Reconstitute each 250,000 IU vial of Abbokinase by adding 5 mL sterile water for injection (NOT bacteriostatic) to yield 50,000 IU/mL. Roll or tilt vial to mix; avoid agitating or shaking to prevent foaming and filament formation. May be terminally filtered through a 0.45 micron or smaller cellulose membrane. Reconstitute as many vials as needed to achieve the required dose. Further dilute by adding the contents of each vial to enough NS or D5W to produce a final volume of 195 mL for infusion. Use immediately. **For Coronary Artery Thrombosis** – Reconstitute three vials of Abbokinase as described above. Further dilute by adding the contents of the three vials to 500 mL of D5W. Use immediately.

ADMINISTER: **Direct:** Follow direction given under "Route & Dosage." **IV Infusion:** Give through in-line 0.22- or 0.45-micron filter using a constant infusion pump according to the rate indicated under "Route & Dosage" above.

- Discard unused portion because the product contains no preservatives.
- Store unopened vials at 2°–8° C (36°–46° F).

ADVERSE EFFECTS (≥1%) **Body as a Whole:** Hypersensitivity (bronchospasm, periorbital swelling, angioneurotic edema, anaphylaxis); headache, musculoskeletal pain, flushing, pyrexia. **Hematologic:** Phlebitis, *bleeding or oozing at sites* *of percutaneous trauma;* prolonged systemic hypocoagulability; spontaneous bleeding (GU, GI, retroperitoneal); **CV:** Unstable blood pressure; reperfusion atrial or ventricular dysrhythmias. **Skin:** Urticaria, itching. **GI:** Nausea.

INTERACTIONS Drug: ANTICOAGULANTS, NSAIDS, **aspirin** increase risk of bleeding; **aminocaproic acid** reverses the action of urokinase. **Herbal: Feverfew, garlic, ginger, ginkgo** may increase risk of bleeding.

PHARMACOKINETICS Absorption: Rapidly cleared from circulation. **Peak:** 3–4 h. **Elimination:** Small amount excreted in urine and bile. **Half-Life:** 10–20 min.

NURSING IMPLICATIONS

Assessment & Drug Effects

- Monitor for therapeutic effectiveness: Measurable signs of clinical response may not occur for 6–8 h after therapy is started.
- Note: Anticoagulant therapy with heparin is reinstituted at end of urokinase therapy and when thrombin time has decreased to less than twice normal control value (usually within 3–4 h).
- Be aware that severe spontaneous bleeding, including fatality from cerebral hemorrhage, has occurred during urokinase treatment. Risk is estimated to be twice that associated with heparin therapy.
- See streptokinase for additional nursing implications.

Patient & Family Education

- Report any of the following to physician immediately: Evidence or suspicion of bleeding, fever, chills, itching, difficulty breathing, back or chest pain.
- Do not breast feed while taking this drug.

VALACYCLOVIR HYDROCHLORIDE

(val-a-cy′clo-vir)

Valtrex

Classifications: ANTI-INFECTIVE; ANTIVIRAL

Prototype: Acyclovir

Pregnancy Category: B

AVAILABILITY 500 mg tablets

ACTIONS An antiviral agent hydrolyzed in the intestinal wall or liver to acyclovir; interferes with viral DNA synthesis. Because of increased GI absorption, the plasma level of this drug is substantially higher than that of acyclovir when both are taken orally.

THERAPEUTIC EFFECTS Active against *Herpes simplex* virus types 1 (HSV-1) and 2 (HSV-2), *Varicella zoster* virus, and *cytomegalovirus.* Inhibits viral replication.

USES *Herpes zoster* (shingles) in immunocompetent adults. Treatment and suppression of recurrent genital herpes; suppression of recurrent herpes in HIV-positive patients; treatment of cold sores.

CONTRAINDICATIONS Hypersensitivity to or intolerance of valacyclovir or acyclovir; pregnancy (category B).

CAUTIOUS USE Renal impairment, patients receiving nephrotoxic drugs, advanced HIV disease, allogeneic bone marrow transplant and renal transplant recipients, treatment of disseminated herpes zoster, immunocompromised patients, lactation. Safety and efficacy in children are not established.

V

ROUTE & DOSAGE

Herpes Zoster

Adult: **PO** 1 g (2 × 500 mg) t.i.d. for 7 d, start within 48 h of onset of zoster rash

Renal Impairment

Cl_{cr} 30–49 mL/min: 1 g q12h 10–29 mL/min: 1 g q24h <10 mL/min: 500 mg q24h

Treatment of Recurrent Genital Herpes

Adult: **PO** 500 mg b.i.d. × 3 d

Renal Impairment

Cl_{cr} ≤29 mL/min: 500 mg q.d.

Suppression of Recurrent Genital Herpes

Adult: **PO** 1 g q.d.

Treatment of Cold Sores

Adult: **PO** 2 g 12 h × 2 doses

ADMINISTRATION

Oral

- Start drug as soon as possible after diagnosis of herpes zoster, preferably within 48 h of onset of rash.
- Note: Dosage reduction is recommended for patients with renal impairment.
- Give valacyclovir after hemodialysis.
- Store at 15°–30° C (59°–86° F).

ADVERSE EFFECTS (≥1%) **CNS:** *Headache,* weakness, somnolence, dizziness, fatigue, lethargy, confusion. **GI:** *Nausea, vomiting, diarrhea,* abdominal pain, dyspepsia, flatulence. **Urogenital:** Glomerulonephritis, renal tubular damage, acute renal failure. **Skin:** Rash, urticaria, pruritus.

INTERACTIONS Drug: Probenecid, cimetidine decrease valacyclovir elimination. **Zidovudine** may cause increased drowsiness and lethargy.

PHARMACOKINETICS Absorption: Rapidly absorbed from GI tract; 54% reaches systemic circulation as acyclovir. **Peak:** 1.5 h. **Distribution:** 13.5%–17.9% bound to plasma proteins; distributes into plasma, cerebrospinal fluid, saliva, and major body organs; crosses placenta; excreted in breast milk. **Metabolism:** Rapidly converted to acyclovir during first pass through intestine and liver. **Elimination:** 40%–50% excreted in urine. **Half-Life:** 2.5–3.3 h.

NURSING IMPLICATIONS

Assessment & Drug Effects

- Monitor kidney function in patients with kidney impairment or those receiving potentially nephrotoxic drugs.
- Monitor for S&S of hypersensitivity; if present, withhold drug and notify physician.

Patient & Family Education

- Be aware of potential adverse effects and do not discontinue drug until full course is completed.
- Note: Post-herpes pain is likely to be present for several months after completion of therapy.
- Do not breast feed while taking this drug.

VALDECOXIB

(val-de-cox'ib)

Bextra

Classifications: CENTRAL NERVOUS SYSTEM AGENT; ANALGESIC; NONSTEROIDAL ANTIINFLAMMATORY DRUG (NSAID); CYCLOOXYGENASE-2 (COX-2) INHIBITOR

Prototype: Celecoxib

Pregnancy Category: C

AVAILABILITY 10 mg, 20 mg tablets

ACTIONS Inhibits prostaglandin synthesis primarily through inhibition of cyclooxygenase-2 (COX-2). At therapeutic plasma concentrations, does not inhibit cyclooxygenase-1 (COX-1).

THERAPEUTIC EFFECTS Exhibits anti-inflammatory, analgesic, and antipyretic properties.

USES Treatment of pain and inflammation associated with osteoarthritis, rheumatoid arthritis, primary dysmenorrhea.

CONTRAINDICATIONS Severe hepatic dysfunction; advanced renal failure; hypersensitivity to valdecoxib; history of asthma, urticaria, or allergic-type reactions after taking aspirin or NSAIDS; gastric ulcers; history of GI bleeding; pregnancy (category C); lactation.

CAUTIOUS USE Mild to moderate hepatic dysfunction; renal impairment. Safety and effectiveness in pediatric patients <18 y have not been evaluated.

ROUTE & DOSAGE

Osteoarthritis, Rheumatoid Arthritis

Adult: **PO** 10 mg q.d.

Primary Dysmenorrhea

Adult: **PO** 20 mg q.d. prn

ADMINISTRATION

Oral

- Do not administer to seriously dehydrated patients without first rehydrating. Consult physician.
- Store at 15°–30° C (59°–86° F).

ADVERSE EFFECTS (≥1%) **Body as a Whole:** Back pain, peripheral edema, flu-like symptoms, anaphylaxis (rare), angioedema (rare). **CNS:** Dizziness, headache. **CV:** Hypertension. **GI:** Nausea, vomiting, diarrhea, flatulence, abdominal pain and fullness. **Musculoskeletal:** Myalgia. **Respiratory:** Sinusitis, upper respiratory infection. **Skin:** Rash, serious skin reactions (rare) including Stevens-Johnson syndrome, exfoliative dermatitis, and toxic epidermal necrolysis.

INTERACTIONS Drug: Aspirin may increase risk of GI ulceration; may increase **lithium, warfarin** levels; **fluconazole, ketoconazole** may increase valdecoxib levels.

PHARMACOKINETICS Absorption: 83% of dose reaches systemic circulation. Food has no effect on absorption **Peak:** 3 h. **Metabolism:** Metabolized in liver by CYP3A4 and 2C9 and by glucuronidation. **Elimination:** Metabolites primarily excreted in urine (70%) and 30% in feces. **Half-Life:** 8–11 h.

NURSING IMPLICATIONS

Assessment & Drug Effects

- Monitor BP periodically, and monitor for fluid retention and edema especially in those with a history of hypertension or CHF.
- Lab tests: Monitor baseline and periodic LFTs; monitor renal functions especially with any chronic renal disease; periodically monitor Hct and Hgb and serum electrolytes.
- Concurent drugs: Monitor PT/INR with warfarin therapy and adjust warfarin as needed. Monitor lithium levels and assess for symptoms of toxicity.
- Monitor closely patients with preexisting renal disease for worsening of renal function.
- Monitor asthmatics and report increased frequency of attacks.

Patient & Family Education

- Avoid using valdecoxib during the third trimester of pregnancy.

- Stop taking valdecoxib and promptly report to physician if any of the following occur: S&S of GI ulceration including black, tarry stools and upper GI distress; unexplained weight gain, edema, skin rash; S&S of liver dysfunction including nausea, fatigue, lethargy, itching, jaundice, abdominal pain, and flu-like symptoms.
- Do not breast feed while taking this drug without consulting physician.

VALGANCICLOVIR HYDROCHLORIDE

(val-gan-ci'clo-vir)
Valcyte
Classifications: ANTIINFECTIVE; ANTIVIRAL AGENT
Prototype: Acyclovir
Pregnancy Category: C

AVAILABILITY 450 mg tablets

ACTIONS Rapidly converted to ganciclovir after oral administration by intestinal and hepatic enzymes. In cells infected with cytomegalovirus (CMV) ganciclovir is phosphorylated to ganciclovir triphosphate that inhibits viral DNA synthesis.
THERAPEUTIC EFFECTS Antiviral drug active against cytomegalovirus (CMV). Prevents replication CMV DNA, thus inhibiting replication of the virus.

USES Treatment of CMV retinitis; prevention of CMV disease in high-risk kidney, kidney-pancreas, and heart transplant patients (not effective in liver transplants).

CONTRAINDICATIONS Hypersensitivity to valganciclovir, ganciclovir, or acyclovir. Not recommended for persons on hemodialysis; renal failure; dental work; antimicrobial resistance; neutropenia, thrombocytopenia; pregnancy (category C), females of childbearing age; lactation.
CAUTIOUS USE Impaired kidney function; older adults; dental disease; anemia; leukopenia; bone marrow depression; concomitant use of myelosuppressive drugs; irradiation. Safety and efficacy in children are not established.

ROUTE & DOSAGE

Cytomegalovirus Prophylaxis
Adult: **PO** 900 mg once daily with food, starting within 10 d of transplantation until 100 d post-transplantation

Cytomegalovirus Retinitis Induction
Adult: **PO** 900 mg b.i.d. with food times 21 d

Cytomegalovirus Retinitis Maintenance
Adult: **PO** 900 mg q.d. with food

Renal Impairment
Cl_{cr} 40–59 mL/min: 450 mg b.i.d. (induction) or q.d. (maintenance) 25–39 mL/min: 450 mg q.d. (induction) or q2d (maintenance) 10–24 mL/min: 450 mg q2d (induction) or twice weekly (maintenance)

ADMINISTRATION

Oral
- Exercise caution in handling tablets. Do not crush or break tablets. Avoid direct contact of crushed or broken tablets with skin or mucous membranes.
- Give with food.
- Do not give to patients on hemodialysis.
- Store at 25°–30° C (77°–86° F).

ADVERSE EFFECTS (≥1%) **Body as a Whole:** *Fever,* local and systemic infections, hypersensitivity reactions. **CNS:** *Headache, insomnia,* peripheral neuropathy, paresthesia, convulsions, psychosis, confusion, hallucinations, agitation. **GI:** *Diarrhea, nausea, vomiting, abdominal pain.* **Hematologic:** *Neutropenia, anemia,* <u>thrombocytopenia</u>, pancytopenia, <u>bone marrow suppression, aplastic anemia</u>. **Special Senses:** *Retinal detachment.*

INTERACTIONS Drug: ANTINEOPLASTIC AGENTS, **amphotericin B, didanosine, trimethoprim-sulfamethoxazole (TMP-SMZ), dapsone, pentamidine, probenecid, zidovudine** may increase bone marrow suppression and other toxic effects of valganciclovir; may increase risk of nephrotoxicity from **cyclosporine;** ANTIRETROVIRAL AGENTS may decrease valganciclovir levels; valganciclovir may increase levels and toxicity of ANTIRETROVIRAL AGENTS; may increase risk of seizures due to **imipenem-cilastatin.**

PHARMACOKINETICS Absorption: Well absorbed from GI tract, 60% reaches systemic circulation as ganciclovir. **Onset:** 3–8 d. **Peak:** 1–3 h. **Duration:** Clinical relapse can occur 14 d to 3.5 mo after stopping therapy; positive blood and urine cultures recur 12–60 d after therapy. **Distribution:** Distributes throughout body including CSF, eye, lungs, liver, and kidneys; crosses placenta in animals; not known if distributed into breast milk. **Metabolism:** Metabolized in intestinal wall to ganciclovir, ganciclovir is not metabolized. **Elimination:** 94%–99% of dose is excreted unchanged in urine. **Half-Life:** 4 h.

NURSING IMPLICATIONS

Assessment & Drug Effects

- Withhold drug and notify physician for any of the following: Absolute neutrophil count <500 cells/mm^3, platelet count <25,000/mm^3, hemoglobin <8 g/dL, declining creatinine clearance.
- Monitor for S&S of bronchospasm in asthma patients; notify physician immediately.
- Lab tests: Baseline and frequent serum creatinine or creatinine clearance, CBC with differential, platelet count, Hct & Hgb.

Patient & Family Education

- Schedule ophthalmologic follow-up examinations at least every 4–6 wks while being treated with valganciclovir.
- Keep all scheduled appointments for laboratory tests.
- Do not drive or engage in potentially hazardous activities until response to drug is known.
- Report any of the following immediately: unexpected bleeding, infection.
- Use effective methods of contraception (barrier and other types) during and for at least 90 days following treatment.
- Discontinue drug and notify physician immediately in the event of pregnancy.
- Do not breast feed while taking this drug.

VALPROIC ACID (DIVALPROEX SODIUM, SODIUM VALPROATE) Pr

(val-proe'ic)

Depacon, Depakene, Depakote, Depakote ER, Depakote Sprinkle, Epival ♣, Zalkote

Classifications: CENTRAL NERVOUS SYSTEM (CNS) AGENT; ANTICONVULSANT; GABA INHIBITOR

Pregnancy Category: D

AVAILABILITY 250 mg capsules; 125 mg sprinkle capsules; 125 mg,

250 mg, 500 mg delayed-release tablets; 500 mg sustained-release tablets; 250 mg/5 mL syrup; 100 mg/mL injection

ACTIONS Anticonvulsant unrelated chemically to other drugs used to treat seizure disorders. Mechanism of action unknown; may be related to increased bioavailability of the inhibitory neurotransmitter gamma-aminobutyric acid (GABA) to brain neurons. Inhibits secondary phase of platelet aggregation.

THERAPEUTIC EFFECTS Depresses abnormal neuron discharges in the CNS, thus decreasing seizure activity.

USES Alone or with other anticonvulsants in management of absence (petit mal) and mixed seizures; mania; migraine headache prophylaxis.

UNLABELED USES Status epilepticus refractory to IV diazepam, petit mal variant seizures, febrile seizures in children, other types of seizures including psychomotor (temporal lobe), myoclonic, akinetic and tonic-clonic seizures, photosensitivity seizures, and those refractory to other anticonvulsants.

CONTRAINDICATIONS Hypersensitivity to valproate sodium; thrombocytopenia, patient with bleeding disorders or liver dysfunction or disease; cirrhosis, pancreatitis; congenital metabolic disorders, those with severe seizures, or on multiple anticonvulsant drugs; AIDS; pregnancy (category D), lactation; child <2 y; children <18 y for treatment of mania.

CAUTIOUS USE History of kidney disease, renal impairment or failure; adjunctive treatment with other anticonvulsants; congenital metabolic disorders, those with severe epilepsy, use as sole anticonvulsant drug; hypoalbuminemia; organic brain syndrome; children <2 y especially in first 6 mo of therapy.

ROUTE & DOSAGE

Note: May need to increase dose when converting from immediate release to extended-release products

Management of Seizures, Mania

Adult/Child: **PO/IV** 15 mg/kg/d in divided doses when total daily dose >250 mg, increase at 1 wk intervals by 5–10 mg/kg/d until seizures are controlled or adverse effects develop (max: 60 mg/kg/d)

Migraine Headache Prophylaxis

Adult: **PO** 250 mg b.i.d. (max: 1000 mg/d) or **Depakote ER** 500 mg q.d. × 1 wk, may increase to 1000 mg q.d.

Mania

Adult: **PO** 250 mg t.i.d. (max: 60 mg/kg/d)

ADMINISTRATION

Oral

- Give tablets and capsules whole; instruct patient to swallow whole & not to chew. Instruct to swallow sprinkle capsules whole or sprinkle entire contents on teaspoonful of soft food, and instruct to not chew food.
- Avoid using a carbonated drink as diluent for the syrup because it will release drug from delivery vehicle; free drug painfully irritates oral and pharyngeal membranes.
- Reduce gastric irritation by administering drug with food because serious GI adverse effects can lead to discontinuation of therapy. Enteric-coated tablet or syrup formulation is usually well tolerated.

Intravenous

PREPARE: **IV Infusion:** Dilute each dose in 50 mL or more of D5W, NS, or RL.

V

ADMINISTER: **IV Infusion:** Give a single dose over at least 60 min (≤20 mg/min). Avoid rapid infusion.

INCOMPATIBILITIES **Solution/additive:** No compatibility data available. Should avoid mixing with other drugs.

ADVERSE EFFECTS (≥1%) **CNS:** Breakthrough seizures, *sedation, drowsiness,* dizziness, increased alertness, hallucinations, emotional upset, aggression; deep coma, death (with overdose). **GI:** *Nausea, vomiting, indigestion (transient),* hypersalivation, anorexia with weight loss, increased appetite with weight gain, abdominal cramps, diarrhea, constipation, liver failure, pancreatitis. **Hematologic:** *Prolonged bleeding time,* leukopenia, lymphocytosis, thrombocytopenia, hypofibrinogenemia, bone marrow depression, anemia. **Skin:** Skin rash, photosensitivity, transient hair loss, curliness or waviness of hair. **Endocrine:** Irregular menses, secondary amenorrhea. **Metabolic:** Hyperammonemia (usually asymptomatic) hyperammonemic encephalopathy in patients with urea cycle disorders. **Respiratory:** Pulmonary edema (with overdose).

DIAGNOSTIC TEST INTERFERENCE Valproic acid produces false-positive results for ***urine ketones,*** elevated ***AST, ALT, LDH,*** and ***serum alkaline phosphatase,*** prolonged ***bleeding time,*** altered ***thyroid function tests.***

INTERACTIONS Drug: Alcohol and other CNS DEPRESSANTS potentiate depressant effects; other ANTICONVULSANTS, BARBITURATES increase or decrease anticonvulsant and BARBITURATE levels; **haloperidol, loxapine, maprotiline,** MAOIS, PHENOTHIAZINES, THIOXANTHENES, TRICYCLIC ANTIDEPRESSANTS can increase CNS depression or lower seizure threshold; **aspirin, dipyridamole, warfarin** increase risk of spontaneous bleeding and decrease clotting; **clonazepam** may precipitate absence seizures; SALICYLATES, **cimetidine** may increase valproic acid levels and toxicity. **Mefloquine** can decrease valproic acid levels; **isoniazid** may increase valproic acid levels and hepatotoxicity; **meropenem** may decrease valproic acid levels; **cholestyramine** may decrease absorption. **Herbal: Ginkgo** may decrease anticonvulsant effectiveness.

PHARMACOKINETICS Absorption: Readily absorbed from GI tract. **Peak:** 1–4 h valproic acid; 3–5 h divalproex. **Therapeutic Range:** 50–100 g/mL. **Distribution:** Crosses placenta; distributed into breast milk. **Metabolism:** Metabolized in liver. **Elimination:** Excreted primarily in urine; small amount excreted in feces and expired air. **Half-Life:** 5–20 h.

NURSING IMPLICATIONS

Assessment & Drug Effects

- Monitor for therapeutic effectiveness achieved with serum levels of valproic acid at 50–100 mcg/mL.
- Monitor patient alertness especially with multiple drug therapy for seizure control. Evaluate plasma levels of the adjunctive anticonvulsants periodically as indicators for possible neurologic toxicity.
- Monitor patient carefully during dose adjustments and promptly report presence of adverse effects. Increased dosage is associated with frequency of adverse effects.
- Lab tests: Perform baseline platelet counts, bleeding time, and serum ammonia, then repeat at least q2mo, especially during the first 6 mo of therapy.
- Multiple drugs for seizure control increase the risk of hyperam-

monemia, marked by lethargy, anorexia, asterixis, increased seizure frequency, and vomiting. Report such symptoms promptly to physician. If they persist with decreased dosage, the drug will be discontinued.

Patient & Family Education

- Do not discontinue therapy abruptly; such action could result in loss of seizure control. Consult physician before you stop or alter dosage regimen.
- Note to diabetic patients: Drug may cause a false-positive test for urine ketones. Notify physician if this occurs; a differential diagnostic blood test may be indicated.
- Notify physician promptly if spontaneous bleeding or bruising occurs (e.g., petechiae, ecchymotic areas, otorrhagia, epistaxis, melena).
- Withhold dose and notify physician for following symptoms: visual disturbances, rash, jaundice, light-colored stools, protracted vomiting, diarrhea. Fatal liver failure has occurred in patients receiving this drug.
- Avoid alcohol and self-medication with other depressants during therapy.
- Consult physician before using any OTC drugs during anticonvulsant therapy. Combination drugs containing aspirin, sedatives, and medications for hay fever or other allergies are particularly UNSAFE.
- Do not drive or engage in potentially hazardous activities until response to drug is known.
- Inform doctor or dentist before any kind of surgery that you are taking valproic acid.
- Carry medical identification card at all times. It needs to indicate medical diagnosis, medication(s), physician's name, address, and telephone number.
- Do not breast feed while taking this drug.

VALRUBICIN

(val-roo'bi-sin)

Valstar

Classifications: ANTINEOPLASTIC; ANTIBIOTIC

Prototype: Doxorubicin Hydrochloride

Pregnancy Category: C

AVAILABILITY 200 mg/5 mL vials

ACTIONS Semisynthetic analog of doxorubicin. It is a cytotoxic antibiotic agent that inhibits the incorporation of nucleosides in DNA and RNA, which results in extensive chromosomal damage. Valrubicin interferes with DNA topoisomerase II, which is responsible for the normal DNA separation of strands and the resealing of DNA strands.
THERAPEUTIC EFFECTS Valrubicin has higher antitumor efficacy and lower toxicity than doxirubicin.

USES Intravesical therapy of BCG-refractory carcinoma *in situ* of the urinary bladder.

CONTRAINDICATIONS Hypersensitivity to valrubicin, doxirubicin; patients with a perforated bladder, concurrent UTI, active infection; severe irritable bladder symptoms; severe myelosuppression; pregnancy (category C); lactation.
CAUTIOUS USE Within 2 wk of a transureteral resection; compromised bladder mucosa; mild-to-moderate myelosuppression; concurrent use of anticoagulants, or history of bleeding disorders; GI disorders, renal impairment.

ROUTE & DOSAGE

BCG-Refractory Bladder Carcinoma *in situ*
Adult: **Intravesically** 800 mg once per wk × 6 wk.

ADMINISTRATION

Instillation

- Avoid skin reactions by using gloves during preparation/administration.
- Use only glass, polypropylene, or polyolefin containers and tubing.

PREPARE: Slowly warm 4 vials (5 mL each) to room temperature. When a precipitate is initially present, warm vials in hands until solution clears. Add contents of 4 vials to 55 mL of 0.9% NaCl injection to yield 75 mL of diluted solution.

INSTILL: Aseptically insert a urethral catheter and drain the bladder. Use gravity drainage to instill valrubicin slowly over several min. Withdraw catheter; instruct patient not to void for 2 h. Note: Do not leave a clamped catheter in place.

- Refrigerate. Do not freeze.

ADVERSE EFFECTS (≥1%) **Body as a Whole:** Abdominal pain, asthenia, back pain, fever, headache, malaise, myalgia. **CNS:** Dizziness. **CV:** Vasodilation. **GI:** Diarrhea, flatulence, nausea, vomiting. **Urogenital:** *Urinary frequency, urgency, dysuria, bladder spasm, hematuria, bladder pain, incontinence, cystitis, UTI,* nocturia, local burning, urethral pain, pelvic pain, gross hematuria, urinary retention. **Respiratory:** Pneumonia. **Skin:** Rash. **Other:** Anemia, hyperglycemia, peripheral edema.

INTERACTIONS Drug: No clinically significant interactions established.

PHARMACOKINETICS Absorption: Not absorbed from bladder. **Distribution:** Penetrates bladder wall. **Metabolism:** Not metabolized. **Elimination:** Almost completely excreted by voiding the instillate.

NURSING IMPLICATIONS

Assessment & Drug Effects

- Therapeutic effectiveness: Indicated by regression of the bladder tumor.
- Notify physician if bladder spasms with spontaneous discharge of valrubicin occur during/shortly after instillation.

Patient & Family Education

- Expect red-tinged urine during the first 24 h after administration.
- Report prolonged passage of red-colored urine or prolonged bladder irritation.
- Drink plenty of fluids during 48 h period following administration.
- Use reliable contraception during therapy period (approximately 6 wk).
- Do not breast feed infants during therapy period (approximately 6 wk).

VALSARTAN

(val-sar'tan)
Diovan
Classifications: CARDIOVASCULAR AGENT; ANGIOTENSIN II-RECEPTOR (TYPE AT_1) ANTAGONIST; ANTIHYPERTENSIVE
Prototype: Losartan
Pregnancy Category: C (first trimester); D (second and third trimesters)

AVAILABILITY 40 mg, 80 mg, 160 mg capsules

ACTIONS An angiotensin II receptor (type AT_1 antagonist; blocks the binding of angiotensin II to the AT_1 receptors found in many tissues (e.g., vascular smooth muscle, adrenal glands). Angiotensin II is a potent vasoconstrictor and primary vasoactive hormone of the renin–angiotensin–aldosterone system.

THERAPEUTIC EFFECTS Blocks angiotensin II, which results in vasodilation and blocking of the aldosterone-secreting effects of angiotensin II, thus resulting in an antihypertensive effect.

USES Treatment of hypertension, heart failure.

CONTRAINDICATIONS Hypersensitivity to valsartan or losartan; pregnancy [(category C) first trimester, (category D) second and third trimesters], lactation; severe heart failure with compromised renal function.

CAUTIOUS USE Severe renal or hepatic impairment; congestive heart failure. Safety and efficacy in children <18 y are not established.

ROUTE & DOSAGE

Hypertension

Adult: **PO** 80 mg q.d. (max: 320 mg q.d.)

Heart Failure

Adult: **PO** Start with 40 mg b.i.d. and titrate up to 160 mg b.i.d.

ADMINISTRATION

Oral

- Give on an empty stomach.
- Correct volume depletion prior to initiation of therapy to prevent hypotension.
- Reduce dosage with severe hepatic or renal impairment.
- Note: Daily dose may be titrated up to 320 mg.
- Store at 15°–30° C (59°–86° F).

ADVERSE EFFECTS (≥1%) **Body as a Whole:** Arthralgia. **CNS:** Headache, dizziness. **GI:** Diarrhea, nausea. **Respiratory:** Cough, sinusitis. **Metabolic:** Hyperkalemia.

INTERACTIONS No clinically significant interactions established.

PHARMACOKINETICS Absorption: Rapidly absorbed from GI tract, 25% bioavailability. **Onset:** Blood pressure decreased in 2 wk. **Peak:** Plasma levels, 2–4 h; blood pressure effect 4 wk. **Distribution:** 99% protein bound. **Metabolism:** Metabolized in the liver. **Elimination:** Excreted primarily in feces. **Half-Life:** 6 h.

NURSING IMPLICATIONS

Assessment & Drug Effects

- Monitor BP periodically; take trough readings, just prior to the next scheduled dose, when possible.
- Lab tests: Monitor liver function tests, BUN and creatinine, serum potassium, and CBC with differential, periodically.

Patient & Family Education

- Inform physician immediately if you become pregnant.
- Note: Maximum pressure lowering effect is usually evident between 2 and 4 wk after initiation of therapy.
- Notify physician of episodes of dizziness, especially those that occur when making position changes.
- Do not breast feed while taking this drug.

V

VANCOMYCIN HYDROCHLORIDE

(van-koe-mye′sin)

Vancocin

Classifications: ANTI-INFECTIVE; ANTIBIOTIC

Pregnancy Category: B

AVAILABILITY 125 mg, 250 mg capsules; 1 g, 10 g oral powder; 500 mg, 1 g injection

ACTIONS Prepared from *Streptomyces orientalis,* with bactericidal and bacteriostatic actions. Acts by interfering with cell membrane synthesis in multiplying organisms.

THERAPEUTIC EFFECTS Active against many gram-positive organisms, including group A *beta-hemolytic Streptococci, Staphylococci, Pneumococci, Enterococci, Clostridia,* and *Corynebacteria.* Gram-negative organisms, mycobacteria, and fungi are highly resistant.

USES Parenterally for potentially life-threatening infections in patients allergic, nonsensitive, or resistant to other less toxic antimicrobial drugs. Used orally only in *Clostridium difficile* colitis (not effective by oral route for treatment of systemic infections).

CONTRAINDICATIONS Known hypersensitivity to vancomycin, allergy to corn or corn products, previous hearing loss, concurrent or sequential use of other ototoxic or nephrotoxic agents, IM administration.

CAUTIOUS USE Neonates; children; older adults; impaired kidney function, renal failure, renal impairment, concomitant administration of aminoglycosides; hearing impairment; colitis, inflammatory disorders of the intestine; pregnancy (category B), lactation.

ROUTE & DOSAGE

Systemic Infections

Adult: **IV** 500 mg q6h or 1 g q12h, infuse over 60–90 min
Child: **IV** 40 mg/kg/d divided q6h, infuse over 60–90 min
Neonate: **IV** 10 mg/kg/d divided q8–12h, infuse over 60–90 min

***Clostridium difficile* Colitis**

Adult: **PO** 125–500 mg q6h
Child: **PO** 40 mg/kg/d divided q6h (max: 2 g/d)

ADMINISTRATION

Oral

- Oral solution is prepared by adding to 10 g oral powder 115 mL of distilled water. The solution may be further diluted in 10 g of water.

Intravenous

PREPARE: **Intermittent:** Reconstitute 500 mg vial or 1 g vial with 10 mL or 20 mL, respectively, of sterile water for injection to yield 50 mg/mL. Further dilute each 1 g with at least 200 mL of D5W, NS, or RL.

ADMINISTER: **Intermittent:** Give a single dose at a rate of 10 mg/min or over NOT LESS than 60 min. Avoid rapid infusion, which may cause sudden hypotension. Monitor IV site closely; necrosis and tissue sloughing will result from extravasation.

INCOMPATIBILITIES **Solution/additive: Aminophylline,** BARBITURATES, **cefotaxime, chloramphenicol, chlorothiazide, dexamethasone, heparin, sodium bicarbonate, warfarin. Y-site: albumin, aztreonam, cefepime, cefotaxime, cefotetan, cefoxitin, ceftazidime, ceftriaxone, cefuroxime, foscarnet, heparin, idarubicin, naf-**

V

cillin, omeprazole, piperacillin/tazobactam, ticarcillin, ticarcillin/clavulanate, warfarin.

▪ Store oral and parenteral solutions in refrigerator for up to 14 d; after further dilution, parenteral solution is stable 24 h at room temperature.

ADVERSE EFFECTS (≥1%) **Special Senses:** Ototoxicity (auditory portion of eighth cranial nerve). **Urogenital:** Nephrotoxicity leading to uremia. **Body as a Whole:** Hypersensitivity reactions (chills, fever, skin rash, urticaria, shock-like state), anaphylactoid reaction with vascular collapse, superinfections, severe pain, thrombophlebitis at injection site, generalized tingling following rapid IV infusion. **Hematologic:** Transient leukopenia, eosinophilia. **GI:** Nausea, warmth. **Other:** Injection reaction that includes *hypotension accompanied by flushing and erythematous rash on face and upper body* ("red-neck syndrome") following rapid IV infusion.

INTERACTIONS Drug: Adds to toxicity of OTOTOXIC and NEPHROTOXIC DRUGS (AMINOGLYCOSIDES, **amphotericin B, colistin, capreomycin; cidofovir; cisplatin; cyclosporine; foscarnet; ganciclovir; IV pentamidine; polymyxin B; streptozocin; tacrolimus**). **Cholestyramine, colestipol** can decrease absorption of oral vancomycin; may increase risk of lactic acidosis with **metformin.**

PHARMACOKINETICS Absorption: Not absorbed from GI tract. **Peak:** 30 min after end of infusion. **Distribution:** Diffuses into pleural, ascitic, pericardial, and synovial fluids; small amount penetrates CSF if meninges are inflamed; crosses placenta. **Elimination:** 80%–90% of IV dose excreted in urine within 24 h; PO dose excreted in feces. **Half-Life:** 4–8 h.

NURSING IMPLICATIONS

Assessment & Drug Effects

- Monitor BP and heart rate continuously through period of drug administration.
- Lab tests: Monitor urinalysis, kidney & liver functions, and hematologic studies periodically.
- Monitor serial tests of vancomycin blood levels (peak and trough) in patients with borderline kidney function, in infants and neonates, and in patients >60 y.
- Assess hearing. Drug may cause damage to auditory branch (not vestibular branch) of eighth cranial nerve, with consequent deafness, which may be permanent.
- Be aware that serum levels of 60–80 mcg/mL are associated with ototoxicity. Tinnitus and high-tone hearing loss may precede deafness, which may progress even after drug is withdrawn. Older adults and those on high doses are especially susceptible.
- Monitor I&O: Report changes in I&O ratio and pattern. Oliguria or cloudy or pink urine may be a sign of nephrotoxicity (also manifested by transient elevations in BUN, albumin, and hyaline and granular casts in urine).

Patient & Family Education

- Notify physician promptly of ringing in ears.
- Adhere to drug regimen (i.e., do not increase, decrease, or interrupt dosage. The full course of prescribed drug therapy must be completed).
- Do not breast feed while taking this drug.

VARDENAFIL HYDROCHLORIDE

(var-den'a-fil hy-dro-chlo'ride)
Levitra
Classifications: IMPOTENCE AGENT; PHOSPHODIESTERASE (PDE) INHIBITOR; VASODILATOR
Prototype: Sildenafil
Pregnancy Category: B

AVAILABILITY 2.5 mg, 5 mg, 10 mg, 20 mg tablets

ACTIONS A selective phosphodiesterase (PDE) type 5 inhibitor similar to sildenafil. The physiologic mechanism of erection of the penis involves release of nitric oxide (NO) in the corpus cavernosum during sexual stimulation. Nitric oxide then activates an enzyme that results in increased levels of cyclic guanosine monophosphate (cGMP). Cyclic GMP causes smooth muscle relaxation in the corpus cavernosum, thereby allowing inflow of blood into the penis. PDE type 5 is responsible for degradation of cGMP in the corpus cavernosum. Vardenafil enhances the effect of NO as well as inhibits PDE type 5.

THERAPEUTIC EFFECTS Vardenafil is a selective inhibitor of cGMP-specific PDE type 5, thereby raising concentration of cGMP in the corpus cavernosum, and resulting in a sustained erection.

USES Treatment of erectile dysfunction.

CONTRAINDICATIONS Hypersensitivity to vardenafil or sildenafil; concurrent administration of nitrates or nitroglycerin; QT prolongation, renal failure, severe renal impairment; retinitis pigmentosa; not recommended for women or children; lactation.

CAUTIOUS USE CAD, MI, or stroke within 6 mo; hypotension, or hypertension; risk factors for CVA; anatomic deformity of the penis; subaortic stenosis; sickle cell anemia, leukemia; multiple myeloma; leukemia; coagulopathy; active bleeding or a peptic ulcer; GERD; hepatitis, cirrhosis; older adults; concurrent use with other medicines for penile dysfunction; pregnancy (category B).

ROUTE & DOSAGE

Erectile Dysfunction
Adult: **PO** 10 mg approximately 60 min before sexual activity. May increase to max 20 mg/d if needed. If taking ritonavir, max dose is 2.5 mg/72 h. If taking erythromycin, indinavir, itraconazole, ketoconazole, max dose is 2.5–5 mg/24 h
Geriatric: **PO** Start with 5 mg 60 min before sexual activity (max: 20 mg/d)

Hepatic Impairment
Moderate impairment: reduce dose to 5 mg (max: 10 mg/d)

ADMINISTRATION

Oral
- Take approximately 1 h before expected intercourse, but preferably not after a heavy or high-fat meal.
- Store at 15°–30° C (59°–86° F).

ADVERSE EFFECTS (≥1%) **Body as a Whole:** *Flushing,* flu-like syndrome, back pain, anaphylactoid reactions, asthenia, facial edema, pain, paresthesias. **CNS:** *Headache,* dizziness, insomnia, somnolence, vertigo. **CV:** Angina, hypertension, hypotension, MI, orthostatic hypotension, palpitations, syncope, sinus tachycardia. **GI:** Dyspepsia, nausea, vomiting, abdominal pain, abnormal liver function tests, diarrhea,

V

dysphagia, esophagitis, gastritis, GERD, xerostomia. **Metabolic:** Increased creatine kinase. **Musculoskeletal:** Arthralgia, myalgia, hypertonia, hyperesthesia. **Respiratory:** Rhinitis, sinusitis, dyspnea, epistaxis, pharyngitis. **Skin:** Photosensitivity, rash, pruritus, sweating. **Special Senses:** Tinnitus. **Urogenital:** Ejaculation dysfunction.

INTERACTIONS Drug: May potentiate hypotensive effects of NITRATES, **alfuzosin, doxazosin, prazosin, tamsulosin, terazosin; amiodarone, dofetilide, procainamide, quinidine, sotalol** may increase QTc interval leading to arrhythmias; **erythromycin** (and other MACROLIDES), **indinavir, itraconazole, ketoconazole,** PROTEASE INHIBITORS, **ritonavir, voriconazole** may increase level and toxicity of vardenafil.

PHARMACOKINETICS Absorption: Rapidly absorbed, 15% reaches systemic circulation. **Onset:** Within 1 h. **Peak:** 0.5–2 h. **Metabolism:** Metabolized in liver by CYP3A4. **Elimination:** Primarily excreted in feces (90–95%). **Half-Life:** 4–5 h.

NURSING IMPLICATIONS

Assessment & Drug Effects

- Monitor CV status and report angina or other S&S of cardiac dysfunction.
- Lab tests: Baseline and periodic LFTs.

Patient & Family Education

- Do not take more than once a day and never take more than the prescribed dose.
- Do not take this drug without consulting physician if you are taking drugs called "alpha blockers" or "nitrates" or any other drugs for high blood pressure, chest pain, or enlarged prostate.
- Report promptly any of the following: palpitations, chest pain, back pain, difficulty breathing, or shortness of breath; dizziness or fainting; changes in vision; dizziness; swollen eyelids; muscle aches; painful or prolonged erection (lasting longer than 4 h); skin rash, or itching.

VARICELLA VACCINE

(var-i-cel'la)

Varivax

Classifications: ANTIINFECTIVE; VACCINE; VIRAL

Prototype: Hepatitis B

Pregnancy Category: C

AVAILABILITY 1350 PFU/vial

ACTIONS A live attenuated vaccine that acts against both chickenpox and shingles, both of which are caused by *Varicella zoster* infection.

THERAPEUTIC EFFECTS Protects healthy children and adults from varicella effectively.

USES Vaccination against varicella in individuals ≥12 mo.

CONTRAINDICATIONS Hypersensitivity to any component of the vaccine; history of anaphylactoid reaction to neomycin; individuals with blood dyscrasia, leukemia, lymphomas, bone marrow or lymphatic system malignancies, concomitant immunosuppression therapy; individuals with primary or acquired immunodeficient states; active untreated tuberculosis; any febrile respiratory illness or other febrile infections; lactation; pregnancy (category C); children <1 y.

CAUTIOUS USE Acute lymphoblastic leukemia in remission.

ROUTE & DOSAGE

Varicella Protection

Adult: **SC** Primary immunization of 0.5 mL followed by 0.5 mL 4–8 wk after first dose, may need to revaccinate 3 mo after initial series if patient fails to seroconvert
Child: **SC** *12 mo–12 y,* Single dose of 0.5 mL

ADMINISTRATION

Subcutaneous

- Reconstitute vaccine with 0.7 mL of supplied diluent; gently agitate the vial to mix. Withdraw entire contents of vial (0.5 mL) into syringe for injection. Change needle on syringe and administer immediately or within 30 min of reconstitution.
- Give SC into the outer aspect of the deltoid. Exercise caution not to inject IV.
- Store powder vaccine in frost-free freezer at –15° C (+5° F) or colder. Store diluent separately at room temperature or in the refrigerator.

ADVERSE EFFECTS (≥1%) **CNS:** Headache, fever. **Hematologic:** Mild thrombocytopenia. **Skin:** *Redness, swelling, or rash at injection site.* **Other:** Herpes zoster infection (rare).

INTERACTIONS Drug: Acyclovir decreases vaccine's effectiveness. It is recommended that **yellow fever vaccine** be given at least 1 mo apart from varicella or any other live virus vaccine. Avoid **salicylates** for 6 wk after vaccination to decrease risk of developing Reye's syndrome.

PHARMACOKINETICS Onset: Seroconversion approximately 42 d after vaccination. **Duration:** >5–10 y in healthy children. **Distribution:** Crosses placenta; distributed into breast milk.

NURSING IMPLICATIONS

Assessment & Drug Effects

- Withhold vaccine and notify physician if patient has a history of hypersensitivity to neomycin or a current febrile infection.
- Monitor for signs and symptoms of hypersensitivity (see Appendix F) and administer epinephrine if an anaphylactoid reaction occurs.

Patient & Family Education

- Avoid use of salicylates (e.g., acetylsalicylic acid) for 6 wk after vaccination, especially with children and adolescents.
- Notify physician about all adverse reactions (i.e., fever, rash, respiratory illness).
- Do not breast feed after taking this drug.

VASOPRESSIN INJECTION (Pr)

(vay-soe-press'in)

Pitressin

Classifications: HORMONES AND SYNTHETIC SUBSTITUTES; PITUITARY (ANTIDIURETIC)

Pregnancy Category: X

AVAILABILITY 20 pressor units/mL injection

ACTIONS Polypeptide hormone extracted from animal posterior pituitaries. Possesses pressor and antidiuretic (ADH) properties, but is relatively free of oxytocic properties. Produces concentrated urine by increasing tubular reabsorption of water (ADH activity), thus preserving up to 90% of water.

THERAPEUTIC EFFECTS May increase sodium and decrease potassium reabsorption but plays no causative role in edema formation.

V

Small doses may produce anginal pain; large doses may precipitate MI, decrease heart rate and cardiac output, and increase pulmonary arterial pressure and BP. The tannate (in peanut oil) is preferred for chronic therapy; intranasal aqueous vasopressin is effective for daily maintenance of mild diabetes insipidus. Effective in the treatment of antidiuresis caused by diabetes insipidus.

USES Antidiuretic to treat diabetes insipidus, to dispel gas shadows in abdominal roentgenography, and as prevention and treatment of postoperative abdominal distension. Also given to treat transient polyuria due to ADH deficiency (related to head injuries or to neurosurgery).

UNLABELED USES Test for differential diagnosis of nephrogenic, psychogenic, and neurohypophyseal diabetes insipidus; test to elevate ability of kidney to concentrate urine, and provocative test for pituitary release of corticotropin and growth hormone; emergency and adjunct pressor agent in the control of massive GI hemorrhage (e.g., esophageal varices).

CONTRAINDICATIONS Chronic nephritis accompanied by nitrogen retention; ischemic heart disease, PVCs, advanced arteriosclerosis; pregnancy (category X); during first stage of labor.

CAUTIOUS USE Epilepsy; migraine; asthma; heart failure, angina pectoris; any state in which rapid addition to extracellular fluid may be hazardous; vascular disease; preoperative and postoperative polyuric patients, kidney disease; goiter with cardiac complications; older adult patients, children, lactation.

V

ROUTE & DOSAGE

Diabetes Insipidus

Adult: **IM/SC** 5–10 U aqueous solution 2–4 times/d (5–60 U/d) or 1.25–2.5 U in oil q2–3d **Intranasal** Apply to cotton pledget or intranasal spray

Child: **IM/SC** 2.5–10 U aqueous solution 2–4 times/d

Abdominal Distention, Abdominal Radiographic Procedures

Adult: **IM/SC** 5 U with 5–10 U q3–4h prn or 5–15 U 2 h and 30 min prior to procedure

GI Hemorrhage

Adult: **IV** 0.1–1 U/mL at 0.2–0.4 U/min up to 0.9 U/min

ADMINISTRATION

Intramuscular/Subcutaneous

- Give 1–2 glasses of water with vasopressin to reduce adverse effects of tannate and improve therapeutic response.
- Do NOT administer vasopressin tannate via IV. Warm ampul to body temperature and shake vigorously to disperse active principle before withdrawing drug for IM administration.
- The tannate injection is often painful, and allergic reactions may develop. It is preferred for use in chronic therapy because of its longer duration of action.

Intravenous

PREPARE: **IV Infusion:** Give vasopressin aqueous injection by continuous IV. Dilute with NS or D5W to a concentration of 0.1–1 U/mL.

ADMINISTER: **IV Infusion:** Titrate dose and rate to patient's response.

ADVERSE EFFECTS (≥1%) **Skin:** Rash, urticaria. **Body as a Whole:** Anaphylaxis; *tremor,* sweating, bronchoconstriction, *circumoral and facial pallor,* angioneurotic edema, *pounding in head, water intoxication* (especially with tannate), gangrene at injection site with intraarterial infusion. **GI:** *Eructations, passage of gas, nausea, vomiting,* heartburn, abdominal cramps, increased bowel movements secondary to excessive use. **CV:** Angina (in patient with coronary vascular disease); cardiac arrest, hypertension, bradycardia, minor arrhythmias, premature atrial contraction, heart block, peripheral vascular collapse, coronary insufficiency, MI; cardiac arrhythmia, pulmonary edema, bradycardia (with intraarterial infusion). **Urogenital:** Uterine cramps. **Respiratory:** Congestion, rhinorrhea, irritation, mucosal ulceration and pruritus, postnasal drip. **Special Senses:** Conjunctivitis.

DIAGNOSTIC TEST INTERFERENCE Vasopressin increases ***plasma cortisol*** levels.

INTERACTIONS Drug: Alcohol, demeclocycline, epinephrine, heparin, lithium, phenytoin may decrease antidiuretic effects of vasopressin; **guanethidine, neostigmine** increase vasopressor actions; **chlorpropamide, clofibrate, carbamazepine,** THIAZIDE DIURETICS may increase antidiuretic activity.

PHARMACOKINETICS Duration: 2–8 h in aqueous solution, 48–72 h in oil, 30–60 min IV infusion. **Distribution:** Extracellular fluid. **Metabolism:** Metabolized in liver and kidneys. **Elimination:** Excreted in urine. **Half-Life:** 10–20 min.

NURSING IMPLICATIONS

Assessment & Drug Effects

- Monitor infants and children closely. They are more susceptible to volume disturbances (such as sudden reversal of polyuria) than adults.
- Establish baseline data of BP, weight, I&O pattern and ratio. Monitor BP and weight throughout therapy. (Dose used to stimulate diuresis has little effect on BP.) Report sudden changes in pattern to physician.
- Be alert to the fact that even small doses of vasopressin may precipitate MI or coronary insufficiency, especially in older adult patients. Keep emergency equipment and drugs (antiarrhythmics) readily available.
- Check patient's alertness and orientation frequently during therapy. Lethargy and confusion associated with headache may signal onset of water intoxication, which, although insidious in rate of development, can lead to convulsions and terminal coma.
- Monitor urine output, specific gravity, and serum osmolality while patient is hospitalized.
- Withhold vasopressin, restrict fluid intake, and notify physician if urine-specific gravity is <1.015.

Patient & Family Education

- Be prepared for possibility of anginal attack and have coronary vasodilator available (e.g., nitroglycerin) if there is a history of coronary artery disease. Report to physician.
- Measure and record data related to polydipsia and polyuria. Learn how to determine specific gravity and how to keep an accurate record of output. Understand that treatment should diminish intense

V

thirst and restore undisturbed normal sleep.
- Avoid concentrated fluids (e.g., undiluted syrups), since these increase urine volume.
- Do not breast feed while taking this drug without consulting physician.

VECURONIUM

(vek-yoo-roe'nee-um)
Norcuron
Classifications: AUTONOMIC NERVOUS SYSTEM AGENT; NONDEPOLARIZING SKELETAL MUSCLE RELAXANT
Prototype: Tubocurarine
Pregnancy Category: C

AVAILABILITY 10 mg, 20 mg vials

ACTIONS Intermediate-acting nondepolarizing skeletal muscle relaxant structurally similar to pancuronium. Demonstrates negligible histamine release and therefore has minimal direct effect on cardiovascular system, unlike older neuromuscular blocking agents.
THERAPEUTIC EFFECTS Inhibits neuromuscular transmission by competitively binding with acetylcholine to motor endplate receptors (common also with other drugs of this class). Results in skeletal muscular relaxation. Given ONLY after induction of general anesthesia.

USES Adjunct for general anesthesia to produce skeletal muscle relaxation during surgery. Especially useful for patients with severe kidney disease, limited cardiac reserve, and history of asthma or allergy. Also to facilitate endotracheal intubation.
UNLABELED USES Continuous infusion for facilitation of mechanical ventilation.

CONTRAINDICATIONS Safe use during pregnancy (category C), lactation, is not established.
CAUTIOUS USE Severe liver disease; impaired acid–base, fluid and electrolyte balance; severe obesity; adrenal or neuromuscular disease (myasthenia gravis, Eaton-Lambert syndrome); patients with slow circulation time (cardiovascular disease, old age, edematous states); malignant hyperthermia.

ROUTE & DOSAGE

Skeletal Muscle Relaxation
Adult/Child: **IV** ≥*1 y,* 0.04–0.1 mg/kg initially, then after 25–40 min, 0.01–0.15 mg/kg q12–15 min or 0.001 mg/kg/min by continuous infusion
Neonate: **IV** 0.1 mg/kg, followed by 0.03–0.15 mg/kg q1–2h prn

ADMINISTRATION

Note: Vecuronium is administered only by qualified clinicians.

Intravenous

PREPARE: **Direct:** Dilute 10–20 mg with 50 mL sterile water for injection (supplied). **Continuous:** Further dilute with up to 100 mL D5W, NS, or RL to yield 0.1–0.2 mg/mL.
ADMINISTER: **Direct:** Give a bolus dose over 30 sec. **Continuous:** Give at the required rate.
INCOMPATIBILITIES **Y-site: amphotericin B cholesteryl complex, diazepam, etomidate, furosemide, thiopental.**

- Refrigerate after reconstitution below 30° C (86° F), unless otherwise directed. Discard solution after 24 h.

ADVERSE EFFECTS (≥1%) **Body as a Whole:** Skeletal muscle weakness, malignant hyperthermia. **Respiratory:** Respiratory depression.

INTERACTIONS Drug: GENERAL ANESTHETICS increase neuromuscular blockade and duration of action; AMINOGLYCOSIDES, **bacitracin, polymyxin B, clindamycin, lidocaine, parenteral magnesium, quinidine, quinine, trimethaphan, verapamil** increase neuromuscular blockade; DIURETICS may increase or decrease neuromuscular blockade; **lithium** prolongs duration of neuromuscular blockade; NARCOTIC ANALGESICS increase possibility of additive respiratory depression; **succinylcholine** increases onset and depth of neuromuscular blockade; **phenytoin** may cause resistance to or reversal of neuromuscular blockade.

PHARMACOKINETICS Onset: <1 min. **Peak:** 3–5 min. **Duration:** 25–40 min. **Distribution:** Well distributed to tissues and extracellular fluids; crosses placenta; distribution into breast milk unknown. **Metabolism:** Rapid nonenzymatic degradation in bloodstream. **Elimination:** 30%–35% excreted in urine, 30%–35% in bile. **Half-Life:** 30–80 min.

NURSING IMPLICATIONS

Assessment & Drug Effects

- Lab tests: Baseline serum electrolytes, acid–base balance, and kidney & liver functions.
- Use peripheral nerve stimulator during and following drug administration to avoid risk of overdosage and to identify residual paralysis during recovery period. This is especially indicated when cautious use of drug is specified.
- Monitor vital signs at least q15 min until stable, then every 30 min for the next 2 h. Also monitor airway patency until assured that patient has fully recovered from drug effects. Note rate, depth, and pattern of respirations. Obese patients and patients with myasthenia gravis or other neuromuscular disease may have ventilation problems.
- Evaluate patients for recovery from neuromuscular blocking (curare-like) effects as evidenced by ability to breathe naturally or take deep breaths and cough, to keep eyes open, and to lift head keeping mouth closed and by adequacy of hand grip strength. Notify physician if recovery is delayed.
- Note: Recovery time may be delayed in patients with cardiovascular disease, edematous states, and in older adults.

VENLAFAXINE (Pr)

(ven-la-fax′een)

Effexor, Effexor XR

Classifications: CENTRAL NERVOUS SYSTEM (CNS) AGENT; PSYCHOTHERAPEUTIC AGENT; ANTIDEPRESSANT; SEROTONIN NOREPINEPHRINE REUPTAKE INHIBITOR (SNRI)

Pregnancy Category: C

AVAILABILITY 25 mg, 37.5 mg, 50 mg, 75 mg, 100 mg tablets; 37.5 mg, 75 mg, 150 mg sustained-release capsules

ACTIONS Selectively inhibits neuronal uptake of serotonin, norepinephrine, and dopamine in decreasing order of potency. A bicyclic "second-generation" antidepressant, drug is chemically unrelated to tricyclic, tetracyclic, or other antidepressants.

THERAPEUTIC EFFECTS Antidepressant effect is presumed to be linked to its inhibition of CNS presynaptic neuronal uptake of serotonin. Drug does not cause anticholinergic, sedative, or cardiovascular effects.

V

USES Depression, generalized anxiety disorder; social anxiety disorder.
UNLABELED USES Obsessive-compulsive disorder.

CONTRAINDICATIONS Hypersensitivity to venlafaxine, or other SNRI drugs; concurrent administration with MAO inhibitors; abrupt discontinuation; neonates; pregnancy (category C), lactation.
CAUTIOUS USE Renal and hepatic impairment, renal failure; anorexia nervosa, history of mania, suicidal ideations; elevated intraocular pressure, acute closed-angle glaucoma; cardiac disorders, recent MI, heart failure; hypertension; hyperthyroidism; concomitant administration with CNS drugs, CNS depression; history of seizures or seizure disorders; older adults. Safety in children <18 y is not established.

ROUTE & DOSAGE

Depression

Adult: **PO** 25–125 mg t.i.d.
Geriatric: **PO** Start with lower doses in older adults

Anxiety

Adult: **PO** Start with 37.5 mg sustained-release q.d. and increase to 75–225 mg sustained-release per day

Renal Impairment

Cl_{cr} 10–70 mL/min: reduce total daily dose by 25%–50%; <10 mL/min: reduce total daily dose by 50%

ADMINISTRATION

Oral

- Give with food. Sustained-release capsules must be swallowed whole, must not be opened or chewed.
- Dosage increments of up to 75 mg/d are usually made at 4 d or longer intervals.
- Allow 14 d interval after discontinuing an MAO inhibitor before starting venlafaxine.
- Do not abruptly withdraw drug after 1 wk or more of therapy.
- Store at room temperature, 15°–30° C (59°–86° F).

ADVERSE EFFECTS (≥1%) **CV:** *Increased blood pressure and heart rate,* palpitations. **CNS:** *Dizziness,* fatigue, headache, anxiety, insomnia, *somnolence.* **Endocrine:** Small but statistically significant increase in serum cholesterol, weight loss (approximately 3 lb). **GI:** *Nausea, vomiting, dry mouth,* constipation. **Urogenital:** Sexual dysfunction, erectile failure, delayed orgasm, anorgasmia, impotence, abnormal ejaculation. **Special Senses:** Blurred vision. **Body as a Whole:** *Sweating,* asthenia.

INTERACTIONS Drug: Cimetidine, MAO INHIBITORS, **desipramine, haloperidol** may increase venlafaxine levels and toxicity. Should not use in combination with MAO INHIBITORS: do not start until >14 d after stopping MAO INHIBITOR; do not start MAO INHIBITOR until 7 d after stopping venlafaxine. **Trazodone** may lead to **serotonin** syndrome. **Herbal: St. John's wort** may cause **serotonin** syndrome.

PHARMACOKINETICS Absorption: Well absorbed from GI tract. **Onset:** 2 wk. **Peak:** Venlafaxine 1–2 h; metabolite 3–4 h. **Duration:** Approximately 30% protein bound, but extensively tissue bound. **Metabolism:** Undergoes substantial first-pass metabolism to its major active metabolite, *O*-desmethylvenlafaxine, with similar activity to venlafaxine. **Elimination:** Approximately 60% excreted in urine as parent compound and metabolites. **Half-Life:** Venlafaxine 3–4 h, *O*-desmethylvenlafaxine 10 h.

NURSING IMPLICATIONS

Assessment & Drug Effects

- Monitor for worsening of depression or emergence of suicidal ideation.
- Monitor cardiovascular status periodically with measurements of HR and BP.
- Lab tests: Periodic lipid profile.
- Monitor neurologic status and report excessive anxiety, nervousness, and insomnia.
- Monitor weight periodically and report excess weight loss.
- Assess safety, as dizziness and sedation are common.

Patient & Family Education

- Be aware of potential adverse effects and notify physician of those that are bothersome.
- Do not drive or engage in potentially hazardous activities until response to drug is known.
- Avoid using alcohol while on venlafaxine.
- Do not use herbal medications without consulting physician.
- Do not breast feed while taking this drug without consulting physician.

VERAPAMIL HYDROCHLORIDE

(ver-ap′a-mill)

Calan, Calan SR, Covera-HS, Isoptin, Isoptin SR, Verelan, Verelan PM

Classifications: CARDIOVASCULAR AGENT; CALCIUM CHANNEL BLOCKER; ANTIARRHYTHMIC

Prototype: Nifedipine

Pregnancy Category: C

AVAILABILITY 40 mg, 80 mg, 120 mg tablets; 120 mg, 180 mg, 240 mg sustained-release tablets; 100 mg, 120 mg, 180 mg, 200 mg, 240 mg, 300 mg sustained-release capsules; 5 mg/2 mL injection

ACTIONS Inhibits calcium ion influx through slow channels into cells of myocardial and arterial smooth muscle. Dilates coronary arteries and arterioles and inhibits coronary artery spasm. Decreases and slows SA and AV node conduction without affecting normal arterial action potential or intraventricular conduction. Associated vasodilation of arterioles decreases total peripheral vascular resistance and reduces arterial BP at rest. May slightly decrease heart rate.

THERAPEUTIC EFFECTS Dilates coronary arteries and inhibits coronary artery spasm, which increases myocardial oxygen delivery and produces an antianginal effect. Also decreases nodal conduction, which results in an antiarrhythmic effect.

USES Supraventricular tachyarrhythmias; Prinzmetal's (variant) angina, chronic stable angina; unstable, crescendo or preinfarctive angina and essential hypertension.

UNLABELED USES Paroxysmal supraventricular tachycardia, atrial fibrillation; prophylaxis of migraine headache; and as alternate therapy in manic depression.

CONTRAINDICATIONS Severe hypotension (diastolic <90 mm Hg), cardiogenic shock, cardiomegaly, digitalis toxicity, second- or third-degree AV block; Wolff-Parkinson-White syndrome including atrial flutter and fibrillation; accessory AV pathway, left ventricular dysfunction, severe CHF, sinus node disease, sick sinus syndrome (except in patients with functioning ventricu-

lar pacemaker). Safe use during pregnancy (category C), lactation, or in children (oral) is not established.
CAUTIOUS USE Duchenne's muscular dystrophy; hepatic and renal impairment; MI followed by coronary occlusion, aortic stenosis.

ROUTE & DOSAGE

Angina

Adult: **PO** 80 mg q6–8h, may increase up to 320–480 mg/d in divided doses (Note: Covera-HS must be given once daily h.s.)

Hypertension

Adult: **PO** 40–80 mg t.i.d. or 90–240 mg sustained-release 1–2 times/d up to 480 mg/d (Note: Covera-HS must be given once daily h.s.)

Supraventricular Tachycardia, Atrial Fibrillation

Adult: **PO** 240–480 mg/d in divided doses **IV** 5–10 mg IV direct, may repeat in 15–30 min if needed
Child: **IV** *<1 y,* 0.1–0.2 mg/kg; *1–15 y,* 0.1–0.3 mg/kg (2–5 mg)

ADMINISTRATION

Oral

- Give with food to reduce gastric irritation.
- Capsules can be opened and contents sprinkled on food. Do NOT dissolve or chew capsule contents.
- Give Covera-HS once a day in the evening.
- Do not withdraw abruptly; may increase and extend duration of pain in the angina patient.

Intravenous

PREPARE: **IV Direct:** Given undiluted or diluted in 5 mL of sterile water for injection. Inspect parenteral drug preparation before administration. Make sure solution is clear and colorless.
ADMINISTER: **Direct:** Give a single dose over 2–3 min.
INCOMPATIBILITIES **Solution/additive: albumin, aminophylline, amphotericin B, hydralazine, cotrimoxazole. Y-site: albumin, amphotericin B cholesteryl complex, ampicillin, mezlocillin, nafcillin, oxacillin, propofol, sodium bicarbonate.**

- Store at 15°–30° C (59°–86° F) and protect from light.

ADVERSE EFFECTS (≥1%) **CNS:** Dizziness, vertigo, *headache,* fatigue, sleep disturbances, depression, syncope. **CV:** *Hypotension,* congestive heart failure, bradycardia, severe tachycardia, peripheral edema, <u>AV block</u>. **GI:** Nausea, abdominal discomfort, *constipation,* elevated liver enzymes. **Body as a Whole:** Flushing, pulmonary edema, muscle fatigue, diaphoresis. **Skin:** Pruritus.

DIAGNOSTIC TEST INTERFERENCE Verapamil may cause elevations of serum ***AST, ALT, alkaline phosphatase.***

INTERACTIONS Drug: BETA BLOCKERS increase risk of CHF, bradycardia, or heart block; significantly increased levels of **digoxin** and **carbamazepine** and toxicity; potentiates hypotensive effects of HYPOTENSIVE AGENTS; levels of **lithium** and **cyclosporine** may be increased, increasing their toxicity; **calcium salts** (IV) may antagonize verapamil effects. **Food: Grapefruit juice** may increase verapamil levels. **Herbal: Hawthorne** may have additive hypotensive effects.

PHARMACOKINETICS Absorption: 90% absorbed, but only 25%–30% reaches systemic circulation (first pass metabolism). **Peak:** 1–2 h PO;

4–8 h sustained release; 5 min IV. **Distribution:** Widely distributed, including CNS; crosses placenta; present in breast milk. **Metabolism:** Metabolized in liver. **Elimination:** 70% excreted in urine; 16% in feces. **Half-Life:** 2–8 h.

NURSING IMPLICATIONS

Assessment & Drug Effects

- Monitor therapeutic effectiveness. Drug should decrease angina frequency, nitroglycerin consumption, and episodes of ST segment deviation.
- Establish baseline data and periodically monitor: BP and pulse.
- Lab tests: Baseline and periodic liver and kidney functions.
- Instruct patient to remain in recumbent position for at least 1 h after dose is given to diminish subjective effects of transient asymptomatic hypotension that may accompany infusion.
- Monitor for AV block or excessive bradycardia when infusion is given concurrently with digitalis.
- Monitor I&O ratio during IV and early oral maintenance therapy. Renal impairment prolongs duration of action, increasing potential for toxicity and incidence of adverse effects. Advise patient to report gradual weight gain and evidence of edema.
- Monitor ECG continuously during IV administration. Essential because drug action may be prolonged and incidence of adverse reactions is highest during IV administration in older adults, patients with impaired kidney function, and patients of small stature.
- Check BP shortly before administration of next dose to evaluate degree of control during early treatment for hypertension.

Patient & Family Education

- Monitor radial pulse before each dose, notify physician of an irregular pulse or one slower than established guideline.
- Adhere to established guidelines for exercise program.
- Do not drive or engage in potentially hazardous activities until response to drug is known.
- Decrease intake of caffeine-containing beverage (i.e., coffee, tea, chocolate).
- Change positions slowly from lying down to standing to prevent falls because of drug-related vertigo until tolerance to reduced BP is established.
- Notify physician of easy bruising, petechiae, unexplained bleeding.
- Do not use OTC drugs, especially aspirin, unless they are specifically prescribed by physician.
- Do not breast feed while taking this drug without consulting physician.

VIDARABINE

(vye-dare′a-been)

Adenine Arabinoside, ARA-A, Vira-A

Classifications: ANTIINFECTIVE; ANTIVIRAL

Prototype: Zidovudine

Pregnancy Category: C

AVAILABILITY 3% ointment

ACTIONS A pyrimidine nucleoside obtained from *Streptomyces antibioticus*. Mechanism of action is not known but appears to block early stages of DNA synthesis by inhibiting DNA polymerase.

THERAPEUTIC EFFECTS Active against *Herpes simplex* virus types 1 and 2, *Varicella zoster*, vaccinia, *Cytomegalovirus, Hepatitis B* virus, and *Epstein-Barr* virus. Not active against smallpox, adenovirus, DNA or RNA viruses, bacteria, and fungi.

USES Used topically (ophthalmic) for treatment of acute keratoconjunctivitis and recurrent epithelial keratitis caused by *Herpes simplex* virus types 1 and 2. Topical antibiotics and topical corticosteroids may be used concurrently.

CONTRAINDICATIONS Safe use during pregnancy (category C) and lactation is not established.
CAUTIOUS USE Impaired kidney or liver function; patients susceptible to fluid overload or cerebral edema.

ROUTE & DOSAGE

Herpes Keratitis
Adult: **Ophthalmic** Instill 1 cm (1/2 in) ribbon of ointment into lower conjunctival sac q3h 5 times/d

ADMINISTRATION

Instillation
- Instill ribbon of ointment into lower conjunctival sac as prescribed.

ADVERSE EFFECTS ($\geq$1%) **Special Senses** Burning, itching, mild irritation, lacrimation, foreign body sensation, pain, photophobia, punctal occlusion, superficial punctate keratitis.

INTERACTIONS No clinically significant interactions established.

PHARMACOKINETICS Distribution: Widely distributed in body tissues and fluid; crosses blood–brain barrier; trace amounts of ophthalmic application found in aqueous humor; crosses placenta. **Metabolism:** Rapidly deaminated to ara-hypoxanthine (Ara-Hx), a less active metabolite. **Elimination:** Excreted primarily in urine. **Half-Life:** 1.5 h vidarabine, 3.3 h Ara-Hx.

NURSING IMPLICATIONS

Patient & Family Education
- Do not exceed recommended dose, frequency, and duration of treatment.
- Wash hands before and after treatment.
- Vision may be temporarily hazy following instillation; avoid potentially hazardous activities until vision clears.
- Use sunglasses as necessary; drug may cause sensitivity to bright light.
- Do not breast feed while using this drug without consulting physician.

VINBLASTINE SULFATE

(vin-blast′een)
Velban, Velbe A, VLB
Classifications: ANTINEOPLASTIC; MITOTIC INHIBITOR
Prototype: Vincristine
Pregnancy Category: D

AVAILABILITY 10 mg powder for injection; 1 mg/mL vial

ACTIONS Cell cycle-specific alkaloid, extracted from periwinkle plant *Vinca rosea*. Arrests mitosis in metaphase by combining with microtubule proteins; may also interfere with other microtubular functions such as phagocytosis and cell mobility. Spectrum of activity is not completely established.
THERAPEUTIC EFFECTS Interferes with nucleic acid synthesis by arresting proliferating cells in metaphase. Exhibits potent myelosuppressive and immunosuppressive properties, but produces less neurotoxicity, in contrast to vincristine.

USES Palliative treatment of Hodgkin's disease and non-Hodgkin's lymphomas, choriocarcinoma, lymphosarcoma, neuroblastoma, mycosis fungoides, advanced testicular germinal cell cancer, histiocytosis, and other malignancies resistant to other chemotherapy. Used singly or in combination with other chemotherapeutic drugs.

CONTRAINDICATIONS Leukopenia, bacterial infection, pregnancy (category D), lactation, men and women of childbearing potential, older adult patients with cachexia or skin ulcers.

CAUTIOUS USE Malignant cell infiltration of bone marrow; obstructive jaundice, hepatic impairment; history of gout; use of small amount of drug for long periods; use in eyes.

ROUTE & DOSAGE

Antineoplastic

Adult: **IV** 3.7 mg/m^2 infused over 1 min q wk, may increase up to 18.5 mg/m^2 if tolerated

Child: **IV** 2.5 mg/m^2 infused over 1 min q wk, may increase up to 12.5 mg/m^2 if tolerated

ADMINISTRATION

Intravenous

PREPARE: **Direct:** Add 10 mL NS to 10 mg of drug (yields 1 mg/mL). Do not use other diluents. Avoid contact with eyes. Severe irritation and persisting corneal changes may occur. Flush immediately and thoroughly with copious amounts of water. Wash both eyes; do not assume one eye escaped contamination.

ADMINISTER: **Direct:** Drug is usually injected into tubing of running IV infusion of NS or D5W over period of 1 min. Stop injection promptly if extravasation occurs. Use applications of moderate heat and local injection of hyaluronidase to help disperse extravasated drug. Restart infusion in another vein. Observe injection site for sloughing.

INCOMPATIBILITIES **Solution/additive: furosemide, heparin. Y-site: cefepime, furosemide.**

- Refrigerate reconstituted solution in tight, light-resistant containers up to 30 d without loss of potency.

ADVERSE EFFECTS (≥1%) **Body as a Whole:** Fever, weight loss, muscular pains, weakness, parotid gland pain and tenderness, tumor site pain, Raynaud's phenomenon. **CNS:** Mental depression, peripheral neuritis, numbness and paresthesias of tongue and extremities, loss of deep tendon reflexes, headache, convulsions. **GI:** Vesiculation of mouth, stomatitis, pharyngitis, anorexia, *nausea, vomiting,* diarrhea, ileus, abdominal pain, constipation, rectal bleeding, <u>hemorrhagic enterocolitis</u>, bleeding of old peptic ulcer. **Hematologic:** <u>Leukopenia</u>, thrombocytopenia and anemia. **Skin:** *Alopecia (reversible),* vesiculation, photosensitivity, phlebitis, cellulitis, and sloughing following extravasation (at injection site). **Urogenital:** Urinary retention, *hyperuricemia,* aspermia. **Respiratory:** <u>Bronchospasm</u>.

INTERACTIONS Drug: Mitomycin may cause acute shortness of breath and severe bronchospasm; may decrease **phenytoin** levels; ALFA INTERFERONS, **erythromycin, itraconazole** may increase vinblastine toxicity.

PHARMACOKINETICS Distribution: Concentrates in liver, platelets, and leukocytes; poor penetration of blood–brain barrier. **Metabolism:** Partially metabolized in liver. **Elimi-**

V

nation: Excreted in feces and urine. **Half-Life:** 24 h.

NURSING IMPLICATIONS

Assessment & Drug Effects

- Lab tests: Monitor WBC count. Recovery from leukopenic nadir occurs usually within 7–14 d. With high doses, total leukocyte count may not return to normal for 3 wk.
- Do not administer drug unless WBC count has returned to at least 4000/mm^3, even if 7 d have passed.
- Monitor for unexplained bruising or bleeding, which should be promptly reported, even though thrombocyte reduction seldom occurs unless patient has had prior treatment with other antineoplastics.
- Adverse reactions seldom persist beyond 24 h with exception of epilation, leukopenia, and neurologic adverse effects.
- Monitor bowel elimination pattern and bowel sounds to recognize severe constipation or paralytic ileus. A stool softener may be necessary.
- Inspect skin surfaces over pressure areas daily if patient is not ambulating. Note condition of skin of older adults especially.
- Stop drug if oral tissues break down.

Patient & Family Education

- Keep all appointments so that course of treatment is not interrupted.
- Be aware that temporary mental depression sometimes occurs on second or third day after treatment begins.
- Avoid exposure to infection, injury to skin or mucous membranes, and excessive physical stress, especially during leukocyte nadir period.
- Notify physician promptly about onset of symptoms of agranulocytosis (see Appendix F). Do not delay seeking appropriate treatment.
- Avoid exposure to sunlight unless protected with sunscreen lotion (SPF >12) and clothing.
- Do not breast feed while taking this drug.

VINCRISTINE SULFATE (Pr)

(vin-kris′teen)

Oncovin, VCR

Classifications: ANTINEOPLASTIC; MITOTIC INHIBITOR

Pregnancy Category: D

AVAILABILITY 1 mg/mL injection

ACTIONS Cell cycle-specific vinca alkaloid (obtained from periwinkle plant *Vinca rosea*); analog of vinblastine. Arrests mitosis at metaphase, thereby, inhibiting cell division. Antineoplastic mechanism unclear.

THERAPEUTIC EFFECTS In contrast to vinblastine, exhibits relatively low toxic effect on normal cells and thus produces minimal myelosuppression; however, neurologic and neuromuscular effects are more severe.

USES Acute lymphoblastic and other leukemias, Hodgkin's disease, lymphosarcoma, neuroblastoma, Wilms' tumor, lung and breast cancer, reticular cell carcinoma, and osteogenic and other sarcomas.

UNLABELED USES Idiopathic thrombocytopenic purpura, alone or adjunctively with other antineoplastics.

CONTRAINDICATIONS Obstructive jaundice; pregnancy (category D), lactation, men and women of childbearing potential; patient with demyelinating form of Charcot-Marie-Tooth syndrome.

CAUTIOUS USE Leukopenia; preexisting neuromuscular disease; hypertension; infection; patients receiving drugs with neurotoxic potential.

ROUTE & DOSAGE

Antineoplastic
Adult: **IV** 1.4 mg/m^2 (max: 2 mg/m^2) at weekly intervals
Child: **IV** 2 mg/m^2 at weekly intervals

ADMINISTRATION

Intravenous

PREPARE: **Direct:** Reconstitute with provided solution (bacteriostatic NaCl), sterile water, or NS to concentrations of 0.01 to 1.0 mg/mL. Note: Vincristine is available in solution form, which does not require reconstitution. Avoid contact with eyes. Severe irritation and persisting corneal changes may occur. Flush immediately and thoroughly with copious amounts of water. Wash both eyes; do not assume one eye escaped contamination.

ADMINISTER: **Direct:** Drug is usually injected into tubing of running infusion over a 1 min period. Stop injection promptly if extravasation occurs. Use applications of moderate heat and local injection of hyaluronidase to help disperse extravasated drug. Restart infusion in another vein. Observe injection site for sloughing.

INCOMPATIBILITIES **Solution/additive: furosemide. Y-site: cefepime, furosemide, idarubicin, sodium bicarbonate.**

- Store solution in the refrigerator.

ADVERSE EFFECTS (≥1%) **CNS:** *Peripheral neuropathy,* neuritic pain, *paresthesias, especially of hands and feet;* foot and hand drop, sensory loss, athetosis, ataxia, loss of deep tendon reflexes, muscle atrophy, dysphagia, weakness in larynx and extrinsic eye muscles, ptosis, diplopia, mental depression. **Special Senses:** Optic atrophy with blindness; transient cortical blindness, ptosis, diplopia, photophobia. **GI:** Stomatitis, pharyngitis, anorexia, nausea, vomiting, diarrhea, abdominal cramps, *severe constipation (upper-colon impaction), paralytic ileus (especially in children),* rectal bleeding; <u>hepatotoxicity</u>. **Urogenital:** Urinary retention, polyuria, dysuria, SIADH (high urinary sodium excretion, hyponatremia, dehydration, hypotension); uric acid nephropathy. **Skin:** Urticaria, rash, *alopecia,* cellulitis and phlebitis following extravasation (at injection site). **Body as a Whole:** Convulsions with hypertension, malaise, fever, headache, pain in parotid gland area, weight loss. **Metabolic:** Hyperuricemia, hyperkalemia. **CV:** Hypertension, hypotension. **Respiratory:** Bronchospasm.

INTERACTIONS Drug: Mitomycin may cause acute shortness of breath and severe bronchospasm; may decrease **digoxin, phenytoin** levels.

PHARMACOKINETICS Distribution: Concentrates in liver, platelets, and leukocytes; poor penetration of blood–brain barrier. **Metabolism:** Partially metabolized in liver. **Elimination:** Excreted primarily in feces. **Half-Life:** 10–155 h.

NURSING IMPLICATIONS

Assessment & Drug Effects

- Monitor I&O ratio and pattern, BP, and temperature daily.

V

- Weigh patient under standard conditions weekly or more often if ordered. In the presence of edema or ascites, patient's ideal weight is used to determine dosage. Report a steady gain or sudden weight change to physician.
- Lab tests: Monitor serum electrolytes and CBC with differential. Complete bone marrow remission in leukemia varies widely and may not occur for as long as 100 d after therapy is started.
- Be aware that neuromuscular adverse effects, most apt to appear in the patient with preexisting neuromuscular disease, usually disappear after 6 wk of treatment. Children are especially susceptible to neuromuscular adverse effects.
- Assess for hand muscular weakness, and check deep tendon reflexes (depression of Achilles reflex is the earliest sign of neuropathy). Also observe for and report promptly: Mental depression, ptosis, double vision, hoarseness, paresthesias, neuritic pain, and motor difficulties.
- Provide special protection against infection or injury during leukopenic days. Leukopenia occurs in a significant number of patients; leukocyte count in children usually reaches nadir on fourth day and begins to rise on fifth day after drug administration.
- Avoid use of rectal thermometer or intrusive tubing to prevent injury to rectal mucosa.
- Check patient's ability to ambulate and supply support if necessary. Walking may be impaired.
- Take care to distinguish between the depression associated with realization of neoplastic disease and that which is drug-induced.

Patient & Family Education

- Notify physician promptly of stomach, bone, or joint pain, and swelling of lower legs and ankles.
- Start a prophylactic regimen against constipation and paralytic ileus (adequate fluids, high-fiber diet, laxatives) at beginning of treatment and report changes in bowel habit to health care providers as soon as manifested (paralytic ileus is most likely to occur in young children).
- Reversible hair loss is reportedly the most common adverse reaction and may persist for the duration of therapy. Regrowth may start before end of treatment. This is a distressing adverse effect because the scalp hair will drop out in large clumps.
- Do not breast feed while taking this drug.

VINORELBINE TARTRATE

(vin-o-rel'been)

Navelbine

Classifications: ANTINEOPLASTIC AGENT; MITOTIC INHIBITOR

Prototype: Vincristine

Pregnancy Category: D

AVAILABILITY 10 mg/mL injection

ACTIONS A semisynthetic vinca alkaloid with antineoplastic activity. Inhibits polymerization of tubules into microtubules, which disrupts mitotic spindle formation. Neurotoxicity is less than with other vinca alkaloids (e.g., vincristine).

THERAPEUTIC EFFECTS Arrests mitosis at metaphase, thereby, inhibiting cell division in cancer cells.

USES Non-small cell lung cancer.

UNLABELED USES Breast cancer, ovarian cancer, Hodgkin's disease.

CONTRAINDICATIONS Hypersensitivity to vinorelbine, pregnancy (category D), lactation.

CAUTIOUS USE Hypersensitivity to vincristine or vinblastine; infection, leukopenia, or other indicator(s) of bone marrow suppression; chickenpox or *Herpes zoster* infection; hepatic insufficiency; preexisting neurologic or neuromuscular disorders. Safety and efficacy in children are not established.

ROUTE & DOSAGE

Non-Small Cell Lung Cancer, Breast Cancer
Adult: **IV** 30 mg/m^2 weekly

ADMINISTRATION

Intravenous

- Use caution to prevent contact with skin, mucous membranes, or eyes during preparation.

PREPARE: **Direct:** Dilute each 10 mg in a syringe with either 2 or 5 mL of D5W or NS to yield 3 mg/mL or 1.5 mg/L, respectively. **IV Infusion:** Dilute the 10 mg/mL dose in an IV bag with D5W, NS, or RL to a final concentration of 0.5–2 mg/mL (example: 10 mg diluted in 19 mL yields 0.5 mg/mL).
ADMINISTER: **IV Infusion:** Give diluted solution over 6–10 min into the side port closest to an IV bag with free-flowing IV solution; follow by flushing with at least 75–125 mL of IV solution over 10 min. Take every precaution to avoid extravasation. If suspected, discontinue IV immediately and begin in a different site.
INCOMPATIBILITIES **Solution/additive: acyclovir, aminophylline/theophylline, amphotericin B, ampicillin, cefoperazone, ceforanide, cefotetan, ceftriaxone, fluorouracil, furosemide, ganciclovir, methylprednisolone, mitomycin, piperacillin, sodium bicarbonate, thiotepa, trimethoprim–sulfamethoxazole. Y-site: acyclovir, allopurinol, aminophylline/theophylline, amphotericin B, amphotericin B cholesteryl complex, ampicillin, cefazolin, cefoperazone, ceforanide, cefotetan, ceftriaxone, fluorouracil, furosemide, ganciclovir, methylprednisolone, mitomycin, piperacillin, sodium bicarbonate, thiotepa, trimethoprim–sulfamethoxazole.**

- Store at 2°–8° C (36°–46° F).

ADVERSE EFFECTS (≥1%) **CNS:** *Decreased deep tendon reflexes, paresthesia, fatigue, asthenia, peripheral neuropathy,* myalgia, jaw pain. **Hematologic:** *Anemia,* *neutropenia, granulocytopenia*, thrombocytopenia. **GI:** Paralytic ileus, *constipation, nausea, vomiting, diarrhea,* stomatitis, mucositis, hepatotoxicity *(elevated LFT).* **Body as a Whole:** *Pain on injection,* venous pain, thrombophlebitis, *alopecia,* myalgia, muscle weakness.

INTERACTIONS Drug: Increased severity of granulocytopenia in combination with **cisplatin;** increased risk of acute pulmonary reactions in combination with **mitomycin; paclitaxel** may increase neuropathy.

PHARMACOKINETICS Distribution: 60%–80% bound to plasma proteins (including platelets and lymphocytes); sequestered in tissues, especially lung, spleen, liver, and kidney, and released slowly. **Metabolism:** Metabolized in liver. **Elimination:** Excreted primarily in bile and feces (50%), 10% excreted in urine. **Half-Life:** 42–45 h.

NURSING IMPLICATIONS

Assessment & Drug Effects

- Lab tests: Monitor CBC with differential throughout therapy and

V

on the day of treatment prior to each infusion. Monitor kidney & liver functions and serum electrolytes periodically.

- Withhold drug and notify physician if the granulocyte count is below 1000 cells/mm^3.
- Monitor for S&S of infection, especially during period of granulocyte nadir 7–10 d after dosing.

Patient & Family Education

- Be aware of potential and inevitable adverse effects.
- Notify physician of distressing adverse effects, especially symptoms of leukopenia (e.g., chills, fever, cough) and peripheral neuropathy.
- Do not breast feed while taking this drug.

VITAMIN A

(vye′ta-min)

Aquasol A, Del-Vi-A

Classification: VITAMIN

Pregnancy Category: A (X if >RDA)

AVAILABILITY 5,000 IU tablets 10,000 IU, 15,000 IU, 25,000 IU capsules; 50,000 IU/mL injection

ACTIONS Essential for normal growth and development of bones and teeth, for integrity of epithelial and mucosal surfaces, and for synthesis of visual purple necessary for visual adaptation to the dark. Synthetic fat-soluble vitamin available for clinical use as retinol or retinol esters. Formulation includes vitamin A as well as its precursors.

THERAPEUTIC EFFECTS Replacement therapy using Aquasol A. Used also to stimulate healing of cortisone-retarded wounds when applied topically.

USES Vitamin A deficiency and as dietary supplement during periods of increased requirements, such as pregnancy, lactation, infancy, and infections. Used as replacement therapy in conditions that affect absorption, mobilization, or storage of vitamin A (e.g., steatorrhea, severe biliary obstruction, liver cirrhosis, total gastrectomy). Used in skin disorders [e.g., folliculosis keratosis (Darier's disease), psoriasis]; however, other retinoids are being preferentially selected. Also used as a screening test for fat malabsorption.

CONTRAINDICATIONS History of sensitivity to vitamin A or to any ingredient in formulation, hypervitaminosis A, oral administration to patients with malabsorption syndrome. Safe use in amounts exceeding 6000 IU during pregnancy [category A (category X if >RDA)] is not established.

CAUTIOUS USE Women on oral contraceptives, lactation (high doses).

ROUTE & DOSAGE

Severe Deficiency

Adult: **PO** 500,000 IU/d for 3 d followed by 50,000 IU/d for 2 wk, then 10,000–20,000 IU/d for 2 mo **IM** 100,000 IU/d for 3 d followed by 50,000 IU/d for 2 wk

Child: **PO/IM** *<1 y,* 10,000 IU/kg/d for 3 d followed by 7500–15,000 IU/d for 10 d; *1–8 y,* 10,000 IU/kg/d for 3 d followed by 17,000–35,000 IU/d for 2 wk; *>8 y,* same as for adult

Dietary Supplement

Child: **PO** *<4 y,* 10,000 IU/d; *4–8 y,* 15,000 IU/d

ADMINISTRATION

Oral

- Give on an empty stomach or following food or milk if GI upset occurs.
- Store in tight, light-resistant containers.

ADVERSE EFFECTS (≥1%) **CNS:** Irritability, headache, intracranial hypertension (pseudotumor cerebri), increased intracranial pressure, bulging fontanelles, papilledema, exophthalmos, miosis, nystagmus. **Metabolic:** Hypervitaminosis A syndrome (malaise, lethargy, abdominal discomfort, anorexia, vomiting), hypercalcemia. **Musculoskeletal:** Slow growth; deep, tender, hard lumps (subperiosteal thickening) over radius, tibia, occiput; migratory arthralgia; retarded growth; premature closure of epiphyses. **Skin:** Gingivitis, lip fissures, excessive sweating, drying or cracking of skin, pruritus, increase in skin pigmentation, massive desquamation, brittle nails, alopecia. **Urogenital:** Hypomenorrhea, **GI:** Hepatosplenomegaly, jaundice. **Endocrine:** Polydipsia, polyurea. **Hematologic:** Leukopenia, hypoplastic anemias, vitamin A plasma levels >1200 IU/dL, elevations of sedimentation rate and prothrombin time. **Body as a Whole:** Anaphylaxis, death (after IV use).

DIAGNOSTIC TEST INTERFERENCE Vitamin A may falsely increase ***serum cholesterol*** determinations ***(Zlatkis-Zak reaction);*** may falsely elevate ***bilirubin*** determination (with ***Ehrlich's reagent***).

INTERACTIONS Drug: Mineral oil, cholestyramine may decrease absorption of vitamin A.

PHARMACOKINETICS Absorption: Readily absorbed from GI tract in presence of bile salts, pancreatic lipase, and dietary fat. **Distribution:** Stored mainly in liver; small amounts also found in kidney and body fat; distributed into breast milk. **Metabolism:** Metabolized in liver. **Elimination:** Excreted in feces and urine.

NURSING IMPLICATIONS

Assessment & Drug Effects

- Evaluate dosage with consideration of patient's average daily intake of vitamin A. Take dietary and drug history (e.g., intake of fortified foods, dietary supplements, self-administration or prescription drug sources). Women taking oral contraceptives tend to have significantly high plasma vitamin A levels.
- Monitor therapeutic effectiveness. Vitamin A deficiency is often associated with protein malnutrition as well as other vitamin deficiencies. It may manifest as night blindness, restriction of growth and development, epithelial alterations, susceptibility to infection, abnormal dryness of skin, mouth, and eyes (xerophthalmia) progressing to keratomalacia (ulceration and necrosis of cornea and conjunctiva), and urinary tract calculi.

Patient & Family Education

- Avoid use of mineral oil while on vitamin A therapy.
- Notify physician of symptoms of overdosage (e.g., nausea, vomiting, anorexia, drying and cracking of skin or lips, headache, loss of hair).
- Do not breast feed while taking this drug in high doses without consulting physician.

VITAMIN B_1
See Thiamine HCl.

VITAMIN B_2
See Riboflavin.

VITAMIN B_3
See Niacin.

VITAMIN B_6
See Pyridoxine.

VITAMIN B_9
See Folic acid.

VITAMIN B_{12}
See Cyanocobalamin.

VITAMIN B_{12a}
See Hydroxocobalamin.

VITAMIN C
See Ascorbic acid.

VITAMIN D
See Calcitriol.

VITAMIN E (TOCOPHEROL)
(vit′a-min E)
Aquasol E, Vita-Plus E, Vitec
Classification: VITAMIN
Pregnancy Category: A

AVAILABILITY 100 IU, 200 IU, 400 IU, 500 IU, 800 IU tablets; 100 IU, 200 IU, 400 IU, 1000 IU capsules; 15 IU/0.3 mL, 15 IU/30 mL liquid

ACTIONS A group of naturally occurring fat-soluble substances known as tocopherols. Alpha tocopherol, comprising 90% of the tocopherols, is the most biologically potent and has been synthesized. An antioxidant, it prevents peroxidation, a process that gives rise to free radicals (highly reactive chemical structures that damage cell membranes and alter nuclear proteins).

THERAPEUTIC EFFECTS Prevents cell membrane and protein damage and is essential to the digestion and metabolism of polyunsaturated fats. Maintains the integrity of cell membranes, protects against blood clot formation by decreasing platelet aggregation, enhances vitamin A utilization, and promotes normal growth, development, and tone of muscles. Deficiency causes no specific disease in humans but has been associated with increased susceptibility of RBC to hemolysis.

USES To treat and prevent hemolytic anemia due to vitamin E deficiency in premature neonates; to prevent retrolental fibroplasia secondary to oxygen treatment in neonates, and in treatment of diseases with secondary erythrocyte membrane abnormalities (e.g., sickle cell anemia, and G6PD deficiency and as supplement in malabsorption syndromes). Used in patients on diets containing large amounts of polyunsaturated fats for long periods and in the patient who abruptly discontinues such a diet. Also used topically for dry or chapped skin and minor skin disorders.

UNLABELED USES Muscular dystrophy and a number of other conditions with no conclusive evidence of value. A component of many multivitamin formulations and of topical deodorant preparations as an antioxidant.

CONTRAINDICATIONS No clinically significant contraindications established.

CAUTIOUS USE Large doses may exacerbate iron deficiency anemia.

V

ROUTE & DOSAGE

Vitamin E Deficiency
Adult: **PO/IM** 60–75 IU/d
Child: **PO** 1 IU/kg/d

Prophylaxis for Vitamin E Deficiency
Adult: **PO** 12–15 IU/d
Child: **PO** 7–10 IU/d
Neonate: **PO** 5 IU/d

ADMINISTRATION

Oral
- Give on an empty stomach or following food or milk if GI upset occurs.
- Store in tight containers protected from light.

ADVERSE EFFECTS (≥1%) **Body as a Whole:** Skeletal muscle weakness, headache, fatigue (with excessive doses). **GI:** Nausea, diarrhea, intestinal cramps. **Urogenital:** Gonadal dysfunction. **Metabolic:** Increased serum creatine kinase, cholesterol, triglycerides; decreased serum thyroxine and triiodothyronine; increased urinary estrogens, androgens; creatinuria. **Skin:** Sterile abscess, thrombophlebitis, contact dermatitis. **Special Senses:** Blurred vision.

INTERACTIONS Herbal: Mineral oil, cholestyramine may decrease absorption of vitamin E; may enhance anticoagulant activity of **warfarin.**

PHARMACOKINETICS Absorption: 20%–60% absorbed from GI tract if fat absorption is normal; enters blood via lymph. **Distribution:** Stored mainly in adipose tissue; crosses placenta. **Metabolism:** Metabolized in liver. **Elimination:** Excreted primarily in bile.

NURSING IMPLICATIONS

Patient & Family Education
- If taking a large dose of iron, the RDA of vitamin E may be increased.
- Natural sources of vitamin E are found in wheat germ (the richest source) as well as in vegetable oils (sunflower, corn, soybean, cottonseed), green leafy vegetables, nuts, dairy products, eggs, cereals, meat, and liver.

VORICONAZOLE

(vor-i-con′a-zole)
Vfend
Classifications: ANTIINFECTIVE; ANTIBIOTIC; AZOLE ANTIFUNGAL
Prototype: Fluconazole
Pregnancy Category: D

AVAILABILITY 50 mg, 200 mg tablets; 200 mg injection

ACTIONS Inhibits fungal cytochrome P-450 enzymes used for an essential step in fungal ergosterol biosynthesis. The subsequent loss of ergosterol in the fungal cell wall may be responsible for the antifungal activity of voriconazole.
THERAPEUTIC EFFECTS Voriconazole is active against *Aspergillus fumigatus* as well as *A. flavus, A. niger* and *A. terreus*. Variable activity against *Scedosporium apiospermum* and *Fusarium spp.*, including *Fusarium solani,* has been seen.

V

USES Treatment of invasive *Aspergillosis,* esophageal candidiasis.
UNLABELED USES Treatment of other refractory fungal infections, including *Candida* infections.

CONTRAINDICATIONS Known hypersensitivity to voriconazole; intravenous voriconazole should be avoided in moderate or severe renal

impairment (Cl_{cr} <50 mL/min); severe hepatic impairment; children <2 y; history of galactose intolerance; Lapp lactase deficiency or glucose-galactose malabsorption; concurrent use of sirolimus; coadministration of the CYP3A4 substrates terfenadine, astemizole, cisapride, pimozide or quinidine; concurrent use of rifampin, rifabutin, carbamazepine and long-acting barbiturates, ergot alkaloids; sunlight (UV) exposure; pregnancy (category D); lactation.
CAUTIOUS USE Mild to moderate hepatic cirrhosis, hepatitis, hepatic disease; renal disease, renal impairment; ocular disease; hypersensitivity to other azole antifungal agents such as fluconazole; children >2 y and <12 y.

ROUTE & DOSAGE

Aspergillosis
Adult/Geriatric: **IV** 6 mg/kg q12h day 1, then 4 mg/kg q12h. May reduce to 3 mg/kg q12h if not tolerated **PO** *>40 kg,* 400 mg q12h day 1, then 200 mg q12h. May increase to 300 mg q12h if inadequate response. *<40 kg,* 400 mg q12h day 1, then 100 mg q12h. May increase to 150 mg q12h if inadequate response

Esophageal Candidiasis
Adult/Geriatric: **PO** *>40 kg,* 200 mg q12h for a minimum of 14 d and for at least 7 d after resolution of symptoms; *<40 kg,* 100 mg q12h for a minimum of 14 d and for at least 7 d after resolution of symptoms.

Dose adjustment for concomitant fosphenytoin or phenytoin
Adult/Geriatric: **IV** 6 mg/kg q12h day 1, then 5 mg/kg q12h. **PO** *>40 kg,* 400 mg q12h day 1, then 400 mg q12h. *<40 kg,* 400 mg q12h day 1, then 200 mg q12h

ADMINISTRATION

Oral
- Give at least 1 h before or 1 h following a meal.
- Manufacturer recommendation: maintenance dose to be halved in patients with mild to moderate hepatic cirrhosis. Consult physician.
- Store tablets at 15°–30° C (59°–86° F).

Intravenous
- IV voriconazole should be avoided in patients with moderate or severe renal impairment.

PREPARE: **Intermittent:** Use a 20 mL syringe to reconstitute powder with exactly 19 mL of sterile water for injection to yield 10 mg/mL. Discard vial if a vacuum does not pull the diluent into vial. Shake until completely dissolved. From an IV infusion bag of NS, D5W, D5/NS, D5/.45NS, RL or other suitable diluent withdraw and discard a volume of IV solution adequate to produce final voriconazole concentration within the range of 0.5–5 mg/mL. Inject the calculated dose of voriconazole into the IV bag. Discard unused voriconazole. Infuse IV solution immediately.
ADMINISTER: **Intermittent:** Infuse over 1–2 h at a maximum rate of 3 mg/kg per h. DO NOT give a bolus dose.
INCOMPATIBILITIES **Solution/additive:** Do not dilute with **sodium bicarbonate;** do not mix with any other drugs. **Y-site:** Do not infuse with other drugs.

- Store unreconstituted vials at 15°–30° C (59°–86° F).

ADVERSE EFFECTS (≥1%) **Body as a Whole:** Peripheral edema, fever, chills. **CNS:** Headache, hallucinations, dizziness. **CV:** Tachycardia, hypotension, hypertension, vasodilation. **GI:** Nausea, vomiting, abdominal pain, abnormal LFTs, diarrhea, cholestatic jaundice, dry mouth. **Metabolic:** Increased alkaline phosphatase, AST, ALT, hypokalemia, hypomagnesemia. **Skin:** Rash, pruritus. **Special Senses:** *Abnormal vision (enhanced brightness, blurred vision, or color vision changes),* photophobia.

INTERACTIONS Drug: Due to significant increased toxicity or decreased activity, the following drugs are contraindicated with voriconazole: BARBITURATES, **carbamazepine, cisapride, efavirenz,** ERGOT ALKALOIDS, **pimozide, quinidine, rifabutin, sirolimus; fosphenytoin, phenytoin, rifampin, ritonavir** may significantly decrease voriconazole levels. PROTEASE INHIBITORS (except **indinavir**) may increase voriconazole toxicity; voriconazole may increase the toxicity of BENZODIAZEPINES, **cyclosporine,** PROTEASE INHIBITORS (except **indinavir**), NONNUCLEOSIDE REVERSE TRANSCRIPTASE INHIBITORS, **omeprazole, tacrolimus, vinblastine, vincristine, warfarin;** NONNUCLEOSIDE REVERSE TRANSCRIPTASE INHIBITORS may increase or decrease voriconazole levels. **Food:** Absorption reduced with high-fat meals.

PHARMACOKINETICS Absorption: 96% absorbed PO. Has a non-linear pharmacokinetic profile, a small change in dose may cause a large change in serum levels. Steady state not achieved until day 5–6 if no loading dose is given. **Peak:** 1–2 h. **Metabolism:** Metabolized in liver by (and is an inhibitor of) CYP3A4, 2C9 and 2C19. **Elimination:** Primarily excreted in urine. **Half-Life:** 6 h–6 d depending on dose.

NURSING IMPLICATIONS

Assessment & Drug Effects

- Monitor visual acuity, visual field, and color perception if treatment continues beyond 28 days.
- Withhold drug and notify physician if skin rash develops.
- Monitor cardiovascular status especially with preexisting CV disease.
- Lab tests: Monitor baseline and periodic LFTs including bilirubin; patients who develop abnormal liver function tests during therapy should be monitored for the development of more severe hepatic injury. Monitor frequently renal function tests, especially serum creatinine. Monitor periodic CBC with platelet count, Hct & Hgb, serum electrolytes, alkaline phosphatase, blood glucose, and lipid profile.
- Concurrent drugs: Monitor PT/INR closely with warfarin as dose adjustments of warfarin may be needed. Monitor frequently blood glucose levels with sulfonylurea drugs as reduction in the sulfonylurea dosage may be needed. Monitor for and report any of the following: S&S of rhabdomyolysis in patient receiving a statin drug; prolonged sedation in patient receiving a benzodiazepine; S&S of heart block, bradycardia, or CHF in patient receiving a calcium channel blocker.

Patient & Family Education

- Use reliable means of birth control to prevent pregnancy. If you suspect you are pregnant, contact physician immediately.
- Do not drive at night while taking voriconazole as the drug may cause blurred vision and photophobia.
- Do not drive or engage in other potentially hazardous activities until reaction to drug is known.

- Avoid strong, direct sunlight while taking voriconazole.
- Do not breast feed while taking this drug.

WARFARIN SODIUM

(war'far-in)

Coumadin Sodium, Panwarfin, Warfilone ♣

Classifications: BLOOD FORMERS, COAGULATORS, AND ANTICOAGULANTS; ORAL ANTICOAGULANT

Pregnancy Category: X

AVAILABILITY 1 mg, 2 mg, 2.5 mg, 3 mg, 4 mg, 5 mg, 6 mg, 7.5 mg, 10 mg tablets; 2 mg injection

ACTIONS Indirectly interferes with blood clotting by depressing hepatic synthesis of vitamin K-dependent coagulation factors: II, VII, IX, and X.

THERAPEUTIC EFFECTS Deters further extension of existing thrombi and prevents new clots from forming. Unlike heparin, its action is cumulative and more prolonged. Warfarin is not cross allergenic with other coumarin derivatives. Does not reverse ischemic tissue damage and has no effect on platelets. Has no effect on already synthesized circulating coagulation factors or on circulating thrombi.

USES Prophylaxis and treatment of deep vein thrombosis and its extension, pulmonary embolism; treatment of atrial fibrillation with embolization. Also used as adjunct in treatment of coronary occlusion, cerebral transient ischemic attacks (TIAs), and as a prophylactic in patients with prosthetic cardiac valves. Used extensively as rodenticide.

CONTRAINDICATIONS Hemorrhagic tendencies, vitamin C or K deficiency, hemophilia, coagulation factor deficiencies, dyscrasias; active bleeding; open wounds, active peptic ulcer, visceral carcinoma, esophageal varices, malabsorption syndrome; hypertension (diastolic BP >110 mm Hg), cerebral vascular disease; heparin-induced thrombocytopenia (HIT); pericarditis with acute MI; severe hepatic or renal disease; continuous tube drainage of any orifice; subacute bacterial endocarditis; recent surgery of brain, spinal cord, or eye; regional or lumbar block anesthesia; threatened abortion; unreliable patients; pregnancy (category X).

CAUTIOUS USE Alcoholism, allergic disorders, during menstruation, older adults, senility, psychosis; debilitated patients. Endogenous factors that may increase prothrombin time response (enhance anticoagulant effect): carcinoma, CHF, collagen diseases, hepatic and renal insufficiency, diarrhea, fever, pancreatic disorders, malnutrition, vitamin K deficiency. Endogenous factors that may decrease prothrombin time response (decrease anticoagulant response): edema, hypothyroidism, hyperlipidemia, hypercholesterolemia, chronic alcoholism, hereditary resistance to coumarin therapy.

ROUTE & DOSAGE

Anticoagulant

Adult: **PO/IV** 10–15 mg/d for 2–5 d, then 2–10 mg once/d with dose adjusted to maintain a PT 1.2–2 times control or INR of 2–3

Child: **PO** 0.1–0.3 mg/kg/d, adjust to maintain INR of 2–3

ADMINISTRATION

Note: Antidote for bleeding—anticoagulant effect usually is reversed by omitting 1 or more doses of warfarin and by administration of specific antidote phytonadione (vitamin K1) 2.5–10 mg orally. Physician may advise patient to carry vitamin K1 at all times, but not to take it until after consultation. If bleeding persists or progresses to a severe level, vitamin K 15–25 mg IV is given, or a fresh whole blood transfusion may be necessary.

Oral

- Give tablet whole or crushed with fluid of patient's choice.

Intravenous

***PREPARE:* Direct:** Add 2 mL of supplied diluent to 50 mg of warfarin powder.

***ADMINISTER:* Direct:** Give immediately by direct IV at a rate of 25 mg (1 mL)/min.

***INCOMPATIBILITIES* Solution/additive: Ammonium chloride, 5% dextrose, Ringer's lactate,** AMINOGLYCOSIDES, **ascorbic acid, epinephrine, metaraminol, oxytocin, promazine, tetracycline, vancomycin, vitamin B complex with C.**

- Store at 15°–30° C (59°–86° F). Discard discolored or precipitated solutions. Protect all preparations from light and moisture.

ADVERSE EFFECTS (≥1%) **Body as a Whole:** Major or minor hemorrhage from any tissue or organ; hypersensitivity (dermatitis, urticaria, pruritus, fever). **GI:** Anorexia, nausea, vomiting, abdominal cramps, diarrhea, steatorrhea, stomatitis. **Other:** Increased serum transaminase levels, hepatitis, jaundice, burning sensation of feet, transient hair loss. **Overdosage:** Internal or external bleeding, paralytic ileus; skin necrosis of toes (purple toes syndrome), tip of nose, buttocks, thighs, calves, female breast, abdomen, and other fat-rich areas.

DIAGNOSTIC TEST INTERFERENCE Warfarin (coumarins) may cause alkaline urine to be red-orange; may enhance ***uric acid*** excretion, cause elevation of ***serum transaminases,*** and may increase ***lactic dehydrogenase*** activity.

INTERACTIONS Drug: In addition to the drugs listed below, many other drugs have been reported to alter the expected response to warfarin; however, clinical importance of these reports has not been substantiated. The addition or withdrawal of any drug to an established drug regimen should be made cautiously, with more frequent INR determinations than usual and with careful observation of the patient and dose adjustment as indicated. ■ The following may enhance the anticoagulant effects of warfarin: **Acetohexamide, acetaminophen,** ALKYLATING AGENTS, **allopurinol,** AMINOGLYCOSIDES, **aminosalicylic acid, amiodarone,** ANABOLIC STEROIDS, ANTIBIOTICS (ORAL), ANTIMETABOLITES, ANTIPLATELET DRUGS, **aspirin, asparaginase, capecitabine, celecoxib, chloramphenicol, chlorpropamide, chymotrypsin, cimetidine, clofibrate, co-trimoxazole, danazol, dextran, dextrothyroxine, diazoxide, disulfiram, erythromycin, ethacrynic acid, fluconazole, glucagons, guanethidine,** HEPATOTOXIC DRUGS, **influenza vaccine, isoniazid, itraconazole, ketoconazole,** MAO INHIBITORS, **meclofenamate, mefenamic acid, methyldopa, methylphenidate, metronidazole, miconazole, mineral oil, nalidixic acid, neomycin (oral),** NONSTEROIDAL ANTI-INFLAMMATORY DRUGS, **oxandrolone, plicamycin,** POTASSIUM PRODUCTS, **propoxyphene, propylthiouracil, quinidine, quinine, rofecoxib, salicylates, streptokinase, sulindac,** SULFONAMIDES,

SULFONYLUREAS, TETRACYCLINES, THIAZIDES, THYROID DRUGS, **tolbutamide, tricyclic antidepressants, urokinase, vitamin E, zileuton.** ▪ The following may increase or decrease the anticoagulant effects of warfarin: **Alcohol** (acute intoxication may increase, chronic alcoholism may decrease effects), **chloral hydrate,** DIURETICS. ▪ The following may decrease the anticoagulant effects of warfarin: **barbiturates, carbamazepine, cholestyramine,** CORTICOSTEROIDS, **corticotropin, ethchlorvynol, glutethimide, griseofulvin,** LAXATIVES, **mercaptopurine,** ORAL CONTRACEPTIVES, **rifampin, spironolactone, vitamin C, vitamin K. Herbal: Capsicum, celery, chamomile, clove, Devil's claw, Dong quai, Echinacea, fenugreek, feverfew, garlic, ginger, ginkgo, horse chestnut, licorice root, passionflower herb, tumeric, willow bark** may increase risk of bleeding; **ginseng, green tea, St. John's wort** may decrease effectiveness of warfarin. **Food: Cranberry juice** may increase INR.

PHARMACOKINETICS Absorption: Well absorbed from GI tract. **Onset:** 2–7 d. **Peak:** 0.5–3 d. **Distribution:** 97% protein bound; crosses placenta. **Metabolism:** Metabolized in liver. **Elimination:** Excreted in urine and bile. **Half-Life:** 0.5–3 d.

NURSING IMPLICATIONS

Assessment & Drug Effects

- Determine PT/INP prior to initiation of therapy and then daily until maintenance dosage is established.
- Obtain a CAREFUL medication history prior to start of therapy and whenever altered responses to therapy require interpretation; extremely IMPORTANT since many drugs interfere with the activity of anticoagulant drugs (see INTERACTIONS).
- Adjust dose to maintain PT at 11/2–21/2 times the control (12–15 s), or 15%–35% of normal prothrombin activity, or an INR of 2–4 depending on diagnosis.
- Lab tests: For maintenance dosage, PT/INR determinations at 1–4-wk intervals depending on patient's response; periodic urinalyses, stool guaiac, and liver function tests. Blood samples should be drawn at 12–18 h after last dose (optimum).
- Monitor closely older adult, psychotic, or alcoholic patients because they present serious noncompliance problems.
- Note: Patients at greatest risk of hemorrhage include those whose PT/INR are difficult to regulate, who have an aortic valve prosthesis, who are receiving long-term anticoagulant therapy, and older adult and debilitated patients.

Patient & Family Education

- Understand that bleeding can occur even though PT/INR are within therapeutic range. Stop drug and notify physician immediately if bleeding or signs of bleeding appear: Blood in urine, bright red or black tarry stools, vomiting of blood, bleeding with tooth brushing, blue or purple spots on skin or mucous membrane, round pinpoint purplish red spots (often occur in ankle areas), nosebleed, bloody sputum; chest pain; abdominal or lumbar pain or swelling, profuse menstrual bleeding, pelvic pain; severe or continuous headache, faintness or dizziness; prolonged oozing from any minor injury (e.g., nicks from shaving).
- Stop drug and report immediately any symptoms of hepatitis (dark urine, itchy skin, jaundice, ab-

dominal pain, light stools) or hypersensitivity reaction (see Appendix F).

- Avoid brand interchange, take drug at same time each day, and do NOT alter dose.
- Notify physician if there is an unusual increase in menstrual bleeding (slightly increased or prolonged). Note: PT/INR are checked at least monthly in menstruating women.
- Risk of bleeding is increased for up to 1 mo after receiving the influenza vaccine.
- Fever, prolonged hot weather, malnutrition, and diarrhea lengthen PT/INR (enhanced anticoagulant effect).
- A high-fat diet, sudden increase in vitamin K-rich foods (cabbage, cauliflower, broccoli, asparagus, lettuce, turnip greens, onions, spinach, kale, fish, liver), coffee or green tea (caffeine), or by tube feedings with high vitamin K content shorten PT/INR.
- Maintain a well-balanced diet and avoid excess intake of alcohol.
- Inform dentist or any new physician about anticoagulant therapy and duration of treatment.
- Use a soft toothbrush and floss teeth gently with waxed floss.
- Use barrier contraceptive measures; if you become pregnant while on anticoagulant therapy the fetus is at great potential risk of congenital malformations.
- Do not take any other prescription or OTC drug unless specifically approved by physician or pharmacist. Carry medical identification at all times. It needs to indicate medical diagnosis, medication(s), physician's name, address, and telephone number.
- Do not breast feed while taking this drug without consulting physician.

XYLOMETAZOLINE HYDROCHLORIDE

(zye-loe-met-az′oh-leen)

Neo-Synephrine II, Otrivin

Classifications: NASAL DECONGESTANT; VASOCONSTRICTOR

Prototype: Naphazoline

Pregnancy Category: C

AVAILABILITY 0.05%, 0.1% nasal solution

ACTIONS Markedly constricts dilated arterioles of nasal membrane. Has little or no beta-adrenergic activity. Structurally related to naphazoline.

THERAPEUTIC EFFECTS Decreases fluid exudate and mucosal engorgement associated with rhinitis and may open up obstructed eustachian ostia in patient with ear inflammation.

USES Temporary relief of nasal congestion associated with common cold, sinusitis, acute and chronic rhinitis, and hay fever and other allergies.

CONTRAINDICATIONS Sensitivity to adrenergic substances; angle-closure glaucoma; concurrent therapy with MAO inhibitors or tricyclic antidepressants; lactation, and infants. Safe use during pregnancy (category C) is not established.

CAUTIOUS USE Hypertension; hyperthyroidism; heart disease, including angina; advanced arteriosclerosis, older adults, and children.

ROUTE & DOSAGE

Nasal Congestion

Adult: **Nasal** 1–2 sprays or 1–2 drops of 0.1% solution in each nostril q8–10h (max: 3 doses/d)

Child: **Nasal** <6 *mo,* 1 drop of 0.05% solution in each nostril q6h (max: 3 doses/d); *6 mo–12 y,* 1 spray or 2–3 drops of 0.05% solution in each nostril q8–10h (max: 3 doses/d)

ADMINISTRATION

Instillation

- Have patient clear each nostril gently before administering spray or drops.
- Spray: Do not shake container. Hold tube vertically (spray end up) so that solution is delivered in a fine spray. Head should be erect; spray into each nostril; 3–5 min later, clear (blow) nose thoroughly.
- Drops: Patient should be in a lateral, head-low position to permit application of drops to lower nostril surface. Have patient remain in this position for 5 min, then apply drops to opposite nostril surface in same manner; or drops may be instilled with patient in reclining position with head tilted back as far as possible.
- Store at 15°–30° C (59°–86° F) in a tight, light-resistant container.

ADVERSE EFFECTS (≥1%) **All:** Usually mild and infrequent; local stinging, burning, dryness and ulceration, sneezing, headache, insomnia, drowsiness. **With excessive use:** *Rebound nasal congestion* and vasodilation, tremulousness, hypertension, palpitations, tachycardia, arrhythmia, somnolence, sedation, <u>coma</u>.

INTERACTIONS Drug: May cause increase BP with **guanethidine, methyldopa,** MAO INHIBITORS; PHENOTHIAZINES may decrease effectiveness of nasal decongestant.

PHARMACOKINETICS Onset: 5–10 min. **Duration:** 5–6 h.

NURSING IMPLICATIONS

Assessment & Drug Effects

- Evaluate for development of rebound congestion (see ADVERSE EFFECTS).

Patient & Family Education

- Prevent contamination of nasal solution and spread of infection by rinsing dropper and tip of nasal spray in hot water after each use; restrict use to the individual patient.
- Note: Prolonged use can cause rebound congestion and chemical rhinitis. Do NOT exceed prescribed dosage and report to physician if drug fails to provide relief within 3–4 d.
- Do NOT self-medicate with OTC drugs, sprays, or drops without physician's approval.
- Note: Excessive use by a child may lead to CNS depression.
- Do not breast feed while taking this drug.

ZAFIRLUKAST Pr

(za-fir-lu'kast)

Accolate

Classifications: BRONCHODILATOR (RESPIRATORY SMOOTH MUSCLE RELAXANT); LEUKOTRIENE RECEPTOR ANTAGONIST

Pregnancy Category: B

AVAILABILITY 10 mg, 20 mg tablets

ACTIONS Selective peptide leukotriene receptor antagonist (LTRA) of leukotriene D_4 and E_4, thus inhibiting bronchoconstriction. Leukotriene production and receptor affinity have been correlated with the pathogenesis of asthma.

THERAPEUTIC EFFECTS Zafirlukast helps to prevent the signs and symptoms of asthma including airway edema, smooth muscle con-

Z

striction, and altered cellular activity due to inflammation.

USES Prophylaxis and chronic treatment of asthma in adults and children >5 y (not for acute bronchospasm).

CONTRAINDICATIONS Hypersensitivity to zafirlukast; acute asthma attacks, including status asthmaticus, acute bronchospasm; lactation, children <5 y.

CAUTIOUS USE Hepatic impairment, hepatic disease; patients ≥65 y, pregnancy (category B).

ROUTE & DOSAGE

Asthma

Adult: **PO** 20 mg b.i.d. 1 h before or 2 h after meals
Child: **PO** *>5 y,* 10 mg b.i.d.

ADMINISTRATION

Oral

- Give 1 h before or 2 h after meals.
- Store at 20°–25° C (68°–77° F); protect from light and moisture.

ADVERSE EFFECTS (≥1%) **Body as a Whole:** Generalized pain, asthenia, myalgia, fever, back pain. **CNS:** *Headache,* dizziness. **GI:** Nausea, diarrhea, abdominal pain, vomiting, dyspepsia; liver dysfunction, increased liver function tests, hepatic failure. **Other:** Churg-Strauss syndrome (fever, muscle aches and pains, weight loss).

INTERACTIONS Drug: May increase prothrombin time (PT) in patients on **warfarin. Erythromycin** decreases bioavailability of zafirlukast.

PHARMACOKINETICS Absorption: Rapidly absorbed from GI tract, bioavailability significantly reduced by food. **Onset:** 1 wk. **Peak:** 3 h. **Distribution:** >99% protein bound; secreted into breast milk. **Metabolism:** Metabolized in liver via cytochrome P450 2C9 (CYP2C9) and possibly CYP3A4. **Elimination:** 90% excreted in feces, 10% in urine. **Half-Life:** 10 h.

NURSING IMPLICATIONS

Assessment & Drug Effects

- Assess respiratory status and airway function regularly.
- Lab tests: Periodic liver function tests.
- Monitor closely PT and INR with concurrent warfarin therapy.
- Monitor closely phenytoin level with concurrent phenytoin therapy.

Patient & Family Education

- Taking medication regularly, even during symptom-free periods.
- Note: Drug is not intended to treat acute episodes of asthma.
- Report S&S of hepatic toxicity (see Appendix F) or flu-like symptoms to physician. Follow-up lab work is very important.
- Notify physician immediately if condition worsens while using prescribed doses of all antiasthmatic medications.
- Do not breast feed while taking this drug.

ZALCITABINE (DDC, DIDEOXYCYTIDINE)

(zal-cit'a-been)
Hivid
Classifications: ANTIINFECTIVE; ANTIVIRAL
Prototype: Zidovudine
Pregnancy Category: C

AVAILABILITY 0.375 mg, 0.75 mg tablets

ACTIONS A synthetic pyrimidine nucleotide that inhibits the replication of HIV by inhibition of viral DNA synthesis. It appears to act by becoming incorporated into the DNA chains of the HIV virus during viral replication.

THERAPEUTIC EFFECTS Zalcitabine is able to decrease the HIV viral load by its antiviral properties.

USES Combination therapy with zidovudine for AIDS. Second-line monotherapy for AIDS.

UNLABELED USES Can be used in children.

CONTRAINDICATIONS Hypersensitivity to zalcitabine.

CAUTIOUS USE Moderate to severe neuropathy; history of pancreatitis; CHF, cardiomyopathy; renal impairment, hepatic impairment, alcohol abuse; pregnancy (category C). It is not known if zalcitabine is excreted in breast milk. Safety and effectiveness in HIV-infected children <13 y are not established.

ROUTE & DOSAGE

Combination Therapy for HIV
Adult: **PO** 0.75 mg q8h given with zidovudine 200 mg q8h
Child: **PO** 0.015 to 0.04 mg/kg q6h for 8 wk, after 8 wk of monotherapy an alternating regimen of zalcitabine and zidovudine is begun (4-wk cycle of zidovudine for 3 wk and zalcitabine for 1 wk)

Monotherapy for HIV
Adult: **PO** 0.01 mg/kg q8h

ADMINISTRATION

Oral
- Give on an empty stomach.
- Store at 15°–30° C (56°–86° F).

ADVERSE EFFECTS (≥1%) **CV:** May exacerbate existing CHF and cardiomyopathy. **CNS:** *Peripheral neuropathy,* numbness. **GI:** Diarrhea, mouth and esophageal ulcers, pancreatitis, may exacerbate existing hepatic dysfunction. **Hematologic:** Neutropenia, thrombocytopenia. **Skin:** *Transient symptom complex of cutaneous eruptions (maculovesicular in nature), fever, malaise, and aphthous mouth ulcers,* arthralgia, urticaria, anaphylaxis.

INTERACTIONS Drug: May cause additive peripheral neuropathy with **didanosine.**

PHARMACOKINETICS Absorption: Readily absorbed from GI tract. **Onset:** 2 wk. **Distribution:** Distributes somewhat into CSF. **Metabolism:** Does not appear to be metabolized. **Elimination:** 62% excreted unchanged in urine. **Half-Life:** 1.2–1.8 h.

NURSING IMPLICATIONS

Assessment & Drug Effects
- Discontinue drug and promptly notify physician if patient experiences numbness, tingling, burning, or pain in extremities.
- Lab tests: Baseline and periodic tests for serum amylase, serum glucose, triglycerides, and serum calcium levels; monitor closely in patients with history of pancreatitis or elevated serum amylase.

Patient & Family Education
- Report to physician promptly S&S of pancreatitis and peripheral neuropathy (see Appendix F).
- Use contraception while taking zalcitabine.
- Do not breast feed while taking this drug without consulting physician.

Common adverse effects in *italic*, life-threatening effects underlined; generic names in **bold**; classifications in SMALL CAPS; ♣ Canadian drug name; ⊕ Prototype drug

ZALEPLON

(zal′ep-lon)

Sonata

Classifications: CENTRAL NERVOUS SYSTEM AGENT; ANXIOLYTIC; SEDATIVE-HYPNOTIC; NONBENZODIAZEPINE

Prototype: Zolpidem

Pregnancy Category: C

Controlled Substance: Schedule IV

AVAILABILITY 5 mg, 10 mg capsules.

ACTIONS Short acting nonbenzodiazepine with sedative-hypnotic, muscle relaxant, and anticonvulsant activity.

THERAPEUTIC EFFECTS Effectiveness is indicated by less difficulty in initially falling asleep. Preserves deep sleep (stage 3 through stage 4) at hypnotic dose with minimal-to-absent rebound insomnia when discontinued.

USES Short-term treatment of insomnia.

CONTRAINDICATIONS Hypersensitivity to zaleplon.

CAUTIOUS USE Concurrent use of other CNS depressants (e.g., benzodiazepines, alcohol); history of drug abuse; hepatic or renal impairment; pulmonary disease; pregnancy (category C); lactation.

ROUTE & DOSAGE

Insomnia

Adult: **PO** 10 mg h.s. (max: 20 mg h.s.)
Geriatric: **PO** 5 mg h.s. (max: 10 mg h.s.)

ADMINISTRATION

Oral

- Give immediately before bedtime; not while patient is still ambulating.
- Give lower dose of 5 mg to older adult or debilitated patients.
- Store at 20°–25° C (68°–77° F).

ADVERSE EFFECTS (≥1%) **Body as a Whole:** Asthenia, fever, *headache,* migraine, myalgia, back pain. **CNS:** Amnesia, dizziness, paresthesia, somnolence, tremor, vertigo, depression, hypertonia, nervousness, difficulty concentrating. **GI:** Abdominal pain, dyspepsia, nausea, constipation, dry mouth. **Respiratory:** Bronchitis. **Skin:** Pruritus, rash. **Special Senses:** Eye pain, hyperacusis, conjunctivitis. **Urogenital:** Dysmenorrhea.

INTERACTIONS Drug: Alcohol, imipramine, thioridazine may cause additive CNS impairment; **rifampin** increases metabolism of **zaleplon; cimetidine** increases serum levels of **zaleplon. Herbal: Valerian, melatonin** may produce additive sedative effects.

PHARMACOKINETICS Absorption: Rapidly and completely absorbed, 30% reaches systemic circulation. **Onset:** 15–20 min. **Peak:** 1 h. **Duration:** 3–4 h. **Distribution:** 60% protein bound. **Metabolism:** Extensively metabolized in liver to inactive metabolites. CYP3A4 is one of its metabolic pathways. **Elimination:** 70% excreted in urine, 17% in feces. **Half-Life:** 1 h.

NURSING IMPLICATIONS

Assessment & Drug Effects

- Monitor behavior and notify physician for significant changes. Use extra caution with preexisting clinical depression.
- Provide safe environment and monitor ambulation after drug is ingested.
- Monitor respiratory status with preexisting compromised pulmonary function.

Patient & Family Education

- Exercise caution when walking; avoid all hazardous activities after taking zaleplon.
- Do not take in combination with alcohol or any other sleep medication.
- Note: Exhibits altered effectiveness if taken with/immediately after high fat meal.
- Do not use longer than 2–3 wk.
- Expect possible mild/brief rebound insomnia after discontinuing regimen.
- Report use of OTC medications to physician (e.g., cimetidine).
- Report pregnancy to physician immediately.
- Do not breast feed while taking this drug.

ZANAMIVIR

(zan′a-mi-vir)

Relenza

Classifications: ANTIINFECTIVE; ANTIVIRAL

Prototype: Acyclovir

Pregnancy Category: B

AVAILABILITY 5 mg/Rotadisk blister

ACTIONS Inhibitor of influenza A and B viral enzyme; does not permit the release of newly formed viruses from the surface of the infected cells.

THERAPEUTIC EFFECTS Indicated by relief of flu-like symptoms. The inhibition of the viral neuroaminidase enzyme prevents the viral spread across the mucus lining of the respiratory tract, and inhibits the replication of influenza A and B virus.

USES Uncomplicated acute influenza in patients symptomatic <2 d.

CONTRAINDICATIONS Hypersensitivity to zanamivir.

CAUTIOUS USE Concurrent use of inhaled medication with inhaled zanamivir; pregnancy (category B), lactation. Safety and efficacy in children <7 y are unknown.

ROUTE & DOSAGE

Acute Influenza

Adult/Child >7 y: **Inhaled** 2 inhalations (one 5 mg blister/inhalation) b.i.d. (approximately 12 h apart) times 5 d

ADMINISTRATION

Inhalation

- Initiate within 48 h of onset of flu-like symptoms.
- Give scheduled inhaled bronchodilator before zanamivir.
- Store at 25° C (77° F).

ADVERSE EFFECTS (≥1%) **Body as a Whole:** Headache. **CNS:** Dizziness. **GI:** Nausea, diarrhea, vomiting. **Respiratory:** Nasal symptoms, bronchitis, cough, sinusitis; ear, nose, throat infection.

INTERACTIONS Drug: No clinically significant interactions established.

PHARMACOKINETICS Absorption: 4%–17% of inhaled dose is systemically absorbed. **Peak:** 1–2 h. **Distribution:** <10% protein bound. **Metabolism:** Not metabolized. **Elimination:** Excreted in urine. **Half-Life:** 2.5–5.1 h.

NURSING IMPLICATIONS

Patient & Family Education

- Start within 48 h of onset of flu-like symptoms for most effective response.
- Use any scheduled inhaled bronchodilator first; then use zanamivir.
- Do not breast feed while taking this drug.

ZIDOVUDINE (AZIDOTHYMIDINE, AZT) Pr

(zye-doe'vyoo-deen)

Retrovir

Classifications: ANTIINFECTIVE; ANTIVIRAL

Pregnancy Category: C

AVAILABILITY 300 mg tablets; 100 mg capsules; 50 mg/5 mL syrup; 10 mg/mL injection

ACTIONS Analog of thymidine (a major nucleoside in DNA). On entering host cell, zidovudine is converted to a triphosphate (the active form) by endogenous thymidine kinase and other cellular enzymes. Appears to act by being incorporated into growing DNA chains by viral reverse transcriptase, thereby terminating viral replication.

THERAPEUTIC EFFECTS Zidovudine has antiviral action against HIV (human immunodeficiency virus), the causative agent of AIDS (acquired immune deficiency syndrome), LAV (lymphadenopathy-associated virus), and ARV (AIDS-associated retrovirus).

USES Patients who are HIV positive and have a CD_4 count ≤500/mm^3, asymptomatic HIV infection, early and late symptomatic HIV disease, prevention of perinatal transfer of HIV during pregnancy.

UNLABELED USES Pediatric patients, postexposure chemoprophylaxis.

CONTRAINDICATIONS Life-threatening allergic reactions to any of the components of the drug. Safe use during pregnancy (category C), lactation, is not established.

CAUTIOUS USE Impaired renal or hepatic function, bone marrow depression.

ROUTE & DOSAGE

Symptomatic HIV Infection

Adult: **PO** 200 mg q4h (1200 mg/d), after 1 mo may reduce to 100 mg q4h (600 mg/d) **IV** 1–2 mg/kg q4h (1200 mg/d)
Child: **PO/IV** *3 mo–13 y,* 100–180 mg/m^2 q6h

Asymptomatic HIV Infection, Post-exposure Prophylaxis

Adult: **PO** 100 mg q4h while awake, 5 times/d

Prevention of Maternal-Fetal Transmission

Neonate: **PO** 2 mg/kg q6h for 6 wk beginning within 12 h after birth

ADMINISTRATION

Oral

- Do not expose capsules and syrup to light during drug preparation.

Intravenous

PREPARE: **Intermittent:** Withdraw required dose from vial and dilute with D5W to a concentration not to exceed 4 mg/mL.

ADMINISTER: **Intermittent:** Give calculated dose at a constant rate over 60 min; avoid rapid infusion.

- Store at 15°–25° C (59°–77° F) and protected from light unless otherwise directed.

ADVERSE EFFECTS (≥1%) **Body as a Whole:** *Fever,* dyspnea, *malaise,* weakness, *myalgia,* myopathy. **CNS:** *Headache,* insomnia, dizziness, paresthesias, mild confusion, anxiety, restlessness, agitation. **GI:** *Nausea,* diarrhea, *vomiting, anorexia,* GI pain. **Hematologic:** *Bone marrow depression, granulocytopenia, anemia.* **Respiratory:** *Cough,*

Z

wheezing. **Skin:** *Rash,* itching, diaphoresis.

INTERACTIONS Drug: Acetaminophen ganciclovir, interferon-alfa may enhance bone marrow suppression; **Atovaquone, amphotericin B, aspirin, dapsone, doxorubicin, fluconazole, flucytosine, indomethacin, interferon alfa, methadone, pentamidine, vincristine, valproic acid** may increase risk of AZT toxicity; **probenecid** will decrease AZT elimination, resulting in increased serum levels and thus toxicity. **Nelfinavir, rifampin, ritonavir** may decrease zidovodine (AZT) concentrations; other ANTIRETROVIRAL AGENTS may cause lactic acidosis and severe hepatomegaly with steatosis; **stavudine, doxorubicin** may antagonize AZT effects.

PHARMACOKINETICS Absorption: Readily absorbed from GI tract; 60%–70% reaches systemic circulation (first-pass metabolism). **Peak:** 0.5–1.5 h. **Distribution:** Crosses blood–brain barrier and placenta. **Metabolism:** Metabolized in liver. **Elimination:** 63%–95% excreted in urine. **Half-Life:** 1 h.

NURSING IMPLICATIONS

Assessment & Drug Effects

- Evaluate patient at least weekly during the first month of therapy.
- Lab tests: Baseline and frequent (at least q2wk) blood counts, CD_4 (T_4) lymphocyte count, Hgb, and granulocyte count to detect hematologic toxicity.
- Myelosuppression results in anemia, which commonly occurs after 4–6 wk of therapy, and granulocytopenia in 6–8 wk. Frequently, both respond to dosage adjustment. Significant anemia (Hgb <7.5 g/dL or reduction >25% of baseline value), or granulocyte count <750/mm^3 (or reduction >50% of baseline) may require temporary interruption of therapy and transfusions.
- Monitor for common adverse effects, especially severe headache, nausea, insomnia, and myalgia.

Patient & Family Education

- Contact physician promptly if health status worsens or any unusual symptoms develop.
- Understand that this drug is not a cure for HIV infection; you will continue to be at risk for opportunistic infections.
- Do not share drug with others; take drug exactly as prescribed.
- Drug does NOT reduce the risk of transmission of HIV infection through body fluids.
- Do not breast feed while taking this drug; it is not known if the drug is secreted in human milk.

ZILEUTON

(zi-leu'ton)

Leutrol, Zyflo

Classifications: BRONCHODILATOR (RESPIRATORY SMOOTH MUSCLE RELAXANT); LEUKOTRIENE RECEPTOR ANTAGONIST

Prototype: Zafirlukast

Pregnancy Category: C

AVAILABILITY 600 mg tablets

ACTIONS Inhibits 5-lipoxygenase, the enzyme needed to start the conversion of arachidonic acid to leukotrienes. Leukotrienes are considered more important than prostaglandins as inflammatory agents; they induce bronchoconstriction and mucus production. Elevated sputum and blood levels of leukotrienes have been documented during acute asthma attacks.

Common adverse effects in *italic*, life-threatening effects <u>underlined</u>; generic names in **bold**; classifications in SMALL CAPS; ♣ Canadian drug name; ⊕ Prototype drug

THERAPEUTIC EFFECTS Zileuton helps to prevent the signs and symptoms of asthma including airway edema, smooth muscle constriction, and altered cellular activity due to inflammation.

USES Prophylaxis and chronic treatment of asthma in adults and children >12 y.

CONTRAINDICATIONS Hypersensitivity to zileuton or zafirlukast, active liver disease, lactation, pregnancy (category C).
CAUTIOUS USE Hepatic insufficiency. Safety and effectiveness in children >12 y are not established.

ROUTE & DOSAGE

Asthma
Adult/Child: **PO** >12 y, 600 mg q.i.d.

ADMINISTRATION

Oral

- Give at meals and bedtime.
- Store at room temperature, 15°–30° C (59°–86° F); protect from light.

ADVERSE EFFECTS (≥1%) **Body as a Whole:** Pain, asthenia, myalgia, arthralgia, fever, malaise, neck pain/rigidity. **CNS:** *Headache,* dizziness, insomnia, nervousness, somnolence. **CV:** Chest pain. **GI:** Abdominal pain, *dyspepsia,* nausea, constipation, flatulence, vomiting, elevated liver function tests, asymptomatic hepatitis. **Skin:** Pruritus. **Other:** Conjunctivitis, hypertonia, lymphadenopathy, vaginitis, UTI, leukopenia.

INTERACTIONS Drug: May double **theophylline** levels and increase toxicity. Increases hypoprothrombinemic effects of **warfarin.** May increase levels of BETA BLOCKERS (especially **propranolol**), leading to hypotension and bradycardia. May increase **terfenadine** levels, leading to prolongation of QT_C interval.

PHARMACOKINETICS Absorption: Rapidly absorbed from GI tract. **Peak:** 1.7 h. **Duration:** 5–8 h. **Distribution:** 93% protein bound; secreted in the breast milk of rats. **Metabolism:** Metabolized in liver primarily via glucuronide conjugation. **Elimination:** Excreted primarily in urine (94%). **Half-Life:** 2.5 h.

NURSING IMPLICATIONS

Assessment & Drug Effects

- Assess respiratory status and airway function regularly.
- Lab tests: Periodic CBC and routine blood chemistry; monthly liver function tests for 3 mo, then every 2–3 mo for rest of first year, then periodically.
- Instructions for CONCURRENT THERAPIES: Reduce theophylline dose and closely monitor theophylline levels; closely monitor PT and INR with warfarin therapy; closely monitor phenytoin level with phenytoin therapy; closely monitor HR and BP for excessive beta blockade with propranolol therapy.

Patient & Family Education

- Take medication regularly even during symptom-free periods.
- Drug is not intended to treat acute episodes of asthma.
- Report to physician promptly S&S of hepatic toxicity (see Appendix F) or flu-like symptoms. Follow-up lab work is very important.
- Notify physician if condition worsens while using prescribed doses of all antiasthmatic medications.
- Do not breast feed while taking this drug.

ZIPRASIDONE HYDROCHLORIDE

(zip-ra-si'done)

Geodon

Classifications: CENTRAL NERVOUS SYSTEM (CNS) AGENT; PSYCHOTHERAPEUTIC AGENT; ANTIPSYCHOTIC; ATYPICAL

Prototype: Clozapine

Pregnancy Category: C

AVAILABILITY 20 mg, 40 mg, 60 mg, 80 mg capsules; 20 mg/mL injection

ACTIONS Unrelated to phenothiazine or butrophenone antipsychotic agents. Exhibits high *in vitro* binding affinity for the following receptors: dopamine D_2 and D_3, serotonin $5HT_{2A}$, $5HT_{2C}$, $5HT_{1A}$, $5HT_{1D}$, and the alpha-1-adrenergic receptors, and moderate affinity for the histamine H_1 receptor. Antagonist at the D_2, $5HT_{2A}$ and $5HT_{1D}$ receptors, and an agonist at the $5HT_{1A}$ receptor. Additionally, inhibits synaptic reuptake of serotonin and norepinephrine. Antagonism at other receptors may explain some of the other therapeutic and adverse effects (e.g., orthostatic hypotension).

THERAPEUTIC EFFECTS Mechanism of action is unknown; probably related to inhibition of synaptic reuptake of serotonin and norepinephrine through antagonism of dopamine type 2 (D_2) and serotonin type 2 ($5HT_2$) antagonism.

USES Treatment of schizophrenia, acute bipolar mania.

UNLABELED USES Tourette's syndrome.

CONTRAINDICATIONS Hypersensitivity to ziprasidone; history of QT prolongation including congenital long QT syndrome or with other drugs known to prolong the QT interval; AV block, bundle branch block, cardiac arrhythmias, congenital heart disease, recent MI or uncompensated heart failure; bradycardia, hypokalemia or hypomagnesemia; intravenous administration; neuroleptic malignant syndrome and tardive dyskinesia; dehydration or hypovolemia; UV exposure and tanning beds; pregnancy (category C), lactation. Safety and efficacy in children are not established.

CAUTIOUS USE History of seizures, CVA, dementia, Parkinson's disease, or Alzheimer disease; known cardiovascular disease, conduction abnormalities, treatment with antihypertensive drugs; cerebrovascular disease; hepatic impairment; seizure disorder, seizures; breast cancer; risk factors for elevated core body temperature; esophageal motility disorders and risk of aspiration pneumonia; suicide potential; children >7 y for use in Tourette's syndrome only.

ROUTE & DOSAGE

Schizophrenia

Adult: **PO** Start with 20 mg b.i.d. with food, may increase q2d up to 80 mg b.i.d. if needed. **IM** 10 mg q2h or 20 mg q4h up to max of 40 mg/d

Acute Mania

Adult: **PO** Start with 40 mg b.i.d. with food; may increase q2d up to 80 mg b.i.d. if needed

ADMINISTRATION

Note: CONTRAINDICATIONS for this drug. Do NOT administer to anyone with a history of cardiac arrhythmias or other cardiac disease, hypokalemia, hypomagnesemia, prolonged QT/QTc interval, or to anyone on other drugs known to prolong the

Z

QTc interval. Withhold drug and consult physician if any of the foregoing conditions are present.

Oral

- Give with food.
- Make dosage adjustments at intervals of ≥2 days.

Intramuscular

- Give deep IM into a large muscle.
- Store at 15°–30° C (59°–86° F).

ADVERSE EFFECTS (≥1%) **Body as a Whole:** Asthenia, myalgia, weight gain, flu-like syndrome, face edema, chills, hypothermia. **CNS:** *Somnolence,* akathisia, dizziness, extrapyramidal effects, dystonia, hypertonia, agitation, tremor, dyskinesias, hostility, paresthesia, confusion, vertigo, hypokinesia, hyperkinesias, abnormal gait, oculogyric crisis, hypesthesia, ataxia, amnesia, cogwheel rigidity, delirium, hypotonia, akinesia, dysarthria, withdrawal syndrome, buccoglossal syndrome, choreoathetosis, diplopia, incoordination, neuropathy. **CV:** Tachycardia, postural hypotension, prolonged QTc interval, hypertension. **GI:** *Nausea,* constipation, dyspepsia, diarrhea, dry mouth, anorexia, abdominal pain, vomiting. **Metabolic:** Hyperglycemia, diabetes mellitus. **Respiratory:** Rhinitis, increased cough, dyspnea. **Skin:** Rash, fungal dermatitis, photosensitivity. **Special Senses:** Abnormal vision.

INTERACTIONS Drug: Carbamazepine may decrease **ziprasidone** levels; **ketoconazole** may increase **ziprasidone** levels; may enhance hypotensive effects of ANTIHYPERTENSIVE AGENTS; may antagonize effects of **levodopa;** increased risk of arrhythmias and heart block due to prolonged QTc interval with ANTIARRHYTHMIC AGENTS, **amoxapine, arsenic trioxide, cisapride, chlorpromazine, clarithromycin, daunorubicin, diltiazem, dolasetron, doxorubicin, droperidol, erythromycin, halofantrine, indapamide, levomethadyl,** LOCAL ANESTHETICS, **maprotiline, mefloquine, mesoridazine, octreotide, pentamidine, pimozide, probucol, gatifloxacin, grepafloxacin, levofloxacin, moxifloxacin, sparfloxacin,** TRICYCLIC ANTIDEPRESSANTS, **tacrolimus, thioridazine, troleandomycin;** additive CNS depression with SEDATIVE-HYPNOTICS, ANXIOLYTICS, **ethanol,** OPIATE AGONISTS.

PHARMACOKINETICS Absorption: Well absorbed with 60% reaching systemic circulation. **Peak:** 6–8 h. **Metabolism:** Extensively metabolized in the liver. **Elimination:** 20% of metabolites excreted in urine, 66% of metabolites excreted in bile. **Half-Life:** 7 h.

NURSING IMPLICATIONS

Assessment & Drug Effects

- Lab tests: Baseline and periodic ECG, serum potassium and serum magnesium, especially with concomitant diuretic therapy. Periodically monitor blood glucose.
- Monitor diabetics for loss of glycemic control.
- Monitor for S&S of torsade de pointes (e.g., dizziness, palpitations, syncope), tardive dyskinesia (see Appendix F) especially in older adult women and with prolonged therapy, and the appearance of an unexplained rash. Withhold drug and report to physician immediately if any of these develop.
- Monitor I&O ratio and pattern: Notify physician if diarrhea, vomiting or any other conditions develops which may cause electrolyte imbalance.
- Monitor BP lying, sitting, and standing. Report orthostatic hypotension to physician.

Z

- Monitor cognitive status and take appropriate precautions.
- Monitor for loss of seizure control, especially with a history of seizures or dementia.

Patient & Family Education

- Carefully monitor blood glucose levels if diabetic.
- Be aware that therapeutic effect may not be evident for several weeks.
- Report any of the following to a health care provider immediately: Palpitations, faintness or loss of consciousness, rash, abnormal muscle movements, vomiting or diarrhea.
- Do not drive or engage in potentially hazardous activities until response to drug is known.
- Make position changes slowly and in stages to prevent dizziness upon arising.
- Avoid strenuous exercise, exposure to extreme heat, or other activities that may cause dehydration.
- Do not breast feed while taking this drug.

ZOLEDRONIC ACID

(zo-le-dron'ic)
Zometa
Classifications: BISPHOSPHONATE; REGULATOR, BONE METABOLISM
Prototype: Etidronate Disodium
Pregnancy Category: D

AVAILABILITY 4 mg vial

ACTIONS Zoledronic acid inhibits bone resorption by inhibiting osteoclastic activity and inducing osteoclast apoptosis. Zoledronic acid also blocks osteoclastic resorption of bone and cartilage. It inhibits various stimulatory factors of osteoclastic activity by bone tumors.

THERAPEUTIC EFFECTS Zoledronic acid inhibits osteoclastic activity and sketetal calcium release induced by various stimulatory factors released by bone tumors.

USES Treatment of hypercalcemia of malignancy, multiple myeloma, and bony metastases from solid tumors.
UNLABELED USES Paget's disease.

CONTRAINDICATIONS Hypersensitivity to zoledronic acid or other bisphosphonates; preexisting hypocalcemia; serum creatinine of 0.5 mg/dL; pregnancy (category D).
CAUTIOUS USE Lactation, renal, and/or hepatic impairment; dental work; concurrent administration of aminoglycosides, or loop diuretics; older adults. Safety and effectiveness of zoledronic acid in pediatric patients have not been established.

ROUTE & DOSAGE

Hypercalcemia of Malignancy
Adult: **IV** 4 mg over a minimum of 15 min. May consider retreatment if serum calcium has not returned to normal, may repeat after 7 d

Multiple Myeloma and Bony Metastases from Solid Tumors
Adult: **IV** 4 mg over a minimum of 15 min q 3–4 wk

Paget's Disease
Adult: **IV** A single dose of 200 mcg or 400 mcg

Renal Impairment
Use in patients with hypercalcemia of malignancy with Scr ≥4.5 mg/dL, only if the benefit of treatment outweighs the risk of nephrotoxicity. Not recommended in patients with bone metastases if serum (S)Cr >3 mg/dL

Z

ADMINISTRATION

Intravenous

- Do not administer to anyone who is dehydrated or suspected of being dehydrated. Consult physician.
- Do not administer zoledronic acid unless patient is adequately rehydrated.
- Do not administer until serum creatinine values have been evaluated by the physician.

PREPARE: **IV Infusion:** Reconstitute by adding 5 mL of sterile water for injection to each vial. Withdraw the entire contents of the vial (4 mg) and further dilute in 100 mL of D5W or NS. Do not use Lactated Ringer's solution. If not used immediately, refrigerate. The total time between reconstitution and end of infusion must not exceed 24 h.

ADMINISTER: **IV Infusion:** Infuse 4 mg (NEVER MORE) over NO LESS than 15 min.

INCOMPATIBILITIES **Solution/additive and Y-site:** do not mix or infuse with **calcium**-containing solutions (e.g., **Ringers Lactate**).

- Store at 2°–8° C (36°–46° F) follow reconstitution. Must be completely infused within 24 h of reconstitution.

ADVERSE EFFECTS (≥1%) **Body as a Whole:** *Fever,* flu-like syndrome, redness and swelling at injection site, asthenia, chest apin, leg edema, mucositis, rigors. **CNS:** *Insomnia, anxiety, confusion, agitation,* headache, somnolence. **CV:** *Hypotension.* **GI:** *Nausea, vomiting, constipation, abdominal pain, anorexia,* dysphagia. **Hematologic:** *Anemia,* granulocytopenia, thrombocytopenia, <u>pancytopenia</u>. **Metabolic:** *Hypophosphatemia, hypokalemia, hypomagnesemia,* hypocalcemia, dehydration. **Musculoskeletal:** Skeletal pain, arthralgias, osteonecrosis of the jaw in cancer patients. **Respiratory:** *Dyspnea, cough,* pleural effusion. **Skin:** Alopecia, dermatitis. **Urogenital:** Renal deterioration [increase in serum creatinine (SCr)].

INTERACTIONS Drug: LOOP DIURETICS may increase risk of hypocalcemia; **thalidomide** and other NEPHROTOXIC DRUGS may increase risk of renal toxicity.

PHARMACOKINETICS Onset: 4–10 d. **Duration:** 3–4 wks. **Metabolism:** Not metabolized. **Elimination:** Excreted in urine. **Half-Life:** 146 hr.

NURSING IMPLICATIONS

Assessment & Drug Effects

- Lab tests: Baseline renal function tests prior to each dose and periodically thereafter; periodic ionized calcium or corrected serum calcium (CSC) levels, serum phosphate and magnesium, electrolytes, CBC with differential, Hct and Hgb.
- Notify physician immediately of deteriorating renal function as indicated by rising serum creatinine levels over baseline value.
- Withhold subsequent doses of zoledronic acid if serum creatinine is not within 10% of the baseline value. Consult physician.
- Monitor closely patient's hydration status. Note that loop diuretics should be used with caution due to the risk of hypocalcemia.
- Monitor for S&S of bronchospasm in aspirin-sensitive asthma patients; notify physician immediately.

Patient & Family Education

- Maintain adequate daily fluid intake. Consult with physician for guidelines.

Z

- Report unexplained weakness, tiredness, irritation, muscle pain, insomnia, or flu-like symptoms.
- Do not breast feed without consulting physician.

ZOLMITRIPTAN

(zol-mi-trip′tan)

Zomig, Zomig ZMT, Zomig Nasal Spray

Classifications: AUTONOMIC NERVOUS SYSTEM AGENT; ALPHA-ADRENERGIC ANTAGONIST (SYMPATHOLYTIC); SEROTONIN 5-$HT_{1B/1D}$ RECEPTOR AGONIST; ERGOT ALKALOID

Prototype: Sumatriptan

Pregnancy Category: C

AVAILABILITY 2.5 mg, 5 mg tablets orally disintegrating tablets; 5 mg nasal spray

ACTIONS Selective serotonin (5-$HT_{1B/1D}$) receptor agonist. The agonist effects at 5-$HT_{1B/1D}$ reverse the vasodilation of cranial blood vessels associated with a migraine.

THERAPEUTIC EFFECTS Activation of these receptors also reduces the pain pathways associated with migraine headache in addition to causing vasoconstriction of the cranial blood vessels.

USES Acute migraine headaches with or without aura.

CONTRAINDICATIONS Hypersensitivity to zolmitriptan; ischemic heart disease (angina pectoris, arteriosclerosis, ECG changes, history of MI or Prinzmetal's angina); cardiac arrhythmias, symptomatic Wolff-Parkinson-White syndrome, uncontrolled hypertension; hemiplegia or basilar migraine; concurrent administration of ergotamine or sumatriptan; PKU; adults >65 y; pregnancy (category C); children <18 y.

CAUTIOUS USE Men >40 y; postmenopausal women; patients with other cardiac risk factors, such as diabetes, obesity, cigarette smoking, high cholesterol levels, strong family history of CAD; GI disease, PVD, ischemic colitis, Raynaud's disease, cerebrovascular disease, stroke, intracranial bleeding; lactation.

ROUTE & DOSAGE

Acute Migraine

Adult: **PO** 2.5–5 mg, may repeat in 2 h if necessary (max: 10 mg/24 h) **Nasal Spray** One spray into one nostril

ADMINISTRATION

Oral

- Give any time after symptoms of migraine appear. Give ≤2.5 mg by breaking a 5 mg tablet in half. If headache returns, may repeat q2h up to 10 mg in 24 h.
- Do NOT give zolmitriptan within 24 h of an ergot-containing drug or other 5-HT_1 agonist.
- Discard unused tablets that have been removed from the packaging.

Intranasal

- Unit-dose spray device delivers a 5 mg dose. Do not exceed the maximum dose of 10 mg in 24 h.
- Store at 2°–25° C (36°–77° F) and protect from light.

ADVERSE EFFECTS (≥1%) **Body as a Whole:** Asthenia, fatigue, malaise, pain, pressure sensation, paresthesia, throat pressure, warm/cold sensations, hypesthesia. **CNS:** Somnolence, dizziness, drowsiness, headache, hypesthesia, decreased mental acuity, euphoria, tremor. **CV:** Coronary artery vasospasm, transient myocardial ischemia, <u>MI</u>, ventricular tachycardia, ventricular fibrillation, chest pain/tightness/heaviness, palpitations. **GI:** Dry mouth, nausea, vomiting. **Respiratory:** Dyspnea. **Skin:** Flushing. **Other:** Hot flushes.

INTERACTIONS Drug: Dihydroergotamine, methysergide, other 5-HT_1 AGONISTS may cause prolonged vasospastic reactions; SSRIS have rarely caused weakness, hyperreflexia, and incoordination; MAOIS should not be used with 5-HT_1 agonists; **cimetidine** increases half-life of zolmitriptan. **Herbal: Gingko, ginseng, echinacea, St. John's wort** may increase triptan toxicity.

PHARMACOKINETICS Absorption: Rapidly absorbed, 40% bioavailability. **Peak:** 2–3 h. **Distribution:** 25% protein bound. **Metabolism:** Metabolized in liver to active metabolite. **Elimination:** Excreted primarily in urine (65%), 30% excreted in feces. **Half-Life:** 3 h.

NURSING IMPLICATIONS

Assessment & Drug Effects

- Monitor for therapeutic effectiveness: Relief or reduction of migraine pain within 1–4 h.
- Monitor cardiovascular status carefully following first dose in patients at risk for CAD (e.g., postmenopausal women, men >40 y, persons with known CAD risk factors) or coronary artery vasospasms.
- Perform periodic cardiovascular evaluation and ECG with long-term use.
- Report to physician immediately chest pain, nausea, or tightness in chest or throat that is severe or does not quickly resolve.

Patient & Family Education

- Carefully review patient information insert and guidelines for taking drug.
- Do NOT take zolmitriptan during the aura phase, but as early as possible after onset of migraine.
- Concurrent oral contraceptive use may increase incidence of adverse effects.
- Contact physician immediately if any of the following occur after zolmitriptan use: Symptoms of angina (e.g., severe or persistent pain or tightness in chest or throat, sudden nausea), hypersensitivity (e.g., wheezing, facial swelling, skin rash, hives), fainting, or abdominal pain.
- Report any other adverse effects (e.g., tingling, flushing, dizziness) at next physician visit.
- Do not breast feed while taking this drug without consulting physician.

ZOLPIDEM (Pr)

(zol'-pi-dem)
Ambien
Classifications: CENTRAL NERVOUS SYSTEM AGENT; ANXIOLYTIC; SEDATIVE-HYPNOTIC; NON-BENZODIAZEPINE
Pregnancy Category: B
Controlled Substance: Schedule IV

AVAILABILITY 5 mg, 10 mg tablets

ACTIONS Nonbenzodiazepine hypnotic. Does not have muscle relaxant or anticonvulsant effects.
THERAPEUTIC EFFECTS Preserves deep sleep (stages 3 and 4) at hypnotic doses.

USES Short-term treatment of insomnia.

CONTRAINDICATIONS Lactation.
CAUTIOUS USE Depressed patients, hepatic/renal impairment, older adults, pregnancy (category B), patients with compromised respiratory status. Safety and efficacy in children <18 y are not established.

Z

ROUTE & DOSAGE

Short-Term Treatment of Insomnia
Adult: **PO** 5–10 mg h.s. limited to 7–10 d
Geriatric: **PO** start with 5 mg h.s. limited to 7–10 d

ADMINISTRATION

Oral

- Give immediately before bedtime; for more rapid sleep onset, do NOT give with or immediately after a meal.
- Use reduced dosage of 5 mg in older adult or debilitated patients.
- Store at room temperature, 15°–30° C (59°–86° F).

ADVERSE EFFECTS (≥1%) **CNS:** Headache on awakening, drowsiness or fatigue, lethargy, drugged feeling, depression, anxiety, irritability, dizziness, double vision. Confusion and falls reported in elderly. Doses >10 mg may be associated with anterograde amnesia or memory impairment. **GI:** Dyspepsia, nausea, vomiting. **Other:** Myalgia.

INTERACTIONS Drug: CNS DEPRESSANTS, **alcohol,** PHENOTHIAZINES by augmenting CNS depression. **Food:** Extent and rate of absorption of zolpidem is significantly decreased.

PHARMACOKINETICS Absorption: Readily absorbed from GI tract. 70% reaches systemic circulation. Food decreases rate and extent of absorption. **Onset:** 7–27 min. **Peak:** 0.5–2.3h. **Duration:** 6–8 h. **Distribution:** Highly protein bound. Lowest concentrations in CNS, highest concentrations in glandular tissue and fat. Crosses placenta, very small amounts (<0.02%) distributed into breast milk. **Metabolism:** Metabolized in the liver to 3 inactive metabolites. **Elimination:** 79%–96% of dose appears as metabolites in the bile, urine, and feces. **Half-Life:** 1.7–2.5 h.

NURSING IMPLICATIONS

Assessment & Drug Effects

- Assess respiratory function in patients with compromised respiratory status. Report immediately to physician significantly depressed respiratory rate (less than 12/min).
- Monitor patients for S&S of depression (see Appendix F); zolpidem may increase level of depression.
- Monitor older adult or debilitated patients closely for impaired cognitive or motor function and unusual sensitivity to the drug's effects.

Patient & Family Education

- Avoid taking alcohol or other CNS depressants while on zolpidem.
- Do not drive or engage in other potentially hazardous activities until response to drug is known.
- Report vision changes to physician.
- Note: Onset of drug is more rapid when taken on an empty stomach.
- Do not breast feed while taking this drug.

ZONISAMIDE Pr

(zon-i'sa-mide)
Zonegran
Classifications: CENTRAL NERVOUS SYSTEM AGENT; ANTICONVULSANT; SULFONAMIDE
Pregnancy Category: C

AVAILABILITY 25 mg, 50 mg, 100 mg capsules

ACTIONS Anticonvulsant effective against a variety of seizure types. A sulfonamide derivative and a broad spectrum anticonvulsant that does not potentiate the activity of gamma-

Z

aminobutyric acid (GABA) in the synapses of the neurons. It does, however, facilitate dopaminergic and serotonergic neurotransmission.
THERAPEUTIC EFFECTS Suppresses focal spike discharges and electroshock seizures.

USES Adjunctive therapy for partial seizures in adults.

CONTRAINDICATIONS Hypersensitivity to sulfonamides or zonisamide; pregnancy (category C), lactation.
CAUTIOUS USE Children <6 y; renal or hepatic insufficiency, concomitant administration of drugs that induce or inhibit CYP3A4; older adults.

ROUTE & DOSAGE

Partial Seizures
Adult: **PO** start at 100 mg q.d., may increase after 2 wk to 200 mg/d, may then increase q2wk, if necessary (max: 400 mg/d in 1–2 divided doses

ADMINISTRATION

Oral
- Do not crush or break capsules; ensure capsules are swallowed whole with adequate fluid.
- Withdraw drug gradually when discontinued to minimize seizure potential.
- Store at 25° C (77° F); room temperature permitted. Protect from light and moisture.

ADVERSE EFFECTS (≥1%) **Body as a Whole:** Flu-like syndrome, weight loss. **CNS:** Agitation, irritability, anxiety, ataxia, confusion, depression, difficulty concentrating, difficulty with memory, *dizziness,* fatigue, *headache,* insomnia, mental slowing, nervousness, nystagmus, paresthesia, schizophrenic behavior, *somnolence,* tiredness, tremor, convulsion, abnormal gait, hyperesthesia, incoordination. **GI:** Abdominal pain, *anorexia,* constipation, diarrhea, dyspepsia, nausea, dry mouth, flatulence, gingivitis, gum hyperplasia, gastritis, stomatitis, cholelithiasis, glossitis, melena, rectal hemorrhage, ulcerative stomatitis, ulcer, dysphagia. **Metabolic:** Oligohidrosis, sometimes resulting in heat stroke and hyperthermia in children. **Respiratory:** Rhinitis, pharyngitis, cough. **Skin:** Ecchymosis, rash, pruritus. **Special Senses:** Difficulties in verbal expression, diplopia, speech abnormalities, taste perversion, amblyopia, tinnitus. **Urogenital:** Kidney stones.

INTERACTIONS Drug: Phenytoin, carbamazepine, phenobarbital, valproic acid may decrease half-life of zonisamide.

PHARMACOKINETICS Peak: 2–6 h. **Distribution:** 40% protein bound, extensively binds to erythrocytes. **Metabolism:** Acetylated in liver by CYP3A4. **Elimination:** Excreted primarily in urine. **Half-Life:** 63–105 h.

NURSING IMPLICATIONS

Assessment & Drug Effects
- Withhold drug and notify physician if an unexplained rash or S&S of hypersensitivity appear (see Appendix F).
- Monitor for and report S&S of CNS impairment (somnolence, excessive fatigue, cognitive deficits, speech or language problems, incoordination, gait disturbances); oligohidrosis (lack of sweating) and hyperthermia in pediatric patients.
- Lab tests: Periodic BUN and serum creatinine, and CBC with differential.

Patient & Family Education

- Do not abruptly stop taking this medication.
- Increase daily fluid intake to minimize risk of renal stones. Notify physician immediately of S&S of renal stones: sudden back or abdominal pain, and blood in urine.
- Report any of the following: dizziness, excess drowsiness, frequent headaches, malaise, double vision, lack of coordination, persistent nausea, sore throat, fever, mouth ulcers, or easy bruising.
- Exercise special caution with concurrent use of alcohol or CNS depressants.
- Do not drive or engage in other potentially hazardous activities until response to drug is known.
- Do not breast feed while taking this drug.

APPENDIXES

(Generic names are in **bold**)

APPENDIX A-1
OCULAR MEDICATIONS:

BETA-ADRENERGIC BLOCKERS Prototype for classification: Propranolol HCl Use: Intraocular hypertension and chronic open-angle glaucoma.

Betaxolol HCl 0.25%, 0.5% soln Betoptic, Betoptic S	*Adult:* **Topical** 1 drop of 0.5% solution or 0.25% suspension in affected eye twice daily.
Carteolol HCl 1% soln Ocupress	*Adult:* **Topical** 1 drop b.i.d.
Levobetaxolol 0.5% susp Betaxon	*Adult:* **Topical** 1 drop b.i.d.
Levobunolol 0.25%, 0.5% soln Betagan	*Adult:* **Topical** 1–2 drops 1–2 times/d.
Metipranolol HCl 0.3% soln OptiPranolol	*Adult:* **Topical** 1 drop b.i.d.
Timolol maleate 0.25%, 0.5% soln Betimol, Timoptic, Timoptic XE, Istalol	*Adult:* **Topical** 1 drop of 0.25–0.5% solution b.i.d.; may decrease to q.d. Apply gel q.d. Apply Istalol solution once daily.

Adverse Effects/Clinical Implications: May cause *mild ocular stinging* and discomfort; tearing; may also have the adverse effects of systemic beta blockers. May mask symptoms of acute hypoglycemia in diabetic patients (tachycardia, tremor, but not sweating). May precipitate thyroid storm in patients with hyperthyroidism. Patients with impaired cardiac function and the elderly should report to physician signs and symptoms of CHF (see Appendix G). Monitor BP for hypotension and heart rate for bradycardia.

MIOTICS Prototype for classification: Pilocarpine HCl Use: Open-angle and angle-closure glaucomas; to reduce IOP and to protect the lens during surgery and laser iridotomy; to counteract effects of mydriatics and cycloplegics following surgery or ophthalmoscopic examination.

Apraclonidine HCl Iopidine	**Intraoperative and Post-surgical Increase in IOP:** *Adult:* **Topical** 1 drop of 1% solution in affected eye 1 h before surgery and 1 drop in same eye immediately after surgery. **Open-angle Glaucoma:** *Adult:* **Topical** 1 drop of 0.5% solution in affected eye q12h.

Brimonidine tartrate Alphagan P	**Glaucoma:** *Adult:* **Topical** 1 drop in affected eye(s) t.i.d. approximately 8 h apart.
Brinzolamide Azopt	**Ocular Hypertension or Open-angle Glaucoma:** *Adult:* **Topical** 1 drop in affected eye(s) t.i.d.
Carbachol Isopto, Carbachol, Miostat	*Adult:* **Topical** 1–2 drops of 0.75–3% solution in lower conjunctival sac q4–8h. **Intraocular** 0.5 ml of 0.01% solution injected into anterior chamber of eye.
Demecarium bromide Humorsol	**Glaucoma:** *Adult:* **Topical** 1–2 drops of 0.125–0.25% solution 2 times/wk up to b.i.d. **Convergent Strabismus:** *Child:* 1 drop of 0.125% solution in each eye daily for 2–3 wk; then decrease to 1 drop q.o.d. for 2–8 wk; then 1 drop 2 times/wk.
Dorzolamide Trusopt	**Ocular Hypertension or Open-angle Glaucoma:** *Adult/Child:* **Topical** 1 drop in affected eye(s) t.i.d.
Echothiophate iodide Phospholine Iodide	**Glaucoma:** *Adult:* **Topical** 1 drop of 0.03–0.25% solution in conjunctival sac 1–2 times/d. **Accommodative Esotropia:** *Adult:* **Topical** ***Diagnosis:*** 1 drop of 0.125% solution in both eyes once/d at bedtime for 2–3 wk. ***Treatment:*** 1 drop of 0.125% solution q.o.d. or 1 drop of 0.06% solution daily (max: 1 drop 0.125% solution daily).
Pilocarpine HCl Adsorbocarpine, Isopto Carpine, Minims, Pilocarpine, Miocarpine, Ocusert, Pilo	**Acute Glaucoma:** *Adult:* **Topical** 1 drop of 1–2% solution in affected eye q5–10min for 3–6 doses, then 1 drop q1–3h until IOP is reduced. **Chronic Glaucoma:** *Adult:* **Topical** 1 drop of 0.5–4% solution in affected eye q4–12h or 1 ocular system (Ocusert) q7d **Miotic:** *Adult:* **Topical** 1 drop of 1% solution in affected eye.

Adverse Effects/Clinical Implications: Ocular: Ciliary spasm with browache, twitching of eyelids, eye pain with change in eye focus, miosis, *diminished vision in poorly illuminated areas,* blurred vision, reduced visual acuity, sensitivity, contact allergy, lacrimation, follicular conjunctivitis, conjunctival irritation, cataract, retinal detachment. **CNS:** *Headache, drowsiness,* depression, syncope. **GI:** Abnormal taste, dry mouth. **Clinical Implications:** Wait 15 min after instillation before inserting soft contact lenses to avoid staining the lenses. Use with MAO inhibitors may have increased risk of hypertensive emergency. May increase the effects of beta blockers and other antihypertensives on blood pressure and heart rate. TCAs may reduce the effects of **brimonidine. Brinzolamide** is a carbonic anhydrase inhibitor (prototype: acetazolamide) and is a sulfonamide. It should not be used by patients with sulfa allergies. **Demecarium bromide** is capable of producing cumulative systemic effects. It is essential to adhere precisely to prescribed drug concentration, dosage schedule, and technique of administration. Reconstituted solutions of **echothiophate** remain stable for

1 mo at room temperature. Expiration date should appear on label. The length of time solutions remain stable under refrigeration varies with manufacturer. **Echothiophate** therapy is generally discontinued 2–6 wk before surgery. If necessary, alternate miotic therapy is substituted. Medication should be given in the evening. Give at least 5 min apart from other topical ophthalmic drugs. The patient with brown or hazel eyes may require a stronger ophthalmic solution or more frequent instillation of **physostigmine** for desired effects than the patient with blue eyes.

PROSTAGLANDINS Prototype for classification: Latanoprost
Use: Open-angle glaucoma and intraocular hypertension.

Bimatoprost Lumigan	*Adult:* **Topical** 1 drop in affected eye(s) once daily in the evening.
Latanoprost Xalatan	*Adult:* **Topical** 1 drop (1.5 mg) in affected eye(s) once daily in the evening.
Travaprost Travatan	*Adult:* **Topical** 1 drop in affected eye(s) once daily in the evening.
Unoprostone isopropyl Rescula	*Adult:* **Topical** 1 drop in affected eye(s) b.i.d.

Adverse Effects: Ocular: *Conjunctival hyperemia, growth of eyelashes, ocular pruritus,* ocular dryness, visual disturbance, ocular burning, foreign body sensation, eye pain, pigmentation of the periocular skin, blepharitis, cataract, superficial punctate keratitis, eyelid erythema, ocular irritation, eyelash darkening, eye discharge, tearing, photophobia, allergic conjunctivitis, increases in iris pigmentation (brown pigment), conjunctival edema. **Body as a Whole:** Headaches, abnormal liver function tests, asthenia, and hirsutism. **Clinical Implications:** Should instill in the evening. Wait 15 min after instillation before inserting soft contact lenses to avoid staining the lenses. Give at least 5 min apart from other topical ophthalmic drugs.

MYDRIATIC Prototype for classification: Homatropine HBr Use: Mydriatic for ocular examination and as cycloplegic to measure errors of refraction. Also inflammatory conditions of uveal tract, ciliary spasm, as a cycloplegic and mydriatic in preoperative and postoperative conditions, and as an optical aid in select patients with axial lens opacities.

Cyclopentolate HCl AK-Pentolate, Cyclogyl, Pentalair	**Cycloplegic Refraction:** *Adult:* **Topical** 1 drop of 1% solution in eye 40–50 min before procedure, followed by 1 drop in 5 min; may need 2% solution in patients with darkly pigmented eyes. *Child:* **Topical** 1 drop of 0.5–1% solution in eye 40–50 min before procedure, followed by 1 drop in 5 min; may need 2% solution in patients with darkly pigmented eyes.
Dipivefrin HCl Propine	**Glaucoma:** *Adult:* **Topical** 1 drop in eye q12h.

Epinephryl borate Epinal, Eppy/N	*Adult:* **Topical** 1–2 drops as needed.
Homatropine HBr AK-Homatropine, Homatrine, Isopto Homatropine	**Cycloplegic Refraction:** *Adult:* **Topical** 1–2 drops of 2% or 5% solution in eye repeated in 5–10 min if necessary. **Ocular Inflammation:** *Adult:* **Topical** 1–2 drops of 2% or 5% solution in eye up to q3–4h.
Hydroxyamphetamine HBr Paredrine	
Hydroxyamphetamine HBr/ Tropicamide Paremyd	**Dilation of pupil:** *Adult:* **Topical** 1–2 drops in conjunctival sac.
Phenylephrine HCl AK-Dilate Ophthalmic, Alconefrin, Isopto Frin, Mydfrin, Neo-Synephrine, Prefrin Liquifilm, Vacon	**Ophthalmoscopy:** *Adult:* **Topical** 1 drop of 2.5% or 10% solution before examination. *Child:* **Topical** 1 drop of 2.5% solution before examination. **Vasoconstrictor:** *Adult:* **Topical** 2 drops of 0.12–0.15% solution q3–4h as necessary.
Tropicamide Mydriacyl, Tropicacyl	**Refraction:** *Adult:* **Topical** 1–2 drops of 1% solution in each eye, repeat in 5 min; if patient is not seen within 20–30 min, an additional drop may be instilled. **Examination of Fundus:** *Adult:* **Topical** 1–2 drops of 0.5% solution in each eye 15–20 min prior to examination; may repeat q30min if necessary.

Contraindicated in: Primary (narrow-angle) glaucoma or predisposition to glaucoma; children <6 y. **Cautious use in:** Increased IOP, infants, children, pregnancy (category C), the elderly or debilitated; hypertension; hyperthyroidism; diabetes; cardiac disease. **Adverse Effects:** Increased IOP, *blurred vision, photophobia*. **Prolonged use:** Local irritation, congestion, edema, eczema, follicular conjunctivitis. **Excessive dosage/systemic absorption:** Symptoms of atropine poisoning (flushing, dry skin, mouth, nose; decreased sweating; fever, rash, rapid/irregular pulse; abdominal and bladder distension; hallucinations, confusion). **CNS:** Psychotic reaction, behavior disturbances, ataxia, incoherent speech, restlessness, hallucinations, somnolence, disorientation, failure to recognize people, grand mal seizures. **Clinical Implications:** Carefully monitor **cyclopentolate** patients with seizure disorders, since systemic absorption may precipitate a seizure. Photophobia associated with mydriasis may require patient to wear dark glasses. Since drug causes blurred vision, supervision of activity may be indicated.

VASOCONSTRICTOR; DECONGESTANT Prototype for classification: Naphazoline HCl Use: Ocular vasoconstrictor.

Naphazoloine HCl AK-Con, Albalon, Allerest, Clear Eyes, Comfort, Degest-2, Muro's Opcon, Nafazair, Naphcon, Privine, VasoClear, Vasocon	*Adult:* **Topical** 1–3 drops of 0.1% solution q3–4h prn or 1–2 drops of a 0.01–0.03% solution q4h prn.
Tetrahydrozoline HCl Collyrium, Mallazine, Murine Plus, Optigene, Soothe, Tyzine, Visine	*Adult:* **Topical** 1–2 drops of 0.05% solution in eye b.i.d. or t.i.d.

Contraindicated in: Narrow-angle glaucoma; concomitant use with MAO INHIBITORS or TRICYCLIC ANTIDEPRESSANTS **Cautious use in:** Hypertension, cardiac irregularities, advanced arteriosclerosis; diabetes; hyperthyroidism; elderly patients. **Adverse Effects:** Pupillary dilation, increased intraocular pressure, rebound redness of the eye, headache, hypertension, nausea, weakness, sweating. **Overdosage:** Drowsiness, hypothermia, bradycardia, shocklike hypotension, coma.

CORTICOSTEROID, ANTI-INFLAMMATORY **Prototype for classification: Hydrocortisone** **Use:** Inflammation. **Unlabeled use:** Anterior uveitis.

Dexamethasone sodium phosphate Decadron Phosphate, Maxidex Ophthalmic	*Adult:* **Topical** 1–2 drops in conjunctival sac up to 4–6 times/d; may instill hourly for severe disease.
Fluorometholone Fluor-Op, FML Forte, FML Liquifilm	*Adult and Child >2 y:* **Topical** 1–2 drops of suspension in conjunctival sac q.h. for the first 24–48 h; then b.i.d. to q.i.d.; or a thin strip of ointment q4h for the first 24–48 h; then 1–3 times/d.
Loteprednol etabonate Alrex, Lotemax	*Adult:* **Topical** 1–2 drops in conjunctival sac q.i.d. during initial treatment, may increase to q1h if necessary.
Prednisolone sodium phosphate Inflamase, Inflamase Mild, Pred Mild, Inflamase Forte	*Adult:* **Topical** 1–2 drops in conjunctival sac q.h. during the day; then q2h at night; may decrease to 1 drop t.i.d. or q.i.d.
Rimexolone Vexol	**Postoperative Ocular Inflammation:** *Adult:* **Topical** 1–2 drops q.i.d. beginning 24 h after surgery, continue through first 2 wk postoperatively. **Anterior Uveitis:** *Adult:* **Topical** 1–2 drops in affected eye every hour while awake for first week, then q2h for second week, then taper frequency until uveitis resolves.

Contraindicated in: Ocular fungal diseases, *herpes simplex* keratitis, ocular infections, ocular mycobacterial infections, viral disease of cornea or conjunctiva such as vaccina, varicella. **Adverse Effects: Ocular:** Blurred vision, photophobia, conjunctival edema, corneal edema, erosion, eye discharge, dryness, irritation, pain; prolonged use: glaucoma, ocular hypertension, damage to optic nerve, defects in visual acuity and visual fields, posterior subcapsular cataract formation, secondary ocular infections. **Other:** Headache, taste perversion. **Clinical Implications:** Shake all products well before use.

OCULAR ANTIHISTAMINES **Use:** Relief of signs and symptoms of allergic conjunctivitis.

Azelastine HCl OPTIVAR	*Adult and Child >3 y:* **Topical** 1 drop in affected eye(s) b.i.d.
Cromolyn Sodium Crolom, Opticrom	*Adult:* **Topical** 1–2 drops in each eye 4–6 times/d.
Emedastine difumarate Emadine	*Adult and Child >3 y:* **Topical** 1 drop in affected eye(s) up to q.i.d.
Epinastine hydrochloride Elestat	*Adult and Child >3 y:* **Topical** 1 drop in affected eye(s) up to b.i.d.
Ketotifen fumarate Zaditor	*Adult:* **Topical** 1 drop in affected eye(s) q8–12h.
Levocabastine HCl Livostin	*Adult:* **Topical** 1 drop in affected eye(s) q.i.d., shake well before using.
Lodoxamide Alomide	*Adult and Child >2 mo:* **Topical** 1–2 drop in affected eye(s) q.i.d. for up to 3 mo.
Nedocromil sodium Alocril	*Adult and Child >3 y:* **Topical** 1–2 drops in affected eye(s) b.i.d.
Olopatadine HCl Patanol	*Adult and Child >3 y:* **Topical** 1–2 drops in affected eye(s) b.i.d. at least 6–8 h apart.
Pemirolast potassium Alamast	*Adult:* **Topical** 1–2 drops in affected eye(s) q.i.d.

Adverse Effects: Ocular: Allergic reactions, *burning, stinging,* discharge, dry eyes, eye pain, eyelid disorder, itching keratitis, lacrimation disorder, mydriasis, photophobia, rash. **CNS:** Drowsiness, fatigue, headache. **Other:** Dry mouth, cold syndrome, pharyngitis, rhinitis, sinusitis, taste perversion. **Clinical Implications:** Wait 10 min after instilling **emedastine** before inserting soft contact lenses; do not use **levocabastine, olopatadine** with soft contact lenses.

APPENDIX A-2
LOW MOLECULAR WEIGHT HEPARINS:

ANTICOAGULANT, LOW MOLECULAR WEIGHT HEPARIN Prototype for classification: Enoxaparin **Use:** Prevention and treatment of DVT following hip or knee replacement or abdominal surgery, unstable angina, acute coronary syndromes.

Dalteparin sodium Fragmin	**DVT Prophylaxis, Abdominal Surgery:** *Adult:* **SC** 2500 IU (16 mg) q.d. starting 1–2 h prior to surgery and continuing for 5–10 d postoperatively **DVT Prophylaxis, Total Hip Arthroplasty:** *Adult:* **SC** 2500–5000 IU q.d. starting 1–2 h prior to surgery and continuing for 5–14 d postoperatively **Acute Thromboembolism:** *Adult:* **SC** 120 IU/kg b.i.d. for at least 5 d. **Recurrent Thromboembolism:** *Adult:* **SC** 5000 IU b.i.d. for 3–6 mo. **Unstable angina/non Q-wave MI:** *Adult:* **SC** 120 IU/kg (max 10,000 IU) q12h. **DVT prophylaxis with risk of PE:** *Adult:* **SC** 5000 IU once daily for 12–14 d.
Enoxaparin Lovenox	**Prevention of DVT after Hip or Knee Surgery:** *Adult:* **SC** 30 mg SC b.i.d. for 10–14 d starting 12–24 h post-surgery. **Prevention of DVT after Abdominal Surgery:** *Adult:* **SC** 40 mg q.d. starting 2 h before surgery and continuing for 7–10 d (max 12 d) **Treatment of DVT and Pulmonary Embolus:** *Adult:* **SC** 1 mg/kg b.i.d.; monitor anti-Xa activity to determine appropriate dose. **Acute Coronary Syndrome:** *Adult:* **SC** 1 mg/kg q12h × 2–8 d. Give concurrently with aspirin 100–325 mg/d.
Tinzaparin sodium Innohep	**Treatment of DVT:** *Adult:* **SC** 175 anti-Xa IU/kg q.d. × at least 6 d.

Contraindicated in: Hypersensitivity to ardeparin, other low molecular weight heparins, pork products, or parabens; active major bleeding, thrombocytopenia that is positive for antiplatelet antibodies with ardeparin; uncontrolled hypertension; nursing mothers. **Cautious use in:** Hypersensitivity to heparin; history of heparin-induced thrombocytopenia; bacterial endocarditis; severe and uncontrolled hypertension, cerebral aneurysm or hemorrhagic stroke, bleeding disorders, recent GI bleeding or associated GI disorders (e.g., ulcerative colitis), thrombocytopenia, or platelet disorders; severe liver or renal disease, diabetic retinopathy, hypertensive retinopathy, invasive procedures; pregnancy (category C). **Adverse Effects: Body as a Whole:** Allergic reactions (rash, urticaria), arthralgia, pain and inflammation at injection site, peripheral edema, fever. **CNS:** CVA, dizziness, headache, insomnia. **CV:** Chest pain. **GI:** Nausea, vomiting. **Hematologic:** *Hemorrhage,* thrombocytopenia, ecchymoses, anemia. **Respiratory:** Dyspnea **Skin:** Rash, pruritus. **Drug Interactions:** Aspirin, NSAIDs, **warfarin** can increase risk of hemorrhage **Clinical Implications:** Alternate injection sites using the abdomen, anterior thigh, or outer aspect of upper arms. **Lab tests:** CBC with platelet count, urinalysis, and stool for occult blood should be tested throughout therapy. Routine coagulation tests are not required. Carefully monitor for and immediately report S&S of excessive anticoagulation (e.g., bleeding at venipuncture sites or surgical site) or hemorrhage (e.g., drop in BP or Hct). Patients on oral anticoagulants, platelet inhibitors, or with impaired renal function must be very carefully monitored for hemorrhage. Patient should be sitting or lying supine for injection. Inject deep SC with entire length of needle inserted into skin fold. Hold skin fold gently throughout injection and do not rub site after injection.

APPENDIX A-3
INHALED CORTICOSTEROIDS (ORAL AND NASAL INHALATIONS):

CORTICOSTEROID, ANTI-INFLAMMATORY **Prototype for classification: Hydrocortisone** **Use:** Oral inhalation to treat steroid-dependent asthma, nasal inhalation for the management of the symptoms of seasonal or perennial rhinitis.

Beclomethasone diproprionate Beclovent, Beconase Nasal Inhaler, QVAR, Vancenase Nasal Inhaler, Vanceril, Vanceril D, Vancenase AQ	**Asthma:** *Adult:* **Oral inhaler** 2 inhalations t.i.d. or q.i.d. up to 20 inhalations/d; may try to reduce systemic steroids after 1 wk of concomitant therapy; QVAR 40–80 mcg b.i.d. (max 320 mcg/d). *Child 6–12 y:* **Oral inhaler** 1–2 inhalations t.i.d. or q.i.d. up to 10 inhalations/d; QVAR 5–11 y, 40–80 mcg b.i.d. (max 160 mcg/d). **Allergic Rhinitis:** *Adult:* **Nasal inhaler** 1 spray in each nostril b.i.d. to q.i.d. *Child >6 y:* spray q.d.
Budesonide Pulmicort, Turbuhaler, Pulmicort, Respules, Rhinocort, Rhinocort Aqua, Rhinocort, Turbuhaler	**Asthma, Maintenance Therapy:** *Adult:* **Oral inhalation** 1 or 2 inhalations (200 mcg/inhalation) q.d.–b.i.d. (max 800 mcg b.i.d). *Child ≥6 y:* **Oral inhalation** 1 inhalation (200 mcg/inhalation) q.d.–b.i.d. (max 400 mcg b.i.d.) *Child 12 mo–8 y:* **Nebulization** 0.5 mg/d in 1–2 divided doses. **Rhinitis:** *Adult, Child ≥6 y:* **Intranasal** 2 sprays in each nostril in the morning and evening or 4 sprays in each nostril in the morning. Each actuation releases 32 mg from the nasal adapter.
Dexamethasone Aeroseb-Dex, Decadron, Decaspray	*Adult:* **Oral Inhalation** Up to 3 inhalations t.i.d. or q.i.d. (max 12 inhalations/d). **Intranasal** 2 sprays in each nostril b.i.d. or t.i.d. (max 12 sprays/d) *Child:* **Oral Inhalation** Up to 2 inhalations q.i.d. (max 8 inhalations/d). **Intranasal** 1 or 2 sprays in each nostril b.i.d. (max 8 sprays/d).
Flunisolide AeroBid, Nasalide, Nasarel	**Allergic Rhinitis:** *Adult:* **Inhaled/Intranasal** 2 sprays orally, or intranasally in each nostril, b.i.d.; may increase to t.i.d., if needed. *Child:* **Inhaled/Intranasal** 6–14 y, 1 spray orally, or intranasally in each nostril t.i.d. or 2 sprays b.i.d.
Fluticasone Flonase, Flovent	**Seasonal Allergic Rhinitis:** *Adult:* **Intranasal** 100 mcg (1 inhalation) in each nostril 1–2 times daily (max 4 times daily). **Inhalation** 1–2 inhalations b.i.d. *Child ≥4 y:* **Intranasal** 1 spray in each nostril once daily. May increase to 2 sprays in each nostril once daily if inadequate response, then decrease to 1 spray in each nostril once daily when control is achieved.

Mometasone furoate monohydrate Nasonex	*Adult:* **Intranasal** 2 sprays (50 mcg each) in each nostril once daily. *Child ≥2 y:* **Intranasal** 1 spray in each nostril once daily.
Triamcinolone acetonide Azmacort, Tri-Nasal	*Adult:* **Inhalation** 2 puffs 3–4 times/d (max 16 puffs/d) or 4 puffs b.i.d. **Nasal spray** 2 spray/ nostril once daily (max 8 sprays/d) *Child 6–12 y:* **Inhalation** 1–2 sprays t.i.d. or q.i.d. (max 12 sprays/d) or 2–4 sprays b.i.d.

Contraindicated in: Nonasthmatic bronchitis, primary treatment of status asthmaticus, acute attack of asthma. **Cautious use in:** Patients receiving systemic corticosteroids; use with extreme caution if at all in respiratory tuberculosis, untreated fungal, bacterial, or viral infections, and ocular herpes simplex; nasal inhalation therapy for nasal septal ulcers, nasal trauma, or surgery. **Adverse Effects: Oral inhalation:** *Candidal infection of oropharynx* and occasionally larynx, hoarseness, dry mouth, sore throat, sore mouth. **Nasal (inhaler):** *Transient nasal irritation, burning, sneezing,* epistaxis, bloody mucous, nasopharyngeal itching, dryness, crusting, and ulceration; headache, nausea, vomiting. **Other:** With excessive doses, symptoms of hypercorticism. Increase risk of adverse effects if Advair is used with other long-acting beta-agonists. **Clinical Implications:** Note that oral inhalation and nasal inhalation products are not to be used interchangeably. **Oral inhaler:** Emphasize the following: (1) Shake inhaler well before using. (2) After exhaling fully, place mouthpiece well into mouth with lips closed firmly around it. (3) Inhale slowly through mouth while activating the inhaler. (4) Hold breath 5–10 sec, if possible, then exhale slowly. (5) Wait 1 min between puffs. Clean inhaler daily. Separate parts as directed in package insert, rinse them with warm water, and dry them thoroughly. Rinsing mouth and gargling with warm water after each oral inhalation removes residual medication from oropharyngeal area. Mouth care may also delay or prevent onset of oral dryness, hoarseness, and candidiasis. **Nasal inhaler:** Directions for use of nasal inhaler provided by manufacturer should be carefully reviewed with patient. Emphasize the following points: (1) Gently blow nose to clear nostrils. (2) Shake inhaler well before using. (3) If 2 sprays in each nostril are prescribed, direct one spray toward upper, and the other toward lower part of nostril. (4) Wash cap and plastic nosepiece daily with warm water; dry thoroughly. Inhaled steroids do not provide immediate symptomatic relief and are not prescribed for this purpose.

APPENDIX A-4

TOPICAL CORTICOSTEROIDS:

CORTICOSTEROID, ANTI-INFLAMMATORY **Prototype for classification: Hydrocortisone** **Use:** As a topical corticosteroid, the drug is used for the relief of the inflammatory and pruritic manifestations of corticosteroid-responsive dermatoses.

Hydrocortisone Aeroseb-HC, Alphaderm, Cetacort, Cortaid, Cort-Dome, Cortenema, Cortril, Dermacort, Dermolate, Hydrocortone, Hytone, Proctocort, Rectocort, Synacort Anusol HC, CaldeCort	*Adult:* **Topical** Apply a small amount to the affected area 1–4 times/d. **PR** Insert 1% cream, 10% foam, 10–25 mg suppository, or 100 mg enema nightly.
Hydrocortisone acetate Carmol HC, Colifoam, Cortaid, Cortamed, Cort-Dome, Cortef Acetate, Corticaine, Cortifoam, Cortiment A, Epifoam, Hydrocortone Acetate	
Alclometasone diproprionate Alclovate	*Adult:* **Topical** 0.05% cream or ointment applied sparingly b.i.d. or t.i.d.; may use occlusive dressing for resistant dermatoses.
Amcinonide Cyclocort	*Adult:* **Topical** Apply thin film b.i.d. or t.i.d.
Betamethasone dipropionate Diprolene, Diprolene AF, Diprosone, Maxivate, Alphatrex, Teladar	
Betamethasone valerate Betatrex, Luxiq, Valisone, Psorion, Beta-Val	*Adult:* **Topical** Apply sparingly b.i.d.
Clobetasol propionate Dermovate, Temovate	*Adult:* **Topical** Apply sparingly b.i.d. (max 50 g/wk), or b.i.d. 3d/wk or 1–2 times/wk for up to 6 mo.
Clocortolone pivalate Cloderm	*Adult:* **Topical** Apply thin layer 1–4 times/d.
Desonide DesOwen, Tridesilon	*Adult:* **Topical** Apply thin layer b.i.d. to q.i.d.
Desoximetasone Topicort, Topicort-LP	*Adult:* **Topical** Apply thin layer b.i.d.
Dexamethasone Sodium Phosphate Decaderm	*Adult:* **Topical** Apply thin layer t.i.d. or q.i.d.

Diflorasone diacetate Florone, Florone E, Maxiflor, Psorcon	*Adult:* **Topical** Apply thin layer of ointment 1–3 times/d or cream 2–4 times/d.
Fluocinolone acetonide Fluoderm, Fluolar, Fluonid, Flurosyn, Synalar, Synalar-HP, Synemol	*Adult:* **Topical** Apply thin layer b.i.d. to q.i.d.
Fluocinonide Lidemol, Lidex, Lidex-E, Lyderm, Topsyn	*Adult:* **Topical** Apply thin layer b.i.d. to q.i.d.
Flurandrenolide Cordran, Cordran SP, Drenison	*Adult:* **Topical** Apply thin layer b.i.d. or t.i.d.; apply tape 1–2 times/d at 12 h intervals. *Child:* **Topical** Apply thin layer 1–2 times/d; apply tape once/d.
Fluticasone Cutivate	*Adult, Child >3 mo:* **Topical** Apply a thin film of cream or ointment to affected area once or twice daily.
Halcinonide Halog	*Adult:* **Topical** Apply thin layer b.i.d. or t.i.d. *Child:* **Topical** Apply thin layer once/d.
Mometasone furoate Elocon	*Adult:* **Topical** Apply a thin film of cream or ointment or a few drops of lotion to affected area once/d.
Triamcinolone Aristocort, Atolone, Kenacort, Kenalog, Kenalog-E	*Adult:* **Topical** Apply sparingly b.i.d. or t.i.d.

Contraindicated in: Topical steroids contraindicated in presence of varicella, vaccinia, on surfaces with compromised circulation, and in children <2 y. **Cautious use in:** Children; diabetes mellitus; stromal *herpes simplex;* glaucoma, tuberculosis of eye; osteoporosis; untreated fungal, bacterial, or viral infections **Adverse Effects: Skin:** Skin thinning and atrophy, *acne, impaired wound healing;* petechiae, ecchymosis, easy bruisings; suppression of skin test reaction; hypopigmentation or hyperpigmentation, hirsutism, acneiform eruptions, subcutaneous fat atrophy; allergic dermatitis, urticaria, angioneurotic edema, increased sweating. **Clinical Implications:** Administer retention enema preferably after a bowel movement. The enema should be retained at least 1 h or all night if possible. If an occlusive dressing is to be used, apply medication sparingly, rub until it disappears, and then reapply, leaving a thin coat over lesion. Completely cover area with transparent plastic or other occlusive device or vehicle. Avoid covering a weeping or exudative lesion. Usually, occlusive dressings are not applied to face, scalp, scrotum, axilla, and groin. Inspect skin carefully between applications for ecchymotic, petechial, and purpuric signs, maceration, secondary infection, skin atrophy, striae or milaria; if present, stop medication and notify physician. Warn patient not to self-dose with OTC topical preparations of a corticosteroid more than 7 d. They should not be used for children <2 y. If symptoms do not abate, consult physician. Usually, topical preparations are applied after a shower or bath when skin is damp or wet. Cleansing and application of prescribed preparation should be done with extreme gentleness because of fragility, easy bruisability, and poor-healing skin. Hazard of systemic toxicity is higher in small children because of the greater ratio of skin surface area to body weight. Apply sparingly. Urge patient on long-term therapy with topical corticosterone to check expiration date.

Schedule I

High potential for abuse and of no currently accepted medical use. Examples: heroin, LSD, marijuana, mescaline, peyote. Not obtainable by prescription but may be legally procured for research, study, or instructional use.

Schedule II

High abuse potential and high liability for severe psychological or physical dependence. Prescription required and cannot be renewed.[a] Includes opium derivatives, other opioids, and short-acting barbiturates. Examples: amphetamine, cocaine, meperidine, morphine, secobarbital.

Schedule III

Potential for abuse is less than that for drugs in Schedules I and II. Moderate to low physical dependence and high psychological dependence. Includes certain stimulants and depressants not included in the above schedules and preparations containing limited quantities of certain opioids. Examples: chlorphentermine, glutethimide, mazindol, paregoric, phendimetrazine. Prescription required.[b]

Schedule IV

Lower potential for abuse than Schedule III drugs. Examples: certain psychotropics (tranquilizers), chloral hydrate, chlordiazepoxide, diazepam, meprobamate, phenobarbital. Prescription required.[a]

Schedule V

Abuse potential less than that for Schedule IV drugs. Preparations contain limited quantities of certain narcotic drugs; generally intended for antitussive and antidiarrheal purposes and may be distributed without a prescription provided that:

1. Such distribution is made only by a pharmacist.
2. Not more than 240 mL or not more than 48 solid dosage units of any substance containing opium, nor more than 120 mL or not more than 24 solid dosage units of any other controlled substance may be distributed at retail to the same purchaser in any given 48-hour period without a valid prescription order.
3. The purchaser is at least 18 years old.
4. The pharmacist knows the purchaser or requests suitable identification.
5. The pharmacist keeps an official written record of: name and address of purchaser, name and quantity of controlled substance purchased, date of sale, initials of dispensing pharmacist. This record is to be made available for inspection and copying by U.S. officers authorized by the Attorney General.

6. Other federal, state, or local law does not require a prescription order.

Under jurisdiction of the Federal Controlled Substances Act:
[a]Except when dispensed directly by a practitioner, other than a pharmacist, to an ultimate user, no controlled substance in Schedule II may be dispensed without a *written* prescription, except that in emergency situations such drug may be dispensed upon oral prescription and a written prescription must be obtained within the time frame prescribed by law. No prescription for a controlled substance in Schedule II may be refilled.
[b]Refillable up to 5 times within 6 mo, but only if so indicated by physician.

◆ APPENDIX C FDA PREGNANCY CATEGORIES

The FDA requires that all prescription drugs absorbed systemically or known to be potentially harmful to the fetus be classified according to one of five pregnancy categories (A, B, C, D, X). The identifying letter signifies the level of risk to the fetus and is to appear in the precautions section of the package insert. The categories described by the FDA are as follows:

Category A

Controlled studies in women fail to demonstrate a risk to the fetus in the first trimester (and there is no evidence of risk in later trimesters), and the possibility of fetal harm appears remote.

Category B

Either animal-reproduction studies have not demonstrated a fetal risk but there are no controlled studies in pregnant women, or animal-reproduction studies have shown an adverse effect (other than a decrease in fertility) that was not confirmed in controlled studies in women in the first trimester (and there is no evidence of a risk in later trimesters).

Category C

Either studies in animals have revealed adverse effects on the fetus (teratogenic or embryocidal effects or other) and there are no controlled studies in women, or studies in women and animals are not available. Drugs should be given only if the potential benefit justifies the potential risk to the fetus.

Category D

There is positive evidence of human fetal risk, but the benefits from use in pregnant women may be acceptable despite the risk (e.g., if the drug is needed in a life-threatening situation or for a serious disease for which safer drugs cannot be used or are ineffective). There will be an appropriate statement in the "warnings" section of the labeling.

Category X

Studies in animals or human beings have demonstrated fetal abnormalities or there is evidence of fetal risk based on human experience, or both, and the risk of the use of the drug in pregnant women clearly outweighs any possible benefit. The drug is contraindicated in women who are or may become pregnant. There will be an appropriate statement in the "contraindications" section of the labeling.

◆ APPENDIX D ORAL DOSAGE FORMS THAT SHOULD NOT BE CRUSHED

Some oral dosage forms should not be crushed or chewed. These dosage forms have been specially designed to release the drug slowly over several hours, to protect the drug from the low pH of the stomach, and/or to protect the stomach from the irritating effects of the drug.

Drugs may have an **enteric coating** which is designed to allow the drug to pass through the stomach intact with the drug being released in the intestines. This protects the stomach from the irritating effects of the drug, protects the drug from being destroyed by the acid pH of the stomach, and can delay the onset of action.

Extended-release (slow release, SR) formulations are designed to release the drug over an extended period of time. These formulations can include multiple-layer compressed tablets where drug is released as each layer dissolves, mixed-release pellets that dissolve at different time intervals, and special tablets that are themselves inert but are designed to release drug slowly from the formulation. Some extended-release dosage forms are scored and may be broken in half without affecting the release mechanism but still should not be crushed or chewed. Some mixed-release capsule formulations can be opened and the contents sprinkled on food. However, the pellets should not be crushed or chewed. Some extended-release formulations can be identified by common abbreviations used in their brand names. These abbreviations include: CR (controlled release), CRT (controlled-release tablet), LA (long acting), SR (sustained release), TR (time release), SA (sustained action), and XL or XR (extended release).

Occasionally, drugs should not be crushed because they are oral mucosa irritants, are extremely bitter, or contain dyes that may stain teeth or mucosal tissue.

The table contains a list of drugs found in the Guide that should not be crushed or chewed. A liquid dosage form may be available for many of these drugs. However, the dose or frequency of administration may be different from the slow-release product. Check with your pharmacist for liquid availability and dosing conversions.

	Generic Name	Comments
Accutane	isotretinoin	mucous membrane irritant
Acutrim	phenylpropanolamine	slow release
Adalat CC	nifedipine	slow release
Allerest 12 Hour	chlorpheniramine phenylpropanolamine	slow release
Artane Sequels	trihexyphenidyl	slow release; capsules may be opened and contents taken without chewing or crushing
Azulfidine Entabs	sulfasalazine	enteric coated

	Generic Name	Comments
Bayer Extra Strength Enteric 500	aspirin, enteric coated	enteric coated; slow release
Bayer Low Adult 81 mg	aspirin, enteric coated	enteric coated
Bayer Caplet	aspirin, enteric coated	enteric coated
Biphetamine	amphetamine, dextroamphetamine	slow release
Bisacodyl	bisacodyl	enteric coated
BiscoLax	bisacodyl	enteric coated
Bromfed, Bromfed-PD	brompheniramine, pseudoephedrine	slow release
Calan SR	verapamil	slow release
Cama Arthritis Strength	aspirin, magnesium oxide, aluminum hydroxide	special table formulation
Cardizem, Cardizem CD, Cardizem SR	diltiazem	slow release; capsules may be opened and contents taken without chewing or crushing
Chloral Hydrate	chloral hydrate	liquid-filled capsule
Chlor-Trimeton Repetab	chlorpheniramine	slow release
Choledyl SA	oxtriphylline	slow release
Compazine Spansule	prochlorperazine	slow release; capsules may be opened and contents taken without chewing or crushing
Constant T	theophylline	slow release; capsules may be opened and contents taken without chewing or crushing
Contac	chlorpheniramine, phenylpropanolamine	slow release; capsules may be opened and contents taken without chewing or crushing
Cotazym S	pancrelipase	enteric coated; capsules may be opened and contents taken without chewing or crushing
Covera-HS	verapamil	slow release
Deconamine SR	chlorpheniramine, pseudoephedrine	slow release
Depakene	valproic acid	slow release; mucous membrane irritant
Depakote	valproate disodium	enteric coated

	Generic Name	Comments
Desoxyn Gradumets	methamphetamine	slow release
Dexatrim Max Strength	phenylpropanolamine	slow release
Dexedrine Spansule	dextroamphetamine	slow release
Diamox Sequels	acetazolamide	slow release
Dilacor XR	diltiazem	slow release
Dilatrate-SR	isosorbide dinitrate	slow release
Dimetane Extentab	brompheniramine, phenylephrine	slow release
Disophrol Chronotab	dexbrompheniramine, pseudoephedrine	slow release
Donnatal Extentab	atropine, scopolamine, hyoscyamine, phenobarbital	slow release
Donnazyme	pancreatin, pepsin, bile salts, atropine, scopolamine, hyoscyamine, phenobarbital	slow release
Drixoral	dexbrompheniramine, pseudoephedrine	slow release
Dulcolax	bisacodyl	enteric coated
Easprin	aspirin	enteric coated
Ecotrin	aspirin	enteric coated
E.E.S 400	erythromycin ethylsuccinate	enteric coated
Elixophyllin SR	theophylline	slow release; capsules may be opened and contents taken without chewing or crushing
E-Mycin	erythromycin	enteric coated
Ergostat	ergotamine	sublingual tablet
Eryc	erythromycin	enteric coated; capsules may be opened and contents taken without chewing or crushing
Ery-tab	erythromycin	enteric coated
Erythrocin Stearate	erythromycin	enteric coated
Erythromycin Base	erythromycin	enteric coated
Eskalith CR	lithium	slow release

	Generic Name	Comments
Fedahist Timecaps	chlorpheniramine, pseudoephedrine	slow release
Feldene	piroxicam	mucous membrane irritant
Feosol	ferrous sulfate	enteric coated
Feosol Spansule	ferrous sulfate	slow release; capsules may be opened and contents taken without chewing or crushing
Fergon	ferrous gluconate	slow release; capsules may be opened and contents taken without chewing or crushing
Ferro-Sequels	ferrous fumarate, docusate	slow release
Fero-Gradumet	ferrous sulfate	slow release
Festal II	pancrelipase	enteric coated
Glucotrol XL	glipizide	slow release
Gris-Peg	griseofulvin ultramicrosize	crushing may result in precipitation of drug as larger particles
Ilotycin	erythromycin	enteric coated
Inderal LA	propranolol	slow release
Inderide LA	propranolol, hydrochlorothiazide	slow release
Indocin SR	indomethacin	slow release; capsules may be opened and contents taken without chewing or crushing
Isoptin SR	verapamil	slow release
Isordil Tembid	isosorbide dinitrate	slow release
Iso-Bid	isosorbide dinitrate	slow release
Isosorbide dinitrate SR	isosorbide dinitrate	slow release
Isuprel Glossets	isoproterenol	sublingual
Kaon CL 10	potassium chloride	slow release
Klor-Con	potassium chloride	slow release
Klotrix	potassium chloride	slow release
K-Tab	potassium chloride	slow release
Levsinex Timecaps	hyoscyamine	slow release
Lithobid	lithium	slow release

	Generic Name	Comments
Meprospan	meprobamate	slow release; capsules may be opened and contents taken without chewing or crushing
Mestinon Timespan	pyridostigmine	slow release
Micro K	potassium chloride	slow release
MS Contin	morphine	slow release
Naldecon	phenylephrine, phenylpropanolamine, chlorpheniramine, phenyltoloxamine	slow release
Nico-400	niacin	slow release
Nicobid	niacin	slow release
Nitro Bid	nitroglycerin	slow release; capsules may be opened and contents taken without chewing or crushing
Nitroglyn	nitroglycerin	slow release; capsules may be opened and contents taken without chewing or crushing
Nitrong SR	nitroglycerin	slow release
Nolamine	phenylpropanolamine, chlorpheniramine, phenindamine	slow release
Norflex	orphenadrine	slow release
Norpace CR	disopyramide	slow release
Novafed A	pseudoephedrine, chlorpheniramine	slow release
Oramorph SR	morphine	slow release
Ornade Spansule	phenylpropanolamine, chlorpheniramine	slow release
Pancrease	pancrelipase	enteric coated
Papaverine Sustained Action	papaverine	slow release
Pavabid	papaverine	slow release
Pavabid Plateau	papaverine	slow release; capsules may be opened and contents taken without chewing or crushing
PBZ-SR	tripelennamine hydrochloride	slow release

	Generic Name	Comments
Perdiem	psyllium hydrophilic mucioid	wax coated
Peritrate SA	pentaerythritol tetranitrate	slow release
Permitil Chronotab	fluphenazine	slow release
Phazyme Phazyme 95	simethicone	slow release
Phyllocontin	aminophylline	slow release
Plendil	felodipine	slow release
Polaramine Repetabs	dexchlorpheniramine	slow release
Prevacid	lansoprazole	slow release; capsules may be opened and contents taken without chewing or crushing
Prilosec	omeprazole	slow release
Procainamide HCl SR	procainamide	slow release
Procan SR	procainamide	slow release
Procardia XL	nifedipine	slow release
Pronestyl SR	procainamide	slow release
Proventil Repetabs	albuterol	slow release
Prozac	fluoxetine	slow release; capsules may be opened and contents taken without chewing or crushing
Quibron-T SR	theophylline	slow release
Quinaglute Dura Tabs	quinidine gluconate	slow release
Quinidex Extentabs	quinidine sulfate	slow release
Respid	theophylline	slow release
Ritalin SR	methylphenidate	slow release
Robimycin Robitab	erythromycin	enteric coated
Rondec TR	pseudoephedrine, carbinoxamine	slow release
Roxanol SR	morphine	slow release
Sinemet CR	levodopacarbidopa	slow release; tablet is scored and may be broken in half

	Generic Name	Comments
Slo-Bid Gyrocaps	theophylline	slow release; capsules may be opened and contents taken without chewing or crushing
Slo-Phyllin Gyrocaps	theophylline	slow release; capsules may be opened and contents taken without chewing or crushing
Slow-Fe	ferrous sulfate	slow release
Slow-K	potassium chloride	slow release
Sorbitrate SA	isosorbide dinitrate	slow release
Sudafed 12 hour	pseudoephedrine	slow release
Tavist-D	phenylpropanolamine, clemastine	multiple compressed tablet
Teldrin	chlorpheniramine	slow release; capsules may be opened and contents taken without chewing or crushing
Tepanil Ten-Tab	diethylpropion	slow release
Tessalon Perles	benzonatate	slow release
Theo-24	theophylline	slow release
Theobid Theobid Jr.	theophylline	slow release
Theo-Dur	theophylline	slow release
Theo-Dur Sprinkle	theophylline	slow release; capsules may be opened and contents taken without chewing or crushing
Theolair SR	theophylline	slow release
Thorazine Spansule	chlorpromazine	slow release
Toprol XL	metaprolol	slow release
Trental	pentoxifylline	slow release
Triaminic	phenylpropanolamine, chlorpheniramine	enteric coated
Triaminic 12	phenylpropanolamine, chlorpheniramine	slow release
Triaminic TR	phenylpropanolamine, pyrilamine, pheniramine	multiple compressed tablet
Trilafon Repetabs	perphenazine	slow release
Triptone Caplets	scopolamine	slow release
Uniphyl	theophylline	slow release
Valrelease	diazepam	slow release

	Generic Name	Comments
Verelan	verapamil	slow release; capsules may be opened and contents taken without chewing or crushing
Volmax	albuterol	slow release
Welbutrin SR	bupropion	bupropion
ZORprin	aspirin	slow release

◆ APPENDIX E PRESCRIPTION COMBINATION DRUGS*

Accuretic (ANTIHYPERTENSIVE) *tablet:* 10 mg quinapril/12.5 mg hydrochlorothiazide, 20 mg quinapril/12.5 mg hydrochlorothiazide, 20 mg quinapril/25 mg hydrochlorothiazide.

Activelle (HORMONE REPLACEMENT THERAPY) *tablet:* estradiol 1 mg and norethindrone acetate 0.5 mg.

Advair Diskus (BRONCHODILATOR) *Inhalation powder:* fluticasone propionate 100 mcg/salmeterol 50 mcg; fluticasone propionate 250 mcg/salmeterol 50 mcg.

Advicor (ANTILIPEMIC) *Tablets, sustained release:* niacin 500 mg/lovastatin 20 mg; niacin 750 mg/lovastatin 20 mg; niacin 1000 mg/lovastatin 20 mg.

Aggrenox (ANTIPLATELET) *extended release capsule:* dipyridamole 200 mg/aspirin 25 mg. 1 capsule b.i.d.

Aladrine (ANTIASTHMATIC) *tablet:* ephedrine sulfate 8.1 mg, secobarbital sodium 16.2 mg.

Alazide (DIURETIC) *tablet:* spironolactone 25 mg, hydrochlorothiazide 25 mg.

Aldactazide 25/25 (DIURETIC) *tablet:* spironolactone 25 mg, hydrochlorothiazide 25 mg.

Aldactazide 50/50 (DIURETIC) *tablet:* spironolactone 50 mg, hydrochlorothiazide 50 mg.

Aldoclor-150 (ANTIHYPERTENSIVE) *tablet:* chlorothiazide 150 mg, methyldopa 250 mg.

Aldoclor-250 (ANTIHYPERTENSIVE) *tablet:* chlorothiazide 250 mg, methyldopa 250 mg.

Aldoril-15 (ANTIHYPERTENSIVE) *tablet:* hydrochlorothiazide 15 mg, methyldopa 250 mg.

Aldoril-25 (ANTIHYPERTENSIVE) *tablet:* hydrochlorothiazide 25 mg, methyldopa 250 mg.

Aldoril D30 (ANTIHYPERTENSIVE) *tablet:* hydrochlorothiazide 30 mg, methyldopa 500 mg.

Aldoril D50 (ANTIHYPERTENSIVE) *tablet:* hydrochlorothiazide 50 mg, methyldopa 500 mg.

Amacodone C (NARCOTIC AGONIST ANALGESIC [schedule III]) *tablet:* hydrocodone bitartrate 5 mg, acetaminophen 500 mg.

Amaphen (NONNARCOTIC AGONIST ANALGESIC) *capsule:* acetaminophen 325 mg, caffeine 40 mg, butalbital 50 mg.

Amaphen with Codeine (NARCOTIC AGONIST ANALGESIC [schedule III]) *capsule:* codeine phosphate 30 mg, acetaminophen 325 mg, caffeine 40 mg, butalbital 50 mg.

Ambenyl Cough Syrup (ANTITUSSIVE) *syrup:* bromodiphenhydramine hydrochloride 12.5 mg, codeine phosphate 10 mg, alcohol 5%.

Anexsia 5/500 (NARCOTIC ANALGESIC [schedule III]) hydrocodone 5 mg, acetaminophen 500 mg.

Anexsia 7.5/650 (NARCOTIC ANALGESIC [schedule III]) hydrocodone 7.5 mg, acetaminophen 650 mg.

Anodynos-DHC (NARCOTIC ANALGESIC [schedule III]) hydrocodone 5 mg, acetaminophen 500 mg.

Anoquan (NONNARCOTIC AGONIST ANALGESIC) *capsule:* acetaminophen 325 mg, caffeine 40 mg, butalbital 50 mg.

Antrocol (GASTROINTESTINAL ANTICHOLINERGIC, SEDATIVE) *capsule, tablet:* atropine sulfate 0.195 mg, phenobarbital 16 mg.

Apresazide 25/25 (ANTHIHYPERTENSIVE) *capsule:* hydralazine hydrochloride 25 mg, hydrochlorothiazide 25 mg.

*For a complete list that includes non-prescription drugs, please see our companion website at www.prenhall.com/.

Apresazide 50/50 (ANTIHYPERTENSIVE) *capsule:* hydralazine hydrochloride 50 mg, hydrochlorothiazide 50 mg.

Apresazide 100/50 (ANTIHYPERTENSIVE) *capsule:* hydralazine hydrochloride 100 mg, hydrochlorothiazide 50 mg.

Apresodex (ANTIHYPERTENSIVE) *tablet:* hydralazine hydrochloride 25 mg, hydrochlorothiazide 15 mg.

Apresoline-Esidrex (ANTIHYPERTENSIVE) *tablet:* hydralazine hydrochloride 25 mg, hydrochlorothiazide 15 mg.

Aprozide 25/25 (ANTIHYPERTENSIVE) hydralazine 25 mg, hydrochlorothiazide 25 mg.

Aprozide 50/50 (ANTIHYPERTENSIVE) hydralazine 50 mg, hydrochlorothiazide 50 mg.

Aprozide 100/50 (ANTIHYPERTENSIVE) hydralazine 100 mg, hydrochlorothiazide 50 mg.

Aralen Phosphate with Primaquine Phosphate (ANTIMALARIAL) *tablet:* chloroquine phosphate 500 mg (300 mg base), primaquine phosphate 79 mg (45 mg base).

Arthrotec 50 (NSAID) *tablet:* diclofenac sodium 50 mg, misoprostol 200 μg.

Arthrotec 75 (NSAID) *tablet:* diclofenac sodium 75 mg, misoprostol 200 μg.

Atacand HCT (ANTIHYPERTENSIVE) *tablet:* candesartan 32 mg/hydrochlorothiazide 12.5 mg; candesartan 16 mg/hydrochlorothiazide 12.5 mg

Auralgan Otic (OTIC PREPARATION: DECONGESTANT, ANALGESIC) *solution:* benzocaine 1.4%, antipyrine 5.4%, glycerin, oxyquinoline sulfate.

Avalide (ANTIHYPERTENSIVE) *tablet:* irbesartan 150 mg/hydrochlorothiazide 12.5 mg; irbesartan 300 mg/hydrochlorothiazide 12.5 mg.

Avandamet (HYPOGLYCEMIC AGENT) *tablet:* 1 mg rosiglitazone maleate/500 mg metformin HCl; 2 mg rosiglitazone/500 mg metformin; 4 mg rosiglitazone/500 mg metformin; 2 mg rosiglitazone/1000 mg metformin; 4 mg rosiglitazone/1000 mg metformin

Axotal (NONNARCOTIC AGONIST ANALGESIC) *tablet:* aspirin 650 mg, butalbital 50 mg.

Azdone (NARCOTIC AGONIST ANALGESIC [schedule III]) *tablet:* hydrocodone bitartrate 5 mg, aspirin 500 mg.

Azo Gantanol (URINARY ANTIINFECTIVE, ANALGESIC) *tablet:* sulfamethoxazole 500 mg, phenazopyridine hydrochloride 100 mg.

Azo Gantrisin (URINARY ANTIINFECTIVE, ANALGESIC) *tablet:* sulfisoxazole 500 mg, phenazopyridine hydrochloride 50 mg.

B-A-C (ANALGESIC) acetaminophen 650 mg, caffeine 40 mg, butalbital 50 mg.

Bacticort Ophthalmic (ANTIINFLAMMATORY) *suspension:* hydrocortisone 1%, neomycin sulfate 0.35%, polymyxin B 10,000 units.

Bancap (NONNARCOTIC AGONIST ANALGESIC) *capsule:* acetaminophen 325 mg, butalbital 50 mg.

Bancap HC (NARCOTIC AGONIST ANALGESIC [schedule III]) *capsule:* hydrocodone bitartrate 5 mg, acetaminophen 500 mg.

Barbidonna Elixir (GASTROINTESTINAL ANTICHOLINERGIC, SEDATIVE) *syrup:* atropine sulfate 0.034 mg, scopolamine hydrobromide 0.01 mg, hyoscyamine hydrobromide or sulfate 0.174 mg, phenobarbital 21.6 mg per 5 mL, alcohol 15%.

Barbidonna Tablets (GASTROINTESTINAL ANTICHOLINERGIC, SEDATIVE) *tablet:* atropine sulfate 0.025 mg, scopolamine hydrobromide 0.0074 mg, hyoscyamine hydrobromide or sulfate 0.1286 mg, phenobarbital 16 mg/tablet.

Barbidonna #2 Tablets (GASTROINTESTINAL ANTICHOLINERGIC, SEDATIVE) *tablet:* atropine sulfate 0.025 mg, scopolamine hydrobromide 0.0074 mg, hyoscyamine hydrobromide or sulfate 0.1286 mg, phenobarbital 32 mg/tablet.

Bellafoline (GASTROINTESTINAL ANTICHOLINERGIC, SEDATIVE) *tablet:* levorotatory alkaloids of belladonna 0.25 mg; *injection:* levorotatory alkaloids of belladonna 0.5 mg/mL.

Bellergal-S (GASTROINTESTINAL ANTICHOLINERGIC, SEDATIVE) *tablet:* l-alkaloids of belladonna 0.2 mg, phenobarbital 40 mg, ergotamine tartrate 0.6 mg, *tartrazine.*

Benicar HCT (ANTIHYPERTENSIVE) *tablet:* 20 mg olmesartan medoxomil/12.5 mg hydrochlorothiazide; 40 mg olmesartan medoxomil/ 12.5 mg hydrochlorothiazide; 40 mg olmesartan medoxomil/25 mg hydrochlorothiazide

Betoptic Pilo Suspension (ANTIGLAUCOMA) Betaxolol 0.25%, pilocarpine 1.75%.

Biphetamine 12 1/2 (AMPHETAMINE [schedule II]) *capsule:* dextroamphetamine 6.25 mg, amphetamine 6.25 mg.

Biphetamine 20 (AMPHETAMINE [schedule II]) *capsule:* dextroamphetamine 10 mg, amphetamine 10 mg.

Blephamide (OPHTHALMIC STEROID, SULFONAMIDE) *suspension:* prednisolone acetate 0.2%, sodium sulfacetamide 10%, EDTA, polyvinyl alcohol 1.4%, polysorbate 80, sodium thiosulfate, benzalkonium chloride.

Blephamide S.O.P. (OPHTHALMIC STEROID, SULFONAMIDE) *ointment:* prednisolone acetate 0.2%, sodium sulfacetamide 10%, phenylmercuric acetate, mineral oil, white petrolatum, nonionic lanolin derivatives.

Brevicon (MONOPHASIC ORAL CONTRACEPTIVE [ESTROGEN, PROGESTIN]) *tablet:* estrogen: ethinyl estradiol 35 μg; progestin: norethindrone 0.5 mg.

Bromfed (DECONGESTANT, ANTIHISTAMINE) *sustained-released capsule:* pseudoephedrine hydrochloride 120 mg, brompheniramine maleate 12 mg.

Bromfed-PD (DECONGESTANT, ANTIHISTAMINE) *sustained-release capsule:* pseudoephedrine hydrochloride 60 mg, brompheniramine maleate 6 mg.

Bronchial Capsules (ANTIASTHMATIC) *capsule:* theophylline 150 mg, guaifenesin 90 mg/capsule.

Brondecon (ANTIASTHMATIC) *tablet:* oxtriphylline 200 mg, guaifenesin 100 mg, saccharin.

Butace (ANALGESIC) acetaminophen 325 mg, caffeine 40 mg, butalbital 50 mg.

Butibel (GASTROINTESTINAL ANTICHOLINERGIC, SEDATIVE) *elixir:* belladonna extract 15 mg, butabarbital sodium 15 mg, alcohol 7% per 5 mL; *tartrazine; tablet:* belladonna extract 15 mg, butabarbital sodium 15 mg.

Caduet (ANTIHYPERTENSIVE/ANTILIPEMIC) *tablet:* 5 mg amlodipine, 10 mg atorvastatin; 10 mg amlodipine, 10 mg atorvastatin; 5 mg amlodipine, 20 mg atorvastatin; 10 mg amlodipine, 20 mg atorvastatin; 5 mg amlodipine, 40 mg atorvastatin; 10 mg amlodipine, 40 mg atorvastatin; 5 mg amlodipine, 80 mg atorvastatin; 10 mg amlodipine, 80 mg atorvastatin.

Cafergot Suppositories (ANTIMIGRAINE) *suppository:* ergotamine tartrate 2 mg, caffeine 100 mg/ suppository.

Cafergot P-B Suppositories (ANTIMIGRAINE) *suppository:* ergotamine tartrate 2 mg, caffeine 100 mg, l-alkaloids of belladonna 0.25 mg, pentobarbital 60 mg/suppository.

Calcidrine Syrup (ANTITUSSIVE [schedule V]) *syrup:* codeine 8.4 mg, calcium iodide 152 mg, alcohol 6%.

Cam-ap-es (ANTIHYPERTENSIVE) *suspension, tablet:* hydrochlorothiazide 15 mg, reserpine 0.1 mg, hydralazine hydrochloride 25 mg.

Capital with Codeine (NARCOTIC ANALGESIC [schedule V]) *suspension:* codeine phosphate 12 mg, acetaminophen 120 mg/5 mL.

Capozide 25/15 (ANTIHYPERTENSIVE) *tablet:* captopril 25 mg, hydrochlorothiazide 15 mg.

Capozide 25/25 (ANTIHYPERTENSIVE) *tablet:* captopril 25 mg, hydrochlorothiazide 25 mg.

Capozide 50/15 (ANTIHYPERTENSIVE) *tablet:* captopril 50 mg, hydrochlorothiazide 15 mg.

Capozide 50/25 (ANTIHYPERTENSIVE) *tablet:* captopril 50 mg, hydrochlorothiazide 25 mg.

Carisoprodol Compound (SKELETAL MUSCLE RELAXANT, ANALGESIC) *tablet:* carisoprodol 200 mg, aspirin 325 mg.

Carmol HC (ANTIINFLAMMATORY) *cream:* hydrocortisone acetate 1%, urea 10%.

Celestone-Soluspan (GLUCOCORTICOID) *injection (suspension):* betamethasone acetate 3 mg, betamethasone sodium phosphate 3 mg/mL.

Cetacaine (TOPICAL ANESTHETIC) *gel, liquid, ointment, aerosol:* benzocaine 14%, tetracaine hydrochloride 2%, butamben 2%, benzalkonium chloride 0.5% with cetyldimethylethylammonium bromide.

Cetapred (STEROID, SULFONAMIDE) *ophthalmic ointment:* prednisolone acetate 0.25%, sodium sulfacetamide 10%, mineral oil, white petrolatum, liquid lanolin, parabens.

Chardonna-2 (GASTROINTESTINAL ANTICHOLINERGIC, SEDATIVE) *tablet:* belladonna extract 15 mg, phenobarbital 15 mg.

Cheracol Syrup (NARCOTIC ANTITUSSIVE, EXPECTORANT [schedule V]) *syrup:* codeine phosphate 10 mg, guaifenesin 100 mg/5 mL, alcohol 4.75%.

Chloromycetin Hydrocortisone (OPHTHALMIC STEROID, ANTIBIOTIC) *solution:* hydrocortisone acetate 8.5%, chloramphenicol 0.25%, cholesterol, methylcellulose, benzethonium chloride 0.01%.

Chloroserpine (ANTIHYPERTENSIVE) chlorothiazide 500 mg, reserpine 0.125 mg.

Chlorzoxazone with APAP (SKELETAL MUSCLE RELAXANT, ANALGESIC) *tablet:* chlorzoxazone 250 mg, acetaminophen 300 mg.

Ciprodex Otic (ANTIINFECTIVE/ANTIINFLAMMATORY) *topical:* ciprofloxacin 0.3%/dexamethasone 0.1% otic suspension

Claritin D (ANTIHISTAMINE, DECONGESTANT) loratidine, 5 mg, pseudoephedrine 120 mg, loratidine 10 mg, pseudoephedrine 240 mg.

Climara Pro (HORMONE REPLACEMENT THERAPY) *transdermal patch:* estradiol 0.045 mg/levonorgestrel acetate 0.015 mg.

Clindex (ANTISPASMODIC) clidinium 2.5 mg, chlordiazepoxide 5 mg.

Clinoxide (ANTISPASMODIC) clidinium 2.5 mg, chlordiazepoxide 5 mg.

Clipoxide (ANTISPASMODIC) clidinium 2.5 mg, chlordiazepoxide 5 mg.

Codamine Syrup (ANTITUSSIVE [schedule III]) *syrup:* phenylpropanolamine 25 mg, hydrocodone 5 mg.

Codiclear DH Syrup (ANTITUSSIVE [schedule III]) *syrup:* hydrocodone 5 mg, guaifenesin 100 mg, alcohol 10%.

Codimal DH (ANTITUSSIVE [schedule III]) *syrup:* phenylephrine hydrochloride 5 mg, pyrilamine maleate 8.33 mg, hydrocodone bitartrate 1.66 mg/5 mL.

Codimal LA (ANTIHISTAMINE, DECONGESTANT) pseudoephedrine 120 mg, chlorpheniramine 8 mg.

Co-Gesic (NARCOTIC ANALGESIC [schedule III]) hydrocodone 5 mg, acetaminophen 500 mg.

Colabid (ANTIGOUT) probenecid 500 mg, colchicine 0.5 mg.

ColBenemid (ANTIGOUT) *tablet:* probenecid 500 mg, colchicine 0.5 mg.

Col-Probenecid (ANTIGOUT) *tablet:* probenecid 500 mg, colchicine 0.5 mg.

Coly-Mycin S Otic (OTIC: STEROID, ANTIBIOTIC) *suspension:* hydrocortisone acetate 1%, neomycin sulfate 3.3 mg, colistin sulfate 3 mg, thonzonium bromide 0.05%/mL, polysorbate 80, acetic acid, sodium acetate, thimerosal.

Combipatch (HORMONE REPLACEMENT THERAPY) *transdermal patch:* estradiol 0.05 mg/norethindrone acetate 0.14 mg; estradiol 0.25 mg/norethindrone acetate 0.14 mg

Combipres 0.1 (ANTIHYPERTENSIVE) *tablet:* chlorthalidone 15 mg, clonidine hydrochloride 0.1 mg.

Combipres 0.2 (ANTIHYPERTENSIVE) *tablet:* chlorthalidone 15 mg, clonidine hydrochloride 0.2 mg.

Combipres 0.3 (ANTIHYPERTENSIVE) *tablet:* chlorthalidone 15 mg, clonidine hydrochloride 0.3 mg.

Combivir (ANTIVIRAL) zidovudine 300 mg, lamivudine 150 mg.

Condrin-LA (DECONGESTANT, ANTIHISTAMINE) *capsule:* phenylpropanolamine hydrochloride 75 mg, chlorpheniramine maleate 12 mg.

Cordran-N (CORTICOSTEROID, ANTIBIOTIC) *cream, ointment:* neomycin sulfate 0.5%, flurandrenolide 0.05%.

Cortisporin (OPHTHALMIC STEROID, ANTIBIOTIC) *suspension:* hydrocortisone 1%, neomycin sulfate equivalent to 0.35% neomycin base, polymyxin B sulfate 10,000 units/mL, thimerosal cetyl alcohol 0.001%, glyceryl monostearate, polyoxyl 40 stearate, propylene glycol, mineral oil.

Cortisporin Ointment (OPHTHALMIC STEROID, ANTIBIOTIC) *ointment:* hydrocortisone 1%, neomycin sulfate equivalent to 0.35% neomycin base, bacitracin zinc 400 units, polymyxin B sulfate 10,000 units/g, white petrolatum.

Corzide 40/5 (ANTIHYPERTENSIVE) *tablet:* nadolol 40 mg, bendroflumethiazide 5 mg.

Corzide 80/5 (ANTIHYPERTENSIVE) *tablet:* nadolol 80 mg, bendroflumethiazide 5 mg.

Cosopt (OPHTHALMIC, GLAUCOMA) dorzolamide, timolol.

Cotrim (ANTIINFECTIVE) *tablet:* trimethoprim 80 mg, sulfamethoxazole 400 mg.

Cotrim DS (Double Strength) (ANTIINFECTIVE) *tablet:* trimethoprim 160 mg, sulfamethoxazole 800 mg.

Cotrim Pediatric (ANTIINFECTIVE) *suspension:* trimethoprim 40 mg, sulfamethoxazole 200 mg/5 mL.

Cyclomydril (OPHTHALMIC DECONGESTANT) *ophthalmic solution:* cyclopentolate hydrochloride 0.2%, phenylephrine hydrochloride 0.1%.

Damason-P (NARCOTIC ANALGESIC [schedule III]) hydrocodone 5 mg, aspirin 224 mg, caffeine 32 mg.

Darvocet-A 500 (NARCOTIC AGONIST ANALGESIC [schedule IV]) *tablet:* propoxyphene napsylate 100 mg, acetaminophen 500 mg.

Darvocet-N 50 (NARCOTIC AGONIST ANALGESIC [schedule IV]) *tablet:* propoxyphene napsylate 50 mg, acetaminophen 325 mg.

Darvocet-N 100 (NARCOTIC AGONIST ANALGESIC [schedule IV]) *tablet:* propoxyphene napsylate 100 mg, acetaminophen 650 mg.

Darvon Compound-65 (NARCOTIC AGONIST ANALGESIC [schedule IV]) *pulvule (capsule):* propoxyphene hydrochloride 65 mg, aspirin 389 mg, caffeine 32.4 mg.

Decadron with Xylocaine (GLUCOCORTICOID) *injection:* dexamethasone sodium phosphate 4 mg, lidocaine hydrochloride 10 mg/mL, EDTA, parabens, sodium bisulfite.

Deconamine (DECONGESTANT, ANTIHISTAMINE) *syrup:* pseudoephedrine hydrochloride 30 mg, chlorpheniramine maleate 2 mg/5 mL, sorbitol; *tablet:* pseudoephedrine hydrochloride 60 mg, chlorpheniramine maleate 4 mg.

Demerol APAP (NARCOTIC AGONIST ANALGESIC [schedule II]) *tablet:* meperidine hydrochloride 50 mg, acetaminophen 300 mg.

Demi-Regroton (ANTIHYPERTENSIVE) *injection:* chlorthalidone 25 mg, reserpine 0.125 mg.

Demulen 1/50 (ORAL CONTRACEPTIVE) ethinyl estradiol 50 μg, norethindrone 1 mg.

Depo-Testadiol (ESTROGEN, ANDROGEN) *injection:* estradiol cypionate 2 mg, testosterone cypionate 50 mg/mL, chlorobutanol in cottonseed oil.

Deprol (PSYCHOTHERAPEUTIC [schedule IV]) *tablet:* meprobamate 400 mg, benactyzine hydrochloride 1 mg, *tartrazine.*

Dilantin with Phenobarbital (ANTICONVULSANT) *capsule:* phenytoin 100 mg, phenobarbital 16 or 32 mg.

Dilaudid Cough Syrup (NARCOTIC ANTITUSSIVE [schedule II]) *syrup:* hydromorphone 1 mg, guaifenesin 100 mg, alcohol 5%.

Dilor G (ANTIASTHMATIC) *tablet:* dyphylline 200 mg, guaifenesin 200 mg; *liquid:* dyphylline 100 mg, guaifenesin 100 mg/5 mL, saccharin, sorbitol.

Diupres 250 (ANTIHYPERTENSIVE) *tablet:* chlorothiazide 250 mg, reserpine 0.125 mg.

Diupres 500 (ANTIHYPERTENSIVE) *tablet:* chlorothiazide 500 mg, reserpine 0.125 mg.

Diurese-R (ANTIHYPERTENSIVE) *tablet:* trichlormethiazide 4 mg, reserpine 0.1 mg.

Diurigen with Reserpine (ANTIHYPERTENSIVE) chlorothiazide 250 mg, reserpine 0.125 mg.

Diutensin-R (ANTIHYPERTENSIVE) *tablet:* methyclothiazide 2.5 mg, reserpine 0.1 mg.

Dolacet (NARCOTIC AGONIST ANALGESIC [schedule III]) *capsule:* hydrocodone bitartrate 5 mg, acetaminophen 500 mg.

Dolene AP-65 (NARCOTIC AGONIST ANALGESIC [schedule IV]) *tablet:* propoxyphene hydrochloride 65 mg, acetaminophen 650 mg.

Dolene Compound-65 (NARCOTIC AGONIST ANALGESIC [schedule IV]) *capsule:* propoxyphene hydrochloride 65 mg, aspirin 389 mg, caffeine 32.4 mg.

Donnagel-PG (ANTIDIARRHEAL [schedule V]) *suspension:* powdered opium 24 mg, kaolin 6 g, pectin 142.8 mg, hyoscyamine sulfate 0.1037 mg, atropine sulfate 0.0194 mg, scopolamine hydrobromide 0.0065 mg/30 mL, alcohol 5%.

Donnatal (GASTROINTESTINAL ANTICHOLINERGIC, SEDATIVE) *capsule, tablet, elixir:* atropine sulfate 0.0194 mg, scopolamine hydrobromide 0.0065 mg, hyoscyamine hydrobromide or sulfate 0.1037 mg, phenobarbital 16.2 mg; the elixir contains alcohol 23%/5 mL.

Donnatal Extentab (GASTROINTESTINAL ANTICHOLINERGIC, SEDATIVE) *tablet:* atropine sulfate 0.0582 mg, scopolamine hydrobromide 0.0195 mg, hyoscyamine sulfate 0.3111 mg, phenobarbital 48.6 mg.

Donnatal No. 2 (GASTROINTESTINAL ANTICHOLINERGIC, SEDATIVE) *tablet:* atropine sulfate 0.0194 mg, scopolamine hydrobromide 0.0065 mg, hyoscyamine hydrobromide or sulfate 0.1037 mg, phenobarbital 32.4 mg.

Donnazyme (DIGESTIVE AID) *elixir:* pancreatin 300 mg, pepsin 150 mg, bile salts 150 mg, hyoscyamine sulfate 0.0518 mg, atropine sulfate 0.0097 mg, scopolamine hydrobromide 0.0033 mg, phenobarbital 8.1 mg.

Drize (DECONGESTANT, ANTIHISTAMINE) *capsule:* phenylpropanolamine hydrochloride 75 mg, chlorpheniramine maleate 12 mg.

Duac (ANTIACNE) *gel:* clindamycin 1%/benzoyl peroxide 5%

Duo-Medihaler (BRONCHODILATOR [ADRENERGIC]) *aerosol:* each valve actuation delivers isoproterenol hydrochloride 0.16 mg, phenylephrine bitartrate 0.24 mg.

DuoNeb (BETA-AGONIST/ANTICHOLINERGIC BRONCHODILATOR) *inhalation solution:* 3 mg albuterol sulfate/0.5 mg ipratropium bromide per 3 mL

Duradyne DHC (NARCOTIC AGONIST ANALGESIC [schedule III]) *tablet:* hydrocodone bitartrate 5 mg, acetaminophen 500 mg.

Dyazide (DIURETIC) *capsule:* triamterene 37.5 mg, hydrochlorothiazide 25 mg.

Dyflex-G (ANTIASTHMATIC) *tablet:* dyphylline 200 mg, guaifenesin 200 mg.

Dyline-GG (ANTIASTHMATIC) *tablet:* dyphylline 200 mg, guaifenesin 200 mg.

Elase (TOPICAL ENZYME) *ointment:* fibrinolysin 1 unit, desoxyribonuclease (from bovine pancreas) 666.6 units/g in a liquid petrolatum and polyethylene base.

Elase-Chloromycetin (TOPICAL ENZYME) *ointment:* chloramphenicol 10 mg, fibrinolysin 1 unit, desoxyribonuclease (from bovine pancreas) 666.6 units/g in a liquid petrolatum and polyethylene base.

Elixophyllin-GG (ANTIASTHMATIC) theophylline 100 mg, guaifenesin 100 mg.

Empirin with Codeine No. 2 (NARCOTIC AGONIST ANALGESIC [schedule III]) *tablet:* codeine phosphate 15 mg, aspirin 325 mg.

Empirin with Codeine No. 3 (NARCOTIC AGONIST ANALGESIC [schedule III]) *tablet:* codeine phosphate 30 mg, aspirin 325 mg.

Empirin with Codeine No. 4 (NARCOTIC AGONIST ANALGESIC [schedule III]) *tablet:* codeine phosphate 60 mg, aspirin 325 mg.

Endolor (ANALGESIC) acetaminophen 325 mg, caffeine 40 mg, butalbital 50 mg.

Enduronyl (ANTIHYPERTENSIVE) *tablet:* methyclothiazide 5 mg, deserpidine 0.25 mg; inactive ingredients: corn starch D&C Yellow No. 10, FD&C Yellow No. 6, lactose, magnesium, stearate, talc, others.

Enduronyl Forte (ANTIHYPERTENSIVE) *tablet:* methyclothiazide 5 mg, deserpidine 0.5 mg; inactive ingredients: corn starch, iron oxide, lactose, magnesium, stearate, talc, others.

Entozyme (DIGESTIVE AID) *tablet:* pepsin 250 mg in outer core, pancreatin 300 mg and bile salts 150 mg in enteric-coated inner core.

E-Pilo-1 (ANTIGLAUCOMA) pilocarpine 1%, epinephrine bitartrate 1%.

E-Pilo-2 (ANTIGLAUCOMA) pilocarpine 2%, epinephrine bitartrate 1%.

E-Pilo-3 (ANTIGLAUCOMA) pilocarpine 3%, epinephrine bitartrate 1%.

E-Pilo-4 (ANTIGLAUCOMA) pilocarpine 4%, epinephrine bitartrate 1%.

E-Pilo-6 (ANTIGLAUCOMA) pilocarpine 6%, epinephrine bitartrate 1%.

Epzicom (ANTIRETROVIRAL AGENT) *tablet:* abacavir 600 mg, lamivudine 300 mg. Dosed once daily.

Equagesic (NARCOTIC AGONIST ANALGESIC [schedule IV]) *tablet:* aspirin 325 mg, meprobamate 200 mg.

Equazine-M (ANALGESIC) aspirin 325 mg, meprobamate 200 mg.

Ergo Caff (ANTIMIGRAINE) *tablet:* ergotamine tartrate 1 mg, caffeine 100 mg.

Esgic (NONNARCOTIC AGONIST ANALGESIC) *capsule, tablet:* acetaminophen 325 mg, caffeine 40 mg, butalbital 50 mg.

Esimil (ANTIHYPERTENSIVE) *tablet:* hydrochlorothiazide 25 mg, guanethidine monosulfate 10 mg.

Estratest (ESTROGEN, ANDROGEN) *tablet:* esterified estrogens 1.25 mg, methyltestosterone 2.5 mg.

Estratest H.S. (ESTROGEN, ANDROGEN) *tablet:* esterified estrogens 0.625 mg, methyltestosterone 1.25 mg.

Etrafon (PSYCHOTHERAPEUTIC) *tablet:* perphenazine 2 mg, amitriptyline 25 mg; sugar coated.

Etrafon-A (PSYCHOTHERAPEUTIC) *tablet:* perphenazine 4 mg, amitriptyline 10 mg; sugar coated.

Etrafon-Forte (PSYCHOTHERAPEUTIC) *tablet:* perphenazine 4 mg, amitriptyline 25 mg; sugar coated.

Etrafon 2–10 (PSYCHOTHERAPEUTIC) *tablet:* perphenazine 2 mg, amitriptyline 10 mg; sugar coated.

Fedahist (DECONGESTANT, ANTIHISTAMINE) *tablet:* pseudoephedrine hydrochloride 60 mg, chlorpheniramine maleate 4 mg.

Femcet (ANALGESIC) acetaminophen 325 mg, caffeine 40 mg, butalbital 50 mg.

Fergon Plus (IRON SUPPLEMENT) ferrous gluconate 58 mg, ascorbic acid 75 mg.

Fioricet (NONNARCOTIC AGONIST ANALGESIC) *tablet:* acetaminophen 325 mg, butalbital 50 mg, caffeine 40 mg.

Fiorinal (NONNARCOTIC AGONIST ANALGESIC [schedule III]) *capsule, tablet:* aspirin 325 mg, butalbital 50 mg, caffeine 40 mg.

Fiorinal with Codeine No. 1 (NARCOTIC AGONIST ANALGESIC [schedule III]) *capsule:* codeine phosphate 7.5 mg, aspirin 325 mg, caffeine 40 mg, butalbital 50 mg.

Fiorinal with Codeine No. 2 (NARCOTIC AGONIST ANALGESIC [schedule III]) *capsule:* codeine phosphate 15 mg, aspirin 325 mg, caffeine 40 mg, butalbital 50 mg.

Fiorinal with Codeine No. 3 (NARCOTIC AGONIST ANALGESIC [schedule III]) *capsule* codeine phosphate 30 mg, aspirin 325 mg, caffeine 40 mg, butalbital 50 mg.

Flexaphen (SKELETAL MUSCLE RELAXANT) *capsule:* chlorzoxazone 250 mg, acetaminophen 300 mg.

Fluress (OPHTHALMIC ANESTHETIC) *ophthalmic solution:* benoxinate hydrochloride 0.4%, fluorescein sodium with providone 0.25%, chlorobutanol 1%.

Genora 0.5/35 (ORAL CONTRACEPTIVE) ethinyl estradiol 35 μg, norethindrone 0.5 mg

Genora 1/35 (ORAL CONTRACEPTIVE) ethinyl estradiol 35 μg, norethindrone 1 mg.

Genora 1/50 (ORAL CONTRACEPTIVE) mestranol 50 μg, norethindrone 1 mg.

Glucovance (ANTIDIABETIC) *tablet:* glyburide 1.25 mg/metformin 250 mg; glyburide 2.5 mg/metformin 500 mg; glyburide 5 mg/metformin 500 mg.

Glyceryl-T (ANTIASTHMATIC) *capsule, liquid (per 5 mL):* theophylline 150 mg, guaifenesin 90 mg.

Granulex (TOPICAL ENZMYE) *aerosol:* trypsin 0.1 mg, balsam Peru 72.5 mg, castor oil 650 mg/0.82 mL.

Helidac (ANTIULCER, ANTIINFECTIVE) *tablet:* bismuth subsalicylate 262.4 mg, metronidazole 250 mg, tetracycline 500 mg.

Hexalol (URINARY ANTIINFECTIVE) *tablet:* methenamine 40.8 mg, phenyl salicylate 18.1 mg, atropine sulfate 0.03 mg, hyoscyamine 0.03 mg, benzoic acid 4.5 mg, methylene blue 5.4 mg.

Hycodan (ANTITUSSIVE [schedule III]) *tablet:* hydrocodone bitartrate 5 mg, homatropine methylbromide 1.5 mg.

Hycomine Compound (ANTITUSSIVE [schedule III]) *tablet:* phenylephrine hydrochloride 10 mg, chlorpheniramine maleate 2 mg, hydrocodone bitartrate 5 mg, acetaminophen 250 mg, caffeine 30 mg.

Hycomine Pediatric (ANTITUSSIVE [schedule III]) *syrup:* phenylpropanolamine hydrochloride 12.5 mg, hydrocodone bitartrate 2.5 mg/5 mL, saccharin, sorbitol.

Hycomine Syrup (ANTITUSSIVE [schedule III]) *syrup:* phenylpropanolamine hydrochloride 25 mg, hydrocodone bitartrate 5 mg/5 mL.

Hycotuss Expectorant (ANTITUSSIVE [schedule III]) guaifenesin 100 mg, hydrocodone 5 mg.

Hydrazide 25/25 (ANTIHYPERTENSIVE) hydralazine 25 mg, hydrochlorothiazide 25 mg.

Hydrazide 50/50 (ANTIHYPERTENSIVE) hydralazine 50 mg, hydrochlorothiazide 50 mg.

Hydrocet (NARCOTIC ANALGESIC [schedule III]) hydrocodone 5 mg, acetaminophen 500 mg.

Hydrogesic (NARCOTIC ANALGESIC [schedule III]) hydrocodone 5 mg, acetaminophen 500 mg.

Hydromox R (ANTIHYPERTENSIVE) *tablet:* quinethazone 50 mg, reserpine 0.125 mg.

Hydrophed (ANTIASTHMATIC) *tablet:* theophylline 130 mg, ephedrine sulfate 25 mg, hydroxyzine hydrochloride 10 mg.

Hydropres 25 (ANTIHYPERTENSIVE) *tablet:* hydrochlorothiazide 25 mg, reserpine 0.125 mg.

Hydropres 50 (ANTIHYPERTENSIVE) *tablet:* hydrochlorothiazide 50 mg, reserpine 0.125 mg.

Hydro-Serp (ANTIHYPERTENSIVE) *tablet:* hydrochlorothiazide 50 mg, reserpine 0.125 mg.

Hydroserpine (ANTIHYPERTENSIVE) *tablet:* hydrochlorothiazide 50 mg, reserpine 0.125 mg.

Hydrosine 25 (ANTIHYPERTENSIVE) hydrochlorothiazide 25 mg, reserpine 0.125 mg.

Hydrosine 50 (ANTIHYPERTENSIVE) hydrochlorothiazide 50 mg, reserpine 0.125 mg.

Hyzaar (ANTIHYPERTENSIVE) losartan 50 mg, hydrochlorothiazide 12.5 mg.

Ilopan-Choline (GI STIMULANT) *tablet:* dexpanthenol 50 mg, choline bitartrate 25 mg.

Inderide 40/25 (ANTIHYPERTENSIVE) *tablet:* propranolol hydrochloride 40 mg, hydrochlorothiazide 25 mg.

Inderide 80/25 (ANTIHYPERTENSIVE) *tablet:* propranolol hydrochloride 80 mg, hydrochlorothiazide 25 mg.

Inderide LA 80/50 (ANTIHYPERTENSIVE) *long-acting capsule:* propranolol hydrochloride 80 mg, hydrochlorothiazide 50 mg.

Inderide LA 120/50 (ANTIHYPERTENSIVE) *long-acting capsule:* propranolol hydrochloride 120 mg, hydrochlorothiazide 50 mg.

Inderide LA 160/50 (ANTIHYPERTENSIVE) *long-acting capsule:* propranolol hydrochloride 160 mg, hydrochlorothiazide 50 mg.

Innovar (ANESTHETIC ADJUNCT [schedule II]) *injection:* fentanyl (citrate) 0.05 mg, droperidol 2.5 mg/mL.

Isopto P-ES (ANTIGLAUCOMA) *solution:* pilocarpine hydrochloride 2%, physostigmine salicylate 0.25%

Kapectolin PG (ANTIDIARRHEAL [schedule V]) powdered opium 24 mg, kaolin 6 g, pectin 142.8 mg, hyoscyamine 0.1037 mg, atropine 0.0194 mg, scopolamine 0.0065 mg.

Kinesed (GASTROINTESTINAL ANTICHOLINERGIC, SEDATIVE) *chewable tablet:* atropine sulfate 0.02 mg, scopolamine hydrobromide 0.007 mg, hyoscyamine hydrobromide or sulfate 0.1 mg, phenobarbital 16 mg, saccharin.

Lanophyllin-GG (ANTIASTHMATIC) *capsule:* theophylline 150 mg, guaifenesin 90 mg.

Levlen (ORAL CONTRACEPTIVE) ethinyl estradiol 30 μg, levonorgestrel 0.15 mg.

Lexxel (ANTIHYPERTENSIVE) *tablet:* enalapril 5 mg, felodipine 5 mg.

Librax (GASTROINTESTINAL ANTICHOLINERGIC) *capsule:* clidinium bromide 2.5 mg, chlordiazepoxide hydrochloride 5 mg.

LidoSite (LOCAL ANESTHETIC) *transdermal patch:* lidocaine 10%, epinephrine 0.1%.

Lidox (ANTISPASMODIC) clidinium bromide 2.5 mg, chloridazepoxide 5 mg.

Limbitrol 5–12.5 (PSYCHOTHERAPEUTIC [schedule IV]) *tablet:* chlordiazepoxide 5 mg, amitriptyline (as hydrochloride) 12.5 mg.

Limbitrol DS 10–25 (PSYCHOTHERAPEUTIC [schedule IV]) *tablet:* chlordiazepoxide 10 mg, amitriptyline (as hydrochloride) 25 mg.

Lobac (SKELETAL MUSCLE RELAXANT, ANALGESIC) *capsule:* chlorzoxazone 250 mg, acetaminophen 300 mg.

Loestrin 1/20 (ORAL CONTRACEPTIVE) *tablet:* ethinyl estradiol 20 μg, norethindrone acetate 1 mg.

Loestrin 1/20 Fe (ORAL CONTRACEPTIVE) *tablet:* ethinyl estradiol 20 μg, norethindrone acetate 1 mg, ferrous fumarate 75 mg in last 7 tablets.

Loestrin 1.5/30 (ORAL CONTRACEPTIVE) *tablet:* ethinyl estradiol 30 μg, norethindrone acetate 1.5 mg.

Loestrin 1.5/30 Fe (ORAL CONTRACEPTIVE) *tablet:* ethinyl estradiol 30 μg, norethindrone acetate 1.5 mg, ferrous fumarate 75 mg in last 7 tablets.

Lo/Ovral (ORAL CONTRACEPTIVE) *tablet:* ethinyl estradiol 30 μg, norgestrel 0.3 mg.

Lopressor HCT 50/25 (ANTIHYPERTENSIVE) *tablet:* metoprolol tartrate 50 mg, hydrochlorothiazide 25 mg.

Lopressor HCT 100/25 (ANTIHYPERTENSIVE) *tablet:* metoprolol tartrate 100 mg, hydrochlorothiazide 25 mg.

Lopressor HCT 100/50 (ANTIHYPERTENSIVE) *tablet:* metoprolol tartrate 100 mg, hydrochlorothiazide 50 mg.

Lorcet (NARCOTIC ANALGESIC [schedule III]) hydrocodone 5 mg, acetaminophen 500 mg.

Lorcet-HD (NARCOTIC ANALGESIC [schedule III]) hydrocodone 5 mg, acetaminophen 500 mg.

Lortab 5 (NARCOTIC ANALGESIC [schedule III]) hydrocodone 5 mg, acetaminophen 500 mg.

Lortab 7.5/500 (NARCOTIC ANALGESIC [schedule III]) hydrocodone 7.5 mg, acetaminophen 500 mg.

Lotrel (ANTIHYPERTENSIVE) amlodipine 5 mg, benazepril 10 mg, *or* amlodipine 10 mg/benazepril 20 mg.

Lotrisone (CORTICOSTEROID, ANTIFUNGAL) *cream:* betamethasone (as dipropionate) 0.05%, clotrimazole 1% in a hydrophilic emollient base with mineral oil and white petrolatum.

Lufyllin-EPG (BRONCHODILATOR) dyphylline 100 mg, ephedrine 16 mg, guaifenesin 200 mg, phenobarbital 16 mg.

Lufyllin-GG (BRONCHODILATOR) dyphylline 100 mg, guaifenesin 100 mg, alcohol 17%.

Malarone (ANTIMALARIAL) *tablet:* atovaquone 250 mg/proguanil HCl 100 mg; atovaquone 62.5 mg/proguanil HCl 25 mg. Dose: *Adult:* PO 1 tablet q.d.; *Child:* PO 11–20 kg: 1 pediatric tablet q.d.; 21–30 kg: 2 ped tabs q.d.; 31–40 kg: 3 ped tabs q.d.; >40 kg 1 adult tablet q.d.

Marax (ANTIASTHMATIC, BRONCHODILATOR) *tablet:* theophylline 130 mg, ephedrine sulfate 25 mg, hydroxyzine hydrochloride 10 mg.

Marnal (ANALGESIC [schedule III]) aspirin 325 mg, caffeine 40 mg, butalbital 50 mg.

Maxitrol (OPHTHALMIC STEROID, ANTIBIOTIC) *ointment, ophthalmic suspension:* dexamethasone 0.1%, neomycin sulfate equivalent to 0.35% neomycin base, polymyxin B sulfate 10,000 units.

Maxzide (DIURETIC) *tablet:* triamterene 75 mg, hydrochlorothiazide 50 mg.

Mediatric (HORMONE, MULTIVITAMIN [schedule III]) *capsule, tablet:* conjugated estrogens 0.25 mg, methyltestosterone 2.5 mg, methamphetamine hydrochloride 1 mg, vitamin B1 10 mg, B2 5 mg, B3 50 mg, B5 20 mg, B6 3 mg, B12 2.5 μg, ascorbic acid 100 mg, ferrous sulfate 9 mg.

Medigesic (ANALGESIC) acetaminophen 325 mg, caffeine 40 mg, butalbital 50 mg.

Menrium 5–2 (ESTROGEN, PSYCHOTHERAPEUTIC) *tablet:* chlordiazepoxide 5 mg, esterified estrogens 0.2 mg.

Menrium 5–4 (ESTROGEN, PSYCHOTHERAPEUTIC) *tablet:* chlordiazepoxide 5 mg, esterified estrogens 0.4 mg.

Menrium 10–4 (ESTROGEN, PSYCHOTHERAPEUTIC) *tablet:* chlordiazepoxide 10 mg, esterified estrogens 0.4 mg.

Mepergan (NARCOTIC ANALGESIC [schedule II]) meperidine 25 mg, promethazine 25 mg.

Mepergan Fortis (NARCOTIC ANALGESIC [schedule II]) meperidine 50 mg, promethazine 25 mg.

Metaglip (HYPOGLYCEMIC AGENT) *tablet:* glipizide 2.5 mg/metformin HCl 250 mg; glipizide 2.5

mg/metformin 500 mg; glipizide 5 mg/metformin 500 mg

Metatensin #2 (ANTIHYPERTENSIVE) *tablet:* trichlormethiazide 2 mg, reserpine 0.1 mg, *tartrazine.*

Metatensin #4 (ANTIHYPERTENSIVE) *tablet:* trichlormethiazide 4 mg, reserpine 0.1 mg.

Metimyd (STEROID, SULFONAMIDE) *suspension:* prednisolone acetate 0.5%, sodium sulfacetamide 10%, phenylethyl alcohol 0.5%, benzalkonium chloride 0.025%, sodium thiosulfate, EDTA, tyloxapol.

Micardis HCT (ANTIHYPERTENSIVE) *tablet:* telmisartan 40 mg/hydrochlorothiazide 12.5 mg; telmisartan 80 mg/hydrochlorothiazide 12.5 mg.

Micrainin (NARCOTIC AGONIST ANALGESIC [schedule IV]) *tablet:* aspirin 325 mg, meprobamate 200 mg.

Minizide 1 (ANTIHYPERTENSIVE) *capsule:* polythiazide 0.5 mg, prazosin hydrochloride 1 mg.

Minizide 2 (ANTIHYPERTENSIVE) *capsule:* polythiazide 0.5 mg, prazosin hydrochloride 2 mg.

Minizide 5 (ANTIHYPERTENSIVE) *capsule:* polythiazide 0.5 mg, prazosin hydrochloride 5 mg.

Modicon (ORAL CONTRACEPTIVE) ethinyl estradiol 35 μg, norethindrone 0.5 mg.

Moduretic (DIURETIC) *tablet:* amiloride hydrochloride 5 mg, hydrochlorothiazide 50 mg.

Murocoll-2 (MYDRIATIC) *ophthalmic drops:* scopolamine hydrobromide 0.3%, phenylephrine hydrochloride 10%/5 mL, benzalkonium chloride 0.01%, sodium metabisulfite, EDTA.

Mus-Lax (SKELETAL MUSCLE RELAXANT) *capsule:* chlorzoxazone 250 mg, acetaminophen 300 mg.

Mycitracin (OPHTHALMIC ANTIINFECTIVE) *ophthalmic ointment:* polymyxin B sulfate 10,000 units, neomycin sulfate 3.5 mg, bacitracin 500 units/g; in a lanolin, mineral oil, and white petrolatum base with chlorobutanol 0.65%.

Mycolog II (CORTICOSTEROID, ANTIFUNGAL) *cream, ointment:* triamcinolone acetonide 0.1%, nystatin 100,000 units/g.

Naldecon (DECONGESTANT, ANTIHISTAMINE) *sustained-release tablet:* phenylpropanolamine hydrochloride 40 mg, phenylephrine hydrochloride 10 mg, chlorpheniramine maleate 5 mg, phenyltoloxamine citrate 15 mg; *syrup:* phenylpropanolamine hydrochloride 20 mg, phenylephrine hydrochloride 5 mg, chlorpheniramine maleate 2.5 mg, phenyltoloxamine citrate 7.5 mg.

Naldecon Senior DX (ANTITUSSIVE) dextromethorphan 10 mg, guaifenesin 200 mg.

Nelova 0.5/35 E (ORAL CONTRACEPTIVE) ethinyl estradiol 35 μg, norethindrone 0.5 mg.

Nelova (ORAL CONTRACEPTIVE) ethinyl estradiol 35 μg, norethindrone 1 mg.

Nelova 1/50 M (ORAL CONTRACEPTIVE) mestranol 50 μg, norethindrone 1 mg.

Nelova 10/11 (ORAL CONTRACEPTIVE) ethinyl estradiol 35 μg, norethindrone 0.5 mg|×|10 tablets and 1 mg|×|11 tablets.

Neo-Cortef (CORTICOSTEROID ANTIBIOTIC) *water-soluble cream, topical ointment:* hydrocortisone acetate 1%, neomycin sulfate 0.5%; ointment has white petrolatum mineral base.

NeoDecadron (CORTICOSTEROID ANTIBIOTIC, OPHTHALMIC CORTICOSTEROID ANTIBIOTIC) *topical cream:* dexamethasone phosphate 0.1%, neomycin sulfate 0.5% in a greaseless base; *ophthalmic solution:* dexamethasone sodium phosphate 0.1%, neomycin sulfate equivalent to 0.35% base, benzalkonium chloride 0.02%, sodium bisulfite 0.01%; *ophthalmic ointment:* dexamethasone sodium phosphate 0.05%, neomycin sulfate equivalent to 0.35% base in white petrolatum and mineral oil.

Neosporin (OPHTHALMIC ANTIINFECTIVE) *ophthalmic drops:* polymyxin B sulfate 10,000 units, neomycin sulfate 1.75 mg, gramicidin 0.025 mg/mL; *ophthalmic ointment:* polymyxin B sulfate 10,000 units, neomycin sulfate 3.5 mg, bacitracin zinc 400 units/g in a white petrolatum base.

Neosporin G.U. Irrigant (ANTI-INFECTIVE) *solution:* neomycin sulfate 40 mg, polymyxin B sulfate 200,000 units/mL, methylparaben.

Neotal (OPHTHALMIC ANTIINFECTIVE) *ophthalmic ointment:* polymyxin B sulfate 5000 units, neomycin sulfate 5 mg, bacitracin zinc 400 units/g in a white petrolatum and mineral oil base.

Neothylline-GG (BRONCHODILATOR EXPECTORANT) *tablet:* dyphylline 200 mg, guaifenesin 200 mg.

Neutra-Phos (PHOSPHORUS REPLACEMENT) *capsule, powder:* phosphorous 250 mg, potassium 278 mg, sodium 164 mg; combination of monobasic, dibasic, sodium, and potassium phosphate.

Nolamine (DECONGESTANT, ANTIHISTAMINE) *tablet:* phenylpropanolamine hydrochloride 50 mg, chlorpheniramine maleate 4 mg, phenindamine tartrate 24 mg.

Norcet (NARCOTIC ANALGESIC [schedule III]) hydrocodone 5 mg, acetaminophen 500 mg.

Norco (NARCOTIC AGONIST ANALGESIC [schedule III]) *tablet:* hydrocodone bitartrate 10 mg, acetaminophen 325 mg.

Nordette (ORAL CONTRACEPTIVE) ethinyl estradiol 30 μg, levonorgestrel 0.15 mg.

Norethin 1/35 E (ORAL CONTRACEPTIVE) ethinyl estradiol 35 μg, norethindrone 1 mg.

Norethin 1/50 M (ORAL CONTRACEPTIVE) mestranol 50 μg, norethindrone 1 mg.

Norgesic (SKELETAL MUSCLE RELAXANT) *tablet:* orphenadrine citrate 25 mg, aspirin 385 mg, caffeine 30 mg.

Norgesic Forte (SKELETAL MUSCLE RELAXANT, ANALGESIC) *tablet:* orphenadrine citrate 50 mg, aspirin 700 mg, caffeine 60 mg.

Norinyl 1+35 (ORAL CONTRACEPTIVE) ethinyl estradiol 35 μg, norethindrone 1 mg.

Norinyl 1+50 (ORAL CONTRACEPTIVE) mestranol 50 μg, norethindrone 1 mg.

Norlestrin 1/50 (ORAL CONTRACEPTIVE) ethinyl estradiol 50 μg, norethindrone 1 mg.

Norlestrin 2.5/50 (ORAL CONTRACEPTIVE) ethinyl estradiol 50 μg, norethindrone 2.5 mg.

Normozide 100/25 (ANTIHYPERTENSIVE) labetalol 100 mg, hydrochlorothiazide 25 mg.

Normozide 200/25 (ANTIHYPERTENSIVE) labetalol 200 mg, hydrochlorothiazide 25 mg.

Normozide 300/25 (ANTIHYPERTENSIVE) labetalol 300 mg, hydrochlorothiazide 25 mg.

Novafed A (DECONGESTANT, ANTIHISTAMINE) *capsule:* pseudoephedrine hydrochloride 120 mg, chlorpheniramine maleate 8 mg.

Novahistine DH (ANTITUSSIVE, DECONGESTANT, ANTIHISTAMINE [schedule V]) *liquid:* codeine phosphate 10 mg, pseudoephedrine hydrochloride 30 mg, chlorpheniramine maleate 2 mg/5 mL, alcohol 5%, saccharin, sorbitol.

Novahistine Expectorant (ANTITUSSIVE, DECONGESTANT, EXPECTORANT [schedule V]) *liquid:* codeine phosphate 10 mg, pseudoephedrine hydrochloride 30 mg, guaifenesin 100 mg/5 mL, alcohol 7.5%.

Ophtha P/S (CORTICOSTEROID, SULFONAMIDE) *ophthalmic suspension:* prednisolone acetate 0.5%, sodium sulfacetamide 10%, benzalkonium chloride 0.025%.

Ophthocort (CORTICOSTEROID, ANTIBIOTIC) *ophthalmic ointment:* hydrocortisone acetate 0.5%, chloramphenicol 1%, polymyxin B sulfate 10,000 units/g, liquid petrolatum and polyethylene.

Optimyd (CORTICOSTEROID, SULFONAMIDE) *ophthalmic solution:* prednisolone sodium phosphate 0.5%, sodium sulfacetamide 10%, benzalkonium chloride 0.025%, phenylethyl alcohol 0.5%.

Optised (DECONGESTANT) phenylephrine 0.12%, zinc sulfate 0.25%.

Oreticyl 25 (ANTIHYPERTENSIVE) *tablet:* hydrochlorothiazide 25 mg, deserpidine 0.125 mg.

Oreticyl 50 (ANTIHYPERTENSIVE) *tablet:* hydrochlorothiazide 50 mg, deserpidine 0.125 mg.

Oreticyl Forte (ANTIHYPERTENSIVE) *tablet:* hydrochlorothiazide 25 mg, deserpidine 0.25 mg.

Ornade Spansules (DECONGESTANT, ANTIHISTAMINE) *sustained-release capsule:* phenylpropanolamine hydrochloride 75 mg, chlorpheniramine maleate 12 mg.

Parafon Forte (SKELETAL MUSCLE RELAXANT) *tablet:* chlorzoxazone 250 mg, acetaminophen 300 mg.

Paremyd (MYDRIATIC/CYCLOPLEGIC) *ophthalmic solution:* 1% hydroxyamphetamine, 0.25% tropicamide.

Parepectolin (ANTIDIARRHEAL [schedule V]) *suspension:* opium 15 mg (equivalent to paregoric 3.7 mL), kaolin 5.5 g, pectin 162 mg/30 mL, alcohol 0.69%, saccharin.

P_1E_1, $P2E_1$, P_3E_1, P_6E_1 (ANTIGLAUCOMA) *ophthalmic solution:* epinephrine bitartrate 1%, pilocarpine hydrochloride 1%, 2%, 3%, 4%, or 6%, benzalkonium chloride 0.01%, polyethylene glycol, *sodium bisulfite.*

Percocet (NARCOTIC ANALGESIC [schedule II]) *tablet:* oxycodone 7.5 mg/acetaminophen 325 mg; oxycodone 10 mg/acetaminophen 325 mg.

Percodan (NARCOTIC ANALGESIC [schedule II]) *tablet:* oxycodone hydrochloride 4.5 mg, oxycodone terephthalate 0.38 mg, aspirin 325 mg.

Percodan-Demi (NARCOTIC ANALGESIC [schedule II]) *tablet:* oxycodone hydrochloride 2.25 mg, oxycodone terephthalate 0.19 mg, aspirin 325 mg.

Phenaphen-650 with Codeine (NARCOTIC ANALGESIC [schedule III]) *tablet:* codeine phosphate 30 mg, acetaminophen 650 mg, *sodium bisulfite.*

Phenaphen with Codeine No. 3 (NARCOTIC ANALGESIC [schedule III]) *capsule:* codeine phosphate 30 mg, acetaminophen 325 mg.

Phenaphen with Codeine No. 4 (NARCOTIC ANALGESIC [schedule III]) *tablet:* codeine phosphate 60 mg, acetaminophen 325 mg.

Phenergan with Codeine (ANTITUSSIVE [schedule V]) promethazine 6.25 mg, codeine 10 mg.

Phenergan-D (DECONGESTANT, ANTIHISTAMINE) *tablet:* pseudoephedrine hydrochloride 60 mg, promethazine hydrochloride 6.25 mg, saccharin.

Phrenilin (NONNARCOTIC AGONIST ANALGESIC) *tablet:* acetaminophen 325 mg, butalbital 50 mg.

Phrenilin Forte (NONNARCOTIC AGONIST ANALGESIC) *capsule:* acetaminophen 650 mg, butalbital 50 mg.

PMB 200 (ESTROGEN, ANXIOLYTIC) *tablet:* conjugated estrogens 0.45 mg, meprobamate 200 mg.

PMB 400 (ESTROGEN, ANXIOLYTIC) *tablet:* conjugated estrogens 0.45 mg, meprobamate 400 mg.

Polaramine Expectorant (DECONGESTANT, ANTIHISTAMINE, EXPECTORANT) *liquid:* pseudoephedrine sulfate 20 mg, dexchlorpheniramine maleate 3 mg, guaifenesin 100 mg/5 mL, alcohol 7.2%.

Polycillin-PRB (ANTIBIOTIC) *oral suspension:* ampicillin trihydrate 3.5 g, probenecid 1 g/bottle.

Poly-Histine D (ANTIHISTAMINE, DECONGESTANT) phenylpropanolamine 50 mg, phenyltoloxamine 16 mg, pyrilamine 16 mg, pheniramine 16 mg.

Polysporin Ointment (ANTIINFECTIVE [OPHTHALMIC]) *ophthalmic ointment:* polymyxin B sulfate 10,000 units, bacitracin zinc 500 units/g, white petrolatum, mineral oil.

Pravigard (LIPID-LOWERING AGENT) *tablet:* pravastatin 20 mg/buffered aspirin 81 mg; pravastatin 20 mg/buffered aspirin 325 mg; pravastatin 40 mg/aspirin 81 mg; pravastatin 40 mg/buffered aspirin 325 mg; pravastatin 80 mg/buffered aspirin 81 mg; pravastatin 80 mg/buffered aspirin 325 mg.

Prefrin-A (OPHTHALMIC DECONGESTANT) *ophthalmic solution:* phenylephrine hydrochloride 0.12%, pyrilamine maleate 0.1%, antipyrine 0.1%, benzalkonium chloride, EDTA, sodium bisulfite.

Premarin with Methyltestosterone (ESTROGEN, ANDROGEN) *tablet:* conjugated estrogens 0.625 mg, methyltestosterone 5 mg.

Premphase (ESTROGEN, PROGESTERONE) *tablet:* conjugated estrogen 0.625 mg, medroxyprogesterone acetate 5 mg.

PremPro (ESTROGEN, PROGESTIN) *tablet:* conjugated estrogen 0.3 mg/medroxyprogesterone 1.5 mg; conjugated estrogen 0.45 mg/medroxyprogesterone 1.5 mg; conjugated estrogen 0.625 mg, medroxyprogesterone 2.5 mg; conjugated estrogen 0.625 mg, medroxyprogesterone 5 mg.

Prevacid NapraPac (PROTON PUMP INHIBITOR/ANTIINFLAMMATORY) *capsules & tablets:* lansoprazole 15 mg capsule, naproxen sodium 375 mg tablet; lansoprazole 15 mg capsule, naproxen sodium 500 mg tablet.

Prevpac (ANTIBIOTIC/ANTISECRETORY) *capsules & tablets:* amoxicillin 500 mg capsules, clarithromycin 500 mg tablets, lansoprazole 30 mg capsules.

Probampacin (ANTIBIOTIC) *suspension:* ampicillin trihydrate 3.5 g, probenecid 1 g/bottle.

Proben-C (ANTIGOUT) *tablet:* probenecid 500 mg, colchicine 0.5 mg.

Probenecid with Colchicine (ANTIGOUT) *tablet:* probenecid 500 mg, colchicine 0.5 mg.

Propacet (NARCOTIC ANALGESIC) propoxyphene napsalate 100 mg, acetaminophen 650 mg (CIV).

Pseudo-Chlor (ANTIHISTAMINE, DECONGESTANT) pseudoephedrine 120 mg, chlorpheniramine 8 mg.

Pyridium Plus (ANALGESIC) *tablet:* phenazopyridine hydrochloride 150 mg, hyoscyamine hydrobromide 0.3 mg, butalbital 15 mg.

Quadrinal (BRONCHODILATOR, EXPECTORANT) *tablet:* theophylline calcium salicylate 130 mg (63.5 mg of anhydrous theophylline), ephedrine hydrochloride 24 mg, potassium iodide 320 mg, phenobarbital 24 mg.

Quibron (BRONCHODILATOR, EXPECTORANT) *capsule:* theophylline 150 mg, guaifenesin 90 mg.

Quibron-300 (BRONCHODILATOR, EXPECTORANT) *capsule:* theophylline 300 mg, guaifenesin 180 mg.

Quibron Plus (ANTIASTHMATIC) theophylline 150 mg, ephedrine 25 mg, guaifenesin 100 mg, butabarbital 20 mg.

Rauzide (ANTIHYPERTENSIVE) *tablet:* bendroflumethiazide 4 mg, powdered rauwolfia serpentina 50 mg, tartrazine.

Rebetron (INTERFERON, ANTIVIRAL) ribavirin 200-mg capsule; interferon alfa-2b recombinant 3 mU/0.5 mL injection.

Regroton (ANTIHYPERTENSIVE) *tablet:* chlorthalidone 50 mg, reserpine 0.25 mg.

Renese-R (ANTIHYPERTENSIVE) *tablet:* polythiazide 2 mg, reserpine 0.25 mg.

Repan (ANALGESIC) acetaminophen 325 mg, caffeine 40 mg, butalbital 50 mg.

Rifamate (ANTITUBERCULOSIS) *capsule:* isoniazid 150 mg, rifampin 300 mg.

Rifater (ANTITUBERCULOSIS) rifampin 120 mg, isoniazid 50 mg, pyrazinamide 300 mg.

Rimactane/INH Dual Pack (ANTITUBERCULOSIS) *pack:* thirty isoniazid 300 mg tablets, sixty rifampin 300 mg capsules.

Robaxisal (SKELETAL MUSCLE RELAXANT) *tablet:* methocarbamol 400 mg, aspirin 325 mg.

Robitussin A-C (ANTITUSSIVE, EXPECTORANT [schedule V]) *syrup:* codeine phosphate 10 mg, guaifenesin 100 mg/5 mL, alcohol 3.5%, saccharin.

Robitussin-DAC (ANTITUSSIVE, EXPECTORANT [schedule V]) *syrup:* phenylpropanolamine hydrochloride 30 mg, codeine phosphate 10 mg, guaifenesin 100 mg, alcohol 1.4%, saccharin.

Rondec (DECONGESTANT, ANTIHISTAMINE) *tablet:* pseudoephedrine hydrochloride 60 mg, carbinoxamine maleate 4 mg; *drops:* pseudoephedrine hydrochloride 25 mg, carbinoxamine maleate 2 mg/mL; *syrup:* pseudoephedrine hydrochloride 60 mg, carbinoxamine maleate 4 mg/mL.

Roxicet (NARCOTIC ANALGESIC [schedule II]) oxycodone 5 mg, acetaminophen 325 mg.

Roxiprin (NARCOTIC ANALGESIC [schedule II]) oxycodone 5 mg, aspirin 325 mg.

Salazide (ANTIHYPERTENSIVE) hydroflumethiazide 50 mg, reserpine 0.125 mg.

Salutensin (ANTIHYPERTENSIVE) *tablet:* hydroflumethiazide 50 mg, reserpine 0.125 mg.

Salutensin-Demi (ANTIHYPERTENSIVE) *tablet:* hydroflumethiazide 25 mg, reserpine 0.125 mg.

Sedapap-10 (ANALGESIC) *tablet:* acetaminophen 650 mg, butalbital 50 mg.

Ser-A-Gen (ANTIHYPERTENSIVE) *tablet:* hydrochlorothiazide 15 mg, reserpine 0.1 mg, hydralazine hydrochloride 25 mg.

Seralazide (ANTIHYPERTENSIVE) *tablet:* hydrochlorothiazide 15 mg, reserpine 0.1 mg, hydralazine hydrochloride 25 mg.

Ser-Ap-Es (ANTIHYPERTENSIVE) *tablet:* hydrochlorothiazide 15 mg, reserpine 0.1 mg, hydralazine hydrochloride 25 mg.

Serpasil-Apresoline #1 (ANTIHYPERTENSIVE) *tablet:* reserpine 0.1 mg, hydralazine hydrochloride 25 mg, tartrazine.

Serpasil-Apresoline #2 (ANTIHYPERTENSIVE) *tablet:* reserpine 0.2 mg, hydralazine hydrochloride 50 mg, tartrazine.

Serpasil-Esidrex #1 (ANTIHYPERTENSIVE) *tablet:* hydrochlorothiazide 25 mg, reserpine 0.1 mg.

Serpasil-Esidrex #2 (ANTIHYPERTENSIVE) *tablet:* hydrochlorothiazide 50 mg, reserpine 0.1 mg.

Serpazide (ANTIHYPERTENSIVE) hydrochlorothiazide 15 mg, reserpine 0.1 mg, hydralazine 25 mg.

Soma Compound (SKELETAL MUSCLE RELAXANT) *tablet:* carisoprodol 200 mg, aspirin 325 mg.

Soma Compound with Codeine (SKELETAL MUSCLE RELAXANT [schedule III]) *tablet:* carisoprodol 200 mg, aspirin 325 mg, codeine phosphate 16 mg, sodium meta-bisulfite.

Spironazide (DIURETIC) *tablet:* spironolactone 25 mg, hydrochlorothiazide 25 mg.

Spirozide (DIURETIC) *tablet:* spironolactone 25 mg, hydrochlorothiazide 25 mg.

Stalevo (ANTIPARKINSONS AGENT) *tablet:* 12.5 mg carbidopa/50 mg levodopa/200 mg entacapone; 25 mg carbidopa/100 mg levodopa/200 mg entacapone; 37.5 mg carbidopa/150 mg levodopa/200 mg entacapone

Statrol (OPHTHALMIC ANTIBIOTIC) *ophthalmic ointment:* polymyxin B sulfate 10,000 units, neomycin sulfate 3.5 mg, parabens in a white petrolatum and lanolin base; *ophthalmic solution:* polymyxin B sulfate 16,250 units, neomycin sulfate 3.5 mg/mL, benzalkonium chloride 0.004%, hydroxypropyl methylcellulose 0.5%.

Sulfamide (OCULAR ANTIINFLAMMATORY) prednisolone acetate 0.5%, sulfacetamide 10%.

Sulfoxyl Regular (ANTIACNE) *lotion:* benzoyl peroxide 5%, sulfur 2%.

Sulfoxyl Strong (ANTIACNE) *lotion:* benzoyl peroxide 10%, sulfur 5%.

Symbyax (ATYPICAL ANTIPSYCHOTIC/SSRI) *capsule:* olanzapine 6 mg, fluoxetine 25 mg; olanzapine 6 mg, fluoxetine 50 mg; olanzapine 12 mg, fluoxetine 25 mg; olanzapine 12 mg, fluoxetine 50 mg.

Synalgos-DC (NARCOTIC AGONIST ANALGESIC [schedule III]) *capsule:* dihydrocodeine bitartrate 16 mg, aspirin 356.4 mg, caffeine 30 mg.

Talacen (NARCOTIC AGONIST-ANTIAGONIST ANALGESIC [schedule IV]) *tablet:* pentazocine hydrochloride 25 mg, acetaminophen 625 mg.

Talwin Compound (NARCOTIC ANALGESIC [schedule IV]) pentazocine 12.5 mg, aspirin 325 mg.

Talwin NX (NARCOTIC ANALGESIC [schedule IV]) pentazocine 50 mg, naloxone 0.5 mg.

Tarka (ANTIHYPERTENSIVE) *tablet:* trandolapril 2 mg, verapamil HCl 180 mg; trandolapril 4 mg; verapamil HCl 240 mg; trandolapril 1 mg, verapamil HCl 240 mg, trandolapril 2 mg, verapamil HCl 240 mg.

Tavist-D (DECONGESTANT, ANTIHISTAMINE) *tablet:* phenylpropanolamine hydrochloride 75 mg, clemastine fumarate 1.34 mg.

Teczem (ANTIHYPERTENSIVE) *tablet:* enalapril 5 mg, diltiazem 180 mg.

Tedral SA (ANTIASTHMATIC, BRONCHODILATOR) *sustained-action*

tablet: theophylline 180 mg, ephedrine hydrochloride 48 mg, phenobarbital 25 mg.

Teebaconin and Vitamin B_6 (ANTITUBERCULOSIS) *tablet:* isoniazid 300 mg (or 100 mg), pyridoxine hydrochloride 30 mg (or 10 mg), tartrazine.

Tega-Tussin Syrup (ANTITUSSIVE [schedule III]) *syrup:* phenylephrine 5 mg, chlorpheniramine 2 mg, hydrocodone 5 mg.

Tenoretic 50 (ANTIHYPERTENSIVE) *tablet:* chlorthalidone 25 mg, atenolol 50 mg.

Tenoretic 100 (ANTIHYPERTENSIVE) *tablet:* chlorthalidone 25 mg, atenolol 100 mg.

Terra-Cortril Suspension (OCULAR STEROID AND ANTIBIOTIC) *suspension:* hydrocortisone acetate 1.5%, oxytetracycline 0.5%.

Teveten HCT (ANTIHYPERTENSIVE) *tablet:* eprosartan mesylate 600 mg/hydrochlorothiazide 12.5 mg; eprosartan 600 mg/hydrochlorothiazide 25 mg

T-Gesic (NARCOTIC ANALGESIC [schedule III]) hydrocodone 5 mg, acetaminophen 500 mg.

Theolair-Plus (ANTIASTHMATIC) *liquid:* theophylline 125 mg, guaifenesin 100 mg/15 mL, menthol; *250 mg tablet :* theophylline 250 mg, guaifenesin 200 mg; *125 mg tablet:* theophylline 125 mg, guaifenesin 100 mg.

Timolide (ANTIHYPERTENSIVE) *tablet:* hydrochlorothiazide 25 mg, timolol maleate 10 mg.

Trandate HCT 100/25 (ANTIHYPERTENSIVE) labetalol 100 mg, hydrochlorothiazide 25 mg.

Trandate HCT 200/25 (ANTIHYPERTENSIVE) labetalol 200 mg, hydrochlorothiazide 25 mg.

Trandate HCT 300/25 (ANTIHYPERTENSIVE) labetalol 300 mg, hydrochlorothiazide 25 mg.

Triacin-C Cough Syrup (ANTITUSSIVE [schedule V]) *syrup:* pseudoephedrine 30 mg, triprolidine 1.25 mg, codeine 10 mg.

Triad (ANALGESIC) acetaminophen 325 mg, caffeie 40 mg, butalbital 50 mg.

Triaminic Expectorant DH (DECONGESTANT, ANTIHISTAMINE, ANTITUSSIVE, EXPECTORANT [schedule III]) *liquid:* phenylpropanolamine hydrochloride 12.5 mg, pyrilamine maleate 6.25 mg, pheniramine maleate 6.25 mg, hydrocodone bitartrate 1.67 mg, guaifenesin 100 mg/5 mL, alcohol 5%, saccharin, sorbitol.

Triaminic Expectorant with Codeine (DECONGESTANT, ANTITUSSIVE, EXPECTORANT [schedule V]) *liquid:* phenylpropanolamine hydrochloride 12.5 mg, codeine phosphate 10 mg, guaifenesin 100 mg/5 mL, alcohol 5%, saccharin, sorbitol.

Triaminic Oral Infant Drops (DECONGESTANT, ANTIHISTAMINE) *liquid:* phenylpropanolamine hydrochloride 20 mg, pyrilamine maleate 10 mg, pheniramine maleate 10 mg/mL, saccharin, sorbitol.

Triaminic TR Tablets (DECONGESTANT, ANTIHISTAMINE [schedule V]) *timed-release tablet:* phenylpropanolamine hydrochloride 50 mg, pyrilamine maleate 25 mg, pheniramine maleate 25 mg.

Triaprin (ANALGESIC) acetaminophen 325 mg, butalbital 50 mg.

Triavil (PSYCHOTHERAPEUTIC) *2–10 tablet:* perphenazine 2 mg, amitriptyline 10 mg; *2–25 tablet:* perphenazine 2 mg, amitriptyline 25 mg; *4–10 tablet:* perphenazine 4 mg, amitriptyline 10 mg; *4–25 tablet:* perphenazine 4 mg, amitriptyline 25 mg; *4–50 tablet:* perphenazine 4 mg, amitriptyline 50 mg.

Tri-Barbs (SEDATIVE-HYPNOTIC [schedule II]) *capsule:* phenobarbital 32 mg, butabarbital sodium 32 mg, secobarbital sodium 32 mg.

Tri-Hydroserpine (ANTIHYPERTENSIVE) *tablet:* hydrochlorothiazide 15 mg, reserpine 0.1 mg, hydralazine hydrochloride 25 mg.

Tri-Levlen (ORAL CONTRACEPTIVE) ethinyl estradiol 30 μg|×|6 d, 40 μg|×|5 d, 30 μg|×|10 d, levonorgestrel 0.05 mg|×|6 d, 0.075 mg|×|5 d, 0.125 mg|×|10 d.

Tri-Luma Cream (STEROID) *cream:* hydroquinone, tretinoin, fluocinolone acetonide

Trinalin Repetabs (DECONGESTANT, ANTIHISTAMINE) *tablet:* pseudoephedrine sulfate 120 mg, azatadine maleate 1 mg; sugar coated.

Tri-Norinyl (ORAL CONTRACEPTIVE) ethinyl estradiol 35 μg, norethindrone 0.5 mg|×|7 d, 1 mg|×|9 d, 0.5 mg|×|5 d.

Triphasil (ORAL CONTRACEPTIVE) ethinyl estradiol 30 μg|×|6 d, 40 μg|×|5 d, 30 μg|×|10 d, levonorgestrel 0.05 mg|×|6 d, 0.075 mg|×|5 d, 0.125 mg|×|10 d.

Triple Antibiotic (OPHTHALMIC ANTIINFECTIVE) *ophthalmic ointment:* hydrocortisone 1%, neomycin sulfate 0.5%, bacitracin zinc 400 units, polymyxin B sulfate 10,000 units/g.

Triple Sulfa (ANTIINFECTIVE) *tablet:* sulfadiazine 167 mg, sulfamerazine 167 mg, sulfamethazine 167 mg.

Triple Sulfa No. 2 (ANTIINFECTIVE) *tablet:* sulfadiazine 162 mg, sulfamerazine 162 mg, sulfamethazine 162 mg.

Trizivir (REVERSE TRANSCRIPTASE INHIBITOR) *tablets:* abacavir 300 mg, lamivudine 150 mg, zidovudine 300 mg.

Truvada (NUCLEOSIDE REVERSE TRANSCRIPTASE INHIBITOR) *tablets:* emtricitabine 200 mg, tenofovir disproxil fumarate 300 mg.

Tuinal 100 mg Pulvules (SEDATIVE-HYPNOTIC [schedule II]) *capsule:* amobarbital sodium 50 mg, secobarbital sodium 50 mg.

Tuinal 200 mg Pulvules (SEDATIVE-HYPNOTIC [schedule II]) *capsule:* amobarbital sodium 100 mg, secobarbital sodium 100 mg.

Tussionex (ANTITUSSIVE [schedule III]) chlorpheniramine 8 mg, hydrocodone 10 mg.

Twinrix (VACCINE) *injection:* Hepatitis A vaccine 720 ELU/ Hepatitis B recombinant vaccine 20 mcg per single dose vial. Dose: *Adult:* IM dose at 0-, 1-, and 6-mo schedule.

Tylenol with Codeine No. 1 (NARCOTIC AGONIST ANALGESIC [schedule III]) *tablet:* acetaminophen 300 mg, codeine phosphate 7.5 mg, sodium metabisulfite.

Tylenol with Codeine No. 2 (NARCOTIC AGONIST ANALGESIC [schedule III]) *tablet:* acetaminophen 300 mg, codeine phosphate 15 mg, sodium metabisulfite.

Tylenol with Codeine No. 3 (NARCOTIC AGONIST ANALGESIC [schedule III]) *tablet:* acetaminophen 300 mg, codeine phosphate 30 mg, sodium metabisulfite.

Tylenol with Codeine No. 4 (NARCOTIC AGONIST ANALGESIC [schedule III]) *tablet:* acetaminophen 300 mg, codeine phosphate 60 mg, sodium metabisulfite.

Tylox (NARCOTIC AGONIST ANALGESIC [schedule II]) *capsule:* oxycodone hydrochloride 5 mg, acetaminophen 500 mg, sodium metabisulfite.

Ty-Tab #3 (NARCOTIC AGONIST ANALGESIC [schedule III]) *tablet:* codeine phosphate 30 mg, acetaminophen 300 mg.

Ultracet (ANALGESIC/ANTIPYRETIC) *tablet:* tramadol 37.5 mg/acetaminophen 325 mg

Unipres (ANTIHYPERTENSIVE) *tablet:* hydrochlorothiazide 15 mg, reserpine 0.1 mg, hydralazine hydrochloride 25 mg.

Uniretic (ANTIHYPERTENSIVE) moexipril 7.5 mg, hydrochlorothiazide 12.5 mg, moexipril 15 mg, hydrochlorothiazide 25 mg.

Urobiotic-250 (URINARY ANTIINFECTIVE) *capsule:* oxytetracycline hydrochloride 250 mg, sulfamethizole 250 mg, phenazopyridine hydrochloride 50 mg.

Uro-Phosphate (URINARY ANTIINFECTIVE) *tablet:* methenamine 300 mg, sodium acid phosphate 500 mg; sugar coated.

Uroquid-Acid (URINARY ANTIINFECTIVE) *tablet:* methenamine mandelate 350 mg, sodium acid phosphate 200 mg; sugar coated.

Uroquid-Acid No. 2 (URINARY ANTIINFECTIVE) *tablet:* methenamine mandelate 500 mg, sodium acid phosphate 500 mg.

Vanoxide-HC (ANTIACNE) *water-washable lotion:* benzoyl peroxide 5%, hydrocortisone 0.5%, mineral oil, propylene glycol, cetyl alcohol, parabens.

Vaseretic (ANTIHYPERTENSIVE) *tablet:* enalapril maleate 10 mg, hydrochlorothiazide 25 mg.

Vasocidin (OPHTHALMIC CORTICOSTEROID, ANTIINFECTIVE) *ophthalmic solution:* prednisolone sodium phosphate 0.25%, sodium sulfacetamide 10%, EDTA, thimerosal 0.001%, polaxamer 407; *ophthalmic ointment:* prednisolone acetate 0.5%, sodium sulfacetamide 10%, mineral oil, white petrolatum.

Vasocon-A (OPHTHALMIC DECONGESTANT) *ophthalmic solution:* naphazoline hydrochloride 0.05%, antazoline phosphate 0.5%, benzalkonium chloride 0.01%, PEG-8000 polyvinyl alcohol, povidone.

Vasosulf (SULFONAMIDE DECONGESTANT) *ophthalmic solution:* sodium sulfacetamide 15%, phenylephrine hydrochloride 0.125%.

Veltap (ANTIHISTAMINE, DECONGESTANT) phenylpropanolamine 5 mg, brompheniramine 4 mg, alcohol 3%.

Vicodin (NARCOTIC AGONIST ANALGESIC [schedule III]) *tablet:* hydrocodone bitartrate 5 mg, acetaminophen 500 mg.

Vicodin HP (NARCOTIC AGONIST ANALGESIC [schedule III]) *tablet:* hydrocodone 10 mg, acetaminophen 660 mg.

Vicoprofen (NARCOTIC AGONIST ANALGESIC C-III) hydrocodone bitartrate 7.5 mg, ibuprofen 200 mg.

Vytorin (ANTILIPEMIC AGENT) *tablet:* ezetimibe 10 mg, simvastatin 10 mg; ezetimibe 10 mg, simvastatin 20 mg; ezetimibe 10 mg, simvastatin 40 mg; ezetimibe 10 mg, simvastatin 80 mg.

Wigraine (ANTIMIGRAINE) *tablet:* ergotamine tartrate 1 mg, caffeine 100 mg, lactose, magnesium stearate, microcrystalline cellulose, starch; *suppository:* ergotamine tartrate 2 mg, caffeine 100 mg, tartaric acid 21.5 mg, synthetic cocoa butter base.

Wygesic (NARCOTIC AGONIST ANALGESIC [schedule IV]) *tablet:* propoxyphene hydrochloride 65 mg, acetaminophen 650 mg.

Xalcom (ANTIGLAUCOMA AGENT) *ocular solution:* latanoprost 0.005%/ timolol 0.5%.

Ziac (ANTIHYPERTENSIVE) *tablet:* bisoprolol 2.5 mg, hydrochlorothiazide 6.25 mg; bisoprolol 5 mg, hydrochlorothiazide 6.25 mg; bisoprolol 10 mg, hydrochlorothiazide 6.25 mg.

Zincfrin (OPHTHALMIC DECONGESTANT) *solution:* phenylephrine hydrochloride 0.12%, zinc sulfate 0.25%, benzalkonium chloride 0.01%.

Zydone (NARCOTIC AGONIST ANALGESIC [schedule III]) *capsule:* hydrocodone bitartrate 5 mg, acetaminophen 500 mg.

Zyrtec-D (ANTIHISTAMINE/DECONGESTANT) *tablet, sustained release:* cetirizine 5 mg/pseudoephedrine 120 mg.

◆ APPENDIX F GLOSSARY OF KEY TERMS, CLINICAL CONDITIONS, AND ASSOCIATED SIGNS AND SYMPTOMS

acute dystonia extrapyramidal symptom manifested by abnormal posturing, grimacing, spastic torticollis (neck torsion), and oculogyric (eyeball movement) crisis.

adverse effect unintended, unpredictable, and nontherapeutic response to drug action. Adverse effects occur at doses used therapeutically or for prophylaxis or diagnosis. They generally result from drug toxicity, idiosyncrasies, or hypersensitivity reactions caused by the drug itself or by ingredients added during manufacture, e.g., preservatives, dyes, or vehicles.

afterload resistance that ventricles must work against to eject blood into the aorta during systole.

agranulocytosis sudden drop in leukocyte count; often followed by a severe infection manifested by high fever, chills, prostration, and ulcerations of mucous membrane such as in the mouth, rectum, or vagina.

akathisia extrapyramidal symptom manifested by a compelling need to move or pace, without specific pattern, and an inability to be still.

analeptic restorative medication that enhances excitation of the CNS without affecting inhibitory impulses.

anaphylactoid reaction excessive allergic response manifested by wheezing, chills, generalized pruritic urticaria, diaphoresis, sense of uneasiness, agitation, flushing, palpitations, coughing, difficulty breathing, and cardiovascular collapse.

anticholinergic actions inhibition of parasympathetic response manifested by dry mouth, decreased peristalsis, constipation, blurred vision, and urinary retention.

bioavailability fraction of active drug that reaches its action sites after administration by any route. Following an IV dose, bioavailability is 100%; however, such factors as first-pass effect, enterohepatic cycling, and biotransformation reduce bioavailability of an orally administered drug.

blood dyscrasia pathological condition manifested by fever, sore mouth or throat, unexplained fatigue, easy bruising or bleeding.

cardiotoxicity impairment of cardiac function manifested by one or more of the following: hypotension, arrhythmias, precordial pain, dyspnea, electrocardiogram (ECG) abnormalities, cardiac dilation, congestive failure.

cholinergic response stimulation of the parasympathetic response manifested by lacrimation, diaphoresis, salivation, abdominal cramps, diarrhea, nausea, and vomiting.

circulatory overload excessive vascular volume manifested by increased central venous pressure (CVP), elevated blood pressure, tachycardia, distended neck veins, peripheral edema, dyspnea, cough, and pulmonary rales.

CNS stimulation excitement of the CNS manifested by hyperactivity, excitement, nervousness, insomnia, and tachycardia.

CNS toxicity impairment of CNS function manifested by ataxia, tremor, incoordination, paresthesias, numbness, impairment of pain or touch sensation, drowsiness, confusion, headache, anxiety, tremors, and behavior changes.

congestive heart failure (CHF) impaired pumping ability of the heart manifested by paroxysmal nocturnal dyspnea, cough, fatigue or dyspnea on exertion, tachycardia, peripheral or pulmonary edema, and weight gain.

Cushing's syndrome fatty swellings in the interscapular area (buffalo hump) and in the facial area (moon face), distension of the abdomen, ecchymoses following even minor trauma, impotence, amenorrhea, high blood pressure, general weakness, loss of muscle mass, osteoporosis, and psychosis.

dehydration decreased intracellular or extracellular fluid manifested by elevated temperature, dry skin and mucous membranes, decrease tissue turgor, sunken eyes, furrowed tongue, low blood pressure, diminished or irregular pulse, muscle or abdominal cramps, thick secretions, hard feces and impaction, scant urinary output, urine specific gravity above 1.030, an elevated hemoglobin.

disulfiram-type reaction Antabuse-type reaction manifested by facial flushing, pounding headache, sweating, slurred speech, abdominal cramps, nausea, vomiting, tachycardia, fever, palpitations, drop in blood pressure, dyspnea, and sense of chest constriction. Symptoms may last up to 24 hours.

enzyme induction stimulation of microsomal enzymes by a drug resulting in its accelerated metabolism and decreased activity. If reactive intermediates are formed, drug-mediated toxicity may be exacerbated.

first-pass effect reduced bioavailability of an orally administered drug due to metabolism in GI epithelial cells and liver or to biliary excretion. Effect may be avoided by use of sublingual tablets or rectal suppositories.

fixed drug eruption drug-induced circumscribed skin lesion that persists or recurs in the same site. Residual pigmentation may remain following drug withdrawal.

half-life ($t_{1/2}$) time required for concentration of a drug in the body to decrease by 50%. Half-life also represents the time necessary to reach steady state or to decline from steady state after a change (i.e., starting or stopping) in the dosing regimen. Half-life may be affected by a disease state and age of the drug user.

heat stroke a life-threatening condition manifested by absence of sweating; red, dry, hot skin; dilated pupils; dyspnea; full bounding pulse; temperature above 40° C (105° F); and mental confusion.

hepatic toxicity impairment of liver function manifested by jaundice, dark urine, pruritus, lightcolored stools, eosinophilia, itchy skin or rash, and persistently high elevations of alanine amino-transferase (ALT) and aspartate aminotransferase (AST).

hyperammonemia elevated level of ammonia or ammonium in the blood manifested by lethargy, decreased appetite, vomiting, asterixis (flapping tremor), weak pulse, irritability, decreased responsiveness, and seizures.

hypercalcemia elevated serum calcium manifested by deep bone and flank pain, renal calculi, anorexia, nausea, vomiting, thirst, constipation, muscle hypotonicity, pathologic fracture, bradycardia, lethargy, and psychosis.

hyperglycemia elevated blood glucose manifested by flushed, dry skin, low blood pressure and elevated pulse, tachypnea, Kussmaul's respirations, polyuria, polydipsia; polyphagia, lethargy, and drowsiness.

hyperkalemia excessive potassium in blood, which may produce lifethreatening cardiac arrhythmias, including bradycardia and heart block, unusual fatigue, weakness or heaviness of limbs, general muscle weakness, muscle cramps, paresthesias, flaccid paralysis of extremities, shortness of breath, nervousness, confusion, diarrhea, and GI distress.

hypermagnesemia excessive magnesium in blood, which may produce cathartic effect, profound thirst, flushing, sedation, confusion, depressed deep tendon reflexes (DTRs), muscle weakness, hypotension, and depressed respirations.

hypernatremia excessive sodium in blood, which may produce confusion, neuromuscular excitability, muscle weakness, seizures, thirst, dry and flushed skin, dry mucous membranes, pyrexia, agitation, and oliguria or anuria.

hypersensitivity reactions excessive and abnormal sensitivity to given agent manifested by urticaria, pruritus, wheezing, edema, redness, and anaphylaxis.

hyperthyroidism excessive secretion by the thyroid glands, which increases basal metabolic rate, resulting in warm, flushed, moist skin; tachycardia, exophthalmos; infrequent lid blinking; lid edema; weight loss despite increased appetite; frequent urination; menstrual irregularity; breathlessness; hypoventilation; congestive heart failure; excessive sweating.

hyperuricemia excessive uric acid in blood, resulting in pain in flank; stomach, or joints, and changes in intake and output ratio and pattern.

hypocalcemia abnormally low calcium level in blood, which may result in depression; psychosis; hyperreflexia; diarrhea; cardiac arrhythmias; hypotension; muscle spasms; paresthesias of feet, fingers, tongue; positive Chvostek's sign. Severe deficiency (tetany) may result in carpopedal spasms, spasms of face muscle, laryngospasm, and generalized convulsions.

hypoglycemia abnormally low glucose level in the blood, which may result in acute fatigue, restlessness, malaise, marked irritability and weakness, cold sweats, excessive hunger, headache, dizziness, confusion, slurred speech, loss of consciousness, and death.

hypokalemia abnormally low level of potassium in blood, which may result in malaise, fatigue, paresthesias, depressed reflexes, muscle weakness and cramps, rapid, irregular pulse, arrhythmias, hypotension, vomiting, paralytic ileus, mental confusion, depression, delayed thought process, abdominal distension, polyuria, shallow breathing, and shortness of breath.

hypomagnesemia abnormally low level of magnesium in

blood, resulting in nausea, vomiting, cardiac arrhythmias, and neuromuscular symptoms (tetany, positive Chvostek's and Trousseau's signs, seizures, tremors, ataxia, vertigo, nystagmus, muscular fasciculations).

hypophosphatemia abnormally low level of phosphates in blood, resulting in muscle weakness, anorexia, malaise, absent deep tendon reflexes, bone pain, paresthesias, tremors, negative calcium balance, osteomalacia, osteoporosis.

hypothyroidism condition caused by thyroid hormone deficiency that lowers basal metabolic rate and may result in periorbital edema, lethargy, puffy hands and feet, cool, pale skin, vertigo, nocturnal cramps, decreased GI motility, constipation, hypotension, slow pulse, depressed muscular activity, and enlarged thyroid gland.

hypoxia insufficient oxygenation in the blood manifested by dyspnea, tachypnea, headache, restlessness, cyanosis, tachycardia, dysrhythmias, confusion, decreased level of consciousness, and euphoria or delirium.

international normalizing ratio measurement that normalizes for the differences obtained from various laboratory readings in the value for thromboplastin blood level.

leukopenia abnormal decrease in number of white blood cells, usually below 5000 per cubic millimeter, resulting in fever, chills, sore mouth or throat, and unexplained fatigue.

liver toxicity manifested by anorexia, nausea, fatigue, lethargy, itching, jaundice, abdominal pain, dark-colored urine, and flu-like symptoms.

metabolic acidosis decrease in pH value of the extracellular fluid caused by either an increase in hydrogen ions or a decrease in bicarbonate ions. It may result in one or more of the following: lethargy, headache, weakness, abdominal pain, nausea, vomiting, dyspnea, hyperpnea progressing to Kussmaul breathing, dehydration, thirst, weakness, flushed face, full bounding pulse, progressive drowsiness, mental confusion, combativeness.

metabolic alkalosis increase in pH value of the extracellular fluid caused by either a loss of acid from the body (e.g., through vomiting) or an increased level of bicarbonate ions (e.g., through ingestion of sodium bicarbonate). It may result in muscle weakness, irritability, confusion, muscle twitching, slow and shallow respirations, and convulsive seizures.

microsomal enzymes drug-metabolizing enzymes located in the endoplasmic reticulum of the liver and other tissues chiefly responsible for oxidative drug metabolism, e.g., cytochrome P450.

myopathy any disease or abnormal condition of striated muscles manifested by muscle weakness, myalgia, diaphoresis, fever, and reddish-brown urine (myoglobinuria) or oliguria.

nephrotoxicity impairment of the nephrons of the kidney manifested by one or more of the following: oliguria, urinary frequency, hematuria, cloudy urine, rising BUN and serum creatinine, fever, graft tenderness or enlargement.

neuroleptic malignant syndrome (NMS) potentially fatal complication associated with antipsychotic drugs manifested by hyperpyrexia, altered mental status, muscle rigidity, irregular pulse, fluctuating BP, diaphoresis, and tachycardia.

orphan drug (as defined by the Orphan Drug Act, an amendment of the Federal Food, Drug, and Cosmetic Act which took effect in January 1983): drug or biological product used in the treatment, diagnosis, or prevention of a rare disease. A rare disease or condition is one that affects fewer than 200,000 persons in the United States, or affects more than 200,000 persons but for which there is no reasonable expectation that drug research and development costs can be recovered from sales within the United States.

ototoxicity impairment of the ear manifested by one or more of the following: headache, dizziness or vertigo, nausea and vomiting with motion, ataxia, nystagmus.

prodrug inactive drug form that becomes pharmacologically active through biotransformation.

protein binding reversible interaction between protein and drug resulting in a drug-protein complex (bound drug) which is in equilibrium with free (active) drug in plasma and tissues. Since only free drug can diffuse to action sites, factors that influence drug-binding (e.g., displacement of bound drug by another drug, or decreased albumin concentration) may potentiate pharmacological effect.

pseudomembranous enterocolitis life-threatening superinfection characterized by severe diarrhea and fever.

pseudoparkinsonism extrapyramidal symptom manifested by slowing of volitional movement (akinesia), mask facies, rigidity and tremor at rest (especially of upper extremities); and pill rolling motion.

pulmonary edema excessive fluid in the lung tissue manifestied by one or more of the following: shortness of breath, cyanosis, persistent productive cough (frothy sputum may be blood tinged), expiratory rales, restlessness, anxiety, increased heart rate, sense of chest pressure.

renal insufficiency reduced capacity of the kidney to perform its functions as manifested by one or more of the following: dysuria, oliguria, hematuria, swelling of lower legs and feet.

serotonin syndrome manifested by restlessness, myoclonus, mental status changes, hyperreflexia, diaphoresis, shivering, and tremor.

Somogyi effect rebound phenomenon clinically manifested by fasting hyperglycemia and worsening of diabetic control due to unnecessarily large p.m. insulin doses. Hormonal response to unrecognized hypoglycemia (i.e., release of epinephrine, glucagon, growth hormone, cortisol) causes insensitivity to insulin. Increasing the amount of insulin required to treat the hyperglycemia intensifies the hypoglycemia.

superinfection new infection by an organism different from the initial infection being treated by antimicrobial therapy manifested by one or more of the following: black, hairy tongue; glossitis, stomatitis; anal itching; loose, foul-smelling stools; vaginal itching or discharge; sudden fever; cough.

tachyphylaxis rapid decrease in response to a drug after administration of a few doses. Initial drug response cannot be restored by an increase in dose.

tardive dyskinesia extrapyramidal symptom manifested by involuntary rhythmic, bizarre movements of face, jaw, mouth, tongue, and sometimes extremities.

vasovagal symptoms transient vascular and neurogenic reaction marked by pallor, nausea, vomiting, bradycardia, and rapid fall in arterial blood pressure.

water intoxication (dilutional hyponatremia) less than normal concentration of sodium in the blood resulting from excess extracellular and intracellular fluid and producing one or more of the following: lethargy, confusion, headache, decreased skin turgor, tremors, convulsions, coma, anorexia, nausea, vomiting, diarrhea, sternal fingerprinting, weight gain, edema, full bounding pulse, jugular vein distension, rales, signs and symptoms of pulmonary edema.

◆ APPENDIX G ABBREVIATIONS

ABGs	arterial blood gases
a.c.	before meals (*ante cibum*)
ACD	acid–citrate–dextrose
ACE	angiotensin-converting enzyme
ACh	acetylcholine
ACIP	Advisory Committee on Immunization Practices
ACLS	advanced cardiac life support
ACS	acute coronary syndrome
ACT	activated clotting time
ACTH	adrenocorticotropic hormone
AD	Alzheimer's disease
ADD	attention deficit disorder
ADH	antidiuretic hormone
ADLs	activities of daily living
ad lib	as desired (*ad libitum*)
ADP	adenosine diphosphate
ADT	alternate-day drug (administration)
AIDS	acquired immunodeficiency syndrome
alpha1-PI	alpha1-proteinase inhibitor
ALS	amyotrophic lateral sclerosis
ALT	alanine aminotransferase (formerly SGPT)
AML	acute myelogenous leukemia
AMP	adenosine monophosphate
ANA	antinuclear antibody(ies)
ANC	acid neutralizing capacity
aPTT	activated partial thromboplastin time
ARC	AIDS related complex
ARDS	adult respiratory distress syndrome
ASHD	arteriosclerotic heart disease
AST	aspartate aminotransferase (formerly SGOT)
AT_1	angiotensin II receptor subtype I
AT_2	angiotensin II receptor subtype II
ATP	adenosine triphosphate
AV	atrioventricular
b.i.d.	two times a day
BMD	bone mineral density
BMI	body mass index
BMR	basal metabolic rate
BP	blood pressure
BPH	benign prostatic hypertrophy
bpm	beats per minute
BSA	body surface area
BSE	breast self-exam
BSP	bromsulphalein
BT	bleeding time
BUN	blood urea nitrogen
C	centigrade, Celsius

CAD	coronary artery disease
cAMP	cyclic adenosine monophosphate
CBC	complete blood count
cc	cubic centimeter
CDC	Centers for Disease Control
CF	cystic fibrosis
cGMP	cyclic guanosine monophosphate
CHF	congestive heart failure
Cl_{cr}	creatinine clearance
CLL	chronic lymphocytic leukemia
cm	centimeter
CMV	cytomegalovirus-I
CNS	central nervous system
Coll	collyrium (eye wash)
COMT	catecholamine-*o*-methyl transferase
COPD	chronic obstructive pulmonary disease
COX-2	cyclooxygenase-2
CPK	creatinine phosphokinase
CPR	cardiopulmonary resuscitation
CRF	chronic renal failure
CRFD	chronic renal failure disease
C&S	culture and sensitivity
CSF	cerebrospinal fluid
CSP	cellulose sodium phosphate
CT	clotting time
CTZ	chemoreceptor trigger zone
CV	cardiovascular
CVA	cerebrovascular accident
CVP	central venous pressure
d	day
D5W	5% dextrose in water
D&C	dilation and curettage
DIC	disseminated intravascular coagulation
DKA	diabetic keto-acidosis
dl	deciliter (100 ml or 0.1 liter)
DM	diabetes mellitus
DNA	deoxyribonucleic acid
DPD	dihydropyrimidine dehydrogenase
DTRs	deep tendon reflexes
DVT	deep venous thrombosis
ECG, EKG	electrocardiogram
ECT	electroconvulsive therapy
EEG	electroencephalogram
EENT	eye, ear, nose, throat
e.g.	for example (*exempli gratia*)
EGFR	epidermal growth factor receptor
ENT	ear, nose, throat
EPS	extrapyramidal symptoms (or syndrome)
ER	estrogen receptor
F	Fahrenheit

FBS	fasting blood sugar
FDA	Food and Drug Administration
FSH	follicle-stimulating hormone
FTI	free thyroxine index
5-FU	5-fluorouracil
FUO	fever of unknown origin
g	gram
G6PD	glucose-6-phosphate dehydrogenase
GABA	gamma-aminobutyric acid
GERD	gastroesophageal reflux disease
GM-CSF	granulocyte-macrophage colony-stimulating factor
GnRH	gonadotropic releasing hormone
GFR	glomerular filtration rate
GH	growth hormone
GI	gastrointestinal
GPIIb/IIIa	glycoprotein IIb/IIIa
GU	genitourinary
h	hour
HACA	human antichimeric antibody
HbA_{1c}	glycosylated hemoglobin
HBV	viral hepatitis B
HCG	human chorionic gonadotropin
Hct	hematocrit
HDL	high density lipoprotein
HDL-C	high-density-lipoprotein cholesterol
HER	human epidermal growth factor
Hgb	hemoglobin
5-HIAA	5-hydroxyindoleacetic acid
HIT	heparin-induced thrombocytopenia
HIV	human immunodeficiency virus
HMG-CoA	3-hydroxy-3-methyl-glutaryl coenzyme A
HPA	hypothalamic–pituitary–adrenocortical (axis)
HPV	human papillomavirus
HR	heart rate
h.s.	nightly or at bedtime (*hora somni*)
HSV-1	herpes simplex virus type 1
HSV-2	herpes simplex virus type 2
5-HT	5-hydroxytryptamine (serotonin receptor)
IBW	ideal body weight
IC	intracoronary
ICP	intracranial pressure
ICU	intensive care unit
ID	intradermal
IFN	interferon
Ig	immunoglobulin
IGF-1	insulin-like growth factor 1
IL	interleukin
IM	intramuscular
INR	international normalizing ratio
IOP	intraocular pressure

IPPB	intermittent positive pressure breathing
iPTH	idiopathic parathyroid hormone
ITP	idiopathic thrombocytopenia purpura
IU	international unit
IV	intravenous
JRA	juvenile rheumatoid arthritis
kg	kilogram
17-KGS	17-ketogenic steroids
17-KS	17-ketosteroids
KVO	keep vein open
L	liter
LDH	lactic dehydrogenase
LDL	low density lipoprotein
LDL-C	low-density-lipoprotein cholesterol
LE	lupus erythematosus
LFT	liver function test
LH	luteinizing hormone
LSD	lysergic acid diethylamide
LTRA	leukotriene receptor antagonist
LVEDP	left ventricular end diastolic pressure
M	molar (strength of a solution)
m^2	square meter (of body surface area)
MAO	monoamine oxidase
MAOI	monoamine oxidase inhibitor
MBD	minimal brain dysfunction
MCH	mean corpuscular hemoglobin
MCHC	mean corpuscular hemoglobin concentration
mCi	millicurie
μg, mcg	microgram (1/1000 of a milligram)
μm	micrometer
MDI	metered dose inhaler
MDR	minimum daily requirements
mEq	milliequivalent
mg	milligram
min	minute
MI	myocardial infarction
MIC	minimum inhibitory concentration
ml	milliliter (0.001 liter)
mm	millimeter
mo	month
MPS I	mucopolysaccharidosis I
MRSA	methicillin-resistant *Staphylococcus aureus*
MS	multiple sclerosis
N	normal (strength of a solution)
NADH	reduced form of nicotine adenine dinucleotide
NAPA	*N*-acetyl procainamide
nb	note well (*nota bene*)
ng	nanogram (1/1000 of a microgram)
NMS	neuroleptic malignant syndrome
NNRTI	nonnucleoside reverse transcriptase inhibitor

NPN	nonprotein nitrogen
NPO	nothing by mouth
NRTI	nucleoside reverse transcriptase inhibitor
NS	normal saline
NSAID	nonsteroidal antiinflammatory drug
NSCLC	non-small cell lung cancer
NSR	normal sinus rhythm
OAB	overactive bladder
OC	oral contraceptive
ODT	oral disintegrating tablet
17-OHCS	17-hydroxycorticosteroids
OTC	over the counter (nonprescription)
PABA	*para*-aminobenzoic acid
PAS	*para*-aminosalicylic acid
PAWP	pulmonary artery wedge pressure
PBI	protein-bound iodine
PBP	penicillin-binding protein
p.c.	after meals (*post cibum*)
PCI	percutaneous coronary intervention
PCWP	pulmonary capillary wedge pressure
PE	pulmonary embolism
PDE	phosphodiesterase
PERLA	pupils equal, react to light and accommodation
PG	prostaglandin
PGE2	prostaglandin E2
pH	hydrogen ion concentration
PID	pelvic inflammatory disease
PKU	phenylketonuria
PMDD	premenstrual dysphoric disorder
PND	paroxysmal nocturnal dyspnea
PO	by mouth or orally (*per os*)
PPI	proton pump inhibitor
PPM	parts per million
PR	rectally (*per rectum*)
prn	when required (*pro re nata*)
PSA	prostate-specific antigen
PSP	phenolsulfonphthalein
PSVT	paroxysmal supraventricular tachycardia
PT	prothrombin time
PTH	parathyroid hormone
PTT	partial thromboplastin time
PUD	peptic ulcer disease
PVC	premature ventricular contraction
PVD	peripheral vascular disease
PZI	protamine zinc insulin
q.d.	every day
q.i.d.	four times daily
q.o.d.	every other day
RA	rheumatoid arthritis
RAI	radioactive iodine

RAST	radioallergosorbent test
RBC	red blood (cell) count
RDA	recommended (daily) dietary allowance
RDS	respiratory distress syndrome
REM	rapid eye movement
rem	radiation equivalent man
RES	reticuloendothelial system
RIA	radioimmunoassay
RL	Ringer's lactate
RNA	ribonucleic acid
ROM	range of motion
RSV	respiratory syncytial virus
RT	reverse transcriptase
RT_3U	total serum thyroxine concentration
s	second
S&S	signs and symptoms
SA	sinoatrial
SBE	subacute bacterial endocarditis
SC	subcutaneous
S_{cr}	serum creatinine
SGGT	serum gamma-glutamyl transferase
SGOT	serum glutamic–oxaloacetic transaminase (*see* AST)
SGPT	serum glutamic–pyruvic transaminase (*see* ALT)
SIADH	syndrome of inappropriate antidiuretic hormone
SI Units	International System of Units
SK	streptokinase
SL	sublingual
SLE	systemic lupus erythematosus
SMA	sequential multiple analysis
SNRI	serotonin norepinephrine reuptake inhibitor
SOS	if necessary (*si opus cit*)
sp	species
SPF	sun protection factor
sq	square
SR	sedimentation rate
SRS-A	slow-reactive substance of anaphylaxis
SSRI	selective serotonin reuptake inhibitor
stat	immediately
STD	sexually transmitted disease
SVT	supraventricular tachyarrhythmias
$t_{1/2}$	half-life
T_3	triiodothyronine
T_4	thyroxine
TCA	tricyclic antidepressant
TG	total triglycerides
TIA	transient ischemic attack
t.i.d.	three times a day (*ter in die*)
TNF	tumor necrosis factor
tPA	tissue plasminogen activator
TPN	total parenteral nutrition

TPR	temperature, pulse, respirations
TSH	thyroid-stimulating hormone
TSS	toxic shock syndrome
TT	thrombin time
URI	upper respiratory infection
USP	United States Pharmacopeia
USPHS	United States Public Health Service
UTI	urinary tract infection
UV-A, UVA	ultraviolet A wave
VDRL	venereal disease research laboratory
VEGF	vascular endothelial growth factor
VLDL	very low density lipoprotein
VMA	vanillylmandelic acid
VREF	vancomycin resistant *Enterococcus faecium*
VRSA	vancomycin resistance *Staphylococcus aureus*
VS	vital signs
wk	week
WBC	white blood (cell) count
WBCT	whole blood clotting time
y	year

BIBLIOGRAPHY

American Hospital Formulary Service (AHFS) Drug Information. 05. Bethesda, MD: American Society of Health-System Pharmacists. 2005.

Bindler R, Howry L, Prentice Hall Pediatric Drug Guide with Nursing Implications. *Upper Saddle River, NJ: Prentice Hall Health*. 2005.

Cada DJ, Baker DE, Levien T, Quinupristin/Dalfopristin. *Hospital Pharmacy*. 2000; 35(1):177–193.

Drug Facts and Comparisons. St. Louis: Wolters Kluwer Health. 2005.

Gelman CR, Rumack BH, Eds. *Micromedex*. Stamford, CT: Thompson Healthcare. 2005.

Gold Standard Media. http://www.gsm.com: *Clinical Pharmacology*. 2005.

Physicians' Desk Reference. 59th ed. Stamford, CT: Thompson Healthcare. 2005.

Semla TP, Beizer JL, Higbee MD, *Geriatric Dosage Handbook*. 11th ed. Hudson, OH: Lexi-Comp. 2004.

Trissel LA, *Handbook of Injectable Drugs*. 12th ed. Bethesda, MD: American Society of Health-System Pharmacists. 2003.

Trissel LA, Gilbert DK, Williams KY, Compatibility of screening of gatifloxacin during simulated Y-site administration with other drugs. *Hospital Pharmacy*. 1999; 34(12):1409–1416.

Trissel LA, Zhang Y, Xu QA, Incompatibility of erythromycin lactiobionate and sulfamethoxazole/trimethoprim with linezolid injection. *Hospital Pharmacy*. 2000; 35:1192–1196.

USP DI: Advice to Patients. Rockville, MD: US Pharmacopeial Convention. 2005.

USP DI: Drug Information for the Health Care Professional. Rockville, MD: US Pharmacopeial Convention. 2005.

Xu QA, Trissel LA, Williams KY, *Compatibility and stability of linezolid injection admixed with three cephalosporin antibiotics*. Journal of the American Pharmaceutical Association. 2000; 40(40):509–514.

Index

A

Drug categories are in SMALL CAPS. Prototypes in **bold.**
Generic drug names are given in parentheses.

Drug categories are in SMALL CAPS. Prototypes in **bold.**
Generic drug names are given in parentheses.

Drug categories are in SMALL CAPS. Prototypes in **bold.**
Generic drug names are given in parentheses.

Drug categories are in SMALL CAPS. Prototypes in **bold**.
Generic drug names are given in parentheses.

Drug categories are in SMALL CAPS. Prototypes in **bold.**
Generic drug names are given in parentheses.

Drug categories are in SMALL CAPS. Prototypes in **bold.**
Generic drug names are given in parentheses.

Drug categories are in SMALL CAPS. Prototypes in **bold.**
Generic drug names are given in parentheses.

Drug categories are in SMALL CAPS. Prototypes in **bold**.
Generic drug names are given in parentheses.

Drug categories are in SMALL CAPS. Prototypes in **bold.**
Generic drug names are given in parentheses.

Drug categories are in SMALL CAPS. Prototypes in **bold.**
Generic drug names are given in parentheses.

C

Drug categories are in SMALL CAPS. Prototypes in **bold.**
Generic drug names are given in parentheses.

Drug categories are in SMALL CAPS. Prototypes in **bold.**
Generic drug names are given in parentheses.

Drug categories are in SMALL CAPS. Prototypes in **bold.**
Generic drug names are given in parentheses.

Drug categories are in SMALL CAPS. Prototypes in **bold.**
Generic drug names are given in parentheses.

D

Drug categories are in SMALL CAPS. Prototypes in **bold.**
Generic drug names are given in parentheses.

Drug categories are in SMALL CAPS. Prototypes in **bold.**
Generic drug names are given in parentheses.

E

Drug categories are in SMALL CAPS. Prototypes in **bold.**
Generic drug names are given in parentheses.

Drug categories are in SMALL CAPS. Prototypes in **bold.**
Generic drug names are given in parentheses.

F

Drug categories are in SMALL CAPS. Prototypes in **bold.**
Generic drug names are given in parentheses.

Drug categories are in SMALL CAPS. Prototypes in **bold.**
Generic drug names are given in parentheses.

H

Drug categories are in SMALL CAPS. Prototypes in **bold.**
Generic drug names are given in parentheses.

Drug categories are in SMALL CAPS. Prototypes in **bold.**
Generic drug names are given in parentheses.

J

Drug categories are in SMALL CAPS. Prototypes in **bold.**
Generic drug names are given in parentheses.

Drug categories are in SMALL CAPS. Prototypes in **bold.**
Generic drug names are given in parentheses.

Drug categories are in SMALL CAPS. Prototypes in **bold.**
Generic drug names are given in parentheses.

M

Drug categories are in SMALL CAPS. Prototypes in **bold.**
Generic drug names are given in parentheses.

N

Drug categories are in SMALL CAPS. Prototypes in **bold.**
Generic drug names are given in parentheses.

Drug categories are in SMALL CAPS. Prototypes in **bold.**
Generic drug names are given in parentheses.

O

Drug categories are in SMALL CAPS. Prototypes in **bold.**
Generic drug names are given in parentheses.

Drug categories are in SMALL CAPS. Prototypes in **bold.**
Generic drug names are given in parentheses.

Drug categories are in SMALL CAPS. Prototypes in **bold.**
Generic drug names are given in parentheses.

Q

R

Drug categories are in SMALL CAPS. Prototypes in **bold.**
Generic drug names are given in parentheses.

Drug categories are in SMALL CAPS. Prototypes in **bold.**
Generic drug names are given in parentheses.

Drug categories are in SMALL CAPS. Prototypes in **bold.**
Generic drug names are given in parentheses.

U

V

Drug categories are in SMALL CAPS. Prototypes in **bold.**
Generic drug names are given in parentheses.